Drug Information Handbook

5th Edition  *1997-98*

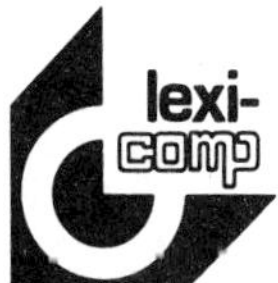

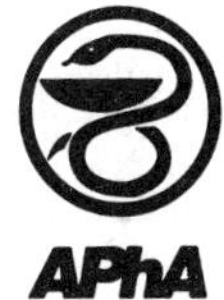

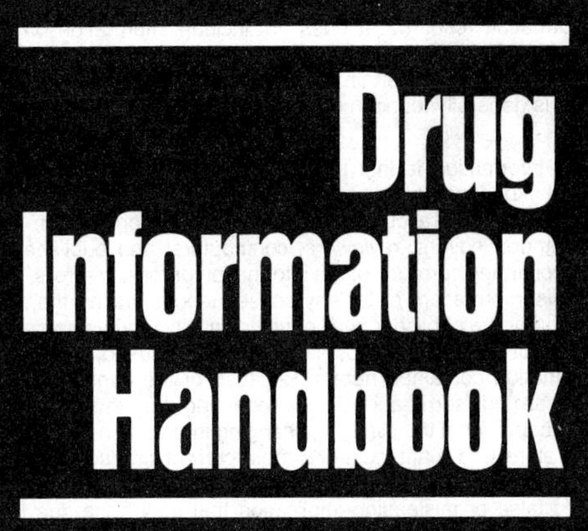

Drug Information Handbook

5th Edition  **1997-98**

Charles Lacy, RPh, PharmD
Drug Information Pharmacist
Cedars-Sinai Medical Center
Los Angeles, California

Lora L. Armstrong, RPh, BSPharm, BCPS
Director of Drug Information Services
The University of Chicago Hospitals
Chicago, Illinois

Naomi B. Ingrim, RPh, PharmD
Specialist in Poison Information
Central Texas Poison Center
Temple, Texas

Leonard L. Lance, RPh, BSPharm
Pharmacist
Lexi-Comp, Inc.
Hudson, Ohio

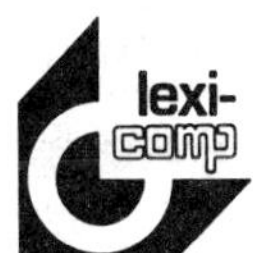

LEXI-COMP INC
Hudson (Cleveland)

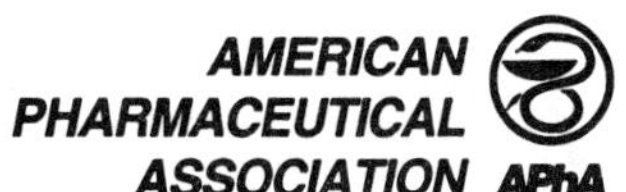

This handbook is intended to serve the user as a handy quick reference and not as a complete drug information resource. It does not include information on every therapeutic agent available. The publication covers 1,029 commonly used drugs and is specifically designed to present certain important aspects of drug data in a more concise format than is generally found in medical literature or product material supplied by manufacturers.

The nature of drug information is that it is constantly evolving because of ongoing research and clinical experience and is often subject to interpretation. While great care has been taken to ensure the accuracy of the information presented, the reader is advised that the authors, editors, reviewers, contributors, and publishers cannot be responsible for the continued currency of the information or for any errors, omissions, or the application of this information, or for any consequences arising therefrom. Therefore, the author(s) and/or the publisher shall have no liability to any person or entity with regard to claims, loss, or damage caused, or alleged to be caused, directly or indirectly, by the use of information contained herein. Because of the dynamic nature of drug information, readers are advised that decisions regarding drug therapy must be based on the independent judgment of the clinician, changing information about a drug (eg, as reflected in the literature and manufacturer's most current product (information), and changing medical practices. The editors are not responsible for any inaccuracy of quotation or for any false or misleading implication that may arise due to the text or formulas as used or due to the quotation of revisions no longer official.

The editors, authors, and contributors have written this book in their private capacities. No official support or endorsement by any federal agency or pharmaceutical company is intended or inferred.

The publishers have made every effort to trace the copyright holders for borrowed material. If they have inadvertently overlooked any, they will be pleased to make the necessary arrangements at the first opportunity.

If you have any suggestions or questions regarding any information presented in this handbook, please contact our drug information pharmacist at

1-800-837-LEXI (5394)

This manual was produced using the FormuLex™ Program — a complete publishing service of Lexi-Comp Inc.

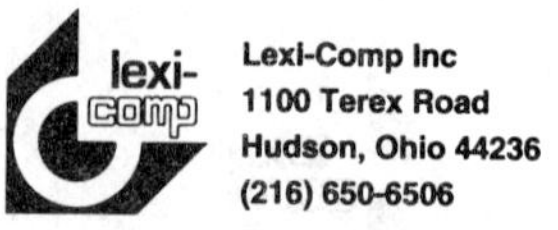

Lexi-Comp Inc
1100 Terex Road
Hudson, Ohio 44236
(216) 650-6506

ISBN 0-916589-56-0

TABLE OF CONTENTS

ABOUT THE AUTHORS

Charles F. Lacy, RPh, PharmD

Dr Lacy received his doctorate from the University of Southern California School of Pharmacy. With over 15 years of clinical experience at one of the nation's largest teaching hospitals, he has developed a reputation as an acknowledged expert in drug information and critical care drug therapy.

In his current capacity as Drug Information Specialist at Cedar-Sinai Medical Center in Los Angeles, Dr Lacy plays an active role in the education and training of the medical, pharmacy, and nursing staff. He coordinates the Drug Information Center, the Medical Center's Intern Pharmacist Clinical Training Program, the Department's Continuing Education Program for Pharmacists; maintains the Medical Center Formulary Program; and is editor of the Medical Center's *Drug Formulary Handbook* and the drug information newsletter — *Prescription.*

Presently, Dr Lacy holds teaching affiliations with the University of Southern California School of Pharmacy, the University of California at San Francisco School of Pharmacy, the University of the Pacific School of Pharmacy and the University of Alberta at Edmonton, School of Pharmacy and Health Sciences.

Dr Lacy is an active member of numerous professional associations including the American Society of Health-System Pharmacists (ASHP), the California Society of Hospital Pharmacists (CSHP), and the American College of Clinical Pharmacy (ACCP).

Lora L. Armstrong, RPh, BSPharm, BCPS

Lora L. Armstrong received her bachelor's degree in pharmacy from Ferris State University. With over 15 years of clinical experience at one of the nation's most prominent teaching institutions, she has developed a reputation as an acknowledged expert in drug information. Her interests involve the areas of critical care, hematology, oncology, infectious disease, and pharmacokinetics. Ms Armstrong is a Board Certified Pharmacotherapy Specialist (BCPS).

In her current capacity as Director of Drug Information at the University of Chicago Hospitals (UCH), Ms Armstrong plays an active role in the education and training of the medical, pharmacy, and nursing staff. She coordinates the Drug Information Center, the medical center's Adverse Drug Reaction Monitoring Program, and the department's Continuing Education Program for Pharmacists. She also maintains the hospital's strict formulary program and is editor of the *UCH Formulary of Accepted Drugs* and the drug information newsletter "Topics in Drug Therapy." Ms. Armstrong also serves on the Editorial Advisory Board of the *Journal of the American Pharmaceutical Association.*

Ms Armstrong is an active member of the American Society of Health-System Pharmacists (ASHP), the American Pharmaceutical Association (APhA), the American College of Clinical Pharmacy (ACCP), and the Society of Critical Care Medicine (SCCM). She is the APhA designated author for this handbook.

Naomi B. Ingrim, PharmD

Dr Ingrim received her PharmD degree from the University of Nebraska Medical Center - Omaha in 1980 and completed two residencies in Hospital Pharmacy Practice and in Drug Information, respectively in 1982 and 1983. Since that time she has held a variety of clinical, teaching, and management positions, broadening her expertise and further strengthening her drug information skills.

From 1984-89, she held positions at Scott and White Hospital in Temple, Texas as Clinical Pharmacist in Drug Information and Pediatrics and as Assistant Professor in Pediatrics with Texas A & M Medical School. During the following four years, she served as Clinical Pharmacy Coordinator at Egleston Children's Hospital at Emory University in Atlanta, Georgia and was cross-appointed with the Emory University Medical School Department of Pediatrics and Mercer University Southern School of Pharmacy. From 1991-93, she additionally served as the Acting Director of Egleston Hospital Pharmacy Department. In this capacity, Dr Ingrim directed the development of an active clinical program and staff, including a supportive drug information service/center. She has had much experience designing ADR, CQI, and DUE programs, teaching and public speaking, serving on hospital/national pharmacy organization committees, writing technical documents, and performing drug-related research.

Dr Ingrim is active in state pharmacy organizations, the American Society of Health-System Pharmacists (ASHP), and the American College of Clinical Pharmacists (ACCP).

Currently, Dr Ingrim serves as a Specialist in Poison Information at the Central Texas Poison Center and as adjunct faculty with Texas A&M University. She is also a freelance consultant in drug information, clinical pharmacy practice, and expert system development.

Leonard L. Lance, RPh, BSPharm

Leonard L. (Bud) Lance has been directly involved in the pharmaceutical industry since receiving his bachelor's degree in pharmacy from Ohio Northern University in 1970. Upon graduation from ONU, Mr Lance spent four years as a navy pharmacist in various military assignments and was instrumental in the development and operation of the first whole hospital I.V. admixture program in a military (Portsmouth Naval Hospital) facility.

After completing his military service, he entered the retail pharmacy field and has managed both an independent and a home I.V. franchise pharmacy operation. Since the late 1970s Mr Lance has focused much of his interest on using computers to improve pharmacy service and to advance the dissemination of drug information to practitioners and other health care professionals.

As a result of his strong publishing interest, he serves in the capacity of pharmacy editor and technical advisor as well as pharmacy (information) database coordinator for Lexi-Comp. Along with the *Drug Information Handbook for the Allied Health Professional* edition, he provides technical support to Lexi-Comp's *Pediatric Dosage Handbook, Laboratory Test Handbook, Diagnostic Procedure Handbook, Infectious Diseases Handbook,Poisoning & Toxicology Handbook*, and *Geriatric Dosage Handbook* publications. Mr Lance has also assisted approximately 120 major hospitals in producing their own formulary (pharmacy) publications through Lexi-Comp's custom publishing service.

Mr Lance is a member and past president (1984) of the Summit Pharmaceutical Association (SPA). He is also a member of the Ohio Pharmacists Association (OPA), the American Pharmaceutical Association (APhA), and the American Society of Health-System Pharmacists (ASHP).

EDITORIAL ADVISORY PANEL

PREFACE

Drug therapy literature is voluminous and of varying quality. Despite the large number of publications available on the subject, it is difficult to compile this data into a logical guide that can best direct therapy for the multitudes of existent disease states. The authors have extensively researched this literature and have arranged the information into this unified compendium. The material is presented in a concise manner designed to ensure consistent presentation of the information and to facilitate the clinician's decisions regarding drug therapy. This format was developed to lend itself for use by all practitioners and students involved in drug therapy decisions. We have tried to emphasize fundamental principles of drug therapy, while paying particular attention to providing new, pertinent, and practical information.

ACKNOWLEDGMENTS

The *Drug Information Handbook* exists in its present form as the result of the concerted efforts of the following individuals: Robert D. Kerscher, publisher and president of Lexi-Comp Inc; James P. Caro, senior vice president of professional resources, American Pharmaceutical Association (APhA); Lynn D. Coppinger, managing editor; and David C. Marcus, systems analyst.

Other members of the Lexi-Comp staff whose contributions deserve special mention include Diane Harbart, MT (ASCP), medical editor; Barbara F. Kerscher, production manager; Alexandra Hart, composition specialist; Jeanne Wilson, Beth Daulbaugh, Julie Katzen, and Leslie Ruggles, project managers; Jennifer Harbart, and Jacqueline L. Mizer, production assistants; Tracey J. Reinecke, graphic designer; Brian B. Vossler, Jerry Reeves, and Marc L. Long, sales managers; Jay L. Katzen, product manager; Kenneth J. Hughes, manager of authoring systems; Kristin M. Thompson, Matthew C. Kerscher, Tina L. Collins, and Mary M. Murphy, sales and marketing representatives; Edmund A. Harbart, vice-president, custom publishing division; Jack L. Stones, vice-president, reference publishing division; Dennis P. Smithers and Sean Conrad, system analysts; and Thury L. O'Connor, vice-president of technology.

Another APhA staff member whose contribution was important is Julian I. Graubart, Director of Books and Electronic Products. A special thanks goes to Chris Lomax, PharmD, director of pharmacy, Children's Hospital, Los Angeles, who played a significant role in bringing APhA and Lexi-Comp together.

Much of the material contained in this book was a result of pharmacy contributors throughout the United States and Canada. Lexi-Comp has assisted many medical institutions to develop hospital-specific formulary manuals that contain clinical drug information as well as dosing. Working with these clinical pharmacists, hospital pharmacy and therapeutics committees, and hospital drug information centers, Lexi-Comp has developed an evolutionary drug database that reflects the practice of pharmacy in these major institutions.

In addition, the authors wish to thank their families, friends, and colleagues who supported them in their efforts to complete this handbook.

USE OF THE DRUG INFORMATION HANDBOOK

The *Drug Information Handbook, 5th Edition* is divided into four sections.

The first section is a compilation of introductory text pertinent to the use of this book.

The drug information section of the handbook, in which all drugs are listed alphabetically, details information pertinent to each drug. Extensive cross-referencing is provided by brand names and synonyms.

The third section is an invaluable appendix section with charts, tables, nomograms, algorithms, and guidelines.

The last section of this handbook is an index listing drugs in their unique therapeutic category.

Alphabetical Listing of Drugs

Drug information is presented in a consistent format and provides the following:

Generic Name	U.S. adopted name
Pronunciation Guide	Phonetic pronunciation
Related Information	Cross-reference to other pertinent drug information found elsewhere in this handbook
Brand Names	U.S. trade names (manufacturer-specific)
Canadian/Mexican Brand Names	Trade names found in Canada or Mexico
Synonyms	Other names or accepted abbreviations of the generic drug
Use	Information pertaining to appropriate indications of the drug. Includes both FDA approved and non-FDA approved indications.
Restrictions	The controlled substance classification from the Drug Enforcement Agency (DEA). U.S. schedules are I-V. Schedules vary by country and sometimes state (ie, Massachusetts uses I-VI)
Pregnancy Risk Factor	Five categories established by the FDA to indicate the potential of a systemically absorbed drug for causing birth defects
Pregnancy Implications	Information pertinent to or associated with the use of the drug as it relates to pregnancy and/or breast feeding
Contraindications	Information pertaining to inappropriate use of the drug
Warnings/Precautions	Hazardous conditions related to use of the drug and disease states or patient populations in which the drug should be cautiously used
Adverse Reactions	Side effects are grouped by percentage of incidence and body system
Overdosage/Toxicology	Comments and/or considerations are offered when appropriate and include signs or symptoms of excess drug and suggested management of the patient
Drug Interactions	Description of the interaction between the drug listed in the monograph and other drugs or drug classes. May include possible mechanisms and effect of combined therapy. May also include a strategy to manage the patient on combined therapy (ie, quinidine).
Stability	Information regarding storage of product or steps for reconstitution. Provides the time and conditions for which a solution or mixture will maintain full potency. For example, some solutions may require refrigeration after reconstitution while stored at room temperature prior to preparation.
Mechanism of Action	How the drug works in the body to elicit a response
Pharmacodynamics/Kinetics	The magnitude of a drug's effect depends on the drug concentration at the site of action. The pharmacodynamics are expressed in terms of onset of action and duration of action. Pharmacokinetics are expressed in terms of absorption, distribution (including appearance in breast milk and crossing of the placenta), protein binding, metabolism, bioavailability, half-life, time to peak serum concentration, and elimination.
Usual Dosage	The amount of the drug to be typically given or taken during therapy for children and adults; also includes any dosing adjustment for renal impairment or hepatic failure
Dietary Considerations	Information is offered, when appropriate, regarding food and/or alcohol considerations

(continued)

Administration	Information regarding the recommended final concentrations, rates of administration for parenteral drugs, or other guidelines when giving the medication
Monitoring Parameters	Laboratory tests and patient physical parameters that should be monitored for safety and efficacy of drug therapy
Reference Range	Therapeutic and toxic serum concentrations listed including peak and trough levels
Test Interactions	Listing of assay interferences when relevant; (B) = Blood; (S) = Serum; (U) = Urine
Patient Information	Specific information pertinent for the patient
Nursing Implications	Includes additional instructions for the administration of the drug and monitoring tips from the nursing perspective
Additional Information	Information about sodium content and/or pertinent information about specific brands
Dosage Forms	Information with regard to form, strength, and availability of the drug
Extemporaneous Preparations	Directions for preparing liquid formulations from solid drug products. May include stability information and references.

Appendix

The appendix offers a compilation of tables, guidelines, nomograms, algorithms, and conversion information which can often be helpful when considering patient care.

Therapeutic Category & Key Word Index

This index provides a useful listing of drugs by their therapeutic classification, as well as controlled substance information.

Canadian/Mexican Brand Name Index

This handy index lists the brand names used in Canada and Mexico.

FDA PREGNANCY CATEGORIES

Throughout this book there is a field labeled Pregnancy Risk Factor (PRF) and the letter A, B, C, D or X immediately following which signifies a category. The FDA has established these five categories to indicate the potential of a systemically absorbed drug for causing birth defects. The key differentiation among the categories rests upon the reliability of documentation and the risk:benefit ratio. Pregnancy Category X is particularly notable in that if any data exists that may implicate a drug as a teratogen and the risk:benefit ratio is clearly negative, the drug is contraindicated during pregnancy.

These categories are summarized as follows:

A	Controlled studies in pregnant women fail to demonstrate a risk to the fetus in the first trimester with no evidence of risk in later trimesters. The possibility of fetal harm appears remote.
B	Either animal-reproduction studies have not demonstrated a fetal risk but there are no controlled studies in pregnant women, or animal-reproduction studies have shown an adverse effect (other than a decrease in fertility) that was not confirmed in controlled studies in women in the first trimester and there is no evidence of a risk in later trimesters.
C	Either studies in animals have revealed adverse effects on the fetus (teratogenic or embryocidal effects or other) and there are no controlled studies in women, or studies in women and animals are not available. Drugs should be given only if the potential benefits justify the potential risk to the fetus.
D	There is positive evidence of human fetal risk, but the benefits from use in pregnant women may be acceptable despite the risk (eg, if the drug is needed in a life-threatening situation or for a serious disease for which safer drugs cannot be used or are ineffective).
X	Studies in animals or human beings have demonstrated fetal abnormalities or there is evidence of fetal risk based on human experience, or both, and the risk of the use of the drug in pregnant women clearly outweighs any possible benefit. The drug is contraindicated in women who are or may become pregnant.

DRUGS IN PREGNANCY

Analgesics

Acceptable: Acetaminophen, meperidine, methadone
Controversial: Codeine, propoxyphene
Unacceptable: Nonsteroidal anti-inflammatory agents, salicylates, phenazopyridine

Antimicrobials

Acceptable: Penicillins, 1st and 2nd generation cephalosporins, erythromycin (base and EES), clotrimazole, miconazole, nystatin, isoniazid*, lindane
Controversial: 3rd generation cephalosporins, aminoglycosides, nitrofurantoin†
Unacceptable: Erythromycin estolate, chloramphenicol, sulfa, metronidazole, tetracyclines, acyclovir

ENT

Acceptable: Diphenhydramine*, dextromethorphan
Controversial: Pseudoephedrine
Unacceptable: Brompheniramine, cyproheptadine, dimenhydrinate

GI

Acceptable: Trimethobenzamide, antacids*, simethicone, other H_2-blockers, psyllium, bisacodyl, docusate
Controversial: Metoclopramide, prochlorperazine

Neurologic

Controversial: Phenytoin, phenobarbital
Unacceptable: Carbamazepine, valproic acid, ergotamine

Pulmonary

Acceptable: Theophylline, metaproterenol, terbutaline, inhaled steroids
Unacceptable: Epinephrine, oral steroids

Psych

Acceptable: Hydroxyzine*, lithium*, haloperidol
Controversial: Benzodiazepines, tricyclics, phenothiazines

Other

Acceptable: Heparin, insulin
Unacceptable: Warfarin, sulfonylureas

*Do not use in first trimester
†Do not use in third trimester

SAFE WRITING

Health professionals and their support personnel frequently produce handwritten copies of information they see in print; therefore, such information is subjected to even greater possibilities for error or misinterpretation on the part of others. Thus, particular care must be given to how drug names and strengths are expressed when creating written healthcare documents.

The following are a few examples of safe writing rules suggested by the Institute for Safe Medication Practices, Inc.*

1. There should be a space between a number and its units as it is easier to read. There should be no periods after the abbreviations mg or mL.

Correct	Incorrect
10 mg	10mg
100 mg	100mg

2. Never place a decimal and a zero after a whole number (2 mg is correct and 2.0 mg is incorrect). If the decimal point is not seen because it falls on a line or because individuals are working from copies where the decimal point is not seen, this causes a tenfold overdose.
3. Just the opposite is true for numbers less than one. Always place a zero before a naked decimal (0.5 mL is correct, .5 mL is **incorrect**).
4. Never abbreviate the word unit. The handwritten U or u, looks like a 0 (zero), and may cause a tenfold overdose error to be made.
5. Q.D. is not a safe abbreviation for once daily, as when the Q is followed by a sloppy dot, it looks like QID which means four times daily.
6. O.D. is not a safe abbreviation for once daily, as it is properly interpreted as meaning "right eye" and has caused liquid medications such as saturated solution of potassium iodide and lugol's solution to be administered incorrectly. There is no safe abbreviation for once daily. It must be written out in full.
7. Do not use chemical names such as 6-mercaptopurine or 6-thioguanine, as sixfold overdoses have been given when these were not recognized as chemical names. The proper names of these drugs are mercaptopurine or thioguanine.
8. Do not abbreviate drug names (5FC, 6MP, 5-ASA, MTX, HCTZ, CPZ, PBZ, etc) as they are misinterpreted and cause error.
9. Do not use the apothecary system or symbols.
10. Do not abbreviate microgram as µg; instead use mcg as there is less likelihood of misinterpretation.
11. When writing an outpatient prescription, write a complete prescription. A complete prescription can prevent the prescriber, the pharmacist, and/or the patient from making a mistake and can eliminate the need for further clarification. The legible prescriptions should contain:
    a. patient's full name
    b. for pediatric or geriatric patients: their age (or weight where applicable)
    c. drug name, dosage form and strength; if a drug is new or rarely prescribed, print this information
    d. number or amount to be dispensed
    e. complete instructions for the patient, including the purpose of the medication
    f. when there are recognized contraindications for a prescribed drug, indicate to the pharmacist that you are aware of this fact (ie, when prescribing a potassium salt for a patient receiving an ACE inhibitor, write "K serum leveling being monitored")

*From "Safe Writing" by Davis NM, PharmD and Cohen MR, MS, Lecturers and Consultants for Safe Medication Practices, 1143 Wright Drive, Huntington Valley, PA 19006. Phone: (215) 947-7566.

ALPHABETICAL LISTING OF DRUGS

A-200™ Shampoo [OTC] *see* Pyrethrins *on page 1079*

Abbokinase® *see* Urokinase *on page 1282*

Abbreviations and Measurements *see page 1330*

Abciximab (ab SIK si mab)

Brand Names ReoPro™

Synonyms C7E3; 7E3

Therapeutic Category Platelet Aggregation Inhibitor

Use Adjunct to percutaneous transluminal coronary angioplasty or atherectomy (PTCA) for the prevention of acute cardiac ischemic complications in patients at high risk for abrupt closure of the treated coronary vessel

Patients at high risk of closure or restenosis:

- Acute evolving myocardial infarction (MI) within 12 hours of onset of symptoms requiring rescue PTCA
- Early postinfarction angina or unstable angina with at least 2 episodes of angina associated with EKG changes during previous 24 hours
- Non-Q-wave myocardial infarction
- Clinical or angiographic characteristic indicating high risk (see "Characteristics of Type A, B, and C Lesions" below)
  - Unfavorable anatomy (ie, 2 or more type B lesions) **or**
  - One or more type B lesions with diabetes **or**
  - One or more type B lesions and a female and over the age of 65 **or**
  - One type C lesion
- Thrombus score is based upon angiographic evidence

Characteristics of Type A, B, and C Lesions

- Type A lesions (minimally complex)
  - Discrete (length <10 mm)
  - Concentric
  - Readily accessible
  - Nonangulated segment (<45°)
  - Smooth contour
  - Little or no calcification
  - Less than totally occlusive
  - Not ostial in location
  - No major side branch involvement
  - No thrombus
- Type B lesions (moderately complex)
  - Tubular (length 10-20 mm)
  - Eccentric
  - Moderate tortuosity of proximal segment
  - Moderate angulated segment (>45°, <90°)
  - Irregular contour
  - Moderate or heavy calcification
  - Total occlusions <3 months old
  - Ostial in location
  - Bifurcation lesions requiring double lead wires
  - Some thrombus present
- Type C lesions (severely complex)
  - Diffuse (length >20 mm)
  - Excessive tortuosity of proximal segment
  - Extremely angulated segments >90°
  - Total occlusions >3 months old and/or bridging collaterals
  - Inability to protect major side branches
  - Degenerated vein grafts with friable lesions

Recent data suggest that abciximab may also benefit patients with a moderate risk of ischemic complication due to unstable angina

Pregnancy Risk Factor C

Pregnancy/Breast-Feeding Implications It is not known whether abciximab can cause fetal harm when administered to a pregnant woman or can affect reproduction capacity

Contraindications

- Active internal hemorrhage or recent (within 6 weeks) clinically significant gastrointestinal or genitourinary bleeding
- History of cerebrovascular accident within 2 years, or cerebrovascular accident with significant neurological deficit
- Bleeding diathesis or administration of oral anticoagulants within 7 days unless prothrombin time (PT) is less than or equal to 1.2 times control PT value
- Thrombocytopenia (<100,000 cells/microliter)
- Recent (within 6 weeks) major surgery or trauma
- Intracranial tumor, arteriovenous malformation, or aneurysm
- Severe uncontrolled hypertension
- History of vasculitis

Use of dextran before PTCA or intent to use dextran during PTCA
Known hypersensitivity to abciximab or to murine proteins

Warnings/Precautions Administration of abciximab is associated with a significantly increased frequency of major bleeding complications including retroperitoneal bleeding, spontaneous GI or GU bleeding and bleeding at the arterial access site

Clinical data indicate that the risk of major bleeding due to abciximab therapy may be elevated in the following settings:
- Patients weighing <75 kilograms
- Elderly patients (>65 years of age)
- History of previous gastrointestinal disease
- Recent thrombolytic therapy

Increased risk of hemorrhage during or following angioplasty is associated with the following factors; these risks may be additive to that associated with abciximab therapy:
- Unsuccessful PTCA
- PTCA procedure >70 minutes duration
- PTCA performed within 12 hours of symptom onset for acute myocardial infarction

There is no data concerning the safety or efficacy of readministration of abciximab; administration of abciximab may result in human antichimeric antibody formation that can cause hypersensitivity reactions (including anaphylaxis), thrombocytopenia, or diminished efficacy. Anticoagulation, such as with heparin, may contribute to the risk of bleeding.

Adverse Reactions

>10%:
- Cardiovascular: Hypotension
- Central nervous system: Pain
- Gastrointestinal: Nausea
- Hematologic: Major bleeding episodes

1% to 10%:
- Cardiovascular: Bradycardia, peripheral edema
- Hematologic: Minor bleeding episodes, thrombocytopenia, anemia
- Respiratory: Pleural effusion

Overdosage/Toxicology Since abciximab is a platelet antiaggregate, patients who bleed following its administration may be best treated with platelet infusions

Drug Interactions

Increased toxicity:
- Bleeding: Heparin, other anticoagulants, thrombolytics, and antiplatelet drugs
- Allergic reactions: Diagnostic or therapeutic monoclonal antibodies

Stability Vials should be stored at 2°C to 8°C, do not freeze; after admixture, the prepared solution is stable for 12 hours; abciximab should be administered in a separate intravenous line; no incompatibilities have been observed with glass bottles or PVC bags

Usual Dosage I.V.: 0.25 mg/kg bolus followed by an infusion of 10 mcg/minute for 12 hours

Administration Abciximab is intended for coadministration with aspirin postangioplasty and heparin infused and weight adjusted to maintain a therapeutic bleeding time (eg, ACT 300-500 seconds)

Bolus dose: Aseptically withdraw the necessary amount of abciximab (2 mg/mL) for the bolus dose through a 0.22-micron filter into a syringe; the bolus should be administered 10-60 minutes before the procedure

Continuous infusion: Aseptically withdraw 4.5 mL (9 mg) of abciximab for the infusion through a 0.22 micron filter into a syringe; inject this into 250 mL of NS or D_5W to make a solution with a final concentration of 30 mcg/mL. Infuse at a rate of 17 mL/hour (10 mcg/minute) for 12 hours via pump; **filter all infusions**.

Monitoring Parameters Prothrombin time, activated partial thromboplastin time, hemoglobin, hematocrit, platelet count, fibrinogen, fibrin split products, transfusion requirements, signs of hypersensitivity reactions, guaiac stools, and Hemastix® urine

Nursing Implications Do not shake the vial; maintain bleeding precautions, avoid unnecessary arterial and venous punctures, use saline or heparin lock for blood drawing, assess sheath insertion site and distal pulses of affected leg every 15 minutes for the first hour and then every 1 hour for the next 6 hours. Observe patient for mental status changes, hemorrhage, assess nose and mouth mucous membranes, puncture sites for oozing, ecchymosis and hematoma formation, and examine urine, stool and emesis for presence of occult or frank blood; gentle care should be provided when removing dressings

Dosage Forms Injection: 2 mg/mL (5 mL)

Abelcet™ Injection *see* Amphotericin B Lipid Complex *on page 84*

ABLC *see* Amphotericin B Lipid Complex *on page 84*

Absorbine® Antifungal [OTC] *see* Tolnaftate *on page 1243*

Absorbine® Antifungal Foot Powder [OTC] *see* Miconazole *on page 834*

Absorbine® Jock Itch [OTC] *see* Tolnaftate *on page 1243*

Absorbine Jr.® Antifungal [OTC] *see* Tolnaftate *on page 1243*

Acarbose (AY car bose)

Related Information

Hypoglycemic Drugs, Comparison of Oral Agents *on page 1411*

Brand Names Precose™

Therapeutic Category Alpha-Glucosidase Inhibitor

Use

Monotherapy, as indicated as an adjunct to diet to lower blood glucose in patients with noninsulin-dependent diabetes mellitus (NIDDM) whose hyperglycemia cannot be managed on diet alone

Combination with a sulfonylurea when diet plus either acarbose or a sulfonylurea do not result in adequate glycemic control

Pregnancy Risk Factor B

Pregnancy/Breast-Feeding Implications It is not known whether acarbose is excreted in human milk

Contraindications Known hypersensitivity to the drug and in patients with diabetic ketoacidosis or cirrhosis; patients with inflammatory bowel disease, colonic ulceration, partial intestinal obstruction or in patients predisposed to intestinal obstruction; patients who have chronic intestinal diseases associated with marked disorders of digestion or absorption and in patients who have conditions that may deteriorate as a result of increased gas formation in the intestine

Warnings/Precautions Hypoglycemia: Acarbose may increase the hypoglycemic potential of sulfonylureas. Oral glucose (dextrose) should be used in the treatment of mild to moderate hypoglycemia. Severe hypoglycemia may require the use of either intravenous glucose infusion or glucagon injection.

Elevated serum transaminase levels: Treatment-emergent elevations of serum transaminases (AST and/or ALT) occurred in 15% of acarbose-treated patients in long-term studies. These serum transaminase elevations appear to be dose related. At doses >100 mg 3 times/day, the incidence of serum transaminase elevations greater than 3 times the upper limit of normal was 2-3 times higher in the acarbose group than in the placebo group. These elevations were asymptomatic, reversible, more common in females, and, in general, were not associated with other evidence of liver dysfunction.

When diabetic patients are exposed to stress such as fever, trauma, infection, or surgery, a temporary loss of control of blood glucose may occur. At such times, temporary insulin therapy may be necessary.

Adverse Reactions

>10%:

Gastrointestinal: Abdominal pain (21%) and diarrhea (33%) tend to return to pretreatment levels over time, and the frequency and intensity of flatulence (77%) tend to abate with time

Hepatic: Elevated liver transaminases

<1%:

Central nervous system: Sleepiness, headache, vertigo

Dermatologic: Erythema, urticaria

Gastrointestinal: Severe gastrointestinal distress

Neuromuscular & skeletal: Weakness

Overdosage/Toxicology An overdose will not result in hypoglycemia; an overdose may result in transient increases in flatulence, diarrhea, and abdominal discomfort which shortly subside

Drug Interactions Decreased effect: Thiazides and other diuretics, corticosteroids, phenothiazines, thyroid products, estrogens, oral contraceptives, phenytoin, nicotinic acid, sympathomimetics, calcium channel-blocking drugs, isoniazid, intestinal adsorbents (eg, charcoal), digestive enzyme preparations (eg, amylase, pancreatin)

Stability Store at <25°C (77°F) and protect from moisture

Mechanism of Action Competitive, reversible inhibition of pancreatic alpha-amylase and membrane-bound intestinal alpha-glucoside hydrolase enzymes to result in delayed glucose absorption and a lowering of postprandial hyperglycemia

Pharmacodynamics/Kinetics

Absorption: <2% absorbed as active drug

Metabolism: Metabolized exclusively within the gastrointestinal tract, principally by intestinal bacteria and by digestive enzymes; ~34% of dose is metabolized, absorbed, and subsequently excreted in the urine; 13 metabolites have been identified

Bioavailability: Low systemic bioavailability of parent compound because acarbose acts locally within the gastrointestinal tract

Elimination: The fraction that is absorbed as intact drug is almost completely excreted by the kidney

Usual Dosage Oral:

Adults: Dosage must be individualized on the basis of effectiveness and tolerance while not exceeding the maximum recommended dose of 100 mg 3 times/day

Initial dose: 25 mg 3 times/day with the first bite of each main meal

Maintenance dose: Should be adjusted at 4- to 8-week intervals based on 1-hour postprandial glucose levels and tolerance. Dosage may be increased from 25 mg 3 times/day to 50 mg 3 times/day. Some patients may benefit from increasing the dose to 100 mg 3 times/day.

Maintenance dose ranges: 50-100 mg 3 times/day.

Maximum dose:

≤60 kg: 50 mg 3 times/day

>60 kg: 100 mg 3 times/day

Patients receiving sulfonylureas: Acarbose given in combination with a sulfonylurea will cause a further lowering of blood glucose and may increase the hypoglycemic potential of the sulfonylurea. If hypoglycemia occurs, appropriate adjustments in the dosage of these agents should be made.

Dosing adjustment in renal impairment: Cl_{cr} <25 mL/minute: Peak plasma concentrations were 5 times higher and AUCs were 6 times larger than in volunteers with normal renal function; however, long term clinical trials in diabetic patients with significant renal dysfunction have not been conducted and treatment of these patients with acarbose is not recommended

Administration Should be administered with the first bite of each main meal

Monitoring Parameters Postprandial glucose, glycosylated hemoglobin levels, serum transaminase levels should be checked every 3 months during the first year of treatment and periodically thereafter

Patient Information Take acarbose 3 times/day at the start (with the first bite) of each main meal. It is important to continue to adhere to dietary instructions, a regular exercise program, and regular testing of urine and/or blood glucose.

The risk of hypoglycemia, its symptoms and treatment, and conditions that predispose to its development should be well understood by patients and responsible family members. A source of glucose (dextrose) should be readily available to treat symptoms of low blood glucose when taking acarbose in combination with a sulfonylurea or insulin. If side effects occur, they usually develop during the first few weeks of therapy and are most often mild to moderate gastrointestinal effects, such as flatulence, diarrhea, or abdominal discomfort and generally diminish in frequency and intensity with time.

Dosage Forms Tablet: 50 mg, 100 mg

Accolate® *see* Zafirlukast *on page 1316*

Accupril® *see* Quinapril *on page 1085*

Accutane® *see* Isotretinoin *on page 686*

ACE *see* Captopril *on page 197*

Acebutolol (a se BYOO toe lole)

Related Information

Beta-Blockers Comparison *on page 1398*

Brand Names Sectral®

Canadian/Mexican Brand Names Monitan® (Canada); Rhotral® (Canada)

Synonyms Acebutolol Hydrochloride

Therapeutic Category Antiarrhythmic Agent, Class II; Antihypertensive; Beta-Adrenergic Blocker

Use Treatment of hypertension, ventricular arrhythmias, angina

Pregnancy Risk Factor B

Contraindications Hypersensitivity to beta-blocking agents, avoid use in uncompensated congestive heart failure; cardiogenic shock; bradycardia or heart block; sinus node dysfunction; A-V conduction abnormalities. Although acebutolol primarily blocks $beta_1$-receptors, high doses can result in $beta_2$-receptor blockage. Use with caution in bronchospastic lung disease and renal dysfunction (especially the elderly).

Warnings/Precautions Abrupt withdrawal of beta-blockers may result in an exaggerated cardiac beta-adrenergic responsiveness. Symptomatology has included reports of tachycardia, hypertension, ischemia, angina, myocardial infarction, and sudden death. It is recommended that patients be tapered gradually off of beta-blockers over a 2-week period rather than via abrupt discontinuation.

Adverse Reactions

>10%: Fatigue

1% to 10%:

Cardiovascular: Chest pain, edema, bradycardia, hypotension

(Continued)

Acebutolol *(Continued)*

Central nervous system: Headache, dizziness, insomnia, depression, abnormal dreams
Dermatologic: Rash
Gastrointestinal: Constipation, diarrhea, dyspepsia, nausea, flatulence
Genitourinary: Polyuria
Neuromuscular & skeletal: Arthralgia, myalgia
Ocular: Abnormal vision
Respiratory: Dyspnea, rhinitis, cough

<1%:
Cardiovascular: Ventricular arrhythmias, heart block, heart failure, facial edema
Gastrointestinal: Xerostomia, anorexia
Genitourinary: Impotence, urinary retention
Miscellaneous: Cold extremities

Overdosage/Toxicology Symptoms of intoxication include cardiac disturbances, CNS toxicity, bronchospasm, hypoglycemia, and hyperkalemia. The most common cardiac symptoms include hypotension and bradycardia; atrioventricular block, intraventricular conduction disturbances, cardiogenic shock, and systole may occur with severe overdose, especially with membrane-depressant drugs (eg, propranolol); CNS effects include convulsions, coma, and respiratory arrest is commonly seen with propranolol and other membrane-depressant and lipid-soluble drugs

Treatment includes symptomatic treatment of seizures, hypotension, hyperkalemia and hypoglycemia; bradycardia and hypotension resistant to atropine, isoproterenol or pacing may respond to glucagon; wide QRS defects caused by the membrane-depressant poisoning may respond to hypertonic sodium bicarbonate; repeat-dose charcoal, hemoperfusion, or hemodialysis may be helpful.

Drug Interactions

Decreased effect of beta-blockers with aluminum salts, barbiturates, calcium salts, cholestyramine, colestipol, NSAIDs, penicillins (ampicillin), rifampin, salicylates, and sulfinpyrazone due to decreased bioavailability and plasma levels; decreased effect of sulfonylureas with beta-blockers

Increased effect/toxicity of beta-blockers with calcium blockers (diltiazem, felodipine, nicardipine), oral contraceptives, flecainide, haloperidol (propranolol, hypotensive effects), H_2-antagonists (metoprolol, propranolol only by cimetidine, possibly ranitidine), hydralazine (metoprolol, propranolol), loop diuretics (propranolol, not atenolol), MAO inhibitors (metoprolol, nadolol, bradycardia), phenothiazines (propranolol), propafenone (metoprolol, propranolol), quinidine (in extensive metabolizers), ciprofloxacin, thyroid hormones (metoprolol, propranolol, when hypothyroid patient is converted to euthyroid state)

Beta-blockers may increase the effect/toxicity of flecainide, haloperidol (hypotensive effects), hydralazine, phenothiazines, acetaminophen, anticoagulants (propranolol, warfarin), benzodiazepines (not atenolol), clonidine (hypertensive crisis after or during withdrawal of either agent), epinephrine (initial hypertensive episode followed by bradycardia), nifedipine and verapamil lidocaine, ergots (peripheral ischemia), prazosin (postural hypotension)

Beta-blockers may affect the action or levels of ethanol, disopyramide, nondepolarizing muscle relaxants and theophylline although the effects are difficult to predict

Mechanism of Action Competitively blocks $beta_1$-adrenergic receptors with little or no effect on $beta_2$-receptors except at high doses; exhibits membrane stabilizing and intrinsic sympathomimetic activity

Pharmacodynamics/Kinetics

Absorption: Oral: Well absorbed (40%)
Protein binding: 5% to 15%
Metabolism: Extensive first-pass
Half-life: 6-7 hours average
Time to peak: 2-4 hours
Elimination: ~55% of dose excreted via bile into feces and 35% excreted into urine

Usual Dosage Oral:

Adults: 400-800 mg/day in 2 divided doses; maximum: 1200 mg/day
Elderly: Initial: 200-400 mg/day; dose reduction due to age related decrease in Cl_{cr} will be necessary; do not exceed 800 mg/day

Dosing adjustment in renal impairment:

Cl_{cr} 25-49 mL/minute/1.73 m^2: Reduce dose by 50%
Cl_{cr} <25 mL/minute/1.73 m^2: Reduce dose by 75%

Dosing adjustment in hepatic impairment: Use with caution

Monitoring Parameters Blood pressure, orthostatic hypotension, heart rate, CNS effects, EKG

Test Interactions ↑ triglycerides, potassium, uric acid, cholesterol (S), glucose; ↓ HDL, ↑ thyroxine (S)

Patient Information Do not discontinue abruptly; consult pharmacist or physician before taking with other adrenergic drugs (eg, cold medications); notify physician if CHF symptoms become worse or if other side effects occur; take at the same time each day; use with caution while driving or performing tasks requiring alertness; may mask signs of hypoglycemia in diabetics; may be taken without regard to meals

Dosage Forms Capsule, as hydrochloride: 200 mg, 400 mg

Acebutolol Hydrochloride *see* Acebutolol *on page 17*

Acel-Imune® *see* Diphtheria, Tetanus Toxoids, and Acellular Pertussis Vaccine *on page 403*

Aceon® *see* Perindopril Erbumine *on page 976*

Acephen® [OTC] *see* Acetaminophen *on this page*

Aceta® [OTC] *see* Acetaminophen *on this page*

Acetaminophen (a seet a MIN oh fen)

Related Information

Acetaminophen Toxicity Nomogram *on page 1555*

Dosing Data for Acetaminophen and NSAIDs *on page 1377*

Brand Names Acephen® [OTC]; Aceta® [OTC]; Anacin-3® [OTC]; Apacet® [OTC]; Banesin® [OTC]; Dapa® [OTC]; Datril® [OTC]; Dorcol® [OTC]; Feverall™ [OTC]; Genapap® [OTC]; Halenol® [OTC]; Neopap® [OTC]; Panadol® [OTC]; Tempra® [OTC]; Tylenol® [OTC]; Valadol® [OTC]

Canadian/Mexican Brand Names 222 AF® (Canada); Abenol® (Canada); Atasol® (Canada); Pediatrix® (Canada); Tantaphen® (Canada); Algitrin® (Mexico); Analphen® (Mexico); Cilag® (Mexico); Febrin® (Mexico); Minofen® (Mexico); Neodol® (Mexico); Sinedol® (Mexico); Sinedol® 500 (Mexico); Temperal® (Mexico); Tylex® 750 (Mexico); Winasorb® (Mexico)

Synonyms APAP; N-Acetyl-P-Aminophenol; Paracetamol

Therapeutic Category Analgesic, Miscellaneous; Antipyretic

Use Treatment of mild to moderate pain and fever; does not have antirheumatic effects (analgesic)

Pregnancy Risk Factor B

Contraindications Patients with known G-6-PD deficiency; hypersensitivity to acetaminophen

Warnings/Precautions May cause severe hepatic toxicity on overdose; use with caution in patients with alcoholic liver disease; chronic daily dosing in adults of 5-8 g of acetaminophen over several weeks or 3-4 g/day of acetaminophen for 1 year have resulted in liver damage

Adverse Reactions

<1%:

Dermatologic: Rash

Gastrointestinal: Nausea, vomiting

Hematologic: Blood dyscrasias (neutropenia, pancytopenia, leukopenia), anemia

Renal: Analgesic nephropathy, nephrotoxicity with chronic overdose

Miscellaneous: Hypersensitivity reactions (rare)

Overdosage/Toxicology Symptoms of overdose include hepatic necrosis, transient azotemia, renal tubular necrosis with acute toxicity, anemia, and GI disturbances with chronic toxicity.

Acetylcysteine 140 mg/kg orally (loading) followed by 70 mg/kg every 4 hours for 17 doses. Therapy should be initiated based upon laboratory analysis suggesting high probability of hepatotoxic potential. Activated charcoal is very effective at binding acetaminophen.

Drug Interactions Cytochrome P-450 1A2 enzyme substrate (minor) and cytochrome P-450 2E enzyme substrate

Decreased effect: Rifampin can interact to reduce the analgesic effectiveness of acetaminophen

Increased toxicity: Barbiturates, carbamazepine, hydantoins, sulfinpyrazone can increase the hepatotoxic potential of acetaminophen; chronic ethanol abuse increases risk for acetaminophen toxicity

Mechanism of Action Inhibits the synthesis of prostaglandins in the central nervous system and peripherally blocks pain impulse generation; produces antipyresis from inhibition of hypothalamic heat-regulating center

Pharmacodynamics/Kinetics

Protein binding: 20% to 50%

Metabolism: At normal therapeutic dosages, the parent compound is metabolized in the liver to sulfate and glucuronide metabolites, while a small amount is

(Continued)

Acetaminophen *(Continued)*

metabolized by microsomal mixed function oxidases to a highly reactive intermediate (acetylimidoquinone) which is conjugated with glutathione and inactivated; at toxic doses (as little as 4 g in a single day) glutathione conjugation becomes insufficient to meet the metabolic demand causing an increase in acetylimidoquinone concentration, which is thought to cause hepatic cell necrosis

Half-life:

Neonates: 2-5 hours

Adults:

Normal renal function: 1-3 hours

End stage renal disease: 1-3 hours

Time to peak serum concentration: Oral: 10-60 minutes after normal doses, may be delayed in acute overdoses

Usual Dosage Oral, rectal (if fever not controlled with acetaminophen alone, administer with full doses of aspirin on an every 4- to 6-hour schedule, if aspirin is not otherwise contraindicated):

Children <12 years: 10-15 mg/kg/dose every 4-6 hours as needed; do **not** exceed 5 doses (2.6 g) in 24 hours; alternatively, the following doses may be used. See table.

Acetaminophen Dosing

Age	Dosage (mg)	Age	Dosage (mg)
0-3 mo	40	4-5 y	240
4-11 mo	80	6-8 y	320
1-2 y	120	9-10 y	400
2-3 y	160	11 y	480

Adults: 325-650 mg every 4-6 hours or 1000 mg 3-4 times/day; do **not** exceed 4 g/day

Dosing interval in renal impairment:

Cl_{cr} 10-50 mL/minute: Administer every 6 hours

Cl_{cr} <10 mL/minute: Administer every 8 hours (metabolites accumulate)

Hemodialysis: Moderately dialyzable (20% to 50%)

Dosing adjustment/comments in hepatic impairment: Appears to be well tolerated in cirrhosis; serum levels may need monitoring with long-term use

Dietary Considerations

Food: May slightly delay absorption of extended-release preparations; rate of absorption may be decreased when given with food high in carbohydrates

Alcohol: Excessive intake of alcohol may increase the risk of acetaminophen-induced hepatotoxicity; avoid or limit alcohol intake

Administration Administer with food

Monitoring Parameters Relief of pain or fever

Reference Range

Therapeutic concentration: 10-30 μg/mL

Toxic concentration: >200 μg/mL

Toxic concentration with probable hepatotoxicity: >200 μg/mL at 4 hours or 50 μg/mL at 12 hours

Test Interactions ↑ chloride, bilirubin, uric acid, glucose, ammonia (B), chloride (S), uric acid (S), alkaline phosphatase (S), chloride (S); ↓ sodium, bicarbonate, calcium (S)

Nursing Implications

Suppositories: Do not freeze

Suspension, oral: Shake well before pouring a dose

Dosage Forms

Caplet: 160 mg, 325 mg, 500 mg

Caplet, extended: 650 mg

Capsule: 80 mg

Drops: 48 mg/mL (15 mL); 60 mg/0.6 mL (15 mL); 80 mg/0.8 mL (15 mL); 100 mg/mL (15 mL, 30 mL)

Elixir: 80 mg/5 mL, 120 mg/5 mL, 160 mg/5 mL, 167 mg/5 mL, 325 mg/5 mL

Liquid, oral: 160 mg/5 mL, 500 mg/15 mL

Solution: 100 mg/mL (15 mL); 120 mg/2.5 mL

Suppository, rectal: 80 mg, 120 mg, 125 mg, 300 mg, 325 mg, 650 mg

Suspension, oral: 160 mg/5 mL

Suspension, oral drops: 80 mg/0.8 mL

Tablet: 325 mg, 500 mg, 650 mg

Tablet, chewable: 80 mg, 160 mg

Acetaminophen and Codeine (a seet a MIN oh fen & KOE deen)

Related Information

Acetaminophen Toxicity Nomogram *on page 1555*

Dose Equivalents for Opioid Analgesics in Opioid-Naive Adults <50 kg *on page 1376*

Dose Equivalents for Opioid Analgesics in Opioid-Naive Adults ≥50 kg *on page 1375*

Brand Names Capital® and Codeine; Phenaphen® With Codeine; Tylenol® With Codeine

Canadian/Mexican Brand Names Atesol® 8, 15, 30 with caffeine (Canada); Empracet® 30, 60 (Canada); Emtec 30®; Lenoltec No 1, 2, 3, 4 (Canada); Novo-Gesic-C8® (Canada); Novo-Gesic-C15® (Canada); Novo-Gesic-C30® (Canada); Tylex® CD (Mexico)

Synonyms Codeine and Acetaminophen

Therapeutic Category Analgesic, Narcotic

Use Relief of mild to moderate pain

Restrictions C-III; C-V

Pregnancy Risk Factor C

Contraindications Hypersensitivity to acetaminophen, codeine phosphate, or similar compounds

Warnings/Precautions Use with caution in patients with hypersensitivity reactions to other phenanthrene derivative opioid agonists (morphine, hydrocodone, hydromorphone, levorphanol, oxycodone, oxymorphone); tablets contain metabisulfite which may cause allergic reactions

Adverse Reactions

>10%:
- Central nervous system: Lightheadedness, dizziness, sedation
- Gastrointestinal: Nausea, vomiting
- Respiratory: Shortness of breath

1% to 10%:
- Central nervous system: Euphoria, dysphoria
- Dermatologic: Pruritus
- Gastrointestinal: Constipation, abdominal pain
- Miscellaneous: Histamine release

<1%:
- Cardiovascular: Palpitations, hypotension, bradycardia, peripheral vasodilation
- Central nervous system: Increased intracranial pressure
- Endocrine & metabolic: Antidiuretic hormone release
- Gastrointestinal: Biliary tract spasm
- Genitourinary: Urinary retention
- Ocular: Miosis
- Respiratory: Respiratory depression
- Miscellaneous: Physical and psychological dependence

Overdosage/Toxicology Symptoms of overdose include hepatic necrosis, blood dyscrasias, respiratory depression

Acetylcysteine 140 mg/kg orally (loading) followed by 70 mg/kg every 4 hours for 17 doses; therapy should be initiated based upon laboratory analysis suggesting high probability of hepatotoxic potential

Naloxone 2 mg I.V. (0.01 mg/kg for children) with repeat administration as necessary up to a total of 10 mg; can also be used to reverse the toxic effects of the opiate. Activated charcoal is effective at binding certain chemicals, and this is especially true for acetaminophen.

Drug Interactions Increased toxicity: CNS depressants, phenothiazines, tricyclic antidepressants, guanabenz, MAO inhibitors (may also decrease blood pressure)

Mechanism of Action Inhibits the synthesis of prostaglandins in the central nervous system and peripherally blocks pain impulse generation; produces antipyresis from inhibition of hypothalamic heat-regulating center; binds to opiate receptors in the CNS, causing inhibition of ascending pain pathways, altering the perception of and response to pain; causes cough supression by direct central action in the medulla; produces generalized CNS depression

Usual Dosage Doses should be adjusted according to severity of pain and response of the patient. Adult doses ≥60 mg codeine fail to give commensurate relief of pain but merely prolong analgesia and are associated with an appreciably increased incidence of side effects. Oral:

Children: Analgesic:
- Codeine: 0.5-1 mg codeine/kg/dose every 4-6 hours
- Acetaminophen: 10-15 mg/kg/dose every 4 hours up to a maximum of 2.6 g/24 hours for children <12 years
  - 3-6 years: 5 mL 3-4 times/day as needed of elixir
  - 7-12 years: 10 mL 3-4 times/day as needed of elixir

(Continued)

Acetaminophen and Codeine *(Continued)*

>12 years: 15 mL every 4 hours as needed of elixir

Adults:

Antitussive: Based on codeine (15-30 mg/dose) every 4-6 hours

Analgesic: Based on codeine (30-60 mg/dose) every 4-6 hours

1-2 tablets every 4 hours to a maximum of 12 tablets/24 hours

Dosing adjustment in renal impairment: Refer to individual monographs for Acetaminophen and Codeine

Monitoring Parameters Relief of pain, respiratory and mental status, blood pressure, bowel function

Patient Information May cause drowsiness; do not exceed recommended dose; do not take for more than 10 days without physician's advice

Nursing Implications Observe patient for excessive sedation, respiratory depression, constipation

Dosage Forms

Capsule:

#2: Acetaminophen 325 mg and codeine phosphate 15 mg (C-III)

#3: Acetaminophen 325 mg and codeine phosphate 30 mg (C-III)

#4: Acetaminophen 325 mg and codeine phosphate 60 mg (C-III)

Elixir: Acetaminophen 120 mg and codeine phosphate 12 mg per 5 mL with alcohol 7% (C-V)

Suspension, oral, alcohol free: Acetaminophen 120 mg and codeine phosphate 12 mg per 5 mL (C-V)

Tablet: Acetaminophen 500 mg and codeine phosphate 30 mg (C-III); acetaminophen 650 mg and codeine phosphate 30 mg (C-III)

Tablet:

#1: Acetaminophen 300 mg and codeine phosphate 7.5 mg (C-III)

#2: Acetaminophen 300 mg and codeine phosphate 15 mg (C-III)

#3: Acetaminophen 300 mg and codeine phosphate 30 mg (C-III)

#4: Acetaminophen 300 mg and codeine phosphate 60 mg (C-III)

Acetaminophen and Hydrocodone *see* Hydrocodone and Acetaminophen *on page 620*

Acetaminophen and Oxycodone *see* Oxycodone and Acetaminophen *on page 938*

Acetaminophen Toxicity Nomogram *see page 1555*

Acetazolamide (a set a ZOLE a mide)

Related Information

Epilepsy Treatment *on page 1531*

Glaucoma Drug Therapy Comparison *on page 1410*

Sulfonamide Derivatives *on page 1420*

Brand Names Diamox®; Diamox Sequels®

Canadian/Mexican Brand Names Acetazolam® (Canada); Apo-Acetazolamide® (Canada); Novo-Zolamide® (Canada)

Therapeutic Category Anticonvulsant; Carbonic Anhydrase Inhibitor; Diuretic, Carbonic Anhydrase Inhibitor

Use Lowers intraocular pressure to treat glaucoma, also as a diuretic, adjunct treatment of refractory seizures and acute altitude sickness; centrencephalic epilepsies (sustained release not recommended for anticonvulsant)

Pregnancy Risk Factor C

Pregnancy/Breast-Feeding Implications Despite widespread usage, no reports linking the use of acetazolamide with congenital defects have been located. The American Academy of Pediatrics considers acetazolamide to be compatible with breast-feeding.

Contraindications Hypersensitivity to sulfonamides or acetazolamide, patients with hepatic disease or insufficiency; patients with decreased sodium and/or potassium levels; patients with adrenocortical insufficiency, hyperchloremic acidosis, severe renal disease or dysfunction, or severe pulmonary obstruction; long-term use in noncongestive angle-closure glaucoma

Warnings/Precautions

Use in impaired hepatic function may result in coma; use with caution in patients with respiratory acidosis and diabetes mellitus; impairment of mental alertness and/or physical coordination may occur

I.M. administration is painful because of the alkaline pH of the drug

Drug may cause substantial increase in blood glucose in some diabetic patients; malaise and complaints of tiredness and myalgia are signs of excessive dosing and acidosis in the elderly

Adverse Reactions

>10%:

Central nervous system: Malaise

Gastrointestinal: Anorexia, diarrhea, metallic taste

Genitourinary: Polyuria
Neuromuscular & skeletal: Muscular weakness
1% to 10%: Central nervous system: Mental depression, drowsiness
<1%:
Central nervous system: Fever, fatigue
Dermatologic: Rash
Endocrine & metabolic: Hyperchloremic metabolic acidosis, hypokalemia, hyperglycemia
Gastrointestinal: Black stools, GI irritation, dryness of the mouth
Genitourinary: Dysuria
Hematologic: Bone marrow suppression, blood dyscrasias
Neuromuscular & skeletal: Paresthesia
Ocular: Myopia
Renal: Renal calculi

Overdosage/Toxicology Symptoms of overdose include low blood sugar, tingling of lips and tongue, nausea, yawning, confusion, agitation, tachycardia, sweating, convulsions, stupor, and coma

Hypoglycemia should be managed with 50 mL I.V. dextrose 50% followed immediately with a continuous infusion of 10% dextrose in water (administer at a rate sufficient enough to approach a serum glucose level of 100 mg/dL). The use of corticosteroids to treat the hypoglycemia is controversial, however, the addition of 100 mg of hydrocortisone to the dextrose infusion may prove helpful.

Drug Interactions

Decreased effect: Increased lithium excretion and altered excretion of other drugs by alkalinization of urine (such as amphetamines, quinidine, procainamide, methenamine, phenobarbital, salicylates); primidone serum concentrations may be decreased

Increased toxicity: Cyclosporine trough concentrations may be increased resulting in possible nephrotoxicity and neurotoxicity; salicylate use may result in carbonic anhydrase inhibitor accumulation and toxicity including CNS depression and metabolic acidosis; digitalis toxicity may occur if hypokalemia is untreated

Stability

Reconstituted solution may be stored under refrigeration (2°C to 8°C) for 1 week
Standard diluent: 500 mg/50 mL D_5W
Minimum volume: 50 mL D_5W
Stability of IVPB solution: 5 days at room temperature (25°C) and 44 days at refrigeration (5°C)
Reconstitute with at least 5 mL sterile water to provide a solution containing not more than 100 mg/mL; further dilution in 50 mL of either D_5W or NS for I.V. infusion administration

Mechanism of Action Reversible inhibition of the enzyme carbonic anhydrase resulting in reduction of hydrogen ion secretion at renal tubule and an increased renal excretion of sodium, potassium, bicarbonate, and water to decrease production of aqueous humor; also inhibits carbonic anhydrase in central nervous system to retard abnormal and excessive discharge from CNS neurons

Pharmacodynamics/Kinetics

Onset of action:
Extended release capsule: 2 hours
I.V.: 2 minutes
Peak effect:
Extended release capsule: 3-6 hours
Tablet: 1-4 hours
I.V.: 15 minutes
Duration:
Extended release capsule: 18-24 hours
Tablet: 8-12 hours
I.V.: 4-5 hours
Distribution: Distributes into erythrocytes, kidneys; crosses blood-brain barrier; crosses placenta and distributes into milk to ~30% of plasma concentrations
Protein binding: 95%
Half-life: 2.4-5.8 hours
Elimination: 70% to 100% of I.V. or tablet dose is excreted unchanged in the urine within 24 hours

Usual Dosage Note: I.M. administration is not recommended because of pain secondary to the alkaline pH

Children:
Glaucoma:
Oral: 8-30 mg/kg/day or 300-900 mg/m^2/day divided every 8 hours
I.M., I.V.: 20-40 mg/kg/24 hours divided every 6 hours, not to exceed 1 g/day
Edema: Oral, I.M., I.V.: 5 mg/kg or 150 mg/m^2 once every day

(Continued)

Acetazolamide *(Continued)*

Epilepsy: Oral: 8-30 mg/kg/day in 1-4 divided doses, not to exceed 1 g/day; sustained release capsule is not recommended for treatment of epilepsy

To slow the progression of hydrocephalus in infants who may not be good candidates for surgery, acetazolamide I.V. or oral doses of 5 mg/kg/dose every 6 hours increased by 25 mg/kg/day to a maximum of 100 mg/kg/day, if tolerated, have been used. Furosemide was used in combination with acetazolamide.

Adults:

Glaucoma:

Chronic simple (open-angle): Oral: 250 mg 1-4 times/day or 500 mg sustained release capsule twice daily

Secondary, acute (closed-angle): I.M., I.V.: 250-500 mg, may repeat in 2-4 hours to a maximum of 1 g/day

Edema: Oral, I.M., I.V.: 250-375 mg once daily

Epilepsy: Oral: 8-30 mg/kg/day in 1-4 divided doses; **sustained release capsule is not recommended for treatment of epilepsy**

Altitude sickness: Oral: 250 mg every 8-12 hours (or 500 mg extended release capsules every 12-24 hours)

Therapy should begin 24-48 hours before and continue during ascent and for at least 48 hours after arrival at the high altitude

Urine alkalinization: Oral: 5 mg/kg/dose repeated 2-3 times over 24 hours

Elderly: Oral: Initial: 250 mg twice daily; use lowest effective dose

Dosing adjustment in renal impairment:

Cl_{cr} 10-50 mL/minute: Administer every 12 hours

Cl_{cr} <10 mL/minute: Avoid use → ineffective

Hemodialysis: Moderately dialyzable (20% to 50%)

Peritoneal dialysis: Supplemental dose is not necessary

Administration Recommended rate of administration: 100-500 mg/minute for I.V. push and 4-8 hours for I.V. infusions

Monitoring Parameters Intraocular pressure, potassium, serum bicarbonate; serum electrolytes, periodic CBC with differential

Test Interactions May cause false-positive results for urinary protein with Albustix®, Labstix®, Albutest®, Bumintest®

Patient Information Report numbness or tingling of extremities to physician; do not crush, chew, or swallow contents of long-acting capsule, but may be opened and sprinkled on soft food; ability to perform tasks requiring mental alertness and/or physical coordination may be impaired; take with food; drug may cause substantial increase in blood glucose in some diabetic patients

Additional Information Sodium content of 500 mg injection: 47.2 mg (2.05 mEq)

Dosage Forms

Capsule, sustained release: 500 mg

Injection: 500 mg

Tablet: 125 mg, 250 mg

Extemporaneous Preparations Tablets may be crushed and suspended in cherry, chocolate, raspberry, or other highly flavored carbohydrate syrup in concentrations of 25-100 mg/mL; simple suspensions are stable for 7 days. For solutions with longer stability, see references Parastampuria and Alexander.

Alexander KS, Haribhakti RP, and Parker GA, "Stability of Acetazolamide in Suspension Compounded From Tablets," *Am J Hosp Pharm*, 1991, 48(6):1241-4.

McEvoy G, ed, AHFS Drug Information 96, Bethesda, MD: American Society of Health-System Pharmacists, 1996.

Parastampuria J and Gupta VD, "Development of Oral Liquid Dosage Forms of Acetazolamide," *J Pharm Sci*, 1990, 79:385-6.

Acetic Acid (a SEE tik AS id)

Brand Names VōSol®

Synonyms Ethanoic Acid

Therapeutic Category Antibacterial, Otic; Antibacterial, Topical

Use Irrigation of the bladder; treatment of superficial bacterial infections of the external auditory canal and vagina

Pregnancy Risk Factor C

Contraindications During transurethral procedures; hypersensitivity to drug or components

Warnings/Precautions Not for internal intake or I.V. infusion; topical use or irrigation use only; use of irrigation in patients with mucosal lesions of urinary bladder may cause irritation; systemic acidosis may result from absorption

Adverse Reactions

<1%:

Endocrine & metabolic: Systemic acidosis

Genitourinary: Urologic pain
Renal: Hematuria

Usual Dosage
Irrigation (note dosage of an irrigating solution depends on the capacity or surface area of the structure being irrigated):
For continuous irrigation of the urinary bladder with 0.25% acetic acid irrigation, the rate of administration will approximate the rate of urine flow; usually 500-1500 mL/24 hours
For periodic irrigation of an indwelling urinary catheter to maintain patency, about 50 mL of 0.25% acetic acid irrigation is required
Otic: Insert saturated wick; keep moist 24 hours; remove wick and instill 5 drops 3-4 times/day

Nursing Implications For continuous or intermittent irrigation of the urinary bladder, urine pH should be checked at least 4 times/day and the irrigation rate adjusted to maintain a pH of 4.5-5

Dosage Forms Solution:
Irrigation: 0.25% (1000 mL)
Otic: Acetic acid 2% in propylene glycol (15 mL, 30 mL, 60 mL)

Acetohexamide (a set oh HEKS a mide)

Related Information
Hypoglycemic Drugs, Comparison of Oral Agents *on page 1411*
Sulfonamide Derivatives *on page 1420*

Brand Names Dymelor®

Therapeutic Category Antidiabetic Agent, Oral; Antihyperglycemic Agent; Hypoglycemic Agent, Oral; Sulfonylurea Agent

Use Adjunct to diet for the management of mild to moderately severe, stable, noninsulin-dependent (type II) diabetes mellitus

Pregnancy Risk Factor D

Pregnancy/Breast-Feeding Implications When administered near term, acetohexamide crosses the placenta and may persist in the neonatal serum for several days; despite lack of evidence of teratogenicity, acetohexamide should not be used in pregnancy

Contraindications Diabetes complicated by ketoacidosis, therapy of type I diabetes, hypersensitivity to sulfonylureas

Warnings/Precautions Advise patient to avoid alcohol or products containing alcohol; monitor for signs and symptoms of hypoglycemia (fatigue, excessive hunger, profuse sweating, or numbness of extremities)

Adverse Reactions
>10%:
Central nervous system: Headache, dizziness
Gastrointestinal: Constipation, diarrhea, heartburn, anorexia, epigastric fullness
1% to 10%: Dermatologic: Rash, urticaria, photosensitivity
<1%:
Endocrine & metabolic: Hypoglycemia
Hematologic: Aplastic anemia, hemolytic anemia, bone marrow suppression, thrombocytopenia, agranulocytosis

Overdosage/Toxicology Symptoms of overdose include low blood sugar, tingling of lips and tongue, nausea, yawning, confusion, agitation, tachycardia, sweating, convulsions, stupor, and coma

Hypoglycemia should be managed with 50 mL I.V. dextrose 50% followed immediately with a continuous infusion of 10% dextrose in water (administer at a rate sufficient enough to approach a serum glucose level of 100 mg/dL). The use of corticosteroids to treat hypoglycemia is controversial, however, the addition of 100 mg of hydrocortisone to the dextrose infusion may prove helpful.

Drug Interactions
Monitor patient closely; large number of drugs interact with sulfonylureas
Decreased effect: Decreases hypoglycemic effect when coadministered with cholestyramine, diazoxide, hydantoins, rifampin, thiazides, loop or thiazide diuretics, and phenylbutazone
Increased effect: Increases hypoglycemia when coadministered with salicylates or beta-adrenergic blockers; MAO inhibitors; oral anticoagulants, NSAIDs, sulfonamides, phenylbutazone, insulin, clofibrate, fenfluramine, fluconazole, gemfibrozil, H_2-antagonists, methyldopa, tricyclic antidepressants

Mechanism of Action Believed to cause hypoglycemia by stimulating insulin release from the pancreatic beta cells; reduces glucose output from the liver (decreases gluconeogenesis); insulin sensitivity is increased at peripheral target sites (alters receptor sensitivity/receptor density); potentiates effects of ADH; may produce mild diuresis and significant uricosuric activity

Pharmacodynamics/Kinetics
Onset of effect: 1 hour
(Continued)

Acetohexamide *(Continued)*

Peak hypoglycemic effects: 8-10 hours
Duration: 12-24 hours, prolonged with renal impairment
Distribution: Into breast milk
Protein binding: ~90% (ionic/nonionic)
Metabolism: In the liver to potent active metabolite
Half-life:
Parent compound: 0.8-2.4 hours
Metabolite: 5-6 hours
Elimination: Urinary excretion <40% as unchanged drug; metabolite, hydroxyhexamide is more potent and is excreted less rapidly; ~80% to 95% of dose excreted in urine within 24 hours; ~15% is excreted in bile

Usual Dosage Adults: Oral (elderly patients may be more sensitive and should be started at a lower dosage initially): 250 mg to 1.5 g/day in 1-2 divided doses; doses >1.5 g/day are not recommended; if dose is ≤1 g, administer as a single daily dose

Dosing adjustment in renal impairment: Cl_{cr} <50 mL/minute: Avoid use; prolonged hypoglycemia occurs in azotemic patients

Dosing adjustment in hepatic impairment: Initiate therapy at lower than recommended doses

Dietary Considerations Alcohol: Avoid use

Monitoring Parameters Fasting blood glucose, urine glucose, hemoglobin A_{1c} or fructosamine

Reference Range Target range: Adults:
Fasting blood glucose: <120 mg/dL
Adults: 80-140 mg/dL
Geriatrics: 100-150 mg/dL
Glycosylated hemoglobin: <7%

Patient Information If nausea or stomach upset occurs, may be taken with food; take at the same time each day; avoid alcohol; avoid hypoglycemia, eat regularly, do not skip meals; keep sugar source with you

Nursing Implications Blood (preferred) and urine glucose concentrations should be monitored when therapy is started; normally takes 7 days to determine therapeutic response; patients who are anorexic or NPO may need to have their dose held to avoid hypoglycemia

Dosage Forms Tablet: 250 mg, 500 mg

Acetophenazine (a set oh FEN a zeen)

Related Information
Antipsychotic Agents Comparison *on page 1396*

Brand Names Tindal®

Synonyms Acetophenazine Maleate

Therapeutic Category Antipsychotic Agent

Use Management of manifestations of psychotic disorders

Pregnancy Risk Factor C

Contraindications Blood dyscrasias and bone marrow suppression, patients in coma or brain damage, known hypersensitivity to acetophenazine

Adverse Reactions
>10%:
Cardiovascular: Hypotension, orthostatic hypotension
Central nervous system: Pseudoparkinsonism, akathisia, dystonias, tardive dyskinesia (persistent), dizziness
Gastrointestinal: Constipation
Ocular: Pigmentary retinopathy
Respiratory: Nasal congestion
Miscellaneous: Diaphoresis (decreased)
1% to 10%:
Dermatologic: Increased sensitivity to sun, rash
Endocrine & metabolic: Changes in menstrual cycle, breast pain, changes in libido
Gastrointestinal: Weight gain, nausea, vomiting, stomach pain
Genitourinary: Dysuria, ejaculatory disturbances
Neuromuscular & skeletal: Trembling fingers
<1%:
Central nervous system: Neuroleptic malignant syndrome (NMS), impairment of temperature regulation, lowering of seizures threshold
Dermatologic: Discoloration of skin (blue-gray)
Endocrine & metabolic: Galactorrhea
Genitourinary: Priapism
Hematologic: Agranulocytosis, leukopenia
Hepatic: Cholestatic jaundice, hepatotoxicity

Ocular: Cornea and lens changes, pigmentary retinopathy

Overdosage/Toxicology

Seizures: I.V.: Diazepam 5-10 mg (adults), 0.25-0.4 mg/kg (children up to 5 years)

Recurrence: Consider phenytoin or phenobarbital

Hypotension: I.V. fluids (10-20 mL/kg); place in Trendelenburg position; dopamine or levarterenol may be infused if no response

Arrhythmias: Lidocaine drip or phenytoin are considered drugs of choice

Documented torsade de pointes: Isoproterenol 2-10 mcg/minute (0.1-1 mcg/minute in children) magnesium sulfate

Mechanism of Action Antagonizes the effects of dopamine in the basal ganglia and limbic areas of the forebrain; this activity appears responsible for the antipsychotic efficacy, as well as the production of extrapyramidal symptoms; increases the secretion of prolactin and has a marked suppressive effect on the chemoreceptor trigger zone; also produces peripheral blockade of cholinergic neurons

Pharmacodynamics/Kinetics

Duration of effect: ~24 hours, permitting daily dosing

Absorption: Tissue saturation, particularly in high lipid tissues such as the central nervous system

Metabolism: Phenothiazines are extensively hepatically metabolized with major routes of metabolism including oxidative processes and glucuronidation

Half-life, elimination: Range: 20-40 hours

Elimination: From the plasma is not significant for the phenothiazines; elimination from tissue saturated sites such as the central nervous system is slow, with metabolites of some phenothiazines detected in urine for several months after discontinuation of the drug

Usual Dosage Adults: Oral: 20 mg 3 times/day up to 60-120 mg/day

Hospitalized schizophrenic patients may require doses as high as 400-600 mg/day

Hemodialysis: Not dialyzable (0% to 5%)

Reference Range Therapeutic plasma levels have not yet been established

Test Interactions ↑ cholesterol (S), glucose; ↓ uric acid (S)

Dosage Forms Tablet, as maleate: 20 mg

Acetophenazine Maleate *see* Acetophenazine *on previous page*

Acetoxymethylprogesterone *see* Medroxyprogesterone Acetate *on page 771*

Acetylcholine (a se teel KOE leen)

Related Information

Glaucoma Drug Therapy Comparison *on page 1410*

Brand Names Miochol®

Synonyms Acetylcholine Chloride

Therapeutic Category Cholinergic Agent, Ophthalmic; Ophthalmic Agent, Miotic

Use Produces complete miosis in cataract surgery, keratoplasty, iridectomy and other anterior segment surgery where rapid miosis is required

Pregnancy Risk Factor C

Pregnancy/Breast-Feeding Implications Acetylcholine is used primarily in the eye and there are no reports of its use in pregnancy; because it is ionized at physiologic pH, transplacental passage would not be expected

Contraindications Hypersensitivity to acetylcholine chloride and any components; acute iritis and acute inflammatory disease of the anterior chamber

Warnings/Precautions Systemic effects rarely occur but can cause problems for patients with acute cardiac failure, bronchial asthma, peptic ulcer, hyperthyroidism, GI spasm, urinary tract obstruction, and Parkinson's disease; open under aseptic conditions only

Adverse Reactions

<1%:

Cardiovascular: Bradycardia, hypotension, flushing

Central nervous system: Headache

Ocular: Altered distance vision, decreased night vision, transient lenticular opacities

Respiratory: Dyspnea

Miscellaneous: Diaphoresis

Overdosage/Toxicology Treatment includes flushing eyes with water or normal saline and supportive measures; if accidentally ingested, induce emesis or perform gastric lavage

Drug Interactions

Decreased effect possible with flurbiprofen and suprofen, ophthalmic

Increased effect may be prolonged or enhanced in patients receiving tacrine

Stability Prepare solution immediately before use and discard unused portion; acetylcholine solutions are unstable

(Continued)

Acetylcholine *(Continued)*

Mechanism of Action Causes contraction of the sphincter muscles of the iris, resulting in miosis and contraction of the ciliary muscle, leading to accommodation spasm

Pharmacodynamics/Kinetics
Onset of miosis: Occurs promptly
Duration: ~10 minutes

Usual Dosage Adults: Intraocular: 0.5-2 mL of 1% injection (5-20 mg) instilled into anterior chamber before or after securing one or more sutures

Patient Information May sting on instillation; use caution while driving at night or performing hazardous tasks; do not touch dropper to eye

Nursing Implications Discard any solution that is not used; open under aseptic conditions only

Dosage Forms Powder, intraocular, as chloride: 1:100 [10 mg/mL] (2 mL, 15 mL)

Acetylcholine Chloride *see* Acetylcholine *on previous page*

Acetylcysteine (a se teel SIS teen)

Related Information
Toxicology Information *on page 1553*

Brand Names Mucomyst®; Mucosil™

Synonyms Acetylcysteine Sodium; Mercapturic Acid; NAC; *N*-Acetylcysteine; *N*-Acetyl-L-cysteine

Therapeutic Category Antidote, Acetaminophen; Mucolytic Agent

Use Adjunctive mucolytic therapy in patients with abnormal or viscid mucous secretions in acute and chronic bronchopulmonary diseases; pulmonary complications of surgery and cystic fibrosis; diagnostic bronchial studies; antidote for acute acetaminophen toxicity

Pregnancy Risk Factor B

Pregnancy/Breast-Feeding Implications There are no adequate and well controlled studies in pregnant women; use if only clearly needed

Contraindications Known hypersensitivity to acetylcysteine

Warnings/Precautions Since increased bronchial secretions may develop after inhalation, percussion, postural drainage and suctioning should follow; if bronchospasm occurs, administer a bronchodilator; discontinue acetylcysteine if bronchospasm progresses

Adverse Reactions
>10%:
- Gastrointestinal: Vomiting
- Miscellaneous: Unpleasant odor during administration

1% to 10%:
- Central nervous system: Drowsiness, chills
- Gastrointestinal: Stomatitis, nausea
- Local: Irritation
- Respiratory: Bronchospasm, rhinorrhea, hemoptysis
- Miscellaneous: Clamminess

<1%: Dermatologic: Skin rash

Overdosage/Toxicology The treatment of acetylcysteine toxicity is usually aimed at reversing anaphylactoid symptoms or controlling nausea and vomiting. The use of epinephrine, antihistamines, and steroids may be beneficial.

Stability Store opened vials in the refrigerator, use within 96 hours; dilutions should be freshly prepared and used within 1 hour; light purple color of solution does **not** affect its mucolytic activity

Mechanism of Action Exerts mucolytic action through its free sulfhydryl group which opens up the disulfide bonds in the mucoproteins thus lowering mucous viscosity. The exact mechanism of action in acetaminophen toxicity is unknown; thought to act by providing substrate for conjugation with the toxic metabolite.

Pharmacodynamics/Kinetics
Oral:
- Peak plasma levels: 1-2 hours
- Distribution: 0.33-0.47 L/kg
- Plasma protein binding: 50%

Onset of action: Inhalation: Mucus liquefaction occurs maximally within 5-10 minutes
Duration: Can persist for >1 hour
Half-life:
- Reduced acetylcysteine: 2 hours
- Total acetylcysteine: 5.5 hours

Usual Dosage
Acetaminophen poisoning: Children and Adults: Oral: 140 mg/kg; followed by 17 doses of 70 mg/kg every 4 hours; repeat dose if emesis occurs within 1 hour of

administration; therapy should continue until all doses are administered even though the acetaminophen plasma level has dropped below the toxic range

Inhalation: Acetylcysteine 10% and 20% solution (Mucomyst®) (dilute 20% solution with sodium chloride or sterile water for inhalation); 10% solution may be used undiluted

Infants: 1-2 mL of 20% solution or 2-4 mL 10% solution until nebulized given 3-4 times/day

Children: 3-5 mL of 20% solution or 6-10 mL of 10% solution until nebulized given 3-4 times/day

Adolescents: 5-10 mL of 10% to 20% solution until nebulized given 3-4 times/day

Note: Patients should receive an aerosolized bronchodilator 10-15 minutes prior to acetylcysteine

Meconium ileus equivalent: Children and Adults: 100-300 mL of 4% to 10% solution by irrigation or orally

Administration For treatment of acetaminophen overdosage, administer orally as a 5% solution

Dilute the 20% solution 1:3 with a cola, orange juice, or other soft drink

Use within 1 hour of preparation; unpleasant odor becomes less noticeable as treatment progresses

Reference Range Determine acetaminophen level as soon as possible, but no sooner than 4 hours after ingestion (to ensure peak levels have been obtained); administer for acetaminophen level >150 μg/mL; toxic concentration with probable hepatotoxicity: >200 μg/mL at 4 hours or 50 μg at 12 hours

Patient Information Clear airway by coughing deeply before aerosol treatment

Nursing Implications Assess patient for nausea, vomiting, and skin rash following oral administration for treatment of acetaminophen poisoning; intermittent aerosol treatments are commonly given when patient arises, before meals, and just before retiring at bedtime

Dosage Forms Solution, as sodium: 10% [100 mg/mL] (4 mL, 10 mL, 30 mL); 20% [200 mg/mL] (4 mL, 10 mL, 30 mL, 100 mL)

Acetylcysteine Sodium *see* Acetylcysteine *on previous page*

Acetylsalicylic Acid *see* Aspirin *on page 106*

Aches-N-Pain® [OTC] *see* Ibuprofen *on page 639*

Achromycin® *see* Tetracycline *on page 1203*

Achromycin® V *see* Tetracycline *on page 1203*

Aciclovir *see* Acyclovir *on next page*

Acidulated Phosphate Fluoride *see* Fluoride *on page 536*

Aclovate® *see* Alclometasone *on page 40*

Acrivastine and Pseudoephedrine

(AK ri vas teen & soo doe e FED rin)

Related Information

Pseudoephedrine *on page 1074*

Brand Names Semprex-D®

Synonyms Pseudoephedrine and Acrivastine

Therapeutic Category Antihistamine, H_1 Blocker; Decongestant

Use Temporary relief of nasal congestion, decongest sinus openings, running nose, itching of nose or throat, and itchy, watery eyes due to hay fever or other upper respiratory allergies

Pregnancy Risk Factor B

Contraindications MAO inhibitor therapy within 14 days of initiating therapy, severe hypertension, severe coronary artery disease, hypersensitivity to pseudoephedrine, acrivastine (or other alkylamine antihistamines), or any component, renal impairment (Cl_{cr} <48 mL/minute)

Warnings/Precautions Use with caution in patients >60 years of age; use with caution in patients with high blood pressure, ischemic heart disease, diabetes, increased intraocular pressure, GI or GU obstruction, asthma, thyroid disease, or prostatic hypertrophy; not recommended for use in children

Adverse Reactions

>10%: Central nervous system: Drowsiness, headache

1% to 10%:

Cardiovascular: Tachycardia, palpitations

Central nervous system: Nervousness, dizziness, insomnia, vertigo, lightheadedness, fatigue

Gastrointestinal: Nausea, vomiting, xerostomia, diarrhea

Genitourinary: Dysuria

Neuromuscular & skeletal: Weakness

Respiratory: Pharyngitis, cough increase

Miscellaneous: Diaphoresis

(Continued)

Acrivastine and Pseudoephedrine *(Continued)*

<1%:
Endocrine & metabolic: Dysmenorrhea
Gastrointestinal: Dyspepsia

Overdosage/Toxicology Symptoms of overdose include trembling, tachycardia, stridor, loss of consciousness, and possible convulsions

There is no specific antidote for pseudoephedrine intoxication, and the bulk of the treatment is supportive. Hyperactivity and agitation usually respond to reduced sensory input, however, with extreme agitation haloperidol (2-5 mg I.M. for adults) may be required.

Hyperthermia is best treated with external cooling measures, or when severe or unresponsive, muscle paralysis with pancuronium may be needed. Hypertension is usually transient and generally does not require treatment unless severe. For diastolic blood pressure >110 mm Hg, a nitroprusside infusion should be initiated. Seizures usually respond to diazepam I.V. and/or phenytoin maintenance regimens.

Drug Interactions
Decreased effect of guanethidine, reserpine, methyldopa, and beta-blockers
Increased toxicity with MAO inhibitors (hypertensive crisis), sympathomimetics, CNS depressants, alcohol (sedation)

Mechanism of Action Refer to Pseudoephedrine monograph; acrivastine is an analogue of triprolidine and it is considered to be relatively less sedating than traditional antihistamines; believed to involve competitive blockade of H_1-receptor sites resulting in the inability of histamine to combine with its receptor sites and exert its usual effects on target cells

Usual Dosage Adults: 1 capsule 3-4 times/day
Dosing comments in renal impairment: Do not use

Dosage Forms Capsule: Acrivastine 8 mg and pseudoephedrine hydrochloride 60 mg

ACT *see* Dactinomycin *on page 337*
ACT® [OTC] *see* Fluoride *on page 536*
Actagen® Syrup [OTC] *see* Triprolidine and Pseudoephedrine *on page 1270*
Actagen® Tablet [OTC] *see* Triprolidine and Pseudoephedrine *on page 1270*
ActHIB® *see Haemophilus* b Conjugate Vaccine *on page 595*
Acticort™ *see* Hydrocortisone *on page 623*
Actidose-Aqua® [OTC] *see* Charcoal *on page 245*
Actidose® With Sorbitol [OTC] *see* Charcoal *on page 245*
Actifed® Allergy Tablet (Day) [OTC] *see* Pseudoephedrine *on page 1074*
Actigall™ *see* Ursodiol *on page 1283*
Actinex® *see* Masoprocol *on page 760*
Actinomycin D *see* Dactinomycin *on page 337*
Activase® *see* Alteplase *on page 53*
Activated Carbon *see* Charcoal *on page 245*
Activated Charcoal *see* Charcoal *on page 245*
Activated Dimethicone *see* Simethicone *on page 1136*
Activated Ergosterol *see* Ergocalciferol *on page 456*
Activated Methylpolysiloxane *see* Simethicone *on page 1136*
Actron® [OTC] *see* Ketoprofen *on page 697*
ACU-dyne® [OTC] *see* Povidone-Iodine *on page 1031*
Acular® *see* Ketorolac Tromethamine *on page 698*
Acutrim® Precision Release® [OTC] *see* Phenylpropanolamine *on page 991*
ACV *see* Acyclovir *on this page*
Acycloguanosine *see* Acyclovir *on this page*

Acyclovir (ay SYE kloe veer)

Related Information
Guidelines for the Prevention of Opportunistic Infections in Persons with HIV *on page 1457*
Treatment of Sexually Transmitted Diseases *on page 1485*

Brand Names Zovirax®

Canadian/Mexican Brand Names Avirax® (Canada); Acifur® (Mexico)

Synonyms Aciclovir; ACV; Acycloguanosine

Therapeutic Category Antiviral Agent, Oral; Antiviral Agent, Parenteral; Antiviral Agent, Topical

Use Treatment of initial and prophylaxis of recurrent mucosal and cutaneous herpes simplex (HSV-1 and HSV-2) infections; herpes simplex encephalitis; herpes zoster; genital herpes infection; varicella-zoster infections in healthy, nonpregnant persons >13 years of age, children >12 months of age who have a chronic skin or lung disorder or are receiving long-term aspirin therapy, and immunocompromised patients; for herpes zoster, acyclovir should be started within 72 hours of the appearance of the rash to be effective; acyclovir will not prevent postherpetic neuralgias

Pregnancy Risk Factor C

Contraindications Hypersensitivity to acyclovir

Warnings/Precautions Use with caution in patients with pre-existing renal disease or in those receiving other nephrotoxic drugs concurrently; maintain adequate urine output during the first 2 hours after I.V. infusion; use with caution in patients with underlying neurologic abnormalities, serious hepatic or electrolyte abnormalities, or substantial hypoxia

Adverse Reactions

>10%:

- Central nervous system: Headache
- Local: Inflammation at injection site

1% to 10%:

- Central nervous system: Lethargy, dizziness, seizures, confusion, agitation, coma
- Dermatologic: Rash
- Gastrointestinal: Nausea, vomiting
- Neuromuscular & skeletal: Tremor
- Renal: Impaired renal function

<1%:

- Central nervous system: Mental depression, insomnia
- Gastrointestinal: Anorexia
- Hepatic: LFT elevation
- Miscellaneous: Sore throat

Overdosage/Toxicology Symptoms of overdose include elevated serum creatinine, renal failure

In the event of an overdose, sufficient urine flow must be maintained to avoid drug precipitation within the renal tubules. Hemodialysis has resulted in up to 60% reductions in serum acyclovir levels.

Drug Interactions Increased CNS side effects with zidovudine and probenecid

Stability Incompatible with blood products and protein-containing solutions; reconstituted solutions remain stable for 24 hours at room temperature; do not refrigerate reconstituted solutions as they may precipitate; in patients who require fluid restriction, a concentration of up to 10 mg/mL has been infused, however, concentrations >10 mg/mL (usual recommended concentration: <7 mg/mL in D_5W) increase the risk of phlebitis

Mechanism of Action Inhibits DNA synthesis and viral replication by competing with deoxyguanosine triphosphate for viral DNA polymerase and being incorporated into viral DNA

Pharmacodynamics/Kinetics

- Absorption: Oral: 15% to 30%; food does not appear to affect absorption
- Distribution: Widely distributed throughout the body including brain, kidney, lungs, liver, spleen, muscle, uterus, vagina, and CSF
- Protein binding: <30%
- Metabolism: Small amount of hepatic metabolism
- Half-life, terminal phase:
  - Neonates: 4 hours
  - Children 1-12 years: 2-3 hours
  - Adults: 3 hours
- Time to peak serum concentration:
  - Oral: Within 1.5-2 hours
  - I.V.: Within 1 hour
- Elimination: Primary route is the kidney (30% to 90% of a dose excreted unchanged); hemodialysis removes ~60% of the dose while removal by peritoneal dialysis is to a much lesser extent (supplemental dose recommended)

Usual Dosage

Dosing weight should be based on the smaller of lean body weight or total body weight

Adult determination of lean body weight (LBW) in kg:

- LBW males: 50 kg + (2.3 kg x inches >5 feet)
- LBW females: 45 kg + (2.3 kg x inches >5 feet)

Treatment of herpes simplex virus infections: Children and Adults: I.V.:

- Mucocutaneous HSV infection: 750 mg/m²/day divided every 8 hours or 5 mg/kg/dose every 8 hours for 5-10 days
- HSV encephalitis: 1500 mg/m²/day divided every 8 hours for 5-10 days

Treatment of herpes simplex virus infections: Adults:

- Oral: Treatment: 200 mg every 4 hours while awake (5 times/day)
- Topical: ½" ribbon of ointment for a 4" square surface area every 3 hours (6 times/day)

(Continued)

Acyclovir *(Continued)*

Treatment of varicella-zoster virus (chickenpox) infections:

Oral:

Children: 10-20 mg/kg/dose (up to 800 mg) 4 times/day for 5 days; begin treatment within the first 24 hours of rash onset

Adults: 600-800 mg/dose every 4 hours while awake (5 times/day) for 7-10 days or 1000 mg every 6 hours for 5 days

I.V.: Children and Adults: 1500 mg/m^2/day divided every 8 hours or 10 mg/kg/dose every 8 hours for 7 days

Treatment of herpes zoster infections:

Oral:

Children (immunocompromised): 250-600 mg/m^2/dose 4-5 times/day for 7-10 days

Adults (immunocompromised): 800 mg every 4 hours (5 times/day) for 7-10 days

I.V.:

Children and Adults (immunocompromised): 10-12 mg/kg/dose every 8 hours

Older Adults (immunocompromised): 7.5 mg/kg/dose every 8 hours

If nephrotoxicity occurs: 5 mg/kg/dose every 8 hours

Prophylaxis in immunocompromised patients:

Varicella zoster or herpes zoster in HIV-positive patients: Adults: Oral: 400 mg every 4 hours (5 times/day) for 7-10 days

Bone marrow transplant recipients: Children and Adults: I.V.:

Autologous patients who are HSV seropositive: 150 mg/m^2/dose (5 mg/kg) every 12 hours; with clinical symptoms of herpes simplex: 150 mg/m^2/dose every 8 hours

Autologous patients who are CMV seropositive: 500 mg/m^2/dose (10 mg/kg) every 8 hours; for clinically symptomatic CMV infection, consider replacing acyclovir with ganciclovir

Prophylaxis of herpes simplex virus infections: Adults: 200 mg 3-4 times/day or 400 mg twice daily

Dosing adjustment in renal impairment:

Oral: HSV/varicella-zoster:

Cl_{cr} 10-25 mL/minute: Administer dose every 8 hours

Cl_{cr} <10 mL/minute: Administer dose every 12 hours

I.V.:

Cl_{cr} 25-50 mL/minute: 5-10 mg/kg/dose: Administer every 12 hours

Cl_{cr} 10-25 mL/minute: 5-10 mg/kg/dose: Administer every 24 hours

Cl_{cr} <10 mL/minute: 2.5-5 mg/kg/dose: Administer every 24 hours

Hemodialysis: Dialyzable (50% to 100%); administer dose postdialysis

Peritoneal dialysis: Dose as for Cl_{cr} <10 mL/minute

Continuous arterio-venous or veno-venous hemofiltration (CAVH/CAVHD) effects: Dose as for Cl_{cr} <10 mL/minute

Administration Infuse over 1 hour; maintain adequate hydration of patient; check and rotate infusion sites for phlebitis

Monitoring Parameters Urinalysis, BUN, serum creatinine, liver enzymes, CBC

Patient Information Patients are contagious only when viral shedding is occurring; recurrences tend to appear within 3 months of original infection; acyclovir is **not** a cure; avoid sexual intercourse when lesions are present; may take with food

Nursing Implications Wear gloves when applying ointment for self-protection

Additional Information Sodium content of 1 g: 4.2 mEq

Dosage Forms

Capsule: 200 mg

Powder for Injection: 500 mg (10 mL); 1000 mg (20 mL)

Ointment, topical: 5% [50 mg/g] (3 g, 15 g)

Suspension, oral (banana flavor): 200 mg/5 mL

Tablet: 400 mg, 800 mg

Adagen™ *see* Pegademase Bovine *on page 955*

Adalat® *see* Nifedipine *on page 901*

Adalat® CC *see* Nifedipine *on page 901*

Adamantanamine Hydrochloride *see* Amantadine *on page 56*

Adapalene (a DAP a leen)

Brand Names Differin™

Therapeutic Category Acne Products

Use Treatment of acne vulgaris

Pregnancy Risk Factor C

Pregnancy/Breast-Feeding Implications

Pregnancy effects: No teratogenic effects were seen in rats at oral doses of adapalene 0.15 to 5 mg/kg/day topically

Breast feeding/lactation: There are no adequate and well controlled studies in pregnant women; it is not known whether adapalene is excreted in breast milk

Contraindications Hypersensitivity to adapalene or any of the components in the vehicle gel

Warnings/Precautions Use with caution in patients with eczema; avoid excessive exposure to sunlight and sunlamps; avoid contact with abraded skin, mucous membranes, eyes, mouth, angles of the nose

Certain cutaneous signs and symptoms such as erythema, dryness, scaling, burning or pruritus may occur during treatment; these are most likely to occur during the first 2-4 weeks and will usually lessen with continued use

Adverse Reactions

>10%: Dermatologic: Erythema, scaling, dryness, pruritus, burning, pruritus or burning immediately after application

≤1% Dermatologic: Skin irritation, stinging sunburn, acne flares

Overdosage/Toxicology Toxic signs of an overdose commonly respond to drug discontinuation, and generally return to normal spontaneously within a few days to weeks; when confronted with signs of increased intracranial pressure, treatment with mannitol (0.25 g/kg I.V. up to 1 g/kg/dose repeated every 5 minutes as needed), dexamethasone (1.5 mg/kg I.V. load followed with 0.375 mg/kg every 6 hours for 5 days), and/or hyperventilation should be employed

Mechanism of Action Retinoid-like compound which is a modulator of cellular differentiation, keratinization and inflammatory processes, all of which represent important features in the pathology of acne vulgaris

Pharmacodynamics/Kinetics

Absorption: Topical: Minimum absorption occurs

Elimination: In bile

Usual Dosage Children >12 years and Adults: Topical: Apply once daily before retiring; therapeutic results should be noticed after 8-12 weeks of treatment

Patient Information Thoroughly wash hands after applying; avoid hydration of skin immediately before application; minimize exposure to sunlight; avoid washing face more frequently than 2-3 times/day; if severe irritation occurs, discontinue medication temporarily and adjust dose when irritation subsides; avoid using topical preparations with high alcoholic content during treatment period; do not exceed prescribed dose

Nursing Implications Observe for signs of hypersensitivity, blistering, excessive dryness; do not apply to mucous membranes

Dosage Forms Gel, topical (alcohol free): 0.1% (15 g, 45 g)

Adapin® Oral *see* Doxepin *on page 424*

Adeflor® *see* Vitamins, Multiple *on page 1310*

Adenine Arabinoside *see* Vidarabine *on page 1300*

Adenocard® *see* Adenosine *on this page*

Adenosine (a DEN oh seen)

Related Information

Adult ACLS Algorithm, Tachycardia *on page 1512*

Antiarrhythmic Drugs *on page 1389*

Brand Names Adenocard®

Synonyms 9-Beta-D-ribofuranosyladenine

Therapeutic Category Antiarrhythmic Agent, Miscellaneous

Use Treatment of paroxysmal supraventricular tachycardia (PSVT) including that associated with accessory bypass tracts (Wolff-Parkinson-White syndrome); when clinically advisable, appropriate vagal maneuvers should be attempted prior to adenosine administration; not effective in atrial flutter, atrial fibrillation, or ventricular tachycardia

Pregnancy Risk Factor C

Pregnancy/Breast-Feeding Implications Case reports (4) on administration during pregnancy have indicated no adverse effects on fetus or newborn attributable to adenosine

Contraindications Known hypersensitivity to adenosine; second or third degree A-V block or sick-sinus syndrome (except in patients with a functioning artificial pacemaker), atrial flutter, atrial fibrillation, and ventricular tachycardia (the drug is not effective in converting these arrhythmias to sinus rhythm)

Warnings/Precautions Patients with pre-existing S-A nodal dysfunction may experience prolonged sinus pauses after adenosine; there have been reports of atrial fibrillation/flutter in patients with PSVT associated with accessory conduction pathways after adenosine; adenosine decreases conduction through the A-V node and may produce a short lasting first, second, or third degree heart block. Because of the very short half-life, the effects are generally self limiting. At the time of conversion to normal sinus rhythm, a variety of new rhythms may appear on the EKG.

(Continued)

Adenosine *(Continued)*

A limited number of patients with asthma have received adenosine and have not experienced exacerbation of their asthma. Be alert to the possibility that adenosine could produce bronchoconstriction in patients with asthma.

Adverse Reactions

>10%:
- Cardiovascular: Facial flushing (18%), palpitations, chest pain, hypotension
- Central nervous system: Headache
- Respiratory: Shortness of breath/dyspnea (12%)
- Miscellaneous: Diaphoresis

1% to 10%:
- Central nervous system: Dizziness
- Gastrointestinal: Nausea (3%)
- Neuromuscular & skeletal: Paresthesia, numbness
- Respiratory: Chest pressure (7%)

<1%:
- Cardiovascular: Hypotension
- Central nervous system: Lightheadedness, headache, dizziness, apprehension, intracranial pressure
- Gastrointestinal: Metallic taste, tightness in throat, pressure in groin
- Neuromuscular & skeletal: Neck and back pain
- Ocular: Blurred vision
- Respiratory: Hyperventilation
- Miscellaneous: Burning sensation, heaviness in arms

Overdosage/Toxicology Since half-life of adenosine is <10 seconds, any adverse effects are rapidly self-limiting. Intoxication is usually short-lived since the half-life of the drug is very short.

Treatment of prolonged effects requires individualization. Theophylline and other methylxanthines are competitive inhibitors of adenosine and may have a role in reversing its toxic effects.

Drug Interactions

Decreased effect: Methylxanthines antagonize effects

Increased effect: Dipyridamole potentiates effects of adenosine

Increased toxicity: Carbamazepine may increase heart block

Stability Do **not** refrigerate, precipitation may occur (may dissolve by warming to room temperature)

Mechanism of Action Slows conduction time through the A-V node, interrupting the re-entry pathways through the A-V node, restoring normal sinus rhythm

Pharmacodynamics/Kinetics

Onset: Clinical effects occur rapidly

Duration: Very brief

Metabolism: In the blood and tissue to inosine then to adenosine monophosphate (AMP) and hypoxanthine

Half-life: <10 seconds, thus adverse effects are usually rapidly self-limiting

Usual Dosage Rapid I.V. push (over 1-2 seconds) via peripheral line:

Neonates: Initial dose: 0.05 mg/kg; if not effective within 2 minutes, increase dose by 0.05 mg/kg increments every 2 minutes to a maximum dose of 0.25 mg/kg or until termination of PSVT

Maximum single dose: 12 mg

Infants and Children: Pediatric advanced life support (PALS): Treatment of SVT: 0.1 mg/kg; if not effective, administer 0.2 mg/kg

Alternatively: Initial dose: 0.05 mg/kg; if not effective within 2 minutes, increase dose by 0.05 mg/kg increments every 2 minutes to a maximum dose of 0.25 mg/kg or until termination of PSVT; medium dose required: 0.15 mg/kg

Maximum single dose: 12 mg

Adults: 6 mg; if not effective within 1-2 minutes, 12 mg may be given; may repeat 12 mg bolus if needed

Maximum single dose: 12 mg

Hemodialysis: Significant drug removal is unlikely based on physiochemical characteristics

Peritoneal dialysis: Significant drug removal is unlikely based on physiochemical characteristics

Note: Patients who are receiving concomitant theophylline therapy may be less likely to respond to adenosine therapy

Note: Higher doses may be needed for administration via peripheral versus central vein

Administration For rapid bolus I.V. use only; administer I.V. push over 1-2 seconds at a peripheral I.V. site closest to patient; follow each bolus with normal saline flush. **Note:** Preliminary results in adults suggest adenosine may be administered via central line at lower doses (eg, adults initial dose: 3 mg)

Monitoring Parameters EKG monitoring, heart rate, blood pressure

Nursing Implications Be alert for possible exacerbation of asthma in asthmatic patients

Dosage Forms Injection, preservative free: 3 mg/mL (2 mL)

ADH *see* Vasopressin *on page 1293*

Adipex-P® *see* Phentermine *on page 987*

Adlone® *see* Methylprednisolone *on page 819*

ADR *see* Doxorubicin *on page 425*

Adrenalin® *see* Epinephrine *on page 448*

Adrenaline *see* Epinephrine *on page 448*

Adrenergic Agonists, Cardiovascular Comparison *see page 1385*

Adriamycin PFS™ *see* Doxorubicin *on page 425*

Adriamycin RDF™ *see* Doxorubicin *on page 425*

Adrucil® *see* Fluorouracil *on page 538*

Adsorbent Charcoal *see* Charcoal *on page 245*

Adsorbocarpine® Ophthalmic *see* Pilocarpine *on page 999*

Adsorbonac® Ophthalmic [OTC] *see* Sodium Chloride *on page 1142*

Adult ACLS Algorithm, Asystole *see page 1511*

Adult ACLS Algorithm, Bradycardia *see page 1514*

Adult ACLS Algorithm, Electrical Conversion *see page 1515*

Adult ACLS Algorithm, Hypotension, Shock *see page 1516*

Adult ACLS Algorithm, Pulseless Electrical Activity *see page 1510*

Adult ACLS Algorithm, Tachycardia *see page 1512*

Adult ACLS Algorithm, V. Fib and Pulseless V. Tach *see page 1509*

Advanced Formula Oxy® Sensitive Gel [OTC] *see* Benzoyl Peroxide *on page 140*

Adverse Events and Vaccination *see page 1439*

Adverse Hematologic Effects, Drugs Associated With *see page 1567*

Advil® [OTC] *see* Ibuprofen *on page 639*

AeroBid®-M Oral Aerosol Inhaler *see* Flunisolide *on page 532*

AeroBid® Oral Aerosol Inhaler *see* Flunisolide *on page 532*

Aerodine® [OTC] *see* Povidone-Iodine *on page 1031*

Aerolate® *see* Theophylline Salts *on page 1207*

Aerolate III® *see* Theophylline Salts *on page 1207*

Aerolate JR® *see* Theophylline Salts *on page 1207*

Aerolate SR® *see* Theophylline Salts *on page 1207*

Aeroseb-Dex® *see* Dexamethasone *on page 356*

Aeroseb-HC® *see* Hydrocortisone *on page 623*

Aerosporin® *see* Polymyxin B *on page 1018*

Afrin® Children's Nose Drops [OTC] *see* Oxymetazoline *on page 940*

Afrin® Nasal Solution [OTC] *see* Oxymetazoline *on page 940*

Afrin® Saline Mist [OTC] *see* Sodium Chloride *on page 1142*

Afrin® Tablet [OTC] *see* Pseudoephedrine *on page 1074*

Aftate® for Athlete's Foot [OTC] *see* Tolnaftate *on page 1243*

Aftate® for Jock Itch [OTC] *see* Tolnaftate *on page 1243*

$AgNO_3$ *see* Silver Nitrate *on page 1135*

Agoral® Plain [OTC] *see* Mineral Oil *on page 841*

AHF *see* Antihemophilic Factor (Human) *on page 94*

A-HydroCort® *see* Hydrocortisone *on page 623*

Airet® *see* Albuterol *on page 38*

Akarpine® Ophthalmic *see* Pilocarpine *on page 999*

AKBeta® *see* Levobunolol *on page 712*

AK-Chlor® *see* Chloramphenicol *on page 250*

AK-Cide® Ophthalmic *see* Sulfacetamide Sodium and Prednisolone *on page 1172*

AK-Con® *see* Naphazoline *on page 879*

AK-Dex® *see* Dexamethasone *on page 356*

AK-Dilate® Ophthalmic Solution *see* Phenylephrine *on page 989*

AK-Fluor *see* Fluorescein Sodium *on page 535*

AK-Homatropine® *see* Homatropine *on page 612*

AK-NaCl® [OTC] *see* Sodium Chloride *on page 1142*

AK-Nefrin® Ophthalmic Solution *see* Phenylephrine *on page 989*

AK-Pentolate® *see* Cyclopentolate *on page 323*

AK-Poly-Bac® Ophthalmic *see* Bacitracin and Polymyxin B *on page 129*

AK-Pred® *see* Prednisolone *on page 1037*

AKPro® Ophthalmic *see* Dipivefrin *on page 406*

AK-Spore H.C.® Ophthalmic Ointment *see* Bacitracin, Neomycin, Polymyxin B, and Hydrocortisone *on page 130*

AK-Spore H.C.® Ophthalmic Suspension *see* Neomycin, Polymyxin B, and Hydrocortisone *on page 890*

AK-Spore H.C.® Otic *see* Neomycin, Polymyxin B, and Hydrocortisone *on page 890*

AK-Spore® Ophthalmic Ointment *see* Bacitracin, Neomycin, and Polymyxin B *on page 129*

AK-Spore® Ophthalmic Solution *see* Neomycin, Polymyxin B, and Gramicidin *on page 889*

AK-Sulf® Ophthalmic *see* Sulfacetamide Sodium *on page 1171*

AK-Taine® *see* Proparacaine *on page 1062*

AKTob® Ophthalmic *see* Tobramycin *on page 1233*

AK-Tracin® *see* Bacitracin *on page 127*

AK-Trol® *see* Neomycin, Polymyxin B, and Dexamethasone *on page 889*

Ala-Cort® *see* Hydrocortisone *on page 623*

Ala-Scalp™ *see* Hydrocortisone *on page 623*

Ala-Tet® *see* Tetracycline *on page 1203*

Alba-Dex® *see* Dexamethasone *on page 356*

Albalon® Liquifilm® *see* Naphazoline *on page 879*

Albendazole (al BEN da zole)

Brand Names Albenza®

Therapeutic Category Anthelmintic

Use Treatment of parenchymal neurocysticercosis and cystic hydatid disease of the liver, lung, and peritoneum; also in the treatment of ascariasis, trichuriasis, enterobiasis, hook worm, strongyloidiasis, giardiasis, and microsporidiosis in patients with HIV; steroid and anticonvulsant therapy should be used concurrently during the first week of therapy for neurocysticercosis to prevent cerebral hypertension

Pregnancy Risk Factor C; although it has been shown to be teratogenic in laboratory animals and should not be used during pregnancy if at all possible

Contraindications Patients with hypersensitivity to albendazole or its components; pregnant women

Warnings/Precautions Corticosteroids should be administered 1-2 days before albendazole therapy in patients with neurocysticercosis to minimize inflammatory reactions

Adverse Reactions

>1%:

Central nervous system: Dizziness, headache, vertigo, fever

Dermatologic: Alopecia, rash, pruritus

Gastrointestinal: Abdominal pain, nausea, vomiting, diarrhea, xerostomia

Hematologic: Eosinophilia, neutropenia, pancytopenia

Hepatic: Increased LFTs, jaundice

Miscellaneous: Allergic reactions

<1%:

Central nervous system: Increased intracranial pressure

Gastrointestinal: Anorexia, constipation, epigastric pain

Drug Interactions

Decreased effect: Carbamazepine may accelerate albendazole metabolism

Increased effect: Dexamethasone increases plasma levels of albendazole metabolites; praziquantel may increase plasma concentrations of albendazole by 50%; albendazole inhibits hepatic cytochrome P-450 1A and may consequently interact by increasing the concentrations of many drugs which are metabolized by this route; food (especially fatty meals) increases the oral bioavailability by 4-5 times

Mechanism of Action Active metabolite, albendazole, causes selective degeneration of cytoplasmic microtubules in intestinal and tegmental cells of intestinal helminths and larvae; glycogen is depleted, glucose uptake and cholinesterase secretion are impaired, and desecratory substances accumulate intracellulary. ATP production decreases causing energy depletion, immobilization, and worm death; albendazole has activity against *Ascaris lumbricoides* (roundworm), *Ancylostoma duodenale* and *Necatory americanus* (hookworms), *Enterobius vermicularis* (pinworm), *Hymeolepsis nana* and *Taenia* sp (tapeworms), *Opisthorchis sinensis* and *Opisthorchis viverrini* (liver flukes), *Stronyloides stercoralis* and *Trichuris trichiura* (whipworm); activity has also been shown against the liver fluke *Clonorchis sinensis, Giardia lamblia, Cysticercus cellulosae, Echinococcus granulosis,* and *Multilocularis,* and *Toxocara* sp.

Pharmacodynamics/Kinetics

Absorption: Oral absorption is poor (<5%); may increase up to 4-5 times when administered with a fatty meal

Distribution: Well distributed inside hydatid cysts; excellent CSF concentrations

Protein binding: 70%
Metabolism: Extensive first-pass metabolism; metabolic pathways include rapid sulfoxidation (major), hydrolysis, and oxidation
Half-life: 8-12 hours
Time to peak serum concentration: 2-2.4 hours
Elimination: Active and inactive metabolites excreted in urine

Usual Dosage Oral:
Children ≤2 years:
Neurocysticercosis: 15 mg/kg for 8 days; repeat as necessary
Hookworm, pinworm, roundworm: 200 mg as a single dose; may be repeated in 3 weeks
Strongyloidiasis and tapeworm: 200 mg/day for 3 days; may be repeated in 3 weeks
Children >2 years and Adults:
Hydatid disease: 800-1200 mg/day in divided doses for 28 days followed by a 2-week drug-free period, then repeated for a duration of therapy ranging from 1-12 months determined by the size, number, and location of cysts
Neurocysticercosis: 15 mg/kg for 8-30 days; repeat as necessary
Roundworm, pinworm, hookworm: 400 mg as a single dose; may be repeated in 3 weeks
Giardiasis: 400 mg/day for 3 days
Strongyloidiasis and tapeworm: 400 mg/day for 3 days; may be repeated in 3 weeks (giardiasis is a single course)

Monitoring Parameters Monitor fecal specimens for ova and parasites for 3 weeks after treatment; if positive, retreat; monitor LFTs, CBC, and clinical signs of hepatotoxicity

Patient Information Take with a high fat diet

Dosage Forms Tablet: 200 mg

Albenza® *see* Albendazole *on previous page*

Albumin (al BYOO min)

Brand Names Albuminar®; Albumisol®; Albutein®; Buminate®; Plasbumin®

Synonyms Albumin (Human); Normal Human Serum Albumin; Normal Serum Albumin (Human); Salt Poor Albumin; SPA

Therapeutic Category Blood Product Derivative; Plasma Volume Expander, Colloid

Use Plasma volume expansion and maintenance of cardiac output in the treatment of certain types of shock or impending shock; may be useful for burn patients, ARDS, and cardiopulmonary bypass; other uses considered by some investigators (but not proven) are retroperitoneal surgery, peritonitis, and ascites; unless the condition responsible for hypoproteinemia can be corrected, albumin can provide only symptomatic relief or supportive treatment; nutritional supplementation is not an appropriate indication for albumin

Pregnancy Risk Factor C

Contraindications Patients with severe anemia or cardiac failure, known hypersensitivity to albumin; avoid 25% concentration in preterm infants due to risk of idiopathic ventricular hypertrophy

Warnings/Precautions Use with caution in patients with hepatic or renal failure because of added protein load; rapid infusion of albumin solutions may cause vascular overload. All patients should be observed for signs of hypervolemia such as pulmonary edema. Use with caution in those patients for whom sodium restriction is necessary. Rapid infusion may cause hypotension.

Adverse Reactions
1% to 10%:
Cardiovascular: Precipitation of congestive heart failure or hypotension, tachycardia, hypervolemia
Central nervous system: Fever, chills
Dermatologic: Rash
Gastrointestinal: Nausea, vomiting
Respiratory: Pulmonary edema

Overdosage/Toxicology Symptoms of overdose include hypervolemia, congestive heart failure, pulmonary edema

Stability Do not use solution if it is turbid or contains a deposit; use within 4 hours after opening vial

Usual Dosage I.V.:
5% should be used in hypovolemic patients or intravascularly-depleted patients
25% should be used in patients in whom fluid and sodium intake must be minimized
Dose depends on condition of patient:
Children:
Emergency initial dose: 25 g
Nonemergencies: 25% to 50% of the adult dose
(Continued)

Albumin *(Continued)*

Adults: Usual dose: 25 g; no more than 250 g should be administered within 48 hours

Hypoproteinemia: 0.5-1 g/kg/dose; repeat every 1-2 days as calculated to replace ongoing losses

Hypovolemia: 0.5-1 g/kg/dose; repeat as needed; maximum dose: 6 g/kg/day

Administration Albumin administration must be completed within 6 hours after entering the 5% container, provided that administration is begun within 4 hours of entering the container; rapid infusion may cause vascular overload; albumin is best administered at a rate of 2-4 mL/minute; 25% albumin may be given at a rate of 1 mL/minute

Test Interactions ↑ alkaline phosphatase (S)

Additional Information Sodium content of 1 L: Both 5% and 25% albumin contain 130-160 mEq

Dosage Forms Injection, as human: 5% [50 mg/mL] (50 mL, 250 mL, 500 mL, 1000 mL); 25% [250 mg/mL] (10 mL, 20 mL, 50 mL, 100 mL)

Albuminar® *see* Albumin *on previous page*

Albumin (Human) *see* Albumin *on previous page*

Albumisol® *see* Albumin *on previous page*

Albutein® *see* Albumin *on previous page*

Albuterol (al BYOO ter ole)

Brand Names Airet®; Proventil®; Proventil® HFA; Ventolin®; Ventolin® Rotocaps®; Volmax®

Canadian/Mexican Brand Names Apo-Salvent® (Canada); Novo-Salmol® (Canada); Sabulin® (Canada); Volmax® (Canada); Salbulin® (Mexico); Salbutalan® (Mexico)

Synonyms Salbutamol

Therapeutic Category $Beta_2$-Adrenergic Agonist Agent; Bronchodilator; Sympathomimetic

Use Bronchodilator in reversible airway obstruction due to asthma or COPD

Pregnancy Risk Factor C

Pregnancy/Breast-Feeding Implications

Clinical effects on the fetus: Crosses the placenta. Tocolytic effects, fetal tachycardia, fetal hypoglycemia secondary to maternal hyperglycemia with oral or intravenous routes reported. Available evidence suggests safe use during pregnancy.

Breast-feeding/lactation: No data on crossing into breast milk or clinical effects on the infant

Contraindications Hypersensitivity to albuterol, adrenergic amines or any ingredients

Warnings/Precautions Use with caution in patients with hyperthyroidism, diabetes mellitus, or sensitivity to sympathomimetic amines; cardiovascular disorders including coronary insufficiency or hypertension; excessive use may result in tolerance

Some adverse reactions may occur more frequently in children 2-5 years of age than in adults and older children

Because of its minimal effect on $beta_1$-receptors and its relatively long duration of action, albuterol is a rational choice in the elderly when a beta agonist is indicated. All patients should utilize a spacer device when using a metered dose inhaler. Oral use should be avoided in the elderly due to adverse effects.

Adverse Reactions

>10%:

Cardiovascular: Tachycardia, palpitations, pounding heartbeat

Gastrointestinal: GI upset, nausea

1% to 10%:

Cardiovascular: Flushing of face, hypertension or hypotension

Central nervous system: Nervousness, CNS stimulation, hyperactivity, insomnia, dizziness, lightheadedness, drowsiness, headache

Gastrointestinal: Xerostomia, heartburn, vomiting, unusual taste

Genitourinary: Dysuria

Neuromuscular & skeletal: Muscle cramping, tremor, weakness

Respiratory: Coughing

Miscellaneous: Diaphoresis (increased)

<1%:

Cardiovascular: Chest pain, unusual pallor

Gastrointestinal: Loss of appetite

Respiratory: Paradoxical bronchospasm

Overdosage/Toxicology Symptoms of overdose include hypertension, tachycardia, angina, hypokalemia;

Hypokalemia and tachyarrhythmias: Prudent use of a cardioselective beta-adrenergic blocker (eg, atenolol or metoprolol); keep in mind the potential for induction of bronchoconstriction in an asthmatic. Dialysis has not been shown to be of value in the treatment of an overdose with this agent.

Drug Interactions

Decreased effect: Beta-adrenergic blockers (eg, propranolol)

Increased therapeutic effect: Inhaled ipratropium may increase duration of bronchodilation, nifedipine may increase FEV-1

Increased toxicity: Cardiovascular effects are potentiated in patients also receiving MAO inhibitors, tricyclic antidepressants, sympathomimetic agents (eg, amphetamine, dopamine, dobutamine), inhaled anesthetics (eg, enflurane)

Mechanism of Action Relaxes bronchial smooth muscle by action on beta$_2$-receptors with little effect on heart rate

Pharmacodynamics/Kinetics

Peak effect:
- Oral: 2-3 hours
- Nebulization/oral inhalation: Within 0.5-2 hours

Duration of action:
- Oral: 4-6 hours
- Nebulization/oral inhalation: 3-4 hours

Metabolism: By the liver to an inactive sulfate, with 28% appearing in the urine as unchanged drug

Half-life:
- Inhalation: 3.8 hours
- Oral: 3.7-5 hours

Elimination: 30% appears in urine as unchanged drug

Usual Dosage

Oral:
- Children:
  - 2-6 years: 0.1-0.2 mg/kg/dose 3 times/day; maximum dose not to exceed 12 mg/day (divided doses)
  - 6-12 years: 2 mg/dose 3-4 times/day; maximum dose not to exceed 24 mg/day (divided doses)
- Children >12 years and Adults: 2-4 mg/dose 3-4 times/day; maximum dose not to exceed 32 mg/day (divided doses)
- Elderly: 2 mg 3-4 times/day; maximum: 8 mg 4 times/day

Inhalation MDI: 90 mcg/spray:
- Children <12 years: 1-2 inhalations 4 times/day using a tube spacer
- Children ≥12 years and Adults: 1-2 inhalations every 4-6 hours; maximum: 12 inhalations/day
- Exercise-induced bronchospasm: 2 inhalations 15 minutes before exercising

Inhalation: Nebulization: 2.5 mg = 0.5 mL of the 0.5% inhalation solution to be diluted in 1-2.5 mL of NS **or** 0.01-0.05 mL/kg of 0.5% solution every 4-6 hours; intensive care patients may require more frequent administration; minimum dose: 0.1 mL; maximum dose: 1 mL diluted in 1-2 mL normal saline
- <5 years: 1.25-2.5 mg every 4-6 hours as needed
- >5 years: 2.5-5 mg every 4-6 hours as needed

Hemodialysis: Not removed by hemodialysis

Monitoring Parameters Heart rate, CNS stimulation, asthma symptoms, arterial or capillary blood gases (if patients condition warrants)

Test Interactions ↑ renin (S), ↑ aldosterone (S)

Patient Information Do not exceed recommended dosage; rinse mouth with water following each inhalation to help with dry throat and mouth; follow specific instructions accompanying inhaler; if more than one inhalation is necessary, wait at least 1 full minute between inhalations. May cause nervousness, restlessness, insomnia; if these effects continue after dosage reduction, notify physician; also notify physician if palpitations, tachycardia, chest pain, muscle tremors, dizziness, headache, flushing or if breathing difficulty persists.

Nursing Implications Before using, the inhaler must be shaken well; assess lung sounds, pulse, and blood pressure before administration and during peak of medication; observe patient for wheezing after administration, if this occurs, call physician

Dosage Forms

Aerosol (Proventil®, Ventolin®): 90 mcg/dose (17 g) [200 doses]

Aerosol, chlorofluorocarbon free (Proventil® HFA): 90 mcg/dose (17 g)

Capsule for oral inhalation (Ventolin® Rotocaps®): 200 mcg [to be used with Rotahaler® inhalation device]

Solution, inhalation: 0.083% (3 mL); 0.5% (20 mL)
- Airet®: 0.083%
- Proventil®: 0.083% (3 mL), 0.5% (20 mL)
- Ventolin®: 0.5% (20 mL)

(Continued)

Albuterol *(Continued)*

Syrup, as sulfate: 2 mg/5 mL (480 mL)
Proventil®, Ventolin®: 2 mg/5 mL (480 mL)
Tablet, as sulfate: 2 mg, 4 mg
Proventil®, Ventolin®: 2 mg, 4 mg
Tablet, extended release:
Proventil® Repetabs®: 4 mg
Volmax®: 4 mg, 8 mg

Alcaine® *see* Proparacaine *on page 1062*

Alclometasone (al kloe MET a sone)

Brand Names Aclovate®

Canadian/Mexican Brand Names Logoderm® (Mexico)

Synonyms Alclometasone Dipropionate

Therapeutic Category Anti-inflammatory Agent; Corticosteroid, Topical (Low Potency)

Use Treats inflammation of corticosteroid-responsive dermatosis (low potency topical corticosteroid)

Pregnancy Risk Factor C

Contraindications Viral, fungal, or tubercular skin lesions, known hypersensitivity to alclometasone or any component

Warnings/Precautions Adverse systemic effects may occur when used on large areas of the body, denuded areas, for prolonged periods of time, with an occlusive dressing, and/or in infants or small children

Adverse Reactions

1% to 10%:
Dermatologic: Itching, erythema, dryness papular rashes
Local: Burning, irritation

<1%: Dermatologic: Hypertrichosis, acneiform eruptions, hypopigmentation, perioral dermatitis, maceration of skin, skin atrophy, striae, miliaria

Overdosage/Toxicology Symptoms of overdose include cushingoid appearance (systemic), muscle weakness (systemic), osteoporosis (systemic) all with long-term use only. When consumed in excessive quantities for prolonged periods, systemic hypercorticism and adrenal suppression may occur; in those cases, discontinuation and withdrawal of the corticosteroid should be done judiciously.

Stability Store between 2°C and 30°C (36°F and 86°F)

Mechanism of Action Stimulates the synthesis of enzymes needed to decrease inflammation, suppress mitotic activity, and cause vasoconstriction

Usual Dosage Topical: Apply a thin film to the affected area 2-3 times/day

Patient Information Before applying, gently wash area to reduce risk of infection; apply a thin film to cleansed area and rub in gently and thoroughly until medication vanishes; avoid exposure to sunlight, severe sunburn may occur

Nursing Implications For external use only; do not use on open wounds; apply sparingly to occlusive dressings; should not be used in the presence of open or weeping lesions

Dosage Forms

Cream, as dipropionate: 0.05% (15 g, 45 g, 60 g)
Ointment, topical, as dipropionate: 0.05% (15 g, 45 g, 60 g)

Alclometasone Dipropionate *see* Alclometasone *on this page*

Alconefrin® Nasal Solution [OTC] *see* Phenylephrine *on page 989*

Aldactone® *see* Spironolactone *on page 1156*

Aldesleukin (al des LOO kin)

Related Information

Cancer Chemotherapy Regimens *on page 1351*

Brand Names Proleukin®

Synonyms IL-2; Interleukin-2

Therapeutic Category Biological Response Modulator

Use Treatment of metastatic renal cell carcinoma; also, investigated in tumors known to have a response to immunotherapy, such as melanoma; has been used in conjunction with LAK cells, TIL cells, IL-1, and interferon

Pregnancy Risk Factor C

Contraindications Known history of hypersensitivity to interleukin-2 or any component; patients with an abnormal thallium stress test or pulmonary function test; patients who have had an organ allograft; retreatment in patients who have experienced sustained ventricular tachycardia (≥5 beats), cardiac rhythm disturbances not controlled or unresponsive to management, recurrent chest pain with EKG changes (consistent with angina or myocardial infarction), intubation required >72 hours, pericardial tamponade; renal dysfunction requiring dialysis

>72 hours, coma or toxic psychosis lasting >48 hours, repetitive or difficult to control seizures, bowel ischemia/perforation, GI bleeding requiring surgery

Warnings/Precautions High-dose IL-2 therapy has been associated with capillary leak syndrome (CLS); CLS results in hypotension and reduced organ perfusion which may be severe and can result in death; therapy should be restricted to patients with normal cardiac and pulmonary functions as defined by thallium stress and formal pulmonary function testing; extreme caution should be used in patients with normal thallium stress tests and pulmonary functions tests who have a history of prior cardiac or pulmonary disease. Postnephrectomy patients must have a serum creatinine of ≤1.5 mg/dL prior to treatment.

Intensive aldesleukin treatment is associated with impaired neutrophil function (reduced chemotaxis) and with an increased risk of disseminated infection, including sepsis and bacterial endocarditis, in treated patients. Consequently, pre-existing bacterial infections should be adequately treated prior to initiation of therapy. Additionally, all patients with indwelling central lines should receive antibiotic prophylaxis effective against *S. aureus*. Antibiotic prophylaxis which has been associated with a reduced incidence of staphylococcal infections in aldesleukin studies includes the use of oxacillin, nafcillin, ciprofloxacin, or vancomycin.

Standard prophylactic supportive care during high-dose IL-2 treatment includes acetaminophen to relieve constitutional symptoms and an H_2-antagonist to reduce the risk of GI ulceration and/or bleeding.

Adverse Reactions

>10%:

Cardiovascular: Sensory dysfunction, sinus tachycardia, arrhythmias, pulmonary congestion; hypotension (dose-limiting toxicity) which may require vasopressor support and hemodynamic changes resembling those seen in septic shock can be seen within 2 hours of administration; angina, acute myocardial infarction, SVT with hypotension has been reported, edema

Central nervous system: Dizziness, pain, fever, chills, cognitive changes, fatigue, malaise, disorientation, somnolence, paranoid delusion, and other behavioral changes; reversible and dose related; however, may continue to worsen for several days even after the infusion is stopped

Dermatologic: Pruritus, erythema, rash, dry skin, exfoliative dermatitis, macular erythema

Gastrointestinal: Nausea, vomiting, weight gain, diarrhea, stomatitis, anorexia, GI bleeding

Hematologic: Anemia, thrombocytopenia, leukopenia, eosinophilia, coagulation disorders

Hepatic: Elevated transaminase and alkaline phosphatase, jaundice

Neuromuscular & skeletal: Weakness, rigors which can be decreased or ameliorated with acetaminophen or a nonsteroidal agent and meperidine

Renal: Oliguria, anuria, proteinuria; renal failure (dose-limiting toxicity) manifested as oliguria noted within 24-48 hours of initiation of therapy; marked fluid retention, azotemia, and increased serum creatinine seen, which may return to baseline within 7 days of discontinuation of therapy; hypophosphatemia

Respiratory: Dyspnea, pulmonary edema

1% to 10%: Cardiovascular: Increase in vascular permeability: Capillary-leak syndrome manifested by severe peripheral edema, ascites, pulmonary infiltration, and pleural effusion; occurs in 2% to 4% of patients and is resolved after therapy ends

<1%:

Cardiovascular: Congestive heart failure

Central nervous system: Coma, seizure

Dermatologic: Alopecia

Endocrine & metabolic: Hypercalcemia, hypocalcemia, hypomagnesemia, hypothyroidism, increased plasma levels of stress-related hormones, acidosis

Gastrointestinal: Pancreatitis

Genitourinary: Polyuria

Neuromuscular & skeletal: Arthritis, muscle spasm

Miscellaneous: Allergic reactions

Overdosage/Toxicology Side effects following the use of aldesleukin are dose related. Administration of more than the recommended dose has been associated with a more rapid onset of expected dose-limiting toxicities. Adverse reactions generally will reverse when the drug is stopped particularly because of its short serum half-life.

Provide supportive treatment of any continuing symptoms. Life-threatening toxicities have been ameliorated by the I.V. administration of dexamethasone, which may result in less of therapeutic effect of aldesleukin.

(Continued)

Aldesleukin *(Continued)*

Drug Interactions

Decreased toxicity: Corticosteroids have been shown to ↓ toxicity of IL-2, but have not been used since there is concern that they may ↓ the efficacy of the lymphokine

Increased toxicity:

- Aldesleukin may affect central nervous function; therefore, interactions could occur following concomitant administration of psychotropic drugs (eg, narcotics, analgesics, antiemetics, sedatives, tranquilizers)
- Concomitant administration of drugs possessing nephrotoxic (eg, aminoglycosides, indomethacin), myelotoxic (eg, cytotoxic chemotherapy), cardiotoxic (eg, doxorubicin), or hepatotoxic (eg, methotrexate, asparaginase) effects with aldesleukin may ↑ toxicity in these organ systems; the safety and efficacy of aldesleukin in combination with chemotherapy agents has not been established
- Beta-blockers and other antihypertensives may potentiate the hypotension seen with Proleukin®
- Iodinated contrast media: Acute reactions including fever, chills, nausea, vomiting, pruritus, rash, diarrhea, hypotension, edema, and oliguria have occurred within hours of contrast infusion; this reaction may occur within 4 weeks or up to several months after IL-2 administration

Stability

Store vials of lyophilized injection in a refrigerator at 2°C to 8°C (36°F to 46°F)

Reconstituted or diluted solution is stable for up to 48 hours at refrigerated and room temperatures 2°C to 25°C (36°F to 77°F); however, since this product contains no preservatives, the reconstituted and diluted solutions should be stored in the refrigerator

- **Compatible** only with D_5W
- Gently swirl, do not shake
- **Note:** As with most biological proteins, solutions containing IL-2 should not be filtered; filtration will result in significant loss of bioactivity; see table.

Recommendations for IL-2 (Aldesleukin - Proleukin™) Dilutions in D_5W*

Concentration (µg/mL)	Concentration (million units/mL)	Stability Recommendation
<60	<1	Human serum albumin must be added to bag **prior to addition** of IL-2; these solutions are stable for 6 days at room temperature†
60-100	1-1.7	**These concentrations should not be utilized as they are unstable**
100-500	1.7-8.4	These solutions are stable for 6 days at room temperature†

*1.3 mg of IL-2 (aldesleukin - Proleukin™) is equivalent to 22 million units.

†Although stability is 6 days, IL-2 does not contain a preservative and 24-hour expiration dating should be used.

Volume of Human Serum Albumin to Be Added to IL-2 (Aldesleukin - Proleukin™) Infusions in D_5W

Volume of I.V. Diluent (mL)	Volume of 5% Human Serum Albumin to Be Added Prior to IL-2 Addition (mL)	Volume of 25% Human Serum Albumin to Be Added Prior to IL-2 Addition (mL)
50	1	0.2
100	2	0.4
150	3	0.6
200	4	0.8
250	5	1
500	10	2

Concentrations of IL-2 which fall into the unstable (60-100 mcg/mL **or** 1-1.7 microunits/mL) range require addition of human serum albumin (final human serum albumin concentration of 0.1%) as shown in the table

Standard aldesleukin I.V. dilutions:

- Dose/50-1000 mL D_5W
- Concentrations <1,000,000 units/mL require the addition of human albumin to PVC bag prior to addition of IL-2

Stable for 48 hours at room temperature or refrigeration (2°C to 8°C); refrigeration is recommended due to lack of preservative

Incompatible with NS

Mechanism of Action IL-2 promotes proliferation, differentiation, and recruitment of T and B cells, natural killer (NK) cells, and thymocytes; IL-2 also causes cytolytic activity in a subset of lymphocytes and subsequent interactions between the immune system and malignant cells; IL-2 can stimulate lymphokine-activated killer (LAK) cells and tumor-infiltrating lymphocytes (TIL) cells. LAK cells (which are derived from lymphocytes from a patient and incubated in IL-2) have the ability to lyse cells which are resistant to NK cells; TIL cells (which are derived from cancerous tissue from a patient and incubated in IL-2) have been shown to be 50% more effective than LAK cells.

Pharmacodynamics/Kinetics

Absorption: Oral: Not absorbed

Distribution: V_d: Has been noted to be 4-7 L; primarily into the plasma and then into a second compartment, the lymphocytes themselves

Bioavailability: I.M.: 37%

Half-life:

Initial: 6-13 minutes

Terminal: 20-120 minutes

Usual Dosage Refer to individual protocols; all orders must be written in million International units (million IU)

Adults: Metastatic renal cell carcinoma (RCC):

Treatment consists of two 5-day treatment cycles separated by a rest period. 600,000 units/kg (0.037 mg/kg)/dose administered every 8 hours by a 15-minute I.V. infusion for a total of 14 doses; following 9 days of rest, the schedule is repeated for another 14 doses, for a maximum of 28 doses per course

Dose modification: In high-dose therapy of RCC, see manufacturer's guidelines for holding and restarting therapy; hold or interrupt a dose - DO NOT DOSE REDUCE; or refer to specific protocol

Retreatment: Patients should be evaluated for response approximately 4 weeks after completion of a course of therapy and again immediately prior to the scheduled start of the next treatment course; additional courses of treatment may be given to patients only if there is some tumor shrinkage or stable disease following the last course and retreatment is not contraindicated. Each treatment course should be separated by a rest period of at least 7 weeks from the date of hospital discharge; tumors have continued to regress up to 12 months following the initiation of therapy

Investigational regimen: S.C.: 11 million Units (flat dose) daily x 4 days per week for 4 consecutive weeks; repeat every 6 weeks

Administration Administer in D_5W only; incompatible with sodium chloride solutions

Management of symptoms related to vascular leak syndrome:

If actual body weight increases >10% above baseline, or rales or rhonchi are audible:

Administer furosemide at dosage determined by patient response

Administer dopamine hydrochloride 2-4 mcg/kg/minute to maintain renal blood flow and urine output

If patient has dyspnea at rest: Administer supplemental oxygen by face mask

If patient has severe respiratory distress: Intubate patient and provide mechanical ventilation; administer ranitidine (as the hydrochloride salt), 50 mg I.V. every 8-12 hours as prophylaxis against stress ulcers

Monitoring Parameters

The following clinical evaluations are recommended for all patients prior to beginning treatment and then daily during drug administration:

Standard hematologic tests including CBC, differential, and platelet counts

Blood chemistries including electrolytes, renal and hepatic function tests

Chest x-rays

Daily monitoring during therapy should include vital signs (temperature, pulse, blood pressure, and respiration rate) and weight; in a patient with a decreased blood pressure, especially <90 mm Hg, constant cardiac monitoring for rhythm should be conducted. If an abnormal complex or rhythm is seen, an EKG should be performed; vital signs in these hypotension patients should be taken hourly and central venous pressure (CVP) checked.

During treatment, pulmonary function should be monitored on a regular basis by clinical examination, assessment of vital signs and pulse oximetry. Patients with dyspnea or clinical signs of respiratory impairment (tachypnea or rales) should be further assessed with arterial blood gas determination. These tests are to be repeated as often as clinically indicated.

Cardiac function is assessed daily by clinical examination and assessment of vital signs. Patients with signs or symptoms of chest pain, murmurs, gallops, irregular rhythm or palpitations should be further assessed with an EKG

(Continued)

Aldesleukin *(Continued)*

examination and CPK evaluation. If there is evidence of cardiac ischemia or congestive heart failure, a repeat thallium study should be done.

Additional Information

1 Cetus Unit = 6 International units
1.1 mg = 18 x 10^6 International units (or 3 x 10^6 Cetus units)
1 Roche Unit (Teceleukin) = 3 International units
Reimbursement Hot Line: 1-800-775-7533
Professional services: 1-800-244-7668

Dosage Forms Powder for injection, lyophilized: 22 x 10^6 IU [18 million IU/mL = 1.1 mg/mL when reconstituted]

Aldomet® *see* Methyldopa *on page 814*

Alendronate (a LEN droe nate)

Brand Names Fosamax™

Synonyms Alendronate Sodium

Therapeutic Category Bisphosphonate Derivative

Use FDA-approved: Osteoporosis in postmenopausal women; Paget's disease of the bone

Pregnancy Risk Factor C

Contraindications Hypersensitivity to bisphosphonates or any component of the product; hypocalcemia; abnormalities of the esophagus which delay esophageal emptying such as stricture or achalasia; inability to stand or sit upright for at least 30 minutes

Warnings/Precautions Use caution in patients with renal impairment; concomitant hormone replacement therapy with alendronate for osteoporosis in postmenopausal women is not recommended; hypocalcemia must be corrected before therapy initiation with alendronate; ensure adequate calcium and vitamin D intake to provide for enhanced needs in patients with Paget's disease in whom the pretreatment rate of bone turnover may be greatly elevated.

Adverse Reactions

Note: Incidence of adverse effects increases significantly in patients treated for Paget's disease at 40 mg/day, mostly GI adverse effects

1% to 10%:
- Central nervous system: Headache (2.6%); pain (4.1%)
- Gastrointestinal: Flatulence (2.6%); acid regurgitation (2%); esophagitis ulcer (1.5%); dysphagia, abdominal distention (1%)

<1%:
- Dermatologic: Rash, erythema (rare)
- Gastrointestinal: Gastritis (0.5%)

Overdosage/Toxicology Symptoms of overdose include hypocalcemia, hypophosphatemia; upper GI adverse events (upset stomach, heartburn, esophagitis, gastritis or ulcer)

Treat with milk or antacids to bind alendronate; dialysis would not be beneficial

Mechanism of Action A bisphosphonate which inhibits bone resorption via actions on osteoclasts or on osteoclast precursors; decreases the rate of bone resorption direction, leading to an indirect decrease in bone formation

Pharmacodynamics/Kinetics

Absorption: Oral:
- Male: 0.6% given in a fasting state
- Female: 0.7%

Protein binding: ~78%
Metabolism: Not metabolized
Bioavailability: Reduced up to 60% with food or drink
Half-life: Terminal: Exceeds 10 years; serum concentrations cleared >95% in 6 hours
Elimination: Renal with unabsorbed drug eliminated in feces

Usual Dosage Oral:

Adults: Patients with osteoporosis or Paget's disease should receive supplemental calcium and vitamin D if dietary intake is inadequate

Osteoporosis in postmenopausal women: 10 mg once daily. Safety of treatment for >4 years has not been studied (extension studies are ongoing).

Paget's disease of bone: 40 mg once daily for 6 months

Retreatment: Relapses during the 12 months following therapy occurred in 9% of patients who responded to treatment. Specific retreatment data are not available. Retreatment with alendronate may be considered, following a 6-month post-treatment evaluation period, in patients who have relapsed based on increases in serum alkaline phosphatase, which should be measured periodically. Retreatment may also be considered in those who failed to normalize their serum alkaline phosphatase.

Elderly: No dosage adjustment is necessary

Dosage adjustment in renal impairment:

Cl_{cr} 30-60 mL/minute: No adjustment necessary

Cl_{cr} <35 mL/minute: Alendronate is not recommended due to lack of experience

Administration It is imperative to administer alendronate 30-60 minutes before the patient takes any food, drink, or other medications orally to avoid interference with absorption. The patient should take alendronate on an empty stomach with a full glass (8 oz) of **plain water** (not mineral water) and avoid lying down for 30 minutes after swallowing tablet to help delivery to stomach.

Monitoring Parameters Alkaline phosphatase should be periodically measured; serum calcium, phosphorus, and possibly potassium due to its drug class; use of absorptiometry may assist in noting benefit in osteoporosis; monitor pain and fracture rate

Reference Range Calcium (total): Adults: 9.0-11.0 mg/dL (2.05-2.54 mmol/L), may slightly decrease with aging; phosphorus: 2.5-4.5 mg/dL (0.81-1.45 mmol/L)

Patient Information Food, beverages (including mineral water), and other medications may significantly reduce the absorption and therefore the effectiveness; take with plain water (6-8 oz) at least 30 minutes before the first food, beverage, or medication of the day; must take supplemental calcium while treated with alendronate

Nursing Implications Patients should be instructed that the expected benefits of alendronate may only be obtained when each tablet is taken with plain water the first thing in the morning and at least 30 minutes before the first food, beverage, or medication of the day. Also instruct them that waiting >30 minutes will improve alendronate absorption. Even dosing with orange juice or coffee markedly reduces the absorption of alendronate.

Instruct patients to take alendronate with a full glass of water (6-8 oz 180-240 mL) and not to lie down (stay fully upright sitting or standing) for at least 30 minutes following administration to facilitate delivery to the stomach and reduce the potential for esophageal irritation.

Patients should be instructed to take supplemental calcium and vitamin D if dietary intake is inadequate. Consider weight-bearing exercise along with the modification of certain behavioral factors, such as excessive cigarette smoking or alcohol consumption if these factors exist.

Dosage Forms Tablet, as sodium: 10 mg, 40 mg

Alendronate Sodium *see* Alendronate *on previous page*

Aleve® [OTC] *see* Naproxen *on page 880*

Alfenta® *see* Alfentanil *on this page*

Alfentanil (al FEN ta nil)

Related Information

Narcotic Agonists Comparison *on page 1414*

Brand Names Alfenta®

Canadian/Mexican Brand Names Alfenta® (Canada); Rapifen® (Mexico)

Synonyms Alfentanil Hydrochloride

Therapeutic Category Analgesic, Narcotic

Use Analgesic adjunct given by continuous infusion or in incremental doses in maintenance of anesthesia with barbiturate or N_2O or a primary anesthetic agent for the induction of anesthesia in patients undergoing general surgery in which endotracheal intubation and mechanical ventilation are required

Restrictions C-II

Pregnancy Risk Factor C

Contraindications Hypersensitivity to alfentanil hydrochloride or narcotics; increased intracranial pressure, severe respiratory depression

Warnings/Precautions Drug dependence, head injury, acute asthma and respiratory conditions; hypotension has occurred in neonates with respiratory distress syndrome; use caution when administering to patients with bradyarrhythmias; rapid I.V. infusion may result in skeletal muscle and chest wall rigidity → impaired ventilation → respiratory distress/arrest; inject slowly over 3-5 minutes; nondepolarizing skeletal muscle relaxant may be required. Alfentanil may produce more hypotension compared to fentanyl, therefore, be sure to administer slowly and ensure patient has adequate hydration.

Adverse Reactions

>10%:

- Cardiovascular: Bradycardia, peripheral vasodilation
- Central nervous system: Drowsiness, sedation, increased intracranial pressure
- Gastrointestinal: Nausea, vomiting, constipation

Endocrine & metabolic: Antidiuretic hormone release

Ocular: Miosis

1% to 10%:

- Cardiovascular: Cardiac arrhythmias, orthostatic hypotension
- Central nervous system: Confusion, CNS depression

(Continued)

Alfentanil *(Continued)*

Ocular: Blurred vision

<1%:

Central nervous system: Convulsions, mental depression, paradoxical CNS excitation or delirium, dizziness, dysesthesia

Dermatologic: Rash, urticaria, itching

Gastrointestinal: Biliary tract spasm

Genitourinary: Urinary tract spasm

Respiratory: Respiratory depression, bronchospasm, laryngospasm

Miscellaneous: Physical and psychological dependence with prolonged use, cold, clammy skin

Overdosage/Toxicology Symptoms of overdose include miosis, respiratory depression, seizures, CNS depression

Naloxone 2 mg I.V. (0.01 mg/kg for children) with repeat administration as necessary up to a total of 10 mg; may precipitate withdrawal

Drug Interactions Cytochrome P-450 3A enzyme substrate

Decreased effect: Phenothiazines may antagonize the analgesic effect of opiate agonists

Increased effect: Dextroamphetamine may enhance the analgesic effect of morphine and other opiate agonists

Increased toxicity: CNS depressants (eg, benzodiazepines, barbiturates, phenothiazines, tricyclic antidepressants), erythromycin, reserpine, beta-blockers

Stability Dilute in D_5W, NS, or LR

Mechanism of Action Binds with stereospecific receptors at many sites within the CNS, increases pain threshold, alters pain perception, inhibits ascending pain pathways; is an ultra short-acting narcotic

Pharmacodynamics/Kinetics

Distribution: V_d:

Newborns, premature: 1 L/kg

Children: 0.163-0.48 L/kg

Adults: 0.46 L/kg

Half-life, elimination:

Newborns, premature: 5.33-8.75 hours

Children: 40-60 minutes

Adults: 83-97 minutes

Usual Dosage Doses should be titrated to appropriate effects; wide range of doses is dependent upon desired degree of analgesia/anesthesia

Children <12 years: Dose not established

Adults: Dose should be based on ideal body weight; see table.

Alfentanil

Indication	Approximate Duration of Anesthesia (min)	Induction Period (Initial Dose) (mcg/kg)	Maintenance Period (Increments/ Infusion)	Total Dose (mcg/kg)	Effects
Incremental injection	≤30	8-20	3-5 mcg/kg or 0.5-1 mcg/kg/min	8-40	Spontaneously breathing or assisted ventilation when required.
	30-60	20-50	5-15 mcg/kg	Up to 75	Assisted or controlled ventilation required. Attenuation of response to laryngoscopy and intubation.
Continuous infusion	>45	50-75	0.5-3.0 mcg/kg/min average infusion rate 1-1.5 mcg/kg/min	Dependent on duration of procedure	Assisted or controlled ventilation required. Some attenuation of response to intubation and incision, with intraoperative stability.
Anesthetic induction	>45	130-245	0.5-1.5 mcg/kg/min or general anesthetic	Dependent on duration of procedure	Assisted or controlled ventilation required. Administer slowly (over three minutes). Concentration of inhalation agents reduced by 30% to 50% for initial hour.

Monitoring Parameters Respiratory rate, blood pressure, heart rate

Reference Range 100-340 ng/mL (depending upon procedure)

Nursing Implications Monitor patient for CNS, respiratory depression, and urticaria

Dosage Forms Injection, preservative free, as hydrochloride: 500 mcg/mL (2 mL, 5 mL, 10 mL, 20 mL)

Alfentanil Hydrochloride *see* Alfentanil *on page 45*
Alferon® N *see* Interferon Alfa-n3 *on page 667*

Alglucerase (al GLOO ser ase)

Brand Names Ceredase®; Cerezyme®

Synonyms Glucocerebrosidase

Therapeutic Category Enzyme, Glucocerebrosidase

Use Orphan drug for treatment of Gaucher's disease

Pregnancy Risk Factor C

Contraindications Hypersensitivity to any component

Warnings/Precautions Prepared from pooled human placental tissue that may contain the causative agents of some viral diseases

Adverse Reactions

>10%: Local: Discomfort, burning, and edema at the site of injection

<1%:

Central nervous system: Fever, chills

Gastrointestinal: Abdominal discomfort, nausea, vomiting

Overdosage/Toxicology No obvious toxicity was detected after single doses of up to 234 units/kg

Stability Refrigerate (4°C), do not shake

Mechanism of Action Glucocerebrosidase is an enzyme prepared from human placental tissue. Gaucher's disease is an inherited metabolic disorder caused by the defective activity of beta-glucosidase and the resultant accumulation of glucosyl ceramide laden macrophages in the liver, bone, and spleen; acts by replacing the missing enzyme associated with Gaucher's disease.

Usual Dosage Usually administered as a 20-60 units/kg I.V. infusion given with a frequency ranging from 3 times/week to once every 2 weeks

Administration Filter during administration

Patient Information Alglucerase should be stored under refrigeration (4°C), solutions should not be shaken

Dosage Forms Injection: 10 units/mL (5 mL); 80 units/mL (5 mL)

Alkaban-AQ® *see* Vinblastine *on page 1300*
Alka-Mints® [OTC] *see* Calcium Carbonate *on page 185*
Alkeran® *see* Melphalan *on page 776*
Allbee® With C *see* Vitamins, Multiple *on page 1310*
Allegra® *see* Fexofenadine *on page 517*
Aller-Chlor® [OTC] *see* Chlorpheniramine *on page 260*
Allercon® Tablet [OTC] *see* Triprolidine and Pseudoephedrine *on page 1270*
Allerest® 12 Hour Nasal Solution [OTC] *see* Oxymetazoline *on page 940*
Allerest® Eye Drops [OTC] *see* Naphazoline *on page 879*
Allerfrin® Syrup [OTC] *see* Triprolidine and Pseudoephedrine *on page 1270*
Allerfrin® Tablet [OTC] *see* Triprolidine and Pseudoephedrine *on page 1270*
AllerMax® Oral [OTC] *see* Diphenhydramine *on page 399*
Allerphed Syrup [OTC] *see* Triprolidine and Pseudoephedrine *on page 1270*

Allopurinol (al oh PURE i nole)

Related Information

Antacid Drug Interactions *on page 1388*
Desensitization Protocols *on page 1496*
Toxicities of Chemotherapeutic Agents *on page 1382*

Brand Names Lopurin®; Zurinol®; Zyloprim®

Canadian/Mexican Brand Names Apo-Allopurinol® (Canada); Novo-purol® (Canada); Purinol® (Canada); Atisuril® (Mexico); Unizuric® 300 (Mexico)

Therapeutic Category Uricosuric Agent

Use Prevention of attack of gouty arthritis and nephropathy; also used to treat secondary hyperuricemia which may occur during treatment of tumors or leukemia, and to prevent recurrent calcium oxalate calculi

Pregnancy Risk Factor C

Pregnancy/Breast-Feeding Implications There are few reports describing the use of allopurinol during pregnancy; no adverse fetal outcomes attributable to allopurinol have been reported in humans

Contraindications Not to be used in pregnancy or lactation, or in patients with a previous severe allergy reaction to allopurinol or any component

Warnings/Precautions Do not use to treat asymptomatic hyperuricemia. Discontinue at first signs of rash; reduce dosage in renal insufficiency, reinstate with caution in patients who have had a previous mild allergic reaction, use with caution in children; monitor liver function and complete blood counts before initiating therapy and periodically during therapy, use with caution in patients taking diuretics concurrently.

(Continued)

Allopurinol *(Continued)*

Adverse Reactions

>10%: Dermatologic: Skin rash (usually maculopapular), exfoliative, urticarial or purpuric lesions, and Stevens-Johnson syndrome have been reported

1% to 10%:

- Central nervous system: Drowsiness, chills, fever
- Dermatologic: Alopecia
- Gastrointestinal: Nausea, vomiting, diarrhea, abdominal pain, gastritis, dyspepsia
- Hepatic: Increased alkaline phosphatase, AST, and ALT, hepatomegaly, hyperbilirubinemia, and jaundice, hepatic necrosis has been reported

<1%:

- Cardiovascular: Vasculitis
- Central nervous system: Headache, somnolence
- Dermatologic: Toxic epidermal necrolysis
- Hematologic: Bone marrow suppression has been reported in patients receiving allopurinol with other myelosuppressive agents
- Local: Thrombophlebitis
- Neuromuscular & skeletal: Peripheral neuropathy, neuritis, paresthesia
- Ocular: Cataracts
- Renal: Renal impairment
- Respiratory: Epistaxis
- Miscellaneous: Idiosyncratic: Reaction characterized by fever, chills, leukopenia, leukocytosis, eosinophilia, arthralgia, skin rash, pruritus, nausea, and vomiting

Overdosage/Toxicology If significant amounts of allopurinol are thought to have been absorbed, it is a theoretical possibility that oxypurinol stones could be formed but no record of such occurrence in overdose exists

Alkalinization of the urine and forced diuresis can help prevent potential xanthine stone formation

Drug Interactions Hepatic enzyme inhibitor

Decreased effect: Alcohol decreases effectiveness

Increased toxicity:

- Inhibits metabolism of azathioprine and mercaptopurine
- Use with ampicillin or amoxicillin may increase the incidence of skin rash
- Urinary acidification with large amounts of vitamin C may increase kidney stone formation
- Thiazide diuretics enhance toxicity, monitor renal function
- Allopurinol prolongs half-life of oral anticoagulants; allopurinol increases serum half-life of theophylline; allopurinol may compete for excretion in renal tubule with chlorpropamide and increases chlorpropamide's serum half-life

Mechanism of Action Allopurinol inhibits xanthine oxidase, the enzyme responsible for the conversion of hypoxanthine to xanthine to uric acid. Allopurinol is metabolized to oxypurinol which is also an inhibitor of xanthine oxidase; allopurinol acts on purine catabolism, reducing the production of uric acid without disrupting the biosynthesis of vital purines.

Pharmacodynamics/Kinetics

Decreases in serum uric acid occur in 1-2 days with nadir achieved in 1-2 weeks

Absorption:

- Oral: ~80% of dose absorbed from GI tract; peak plasma concentrations are seen 30-120 minutes after administration
- Rectal: Poor and erratic

Distribution: V_d ~1.6 L/kg; distributes into breast milk

Protein binding: <1%

Metabolism: ~75% metabolized to active metabolites, chiefly oxypurinol

Half-life:

- Normal renal function:
  - Parent drug: 1-3 hours
  - Oxypurinol: 18-30 hours
- End stage renal disease: Half-life is prolonged

Elimination: Both allopurinol and oxypurinol are dialyzable; 10% may be eliminated by enterohepatic excretion; <10% excreted in urine unchanged; 45% to 65% excreted as oxypurinol

Usual Dosage Oral:

Children ≤10 years: 10 mg/kg/day in 2-3 divided doses **or** 200-300 mg/m²/day in 2-4 divided doses, maximum: 800 mg/24 hours

- Alternative:
  - <6 years: 150 mg/day in 3 divided doses
  - 6-10 years: 300 mg/day in 2-3 divided doses

Children >10 years and Adults: Daily doses >300 mg should be administered in divided doses

Myeloproliferative neoplastic disorders: 600-800 mg/day in 2-3 divided doses for prevention of acute uric acid nephropathy for 2-3 days starting 1-2 days before chemotherapy

Gout:

Mild: 200-300 mg/day

Severe: 400-600 mg/day

Elderly: Initial dose: 100 mg/day, increase until desired uric acid level is obtained

Dosing adjustment in renal impairment: Must be adjusted due to accumulation of allopurinol and metabolites; removed by hemodialysis. See table.

Adult Maintenance Doses of Allopurinol*

Creatinine Clearance (mL/min)	Maintenance Dose of Allopurinol (mg)
140	400 qd
120	350 qd
100	300 qd
80	250 qd
60	200 qd
40	150 qd
20	100 qd
10	100 q2d
0	100 q3d

*This table is based on a standard maintenance dose of 300 mg of allopurinol per day for a patient with a creatinine clearance of 100 mL/min.

Hemodialysis: Administer dose posthemodialysis or administer 50% supplemental dose

Monitoring Parameters CBC, serum uric acid levels, I & O, hepatic and renal function, especially at start of therapy

Reference Range Uric acid, serum: An increase occurs during childhood

Adults:

Male: 3.4-7 mg/dL or slightly more

Female: 2.4-6 mg/dL or slightly more

Values >7 mg/dL are sometimes arbitrarily regarded as hyperuricemia, but there is no sharp line between normals on the one hand, and the serum uric acid of those with clinical gout. Normal ranges cannot be adjusted for purine ingestion, but high purine diet increases uric acid. Uric acid may be increased with body size, exercise, and stress.

Patient Information Take after meals with plenty of fluid (at least 10-12 glasses of fluids per day); discontinue the drug and contact physician at first sign of rash, painful urination, blood in urine, irritation of the eyes, or swelling of the lips or mouth; may cause drowsiness; alcohol decreases effectiveness

Dosage Forms Tablet: 100 mg, 300 mg

Extemporaneous Preparations Crush tablets to make a 5 mg/mL suspension in simple syrup; stable 14 days under refrigeration

Nahata MC and Hipple TF, *Pediatric Drug Formulations*, 1st ed, Harvey Whitney Books Co, 1990.

All-*trans*-Retinoic Acid *see* Tretinoin, Oral *on page 1251*

Alomide® *see* Lodoxamide Tromethamine *on page 736*

Alora® Transdermal *see* Estradiol *on page 468*

Alphagan® *see* Brimonidine *on page 164*

Alphamin® *see* Hydroxocobalamin *on page 629*

Alphamul® [OTC] *see* Castor Oil *on page 216*

AlphaNine® *see* Factor IX Complex (Human) *on page 502*

Alphatrex® *see* Betamethasone *on page 147*

Alprazolam (al PRAY zoe lam)

Related Information

Benzodiazepines Comparison *on page 1397*

Brand Names Xanax®

Canadian/Mexican Brand Names Apo-Alpraz® (Canada); Novo-Aloprazol® (Canada); Nu-Alprax® (Canada); Tafil® (Mexico); Xanax TS™

Therapeutic Category Antianxiety Agent; Benzodiazepine

Use Treatment of anxiety; adjunct in the treatment of depression; management of panic attacks

Restrictions C-IV

Pregnancy Risk Factor D

Contraindications Hypersensitivity to alprazolam or any component, there may be a cross-sensitivity with other benzodiazepines; severe uncontrolled pain, (Continued)

Alprazolam *(Continued)*

narrow-angle glaucoma, severe respiratory depression, pre-existing CNS depression; not to be used in pregnancy or lactation

Warnings/Precautions Withdrawal symptoms including seizures have occurred 18 hours to 3 days after abrupt discontinuation; when discontinuing therapy, decrease daily dose by no more than 0.5 mg every 3 days; reduce dose in patients with significant hepatic disease. Not intended for management of anxieties and minor distresses associated with everyday life.

Adverse Reactions

>10%:

- Cardiovascular: Tachycardia, chest pain
- Central nervous system: Drowsiness, fatigue, ataxia, lightheadedness, memory impairment, insomnia, anxiety, depression, headache
- Dermatologic: Rash
- Endocrine & metabolic: Decreased libido
- Gastrointestinal: Xerostomia, constipation, decreased salivation, nausea, vomiting, diarrhea, increased or decreased appetite
- Neuromuscular & skeletal: Dysarthria
- Ocular: Blurred vision
- Miscellaneous: Diaphoresis

1% to 10%:

- Cardiovascular: Syncope, hypotension
- Central nervous system: Confusion, nervousness, dizziness, akathisia
- Dermatologic: Dermatitis
- Gastrointestinal: Weight gain or loss, increased salivation
- Neuromuscular & skeletal: Rigidity, tremor, muscle cramps
- Otic: Tinnitus
- Respiratory: Nasal congestion, hyperventilation

Overdosage/Toxicology Symptoms of overdose include somnolence, confusion, coma, and diminished reflexes

Treatment for benzodiazepine overdose is supportive. Rarely is mechanical ventilation required; flumazenil has been shown to selectively block the binding of benzodiazepines to CNS receptors, resulting in a reversal of benzodiazepine-induced sedation; however, its use may not alter the course of overdose.

Drug Interactions

Decreased therapeutic effect: Carbamazepine, disulfiram

Increased toxicity: Oral contraceptives, CNS depressants, cimetidine, lithium

Mechanism of Action Binds at stereospecific receptors at several sites within the central nervous system, including the limbic system, reticular formation; effects may be mediated through GABA

Pharmacodynamics/Kinetics

Distribution: V_d: 0.9-1.2 L/kg; distributes into breast milk

Protein binding: 80%

Metabolism: Extensive in the liver; major metabolite is inactive

Half-life: 12-15 hours

Time to peak serum concentration: Within 1-2 hours

Elimination: Excretion of metabolites and parent compound in urine

Usual Dosage Oral:

Children <18 years: Safety and dose have not been established

Adults:

- Anxiety: Effective doses are 0.5-4 mg/day in divided doses; the manufacturer recommends starting at 0.25-0.5 mg 3 times/day; titrate dose upward; maximum: 4 mg/day
- Depression: Average dose required: 2.5-3 mg/day in divided doses
- Alcohol withdrawal: Usual dose: 2-2.5 mg/day in divided doses
- Panic disorder: Many patients obtain relief at 2 mg/day, as much as 6 mg/day may be required

Dosing adjustment in hepatic impairment: Reduce dose by 50% to 60% or avoid in cirrhosis

Note: Treatment >4 months should be re-evaluated to determine the patient's need for the drug

Dietary Considerations Alcohol: May have additive CNS effects, avoid use

Monitoring Parameters Respiratory and cardiovascular status

Test Interactions ↑ alkaline phosphatase

Patient Information Avoid alcohol and other CNS depressants; avoid activities needing good psychomotor coordination until CNS effects are known; drug may cause physical or psychological dependence; avoid abrupt discontinuation after prolonged use

Nursing Implications Assist with ambulation during beginning therapy, raise bed rails and keep room partially illuminated at night; monitor for CNS respiratory depression

Dosage Forms Tablet: 0.25 mg, 0.5 mg, 1 mg, 2 mg

Alprostadil (al PROS ta dill)

Brand Names Caverject® Injection; Muse® Pellet; Prostin VR Pediatric® Injection

Synonyms PGE_1; Prostaglandin E_1

Therapeutic Category Prostaglandin

Use Temporary maintenance of patency of ductus arteriosus in neonates with ductal-dependent congenital heart disease until surgery can be performed. These defects include cyanotic (eg, pulmonary atresia, pulmonary stenosis, tricuspid atresia, Fallot's tetralogy, transposition of the great vessels) and acyanotic (eg, interruption of aortic arch, coarctation of aorta, hypoplastic left ventricle) heart disease; diagnosis and treatment of erectile dysfunction of vasculogenic, psychogenic, or neurogenic etiology; adjunct in the diagnosis of erectile dysfunction

Investigational: Treatment of pulmonary hypertension in infants and children with congenital heart defects with left-to-right shunts

Pregnancy Risk Factor X

Contraindications Hyaline membrane disease or persistent fetal circulation and when a dominant left-to-right shunt is present; respiratory distress syndrome; hypersensitivity to the drug or components; conditions predisposing patients to priapism (sickle cell anemia, multiple myeloma, leukemia); patients with anatomical deformation of the penis, penile implants; use in men for whom sexual activity is inadvisable or contraindicated

Warnings/Precautions Use cautiously in neonates with bleeding tendencies; apnea may occur in 10% to 12% of neonates with congenital heart defects, especially in those weighing <2 kg at birth; apnea usually appears during the first hour of drug infusion; priapism may occur; treat immediately to avoid penile tissue damage and permanent loss of potency; discontinue therapy if signs of penile fibrosis develop (penile angulation, cavernosal fibrosis, or Peyronie's disease)

Adverse Reactions

>10%:

- Cardiovascular: Flushing
- Central nervous system: Fever
- Genitourinary: Penile pain
- Respiratory: Apnea

1% to 10%:

- Cardiovascular: Bradycardia, hypotension, hypertension, tachycardia, cardiac arrest, edema
- Central nervous system: Seizures, headache, dizziness
- Endocrine & metabolic: Hypokalemia
- Gastrointestinal: Diarrhea
- Genitourinary: Prolonged erection, penile fibrosis, penis disorder, penile rash, penile edema
- Hematologic: Disseminated intravascular coagulation
- Local: Injection site hematoma, injection site bruising
- Neuromuscular & skeletal: Back pain
- Respiratory: Upper respiratory infection, flu syndrome, sinusitis, nasal congestion, cough
- Miscellaneous: Sepsis, localized pain in structures other than the injection site

<1%:

- Cardiovascular: Cerebral bleeding, congestive heart failure, second degree heart block, shock, supraventricular tachycardia, ventricular fibrillation, hyperemia
- Central nervous system: Hyperirritability, hypothermia, jitteriness, lethargy
- Endocrine & metabolic: Hypoglycemia, hyperkalemia
- Gastrointestinal: Gastric regurgitation
- Genitourinary: Anuria, balanitis, urethral bleeding, penile numbness, yeast infection, penile pruritus and erythema, abnormal ejaculation
- Hematologic: Anemia, bleeding, thrombocytopenia
- Hepatic: Hyperbilirubinemia
- Neuromuscular & skeletal: Hyperextension of neck, stiffness
- Renal: Hematuria
- Respiratory: Bradypnea, bronchial wheezing
- Miscellaneous: Peritonitis

Overdosage/Toxicology Symptoms of overdose when treating patent ductus arteriosus include apnea, bradycardia, hypotension, and flushing

If hypotension or pyrexia occurs, the infusion rate should be reduced until the symptoms subside, while apnea or bradycardia requires drug discontinuation; if intracavernous overdose occurs, supervise until any systemic effects have resolved or until penile detumescence has occurred

(Continued)

Alprostadil *(Continued)*

Stability

Ductus arteriosus: Refrigerate ampuls; protect from freezing; prepare fresh solutions every 24 hours; **compatible** in D_5W, $D_{10}W$, and NS solutions

Erectile dysfunction: Refrigerate at 2°C to 8°C until dispensed; after dispensing, stable for up to 3 months at or below 25°C; do not freeze; use only the supplied diluent for reconstitution (ie, bacteriostatic/sterile water with benzyl alcohol 0.945%)

Mechanism of Action Causes vasodilation by means of direct effect on vascular and ductus arteriosus smooth muscle; relaxes trabecular smooth muscle by dilation of cavernosal arteries when injected along the penile shaft, allowing blood flow to and entrapment in the lacunar spaces of the penis (ie, corporeal veno-occlusive mechanism)

Pharmacodynamics/Kinetics

Distribution: Nonsignificant amounts distribute peripherally following penile injection

Protein binding, plasma: 81% to albumin

Metabolism: ~75% metabolized by oxidation in one pass through the lungs

Half-life: 5-10 minutes

Elimination: Metabolites excreted in urine (90% within 24 hours)

Usual Dosage

Patent ductus arteriosus (Prostin VR Pediatric®):

I.V. continuous infusion into a large vein, or alternatively through an umbilical artery catheter placed at the ductal opening: 0.05-0.1 mcg/kg/minute with therapeutic response, rate is reduced to lowest effective dosage; with unsatisfactory response, rate is increased gradually; maintenance: 0.01-0.4 mcg/kg/minute

PGE_1 is usually given at an infusion rate of 0.1 mcg/kg/minute, but it is often possible to reduce the dosage to ½ or even $^1/_{10}$ without losing the therapeutic effect. The mixing schedule is shown in the table.

Add 1 Ampul (500 mcg) to:	Concentration (mcg/mL)	Infusion Rate	
		mL/min/kg Needed to Infuse 0.1 mcg/kg/min	mL/kg/24 h
250 mL	2	0.05	72
100 mL	5	0.02	28.8
50 mL	10	0.01	14.4
25 mL	20	0.005	7.2

Therapeutic response is indicated by increased pH in those with acidosis or by an increase in oxygenation (pO_2) usually evident within 30 minutes

Erectile dysfunction

Caverject®:

Vasculogenic, psychogenic, or mixed etiology: Individualize dose by careful titration; usual dose: 2.5-60 mcg (doses >60 mcg are not recommended); initiate dosage titration at 2.5 mcg, increasing by 2.5 mcg to a dose of 5 mcg and then in increments of 5-10 mcg depending on the erectile response until the dose produces an erection suitable for intercourse, not lasting >1 hour; if there is absolutely no response to initial 2.5 mcg dose, the second dose may increased to 7.5 mcg, followed by increments of 5-10 mcg

Neurogenic etiology (eg, spinal cord injury): Initiate dosage titration at 1.25 mcg, increasing to a doses of 2.5 mcg and then 5 mcg; increase further in increments 5 mcg until the dose is reached that produces an erection suitable for intercourse, not lasting >1 hour

Note: Patient must stay in the physician's office until complete detumescence occurs; if there is no response, then the next higher dose may be given within 1 hour; if there is still no response, a 1-day interval before giving the next dose is recommended; increasing the dose or concentration in the treatment of impotence results in increasing pain and discomfort

Muse® Pellet: Intraurethral: Administer as needed to achieve an erection; duration of action is about 30-60 minutes; use only two systems per 24-hour period

Monitoring Parameters Arterial pressure, respiratory rate, heart rate, temperature, degree of penile pain, length of erection, signs of infection

Patient Information Store in refrigerator; if self-injecting for the treatment of impotence, dilute with the supplied diluent and use immediately after diluting; see physician at least every 3 months to ensure proper technique and for dosage adjustment; alternate sides of the penis with each injection; do not inject more than 3 times/week, allowing at least 24 hours between each dose; dispose of the syringe, needle, and vial properly; discard single-use vials after each use; report moderate to severe penile pain or erections lasting >6 hours to a physician immediately; inform a physician as soon as possible if any new penile pain, nodules, hard tissue or signs of infection develop; the risk of transmission of blood-borne diseases is increased with use of alprostadil injections since a small amount of bleeding at the injection site is possible; do not share this medication or needles/syringes

Nursing Implications

Ductus arteriosus: Monitor arterial pressure; assess all vital functions; apnea and bradycardia may indicate overdose, stop infusion if occurring; infuse for the shortest time and at the lowest dose that will produce the desired effects. Flushing is usually a result of catheter malposition; central line preferred for I.V. administration.

Erectile dysfunction: Use a ½", 27- to 30-gauge needle; inject into the dorsolateral aspect of the proximal third of the penis, avoiding visible veins; alternate side of the penis for injections; if the patient is going to be self-injecting at home, carefully assess their aseptic technique for injection and knowledge of proper disposal of the syringe, needle and vial; observe for signs of infection, penile fibrosis, and significant pain or priapism

Dosage Forms

Injection:

- Caverject®: 5 mcg, 10 mcg, 20 mcg
- Prostin VR Pediatric®: 500 mcg/mL (1 mL)

Pellet, urethral: 125 mcg, 250 mcg, 500 mcg, 1000 mcg

AL-R® [OTC] *see* Chlorpheniramine *on page 260*

Altace™ *see* Ramipril *on page 1092*

Alteplase (AL te plase)

Brand Names Activase®

Canadian/Mexican Brand Names Lysatec-rt-PA® (Canada)

Synonyms Alteplase, Recombinant; Alteplase, Tissue Plasminogen Activator, Recombinant; t-PA

Therapeutic Category Thrombolytic Agent

Use Management of acute myocardial infarction for the lysis of thrombi in coronary arteries; management of acute massive pulmonary embolism (PE) in adults

Acute myocardial infarction (AMI): Chest pain ≥20 minutes, ≤12-24 hours; S-T elevation ≥0.1 mV in at least two EKG leads

Acute pulmonary embolism (APE): Age ≤75 years: As soon as possible within 5 days of thrombotic event. Documented massive pulmonary embolism by pulmonary angiography or echocardiography or high probability lung scan with clinical shock.

Acute ischemic stroke (rule out hemorrhagic courses before administering)

Pregnancy Risk Factor C

Contraindications No central venous puncture (CVP line) or noncompressible arterial sticks. BP systolic ≥180, diastolic ≥110 unresponsive to nitrate or calcium antagonist; pregnancy; recent (within 1 month): cerebral-vascular accident or transient ischemic attack, gastrointestinal bleeding, trauma or surgery, prolonged external cardiac massage; intracranial neoplasm, suspected aortic dissection, arteriovenous malformation or aneurysm, bleeding diathesis, severe hepatic or renal disease, hemostatic defects, severe uncontrolled hypertension

Warnings/Precautions Doses >150 mg have been associated with an increase of intracranial hemorrhage

Adverse Reactions

1% to 10%:

- Cardiovascular: Hypotension
- Central nervous system: Fever
- Dermatologic: Bruising
- Gastrointestinal: GI hemorrhage, nausea, vomiting
- Genitourinary: GU hemorrhage

<1%:

- Hematologic: Retroperitoneal hemorrhage, gingival hemorrhage, intracranial hemorrhage rapid lysis of coronary artery thrombi by thrombolytic agents may be associated with reperfusion-related atrial and/or ventricular arrhythmias
- Respiratory: Epistaxis

Overdosage/Toxicology Increased incidence of intracranial bleeding

Drug Interactions Increased effect: Anticoagulants, aspirin, ticlopidine, dipyridamole, and heparin are at least additive

Stability Refrigerate; must be used within 8 hours of reconstitution; alteplase is **incompatible** with dobutamine, dopamine, heparin, and nitroglycerin infusions; physically **compatible** with lidocaine, metoprolol, propranolol when administered via Y site; **compatible** with either D_5W or NS

(Continued)

Alteplase *(Continued)*

Standard dose: 100 mg/100 mL 0.9% NaCl [total volume: 200 mL]

Mechanism of Action Initiates local fibrinolysis by binding to fibrin in a thrombus (clot) and converts entrapped plasminogen to plasmin

Pharmacodynamics/Kinetics Elimination: Cleared rapidly from circulating plasma at a rate of 550-650 mL/minute, primarily by the liver; >50% present in plasma is cleared within 5 minutes after the infusion has been terminated, and ~80% is cleared within 10 minutes

Usual Dosage

Coronary artery thrombi: I.V.: Front loading dose: Total dose is 100 mg over 1.5 hours (for patients who weigh <65 kg, use 1.25 mg/kg/total dose). Add this dose to a 100 mL bag of 0.9% sodium chloride for a total volume of 200 mL. Infuse 15 mg (30 mL) over 1-2 minutes; infuse 50 mg (100 mL) over 30 minutes. Begin heparin 5000-10,000 unit bolus followed by continuous infusion of 1000 units/hour. Infuse 35 mg/hour (70 mL) for next 2 hours.

Acute pulmonary embolism: 100 mg over 2 hours

Acute ischemic stroke: Doses should be given within the first 3 hours of the onset of symptoms. Load with 90 mcg/kg as a bolus, followed by 0.81 mg/kg as a continuous infusion over 60 minutes; maximum total dose should not exceed 90 mg

Administration Do not use bacteriostatic water for reconstitution

Reference Range

Not routinely measured; literature supports therapeutic levels of 0.52-1.8 μg/mL

Fibrinogen: 200-400 mg/dL

Activated partial thromboplastin time (APTT): 22.5-38.7 seconds

Prothrombin time (PT): 10.9-12.2 seconds

Nursing Implications Assess for hemorrhage during first hour of treatment

Dosage Forms Powder for injection, lyophilized (recombinant): 20 mg [11.6 million units] (20 mL); 50 mg [29 million units] (50 mL); 100 mg [58 million units] (100 mL)

Alteplase, Recombinant *see* Alteplase *on previous page*

Alteplase, Tissue Plasminogen Activator, Recombinant *see* Alteplase *on previous page*

ALternaGEL® [OTC] *see* Aluminum Hydroxide *on next page*

Altretamine (al TRET a meen)

Related Information

Toxicities of Chemotherapeutic Agents *on page 1382*

Brand Names Hexalen®

Synonyms Hexamethylmelamine

Therapeutic Category Antineoplastic Agent, Miscellaneous

Use Palliative treatment of persistent or recurrent ovarian cancer following first-line therapy with a cisplatin- or alkylating agent-based combination

Pregnancy Risk Factor D

Contraindications Hypersensitivity to altretamine, pre-existing severe bone marrow suppression or severe neurologic toxicity

Warnings/Precautions The U.S. Food and Drug Administration (FDA) currently recommends that procedures for proper handling and disposal of antineoplastic agents be considered. Peripheral blood counts and neurologic examinations should be done routinely before and after drug therapy. Use with caution in patients previously treated with other myelosuppressive drugs or with pre-existing neurotoxicity; use with caution in patients with renal or hepatic dysfunction; altretamine may be slightly mutagenic.

Adverse Reactions

>10%:

- Central nervous system: Peripheral sensory neuropathy, neurotoxicity
- Gastrointestinal: Nausea, vomiting
- Hematologic: Anemia, thrombocytopenia, leukopenia

1% to 10%:

- Central nervous system: Seizures
- Gastrointestinal: Anorexia, diarrhea, stomach cramps
- Hepatic: Increased alkaline phosphatase

<1%:

- Central nervous system: Dizziness, depression
- Dermatologic: Rash, alopecia
- Hematologic: Myelosuppression
- Hepatic: Hepatotoxicity
- Neuromuscular & skeletal: Tremor

Overdosage/Toxicology Symptoms of overdose include nausea, vomiting, peripheral neuropathy, severe bone marrow suppression; after decontamination, treatment is supportive

Drug Interactions

Decreased effect: Phenobarbital may increase metabolism of altretamine

Increased toxicity: May cause severe orthostatic hypotension when administered with MAO inhibitors; cimetidine may decrease metabolism of altretamine

Mechanism of Action Although altretamine clinical antitumor spectrum resembles that of alkylating agents, the drug has demonstrated activity in alkylator-resistant patients; probably requires hepatic microsomal mixed-function oxidase enzyme activation to become cytotoxic. The drug selectively inhibits the incorporation of radioactive thymidine and uridine into DNA and RNA, inhibiting DNA and RNA synthesis; metabolized to reactive intermediates which covalently bind to microsomal proteins and DNA. These reactive intermediates can spontaneously degrade to demethylated melamines and formaldehyde which are also cytotoxic.

Pharmacodynamics/Kinetics

Absorption: Oral: Well absorbed (75% to 89%)

Metabolism: Rapid and extensive demethylation in liver; high concentrations in liver and kidney, but low concentrations in other organs

Half-life: 13 hours

Peak plasma levels: 0.5-3 hours after dose

Elimination: In urine (<1% unchanged)

Usual Dosage Adults: Oral (refer to protocol): 4-12 mg/kg/day in 3-4 divided doses for 21-90 days

Alternatively: 240-320 mg/m^2/day in 3-4 divided doses for 21 days, repeated every 6 weeks

Alternatively: 260 mg/m^2/day for 14-21 days of a 28-day cycle in 4 divided doses

Temporarily discontinue (for ≥14 days) & subsequently restart at 200 mg/m^2/day if any of the following occurs:

if GI intolerance unresponsive to symptom measures

WBC <2000/mm^3

granulocyte count <1000/mm^3

platelet count <75,000/mm^3

progressive neurotoxicity

Administration Administer orally; administer total daily dose as 4 divided oral doses after meals and at bedtime

Patient Information Report any numbness or tingling in extremities to physician; nausea and vomiting may occur and even begin up to weeks after therapy is stopped

Dosage Forms Capsule: 50 mg

Alu-Cap® [OTC] *see* Aluminum Hydroxide *on this page*

Aluminum Hydroxide (a LOO mi num hye DROKS ide)

Brand Names ALternaGEL® [OTC]; Alu-Cap® [OTC]; Alu-Tab® [OTC]; Amphojel® [OTC]; Dialume® [OTC]; Nephrox Suspension [OTC]

Therapeutic Category Antidote, Hyperphosphatemia

Use Treatment of hyperacidity; hyperphosphatemia

Pregnancy Risk Factor C

Pregnancy/Breast-Feeding Implications

Clinical effects on the fetus: No data available; available evidence suggests safe use during pregnancy and breast-feeding

Breast-feeding/lactation: No data available

Contraindications Hypersensitivity to aluminum salts or drug dry components

Warnings/Precautions Hypophosphatemia may occur with prolonged administration or large doses; aluminum intoxication and osteomalacia may occur in patients with uremia. Use with caution in patients with congestive heart failure, renal failure, edema, cirrhosis, and low sodium diets, and patients who have recently suffered gastrointestinal hemorrhage; uremic patients not receiving dialysis may develop osteomalacia and osteoporosis due to phosphate depletion.

Elderly, due to disease and/or drug therapy, may be predisposed to constipation and fecal impaction. Careful evaluation of possible drug interactions must be done. When used as an antacid in ulcer treatment, consider buffer capacity (mEq/mL) to calculate dose; consider renal insufficiency as predisposition to aluminum toxicity.

Adverse Reactions

>10%: Gastrointestinal: Constipation, chalky taste, stomach cramps, fecal impaction

1% to 10%: Gastrointestinal: Nausea, vomiting, discoloration of feces (white speckles)

<1%: Endocrine & metabolic: Hypophosphatemia, hypomagnesemia

Overdosage/Toxicology Aluminum antacids may cause constipation, phosphate depletion, and bezoar or fecalith formation; in patients with renal failure, aluminum may accumulate to toxic levels

(Continued)

Aluminum Hydroxide *(Continued)*

Deferoxamine, traditionally used as an iron chelator, has been shown to increase urinary aluminum output

Deferoxamine chelation of aluminum has resulted in improvements of clinical symptoms and bone histology; however, remains an experimental treatment for aluminum poisoning and has a significant potential for adverse effects

Drug Interactions Decreased effect: Tetracyclines, digoxin, indomethacin, or iron salts, isoniazid, allopurinol, benzodiazepines, corticosteroids, penicillamine, phenothiazines, ranitidine, ketoconazole, itraconazole

Usual Dosage Oral:

Peptic ulcer disease:

Children: 5-15 mL/dose every 3-6 hours or 1 and 3 hours after meals and at bedtime

Adults: 15-45 mL every 3-6 hours or 1 and 3 hours after meals and at bedtime

Prophylaxis against gastrointestinal bleeding:

Infants: 2-5 mL/dose every 1-2 hours

Children: 5-15 mL/dose every 1-2 hours

Adults: 30-60 mL/dose every hour

Titrate to maintain the gastric pH >5

Hyperphosphatemia:

Children: 50-150 mg/kg/24 hours in divided doses every 4-6 hours, titrate dosage to maintain serum phosphorus within normal range

Adults: 500-1800 mg, 3-6 times/day, between meals and at bedtime; best taken with a meal or within 20 minutes of a meal

Antacid: Adults: 30 mL 1 and 3 hours postprandial and at bedtime

Monitoring Parameters Monitor phosphorous levels periodically when patient is on chronic therapy

Test Interactions Decreases phosphorus, inorganic (S)

Patient Information Dilute dose in water or juice, shake well; chew tablets thoroughly before swallowing with water; do not take oral drugs within 1-2 hours of administration; notify physician if relief is not obtained or if there are any signs to suggest bleeding from the GI tract

Nursing Implications Used primarily as a phosphate binder; dose should be given within 20 minutes of a meal and followed with water

Dosage Forms

Capsule:

Alu-Cap®: 400 mg

Dialume®: 500 mg

Liquid: 600 mg/5 mL

ALternaGEL®: 600 mg/5 mL

Suspension, oral: 320 mg/5 mL; 450 mg/5 mL; 675 mg/5 mL

Amphojel®: 320 mg/5 mL

Tablet:

Amphojel®: 300 mg, 600 mg

Alu-Tab®: 500 mg

Aluminum Sucrose Sulfate, Basic *see* Sucralfate *on page 1168*

Alupent® *see* Metaproterenol *on page 793*

Alu-Tab® [OTC] *see* Aluminum Hydroxide *on previous page*

Amantadine (a MAN ta deen)

Related Information

Guidelines for the Prevention of Opportunistic Infections in Persons with HIV *on page 1457*

Brand Names Symadine®; Symmetrel®

Canadian/Mexican Brand Names Endantadine® (Canada); PMS-Amantadine (Canada)

Synonyms Adamantanamine Hydrochloride; Amantadine Hydrochloride

Therapeutic Category Anti-Parkinson's Agent; Antiviral Agent, Oral

Use Symptomatic and adjunct treatment of parkinsonism; prophylaxis and treatment of influenza A viral infection; treatment of drug-induced extrapyramidal symptoms

Pregnancy Risk Factor C

Contraindications Hypersensitivity to amantadine hydrochloride or any component

Warnings/Precautions Use with caution in patients with liver disease, a history of recurrent and eczematoid dermatitis, uncontrolled psychosis or severe psychoneurosis, seizures and in those receiving CNS stimulant drugs; when treating Parkinson's disease, do not discontinue abruptly. In many patients, the therapeutic benefits of amantadine are limited to a few months. Elderly patients may be more susceptible to the CNS effects (using 2 divided daily doses may minimize this effect).

Adverse Reactions

1% to 10%:

- Cardiovascular: Orthostatic hypotension, peripheral edema
- Central nervous system: Insomnia, depression, anxiety, irritability, dizziness, hallucinations, ataxia, headache, somnolence, nervousness, dream abnormality, agitation, fatigue
- Dermatologic: Livedo reticularis
- Gastrointestinal: Nausea, anorexia, constipation, diarrhea, xerostomia
- Respiratory: Dry nose

<1%:

- Cardiovascular: Congestive heart failure, hypertension
- Central nervous system: Psychosis, slurred speech, euphoria, confusion, amnesia, instances of convulsions
- Dermatologic: Rash, eczematoid dermatitis
- Endocrine & metabolic: Decreased libido
- Genitourinary: Urinary retention
- Gastrointestinal: Vomiting
- Hematologic: Leukopenia, neutropenia
- Neuromuscular & skeletal: Hyperkinesis, weakness
- Ocular: Visual disturbances, oculogyric episodes
- Respiratory: Dyspnea

Overdosage/Toxicology Symptoms of overdose include nausea, vomiting, slurred speech, blurred vision, lethargy, hallucinations, seizures, myoclonic jerking

Treatment should be directed at reducing the CNS stimulation and at maintaining cardiovascular function. Seizures can be treated with diazepam while a lidocaine infusion may be required for the cardiac dysrhythmias.

Drug Interactions

Increased effect: Drugs with anticholinergic or CNS stimulant activity

Increased toxicity/levels: Hydrochlorothiazide plus triamterene, amiloride

Stability Protect from freezing

Mechanism of Action As an antiviral, blocks the uncoating of influenza A virus preventing penetration of virus into host; antiparkinsonian activity may be due to its blocking the reuptake of dopamine into presynaptic neurons and causing direct stimulation of postsynaptic receptors

Pharmacodynamics/Kinetics

Onset of antidyskinetic action: Within 48 hours

Absorption: Well absorbed from GI tract

Distribution: To saliva, tear film, and nasal secretions; in animals, tissue (especially lung) concentrations higher than serum concentrations, crosses blood-brain barrier

- V_d:
  - Normal: 4.4±0.2 L/kg
  - Renal failure: 5.1±0.2 L/kg

Protein binding:

- Normal renal function: ~67%
- Hemodialysis patients: ~59%

Metabolism: Not appreciable, small amounts of an acetyl metabolite identified

Half-life:

- Normal renal function: 2-7 hours
- End stage renal disease: 7-10 days

Time to peak: 1-4 hours

Elimination: 80% to 90% excreted unchanged in urine by glomerular filtration and tubular secretion

Usual Dosage

Children:

- 1-9 years: (<45 kg): 5-9 mg/kg/day in 1-2 divided doses to a maximum of 150 mg/day
- 10-12 years: 100-200 mg/day in 1-2 divided doses
- Prophylaxis: Administer for 10-21 days following exposure if the vaccine is concurrently given or for 90 days following exposure if the vaccine is unavailable or contraindicated and re-exposure is possible

Adults:

- Parkinson's disease: 100 mg twice daily
- Influenza A viral infection: 200 mg/day in 1-2 divided doses
- Prophylaxis: Minimum 10-day course of therapy following exposure if the vaccine is concurrently given or for 90 days following exposure if the vaccine is unavailable or contraindicated and re-exposure is possible

Elderly patients should take the drug in 2 daily doses rather than a single dose to avoid adverse neurologic reactions

(Continued)

Amantadine *(Continued)*

Dosing interval in renal impairment:

Cl_{cr} 50-60 mL/minute: Administer 200 mg alternating with 100 mg/day
Cl_{cr} 30-50 mL/minute: Administer 100 mg/day
Cl_{cr} 20-30 mL/minute: Administer 200 mg twice weekly
Cl_{cr} 10-20 mL/minute: Administer 100 mg 3 times/week
Cl_{cr} <10 mL/minute: Administer 200 mg alternating with 100 mg every 7 days

Hemodialysis: Slightly hemodialyzable (5% to 20%); no supplemental dose is needed

Peritoneal dialysis: No supplemental dose is needed

Continuous arterio-venous or venous-venous hemofiltration (CAVH/CAVHD): No supplemental dose is needed

Monitoring Parameters Renal function, mental status, blood pressure

Patient Information Do not abruptly discontinue therapy, it may precipitate a parkinsonian crisis; may impair ability to perform activities requiring mental alertness or coordination; must take throughout flu season or for at least 10 days following vaccination for effective prophylaxis; take second dose of the day in early afternoon to decrease incidence of insomnia

Nursing Implications If insomnia occurs, the last daily dose should be given several hours before retiring; assess parkinsonian symptoms prior to and throughout course of therapy

Dosage Forms

Capsule, as hydrochloride: 100 mg
Syrup, as hydrochloride: 50 mg/5 mL (480 mL)

Amantadine Hydrochloride *see* Amantadine *on page 56*

Amaphen® *see* Butalbital Compound *on page 176*

Amaryl® *see* Glimepiride *on page 574*

Ambi 10® [OTC] *see* Benzoyl Peroxide *on page 140*

Ambien™ *see* Zolpidem *on page 1326*

Ambi® Skin Tone [OTC] *see* Hydroquinone *on page 628*

Amcinonide (am SIN oh nide)

Related Information

Corticosteroids Comparison *on page 1407*

Brand Names Cyclocort®

Canadian/Mexican Brand Names Visderm® (Mexico)

Therapeutic Category Anti-inflammatory Agent; Corticosteroid, Topical (High Potency)

Use Relief of the inflammatory and pruritic manifestations of corticosteroid-responsive dermatoses (high potency corticosteroid)

Pregnancy Risk Factor C

Contraindications Hypersensitivity to amcinonide or any component; use on the face, groin, or axilla

Warnings/Precautions Adverse systemic effects may occur when used on large areas of the body, denuded areas, for prolonged periods of time, with an occlusive dressing, and/or in infants or small children; occlusive dressings should not be used in presence of infection or weeping lesions

Adverse Reactions

1% to 10%:

Dermatologic: Itching, maceration of skin, skin atrophy, erythema, dryness, papular rashes

Local: Burning, irritation

<1%: Dermatologic: Hypertrichosis, acneiform eruptions, hypopigmentation, perioral dermatitis, striae, miliaria

Overdosage/Toxicology Symptoms of overdose include cushingoid appearance (systemic), muscle weakness (systemic), osteoporosis (systemic) all with long-term use only. When consumed in excessive quantities for prolonged periods, systemic hypercorticism and adrenal suppression may occur; in those cases, discontinuation and withdrawal of the corticosteroid should be done judiciously.

Mechanism of Action Stimulates the synthesis of enzymes needed to decrease inflammation, suppress mitotic activity, and cause vasoconstriction

Pharmacodynamics/Kinetics

Absorption: Adequate through intact skin; increases with skin inflammation or occlusion

Metabolism: In the liver

Elimination: By the kidney and in bile

Usual Dosage Adults: Topical: Apply in a thin film 2-3 times/day

Patient Information Before applying, gently wash area to reduce risk of infection; apply a thin film to cleansed area and rub in gently and thoroughly until medication vanishes; avoid exposure to sunlight, severe sunburn may occur

Nursing Implications Assess for worsening of rash or fever

Dosage Forms

Cream: 0.1% (15 g, 30 g, 60 g)
Lotion: 0.1% (20 mL, 60 mL)
Ointment, topical: 0.1% (15 g, 30 g, 60 g)

Amcort® *see* Triamcinolone *on page 1255*

Amen® *see* Medroxyprogesterone Acetate *on page 771*

Americaine® [OTC] *see* Benzocaine *on page 138*

A-Methapred® *see* Methylprednisolone *on page 819*

Amethocaine Hydrochloride *see* Tetracaine *on page 1202*

Amethopterin *see* Methotrexate *on page 806*

Amfepramone *see* Diethylpropion *on page 380*

Amicar® *see* Aminocaproic Acid *on page 64*

Amidate® *see* Etomidate *on page 496*

Amifostine (am i FOS teen)

Brand Names Ethyol®

Synonyms Ethiofos; Gammaphos

Therapeutic Category Antidote, Cisplatin

Use Reduces the cumulative renal toxicity associated with repeated administration of cisplatin in patients with advanced ovarian cancer or nonsmall cell lung cancer. In these settings, the clinical data do not suggest that the effectiveness of cisplatin-based chemotherapy regimens is altered by amifostine.

Pregnancy Risk Factor C

Contraindications Known hypersensitivity to aminothiol compounds or mannitol

Warnings/Precautions The U.S. Food and Drug Administration (FDA) currently recommends that procedures for proper handling and disposal of antineoplastic agents be considered

Limited data are currently available regarding the preservation of antitumor efficacy when amifostine is administered prior to cisplatin therapy in settings other than advanced ovarian cancer or nonsmall cell lung cancer. Amifostine should therefore not be used in patients receiving chemotherapy for other malignancies in which chemotherapy can produce a significant survival benefit or cure, except in the context of a clinical study.

Patients who are hypotensive or in a state of dehydration should not receive amifostine. Patients receiving antihypertensive therapy that cannot be stopped for 24 hours preceding amifostine treatment also should not receive amifostine. Patients should be adequately hydrated prior to amifostine infusion and kept in a supine position during the infusion. Blood pressure should be monitored every 5 minutes during the infusion. If hypotension requiring interruption of therapy occurs, patients should be placed in the Trendelenburg position and given an infusion of normal saline using a separate I.V. line.

It is recommended that antiemetic medication, including dexamethasone 20 mg I.V. and a serotonin $5HT_3$ receptor antagonist be administered prior to and in conjunction with amifostine.

Reports of clinically relevant hypocalcemia are rare, but serum calcium levels should be monitored in patients at risk of hypocalcemia, such as those with nephrotic syndrome

Adverse Reactions

>10%:

Cardiovascular: Flushing; hypotension (62%) (see Additional Information)
Central nervous system: Chills, dizziness, somnolence
Gastrointestinal: Nausea/vomiting (may be severe)
Respiratory: Sneezing
Miscellaneous: Feeling of warmth/coldness, hiccups

<1%:

Dermatologic: Mild rashes
Endocrine & metabolic: Hypocalcemia
Neuromuscular & skeletal: Rigors

Overdosage/Toxicology Symptoms of overdose include increased nausea and vomiting, hypotension

Treatment includes infusion of normal saline and other supportive measures, as clinically indicated

Drug Interactions Increased toxicity: Special consideration should be given to patients receiving antihypertensive medications or other drugs that could potentiate hypotension

Stability

Store intact vials of lyophilized powder at room temperature (20°C to 25°C/68°F to 77°F)

(Continued)

Amifostine *(Continued)*

Reconstitute with 9.7 mL of sterile 0.9% sodium chloride. The reconstituted solution (500 mg/10 mL) is chemically stable for up to 5 hours at room temperature (25°C) or up to 24 hours under refrigeration (2°C to 8°C).

Amifostine should be further diluted in 0.9% sodium chloride to a concentration of 5-40 mg/mL and is chemically stable for up to 5 hours at room temperature (25°C) or up to 24 hours under refrigeration (2°C to 8°C)

Mechanism of Action Prodrug that is dephosphorylated by alkaline phosphatase in tissues to a pharmacologically active free thiol metabolite that can reduce the toxic effects of cisplatin. The free thiol is available to bind to, and detoxify, reactive metabolites of cisplatin; and can also act as a scavenger of free radicals that may be generated in tissues exposed to cisplatin.

Pharmacodynamics/Kinetics

Absorption: Oral: Poor

Distribution: V_d: 3.5 L

Metabolism: Hepatic dephosphorylation to two metabolites (WR-33278 and WR-1065)

Half-life: 9 minutes

Elimination: Renal; plasma clearance: 2.17 L/minute

Usual Dosage Adults: I.V. (refer to individual protocols): 910 mg/m^2 administered once daily as a 15-minute I.V. infusion, starting 30 minutes prior to chemotherapy

Note: 15-minute infusion is better tolerated than more extended infusions. Further reductions in infusion times have not been systematically investigated. The infusion of amifostine should be interrupted if the systolic blood pressure decreases significantly from the baseline value. See table.

Decrease in Systolic Blood Pressure

Baseline systolic blood pressure (mm Hg)	<100	100–119	120–139	140–179	≥180
Decrease in systolic blood pressure during infusion of amifostine (mm Hg)	20	25	30	40	50

If the blood pressure returns to normal within 5 minutes and the patient is asymptomatic, the infusion may be restarted so that the full dose of amifostine may be administered. If the full dose of amifostine cannot be administered, the dose of amifostine for subsequent cycles should be 740 mg/m^2.

Administration I.V.: Administer over 15 minutes; administration as a longer infusion is associated with a higher incidence of side effects

Monitoring Parameters Blood pressure should be monitored every 5 minutes during the infusion

Additional Information Mean onset of hypotension is 14 minutes into the 15-minute infusion and the mean duration was 6 minutes. Hypotension should be treated with fluid infusion and postural management of the patient (supine or Trendelenburg position). If the blood pressure returns to normal within 5 minutes and the patient is asymptomatic, the infusion may be restarted.

Dosage Forms Injection, vials: 500 mg powder

Amikacin (am i KAY sin)

Related Information

Antimicrobial Drugs of Choice *on page 1468*

Bacterial Meningitis Practical Guidelines for Management *on page 1475*

Brand Names Amikin®

Canadian/Mexican Brand Names Amikin® (Canada); Amikin® (Mexico); Amikafur® (Mexico); Amikayect® (Mexico); Biclin® (Mexico); Gamikal® (Mexico); Yectamid® (Mexico)

Synonyms Amikacin Sulfate

Therapeutic Category Antibiotic, Aminoglycoside

Use Treatment of documented gram-negative enteric infection resistant to gentamicin and tobramycin (bone infections, respiratory tract infections, endocarditis, and septicemia); documented infection of mycobacterial organisms susceptible to amikacin including *Pseudomonas, Proteus, Serratia*, and gram-positive *Staphylococcus*

Pregnancy Risk Factor C

Contraindications Hypersensitivity to amikacin sulfate or any component; cross-sensitivity may exist with other aminoglycosides

Warnings/Precautions Dose and/or frequency of administration must be monitored and modified in patients with renal impairment; drug should be discontinued if signs of ototoxicity, nephrotoxicity, or hypersensitivity occur; ototoxicity is proportional to the amount of drug given and the duration of treatment; tinnitus or vertigo may be indications of vestibular injury and impending bilateral irreversible damage; renal damage is usually reversible

Adverse Reactions

1% to 10%:

Central nervous system: Neurotoxicity

Otic: Ototoxicity (auditory), ototoxicity (vestibular)

Renal: Nephrotoxicity

<1%:

Cardiovascular: Hypotension

Central nervous system: Headache, drowsiness, drug fever

Dermatologic: Rash

Gastrointestinal: Nausea, vomiting

Hematologic: Eosinophilia

Neuromuscular & skeletal: Paresthesia, tremor, arthralgia, weakness

Respiratory: Dyspnea

Overdosage/Toxicology Symptoms of overdose include ototoxicity, nephrotoxicity, and neuromuscular toxicity

Treatment of choice following a single acute overdose appears to be the maintenance of good urine output of at least 3 mL/kg/hour. Dialysis is of questionable value in the enhancement of aminoglycoside elimination. If required, hemodialysis is preferred over peritoneal dialysis in patients with normal renal function.

Drug Interactions

Decreased effect of aminoglycoside: High concentrations of penicillins and/or cephalosporins (*in vitro* data)

Increased toxicity of aminoglycoside: Indomethacin I.V., amphotericin, loop diuretics, vancomycin, enflurane, methoxyflurane; increased toxicity of depolarizing and nondepolarizing neuromuscular blocking agents and polypeptide antibiotics with administration of aminoglycosides

Stability Stable for 24 hours at room temperature and 2 days at refrigeration when mixed in D_5W, $D_5{}^1/_4NS$, $D_5{}^1/_2NS$, NS, LR

Mechanism of Action Inhibits protein synthesis in susceptible bacteria by binding to ribosomal subunits

Pharmacodynamics/Kinetics

Absorption: I.M.: May be delayed in the bedridden patient

Distribution: Crosses the placenta; primarily distributes into extracellular fluid (highly hydrophilic); penetrates the blood-brain barrier when meninges are inflamed

Relative diffusion of antimicrobial agents from blood into cerebrospinal fluid (CSF): Good only with inflammation (exceeds usual MICs); ratio of CSF to blood level (%):

Normal meninges: 10-20

Inflamed meninges: 15-24

Half-life (dependent on renal function):

Infants:

Low birthweight (1-3 days): 7-9 hours

Full term >7 days: 4-5 hours

Children: 1.6-2.5 hours

Adults:

Normal renal function: 1.4-2.3 hours

Anuria: End stage renal disease: 28-86 hours

Time to peak serum concentration:

I.M.: Within 45-120 minutes

I.V.: Within 30 minutes following 30-minute infusion

Elimination: 94% to 98% excreted unchanged in urine via glomerular filtration within 24 hours; clearance dependent on renal function and patient age

Usual Dosage Individualization is critical because of the low therapeutic index

Use of ideal body weight (IBW) for determining the mg/kg/dose appears to be more accurate than dosing on the basis of total body weight (TBW)

In morbid obesity, dosage requirement may best be estimated using a dosing weight of IBW + 0.4 (TBW - IBW)

Initial and periodic peak and trough plasma drug levels should be determined, particularly in critically ill patients with serious infections or in disease states known to significantly alter aminoglycoside pharmacokinetics (eg, cystic fibrosis, burns, or major surgery)

Once daily dosing: Higher peak serum drug concentration to MIC ratios, demonstrated aminoglycoside postantibiotic effect, decreased renal cortex drug uptake, and improved cost-time efficiency are supportive reasons for the use of once daily dosing regimens for aminoglycosides. Current research indicates those regimens to be as effective for nonlife-threatening infections, with no higher incidence of nephrotoxicity, than those requiring multiple daily doses. Doses are determined by calculating the entire day's dose via usual multiple dose calculation techniques and administering this quantity as a single dose.

(Continued)

Amikacin *(Continued)*

Doses are then adjusted to maintain mean serum concentrations above the MIC(s) of the causative organism(s). (Example: 14-35 mg/kg as a single dose/24 hours; peak (maximum) serum concentration may approximate 40-55 mcg/mL and trough (minimum) serum concentration <3 mcg/L). Further research is needed for universal recommendation in all patient populations and gram-negative disease; exceptions may include those with known high clearance (eg, children, patients with cystic fibrosis or burns who may require shorter dosage intervals) and patients with renal function impairment for whom longer than conventional dosage intervals are usually required.

Infants, Children, and Adults: I.M., I.V.: 5-7.5 mg/kg/dose every 8 hours

Dosing interval in renal impairment: Some patients may require larger or more frequent doses if serum levels document the need (ie, cystic fibrosis or febrile granulocytopenic patients)

Cl_{cr} ≥60 mL/minute: Administer every 8 hours
Cl_{cr} 40-60 mL/minute: Administer every 12 hours
Cl_{cr} 20-40 mL/minute: Administer every 24 hours
Cl_{cr} 10-20 mL/minute: Administer every 48 hours
Cl_{cr} <10 mL/minute: Administer every 72 hours

Hemodialysis: Dialyzable (50% to 100%); administer dose postdialysis or administer $^2/_3$ normal dose as a supplemental dose postdialysis and follow levels

Peritoneal dialysis: Dose as Cl_{cr} <10 mL/minute: Follow levels

Continuous arterio-venous or veno-venous hemodiafiltration (CAVH) effects: Dose as Cl_{cr} <10 mL/minute: Follow levels

Administration Administer I.M. injection in large muscle mass; administer around-the-clock rather than 3 times/day, to promote less variation in peak and trough serum levels

Monitoring Parameters Urinalysis, BUN, serum creatinine, appropriately timed peak and trough concentrations, vital signs, temperature, weight, I & O, hearing parameters (audiology testing warranted in extended treatment courses (>10 days))

Reference Range

Sample size: 0.5-2 mL blood (red top tube) or 0.1-1 mL serum (separated)

Therapeutic levels:

Peak:
- Life-threatening infections: 25-30 μg/mL
- Serious infections: 20-25 μg/mL
- Urinary tract infections: 15-20 μg/mL
- Synergy against gram-positive organisms: 15-20 μg/mL

Trough:
- Serious infections: 1-4 μg/mL
- Life-threatening infections: 4-8 μg/mL

Toxic concentration: Peak: >35 μg/mL; Trough: >10 μg/mL

Timing of serum samples: Draw peak 30 minutes after completion of 30-minute infusion or at 1 hour following initiation of infusion or I.M. injection; draw trough immediately before next dose

The presence of fever may decrease peak levels; *in vitro* data indicate the presence of high concentrations of penicillins concurrent with sampling of aminoglycoside levels may result in inactivation (decreased values)

Patient Information Report loss of hearing, ringing or roaring in the ears, or feeling of fullness in head

Nursing Implications Aminoglycoside levels measured from blood taken from Silastic® central catheters can sometimes give falsely high readings (draw levels from alternate lumen or peripheral stick, if possible)

Additional Information Sodium content of 1 g: 29.9 mg (1.3 mEq)

Dosage Forms Injection, as sulfate: 50 mg/mL (2 mL, 4 mL); 250 mg/mL (2 mL, 4 mL)

Amikacin Sulfate *see* Amikacin *on page 60*
Amikin® *see* Amikacin *on page 60*

Amiloride (a MIL oh ride)

Related Information

Heart Failure: Management of Patients With Left-Ventricular Systolic Dysfunction *on page 1533*

Brand Names Midamor®

Synonyms Amiloride Hydrochloride

Therapeutic Category Diuretic, Potassium Sparing

Use Counteracts potassium loss induced by other diuretics in the treatment of hypertension or edematous conditions including CHF, hepatic cirrhosis, and hypoaldosteronism; usually used in conjunction with more potent diuretics such as thiazides or loop diuretics

Investigational: Cystic fibrosis

Pregnancy Risk Factor B

Contraindications Hyperkalemia, potassium supplementation and impaired renal function, hypersensitivity to amiloride or any component

Warnings/Precautions Use cautiously in patients with severe hepatic insufficiency; may cause hyperkalemia (serum levels >5.5 mEq/L) which, if uncorrected, is potentially fatal; medication should be discontinued if potassium level are >6.5 mEq/L

Adverse Reactions

1% to 10%:

- Central nervous system: Headache, fatigue, dizziness
- Endocrine & metabolic: Hyperkalemia, hyperchloremic metabolic acidosis, dehydration, hyponatremia, gynecomastia
- Gastrointestinal: Nausea, diarrhea, vomiting, abdominal pain, gas pain, appetite changes, constipation
- Genitourinary: Impotence
- Neuromuscular & skeletal: Muscle cramps, weakness
- Respiratory: Cough, dyspnea

<1%:

- Cardiovascular: Angina pectoris, orthostatic hypotension, arrhythmias, palpitations, chest pain
- Central nervous system: Vertigo, nervousness, insomnia, depression
- Dermatologic: Rash or dryness, pruritus, alopecia
- Endocrine & metabolic: Decreased libido
- Gastrointestinal: GI bleeding, heartburn, flatulence, dyspepsia
- Genitourinary: Polyuria, bladder spasms, dysuria
- Hepatic: Jaundice
- Neuromuscular & skeletal: Arthralgia, tremor, neck/shoulder pain, back pain
- Ocular: Increased intraocular pressure
- Respiratory: Shortness of breath
- Miscellaneous: Thirst

Overdosage/Toxicology Clinical signs are consistent with dehydration and electrolyte disturbance; large amounts may result in life-threatening hyperkalemia (>6.5 mEq/L)

This can be treated with I.V. glucose (dextrose 25% in water), with rapid-acting insulin, with concurrent I.V. sodium bicarbonate and, if needed, Kayexalate® oral or rectal solutions in sorbitol; persistent hyperkalemia may require dialysis.

Drug Interactions

Decreased effect of amiloride: Nonsteroidal anti-inflammatory agents

Increased risk of amiloride-associated hyperkalemia: Triamterene, spironolactone, angiotensin-converting enzyme (ACE) inhibitors, potassium preparations, indomethacin

Increased toxicity of amantadine and lithium by reduction of renal excretion

Mechanism of Action Interferes with potassium/sodium exchange (active transport) in the distal tubule, cortical collecting tubule and collecting duct by inhibiting sodium, potassium-ATPase; decreases calcium excretion; increases magnesium loss

Pharmacodynamics/Kinetics

Absorption: Oral: ~15% to 25%

- Onset: 2 hours
- Duration: 24 hours

Distribution: V_d: 350-380 L

Protein binding: 23%

Metabolism: No active metabolites

Half-life:

- Normal renal function: 6-9 hours
- End stage renal disease: 8-144 hours

Peak serum concentration: 6-10 hours

Elimination: Unchanged equally in the urine and the feces

Usual Dosage Oral:

Children: Although safety and efficacy have not been established by the FDA in children, a dosage of 0.625 mg/kg/day has been used in children weighing 6-20 kg

Adults: 5-10 mg/day (up to 20 mg)

Elderly: Initial: 5 mg once daily or every other day

Dosing adjustment in renal impairment:

- Cl_{cr} 10-50 mL/minute: Administer at 50% of normal dose
- Cl_{cr} <10 mL/minute: Avoid use

Monitoring Parameters I & O, daily weights, blood pressure, serum electrolytes, renal function

Test Interactions ↑ potassium (S)

(Continued)

Amiloride *(Continued)*

Patient Information Take with food or milk; avoid salt substitutes; because of high potassium content, avoid bananas and oranges; report any muscle cramps, weakness, nausea, or dizziness; use caution operating machinery or performing other tasks requiring alertness

Nursing Implications Assess fluid status via daily weights, I & O ratios, standing and supine blood pressures; observe for hyperkalemia; if ordered once daily, dose should be given in the morning

Dosage Forms Tablet, as hydrochloride: 5 mg

Amiloride Hydrochloride *see* Amiloride *on page 62*

2-Amino-6-Mercaptopurine *see* Thioguanine *on page 1216*

2-Amino-6-Trifluoromethoxy-benzothiazole *see* Riluzole *on page 1108*

Aminobenzylpenicillin *see* Ampicillin *on page 85*

Aminocaproic Acid (a mee noe ka PROE ik AS id)

Brand Names Amicar®

Therapeutic Category Hemostatic Agent

Use Treatment of excessive bleeding from fibrinolysis

Pregnancy Risk Factor C

Contraindications Disseminated intravascular coagulation, hematuria of upper urinary tract

Warnings/Precautions Rapid I.V. administration of the undiluted drug is not recommended; aminocaproic acid may accumulate in patients with decreased renal function; do not use in hematuria of upper urinary tract origin unless possible benefits outweigh risks; use with caution in patients with cardiac, renal or hepatic disease; do not administer without a definite diagnosis of laboratory findings indicative of hyperfibrinolysis; should not be used in nursing women

Adverse Reactions

1% to 10%:

- Cardiovascular: Hypotension, bradycardia, arrhythmia
- Central nervous system: Dizziness, headache, malaise, fatigue
- Dermatologic: Rash
- Gastrointestinal: GI irritation, nausea, cramps, diarrhea
- Hematologic: Decreased platelet function, elevated serum enzymes
- Neuromuscular & skeletal: Myopathy, weakness
- Otic: Tinnitus
- Respiratory: Nasal congestion

<1%:

- Central nervous system: Convulsions
- Genitourinary: Ejaculation problems
- Neuromuscular & skeletal: Rhabdomyolysis
- Renal: Renal failure

Overdosage/Toxicology Symptoms of overdose include nausea, diarrhea, delirium, hepatic necrosis, thromboembolism

Drug Interactions Increased toxic effect with oral contraceptives, estrogens

Mechanism of Action Competitively inhibits activation of plasminogen to plasmin, also, a lesser antiplasmin effect

Pharmacodynamics/Kinetics

Oral:

- Peak effect: Within 2 hours
- Therapeutic effect: Within 1-72 hours after dose

Distribution: Widely distributes through intravascular and extravascular compartments

Metabolism: Minimal hepatic

Half-life: 1-2 hours

Elimination: 68% to 86% excreted as unchanged drug in urine within 12 hours

Usual Dosage In the management of acute bleeding syndromes, oral dosage regimens are the same as the I.V. dosage regimens in adults and children

Chronic bleeding: Oral, I.V.: 5-30 g/day in divided doses at 3- to 6-hour intervals

Acute bleeding syndrome:

- Children: Oral, I.V.: 100 mg/kg or 3 g/m^2 during the first hour, followed by continuous infusion at the rate of 33.3 mg/kg/hour or 1 g/m^2/hour; total dosage should not exceed 18 g/m^2/24 hours
  - Traumatic hyphema: Oral: 100 mg/kg/dose every 6-8 hours
- Adults:
  - Oral: For elevated fibrinolytic activity, administer 5 g during first hour, followed by 1-1.25 g/hour for approximately 8 hours or until bleeding stops
  - I.V.: 4-5 g in 250 mL of diluent during first hour followed by continuous infusion at the rate of 1-1.25 g/hour in 50 mL of diluent, continue for 8 hours or until bleeding stops
  - Maximum daily dose: Oral, I.V.: 30 g

Dosing adjustment in renal impairment: Oliguria or ESRD: Reduce dose by 15% to 25%

Administration Administration by infusion using appropriate I.V. solution (dextrose 5% or 0.9% sodium chloride); rapid I.V. injection (IVP) should be avoided since hypotension, bradycardia, and arrhythmia may result. Aminocaproic acid may accumulate in patients with decreased renal function.

Monitoring Parameters Fibrinogen, fibrin split products, creatine phosphokinase (with long-term therapy)

Reference Range Therapeutic concentration: >130 μg/mL (concentration necessary for inhibition of fibrinolysis)

Test Interactions ↑ potassium, creatine phosphokinase [CPK] (S)

Patient Information Report any signs of bleeding; change positions slowly to minimize dizziness

Dosage Forms

Injection: 250 mg/mL (20 mL, 96 mL, 100 mL)
Syrup: 1.25 g/5 mL (480 mL)
Tablet: 500 mg

Amino-Cerv™ Vaginal Cream *see* Urea *on page 1280*

Aminoglutethimide (a mee noe gloo TETH i mide)

Brand Names Cytadren®

Therapeutic Category Adrenal Steroid Inhibitor; Antiadrenal Agent; Antineoplastic Agent, Miscellaneous

Use Suppression of adrenal function in selected patients with Cushing's syndrome; also used successfully in postmenopausal patients with advanced breast carcinoma and in patients with metastatic prostate carcinoma as salvage (third-line hormonal agent)

Pregnancy Risk Factor D

Pregnancy/Breast-Feeding Implications Suspected of causing virilization when given throughout pregnancy

Contraindications Hypersensitivity to aminoglutethimide or any component and glutethimide

Warnings/Precautions Monitor blood pressure in all patients at appropriate intervals; hypothyroidism may occur; **mineralocorticoid replacement therapy may be necessary in up to 50% of patients** (ie, fludrocortisone); if glucocorticoid replacement therapy is necessary, 20-30 mg of hydrocortisone daily in the morning will replace endogenous secretion (steroid replacement regimen is controversial - high-dose versus low-dose)

Adverse Reactions Most adverse effects will diminish in incidence and severity after the first 2-6 weeks

>10%:

- Central nervous system: Headache, dizziness, drowsiness, and lethargy are frequent at the start of therapy, clumsiness
- Dermatologic: Skin rash
- Gastrointestinal: Nausea, vomiting, anorexia
- Hepatic: Cholestatic jaundice
- Neuromuscular & skeletal: Myalgia
- Renal: Nephrotoxicity
- Respiratory: Pulmonary alveolar damage
- Miscellaneous: Systemic lupus erythematosus

1% to 10%:

- Cardiovascular: Hypotension and tachycardia, orthostatic hypotension
- Central nervous system: Headache
- Dermatologic: Hirsutism in females
- Endocrine & metabolic: Adrenocortical insufficiency
- Hematologic: Rare cases of neutropenia, leukopenia, thrombocytopenia, pancytopenia, and agranulocytosis have been reported
- Neuromuscular & skeletal: Myalgia

<1%: Endocrine & metabolic: Adrenal suppression, lipid abnormalities (hypercholesterolemia), hyperkalemia, hypothyroidism, goiter

Overdosage/Toxicology Symptoms of overdose include ataxia, somnolence, lethargy, dizziness, distress, fatigue, coma, hyperventilation, respiratory depression, hypovolemic shock; treatment is supportive

Drug Interactions

Decreased effect:

- Dexamethasone: Reported to increase metabolism
- Digitoxin: Increases clearance of digitoxin after 3-8 weeks of aminoglutethimide therapy
- Theophylline: Aminoglutethimide increases metabolism of theophylline
- Warfarin: Decreases anticoagulant response to warfarin

Increased toxicity: Propranolol: Case report of enhanced aminoglutethimide toxicity (rash and lethargy)

(Continued)

Aminoglutethimide *(Continued)*

Mechanism of Action Blocks the enzymatic conversion of cholesterol to delta-5-pregnenolone, thereby reducing the synthesis of adrenal glucocorticoids, mineralocorticoids, estrogens, aldosterone, and androgens

Pharmacodynamics/Kinetics

Onset of action (adrenal suppression): 3-5 days

Absorption: Oral: Well absorbed (90%)

Distribution: Crosses the placenta

Protein binding: Minimally bound to plasma proteins (20% to 25%)

Metabolism: Major metabolite is N-acetylaminoglutethimide

Half-life: 7-15 hours; shorter following multiple administrations than following single doses (induces hepatic enzymes increasing its own metabolism)

Elimination: 34% to 50% excreted in urine as unchanged drug and 25% excreted as metabolite

Usual Dosage Adults: Oral: 250 mg every 6 hours may be increased at 1- to 2-week intervals to a total of 2 g/day; administer in divided doses, 2-3 times/day to reduce incidence of nausea and vomiting

Dosing adjustment in renal impairment: Dose reduction may be necessary

Patient Information Masculinization can occur and is reversible after discontinuing treatment; may cause drowsiness or dizziness

Dosage Forms Tablet, scored: 250 mg

Amino-Opti-E® [OTC] *see* Vitamin E *on page 1309*

Aminophyllin™ *see* Theophylline Salts *on page 1207*

Aminophylline *see* Theophylline Salts *on page 1207*

Aminosalicylate Sodium (a MEE noe sa LIS i late SOW dee um)

Brand Names Sodium P.A.S.

Canadian/Mexican Brand Names Tubasal® (Canada); Salofalk® (Mexico)

Synonyms Para-Aminosalicylate Sodium; PAS

Therapeutic Category Anti-inflammatory Agent; Antitubercular Agent; Nonsteroidal Anti-inflammatory Agent (NSAID), Oral

Use Treatment of tuberculosis with combination drugs

Pregnancy Risk Factor C

Contraindications Hypersensitivity to aminosalicylate sodium

Warnings/Precautions Use with caution in patients with hepatic or renal dysfunction, patients with gastric ulcer, patients with CHF, and patients who are sodium restricted

Adverse Reactions

1% to 10%: Gastrointestinal: Nausea, vomiting, diarrhea, abdominal pain

<1%:

- Cardiovascular: Vasculitis
- Central nervous system: Fever
- Dermatologic: Skin eruptions
- Endocrine & metabolic: Goiter with or without myxedema
- Hematologic: Leukopenia, agranulocytosis, thrombocytopenia, hemolytic anemia
- Hepatic: Jaundice, hepatitis

Overdosage/Toxicology Acute overdose results in crystalluria and renal failure, nausea, and vomiting

Alkalinization of the urine with sodium bicarbonate and forced diuresis can prevent crystalluria and nephrotoxicity

Drug Interactions Decreased levels of digoxin and vitamin B_{12}

Mechanism of Action Aminosalicylic acid (PAS) is a highly specific bacteriostatic agent active against *M. tuberculosis*. Most strains of *M. tuberculosis* are sensitive to a concentration of 1 mcg/mL; structurally related to para-aminobenzoic acid (PABA) and its mechanism of action is thought to be similar to the sulfonamides, a competitive antagonism with PABA; disrupts plate biosynthesis in sensitive organisms.

Pharmacodynamics/Kinetics

Absorption: Readily absorbed >90%

Metabolism: >50% acetylated in liver

Elimination: >80% excreted through kidneys as parent drug and metabolites; elimination is reduced with renal dysfunction

Usual Dosage Oral:

Children: 275-420 mg/kg/day in 3-4 equally divided doses

Adults: 150 mg/kg/day in 2-3 equally divided doses (usually 14-16 g/day)

Dosing adjustment in renal impairment:

Cl_{cr} 10-50 mL/minute: Administer 50% to 75% of dose

Cl_{cr} <10 mL/minute: Administer 50% of dose

Administer after hemodialysis CAPD/CAVHD: Dose for Cl_{cr} <10 mL/minute

Administration Administer with food or meals

Patient Information Notify physician if persistent sore throat, fever, unusual bleeding or bruising, persistent nausea, vomiting, or abdominal pain occurs; do not stop taking before consulting your physician; take with food or meals; do not use products that are brown or purple; store in a cool, dry place away from sunlight

Nursing Implications Do not administer if discolored

Dosage Forms Tablet: 500 mg

5-Aminosalicylic Acid *see* Mesalamine *on page 787*

Amiodarone (a MEE oh da rone)

Related Information

Antiarrhythmic Drugs *on page 1389*

Comparative Pharmacokinetic Properties of Antiarrhythmic Agents *on page 1391*

Brand Names Cordarone®

Canadian/Mexican Brand Names Braxan® (Mexico); Cardiorona® (Mexico)

Synonyms Amiodarone Hydrochloride

Therapeutic Category Antiarrhythmic Agent, Class III

Use

Oral: Management of life-threatening recurrent ventricular fibrillation (VF) or hemodynamically unstable ventricular tachycardia (VT)

I.V.: Initiation of treatment and prophylaxis of frequency recurring VF and unstable VT in patients refractory to other therapy. Also, for patients for whom oral amiodarone is indicated but who are unable to take oral medication.

Pregnancy Risk Factor D

Contraindications Hypersensitivity to amiodarone; severe sinus node dysfunction, second and third degree A-V block, marked sinus bradycardia except if pacemaker is placed, thyroid disease, pregnancy and lactation

Warnings/Precautions Not considered first-line antiarrhythmic due to high incidence of significant and potentially fatal toxicity (ie, hypersensitivity pneumonitis or interstitial/alveolar pneumonitis, hepatic failure, heart block, bradycardia or exacerbated arrhythmias), especially with large doses; reserve for use in arrhythmias refractory to other therapy; hospitalize patients while loading dose is administered; use cautiously in elderly due to predisposition to toxicity; due to an extensive tissue distribution and prolonged elimination period, the time at which a life-threatening arrhythmia will recur following discontinued therapy or an interaction with subsequent treatment may occur is unpredictable; patients must be observed carefully and extreme caution taken when other antiarrhythmic agents are substituted after discontinuation of amiodarone

Adverse Reactions With large dosages (≥400 mg/day), adverse reactions occur in ~75% patients and require discontinuance in 5% to 20%

>10%:

Cardiovascular: Hypotension (especially with I.V. form)

Central nervous system: Ataxia, fatigue, malaise, dizziness, headache, insomnia, nightmares

Dermatologic: Photosensitivity

Gastrointestinal: Nausea, vomiting

Neuromuscular & skeletal: Tremor, paresthesias, muscle weakness

Respiratory: Pulmonary fibrosis (cough, fever, dyspnea, malaise), interstitial pneumonitis

Miscellaneous: Alveolitis

1% to 10%:

Cardiovascular: Congestive heart failure, cardiac arrhythmias (atropine-resistant bradycardia, heart block, sinus arrest, paroxysmal ventricular tachycardia), myocardial depression, flushing, edema

Central nervous system: Fever

Endocrine & metabolic: Hypothyroidism or hyperthyroidism (less common), decreased libido

Gastrointestinal: Constipation, anorexia, abdominal pain, abnormal salivation, abnormal taste (oral form)

Hematologic: Coagulation abnormalities

Hepatic: Abnormal liver function tests

Local: Phlebitis with concentrations >3 mg/mL

Ocular: Visual disturbances

Miscellaneous: Abnormal smell (oral form)

<1%:

Cardiovascular: Hypotension (with oral form), vasculitis, atrial fibrillation, increased Q-T interval, ventricular fibrillation

Central nervous system: Pseudotumor cerebri

Dermatologic: Rash, alopecia, discoloration of skin (slate blue), Stevens-Johnson syndrome

(Continued)

Amiodarone *(Continued)*

Endocrine & metabolic: Hyperglycemia, hypertriglyceridemia
Genitourinary: Epididymitis
Hematologic: Thrombocytopenia
Hepatic: Cirrhosis, severe hepatic toxicity (potentially fatal hepatitis), increased ALT and AST
Ocular: Optic neuritis, corneal microdeposits, photophobia

Overdosage/Toxicology Symptoms include extensions of pharmacologic effect, sinus bradycardia and/or heart block, hypotension and Q-T prolongation

Patients should be monitored for several days following ingestion. Intoxication with amiodarone necessitates EKG monitoring; bradycardia may be atropine resistant; injectable isoproterenol or a temporary pacemaker may be required.

Drug Interactions Cytochrome P-450 3A enzyme inhibitor

Amiodarone appears to interfere with the hepatic metabolism of several drugs resulting in significantly increased plasma concentrations; see table.

Amiodarone Common Drug Interactions

Drug	Interaction
Anticoagulants, oral	The effects of the anticoagulant is increased due to inhibition of its metabolism
β-adrenergic receptor antagonists	β-blocker effects are enhanced by amiodarone's inhibition of the β-blocker's hepatic metabolism
Calcium channel antagonists	Additive effects of both drugs resulting in a reduction in cardiac sinus conduction, atrioventricular nodal conduction and myocardial contractility
Digoxin	Digoxin concentrations may be increased with resultant increases in activity and potential for toxicity
Flecainide	Flecainide plasma concentrations are increased
Phenytoin	Phenytoin serum concentrations are increased due to reduction in phenytoin metabolism, with possible symptoms of phenytoin toxicity
Procainamide	Procainamide serum concentrations may be increased
Quinidine	Quinidine serum concentrations may be increased and can potentially cause fatal cardiac dysrhythmias

Stability I.V. infusions >2 hours must be administered in glass or polyolefin bottles; **incompatible** with aminophylline, cefamandole, cefazolin, mezlocillin, heparin, and sodium bicarbonate; store at room temperature; protect from light

Mechanism of Action Class III antiarrhythmic agent which inhibits adrenergic stimulation, prolongs the action potential and refractory period in myocardial tissue; decreases A-V conduction and sinus node function

Pharmacodynamics/Kinetics

Onset of effect: 3 days to 3 weeks after starting therapy
Peak effect: 1 week to 5 months
Duration of effect after discontinuation of therapy: 7-50 days

Note: Mean onset of effect and duration after discontinuation may be shorter in children versus adults

Distribution: V_d: 66 L/kg (range: 18-148 L/kg); crosses placenta; distributes into breast milk in concentrations higher than maternal plasma concentrations
Protein binding: 96%
Metabolism: In liver, major metabolite active
Bioavailability: ~50%
Half-life: Oral chronic therapy: 40-55 days (range: 26-107 days); shortened in children versus adults
Elimination: Via biliary excretion; possible enterohepatic recirculation; <1% excreted unchanged in urine

Usual Dosage

Oral:

Children (calculate doses for children <1 year on body surface area):

Loading dose: 10-15 mg/kg/day or 600-800 mg/1.73 m^2/day for 4-14 days or until adequate control of arrhythmia or prominent adverse effects occur (this loading dose may be given in 1-2 divided doses/day); dosage should then be reduced to 5 mg/kg/day or 200-400 mg/1.73 m^2/day given once daily for several weeks; if arrhythmia does not recur, reduce to lowest effective dosage possible; usual daily minimal dose: 2.5 mg/kg/day; maintenance doses may be given for 5 of 7 days/week

Adults: Ventricular arrhythmias: 800-1600 mg/day in 1-2 doses for 1-3 weeks, then 600-800 mg/day in 1-2 doses for 1 month; maintenance: 400 mg/day; lower doses are recommended for supraventricular arrhythmias

I.V.:

First 24 hours: 1000 mg according to following regimen

Step 1: 150 mg (10 mL) over first 10 minutes (mix 3 mL in 100 mL D_5W)

Step 2: 360 mg (200 mL) over next 6 hours (mix 18 mL in 500 mL D_5W)

Step 3: 540 mg (300 mL) over next 18 hours

After the first 24 hours: 0.5 mg/minute utilizing concentration of 1-6 mg/mL

Breakthrough VF or VT: 150 mg supplemental doses in 100 mL D_5W over 10 minutes

Note: When switching from I.V. to oral therapy, use the following as a guide:

<1-week I.V. infusion → 800-1600 mg/day

1- to 3-week I.V. infusion → 600-800 mg/day

>3-week I.V. infusion → 400 mg

Dosing adjustment in hepatic impairment: Probably necessary in substantial hepatic impairment

Dialysis: Not removed by hemodialysis or peritoneal dialysis (0% to 5%); no supplemental doses required

Administration Administer with food

Monitoring Parameters Monitor heart rate (EKG) and rhythm throughout therapy; assess patient for signs of thyroid dysfunction (thyroid function tests and liver enzymes), lethargy, edema of the hands, feet, weight loss, and pulmonary toxicity (baseline pulmonary function tests)

Reference Range Therapeutic: 0.5-2.5 mg/L (SI: 1-4 µmol/L) (parent); desethyl metabolite is active and is present in equal concentration to parent drug

Test Interactions Thyroid function tests: Amiodarone partially inhibits the peripheral conversion of thyroxine (T_4) to triiodothyronine (T_3); serum T_4 and reverse triiodothyronine (RT_3) concentrations may be increased and serum T_3 may be decreased; most patients remain clinically euthyroid, however, clinical hypothyroidism or hyperthyroidism may occur

Patient Information Take with food; use sunscreen or stay out of sun to prevent burns; skin discoloration is reversible; photophobia may make sunglasses necessary; do not discontinue abruptly; regular blood work for thyroid functions tests and ophthalmologic exams are necessary; notify physician if persistent dry cough or shortness of breath occurs

Nursing Implications Muscle weakness may present a great hazard for ambulation

Dosage Forms

Injection, as hydrochloride: 50 mg/mL with benzyl alcohol (3 mL)

Tablet, scored, as hydrochloride: 200 mg

Extemporaneous Preparations A 5 mg/mL oral suspension has been made from tablets and has an expected stability of 7 days under refrigeration; three 200 mg tablets are crushed in a mortar, 90 mL of methylcellulose 1%, and 10 mL of syrup (syrup NF (85% sucrose in water) or flavored syrup) are added in small amounts and triturated until uniform; purified water USP is used to make a quantity sufficient to 120 mL

Nahata MC and Hipple TF, *Pediatric Drug Formulations*, 2nd ed, Cincinnati, OH: Harvey Whitney Books Co, 1992.

Amiodarone Hydrochloride *see* Amiodarone *on page 67*

Amitone® [OTC] *see* Calcium Carbonate *on page 185*

Amitriptyline (a mee TRIP ti leen)

Related Information

Antidepressant Agents Comparison *on page 1393*

Brand Names Elavil®; Endep®; Enovil®

Canadian/Mexican Brand Names Apo-Amitriptyline® (Canada); Levate® (Canada); Novo-Tryptin® (Canada); Anapsique® (Mexico); Tryptanol® (Mexico)

Synonyms Amitriptyline Hydrochloride

Therapeutic Category Antidepressant, Tricyclic

Use Treatment of various forms of depression, often in conjunction with psychotherapy; analgesic for certain chronic and neuropathic pain, prophylaxis against migraine headaches

Pregnancy Risk Factor D

Contraindications Hypersensitivity to amitriptyline (cross-sensitivity with other tricyclics may occur); patients receiving MAO inhibitors within past 14 days; narrow-angle glaucoma; avoid use during pregnancy and lactation

Warnings/Precautions

Amitriptyline should not be abruptly discontinued in patients receiving high doses for prolonged periods

(Continued)

Amitriptyline *(Continued)*

Use with caution in patients with cardiac conduction disturbances; an EKG prior to initiation of therapy is advised; use with caution in patients with a history of hyperthyroidism, renal or hepatic impairment

The most anticholinergic and sedating of the antidepressants; pronounced effects on the cardiovascular system (hypotension), hence, many psychiatrists agree it is best to avoid in the elderly

Adverse Reactions Anticholinergic effects may be pronounced; moderate to marked sedation can occur (tolerance to these effects usually occurs)

>10%:

Central nervous system: Dizziness, drowsiness, headache

Gastrointestinal: Xerostomia, constipation, increased appetite, nausea, unpleasant taste, weight gain

Neuromuscular & skeletal: Weakness

1% to 10%:

Cardiovascular: Hypotension, postural hypotension, arrhythmias, tachycardia, sudden death

Central nervous system: Nervousness, restlessness, parkinsonian syndrome, insomnia, sedation, fatigue, anxiety, impaired cognitive function, seizures have occurred occasionally, extrapyramidal symptoms are possible

Gastrointestinal: Diarrhea, heartburn

Genitourinary: Sexual dysfunction, urinary retention

Neuromuscular & skeletal: Tremor

Ocular: Eye pain, blurred vision

Miscellaneous: Diaphoresis (excessive)

<1%:

Dermatologic: Alopecia, photosensitivity

Endocrine & metabolic: Breast enlargement, galactorrhea, rarely SIADH

Gastrointestinal: Trouble with gums, decreased lower esophageal sphincter tone may cause GE reflux

Genitourinary: Testicular edema

Hematologic: Leukopenia, eosinophilia, rarely agranulocytosis

Hepatic: Cholestatic jaundice, increased liver enzymes

Ocular: Increased intraocular pressure

Otic: Tinnitus

Miscellaneous: Allergic reactions

Overdosage/Toxicology Symptoms of overdose include agitation, confusion, hallucinations, urinary retention, hypothermia, hypotension, ventricular tachycardia, seizures

Following initiation of essential overdose management, toxic symptoms should be treated. Sodium bicarbonate is indicated when QRS interval is >0.10 seconds or QT_c >0.42 seconds. Ventricular arrhythmias often respond to phenytoin 15-20 mg/kg (adults) with concurrent systemic alkalinization (sodium bicarbonate 0.5-2 mEq/kg I.V.). Arrhythmias unresponsive to this therapy may respond to lidocaine 1 mg/kg I.V. followed by a titrated infusion. Physostigmine (1-2 mg I.V. slowly for adults or 0.5 mg I.V. slowly for children) may be indicated in reversing cardiac arrhythmias that are due to vagal blockade or for anticholinergic effects, but should only be used as a last measure in life-threatening situations. Seizures usually respond to diazepam I.V. boluses (5-10 mg for adults up to 30 mg or 0.25-0.4 mg/kg/dose for children up to 10 mg/dose). If seizures are unresponsive or recur, phenytoin or phenobarbital may be required.

Drug Interactions Cytochrome P-450 1A2 enzyme substrate and cytochrome P-450 2D6 enzyme substrate

Decreased effect: Phenobarbital may increase the metabolism of amitriptyline; amitriptyline blocks the uptake of guanethidine and thus prevents the hypotensive effect of guanethidine

Increased toxicity: Clonidine → hypertensive crisis; amitriptyline may be additive with or may potentiate the action of other CNS depressants such as sedatives or hypnotics; with MAO inhibitors, hyperpyrexia, hypertension, tachycardia, confusion, seizures, and **deaths have been reported**; amitriptyline may increase the prothrombin time in patients stabilized on warfarin; amitriptyline potentiates the pressor and cardiac effects of sympathomimetic agents such as isoproterenol, epinephrine, etc; cimetidine and methylphenidate may decrease the metabolism of amitriptyline; additive anticholinergic effects seen with other anticholinergic agents

Stability Protect injection and Elavil® 10 mg tablets from light

Mechanism of Action Increases the synaptic concentration of serotonin and/or norepinephrine in the central nervous system by inhibition of their reuptake by the presynaptic neuronal membrane

Pharmacodynamics/Kinetics

Onset of therapeutic effect: 7-21 days

Desired therapeutic effect (for depression) may take as long as 3-4 weeks, at that point dosage should be reduced to lowest effective level

When used for migraine headache prophylaxis, therapeutic effect may take as long as 6 weeks; a higher dosage may be required in a heavy smoker, because of increased metabolism

Distribution: Crosses placenta; enters breast milk

Metabolism: In the liver to nortriptyline (active), hydroxy derivatives, and conjugated derivatives; metabolism may be impaired in the elderly

Half-life: Adults: 9-25 hours (15-hour average)

Time to peak serum concentration: Within 4 hours

Elimination: Renal excretion of 18% as unchanged drug; small amounts eliminated in feces by bile

Usual Dosage

Children: Pain management: Oral: Initial: 0.1 mg/kg at bedtime, may advance as tolerated over 2-3 weeks to 0.5-2 mg/day at bedtime

Adolescents: Oral: Initial: 25-50 mg/day; may administer in divided doses; increase gradually to 100 mg/day in divided doses

Adults:

Oral: 30-100 mg/day single dose at bedtime or in divided doses; dose may be gradually increased up to 300 mg/day; once symptoms are controlled, decrease gradually to lowest effective dose

I.M.: 20-30 mg 4 times/day

Dosing interval in hepatic impairment: Use with caution and monitor plasma levels and patient response

Hemodialysis: Nondialyzable

Dietary Considerations Alcohol: Additive CNS effects, avoid use

Monitoring Parameters Monitor blood pressure and pulse rate prior to and during initial therapy; evaluate mental status; monitor weight

Reference Range Therapeutic: Amitriptyline and nortriptyline 100-250 ng/mL (SI: 360-900 nmol/L); nortriptyline 50-150 ng/mL (SI: 190-570 nmol/L); Toxic: >0.5 µg/mL; plasma levels do not always correlate with clinical effectiveness

Test Interactions ↑ glucose

Patient Information Avoid alcohol ingestion; do not discontinue medication abruptly; may cause urine to turn blue-green; may cause drowsiness; full effect may not occur for 3-6 weeks; dry mouth may be helped by sips of water, sugarless gum, or hard candy

Nursing Implications May increase appetite and possibly a craving for sweets

Dosage Forms

Injection, as hydrochloride: 10 mg/mL (10 mL)

Tablet, as hydrochloride: 10 mg, 25 mg, 50 mg, 75 mg, 100 mg, 150 mg

Amitriptyline Hydrochloride *see* Amitriptyline *on page 69*

Amlexanox (am LEKS an oks)

Brand Names Aphthasol®

Therapeutic Category Anti-inflammatory Agent, Locally Applied

Use Treatment of aphthous ulcers (ie, canker sores); has been investigated in many allergic disorders

Pregnancy Risk Factor B

Pregnancy/Breast-Feeding Implications Due to lack of data, avoid use in pregnancy or lactation, if possible

Contraindications Hypersensitivity to amlexanox or components

Warnings/Precautions Discontinue therapy if rash or contact mucositis develops

Adverse Reactions

>1%:

Dermatologic: Allergic contact dermatitis

Gastrointestinal: Oral irritation

<1%: Gastrointestinal: Contact mucositis

Mechanism of Action As a benzopyrano-bipyridine carboxylic acid derivative, amlexanox has anti-inflammatory and antiallergic properties; it inhibits chemical mediatory release of the slow-reacting substance of anaphylaxis (SRS-A) and may have antagonistic effect son interleukin-3

Pharmacodynamics/Kinetics

Absorption: Systemic absorption with swallowing of topical application of oral paste

Metabolism: Metabolized to hydroxylated and conjugated product

Half-life: 3.5 hours

Time to peak serum concentration: 2 hours

Elimination: 17% excreted unchanged

Usual Dosage Administer (0.5 cm - 1/4") directly on ulcers 4 times/day following oral hygiene, after meals, and at bedtime

(Continued)

Amlexanox *(Continued)*

Dosage Forms Paste: 5% (5 g)

Amlodipine (am LOE di peen)

Related Information

Calcium Channel Blockers Comparative Actions *on page 1401*
Calcium Channel Blockers Comparative Pharmacokinetics *on page 1402*
Calcium Channel Blockers FDA-Approved Indications *on page 1403*

Brand Names Norvasc®

Canadian/Mexican Brand Names Norvas® (Mexico)

Therapeutic Category Antihypertensive; Calcium Channel Blocker

Use Treatment of hypertension and angina

Pregnancy Risk Factor C

Pregnancy/Breast-Feeding Implications Teratogenic and embryotoxic effects have been demonstrated in small animals. No well controlled studies have been conducted in pregnant women. Use in pregnancy only when clearly needed and when the benefits outweigh the potential hazard to the fetus.

Clinical effects on the fetus: No data on crossing the placenta
Breast-feeding/lactation: No data on crossing into breast milk

Contraindications Hypersensitivity

Warnings/Precautions Use with caution and titrate dosages for patients with impaired renal or hepatic function; use caution when treating patients with congestive heart failure, sick-sinus syndrome, severe left ventricular dysfunction, hypertrophic cardiomyopathy (especially obstructive), concomitant therapy with beta-blockers or digoxin, edema, or increased intracranial pressure with cranial tumors; do not abruptly withdraw (may cause chest pain); elderly may experience hypotension and constipation more readily.

Adverse Reactions

>10%: Cardiovascular: Peripheral edema

1% to 10%:
- Cardiovascular: Edema, flushing, palpitations
- Central nervous system: Headache, fatigue, dizziness, somnolence
- Dermatologic: Dermatitis, rash
- Endocrine & metabolic: Sexual dysfunction
- Gastrointestinal: Nausea, abdominal pain
- Respiratory: Shortness of breath
- Neuromuscular & skeletal: Muscle cramps

<1%:
- Cardiovascular: Hypotension, bradycardia, arrhythmias, abnormal EKG, ventricular extrasystoles
- Dermatologic: Alopecia, petechiae
- Gastrointestinal: Weight gain, anorexia
- Neuromuscular & skeletal: Joint stiffness
- Respiratory: Nasal congestion, cough, epistaxis
- Miscellaneous: Diaphoresis

Overdosage/Toxicology The primary cardiac symptoms of calcium blocker overdose includes hypotension and bradycardia. The hypotension is caused by peripheral vasodilation, myocardial depression, and bradycardia. Bradycardia results from sinus bradycardia, second- or third-degree atrioventricular block, or sinus arrest with junctional rhythm. Intraventricular conduction is usually not affected so QRS duration is normal (verapamil does prolong the P-R interval and bepridil prolongs the Q-T and may cause ventricular arrhythmias, including torsade de pointes).

The noncardiac symptoms include confusion, stupor, nausea, vomiting, metabolic acidosis, and hyperglycemia. Following initial gastric decontamination, if possible, repeated calcium administration may promptly reverse the depressed cardiac contractility (but not sinus node depression or peripheral vasodilation); glucagon, epinephrine, and amrinone may treat refractory hypotension; glucagon and epinephrine also increase the heart rate (outside the U.S., 4-aminopyridine may be available as an antidote); dialysis and hemoperfusion are not effective in enhancing elimination although repeat-dose activated charcoal may serve as an adjunct with sustained-release preparations.

Drug Interactions Hepatic enzyme inhibitor

Increased effect:
- Amlodipine and benazepril may increase hypotensive effect
- Amlodipine and cyclosporine may increase cyclosporine levels

Mechanism of Action Inhibits calcium ion from entering the "slow channels" or select voltage-sensitive areas of vascular smooth muscle and myocardium during depolarization, producing a relaxation of coronary vascular smooth muscle and coronary vasodilation; increases myocardial oxygen delivery in patients with vasospastic angina

Pharmacodynamics/Kinetics

Onset of action: 30-50 minutes

Peak effect: 6-12 hours

Duration: 24 hours

Absorption: Oral: Well absorbed

Protein binding: 93%

Metabolism: Hepatic, >90% to inactive compound

Bioavailability: 64% to 90%

Half-life: 30-50 hours

Elimination: Metabolite and parent drug excreted renally

Usual Dosage Adults: Oral: Initial dose: 2.5-5 mg once daily; usual dose: 5-10 mg once daily; maximum dose: 10 mg once daily

Dialysis: Hemodialysis and peritoneal dialysis does not enhance elimination; supplemental dose is not necessary

Dosage adjustment in hepatic impairment: 2.5 mg once daily

Patient Information Do not discontinue abruptly; report any dizziness, shortness of breath, palpitations, or edema

Additional Information Although there is some initial data which may show increased risk of myocardial infarction following treatment of hypertension with calcium antagonists, controlled trials (eg, ALL-HAT) are ongoing to examine the long-term effects of not only calcium antagonists but other antihypertensives in preventing heart disease. Until these studies are completed, patients taking calcium antagonists should be encouraged to continue with prescribed antihypertensive regimes, although a switch from high-dose, short-acting agents to sustained release products may be warranted. It is also generally agreed that calcium antagonists should be avoided as the primary treatment for hypertension unless diuretics or beta-blockers are contraindicated and for the primary treatment of angina following acute myocardial infarction.

Dosage Forms Tablet: 2.5 mg, 5 mg, 10 mg

Ammonapse *see* Sodium Phenylbutyrate *on page 1145*

Ammonium Chloride (a MOE nee um KLOR ide)

Therapeutic Category Diuretic, Miscellaneous; Metabolic Alkalosis Agent; Urinary Acidifying Agent

Use Diuretic or systemic and urinary acidifying agent; treatment of hypochloremic states

Pregnancy Risk Factor C

Contraindications Severe hepatic and renal dysfunction; patients with primary respiratory acidosis

Warnings/Precautions Safety and efficacy not established in children, use with caution in infants

Adverse Reactions

1% to 10%:

Cardiovascular: Bradycardia

Central nervous system: Mental confusion, coma, headache

Dermatologic: Rash

Endocrine & metabolic: Metabolic acidosis secondary to hyperchloremia

Gastrointestinal: Gastric irritation, nausea, vomiting

Local: Pain at site of injection

Respiratory: Hyperventilation

Overdosage/Toxicology Symptoms of overdose include acidosis, headache, drowsiness, confusion, hyperventilation, hypokalemia

Administer sodium bicarbonate or lactate to treat acidosis; supplemental potassium for hypokalemia

Mechanism of Action Increases acidity by increasing free hydrogen ion concentration

Pharmacodynamics/Kinetics

Absorption: Rapid from GI tract, complete within 3-6 hours

Metabolism: In the liver

Elimination: In urine

Usual Dosage Metabolic alkalosis: The following equations represent different methods of correction utilizing either the serum HCO_3^-, the serum chloride, or the base excess

Dosing of mEq NH_4Cl via the chloride-deficit method (hypochloremia):

Dose of mEq NH_4Cl = [0.2 L/kg x body weight (kg)] x [103 - observed serum chloride]; administer 100% of dose over 12 hours, then re-evaluate

Note: 0.2 L/kg is the estimated chloride space and 103 is the average normal serum chloride concentration

(Continued)

Ammonium Chloride *(Continued)*

Dosing of mEq NH_4Cl via the bicarbonate-excess method (refractory hypochloremic metabolic alkalosis):

Dose of NH_4Cl = [0.5 L/kg x body weight (kg) x (observed serum HCO_3^- ~24)]; administer 50% of dose over 12 hours, then re-evaluate

Note: 0.5 L/kg is the estimated bicarbonate space and 24 is the average normal serum bicarbonate concentration

Dosing of mEq NH_4Cl via the base-excess method:

Dose of NH_4Cl = [0.3 L/kg x body weight (kg) x measured base excess (mEq/L)]; administer 50% of dose over 12 hours, then re-evaluate

Note: 0.3 L/kg is the estimated extracellular bicarbonate and base excess is measured by the chemistry lab and reported with arterial blood gases

These equations will yield different requirements of ammonium chloride

Equation #1 is inappropriate to use if the patient has severe metabolic alkalosis without hypochloremia or if the patient has uremia

Equation #3 is the most useful for the first estimation of ammonium chloride dosage

Children: Urinary acidifying agents: Oral, I.V.: 75 mg/kg/day in 4 divided doses; maximum daily dose: 6 g

Adults: Urinary acidifying agent/diuretic:

Oral: 2-3 g every 6 hours

I.V.: 1.5 g/dose every 6 hours

Administration Rapid I.V. injection may increase the likelihood of ammonia toxicity; rate should not exceed 1 mEq/kg/hour; 26.75% solution must be diluted prior to administration

Test Interactions ↑ ammonia (B); ↓ potassium (S), sodium (S)

Patient Information Take oral dose after meals

Dosage Forms

Injection: 26.75% [5 mEq/mL] (20 mL)

Tablet: 500 mg

Tablet, enteric coated: 500 mg

Amobarbital (am oh BAR bi tal)

Brand Names Amytal®

Canadian/Mexican Brand Names Amobarbital® (Canada)

Synonyms Amylobarbitone

Therapeutic Category Anticonvulsant; Barbiturate; Hypnotic; Sedative

Use

Oral: Hypnotic in short-term treatment of insomnia, to reduce anxiety and provide sedation preoperatively

I.M., I.V.: Control status epilepticus or acute seizure episodes. Also used in catatonic, negativistic, or manic reactions and in "Amytal® Interviewing" for narcoanalysis.

Restrictions C-II

Pregnancy Risk Factor D

Contraindications Marked liver function impairment or latent porphyria; hypersensitivity to barbiturates; do not administer in presence of chronic or acute pain

Warnings/Precautions Safety has not been established in children <6 years of age; potential for drug dependency exists; avoid alcoholic beverages; use with caution in patients with CHF, hepatic or renal impairment, hypovolemic shock; when administered I.V., respiratory depression and hypotension are possible, have equipment and personnel available; this I.V. medication should be given only to hospitalized patients

Adverse Reactions

>10%:

Central nervous system: Dizziness, lightheadedness, "hangover" effect, drowsiness, CNS depression, fever

Local: Pain at injection site

1% to 10%:

Central nervous system: Confusion, mental depression, unusual excitement, nervousness, faint feeling, headache, insomnia, nightmares

Gastrointestinal: Nausea, vomiting, constipation

<1%:

Cardiovascular: Hypotension

Central nervous system: Hallucinations

Dermatologic: Rash, exfoliative dermatitis, urticaria, Stevens-Johnson syndrome

Hematologic: Agranulocytosis, megaloblastic anemia, thrombocytopenia

Local: Thrombophlebitis

Respiratory: Respiratory depression, apnea, laryngospasm

Overdosage/Toxicology Symptoms of overdose include unsteady gait, slurred speech, confusion, jaundice, hypothermia, fever, hypotension

If hypotension occurs, administer I.V. fluids and place the patient in the Trendelenburg position. If unresponsive, an I.V. vasopressor (eg, dopamine, epinephrine) may be required. Forced alkaline diuresis is of no value in the treatment of intoxications with short-acting barbiturates. Charcoal hemoperfusion or hemodialysis may be useful in the harder to treat intoxications, especially in the presence of very high serum barbiturate levels.

Drug Interactions

Decreased effect: Cimetidine's tricyclic antidepressants and doxycycline's efficacy may be reduced with amobarbital

Increased toxicity when combined with other CNS depressants or antidepressants, respiratory and CNS depression may be additive

Stability Hydrolyzes when exposed to air; use contents of vial within 30 minutes after constitution; use only clear solution

Mechanism of Action Interferes with transmission of impulses from the thalamus to the cortex of the brain resulting in an imbalance in central inhibitory and facilitatory mechanisms

Pharmacodynamics/Kinetics

Onset of action:
- Oral: Within 1 hour
- I.V.: Within 5 minutes

Distribution: Readily crosses the placenta; small amounts appear in breast milk

Metabolism: Chiefly in the liver by microsomal enzymes

Half-life, biphasic:
- Initial: 40 minutes
- Terminal: 20 hours

Usual Dosage

Children: Oral:
- Sedation: 6 mg/kg/day divided every 6-8 hours
- Insomnia: 2 mg/kg or 70 mg/m^2/day in 4 equally divided doses
- Hypnotic: 2-3 mg/kg

Adults:
- Insomnia: Oral: 65-200 mg at bedtime
- Sedation: Oral: 30-50 mg 2-3 times/day
- Preanesthetic: Oral: 200 mg 1-2 hours before surgery
- Hypnotic:
  - Oral: 65-200 mg at bedtime
  - I.M., I.V.: 65-500 mg, should not exceed 500 mg I.M. or 1000 mg I.V.

Dietary Considerations Alcohol: Avoid use

Administration I.M. injection should be deep to prevent against pain, sterile abscess, and sloughing

Monitoring Parameters Vital signs should be monitored during injection and for several hours after administration

Reference Range

Therapeutic: 1-5 μg/mL (SI: 4-22 μmol/L)

Toxic: >10 μg/mL (SI: >44 μmol/L)

Lethal: >50 μg/mL

Test Interactions ↑ ammonia (B); ↓ bilirubin (S)

Patient Information Avoid alcohol ingestion; physical dependency may result when used for an extended period of time (1-3 months); do not try to get out of bed without assistance, will cause drowsiness

Nursing Implications Raise bed rails at night

Dosage Forms

Capsule, as sodium: 65 mg, 200 mg

Injection, as sodium: 250 mg, 500 mg

Tablet: 30 mg, 50 mg, 100 mg

AMO Vitrax® *see* Sodium Hyaluronate *on page 1144*

Amoxapine (a MOKS a peen)

Related Information

Antidepressant Agents Comparison *on page 1393*

Brand Names Asendin®

Canadian/Mexican Brand Names Demolox® (Mexico)

Therapeutic Category Antidepressant, Tricyclic

Use Treatment of neurotic and endogenous depression and mixed symptoms of anxiety and depression

Pregnancy Risk Factor C

Contraindications Hypersensitivity to amoxapine; cross-sensitivity with other tricyclics may occur; narrow-angle glaucoma; patients receiving MAO inhibitors within past 14 days

(Continued)

Amoxapine *(Continued)*

Warnings/Precautions Use with caution in patients with seizures, cardiac conduction disturbances, cardiovascular diseases, urinary retention, hyperthyroidism, or those receiving thyroid replacement; do not discontinue abruptly in patients receiving high doses chronically; tolerance develops in 1-3 months in some patients, close medical follow-up is essential

Adverse Reactions

>10%:

- Central nervous system: Drowsiness
- Gastrointestinal: Xerostomia, constipation, nausea, unpleasant taste, weight gain

1% to 10%:

- Central nervous system: Dizziness, headache, confusion, nervousness, restlessness, insomnia, ataxia, excitement
- Dermatologic: Edema, skin rash
- Endocrine: Elevated prolactin levels
- Gastrointestinal: Increased appetite
- Neuromuscular & skeletal: Tremor, weakness
- Ocular: Blurred vision
- Miscellaneous: Diaphoresis

<1%:

- Cardiovascular: Hypotension, tachycardia, pallor
- Central nervous system: Anxiety, seizures, neuroleptic malignant syndrome, tardive dyskinesia
- Dermatologic: Photosensitivity
- Endocrine & metabolic: Breast enlargement, galactorrhea, SIADH, increased or decreased libido, impotence, menstrual irregularity, painful ejaculation
- Gastrointestinal: Epigastric distress, vomiting, flatulence, abdominal pain, abnormal taste, diarrhea
- Genitourinary: Testicular edema, urinary retention
- Hematologic: Agranulocytosis, leukopenia
- Hepatic: Elevated liver enzymes
- Neuromuscular & skeletal: Paresthesia
- Ocular: Increased intraocular pressure, mydriasis, lacrimation
- Otic: Tinnitus
- Miscellaneous: Allergic reactions

Overdosage/Toxicology Symptoms of overdose include grand mal convulsions, acidosis, coma, renal failure

Following initiation of essential overdose management, toxic symptoms should be treated. Sodium bicarbonate is indicated when QRS interval is >0.10 seconds or QT_c >0.42 seconds. Ventricular arrhythmias often respond to phenytoin 15-20 mg/kg (adults) with concurrent systemic alkalinization (sodium bicarbonate 0.5-2 mEq/kg I.V.). Arrhythmias unresponsive to this therapy may respond to lidocaine 1 mg/kg I.V. followed by a titrated infusion. Physostigmine (1-2 mg I.V. slowly for adults or 0.5 mg I.V. slowly for children) may be indicated in reversing cardiac arrhythmias that are due to vagal blockade or for anticholinergic effects, but should only be used as a last measure in life-threatening situations. Seizures usually respond to diazepam I.V. boluses (5-10 mg for adults up to 30 mg or 0.25-0.4 mg/kg/dose for children up to 10 mg/dose). If seizures are unresponsive or recur, phenytoin or phenobarbital may be required.

Drug Interactions

- Decreased effect of clonidine, guanethidine
- Increased effect of CNS depressants, adrenergic agents, anticholinergic agents
- Increased toxicity of MAO inhibitors (hyperpyrexia, tachycardia, hypertension, seizures and death may occur); similar interactions as with other tricyclics may occur

Mechanism of Action Reduces the reuptake of serotonin and norepinephrine and blocks the response of dopamine receptors to dopamine

Pharmacodynamics/Kinetics

- Onset of antidepressant effect: Usually occurs after 1-2 weeks
- Absorption: Oral: Rapidly and well absorbed
- Distribution: V_d: 0.9-1.2 L/kg; distributes into breast milk
- Protein binding: 80%
- Metabolism: Extensive in the liver
- Half-life:
  - Parent drug: 11-16 hours
  - Active metabolite (8-hydroxy): Adults: 30 hours
- Time to peak serum concentration: Within 1-2 hours
- Elimination: Excretion of metabolites and parent compound in urine

Usual Dosage Once symptoms are controlled, decrease gradually to lowest effective dose. Maintenance dose is usually given at bedtime to reduce daytime sedation. Oral:

Children: Not established in children <16 years of age
Adolescents: Initial: 25-50 mg/day; increase gradually to 100 mg/day; may administer as divided doses or as a single dose at bedtime
Adults: Initial: 25 mg 2-3 times/day, if tolerated, dosage may be increased to 100 mg 2-3 times/day; may be given in a single bedtime dose when dosage <300 mg/day
Elderly: Initial: 25 mg at bedtime increased by 25 mg weekly for outpatients and every 3 days for inpatients if tolerated; usual dose: 50-150 mg/day, but doses up to 300 mg may be necessary

Maximum daily dose:
Inpatient: 600 mg
Outpatient: 400 mg

Dietary Considerations Alcohol: Avoid use

Monitoring Parameters Monitor blood pressure and pulse rate prior to and during initial therapy evaluate mental status; monitor weight

Reference Range Therapeutic: Amoxapine: 20-100 ng/mL (SI: 64-319 nmol/L); 8-OH amoxapine: 150-400 ng/mL (SI: 478-1275 nmol/L); both: 200-500 ng/mL (SI: 637-1594 nmol/L)

Test Interactions ↑ glucose

Patient Information Dry mouth may be helped by sips of water, sugarless gum, or hard candy; avoid alcohol; very important to maintain established dosage regimen; photosensitivity to sunlight can occur, do not discontinue abruptly; full effect may not occur for 3-4 weeks; full dosage may be taken at bedtime to avoid daytime sedation

Nursing Implications May increase appetite and possibly a craving for sweets; recognize signs of neuroleptic malignant syndrome and tardive dyskinesia

Dosage Forms Tablet: 25 mg, 50 mg, 100 mg, 150 mg

Amoxicillin (a moks i SIL in)

Related Information

Animal and Human Bites Guidelines *on page 1463*
Antimicrobial Drugs of Choice *on page 1468*
Helicobacter pylori Treatment *on page 1534*
Prevention of Bacterial Endocarditis *on page 1449*
Treatment of Sexually Transmitted Diseases *on page 1485*

Brand Names Amoxil®; Biomox®; Polymox®; Trimox®; Wymox®

Canadian/Mexican Brand Names Apo-Amoxi® (Canada); Novamoxin® (Canada); Nu-Amoxi® (Canada); Pro-Amox® (Canada); Acimox® (Mexico); Amoxifur® (Mexico); Amoxisol® (Mexico); Amoxivet® (Mexico); Gimalxina® (Mexico); Grunicina® (Mexico); Hidramox® (Mexico)

Synonyms Amoxycillin; *p*-Hydroxyampicillin

Therapeutic Category Antibiotic, Penicillin

Use Treatment of otitis media, sinusitis, and infections caused by susceptible organisms involving the respiratory tract, skin, and urinary tract; prophylaxis of bacterial endocarditis

Pregnancy Risk Factor B

Contraindications Hypersensitivity to amoxicillin, penicillin, or any component

Warnings/Precautions In patients with renal impairment, doses and/or frequency of administration should be modified in response to the degree of renal impairment; a high percentage of patients with infectious mononucleosis have developed rash during therapy with amoxicillin; a low incidence of cross-allergy with other beta-lactams and cephalosporins exists

Adverse Reactions

1% to 10%:
Central nervous system: Fever
Dermatologic: Urticaria
Miscellaneous: Allergic reactions

<1%:
Central nervous system: Seizures, anxiety, confusion, hallucinations, depression
Gastrointestinal: Nausea, vomiting
Hematologic: Leukopenia, neutropenia, thrombocytopenia
Hepatic: Jaundice

Overdosage/Toxicology Symptoms of penicillin overdose include neuromuscular hypersensitivity (agitation, hallucinations, asterixis, encephalopathy, confusion, and seizures) and electrolyte imbalance with potassium or sodium salts, especially in renal failure

Hemodialysis may be helpful to aid in the removal of the drug from the blood, otherwise most treatment is supportive or symptom directed

Drug Interactions

Decreased effect: Efficacy of oral contraceptives may be reduced
Increased effect: Disulfiram, probenecid may increase amoxicillin levels
(Continued)

Amoxicillin *(Continued)*

Increased toxicity: Allopurinol theoretically has an additive potential for amoxicillin rash

Stability Oral suspension remains stable for 7 days at room temperature or 14 days if refrigerated; unit dose antibiotic oral syringes are stable for 48 hours

Mechanism of Action Interferes with bacterial cell wall synthesis during active multiplication, causing cell wall death and resultant bactericidal activity against susceptible bacteria

Pharmacodynamics/Kinetics

Absorption: Oral: Rapid and nearly complete; food does not interfere

Protein binding: 17% to 20%

Ratio of CSF to blood:

Normal meninges: <1%

Inflamed meninges: 8% to 90%

Metabolism: Partial; renal excretion (80% as unchanged drug); lower in neonates

Half-life:

Neonates, full-term: 3.7 hours

Infants and Children: 1-2 hours

Adults with normal renal function: 0.7-1.4 hours

Patients with Cl_{cr} <10 mL/minute: 7-21 hours

Time to peak: 2 hours (capsule) and 1 hour (suspension)

Elimination: Renal excretion (80% as unchanged drug); lower in neonates

Usual Dosage Oral:

Children: 20-50 mg/kg/day in divided doses every 8 hours

Uncomplicated gonorrhea: ≥2 years: 50 mg/kg plus probenecid 25 mg/kg in a single dose; do not use this regimen in children <2 years of age, probenecid is contraindicated in this age group

Subacute bacterial endocarditis prophylaxis: 50 mg/kg 1 hour before procedure and 25 mg/kg 6 hours later

Adults: 250-500 mg every 8 hours; maximum dose: 2-3 g/day

Uncomplicated gonorrhea: 3 g plus probenecid 1 g in a single dose

Endocarditis prophylaxis: 3 g 1 hour before procedure and 1.5 g 6 hours later

Helicobacter pylori: Clinically effective treatment regimens include triple therapy with amoxicillin or tetracycline, metronidazole, and bismuth subsalicylate; amoxicillin, metronidazole, and an H_2-receptor antagonist. Adult dose: Oral: 250-500 mg 3 times/day

Dosing interval in renal impairment:

Cl_{cr} 10-50 mL/minute: Administer every 12 hours

Cl_{cr} <10 mL/minute: Administer every 24 hours

Dialysis: Moderately dialyzable (20% to 50%) by hemo- or peritoneal dialysis; approximately 50 mg of amoxicillin per liter of filtrate is removed by continuous arterio-venous or veno-venous hemofiltration (CAVH); dose as per Cl_{cr} <10 mL/minute guidelines

Dietary Considerations Food: May be taken with food

Administration Administer around-the-clock rather than 3 times/day to promote less variation in peak and trough serum levels

Monitoring Parameters With prolonged therapy, monitor renal, hepatic, and hematologic function periodically; assess patient at beginning and throughout therapy for infection

Test Interactions ↑ AST, ALT, protein

Patient Information Report diarrhea promptly; entire course of medication (10-14 days) should be taken to ensure eradication of organism; should be taken in equal intervals around-the-clock to maintain adequate blood levels; may interfere with oral contraceptives; females should report symptoms of vaginitis; pediatric drops may be placed on child's tongue or added to formula, milk, etc

Nursing Implications Obtain specimens for culture and sensitivity before the first dose

Dosage Forms

Capsule: 250 mg, 500 mg

Powder for oral suspension: 125 mg/5 mL (5 mL, 80 mL, 100 mL, 150 mL, 200 mL); 250 mg/5 mL (5 mL, 80 mL, 100 mL, 150 mL, 200 mL)

Powder for oral suspension, drops: 50 mg/mL (15 mL, 30 mL)

Tablet, chewable: 125 mg, 250 mg

Amoxicillin and Clavulanate Potassium

(a moks i SIL in & klav yoo LAN ate poe TASS ee um)

Related Information

Animal and Human Bites Guidelines *on page 1463*

Antimicrobial Drugs of Choice *on page 1468*

Brand Names Augmentin®

Canadian/Mexican Brand Names Clavulin® (Canada); Clavulin® (Mexico)

Synonyms Amoxicillin and Clavulanic Acid

Therapeutic Category Antibiotic, Penicillin

Use Treatment of otitis media, sinusitis, and infections caused by susceptible organisms involving the lower respiratory tract, skin and skin structure, and urinary tract; spectrum same as amoxicillin with additional coverage of beta-lactamase producing *B. catarrhalis*, *H. influenzae*, *N. gonorrhoeae*, and *S. aureus* (not MRSA). The expanded coverage of this combination makes it a useful alternative when amoxicillin resistance is present and patients cannot tolerate alternative treatments.

Pregnancy Risk Factor B

Contraindications Known hypersensitivity to amoxicillin, clavulanic acid, or penicillin; concomitant use of disulfiram

Warnings/Precautions In patients with renal impairment, doses and/or frequency of administration should be modified in response to the degree of renal impairment; high percentage of patients with infectious mononucleosis have developed rash during therapy; a low incidence of cross-allergy with cephalosporins exists; incidence of diarrhea is higher than with amoxicillin alone

Adverse Reactions

1% to 10%:
- Dermatologic: Rash, urticaria
- Gastrointestinal: Nausea, vomiting, diarrhea
- Genitourinary: Vaginitis

<1%:
- Central nervous system: Headache
- Gastrointestinal: Abdominal discomfort, flatulence

Overdosage/Toxicology Symptoms of penicillin overdose include neuromuscular hypersensitivity (agitation, hallucinations, asterixis, encephalopathy, confusion, and seizures) and electrolyte imbalance with potassium or sodium salts, especially in renal failure

Hemodialysis may be helpful to aid in the removal of the drug from the blood, otherwise most treatment is supportive or symptom directed

Drug Interactions

Decreased effect: Efficacy of oral contraceptives may be reduced

Increased effect: Disulfiram, probenecid may increase amoxicillin levels, increased effect of anticoagulants

Increased toxicity: Allopurinol theoretically has an additive potential for amoxicillin rash

Stability Discard unused suspension after 10 days; reconstituted oral suspension should be kept in refrigerator; unit dose antibiotic oral syringes are stable for 48 hours

Mechanism of Action Interferes with bacterial cell wall synthesis during active multiplication, causing cell wall death and resultant bactericidal activity against susceptible bacteria. Clavulanic acid binds and inhibits beta-lactamases that inactivate amoxicillin resulting in amoxicillin having an expanded spectrum of activity.

Pharmacodynamics/Kinetics Amoxicillin pharmacokinetics are not affected by clavulanic acid

Absorption: Oral: Rapid and nearly complete; food does not interfere

Protein binding: 17% to 20%

Metabolism: Partial (Clavulanic acid is hepatically metabolized)

Half-life:
- Neonates, full-term: 3.7 hours
- Infants and Children: 1-2 hours
- Adults with normal renal function: ~1 hour for both agents
- Patients with Cl_{cr} <10 mL/minute: 7-21 hours

Time to peak: 2 hours (capsule) and 1 hour (suspension)

Elimination: Amoxicillin excreted primarily (60%) unchanged and clavulanic acid is excreted 30% to 40% unchanged in the urine (lower in neonates)

Usual Dosage Oral:

Children ≤40 kg: 20-40 mg (amoxicillin)/kg/day in divided doses every 8 hours

Children >40 kg and Adults: 250-500 mg every 8 hours or 875 mg every 12 hours

Note: Augmentin® 200 suspension or chewable tablets 200 mg dosed every 12 hours is considered equivalent to Augmentin® "125" dosed every 8 hours; Augmentin® 400 suspension and chewable tablets may be similarly dosed every 12 hours and are equivalent to Augmentin® "250" every 8 hours

Dosing interval in renal impairment:
- Cl_{cr} 10-30 mL/minute: Administer every 12 hours
- Cl_{cr} <10 mL/minute: Administer every 24 hours

Hemodialysis: Moderately dialyzable (20% to 50%)
- Amoxicillin/clavulanic acid: Administer dose after dialysis

Peritoneal dialysis: Moderately dialyzable (20% to 50%)
- Amoxicillin: Administer 250 mg every 12 hours
- Clavulanic acid: Dose for Cl_{cr} <10 mL/minute

(Continued)

Amoxicillin and Clavulanate Potassium *(Continued)*

Continuous arterio-venous or veno-venous hemofiltration (CAVH) effects:
- Amoxicillin: ~50 mg of amoxicillin/L of filtrate is removed
- Clavulanic acid: Dose for Cl_{cr} <10 mL/minute

Administration Administer around-the-clock rather than twice or 3 times/day to promote less variation in peak and trough serum levels

Monitoring Parameters Assess patient at beginning and throughout therapy for infection; with prolonged therapy, monitor renal, hepatic, and hematologic function periodically

Test Interactions Urinary glucose (Benedict's solution, Clinitest®)

Patient Information Report diarrhea promptly; entire course of medication (10-14 days) should be taken to ensure eradication of organism; should be taken in equal intervals around-the-clock to maintain adequate blood levels; females should report onset of symptoms of candidal vaginitis; may interfere with the effects of oral contraceptives

Nursing Implications Two 250 mg tablets are not equivalent to a 500 mg tablet (both tablet sizes contain equivalent clavulanate); potassium content: 0.16 mEq of potassium per 31.25 mg of clavulanic acid

Dosage Forms

Suspension, oral:
- 125 (banana flavor): Amoxicillin trihydrate 125 mg and clavulanate potassium 31.25 mg per 5 mL (75 mL, 150 mL)
- 200: Amoxicillin 200 mg and clavulanate potassium 28.5 mg per 5 mL (50 mL, 75 mL, 100 mL)
- 250 (orange flavor): Amoxicillin trihydrate 250 mg and clavulanate potassium 62.5 mg per 5 mL (75 mL, 150 mL)
- 400: Amoxicillin 400 mg and clavulanate potassium 57 mg per 5 mL (50 mL, 75 mL, 100 mL)

Tablet:
- 250: Amoxicillin trihydrate 250 mg and clavulanate potassium 125 mg
- 500: Amoxicillin trihydrate 500 mg and clavulanate potassium 125 mg
- 875: Amoxicillin trihydrate 875 mg and clavulanate potassium 125 mg

Tablet, chewable:
- 125: Amoxicillin trihydrate 125 mg and clavulanate potassium 31.25 mg
- 250: Amoxicillin trihydrate 250 mg and clavulanate potassium 62.5 mg

Amoxicillin and Clavulanic Acid *see* Amoxicillin and Clavulanate Potassium *on page 78*

Amoxil® *see* Amoxicillin *on page 77*

Amoxycillin *see* Amoxicillin *on page 77*

Amphetamine (am FET a meen)

Synonyms Amphetamine Sulfate; Racemic Amphetamine Sulfate

Therapeutic Category Amphetamine; Central Nervous System Stimulant, Amphetamine

Use Treatment of narcolepsy; exogenous obesity; abnormal behavioral syndrome in children (minimal brain dysfunction); attention deficit hyperactive disorder (ADHD)

Restrictions C-II

Pregnancy Risk Factor C

Contraindications Patients with advanced arteriosclerosis, symptomatic cardiovascular disease, moderate to severe hypertension, hyperthyroidism, glaucoma, hypersensitivity, diabetes mellitus, agitated states, patients with a history of drug abuse, and during or within 14 days following MAO inhibitor therapy. Stimulant medications are contraindicated for use in children with attention deficit disorders and concomitant Tourette's syndrome or tics.

Warnings/Precautions Cardiovascular disease, nephritis, angina pectoris, hypertension, glaucoma, patients with a history of drug abuse, known hypersensitivity to amphetamine

Adverse Reactions

>10%:
- Cardiovascular: Arrhythmia
- Central nervous system: False feeling of well being, nervousness, restlessness, insomnia

1% to 10%:
- Cardiovascular: Hypertension
- Central nervous system: Mood or mental changes, dizziness, lightheadedness, headache
- Endocrine & metabolic: Changes in libido
- Gastrointestinal: Diarrhea, nausea, vomiting, stomach cramps, constipation, anorexia, weight loss, xerostomia
- Ocular: Blurred vision
- Miscellaneous: Diaphoresis (increased)

<1%:
- Cardiovascular: Chest pain
- Central nervous system: CNS stimulation (severe), Tourette's syndrome, hyperthermia, seizures, paranoia
- Dermatologic: Rash, urticaria
- Miscellaneous: Tolerance and withdrawal with prolonged use

Overdosage/Toxicology There is no specific antidote for amphetamine intoxication and the bulk of the treatment is supportive. Hyperactivity and agitation usually respond to reduced sensory input; however, with extreme agitation, haloperidol (2-5 mg I.M. for adults) may be required. Hyperthermia is best treated with external cooling measures, or when severe or unresponsive, muscle paralysis with pancuronium may be needed. Hypertension is usually transient and generally does not require treatment unless severe. For diastolic blood pressures >110 mm Hg, a nitroprusside infusion should be initiated. Seizures usually respond to diazepam IVP and/or phenytoin maintenance regimens.

Drug Interactions Increased toxicity of MAO inhibitors (hyperpyrexia, hypertension, arrhythmias, seizures, cerebral hemorrhage, and death has occurred)

Mechanism of Action The amphetamines are noncatechol sympathomimetic amines with pharmacologic actions similar to ephedrine. They require breakdown by monoamine oxidase for inactivation; produce central nervous system and respiratory stimulation, a pressor response, mydriasis, bronchodilation, and contraction of the urinary sphincter; thought to have a direct effect on both alpha- and beta-receptor sites in the peripheral system, as well as release stores of norepinephrine in adrenergic nerve terminals. The central nervous system action is thought to occur in the cerebral cortex and reticular-activating system. The anorexigenic effect is probably secondary to the CNS-stimulating effect; the site of action is probably the hypothalamic feeding center.

Usual Dosage Oral:

Narcolepsy:
- Children:
  - 6-12 years: 5 mg/day, increase by 5 mg at weekly intervals
  - >12 years: 10 mg/day, increase by 10 mg at weekly intervals
- Adults: 5-60 mg/day in 2-3 divided doses

Attention deficit disorder: Children:
- 3-5 years: 2.5 mg/day, increase by 2.5 mg at weekly intervals
- >6 years: 5 mg/day, increase by 5 mg at weekly intervals not to exceed 40 mg/day

Short-term adjunct to exogenous obesity: Children >12 years and Adults: 10 mg or 15 mg long-acting capsule daily, up to 30 mg/day; or 5-30 mg/day in divided doses (immediate release tablets only)

Reference Range Therapeutic: 20-30 ng/mL; Toxic: >200 ng/mL

Patient Information Take during day to avoid insomnia; do not discontinue abruptly, may cause physical and psychological dependence with prolonged use

Nursing Implications Monitor CNS, dose should not be given in evening or at bedtime

Dosage Forms Tablet, as sulfate: 5 mg, 10 mg

Amphetamine Sulfate *see* Amphetamine *on previous page*

Amphojel® [OTC] *see* Aluminum Hydroxide *on page 55*

Amphotec® *see* Amphotericin B Colloidal Dispersion *on page 83*

Amphotericin B (am foe TER i sin bee)

Related Information

Antifungal Agents *on page 1395*

Desensitization Protocols *on page 1496*

Guidelines for the Prevention of Opportunistic Infections in Persons with HIV *on page 1457*

Brand Names Fungizone®

Therapeutic Category Antifungal Agent, Systemic; Antifungal Agent, Topical

Use Treatment of severe systemic infections and meningitis caused by susceptible fungi such as *Candida* species, *Histoplasma capsulatum, Cryptococcus neoformans, Aspergillus* species, *Blastomyces dermatitidis, Torulopsis glabrata,* and *Coccidioides immitis*; fungal peritonitis; irrigant for bladder fungal infections; and topically for cutaneous and mucocutaneous candidal infections

Pregnancy Risk Factor B

Contraindications Hypersensitivity to amphotericin or any component

Warnings/Precautions Avoid additive toxicity with other nephrotoxic drugs; monitor BUN and serum creatinine levels frequently while therapy is increased and at least weekly thereafter. I.V. amphotericin is used primarily for the treatment of patients with progressive and potentially fatal fungal infections; topical preparations may stain clothing.

(Continued)

Amphotericin B *(Continued)*

Adverse Reactions

>10%:

Central nervous system: Fever, chills, headache, malaise, generalized pain
Endocrine & metabolic: Hypokalemia, hypomagnesemia
Gastrointestinal: Anorexia
Hematologic: Anemia
Renal: Nephrotoxicity

1% to 10%:

Cardiovascular: Hypotension, hypertension, flushing
Central nervous system: Delirium, arachnoiditis, pain along lumbar nerves
Gastrointestinal: Nausea, vomiting
Genitourinary: Urinary retention
Hematologic: Leukocytosis, bone marrow suppression
Local: Thrombophlebitis
Neuromuscular & skeletal: Paresthesia (especially with I.T. therapy)
Renal: Renal tubular acidosis, renal failure

<1%:

Cardiovascular: Cardiac arrest
Central nervous system: Convulsions
Dermatologic: Maculopapular rash
Hematologic: Coagulation defects, thrombocytopenia, agranulocytosis, leukopenia
Hepatic: Acute liver failure
Ocular: Vision changes
Otic: Hearing loss
Renal: Anuria
Respiratory: Dyspnea

Overdosage/Toxicology Symptoms of overdose include renal dysfunction, anemia, thrombocytopenia, granulocytopenia, fever, nausea, and vomiting; treatment is supportive

Drug Interactions Increased toxicity: Cyclosporine and aminoglycosides (nephrotoxicity), corticosteroids (hypokalemia)

Stability

Reconstitute only with sterile water without preservatives, not bacteriostatic water. **Benzyl alcohol, sodium chloride, or other electrolyte solutions may cause precipitation.**

For I.V. infusion, an in-line filter (>1 micron mean pore diameter) may be used

Short-term exposure (<24 hours) to light during I.V. infusion does **not** appreciably affect potency

Reconstituted solutions with sterile water for injection and kept in the dark remain stable for 24 hours at room temperature and 1 week when refrigerated

Stability of parenteral admixture at room temperature (25°C): 24 hours; at refrigeration (4°C): 2 days

Standard diluent: Dose/500 mL D_5W

Minimum volume: 250 mL D_5W (concentrations should not exceed 0.1 mg/mL for peripheral administration or 1 mg/mL for central administration)

Mechanism of Action Binds to ergosterol altering cell membrane permeability in susceptible fungi and causing leakage of cell components with subsequent cell death

Pharmacodynamics/Kinetics

Distribution: Minimal amounts enter the aqueous humor, bile, CSF (inflamed or noninflamed meninges), amniotic fluid, pericardial fluid, pleural fluid, and synovial fluid

Protein binding, plasma: 90% infusion

Half-life, biphasic:

Initial: 15-48 hours
Terminal: 15 days

Time to peak: Within 1 hour following a 4- to 6-hour dose

Usual Dosage

I.V.:

Infants and Children:

Test dose (not required): I.V.: 0.1 mg/kg/dose to a maximum of 1 mg; infuse over 30-60 minutes

Initial therapeutic dose: 0.25 mg/kg gradually increased, usually in 0.25 mg/kg increments on each subsequent day, until the desired daily dose is reached

Maintenance dose: 0.25-1 mg/kg/day given once daily; infuse over 2-6 hours. Once therapy has been established, amphotericin B can be administered on an every other day basis at 1-1.5 mg/kg/dose; cumulative dose: 1.5-2 g over 6-10 week

Adults:

Test dose (not required): 1 mg infused over 20-30 minutes

Initial dose: 0.25 mg/kg administered over 2-6 hours, gradually increased on subsequent days to the desired level by 0.25 mg/kg increments per day; in critically ill patients, may initiate with 1-1.5 mg/kg/day with close observation

Maintenance dose: 0.25-1 mg/kg/day or 1.5 mg/kg over 4-6 hours every other day; do not exceed 1.5 mg/kg/day; cumulative dose: 1-4 g over 4-10 weeks

Duration of therapy varies with nature of infection: Histoplasmosis, *Cryptococcus*, or blastomycosis may be treated with total dose of 2-4 g

I.T.:

Children.: 25-100 mcg every 48-72 hours; increase to 500 mcg as tolerated

Adults: 25-300 mcg every 48-72 hours; increase to 500 mcg to 1 mg as tolerated

Oral: 1 mL (100 mg) 4 times daily

Topical: Apply to affected areas 2-4 times/day for 1-4 weeks of therapy depending on nature and severity of infection

Dosing adjustment in renal impairment: If renal dysfunction is due to the drug, the daily total can be decreased by 50% or the dose can be given every other day; I.V. therapy may take several months

Dialysis: Poorly dialyzed; no supplemental dosage necessary when using hemo- or peritoneal dialysis or CAVH/CAVHD

Administration in dialysate: Children and Adults: 1-2 mg/L of peritoneal dialysis fluid either with or without low-dose I.V. amphotericin B (a total dose of 2-10 mg/kg given over 7-14 days)

Administration via bladder irrigation: Children and Adults: 50 mg/day in 1 L of sterile water irrigation solution instilled over 24 hours for 2-7 days or until cultures are clear

Monitoring Parameters Electrolytes (especially potassium and magnesium), BUN, serum creatinine, liver function tests, temperature, CBC; monitor input and output; monitor for signs of hypokalemia (muscle weakness, cramping, drowsiness, EKG changes, etc)

Reference Range Therapeutic: 1-2 μg/mL (SI: 1-2.2 μmol/L)

Test Interactions ↑ BUN (S); ↓ magnesium, potassium (S)

Patient Information Amphotericin cream may slightly discolor skin and stain clothing; good personal hygiene may reduce the spread and recurrence of lesions; avoid covering topical applications with occlusive bandages; most skin lesions require 1-3 weeks of therapy; report any cramping, muscle weakness, or pain at or near injection site

Nursing Implications May premedicate patients with acetaminophen and diphenhydramine 30 minutes prior to the amphotericin infusion; meperidine (Demerol®) may help to reduce rigors; avoid rapid injection (usually 4- to 6-hour infusion required)

Dosage Forms

Cream: 3% (20 g)

Lotion: 3% (30 mL)

Ointment, topical: 3% (20 g)

Powder for injection, lyophilized: 50 mg

Suspension, oral: 100 mg/mL (24 mL with dropper)

Amphotericin B Colloidal Dispersion

(am foe TER i sin bee koe LOY dal dis PER shun)

Brand Names Amphotec®

Therapeutic Category Antifungal Agent, Systemic

Use Effective in the treatment of invasive mycoses in patient refractory to or intolerant of conventional amphotericin B

Pregnancy Risk Factor B

Pregnancy/Breast-Feeding Implications Due to limited data, consider discontinuing nursing during therapy

Contraindications Hypersensitivity to amphotericin B or its components

Warnings/Precautions Anaphylaxis has been reported; facilities for cardiopulmonary resuscitation should be available; infusion reactions, sometimes, severe, usually subside with continued therapy

Adverse Reactions

1% to 10%:

Cardiovascular: Hypotension, tachycardia

Central nervous system: Headache, chills, fever

Dermatologic: Rash

Endocrine & metabolic: Hypokalemia, hypomagnesemia

Gastrointestinal: Nausea, diarrhea, abdominal pain

Hematologic: Thrombocytopenia

(Continued)

Amphotericin B Colloidal Dispersion *(Continued)*

Hepatic: LFT change
Neuromuscular & skeletal: Rigors
Respiratory: Dyspnea

Note: Amphotericin B colloidal dispersion has an improved therapeutic index compared to conventional amphotericin B, and has been used safely in patients with amphotericin B-related nephrotoxicity; however, continued decline of renal function has occurred in some patients

Overdosage/Toxicology Symptoms of overdose include renal dysfunction, anemia, thrombocytopenia, granulocytopenia, fever, nausea, vomiting; treatment is supportive

Drug Interactions Increased toxicity: Cyclosporine and aminoglycosides (nephrotoxicity), corticosteroids (hypokalemia)

Mechanism of Action Binds to ergosterol altering cll membrane permeability in susceptible fungi and causing leakage of cell components with subsequent cell death

Pharmacodynamics/Kinetics

Distribution: V_d: Total amphotericin B increases with increasing doses of total amphotericin B (with 4 mg/kg/day = 4 L/kg); predominantly distributed in the liver; concentrations in kidneys and other tissues are lower than observed with conventional amphotericin B

Half-life: 28-29 hours

Plasma concentration: Total amphotericin B remains between 1-3 mcg/mL

Elimination: Clearance: 0.1 L/hour/kg (with 4 mg/kg/day)

Usual Dosage Children and Adults: 3-4 mg/kg/day I.V. (infusion of 1 mg/kg/hour); maximum: 7.5 mg/kg/day; duration of therapy is often <6 weeks

Monitoring Parameters Liver function tests, electrolytes, BUN, Cr, temperature, CBC, I/O, signs of hypokalemia (muscle weakness, cramping, drowsiness, EKG changes)

Nursing Implications May premedicate with acetaminophen and diphenhydramine 30 minutes prior to infusion; meperidine may help reduce rigors; avoid injection faster than 1 mg/kg/hour

Dosage Forms Suspension for injection: 50 mg, 100 mg (reconstituted to 5 mg/mL before further dilution)

Amphotericin B Lipid Complex

(am foe TER i sin bee LIP id KOM pleks)

Brand Names Abelcet™ Injection

Synonyms ABLC

Therapeutic Category Antifungal Agent, Systemic

Use Treatment of aspergillosis or any type of progressive fungal infection in patients who are refractory to or intolerant of conventional amphotericin B therapy; orphan drug status for cryptococcal meningitis

Pregnancy Risk Factor B

Pregnancy/Breast-Feeding Implications Due to limited data, consider discontinuing nursing during therapy

Contraindications Hypersensitivity to amphotericin or any component in the formulation

Warnings/Precautions Anaphylaxis has been reported with amphotericin B desoxycholate and other amphotericin B-containing drugs. Facilities for cardiopulmonary resuscitation should be available during administration due to the possibility of anaphylactic reaction. If severe respiratory distress occurs, the infusion should be immediately discontinued and the patient should not receive further infusions. During the initial dosing, the drug should be administered intravenously and under close clinical observation by medically trained personnel. Acute reactions (including fever and chills) may occur 1-2 hours after starting an intravenous infusion. These reactions are usually more common with the first few doses and generally diminish with subsequent doses.

Adverse Reactions Reduced nephrotoxicity as well as frequent infusion related side effects have been reported with this formulation

>10%:

Central nervous system: Chills, fever
Renal: Increased serum creatinine
Miscellaneous: Multiple organ failure

1% to 10%:

Cardiovascular: Hypotension, cardiac arrest
Central nervous system: Headache, pain
Dermatologic: Rash
Endocrine & metabolic: Bilirubinemia, hypokalemia, acidosis
Gastrointestinal: Nausea, vomiting, diarrhea, gastrointestinal hemorrhage, abdominal pain

Renal: Renal failure

Respiratory: Respiratory failure, dyspnea, pneumonia

Drug Interactions Increased toxicity: Toxic effect of nephrotoxic drugs may be additive; corticosteroids may increase potassium depletion caused by amphotericin; may predispose patients receiving cardiac glycosides or skeletal muscle relaxants to toxicity secondary to hypokalemia

Mechanism of Action As a modification of dimyristoyl phosphatidylcholine:dimyristoyl phosphatidylglycerol 7:3 (DMPC:DMPG) liposome, amphotericin B lipid-complex has a higher drug to lipid ratio and the concentration of amphotericin B is 33 M; ABLC is a ribbon-like structure, not a liposome; mechanism is like amphotericin - includes binding to ergosterol altering cell membrane permeability in susceptible fungi and causing leakage of cell components with subsequent cell death

Usual Dosage

Children and Adults: I.V.: 2.5-5 mg/kg/day as a single infusion **Note:** Significantly higher dose of ABLC are tolerated; it appears that attaining higher doses with ABLC produce more rapid fungicidal activity *in vivo* than standard amphotericin B preparations

Dosing adjustment in renal impairment: None necessary; effects of renal impairment are not currently known

Hemodialysis: No supplemental dosage necessary

Peritoneal dialysis: No supplemental dosage necessary

Continuous arterio-venous or veno-venous hemofiltration (CAVH/CAVHD): No supplemental dosage necessary

Monitoring Parameters

BUN and serum creatinine levels should be determined every other day while therapy is increased and at least weekly thereafter; monitor input and output

Serum potassium and magnesium should be monitored closely; monitor for signs of hypokalemia (muscle weakness, cramping, drowsiness, EKG changes, etc)

Monitor electrolytes, liver function, hematocrit, CBC, blood pressure, and temperature regularly

Patient Information I.V. therapy may take several months; personal hygiene is very important to help reduce the spread and recurrence of lesions; most skin lesions require 1-3 weeks of therapy; report any hearing loss

Dosage Forms Injection: 5 mg (20 mL)

Ampicillin (am pi SIL in)

Related Information

Animal and Human Bites Guidelines *on page 1463*

Antibiotic Treatment of Adults With Infectious Endocarditis *on page 1465*

Antimicrobial Drugs of Choice *on page 1468*

Bacterial Meningitis Practical Guidelines for Management *on page 1475*

Desensitization Protocols *on page 1496*

Prevention of Bacterial Endocarditis *on page 1449*

Brand Names Marcillin®; Omnipen®; Omnipen®-N; Polycillin®; Polycillin-N®; Principen®; Totacillin®; Totacillin®-N

Canadian/Mexican Brand Names Ampicin® [Sodium] (Canada); Apo-Ampi® [Trihydrate] (Canada); Jaa Amp® [Trihydrate] (Canada); Nu-Ampi® [Trihydrate] (Canada); Pro-Ampi® [Trihydrate] (Canada); Taro-Ampicillin® [Trihydrate] (Canada); Anglopen® (Mexico); Binotal® (Mexico); Dibacilina® (Mexico); Flamicina® (Mexico); Lampicin® (Mexico); Marovilina® (Mexico); Pentrexyl® (Mexico); Sinaplin® (Mexico)

Synonyms Aminobenzylpenicillin; Ampicillin Sodium; Ampicillin Trihydrate

Therapeutic Category Antibiotic, Penicillin

Use Treatment of susceptible bacterial infections (nonbeta-lactamase-producing organisms); susceptible bacterial infections caused by streptococci, pneumococci, nonpenicillinase-producing staphylococci, *Listeria*, meningococci; some strains of *H. influenzae, Salmonella, Shigella, E. coli, Enterobacter*, and *Klebsiella*

Pregnancy Risk Factor B

Contraindications Known hypersensitivity to ampicillin or other penicillins

Warnings/Precautions Dosage adjustment may be necessary in patients with renal impairment; a low incidence of cross-allergy with other beta-lactams exists; high percentage of patients with infectious mononucleosis have developed rash during therapy with ampicillin. Appearance of a rash should be carefully evaluated to differentiate a nonallergic ampicillin rash from a hypersensitivity reaction. Ampicillin rash occurs in 5% to 10% of children receiving ampicillin and is a generalized dull red, maculopapular rash, generally appearing 3-14 days after the start of therapy. It normally begins on the trunk and spreads over most of the body. It may be most intense at pressure areas, elbows, and knees.

(Continued)

Ampicillin *(Continued)*

Adverse Reactions

>10%:

Central nervous system: Pain

Dermatologic: Rash (appearance of a rash should be carefully evaluated to differentiate a nonallergic ampicillin rash from a hypersensitivity reaction; incidence is higher in patients with viral infections, *Salmonella* infections, lymphocytic leukemia, or patients that have hyperuricemia)

Gastrointestinal: Diarrhea, vomiting, oral candidiasis

1% to 10%: Gastrointestinal: Severe abdominal or stomach cramps

<1%:

Central nervous system: Penicillin encephalopathy, seizures

Hematologic: Lymphocytic leukemia

Overdosage/Toxicology Symptoms of penicillin overdose include neuromuscular hypersensitivity (agitation, hallucinations, asterixis, encephalopathy, confusion, and seizures) and electrolyte imbalance with potassium or sodium salts, especially in renal failure

Hemodialysis may be helpful to aid in the removal of the drug from the blood, otherwise most treatment is supportive or symptom directed

Drug Interactions

Decreased effect: Efficacy of oral contraceptives may be reduced

Increased effect: Disulfiram, probenecid may increase penicillin levels, increased effect of anticoagulants

Increased toxicity: Allopurinol theoretically has an additive potential for amoxicillin (ampicillin) rash

Stability Oral suspension is stable for 7 days at room temperature or for 14 days under refrigeration; solutions for I.M. or direct I.V. should be used within 1 hour; solutions for I.V. infusion will be inactivated by dextrose at room temperature; if dextrose-containing solutions are to be used, the resultant solution will only be stable for 2 hours versus 8 hours in the 0.9% sodium chloride injection. D_5W has limited stability.

Minimum volume: Concentration should not exceed 30 mg/mL due to concentration-dependent stability restrictions. Manufacturer may supply as either the anhydrous or the trihydrate form.

Stability of parenteral admixture in NS at room temperature (25°C): 8 hours

Stability of parenteral admixture in NS at refrigeration temperature (4°C): 2 days

Standard diluent: 500 mg/50 mL NS; 1 g/50 mL NS; 2 g/100 mL NS

Mechanism of Action Interferes with bacterial cell wall synthesis during active multiplication, causing cell wall death and resultant bactericidal activity against susceptible bacteria

Pharmacodynamics/Kinetics

Absorption: Oral: 50%

Distribution: Distributes into bile; penetration into CSF occurs with inflamed meninges only, good only with inflammation (exceeds usual MICs)

Normal meninges: Nil

Inflamed meninges: 5-10

Protein binding: 15% to 25%

Half-life:

Neonates:

2-7 days: 4 hours

8-14 days: 2.8 hours

15-30 days: 1.7 hours

Children and Adults: 1-1.8 hours

Anuria/end stage renal disease: 7-20 hours

Time to peak: Oral: Within 1-2 hours

Elimination: ~90% of the drug excreted unchanged in the urine within 24 hours

Usual Dosage

Infants and Children: I.M., I.V.: 100-400 mg/kg/day in doses divided every 4-6 hours

Meningitis: 200 mg/kg/day in doses divided every 4-6 hours; maximum dose: 12 g/day

Children: Oral: 50-100 mg/kg/day in doses divided every 6 hours; maximum dose: 2-3 g/day

Adults:

Oral: 250-500 mg every 6 hours

I.M.: 500 mg to 1.5 g every 4-6 hours

I.V.: 500 mg to 3 g every 4-6 hours; maximum dose: 12 g/day

Sepsis/meningitis: 150-250 mg/kg/24 hours divided every 3-4 hours

Dosing interval in renal impairment:

Cl_{cr} 30-50 mL/minute: Administer every 6-8 hours

Cl_{cr} 10-30 mL/minute: Administer every 8-12 hours

Cl_{cr} <10 mL/minute: Administer every 12 hours

Hemodialysis: Moderately dialyzable (20% to 50%); administer dose after dialysis

Peritoneal dialysis: Moderately dialyzable (20% to 50%)

Administer 250 mg every 12 hours

Continuous arterio-venous or veno-venous hemofiltration (CAVH) effects: ~50 mg of ampicillin/L of filtrate is removed

Dietary Considerations Food: Decreases drug absorption rate; decreases drug serum concentration. Take on an empty stomach 1 hour before or 2 hours after meals.

Administration Administer around-the-clock rather than 4 times/day to promote less variation in peak and trough serum levels; administer orally on an empty stomach (ie, 1 hour prior to, or 2 hours after meals) to increase total absorption

Test Interactions ↑ protein; urinary glucose (Benedict's solution, Clinitest®); ↑ positive Coombs' [direct]

Patient Information Refrigerate at 2°C to 8°C (36°F to 46°F); do not freeze

Nursing Implications Ampicillin and gentamicin should not be mixed in the same I.V. tubing or administered concurrently

Additional Information

Sodium content of 5 mL suspension (250 mg/5 mL): 10 mg (0.4 mEq)

Sodium content of 1 g: 66.7 mg (3 mEq)

Dosage Forms

Capsule, as anhydrous: 250 mg, 500 mg

Capsule, as trihydrate: 250 mg, 500 mg

Powder for injection, as sodium: 125 mg, 250 mg, 500 mg, 1 g, 2 g, 10 g

Powder for oral suspension, as trihydrate: 125 mg/5 mL (5 mL unit dose, 80 mL, 100 mL, 150 mL, 200 mL); 250 mg/5 mL (5 mL unit dose, 80 mL, 100 mL, 150 mL, 200 mL); 500 mg/5 mL (5 mL unit dose, 100 mL)

Powder for oral suspension, drops, as trihydrate: 100 mg/mL (20 mL)

Ampicillin and Sulbactam (am pi SIL in & SUL bak tam)

Related Information

Animal and Human Bites Guidelines *on page 1463*

Antimicrobial Drugs of Choice *on page 1468*

Brand Names Unasyn®

Canadian/Mexican Brand Names Unasyna® (Mexico); Unasyna® Oral (Mexico)

Synonyms Sulbactam and Ampicillin

Therapeutic Category Antibiotic, Penicillin

Use Treatment of susceptible bacterial infections involved with skin and skin structure, intra-abdominal infections, gynecological infections; spectrum is that of ampicillin plus organisms producing beta-lactamases such as *S. aureus, H. influenzae, E. coli, Klebsiella, Acinetobacter, Enterobacter,* and anaerobes

Pregnancy Risk Factor B

Contraindications Hypersensitivity to ampicillin, sulbactam or any component, or penicillins

Warnings/Precautions Dosage adjustment may be necessary in patients with renal impairment; a low incidence of cross-allergy with other beta-lactams exists; high percentage of patients with infectious mononucleosis have developed rash during therapy with ampicillin. Appearance of a rash should be carefully evaluated to differentiate a nonallergic ampicillin rash from a hypersensitivity reaction. Ampicillin rash occurs in 5% to 10% of children receiving ampicillin and is a generalized dull red, maculopapular rash, generally appearing 3-14 days after the start of therapy. It normally begins on the trunk and spreads over most of the body. It may be most intense at pressure areas, elbows, and knees.

Adverse Reactions

>10%: Local: Pain at injection site (I.M.)

1% to 10%:

Dermatologic: Rash

Gastrointestinal: Diarrhea

Local: Pain at injection site (I.V.)

<1%:

Cardiovascular: Chest pain

Central nervous system: Fatigue, malaise, headache, chills

Dermatologic: Itching

Gastrointestinal: Nausea, vomiting, enterocolitis, pseudomembranous colitis, hairy tongue

Genitourinary: Dysuria

Hematologic: Decreased WBC, neutrophils, platelets, hemoglobin, and hematocrit

Hepatic: Increased liver enzymes

Local: Thrombophlebitis

Renal: Increased BUN/creatinine

(Continued)

Ampicillin and Sulbactam *(Continued)*

Miscellaneous: Hypersensitivity reactions, candidiasis

Overdosage/Toxicology Symptoms of penicillin overdose include neuromuscular hypersensitivity (agitation, hallucinations, asterixis, encephalopathy, confusion, and seizures) and electrolyte imbalance with potassium or sodium salts, especially in renal failure

Hemodialysis may be helpful to aid in the removal of the drug from the blood, otherwise most treatment is supportive or symptom directed

Drug Interactions

Decreased effect: Efficacy of oral contraceptives may be reduced

Increased effect: Disulfiram, probenecid results in increased ampicillin levels

Increased toxicity: Allopurinol theoretically has an additive potential for ampicillin rash

Stability I.M. and direct I.V. administration: Use within 1 hour after preparation; reconstitute with sterile water for injection or 0.5% or 2% lidocaine hydrochloride injection (I.M.); sodium chloride 0.9% (NS) is the diluent of choice for I.V. piggyback use, solutions made in NS are stable up to 72 hours when refrigerated whereas dextrose solutions (same concentration) are stable for only 4 hours

Mechanism of Action Interferes with bacterial cell wall synthesis during active multiplication, causing cell wall death and resultant bactericidal activity against susceptible bacteria; addition of sulbactam, a beta-lactamase inhibitor, to ampicillin extends the spectrum of ampicillin to include beta-lactamase producing organisms

Pharmacodynamics/Kinetics

Distribution: Into bile, blister and tissue fluids; poor penetration into CSF with uninflamed meninges; higher concentrations attained with inflamed meninges

Protein binding:

- Ampicillin: 28%
- Sulbactam: 38%

Half-life: Ampicillin and sulbactam are similar: 1-1.8 hours and 1-1.3 hours, respectively in patients with normal renal function

Elimination: ~75% to 85% of both drugs are excreted unchanged in the urine within 8 hours following administration

Usual Dosage Unasyn® (ampicillin/sulbactam) is a combination product. Each 3 g vial contains 2 g of ampicillin and 1 g of sulbactam. Sulbactam has very little antibacterial activity by itself, but effectively extends the spectrum of ampicillin to include beta-lactamase producing strains that are resistant to ampicillin alone. Therefore, dosage recommendations for Unasyn® are based on the ampicillin component.

I.M., I.V.:

- Children (3 months to 12 years): 100-200 mg ampicillin/kg/day (150-300 mg Unasyn®) divided every 6 hours; maximum dose: 8 g ampicillin/day (12 g Unasyn®)
- Adults: 1-2 g ampicillin (1.5-3 g Unasyn®) every 6-8 hours; maximum dose: 8 g ampicillin/day (12 g Unasyn®)

Dosing interval in renal impairment:

- Cl_{cr} 15-29 mL/minute: Administer every 12 hours
- Cl_{cr} 5-14 mL/minute: Administer every 24 hours

Administration Administer around-the-clock rather than 4 times/day to promote less variation in peak and trough serum levels

Monitoring Parameters With prolonged therapy, monitor hematologic, renal, and hepatic function

Test Interactions False-positive urinary glucose levels (Benedict's solution, Clinitest®)

Nursing Implications Ampicillin and gentamicin should not be mixed in the same I.V. tubing or administered concurrently

Dosage Forms Powder for injection: 1.5 g [ampicillin sodium 1 g and sulbactam sodium 0.5 g]; 3 g [ampicillin sodium 2 g and sulbactam sodium 1 g]

Ampicillin Sodium *see* Ampicillin *on page 85*

Ampicillin Trihydrate *see* Ampicillin *on page 85*

AMPT *see* Metyrosine *on page 831*

Amrinone (AM ri none)

Related Information

Adrenergic Agonists, Cardiovascular Comparison *on page 1385*

Adult ACLS Algorithm, Hypotension, Shock *on page 1516*

Cardiovascular Agents Comparison *on page 1405*

Brand Names Inocor®

Synonyms Amrinone Lactate

Therapeutic Category Phosphodiesterase Enzyme Inhibitor

Use Treatment of low cardiac output states (sepsis, congestive heart failure); adjunctive therapy of pulmonary hypertension; normally prescribed for patients who have not responded well to therapy with digitalis, diuretics, and vasodilators

Pregnancy Risk Factor C

Contraindications Hypersensitivity to amrinone lactate or sulfites (contains sodium metabisulfite)

Warnings/Precautions Diuresis may result from improvement in cardiac output and may require dosage reduction of diuretics

Adverse Reactions

1% to 10%:

Cardiovascular: Arrhythmias, hypotension (may be infusion rate-related), ventricular and supraventricular arrhythmias

Gastrointestinal: Nausea

Hematologic: Thrombocytopenia (may be dose-related)

<1%:

Cardiovascular: Chest pain

Central nervous system: Fever

Gastrointestinal: Vomiting, abdominal pain, anorexia

Hepatic: Hepatotoxicity

Local: Pain or burning at injection site

Overdosage/Toxicology Symptoms of overdose includes hypotension (sometimes severe); there is no specific antidote for amrinone intoxication; treatment is supportive

Drug Interactions When furosemide is admixed with amrinone, a precipitate immediately forms; diuretics may cause significant hypovolemia and decrease filling pressure

Stability May be administered undiluted for I.V. bolus doses. For continuous infusion: Dilute with 0.45% or 0.9% sodium chloride to final concentration of 1-3 mg/mL; use within 24 hours; do not directly dilute with dextrose-containing solutions, chemical interaction occurs; may be administered I.V. into running dextrose infusions. Furosemide forms a precipitate when injected in I.V. lines containing amrinone.

Mechanism of Action Inhibits myocardial cyclic adenosine monophosphate (cAMP) phosphodiesterase activity and increases cellular levels of cAMP resulting in a positive inotropic effect and increased cardiac output; also possesses systemic and pulmonary vasodilator effects resulting in pre- and afterload reduction; slightly increases atrioventricular conduction

Pharmacodynamics/Kinetics

Onset of action: I.V.: Within 2-5 minutes

Peak effect: Within 10 minutes

Duration: Dose dependent (~30 minutes low dose, ~2 hours higher doses)

Distribution: V_d: 1.2 L/kg

Protein binding: 10% to 49%

Metabolism: Hepatic

Half-life:

Neonates 1-2 weeks: 22.2 hours

Infants 6-38 weeks: 6.8 hours; negative correlation of age with half-life in infants 4-38 weeks of age

Adults, normal volunteers: 3.6 hours

Adults with CHF: 5.8 hours

Elimination: 60% to 90% excreted as metabolites in urine within 24 hours

Usual Dosage Dosage is based on clinical response

Note: Dose should not exceed 10 mg/kg/24 hours

Children and Adults: 0.75 mg/kg I.V. bolus over 2-3 minutes followed by maintenance infusion of 5-10 mcg/kg/minute; I.V. bolus may need to be repeated in 30 minutes

Dosing adjustment in renal failure: Cl_{cr} <10 mL/minute: Administer 50% to 75% of dose

Administration Should be administered solely via an I.V. pump

Monitoring Parameters Patients should be carefully monitored for hemodynamic response (hypotension) and potential adverse effects (ie, thrombocytopenia, hepatotoxicity, and GI effects); monitor cardiac index, stroke volume, systemic vascular resistance, and pulmonary vascular resistance (if Swan-Ganz catheter available); CVP, blood pressure and heart rate (every 5 minutes during infusion), fluids and electrolytes (especially potassium), fluid status, platelet count, CBC, liver function and renal function tests

Patient Information Make position changes slowly because of postural hypotension

Dosage Forms Injection, as lactate: 5 mg/mL (20 mL)

Amrinone Lactate *see* Amrinone *on previous page*

Amvisc® *see* Sodium Hyaluronate *on page 1144*

Amvisc® Plus *see* Sodium Hyaluronate *on page 1144*

Amyl Nitrite (AM il NYE trite)

Synonyms Isoamyl Nitrite

Therapeutic Category Antidote, Cyanide; Vasodilator, Coronary

Use Coronary vasodilator in angina pectoris; adjunct in treatment of cyanide poisoning; used to produce changes in the intensity of heart murmurs

Pregnancy Risk Factor X

Contraindications Severe anemia; hypersensitivity to nitrates

Warnings/Precautions Use with caution in patients with increased intracranial pressure, low systolic blood pressure, and coronary artery disease

Adverse Reactions

1% to 10%:

- Cardiovascular: Postural hypotension, cutaneous flushing of head, neck, and clavicular area
- Central nervous system: Headache

<1%:

- Dermatologic: Rash
- Hematologic: Hemolytic anemia

Overdosage/Toxicology Symptoms of overdose include hypotension; treatment includes general supportive measures for transient hypotension; I.V. fluids; Trendelenburg position, vasopressors

Drug Interactions Increased toxicity: Alcohol

Stability Store in cool place; protect from light

Pharmacodynamics/Kinetics

Onset of action: Angina relieved within 30 seconds

Duration: 3-15 minutes

Usual Dosage Adults: 1-6 inhalations from one capsule are usually sufficient to produce the desired effect

Administration Administer nasally; patient should not be sitting; crush ampul in woven covering between fingers and then hold under patient's nostrils

Monitoring Parameters Monitor blood pressure during therapy

Patient Information Lie down during administration, crush ampul between fingers and then inhale through nostrils; may cause dizziness; call paramedics or have someone take you to the hospital immediately if pain is not relieved after 3 doses

Dosage Forms Inhalant, crushable glass perles: 0.18 mL, 0.3 mL

Amylobarbitone *see* Amobarbital *on page 74*

Amytal® *see* Amobarbital *on page 74*

Anacin® [OTC] *see* Aspirin *on page 106*

Anacin-3® [OTC] *see* Acetaminophen *on page 19*

Anadrol® *see* Oxymetholone *on page 941*

Anafranil® *see* Clomipramine *on page 296*

Anaprox® *see* Naproxen *on page 880*

Anaspaz® *see* Hyoscyamine *on page 635*

Anastrozole (an AS troe zole)

Brand Names Arimidex®

Therapeutic Category Antineoplastic Agent, Hormone (Antiestrogen)

Use Treatment of advanced breast cancer in postmenopausal women with disease progression following tamoxifen therapy. Patients with ER-negative disease and patients who did not respond to tamoxifen therapy rarely responded to anastrozole.

Pregnancy Risk Factor C

Pregnancy/Breast-Feeding Implications Anastrozole can cause fetal harm when administered to a pregnant woman

Contraindications Hypersensitivity to any component

Warnings/Precautions Use with caution in patients with hyperlipidemias; mean serum total cholesterol and LDL cholesterol occurs in patients receiving anastrozole

Adverse Reactions

>5%:

- Cardiovascular: Flushing
- Gastrointestinal: Little to mild nausea (10%), vomiting
- Neuromuscular & skeletal: Increased bone and tumor pain

2% to 5%:

- Cardiovascular: Hypertension
- Central nervous system: Somnolence, confusion, insomnia, anxiety, nervousness, fever, malaise, accidental injury
- Dermatologic: Hair thinning, pruritus
- Endocrine & metabolic: Breast pain

Gastrointestinal: Weight loss
Genitourinary: Urinary tract infection
Local: Thrombophlebitis
Neuromuscular & skeletal: Myalgia, arthralgia, pathological fracture, neck pain
Respiratory: Sinusitis, bronchitis, rhinitis
Miscellaneous: Flu-like syndrome, infection

Overdosage/Toxicology Symptoms of overdose include severe irritation to the stomach (necrosis, gastritis, ulceration and hemorrhage)

There is no specific antidote; treatment must be symptomatic. Vomiting may be induced if the patient is alert. Dialysis may be helpful because anastrozole is not highly protein bound. General supportive care, including frequent monitoring of all vital signs and close observation.

Drug Interactions

Cytochrome P-450 1A2 substrate
Cytochrome P-450 2C8/9 substrate
Cytochrome P-450 3A4 substrate

Anastrozole inhibited *in vitro* metabolic reactions catalyzed by cytochromes P-450 1A2, 2C8/9, and 3A4, but only at relatively high concentrations. It is unlikely that coadministration of anastrozole with other drugs will result in clinically significant inhibition of cytochrome P-450-mediated metabolism of other drugs.

Mechanism of Action Potent and selective nonsteroidal aromatase inhibitor. It significantly lowers serum estradiol concentrations and has not detectable effect on formation of adrenal corticosteroids or aldosterone. In postmenopausal women, the principal source of circulating estrogen is conversion of adrenally generated androsternedione to estrone by aromatase in peripheral tissues.

Pharmacodynamics/Kinetics

Absorption: Well absorbed from GI tract; food does not affect absorption
Protein binding, plasma: 40%
Metabolism: Extensively in the liver
Half-life: 50 hours
Elimination: Primarily via hepatic metabolism (85%) and to a lesser extent renal excretion (11%)

Usual Dosage Breast cancer: Adults: Oral (refer to individual protocols): 1 mg once daily

Dosage adjustment in renal impairment: Because only about 10% is excreted unchanged in the urine, dosage adjustment in patients with renal insufficiency is not necessary

Dosage adjustment in hepatic impairment: Plasma concentrations in subjects with hepatic cirrhosis were within the range concentrations in normal subjects across all clinical trials; therefore, no dosage adjustment is needed

Test Interactions Lab test abnormalities: GGT, AST, ALT, alkaline phosphatase, total cholesterol and LDL increased; three-fold elevations of mean serum GGT levels have been observed among patients with liver metastases. These changes were likely related to the progression of liver metastases in these patients, although other contributing factors could not be ruled out. Mean serum total cholesterol levels increased by 0.5 mmol/L among patients.

Dosage Forms Tablet: 1 mg

Anbesol® [OTC] *see* Benzocaine *on page 138*
Anbesol® Maximum Strength [OTC] *see* Benzocaine *on page 138*
Ancef® *see* Cefazolin *on page 220*
Ancobon® *see* Flucytosine *on page 526*
Androderm® Transdermal System *see* Testosterone *on page 1198*
Android® *see* Methyltestosterone *on page 821*
Andro-L.A.® Injection *see* Testosterone *on page 1198*
Androlone® *see* Nandrolone *on page 878*
Androlone®-D *see* Nandrolone *on page 878*
Andropository® Injection *see* Testosterone *on page 1198*
Anectine® Chloride *see* Succinylcholine *on page 1166*
Anectine® Flo-Pack® *see* Succinylcholine *on page 1166*
Anergan® *see* Promethazine *on page 1058*
Anestacon® *see* Lidocaine *on page 723*
Aneurine Hydrochloride *see* Thiamine *on page 1214*
Anexsia® *see* Hydrocodone and Acetaminophen *on page 620*
Angiotensin-Converting Enzyme Inhibitors Comparison *see page 1386*
Animal and Human Bites Guidelines *see page 1463*

Anisotropine (an iss oh TROE peen)

Brand Names Valpin® 50

Canadian/Mexican Brand Names Miradon® (Canada)

(Continued)

Anisotropine *(Continued)*

Synonyms Anisotropine Methylbromide

Therapeutic Category Anticholinergic Agent

Use Adjunctive treatment of peptic ulcer

Pregnancy Risk Factor C

Contraindications Narrow-angle glaucoma, obstructive GI tract or uropathy, severe ulcerative colitis, myasthenia gravis, intestinal atony, hepatic disease, hypersensitivity

Warnings/Precautions Drug-induced heatstroke can develop in hot or humid climates

Adverse Reactions

>10%:
- Cardiovascular: Palpitations
- Dermatologic: Dry skin
- Gastrointestinal: Constipation, dry throat, xerostomia
- Respiratory: Dry nose
- Miscellaneous: Diaphoresis (decreased)

1% to 10%:
- Endocrine & metabolic: Decreased flow of breast milk
- Gastrointestinal: Decreased salivary secretion

<1%:
- Cardiovascular: Orthostatic hypotension,
- Central nervous system: Confusion, drowsiness, headache, loss of memory, fatigue
- Dermatologic: Rash
- Gastrointestinal: Bloated feeling, nausea, vomiting
- Genitourinary: Decreased urination
- Neuromuscular & skeletal: Weakness
- Ocular: Increased intraocular pain, blurred vision, increased sensitivity to light

Overdosage/Toxicology Symptoms of overdose include blurred vision, dysphagia, urinary retention, tachycardia, hypertension

Anisotropine toxicity is caused by strong binding of the drug to cholinergic receptors. Anticholinesterase inhibitors reduce acetylcholinesterase, the enzyme that breaks down acetylcholine and thereby allows acetylcholine to accumulate and compete for receptor binding with this offending anticholinergic. For an overdose with severe life-threatening symptoms, physostigmine 1-2 mg (0.5 or 0.02 mg/kg for children) S.C. or I.V., slowly may be given to reverse these effects.

Mechanism of Action Blocks the action of acetylcholine at parasympathetic sites in smooth muscle, secretory glands, and the CNS; increases cardiac output, dries secretions, antagonizes histamine and serotonin

Pharmacodynamics/Kinetics

Absorption: Poor (~10%) from GI tract

Elimination: Principally in urine as unchanged drug and metabolites

Usual Dosage Adults: Oral: 50 mg 3 times/day

Administration Administer 30-60 minutes before meals

Monitoring Parameters Monitor patient's vital signs and I & O

Patient Information Dry mouth can be relieved by sugarless gum or hard candy; drink plenty of fluids

Dosage Forms Tablet, as methylbromide: 50 mg

Anisotropine Methylbromide *see* Anisotropine *on previous page*

Anisoylated Plasminogen Streptokinase Activator Complex *see* Anistreplase *on this page*

Anistreplase (a NISS tre plase)

Brand Names Eminase®

Synonyms Anisoylated Plasminogen Streptokinase Activator Complex; APSAC

Therapeutic Category Thrombolytic Agent

Use Management of acute myocardial infarction (AMI) in adults; lysis of thrombi obstructing coronary arteries, reduction of infarct size; and reduction of mortality associated with AMI

Pregnancy Risk Factor C

Contraindications Active internal bleeding, history of CVA, intracranial neoplasma, known hypersensitivity to anistreplase or other kinases (streptokinase); history of cerebrovascular accident; recent intracranial surgery or trauma; arteriovenous malformation or aneurysm; severe uncontrolled hypertension

Adverse Reactions

>10%:
- Cardiovascular: Arrhythmias, hypotension, perfusion arrhythmias
- Hematologic: Bleeding or oozing from cuts

1% to 10%: Miscellaneous: Anaphylactic reaction

<1%:
- Central nervous system: Headache, chills
- Dermatologic: Rash
- Gastrointestinal: Nausea, vomiting
- Hematologic: Anemia
- Ocular: Eye hemorrhage
- Respiratory: Bronchospasm, epistaxis
- Miscellaneous: Diaphoresis

Drug Interactions Increased efficacy and bleeding potential: Anticoagulants (heparin, warfarin), antiplatelet agents (aspirin)

Stability Discard solution 30 minutes after reconstitution if not administered; do not shake solution

Mechanism of Action Activates the conversion of plasminogen to plasmin by forming a complex exposing plasminogen-activating site and cleavage of a peptide bond that converts plasminogen to plasmin; plasmin being capable of thrombolysis, by degrading fibrin, fibrinogen and other procoagulant proteins into soluble fragments, effective both outside and within the formed thrombus/embolus

Pharmacodynamics/Kinetics

Duration of action: Fibrinolytic effect persists for 4-6 hours following administration

Metabolism: Anistreplase is an acylated complex of streptokinase with lys-plasminogen; one of the purposes of this acylation is to extend the serum circulating time of anistreplase; because deacylation of the complex occurs more rapidly than dissociation, fibrinolytic activity is controlled by the rate of deacylation rather than of dissociation

Half-life: 70-120 minutes

Usual Dosage Adults: I.V.: 30 units injected over 2-5 minutes as soon as possible after onset of symptoms

Administration Can be given as a bolus; avoid I.M. injections and nonessential handling of patient after administration of drug

Nursing Implications Drug should not be used for any condition in which bleeding constitutes a significant hazard or would be particularly difficult to manage

Dosage Forms Powder for injection, lyophilized: 30 units

Anodynos-DHC® *see* Hydrocodone and Acetaminophen *on page 620*

Anoquan® *see* Butalbital Compound *on page 176*

Ansaid® *see* Flurbiprofen *on page 547*

Ansamycin *see* Rifabutin *on page 1105*

Antabuse® *see* Disulfiram *on page 411*

Antacid Drug Interactions *see page 1388*

Anthra-Derm® *see* Anthralin *on this page*

Anthralin (AN thra lin)

Brand Names Anthra-Derm®; Drithocreme®; Drithocreme® HP 1%; Dritho-Scalp®; Lasan™; Lasan HP-1™

Canadian/Mexican Brand Names Anthraforte® (Canada); Anthranol® (Canada); Anthrascalp® (Canada); Anthranol® (Mexico)

Therapeutic Category Antipsoriatic Agent, Topical; Keratolytic Agent

Use Treatment of psoriasis (quiescent or chronic psoriasis)

Pregnancy Risk Factor C

Contraindications Hypersensitivity to anthralin or any component, acute psoriasis (acutely or actively inflamed psoriatic eruptions); use on the face

Warnings/Precautions If redness is observed, reduce frequency of dosage or discontinue application; avoid eye contact; should generally not be applied to intertriginous skin areas and high strengths should not be used on these sites; do not apply to face or genitalia; use caution in patients with renal disease and in those having extensive and prolonged applications; perform periodic urine tests for albuminuria.

Adverse Reactions

1% to 10%: Dermatologic: Transient primary irritation of uninvolved skin; temporary discoloration of hair and fingernails, may stain skin, hair, or fabrics

<1%: Dermatologic: Rash, excessive irritation

Drug Interactions Increased toxicity: Long-term use of topical corticosteroids may destabilize psoriasis, and withdrawal may also give rise to a "rebound" phenomenon, allow an interval of at least 1 week between the discontinuance of topical corticosteroids and the commencement of therapy

Mechanism of Action Reduction of the mitotic rate and proliferation of epidermal cells in psoriasis by inhibiting synthesis of nucleic protein from inhibition of DNA synthesis to affected areas

(Continued)

Anthralin *(Continued)*

Usual Dosage Adults: Topical: Generally, apply once a day or as directed. The irritant potential of anthralin is directly related to the strength being used and each patient's individual tolerance. Always commence treatment for at least one week using the lowest strength possible.

Skin application: Apply sparingly only to psoriatic lesions and rub gently and carefully into the skin until absorbed. Avoid applying an excessive quantity which may cause unnecessary soiling and staining of the clothing or bed linen.

Scalp application: Comb hair to remove scalar debris and, after suitably parting, rub cream well into the lesions, taking care to prevent the cream from spreading onto the forehead

Remove by washing or showering; optimal period of contact will vary according to the strength used and the patient's response to treatment. Continue treatment until the skin is entirely clear (ie, when there is nothing to feel with the fingers and the texture is normal)

Patient Information For external use only; may discolor skin, hair, or fabrics; avoid sunlight to treated areas

Nursing Implications Wear gloves; can discolor skin, hair, or clothes

Dosage Forms

Cream: 0.1% (50 g, 65 g); 0.2% (65 g); 0.25% (50 g); 0.4% (65 g); 0.5% (50 g); 1% (50 g, 65 g)

Ointment, topical: 0.1% (42.5 g); 0.25% (42.5 g); 0.4% (60 g); 0.5% (42.5 g); 1% (42.5 g)

Antiarrhythmic Drugs *see page 1389*

AntibiOtic® Otic *see* Neomycin, Polymyxin B, and Hydrocortisone *on page 890*

Antibiotic Treatment of Adults With Infectious Endocarditis *see page 1465*

Anticonvulsants by Seizure Type *see page 1392*

Antidepressant Agents Comparison *see page 1393*

Antidigoxin Fab Fragments *see* Digoxin Immune Fab *on page 389*

Antidiuretic Hormone *see* Vasopressin *on page 1293*

Antiemetics for Chemotherapy Induced Nausea and Vomiting *see page 1348*

Antifungal Agents *see page 1395*

Antihemophilic Factor (Human)

(an tee hee moe FIL ik FAK tor HYU man)

Brand Names Hemofil® M; Humate-P®; Koāte®-HP; Koāte®-HS; Monoclate-P®; Profilate® OSD; Profilate® SD

Synonyms AHF; Factor VIII

Therapeutic Category Antihemophilic Agent; Blood Product Derivative

Use Management of hemophilia A in patients whom a deficiency in factor VIII has been demonstrated. Can be of significant therapeutic value in patients with acquired factor VII inhibitors not exceeding 10 Bethesda units/mL.

Orphan drug status: Von Willebrand disease and prevention of bleeding from surgery in hemophilia A

Pregnancy Risk Factor C

Contraindications Hypersensitivity to mouse protein (Monoclate-P®; Hemofil® M, Method M, Monoclonal Purified) and Antihemophilic Factor (Human); Method M, Monoclonal Purified contain trace amounts of mouse protein

Warnings/Precautions Risk of viral transmission is not totally eradicated. Risk of hepatitis: Because antihemophilic factor is prepared for pooled plasma, it may contain the causative agent of viral hepatitis. Antihemophilic factor contains trace amounts of blood groups A and B isohemagglutinins; when large or frequently repeated doses are given to individuals with blood groups A, B, and AB, the patient should be monitored for signs of progressive anemia and the possibility of intravascular hemolysis should be considered.

Adverse Reactions

<1%:

Cardiovascular: Flushing, tachycardia

Central nervous system: Headache

Gastrointestinal: Nausea, vomiting

Neuromuscular & skeletal: Paresthesia

Sensitivity reactions: Allergic vasomotor reactions, tightness in neck or chest

Overdosage/Toxicology Intravascular hemolysis

Stability Dried concentrate should be refrigerated (2°C to 8°C/36°F to 46°F) but may be stored at room temperature for up to 6 months depending upon specific product; if refrigerated, the dried concentrate and diluent should be warmed to room temperature before reconstitution; gently agitate or rotate vial after adding diluent, do not shake vigorously; do **not** refrigerate after reconstitution, a precipitation may occur; Method M, monoclonal purified products should be administered within 1 hour after reconstitution

Stability of parenteral admixture at room temperature (25°C): 24 hours, but it is recommended to administer within 3 hours after reconstitution

Mechanism of Action Protein (factor VIII) in normal plasma which is necessary for clot formation and maintenance of hemostasis; activates factor X in conjunction with activated factor IX; activated factor X converts prothrombin to thrombin, which converts fibrinogen to fibrin and with factor XIII forms a stable clot

Pharmacodynamics/Kinetics

Distribution: Does not readily cross the placenta

Half-life, biphasic: 4-24 hours with a mean of 12 hours (biphasic: 12 hours is usually used for dosing interval estimates)

Usual Dosage I.V.: Individualize dosage based on coagulation studies performed prior to and during treatment at regular intervals. One AHF unit is the activity present in 1 mL of normal pooled human plasma; dosage should be adjusted to actual vial size currently stocked in the pharmacy.

Hospitalized patients: 20-50 units/kg/dose; may be higher for special circumstances. Dose can be given every 12-24 hours and more frequently in special circumstances.

Formula to approximate percentage increase in plasma antihemophilic factor:

Units required = desired level increase (desired level - actual level) x plasma volume (mL)

Total blood volume (mL blood/kg) = 70 mL/kg (adults); 80 mL/kg (children)

Plasma volume = total blood volume (mL) x [1 - Hct (in decimals)]

Example: For a 70 kg adult with a Hct = 40% : plasma volume = [70 kg x 70 mL/kg] x [1 - 0.4] = 2940 mL

To calculate number of units of factor VIII needed to increase level to desired range (highly individualized and dependent on patient's condition):

Number of units = desired level increase [desired level - actual level] x plasma volume (in mL)

Example: For a 100% level in the above patient who has an actual level of 20% the number of units needed = [1 (for a 100% level) - 0.2] x 2940 mL = 2352 units

Administration I.V. administration only; maximum rate of administration is product dependent: Monoclate-P® 2 mL/minute; Humate-P® 4 mL/minute; administration of other products should not exceed 10 mL/minute; use filter needle to draw product into syringe

Monitoring Parameters Heart rate (before and during I.V. administration); antihemophilic factor levels prior to and during treatment; in patients with circulating inhibitors, the inhibitor level should be monitored

Reference Range

Average normal antihemophilic factor plasma activity ranges 50% to 150%

Level to prevent spontaneous hemorrhage: 5%

Required peak postinfusion AHF activity in blood (as % of normal or units/dL plasma):

Early hemarthrosis or muscle bleed or oral bleed: 20% to 40%

More extensive hemarthrosis, muscle bleed, or hematoma: 30% to 60%

Life-threatening bleeds, such as head injury, throat bleed, severe abdominal pain

Minor surgery, including tooth extraction: 60% to 80%

Major surgery: 80% to 100% (pre- and postoperative)

Nursing Implications Reduce rate of administration or temporarily discontinue if patient becomes tachycardiac

Dosage Forms Injection: 10 mL, 20 mL, 30 mL

Antihemophilic Factor (Porcine)

(an tee hee moe FIL ik FAK ter POR seen)

Brand Names Hyate®:C

Therapeutic Category Antihemophilic Agent; Blood Product Derivative

Use Treatment of congenital hemophiliacs with antibodies to human factor VIII:C and also for previously nonhemophiliac patients with spontaneously acquired inhibitors to human factor VIII:C; patients with inhibitors who are bleeding or who are to undergo surgery

Pregnancy Risk Factor C

Contraindications Should not be used to treat patients who have previously suffered acute allergic reaction to antihemophilic factor (porcine)

Warnings/Precautions Rarely administration has been associated with anaphylaxis; adrenaline, hydrocortisone, and facilities for cardiopulmonary resuscitation should be available in case such a reaction occurs; infusion may be followed by a

(Continued)

Antihemophilic Factor (Porcine) *(Continued)*

rise in plasma levels of antibody to both human and porcine factor VIII:C; inhibitor levels should be monitored both during and after treatment

Adverse Reactions Reactions tend to lessen in frequency and severity as further infusions are given; hydrocortisone and/or antihistamines may help to prevent or alleviate side effects and may be prescribed as precautionary measures

1% to 10%:

Central nervous system: Fever, headache, chills

Dermatologic: Rashes

Gastrointestinal: Nausea, vomiting

Stability Store at temperature of -15°C to <20°C; use before expiration date; reconstituted Hyate®:C must not be stored, stable for 24 hours at room temperature

Mechanism of Action Factor VIII:C is the coagulation portion of the factor VIII complex in plasma. Factor VIII:C acts as a cofactor for factor IX to activate factor X in the intrinsic pathway of blood coagulation.

Usual Dosage Clinical response should be used to assess efficacy rather than relying upon a particular laboratory value for recovery of factor VIII:C.

Initial dose:

Antibody level to human factor VIII:C <50 Bethesda units/mL: 100-150 porcine units/kg (body weight) is recommended

Antibody level to human factor VIII:C >50 Bethesda units/mL: Activity of the antibody to porcine factor VIII:C should be determined; **an antiporcine antibody level** >20 Bethesda units/mL indicates that the patient is unlikely to benefit from treatment; for lower titers, a dose of 100-150 porcine units/kg is recommended

If a patient has previously been treated with Hyate®:C, this may provide a guide to his likely response and, therefore, assist in estimation of the preliminary dose

Subsequent doses: Following administration of the initial dose, if the recovery of factor VIII:C in the patient's plasma is not sufficient, a further higher dose should be administered; if recovery after the second dose is still insufficient, a third and higher dose may prove effective

Administration Administer by I.V. route only; infusion rate should be <10 mL/minute

Reference Range Treatment is not normally indicated in patients with an antibody titer <5 Bethesda units/mL (BU/mL) against human factor VIII:C and is likely to be ineffective in patients with an antibody titer >50 Bethesda units/mL against human factor VIII:C

If a patient has an antibody titer >50 Bethesda units/mL against human factor VIII:C, the activity of the antibody against porcine factor VIII should be determined

An antibody titer <15-20 Bethesda units/mL against porcine factor VIII:C indicates suitability for treatment with antihemophilic factor (Porcine)-Hyate®:C

Factor VIII levels: 50% to 150%, draw 6-8 hours after dose administration

Additional Information Sodium ion concentration is not more than 200 mmol/L; the assayed amount of activity is stated on the label, but may vary depending on the type of assay and hemophilic substrate plasma used

Dosage Forms Powder for injection, lyophilized: 400-700 porcine units to be reconstituted with 20 mL sterile water

Antihist-1® [OTC] *see* Clemastine *on page 289*

Anti-Inhibitor Coagulant Complex

(an tee-in HI bi tor coe AG yoo lant KOM pleks)

Brand Names Autoplex T®; Feiba VH Immuno®

Synonyms Coagulant Complex Inhibitor

Therapeutic Category Antihemophilic Agent; Blood Product Derivative

Use Patients with factor VIII inhibitors who are to undergo surgery or those who are bleeding

Pregnancy Risk Factor C

Contraindications Disseminated intravascular coagulation; patients with normal coagulation mechanism

Warnings/Precautions Products are prepared from pooled human plasma; such plasma may contain the causative agents of viral diseases. Tests used to control efficacy such as APTT, WBCT, and TEG do not correlate with clinical efficacy. Dosing to normalize these values may result in DIC. Identification of the clotting deficiency as caused by factor VIII inhibitors is essential prior to starting therapy. Use with extreme caution in patients with impaired hepatic function.

Adverse Reactions

<1%:

Cardiovascular: Hypotension, flushing
Central nervous system: Fever, headache, chills
Dermatologic: Rash, urticaria
Hematologic: Disseminated intravascular coagulation
Miscellaneous: Anaphylaxis, indications of protein sensitivity

Overdosage/Toxicology Rapid infusion may cause hypotension, excessive administration can cause DIC

Stability Store at 2°C to 8°C (36°F to 46°F); use within 1-3 hours after reconstitution

Usual Dosage Dosage range: 25-100 factor VIII correctional units per kg depending on the severity of hemorrhage

Test Interactions ↑ ↓ PT, ↑ ↓ PTT, ↓ WBCT, ↓ fibrin, ↓ platelets, ↑ fibrin split products

Nursing Implications Monitor for hypotension, may reinitiate infusion at a slower rate; have epinephrine ready to treat hypersensitivity reactions

Dosage Forms Injection:

Autoplex T®, with heparin 2 units: Each bottle is labeled with correctional units of Factor VIII

Feiba VH Immuno®, heparin free: Each bottle is labeled with correctional units of Factor VIII

Antilirium® *see* Physostigmine *on page 997*
Antimicrobial Drugs of Choice *see page 1468*
Antimicrobial Prophylaxis *see page 1445*
Antiminth® [OTC] *see* Pyrantel Pamoate *on page 1076*
Antipsychotic Agents Comparison *see page 1396*
Antispas® Injection *see* Dicyclomine *on page 376*

Antithrombin III (an tee THROM bin three)

Brand Names ATnativ®; Thrombate III®

Synonyms ATIII; Heparin Cofactor I

Therapeutic Category Anticoagulant; Blood Product Derivative

Use Agent for hereditary antithrombin III deficiency

Unlabeled use: Has been used effectively for acquired antithrombin III deficiencies related to DIC, pre-eclampsia, liver disease, shock and surgery complicated by DIC

Pregnancy Risk Factor C

Contraindications Hypersensitivity to any component

Warnings/Precautions Test methods and treatment methods may not totally eradicate HBAg and HIV from pooled plasma used in processing of this product

Adverse Reactions

<1%:

Central nervous system: Dizziness, lightheadedness, fever
Cardiovascular: Chest tightness, chest pain, vasodilatory effects, edema
Dermatologic: Urticaria
Endocrine & metabolic: Fluid overload
Gastrointestinal: Nausea, foul taste in mouth, cramps, bowel fullness
Hematologic: Hematoma formation
Ocular: Film over eye
Renal: Diuretic effects
Respiratory: Shortness of breath

Overdosage/Toxicology Levels of 150% to 200% have been documented in patients with no signs or symptoms of complications

Drug Interactions Increased toxicity: Anticoagulation effect of heparin is enhanced

Stability Reconstitute with 10 mL sterile water for injection, normal saline or D_5W; **do not shake**; stability of I.V. admixture: 24 hours at room temperature; do not refrigerate

Mechanism of Action Antithrombin III is the primary physiologic inhibitor of *in vivo* coagulation. It is an alpha$_2$-globulin. Its principal actions are the inactivation of thrombin, plasmin, and other active serine proteases of coagulation, including factors IXa, Xa, XIa, XIIa, and VIIa. The inactivation of proteases is a major step in the normal clotting process. The strong activation of clotting enzymes at the site of every bleeding injury facilitates fibrin formation and maintains normal hemostasis. Thrombosis in the circulation would be caused by active serine proteases if they were not inhibited by antithrombin III after the localized clotting process. Patients with congenital deficiency are in a prethrombotic state, even if asymptomatic, as evidenced by elevated plasma levels of prothrombin activation fragment, which are normalized following infusions of antithrombin III concentrate.

(Continued)

Antithrombin III *(Continued)*

Usual Dosage After first dose of antithrombin III, level should increase to 120% of normal; thereafter maintain at levels >80%. Generally, achieved by administration of maintenance doses once every 24 hours; initially and until patient is stabilized, measure antithrombin III level at least twice daily, thereafter once daily and always immediately before next infusion. 1 unit = quantity of antithrombin III in 1 mL of normal pooled human plasma; administration of 1 unit/1 kg raises AT-III level by 1% to 2%; assume plasma volume of 40 mL/kg

Initial dosage (units) = [desired AT-III level % - baseline AT-III level %] x body weight (kg) divided by 1%/units/kg, eg, if a 70 kg adult patient had a baseline AT-III level of 57%, the initial dose would be (120% - 57%) x 70/1%/units/kg = 4,410 units

Measure antithrombin III preceding and 30 minutes after dose to calculate *in vivo* recovery rate; maintain level within normal range for 2-8 days depending on type of surgery or procedure

Administration Infuse over 5-10 minutes; rate of infusion is 50 units/minute (1 mL/minute) not to exceed 100 units/minute (2 mL/minute)

Monitoring Parameters Monitor antithrombin III levels during treatment period

Reference Range Maintain antithrombin III level in plasma >80%

Dosage Forms Powder for injection: 500 units (50 mL)

Antithymocyte Globulin (Equine) *see* Lymphocyte Immune Globulin *on page 749*

Antithymocyte Immunoglobulin *see* Lymphocyte Immune Globulin *on page 749*

Anti-Tuss® Expectorant [OTC] *see* Guaifenesin *on page 589*

Antivert® *see* Meclizine *on page 769*

Antrizine® *see* Meclizine *on page 769*

Anturane® *see* Sulfinpyrazone *on page 1178*

Anucort-HC® *see* Hydrocortisone *on page 623*

Anumed HC™ *see* Hydrocortisone *on page 623*

Anusol-HC® [OTC] *see* Hydrocortisone *on page 623*

Anusol® Ointment [OTC] *see* Pramoxine *on page 1033*

Anxanil® *see* Hydroxyzine *on page 634*

Apacet® [OTC] *see* Acetaminophen *on page 19*

APAP *see* Acetaminophen *on page 19*

Aphthasol® *see* Amlexanox *on page 71*

A.P.L.® *see* Chorionic Gonadotropin *on page 272*

Aplisol® *see* Tuberculin Purified Protein Derivative *on page 1276*

Aplitest® *see* Tuberculin Purified Protein Derivative *on page 1276*

Aplonidine *see* Apraclonidine *on this page*

APPG *see* Penicillin G Procaine *on page 964*

Apraclonidine (a pra KLOE ni deen)

Brand Names Iopidine®

Synonyms Aplonidine; Apraclonidine Hydrochloride; p-Aminoclonidine

Therapeutic Category $Alpha_2$-Adrenergic Agonist Agent, Ophthalmic; Sympathomimetic Agent, Ophthalmic

Use Prevention and treatment of postsurgical intraocular pressure elevation

Pregnancy Risk Factor C

Contraindications Known hypersensitivity to apraclonidine or clonidine

Warnings/Precautions Closely monitor patients who develop exaggerated reductions in intraocular pressure; use with caution in patients with cardiovascular disease and in patients with a history of vasovagal reactions

Adverse Reactions

1% to 10%:

- Central nervous system: Lethargy
- Gastrointestinal: Xerostomia
- Ocular: Upper lid elevation, conjunctival blanching, mydriasis, burning and itching eyes, discomfort, conjunctival microhemorrhage, blurred vision
- Respiratory: Dry nose

<1%:

- Sensitivity reactions: Allergic response
- Miscellaneous: Some systemic effects have also been reported including GI, CNS, and cardiovascular symptoms (arrhythmias)

Drug Interactions Increased effect: Topical beta-blockers, pilocarpine → additive ↓ intraocular pressure

Stability Store in tight, light-resistant containers

Mechanism of Action Apraclonidine is a potent alpha-adrenergic agent similar to clonidine; relatively selective for $alpha_2$-receptors but does retain some binding to $alpha_1$-receptors; appears to result in reduction of aqueous humor formation;

its penetration through the blood-brain barrier is more polar than clonidine which reduces its penetration through the blood-brain barrier and suggests that its pharmacological profile is characterized by peripheral rather than central effects.

Pharmacodynamics/Kinetics
Onset of action: 1 hour
Maximum IOP: 3-5 hours

Usual Dosage Adults: Ophthalmic: Instill 1 drop in operative eye 1 hour prior to laser surgery, second drop in eye upon completion of procedure

Monitoring Parameters Closely monitor patients who develop exaggerated reductions in intraocular pressure

Dosage Forms Solution, ophthalmic, as hydrochloride: 0.5% (5 mL); 1% (0.1 mL, 0.25 mL)

Apraclonidine Hydrochloride *see* Apraclonidine *on previous page*

Apresoline® *see* Hydralazine *on page 615*

Aprodine® Syrup [OTC] *see* Triprolidine and Pseudoephedrine *on page 1270*

Aprodine® Tablet [OTC] *see* Triprolidine and Pseudoephedrine *on page 1270*

Aprotinin (a proe TYE nin)

Brand Names Trasylol®

Therapeutic Category Blood Product Derivative; Hemostatic Agent

Use Reduction or prevention of blood loss in patients undergoing coronary artery bypass surgery when a high risk of excessive bleeding exists; this includes open heart reoperation, pre-existing coagulopathies, operations on the great vessels, and when a patient's beliefs prohibit blood transfusions

Pregnancy Risk Factor C

Contraindications Hypersensitivity to aprotinin or any component, patients with thromboembolic disease requiring anticoagulants or blood factor administration

Warnings/Precautions Patients with a previous exposure to aprotinin are at an increased risk of hypersensitivity reactions

Adverse Reactions
1% to 10%
Cardiovascular: Atrial fibrillation, myocardial infarction, heart failure, atrial flutter, ventricular tachycardia, hypotension
Central nervous system: Fever, mental confusion
Local: Phlebitis
Renal: Increased potential for postoperative renal dysfunction
Respiratory: Dyspnea, bronchoconstriction
<1%:
Cardiovascular: Cerebral embolism, cerebrovascular events
Central nervous system: Convulsions
Hematologic: Hemolysis
Hepatic: Liver damage
Respiratory: Pulmonary edema
Miscellaneous: Anaphylactic reactions have been reported in <0.5% of recipients, such reactions are more likely with repeated administration

Overdosage/Toxicology Maximum amount of aprotinin that can safely be given has not yet been determined. One case report of aprotinin overdose was associated with the development of hepatic and renal failure and eventually death. Autopsy demonstrated severe hepatic necrosis and extensive renal tubular and glomerular necrosis. The relationship with these findings and aprotinin remains unclear.

Drug Interactions
Decreased effect: Fibrinolytic effects of streptokinase or anistreplase decrease effects of captopril
Increased effect: Heparin's whole blood clotting time may be prolonged; use with succinylcholine can produce prolonged or recurring apnea

Stability Vials should be stored between 2°C and 25°C and protected from freezing; it is **incompatible** with corticosteroids, heparin, tetracyclines, amino acid solutions, and fat emulsion

Mechanism of Action Serine protease inhibitor; inhibits plasmin, kallikrein, and platelet activation producing antifibrinolytic effects; a weak inhibitor of plasma pseudocholinesterase. It also inhibits the contact phase activation of coagulation and preserves adhesive platelet glycoproteins making them resistant to damage from increased circulating plasmin or mechanical injury occurring during bypass

Pharmacodynamics/Kinetics
Half-life: 150 minutes
Elimination: By the kidney

Usual Dosage
Test dose: **All** patients should receive a 1 mL I.V. test dose at least 10 minutes prior to the loading dose to assess the potential for allergic reactions
Regimen A (standard dose):
2 million units (280 mg) loading dose I.V. over 20-30 minutes
(Continued)

Aprotinin *(Continued)*

2 million units (280 mg) into pump prime volume
500,000 units/hour (70 mg/hour) I.V. during operation

Regimen B (low dose):

1 million units (140 mg) loading dose I.V. over 20-30 minutes
1 million units (140 mg) into pump prime volume
250,000 units/hour (35 mg/hour) I.V. during operation

Administration All intravenous doses should be administered through a central line

Monitoring Parameters Bleeding times, prothrombin time, activated clotting time, platelet count, red blood cell counts, hematocrit, hemoglobin and fibrinogen degradation products; for toxicity also include renal function tests and blood pressure

Reference Range Antiplasmin effects occur when plasma aprotinin concentrations are 125 KIU/mL and antikallikrein effects occur when plasma levels are 250-500 KIU/mL; it remains unknown if these plasma concentrations are required for clinical benefits to occur during cardiopulmonary bypass

Test Interactions Aprotinin prolongs whole blood clotting time of heparinized blood as determined by the Hemochrom® method or similar surface activation methods. Patients may require additional heparin even in the presence of activated clotting time levels that appear to represent adequate anticoagulation.

Dosage Forms Injection: 1.4 mg/mL [10,000 units/mL] (100 mL, 200 mL)

APSAC *see* Anistreplase *on page 92*

Aquacare® [OTC] *see* Urea *on page 1280*

Aquachloral® Supprettes® *see* Chloral Hydrate *on page 247*

AquaMEPHYTON® *see* Phytonadione *on page 998*

Aquaphyllin® *see* Theophylline Salts *on page 1207*

Aquasol A® *see* Vitamin A *on page 1307*

Aquasol E® [OTC] *see* Vitamin E *on page 1309*

Aquatag® *see* Benzthiazide *on page 141*

Aquatensen® *see* Methyclothiazide *on page 813*

Aqueous Procaine Penicillin G *see* Penicillin G Procaine *on page 964*

Aqueous Testosterone *see* Testosterone *on page 1198*

Aquest® *see* Estrone *on page 474*

Ara-A *see* Vidarabine *on page 1300*

Arabinofuranosyladenine *see* Vidarabine *on page 1300*

Arabinosylcytosine *see* Cytarabine *on page 332*

Ara-C *see* Cytarabine *on page 332*

Aralen® Phosphate *see* Chloroquine Phosphate *on page 256*

Aralen® Phosphate With Primaquine Phosphate *see* Chloroquine and Primaquine *on page 255*

Aramine® *see* Metaraminol *on page 794*

Arduan® *see* Pipecuronium *on page 1003*

Aredia™ *see* Pamidronate *on page 947*

Argesic®-SA *see* Salsalate *on page 1122*

Arginine (AR ji neen)

Brand Names R-Gene®

Synonyms Arginine Hydrochloride

Therapeutic Category Diagnostic Agent, Pituitary Function; Metabolic Alkalosis Agent

Use Pituitary function test (growth hormone); management of severe, uncompensated, metabolic alkalosis (pH ≥7.55) **after** optimizing therapy with sodium and potassium supplements

Pregnancy Risk Factor C

Contraindications Known hypersensitivity to arginine; renal or hepatic failure

Warnings/Precautions Arginine may elevate blood urea nitrogen and cause severe hyperkalemia (due to rapid intracellular potassium displacement) in patients with renal dysfunction; serum potassium concentrations must be monitored during arginine administration. Arginine hydrochloride can be metabolized to nitrogen containing products for excretion; temporary effect of a high nitrogen load on the kidneys should be evaluated. Administer with caution due to high chloride (0.475 mEq/mL) content; have agents available (antihistamines) in the event of an allergic reaction; rapid I.V. infusion may produce local irritation, flushing, nausea or vomiting.

Adverse Reactions

1% to 10%:

Cardiovascular: Rapid I.V. infusion may produce flushing
Central nervous system: Headache

Gastrointestinal: Nausea, vomiting
Local: Venous irritation
Neuromuscular & skeletal: Numbness

<1%:
Endocrine & metabolic: Hyperglycemia, hyperkalemia, increased serum gastrin concentration, hyperchloremia
Gastrointestinal: Abdominal pain, bloating

Drug Interactions

Increased toxicity:
Estrogen-progesterone combinations (↑ growth hormone response and ↓ glucagon and insulin effects)
Spironolactone (potentially fatal hyperkalemia has been reported)

Stability Store at room temperature

Mechanism of Action

Stimulates pituitary release of growth hormone and prolactin through origins in the hypothalamus; patients with impaired pituitary function have lower or no increase in plasma concentrations of growth hormone after administration of arginine. Arginine hydrochloride has been used for severe metabolic alkalosis due to its high chloride content.

Arginine hydrochloride has been used investigationally to treat metabolic alkalosis. Arginine contains 475 mEq of hydrogen ions and 475 mEq of chloride ions/L. Arginine is metabolized by the liver to produce hydrogen ions. It may be used in patients with relative hepatic insufficiency because arginine combines with ammonia in the body to produce urea.

Pharmacodynamics/Kinetics

Absorption: Oral: Well absorbed
Time to peak serum concentration: Within 2 hours

Usual Dosage I.V.:

Pituitary function test:
Children: 500 mg kg/dose administered over 30 minutes
Adults: 30 g (300 mL) administered over 30 minutes

Metabolic alkalosis: Children and Adults: Arginine hydrochloride is a fourth-line treatment for uncompensated metabolic alkalosis after sodium chloride, potassium chloride, and ammonium chloride supplementation has been optimized.
Arginine dose (G) = weight (kg) x 0.1 x ($HC03^-$ - 24) where $HC03^-$ = the patient's serum bicarbonate concentration in mEq/L
Administer ½ to ⅓ dose calculated then re-evaluate
Note: Arginine hydrochloride should never be used as an alternative to chloride supplementation but used in the patient who is unresponsive to sodium chloride or potassium chloride supplementation

Hypochloremia: Children and Adults: Arginine dose (mL) = 0.4 x weight (kg) x (103-Cl^-) where Cl^- = the patient's serum chloride concentration in mEq/L
Give ½ to ⅓ dose calculated then re-evaluate

Administration Administer by central line only

Monitoring Parameters Acid-base status (arterial or capillary blood gases), serum electrolytes (sodium, potassium, chloride, HCO_3), BUN, glucose. Arginine may elevate blood urea nitrogen and cause severe hyperkalemia (due to rapid intracellular potassium displacement) in patients with renal dysfunction. Serum potassium concentrations must be monitored during arginine administration.

Nursing Implications Leakage of I.V. arginine may cause necrosis and phlebitis

Additional Information Chloride content: 47.5 mEq/100 mL; 950 mOsmol/L

Dosage Forms Injection, as hydrochloride: 10% [100 mg/mL = 950 mOsm/L] (500 mL)

Arginine Hydrochloride *see* Arginine *on previous page*
8-Arginine Vasopressin *see* Vasopressin *on page 1293*
Aricept® *see* Donepezil *on page 416*
Arimidex® *see* Anastrozole *on page 90*
Aristocort® *see* Triamcinolone *on page 1255*
Aristocort® A *see* Triamcinolone *on page 1255*
Aristocort® Forte *see* Triamcinolone *on page 1255*
Aristocort® Intralesional *see* Triamcinolone *on page 1255*
Aristospan® Intra-Articular *see* Triamcinolone *on page 1255*
Aristospan® Intralesional *see* Triamcinolone *on page 1255*
Arm-a-Med® Isoetharine *see* Isoetharine *on page 678*
Arm-a-Med® Isoproterenol *see* Isoproterenol *on page 681*
Arm-a-Med® Metaproterenol *see* Metaproterenol *on page 793*
Armour® Thyroid *see* Thyroid *on page 1223*
Arrestin® *see* Trimethobenzamide *on page 1265*
Artane® *see* Trihexyphenidyl *on page 1263*
Artha-G® *see* Salsalate *on page 1122*

Arthropan® [OTC] *see* Choline Salicylate *on page 271*
Articulose-50® *see* Prednisolone *on page 1037*
ASA *see* Aspirin *on page 106*
A.S.A. [OTC] *see* Aspirin *on page 106*
5-ASA *see* Mesalamine *on page 787*
Asacol® *see* Mesalamine *on page 787*

Ascorbic Acid (a SKOR bik AS id)

Brand Names Ascorbicap® [OTC]; C-Crystals® [OTC]; Cebid® Timecelles® [OTC]; Cecon® [OTC]; Cevalin® [OTC]; Cevi-Bid® [OTC]; Ce-Vi-Sol® [OTC]; Dull-C® [OTC]; Flavorcee® [OTC]; N'ice® Vitamin C Drops [OTC]; Vita-C® [OTC]

Canadian/Mexican Brand Names Apo-C® (Canada); Ascorbic® 500 (Canada); Redoxon® (Canada); Revitalose® C-1000® (Canada); Ce-Vi-Sol® (Mexico); Redoxon® Forte (Mexico)

Synonyms Vitamin C

Therapeutic Category Urinary Acidifying Agent; Vitamin, Water Soluble

Use Prevention and treatment of scurvy and to acidify the urine

Investigational: In large doses to decrease the severity of "colds"; dietary supplementation; a 20-year study was recently completed involving 730 individuals which indicates a possible decreased risk of death by stroke when ascorbic acid at doses of ≥45 mg/day was administered

Pregnancy Risk Factor A (C if used in doses above RDA recommendation)

Contraindications Large doses during pregnancy

Warnings/Precautions Diabetics and patients prone to recurrent renal calculi (eg, dialysis patients) should not take excessive doses for extended periods of time

Adverse Reactions

1% to 10%: Renal: Hyperoxaluria

<1%:

- Cardiovascular: Flushing
- Central nervous system: Faintness, dizziness, headache, fatigue
- Gastrointestinal: Nausea, vomiting, heartburn, diarrhea
- Neuromuscular & skeletal: Flank pain

Overdosage/Toxicology Symptoms of overdose include renal calculi, nausea, gastritis, diarrhea; diuresis with forced fluids may be useful following a massive ingestion

Drug Interactions

Decreased effect:

- Ascorbic acid decreases propranolol peak (maximum) serum concentration and AUC and increases the T_{max} significantly, resulting in increased bradycardia, possibly due to decreased absorption and first-pass metabolism (n=5)
- Aspirin decreases ascorbate levels, increases aspirin
- Fluphenazine decreases fluphenazine levels
- Warfarin decreases effect

Increased effect: Iron enhances absorption; oral contraceptives increase contraceptive effect

Stability Injectable form should be stored under refrigeration (2°C to 8°C); protect oral dosage forms from light; is rapidly oxidized when in solution in air and alkaline media

Mechanism of Action Not fully understood; necessary for collagen formation and tissue repair; involved in some oxidation-reduction reactions as well as other metabolic pathways, such as synthesis of carnitine, steroids, and catecholamines and conversion of folic acid to folinic acid

Pharmacodynamics/Kinetics

Absorption: Oral: Readily absorbed; an active process and is thought to be dose-dependent

Distribution: Widely distributed

Metabolism: In the liver by oxidation and sulfation

Elimination: In urine; there is an individual specific renal threshold for ascorbic acid; when blood levels are high, ascorbic acid is excreted in the urine; whereas when the levels are subthreshold, very little if any ascorbic acid is cleared into the urine

Usual Dosage Oral, I.M., I.V., S.C.:

Recommended daily allowance (RDA):

- <6 months: 30 mg
- 6 months to 1 year: 35 mg
- 1-3 years: 40 mg
- 4-10 years: 45 mg
- 11-14 years: 50 mg
- >14 years and Adults: 60 mg

Children:
- Scurvy: 100-300 mg/day in divided doses for at least 2 weeks
- Urinary acidification: 500 mg every 6-8 hours
- Dietary supplement: 35-100 mg/day

Adults:
- Scurvy: 100-250 mg 1-2 times/day for at least 2 weeks
- Urinary acidification: 4-12 g/day in 3-4 divided doses
- Prevention and treatment of colds: 1-3 g/day
- Dietary supplement: 50-200 mg/day

Administration Avoid rapid I.V. injection

Monitoring Parameters Monitor pH of urine when using as an acidifying agent

Test Interactions False-positive urinary glucose with cupric sulfate reagent, false-negative urinary glucose with glucose oxidase method; false-negative stool occult blood 48-72 hours after ascorbic acid ingestion

Patient Information Do not take more than the recommended dose; take with plenty of water; report any pain on urination

Additional Information Sodium content of 1 g: ~5 mEq

Dosage Forms

Capsule, timed release: 500 mg
Crystals: 4 g/teaspoonful (100 g, 500 g); 5 g/teaspoonful (180 g)
Injection: 250 mg/mL (2 mL, 30 mL); 500 mg/mL (2 mL, 50 mL)
Liquid, oral: 35 mg/0.6 mL (50 mL)
Lozenges: 60 mg
Powder: 4 g/teaspoonful (100 g, 500 g)
Solution, oral: 100 mg/mL (50 mL)
Syrup: 500 mg/5 mL (5 mL, 10 mL, 120 mL, 480 mL)
Tablet: 25 mg, 50 mg, 100 mg, 250 mg, 500 mg, 1000 mg
Tablet:
- Chewable: 100 mg, 250 mg, 500 mg
- Timed release: 500 mg, 1000 mg, 1500 mg

Ascorbicap® [OTC] *see* Ascorbic Acid *on previous page*
Ascriptin® [OTC] *see* Aspirin *on page 106*
Asendin® *see* Amoxapine *on page 75*
Asmalix® *see* Theophylline Salts *on page 1207*

Asparaginase (a SPIR a ji nase)

Related Information

Antiemetics for Chemotherapy Induced Nausea and Vomiting *on page 1348*
Cancer Chemotherapy Regimens *on page 1351*
Toxicities of Chemotherapeutic Agents *on page 1382*

Brand Names Elspar®; Erwiniar®

Synonyms L-asparaginase

Therapeutic Category Antineoplastic Agent, Miscellaneous; Protein Synthesis Inhibitor

Use Treatment of acute lymphocytic leukemia, lymphoma; used for induction therapy

Pregnancy Risk Factor C

Pregnancy/Breast-Feeding Implications Based on limited reports in humans, the use of asparaginase does not seem to pose a major risk to the fetus when used in the 2nd and 3rd trimesters, or when exposure occurs prior to conception in either females or males. Because of the teratogenicity observed in animals and the lack of human data after 1st trimester exposure, asparaginase should be used cautiously, if at all, during this period.

Contraindications Pancreatitis (active or any history of), hypersensitivity to asparaginase or any component; if a reaction occurs to Elspar®, obtain **Erwinia L-asparaginase** and use with caution

Warnings/Precautions The U.S. Food and Drug Administration (FDA) currently recommends that procedures for proper handling and disposal of antineoplastic agents be considered; monitor for severe allergic reactions; risk for hypersensitivity increases with successive doses

The following precautions should be taken when administering:

- Only administer in hospital setting
- Monitor blood pressure every 15 minutes for 1 hour
- Administer a small test dose first; the intradermal skin test is commonly given prior to the initial injection, using a dose of 0.1 mL of 20 unit/mL dilute solution (~2 units); the skin test site should be observed for at least 1 hour for a wheal or erythema; note that a negative skin test does not preclude the possibility of an allergic reaction; desensitization should be performed in patients who have been found to be hypersensitive by the intradermal skin test or who have received previous courses of therapy with the drug
- Have epinephrine, diphenhydramine, and hydrocortisone at the bedside

(Continued)

Asparaginase *(Continued)*

Have a running I.V. in place
A physician should be readily accessible
Avoid administering at night

Adverse Reactions

>10%:

Immediate effects: Fever, chills, nausea, and vomiting occur in 50% to 60% of patients

Gastrointestinal: Pancreatitis: Occurs in <15% of patients, but may progress to severe hemorrhagic pancreatitis

Emetic potential: Moderate (30% to 60%)

Renal: Prerenal azotemia

Miscellaneous: Hypersensitivity effects: Hypersensitivity and anaphylactic reactions occur in ~10% to 40% of patients and can be fatal; this reaction is more common in patients receiving asparaginase alone or by I.V. administration; hypersensitivity appears rarely with the first dose and more commonly after the second or third treatment; hypersensitivity may be treated with antihistamines and/or steroids; if an anaphylactic reaction occurs, a change in treatment to the *Erwinia* preparation may be made, since this preparation does not share antigenic cross-reactivity with the *E. coli* preparation; note that allergic reactions to the *Erwinia* preparation may also occur and ultimately develop in 5% to 20% of patients

1% to 10%:

Endocrine & metabolic: Hyperuricemia

Gastrointestinal: Mouth sores

<1%:

Cardiovascular: Hypotension, leg vein thrombosis

Central nervous system: Chills, malaise, disorientation, drowsiness, seizures, and coma which may be due to elevated NH_4 levels; hyperthermia, drowsiness, fever, hallucinations

Dermatologic: Rash, pruritus, urticaria

Endocrine & metabolic: Transient diabetes mellitus

Gastrointestinal: Weight loss

Hematologic: Inhibition of protein synthesis will cause a decrease in production of albumin, insulin (resulting in hyperglycemia), serum lipoprotein, antithrombin III, and clotting factors II, V, VII, VIII, IX, and X; the loss of the later two proteins may result in either thrombotic or hemorrhagic events; these protein losses occur in 100% of patients

Myelosuppressive effects: Myelosuppression is uncommon
WBC: Mild
Platelets: Mild
Onset (days): 7
Nadir (days): 14
Recovery (days): 21

Hepatic: Increases in serum bilirubin, SGOT, SGPT, alkaline phosphatase, and possible decrease in mobilization of lipids

Renal: Azotemia

Respiratory: Laryngeal spasm, coughing

Overdosage/Toxicology Symptoms of overdose include nausea, diarrhea

Drug Interactions

Decreased effect: Methotrexate: Asparaginase terminates methotrexate action by inhibition of protein synthesis and prevention of cell entry into the S phase

Increased toxicity:

Vincristine and prednisone: An ↑ toxicity has been noticed when asparaginase is administered with VCR and prednisone
Cyclophosphamide (↓ metabolism)
Mercaptopurine (↑ hepatotoxicity)
Vincristine (↑ neuropathy)
Prednisone (↑ hyperglycemia)

Stability Intact vials of powder should be refrigerated (<8°C); lyophilized powder should be reconstituted with 1-5 mL sterile water for I.V. administration or NS for I.M. use, reconstituted solutions are stable 1 week at room temperature; shake well but not too vigorously; use of a 5 micron in-line filter is recommended to remove fiber-like particles in the solution (not 0.2 micron filter - has been associated with some loss of potency)

Standard I.M. dilution:

5000 IU/mL: 2 mL/syringe

Usually no >2 mL/injection site, however, contact RN first to clarify administration route.

Standard I.V. dilution:

Dose/50-250 mL NS or D_5W

Stable for 8 hours at room temperature or refrigeration

Mechanism of Action Some malignant cells (ie, lymphoblastic leukemia cells and those of lymphocyte derivation) must acquire the amino acid asparagine from surrounding fluid such as blood, whereas normal cells can synthesize their own asparagine. Asparaginase is an enzyme that deaminates asparagine to aspartic acid and ammonia in the plasma and extracellular fluid and therefore deprives tumor cells of the amino acid for protein synthesis.

There are two purified preparations of the enzyme: one from *Escherichia coli* and one from *Erwinia carotovora.* These two preparations vary slightly in the gene sequencing and have slight differences in enzyme characteristics. Both are highly specific for asparagine and have less than 10% activity for the D-isomer. The preparation from *E. coli* has had the most use in clinical and research practice.

Pharmacodynamics/Kinetics

Absorption: Not absorbed from GI tract, therefore, requires parenteral administration; I.M. administration produces peak blood levels 50% lower than those from I.V. administration (I.M. may be less immunogenic)

Distribution: V_d: 4-5 L/kg; 70% to 80% of plasma volume; does not penetrate the CSF

Metabolism: Systemically degraded, only trace amounts are found in the urine

Half-life: 8-30 hours

Elimination: Clearance unaffected by age, renal function, or hepatic function

Usual Dosage Refer to individual protocols; dose must be individualized based upon clinical response and tolerance of the patient

I.M. administration is **preferred** over I.V. administration; I.M. administration may decrease the risk of anaphylaxis

Asparaginase is available from 2 different microbiological sources: One is from *Escherichia coli* and the other is from *Erwinia carotovora*; the *Erwinia* is restricted to patients who have sustained allergic reactions to the *E. coli* preparation

I.M., I.V.: 6000 units/m^2 every other day for 3-4 weeks or daily doses of 1000-20,000 units/m^2 for 10-20 days; other induction regimens have been utilized

Hemodialysis: Significant drug removal is unlikely based on physiochemical characteristics

Peritoneal dialysis: Significant drug removal is unlikely based on physiochemical characteristics

Desensitization should be performed before administering the first dose of asparaginase to patients who developed a positive reaction to the intradermal skin test or who are being retreated; one schedule begins with a total of 1 unit given I.V. and doubles the dose every 10 minutes until the total amount given in the planned dose for that day

Asparaginase Desensitization

Injection No.	Elspar Dose (IU)	Accumulated Total Dose
1	1	1
2	2	3
3	4	7
4	8	15
5	16	31
6	32	63
7	64	127
8	128	255
9	256	511
10	512	1,023
11	1,024	2,047
12	2,048	4,095
13	4,096	8,191
14	8,192	16,383
15	16,384	32,767
16	32,768	65,535
17	65,536	131,071
18	131,072	262,143

For example, if a patient was to receive a total dose of 4000 units, he/she would receive injections 1 through 12 during the desensitization

Administration Must only be given as a deep intramuscular injection into a large muscle; use two injection sites for I.M. doses >2 mL

(Continued)

Asparaginase *(Continued)*

May be administered I.V. infusion in 50 mL of D_5W or NS over more than 30 minutes; a small test dose (0.1 mL of a dilute 20 unit/mL solution) should be given first

Occasionally, gelatinous fiber-like particles may develop on standing; filtration through a 5 micron filter during administration will remove the particles with no loss of potency; some loss of potency has been observed with the use of a 0.2 micron filter

Monitoring Parameters Vital signs during administration, CBC, urinalysis, amylase, liver enzymes, prothrombin time, renal function tests, urine dipstick for glucose, blood glucose, uric acid

Test Interactions ↓ thyroxine and thyroxine-binding globulin

Patient Information Drowsiness may occur during therapy; nausea or vomiting may interrupt dosing schedule initially

Nursing Implications Appropriate agents for maintenance of an adequate airway and treatment of a hypersensitivity reaction (antihistamine, epinephrine, oxygen, I.V. corticosteroids) should be readily available. Be prepared to treat anaphylaxis at each administration; monitor for onset of abdominal pain and mental status changes.

Dosage Forms Injection:
10,000 units/10 mL
10,000 units/vial (*Erwinia*)

A-Spas® S/L *see* Hyoscyamine *on page 635*

Aspergum® [OTC] *see* Aspirin *on this page*

Aspirin (AS pir in)

Related Information

Dosing Data for Acetaminophen and NSAIDs *on page 1377*

Brand Names Anacin® [OTC]; A.S.A. [OTC]; Ascriptin® [OTC]; Aspergum® [OTC]; Bayer® Aspirin [OTC]; Bufferin® [OTC]; Easprin®; Ecotrin® [OTC]; Empirin® [OTC]; Measurin® [OTC]; Synalgos® [OTC]; ZORprin®

Canadian/Mexican Brand Names ASA® (Canada); Apo-ASA® (Canada); Asaphen® (Canada); Entrophen® (Canada); MSD® Enteric Coated ASA (Canada); Novasen (Canada)

Synonyms Acetylsalicylic Acid; ASA

Therapeutic Category Analgesic, Salicylate; Anti-inflammatory Agent; Antipyretic; Nonsteroidal Anti-inflammatory Agent (NSAID), Oral; Salicylate

Use Treatment of mild to moderate pain, inflammation, and fever; may be used as a prophylaxis of myocardial infarction and transient ischemic episodes; management of rheumatoid arthritis, rheumatic fever, osteoarthritis, and gout (high dose)

Pregnancy Risk Factor C (D if full-dose aspirin in 3rd trimester)

Contraindications Bleeding disorders (factor VII or IX deficiencies), hypersensitivity to salicylates or other NSAIDs, tartrazine dye and asthma

Warnings/Precautions Use with caution in patients with platelet and bleeding disorders, renal dysfunction, erosive gastritis, or peptic ulcer disease, previous nonreaction does not guarantee future safe taking of medication; do not use aspirin in children <16 years of age for chickenpox or flu symptoms due to the association with Reye's syndrome

Otic: Discontinue use if dizziness, tinnitus, or impaired hearing occurs; surgical patients: avoid ASA if possible, for 1 week prior to surgery because of the possibility of postoperative bleeding; use with caution in impaired hepatic function

Elderly are a high-risk population for adverse effects from nonsteroidal anti-inflammatory agents. As much as 60% of elderly with GI complications to NSAIDs can develop peptic ulceration and/or hemorrhage asymptomatically. Also, concomitant disease and drug use contribute to the risk for GI adverse effects. Use lowest effective dose for shortest period possible. Consider renal function decline with age. Use of NSAIDs can compromise existing renal function especially when Cl_{cr} is <30 mL/minute. Tinnitus may be a difficult and unreliable indication of toxicity due to age-related hearing loss or eighth cranial nerve damage. CNS adverse effects such as confusion, agitation, and hallucination are generally seen in overdose or high-dose situations, but elderly may demonstrate these adverse effects at lower doses than younger adults.

Adverse Reactions

>10%: Gastrointestinal: Nausea, vomiting, dyspepsia, epigastric discomfort, heartburn, stomach pains

1% to 10%:
Central nervous system: Fatigue
Dermatologic: Rash, urticaria
Gastrointestinal: Gastrointestinal ulceration

Hematologic: Hemolytic anemia
Neuromuscular & skeletal: Weakness
Respiratory: Dyspnea
Miscellaneous: Anaphylactic shock

<1%:
Central nervous system: Insomnia, nervousness, jitters
Endocrine & metabolic: Iron deficiency
Hematologic: Occult bleeding, prolongation of bleeding time, leukopenia, thrombocytopenia, anemia
Hepatic: Hepatotoxicity
Renal: Impaired renal function
Respiratory: Bronchospasm

Overdosage/Toxicology Symptoms of overdose include tinnitus, headache, dizziness, confusion, metabolic acidosis, hyperpyrexia, hypoglycemia, coma. Treatment should also be based upon symptomatology.

Salicylates

Toxic Symptoms	Treatment
Overdose	Induce emesis with ipecac, and/or lavage with saline, followed with activated charcoal
Dehydration	I.V. fluids with KCl (no D_5W only)
Metabolic acidosis (must be treated)	Sodium bicarbonate
Hyperthermia	Cooling blankets or sponge baths
Coagulopathy/hemorrhage	Vitamin K I.V.
Hypoglycemia (with coma, seizures, or change in mental status)	Dextrose 25 g I.V.
Seizures	Diazepam 5-10 mg I.V.

Drug Interactions
Decreased effect: Possible decreased serum concentration of NSAIDs; aspirin may antagonize effects of probenecid
Increased toxicity: Aspirin may increase methotrexate serum levels and may displace valproic acid from binding sites which can result in toxicity; warfarin and aspirin may increase bleeding; NSAIDs and aspirin may increase GI adverse effects

Stability Keep suppositories in refrigerator, do not freeze; hydrolysis of aspirin occurs upon exposure to water or moist air, resulting in salicylate and acetate, which possess a vinegar-like odor; do not use if a strong odor is present

Mechanism of Action Inhibits prostaglandin synthesis, acts on the hypothalamus heat-regulating center to reduce fever, blocks prostaglandin synthetase action which prevents formation of the platelet-aggregating substance thromboxane A_2

Pharmacodynamics/Kinetics
Absorption: From stomach and small intestine
Distribution: Readily distributes into most body fluids and tissues
Metabolism: Hydrolyzed to salicylate (active) by esterases in the GI mucosa, red blood cells, synovial fluid and blood; metabolism of salicylate occurs primarily by hepatic microsomal enzymes; metabolic pathways are saturable
Half-life:
Parent drug: 15-20 minutes
Salicylates (dose-dependent): From 3 hours at lower doses (300-600 mg), to 5-6 hours (after 1 g) to 10 hours with higher doses
Time to peak serum concentration: ~1-2 hours

Usual Dosage
Children:
Analgesic and antipyretic: Oral, rectal: 10-15 mg/kg/dose every 4-6 hours, up to a total of 60-80 mg/kg/24 hours
Anti-inflammatory: Oral: Initial: 60-90 mg/kg/day in divided doses; usual maintenance: 80-100 mg/kg/day divided every 6-8 hours, maximum dose: 3.6 g/day; monitor serum concentrations
Kawasaki disease: Oral: 80-100 mg/kg/day divided every 6 hours; after fever resolves: 8-10 mg/kg/day once daily; monitor serum concentrations
Antirheumatic: Oral: 60-100 mg/kg/day in divided doses every 4 hours

Adults:
Analgesic and antipyretic: Oral, rectal: 325-650 mg every 4-6 hours up to 4 g/day
Anti-inflammatory: Oral: Initial: 2.4-3.6 g/day in divided doses; usual maintenance: 3.6-5.4 g/day; monitor serum concentrations
TIA: Oral: 1.3 g/day in 2-4 divided doses
Myocardial infarction prophylaxis: 160-325 mg/day

Dosing adjustment in renal impairment: Cl_{cr} <10 mL/minute: Avoid use

(Continued)

Aspirin *(Continued)*

Hemodialysis: Dialyzable (50% to 100%)

Dosing adjustment in hepatic disease: Avoid use in severe liver disease

Dietary Considerations

Alcohol: Combination causes GI irritation, possible bleeding; avoid or limit alcohol. Patients at increased risk include those prone to hypoprothrombinemia, vitamin K deficiency, thrombocytopenia, thrombotic thrombocytopenia purpura, severe hepatic impairment, and those receiving anticoagulants.

Food: May decrease the rate but not the extent of oral absorption. Drug may cause GI upset, bleeding, ulceration, perforation. Take with food or large volume of water or milk to minimize GI upset.

Folic acid: Hyperexcretion of folate; folic acid deficiency may result, leading to macrocytic anemia. Supplement with folic acid if necessary.

Iron: With chronic use and at doses of 3-4 g/day, iron deficiency anemia may result; supplement with iron if necessary

Sodium: Hypernatremia resulting from buffered aspirin solutions or sodium salicylate containing high sodium content. Avoid or use with caution in CHF or any condition where hypernatremia would be detrimental.

Curry powder, paprika, licorice, Benedictine liqueur, prunes, raisins, tea and gherkins: Potential salicylate salicylate accumulation. These foods contain 6 mg salicylate/100 g. An ordinarily American diet contains 10-200 mg/day of salicylate. Foods containing salicylates may contribute to aspirin hypersensitivity. Patients at greatest risk for aspirin hypersensitivity include those with asthma, nasal polyposis or chronic urticaria.

Fresh fruits containing vitamin C: Displaces drug from binding sites, resulting in increased urinary excretion of aspirin. Educate patients regarding the potential for a decreased analgesic effect of aspirin with consumption of foods high in vitamin C.

Administration Administer with food or a full glass of water to minimize GI distress

Reference Range Timing of serum samples: Peak levels usually occur 2 hours after ingestion. Salicylate serum concentrations correlate with the pharmacological actions and adverse effects observed. See table.

Serum Salicylate: Clinical Correlations

Serum Salicylate Concentration (mcg/mL)	Desired Effects	Adverse Effects/Intoxication
~100	Antiplatelet Antipyresis Analgesia	GI intolerance and bleeding, hypersensitivity, hemostatic defects
150-300	Anti-inflammatory	Mild salicylism
250-400	Treatment of rheumatic fever	Nausea/vomiting, hyperventilation, salicylism, flushing, sweating, thirst, headache, diarrhea, and tachycardia
>400-500		Respiratory alkalosis, hemorrhage, excitement, confusion, asterixis, pulmonary edema, convulsions, tetany, metabolic acidosis, fever, coma, cardiovascular collapse, renal and respiratory failure

Test Interactions False-negative results for glucose oxidase urinary glucose tests (Clinistix®); false-positives using the cupric sulfate method (Clinitest®); also, interferes with Gerhardt test, VMA determination; 5-HIAA, xylose tolerance test and T_3 and T_4

Patient Information Watch for bleeding gums or any signs of GI bleeding; take with food or milk to minimize GI distress, notify physician if ringing in ears or persistent GI pain occurs; avoid other concurrent aspirin or salicylate-containing products

Nursing Implications Do not crush sustained release or enteric coated tablet

Dosage Forms

Capsule: 356.4 mg and caffeine 30 mg

Suppository, rectal: 60 mg, 120 mg, 125 mg, 130 mg, 195 mg, 200 mg, 300 mg, 325 mg, 600 mg, 650 mg, 1.2 g

Tablet: 65 mg, 75 mg, 81 mg, 325 mg, 500 mg

Tablet: 400 mg and caffeine 32 mg

Tablet:

Buffered: 325 mg and magnesium-aluminum hydroxide 150 mg; 325 mg, magnesium hydroxide 75 mg, aluminum hydroxide 75 mg, buffered with calcium carbonate; 325 mg and magnesium-aluminum hydroxide 75 mg

Chewable: 81 mg
Controlled release: 800 mg
Delayed release: 81 mg
Enteric coated: 81 mg, 325 mg, 500 mg, 650 mg, 975 mg
Gum: 227.5 mg
Timed release: 650 mg

Aspirin and Codeine (AS pir in & KOE deen)

Related Information

Dose Equivalents for Opioid Analgesics in Opioid-Naive Adults <50 kg *on page 1376*

Dose Equivalents for Opioid Analgesics in Opioid-Naive Adults ≥50 kg *on page 1375*

Brand Names Empirin® With Codeine

Canadian/Mexican Brand Names Coryphen® Codeine (Canada); 222® Tablets (Canada); 282® Tablets (Canada); 292® Tablets (Canada)

Synonyms Codeine and Aspirin

Therapeutic Category Analgesic, Narcotic

Use Relief of mild to moderate pain

Restrictions C-III

Pregnancy Risk Factor D

Contraindications Hypersensitivity to aspirin, codeine or any component; premature infants or during labor for delivery of a premature infant

Warnings/Precautions Use with caution in patients with impaired renal function, erosive gastritis, or peptic ulcer disease; children and teenagers should not use for chickenpox or flu symptoms before a physician is consulted about Reye's syndrome

Adverse Reactions

>10%:

- Central nervous system: Lightheadedness, dizziness, sedation
- Gastrointestinal: Nausea, heartburn, stomach pains, dyspepsia, epigastric discomfort, vomiting
- Respiratory: Shortness of breath

1% to 10%:

- Central nervous system: Fatigue, euphoria, dysphoria
- Dermatologic: Rash, pruritus
- Gastrointestinal: Gastrointestinal ulceration, constipation
- Hematologic: Hemolytic anemia
- Neuromuscular & skeletal: Weakness
- Respiratory: Dyspnea
- Miscellaneous: Anaphylactic shock

<1%:

- Cardiovascular: Palpitations, hypotension, bradycardia, peripheral vasodilation
- Central nervous system: Insomnia, nervousness, jitters, increased intracranial pressure
- Endocrine & metabolic: Antidiuretic hormone release, iron deficiency
- Gastrointestinal: Biliary tract spasm
- Genitourinary: Urinary retention
- Hematologic: Occult bleeding, prolongation of bleeding time, leukopenia, thrombocytopenia, anemia
- Hepatic: Hepatotoxicity
- Ocular: Miosis
- Renal: Impaired renal function
- Respiratory: Bronchospasm, respiratory depression
- Miscellaneous: Physical and psychological dependence

Overdosage/Toxicology Antidote is naloxone for codeine. Naloxone 2 mg I.V. (0.01 mg/kg for children) with repeat administration as necessary up to a total of 10 mg; see Aspirin monograph for treatment of aspirin toxicity.

Drug Interactions Refer to individual monographs for Aspirin and Codeine

Mechanism of Action Inhibits prostaglandin synthesis, acts on the hypothalamus heat-regulating center to reduce fever, blocks prostaglandin synthetase action which prevents formation of the platelet-aggregating substance thromboxane A_2; binds to opiate receptors in the CNS, causing inhibition of ascending pain pathways, altering the perception of and response to pain; causes cough supression by direct central action in the medulla; produces generalized CNS depression

Usual Dosage Oral:

Children:

- Aspirin: 10 mg/kg/dose every 4 hours
- Codeine: 0.5-1 mg/kg/dose every 4 hours

Adults: 1-2 tablets every 4-6 hours as needed for pain

(Continued)

Aspirin and Codeine *(Continued)*

Dosing adjustment in renal impairment:

Cl_{cr} 10-50 mL/minute: Administer 75% of dose

Cl_{cr} <10 mL/minute: Avoid use

Dosing interval in hepatic disease: Avoid use in severe liver disease

Dietary Considerations Alcohol: Additive CNS effects, avoid use

Administration Administer with food or a full glass of water to minimize GI distress

Monitoring Parameters Observe patient for excessive sedation, respiratory depression, pain relief, blood pressure, mental status

Test Interactions Urine glucose, urinary 5-HIAA, serum uric acid

Patient Information May cause drowsiness; avoid alcohol; watch for bleeding gums or any signs of GI bleeding; take with food or milk to minimize GI distress; notify physician if ringing in ears or persistent GI pain occurs

Dosage Forms Tablet:

#2: Aspirin 325 mg and codeine phosphate 15 mg

#3: Aspirin 325 mg and codeine phosphate 30 mg

#4: Aspirin 325 mg and codeine phosphate 60 mg

Assessment of Liver Function *see page 1343*

Assessment of Renal Function *see page 1344*

Astemizole (a STEM mi zole)

Brand Names Hismanal®

Canadian/Mexican Brand Names Adistan® (Mexico); Antagon-1® (Mexico); Astemina® (Mexico)

Therapeutic Category Antihistamine, H_1 Blocker; Antihistamine, H_1 Blocker, Nonsedating

Use Perennial and seasonal allergic rhinitis and other allergic symptoms including urticaria

Pregnancy Risk Factor C

Contraindications Hypersensitivity to astemizole or any component, concurrent use of erythromycin, quinine, ketoconazole or itraconazole, significant hepatic dysfunction

Warnings/Precautions Use with caution in patients receiving drugs which prolong QRS or Q-T interval; rare cases of severe cardiovascular events (cardiac arrest, arrhythmias) have been reported in the following situations: overdose (even as low as 20-30 mg/day), significant hepatic dysfunction, when used in combination with quinine, erythromycin, ketoconazole, or itraconazole; safety and efficacy in children <12 years of age have not been established; discontinue therapy immediately with signs of cardiotoxicity including syncope

Adverse Reactions

1% to 10%:

Central nervous system: Drowsiness, headache, fatigue, nervousness, dizziness

Gastrointestinal: Appetite increase, weight gain, nausea, diarrhea, abdominal pain, xerostomia

Neuromuscular & skeletal: Arthralgia

Respiratory: Pharyngitis

<1%:

Cardiovascular: Palpitations, edema

Central nervous system: Depression

Dermatologic: Angioedema, photosensitivity, rash

Hepatic: Hepatitis

Neuromuscular & skeletal: Myalgia, paresthesia

Respiratory: Bronchospasm, epistaxis

Miscellaneous: Thickening of mucous

Overdosage/Toxicology Symptoms of overdose include sedation, apnea, diminished mental alertness, ventricular tachycardia, torsade de pointes

There is not a specific treatment for an antihistamine overdose, however most of its clinical toxicity is due to anticholinergic effects. Anticholinesterase inhibitors including physostigmine, neostigmine, pyridostigmine and edrophonium may be useful for the overdose with severe life-threatening symptoms. Physostigmine 1-2 mg (0.5 or 0.02 mg/kg for children) I.V., slowly may be given to reverse the anticholinergic effects. Cases of ventricular arrhythmias following dosages >200 mg have been reported, however, overdoses of up to 500 mg have been reported without ill effect. Patients should be carefully observed with EKG monitoring in cases of suspected overdose. Magnesium may be helpful for torsade de pointes or a lidocaine bolus followed by a titrated infusion.

Drug Interactions Increased toxicity: CNS depressants (sedation), triazole antifungals, macrolide antibiotics and quinine may inhibit the metabolism of astemizole resulting in potentially life-threatening arrhythmias (torsade de pointes, etc.)

Mechanism of Action Competes with histamine for H_1-receptor sites on effector cells in the gastrointestinal tract, blood vessels, and respiratory tract; binds to lung receptors significantly greater than it binds to cerebellar receptors, resulting in a reduced sedative potential

Pharmacodynamics/Kinetics Long-acting, with steady-state plasma levels seen within 4-8 weeks following initiation of chronic therapy

Distribution: Nonsedating action reportedly due to the drug's low lipid solubility and poor penetration through the blood-brain barrier

Protein binding: 97%

Metabolism: Undergoes exclusive first-pass metabolism

Half-life: 20 hours

Time to peak serum concentration: Oral: Long-acting, with steady-state plasma levels of parent compound and metabolites seen within 4-8 weeks following initiation of chronic therapy; peak plasma levels appear in 1-4 hours following administration

Elimination: By metabolism in the liver to active and inactive metabolites, which are thereby excreted in feces and to a lesser degree in urine

Usual Dosage Oral:

Children:

- <6 years: 0.2 mg/kg/day
- 6-12 years: 5 mg/day

Children >12 years and Adults: 10-30 mg/day; administer 30 mg on first day, 20 mg on second day, then 10 mg/day in a single dose

Patient Information Take on an empty stomach at least 2 hours after a meal or 1 hour before a meal; may cause drowsiness; do not exceed recommended dose; notify physician or pharmacist if taking any heart medications. Because of its delayed onset, astemizole is useful for prophylaxis of allergic symptoms, rather than for acute relief.

Nursing Implications Raise bed rails at night; may need assistance with ambulation; administer on an empty stomach

Dosage Forms Tablet: 10 mg

Asthma, Guidelines for the Diagnosis and Management of *see page 1518*

AsthmaHaler® *see* Epinephrine *on page 448*

AsthmaNefrin® [OTC] *see* Epinephrine *on page 448*

Astramorph™ PF *see* Morphine Sulfate *on page 858*

Atarax® *see* Hydroxyzine *on page 634*

Atenolol (a TEN oh lole)

Related Information

Beta-Blockers Comparison *on page 1398*

Brand Names Tenormin®

Canadian/Mexican Brand Names Apo-Atenol® (Canada); Novo-Atenol® (Canada); Nu-Atenol® (Canada); Taro-Atenol® (Canada)

Therapeutic Category Antianginal Agent; Antihypertensive; Beta-Adrenergic Blocker

Use Treatment of hypertension, alone or in combination with other agents; management of angina pectoris, postmyocardial infarction patients

Unlabeled use: Acute alcohol withdrawal, supraventricular and ventricular arrhythmias, and migraine headache prophylaxis

Pregnancy Risk Factor C

Pregnancy/Breast-Feeding Implications

Clinical effects on the fetus: Crosses the placenta; persistent beta-blockade, bradycardia, IUGR; IUGR probably related to maternal hypertension. Available evidence suggest safe use during pregnancy and breast-feeding. Monitor breast-fed infant for symptoms of beta-blockade.

Breast-feeding/lactation: Crosses into breast milk.

Clinical effects on the infant: 1 report of symptoms of beta-blockade including cyanosis, hypothermia, bradycardia. American Academy of Pediatrics considers COMPATIBLE with breast-feeding.

Contraindications Hypersensitivity to beta-blocking agents, pulmonary edema, cardiogenic shock, bradycardia, heart block without a pacemaker, uncompensated congestive heart failure, sinus node dysfunction, A-V conduction abnormalities, diabetes mellitus

Warnings/Precautions Safety and efficacy in children have not been established; administer with caution to patients (especially the elderly) with bronchospastic disease, CHF, renal dysfunction, severe peripheral vascular disease, myasthenia gravis, diabetes mellitus, hyperthyroidism. **Abrupt withdrawal of the drug should be avoided,** drug should be discontinued over 1-2 weeks; may

(Continued)

Atenolol *(Continued)*

potentiate hypoglycemia in a diabetic patient and mask signs and symptoms; modify dosage in patients with renal impairment.

Adverse Reactions

1% to 10%:

Cardiovascular: Persistent bradycardia, hypotension, chest pain, edema, heart failure, second or third degree A-V block, Raynaud's phenomenon

Central nervous system: Dizziness, fatigue, insomnia, lethargy, confusion, mental impairment, depression, headache, nightmares

Gastrointestinal: Constipation, diarrhea, nausea

Genitourinary: Impotence

<1%:

Respiratory: Dyspnea (especially with large doses), wheezing

Miscellaneous: Cold extremities

Overdosage/Toxicology Symptoms of intoxication include cardiac disturbances, CNS toxicity, bronchospasm, hypoglycemia and hyperkalemia. The most common cardiac symptoms include hypotension and bradycardia; atrioventricular block, intraventricular conduction disturbances, cardiogenic shock, and systole may occur with severe overdose, especially with membrane-depressant drugs (eg, propranolol); CNS effects include convulsions, coma, and respiratory arrest (commonly seen with propranolol and other membrane-depressant and lipid-soluble drugs).

Treatment includes symptomatic treatment of seizures, hypotension, hyperkalemia, and hypoglycemia; bradycardia and hypotension resistant to atropine, isoproterenol, or pacing may respond to glucagon; wide QRS defects caused by the membrane-depressant poisoning may respond to hypertonic sodium bicarbonate; repeat-dose charcoal, hemoperfusion, or hemodialysis may be helpful in removal of only those beta-blockers with a small V_d, long half-life, or low intrinsic clearance (acebutolol, atenolol, nadolol, sotalol)

Drug Interactions

Decreased effect of beta-blockers with aluminum salts, barbiturates, calcium salts, cholestyramine, colestipol, NSAIDs, penicillins (ampicillin), rifampin, salicylates, and sulfinpyrazone due to decreased bioavailability and plasma levels

Beta-blockers may decrease the effect of sulfonylureas

Increased effect/toxicity of beta-blockers with calcium blockers (diltiazem, felodipine, nicardipine), contraceptives, flecainide, haloperidol (propranolol, hypotensive effects), H_2-antagonists (metoprolol, propranolol only by cimetidine, possibly ranitidine), hydralazine (metoprolol, propranolol), MAO inhibitors (metoprolol, nadolol, bradycardia), phenothiazines (propranolol), propafenone (metoprolol, propranolol), quinidine (in extensive metabolizers), ciprofloxacin, thyroid hormones (metoprolol, propranolol, when hypothyroid patient is converted to euthyroid state)

Beta-blockers may increase the effect/toxicity of flecainide, haloperidol (hypotensive effects), hydralazine, phenothiazines, acetaminophen, anticoagulants (propranolol, warfarin), benzodiazepines (not atenolol), clonidine (hypertensive crisis after or during withdrawal of either agent), epinephrine (initial hypertensive episode followed by bradycardia), nifedipine and verapamil lidocaine, ergots (peripheral ischemia), prazosin (postural hypotension)

Beta-blockers may affect the action or levels of ethanol, disopyramide, nondepolarizing muscle relaxants and theophylline although the effects are difficult to predict

Mechanism of Action Competitively blocks response to beta-adrenergic stimulation, selectively blocks $beta_1$-receptors with little or no effect on $beta_2$-receptors except at high doses

Pharmacodynamics/Kinetics

Absorption: Incomplete from GI tract

Distribution: Low lipophilicity; does **not** cross the blood-brain barrier

Protein binding: Low at 3% to 15%

Metabolism: Partial hepatic

Half-life, beta:

Neonates: Mean: 16 hours, up to 35 hours

Children: 4.6 hours; children >10 years of age may have longer half-life (>5 hours) compared to children 5-10 years of age (<5 hours)

Adults:

Normal renal function: 6-9 hours, longer in those with renal impairment

End stage renal disease: 15-35 hours

Time to peak: Oral: Within 2-4 hours

Elimination: 40% excreted as unchanged drug in urine, 50% in feces

Usual Dosage

Oral:

Children: 1-2 mg/kg/dose given daily

Adults:

Hypertension: 50 mg once daily, may increase to 100 mg/day; doses >100 mg are unlikely to produce any further benefit

Angina pectoris: 50 mg once daily, may increase to 100 mg/day; some patients may require 200 mg/day

Postmyocardial infarction: Follow I.V. dose with 100 mg/day or 50 mg twice daily for 6-9 days postmyocardial infarction

I.V.: Postmyocardial infarction: Early treatment: 5 mg slow I.V. over 5 minutes; may repeat in 10 minutes; if both doses are tolerated, may start oral atenolol 50 mg every 12 hours or 100 mg/day for 6-9 days postmyocardial infarction

Dosing interval in renal impairment:

Cl_{cr} 15-35 mL/minute: Administer 50 mg/day maximum

Cl_{cr} <15 mL/minute: Administer 50 mg every other day maximum

Hemodialysis: Moderately dialyzable (20% to 50%) via hemodialysis; administer dose postdialysis or administer 25-50 mg supplemental dose

Peritoneal dialysis: Elimination is not enhanced; supplemental dose is not necessary

Administration Administer I.V. at 1 mg/minute; intravenous administration requires a cardiac monitor and blood pressure monitor

Monitoring Parameters Monitor blood pressure, apical and radial pulses, fluid I & O, daily weight, respirations, and circulation in extremities before and during therapy

Test Interactions ↑ glucose; ↓ HDL

Patient Information Adhere to dosage regimen; watch for postural hypotension; **abrupt withdrawal of the drug should be avoided;** take at the same time each day; may mask diabetes symptoms; notify physician if any adverse effects occur; use with caution while driving or performing tasks requiring alertness; may be taken without regard to meals

Dosage Forms

Injection: 0.5 mg/mL (10 mL)

Tablet: 25 mg, 50 mg, 100 mg

Extemporaneous Preparations A 2 mg/mL atenolol oral liquid compounded from tablets and a commercially available oral diluent was found to be stable for up to 40 days when stored at 5°C or 25°C

Garner SS, Wiest DB, and Reynolds ER, "Stability of Atenolol in an Extemporaneously Compounded Oral Liquid," *Am J Hosp Pharm*, 1994, 51(4):508-11.

ATG *see* Lymphocyte Immune Globulin *on page 749*

Atgam® *see* Lymphocyte Immune Globulin *on page 749*

ATIII *see* Antithrombin III *on page 97*

Ativan® *see* Lorazepam *on page 742*

ATnativ® *see* Antithrombin III *on page 97*

Atolone® *see* Triamcinolone *on page 1255*

Atorvastatin (a TORE va sta tin)

Related Information

Lipid-Lowering Agents *on page 1413*

Brand Names Lipitor®

Therapeutic Category Antilipemic Agent; HMG-CoA Reductase Inhibitor

Use Adjunct to diet for the reduction of elevated total and LDL-cholesterol levels in patients with hypercholesterolemia (Type IIa, IIb, and IIc); used in hypercholesterolemic patients without clinically evident heart disease to reduce the risk of myocardial infarction, to reduce the risk for revascularization, and reduce the risk of death due to cardiovascular causes

Pregnancy Risk Factor X

Contraindications Hypersensitivity to atorvastatin or its components (may have cross-sensitivity with other HMG-CoA reductase inhibitors); patients with active liver disease; pregnancy or lactation

Warnings/Precautions Discontinue therapy if symptoms of myopathy or renal failure due to rhabdomyolysis develop; use with caution in patients with history of liver disease or who consume excessive amounts of alcohol

Adverse Reactions

>1%:

Central nervous system: Headache

Gastrointestinal: Diarrhea, flatulence, abdominal pain (2% to 3%)

Neuromuscular & skeletal: Myalgia (1% to 5%)

<1%:

Central nervous system: Giddiness, euphoria, mild confusion, impaired short-torm memory

Hepatic: Mild LFT increases

Respiratory: Pharyngitis, rhinitis

Overdosage/Toxicology Few symptoms anticipated; treatment is supportive

(Continued)

Atorvastatin *(Continued)*

Drug Interactions

Increased toxicity: Gemfibrozil (musculoskeletal effects such as myopathy, myalgia and/or muscle weakness accompanied by markedly elevated CK concentrations, rash and/or pruritus); clofibrate, niacin (myopathy), erythromycin, cyclosporine, oral anticoagulants (elevated PT)

Increased effect/toxicity of levothyroxine

Concurrent use of erythromycin and atorvastatin may result in rhabdomyolysis

Mechanism of Action Inhibitor of 3-hydroxy-3-methylglutaryl coenzyme A (HMG-CoA) reductase, the rate limiting enzyme in cholesterol synthesis (reduces the production of mevalonic acid from HMG-CoA); this then results in a compensatory increase in the expression of LDL receptors on hepatocyte membranes and a stimulation of LDL catabolism

Pharmacodynamics/Kinetics

Absorption: Rapid

Protein binding: 98%

Metabolism: Undergoes enterohepatic recycling; not a prodrug; metabolized to active ortho- and parahydroxylated derivates and an inactive beta-oxidation product

Half-life: 14 hours (parent)

Time to peak serum concentration: 1-2 hours (maximal reduction in plasma cholesterol and triglycerides in 2 weeks)

Elimination: 2% excreted as unchanged drug in the urine

Usual Dosage Adults: Oral: Initial: 10 mg once daily, titrate up to 80 mg/day if needed

Dosing adjustment in renal impairment: No dosage adjustment necessary

Dosing adjustment in hepatic impairment: Decrease dosage with severe disease (eg, chronic alcoholic liver disease)

Monitoring Parameters Lipid levels after 2-4 weeks; LFTs, CPK

Patient Information May take with food if desired; may take without regard to time of day

Dosage Forms Tablet: 10 mg, 20 mg, 40 mg

Atovaquone (a TOE va kwone)

Brand Names Mepron™

Therapeutic Category Antiprotozoal

Use Acute oral treatment of mild to moderate *Pneumocystis carinii* pneumonia (PCP) in patients who are intolerant to co-trimoxazole (ie, not as effective as co-trimoxazole, however, much fewer treatment-limiting adverse effects); orphan drug status for AIDS-associated PCP, prevention of PCP in high-risk, HIV-infected patients (defined by one or more episodes of PCP or a peripheral CD4+ lymphocyte count ≤200/mm^3); treatment/suppression of *Toxoplasma gondii* encephalitis, primary prophylaxis of HIV-infected persons at high risk for developing *Toxoplasma gondii* encephalitis

Pregnancy Risk Factor C

Contraindications Life-threatening allergic reaction to the drug or formulation

Warnings/Precautions Has only been used in mild to moderate PCP; use with caution in elderly patients due to potentially impaired renal, hepatic, and cardiac function

Adverse Reactions

>10%:

- Central nervous system: Headache, fever, insomnia, anxiety
- Dermatologic: Rash
- Gastrointestinal: Nausea, diarrhea, vomiting
- Respiratory: Cough

1% to 10%:

- Central nervous system: Dizziness
- Dermatologic: Pruritus
- Endocrine & metabolic: Hypoglycemia, hyponatremia
- Gastrointestinal: Abdominal pain, constipation, anorexia, dyspepsia
- Hematologic: Anemia, neutropenia, leukopenia
- Hepatic: Elevated amylase and liver enzymes
- Neuromuscular & skeletal: Weakness
- Renal: Elevated BUN/creatinine
- Respiratory: Cough
- Miscellaneous: Oral *Monilia*

Drug Interactions

Decreased effect: Rifamycins used concurrently decrease the steady-state plasma concentrations of atovaquone; coadministration with TMP-SMZ results in clinically insignificant decreases in TMP-SMZ plasma concentrations

Increased effect: Increased zidovudine levels occur due to decreased metabolism, however unlikely to produce clinically significant effects

Note: Possible increased toxicity with other highly protein bound drugs

Stability Do not freeze

Mechanism of Action Has not been fully elucidated; may inhibit electron transport in mitochondria inhibiting metabolic enzymes

Pharmacodynamics/Kinetics

Absorption: Decreased significantly in single doses >750 mg; increased threefold when administered with a high-fat meal

Distribution: Enterohepatically recirculated

Protein binding: >99.9%

Bioavailability: ~30%

Half-life: 2.9 days

Elimination: In feces

Usual Dosage Adults: Oral: 750 mg 2 times/day with food for 21 days

Patient Information Take only prescribed dose; take each dose with a meal, preferably one with high fat content

Dosage Forms Suspension, oral (citrus flavor): 750 mg/5 mL (210 mL)

Atozine® *see* Hydroxyzine *on page 634*

Atracurium (a tra KYOO ree um)

Related Information

Neuromuscular Blocking Agents Comparison *on page 1417*

Brand Names Tracrium®

Synonyms Atracurium Besylate

Therapeutic Category Neuromuscular Blocker Agent, Nondepolarizing; Skeletal Muscle Relaxant

Use Drug of choice for neuromuscular blockade in patients with renal and/or hepatic failure; eases endotracheal intubation as an adjunct to general anesthesia and relaxes skeletal muscle during surgery or mechanical ventilation; does not relieve pain

Pregnancy Risk Factor C

Contraindications Hypersensitivity to atracurium besylate or any component

Warnings/Precautions Reduce initial dosage in patients in whom substantial histamine release would be potentially hazardous (eg, patients with clinically important cardiovascular disease); maintenance of an adequate airway and respiratory support is critical

Adverse Reactions Mild, rare, and generally suggestive of histamine release

1% to 10%: Cardiovascular: Flushing

<1%:

- Cardiovascular: Effects are minimal and transient
- Dermatologic: Erythema, itching, urticaria
- Respiratory: Wheezing, bronchial secretions

Causes of prolonged neuromuscular blockade:

- Excessive drug administration
- Cumulative drug effect, decreased metabolism/excretion (hepatic and/or renal impairment)
- Accumulation of active metabolites
- Electrolyte imbalance (hypokalemia, hypocalcemia, hypermagnesemia, hypernatremia)
- Hypothermia
- Drug interactions
- Increased sensitivity to muscle relaxants (eg, neuromuscular disorders such as myasthenia gravis or polymyositis)

Overdosage/Toxicology Symptoms of overdose include respiratory depression, cardiovascular collapse

Neostigmine 1-3 mg slow I.V. push in adults (0.5 mg in children) antagonizes the neuromuscular blockade, and should be administered with or immediately after atropine 1-1.5 mg I.V. push (adults). This may be especially useful in the presence of bradycardia.

Drug Interactions Prolonged neuromuscular blockade:

Inhaled anesthetics:

- Halothane has only a marginal effect, enflurane and isoflurane increases the potency and prolong duration of neuromuscular blockade induced by atracurium by 35% to 50%
- Dosage should be reduced by 33% in patients receiving isoflurane or enflurane and by 20% in patients receiving halothane
- Local anesthetics
- Calcium channel blockers
- Corticosteroids
- Antiarrhythmics (eg, quinidine or procainamide)
- Antibiotics (eg, aminoglycosides, tetracyclines, vancomycin, clindamycin)
- Immunosuppressants (eg, cyclosporine)

(Continued)

Atracurium *(Continued)*

Stability Refrigerate; unstable in alkaline solutions; **compatible** with D_5W, D_5NS, and NS; do not dilute in LR

Mechanism of Action Blocks neural transmission at the myoneural junction by binding with cholinergic receptor sites

Pharmacodynamics/Kinetics

Onset of action: I.V.: 2 minutes

Peak effect: Within 3-5 minutes

Duration: Recovery begins in 20-35 minutes when anesthesia is balanced

Metabolism: Some metabolites are active; undergoes rapid nonenzymatic degradation in the blood stream, additional metabolism occurs via ester hydrolysis

Half-life, biphasic: Adults:

Initial: 2 minutes

Terminal: 20 minutes

Usual Dosage I.V. (not to be used I.M.):

Children 1 month to 2 years: 0.3-0.4 mg/kg initially followed by maintenance doses of 0.3-0.4 mg/kg as needed to maintain neuromuscular blockade

Atracurium Besylate Infusion Chart

Drug Delivery Rate (mcg/kg/min)	Infusion Rate (mL/min) 0.2 mg/mL (20 mg/100 mL)	Infusion Rate (mL/min) 0.5 mg/mL (50 mg/100 mL)
5	0.025	0.01
6	0.03	0.012
7	0.035	0.014
8	0.04	0.016
9	0.045	0.018
10	0.05	0.02

Children >2 years to Adults: 0.4-0.5 mg/kg then 0.08-0.1 mg/kg 20-45 minutes after initial dose to maintain neuromuscular block

Infusions (requires use of an infusion pump): 0.2 mg/mL or 0.5 mg/mL in D_5W or NS, see table.

Continuous infusion: Initial: 9-10 mcg/kg/minute followed by 5-9 mcg/kg/minute maintenance

Dosage adjustment for hepatic or renal impairment is not necessary

Administration Administer undiluted as a bolus injection; not for I.M. inject, too much tissue irritation; administration requires the use of an infusion pump

Monitoring Parameters Vital signs (heart rate, blood pressure, respiratory rate)

Patient Information May be difficult to talk because of head and neck muscle blockade

Dosage Forms

Injection, as besylate: 10 mg/mL (5 mL, 10 mL)

Injection, preservative-free, as besylate: 10 mg/mL (5 mL)

Atracurium Besylate *see* Atracurium *on previous page*

Atrofen™ *see* Baclofen *on page 130*

Atromid-S® *see* Clofibrate *on page 294*

Atropair® *see* Atropine *on this page*

Atropine (A troe peen)

Related Information

Adult ACLS Algorithm, Asystole *on page 1511*

Adult ACLS Algorithm, Bradycardia *on page 1514*

Adult ACLS Algorithm, Pulseless Electrical Activity *on page 1510*

Cycloplegic Mydriatics Comparison *on page 1409*

Pediatric ALS Algorithm, Bradycardia *on page 1506*

Brand Names Atropair®; Atropine-Care®; Atropisol®; Isopto® Atropine; I-Tropine®; Ocu-Tropine®

Canadian/Mexican Brand Names Tropyn® Z (Mexico)

Synonyms Atropine Sulfate

Therapeutic Category Anticholinergic Agent; Anticholinergic Agent, Ophthalmic; Antidote, Organophosphate Poisoning; Antispasmodic Agent, Gastrointestinal; Bronchodilator; Ophthalmic Agent, Mydriatic

Use Preoperative medication to inhibit salivation and secretions; treatment of sinus bradycardia; management of peptic ulcer; treat exercise-induced bronchospasm;

antidote for organophosphate pesticide poisoning; produce mydriasis and cycloplegia for examination of the retina and optic disc and accurate measurement of refractive errors; uveitis

Pregnancy Risk Factor C

Contraindications Hypersensitivity to atropine sulfate or any component; narrow-angle glaucoma; tachycardia; thyrotoxicosis; obstructive disease of the GI tract; obstructive uropathy

Warnings/Precautions Use with caution in children with spastic paralysis; use with caution in elderly patients. Low doses cause a paradoxical decrease in heart rates. Some commercial products contain sodium metabisulfite, which can cause allergic-type reactions. May accumulate with multiple inhalational administration, particularly in the elderly. Heat prostration may occur in hot weather. Use with caution in patients with autonomic neuropathy, prostatic hypertrophy, hyperthyroidism, congestive heart failure, cardiac arrhythmias, chronic lung disease, biliary tract disease; anticholinergic agents are generally not well tolerated in the elderly and their use should be avoided when possible; atropine is rarely used except as a preoperative agent or in the acute treatment of bradyarrhythmias.

Adverse Reactions

>10%:

- Dermatologic: Dry, hot skin
- Gastrointestinal: Impaired GI motility, constipation, dry throat, xerostomia
- Local: Irritation at injection site
- Respiratory: Dry nose
- Miscellaneous: Diaphoresis (decreased)

1% to 10%:

- Dermatologic: Increased sensitivity to light
- Endocrine & metabolic: Decreased flow of breast milk
- Gastrointestinal: Dysphagia

<1%:

- Cardiovascular: Orthostatic hypotension, tachycardia, palpitations, ventricular fibrillation
- Central nervous system: Confusion, drowsiness, ataxia, fatigue, delirium, headache, loss of memory, restlessness; the elderly may be at increased risk for confusion and hallucinations
- Dermatologic: Rash
- Gastrointestinal: Bloated feeling, nausea, vomiting
- Genitourinary: Dysuria
- Neuromuscular & skeletal: Tremor, weakness
- Ocular: Increased intraocular pain, blurred vision, mydriasis

Overdosage/Toxicology Symptoms of overdose include dilated, unreactive pupils; blurred vision; hot, dry flushed skin; dryness of mucous membranes; difficulty in swallowing, foul breath, diminished or absent bowel sounds, urinary retention, tachycardia, hyperthermia, hypertension, increased respiratory rate

Anticholinergic toxicity is caused by strong binding of the drug to cholinergic receptors. Anticholinesterase inhibitors reduce acetylcholinesterase, the enzyme that breaks down acetylcholine and thereby allows acetylcholine to accumulate and compete for receptor binding with the offending anticholinergic. For anticholinergic overdose with severe life-threatening symptoms, physostigmine 1-2 mg (0.5 or 0.02 mg/kg for children) S.C. or I.V., slowly may be given to reverse these effects.

Drug Interactions

- Decreased effect: Phenothiazines, levodopa, antihistamines with cholinergic mechanisms decrease anticholinergic effects of atropine
- Increased toxicity: Amantadine increases anticholinergic effects, thiazides increase effect

Stability Store injection at <40°C, avoid freezing

Mechanism of Action Blocks the action of acetylcholine at parasympathetic sites in smooth muscle, secretory glands and the CNS; increases cardiac output, dries secretions, antagonizes histamine and serotonin

Pharmacodynamics/Kinetics

- Absorption: Well absorbed from all dosage forms
- Distribution: Widely distributes throughout the body; crosses the placenta; trace amounts appear in breast milk; crosses the blood-brain barrier
- Metabolism: In the liver
- Half-life: 2-3 hours
- Elimination: Both metabolites and unchanged drug (30% to 50%) are excreted into urine

Usual Dosage

Children:

Preanesthetic: I.M., I.V., S.C.:

- ≤5 kg: 0.02 mg/kg/dose 30-60 minutes preop then every 4-6 hours as needed
- >5 kg: 0.01-0.02 mg/kg/dose to a maximum 0.4 mg 30-60 minutes preop; minimum dose: 0.1 mg

(Continued)

Atropine *(Continued)*

Bradycardia: I.V., intratracheal: 0.02 mg/kg every 5 minutes
Minimum dose: 0.1 mg (if administered via endotracheal tube, dilute to 1-2 mL with normal saline prior to endotracheal administration)
Maximum single dose: 0.5 mg (adolescents: 1 mg)
Total maximum dose: 1 mg (adolescents: 2 mg)
When using to treat bradycardia in neonates, reserve use for those patients unresponsive to improved oxygenation
Organophosphate or carbamate poisoning: I.V.: 0.02-0.05 mg/kg every 10-20 minutes until atropine effect (dry flushed skin, tachycardia, mydriasis, fever) is observed then every 1-4 hours for at least 24 hours
Bronchospasm: Inhalation: 0.03-0.05 mg/kg/dose 3-4 times/day; maximum: 1 mg
Ophthalmic, 0.5% solution: Instill 1-2 drops twice daily for 1-3 days before the procedure

Adults (doses <0.5 mg have been associated with paradoxical bradycardia):
Asystole: I.V.: 1 mg; may repeat every 3-5 minutes as needed; may administer intratracheal in 1 mg/10 mL dilution only, intratracheal dose should be 2-2.5 times the I.V. dose
Preanesthetic: I.M., I.V., S.C.: 0.4-0.6 mg 30-60 minutes preop and repeat every 4-6 hours as needed
Bradycardia: I.V.: 0.5-1 mg every 5 minutes, not to exceed a total of 3 mg or 0.04 mg/kg; may administer intratracheal in 1 mg/10 mL dilution only, intratracheal dose should be 2-2.5 times the I.V. dose
Neuromuscular blockade reversal: I.V.: 25-30 mcg/kg 30 seconds before neostigmine or 10 mcg/kg 30 seconds before edrophonium
Organophosphate or carbamate poisoning: I.V.: 1-2 mg/dose every 10-20 minutes until atropine effect (dry flushed skin, tachycardia, mydriasis, fever) is observed, then every 1-4 hours for at least 24 hours; up to 50 mg in first 24 hours and 2 g over several days may be given in cases of severe intoxication
Bronchospasm: Inhalation: 0.025-0.05 mg/kg/dose every 4-6 hours as needed (maximum: 5 mg/dose)
Ophthalmic solution: 1%: Instill 1-2 drops 1 hour before the procedure
Uveitis: Instill 1-2 drops 4 times/day
Ophthalmic ointment: Apply a small amount in the conjunctival sac up to 3 times/day; compress the lacrimal sac by digital pressure for 1-3 minutes after instillation

Monitoring Parameters Heart rate, blood pressure, pulse, mental status; intravenous administration requires a cardiac monitor

Patient Information Maintain good oral hygiene habits because lack of saliva may increase chance of cavities. Observe caution while driving or performing other tasks requiring alertness, as drug may cause drowsiness, dizziness, or blurred vision. Notify physician if rash, flushing, or eye pain occurs, or if difficulty in urinating, constipation, or sensitivity to light becomes severe or persists. Do not allow dropper bottle or tube to touch eye during administration.

Nursing Implications Observe for tachycardia if patient has cardiac problems

Dosage Forms
Injection, as sulfate: 0.1 mg/mL (5 mL, 10 mL); 0.3 mg/mL (1 mL, 30 mL); 0.4 mg/mL (1 mL, 20 mL, 30 mL); 0.5 mg/mL (1 mL, 5 mL, 30 mL); 0.8 mg/mL (0.5 mL, 1 mL); 1 mg/mL (1 mL, 10 mL)
Ointment, ophthalmic, as sulfate: 0.5%, 1% (3.5 g)
Solution, ophthalmic, as sulfate: 0.5% (1 mL, 5 mL); 1% (1 mL, 2 mL, 5 mL, 15 mL); 2% (1 mL, 2 mL); 3% (5 mL)
Tablet, as sulfate: 0.4 mg

Atropine and Diphenoxylate *see* Diphenoxylate and Atropine *on page 400*
Atropine-Care® *see* Atropine *on page 116*
Atropine Sulfate *see* Atropine *on page 116*
Atropisol® *see* Atropine *on page 116*
Atrovent® *see* Ipratropium *on page 672*

Attapulgite (at a PULL gite)

Brand Names Children's Kaopectate® [OTC]; Diasorb® [OTC]; Kaopectate® Advanced Formula [OTC]; Kaopectate® Maximum Strength Caplets; Rheaban® [OTC]

Canadian/Mexican Brand Names Kaopectate® (Canada)

Therapeutic Category Antidiarrheal

Use Symptomatic treatment of diarrhea

Contraindications Hypersensitivity to any component

Warnings/Precautions Use with caution in patients <3 years or >60 years of age or in presence of high fever

Adverse Reactions The powder, if chronically inhaled, can cause pneumoconiosis, since it contains large amounts of silica

1% to 10%: Gastrointestinal: Constipation (dose related)

<1%: Gastrointestinal: Fecal impaction

Overdosage/Toxicology Attapulgite is physiologically inert; upon oral ingestion it swells into a mass that can be up to 12 times the volume of the dry powder, which may cause intestinal obstruction. With an oral ingestion of the dry powder, dilution with 4-8 oz of water for adults (no more than 15 mL/kg in children) along with saline catharsis (magnesium citrate 4 mL/kg) usually prevents any powder-induced intestinal obstruction.

Drug Interactions Decreased GI absorption of orally administered clindamycin, tetracyclines, penicillamine, digoxin

Mechanism of Action Controls diarrhea because of its absorbent action

Pharmacodynamics/Kinetics Absorption: Not absorbed from GI tract

Usual Dosage Oral:

Children:

- <3 years: Not recommended
- 3-6 years: 750 mg/dose up to 2250 mg/24 hours
- 6-12 years: 1200-1500 mg/dose up to 4500 mg/24 hours

Adults: 1200-1500 mg after each loose bowel movement or every 2 hours; 15-30 mL up to 8 times/day, up to 9000 mg/24 hours

Patient Information If diarrhea is not controlled in 48 hours, contact a physician

Nursing Implications Shake well before giving, dilute accordingly

Dosage Forms

Liquid, oral concentrate: 600 mg/15 mL (180 mL, 240 mL, 360 mL, 480 mL); 750 mg/15 mL (120 mL)

Tablet: 750 mg

Tablet, chewable: 300 mg, 600 mg

Attenuvax® *see* Measles Virus Vaccine, Live *on page 764*

Augmentin® *see* Amoxicillin and Clavulanate Potassium *on page 78*

Auranofin (au RANE oh fin)

Brand Names Ridaura®

Therapeutic Category Gold Compound

Use Management of active stage of classic or definite rheumatoid arthritis in patients that do not respond to or tolerate other agents; psoriatic arthritis; adjunctive or alternative therapy for pemphigus

Pregnancy Risk Factor C

Contraindications Renal disease, history of blood dyscrasias, congestive heart failure, exfoliative dermatitis, necrotizing enterocolitis, history of anaphylactic reactions

Warnings/Precautions NSAIDs and corticosteroids may be discontinued after starting gold therapy; therapy should be discontinued if platelet count falls to <100,000/mm³; WBC <4000, granulocytes <1500/mm³, explain possibility of adverse effects and their manifestations; use with caution in patients with renal or hepatic impairment

Adverse Reactions

>10%:

- Dermatologic: Itching, rash
- Gastrointestinal: Stomatitis
- Ocular: Conjunctivitis
- Renal: Proteinuria

1% to 10%:

- Dermatologic: Urticaria, alopecia
- Gastrointestinal: Glossitis
- Hematologic: Eosinophilia, leukopenia, thrombocytopenia
- Renal: Hematuria

<1%:

- Dermatologic: Angioedema
- Gastrointestinal: Ulcerative enterocolitis, GI hemorrhage, gingivitis, dysphagia, metallic taste
- Hematologic: Agranulocytosis, anemia, aplastic anemia
- Hepatic: Hepatotoxicity
- Neuromuscular & skeletal: Peripheral neuropathy
- Respiratory: Interstitial pneumonitis

Overdosage/Toxicology Symptoms of overdose include hematuria, proteinuria, fever, nausea, vomiting, diarrhea; signs of gold toxicity include decrease in hemoglobin, leukopenia, granulocytes and platelets, proteinuria, hematuria, pruritus, stomatitis or persistent diarrhea; advise patients to report any symptoms of toxicity; metallic taste may indicate stomatitis

(Continued)

Auranofin *(Continued)*

Mild gold poisoning: Dimercaprol 2.5 mg/kg 4 times/day for 2 days or for more severe forms of gold intoxication, dimercaprol 3 mg/kg every 4 hours for 2 days, should be initiated; after 2 days the initial dose should be repeated twice daily on the third day and once daily thereafter for 10 days; other chelating agents have been used with some success

Drug Interactions Increased toxicity: Penicillamine, antimalarials, hydroxychloroquine, cytotoxic agents, immunosuppressants

Stability Store in tight, light-resistant containers at 15°C to 30°C

Mechanism of Action The exact mechanism of action of gold is unknown; gold is taken up by macrophages which results in inhibition of phagocytosis and lysosomal membrane stabilization; other actions observed are decreased serum rheumatoid factor and alterations in immunoglobulins. Additionally, complement activation is decreased, prostaglandin synthesis is inhibited, and lysosomal enzyme activity is decreased.

Usual Dosage Oral:

Children: Initial: 0.1 mg/kg/day divided daily; usual maintenance: 0.15 mg/kg/day in 1-2 divided doses; maximum: 0.2 mg/kg/day in 1-2 divided doses

Adults: 6 mg/day in 1-2 divided doses; after 3 months may be increased to 9 mg/day in 3 divided doses; if still no response after 3 months at 9 mg/day, discontinue drug

Dosing adjustment in renal impairment:

Cl_{cr} 50-80 mL/minute: Reduce dose to 50%

Cl_{cr} <50 mL/minute: Avoid use

Monitoring Parameters Monitor urine for protein; CBC and platelets; monitor for mouth ulcers and skin reactions; may monitor auranofin serum levels

Reference Range Gold: Normal: 0-0.1 µg/mL (SI: 0-0.0064 µmol/L); Therapeutic: 1-3 µg/mL (SI: 0.06-0.18 µmol/L); Urine: <0.1 µg/24 hours

Test Interactions May enhance the response to a tuberculin skin test

Patient Information Minimize exposure to sunlight; benefits from drug therapy may take as long as 3 months to appear; notify physician of pruritus, rash, sore mouth; metallic taste may occur; take shortly after a meal or light snack, can be given as bedtime dose if drowsiness occurs; optimum effect may take 2-4 weeks to be achieved; avoid alcohol; be aware of possible photosensitivity reaction; may cause painful erections; avoid sudden changes in position

Nursing Implications Discontinue therapy if platelet count falls <100,000/mm^3

Dosage Forms Capsule: 3 mg [29% gold]

Aureomycin® *see* Chlortetracycline *on page 265*

Auro® Ear Drops [OTC] *see* Carbamide Peroxide *on page 203*

Aurolate® *see* Gold Sodium Thiomalate *on page 582*

Aurothioglucose (aur oh thye oh GLOO kose)

Brand Names Solganal®

Therapeutic Category Gold Compound

Use Adjunctive treatment in adult and juvenile active rheumatoid arthritis; alternative or adjunct in treatment of pemphigus; psoriatic patients who do not respond to NSAIDs

Pregnancy Risk Factor C

Contraindications Renal disease, history of blood dyscrasias, congestive heart failure, exfoliative dermatitis, hepatic disease, SLE, history of hypersensitivity

Warnings/Precautions Use with caution in patients with impaired renal or hepatic function; NSAIDs and corticosteroids may be discontinued over time after initiating gold therapy; explain the possibility of adverse reactions before initiating therapy; pregnancy should be ruled out before therapy is started; therapy should be discontinued if platelet counts fall to <100,000/mm^3, WBC <4000, granulocytes <1500/mm^3

Adverse Reactions

>10%:

Dermatologic: Itching, rash, exfoliative dermatitis, reddened skin

Gastrointestinal: Gingivitis, glossitis, metallic taste, stomatitis

1% to 10%: Renal: Proteinuria

<1%:

Central nervous system: Encephalitis, EEG abnormalities, fever

Dermatologic: Alopecia

Gastrointestinal: Ulcerative enterocolitis

Genitourinary: Vaginitis

Hematologic: Agranulocytosis, aplastic anemia, eosinophilia, leukopenia, thrombocytopenia

Hepatic: Hepatotoxicity

Respiratory: Pharyngitis, bronchitis, pulmonary fibrosis, interstitial pneumonitis

Neuromuscular & skeletal: Peripheral neuropathy
Ocular: Conjunctivitis, corneal ulcers, iritis
Renal: Glomerulitis, hematuria, nephrotic syndrome
Miscellaneous: Anaphylactic shock, allergic reaction (severe)

Overdosage/Toxicology Symptoms of overdose include hematuria, proteinuria, fever, nausea, vomiting, diarrhea; signs of gold toxicity include decrease in hemoglobin, leukopenia, granulocytes and platelets; proteinuria, hematuria, pruritus, stomatitis, persistent diarrhea, rash, or metallic taste; advise patients to report any symptoms of toxicity.

For mild gold poisoning, dimercaprol 2.5 mg/kg 4 times/day for 2 days or for more severe forms of gold intoxication, dimercaprol 3-5 mg/kg every 4 hours for 2 days, should be initiated; then after 2 days the initial dose should be repeated twice daily on the third day, and once daily thereafter for 10 days; other chelating agents have been used with some success

Drug Interactions Increased toxicity: Penicillamine, antimalarials, hydroxychloroquine, cytotoxic agents, immunosuppressants

Stability Protect from light and store at 15°C to 30°C

Mechanism of Action Unknown, may decrease prostaglandin synthesis or may alter cellular mechanisms by inhibiting sulfhydryl systems

Pharmacodynamics/Kinetics

Absorption: I.M.: Erratic and slow
Distribution: Crosses placenta; appears in breast milk
Protein binding: 95% to 99%
Half-life: 3-27 days (half-life dependent upon single or multiple dosing)
Time to peak serum concentration: Within 4-6 hours
Elimination: 70% renal excretion; 30% fecal

Usual Dosage I.M.: Doses should initially be given at weekly intervals

Children 6-12 years: Initial: 0.25 mg/kg/dose first week; increment at 0.25 mg/kg/dose increasing with each weekly dose; maintenance: 0.75-1 mg/kg/dose weekly not to exceed 25 mg/dose to a total of 20 doses, then every 2-4 weeks

Adults: 10 mg first week; 25 mg second and third week; then 50 mg/week until 800 mg to 1 g cumulative dose has been given; if improvement occurs without adverse reactions, administer 25-50 mg every 2-3 weeks, then every 3-4 weeks

Administration Administer by deep I.M. injection into the upper outer quadrant of the gluteal region

Monitoring Parameters CBC with differential, platelet count, urinalysis, baseline renal and liver function tests

Reference Range Gold: Normal: 0-0.1 μg/mL (SI: 0-0.0064 μmol/L); Therapeutic: 1-3 μg/mL (SI: 0.06-0.18 μmol/L); Urine: <0.1 μg/24 hours

Patient Information Minimize exposure to sunlight; benefits from drug therapy may take as long as 3 months to appear; notify physician of pruritus, rash, sore mouth; metallic taste may occur

Nursing Implications Therapy should be discontinued if platelet count falls <100,000/mm^3; vial should be thoroughly shaken before withdrawing a dose; explain the possibility of adverse reactions before initiating therapy; advise patients to report any symptoms of toxicity

Dosage Forms Injection, suspension: 50 mg/mL [gold 50%] (10 mL)

Autoplex T® *see* Anti-Inhibitor Coagulant Complex *on page 96*

AVC™ Cream *see* Sulfanilamide *on page 1176*

AVC™ Suppository *see* Sulfanilamide *on page 1176*

Aventyl® Hydrochloride *see* Nortriptyline *on page 917*

Avitene® *see* Microfibrillar Collagen Hemostat *on page 836*

Avlosulfon® *see* Dapsone *on page 343*

Avonex® *see* Interferon Beta-1a *on page 668*

Axid® *see* Nizatidine *on page 913*

Axid® AR [OTC] *see* Nizatidine *on page 913*

Axotal® *see* Butalbital Compound *on page 176*

Ayr® Saline [OTC] *see* Sodium Chloride *on page 1142*

Azactam® *see* Aztreonam *on page 126*

Azatadine (a ZA ta deen)

Brand Names Optimine®

Canadian/Mexican Brand Names Idulamine® (Mexico)

Synonyms Azatadine Maleate

Therapeutic Category Antihistamine, H_1 Blocker

Use Treatment of perennial and seasonal allergic rhinitis and chronic urticaria

Pregnancy Risk Factor B

(Continued)

Azatadine *(Continued)*

Contraindications Hypersensitivity to azatadine or to other related antihistamines including cyproheptadine; patients taking monoamine oxidase inhibitors should not use azatadine

Warnings/Precautions Sedation and somnolence are the most commonly reported adverse effects

Adverse Reactions

>10%:

Central nervous system: Slight to moderate drowsiness
Respiratory: Thickening of bronchial secretions

1% to 10%:

Central nervous system: Headache, fatigue, nervousness, dizziness
Gastrointestinal: Appetite increase, weight gain, nausea, diarrhea, abdominal pain, xerostomia
Neuromuscular & skeletal: Arthralgia
Respiratory: Pharyngitis

<1%:

Cardiovascular: Palpitations, edema
Central nervous system: Depression
Dermatologic: Angioedema, photosensitivity, rash
Hepatic: Hepatitis
Neuromuscular & skeletal: Myalgia, paresthesia
Respiratory: Bronchospasm, epistaxis

Overdosage/Toxicology Symptoms of overdose include CNS depression or stimulation, dry mouth, flushed skin, fixed and dilated pupils, apnea.

There is no specific treatment for an antihistamine overdose, however, most of its clinical toxicity is due to anticholinergic effects. Anticholinesterase inhibitors may be useful by reducing acetylcholinesterase; anticholinesterase inhibitors include physostigmine, neostigmine, pyridostigmine, and edrophonium. For anticholinergic overdose with severe life-threatening symptoms, physostigmine 1-2 mg (0.5 or 0.02 mg/kg for children) I.V., slowly may be given to reverse these effects.

Drug Interactions Increased effect/toxicity: Procarbazine, CNS depressants, tricyclic antidepressants, alcohol

Mechanism of Action Azatadine is a piperidine-derivative antihistamine; has both anticholinergic and antiserotonin activity; has been demonstrated to inhibit mediator release from human mast cells *in vitro*; mechanism of this action is suggested to prevent calcium entry into the mast cell through voltage-dependent calcium channels

Pharmacodynamics/Kinetics

Absorption: Oral: Rapid and extensive
Half-life, elimination: ~8.7 hours
Elimination: ~20% of dose excreted unchanged in urine over 48 hours

Usual Dosage Children >12 years and Adults: Oral: 1-2 mg twice daily

Dietary Considerations Alcohol: Additive CNS effects, avoid use

Patient Information May cause drowsiness; avoid alcohol; can impair coordination and judgment

Nursing Implications Assist with ambulation

Dosage Forms Tablet, as maleate: 1 mg

Azatadine Maleate *see* Azatadine *on previous page*

Azathioprine (ay za THYE oh preen)

Related Information

Toxicities of Chemotherapeutic Agents *on page 1382*

Brand Names Imuran®

Canadian/Mexican Brand Names Azatrilem® (Mexico)

Synonyms Azathioprine Sodium

Therapeutic Category Antineoplastic Agent, Miscellaneous; Immunosuppressant Agent

Use Adjunct with other agents in prevention of rejection of solid organ transplants; also used in severe active rheumatoid arthritis unresponsive to other agents; other autoimmune diseases (ITP, SLE, MS, Crohn's Disease); **azathioprine is an imidazolyl derivative of 6-mercaptopurine**

Pregnancy Risk Factor D

Contraindications Hypersensitivity to azathioprine or any component; pregnancy and lactation

Warnings/Precautions Chronic immunosuppression increases the risk of neoplasia; has mutagenic potential to both men and women and with possible hematologic toxicities; use with caution in patients with liver disease, renal impairment; monitor hematologic function closely

Adverse Reactions Dose reduction or temporary withdrawal allows reversal

>10%:
- Central nervous system: Fever, chills
- Gastrointestinal: Nausea, vomiting, anorexia, diarrhea
- Hematologic: Thrombocytopenia, leukopenia, anemia
- Miscellaneous: Secondary infection

1% to 10%:
- Dermatologic: Rash
- Hematologic: Pancytopenia
- Hepatic: Hepatotoxicity

<1%:
- Cardiovascular: Hypotension
- Dermatologic: Alopecia, rash, maculopapular rash
- Gastrointestinal: Aphthous stomatitis
- Neuromuscular & skeletal: Arthralgias, which include myalgias, rigors
- Ocular: Retinopathy
- Respiratory: Dyspnea
- Miscellaneous: Rare hypersensitivity reactions

Overdosage/Toxicology Symptoms of overdose include nausea, vomiting, diarrhea, hematologic toxicity

Following initiation of essential overdose management, symptomatic and supportive treatment should be instituted. Dialysis has been reported to remove significant amounts of the drug and its metabolites, and should be considered as a treatment option in those patients who deteriorate despite established forms of therapy.

Drug Interactions

Increased toxicity: Allopurinol (↓ azathioprine dose to 1/3 to 1/4 of normal dose)

Stability

Stability of parenteral admixture at room temperature (25°C): 24 hours

Stability of parenteral admixture at refrigeration temperature (4°C): 16 days

Stable in neutral or acid solutions, but is hydrolyzed to mercaptopurine in alkaline solutions

Mechanism of Action Antagonizes purine metabolism and may inhibit synthesis of DNA, RNA, and proteins; may also interfere with cellular metabolism and inhibit mitosis

Pharmacodynamics/Kinetics

Distribution: Crosses the placenta

Protein binding: ~30%

Metabolism: Extensively by hepatic xanthine oxidase to 6-mercaptopurine (active)

Half-life:
- Parent drug: 12 minutes
- 6-mercaptopurine: 0.7-3 hours
- End stage renal disease: Slightly prolonged

Elimination: Small amounts eliminated as unchanged drug; metabolites eliminated eventually in urine

Usual Dosage I.V. dose is equivalent to oral dose (dosing should be based on ideal body weight):

Children and Adults: Solid organ transplantation: Oral, I.V.: 2-5 mg/kg/day to start, then 1-2 mg/kg/day maintenance

Adults: Rheumatoid arthritis: Oral: 1 mg/kg/day for 6-8 weeks; increase by 0.5 mg/kg every 4 weeks until response or up to 2.5 mg/kg/day

Dosing adjustment in renal impairment:
- Cl_{cr} 10-50 mL/minute: Administer 75% of normal dose daily
- Cl_{cr} <10 mL/minute: Administer 50% of normal dose daily

Hemodialysis: Slightly dialyzable (5% to 20%)
- Administer dose posthemodialysis

CAPD effects: Unknown

CAVH effects: Unknown

Administration Can be administered IVP over 5 minutes at a concentration not to exceed 10 mg/mL **or** azathioprine can be further diluted with normal saline or D_5W and administered by intermittent infusion over 15-60 minutes

Monitoring Parameters CBC, platelet counts, total bilirubin, alkaline phosphatase

Patient Information Response in rheumatoid arthritis may not occur for up to 3 months; do not stop taking without the physician's approval, do not have any vaccinations before checking with your physician; check with your physician if you have a persistent sore throat, unusual bleeding or bruising, or fatigue

Dosage Forms

Injection, as sodium: 100 mg (20 mL)

Tablet (scored): 50 mg

Extemporaneous Preparations A 50 mg/mL suspension compounded from twenty 50 mg tablets, distilled water, Cologel® 5 mL, and then adding 2:1 simple

(Continued)

Azathioprine *(Continued)*

syrup/cherry syrup mixture to a total volume of 20 mL, was stable for 8 weeks when stored in the refrigerator

Handbook on Extemporaneous Formulations, Bethesda, MD: American Society of Hospital Pharmacists, 1987.

Azathioprine Sodium *see* Azathioprine *on page 122*

Azdone® *see* Hydrocodone and Aspirin *on page 621*

Azelaic Acid (a zeh LAY ik AS id)

Brand Names Azelex®

Therapeutic Category Topical Skin Product, Acne

Use *Acne vulgaris*: Topical treatment of mild to moderate inflammatory acne vulgaris

Pregnancy Risk Factor B

Pregnancy/Breast-Feeding Implications Since <4% of a topically applied dose is systemically absorbed, the uptake of azelaic acid into breast milk is not expected to cause a significant change from baseline azelaic acid levels in the milk. However, exercise caution when administering to a nursing mother.

Contraindications Known hypersensitivity to any of components

Warnings/Precautions For external use only; not for ophthalmic use; there have been isolated reports of hypopigmentation after use. If sensitivity or severe irritation develops, discontinue treatment and institute appropriate therapy.

Adverse Reactions

1% to 10%:
- Dermatologic: Pruritus, stinging
- Local: Burning
- Neuromuscular & skeletal: Paresthesia

<1%:
- Dermatologic: Erythema, dryness, rash, peeling, dermatitis, contact dermatitis
- Local: Irritation

Mechanism of Action Exact mechanism is not known; *in vitro*, azelaic acid possesses antimicrobial activity against *Propionibacteriaceae acnes* and *Staphylococcus epidermis*; may decrease micromedo formation

Pharmacodynamics/Kinetics

Absorption: ~3% to 5% penetrates the stratum corneum; up to 10% is found in the epidermis and dermis; 4% is systemically absorbed

Half-life: Healthy subjects: 12 hours after topical dosing

Elimination: Mainly excreted unchanged in the urine

Usual Dosage Adults: Topical: After skin is thoroughly washed and patted dry, gently but thoroughly massage a thin film of azelaic acid cream into the affected areas twice daily, in the morning and evening. The duration of use can vary and depends on the severity of the acne. In the majority of patients with inflammatory lesions, improvement of the condition occurs within 4 weeks.

Patient Information Use for the full prescribed treatment period. Avoid the use of occlusive dressings or wrappings. Keep away from the mouth, eyes and other mucous membranes. If it does come in contact with the eyes, wash eyes with large amounts of water and consult a physician if eye irritation persists. If patients have dark complexions, they should report abnormal changes in skin color to their physician. Due in part to the low pH of azelaic acid, temporary skin irritation (pruritus, burning or stinging) may occur when azelaic acid is applied to broken or inflamed skin, usually at the start of treatment. However, this irritation commonly subsides if treatment is continued. If it continues, apply only once a day, or stop the treatment until these effects have subsided. If troublesome irritation persists, discontinue use and consult the physician.

Nursing Implications Wash hands following application

Dosage Forms Cream: 20% (30 g)

Azelex® *see* Azelaic Acid *on this page*

Azidothymidine *see* Zidovudine *on page 1320*

Azithromycin (az ith roe MYE sin)

Related Information

Antimicrobial Drugs of Choice *on page 1468*

Guidelines for the Prevention of Opportunistic Infections in Persons with HIV *on page 1457*

Treatment of Sexually Transmitted Diseases *on page 1485*

Brand Names Zithromax™

Synonyms Azithromycin Dihydrate

Therapeutic Category Antibiotic, Macrolide

Use

Children: Treatment of acute otitis media due to *H. influenzae, M. catarrhalis*, or *S. pneumoniae*; pharyngitis/tonsillitis due to *S. pyogenes*

Adults: Treatment of mild to moderate upper and lower respiratory tract infections, infections of the skin and skin structure, and sexually transmitted diseases due to susceptible strains of *C. trachomatis*, *M. catarrhalis*, *H. influenzae*, *S. aureus*, *S. pneumoniae*, *Mycoplasma pneumoniae*, and *C. psittaci*

Also for prevention of disseminated *Mycobacterium avium* complex in patients with advanced HIV infection

Note: Penicillin I.M. is the usual drug of choice in the treatment of *S. pyogenes* infections and the prophylaxis of rheumatic fever; azithromycin is often effective in its eradication in the nasopharynx; perform susceptibility tests when patients are treated with azithromycin

Pregnancy Risk Factor B

Contraindications Hepatic impairment, known hypersensitivity to azithromycin, other macrolide antibiotics, or any Zithromax™ components; use with pimozide

Warnings/Precautions Use with caution in patients with hepatic dysfunction; hepatic impairment with or without jaundice has occurred chiefly in older children and adults; it may be accompanied by malaise, nausea, vomiting, abdominal colic, and fever; discontinue use if these occur; may mask or delay symptoms of incubating gonorrhea or syphilis, so appropriate culture and susceptibility tests should be performed prior to initiating azithromycin; pseudomembranous colitis has been reported with use of macrolide antibiotics; safety and efficacy have not been established in children <6 months of age with acute otitis media and in children <2 years of age with pharyngitis/tonsillitis

Adverse Reactions

1% to 10%: Gastrointestinal: Diarrhea, nausea, abdominal pain, cramping, vomiting

<1%:

Cardiovascular: Ventricular arrhythmias
Central nervous system: Fever headache, dizziness
Dermatologic: Rash, angioedema
Gastrointestinal: Hypertrophic pyloric stenosis
Genitourinary: Vaginitis
Hematologic: Eosinophilia
Hepatic: Elevated LFTs, cholestatic jaundice
Local: Thrombophlebitis
Otic: Ototoxicity
Renal: Nephritis
Miscellaneous: Allergic reactions

Overdosage/Toxicology Symptoms of overdose include nausea, vomiting, diarrhea, prostration; treatment is supportive and symptomatic

Drug Interactions

Decreased peak serum levels: Aluminum- and magnesium-containing antacids by 24% but not total absorption

Increased effect/toxicity: Azithromycin increases levels of tacrolimus, alfentanil, astemizole, terfenadine, loratadine, bromocriptine, carbamazepine, cyclosporine, digoxin, disopyramide, and triazolam; azithromycin did not affect the response to warfarin or theophylline although caution is advised when administered together

Mechanism of Action Inhibits RNA-dependent protein synthesis at the chain elongation step; binds to the 50S ribosomal subunit resulting in blockage of transpeptidation

Pharmacodynamics/Kinetics

Absorption: Rapid from the GI tract
Distribution: Extensive tissue distribution
Protein binding: 7% to 50% (concentration-dependent)
Metabolism: In the liver
Bioavailability: 37%, decreased by food
Half-life, terminal: 68 hours
Peak serum concentration: 2.3-4 hours
Elimination: 4.5% to 12% of dose is excreted in urine; 50% of dose is excreted unchanged in bile

Usual Dosage Oral:

Children ≥6 months: Otitis media: 10 mg/kg on day 1 (maximum: 500 mg/day) followed by 5 mg/kg/day once daily on days 2-5 (maximum: 250 mg/day)

Children ≥2 years: Pharyngitis, tonsillitis: 12 mg/kg/day once daily for 5 days (maximum: 500 mg/day)

Children: *M. avium*-infected patients with acquired immunodeficiency syndrome: Not currently FDA approved for use; 10-20 mg/kg/day once daily (maximum: 40 mg/kg/day) has been used in clinical trials; prophylaxis for first episode of MAC: 5-12 mg/kg/day once daily (maximum: 500 mg/day)

Adolescents ≥16 years and Adults:

Respiratory tract, skin and soft tissue infections: 500 mg on day 1 followed by 250 mg/day on days 2-5 (maximum: 500 mg/day)

Uncomplicated chlamydial urethritis or cervicitis: Single 1 g dose

(Continued)

Azithromycin *(Continued)*

Prophylaxis of disseminated *M. avium* complex disease in patient with advanced HIV infection: 1200 mg once weekly

Dietary Considerations Food: Rate and extent of GI absorption decreased; take on an empty stomach

Monitoring Parameters Liver function tests, CBC with differential

Patient Information Take capsule 1 hour prior to a meal or 2 hours after; do not take with aluminum- or magnesium-containing antacids; tablet form may be taken with food to decrease GI effects

Dosage Forms

Capsule, as dihydrate: 250 mg

Powder for oral suspension, as dihydrate: 100 mg/5 mL (15 mL); 200 mg/5 mL (15 mL, 22.5 mL); 1 g (single-dose packet)

Tablet, as dihydrate: 250 mg, 600 mg

Azithromycin Dihydrate *see* Azithromycin *on page 124*

Azmacort™ *see* Triamcinolone *on page 1255*

Azo Gantrisin® *see* Sulfisoxazole and Phenazopyridine *on page 1180*

Azo-Standard® [OTC] *see* Phenazopyridine *on page 981*

AZT *see* Zidovudine *on page 1320*

Azthreonam *see* Aztreonam *on this page*

Aztreonam (AZ tree oh nam)

Related Information

Antimicrobial Drugs of Choice *on page 1468*

Bacterial Meningitis Practical Guidelines for Management *on page 1475*

Brand Names Azactam®

Synonyms Azthreonam

Therapeutic Category Antibiotic, Miscellaneous

Use Treatment of patients with documented aerobic gram-negative bacillary infection in which beta-lactam therapy is contraindicated (eg, penicillin or cephalosporin allergy); used for urinary tract infections, lower respiratory tract infections, septicemia, skin/skin structure infections, intra-abdominal infections, and gynecological infections; as part of a multiple-drug regimen for the empirical treatment of neutropenic fever in persons with a history of beta-lactam allergy or with known multidrug-resistant organisms

Pregnancy Risk Factor B

Contraindications Hypersensitivity to aztreonam or any component

Warnings/Precautions Check hypersensitivity to other beta-lactams; may have cross-allergenicity to penicillins and cephalosporins; requires dosage reduction in renal impairment

Adverse Reactions

1% to 10%:

Dermatologic: Rash

Gastrointestinal: Diarrhea, nausea, vomiting

Local: Thrombophlebitis, pain at injection site

<1%:

Cardiovascular: Hypotension

Central nervous system: Seizures, confusion, headache, vertigo, insomnia, dizziness, fever

Endocrine & metabolic: Breast tenderness

Gastrointestinal: Pseudomembranous colitis, aphthous ulcer, abnormal taste, halitosis, numb tongue

Genitourinary: Vaginitis

Hepatic: Hepatitis, jaundice, elevation of liver enzymes

Hematologic: Thrombocytopenia, eosinophilia, leukopenia, neutropenia

Neuromuscular & skeletal: Myalgia, weakness

Ocular: Diplopia

Otic: Tinnitus

Respiratory: Sneezing

Miscellaneous: Anaphylaxis

Overdosage/Toxicology Symptoms of overdose include seizures; if necessary, dialysis can reduce the drug concentration in the blood

Stability Reconstituted solutions are colorless to light yellow straw and may turn pink upon standing without affecting potency; use reconstituted solutions and I.V. solutions (in NS and D_5W) within 48 hours if kept at room temperature or 7 days if kept in refrigerator

Stability of I.V. infusion solution: 48 hours at room temperature (25°C) and 7 days at refrigeration (4°C)

Mechanism of Action Monobactam which is active only against gram-negative bacilli (unlikely cross-allergenicity with other beta-lactams); inhibits bacterial cell wall synthesis during active multiplication, causing cell wall destruction

Pharmacodynamics/Kinetics

Absorption: I.M.: Well absorbed; I.M. and I.V. doses produce comparable serum concentrations

Distribution: Relative diffusion of antimicrobial agents from blood into cerebrospinal fluid (CSF): Good only with inflammation (exceeds usual MICs)

V_d:

Neonates: 0.26-0.36 L/kg

Children: 0.2-0.29 L/kg

Adults: 0.2 L/kg

Ratio of CSF to blood level (%):

Inflamed meninges: 8-40

Normal meninges: ~1

Protein binding: 56%

Metabolism: Partial

Half-life:

Neonates:

<7 days, ≤2.5 kg: 5.5-9.9 hours

<7 days, >2.5 kg: 2.6 hours

1 week to 1 month: 2.4 hours

Children 2 months to 12 years: 1.7 hours

Normal renal function: 1.7-2.9 hours

End stage renal disease: 6-8 hours

Time to peak: Within 60 minutes (I.M., I.V. push) and 90 minutes (I.V. infusion)

Elimination: 60% to 70% excreted unchanged in urine and partially in feces

Usual Dosage

Children >1 month: I.M., I.V.: 90-120 mg/kg/day divided every 6-8 hours

Cystic fibrosis: 50 mg/kg/dose every 6-8 hours (ie, up to 200 mg/kg/day); maximum: 6-8 g/day

Adults:

Urinary tract infection: I.M., I.V.: 500 mg to 1 g every 8-12 hours

Moderately severe systemic infections: 1 g I.V. or I.M. or 2 g I.V. every 8-12 hours

Severe systemic or life-threatening infections (especially caused by *Pseudomonas aeruginosa*): I.V.: 2 g every 6-8 hours; maximum: 8 g/day

Dosing adjustment in renal impairment:

Cl_{cr} 30-50 mL/minute: Administer every 12 hours

Cl_{cr} 10-30 mL/minute: Administer every 24 hours

Cl_{cr} <10 mL/minute: Administer every 48 hours

Hemodialysis: Moderately dialyzable (20% to 50%); administer dose postdialysis or supplemental dose of 500 mg after dialysis

Peritoneal dialysis: Administer as for Cl_{cr} <10 mL/minute

Continuous arterio-venous or veno-venous hemofiltration (CAVH/CAVHD): Removes 50 mg of aztreonam per liter of filtrate per day

Administration Administer by IVP over 3-5 minutes or by intermittent infusion over 20-60 minutes at a final concentration not to exceed 20 mg/mL; administer around-the-clock rather than 3 times/day to promote less variation in peak and trough serum levels

Monitoring Parameters Periodic liver function test

Test Interactions Urine glucose (Clinitest®)

Nursing Implications Obtain specimens for culture and sensitivity before the first dose

Dosage Forms Powder for injection: 500 mg (15 mL, 100 mL); 1 g (15 mL, 100 mL); 2 g (15 mL, 100 mL)

Azulfidine® *see* Sulfasalazine *on page 1177*

Azulfidine® EN-tabs® *see* Sulfasalazine *on page 1177*

Babee Teething® [OTC] *see* Benzocaine *on page 138*

B-A-C® *see* Butalbital Compound *on page 176*

Bacid® [OTC] *see Lactobacillus acidophilus* and *Lactobacillus bulgaricus on page 702*

Baciguent® [OTC] *see* Bacitracin *on this page*

Baci-IM® *see* Bacitracin *on this page*

Bacillus Calmette-Guérin (BCG) Live *see* BCG Vaccine *on page 132*

Bacitracin (bas i TRAY sin)

Related Information

Antimicrobial Drugs of Choice *on page 1468*

Brand Names AK-Tracin®; Baciguent® [OTC]; Baci-IM®

Canadian/Mexican Brand Names Bacitin® (Canada)

Therapeutic Category Antibiotic, Ophthalmic; Antibiotic, Topical; Antibiotic, Miscellaneous

(Continued)

Bacitracin *(Continued)*

Use Treatment of susceptible bacterial infections (staphylococcal pneumonia and empyema); due to toxicity risks, systemic and irrigant uses of bacitracin should be limited to situations where less toxic alternatives would not be effective; oral administration has been successful in antibiotic-associated colitis

Pregnancy Risk Factor C

Contraindications Hypersensitivity to bacitracin or any component; I.M. use is contraindicated in patients with renal impairment

Warnings/Precautions Prolonged use may result in overgrowth of nonsusceptible organisms; I.M. use may cause renal failure due to tubular and glomerular necrosis; **do not administer intravenously** because severe thrombophlebitis occurs

Adverse Reactions

1% to 10%:

- Cardiovascular: Hypotension, edema of the face/lips, tightness of chest
- Central nervous system: Pain
- Dermatologic: Rash, itching
- Gastrointestinal: Anorexia, nausea, vomiting, diarrhea, rectal itching
- Hematologic: Blood dyscrasias
- Miscellaneous: Diaphoresis

Overdosage/Toxicology Symptoms of overdose include nephrotoxicity (parenteral), nausea, vomiting (oral)

Drug Interactions

Increased toxicity: Nephrotoxic drugs, neuromuscular blocking agents, and anesthetics (↑ neuromuscular blockade)

Stability For I.M. use; bacitracin sterile powder should be dissolved in 0.9% sodium chloride injection containing 2% procaine hydrochloride; once reconstituted, bacitracin is stable for 1 week under refrigeration (2°C to 8°C); sterile powder should be stored in the refrigerator; do not use diluents containing parabens

Mechanism of Action Inhibits bacterial cell wall synthesis by preventing transfer of mucopeptides into the growing cell wall

Pharmacodynamics/Kinetics

Duration of action: 6-8 hours

Absorption: Poor from mucous membranes and intact or denuded skin; rapidly absorbed following I.M. administration; not absorbed by bladder irrigation, but absorption can occur from peritoneal or mediastinal lavage

Distribution: Relative diffusion of antimicrobial agents from blood into cerebrospinal fluid (CSF): Nil even with inflammation

Protein binding: Minimally bound to plasma proteins

Time to peak serum concentration: I.M.: Within 1-2 hours

Elimination: Slow elimination into urine with 10% to 40% of dose excreted within 24 hours

Usual Dosage Children and Adults (**do not administer I.V.**):

Infants: I.M.:

- ≤2.5 kg: 900 units/kg/day in 2-3 divided doses
- >2.5 kg: 1000 units/kg/day in 2-3 divided doses

Children: I.M.: 800-1200 units/kg/day divided every 8 hours

Adults: Antibiotic-associated colitis: Oral: 25,000 units 4 times/day for 7-10 days

Topical: Apply 1-5 times/day

Ophthalmic, ointment: Instill 1/4" to 1/2" ribbon every 3-4 hours into conjunctival sac for acute infections, or 2-3 times/day for mild to moderate infections for 7-10 days

Irrigation, solution: 50-100 units/mL in normal saline, lactated Ringer's, or sterile water for irrigation; soak sponges in solution for topical compresses 1-5 times/day or as needed during surgical procedures

Administration For I.M. administration, confirm any orders for parenteral use; pH of urine should be kept >6 by using sodium bicarbonate; bacitracin sterile powder should be dissolved in 0.9% sodium chloride injection containing 2% procaine hydrochloride; do not use diluents containing parabens

Monitoring Parameters I.M.: Urinalysis, renal function tests

Patient Information Ophthalmic ointment may cause blurred vision; do not share eye medications with others

Ophthalmic administration: Tilt head back, place medication in conjunctival sac and close eyes; apply light finger pressure on lacrimal sac for 1 minute following instillation

Topical bacitracin should not be used for longer than 1 week unless directed by a physician

Additional Information 1 unit is equivalent to 0.026 mg

Dosage Forms
Injection: 50,000 units
Ointment:
Ophthalmic: 500 units/g (1 g, 3.5 g, 3.75 g)
Topical: 500 units/g (0.94 g, 15 g, 30 g, 454 g)

Bacitracin and Polymyxin B (bas i TRAY sin & pol i MIKS in bee)

Brand Names AK-Poly-Bac® Ophthalmic; Betadine® First Aid Antibiotics + Moisturizer [OTC]; Polysporin® Ophthalmic; Polysporin® Topical

Canadian/Mexican Brand Names Bioderm® (Canada); Polytopic® (Canada)

Therapeutic Category Antibiotic, Ophthalmic; Antibiotic, Topical

Use Treatment of superficial infections caused by susceptible organisms

Pregnancy Risk Factor C

Contraindications Hypersensitivity to polymyxin, bacitracin, or any component; epithelial herpes simplex keratitis, mycobacterial or fungal infections; topical ointments for external use only

Warnings/Precautions Prolonged use may result in overgrowth of nonsusceptible organisms

Adverse Reactions
1% to 10%:
Cardiovascular: Edema
Dermatologic: Rash
Local: Itching, burning
Ocular: Conjunctival erythema
Miscellaneous: Anaphylactoid reactions

Mechanism of Action Refer to individual monographs for Bacitracin and Polymyxin B

Usual Dosage Children and Adults:
Ophthalmic ointment: Instill ½" ribbon in the affected eye(s) every 3-4 hours for acute infections or 2-3 times/day for mild to moderate infections for 7-10 days
Topical ointment/powder: Apply to affected area 1-4 times/day; may cover with sterile bandage if needed

Patient Information Ophthalmic ointment may cause blurred vision; do not share eye medications with others
Ophthalmic administration: Tilt head back, place medication in conjunctival sac and close eyes; apply light finger pressure on lacrimal sac for 1 minute following instillation

Dosage Forms
Ointment:
Ophthalmic: Bacitracin 500 units and polymyxin B sulfate 10,000 units per g (3.5 g)
Topical: Bacitracin 500 units and polymyxin B sulfate 10,000 units per g in white petrolatum (15 g, 30 g)
Powder: Bacitracin 500 units and polymyxin B sulfate 10,000 units per g (10 g)

Bacitracin, Neomycin, and Polymyxin B
(bas i TRAY sin, nee oh MYE sin & pol i MIKS in bee)

Brand Names AK-Spore® Ophthalmic Ointment; Medi-Quick® Topical Ointment [OTC]; Mycitracin® Topical [OTC]; N-B-P® Ointment [OTC]; Neomixin® Topical [OTC]; Neosporin® Ophthalmic Ointment; Neosporin® Topical Ointment [OTC]; Ocutricin® Topical Ointment; Septa® Topical Ointment [OTC]; Triple Antibiotic® Topical

Canadian/Mexican Brand Names Neotopic® (Canada)

Therapeutic Category Antibiotic, Ophthalmic; Antibiotic, Topical

Use Helps prevent infection in minor cuts, scrapes and burns; short-term treatment of superficial external ocular infections caused by susceptible organisms

Pregnancy Risk Factor C

Contraindications Known hypersensitivity to neomycin, polymyxin B, or zinc bacitracin; epithelial herpes simplex keratitis, mycobacterial or fungal infections; topical ointments for external use only

Warnings/Precautions Symptoms of neomycin sensitization include itching, reddening, edema, failure to heal; do not use topical formulation in eyes or in external ear canal if ear drum is perforated. Prolonged use may result in overgrowth of nonsusceptible organisms. Use neomycin with care in treating extensive burns (>20% body surface area) as absorption is possible which may result in nephrotoxicity and ototoxicity. Ophthalmic ointments may retard corneal healing; do not use topical ointment in or near the eyes.

Adverse Reactions
1% to 10%:
Cardiovascular: Edema
Dermatologic: Reddening, allergic contact dermatitis
Local: Itching, failure to heal

(Continued)

Bacitracin, Neomycin, and Polymyxin B *(Continued)*

Mechanism of Action Refer to individual monographs for Bacitracin, Neomycin, and Polymyxin B

Usual Dosage Children and Adults:

Ophthalmic:

Ointment: Apply 1/2" into the conjunctival sac every 3-4 hours for 7-10 days for acute infections; apply 1/2" 2-3 times/day for mild to moderate infections for 7-10 days

Solution: Instill 1-2 drops every 15-30 minutes for acute infections; 1-2 drops for mild to moderate infections

Topical: Apply 1-5 times/day to infected area and cover with sterile bandage as needed

Patient Information Ophthalmic ointment may cause blurred vision; do not share eye medications with others

Ophthalmic administration: Tilt head back, place medication in conjunctival sac and close eyes; apply light finger pressure on lacrimal sac for 1 minute following instillation

Dosage Forms

Ophthalmic:

Ointment: Bacitracin 400 units, neomycin sulfate 3.5 mg, and polymyxin B sulfate 10,000 units and per g (3.5 g)

Solution, ophthalmic: Gramicidin 0.025 mg, neomycin sulfate 1.75 mg, polymyxin B sulfate 10,000 units per mL (10 mL bottle)

Topical: Ointment: Bacitracin 400 units, neomycin sulfate 3.5 mg, and polymyxin B sulfate 5000 units per g (0.9 g, 30 g)

Bacitracin, Neomycin, Polymyxin B, and Hydrocortisone

(bas i TRAY sin, nee oh MYE sin, pol i MIKS in bee & hye droe KOR ti sone)

Related Information

Neomycin, Polymyxin B, and Hydrocortisone *on page 890*

Brand Names AK-Spore H.C.® Ophthalmic Ointment; Cortisporin® Ophthalmic Ointment; Cortisporin® Topical Ointment; Neotricin HC® Ophthalmic Ointment

Therapeutic Category Antibiotic, Ophthalmic; Antibiotic, Otic; Antibiotic, Topical; Corticosteroid, Ophthalmic; Corticosteroid, Otic; Corticosteroid, Topical (Low Potency)

Use Prevention and treatment of susceptible superficial topical infections

Pregnancy Risk Factor C

Contraindications Hypersensitivity to polymyxin B, bacitracin, neomycin, hydrocortisone or any component

Warnings/Precautions Prolonged use may result in overgrowth of nonsusceptible organisms

Adverse Reactions

1% to 10%:

Dermatologic: Rash, generalized itching

Respiratory: Apnea

Mechanism of Action Refer to individual monographs for Bacitracin, Neomycin, Polymyxin B, and Hydrocortisone

Usual Dosage Children and Adults:

Ophthalmic ointment: Instill 1/2" ribbon to inside of lower lid every 3-4 hours until improvement occurs

Topical: Apply sparingly 2-4 times/day

Patient Information Ophthalmic ointment may cause blurred vision; do not share eye medications with others

Ophthalmic administration: Tilt head back, place medication in conjunctival sac and close eyes; apply light finger pressure on lacrimal sac for 1 minute following instillation

Dosage Forms Ointment:

Ophthalmic: Bacitracin 400 units, neomycin sulfate 3.5 mg, polymyxin B sulfate 10,000 units, and hydrocortisone 10 mg per g (3.5 g)

Topical: Bacitracin 400 units, neomycin sulfate 3.5 mg, polymyxin B sulfate 10,000 units, and hydrocortisone 10 mg per g (15 g)

Baclofen (BAK loe fen)

Brand Names Atrofen™; Lioresal®

Canadian/Mexican Brand Names Alpha-Baclofen® (Canada); PMS-Baclofen (Canada)

Therapeutic Category Skeletal Muscle Relaxant

Use Treatment of reversible spasticity associated with multiple sclerosis or spinal cord lesions

There are a number of unlabeled uses for baclofen including, intractable hiccups, intractable pain relief, and bladder spasticity

Pregnancy Risk Factor C

Contraindications Hypersensitivity to baclofen or any component

Warnings/Precautions Use with caution in patients with seizure disorder, impaired renal function; avoid abrupt withdrawal of the drug; elderly are more sensitive to the effects of baclofen and are more likely to experience adverse CNS effects at higher doses.

Adverse Reactions

>10%:

Central nervous system: Drowsiness, vertigo, dizziness, psychiatric disturbances, insomnia, slurred speech, ataxia, hypotonia

Neuromuscular & skeletal: Weakness

1% to 10%:

Cardiovascular: Hypotension

Central nervous system: Fatigue, confusion, headache, insomnia

Dermatologic: Rash

Gastrointestinal: Nausea, constipation

Genitourinary: Polyuria

<1%:

Cardiovascular: Palpitations, chest pain, syncope

Central nervous system: Euphoria, excitement, depression, hallucinations

Gastrointestinal: Xerostomia, anorexia, abnormal taste, abdominal pain, vomiting, diarrhea

Genitourinary: Enuresis, urinary retention, dysuria, impotence, inability to ejaculate, nocturia

Neuromuscular & skeletal: Paresthesia

Renal: Hematuria

Respiratory: Dyspnea

Overdosage/Toxicology Symptoms of overdose include vomiting, muscle hypotonia, salivation, drowsiness, coma, seizures, respiratory depression

Atropine has been used to improve ventilation, heart rate, blood pressure, and core body temperature. Following initiation of essential overdose management, symptomatic and supportive treatment should be instituted.

Drug Interactions

Increased effect: Opiate analgesics, benzodiazepines, hypertensive agents

Increased toxicity: CNS depressants and alcohol (sedation), tricyclic antidepressants (short-term memory loss), clindamycin (neuromuscular blockade), guanabenz (sedation), MAO inhibitors (decrease blood pressure, CNS, and respiratory effects)

Mechanism of Action Inhibits the transmission of both monosynaptic and polysynaptic reflexes at the spinal cord level, possibly by hyperpolarization of primary afferent fiber terminals, with resultant relief of muscle spasticity

Pharmacodynamics/Kinetics

Onset of action: Muscle relaxation effect requires 3-4 days

Peak effect: Maximal clinical effect is not seen for 5-10 days

Absorption: Oral: Rapid; absorption from GI tract is thought to be dose dependent

Protein binding: 30%

Metabolism: Minimally in the liver

Half-life: 3.5 hours

Time to peak serum concentration: Oral: Within 2-3 hours

Elimination: 85% of oral dose excreted in urine and feces as unchanged drug

Usual Dosage

Oral:

Children:

2-7 years: Initial: 10-15 mg/24 hours divided every 8 hours; titrate dose every 3 days in increments of 5-15 mg/day to a maximum of 40 mg/day

≥8 years: Maximum: 60 mg/day in 3 divided doses

Adults: 5 mg 3 times/day, may increase 5 mg/dose every 3 days to a maximum of 80 mg/day

Hiccups: Usual effective dose: 10-20 mg 2-3 times/day

Intrathecal:

Test dose: 50-100 mcg, doses >50 mcg should be given in 25 mcg increments, separated by 24 hours

Maintenance: After positive response to test dose, a maintenance intrathecal infusion can be administered via an implanted intrathecal pump. Initial dose via pump: Infusion at a 24-hourly rate dosed at twice the test dose.

Dosing adjustment in renal impairment: May be necessary to reduce dosage

Test Interactions ↑ alkaline phosphatase, AST, glucose, ammonia (B); ↓ bilirubin (S)

(Continued)

Baclofen *(Continued)*

Patient Information Take with food or milk; abrupt withdrawal after prolonged use may cause anxiety, hallucinations, tachycardia or spasticity; may cause drowsiness and impair coordination and judgment

Nursing Implications Epileptic patients should be closely monitored; supervise ambulation; avoid abrupt withdrawal of the drug

Dosage Forms

Injection, intrathecal, preservative free: 500 mcg/mL (20 mL); 2000 mcg/mL (5 mL)

Tablet: 10 mg, 20 mg

Extemporaneous Preparations Make a 5 mg/mL suspension by crushing fifteen 20 mg tablets; wet with glycerin, gradually add 45 mL simple syrup in 3 x 5 mL aliquots to make a total volume of 60 mL; refrigerate; stable 35 days

Johnson CE and Hart SM, "Stability of an Extemporaneously Compounded Baclofen Oral Liquid," *Am J Hosp Phar*, 1993, 50:2353-5.

Bacterial Meningitis Practical Guidelines for Management *see page 1475*

Bacticort® Otic *see* Neomycin, Polymyxin B, and Hydrocortisone *on page 890*

Bactine™ Maximum Strength [OTC] *see* Hydrocortisone *on page 623*

Bactocill® *see* Oxacillin *on page 931*

BactoShield® Topical [OTC] *see* Chlorhexidine Gluconate *on page 253*

Bactrim™ *see* Co-Trimoxazole *on page 315*

Bactrim™ DS *see* Co-Trimoxazole *on page 315*

Bactroban® *see* Mupirocin *on page 862*

Baking Soda *see* Sodium Bicarbonate *on page 1140*

BAL *see* Dimercaprol *on page 397*

Baldex® *see* Dexamethasone *on page 356*

BAL in Oil® *see* Dimercaprol *on page 397*

Bancap® *see* Butalbital Compound *on page 176*

Bancap HC® *see* Hydrocodone and Acetaminophen *on page 620*

Banesin® [OTC] *see* Acetaminophen *on page 19*

Banophen® Oral [OTC] *see* Diphenhydramine *on page 399*

Barbidonna® *see* Hyoscyamine, Atropine, Scopolamine, and Phenobarbital *on page 637*

Barbita® *see* Phenobarbital *on page 984*

Barc™ Liquid [OTC] *see* Pyrethrins *on page 1079*

Baridium® [OTC] *see* Phenazopyridine *on page 981*

Barophen® *see* Hyoscyamine, Atropine, Scopolamine, and Phenobarbital *on page 637*

Base Ointment *see* Zinc Oxide *on page 1324*

Bayer® Aspirin [OTC] *see* Aspirin *on page 106*

BCG Vaccine (bee see jee vak SEEN)

Brand Names TheraCys™; TICE® BCG

Synonyms Bacillus Calmette-Guérin (BCG) Live

Therapeutic Category Biological Response Modulator; Vaccine, Live Bacteria

Use Immunization against tuberculosis and immunotherapy for cancer; treatment of bladder cancer

BCG vaccine is not routinely recommended for use in the U.S. for prevention of tuberculosis

BCG vaccine is strongly recommended for infants and children with negative tuberculin skin tests who:

- are at high risk of intimate and prolonged exposure to persistently untreated or ineffectively treated patients with infectious pulmonary tuberculosis, and cannot be removed from the source of exposure, and
- cannot be placed on long-term preventive therapy
- are continuously exposed with tuberculosis who have bacilli resistant to isoniazid and rifampin

BCG is also recommended for tuberculin-negative infants and children in groups in which the rate of new infections exceeds 1% per year and for whom the usual surveillance and treatment programs have been attempted but are not operationally feasible

BCG should be administered with caution to persons in groups at high risk for HIV infection or persons known to be severely immunocompromised. Although limited data suggest that the vaccine may be safe for use in asymptomatic children infected with HIV, BCG vaccination is not recommended for HIV infected adults or for persons with symptomatic disease. Until further research can clearly define the risks and benefits of BCG vaccination for this population, vaccination should be restricted to persons at exceptionally high risk for tuberculosis infection. HIV infected persons thought to be infected with *Mycobacterium tuberculosis* should be strongly recommended for tuberculosis preventive therapy.

Pregnancy Risk Factor C

Contraindications Tuberculin-positive individual, hypersensitivity to BCG vaccine or any component, immunocompromized, AIDS and burn patients

Warnings/Precautions Protection against tuberculosis is only relative, not permanent, nor entirely predictable; for live bacteria vaccine, proper aseptic technique and disposal of all equipment in contact with BCG vaccine as a biohazardous material is recommended; systemic reactions have been reported in patients treated as immunotherapy for bladder cancer

Adverse Reactions

1% to 10%:

Genitourinary: Bladder infection, dysuria, polyuria, prostatitis

Miscellaneous: Flu-like syndrome

<1%:

Dermatologic: Skin ulceration, abscesses

Renal: Hematuria

Miscellaneous: Rarely anaphylactic shock in infants, lymphadenitis, tuberculosis in immunosuppressed patients

Drug Interactions Decreased effect: Antimicrobial or immunosuppressive drugs may impair response to BCG or increase risk of infection; antituberculosis drugs

Stability Refrigerate, protect from light, use within 2 (TICE® BCG) hours of mixing

Mechanism of Action BCG live is an attenuated strain of Bacillus Calmette-Guérin used as a biological response modifier; BCG live, when used intravesicular for treatment of bladder carcinoma *in situ*, is thought to cause a local, chronic inflammatory response involving macrophage and leukocyte infiltration of the bladder. By a mechanism not fully understood, this local inflammatory response leads to destruction of superficial tumor cells of the urothelium. Evidence of systemic immune response is also commonly seen, manifested by a positive PPD tuberculin skin test reaction, however, its relationship to clinical efficacy is not well-established. BCG is active immunotherapy which stimulates the host's immune mechanism to reject the tumor.

Usual Dosage Children >1 month and Adults:

Immunization against tuberculosis: 0.2-0.3 mL percutaneous; initial lesion usually appears after 10-14 days consisting of small red papule at injection site and reaches maximum diameter of 3 mm in 4-6 weeks; conduct postvaccinal tuberculin test in 2-3 months; if test is negative, repeat vaccination

Immunotherapy for bladder cancer: TICE® BCG vaccine 6 x 10^8 viable organisms in 50 mL NS (preservative free) instilled into bladder and retained for 2 hours weekly for 6 weeks

Administration Should only be given intravesicularly or percutaneously; **do not administer I.V., S.C., or intradermally;** can be used for bladder irrigation

Test Interactions PPD intradermal test

Patient Information Notify physician of persistent pain on urination or blood in urine

Dosage Forms Freeze-dried suspension for reconstitution

Injection: 50 mg (2 mL)

Injection, intravesical: 27 mg (3 vials)

BCNU *see* Carmustine *on page 210*

B Complex *see* Vitamins, Multiple *on page 1310*

B Complex With C *see* Vitamins, Multiple *on page 1310*

Beclomethasone (be kloe METH a sone)

Related Information

Asthma, Guidelines for the Diagnosis and Management of *on page 1518*

Estimated Clinical Comparability of Doses for Inhaled Corticosteroids *on page 1522*

Brand Names Beclovent®; Beconase®; Beconase AQ®; Vancenase®; Vancenase® AQ; Vanceril®

Canadian/Mexican Brand Names Beclodisk® (Canada); Becloforte® (Canada); Propaderm® (Canada); Aerobec® (Mexico); Beconase® Aqua (Mexico); Becotide® 100 (Mexico); Becotide® 250 (Mexico); Becotide® Aerosol (Mexico)

Synonyms Beclomethasone Dipropionate

Therapeutic Category Anti-inflammatory Agent, Inhalant; Corticosteroid, Inhalant; Corticosteroid, Intranasal

Use

Oral inhalation: Treatment of bronchial asthma in patients who require chronic administration of corticosteroids

Nasal aerosol: Symptomatic treatment of seasonal or perennial rhinitis and nasal polyposis

Pregnancy Risk Factor C

(Continued)

Beclomethasone *(Continued)*

Pregnancy/Breast-Feeding Implications Data does not support an association between drug and congenital defects in humans

Clinical effects on fetus: No data on crossing the placenta or effects on the fetus

Breast-feeding/lactation: No data on crossing into breast milk or effects on the infant

Contraindications Status asthmaticus; hypersensitivity to the drug or fluorocarbons, oleic acid in the formulation, systemic fungal infections

Warnings/Precautions Not to be used in status asthmaticus; safety and efficacy in children <6 years of age have not been established; avoid using higher than recommended dosages since suppression of hypothalamic, pituitary, or adrenal function may occur

Adverse Reactions

>10%:

- Local: Growth of *Candida* in the mouth, irritation and burning of the nasal mucosa
- Respiratory: Cough, hoarseness

1% to 10%:

- Gastrointestinal: Xerostomia
- Local: Nasal ulceration
- Respiratory: Epistaxis

<1%:

- Central nervous system: Headache
- Dermatologic: Rash
- Gastrointestinal: Dysphagia
- Respiratory: Bronchospasm, rhinorrhea, nasal congestion, sneezing, nasal septal perforations

Overdosage/Toxicology Symptoms of overdose include irritation and burning of the nasal mucosa, sneezing, intranasal and pharyngeal *Candida* infections, nasal ulceration, epistaxis, rhinorrhea, nasal stuffiness, headache. When consumed in excessive quantities, systemic hypercorticism and adrenal suppression may occur, in those cases discontinuation and withdrawal of the corticosteroid should be done judiciously.

Stability Do not store near heat or open flame

Mechanism of Action Controls the rate of protein synthesis, depresses the migration of polymorphonuclear leukocytes, fibroblasts, reverses capillary permeability, and lysosomal stabilization at the cellular level to prevent or control inflammation

Pharmacodynamics/Kinetics

Therapeutic effect: Within 1-4 weeks of use

Inhalation:

- Absorption: Readily absorbed; quickly hydrolyzed by pulmonary esterases prior to absorption
- Distribution: 10% to 25% of dose reaches respiratory tract

Oral:

- Absorption: 90%
- Distribution: Secreted into breast milk
- Protein binding: 87%
- Metabolism: Hepatic
- Half-life:
  - Initial: 3 hours
  - Terminal: 15 hours
- Elimination: Renal

Usual Dosage Nasal inhalation and oral inhalation dosage forms are not to be used interchangeably

Nasal:

- Children 6-12 years: 1 spray in each nostril 3 times/day
- Adults: 1 spray in each nostril 2-4 times/day

Oral inhalation:

- Children 6-12 years: 1-2 inhalations 3-4 times/day; alternatively 2-4 inhalations twice daily; do not exceed 10 inhalations/day
- Adults: 2 inhalations 3-4 times/day; alternatively 2-4 inhalations twice daily; do not exceed 20 inhalations/day; patients with severe asthma should be started on 12-16 inhalations/day (divided 3-4 times/day) and dose should be adjusted downward according to the patient's response

Patient Information Rinse mouth and throat after use to prevent *Candida* infection, report sore throat or mouth lesions to physician. Inhaled beclomethasone makes many asthmatics cough, to reduce chance, inhale drug slowly or use prescribed inhaled bronchodilator 5 minutes before beclomethasone is used; keep inhaler clean and unobstructed, wash in warm water and dry thoroughly; shake thoroughly before using.

Nursing Implications Take drug history of patients with perennial rhinitis, may be drug related; check mucous membranes for signs of fungal infection

Dosage Forms

Nasal, as dipropionate:

Inhalation: (Beconase®, Vancenase®): 42 mcg/inhalation [200 metered doses] (16.8 g)

Spray, as dipropionate (Vancenase® AQ Nasal): 0.084% [120 actuations] (19 g)

Spray, aqueous, nasal, as dipropionate (Beconase AQ®, Vancenase® AQ): 42 mcg/inhalation [≥200 metered doses] (25 g); 84 mcg/inhalation [≥200 metered doses] (25 g)

Oral: Inhalation, as dipropionate:

Beclovent®, Vanceril®: 42 mcg/inhalation [200 metered doses] (16.8 g)

Vanceril® Double Strength: 84 mcg/inhalation (5.4 g - 40 metered doses, 12.2 g - 120 metered doses)

Beclomethasone Dipropionate *see* Beclomethasone *on page 133*

Beclovent® *see* Beclomethasone *on page 133*

Beconase® *see* Beclomethasone *on page 133*

Beconase AQ® *see* Beclomethasone *on page 133*

Becotin® Pulvules® *see* Vitamins, Multiple *on page 1310*

Beepen-VK® *see* Penicillin V Potassium *on page 965*

Belix® Oral [OTC] *see* Diphenhydramine *on page 399*

Belladonna and Opium (bel a DON a & OH pee um)

Brand Names B&O Supprettes®

Canadian/Mexican Brand Names PMS-Opium & Beladonna (Canada)

Synonyms Opium and Belladonna

Therapeutic Category Analgesic, Narcotic

Use Relief of moderate to severe pain associated with rectal or bladder tenesmus that may occur in postoperative states and neoplastic situations; pain associated with ureteral spasms not responsive to non-narcotic analgesics and to space intervals between injections of opiates

Restrictions C-II

Pregnancy Risk Factor C

Contraindications Glaucoma, severe renal or hepatic disease, bronchial asthma, respiratory depression, convulsive disorders, acute alcoholism, premature labor

Warnings/Precautions Usual precautions of opiate agonist therapy should be observed; infants <3 months of age are more susceptible to respiratory depression, use with caution and generally in reduced doses in this age group

Adverse Reactions

>10%:

Dermatologic: Dry skin

Gastrointestinal: Constipation, dry throat, xerostomia

Local: Irritation at injection site

Respiratory: Dry nose

Miscellaneous: Diaphoresis (decreased)

1% to 10%:

Dermatologic: Increased sensitivity to light

Endocrine & metabolic: Decreased flow of breast milk

Gastrointestinal: Dysphagia

<1%:

Cardiovascular: Orthostatic hypotension, ventricular fibrillation, tachycardia, palpitations

Central nervous system: Confusion, drowsiness, headache, loss of memory, fatigue, ataxia, CNS depression

Dermatologic: Rash

Endocrine & metabolic: Antidiuretic hormone release

Gastrointestinal: Bloated feeling, nausea, vomiting, constipation, biliary tract spasm

Genitourinary: Dysuria, urinary retention, urinary tract spasm

Ocular: Increased intraocular pain, blurred vision

Neuromuscular & skeletal: Weakness

Respiratory: Respiratory depression

Miscellaneous: Histamine release, physical and psychological dependence, diaphoresis

Overdosage/Toxicology Primary attention should be directed to ensuring adequate respiratory exchange; opiate agonist-induced respiratory depression may be reversed with parenteral naloxone hydrochloride

Anticholinergic toxicity may be caused by strong binding of a belladonna alkaloid to cholinergic receptors

(Continued)

Belladonna and Opium *(Continued)*

Anticholinesterase inhibitors reduce acetylcholinesterase, the enzyme that breaks down acetylcholine and thereby allows acetylcholine to accumulate and compete for receptor binding with the offending anticholinergic

For an overdose with severe life-threatening symptoms, physostigmine 1-2 mg (0.5 or 0.02 mg/kg for children) S.C. or I.V., slowly may be given to reverse these effects

Drug Interactions

Decreased effect: Phenothiazines

Increased effect/toxicity: CNS depressants, tricyclic antidepressants

Stability Store at 15°C to 30°C (avoid freezing)

Mechanism of Action Anticholinergic alkaloids act primarily by competitive inhibition of the muscarinic actions of acetylcholine on structures innervated by postganglionic cholinergic neurons and on smooth muscle; resulting effects include antisecretory activity on exocrine glands and intestinal mucosa and smooth muscle relaxation. Contains many narcotic alkaloids including morphine; its mechanism for gastric motility inhibition is primarily due to this morphine content; it results in a decrease in digestive secretions, an increase in GI muscle tone, and therefore a reduction in GI propulsion.

Pharmacodynamics/Kinetics

Onset of action:

- Belladonna: 1-2 hours
- Opium: Within 30 minutes

Metabolism: Opium metabolized in the liver with formation of glucuronide metabolites

Elimination: Belladonna is excreted unchanged in urine

Usual Dosage Adults: Rectal: 1 suppository 1-2 times/day, up to 4 doses/day

Test Interactions ↑ aminotransferase [ALT (SGPT)/AST (SGOT)] (S)

Patient Information May cause drowsiness and blurred vision

Nursing Implications Prior to rectal insertion, the finger and suppository should be moistened; assist with ambulation, monitor for CNS depression

Dosage Forms Suppository:

#15 A: Belladonna extract 15 mg and opium 30 mg

#16 A: Belladonna extract 15 mg and opium 60 mg

Benadryl® Injection *see* Diphenhydramine *on page 399*

Benadryl® Oral [OTC] *see* Diphenhydramine *on page 399*

Benadryl® Topical *see* Diphenhydramine *on page 399*

Ben-Allergin-50® Injection *see* Diphenhydramine *on page 399*

Ben-Aqua® [OTC] *see* Benzoyl Peroxide *on page 140*

Benazepril (ben AY ze pril)

Related Information

Angiotensin-Converting Enzyme Inhibitors Comparison *on page 1386*

Brand Names Lotensin®

Synonyms Benazepril Hydrochloride

Therapeutic Category Angiotensin-Converting Enzyme (ACE) Inhibitors; Antihypertensive

Use Treatment of hypertension, either alone or in combination with other antihypertensive agents

Pregnancy Risk Factor D

Pregnancy/Breast-Feeding Implications It is not known whether benazepril is excreted in human milk

Clinical effects on the fetus: No data available on crossing the placenta. Cranial defects, hypocalvaria/acalvaria, oligohydramnios, persistent anuria following delivery, hypotension, renal defects, renal dysgenesis/dysplasia, renal failure, pulmonary hypoplasia, limb contractures secondary to oligohydramnios and stillbirth reported. ACE inhibitors should be avoided during pregnancy.

Breast-feeding/lactation: Crosses into breast milk. American Academy of Pediatrics considers COMPATIBLE with breast-feeding.

Contraindications Hypersensitivity to benazepril or any component or other ACE inhibitors

Warnings/Precautions Use with caution in patients with collagen vascular disease, hypovolemia, valvular stenosis, hyperkalemia, recent anesthesia; modify dosage in patients with renal impairment (especially renal artery stenosis), severe congestive heart failure, or with coadministered diuretic therapy; experience in children is limited; severe hypotension may occur in patients who are sodium and/or volume depleted; initiate lower doses and monitor closely when starting therapy in these patients

Adverse Reactions

1% to 10%:

Central nervous system: Headache, dizziness, fatigue, somnolence, postural dizziness

Gastrointestinal: Nausea

Respiratory: Transient cough

<1%:

Cardiovascular: Hypotension, tachycardia

Central nervous system: Anxiety, insomnia, nervousness

Dermatologic: Rash, photosensitivity, angioedema

Endocrine & metabolic: Hyperkalemia

Gastrointestinal: Constipation, gastritis, vomiting, melena

Genitourinary: Impotence, urinary tract infection

Neuromuscular & skeletal: Hypertonia, paresthesia, arthralgia, arthritis, myalgia, weakness

Respiratory: Asthma, bronchitis, dyspnea, sinusitis

Miscellaneous: Diaphoresis

Overdosage/Toxicology Mild hypotension has been the only toxic effect seen with acute overdose. Bradycardia may also occur; hyperkalemia occurs even with therapeutic doses, especially in patients with renal insufficiency and those taking NSAIDs.

Following initiation of essential overdose management, toxic symptom treatment and supportive treatment should be initiated. Hypotension usually responds to I.V. fluids or Trendelenburg positioning.

Drug Interactions See table.

Drug-Drug Interactions With ACEIs

Precipitant Drug	Drug (Category) and Effect	Description
Antacids	ACE Inhibitors: decreased	Decreased bioavailability of ACEIs. May be more likely with captopril. Separate administration times by 1-2 hours.
NSAIDs (indomethacin)	ACEIs: decreased	Reduced hypotensive effects of ACEIs. More prominent in low renin or volume dependent hypertensive patients.
Phenothiazines	ACEIs: increased	Pharmacologic effects of ACEIs may be increased.
ACEIs	Allopurinol: increased	Higher risk of hypersensitivity reaction possible when given concurrently. Three case reports of Stevens-Johnson syndrome with captopril.
ACEIs	Digoxin: increased	Increased plasma digoxin levels.
ACEIs	Lithium: increased	Increased serum lithium levels and symptoms of toxicity may occur.
ACEIs	Potassium preps/ potassium sparing diuretics increased	Coadministration may result in elevated potassium levels.

Mechanism of Action Competitive inhibition of angiotensin I being converted to angiotensin II, a potent vasoconstrictor, through the angiotensin I-converting enzyme (ACE) activity, with resultant lower levels of angiotensin II which causes an increase in plasma renin activity and a reduction in aldosterone secretion

Pharmacodynamics/Kinetics

Reduction in plasma angiotensin-converting enzyme activity: Oral:

Peak effect: 1-2 hours after administration of 2-20 mg dose

Duration of action: >90% inhibition for 24 hours has been observed after 5-20 mg dose

Reduction in blood pressure:

Peak effect after single oral dose: 2-6 hours

Maximum response With continuous therapy: 2 weeks

Absorption: Rapid (37% of each oral dose); food does not alter significantly; metabolite (benazeprilat) itself unsuitable for oral administration due to poor absorption

Distribution: V_d: ~8.7 L

Metabolism: Rapid and extensive in the liver to its active metabolite, benazeprilat, via enzymatic hydrolysis; undergoes significant first-pass metabolism and is completely eliminated from plasma in 4 hours

Half-life:

Parent drug: 0.6 hour

Metabolite elimination: 22 hours (from 24 hours after dosing onward)

Metabolite: 1.5-2 hours after fasting or 2-4 hours after a meal

Time to peak: 1-1.5 hours (unchanged parent drug)

(Continued)

Benazepril *(Continued)*

Elimination: Nonrenal clearance (ie, biliary, metabolic) appears to contribute to the elimination of benazeprilat (11% to 12%), particularly in patients with severe renal impairment; hepatic clearance is the main elimination route of unchanged benazepril

Dialysis: ~6% of metabolite was removed by 4 hours of dialysis following 10 mg of benazepril administered 2 hours prior to procedure; parent compound was not found in the dialysate

Usual Dosage Adults: Oral: 20-40 mg/day as a single dose or 2 divided doses; maximum daily dose: 80 mg

Dosing interval in renal impairment: Cl_{cr} <30 mL/minute: Administer 5 mg/day initially; maximum daily dose: 40 mg

Hemodialysis: Moderately dialyzable (20% to 50%); administer dose postdialysis or administer 25% to 35% supplemental dose

Peritoneal dialysis: Supplemental dose is not necessary

Patient Information May be taken in disregard to meals; notify physician of persistent cough or other side effects; do not stop therapy except under prescriber advice; may cause dizziness, fainting, and lightheadedness, especially in first week of therapy; sit and stand up slowly; may cause changes in taste or rash; do not add a salt substitute (potassium) without advice of physician

Nursing Implications Watch for hypotensive effect within 1-3 hours of first dose or new higher dose; discontinue therapy immediately if angioedema of the face, extremities, lips, tongue, or glottis occurs

Dosage Forms Tablet, as hydrochloride: 5 mg, 10 mg, 20 mg, 40 mg

Benazepril Hydrochloride *see* Benazepril *on page 136*

Benemid® *see* Probenecid *on page 1044*

Benoxyl® *see* Benzoyl Peroxide *on page 140*

Bentyl® Hydrochloride Injection *see* Dicyclomine *on page 376*

Bentyl® Hydrochloride Oral *see* Dicyclomine *on page 376*

Benylin® Cough Syrup [OTC] *see* Diphenhydramine *on page 399*

Benylin® DM [OTC] *see* Dextromethorphan *on page 366*

Benylin® Expectorant [OTC] *see* Guaifenesin and Dextromethorphan *on page 591*

Benzac AC® Gel *see* Benzoyl Peroxide *on page 140*

Benzac AC® Wash *see* Benzoyl Peroxide *on page 140*

Benzac W® Gel *see* Benzoyl Peroxide *on page 140*

Benzac W® Wash *see* Benzoyl Peroxide *on page 140*

5-Benzagel® *see* Benzoyl Peroxide *on page 140*

10-Benzagel® *see* Benzoyl Peroxide *on page 140*

Benzashave® Cream *see* Benzoyl Peroxide *on page 140*

Benzathine Benzylpenicillin *see* Penicillin G Benzathine *on page 961*

Benzathine Penicillin G *see* Penicillin G Benzathine *on page 961*

Benzazoline Hydrochloride *see* Tolazoline *on page 1239*

Benzene Hexachloride *see* Lindane *on page 728*

Benzhexol Hydrochloride *see* Trihexyphenidyl *on page 1263*

Benzmethyzin *see* Procarbazine *on page 1049*

Benzocaine (BEN zoe kane)

Brand Names Americaine® [OTC]; Anbesol® [OTC]; Anbesol® Maximum Strength [OTC]; Babee Teething® [OTC]; Benzocol® [OTC]; Benzodent® [OTC]; Chigger-Tox® [OTC]; Cylex® [OTC]; Dermoplast® [OTC]; Foille Medicated First Aid® [OTC]; Foille® [OTC]; Hurricaine®; Lanacane® [OTC]; Maximum Strength Anbesol® [OTC]; Maximum Strength Orajel® [OTC]; Mycinettes® [OTC]; Numzitdent® [OTC]; Numzit Teething® [OTC]; Orabase®-B [OTC]; Orabase®-O [OTC]; Orajel® Brace-Aid Oral Anesthetic [OTC]; Orajel® Mouth-Aid [OTC]; Orajel® Maximum Strength [OTC]; Orasept® [OTC]; Orasol® [OTC]; Oratect® [OTC]; Rhulicaine® [OTC]; Rid-A-Pain® [OTC]; Slim-Mint® [OTC]; Solarcaine® [OTC]; Spec-T® [OTC]; Tanac® [OTC]; Unguentine® [OTC]; Vicks Children's Chloraseptic® [OTC]; Vicks Chloraseptic® Sore Throat [OTC]; ZilaDent® [OTC]

Canadian/Mexican Brand Names Graneodin-B® (Mexico)

Synonyms Ethyl Aminobenzoate

Therapeutic Category Local Anesthetic, Ester Type; Local Anesthetic, Oral; Local Anesthetic, Otic; Local Anesthetic, Topical

Use Temporary relief of pain associated with local anesthetic for pruritic dermatosis, pruritus, minor burns, acute congestive and serious otitis media, swimmer's ear, otitis externa, toothache, minor sore throat pain, canker sores, hemorrhoids, rectal fissures, anesthetic lubricant for passage of catheters and endoscopic tubes; nonprescription diet aide

Pregnancy Risk Factor C

Contraindications Children <1 year of age; secondary bacterial infection of area; ophthalmic use; known hypersensitivity to benzocaine or other ester type local anesthetics

Warnings/Precautions Not intended for use when infections are present

Adverse Reactions Dose-related and may result in high plasma levels

1% to 10%:

Dermatologic: Angioedema, contact dermatitis

Local: Burning, stinging

<1%:

Cardiovascular: Edema

Dermatologic: Urticaria

Genitourinary: Urethritis

Hematologic: Methemoglobinemia in infants

Local: Tenderness

Overdosage/Toxicology Methemoglobinemia has been reported with benzocaine in oral overdose. Treatment is primarily symptomatic and supportive; termination of anesthesia by pneumatic tourniquet inflation should be attempted when the agent is administered by infiltration or regional injection. Seizures commonly respond to diazepam, while hypotension responds to I.V. fluids and Trendelenburg positioning. Bradyarrhythmias (when the heart rate is <60) can be treated with I.V., I.M., or S.C. atropine 15 mcg/kg. With the development of metabolic acidosis, I.V. sodium bicarbonate 0.5-2 mEq/kg and ventilatory assistance should be instituted.

Mechanism of Action Ester local anesthetic blocks both the initiation and conduction of nerve impulses by decreasing the neuronal membrane's permeability to sodium ions, which results in inhibition of depolarization with resultant blockade of conduction

Pharmacodynamics/Kinetics

Absorption: Topical: Poorly absorbed after administration to intact skin, but well absorbed from mucous membranes and traumatized skin

Metabolism: Hydrolyzed in the plasma and, to a lesser extent, the liver by cholinesterase

Elimination: Metabolites excreted in urine

Usual Dosage

Children and Adults:

Mucous membranes: Dosage varies depending on area to be anesthetized and vascularity of tissues

Oral mouth/throat preparations: Do not administer for >2 days or in children <2 years of age, unless directed by a physician; refer to specific package labeling

Topical: Apply to affected area as needed

Adults: Nonprescription diet aid: 6-15 mg just prior to food consumption, not to exceed 45 mg/day

Patient Information Do not eat for 1 hour after application to oral mucosa; chemical burns should be neutralized before application of benzocaine; avoid application to large areas of broken skin, especially in children

Dosage Forms

Topical for mucous membranes:

Gel: 6% (7.5 g); 20% (2.5 g, 3.75 g, 7.5 g, 30 g)

Liquid: 20% (3.75 mL, 9 mL, 13.3 mL, 30 mL)

Topical for skin disorders:

Aerosol, external use: 5% (92 mL, 105 g); 20% (82.5 mL, 90 mL, 92 mL, 150 mL)

Cream: (30 g, 60 g); 5% (30 g, 1 lb); 6% (28.4 g)

Lotion: (120 mL); 8% (90 mL)

Ointment: 5% (3.5 g, 28 g)

Spray: 5% (97.5 mL); 20% (20 g, 60 g, 120 g, 13.3 mL, 120 mL)

Mouth/throat preparations:

Cream: 5% (10 g)

Gel: 6.3% (7.5 g); 7.5% (7.2 g, 9.45 g, 14.1 g); 10% (6 g, 9.45 g, 10 g, 15 g); 15% (10.5 g); 20% (9.45 g, 14.1 g)

Liquid: (3.7 mL); 5% (8.8 mL); 6.3% (9 mL, 22 mL, 14.79 mL); 10% (13 mL); 20% (13.3 mL)

Lotion: 0.2% (15 mL); 2.5% (15 mL)

Lozenges: 5 mg, 6 mg, 10 mg, 15 mg

Ointment: 20% (30 g)

Paste: 20% (5 g, 15 g)

Nonprescription diet aid:

Candy: 6 mg

Gum: 6 mg

Benzocol® [OTC] *see* Benzocaine *on previous page*

Benzodent® [OTC] *see* Benzocaine *on previous page*

Benzodiazepines Comparison *see page 1397*

Benzonatate (ben ZOE na tate)

Brand Names Tessalon® Perles

Canadian/Mexican Brand Names Beknol® (Mexico); Pebegal® (Mexico); Tesalon® (Mexico)

Therapeutic Category Antitussive; Cough Preparation; Local Anesthetic, Oral

Use Symptomatic relief of nonproductive cough

Pregnancy Risk Factor C

Contraindications Known hypersensitivity to benzonatate or related compounds (such as tetracaine)

Adverse Reactions

1% to 10%:

Central nervous system: Sedation, headache, dizziness
Dermatologic: Rash
Gastrointestinal: GI upset
Neuromuscular & skeletal: Numbness in chest
Ocular: Burning sensation in eyes
Respiratory: Nasal congestion

Overdosage/Toxicology Symptoms of overdose include restlessness, tremor, CNS stimulation. The drug's local anesthetic activity can reduce the patient's gag reflex and, therefore, may contradict the use of ipecac following ingestion, this is especially true when the capsules are chewed.

Gastric lavage may be indicated if initiated early on following an acute ingestion or in comatose patients. The remaining treatment is supportive and symptomatic.

Mechanism of Action Tetracaine congener with antitussive properties; suppresses cough by topical anesthetic action on the respiratory stretch receptors

Pharmacodynamics/Kinetics

Onset of action: Therapeutic: Within 15-20 minutes
Duration: 3-8 hours

Usual Dosage Children >10 years and Adults: Oral: 100 mg 3 times/day or every 4 hours up to 600 mg/day

Monitoring Parameters Monitor patient's chest sounds and respiratory pattern

Patient Information Swallow capsule whole (do not break or chew capsule); use of hard candy may increase saliva flow to aid in protecting pharyngeal mucosa

Nursing Implications Change patient position every 2 hours to prevent pooling of secretions in lung; capsules are not to be crushed

Dosage Forms Capsule: 100 mg

Benzoyl Peroxide (BEN zoe il peer OKS ide)

Brand Names Advanced Formula Oxy® Sensitive Gel [OTC]; Ambi 10® [OTC]; Ben-Aqua® [OTC]; Benoxyl®; Benzac AC® Gel; Benzac AC® Wash; Benzac W® Gel; Benzac W® Wash; 5-Benzagel®; 10-Benzagel®; Benzashave® Cream; BlemErase® Lotion [OTC]; Brevoxyl® Gel; Clear By Design® Gel [OTC]; Clearsil® Maximum Strength [OTC]; Del Aqua-5® Gel; Del Aqua-10® Gel; Dermoxyl® Gel [OTC]; Desquam-E® Gel; Desquam-X® Gel; Desquam-X® Wash; Dryox® Gel [OTC]; Dryox® Wash [OTC]; Exact® Cream [OTC]; Fostex® 10% BPO Gel [OTC]; Fostex® 10% Wash [OTC]; Fostex® Bar [OTC]; Loroxide® [OTC]; Neutrogena® Acne Mask [OTC]; Oxy-5® Advanced Formula for Sensitive Skin [OTC]; Oxy-5® Tinted [OTC]; Oxy-10® Advanced Formula for Sensitive Skin [OTC]; Oxy 10® Wash [OTC]; PanOxyl®-AQ; PanOxyl® Bar [OTC]; Perfectoderm® Gel [OTC]; Peroxin A5®; Peroxin A10®; Persa-Gel®; Theroxide® Wash [OTC]; Vanoxide® [OTC]

Canadian/Mexican Brand Names Acetoxyl® (Canada); Acnomel® B.P.5 (Canada); H_2Oxyl® (Canada); Oxyderm® (Canada); Solugel® (Canada)

Therapeutic Category Acne Products; Topical Skin Product, Acne

Use Adjunctive treatment of mild to moderate acne vulgaris and acne rosacea

Pregnancy Risk Factor C

Pregnancy/Breast-Feeding Implications It is not known whether benzoyl peroxide can cause fetal harm when administered to pregnant women; topical application is generally considered safe for use in pregnancy

Contraindications Known hypersensitivity to benzoyl peroxide, benzoic acid, or any of its components

Warnings/Precautions For external use only; may bleach colored fabrics; avoid contact with eyes, eyelids, lips, and mucous membranes, and highly inflamed or denuded skin; discontinue if burning, swelling, or undue dryness occurs

Adverse Reactions 1% to 10%:

Dermatologic: Contact dermatitis, dryness, erythema, peeling, stinging
Local: Irritation

Overdosage/Toxicology Symptoms of overdose include excessive scaling, erythema, or edema

For treatment, discontinue use; to hasten resolution of adverse effects, use emollients, cool compresses or topical corticosteroids

Drug Interactions Increased toxicity: Benzoyl peroxide potentiates adverse reactions seen with tretinoin

Mechanism of Action Releases free-radical oxygen which oxidizes bacterial proteins in the sebaceous follicles decreasing the number of anaerobic bacteria and irritating free fatty acids; exerts a keratolytic activity and a comedolytic effect

Pharmacodynamics/Kinetics

Absorption: ~5% through the skin; gels are more penetrating than creams
Metabolism: Major metabolite is benzoic acid
Elimination: Major metabolite, benzoic acid, excreted in urine as benzoate

Usual Dosage Children and Adults:

Cleansers: Wash once or twice daily; control amount of drying or peeling by modifying dose frequency or concentration

Topical: Apply sparingly once daily; gradually increase to 2-3 times/day if needed. If excessive dryness or peeling occurs, reduce dose frequency or concentration; if excessive stinging or burning occurs, remove with mild soap and water; resume use the next day.

Patient Information Shake lotion before using; cleanse and make sure skin is dry before applying; may bleach color from fabrics; may be worn under water-based makeup. Improvement should occur within 2 weeks; keep away from eyes, mouth, mucous membranes; expect dryness and peeling; if excessive redness or irritation occurs, discontinue use. Avoid excessive sunlight, sun lamps, or other topical medication unless directed by a physician.

Nursing Implications Watch for signs of systemic infection; granulation may indicate effectiveness

Dosage Forms

Bar: 5% (113 g); 10% (106 g, 113 g)
Cream: 5% (18 g, 113.4 g); 10% (18 g, 28 g, 113.4 g)
Gel: 2.5% (30 g, 42.5 g, 45 g, 57 g, 60 g, 90 g, 113 g); 5% (42.5 g, 45 g, 60 g, 80 g, 90 g, 113.4 g); 10% (30 g, 42.5 g, 45 g, 56.7 g, 60 g, 90 g, 113.4 g, 120 g); 20% (30 g, 60 g)
Liquid: 5% (120 mL, 150 mL, 240 mL); 10% (120 mL, 150 mL, 240 mL)
Lotion: 5% (25 mL, 30 mL); 5.5% (25 mL); 10% (12 mL, 29 mL, 30 mL, 60 mL)
Mask: 5% (30 mL, 60 mL, 60 g)

Benzthiazide (benz THYE a zide)

Related Information

Sulfonamide Derivatives *on page 1420*

Brand Names Aquatag®; Exna®; Hydrex®; Marazide®; Proaqua®

Therapeutic Category Antihypertensive; Diuretic, Thiazide

Use Management of mild to moderate hypertension; treatment of edema in congestive heart failure and nephrotic syndrome

Pregnancy Risk Factor D

Contraindications Anuria, renal decompensation, hypersensitivity to benzthiazide or any component, cross-sensitivity with other thiazides and sulfonamide derivatives

Warnings/Precautions Hypokalemia, renal disease, hepatic disease, gout, lupus erythematosus, diabetes mellitus; use with caution in severe renal diseases

Adverse Reactions

1% to 10%:
- Cardiovascular: Orthostatic hypotension
- Endocrine & metabolic: Hyponatremia, hypokalemia
- Gastrointestinal: Anorexia, upset stomach, diarrhea

<1%:
- Central nervous system: Drowsiness
- Endocrine & metabolic: Hyperuricemia
- Gastrointestinal: Nausea, vomiting
- Genitourinary: Polyuria
- Hematologic: Aplastic anemia, hemolytic anemia, leukopenia, agranulocytosis, thrombocytopenia
- Hepatic: Hepatitis, hepatic function impairment
- Neuromuscular & skeletal: Paresthesia
- Renal: Uremia
- Miscellaneous: Allergic reactions

Overdosage/Toxicology Symptoms of overdose include hypermotility, diuresis, lethargy, confusion, muscle weakness; following GI decontamination, therapy is supportive with I.V. fluids, electrolytes, and I.V. pressors if needed

Drug Interactions

Decreased effect of oral hypoglycemics, decreased absorption with cholestyramine and colestipol

Increased effect with furosemide and other loop diuretics

(Continued)

Benzthiazide *(Continued)*

Increased toxicity/levels of lithium

Pharmacodynamics/Kinetics

Onset of action: Within 2 hours
Duration: 12 hours

Usual Dosage Oral:

Children: 1-4 mg/kg/day in 3 divided doses
Adults: 50-200 mg/day

Monitoring Parameters Assess weight, I & O reports daily to determine fluid loss; blood pressure, serum electrolytes, BUN, creatinine

Patient Information May be taken with food or milk; take early in day to avoid nocturia; take the last dose of multiple doses no later than 6 PM unless instructed otherwise. A few people who take this medication become more sensitive to sunlight and may experience skin rash, redness, itching, or severe sunburn, especially if sun block SPF ≥15 is not used on exposed skin areas.

Nursing Implications Take blood pressure with patient lying down and standing

Dosage Forms Tablet: 50 mg

Benztropine (BENZ troe peen)

Brand Names Cogentin®

Canadian/Mexican Brand Names PMS-Benztropine (Canada)

Synonyms Benztropine Mesylate

Therapeutic Category Anticholinergic Agent; Anti-Parkinson's Agent

Use Adjunctive treatment of Parkinson's disease; also used in treatment of drug-induced extrapyramidal effects (except tardive dyskinesia) and acute dystonic reactions

Pregnancy Risk Factor C

Contraindications Children <3 years of age, use with caution in older children (dosage not established); patients with narrow-angle glaucoma; hypersensitivity to any component; pyloric or duodenal obstruction, stenosing peptic ulcers; bladder neck obstructions; achalasia; myasthenia gravis

Warnings/Precautions Use with caution in hot weather or during exercise. Elderly patients frequently develop increased sensitivity and require strict dosage regulation - side effects may be more severe in elderly patients with atherosclerotic changes. Use with caution in patients with tachycardia, cardiac arrhythmias, hypertension, hypotension, prostatic hypertrophy (especially in the elderly) or any tendency toward urinary retention, liver or kidney disorders and obstructive disease of the GI or GU tract. When given in large doses or to susceptible patients, may cause weakness and inability to move particular muscle groups.

Adverse Reactions

>10%:

- Dermatologic: Dry skin
- Gastrointestinal: Constipation, dry throat, xerostomia
- Respiratory: Dry nose
- Miscellaneous: Diaphoresis (decreased)

1% to 10%:

- Dermatologic: Increased sensitivity to light
- Endocrine & metabolic: Decreased flow of breast milk
- Gastrointestinal: Dysphagia

<1%:

- Cardiovascular: Tachycardia, orthostatic hypotension, ventricular fibrillation, palpitations
- Central nervous system: Coma, drowsiness, nervousness, hallucinations; the elderly may be at increased risk for confusion and hallucinations, headache, loss of memory, fatigue, ataxia
- Dermatologic: Rash
- Gastrointestinal: Nausea, vomiting, bloated feeling
- Genitourinary: Dysuria
- Ocular: Blurred vision, mydriasis, increased intraocular pain
- Neuromuscular & skeletal: Weakness

Overdosage/Toxicology Symptoms of overdose include CNS depression, confusion, nervousness, hallucinations, dizziness, blurred vision, nausea, vomiting, hyperthermia

For anticholinergic overdose with severe life-threatening symptoms, physostigmine 1-2 mg (0.5 or 0.02 mg/kg for children) S.C. or I.V., slowly may be given to reverse these effects. Anticholinergic toxicity is caused by strong binding of the drug to cholinergic receptors. Anticholinesterase inhibitors reduce acetylcholinesterase, the enzyme that breaks down acetylcholine and thereby allows acetylcholine to accumulate and compete for receptor binding with the offending anticholinergic.

Drug Interactions

Decreased effect: May increase gastric degradation of levodopa and decrease the amount of levodopa absorbed by delaying gastric emptying - the opposite may be true for digoxin

Increased toxicity: Central anticholinergic syndrome can occur when administered with narcotic analgesics, phenothiazines and other antipsychotics, tricyclic antidepressants, quinidine and some other antiarrhythmics, and antihistamines

Mechanism of Action Thought to partially block striatal cholinergic receptors to help balance cholinergic and dopaminergic activity

Pharmacodynamics/Kinetics

Onset of action:

Oral: Within 1 hour

Parenteral: Within 15 minutes

Duration of action: 6-48 hours (wide range)

Usual Dosage Use in children <3 years of age should be reserved for life-threatening emergencies

Drug-induced extrapyramidal reaction: Oral, I.M., I.V.:

Children >3 years: 0.02-0.05 mg/kg/dose 1-2 times/day

Adults: 1-4 mg/dose 1-2 times/day

Acute dystonia: Adults: I.M., I.V.: 1-2 mg

Parkinsonism: Oral:

Adults: 0.5-6 mg/day in 1-2 divided doses; if one dose is greater, administer at bedtime; titrate dose in 0.5 mg increments at 5- to 6-day intervals

Elderly: Initial: 0.5 mg once or twice daily; increase by 0.5 mg as needed at 5-6 days; maximum: 6 mg/day

Dietary Considerations Alcohol: Additive CNS effects, avoid use

Patient Information Take after meals or with food if GI upset occurs; do not discontinue drug abruptly; notify physician if adverse GI effects, rapid or pounding heartbeat, confusion, eye pain, rash, fever, or heat intolerance occurs. Observe caution when performing hazardous tasks or those that require alertness such as driving, as may cause drowsiness. Avoid alcohol and other CNS depressants. May cause dry mouth - adequate fluid intake or hard sugar-free candy may relieve. Difficult urination or constipation may occur - notify physician if effects persist; may increase susceptibility to heat stroke.

Nursing Implications No significant difference in onset of I.M. or I.V. injection, therefore, there is usually no need to use the I.V. route. Improvement is sometimes noticeable a few minutes after injection.

Dosage Forms

Injection, as mesylate: 1 mg/mL (2 mL)

Tablet, as mesylate: 0.5 mg, 1 mg, 2 mg

Benztropine Mesylate *see* Benztropine *on previous page*

Benzylpenicillin Benzathine *see* Penicillin G Benzathine *on page 961*

Benzylpenicillin Potassium *see* Penicillin G, Parenteral, Aqueous *on page 962*

Benzylpenicillin Sodium *see* Penicillin G, Parenteral, Aqueous *on page 962*

Benzylpenicilloyl-polylysine (BEN zil pen i SIL oyl pol i LIE seen)

Related Information

Skin Tests *on page 1501*

Brand Names Pre-Pen®

Synonyms Penicilloyl-polylysine; PPL

Therapeutic Category Diagnostic Agent, Penicillin Allergy Skin Test

Use Adjunct in assessing the risk of administering penicillin (penicillin or benzylpenicillin) in adults with a history of clinical penicillin hypersensitivity

Pregnancy Risk Factor C

Contraindications Patients known to be extremely hypersensitive to penicillin

Warnings/Precautions PPL test alone does not identify those patients who react to a minor antigenic determinant and does not appear to predict reliably the occurrence of late reactions. A negative skin test is associated with an incidence of allergic reactions <5% after penicillin administration and a positive skin test is associated with a >20% incidence of allergic reaction after penicillin administration; have epinephrine 1:1000 available.

Adverse Reactions

1% to 10%: Local: Intense local inflammatory response at skin test site

<1%:

Cardiovascular: Edema

Dermatologic: Pruritus, erythema, urticaria

Local: Wheal

Sensitivity reactions: Systemic allergic reactions occur rarely

(Continued)

Benzylpenicilloyl-polylysine *(Continued)*

Drug Interactions
Decreased effect: Corticosteroids and other immunosuppressive agents may inhibit the immune response to the skin test

Stability Refrigerate; discard if left at room temperature for longer than one day

Mechanism of Action Elicits IgE antibodies which produce type I accelerate urticarial reactions to penicillins

Usual Dosage PPL is administered by a scratch technique or by intradermal injection. For initial testing, PPL should always be applied via the scratch technique. **Do not administer intradermally to patients who have positive reactions to a scratch test.** PPL test alone does not identify those patients who react to a minor antigenic determinant and does not appear to predict reliably the occurrence of late reactions.

Scratch test: Use scratch technique with a 20-gauge needle to make 3-5 mm nonbleeding scratch on epidermis, apply a small drop of solution to scratch, rub in gently with applicator or toothpick. A positive reaction consists of a pale wheal surrounding the scratch site which develops within 10 minutes and ranges from 5-15 mm or more in diameter.

Intradermal test: Use intradermal test with a tuberculin syringe with a 26- to 30-gauge short bevel needle; a dose of 0.01-0.02 mL is injected intradermally. A control of 0.9% sodium chloride should be injected at least 1.5" from the PPL test site. Most skin responses to the intradermal test will develop within 5-15 minutes.

Interpretation:
(-) Negative: No reaction
(±) Ambiguous: Wheal only slightly larger than original bleb with or without erythematous flare and larger than control site
(+) Positive: Itching and marked increase in size of original bleb
Control site should be reactionless

Nursing Implications Always use scratch test for initial testing

Dosage Forms Solution: 0.25 mL

Bepridil (BE pri dil)

Related Information
Calcium Channel Blockers Comparative Actions *on page 1401*
Calcium Channel Blockers Comparative Pharmacokinetics *on page 1402*
Calcium Channel Blockers FDA-Approved Indications *on page 1403*

Brand Names Vascor®

Canadian/Mexican Brand Names Bapadin® (Canada)

Synonyms Bepridil Hydrochloride

Therapeutic Category Antianginal Agent; Calcium Channel Blocker

Use Treatment of chronic stable angina; due to side effect profile, reserve for patients who have been intolerant of other antianginal therapy; bepridil may be used alone or in combination with nitrates or beta-blockers

Pregnancy Risk Factor C

Contraindications History of serious ventricular or atrial arrhythmias (especially tachycardia or those associated with accessory conduction pathways), sick-sinus syndrome, or second or third degree A-V block (without a functioning pacemaker), cardiogenic shock, hypotension, uncompensated cardiac insufficiency, congenital Q-T interval prolongation, patients taking other drugs that prolong the Q-T interval, history of hypersensitivity to bepridil or any component, calcium channel blockers, or adenosine

Warnings/Precautions Use with great caution in patients with history of serious ventricular arrhythmias, IHSS, congenital Q-T interval prolongation, or other drugs that prolong Q-T interval; reserve for patients in whom other antianginals have failed. Carefully titrate dosages for patients with impaired renal or hepatic function; use caution when treating patients with congestive heart failure, sick-sinus syndrome, severe left ventricular dysfunction, hypertrophic cardiomyopathy (especially obstructive), concomitant therapy with beta-blockers or digoxin, edema, or increased intracranial pressure with cranial tumors; do not abruptly withdraw (may cause chest pain); elderly may experience hypotension and constipation more readily.

Adverse Reactions
>10%:
Central nervous system: Dizziness, headache
Gastrointestinal: Nausea, dyspepsia, abdominal pain, GI distress
Neuromuscular & skeletal: Weakness

1% to 10%:
Cardiovascular: Bradycardia, palpitations
Central nervous system: Nervousness
Gastrointestinal: Diarrhea, anorexia, xerostomia
Miscellaneous: Flu syndrome

<1%:

Cardiovascular: Ventricular premature contractions, hypertension, torsade de pointes, edema, syncope, prolonged Q-T intervals
Central nervous system: Fever, psychotic behavior, akathisia
Dermatologic: Rash
Gastrointestinal: Abnormal taste
Genitourinary: Sexual dysfunction
Hematologic: Agranulocytosis
Neuromuscular & skeletal: Tremor, myalgia, arthritis
Ocular: Blurred vision
Respiratory: Nasal congestion, cough, pharyngitis
Miscellaneous: Diaphoresis

Overdosage/Toxicology The primary cardiac symptoms of calcium blocker overdose includes hypotension and bradycardia. The hypotension is caused by peripheral vasodilation, myocardial depression, and bradycardia. Bradycardia results from sinus bradycardia, second- or third-degree atrioventricular block, or sinus arrest with junctional rhythm. Intraventricular conduction is usually not affected so QRS duration is normal (verapamil does prolong the P-R interval and bepridil prolongs the Q-T and may cause ventricular arrhythmias, including torsade de pointes).

The noncardiac symptoms include confusion, stupor, nausea, vomiting, metabolic acidosis and hyperglycemia. Following initial gastric decontamination, if possible, repeated calcium administration may promptly reverse the depressed cardiac contractility (but not sinus node depression or peripheral vasodilation); glucagon, epinephrine, and amrinone may treat refractory hypotension; glucagon and epinephrine also increase the heart rate (outside the U.S., 4-aminopyridine may be available as an antidote); dialysis and hemoperfusion are not effective in enhancing elimination although repeat-dose activated charcoal may serve as an adjunct with sustained-release preparations.

Drug Interactions

Increased toxicity/effect/levels:

Bepridil and cyclosporine may increase cyclosporine levels (other calcium channel blockers have been shown to interact)
Bepridil and digitalis glycoside may increase digitalis glycoside levels

Mechanism of Action Bepridil, a type 4 calcium antagonist, possesses characteristics of the traditional calcium antagonists, inhibiting calcium ion from entering the "slow channels" or select voltage-sensitive areas of vascular smooth muscle and myocardium during depolarization and producing a relaxation of coronary vascular smooth muscle and coronary vasodilation. However, bepridil may also inhibit fast sodium channels (inward), which may account for some of its side effects (eg, arrhythmias); a direct bradycardia effect of bepridil has been postulated via direct action on the S-A node.

Pharmacodynamics/Kinetics

Onset of action: 1 hour
Absorption: Oral: 100%
Distribution: Protein binding: >99%
Metabolism: Hepatic
Bioavailability: 60%
Half-life: 24 hours
Time to peak: 2-3 hours
Elimination: Metabolites renally excreted

Usual Dosage Adults: Oral: Initial: 200 mg/day, then adjust dose at 10-day intervals until optimal response is achieved; maximum daily dose: 400 mg

Monitoring Parameters EKG and serum electrolytes, blood pressure, signs and symptoms of congestive heart failure; elderly may need very close monitoring due to underlying cardiac and organ system defects

Reference Range 1-2 ng/mL

Test Interactions ↑ aminotransferases, ↑ CPK, LDH

Patient Information May cause cardiac arrhythmias if potassium is low; can be taken with food or meals, maintain potassium supplementation as directed, routine EKGs will be necessary during start of therapy or dosage changes; notify physician if the following occur: irregular heartbeat, shortness of breath, pronounced dizziness, constipation, or hypotension

Nursing Implications EKG required; patient should be hospitalized during initiation or escalation of therapy

Additional Information Although there is some initial data which may show increased risk of myocardial infarction following treatment of hypertension with calcium antagonists, controlled trials (eg, ALL-HAT) are ongoing to examine the long-term effects of not only calcium antagonists but other antihypertensives in preventing heart disease. Until these studies are completed, patients taking calcium antagonists should be encouraged to continue with prescribed antihypertensive regimes, although a switch from high-dose, short-acting agents to

(Continued)

Bepridil *(Continued)*

sustained release products may be warranted. It is also generally agreed that calcium antagonists should be avoided as the primary treatment for hypertension unless diuretics or beta-blockers are contraindicated and for the primary treatment of angina following acute myocardial infarction.

Dosage Forms Tablet, as hydrochloride: 200 mg, 300 mg, 400 mg

Bepridil Hydrochloride *see* Bepridil *on page 144*

Beractant (ber AKT ant)

Brand Names Survanta®

Synonyms Bovine Lung Surfactant; Natural Lung Surfactant

Therapeutic Category Lung Surfactant

Use Prevention and treatment of respiratory distress syndrome (RDS) in premature infants

Prophylactic therapy: Body weight <1250 g in infants at risk for developing or with evidence of surfactant deficiency

Rescue therapy: Treatment of infants with RDS confirmed by x-ray and requiring mechanical ventilation (administer as soon as possible - within 8 hours of age)

Warnings/Precautions Rapidly affects oxygenation and lung compliance and should be restricted to a highly supervised use in a clinical setting with immediate availability of clinicians experienced with intubation and ventilatory management of premature infants. If transient episodes of bradycardia and decreased oxygen saturation occur, discontinue the dosing procedure and initiate measures to alleviate the condition; produces rapid improvements in lung oxygenation and compliance that may require immediate reductions in ventilator settings and FiO_2.

Adverse Reactions During the dosing procedure:

Cardiovascular: Transient bradycardia, vasoconstriction, hypotension, hypertension, pallor

Respiratory: Oxygen desaturation, endotracheal tube blockage, hypocarbia, hypercarbia, apnea, pulmonary air leaks, pulmonary interstitial emphysema

Miscellaneous: Increased probability of post-treatment nosocomial sepsis

Stability Refrigerate; protect from light, prior to administration warm by standing at room temperature for 20 minutes or held in hand for 8 minutes; **artificial warming methods should not be used**; unused, unopened vials warmed to room temperature may be returned to the refrigerator within 8 hours of warming only once

Mechanism of Action Replaces deficient or ineffective endogenous lung surfactant in neonates with respiratory distress syndrome (RDS) or in neonates at risk of developing RDS. Surfactant prevents the alveoli from collapsing during expiration by lowering surface tension between air and alveolar surfaces.

Pharmacodynamics/Kinetics Alveolar clearance is rapid

Usual Dosage

Prophylactic treatment: Administer 100 mg phospholipids (4 mL/kg) intratracheal as soon as possible; as many as 4 doses may be administered during the first 48 hours of life, no more frequently than 6 hours apart. The need for additional doses is determined by evidence of continuing respiratory distress; if the infant is still intubated and requiring at least 30% inspired oxygen to maintain a PaO_2 $\leq$80 torr.

Rescue treatment: Administer 100 mg phospholipids (4 mL/kg) as soon as the diagnosis of RDS is made; may repeat if needed, no more frequently than every 6 hours to a maximum of 4 doses

Administration

For intratracheal administration only

Suction infant prior to administration; inspect solution to verify complete mixing of the suspension

Administer intratracheally by instillation through a 5-French end-hole catheter inserted into the infant's endotracheal tube

Administer the dose in four 1 mL/kg aliquots. Each quarter-dose is instilled over 2-3 seconds; each quarter-dose is administered with the infant in a different position; slightly downward inclination with head turned to the right, then repeat with head turned to the left; then slightly upward inclination with head turned to the right, then repeat with head turned to the left.

Monitoring Parameters Continuous EKG and transcutaneous O_2 saturation should be monitored during administration; frequent arterial blood gases are necessary to prevent postdosing hyperoxia and hypocarbia

Nursing Implications Do not shake; if settling occurs during storage, swirl gently

Additional Information Each mL contains 25 mg phospholipids suspended in 0.9% sodium chloride solution. Contents of 1 mL: 0.5-1.75 mg triglycerides, 1.4-3.5 mg free fatty acids, and <1 mg protein.

Dosage Forms Suspension: 200 mg (8 mL)

Berocca® *see* Vitamins, Multiple *on page 1310*

Berubigen® *see* Cyanocobalamin *on page 319*

Beta-2® *see* Isoetharine *on page 678*

Beta-Blockers Comparison *see page 1398*

Beta-Carotene (BAY tah KARE oh teen)

Brand Names Max-Caro® [OTC]; Provatene® [OTC]; Solatene®

Therapeutic Category Vitamin, Fat Soluble

Use Reduces severity of photosensitivity reactions in patients with erythropoietic protoporphyria (EPP)

Pregnancy Risk Factor C

Contraindications Hypersensitivity to beta-carotene

Warnings/Precautions Use with caution in patients with renal or hepatic impairment; not proven effective as a sunscreen

Adverse Reactions

>10%: Dermatologic: Carotenodermia (yellowing of palms, hands, or soles of feet, and to a lesser extent the face)

<1%:

Central nervous system: Dizziness
Dermatologic: Bruising
Gastrointestinal: Diarrhea
Neuromuscular & skeletal: Arthralgia

Drug Interactions Fulfills vitamin A requirements, do not prescribe additional vitamin A

Mechanism of Action The exact mechanism of action in erythropoietic protoporphyria has not as yet been elucidated; although patient must become carotenemic before effects are observed, there appears to be more than a simple internal light screen responsible for the drug's action. A protective effect was achieved when beta-carotene was added to blood samples. The concentrations of solutions used were similar to those achieved in treated patients. Topically applied beta-carotene is considerably less effective than systemic therapy.

Pharmacodynamics/Kinetics

Metabolism: Prior to absorption, converted to vitamin A in the wall of the small intestine and then further oxidized to retinoic acid and retinol in the presence of fat and bile acids; small amounts are then stored in the liver; retinol (active) is conjugated with glucuronic acid

Elimination: In urine and feces

Usual Dosage Oral:

Children <14 years: 30-150 mg/day
Adults: 30-300 mg/day

Patient Information Take with meals; skin may appear slightly yellow-orange; not a proven sunscreen

Dosage Forms Capsule: 15 mg, 30 mg

Betachron E-R® *see* Propranolol *on page 1067*

Betadine® [OTC] *see* Povidone-Iodine *on page 1031*

Betadine® First Aid Antibiotics + Moisturizer [OTC] *see* Bacitracin and Polymyxin B *on page 129*

9-Beta-D-ribofuranosyladenine *see* Adenosine *on page 33*

Betagan® *see* Levobunolol *on page 712*

Betagen [OTC] *see* Povidone-Iodine *on page 1031*

Betamethasone (bay ta METH a sone)

Related Information

Corticosteroids Comparison *on page 1407*

Brand Names Alphatrex®; Betatrex®; Beta-Val®; Celestone®; Cel-U-Jec®; Diprolene®; Diprolene® AF; Diprosone®; Maxivate®; Selestoject®; Teladar®; Urticort®; Valisone®

Canadian/Mexican Brand Names Betnesol® [Disodium Phosphate] (Canada); Diprolene® Glycol [Dipropionate] (Canada); Occlucort® (Canada); Rhoprolene® (Canada); Rhoprosone® (Canada); Selestoject® [Sodium Phosphate] (Canada); Taro-Sone® (Canada); Topilene® (Canada); Topisone® (Canada)

Synonyms Betamethasone Dipropionate; Betamethasone Dipropionate, Augmented; Betamethasone Sodium Phosphate; Betamethasone Valerate; Flubenisolone

Therapeutic Category Anti-inflammatory Agent; Corticosteroid; Corticosteroid, Systemic; Corticosteroid, Topical (Low Potency); Corticosteroid, Topical (Medium Potency); Corticosteroid, Topical (High Potency); Glucocorticoid

Use Inflammatory dermatoses such as seborrheic or atopic dermatitis, neurodermatitis, anogenital pruritus, psoriasis, inflammatory phase of xerosis

Pregnancy Risk Factor C

(Continued)

Betamethasone *(Continued)*

Pregnancy/Breast-Feeding Implications There are no reports linking the use of betamethasone with congenital defects in the literature; betamethasone is often used in patients with premature labor [26-34 weeks gestation] to stimulate fetal lung maturation

Contraindications Systemic fungal infections; hypersensitivity to betamethasone or any component

Warnings/Precautions Fatalities have occurred due to adrenal insufficiency in asthmatic patients during and after transfer from systemic corticosteroids to aerosol steroids; several months may be required for recovery of this syndrome; during this period, aerosol steroids do **not** provide the systemic steroid needed to treat patients having trauma, surgery, or infections; use with caution in patients with hypothyroidism, cirrhosis, ulcerative colitis; do not use occlusive dressings on weeping or exudative lesions and general caution with occlusive dressings should be observed; discontinue if skin irritation or contact dermatitis should occur; do not use in patients with decreased skin circulation

Adverse Reactions

>10%:
- Central nervous system: Insomnia
- Gastrointestinal: Increased appetite, indigestion
- Ocular: Temporary mild blurred vision

1% to 10%:
- Dermatologic: Erythema, itching
- Endocrine & metabolic: Diabetes mellitus
- Local: Dryness, irritation, papular rashes, burning
- Ocular: Cataracts

<1%:
- Cardiovascular: Hypertension
- Central nervous system: Convulsions, vertigo, confusion, headache
- Dermatologic: Thin fragile skin, hyperpigmentation or hypertrichosis, hypopigmentation, impaired wound healing, acneiform eruptions, perioral dermatitis, maceration of skin, skin atrophy, striae, miliaria
- Endocrine & metabolic: Cushingoid state, sodium retention
- Gastrointestinal: Peptic ulcer
- Local: Sterile abscess
- Neuromuscular & skeletal: Myalgia, osteoporosis
- Ocular: Glaucoma, sudden blindness

Overdosage/Toxicology When consumed in excessive quantities for prolonged periods, systemic hypercorticism and adrenal suppression may occur; in those cases, discontinuation and withdrawal of the corticosteroid should be done judiciously

Drug Interactions

Inducer of cytochrome P-450 enzymes
Cytochrome P-450 3A enzyme substrate
Decreased effect (corticosteroid) by barbiturates, phenytoin, rifampin

Mechanism of Action Controls the rate of protein synthesis, depresses the migration of polymorphonuclear leukocytes, fibroblasts, reverses capillary permeability, and lysosomal stabilization at the cellular level to prevent or control inflammation

Pharmacodynamics/Kinetics

Protein binding: 64%
Metabolism: Extensively in the liver
Half-life: 6.5 hours
Time to peak serum concentration: I.V.: Within 10-36 minutes
Elimination: <5% of dose excreted renally as unchanged drug

Usual Dosage Base dosage on severity of disease and patient response

Children: Use lowest dose listed as initial dose for adrenocortical insufficiency (physiologic replacement)
- Oral: 0.0175-0.25 mg/kg/day divided every 6-8 hours **or** 0.5-7.5 mg/m²/day divided every 6-8 hours
- I.M.: 0.0175-0.125 mg base/kg/day divided every 6-12 hours **or** 0.5-7.5 mg base/m²/day divided every 6-12 hours

Adolescents and Adults:
- Oral: 2.4-4.8 mg/day in 2-4 doses; range: 0.6-7.2 mg/day
- I.M.: Betamethasone sodium phosphate and betamethasone acetate: 0.6-9 mg/day (generally, 1/3 to 1/2 of oral dose) divided every 12-24 hours
- Intrabursal, intra-articular, intradermal: 0.25-2 mL
- Intralesional: Rheumatoid arthritis/osteoarthritis:
  - Very large joints: 1-2 mL
  - Large joints: 1 mL
  - Medium joints: 0.5-1 mL
  - Small joints: 0.25-0.5 mL

Topical: Apply thin film 2-4 times/day

Patient Information Take oral with food or milk; apply topical sparingly to areas and gently rub in until it disappears, not for use on broken skin or in areas of infection; do not apply to face or inguinal areas

Nursing Implications Apply topical sparingly to areas; not for use on broken skin or in areas of infection; do not apply to wet skin unless directed; do not apply to face or inguinal area. Not for alternate day therapy; once daily doses should be given in the morning; do not administer injectable sodium phosphate/acetate suspension I.V.

Dosage Forms

Base (Celestone®), Oral:

Syrup: 0.6 mg/5 mL (118 mL)

Tablet: 0.6 mg

Dipropionate salt (Diprosone®)

Aerosol: 0.1% (85 g)

Cream: 0.05% (15 g, 45 g)

Lotion: 0.05% (20 mL, 30 mL, 60 mL)

Ointment: 0.05% (15 g, 45 g)

Dipropionate salt, augmented (Diprolene®)

Cream: 0.05% (15 g, 45 g)

Gel: 0.05% (15 g, 45 g)

Lotion: 0.05% (30 mL, 60 mL)

Ointment, topical: 0.05% (15 g, 45 g)

Valerate salt (Betatrex®, Valisone®)

Cream: 0.01% (15 g, 60 g); 0.1% (15 g, 45 g, 110 g, 430 g)

Lotion: 0.1% (20 mL, 60 mL)

Ointment: 0.1% (15 g, 45 g)

Valerate salt (Beta-Val®)

Cream: 0.01% (15 g, 60 g); 0.1% (15 g, 45 g, 110 g, 430 g)

Lotion: 0.1% (20 mL, 60 mL)

Injection: Sodium phosphate salt (Celestone Phosphate®, Cel-U-Jec®, Selestoject®): 4 mg betamethasone phosphate/mL (equivalent to 3 mg betamethasone/mL) (5 mL)

Injection, suspension: Sodium phosphate and acetate salt (Celestone® Soluspan®): 6 mg/mL (3 mg of betamethasone sodium phosphate and 3 mg of betamethasone acetate per mL) (5 mL)

Betamethasone Dipropionate *see* Betamethasone *on page 147*

Betamethasone Dipropionate, Augmented *see* Betamethasone *on page 147*

Betamethasone Sodium Phosphate *see* Betamethasone *on page 147*

Betamethasone Valerate *see* Betamethasone *on page 147*

Betapace® *see* Sotalol *on page 1151*

Betapen®-VK *see* Penicillin V Potassium *on page 965*

Betasept® [OTC] *see* Chlorhexidine Gluconate *on page 253*

Betaseron® *see* Interferon Beta-1b *on page 669*

Betatrex® *see* Betamethasone *on page 147*

Beta-Val® *see* Betamethasone *on page 147*

Betaxolol (be TAKS oh lol)

Related Information

Beta-Blockers Comparison *on page 1398*

Glaucoma Drug Therapy Comparison *on page 1410*

Brand Names Betoptic®; Betoptic® S; Kerlone®

Synonyms Betaxolol Hydrochloride

Therapeutic Category Beta-Adrenergic Blocker; Beta-Adrenergic Blocker, Ophthalmic

Use Treatment of chronic open-angle glaucoma and ocular hypertension; management of hypertension

Pregnancy Risk Factor C

Contraindications Bronchial asthma, sinus bradycardia, second and third degree A-V block, cardiac failure (unless a functioning pacemaker present), cardiogenic shock, hypersensitivity to betaxolol or any component

Warnings/Precautions Some products contain sulfites which can cause allergic reactions; diminished response occurs over time; use with caution in patients with decreased renal or hepatic function (dosage adjustment required); patients with a history of asthma, congestive heart failure, diabetes mellitus, or bradycardia appear to be at a higher risk for adverse effects

Adverse Reactions

1% to 10%:

Cardiovascular: Bradycardia, palpitations, edema, congestive heart failure

Central nervous system: Dizziness, fatigue, lethargy, headache

Dermatologic: Erythema, itching

(Continued)

Betaxolol *(Continued)*

Ocular: Mild ocular stinging and discomfort, tearing, photophobia, decreased corneal sensitivity, keratitis
Miscellaneous: Cold extremities
<1%:
Cardiovascular: Chest pain
Central nervous system: Nervousness, depression, hallucinations
Hematologic: Thrombocytopenia

Overdosage/Toxicology Symptoms of significant overdose include bradycardia, hypotension, A-V block, CHF, bronchospasm, hypoglycemia

Sympathomimetics (eg, epinephrine or dopamine), glucagon, or a pacemaker can be used to treat the toxic bradycardia, asystole, and/or hypotension; initially, fluids may be the best treatment for toxic hypotension.

Drug Interactions

Decreased effect of beta-blockers with aluminum salts, barbiturates, calcium salts, cholestyramine, colestipol, NSAIDs, penicillins (ampicillin), rifampin, salicylates and sulfinpyrazone due to decreased bioavailability and plasma levels

Beta-blockers may decrease the effect of sulfonylureas

Increased effect/toxicity of beta-blockers with calcium blockers (diltiazem, felodipine, nicardipine), contraceptives, flecainide, haloperidol (propranolol, hypotensive effects), H_2-antagonists (metoprolol, propranolol only by cimetidine, possibly ranitidine), hydralazine (metoprolol, propranolol), loop diuretics (propranolol, not atenolol), MAO inhibitors (metoprolol, nadolol, bradycardia), phenothiazines (propranolol), propafenone (metoprolol, propranolol), quinidine (in extensive metabolizers), ciprofloxacin, thyroid hormones (metoprolol, propranolol, when hypothyroid patient is converted to euthyroid state)

Beta-blockers may increase the effect/toxicity of flecainide, haloperidol (hypotensive effects), hydralazine, phenothiazines, acetaminophen, anticoagulants (propranolol, warfarin), benzodiazepines (not atenolol), clonidine (hypertensive crisis after or during withdrawal of either agent), epinephrine (initial hypertensive episode followed by bradycardia), nifedipine and verapamil lidocaine, ergots (peripheral ischemia), prazosin (postural hypotension)

Beta-blockers may affect the action or levels of ethanol, disopyramide, nondepolarizing muscle relaxants and theophylline although the effects are difficult to predict

Stability Avoid freezing

Mechanism of Action Competitively blocks $beta_1$-receptors, with little or no effect on $beta_2$-receptors; ophthalmic reduces intraocular pressure by reducing the production of aqueous humor

Pharmacodynamics/Kinetics

Onset of action: 1-1.5 hours
Duration: ≥12 hours
Absorption: Systemically absorbed
Metabolism: Hepatic (multiple metabolites)
Half-life: 12-22 hours
Time to peak: Within 2 hours
Elimination: Renal

Usual Dosage Adults:

Ophthalmic: Instill 1 drop twice daily
Oral: 10 mg/day; may increase dose to 20 mg/day after 7-14 days if desired response is not achieved; initial dose in elderly patients: 5 mg/day

Monitoring Parameters Ophthalmic: Intraocular pressure. Systemic: Blood pressure, pulse

Patient Information Intended for twice daily dosing; keep eye open and do not blink for 30 seconds after instillation; wear sunglasses to avoid photophobic discomfort; apply gentle pressure to lacrimal sac during and immediately following instillation (1 minute)

Nursing Implications Monitor for systemic effect of beta-blockade

Dosage Forms

Solution, ophthalmic, as hydrochloride (Betoptic®): 0.5% (2.5 mL, 5 mL, 10 mL)
Suspension, ophthalmic, as hydrochloride (Betoptic® S): 0.25% (2.5 mL, 10 mL, 15 mL)
Tablet, as hydrochloride (Kerlone®): 10 mg, 20 mg

Betaxolol Hydrochloride *see* Betaxolol *on previous page*

Bethanechol (be THAN e kole)

Brand Names Duvoid®; Myotonachol™; Urabeth®; Urecholine®

Canadian/Mexican Brand Names PMS-Bethanechol Chloride (Canada)

Synonyms Bethanechol Chloride

Therapeutic Category Cholinergic Agent

Use Nonobstructive urinary retention and retention due to neurogenic bladder; treatment and prevention of bladder dysfunction caused by phenothiazines; diagnosis of flaccid or atonic neurogenic bladder; gastroesophageal reflux

Pregnancy Risk Factor C

Contraindications Hypersensitivity to bethanechol; do not use in patients with mechanical obstruction of the GI or GU tract or when the strength or integrity of the GI or bladder wall is in question. It is also contraindicated in patients with hyperthyroidism, peptic ulcer disease, epilepsy, obstructive pulmonary disease, bradycardia, vasomotor instability, atrioventricular conduction defects, hypotension, or parkinsonism; **contraindicated for I.M. or I.V. use due to a likely severe cholinergic reaction**

Warnings/Precautions Potential for reflux infection if the sphincter fails to relax as bethanechol contracts the bladder; use with caution when administering to nursing women, as it is unknown if the drug is excreted in breast milk; safety and efficacy in children <5 years of age have not been established; syringe containing atropine should be readily available for treatment of serious side effects; for S.C. injection only; do not administer I.M. or I.V.

Adverse Reactions

Oral: <1%:

- Cardiovascular: Hypotension, cardiac arrest, flushed skin
- Gastrointestinal: Abdominal cramps, diarrhea, nausea, vomiting, salivation
- Respiratory: Bronchial constriction
- Miscellaneous: Diaphoresis, vasomotor response

Subcutaneous: 1% to 10%:

- Cardiovascular: Hypotension, cardiac arrest, flushed skin
- Gastrointestinal: Abdominal cramps, diarrhea, nausea, vomiting, salivation
- Respiratory: Bronchial constriction
- Miscellaneous: Diaphoresis, vasomotor response

Overdosage/Toxicology Symptoms of overdose include nausea, vomiting, abdominal cramps, diarrhea, involuntary defecation, flushed skin, hypotension, bronchospasm

Atropine is the treatment of choice for intoxications manifesting with significant muscarinic symptoms; atropine I.V. 0.6 mg every 3-60 minutes (or 0.01 mg/kg I.V. every 2 hours if needed for children) should be repeated to control symptoms and then continued as needed for 1-2 days following the acute ingestion. Epinephrine 0.1-1 mg S.C. may be useful in reversing severe cardiovascular or pulmonary sequel.

Drug Interactions

Decreased effect: Procainamide, quinidine

Increased toxicity: Bethanechol and ganglionic blockers → critical fall in blood pressure; cholinergic drugs or anticholinesterase agents

Mechanism of Action Stimulates cholinergic receptors in the smooth muscle of the urinary bladder and gastrointestinal tract resulting in increased peristalsis, increased GI and pancreatic secretions, bladder muscle contraction, and increased ureteral peristaltic waves

Pharmacodynamics/Kinetics

Onset of action:

- Oral: 30-90 minutes
- S.C.: 5-15 minutes

Duration of action:

- Oral: Up to 6 hours
- S.C.: 2 hours

Absorption: Oral: Variable

Metabolism and elimination have not been determined

Usual Dosage

Children:

- Oral:
  - Abdominal distention or urinary retention: 0.6 mg/kg/day divided 3-4 times/day
  - Gastroesophageal reflux: 0.1-0.2 mg/kg/dose given 30 minutes to 1 hour before each meal to a maximum of 4 times/day
- S.C.: 0.15-0.2 mg/kg/day divided 3-4 times/day

Adults:

- Oral: 10-50 mg 2-4 times/day
- S.C.: 2.5-5 mg 3-4 times/day, up to 7.5-10 mg every 4 hours for neurogenic bladder

Administration Do **not** administer I.V. or I.M., a severe cholinergic reaction may occur

Monitoring Parameters Observe closely for side effects

Test Interactions ↑ lipase, AST, amylase (S), bilirubin, aminotransferase [ALT (SGPT)/AST (SGOT)] (S)

(Continued)

Bethanechol *(Continued)*

Patient Information Oral should be taken 1 hour before meals or 2 hours after meals to avoid nausea or vomiting; may cause abdominal discomfort, salivation, diaphoresis, or flushing; notify physician if these symptoms become pronounced; rise slowly from sitting/lying down

Nursing Implications Have bedpan readily available, if administered for urinary retention

Dosage Forms

Injection, as chloride: 5 mg/mL (1 mL)

Tablet, as chloride: 5 mg, 10 mg, 25 mg, 50 mg

Bethanechol Chloride *see* Bethanechol *on page 150*

Betimol® Ophthalmic *see* Timolol *on page 1230*

Betoptic® *see* Betaxolol *on page 149*

Betoptic® S *see* Betaxolol *on page 149*

Biavax®II *see* Rubella and Mumps Vaccines, Combined *on page 1118*

Biaxin™ *see* Clarithromycin *on page 287*

Bicalutamide (bye ka LOO ta mide)

Brand Names Casodex®

Therapeutic Category Antiandrogen; Antineoplastic Agent, Miscellaneous

Use In combination therapy with LHRH agonist analogues in treatment of advanced prostatic carcinoma

Pregnancy Risk Factor X

Contraindications Known hypersensitivity to drug or any components of the product; pregnancy

Warnings/Precautions The U.S. Food and Drug Administration (FDA) currently recommends that procedures for proper handling and disposal of antineoplastic agents be considered. Animal data (based on using doses higher than recommended for humans) produced testicular interstitial cell adenoma. In clinical trials, gynecomastia and breast pain were reported in up to 38% and 39% of patients, respectively.

Adverse Reactions

>10%: Endocrine & metabolic: Hot flashes (49%)

≥2% to <5%:

- Cardiovascular: Angina pectoris, congestive heart failure, edema
- Central nervous system: Anxiety, depression, confusion, somnolence, nervousness, fever, chills
- Dermatologic: Dry skin, pruritus, alopecia
- Endocrine & metabolic: Breast pain, diabetes mellitus, decreased libido, dehydration, gout
- Gastrointestinal: Anorexia, dyspepsia, rectal hemorrhage, xerostomia, melena, weight gain
- Genitourinary: Polyuria, urinary impairment, dysuria, urinary retention, urinary urgency
- Hepatic: Alkaline phosphatase increased
- Neuromuscular & skeletal: Myasthenia, arthritis, myalgia, leg cramps, pathological fracture, neck pain, hypertonia, neuropathy
- Renal: Creatinine increased
- Respiratory: Cough increased, pharyngitis, bronchitis, pneumonia, rhinitis, lung disorder
- Miscellaneous: Sepsis, neoplasma

<1%: Gastrointestinal: Diarrhea (0.5%)

Overdosage/Toxicology Symptoms of overdose include hypoactivity, ataxia, anorexia, vomiting, slow respiration, lacrimation

Treatment is supportive, dialysis not of benefit; induce vomiting

Stability Store at room temperature

Mechanism of Action Pure nonsteroidal antiandrogen that binds to androgen receptors; specifically a competitive inhibitor for the binding of dihydrotestosterone and testosterone; prevents testosterone stimulation of cell growth in prostate cancer

Pharmacodynamics/Kinetics

Absorption: Rapid and complete

Protein binding: 96%

Metabolism: Extensive; stereospecific metabolism

Half-life: Up to 10 days; active enantiomer is 5.8 days

Elimination: Not yet studied

Usual Dosage Adults: Oral: 1 tablet once daily (morning or evening), with or without food. It is recommended that bicalutamide be taken at the same time each day; start treatment with bicalutamide at the same time as treatment with an LHRH analog.

Dosage adjustment in renal impairment: None necessary as renal impairment has no significant effect on elimination

Dosage adjustment in liver impairment: Limited data in subjects with severe hepatic impairment suggest that excretion of bicalutamide may be delayed and could lead to further accumulation. Use with caution in patients with moderate to severe hepatic impairment.

Administration Dose should be taken at the same time each day with or without food; start treatment at the same time as treatment with an LHRH analog

Monitoring Parameters Serum prostate-specific antigen, alkaline phosphatase, acid phosphatase, or prostatic acid phosphatase; prostate gland dimensions; skeletal survey; liver scans; chest x-rays; physical exam every 3 months; bone scan every 3-6 months; CBC, LFTs, EKG, echocardiograms, and serum testosterone and luteinizing hormone (periodically)

Patient Information Take at the same time as treatment with LHRH analog; advise of potential side effects; notify the physician if any visual disturbances or yellow discoloration of the skin or eyes

Dosage Forms Tablet: 50 mg

Bicillin® L-A *see* Penicillin G Benzathine *on page 961*

Bicitra® *see* Sodium Citrate and Citric Acid *on page 1144*

BiCNU® *see* Carmustine *on page 210*

Biltricide® *see* Praziquantel *on page 1035*

Biocal® [OTC] *see* Calcium Carbonate *on page 185*

Biocef *see* Cephalexin *on page 239*

Biodine [OTC] *see* Povidone-Iodine *on page 1031*

Biohist-LA® *see* Carbinoxamine and Pseudoephedrine *on page 204*

Biomox® *see* Amoxicillin *on page 77*

Bio-Tab® Oral *see* Doxycycline *on page 430*

Biozyme-C® *see* Collagenase *on page 311*

Bisac-Evac® [OTC] *see* Bisacodyl *on this page*

Bisacodyl (bis a KOE dil)

Related Information

Laxatives, Classification and Properties *on page 1412*

Brand Names Bisac-Evac® [OTC]; Bisacodyl Uniserts®; Bisco-Lax® [OTC]; Carter's Little Pills® [OTC]; Clysodrast®; Dacodyl® [OTC]; Deficol® [OTC]; Dulcolax® [OTC]; Fleet® Laxative [OTC]; Theralax® [OTC]

Canadian/Mexican Brand Names Apo-Bisacodyl® (Canada); PMS-Bisacodyl (Canada); Dulcolan® (Mexico)

Therapeutic Category Laxative, Stimulant

Use Treatment of constipation; colonic evacuation prior to procedures or examination

Pregnancy Risk Factor C

Contraindications Do not use in patients with abdominal pain, obstruction, nausea or vomiting; do not administer bisacodyl tannex enema to children <10 years of age

Warnings/Precautions Bisacodyl tannex should be used with caution in patients with ulceration of the colon and during pregnancy or lactation; safety of bisacodyl tannex usage in children <10 years of age has not been established

Adverse Reactions

<1%:

- Central nervous system: Vertigo
- Endocrine & metabolic: Electrolyte and fluid imbalance (metabolic acidosis or alkalosis, hypocalcemia)
- Gastrointestinal: Mild abdominal cramps, nausea, vomiting, rectal burning

Overdosage/Toxicology Symptoms of overdose include diarrhea, abdominal pain, electrolyte disturbances

Drug Interactions Decreased effect: Milk, antacids; decreased effect of warfarin

Mechanism of Action Stimulates peristalsis by directly irritating the smooth muscle of the intestine, possibly the colonic intramural plexus; alters water and electrolyte secretion producing net intestinal fluid accumulation and laxation

Pharmacodynamics/Kinetics

Onset of action:

- Oral: 6-10 hours
- Rectal: 0.25-1 hour

Absorption: Oral, rectal: <5% absorbed systemically

Metabolism: In the liver

Elimination: Conjugated metabolites excreted in milk, bile, and urine

Usual Dosage

Children:

- Oral: >6 years: 5-10 mg (0.3 mg/kg) at bedtime or before breakfast

(Continued)

Bisacodyl *(Continued)*

Rectal suppository:
<2 years: 5 mg as a single dose
>2 years: 10 mg
Adults:
Oral: 5-15 mg as single dose (up to 30 mg when complete evacuation of bowel is required)
Rectal suppository: 10 mg as single dose
Tannex:
Enema: 2.5 g in 1000 mL warm water
Barium enema: 2.5-5 g in 1000 mL barium suspension
Do not administer >10 g within 72-hour period

Administration Administer tablets 2 hours prior to, or 4 hours after antacids

Patient Information Swallow tablets whole, do **not** crush or chew; do not take antacid or milk within 1 hour of taking drug

Nursing Implications Increased pH may dissolve the enteric coating leading to GI distress; do not crush enteric coated drug product

Dosage Forms
Powder, as tannex: 2.5 g packets (50 packet/box)
Suppository, rectal: 5 mg, 10 mg
Tablet, enteric coated: 5 mg

Bisacodyl Uniserts® *see* Bisacodyl *on previous page*
Bisco-Lax® [OTC] *see* Bisacodyl *on previous page*
Bismatrol® [OTC] *see* Bismuth *on this page*

Bismuth (BIZ muth)

Related Information
Antimicrobial Drugs of Choice *on page 1468*
Helicobacter pylori Treatment *on page 1534*

Brand Names Bismatrol® [OTC]; Devrom® [OTC]; Pepto-Bismol® [OTC]; Pink Bismuth® [OTC]

Synonyms Bismuth Subgallate; Bismuth Subsalicylate

Therapeutic Category Antidiarrheal

Use Symptomatic treatment of mild, nonspecific diarrhea; indigestion, nausea, control of traveler's diarrhea (enterotoxigenic *Escherichia coli*); as an adjunct with other agents such as metronidazole, tetracycline, and an H_2-antagonist in the treatment of *Helicobacter pylori*-associated duodenal ulcer disease

Pregnancy Risk Factor C (D in 3rd trimester)

Contraindications Do not use subsalicylate in patients with influenza or chickenpox because of risk of Reye's syndrome; do not use in patients with known hypersensitivity to salicylates; history of severe GI bleeding; history of coagulopathy

Warnings/Precautions Subsalicylate should be used with caution if patient is taking aspirin; use with caution in children, especially those <3 years of age and those with viral illness; may be neurotoxic with very large doses

Adverse Reactions
>10%: Gastrointestinal: Discoloration of the tongue (darkening), grayish black stools
<1%:
Central nervous system: Anxiety, confusion, slurred speech, headache, mental depression
Gastrointestinal: Impaction may occur in infants and debilitated patients
Neuromuscular & skeletal: Muscle spasms, weakness
Otic: Hearing loss, tinnitus

Overdosage/Toxicology Symptoms of toxicity: **Subsalicylate**: Hyperpnea, nausea, vomiting, tinnitus, hyperpyrexia, metabolic acidoses/respiratory alkalosis, tachycardia, and confusion; seizures in severe overdose, pulmonary or cerebral edema, respiratory failure, cardiovascular collapse, coma, and death. **Note:** Each 262.4 mg tablet of bismuth subsalicylate contains an equivalent of 130 mg aspirin (150 mg/kg of aspirin is considered to be toxic; serious life-threatening toxicity occurs with >300mg/kg)

Treatment: Gastrointestinal decontamination (activated charcoal for immediate release formulations (10 x dose of ASA in g), whole bowel irrigation for enteric coated tablets or when serially increasing ASA plasma levels indicate the presence of an intestinal bezoar), supportive and symptomatic treatment with emphasis on correcting fluid, electrolyte, blood glucose and acid-base disturbances; elimination is enhanced with urinary alkalinization (sodium bicarbonate infusion with potassium), multiple dose activated charcoal, and hemodialysis.

Symptoms of toxicity: **Bismuth**: Rare with short-term administrations of bismuth salts; encephalopathy, methemoglobinemia, seizures

Treatment: Gastrointestinal decontamination; chelation with dimercaprol in doses of 3 mg/kg or penicillamine 100 mg/kg/day for 5 days can hasten recovery from bismuth-induced encephalopathy; methylene blue 1-2 mg/kg in a 1% sterile aqueous solution I.V. push over 4-6 minutes for methemoglobinemia. This may be repeated within 60 minutes if necessary, up to a total dose of 7 mg/kg. Seizures usually respond to I.V. diazepam.

Drug Interactions

Decreased effect: Tetracyclines and uricosurics

Increased toxicity: Aspirin, warfarin, hypoglycemics

Mechanism of Action Bismuth subsalicylate exhibits both antisecretory and antimicrobial action. This agent may provide some anti-inflammatory action as well. The salicylate moiety provides antisecretory effect and the bismuth exhibits antimicrobial directly against bacterial and viral gastrointestinal pathogens. Bismuth has some antacid properties.

Pharmacodynamics/Kinetics

Absorption: Minimally (<1%) absorbed across the GI tract while the salt (eg, salicylate) may be readily absorbed (80%); bismuth subsalicylate is rapidly cleaved to bismuth and salicylic acid in the stomach

Distribution: Salicylate: Volume of distribution: 170 mL/kg

Protein binding, plasma: Bismuth and salicylate: >90%

Metabolism: Bismuth salts undergo chemical dissociation after oral administration; salicylate is extensively metabolized in the liver

Half-life: Bismuth: Terminal: 21-72 days; Salicylate: Terminal: 2-5 hours

Elimination: Bismuth: Renal, biliary; clearance: 50 mL/minute; Salicylate: Only 10% excreted unchanged

Usual Dosage Oral:

Nonspecific diarrhea: Subsalicylate:

Children: Up to 8 doses/24 hours:

3-6 years: $^1/_3$ tablet or 5 mL every 30 minutes to 1 hour as needed

6-9 years: $^2/_3$ tablet or 10 mL every 30 minutes to 1 hour as needed

9-12 years: 1 tablet or 15 mL every 30 minutes to 1 hour as needed

Adults: 2 tablets or 30 mL every 30 minutes to 1 hour as needed up to 8 doses/24 hours

Prevention of traveler's diarrhea: 2.1 g/day or 2 tablets 4 times/day before meals and at bedtime

Subgallate: 1-2 tablets 3 times/day with meals

Helicobacter pylori: Chew 2 tablets 4 times/day with meals and at bedtime with other agents in selected regiment (eg, an H_2-antagonist, tetracycline and metronidazole) for 14 days

Dosing adjustment in renal impairment: Should probably be avoided in patients with renal failure

Test Interactions ↑ uric acid, ↑ AST; bismuth absorbs x-rays and may interfere with diagnostic procedures of GI tract

Patient Information Chew tablet well or shake suspension well before using; may darken stools; if diarrhea persists for more than 2 days, consult a physician; can turn tongue black; tinnitus may indicate toxicity and use should be discontinued

Nursing Implications Seek causes for diarrhea; monitor for tinnitus; may aggravate or cause gout attack; may enhance bleeding if used with anticoagulants

Dosage Forms

Liquid, as subsalicylate (Pepto-Bismol®, Bismatrol®): 262 mg/15 mL (120 mL, 240 mL, 360 mL, 480 mL); 524 mg/15 mL (120 mL, 240 mL, 360 mL)

Tablet:

Chewable, as subsalicylate (Pepto-Bismol®, Bismatrol®): 262 mg

Chewable, as subgallate (Devrom®): 200 mg

Bismuth Subgallate *see* Bismuth *on previous page*

Bismuth Subsalicylate *see* Bismuth *on previous page*

Bismuth Subsalicylate, Metronidazole, and Tetracycline

(BIZ muth sub sa LIS i late, me troe NI da zole, & tet ra SYE kleen)

Brand Names Helidac®

Therapeutic Category Antidiarrheal

Use In combination with an H_2-antagonist, used to treat and decrease rate of recurrence of active duodenal ulcer associated with *H. pylori* infection

Pregnancy Risk Factor D (tetracycline); B (metronidazole)

Pregnancy/Breast-Feeding Implications Avoid use in lactating females, if possible, since both metronidazole and tetracycline are known to be excreted in breast milk and the potential for tumorigenicity and serious adverse reaction in nursing infants exposed to metronidazole and tetracycline, respectively, exists

(Continued)

Bismuth Subsalicylate, Metronidazole, and Tetracycline *(Continued)*

Contraindications Pregnancy or lactation; children; significant renal/hepatic impairment; hypersensitivity to salicylates, bismuth, metronidazole, tetracycline, or any component

Warnings/Precautions See individual monographs

Adverse Reactions See individual monographs

>1%:

Central nervous system: Dizziness

Gastrointestinal: Nausea, diarrhea, abdominal pain, vomiting, anal discomfort, anorexia

Neuromuscular & skeletal: Paresthesia

<1%:

Central nervous system: Insomnia

Gastrointestinal: Constipation

Neuromuscular & skeletal: Weakness, pain

Respiratory: Upper respiratory infection

Overdosage/Toxicology See individual monographs; the most concerning agent with this combination in overdosage is bismuth subsalicylate due to the salicylate component **Note:** Each 262.4 mg tablet of bismuth subsalicylate contains an equivalent of 130 mg aspirin (150 mg/kg of aspirin is considered to be toxic; serious life-threatening toxicity occurs with >300 mg/kg).

Symptoms of salicylate intoxication: Hyperpnea, nausea, vomiting, tinnitus, hyperpyrexia, metabolic acidosis/ respiratory alkalosis, tachycardia, and confusion; seizures in severe OD, pulmonary or cerebral edema, respiratory failure, cardiovascular collapse, coma, and death

Treatment: Gastrointestinal decontamination (activated charcoal for immediate release formulations (10 x dose of ASA in g), whole bowel irrigation for enteric coated tablets or when serially increasing ASA plasma levels indicate the presence of an intestinal bezoar), supportive and symptomatic treatment with emphasis on correcting fluid, electrolyte, blood glucose, and acid-base disturbances; elimination is enhanced with urinary alkalization (sodium bicarbonate infusion with potassium), multiple-dose activated charcoal, and hemodialysis.

Drug Interactions See individual monographs

Decreased effect: A theoretical reduction in tetracycline systemic absorption due to an interaction with bismuth or calcium carbonate, an excipient of bismuth subsalicylate has, as yet, been unproven to occur or to have any clinical bearing

Mechanism of Action Bismuth subsalicylate, metronidazole, and tetracycline individually have demonstrated *in vitro* activity against most susceptible strains of *H. pylori* isolated from patients with duodenal ulcers. Resistance to metronidazole is increasing in the U.S.; an alternative regimen, not containing metronidazole, if *H. pylori* is not eradicated follow therapy.

Pharmacodynamics/Kinetics No data on combination; see individual monographs

Usual Dosage Adults: Chew 2 bismuth subsalicylate 262.4 mg tablets, swallow 1 metronidazole 250 mg tablet, and swallow 1 tetracycline 500 mg capsule plus an H_2-antagonist 4 times/day at meals and bedtime for 14 days; follow with 8 oz of water

Monitoring Parameters See individual monographs

Patient Information Drink adequate amounts of fluid, particularly with the bedtime tetracycline dose to reduce the risk of esophageal irritation and ulceration; if a dose is missed, continue the normal regimen until the medication is gone; do not take double doses; see your physician if more than 4 doses are missed or if ringing in the ears occur; avoid alcoholic beverages during therapy and for at least 1 day afterward; avoid concurrent use of oral contraceptives (use an alternative method) since tetracyclines may make birth control pills less effective; use protective clothing and avoid prolonged exposure to the sun and ultraviolet light; a temporary and harmless darkening of the tongue and a black stool may occur.

Dosage Forms

Capsule: Tetracycline: 500 mg

Tablet:

Bismuth subsalicylate: Chewable: 262.4 mg

Metronidazole: 250 mg

Bisoprolol (bis OH proe lol)

Related Information

Beta-Blockers Comparison *on page 1398*

Brand Names Zebeta®

Synonyms Bisoprolol Fumarate

Therapeutic Category Beta-Adrenergic Blocker

Use Treatment of hypertension, alone or in combination with other agents

Unlabeled use: Angina pectoris, supraventricular arrhythmias, PVCs

Contraindications Hypersensitivity to beta-blocking agents, uncompensated congestive heart failure; cardiogenic shock; bradycardia or heart block; sinus node dysfunction; A-V conduction abnormalities. Although bisoprolol primarily blocks beta$_1$-receptors, high doses can result in beta$_2$-receptor blockage. Therefore, use with caution in patients (especially elderly) with bronchospastic lung disease and renal dysfunction.

Warnings/Precautions Use with caution in patients with inadequate myocardial function, bronchospastic disease, hyperthyroidism, undergoing anesthesia; and in those with impaired hepatic function; acute withdrawal may exacerbate symptoms (gradually taper over a 2-week period)

Adverse Reactions

>10%: Central nervous system: Fatigue, lethargy

1% to 10%:

Central nervous system: Headache, dizziness, insomnia, confusion, depression, abnormal dreams

Cardiovascular: Hypotension, chest pain, heart failure, Raynaud's phenomenon, heart block, edema, bradycardia

Dermatologic: Rash

Gastrointestinal: Constipation, diarrhea, dyspepsia, nausea, flatulence, anorexia

Genitourinary: Polyuria, impotence, urinary retention

Neuromuscular & skeletal: Arthralgia, myalgia

Ocular: Abnormal vision

Respiratory: Dyspnea, rhinitis, cough

Overdosage/Toxicology Symptoms of overdose include severe hypotension, bradycardia, heart failure, and bronchospasm, hypoglycemia

Sympathomimetics (eg, epinephrine or dopamine), glucagon, or a pacemaker can be used to treat the toxic bradycardia, asystole, and/or hypotension (I.V. fluids-initial treatment); may be removed by hemodialysis; other treatment is symptomatic and supportive.

Drug Interactions

Decreased effect/levels with barbiturates, rifampin, sulfinpyrazone

Increased effect/toxicity/levels of flecainide

Mechanism of Action Selective inhibitor of beta$_1$-adrenergic receptors; competitively blocks beta$_1$-receptors, with little or no effect on beta$_2$-receptors at doses <10 mg

Pharmacodynamics/Kinetics

Absorption: Rapid and almost complete from GI tract

Distribution: Distributed widely to body tissues; highest concentrations in heart, liver, lungs, and saliva; crosses the blood-brain barrier; distributes into breast milk

Protein binding: 26% to 33%

Metabolism: Significant first-pass metabolism; extensively metabolized in the liver

Half-life: 9-12 hours

Time to peak: 1.7-3 hours

Elimination: In urine (3% to 10% as unchanged drug); <2% excreted in feces

Usual Dosage Oral:

Adults: 5 mg once daily, may be increased to 10 mg, and then up to 20 mg once daily, if necessary

Elderly: Initial dose: 2.5 mg/day; may be increased by 2.5-5 mg/day; maximum recommended dose: 20 mg/day

Dosing adjustment in renal/hepatic impairment: Cl_{cr} <40 mL/minute: Initial: 2.5 mg/day; increase cautiously

Hemodialysis: Not dialyzable

Monitoring Parameters Blood pressure, EKG, neurologic status

Test Interactions ↑ thyroxine (S), cholesterol (S), glucose; ↑ triglycerides, uric acid; ↓ HDL

Patient Information Do not discontinue abruptly (angina may be precipitated); notify physician if CHF symptoms become worse or side effects occur; take at the same time each day; may mask diabetes symptoms; consult pharmacist or physician before taking with other adrenergic drugs (eg, cold medications); use with caution while driving or performing tasks requiring alertness; may be taken without regard to meals

Dosage Forms Tablet, as fumarate: 5 mg, 10 mg

Bisoprolol Fumarate *see* Bisoprolol *on previous page*

Bistropamide *see* Tropicamide *on page 1275*

Bitolterol (bye TOLE ter ole)

Brand Names Tornalate®

Synonyms Bitolterol Mesylate

Therapeutic Category Beta$_2$-Adrenergic Agonist Agent; Bronchodilator

Use Prevention and treatment of bronchial asthma and bronchospasm

Pregnancy Risk Factor C

Contraindications Known hypersensitivity to bitolterol

Warnings/Precautions Use with caution in patients with unstable vasomotor symptoms, diabetes, hyperthyroidism, prostatic hypertrophy or a history of seizures; also use caution in the elderly and those patients with cardiovascular disorders such as coronary artery disease, arrhythmias, and hypertension; excessive use may result in cardiac arrest and death; do not use concurrently with other sympathomimetic bronchodilators

Adverse Reactions

>10%: Neuromuscular & skeletal: Trembling

1% to 10%:

- Cardiovascular: Flushing of face, hypertension, pounding heartbeat
- Central nervous system: Dizziness, lightheadedness, nervousness
- Gastrointestinal: Xerostomia, nausea, unpleasant taste
- Respiratory: Bronchial irritation, coughing

<1%:

- Cardiovascular: Chest pain, arrhythmias, tachycardia
- Central nervous system: Insomnia
- Respiratory: Paradoxical bronchospasm

Overdosage/Toxicology Symptoms of overdose include tremor, dizziness, nervousness, headache, nausea, coughing

Treatment is symptomatic/supportive; in cases of severe overdose, supportive therapy should be instituted, and prudent use of a cardioselective beta-adrenergic blocker (eg, atenolol or metoprolol) should be considered, keeping in mind the potential for induction of bronchoconstriction in an asthmatic individual. Dialysis has not been shown to be of value in the treatment of an overdose with this agent.

Drug Interactions

Decreased effect: Beta-adrenergic blockers (eg, propranolol)

Increased effect: Inhaled ipratropium may increase duration of bronchodilation, nifedipine may increase FEV-1

Increased toxicity: MAO inhibitors, tricyclic antidepressants, sympathomimetic agents (eg, amphetamine, dopamine, dobutamine), inhaled anesthetics (eg, enflurane)

Mechanism of Action Selectively stimulates beta$_2$-adrenergic receptors in the lungs producing bronchial smooth muscle relaxation; minor beta$_1$ activity

Pharmacodynamics/Kinetics

Duration of effect: 4-8 hours

Metabolism: Bitolterol, a prodrug, is hydrolyzed to colterol (active) following inhalation

Half-life: 3 hours

Time to peak serum concentration (colterol): Inhalation: Within 1 hour

Elimination: In urine and feces

Usual Dosage Children >12 years and Adults:

Bronchospasm: 2 inhalations at an interval of at least 1-3 minutes, followed by a third inhalation if needed

Prevention of bronchospasm: 2 inhalations every 8 hours; do not exceed 3 inhalations every 6 hours or 2 inhalations every 4 hours

Administration Administer around-the-clock rather than 3 times/day, to promote less variation in peak and trough serum levels

Monitoring Parameters Assess lung sounds, pulse, and blood pressure before administration and during peak of medication; observe patient for wheezing after administration

Patient Information Do not exceed recommended dosage, excessive use may lead to adverse effects or loss of effectiveness; shake canister well before use; administer pressurized inhalation during the second half of inspiration, as the airways are open, water and the aerosol distribution is more extensive. If more than one inhalation per dose is necessary, wait at least 1 full minute between inhalations - second inhalation is best delivered after 10 minutes. May cause nervousness, restlessness, and insomnia; if these effects continue after dosage reduction, notify physician. Also notify physician if palpitations, tachycardia, chest pain, muscle tremors, dizziness, headache, flushing, or if breathing difficulty persists.

Nursing Implications Before using, the inhaler must be shaken well

Dosage Forms

Aerosol, oral, as mesylate: 0.8% [370 mcg/metered spray, 300 inhalations] (15 mL)

Solution, inhalation, as mesylate: 0.2% (10 mL, 30 mL, 60 mL)

Bitolterol Mesylate *see* Bitolterol *on previous page*

BlemErase® Lotion [OTC] *see* Benzoyl Peroxide *on page 140*

Blenoxane® *see* Bleomycin *on this page*

Bleo *see* Bleomycin *on this page*

Bleomycin (blee oh MYE sin)

Related Information

Antiemetics for Chemotherapy Induced Nausea and Vomiting *on page 1348*
Cancer Chemotherapy Regimens *on page 1351*
Toxicities of Chemotherapeutic Agents *on page 1382*

Brand Names Blenoxane®

Synonyms Bleo; Bleomycin Sulfate; BLM; NSC 125066

Therapeutic Category Antineoplastic Agent, Antibiotic

Use Treatment of squamous cell carcinomas, melanomas, sarcomas, testicular carcinomas, Hodgkin's lymphoma, and non-Hodgkin's lymphoma; may also be used as a sclerosing agent for malignant pleural effusion

Pregnancy Risk Factor D

Contraindications Hypersensitivity to bleomycin sulfate or any component, severe pulmonary disease

Warnings/Precautions The U.S. Food and Drug Administration (FDA) currently recommends that procedures for proper handling and disposal of antineoplastic agents be considered. Occurrence of pulmonary fibrosis is higher in elderly patients and in those receiving >400 units total and in smokers and patients with prior radiation therapy. A severe idiosyncratic reaction consisting of hypotension, mental confusion, fever, chills and wheezing (similar to anaphylaxis) has been reported in 1% of lymphoma patients treated with bleomycin. Since these reactions usually occur after the first or second dose, careful monitoring is essential after these doses. Check lungs prior to each treatment for fine rales (1st sign). Follow manufacturer recommendations for administering 0_2 during surgery to patients who have received bleomycin.

Adverse Reactions

>10%:

- Cardiovascular: Raynaud's phenomenon
- Central nervous system: Mild febrile reaction, fever, chills, patients may become febrile after intracavitary administration
- Dermatologic: Pruritic erythema
  - Integument: ~50% of patients will develop erythema, induration, and hyperkeratosis and peeling of the skin; hyperpigmentation, alopecia, nailbed changes may occur; this appears to be dose-related and is reversible after cessation of therapy
  - **Irritant chemotherapy**
- Gastrointestinal: Mucocutaneous toxicity, stomatitis, nausea, vomiting, anorexia
  - Emetic potential: Moderately low (10% to 30%)
- Local: Phlebitis, pain at tumor site

1% to 10%:

- Dermatologic: Alopecia
- Gastrointestinal: Weight loss
- Respiratory: Toxicities (usually pneumonitis) occur in 10% of treated patients; 1% of patients progress to pulmonary fibrosis and death
- Miscellaneous: Idiosyncratic: Similar to anaphylaxis and occurs in 1% of lymphoma patients; may include hypotension, confusion, fever, chills, and wheezing. May be immediate or delayed for several hours; symptomatic treatment includes volume expansion, pressor agents, antihistamines, and steroids

<1%:

- Cardiovascular: Myocardial infarction, cerebrovascular accident
- Dermatologic: Skin thickening
- Hematologic: Myelosuppressive:
  - WBC: Rare
  - Platelets: Rare
  - Onset (days): 7
  - Nadir (days): 14
  - Recovery (days): 21
- Hepatic: Hepatotoxicity
- Renal: Renal toxicity
- Respiratory: Dose-related when total dose is >400 units or with single doses >30 units; pathogenesis is poorly understood, but may be related to damage of pulmonary, vascular, or connective tissue, manifested as an acute or chronic interstitial pneumonitis with interstitial fibrosis, hypoxia, and death; symptoms include cough, dyspnea, and bilateral pulmonary infiltrates noted

(Continued)

Bleomycin *(Continued)*

on CXR; it is controversial whether steroids improve symptoms of bleomycin pulmonary toxicity; tachypnea, rales

Overdosage/Toxicology Symptoms of overdose include chills, fever, pulmonary fibrosis, hyperpigmentation

Drug Interactions

Decreased effect:

Digitalis glycosides: May ↓ plasma levels and renal excretion of digoxin

Phenytoin: Results in ↓ phenytoin levels, possibly due to ↓ oral absorption

Increased toxicity: Cisplatin: Results in delayed bleomycin elimination due to ↓ in creatinine clearance secondary to cisplatin

Stability Refrigerate intact vials of powder; reconstitute powder with 1-5 mL SWI or NS which is stable at room temperature for 28 days or in refrigerator for 14 days; may use bacteriostatic agent if prolonged storage is necessary

Incompatible with amino acid solutions, ascorbic acid, cefazolin, furosemide, diazepam, hydrocortisone, mitomycin, nafcillin, penicillin G, aminophylline

Compatible with cyclophosphamide, doxorubicin, mesna, vinblastine, vincristine

Standard I.V. dilution: Dose/50-1000 mL NS or D_5W; stable for 96 hours at room temperature and 14 days under refrigeration

Mechanism of Action Inhibits synthesis of DNA; binds to DNA leading to single- and double-strand breaks; isolated from *Streptomyces verticillus*

Pharmacodynamics/Kinetics

Absorption: I.M. and intrapleural administration produces serum concentrations of 30% of I.V. administration; intraperitoneal and S.C. routes produce serum concentrations equal to those of I.V.

Distribution: V_d: 22 L/m^2; highest concentrations seen in skin, kidney, lung, heart tissues; low concentrations seen in testes and GI tract; does not cross blood-brain barrier

Protein binding: 1%

Metabolism: By several tissue types, including the liver, GI tract, skin, lungs, kidney, and serum

Half-life (biphasic): Dependent upon renal function:

Normal renal function:

Initial: 1.3 hours

Terminal: 9 hours

End stage renal disease:

Initial: 2 hours

Terminal: 30 hours

Time to peak serum concentration: I.M.: Within 30 minutes

Elimination: 50% to 70% of dose excreted in urine as active drug; not removed by hemodialysis

Usual Dosage Refer to individual protocols; 1 unit = 1 mg

May be administered I.M., I.V., S.C., or intracavitary

Children and Adults:

Test dose for lymphoma patients: I.M., I.V., S.C.: Because of the possibility of an anaphylactoid reaction, ≤2 units of bleomycin for the first 2 doses; monitor vital signs every 15 minutes; wait a minimum of 1 hour before administering remainder of dose; if no acute reaction occurs, then the regular dosage schedule may be followed

Single agent therapy:

I.M./I.V./S.C.: Squamous cell carcinoma, lymphoma, testicular carcinoma: 0.25-0.5 units/kg (10-20 units/m^2) 1-2 times/week

CIV: 15 units/m^2 over 24 hours daily for 4 days

Combination agent therapy:

I.M./I.V.: 3-4 units/m^2

I.V.: ABVD: 10 units/m^2 on days 1 and 15

Maximum cumulative lifetime dose: 400 units

Dosing adjustment in renal impairment:

Cl_{cr} 10-50 mL/minute: Administer 75% of normal dose

Cl_{cr} <10 mL/minute: Administer 50% of normal dose

Hemodialysis: None

CAPD effects: None

CAVH effects: None

Adults: Intracavitary injection for malignant pleural effusion: 60 IU in 50-100 mL SWI

Administration I.V. doses should be administered slowly (≤1 unit/minute); I.M. or S.C. may cause pain at injection site

Monitoring Parameters Pulmonary function tests (total lung volume, forced vital capacity, carbon monoxide diffusion), renal function, chest x-ray, temperature initially, CBC with differential and platelet count

Patient Information Hair should reappear after discontinuance of medication; maintain excellent oral hygiene habits; report any coughing, shortness of breath, or wheezing; skin rashes, shaking, chills, or transient high fever may occur following administration

Nursing Implications Patients should be closely monitored for signs of pulmonary toxicity; check body weight at regular intervals

Dosage Forms Powder for injection, as sulfate: 15 units

Bleomycin Sulfate *see* Bleomycin *on page 159*

Bleph®-10 Ophthalmic *see* Sulfacetamide Sodium *on page 1171*

Blephamide® Ophthalmic *see* Sulfacetamide Sodium and Prednisolone *on page 1172*

Blis-To-Sol® [OTC] *see* Tolnaftate *on page 1243*

BLM *see* Bleomycin *on page 159*

Blocadren® Oral *see* Timolol *on page 1230*

Bonine® [OTC] *see* Meclizine *on page 769*

B&O Supprettes® *see* Belladonna and Opium *on page 135*

Botox® *see* Botulinum Toxin Type A *on this page*

Botulinum Toxin Type A (BOT yoo lin num TOKS in type aye)

Replaces Oculinum®

Brand Names Botox®

Therapeutic Category Ophthalmic Agent, Toxin

Use Treatment of strabismus and blepharospasm associated with dystonia (including benign essential blepharospasm or VII nerve disorders in patients ≥12 years of age)

Unlabeled uses: Treatment of hemifacial spasms, spasmodic torticollis (ie, cervical dystonia, clonic twisting of the head), oromandibular dystonia, spasmodic dysphonia (laryngeal dystonia) and other dystonias (ie, writer's cramp, focal task-specific dystonias)

Orphan drug: Treatment of dynamic muscle contracture in pediatric cerebral palsy patients

Pregnancy Risk Factor C

Contraindications Hypersensitivity to botulinum A toxin; relative contraindications to botulinum toxin therapy include diseases of neuromuscular transmission and coagulopathy, including anticoagulant therapy; injections into the central area of the upper eyelid (rapid diffusion of toxin into the levator can occur resulting in a marked ptosis).

Warnings/Precautions Use with caution in patients taking aminoglycosides or any other antibiotic or other drugs that interfere with neuromuscular transmission; do not exceed recommended dose

Adverse Reactions

>10%: Ocular: Dry eyes, lagophthalmos, ptosis, photophobia, vertical deviation

1% to 10%:

- Dermatologic: Diffuse rash
- Ocular: Eyelid edema, blepharospasm

<1%: Ocular: Ectropion, keratitis, diplopia, entropion

Overdosage/Toxicology In the event of an overdosage or injection into the wrong muscle, additional information may be obtained by contacting Allergan Pharmaceuticals at (800)-347-5063 from 8 AM to 4 PM Pacific time, or at (714)-724-5954 at other times

Drug Interactions Increased effect: Botulinum toxin may be potentiated by aminoglycosides

Stability Keep in undiluted vials in freezer (at or below -5°C/23°F); administer within 4 hours after the vial is removed from the freezer and reconstituted; store reconstituted solution in refrigerator (2°C to 8°C/36°F to 46°F)

Mechanism of Action Botulinum A toxin is a neurotoxin produced by *Clostridium botulinum,* spore-forming anaerobic bacillus, which appears to affect only the presynaptic membrane of the neuromuscular junction in humans, where it prevents calcium-dependent release of acetylcholine and produces a state of denervation. Muscle inactivation persists until new fibrils grow from the nerve and form junction plates on new areas of the muscle-cell walls. The antagonist muscle shortens simultaneously ("contracture"), taking up the slack created by agonist paralysis; following several weeks of paralysis, alignment of the eye is measurably changed, despite return of innervation to the injected muscle.

Pharmacodynamics/Kinetics

Strabismus:

- Onset of action: 1-2 days after injection
- Duration of paralysis: 2-6 weeks

(Continued)

Botulinum Toxin Type A *(Continued)*

Blepharospasm:
Onset: 3 days after injection
Peak: 1-2 weeks
Duration of paralysis: 3 months

Usual Dosage
Strabismus: 1.25-5 units (0.05-0.15 mL) injected into any one muscle
Subsequent doses for residual/recurrent strabismus: Re-examine patients 7-14 days after each injection to assess the effect of that dose. Subsequent doses for patients experiencing incomplete paralysis of the target may be increased up to two fold the previously administered dose. Maximum recommended dose as a single injection for any one muscle is 25 units.
Blepharospasm: 1.25-2.5 units (0.05-0.10 mL) injected into the orbicularis oculi muscle
Subsequent doses: Each treatment lasts approximately 3 months. At repeat treatment sessions, the dose may be increased up to twofold if the response from the initial treatment is considered insufficient (usually defined as an effect that does not last >2 months). There appears to be little benefit obtainable from injecting >5 units per site. Some tolerance may be found if treatments are given any more frequently than every 3 months.
The cumulative dose should not exceed 200 units in a 30-day period

Administration Inject using a 27- to 30-gauge needle

Patient Information Patients with blepharospasm may have been extremely sedentary for a long time; caution these patients to resume activity slowly and carefully following administration

Nursing Implications To alleviate spatial disorientation or double vision in strabismic patients, cover the affected eye; have epinephrine ready for hypersensitivity reactions

Dosage Forms Injection: 100 units *Clostridium botulinum* toxin type A

Bovine Lung Surfactant *see* Beractant *on page 146*
Breast-Feeding and Drugs *see page 1569*
Breathe Free® [OTC] *see* Sodium Chloride *on page 1142*
Breezee® Mist Antifungal [OTC] *see* Tolnaftate *on page 1243*
Breonesin® [OTC] *see* Guaifenesin *on page 589*
Brethaire® *see* Terbutaline *on page 1194*
Brethine® *see* Terbutaline *on page 1194*

Bretylium (bre TIL ee um)

Related Information
Adult ACLS Algorithm, Tachycardia *on page 1512*
Adult ACLS Algorithm, V. Fib and Pulseless V. Tach *on page 1509*
Antiarrhythmic Drugs *on page 1389*
Comparative Pharmacokinetic Properties of Antiarrhythmic Agents *on page 1391*
Pediatric ALS Algorithm, Asystole and Pulseless Arrest *on page 1507*

Brand Names Bretylol®

Canadian/Mexican Brand Names Bretylate® (Canada)

Synonyms Bretylium Tosylate

Therapeutic Category Antiarrhythmic Agent, Class III

Use Treatment of ventricular tachycardia and fibrillation; used in the treatment of other serious ventricular arrhythmias resistant to lidocaine

Pregnancy Risk Factor C

Contraindications Digitalis intoxication-induced arrhythmias, hypersensitivity to bretylium or any component

Warnings/Precautions Hypotension, patients with fixed cardiac output (severe pulmonary hypertension or aortic stenosis) may experience severe hypotension due to decrease in peripheral resistance without ability to increase cardiac output; reduce dose in renal failure patients; may have prolonged half-life with aging

Adverse Reactions
>10%: Cardiovascular: Hypotension (both postural and supine)
1% to 10%: Gastrointestinal: Nausea, vomiting
<1%:
Cardiovascular: Transient initial hypertension, increase in PVCs, bradycardia, angina, flushing, syncope
Central nervous system: Vertigo, confusion, hyperthermia
Dermatologic: Rash
Gastrointestinal: Diarrhea, abdominal pain
Neuromuscular & skeletal: Muscle atrophy and necrosis with repeated I.M. injections at same site

Ocular: Conjunctivitis
Renal: Renal impairment
Respiratory: Respiratory depression, nasal congestion
Miscellaneous: Hiccups

Overdosage/Toxicology Symptoms of overdose include significant hypertension followed by severe hypotension

Administration of short-acting hypotensive agent (Nipride®) should be used for the hypertensive response; hypotension should be treated with fluid administration and dopamine or norepinephrine; dialysis is not useful.

Drug Interactions
Increased toxicity: Other antiarrhythmic agents
Additive toxicity or effect by bretylium, pressor catecholamines, digitalis

Stability Standard diluent: 2 g/250 mL D_5W; the premix infusion should be stored at room temperature and protected from freezing

Mechanism of Action Class II antiarrhythmic; after an initial release of norepinephrine at the peripheral adrenergic nerve terminals, inhibits further release by postganglionic nerve endings in response to sympathetic nerve stimulation

Pharmacodynamics/Kinetics
Onset of antiarrhythmic effect:
I.M.: May require 2 hours
I.V.: Within 6-20 minutes
Peak effect: 6-9 hours
Duration: 6-24 hours
Protein binding: 1% to 6%
Metabolism: Not metabolized
Half-life: 7-11 hours; average: 4-17 hours
End stage renal disease: 16-32 hours
Elimination: 70% to 80% excreted over the first 24 hours; excreted unchanged in the urine

Usual Dosage (**Note**: Patients should undergo defibrillation/cardioversion before and after bretylium doses as necessary)

Children:
I.M.: 2-5 mg/kg as a single dose
I.V.: Initial: 5 mg/kg, then attempt electrical defibrillation; repeat with 10 mg/kg if ventricular fibrillation persists at 15-minute intervals to maximum total of 30 mg/kg
Maintenance dose: I.M., I.V.: 5 mg/kg every 6-8 hours

Adults:
Immediate life-threatening ventricular arrhythmias, ventricular fibrillation, unstable ventricular tachycardia: Initial dose: I.V.: 5 mg/kg (undiluted) over 1 minute; if arrhythmia persists, administer 10 mg/kg (undiluted) over 1 minute and repeat as necessary (usually at 15- to 30-minute intervals) up to a total dose of 30-35 mg/kg
Other life-threatening ventricular arrhythmias:
Initial dose: I.M., I.V.: 5-10 mg/kg, may repeat every 1-2 hours if arrhythmia persist; administer I.V. dose (diluted) over 8-10 minutes
Maintenance dose: I.M.: 5-10 mg/kg every 6-8 hours; I.V. (diluted): 5-10 mg/kg every 6 hours; I.V. infusion (diluted): 1-2 mg/minute (little experience with doses >40 mg/kg/day)
2 g/250 mL D_5W (infusion pump should be used for I.V. infusion administration)
Rate of I.V. infusion: 1-4 mg/minute
1 mg/minute = 7 mL/hour
2 mg/minute = 15 mL/hour
3 mg/minute = 22 mL/hour
4 mg/minute = 30 mL/hour

Dosing adjustment in renal impairment:
Cl_{cr} 10-50 mL/minute: Administer 25% to 50% of dose
Cl_{cr} <10 mL/minute: Administer 25% of dose
Dialysis: Not dialyzable (0% to 5%) via hemo- or peritoneal dialysis; supplemental doses are not needed

Administration I.M. injection in adults should not exceed 5 mL volume in any one site

Monitoring Parameters EKG, heart rate, blood pressure; requires a cardiac monitor

Patient Information Anticipate vomiting

Nursing Implications Monitor EKG and blood pressure throughout therapy; onset of action may be delayed 15-30 minutes; rapid infusion may result in nausea and vomiting

Dosage Forms
Injection, as tosylate: 50 mg/mL (10 mL, 20 mL)
(Continued)

Bretylium *(Continued)*

Injection, as tosylate, premixed in D_5W: 1 mg/mL (500 mL); 2 mg/mL (250 mL); 4 mg/mL (250 mL, 500 mL)

Bretylium Tosylate *see* Bretylium *on page 162*

Bretylol® *see* Bretylium *on page 162*

Brevibloc® *see* Esmolol *on page 465*

Brevicon® *see* Ethinyl Estradiol and Norethindrone *on page 486*

Brevital® Sodium *see* Methohexital *on page 806*

Brevoxyl® Gel *see* Benzoyl Peroxide *on page 140*

Bricanyl® *see* Terbutaline *on page 1194*

Brimonidine (bri MOE ni deen)

Brand Names Alphagan®

Synonyms Brimonidine Tartrate

Therapeutic Category $Alpha_2$-Adrenergic Agonist Agent, Ophthalmic; Sympathomimetic

Use Lowering of intraocular pressure in patients with open-angle glaucoma or ocular hypertension

Pregnancy Risk Factor B

Contraindications Known hypersensitivity to brimonidine tartrate or any component of this medication; patients receiving monoamine oxidase (MAO) inhibitor therapy

Warnings/Precautions Exercise caution in treating patients with severe cardiovascular disease. Use with caution in patients with depression, cerebral or coronary insufficiency, Raynaud's phenomenon, orthostatic hypotension or thromboangiitis obliterans

The preservative in brimonidine tartrate, benzalkonium chloride, may be absorbed by soft contact lenses; instruct patients wearing soft contact lenses to wait at least 15 minutes after instilling brimonidine tartrate to insert soft contact lenses

Use with caution in patients with hepatic or renal impairment

Loss of effect in some patients may occur. The IOP-lowering efficacy observed with brimonidine tartrate during the first of month of therapy may not always reflect the long term level of IOP reduction. Routinely monitor IOP.

Adverse Reactions

>10%:
- Central nervous system: Headache, fatigue/drowsiness
- Gastrointestinal: Xerostomia
- Ocular: Ocular hyperemia, burning and stinging, blurring, foreign body sensation, conjunctival follicles, ocular allergic reactions and ocular pruritus

1% to 10%:
- Central nervous system: Dizziness
- Ocular: Corneal staining/erosion, photophobia, eyelid erythema, ocular ache/pain, ocular dryness, tearing, eyelid edema, conjunctival edema, blepharitis, ocular irritation, conjunctival blanching, abnormal vision, lid crusting, conjunctival hemorrhage, abnormal taste, conjunctival discharge
- Respiratory: Upper respiratory symptoms

<1%:
- Sensitivity reactions: Allergic response
- Miscellaneous: Some systemic effects have also been reported including GI, CNS, and cardiovascular symptoms (arrhythmias)

Overdosage/Toxicology

Symptoms of overdose: No information is available on overdosage in humans

Treatment: Maintain a patent airway, supportive and symptomatic therapy

Drug Interactions

Increased effect:
- CNS depressants (eg, alcohol, barbiturates, opiates, sedatives, anesthetics): Additive or potentiating effect
- Topical beta-blockers, pilocarpine → additive decreased intraocular pressure, antihypertensives, cardiac glycosides

Decreased effect: Tricyclic antidepressants can affect the metabolism and uptake of circulating amines

Stability Store at or below 25°C (77°F)

Mechanism of Action Selective for $alpha_2$-receptors; appears to result in reduction of aqueous humor formation and increase uveoscleral outflow

Pharmacodynamics/Kinetics

Onset of action: 1-4 hours

Duration: 12 hours

Usual Dosage Adults: Ophthalmic: Instill 1 drop in affected eye(s) 3 times/day (approximately every 8 hours)

Monitoring Parameters Closely monitor patients who develop fatigue or drowsiness

Patient Information Instruct patients wearing soft contact lenses to wait at least 15 minutes after instilling brimonidine tartrate to insert soft contact lenses. As with other drugs in this class, brimonidine tartrate may cause fatigue or drowsiness in some patients. Caution patients who engage in hazardous activities of the potential for a decrease in mental alertness.

Dosage Forms Solution, ophthalmic, as tartrate: 0.2% (5 mL, 10 mL)

Brimonidine Tartrate *see* Brimonidine *on previous page*

British Anti-Lewisite *see* Dimercaprol *on page 397*

Bromarest® [OTC] *see* Brompheniramine *on next page*

Brombay® [OTC] *see* Brompheniramine *on next page*

Bromocriptine (broe moe KRIP teen)

Brand Names Parlodel®

Canadian/Mexican Brand Names Apo® Bromocriptine (Canada); Cryocriptina® (Mexico); Serocryptin® (Mexico)

Synonyms Bromocriptine Mesylate

Therapeutic Category Anti-Parkinson's Agent; Ergot Alkaloid and Derivative

Use

Usually used with levodopa or levodopa/carbidopa to treat Parkinson's disease - treatment of parkinsonism in patients unresponsive or allergic to levodopa

Prolactin-secreting pituitary adenomas

Acromegaly

Amenorrhea/galactorrhea secondary to hyperprolactinemia in the absence of primary tumor

The indication for prevention of postpartum lactation has been withdrawn voluntarily by Sandoz Pharmaceuticals Corporation

Pregnancy Risk Factor C (See Contraindications)

Contraindications Hypersensitivity to bromocriptine or any component, severe ischemic heart disease or peripheral vascular disorders, pregnancy

Warnings/Precautions Use with caution in patients with impaired renal or hepatic function

Adverse Reactions Incidence of adverse effects is high, especially at beginning of treatment and with dosages >20 mg/day

1% to 10%:

- Cardiovascular: Hypotension, Raynaud's phenomenon
- Central nervous system: Mental depression, confusion, hallucinations
- Gastrointestinal: Nausea, constipation, anorexia
- Neuromuscular & skeletal: Leg cramps
- Respiratory: Nasal congestion

<1%:

- Cardiovascular: Hypertension, myocardial infarction, syncope
- Central nervous system: Dizziness, drowsiness, fatigue, insomnia, headache, seizures
- Gastrointestinal: Vomiting, abdominal cramps

Overdosage/Toxicology Symptoms of overdose include nausea, vomiting, hypotension

Hypotension, when unresponsive to I.V. fluids or Trendelenburg positioning, often responds to norepinephrine infusions started at 0.1-0.2 mcg/kg/minute followed by a titrated infusion

Drug Interactions

Decreased effect: Amitriptyline, butyrophenones, imipramine, methyldopa, phenothiazines, reserpine, → ↓ bromocriptine's efficacy at reducing prolactin

Increased toxicity: Ergot alkaloids (↑ cardiovascular toxicity)

Mechanism of Action Semisynthetic ergot alkaloid derivative with dopaminergic properties; inhibits prolactin secretion and can improve symptoms of Parkinson's disease by directly stimulating dopamine receptors in the corpus stratum

Pharmacodynamics/Kinetics

Protein binding: 90% to 96%

Metabolism: Majority of drug metabolized in the liver

Half-life (biphasic):

- Initial: 6-8 hours
- Terminal: 50 hours

Time to peak serum concentration: Oral: Within 1-2 hours

Elimination: In bile; only 2% to 6% excreted unchanged in urine

Usual Dosage Adults: Oral:

(Continued)

Bromocriptine *(Continued)*

Parkinsonism: 1.25 mg 2 times/day, increased by 2.5 mg/day in 2- to 4-week intervals (usual dose range is 30-90 mg/day in 3 divided doses), though elderly patients can usually be managed on lower doses

Hyperprolactinemia: 2.5 mg 2-3 times/day

Acromegaly: Initial: 1.25-2.5 mg increasing as necessary every 3-7 days; usual dose: 20-30 mg/day

Dosing adjustment in hepatic impairment: No guidelines are available, however, may be necessary

Monitoring Parameters Monitor blood pressure closely as well as hepatic, hematopoietic, and cardiovascular function

Patient Information Take with food or milk; drowsiness commonly occurs upon initiation of therapy; limit use of alcohol; avoid exposure to cold; incidence of side effects is high (68%) with nausea the most common; hypotension occurs commonly with initiation of therapy, usually upon rising after prolonged sitting or lying

Discontinue immediately if pregnant; may restore fertility; women desiring not to become pregnant should use mechanical contraceptive means

Nursing Implications Raise bed rails and institute safety measures; aid patient with ambulation; may cause postural hypotension and drowsiness

Dosage Forms

Capsule, as mesylate: 5 mg

Tablet, as mesylate: 2.5 mg

Bromocriptine Mesylate *see* Bromocriptine *on previous page*

Bromphen® [OTC] *see* Brompheniramine *on this page*

Brompheniramine (brome fen IR a meen)

Brand Names Bromarest® [OTC]; Brombay® [OTC]; Bromphen® [OTC]; Brotane® [OTC]; Chlorphed® [OTC]; Codimal-A®; Cophene-B®; Dehist®; Diamine T.D.® [OTC]; Dimetane® [OTC]; Histaject®; Nasahist B®; ND-Stat®; Oraminic® II; Sinusol-B®; Veltane®

Synonyms Brompheniramine Maleate; Parabromdylamine

Therapeutic Category Antihistamine, H_1 Blocker

Use Perennial and seasonal allergic rhinitis and other allergic symptoms including urticaria

Pregnancy Risk Factor C

Contraindications Narrow-angle glaucoma, bladder neck obstruction, symptomatic prostatic hypertrophy, asthmatic attacks, and stenosing peptic ulcer, hypersensitivity to brompheniramine or any component

Warnings/Precautions Use with caution in patients with heart disease, hypertension, thyroid disease, and asthma; swallow whole, do not crush or chew; antihistamines are more likely to cause dizziness, excessive sedation, syncope, toxic confusional states, and hypotension in the elderly

Adverse Reactions

>10%:

Central nervous system: Slight to moderate drowsiness (compared with other first generation antihistamines, brompheniramine is relatively nonsedating)

Respiratory: Thickening of bronchial secretions

1% to 10%:

Central nervous system: Headache, fatigue, nervousness, dizziness

Gastrointestinal: Appetite increase, weight gain, nausea, diarrhea, abdominal pain, xerostomia

Neuromuscular & skeletal: Arthralgia

Respiratory: Pharyngitis

<1%:

Cardiovascular: Palpitations

Central nervous system: Depression

Dermatologic: Photosensitivity, rash, angioedema

Hepatic: Hepatitis

Neuromuscular & skeletal: Myalgia, paresthesia

Respiratory: Bronchospasm, epistaxis

Overdosage/Toxicology Symptoms of overdose include dry mouth, flushed skin, dilated pupils, CNS depression

There is no specific treatment for an antihistamine overdose, however, most of its clinical toxicity is due to anticholinergic effects; anticholinesterase inhibitors including physostigmine, neostigmine, pyridostigmine, and edrophonium may be useful by reducing acetylcholinesterase; for anticholinergic overdose with severe life-threatening symptoms, physostigmine 1-2 mg (0.5 or 0.02 mg/kg for children) I.V., slowly may be given to reverse these effects

Drug Interactions Increased toxicity: CNS depressants, MAO inhibitors, alcohol, tricyclic antidepressants

Stability Solutions may crystallize if stored at <0°C, crystals will dissolve when warmed

Mechanism of Action Competes with histamine for H_1-receptor sites on effector cells in the gastrointestinal tract, blood vessels, and respiratory tract

Pharmacodynamics/Kinetics

Peak effect: Within 3-9 hours

Time to peak serum concentration: Oral: Within 2-5 hours

Duration of action: Varies with formulation

Metabolism: Extensively by the liver

Half-life: 12-34 hours

Elimination: In urine as inactive metabolites; 2% fecal elimination

Usual Dosage

Oral:

- Children:
  - ≤6 years: 0.125 mg/kg/dose given every 6 hours; maximum: 6-8 mg/day
  - 6-12 years: 2-4 mg every 6-8 hours; maximum: 12-16 mg/day
- Adults: 4 mg every 4-6 hours or 8 mg of sustained release form every 8-12 hours or 12 mg of sustained release every 12 hours; maximum: 24 mg/day
- Elderly: Initial: 4 mg once or twice daily. **Note:** Duration of action may be 36 hours or more, even when serum concentrations are low.

I.M., I.V., S.C.:

- Children ≤12 years: 0.5 mg/kg/24 hours divided every 6-8 hours
- Adults: 10 mg every 6-12 hours, maximum: 40 mg/24 hours

Dietary Considerations Alcohol: Additive CNS effects, avoid use

Patient Information Avoid alcohol; take with food or milk; swallow whole, do not crush or chew extended release products; may cause drowsiness

Nursing Implications Raise bed rails, institute safety measure, aid patient with ambulation

Dosage Forms

Elixir, as maleate: 2 mg/5 mL with 3% alcohol (120 mL, 480 mL, 4000 mL)

Injection, as maleate: 10 mg/mL (10 mL)

Tablet, as maleate: 4 mg, 8 mg, 12 mg

Tablet, sustained release, as maleate: 8 mg, 12 mg

Brompheniramine Maleate *see* Brompheniramine *on previous page*

Bronitin® *see* Epinephrine *on page 448*

Bronkaid® Mist [OTC] *see* Epinephrine *on page 448*

Bronkodyl® *see* Theophylline Salts *on page 1207*

Bronkometer® *see* Isoetharine *on page 678*

Bronkosol® *see* Isoetharine *on page 678*

Brontex® Liquid *see* Guaifenesin and Codeine *on page 590*

Brontex® Tablet *see* Guaifenesin and Codeine *on page 590*

Brotane® [OTC] *see* Brompheniramine *on previous page*

Bucladin®-S Softab® *see* Buclizine *on this page*

Buclizine (BYOO kli zeen)

Brand Names Bucladin®-S Softab®; Vibazine®

Synonyms Buclizine Hydrochloride

Therapeutic Category Antiemetic; Antihistamine, H_1 Blocker

Use Prevention and treatment of motion sickness; symptomatic treatment of vertigo

Pregnancy Risk Factor C

Contraindications Known hypersensitivity to buclizine

Warnings/Precautions Product contains tartrazine; use with caution in patients with angle-closure glaucoma, peptic ulcer, urinary tract obstruction, hyperthyroidism; some preparations contain sodium bisulfite; syrup contains alcohol

Adverse Reactions

>10%: Central nervous system: Drowsiness

<1%:

- Cardiovascular: Hypotension, palpitations
- Central nervous system: Sedation, dizziness, paradoxical excitement, fatigue, insomnia
- Gastrointestinal: Nausea, vomiting
- Genitourinary: Urinary retention
- Neuromuscular & skeletal: Tremor
- Ocular: Blurred vision

Overdosage/Toxicology CNS stimulation or depression; overdose may result in death in infants and children

There is no specific treatment for an antihistamine overdose, however, most of its clinical toxicity is due to anticholinergic effects; anticholinesterase inhibitors

(Continued)

Buclizine *(Continued)*

including physostigmine, neostigmine, pyridostigmine, and edrophonium may be useful by reducing acetylcholinesterase; for anticholinergic overdose with severe life-threatening symptoms, physostigmine 1-2 mg (0.5 or 0.02 mg/kg for children) I.V., slowly may be given to reverse these effects

Drug Interactions Increased toxicity: CNS depressants, MAO inhibitors, tricyclic antidepressants

Mechanism of Action Buclizine acts centrally to suppress nausea and vomiting. It is a piperazine antihistamine closely related to cyclizine and meclizine. It also has CNS depressant, anticholinergic, antispasmodic, and local anesthetic effects, and suppresses labyrinthine activity and conduction in vestibular-cerebellar nerve pathways.

Usual Dosage Adults: Oral:

Motion sickness (prophylaxis): 50 mg 30 minutes prior to traveling; may repeat 50 mg after 4-6 hours

Vertigo: 50 mg twice daily, up to 150 mg/day

Patient Information May cause drowsiness

Nursing Implications Bucladin®-S Softab® may be chewed, swallowed whole, or allowed to dissolve in mouth

Dosage Forms Tablet, chewable, as hydrochloride: 50 mg

Buclizine Hydrochloride *see* Buclizine *on previous page*

Budesonide (byoo DES oh nide)

Related Information

Asthma, Guidelines for the Diagnosis and Management of *on page 1518*

Estimated Clinical Comparability of Doses for Inhaled Corticosteroids *on page 1522*

Brand Names Rhinocort™

Canadian/Mexican Brand Names Entocort® (Canada); Pulmicort® (Canada)

Therapeutic Category Corticosteroid, Intranasal; Corticosteroid, Topical (Medium Potency)

Use

Children and Adults: Management of symptoms of seasonal or perennial rhinitis

Adults: Nonallergic perennial rhinitis

Adverse Reactions

>10%:

- Cardiovascular: Pounding heartbeat
- Central nervous system: Nervousness, headache, dizziness
- Dermatologic: Itching, rash
- Gastrointestinal: GI irritation, bitter taste, oral candidiasis
- Respiratory: Coughing, upper respiratory tract infection, bronchitis, hoarseness
- Miscellaneous: Increased susceptibility to infections, diaphoresis

1% to 10%:

- Central nervous system: Insomnia, psychic changes
- Dermatologic: Acne, urticaria
- Endocrine & metabolic: Menstrual problems
- Gastrointestinal: Anorexia, increase in appetite, xerostomia, dry throat, loss of taste perception
- Ocular: Cataracts
- Respiratory: Epistaxis
- Miscellaneous: Loss of smell

<1%:

- Gastrointestinal: Abdominal fullness
- Respiratory: Bronchospasm, shortness of breath

Drug Interactions Although there have been no reported drug interactions to date, one would expect budesonide could potentially interact with drugs known to interact with other corticosteroids

Usual Dosage

Children <6 years: Not recommended

Children ≥6 years and Adults: Aerosol inhalation: Nasal: Initial: 8 sprays (4 sprays/nostril) per day (256 mcg/day), given as either 2 sprays in each nostril in the morning and evening or as 4 sprays in each nostril in the morning; after symptoms decrease (usually by 3-7 days), reduce dose slowly every 2-4 weeks to the smallest amount needed to control symptoms

Patient Information For intranasal use only; inhaler should be shaken well immediately prior to use; clear nasal passage by blowing nose prior to use; keep inhaler clean and unobstructed; wash in warm water and dry thoroughly; contact physician if symptoms are not improved by 3 weeks of treatment, if condition worsens, or if nasal irritation or burning persists

Dosage Forms Aerosol: 50 mcg released per actuation to deliver ~32 mcg to patient via nasal adapter [200 metered doses] (7 g)

Bufferin® [OTC] *see* Aspirin *on page 106*

Bumetanide (byoo MET a nide)

Related Information

Heart Failure: Management of Patients With Left-Ventricular Systolic Dysfunction *on page 1533*

Sulfonamide Derivatives *on page 1420*

Brand Names Bumex®

Canadian/Mexican Brand Names Burinex® (Canada); Bumedyl® (Mexico)

Therapeutic Category Antihypertensive; Diuretic, Loop

Use Management of edema secondary to congestive heart failure or hepatic or renal disease including nephrotic syndrome; may be used alone or in combination with antihypertensives in the treatment of hypertension; can be used in furosemide-allergic patients; (1 mg = 40 mg furosemide)

Pregnancy Risk Factor D

Contraindications Hypersensitivity to bumetanide or any component; in anuria or increasing azotemia

Warnings/Precautions Loop diuretics are potent diuretics; excess amounts can lead to profound diuresis with fluid and electrolyte loss; close medical supervision and dose evaluation is required

Adverse Reactions

>10%:
- Endocrine & metabolic: Hyperuricemia, hypochloremia, hypokalemia
- Renal: Azotemia

1% to 10%:
- Central nervous system: Dizziness, encephalopathy, headache
- Endocrine & metabolic: Hyponatremia
- Neuromuscular & skeletal: Muscle cramps, weakness

<1%:
- Cardiovascular: Hypotension
- Dermatologic: Rash, pruritus
- Endocrine & metabolic: Hyperglycemia, hyperuricemia
- Gastrointestinal: Cramps, nausea, vomiting
- Hepatic: Alteration of liver function test results
- Otic: Hearing loss
- Renal: Increased serum creatinine

Overdosage/Toxicology Symptoms of overdose include electrolyte depletion, volume depletion; treatment is primarily symptomatic and supportive

Drug Interactions

Decreased effect: Indomethacin and other NSAIDs, probenecid

Increased effect: Other antihypertensive agents; lithium's excretion may be decreased

Stability I.V. infusion solutions should be used within 24 hours after preparation; light sensitive, → discoloration when exposed to light

Mechanism of Action Inhibits reabsorption of sodium and chloride in the ascending loop of Henle and proximal renal tubule, interfering with the chloride-binding cotransport system, thus causing increased excretion of water, sodium, chloride, magnesium, phosphate and calcium; it does not appear to act on the distal tubule

Pharmacodynamics/Kinetics

Onset of effect:
- Oral, I.M.: 0.5-1 hour
- I.V.: 2-3 minutes

Duration of action: 6 hours

Distribution: V_d: 13-25 L/kg

Protein binding: 95%

Metabolism: Partial, occurs in the liver

Half-life:
- Infants <6 months: Possibly 2.5 hours
- Children and Adults: 1-1.5 hours

Elimination: Majority of unchanged drug and metabolites excreted in urine

Usual Dosage

Children:
- <6 months: Dose not established
- >6 months:
  - Oral: Initial: 0.015 mg/kg/dose once daily or every other day; maximum dose: 0.1 mg/kg/day
  - I.M., I.V.: Dose not established

Adults:
- Oral: 0.5-2 mg/dose 1-2 times/day; maximum: 10 mg/day
- I.M., I.V.: 0.5-1 mg/dose; maximum: 10 mg/day
- Continuous I.V. infusions of 0.9-1 mg/hour may be more effective than bolus dosing

(Continued)

Bumetanide *(Continued)*

Administration Administer I.V. slowly, over 1-2 minutes

Monitoring Parameters Blood pressure, serum electrolytes, renal function

Patient Information May be taken with food or milk; rise slowly from a lying or sitting position to minimize dizziness, lightheadedness or fainting; also use extra care when exercising, standing for long periods of time, and during hot weather; take last dose of day early in the evening to prevent nocturia

Nursing Implications Be alert to complaints about hearing difficulty

Dosage Forms

Injection: 0.25 mg/mL (2 mL, 4 mL, 10 mL)

Tablet: 0.5 mg, 1 mg, 2 mg

Bumex® *see* Bumetanide *on previous page*

Buminate® *see* Albumin *on page 37*

Buphenyl® *see* Sodium Phenylbutyrate *on page 1145*

Bupivacaine (byoo PIV a kane)

Brand Names Marcaine®; Sensorcaine®

Synonyms Bupivacaine Hydrochloride

Therapeutic Category Local Anesthetic, Injectable

Use Local anesthetic (injectable) for peripheral nerve block, infiltration, sympathetic block, caudal or epidural block, retrobulbar block

Pregnancy Risk Factor C

Contraindications Hypersensitivity to bupivacaine hydrochloride or any component, para-aminobenzoic acid or parabens

Warnings/Precautions Use with caution in patients with liver disease. Some commercially available formulations contain sodium metabisulfite, which may cause allergic-type reactions. Pending further data, should not be used in children <12 years of age and the solution for spinal anesthesia should not be used in children <18 years of age. **Do not use solutions containing preservatives for caudal or epidural block**; convulsions due to systemic toxicity leading to cardiac arrest have been reported, presumably following unintentional intravascular injection. 0.75% is **not** recommended for obstetrical anesthesia.

Adverse Reactions

1% to 10% (dose related):

- Cardiovascular: Cardiac arrest, hypotension, bradycardia, palpitations
- Central nervous system: Seizures, restlessness, anxiety, dizziness
- Gastrointestinal: Nausea, vomiting
- Neuromuscular & skeletal: Weakness
- Ocular: Blurred vision
- Otic: Tinnitus
- Respiratory: Apnea

Overdosage/Toxicology Treatment is primarily symptomatic and supportive. Termination of anesthesia by pneumatic tourniquet inflation should be attempted when the agent is administered by infiltration or regional injection

Seizures commonly respond to diazepam, while hypotension responds to I.V. fluids and Trendelenburg positioning

Bradyarrhythmias (when the heart rate is <60) can be treated with I.V., or S.C. atropine 15 mcg/kg

With the development of metabolic acidosis, I.V. sodium bicarbonate 0.5-2 mEq/kg and ventilatory assistance should be instituted

Methemoglobinemia should be treated with methylene blue 1-2 mg/kg in a 1% sterile aqueous solution I.V. push over 4-6 minutes repeated up to a total dose of 7 mg/kg.

Drug Interactions

Increased effect: Hyaluronidase

Increased toxicity: Beta-blockers, ergot-type oxytocics, MAO inhibitors, TCAs, phenothiazines, vasopressors

Stability Solutions with epinephrine should be protected from light

Mechanism of Action Blocks both the initiation and conduction of nerve impulses by decreasing the neuronal membrane's permeability to sodium ions, which results in inhibition of depolarization with resultant blockade of conduction

Pharmacodynamics/Kinetics

Onset of anesthesia (dependent on route administered): Within 4-10 minutes generally

Duration of action: 1.5-8.5 hours

Metabolism: In the liver

Half-life (age dependent):

- Neonates: 8.1 hours
- Adults: 1.5-5.5 hours

Elimination: Small amounts (~6%) excreted in urine

Usual Dosage Dose varies with procedure, depth of anesthesia, vascularity of tissues, duration of anesthesia and condition of patient. Metabisulfites (in epinephrine-containing injection); do not use solutions containing preservatives for caudal or epidural block.

Caudal block (with or without epinephrine):
Children: 1-3.7 mg/kg
Adults: 15-30 mL of 0.25% or 0.5%

Epidural block (other than caudal block):
Children: 1.25 mg/kg/dose
Adults: 10-20 mL of 0.25% or 0.5%

Peripheral nerve block: 5 mL dose of 0.25% or 0.5% (12.5-25 mg); maximum: 2.5 mg/kg (plain); 3 mg/kg (with epinephrine); up to a maximum of 400 mg/day

Sympathetic nerve block: 20-50 mL of 0.25% (no epinephrine) solution

Monitoring Parameters Monitor fetal heart rate during paracervical anesthesia

Patient Information Do not chew food in anesthetized region to prevent traumatizing tongue, lip, or buccal mucosa; single dose is usually sufficient in most applications

Dosage Forms

Injection, as hydrochloride: 0.25% (10 mL, 20 mL, 30 mL, 50 mL); 0.5% (10 mL, 20 mL, 30 mL, 50 mL); 0.75% (2 mL, 10 mL, 20 mL, 30 mL)

Injection, as hydrochloride, with epinephrine (1:200,000): 0.25% (10 mL, 30 mL, 50 mL); 0.5% (1.8 mL, 3 mL, 5 mL, 10 mL, 30 mL, 50 mL); 0.75% (30 mL)

Bupivacaine Hydrochloride *see* Bupivacaine *on previous page*

Buprenex® *see* Buprenorphine *on this page*

Buprenorphine (byoo pre NOR feen)

Related Information

Drugs and Routes of Administration Not Recommended for Treatment of Cancer Pain *on page 1378*

Narcotic Agonists Comparison *on page 1414*

Brand Names Buprenex®

Canadian/Mexican Brand Names Temgesic® (Mexico)

Synonyms Buprenorphine Hydrochloride

Therapeutic Category Analgesic, Narcotic

Use Management of moderate to severe pain

Restrictions C-V

Pregnancy Risk Factor C

Contraindications Hypersensitivity to buprenorphine or any component

Warnings/Precautions Use with caution in patients with hepatic dysfunction or possible neurologic injury; may precipitate abstinence syndrome in narcotic-dependent patients

Adverse Reactions

>10%: Central nervous system: Drowsiness

1% to 10%:
Cardiovascular: Hypotension
Central nervous system: Respiratory depression, dizziness, headache
Gastrointestinal: Vomiting, nausea

<1%:
Central nervous system: Euphoria, slurred speech, malaise
Dermatologic: Allergic dermatitis
Genitourinary: Urinary retention
Neuromuscular & skeletal: Paresthesia
Ocular: Blurred vision

Overdosage/Toxicology Symptoms of overdose include CNS depression, pinpoint pupils, hypotension, bradycardia

Treatment of an overdose includes support of the patient's airway, establishment of an I.V. line, and administration of naloxone 2 mg I.V. (0.01 mg/kg for children) with repeat administration as necessary up to a total of 10 mg

Drug Interactions Increased toxicity: Barbiturates, benzodiazepines (increase CNS and respiratory depression)

Stability Protect from excessive heat (>40°C/104°F) and light

Compatible with 0.9% sodium chloride, Lactated Ringer's Solution, 5% dextrose in water, scopolamine, haloperidol, glycopyrrolate, droperidol, and hydroxyzine

Incompatible with diazepam, lorazepam

Mechanism of Action Opiate agonist/antagonist that produces analgesia by binding to kappa and mu opiate receptors in the CNS

Pharmacodynamics/Kinetics

Onset of analgesia: Within 10-30 minutes
Absorption: I.M., S.C.: 30% to 40%
Distribution: V_d: 97-187 L/kg

(Continued)

Buprenorphine *(Continued)*

Protein binding: High
Metabolism: Mainly in the liver; undergoes extensive first-pass metabolism
Half-life: 2.2-3 hours
Elimination: 70% excreted in feces via bile and 20% in urine as unchanged drug

Usual Dosage I.M., slow I.V.:
Children ≥13 years and Adults: 0.3-0.6 mg every 6 hours as needed
Elderly: 0.15 mg every 6 hours; elderly patients are more likely to suffer from confusion and drowsiness compared to younger patients
Long-term use is not recommended

Monitoring Parameters Pain relief, respiratory and mental status, CNS depression, blood pressure

Patient Information May cause drowsiness

Nursing Implications Gradual withdrawal of drug is necessary to avoid withdrawal symptoms

Additional Information 0.3 mg = 10 mg morphine or 75 mg meperidine, has longer duration of action than either agent

Dosage Forms Injection, as hydrochloride: 0.3 mg/mL (1 mL)

Buprenorphine Hydrochloride *see* Buprenorphine *on previous page*

Bupropion (byoo PROE pee on)

Related Information
Antidepressant Agents Comparison *on page 1393*

Brand Names Wellbutrin®; Wellbutrin® SR; Zyban®

Therapeutic Category Antidepressant

Use Treatment of depression; adjunct in smoking cessation

Pregnancy Risk Factor B

Contraindications Seizure disorder, prior diagnosis of bulimia or anorexia nervosa, known hypersensitivity to bupropion, concurrent use of a monoamine oxidase (MAO) inhibitor

Warnings/Precautions The estimated seizure potential is increased many fold in doses in the 450-600 mg/day range; giving a single dose <150 mg will lessen the seizure potential; use in patients with renal or hepatic impairment increases possible toxic effects

Adverse Reactions
>10%:
Central nervous system: Agitation, insomnia, fever, headache, psychosis, confusion, anxiety, restlessness, dizziness, seizures, chills, akathisia
Gastrointestinal: Nausea, vomiting, xerostomia, constipation, weight loss
Genitourinary: Impotence
Neuromuscular & skeletal: Tremor
1% to 10%:
Central nervous system: Hallucinations, fatigue
Dermatologic: Rash
Ocular: Blurred vision
<1%:
Cardiovascular: Syncope
Central nervous system: Drowsiness

Overdosage/Toxicology Symptoms of overdose include labored breathing, salivation, arched back, ataxia, convulsions, sedations, coma, and respiratory depression especially with coingestion of alcohol; bupropion may cause sinus tachycardia and seizures

Treatment is supportive following initial decontamination with activated charcoal (lavage with massive and recent doses). Treat seizures with I.V. benzodiazepines and supportive therapies; dialysis may be of limited value after drug absorption because of slow tissue to plasma diffusion.

Drug Interactions
Decreased effects: Increased clearance: Carbamazepine, phenytoin, cimetidine, phenobarbital
Increased effects: Levodopa, MAO inhibitors

Mechanism of Action Antidepressant structurally different from all other previously marketed antidepressants; like other antidepressants the mechanism of bupropion's activity is not fully understood; weak blocker of serotonin and norepinephrine re-uptake, inhibits neuronal dopamine re-uptake and is **not** a monoamine oxidase A or B inhibitor

Pharmacodynamics/Kinetics
Absorption: Rapidly absorbed from GI tract
Distribution: V_d: 19-21 L/kg
Protein binding: 82% to 88%
Metabolism: Extensively in the liver to multiple metabolites
Half-life: 14 hours

Time to peak serum concentration: Oral: Within 3 hours

Usual Dosage Oral:

Adults:

Depression: 100 mg 3 times/day; begin at 100 mg twice daily; may increase to a maximum dose of 450 mg/day

Smoking cessation: Initiate with 150 mg once daily for 3 days; increase to 150 mg twice daily; treatment should continue for 7-12 weeks

Elderly: Depression: 50-100 mg/day, increase by 50-100 mg every 3-4 days as tolerated; there is evidence that the elderly respond at 150 mg/day in divided doses, but some may require a higher dose

Dosing adjustment/comments in renal or hepatic impairment: Patients with renal or hepatic failure should receive a reduced dosage initially and be closely monitored

Dietary Considerations Alcohol: Additive CNS effects, avoid use

Monitoring Parameters Monitor body weight

Reference Range Therapeutic levels (trough, 12 hours after last dose): 50-100 ng/mL

Test Interactions Decreased prolactin levels

Patient Information Take in equally divided doses 3-4 times/day to minimize the risk of seizures; avoid alcohol; do not take more than recommended dose or more than 150 mg in a single dose; do not discontinue abruptly, may take 3-4 weeks for full effect; may impair driving or other motor or cognitive skills and judgment

Nursing Implications Be aware that drug may cause seizures; dose should not be increased by more than 50 mg/day once weekly

Dosage Forms

Tablet: 75 mg, 100 mg

Tablet, sustained release: 100 mg, 150 mg

BuSpar® *see* Buspirone *on this page*

Buspirone (byoo SPYE rone)

Brand Names BuSpar®

Canadian/Mexican Brand Names Neurosine® (Mexico)

Synonyms Buspirone Hydrochloride

Therapeutic Category Antianxiety Agent; Serotonin Antagonist

Use Management of anxiety; has shown little potential for abuse

Unlabeled use: Panic attacks

Pregnancy Risk Factor B

Contraindications Hypersensitivity to buspirone or any component

Warnings/Precautions Safety and efficacy not established in children <18 years of age; use in hepatic or renal impairment is not recommended; does not prevent or treat withdrawal from benzodiazepines

Adverse Reactions

>10%:

Central nervous system: Dizziness, lightheadedness, headache, restlessness

Gastrointestinal: Nausea

1% to 10%: Central nervous system: Drowsiness

<1%:

Cardiovascular: Chest pain, tachycardia

Central nervous system: Confusion, insomnia, nightmares, sedation, disorientation, excitement, fever, ataxia

Dermatologic: Rash, urticaria

Gastrointestinal: Xerostomia, vomiting, diarrhea, flatulence

Hematologic: Leukopenia, eosinophilia

Neuromuscular & skeletal: Muscle weakness

Ocular: Blurred vision

Otic: Tinnitus

Overdosage/Toxicology Symptoms of overdose include dizziness, drowsiness, pinpoint pupils, nausea, vomiting

There is no known antidote for buspirone, treatment is supportive

Drug Interactions

Increased effects: Cimetidine, food

Increased toxicity: MAO inhibitors, phenothiazines, CNS depressants; increased toxicity of digoxin and haloperidol

Mechanism of Action Selectively antagonizes CNS serotonin 5-HT_1A receptors without affecting benzodiazepine-GABA receptors; may down-regulate postsynaptic 5-HT_2 receptors as do antidepressants

Pharmacodynamics/Kinetics

Protein binding: 95%

Metabolism: In the liver by oxidation and undergoes extensive first-pass metabolism

(Continued)

Buspirone *(Continued)*

Half-life: 2-3 hours

Time to peak serum concentration: Oral: Within 40-60 minutes

Usual Dosage Adults: Oral: 15 mg/day (5 mg 3 times/day); may increase in increments of 5 mg/day every 2-4 days to a maximum of 60 mg/day

Dosing adjustment in renal or hepatic impairment: Dosage should be decreased in patients with severe hepatic insufficiency; anuric patients should be dosed at 25% to 50% of the usual dose

Monitoring Parameters Mental status, symptoms of anxiety; monitor for benzodiazepine withdrawal

Test Interactions ↑ AST, ALT, growth hormone(s), prolactin (S)

Patient Information Take with food; report any change in senses (ie, smelling, hearing, vision); cautious use with alcohol is recommended; cannot be substituted for benzodiazepines unless directed by a physician; takes 2-3 weeks to see the full effect of this medication; if you miss a dose, do **not** double your next dose

Dosage Forms Tablet, as hydrochloride: 5 mg, 10 mg

Buspirone Hydrochloride *see* Buspirone *on previous page*

Busulfan (byoo SUL fan)

Related Information

Antiemetics for Chemotherapy Induced Nausea and Vomiting *on page 1348*
Cancer Chemotherapy Regimens *on page 1351*
Toxicities of Chemotherapeutic Agents *on page 1382*

Brand Names Myleran®

Therapeutic Category Antineoplastic Agent, Alkylating Agent

Use Chronic myelogenous leukemia and bone marrow disorders, such as polycythemia vera and myeloid metaplasia, conditioning regimens for bone marrow transplantation

Pregnancy Risk Factor D

Contraindications Failure to respond to previous courses; should not be used in pregnancy or lactation; hypersensitivity to busulfan or any component

Warnings/Precautions The U.S. Food and Drug Administration (FDA) currently recommends that procedures for proper handling and disposal of antineoplastic agents be considered. May induce severe bone marrow hypoplasia; reduce or discontinue dosage at first sign, as reflected by an abnormal decrease in any of the formed elements of the blood; use with caution in patients recently given other myelosuppressive drugs or radiation treatment. If white blood count is high, hydration and allopurinol should be employed to prevent hyperuricemia.

Adverse Reactions

>10%:

- Cardiovascular: Endocardial fibrosis
- Dermatologic: Skin hyperpigmentation (busulfan tan), urticaria, erythema, alopecia
- Endocrine & metabolic: Ovarian suppression, amenorrhea, sterility
- Genitourinary: Azoospermia, testicular atrophy; malignant tumors have been reported in patients on busulfan therapy
- Hematologic: Severe pancytopenia, leukopenia, thrombocytopenia, anemia, and bone marrow suppression are common and patients should be monitored closely while on therapy; since this is a delayed effect (busulfan affects the stem cells), the drug should be discontinued temporarily at the first sign of a large or rapid fall in any blood element; some patients may develop bone marrow fibrosis or chronic aplasia which is probably due to the busulfan toxicity; in large doses, busulfan is myeloablative and is used for this reason in BMT
- Myelosuppressive:
  - WBC: Moderate
  - Platelets: Moderate
  - Onset (days): 7-10
  - Nadir (days): 14-21
  - Recovery (days): 28

1% to 10%:

- Dermatologic: Hyperpigmentation
- Endocrine & metabolic: Amenorrhea
- Gastrointestinal: Nausea, vomiting, diarrhea; drug has little effect on the GI mucosal lining
  - Emetic potential: Low (<10%)
- Hepatic: Elevated LFTs
- Neuromuscular & skeletal: Weakness
- Ocular: Cataracts

<1%:

Central nervous system: Generalized or myoclonic seizures and loss of consciousness have been associated with high-dose busulfan (4 mg/kg/day)

Endocrine & metabolic: Adrenal suppression, gynecomastia, hyperuricemia

Genitourinary: Isolated cases of hemorrhagic cystitis have been reported

Hepatic: Hepatic dysfunction

Ocular: Cataracts, blurred vision

Respiratory: After long-term or high-dose therapy, a syndrome known as busulfan lung may occur; this syndrome is manifested by a diffuse interstitial pulmonary fibrosis and persistent cough, fever, rales, and dyspnea. May be relieved by corticosteroids

Overdosage/Toxicology Symptoms of overdose include leukopenia, thrombocytopenia

Induction of vomiting or gastric lavage with charcoal is indicated for recent ingestions; the effects of dialysis are unknown

Mechanism of Action Reacts with N-7 position of guanosine and interferes with DNA replication and transcription of RNA. Busulfan has a more marked effect on myeloid cells (and is, therefore, useful in the treatment of CML) than on lymphoid cells. The drug is also very toxic to hematopoietic stem cells (thus its usefulness in high doses in BMT preparative regimens). Busulfan exhibits little immunosuppressive activity. Interferes with the normal function of DNA by alkylation and cross-linking the strands of DNA.

Pharmacodynamics/Kinetics

Absorption: Rapidly and completely from the GI tract

Distribution: V_d: ~1 L/kg; distributed into the CSF and saliva with levels similar to plasma

Protein binding: ~14%

Metabolism: Extensive in the liver (may increase with multiple dosing)

Half-life:

- After first dose: 3.4 hours
- After last dose: 2.3 hours

Time to peak serum concentration:

- Oral: Within 4 hours
- I.V.: Within 5 minutes

Elimination: 10% to 50% excreted in the urine as metabolites within 24 hours; <2% seen as unchanged drug

Usual Dosage Oral (refer to individual protocols):

Children:

For remission induction of CML: 0.06-0.12 mg/kg/day **OR** 1.8-4.6 mg/m^2/day; titrate dosage to maintain leukocyte count above 40,000/mm^3; reduce dosage by 50% if the leukocyte count reaches 30,000-40,000/mm^3; discontinue drug if counts fall to ≤20,000/mm^3

BMT marrow-ablative conditioning regimen: 1 mg/kg/dose (ideal body weight) every 6 hours for 16 doses

Adults:

BMT marrow-ablative conditioning regimen: 1 mg/kg/dose (ideal body weight) every 6 hours for 16 doses

Remission:

Induction of CML: 4-8 mg/day (may be as high as 12 mg/day)

Maintenance doses: Controversial, range from 1-4 mg/day to 2 mg/week; treatment is continued until WBC reaches 10,000-20,000 cells/mm^3 at which time drug is discontinued; when WBC reaches 50,000/mm^3, maintenance dose is resumed

Unapproved uses:

Polycythemia vera: 2-6 mg/day

Thrombocytosis: 4-6 mg/day

Administration Avoid I.M. injection if platelet count falls <100,000/mm^3

Monitoring Parameters CBC with differential and platelet count, hemoglobin, liver function tests

Patient Information Watch for signs of bleeding; excellent oral hygiene is needed to minimize oral discomfort

Dosage Forms Tablet: 2 mg

Butabarbital Sodium (byoo ta BAR bi tal SOW dee um)

Brand Names Butalan®; Buticaps®; Butisol Sodium®

Therapeutic Category Barbiturate; Hypnotic; Sedative

Use Sedative, hypnotic

Restrictions C-III

Pregnancy Risk Factor D

Contraindications Hypersensitivity to butabarbital or any component, presence of acute or chronic pain, latent porphyria, marked liver impairment

(Continued)

Butabarbital Sodium *(Continued)*

Adverse Reactions

>10%: Central nervous system: Dizziness, lightheadedness, drowsiness, "hangover" effect

1% to 10%:

Central nervous system: Confusion, mental depression, unusual excitement, nervousness, faint feeling, headache, insomnia, nightmares

Gastrointestinal: Constipation, nausea, vomiting

<1%:

Cardiovascular: Hypotension

Central nervous system: Hallucinations

Dermatologic: Rash, exfoliative dermatitis, Stevens-Johnson syndrome, angioedema

Hematologic: Agranulocytosis, megaloblastic anemia, thrombocytopenia

Local: Thrombophlebitis

Respiratory: Respiratory depression

Miscellaneous: Dependence

Overdosage/Toxicology Symptoms of overdose include slurred speech, confusion, nystagmus, tachycardia, hypotension

If hypotension occurs, administer I.V. fluids and place the patient in the Trendelenburg position; if unresponsive, an I.V. vasopressor (eg, dopamine, epinephrine) may be required. Forced alkaline diuresis is of no value in the treatment of intoxications with short-acting barbiturates. Charcoal hemoperfusion or hemodialysis may be useful in the harder to treat intoxications, especially in the presence of very high serum barbiturate levels.

Drug Interactions

Decreased effect: Phenothiazines, haloperidol, quinidine, cyclosporine, TCAs, corticosteroids, theophylline, ethosuximide, warfarin, oral contraceptives, chloramphenicol, griseofulvin, doxycycline, beta-blockers

Increased effect/toxicity: Propoxyphene, benzodiazepines, CNS depressants, valproic acid, methylphenidate, chloramphenicol

Mechanism of Action Interferes with transmission of impulses from the thalamus to the cortex of the brain resulting in an imbalance in central inhibitory and facilitatory mechanisms

Pharmacodynamics/Kinetics

Distribution: V_d: 0.8 L/kg

Protein binding: 26%

Metabolism: In the liver

Half-life: 40-140 hours

Time to peak serum concentration: Oral: Within 40-60 minutes

Elimination: In urine as metabolites

Usual Dosage Oral:

Children: Preop: 2-6 mg/kg/dose; maximum: 100 mg

Adults:

Sedative: 15-30 mg 3-4 times/day

Hypnotic: 50-100 mg

Preop: 50-100 mg 1-1½ hours before surgery

Dietary Considerations Alcohol: Additive CNS effects, avoid use

Reference Range Therapeutic: Not established; Toxic: 28-73 µg/mL

Test Interactions ↑ ammonia (B); ↓ bilirubin (S)

Patient Information May cause drowsiness, avoid alcohol or other CNS depressants, may impair judgment and coordination; may cause physical and psychological dependence with prolonged use; do not exceed recommended dose

Nursing Implications Raise bed rails; initiate safety measures; aid with ambulation; monitor for CNS depression

Dosage Forms

Capsule: 15 mg, 30 mg

Elixir, with alcohol 7%: 30 mg/5 mL (480 mL, 3780 mL); 33.3 mg/5 mL (480 mL, 3780 mL)

Tablet: 15 mg, 30 mg, 50 mg, 100 mg

Butace® *see* Butalbital Compound *on this page*

Butalan® *see* Butabarbital Sodium *on previous page*

Butalbital Compound (byoo TAL bi tal KOM pound)

Brand Names Amaphen®; Anoquan®; Axotal®; B-A-C®; Bancap®; Butace®; Endolor®; Esgic®; Femcet®; Fiorgen PF®; Fioricet®; Fiorinal®; G-1®; Isollyl Improved®; Lanorinal®; Marnal®; Medigesic®; Phrenilin®; Phrenilin® Forte; Repan®; Sedapap-10®; Triapin®; Two-Dyne®

Canadian/Mexican Brand Names Tecnal® (Canada)

Therapeutic Category Barbiturate

Use Relief of symptomatic complex of tension or muscle contraction headache

Restrictions C-III (Fiorinal®)

Pregnancy Risk Factor D

Contraindications Patients with porphyria, known hypersensitivity to butalbital or any component

Warnings/Precautions Children and teenagers should not use for chickenpox or flu symptoms before a physician is consulted about Reye's syndrome (Fiorinal®)

Adverse Reactions

>10%:

- Central nervous system: Dizziness, lightheadedness, drowsiness, "hangover" effect
- Gastrointestinal: Nausea, heartburn, stomach pains, dyspepsia, epigastric discomfort

1% to 10%:

- Central nervous system: Confusion, mental depression, unusual excitement, nervousness, faint feeling, headache, insomnia, nightmares, fatigue
- Dermatologic: Rash
- Gastrointestinal: Constipation, vomiting, gastrointestinal ulceration
- Hematologic: Hemolytic anemia
- Neuromuscular & skeletal: Weakness
- Respiratory: Dyspnea
- Miscellaneous: Anaphylactic shock

<1%:

- Cardiovascular: Hypotension
- Central nervous system: Hallucinations, jitters
- Dermatologic: Exfoliative dermatitis, Stevens-Johnson syndrome
- Hematologic: Agranulocytosis, megaloblastic anemia, occult bleeding, prolongation of bleeding time, leukopenia, thrombocytopenia, iron deficiency anemia
- Hepatic: Hepatotoxicity
- Local: Thrombophlebitis
- Renal: Impaired renal function
- Respiratory: Respiratory depression, bronchospasm

Overdosage/Toxicology Symptoms of overdose include slurred speech, confusion, nystagmus, tachycardia, hypotension, tinnitus, headache, dizziness, confusion, metabolic acidosis, hyperpyrexia, hypoglycemia, coma, hepatic necrosis, blood dyscrasias, respiratory depression

Forced alkaline diuresis is of no value in the treatment of intoxications with short-acting barbiturates. Charcoal hemoperfusion or hemodialysis may be useful in the harder to treat intoxications, especially in the presence of very high serum barbiturate levels; see also Acetaminophen for Fioricet® toxicology or Aspirin for Fiorinal® toxicology.

Drug Interactions

- Decreased effect: Phenothiazines, haloperidol, quinidine, cyclosporine, TCAs, corticosteroids, theophylline, ethosuximide, warfarin, oral contraceptives, chloramphenicol, griseofulvin, doxycycline, beta-blockers
- Increased effect/toxicity: Propoxyphene, benzodiazepines, CNS depressants, valproic acid, methylphenidate, chloramphenicol

Mechanism of Action Butalbital, like other barbiturates, has a generalized depressant effect on the central nervous system (CNS). Barbiturates have little effect on peripheral nerves or muscle at usual therapeutic doses. However, at toxic doses serious effects on the cardiovascular system and other peripheral systems may be observed. These effects may result in hypotension or skeletal muscle weakness. While all areas of the central nervous system are acted on by barbiturates, the mesencephalic reticular activating system is extremely sensitive to their effects. Barbiturates act at synapses where gamma-aminobenzoic acid is a neurotransmitter, but they may act in other areas as well.

Usual Dosage Adults: Oral: 1-2 tablets or capsules every 4 hours; not to exceed 6/day

Dosing interval in renal or hepatic impairment: Should be reduced

Dietary Considerations Alcohol: Additive CNS effects, avoid use

Patient Information Children and teenagers should not use this product; may cause drowsiness, avoid alcohol or other CNS depressants, may impair judgment and coordination; may cause physical and psychological dependence with prolonged use; do not exceed recommended dose

Nursing Implications Raise bed rails; initiate safety measures; aid with ambulation; monitor for CNS depression

Dosage Forms

Capsule, with acetaminophen:

- Amaphen®, Anoquan®, Butace®, Endolor®, Esgic®, Femcet®, G-1®, Medigesic®, Repan®, Two-Dyne®: Butalbital 50 mg, caffeine 40 mg, and acetaminophen 325 mg
- Bancap®, Triapin®: Butalbital 50 mg and acetaminophen 325 mg

(Continued)

Butalbital Compound *(Continued)*

Phrenilin® Forte: Butalbital 50 mg and acetaminophen 650 mg

Capsule, with aspirin: (Fiorgen PF®, Fiorinal®, Isollyl Improved®, Lanorinal®, Marnal®): Butalbital 50 mg, caffeine 40 mg, and aspirin 325 mg

Tablet, with acetaminophen:

Esgic®, Fioricet®, Repan®: Butalbital 50 mg, caffeine 40 mg, and acetaminophen 325 mg

Phrenilin®: Butalbital 50 mg and acetaminophen 325 mg

Sedapap-10®: Butalbital 50 mg and acetaminophen 650 mg

Tablet, with aspirin:

Axotal®: Butalbital 50 mg and aspirin 650 mg

B-A-C®: Butalbital 50 mg, caffeine 40 mg, and aspirin 650 mg

Fiorinal®, Isollyl Improved®, Lanorinal®, Marnal®: Butalbital 50 mg, caffeine 40 mg, and aspirin 325 mg

Butenafine (byoo TEN a fine)

Brand Names Mentax®

Synonyms Butenafine Hydrochloride

Therapeutic Category Antifungal Agent, Topical

Use Topical treatment of tinea pedis (athlete's foot) and tinea cruris (jock itch)

Pregnancy Risk Factor B

Contraindications Hypersensitivity to butenafine or components

Adverse Reactions

>1%: Dermatologic: Burning, stinging, irritation, erythema, pruritus (2%)

<1%: Dermatologic: Contact dermatitis

Mechanism of Action Butenafine exerts antifungal activity by blocking squalene epoxidation, resulting in inhibition of ergosterol synthesis (antidermatophyte and *Sporothrix schenckii* activity). In higher concentrations, the drug disrupts fungal cell membranes (anticandidal activity).

Pharmacodynamics/Kinetics

Absorption: Minimal systemic absorption when topically applied

Metabolism: Hepatic; principle metabolite via hydroxylation

Half-life: 35 hours

Time to peak serum concentration: 6 hours (10 ng/mL)

Usual Dosage Children >12 years and Adults: Topical: Apply once daily for 4 weeks

Monitoring Parameters Culture and KOH exam, clinical signs of tinea pedis

Patient Information Report any signs of rash or allergy to your physician immediately; do not apply other topical medications on the same area as butenafine unless directed by your physician

Dosage Forms Cream, as hydrochloride: 1% (2 g, 15 g, 30 g)

Butenafine Hydrochloride *see* Butenafine *on this page*

Buticaps® *see* Butabarbital Sodium *on page 175*

Butisol Sodium® *see* Butabarbital Sodium *on page 175*

Butoconazole (byoo toe KOE na zole)

Related Information

Treatment of Sexually Transmitted Diseases *on page 1485*

Brand Names Femstat®

Canadian/Mexican Brand Names Femstal® (Mexico)

Synonyms Butoconazole Nitrate

Therapeutic Category Antifungal Agent, Imidazole Derivative; Antifungal Agent, Vaginal

Use Local treatment of vulvovaginal candidiasis

Pregnancy Risk Factor C (For use only in 2nd or 3rd trimester)

Contraindications Known hypersensitivity to butoconazole

Warnings/Precautions In pregnancy, use only during second or third trimesters; if irritation or sensitization occurs, discontinue use

Adverse Reactions

1% to 10%: Genitourinary: Vulvar/vaginal burning

<1%: Genitourinary: Vulvar itching, soreness, edema, or discharge; polyuria

Stability Do not store at temperatures >40°C/104°F; avoid freezing

Mechanism of Action Increases cell membrane permeability in susceptible fungi (*Candida*)

Pharmacodynamics/Kinetics

Absorption: Following intravaginal application small amounts of drug are absorbed systemically (25%) within 2-8 hours

Half-life: 21-24 hours

Elimination: Into urine and feces in approximate equal amounts

Usual Dosage Adults:

Nonpregnant: Insert 1 applicatorful (~5 g) intravaginally at bedtime as a single dose; therapy may extend for up to 6 days, if necessary, as directed by physician

Pregnant: **Use only during second or third trimesters**

Patient Information May cause burning or stinging on application; if symptoms of vaginitis persist, contact physician

Dosage Forms Cream, vaginal, as nitrate: 2% with applicator (28 g)

Butoconazole Nitrate *see* Butoconazole *on previous page*

Butorphanol (byoo TOR fa nole)

Related Information

Drugs and Routes of Administration Not Recommended for Treatment of Cancer Pain *on page 1378*

Narcotic Agonists Comparison *on page 1414*

Brand Names Stadol®; Stadol® NS

Synonyms Butorphanol Tartrate

Therapeutic Category Analgesic, Narcotic

Use Management of moderate to severe pain

Pregnancy Risk Factor B (D if used for prolonged periods or in high doses at term)

Contraindications Hypersensitivity to butorphanol or any component; avoid use in opiate-dependent patients who have not been detoxified, may precipitate opiate withdrawal

Warnings/Precautions Use with caution in patients with hepatic/renal dysfunction, may elevate CSF pressure, may increase cardiac workload

Adverse Reactions

>10%: Central nervous system: Drowsiness

1% to 10%:

Cardiovascular: Flushing of the face, hypotension

Central nervous system: Dizziness, lightheadedness, headache

Gastrointestinal: Anorexia, nausea, vomiting

Genitourinary: Decreased urination

Miscellaneous: Diaphoresis (increased)

<1%:

Cardiovascular: Bradycardia or tachycardia, hypertension

Central nervous system: Paradoxical CNS stimulation, confusion, hallucinations, mental depression, false sense of well being, malaise, restlessness, nightmares, CNS depression

Dermatologic: Rash

Gastrointestinal: Stomach cramps, constipation, xerostomia

Genitourinary: Painful urination

Ocular: Blurred vision

Otic: Tinnitus

Neuromuscular & skeletal: Weakness

Respiratory: Shortness of breath, dyspnea, respiratory depression

Miscellaneous: Dependence with prolonged use

Overdosage/Toxicology Symptoms of overdose include respiratory depression, cardiac and CNS depression

Treatment of an overdose includes support of the patient's airway, establishment of an I.V. line and administration of naloxone 2 mg I.V. (0.01 mg/kg for children) with repeat administration as necessary up to a total of 10 mg

Drug Interactions Increased toxicity: CNS depressants, phenothiazines, barbiturates, skeletal muscle relaxants, alfentanil, guanabenz, MAO inhibitors

Stability Store at room temperature, protect from freezing; **incompatible** when mixed in the same syringe with diazepam, dimenhydrinate, methohexital, pentobarbital, secobarbital, thiopental

Mechanism of Action Mixed narcotic agonist-antagonist with central analgesic actions; binds to opiate receptors in the CNS, causing inhibition of ascending pain pathways, altering the perception of and response to pain; produces generalized CNS depression

Pharmacodynamics/Kinetics

Peak effect:

I.M.: Within 0.5-1 hour

I.V.: Within 4-5 minutes

Absorption: Rapidly and well absorbed

Protein binding: 80%

Metabolism: In the liver

Half-life: 2.5-4 hours

Elimination: Primarily in urine

Usual Dosage Adults:

I.M.: 1-4 mg every 3-4 hours as needed

(Continued)

Butorphanol *(Continued)*

I.V.: 0.5-2 mg every 3-4 hours as needed

Nasal spray: Headache: 1 spray in 1 nostril; if adequate pain relief is not achieved within 60-90 minutes, an additional 1 spray in 1 nostril may be given (each spray gives ~1 mg of butorphanol)

Dosing adjustment in renal impairment:

Cl_{cr} 10-50 mL/minute: Administer 75% of dose

Cl_{cr} <10 mL/minute: Administer 50% of dose

Dietary Considerations Alcohol: Additive CNS effects, avoid or limit use; watch for sedation

Monitoring Parameters Pain relief, respiratory and mental status, blood pressure

Reference Range 0.7-1.5 ng/mL

Patient Information May cause drowsiness; avoid alcohol

Nursing Implications Observe for excessive sedation or confusion, respiratory depression; raise bed rails; aid with ambulation

Dosage Forms

Injection, as tartrate: 1 mg/mL (1 mL); 2 mg/mL (1 mL, 2 mL, 10 mL)

Spray, nasal, as tartrate: 10 mg/mL [14-15 doses] (2.5 mL)

Butorphanol Tartrate *see* Butorphanol *on previous page*

BW-430C *see* Lamotrigine *on page 705*

Byclomine® Injection *see* Dicyclomine *on page 376*

Bydramine® Cough Syrup [OTC] *see* Diphenhydramine *on page 399*

C7E3 *see* Abciximab *on page 14*

Cafatine® *see* Ergotamine *on page 459*

Cafatine-PB® *see* Ergotamine *on page 459*

Cafergot® *see* Ergotamine *on page 459*

Cafetrate® *see* Ergotamine *on page 459*

Calan® *see* Verapamil *on page 1297*

Calan® SR *see* Verapamil *on page 1297*

Calci-Chew™ *see* Calcium Carbonate *on page 185*

Calcifediol (kal si fe DYE ole)

Brand Names Calderol®

Synonyms 25-HCC; 25-Hydroxycholecalciferol; 25-Hydroxyvitamin D_3

Therapeutic Category Vitamin, Fat Soluble

Use Treatment and management of metabolic bone disease associated with chronic renal failure

Pregnancy Risk Factor A (D if used in doses above the recommended daily allowance)

Contraindications Hypercalcemia; known hypersensitivity to calcifediol; malabsorption syndrome; hypervitaminosis D; significantly decreased renal function

Warnings/Precautions Adequate (supplemental) dietary calcium is necessary for clinical response to vitamin D; calcium-phosphate product (serum calcium times phosphorus) must not exceed 70; avoid hypercalcemia

Adverse Reactions

1% to 10%:

Cardiovascular: Hypotension, cardiac arrhythmias, hypertension

Central nervous system: Irritability, headache

Dermatologic: Pruritus

Endocrine & metabolic: Polydipsia, hypermagnesemia

Gastrointestinal: Nausea, vomiting, constipation, anorexia, pancreatitis, metallic taste

Genitourinary: Polyuria

Neuromuscular & skeletal: Myalgia, bone pain

Ocular: Conjunctivitis, photophobia

<1%:

Central nervous system: Overt psychosis, seizures

Endocrine & metabolic: Calcification

Gastrointestinal: Weight loss

Hepatic: Elevated AST/ALT

Overdosage/Toxicology Symptoms of overdose include hypercalcemia, hypercalciuria

Following withdrawal of the drug, treatment consists of bed rest, liberal intake of fluids, reduced calcium intake, and cathartic administration. Severe hypercalcemia requires I.V. hydration and forced diuresis. Urine output should be monitored and maintained at >3 mL/kg/hour. I.V. saline can quickly and significantly increase excretion of calcium into urine. Calcitonin, cholestyramine, prednisone, sodium EDTA, biphosphonates, and mithramycin have all been used successfully to treat the more resistant cases of vitamin D-induced hypercalcemia.

Drug Interactions

Decreased effect: Cholestyramine, colestipol

Increased effect: Thiazide diuretics

Additive effect: Antacids (magnesium)

Mechanism of Action Vitamin D analog that (along with calcitonin and parathyroid hormone) regulates serum calcium homeostasis by promoting absorption of calcium and phosphorus in the small intestine; promotes renal tubule resorption of phosphate; increases rate of accretion and resorption in bone minerals

Pharmacodynamics/Kinetics

Absorption: Rapid from the small intestines

Distribution: Activated in the kidneys; stored in liver and fat depots

Half-life: 12-22 days

Time to peak: Within 4 hours (oral)

Elimination: In bile and feces

Usual Dosage Oral: Hepatic osteodystrophy:

Infants: 5-7 mcg/kg/day

Children and Adults: 20-100 mcg/day or every other day; titrate to obtain normal serum calcium/phosphate levels; increase dose at 4-week intervals

Test Interactions ↑ calcium (S), cholesterol (S), magnesium, BUN, AST, ALT; ↓ alk phos

Patient Information Compliance with dose, diet, and calcium supplementation is essential; avoid taking magnesium supplements or magnesium-containing antacids; notify physician if weakness, lethargy, headache, and decreased appetite occur

Dosage Forms Capsule: 20 mcg, 50 mcg

Calciferol™ *see* Ergocalciferol *on page 456*

Calcijex™ *see* Calcitriol *on page 183*

Calcilac® [OTC] *see* Calcium Carbonate *on page 185*

Calcimar® Injection *see* Calcitonin *on this page*

Calci-Mix™ *see* Calcium Carbonate *on page 185*

Calcipotriene (kal si POE try een)

Brand Names Dovonex®

Therapeutic Category Topical Skin Product; Vitamin, Fat Soluble

Use Treatment of moderate plaque psoriasis

Pregnancy Risk Factor C

Contraindications Hypersensitivity to any components of the preparation; patients with demonstrated hypercalcemia or evidence of vitamin D toxicity; use on the face

Warnings/Precautions Use may cause irritations of lesions and surrounding uninvolved skin. If irritation develops, discontinue use. Transient, rapidly reversible elevation of serum calcium has occurred during use. If elevation in serum calcium occurs above the normal range, discontinue treatment until calcium levels are normal. For external use only; not for ophthalmic, oral or intravaginal use.

Adverse Reactions

>10%: Dermatologic: Burning, itching, skin irritation, erythema, dry skin, peeling, rash, worsening of psoriasis

1% to 10%: Dermatologic: Dermatitis

<1%:

Dermatologic: Skin atrophy, hyperpigmentation, folliculitis

Endocrine & metabolic: Hypercalcemia

Mechanism of Action Synthetic vitamin D_3 analog which regulates skin cell production and proliferation

Usual Dosage Adults: Topical: Apply in a thin film to the affected skin twice daily and rub in gently and completely

Patient Information For external use only; avoid contact with the face or eyes; wash hands after application

Nursing Implications Wear gloves

Dosage Forms

Cream: 0.005% (30 g, 60 g, 100 g)

Ointment, topical: 0.005% (30 g, 60 g, 100 g)

Calcitonin (kal si TOE nin)

Brand Names Calcimar® Injection; Cibacalcin® Injection; Miacalcin® Injection; Miacalcin® Nasal Spray; Osteocalcin® Injection; Salmonine® Injection

Canadian/Mexican Brand Names Caltine® (Canada)

Synonyms Calcitonin (Human); Calcitonin (Salmon)

Therapeutic Category Antidote, Hypercalcemia

(Continued)

Calcitonin *(Continued)*

Use

Calcitonin (salmon): Treatment of Paget's disease of bone and as adjunctive therapy for hypercalcemia; also used in postmenopausal osteoporosis and osteogenesis imperfecta

Calcitonin (human): Treatment of Paget's disease of bone

Pregnancy Risk Factor C

Contraindications Hypersensitivity to salmon protein or gelatin diluent

Warnings/Precautions A skin test should be performed prior to initiating therapy of calcitonin salmon; have epinephrine immediately available for a possible hypersensitivity reaction

Adverse Reactions

>10%:

Cardiovascular: Facial flushing

Gastrointestinal: Nausea, diarrhea, anorexia

Local: Edema at injection site

1% to 10%: Genitourinary: Polyuria

<1%:

Cardiovascular: Edema

Central nervous system: Chills, headache, dizziness

Dermatologic: Rash, urticaria

Neuromuscular & skeletal: paresthesia, weakness

Respiratory: Shortness of breath, nasal congestion

Overdosage/Toxicology Symptoms of overdose include nausea, vomiting, hypocalcemia, hypocalcemic tetany

Stability

Salmon calcitonin: Injection: Store under refrigeration at 2°C to 6°C/36°F to 43°F; stable for up to 2 weeks at room temperature; NS has been recommended for the dilution to prepare a skin test

Salmon calcitonin: Nasal: Store unopened bottle under refrigeration at 2°C to 8°C; Once the pump has been activated, store at room temperature

Human calcitonin: Store at ≤25°C/77°F and protect from light

Mechanism of Action Structurally similar to human calcitonin; it directly inhibits osteoclastic bone resorption; promotes the renal excretion of calcium, phosphate, sodium, magnesium and potassium by decreasing tubular reabsorption; increases the jejunal secretion of water, sodium, potassium, and chloride

Pharmacodynamics/Kinetics

Hypercalcemia:

Onset of reduction in calcium: 2 hours

Duration of effect: 6-8 hours

Distribution: Does not cross into the placenta

Metabolism: Rapidly by the kidneys

Half-life: S.C.: 1.2 hours

Elimination: As inactive metabolites in urine

Usual Dosage

Children: Dosage not established

Adults:

Paget's disease:

Salmon calcitonin: I.M., S.C.: 100 units/day to start, 50 units/day or 50-100 units every 1-3 days maintenance dose

Intranasal: 200-400 units (1-2 sprays)/day

Human calcitonin: S.C.: Initial: 0.5 mg/day (maximum: 0.5 mg twice daily); maintenance: 0.5 mg 2-3 times/week or 0.25 mg/day

Hypercalcemia: Initial: Salmon calcitonin: I.M., S.C.: 4 units/kg every 12 hours; may increase up to 8 units/kg every 12 hours to a maximum of every 6 hours

Osteogenesis imperfecta: Salmon calcitonin: I.M., S.C.: 2 units/kg 3 times/week

Postmenopausal osteoporosis: Salmon calcitonin:

I.M., S.C.: 100 units/day

Intranasal: 200 units (1 spray)/day

Monitoring Parameters Serum electrolytes and calcium; alkaline phosphatase and 24-hour urine collection for hydroxyproline excretion (Paget's disease); serum calcium

Reference Range Therapeutic: <19 pg/mL (SI: 19 ng/L) basal, depending on the assay

Patient Information Nasal spray: Notify physician if you develop significant nasal irritation. To activate the pump, hold the bottle upright and depress the two white side arms toward the bottle six times until a faint spray is emitted. The pump is activated once this first faint spray has been emitted; at this point, firmly place the nozzle into the bottle. It is not necessary to reactivate the pump before each daily use. Alternate nostrils with the spray formulation.

Nursing Implications Skin test should be performed prior to administration of salmon calcitonin; refrigerate; I.M. administration is preferred if the volume to injection exceeds 2 mL

Dosage Forms

Injection:

Human (Cibacalcin®): 0.5 mg/vial

Salmon: 200 units/mL (2 mL)

Spray, nasal: **Salmon** (Miacalcin®): 200 units/activation (0.09 mL/dose) (2 mL glass bottle with pump)

Calcitonin (Human) *see* Calcitonin *on page 181*

Calcitonin (Salmon) *see* Calcitonin *on page 181*

Calcitriol (kal si TRYE ole)

Related Information

Antacid Drug Interactions *on page 1388*

Brand Names Calcijex™; Rocaltrol®

Synonyms 1,25 Dihydroxycholecalciferol

Therapeutic Category Vitamin, Fat Soluble

Use Management of hypocalcemia in patients on chronic renal dialysis; reduce elevated parathyroid hormone levels; decrease severity of psoriatic lesions in psoriatic vulgaris

Pregnancy Risk Factor A (D if used in doses above the recommended daily allowance)

Contraindications Hypercalcemia; vitamin D toxicity; abnormal sensitivity to the effects of vitamin D; malabsorption syndrome

Warnings/Precautions Adequate dietary (supplemental) calcium is necessary for clinical response to vitamin D; maintain adequate fluid intake; calcium-phosphate product (serum calcium times phosphorus) must not exceed 70; avoid hypercalcemia or use with renal function impairment and secondary hyperparathyroidism

Adverse Reactions

1% to 10%:

Cardiovascular: Hypotension, cardiac arrhythmias, hypertension

Central nervous system: Irritability, headache

Dermatologic: Pruritus

Endocrine & metabolic: Polydipsia

Gastrointestinal: Nausea, vomiting, constipation, anorexia, pancreatitis, metallic taste

Genitourinary: Polyuria

Neuromuscular & skeletal: Myalgia, bone pain

Ocular: Conjunctivitis, photophobia

<1%:

Central nervous system: Overt psychosis, hyperthermia

Endocrine & metabolic: Hypercalcemia, hypercholesterolemia

Gastrointestinal: Weight loss

Hepatic: Increased LFTs

Respiratory: Rhinorrhea

Overdosage/Toxicology Symptoms of overdose include hypercalcemia, hypercalciuria

Following withdrawal of the drug, treatment consists of bed rest, liberal intake of fluids, reduced calcium intake, and cathartic administration. Severe hypercalcemia requires I.V. hydration and forced diuresis. Urine output should be monitored and maintained at >3 mL/kg/hour. I.V. saline can quickly and significantly increase excretion of calcium into urine. Calcitonin, cholestyramine, prednisone, sodium EDTA, biphosphonates, and mithramycin have all been used successfully to treat the more resistant cases of vitamin D-induced hypercalcemia.

Drug Interactions

Decreased effect/absorption: Cholestyramine, colestipol

Increased effect: Thiazide diuretics

Additive effect: Magnesium-containing antacids

Stability Store in tight, light-resistant container; calcitriol degrades upon prolonged exposure to light

Mechanism of Action Promotes absorption of calcium in the intestines and retention at the kidneys thereby increasing calcium levels in the serum; decreases excessive serum phosphatase levels, parathyroid hormone levels, and decreases bone resorption; increases renal tubule phosphate resorption

Pharmacodynamics/Kinetics

Onset of action: ~2-6 hours

Duration: 3-5 days

Absorption: Oral: Rapid

Metabolism: Primarily to 1,24,25-trihydroxyoholecalciferol and 1,24,25-trihydroxy ergocalciferol

(Continued)

Calcitriol *(Continued)*

Half-life: 3-8 hours

Elimination: Principally in bile and feces with 4% to 6% excreted in urine

Usual Dosage Individualize dosage to maintain calcium levels of 9-10 mg/dL

Renal failure:

Oral:

Children: Initial: 15 ng/kg/day; maintenance: 5-40 ng/kg/day

Adults: 0.25 mcg/day or every other day (may require 0.5-1 mcg/day)

I.V.: Adults: 0.5 mcg (0.01 mcg/kg) 3 times/week; most doses in the range of 0.5-3 mcg (0.01-0.05 mcg/kg) 3 times/week

Hypoparathyroidism/pseudohypoparathyroidism: Oral:

Children:

<1 year: 0.04-0.08 mcg/kg/day

1-6 years: Initial: 0.25 mcg/day, increase at 2- to 4-week intervals

Children >6 years and Adults: 0.5-2 mcg/day

Vitamin D-resistant rickets (familial hypophosphatemia): Oral: 2 mcg/day; initial: 15-20 ng/kg/day; maintenance: 30-60 ng/kg/day

Monitoring Parameters Monitor symptoms of hypercalcemia (weakness, fatigue, somnolence, headache, anorexia, dry mouth, metallic taste, nausea, vomiting, cramps, diarrhea, muscle pain, bone pain and irritability)

Reference Range Calcium (serum) 9-10 mg/dL (4.5-5 mEq/L) but do not include the I.V. dosages; phosphate: 2.5-5 mg/dL

Test Interactions ↑ calcium, cholesterol, magnesium, BUN, AST, ALT, calcium (S), cholesterol (S); ↓ alkaline phosphatase

Patient Information Compliance with dose, diet, and calcium supplementation is essential; notify physician if weakness, lethargy, headache, and decreased appetite occur; avoid taking magnesium supplements or magnesium-containing antacids

Dosage Forms

Capsule: 0.25 mcg, 0.5 mcg

Injection: 1 mcg/mL (1 mL); 2 mcg/mL (1 mL)

Calcium Acetate (KAL see um AS e tate)

Brand Names Phos-Ex®; PhosLo®

Therapeutic Category Antidote, Hyperphosphatemia; Calcium Salt; Electrolyte Supplement, Oral

Use Control of hyperphosphatemia in end stage renal failure; calcium acetate binds phosphorus in the GI tract better than other calcium salts due to its lower solubility and subsequent reduced absorption and increased formation of calcium phosphate; calcium acetate does not promote aluminum absorption

Pregnancy Risk Factor C

Contraindications Hypercalcemia

Warnings/Precautions Calcium carbonate absorption is impaired in achlorhydria (common in elderly - use alternate salt, administer with food); administration is followed by increased gastric acid secretion within 2 hours of administration; while hypercalcemia and hypercalciuria may result when therapeutic replacement amounts are given for prolonged periods, they are most likely to occur in hypoparathyroid patients receiving high doses of vitamin D; avoid concurrent aluminum containing antacids with renal insufficiency and calcium citrate administration.

Adverse Reactions

Mild hypercalcemia (calcium: >10.5 mg/dL) may be asymptomatic or manifest itself as constipation, anorexia, nausea, and vomiting

More severe hypercalcemia (calcium: >12 mg/dL) is associated with confusion, delirium, stupor, and coma

<1%:

Central nervous system: Headache

Endocrine & metabolic: Hypophosphatemia, hypercalcemia

Gastrointestinal: Nausea, anorexia, vomiting, abdominal pain, constipation

Miscellaneous: Thirst

Overdosage/Toxicology Acute single ingestions of calcium salts may produce mild gastrointestinal distress, but hypercalcemia or other toxic manifestations are extremely unlikely; treatment is supportive

Drug Interactions

Decreased effect:

May significantly decrease the bioavailability of tetracyclines

Large intakes of dietary fiber may decrease calcium absorption due to a decreased GI transit time and the formation of fiber-calcium complexes

Mechanism of Action Combines with dietary phosphate to form insoluble calcium phosphate which is excreted in feces

Pharmacodynamics/Kinetics

Absorption: From the GI tract requires vitamin D; minimal absorption unless chronic, high doses are given; calcium is absorbed in soluble, ionized form; solubility of calcium is increased in an acid environment

Distribution: Crosses the placenta; appears in breast milk

Elimination: Mainly in feces as unabsorbed calcium with 20% eliminated by the kidneys

Usual Dosage Adults: Oral: 2 tablets with each meal; dosage may be increased to bring serum phosphate value to <6 mg/dL; most patients require 3-4 tablets with each meal

Reference Range

Serum calcium: 8.4-10.2 mg/dL: Monitor plasma calcium levels if using calcium salts as electrolyte supplements for deficiency

Due to a poor correlation between the serum ionized calcium (free) and total serum calcium, particularly in states of low albumin or acid/base imbalances, direct measurement of ionized calcium is recommended

In low albumin states, the corrected **total** serum calcium may be estimated by: Corrected total calcium = total serum calcium + 0.8 (4.0 - measured serum albumin)

Test Interactions ↑ calcium (S); ↓ magnesium

Patient Information Can take with food; do not take calcium supplements within 1-2 hours of taking other medicine by mouth or eating large amounts of fiber-rich foods; do not use nonprescription antacids or drink large amounts of alcohol, caffeine-containing beverages, or use tobacco

Additional Information 12.7 mEq/g; 250 mg/g elemental calcium (25% elemental calcium); see table.

Elemental Calcium Content of Calcium Salts

Calcium Salt	% Calcium	mEq Ca^{++}/g
Calcium acetate	25	12.6
Calcium carbonate	40	20
Calcium chloride	27.2	13.6
Calcium gluconate	9	4.5

Dosage Forms Elemental calcium listed in brackets

Capsule (Phos-Ex® 125): 500 mg [125 mg]

Tablet:

Phos-Ex® 62.5: 250 mg [62.5 mg]
Phos-Ex® 167: 668 mg [167 mg]
Phos-Ex® 250: 1000 mg [250 mg]
PhosLo®: 667 mg [169 mg]

Calcium Carbonate (KAL see um KAR bun ate)

Brand Names Alka-Mints® [OTC]; Amitone® [OTC]; Biocal® [OTC]; Calci-Chew™; Calcilac® [OTC]; Calci-Mix™; Cal Plus® [OTC]; CalSup® [OTC]; Caltrate® [OTC]; Chooz® [OTC]; Dicarbosil® [OTC]; Glycate® [OTC]; Os-Cal® 250 [OTC]; Os-Cal® 500 [OTC]; Rolaids® Calcium Rich [OTC]; Suplical® [OTC]; Titralac® [OTC]; Tums® [OTC]

Canadian/Mexican Brand Names Apo-Cal® (Canada); Calcite-500® (Canada); Calsan® (Canada); Pharmacal® (Canada)

Therapeutic Category Antacid; Antidote, Hyperphosphatemia; Calcium Salt; Electrolyte Supplement, Oral

Use As an antacid, and treatment and prevention of calcium deficiency or hyperphosphatemia (eg, osteoporosis, osteomalacia, mild/moderate renal insufficiency, hypoparathyroidism, postmenopausal osteoporosis, rickets)

Pregnancy Risk Factor C

Pregnancy/Breast-Feeding Implications

Clinical effects on the fetus: No data available; available evidence suggests safe use during pregnancy and breast-feeding

Breast-feeding/lactation: No data available

Contraindications Hypercalcemia, renal calculi, hypophosphatemia

Warnings/Precautions Calcium carbonate absorption is impaired in achlorhydria (common in elderly - use alternate salt, administer with food); administration is followed by increased gastric acid secretion within 2 hours of administration; while hypercalcemia and hypercalciuria may result when therapeutic replacement amounts are given for prolonged periods, they are most likely to occur in hypoparathyroid patients receiving high doses of vitamin D; avoid concurrent aluminum containing antacids with renal insufficiency and calcium citrate admin istration.

Adverse Reactions

1% to 10%: Gastrointestinal: Constipation, flatulence

(Continued)

Calcium Carbonate *(Continued)*

<1%:

Central nervous system: Mood and mental changes, lethargy

Gastrointestinal: Laxative effect, acid rebound, nausea, vomiting, fecal impaction, anorexia, abdominal pain, xerostomia

Genitourinary: Polyuria

Renal: Renal calculi, hypercalciuria

Overdosage/Toxicology Acute single ingestions of calcium salts may produce mild gastrointestinal distress, but hypercalcemia or other toxic manifestations are extremely unlikely; treatment is supportive

Drug Interactions

Decreased effect:

May significantly decrease the bioavailability of tetracyclines and ciprofloxacin

Large intakes of dietary fiber may decrease calcium absorption due to a decreased GI transit time and the formation of fiber-calcium complexes

Mechanism of Action As dietary supplements to prevent or treat negative calcium balance (eg, osteoporosis), the calcium in calcium salts moderates nerve and muscle performance and allows normal cardiac function; also used to treat hyperphosphatemia in patients with advanced renal insufficiency by combining with dietary phosphate to form insoluble calcium phosphate, which is excreted in feces; calcium salts as antacids neutralize gastric acidity resulting in increased gastric an duodenal bulb pH; they additionally inhibit proteolytic activity of peptic if the pH is increased >4 and increase lower esophageal sphincter tone.

Pharmacodynamics/Kinetics

Absorption: From the GI tract requires vitamin D; minimal absorption unless chronic, high doses are given; calcium is absorbed in soluble, ionized form; solubility of calcium is increased in an acid environment

Distribution: Crosses the placenta; appears in breast milk

Elimination: Mainly in feces as unabsorbed calcium with 20% eliminated by the kidneys

Usual Dosage Oral (dosage is in terms of elemental calcium):

Recommended daily allowance (RDA):

<6 months: 360 mg/day

6-12 months: 540 mg/day

1-10 years: 800 mg/day

10-18 years: 1200 mg/day

Adults: 800 mg/day

Hypocalcemia (dose depends on clinical condition and serum calcium level):

Children: 45-65 mg/kg/day in 4 divided doses

Adults: 1-2 g or more/day

Adults:

Dietary supplementation: 500 mg to 2 g divided 2-4 times/day

To reduce bone loss with aging/osteoporosis: 1000-1500 mg/day (NIH recommendation)

Antacid: 2 tablets or 10 mL every 2 hours, up to 12 times/day

Reference Range

Serum calcium: 8.4-10.2 mg/dL: Monitor plasma calcium levels if using calcium salts as electrolyte supplements for deficiency

Due to a poor correlation between the serum ionized calcium (free) and total serum calcium, particularly in states of low albumin or acid/base imbalances, direct measurement of ionized calcium is recommended

In low albumin states, the corrected **total** serum calcium may be estimated by:

Corrected total calcium = total serum calcium + 0.8 (4.0 - measured serum albumin)

Test Interactions ↑ calcium (S); ↓ magnesium

Patient Information Shake suspension well; chew tablets thoroughly; take with large quantities of water or juice; do not take calcium supplements within 1-2 hours of taking other medicine by mouth or eating large amounts of fiber-rich foods; do not take other antacids or calcium supplements or drink large amounts of alcohol or caffeine-containing beverages; if the maximum dosage of antacids is required for >2 weeks, see your physician

Additional Information 20 mEq calcium/g; 400 mg calcium/g calcium carbonate (40% elemental calcium)

Dosage Forms Elemental calcium listed in brackets

Capsule: 1500 mg [600 mg]

Calci-Mix™: 1250 mg [500 mg]

Florical®: 364 mg [145.6 mg] with sodium fluoride 8.3 mg

Liquid (Tums® Extra Strength): 1000 mg/5 mL (360 mL)

Lozenge (Mylanta® Soothing Antacids): 600 mg [240 mg]

Powder (Cal Carb-HD®): 6.5 g/packet [2.6 g]

Suspension, oral: 1250 mg/5 mL [500 mg]

Tablet: 650 mg [260 mg], 1500 mg [600 mg]
Calciday-667®: 667 mg [267 mg]
Cal-Plus®, Caltrate® 600, Gencalc® 600, Nephro-Calci®: 1500 mg [600 mg]
Os-Cal® 500, Oyst-Cal® 500, Oystercal® 500: 1250 mg [500 mg]
Chewable:
Alka-Mints®: 850 mg [340 mg]
Amitone®: 350 mg [140 mg]
Caltrate, Jr.®: 750 mg [300 mg]
Calci-Chew™, Os-Cal®: 750 mg [300 mg]
Chooz®, Dicarbosil®, Equilet®, Tums®: 500 mg [200 mg]
Mallamint®: 420 mg [168 mg]
Rolaids® Calcium Rich: 550 mg [220 mg]
Tums® E-X Extra Strength: 750 mg [300 mg]
Tums® Ultra®: 1000 mg [400 mg]
Florical®: 364 mg [145.6 mg]with sodium fluoride 8.3 mg

Calcium Channel Blockers Comparative Actions *see page 1401*
Calcium Channel Blockers Comparative Pharmacokinetics *see page 1402*
Calcium Channel Blockers FDA-Approved Indications *see page 1403*

Calcium Chloride (KAL see um KLOR ide)

Related Information
Extravasation Treatment of Other Drugs *on page 1381*

Therapeutic Category Calcium Salt; Electrolyte Supplement, Parenteral

Use Cardiac resuscitation when epinephrine fails to improve myocardial contractions, cardiac disturbances of hyperkalemia, hypocalcemia, or calcium channel blocking agent toxicity; emergent treatment of hypocalcemic tetany, treatment of hypermagnesemia

Pregnancy Risk Factor C

Contraindications In ventricular fibrillation during cardiac resuscitation, hypercalcemia, and in patients with risk of digitalis toxicity, renal or cardiac disease

Warnings/Precautions Avoid too rapid I.V. administration (<1 mL/minute) and extravasation; use with caution in digitalized patients, respiratory failure, or acidosis; hypercalcemia may occur in patients with renal failure, and frequent determination of serum calcium is necessary; avoid metabolic acidosis (ie, administer only 2-3 days then change to another calcium salt)

Adverse Reactions
<1%:
Cardiovascular: Vasodilation, hypotension, bradycardia, cardiac arrhythmias, ventricular fibrillation, syncope
Central nervous system: Lethargy, coma, mania
Dermatologic: Erythema
Endocrine & metabolic: Decreased serum magnesium, hypercalcemia
Gastrointestinal: Elevated serum amylase
Local: Tissue necrosis
Neuromuscular & skeletal: Muscle weakness
Renal: Hypercalciuria

Overdosage/Toxicology Symptoms of overdose include lethargy, nausea, vomiting, coma

Following withdrawal of the drug, treatment consists of bed rest, liberal intake of fluids, reduced calcium intake, and cathartic administration. Severe hypercalcemia requires I.V. hydration and forced diuresis. Urine output should be monitored and maintained at >3 mL/kg/hour. I.V. saline can quickly and significantly increase excretion of calcium into urine.

Drug Interactions
Decreased effect: Calcium may antagonize the effects of calcium channel blockers; concomitant administration with tetracyclines decreases tetracycline bioavailability
Increased toxicity: Administer cautiously to a digitalized patient, may precipitate arrhythmias

Stability
Do not refrigerate solutions; IVPB solutions/I.V. infusion solutions are stable for 24 hours at room temperature
Maximum concentration in parenteral nutrition solutions: 15 mEq/L of calcium and 30 mmol/L of phosphate
Incompatibilities include sodium bicarbonate, carbonates, phosphates, sulfates, and tartrates

Mechanism of Action Moderates nerve and muscle performance via action potential excitation threshold regulation

Pharmacodynamics/Kinetics
Absorption: I.V. calcium salts are absorbed directly into the bloodstream
Distribution: Crosses the placenta; appears in breast milk
(Continued)

Calcium Chloride *(Continued)*

Elimination: Mainly in feces as unabsorbed calcium with 20% eliminated by the kidneys

Usual Dosage Note: Calcium chloride is 3 times as potent as calcium gluconate

Cardiac arrest in the presence of hyperkalemia or hypocalcemia, magnesium toxicity, or calcium antagonist toxicity: I.V.:

Infants and Children: 20 mg/kg; may repeat in 10 minutes if necessary

Adults: 2-4 mg/kg (10% solution), repeated every 10 minutes

Hypocalcemia: I.V.:

Infants and Children: 10-20 mg/kg/dose (infants: <1 mEq; children: 1-7 mEq), repeat every 4-6 hours if needed; doses may be repeated every 1-3 days if needed

Adults: 500 mg to 1 g (7-14 mEq), repeated at 1- to 3-day intervals if necessary

Hypocalcemic tetany: I.V.:

Infants and Children: 10 mg/kg (0.5-0.7 mEq/kg) over 5-10 minutes; may repeat after 6-8 hours or follow with an infusion with a maximum dose of 200 mg/kg/day

Adults: 4.5-16 mEq may be administered until response occurs

Hypocalcemia secondary to citrated blood transfusion: Administer 0.45 mEq **elemental** calcium for each 100 mL citrated blood infused

Reference Range

Serum calcium: 8.4-10.2 mg/dL

Due to a poor correlation between the serum ionized calcium (free) and total serum calcium, particularly in states of low albumin or acid/base imbalances, direct measurement of ionized calcium is recommended

In low albumin states, the corrected **total** serum calcium may be estimated by this equation (assuming a normal albumin of 4 g/dL)

Corrected total calcium = total serum calcium + 0.8 (4.0 - measured serum albumin)

or

Corrected calcium = measured calcium - measured albumin + 4.0

Serum/plasma chloride: 95-108 mEq/L

Test Interactions ↑ calcium (S); ↓ magnesium

Nursing Implications Do not inject calcium chloride I.M. or administer S.C. or use scalp, small hand or foot veins for I.V. administration since severe necrosis and sloughing may occur. Monitor EKG if calcium is infused faster than 2.5 mEq/minute; usual: 0.7-1.5 mEq/minute (0.5-1 mL/minute); **stop the infusion if the patient complains of pain or discomfort.** Warm to body temperature; administer slowly, do not exceed 1 mL/minute (inject into ventricular cavity - not myocardium); **do not infuse calcium chloride in the same I.V. line as phosphate-containing solutions.**

Extravasation treatment:

Hyaluronidase: Add 1 mL NS to 150 unit vial to make 150 units/mL of concentration; mix 0.1 mL of above with 0.9 mL NS in 1 mL syringe to make final concentration = 15 units/mL

Additional Information 14 mEq/g/10 mL; 270 mg elemental calcium/g (27% elemental calcium)

Dosage Forms Elemental calcium listed in brackets

Injection: 10% = 100 mg/mL [27.2 mg/mL] (10 mL)

Calcium Citrate (KAL see um SIT rate)

Brand Names Citracal® [OTC]

Therapeutic Category Calcium Salt

Use As an antacid, and treatment and prevention of calcium deficiency or hyperphosphatemia (eg, osteoporosis, osteomalacia, mild/moderate renal insufficiency, hypoparathyroidism, postmenopausal osteoporosis, rickets)

Pregnancy Risk Factor C

Contraindications Hypercalcemia, renal calculi, ventricular fibrillation

Warnings/Precautions Calcium salt absorption is impaired in achlorhydria (common in elderly - use alternate salt, administer with food); administration is followed by increased gastric acid secretion within 2 hours of administration; while hypercalcemia and hypercalciuria may result when therapeutic replacement amounts are given for prolonged periods, they are most likely to occur in hypoparathyroid patients receiving high doses of vitamin D; avoid concurrent aluminum containing antacids with renal insufficiency and calcium administration.

Adverse Reactions

1% to 10%: Gastrointestinal: Constipation, flatulence

<1%:

Central nervous system: Mood and mental changes, lethargy

Gastrointestinal: Laxative effect, acid rebound, nausea, vomiting, fecal impaction, anorexia, abdominal pain, xerostomia

Genitourinary: Polyuria

Renal: Renal calculi, hypercalciuria

Overdosage/Toxicology Acute single ingestions of calcium salts may produce mild gastrointestinal distress, but hypercalcemia or other toxic manifestations are extremely unlikely; treatment is supportive

Drug Interactions

Decreased effect:

May significantly decrease the bioavailability of tetracyclines and ciprofloxacin

Large intakes of dietary fiber may decrease calcium absorption due to a decreased GI transit time and the formation of fiber-calcium complexes

Mechanism of Action As dietary supplements to prevent or treat negative calcium balance (eg, osteoporosis), the calcium in calcium salts moderates nerve and muscle performance and allows normal cardiac function; also used to treat hyperphosphatemia in patients with advanced renal insufficiency by combining with dietary phosphate to form insoluble calcium phosphate, which is excreted in feces; calcium salts as antacids neutralize gastric acidity resulting in increased gastric an duodenal bulb pH; they additionally inhibit proteolytic activity of peptic if the pH is increased >4 and increase lower esophageal sphincter tone.

Pharmacodynamics/Kinetics

Absorption: From the GI tract requires vitamin D; minimal absorption unless chronic, high doses are given; calcium is absorbed in soluble, ionized form; solubility of calcium is increased in an acid environment

Distribution: Crosses the placenta; appears in breast milk

Elimination: Mainly in feces as unabsorbed calcium with 20% eliminated by the kidneys

Usual Dosage Dosage is in terms of elemental calcium

Recommended daily allowance (RDA):

<6 months: 360 mg/day

6-12 months: 540 mg/day

1-10 years: 800 mg/day

10-18 years: 1200 mg/day

Adults: 1-2 g/day

Reference Range

Serum calcium: 8.4-10.2 mg/dL: Monitor plasma calcium levels if using calcium salts as electrolyte supplements for deficiency

Due to a poor correlation between the serum ionized calcium (free) and total serum calcium, particularly in states of low albumin or acid/base imbalances, direct measurement of ionized calcium is recommended

In low albumin states, the corrected **total** serum calcium may be estimated by:

Corrected total calcium = total serum calcium + 0.8 (4.0 - measured serum albumin)

Test Interactions ↑ calcium (S); ↓ magnesium

Patient Information Chew tablets well, followed by water; do not take calcium supplements within 1-2 hours of taking other medicine by mouth or eating large amounts of fiber-rich foods; do not drink large amounts of alcohol or caffeine-containing beverages or use tobacco

Additional Information 10.6 mEq/g; 211 mg elemental calcium/g (21% elemental calcium)

Dosage Forms Elemental calcium listed in brackets

Tablet: 950 mg [200 mg]

Tablet, effervescent: 2376 mg [500 mg]

Calcium Disodium Edetate *see* Edetate Calcium Disodium *on page 437*

Calcium Disodium Versenate® *see* Edetate Calcium Disodium *on page 437*

Calcium EDTA *see* Edetate Calcium Disodium *on page 437*

Calcium Glubionate (KAL see um gloo BYE oh nate)

Brand Names Neo-Calglucon® [OTC]

Therapeutic Category Calcium Salt

Use Adjunct in treatment and prevention of postmenopausal osteoporosis; treatment and prevention of calcium depletion or hyperphosphatemia (eg, osteoporosis, osteomalacia, mild/moderate renal insufficiency, hypoparathyroidism, rickets)

Pregnancy Risk Factor C

Contraindications Hypercalcemia, renal calculi, ventricular fibrillation

Warnings/Precautions Calcium salt absorption is impaired in achlorhydria (common in elderly - use alternate salt, administer with food); administration is followed by increased gastric acid secretion within 2 hours of administration; while hypercalcemia and hypercalciuria may result when therapeutic replacement amounts are given for prolonged periods, they are most likely to occur in hypoparathyroid patients receiving high doses of vitamin D; avoid concurrent aluminum containing antacids with renal insufficiency and calcium administration

Adverse Reactions

1% to 10%: Gastrointestinal: Constipation, flatulence

(Continued)

Calcium Glubionate *(Continued)*

<1%:

Central nervous system: Mood and mental changes, lethargy

Gastrointestinal: Laxative effect, acid rebound, nausea, vomiting, fecal impaction, anorexia, abdominal pain, xerostomia

Genitourinary: Polyuria

Renal: Renal calculi, hypercalciuria

Overdosage/Toxicology Acute single ingestions of calcium salts may produce mild gastrointestinal distress, but hypercalcemia or other toxic manifestations are extremely unlikely; treatment is supportive

Drug Interactions

Decreased effect:

May significantly decrease the bioavailability of tetracyclines and ciprofloxacin

Large intakes of dietary fiber may decrease calcium absorption due to a decreased GI transit time and the formation of fiber-calcium complexes

Mechanism of Action As dietary supplements, to prevent or treat negative calcium balance (eg, osteoporosis), the calcium in calcium salts moderates nerve and muscle performance and allows normal cardiac function

Pharmacodynamics/Kinetics

Absorption: From the GI tract requires vitamin D; minimal absorption unless chronic, high doses are given; calcium is absorbed in soluble, ionized form; solubility of calcium is increased in an acid environment

Distribution: Crosses the placenta; appears in breast milk

Elimination: Mainly in feces as unabsorbed calcium with 20% eliminated by the kidneys

Usual Dosage Oral:

Recommended daily allowance (RDA) (in terms of elemental calcium):

<6 months: 360 mg/day

6-12 months: 540 mg/day

1-10 years: 800 mg/day

10-18 years: 1200 mg/day

Adults: 800 mg/day

Syrup is a hyperosmolar solution; dosage is in terms of calcium glubionate

Neonatal hypocalcemia: 1200 mg/kg/day in 4-6 divided doses

Maintenance: Infants and Children: 600-2000 mg/kg/day in 4 divided doses up to a maximum of 9 g/day

Adults: 6-18 g/day in divided doses

Reference Range

Serum calcium: 8.4-10.2 mg/dL: Monitor plasma calcium levels if using calcium salts as electrolyte supplements for deficiency

Due to a poor correlation between the serum ionized calcium (free) and total serum calcium, particularly in states of low albumin or acid/base imbalances, direct measurement of ionized calcium is recommended

In low albumin states, the corrected **total** serum calcium may be estimated by: Corrected total calcium = total serum calcium + 0.8 (4.0 - measured serum albumin)

Test Interactions ↑ calcium (S); ↓ magnesium

Patient Information Do not take calcium supplements within 1-2 hours of taking other medicine by mouth or eating large amounts of fiber-rich foods; do not take other calcium-containing products or antacids, drink large amounts of alcohol or caffeine-containing beverages

Additional Information 3.3 mEq/g; 64 mg elemental calcium/g (6% elemental calcium)

Dosage Forms Elemental calcium listed in brackets

Syrup: 1.8 g/5 mL [115 mg/5 mL] (480 mL)

Calcium Gluceptate (KAL see um gloo SEP tate)

Therapeutic Category Calcium Salt; Electrolyte Supplement, Parenteral

Use Treatment of cardiac disturbances of hyperkalemia, hypocalcemia, or calcium channel blocker toxicity; cardiac resuscitation when epinephrine fails to improve myocardial contractions; treatment of hypermagnesemia and hypocalcemia

Pregnancy Risk Factor C

Contraindications In ventricular fibrillation during cardiac resuscitation; patients with risk of digitalis toxicity, renal or cardiac disease; hypercalcemia

Warnings/Precautions Avoid too rapid I.V. administration; avoid extravasation; use with caution in digitalized patients, respiratory failure or acidosis; metabolic acidosis (administer for only 2-3 days then change to another calcium salt)

Adverse Reactions

<1%:

Cardiovascular: Vasodilation, hypotension, bradycardia, cardiac arrhythmias, ventricular fibrillation, syncope

Central nervous system: Lethargy, mania, coma
Dermatologic: Erythema
Endocrine & metabolic: Hypomagnesemia, hypercalcemia
Gastrointestinal: Elevated serum amylase
Local: Tissue necrosis
Neuromuscular & skeletal: Muscle weakness
Renal: Hypercalciuria

Overdosage/Toxicology Symptoms of overdose include lethargy, nausea, vomiting, coma

Following withdrawal of the drug, treatment consists of bed rest, liberal intake of fluids, reduced calcium intake, and cathartic administration. Severe hypercalcemia requires I.V. hydration and forced diuresis with I.V. furosemide (20-40 mg I.V. every 4-6 hours for adults). Urine output should be monitored and maintained at >3 mL/kg/hour. I.V. saline can quickly and significantly increase excretion of calcium into urine. Calcitonin, cholestyramine, prednisone, sodium EDTA, biphosphonates, and mithramycin have all been used successfully to treat the more resistant cases of vitamin D-induced hypercalcemia.

Drug Interactions Administer cautiously to digitalized patients, may precipitate arrhythmias; calcium may antagonize effects of calcium channel blockers

Stability Admixture **incompatibilities** include carbonates, phosphates, sulfates, tartrates

Mechanism of Action Moderates nerve and muscle performance via action potential excitation threshold regulation

Pharmacodynamics/Kinetics

Absorption: I.M. and I.V. calcium salts are absorbed directly into the bloodstream
Distribution: Crosses the placenta; appears in breast milk
Elimination: Mainly in feces as unabsorbed calcium with 20% eliminated by the kidneys

Usual Dosage I.V. (dose expressed in mg of calcium gluceptate):

Cardiac resuscitation in the presence of hypocalcemia, hyperkalemia, magnesium toxicity, or calcium channel blocker toxicity:
- Children: 110 mg/kg/dose
- Adults: 1.1-1.5 g (5-7 mL)

Hypocalcemia:
- Children: 200-500 mg/kg/day divided every 6 hours
- Adults: 500 mg to 1.1 g/dose as needed

After citrated blood administration: Children and Adults: 0.4 mEq/100 mL blood infused

Reference Range

Serum calcium: 8.4-10.2 mg/dL

Due to a poor correlation between the serum ionized calcium (free) and total serum calcium, particularly in states of low albumin or acid/base imbalances, direct measurement of ionized calcium is recommended

In low albumin states, the corrected **total** serum calcium may be estimated by this equation (assuming a normal albumin of 4 g/dL)

Corrected total calcium = total serum calcium + 0.8 (4.0 - measured serum albumin)

or

Corrected calcium = measured calcium - measured albumin + 4.0

Test Interactions ↑ calcium (S); ↓ magnesium

Nursing Implications Warm to body temperature; administer slowly, do not exceed 1 mL/minute (inject into ventricular cavity - not myocardium)

Additional Information 4.1 mEq/g; 82 mg elemental calcium/g (8% elemental calcium)

Dosage Forms Elemental calcium listed in brackets

Injection: 220 mg/mL [18 mg/mL] (5 mL, 50 mL)

Calcium Gluconate (KAL see um GLOO koe nate)

Brand Names Kalcinate®

Therapeutic Category Calcium Salt; Electrolyte Supplement, Oral; Electrolyte Supplement, Parenteral

Use Treatment and prevention of hypocalcemia; treatment of tetany, cardiac disturbances of hyperkalemia, cardiac resuscitation when epinephrine fails to improve myocardial contractions, hypocalcemia, or calcium channel blocker toxicity; calcium supplementation

Pregnancy Risk Factor C

Contraindications In ventricular fibrillation during cardiac resuscitation; patients with risk of digitalis toxicity, renal or cardiac disease, hypercalcemia, renal calculi, hypophosphatemia

Warnings/Precautions Avoid too rapid I.V. administration (1.5-3.3 mL/minute); use with caution in digitalized patients, severe hyperphosphatemia, respiratory (Continued)

Calcium Gluconate *(Continued)*

failure or acidosis; avoid extravasation; may produce cardiac arrest; hypercalcemia may occur in patients with renal failure and frequent determination of serum calcium is necessary; avoid injection into myocardium; the serum calcium level should be monitored twice weekly during the early dose adjustment period; no more than 300-350 mg of elemental calcium should be given at a time

Adverse Reactions

<1%:

Cardiovascular: Vasodilation, hypotension, bradycardia, cardiac arrhythmias, ventricular fibrillation, syncope

Central nervous system: Lethargy, mania, coma

Dermatologic: Erythema

Endocrine & metabolic: Decrease serum magnesium, hypercalcemia

Gastrointestinal: Elevated serum amylase

Local: Tissue necrosis

Neuromuscular & skeletal: Muscle weakness

Renal: Hypercalciuria

Overdosage/Toxicology Acute single oral ingestions of calcium salts may produce mild gastrointestinal distress, but hypercalcemia or other toxic manifestations are extremely unlikely

Treatment is supportive. Severe hypercalcemia following parenteral overdose requires I.V. hydration. Urine output should be monitored and maintained at >3 mL/kg/hour. I.V. saline can quickly and significantly increase excretion of calcium into urine.

Drug Interactions

Decreased effect: Calcium may antagonize the effects of verapamil; concomitant oral administration renders tetracycline antibiotics and ciprofloxacin inactive; large intakes of dietary fiber may decrease calcium absorption due to a decreased GI transit time and the formation of fiber-calcium complexes

Increased toxicity: Administer I.V. form cautiously to a digitalized patient, may precipitate arrhythmias

Stability

Do not refrigerate solutions; IVPB solutions/I.V. infusion solutions are stable for 24 hours at room temperature

Standard diluent: 1 g/100 mL D_5W or NS; 2 g/100 mL D_5W or NS

Maximum concentration in parenteral nutrition solutions is 15 mEq/L of calcium and 30 mmol/L of phosphate

Incompatibilities include sodium bicarbonate, carbonates, phosphates, sulfates, and tartrates

Mechanism of Action When used to prevent or treat negative calcium balance (eg, osteoporosis), the calcium in calcium salts moderates nerve and muscle performance and allows normal cardiac function

Pharmacodynamics/Kinetics

Absorption: From the GI tract requires vitamin D; minimal absorption unless chronic, high doses are given; calcium is absorbed in soluble, ionized form; solubility of calcium is increased in an acid environment

Distribution: Crosses the placenta; appears in breast milk

Elimination: Mainly in feces as unabsorbed calcium with 20% eliminated by the kidneys

Usual Dosage Dosage is in terms of **elemental** calcium

Recommended daily allowance (RDA):

<6 months: 400 mg/day
6-12 months: 600 mg/day
1-10 years: 800 mg/day
10-18 years: 1200 mg/day
Adults: 800 mg/day

Calcium gluconate electrolyte requirement in newborn period:

Premature: 200-1000 mg/kg/24 hours

Term:

0-24 hours: 0-500 mg/kg/24 hours
24-48 hours: 200-500 mg/kg/24 hours
48-72 hours: 200-600 mg/kg/24 hours
>3 days: 200-800 mg/kg/24 hours

Hypocalcemia:

Oral:

Children: 200-500 mg/kg/day divided every 6 hours
Adults: 500 mg to 2 g 2-4 times/day

I.V.:

Infants and Children: 200-500 mg/kg/day (infants <1 mEq/day; children 1-7 mEq/day) as a continuous infusion or in 4 divided doses; doses may be repeated every 1-3 days if necessary

Adults: 2-15 g/24 hours as a continuous infusion or in divided doses, which may be repeated every 1-3 days if necessary

Hypocalcemic tetany: I.V.:

Infants and Children: 100-200 mg/kg/dose (0.5-0.7 mEq/kg/dose) over 5-10 minutes; may repeat every 6-8 hours **or** follow with an infusion of 500 mg/kg/day

Adults: 1-3 g (4.5-16 mEq) may be administered until therapeutic response occurs

Osteoporosis/bone loss: Oral: 1000-1500 mg in divided doses/day

Calcium antagonist toxicity, magnesium intoxication, or cardiac arrest in the presence of hyperkalemia or hypocalcemia: I.V.:

Infants and Children: Calcium chloride is recommended calcium salt; refer to calcium chloride monograph

Adults: 5-8 mL/dose and repeated as necessary at 10-minute intervals, however, calcium chloride is recommended calcium salt; refer to Calcium Chloride monograph

Hypocalcemia secondary to citrated blood infusion: I.V.: Administer 0.45 mEq **elemental** calcium for each 100 mL citrated blood infused

Exchange transfusion: Adults: 300 mg/100 mL of citrated blood exchanged

Maintenance electrolyte requirements for total parenteral nutrition: I.V.: Daily requirements: Adults: 8-16 mEq/1000 kcals/24 hours

Administration I.M. injections should be administered in the gluteal region in adults, usually in volumes <2 mL; avoid I.M. injections in children and adults with muscle mass wasting; do not use scalp veins or small hand or foot veins for I.V. administration; generally, I.V. infusion rates should not exceed 0.7-1.5 mEq/minute (1.5-3.3 mL/minute); **stop the infusion if the patient complains of pain or discomfort**. Warm to body temperature; do not inject into the myocardium when using calcium during advanced cardiac life support.

Reference Range

Serum calcium: 8.4-10.2 mg/dL: Monitor plasma calcium levels if using calcium salts as electrolyte supplements for deficiency

Due to a poor correlation between the serum ionized calcium (free) and total serum calcium, particularly in states of low albumin or acid/base imbalances, direct measurement of ionized calcium is recommended

In low albumin states, the corrected **total** serum calcium may be estimated by: Corrected total calcium = total serum calcium + 0.8 (4.0 - measured serum albumin)

Test Interactions ↑ calcium (S); ↓ magnesium

Patient Information Do not take calcium supplements within 1-2 hours of taking other medicine by mouth or eating large amounts of fiber-rich foods; do not drink large amounts of alcohol or caffeine-containing beverages; take with food

Nursing Implications

Extravasation treatment:

Hyaluronidase: Add 1 mL NS to 150 unit vial to make 150 units/mL of concentration; mix 0.1 mL of above with 0.9 mL NS in 1 mL syringe to make final concentration = 15 units/mL

Do not infuse calcium gluconate solutions in the same I.V. line as phosphate-containing solutions (eg, TPN)

Additional Information 4.5 mEq/g; 90 mg elemental calcium/g (9% elemental calcium)

Dosage Forms Elemental calcium listed in brackets

Injection: 10% = 100 mg/mL [9 mg/mL] (10 mL, 50 mL, 100 mL, 200 mL)

Tablet: 500 mg [45 mg], 650 mg [58.5 mg], 975 mg [87.75 mg], 1 g [90 mg]

Calcium Lactate (KAL see um LAK tate)

Therapeutic Category Calcium Salt

Use Adjunct in prevention of postmenopausal osteoporosis; treatment and prevention of calcium depletion

Pregnancy Risk Factor C

Contraindications Hypercalcemia, renal calculi, ventricular fibrillation

Warnings/Precautions Calcium salt absorption is impaired in achlorhydria (common in elderly - use alternate salt, administer with food); administration is followed by increased gastric acid secretion within 2 hours of administration; while hypercalcemia and hypercalciuria may result when therapeutic replacement amounts are given for prolonged periods, they are most likely to occur in hypoparathyroid patients receiving high doses of vitamin D; avoid concurrent aluminum containing antacids with renal insufficiency and calcium administration

Adverse Reactions

1% to 10%: Gastrointestinal: Constipation, flatulence

<1%:

Central nervous system: Mood and mental changes, lethargy

(Continued)

Calcium Lactate *(Continued)*

Gastrointestinal: Laxative effect, acid rebound, nausea, vomiting, fecal impaction, anorexia, abdominal pain, xerostomia
Genitourinary: Polyuria
Renal: Renal calculi, hypercalciuria

Overdosage/Toxicology Acute single ingestions of calcium salts may produce mild gastrointestinal distress, but hypercalcemia or other toxic manifestations are extremely unlikely; treatment is supportive

Drug Interactions
Decreased effect:
May significantly decrease the bioavailability of tetracyclines and ciprofloxacin
Large intakes of dietary fiber may decrease calcium absorption due to a decreased GI transit time and the formation of fiber-calcium complexes

Mechanism of Action As dietary supplements, to prevent or treat negative calcium balance (eg, osteoporosis), the calcium in calcium salts moderates nerve and muscle performance and allows normal cardiac function

Pharmacodynamics/Kinetics
Absorption: From the GI tract requires vitamin D; minimal absorption unless chronic, high doses are given; calcium is absorbed in soluble, ionized form; solubility of calcium is increased in an acid environment
Distribution: Crosses the placenta; appears in breast milk
Elimination: Mainly in feces as unabsorbed calcium with 20% eliminated by the kidneys

Usual Dosage Oral (in terms of calcium lactate)
Recommended daily allowance (RDA) (in terms of elemental calcium):
<6 months: 360 mg/day
6-12 months: 540 mg/day
1-10 years: 800 mg/day
10-18 years: 1200 mg/day
Adults: 800 mg/day

Infants: 400-500 mg/kg/day divided every 4-6 hours
Children: 500 mg/kg/day divided every 6-8 hours
Maximum daily dose: 9 g
Adults: 1.5-3 g divided every 8 hours

Reference Range
Serum calcium: 8.4-10.2 mg/dL: Monitor plasma calcium levels if using calcium salts as electrolyte supplements for deficiency
Due to a poor correlation between the serum ionized calcium (free) and total serum calcium, particularly in states of low albumin or acid/base imbalances, direct measurement of ionized calcium is recommended
In low albumin states, the corrected **total** serum calcium may be estimated by:
Corrected total calcium = total serum calcium + 0.8 (4.0 - measured serum albumin)

Test Interactions ↑ calcium (S); ↓ magnesium

Patient Information Do not take calcium supplements within 1-2 hours of taking other medicine by mouth or eating large amounts of fiber-rich foods; do not drink large amounts of alcohol or caffeine-containing beverages

Additional Information 6.5 mEq/g; 130 mg elemental calcium/g (13% elemental calcium)

Dosage Forms Elemental calcium listed in brackets
Tablet: 325 mg [42.25 mg], 650 mg [84.5 mg]

Calcium Leucovorin *see* Leucovorin *on page 708*

Calcium Phosphate, Tribasic (KAL see um FOS fate tri BAY sik)

Brand Names Posture® [OTC]

Synonyms Tricalcium Phosphate

Therapeutic Category Calcium Salt

Use Adjunct in prevention of postmenopausal osteoporosis; treatment and prevention of calcium depletion

Pregnancy Risk Factor C

Contraindications Hypercalcemia, renal calculi, ventricular fibrillation

Warnings/Precautions Calcium salt absorption is impaired in achlorhydria (common in elderly - use alternate salt, administer with food); administration is followed by increased gastric acid secretion within 2 hours of administration; while hypercalcemia and hypercalciuria may result when therapeutic replacement amounts are given for prolonged periods, they are most likely to occur in hypoparathyroid patients receiving high doses of vitamin D; avoid concurrent aluminum containing antacids with renal insufficiency and calcium administration

Adverse Reactions
1% to 10%: Gastrointestinal: Constipation, flatulence

<1%:
- Central nervous system: Mood and mental changes, lethargy
- Gastrointestinal: Laxative effect, acid rebound, nausea, vomiting, fecal impaction, anorexia, abdominal pain, xerostomia
- Genitourinary: Polyuria
- Renal: Renal calculi, hypercalciuria

Overdosage/Toxicology Acute single ingestions of calcium salts may produce mild gastrointestinal distress, but hypercalcemia or other toxic manifestations are extremely unlikely; treatment is supportive

Drug Interactions

Decreased effect:
- May significantly decrease the bioavailability of tetracyclines and ciprofloxacin
- Large intakes of dietary fiber may decrease calcium absorption due to a decreased GI transit time and the formation of fiber-calcium complexes

Mechanism of Action As dietary supplements, to prevent or treat negative calcium balance (eg, osteoporosis), the calcium in calcium salts moderates nerve and muscle performance and allows normal cardiac function

Usual Dosage Oral (all doses in terms of elemental calcium):

Recommended daily allowance (RDA) (elemental calcium):
- <6 months: 360 mg/day
- 6-12 months: 540 mg/day
- 1-10 years: 800 mg/day
- 10-18 years: 1200 mg/day
- Adults: 800 mg/day

Children: 45-65 mg/kg/day

Adults: 1-2 g/day

Reference Range

Serum calcium: 8.4-10.2 mg/dL: Monitor plasma calcium levels if using calcium salts as electrolyte supplements for deficiency

Due to a poor correlation between the serum ionized calcium (free) and total serum calcium, particularly in states of low albumin or acid/base imbalances, direct measurement of ionized calcium is recommended

In low albumin states, the corrected **total** serum calcium may be estimated by: Corrected total calcium = total serum calcium + 0.8 (4.0 - measured serum albumin)

Test Interactions ↑ calcium (S); ↓ magnesium

Patient Information Do not take calcium supplements within 1-2 hours of taking other medicine by mouth or eating large amounts of fiber-rich foods; do not drink large amounts of alcohol or caffeine-containing beverages

Additional Information 19.3 mEq/g; 390 mg elemental calcium/g (39% elemental calcium)

Dosage Forms Elemental calcium listed in brackets

Tablet, sugar free: 1565.2 mg [600 mg]

Calcium Polycarbophil (KAL see um pol i KAR boe fil)

Brand Names Equalactin® Chewable Tablet [OTC]; Fiberall® Chewable Tablet [OTC]; FiberCon® Tablet [OTC]; Fiber-Lax® Tablet [OTC]; Mitrolan® Chewable Tablet [OTC]

Therapeutic Category Antidiarrheal; Laxative, Bulk-Producing

Use Treatment of constipation or diarrhea by restoring a more normal moisture level and providing bulk in the patient's intestinal tract; calcium polycarbophil is supplied as the approved substitute whenever a bulk-forming laxative is ordered in a tablet, capsule, wafer, or other oral solid dosage form

Pregnancy Risk Factor C

Adverse Reactions 1% to 10%: Gastrointestinal: Abdominal fullness

Drug Interactions Decreased absorption of oral anticoagulants, digoxin, potassium-sparing diuretics, salicylates, tetracycline, and ciprofloxacin

Usual Dosage Oral:

Children:
- 2-6 years: 500 mg (1 tablet) 1-2 times/day, up to 1.5 g/day
- 6-12 years: 500 mg (1 tablet) 1-3 times/day, up to 3 g/day

Adults: 1 g 4 times/day, up to 6 g/day

Test Interactions ↓ potassium (S)

Patient Information When used as an antacid or for constipation, drink 8 oz of water or other liquid with each dose; diarrhea dose may be repeated every 30 minutes until total dose in achieved

Dosage Forms Tablet:

Sodium free:
- Fiber-Lax®: 625 mg
- FiberCon®: 500 mg

Chewable:
- Equalactin®, Mitrolan®: 500 mg

(Continued)

Calcium Polycarbophil *(Continued)*

Fiberall®: 1250 mg

Caldecort® [OTC] *see* Hydrocortisone *on page 623*

Caldecort® Anti-Itch Spray [OTC] *see* Hydrocortisone *on page 623*

Calderol® *see* Calcifediol *on page 180*

Calm-X® Oral [OTC] *see* Dimenhydrinate *on page 395*

Cal Plus® [OTC] *see* Calcium Carbonate *on page 185*

CalSup® [OTC] *see* Calcium Carbonate *on page 185*

Caltrate® [OTC] *see* Calcium Carbonate *on page 185*

Camphorated Tincture of Opium *see* Paregoric *on page 952*

Camptosar® *see* Irinotecan *on page 673*

Camptothecin-11 *see* Irinotecan *on page 673*

Cancer Chemotherapy Regimens *see page 1351*

Capastat® Sulfate *see* Capreomycin *on this page*

Capital® and Codeine *see* Acetaminophen and Codeine *on page 21*

Capoten® *see* Captopril *on next page*

Capreomycin (kap ree oh MYE sin)

Related Information

Antimicrobial Drugs of Choice *on page 1468*

Brand Names Capastat® Sulfate

Synonyms Capreomycin Sulfate

Therapeutic Category Antibiotic, Miscellaneous; Antitubercular Agent

Use Treatment of tuberculosis in conjunction with at least one other antituberculosis agent

Pregnancy Risk Factor C

Contraindications Known hypersensitivity to capreomycin sulfate

Warnings/Precautions The use of capreomycin in patients with renal insufficiency, pre-existing auditory impairment, and other oto- and nephrotoxic drug (especially other parenteral antituberculous agents) must be undertaken with great caution, and the risk of additional eighth nerve impairment or renal injury should be weighed against the benefits to be derived from therapy

Adverse Reactions

>10%:
- Otic: Ototoxicity
- Renal: Nephrotoxicity

1% to 10%: Hematologic: Eosinophilia

<1%:
- Central nervous system: Vertigo, fever, rash
- Hematologic: Leukocytosis, thrombocytopenia
- Local: Pain, induration, and bleeding at injection site
- Otic: Tinnitus

Overdosage/Toxicology Symptoms of overdose include renal failure, ototoxicity, thrombocytopenia; treatment is supportive

Drug Interactions

Increased effect/duration of nondepolarizing neuromuscular blocking agents

Additive toxicity (nephro- and ototoxicity, respiratory paralysis): Aminoglycosides (eg, streptomycin)

Mechanism of Action Capreomycin is a cyclic polypeptide antimicrobial. It is administered as a mixture of capreomycin IA and capreomycin IB. The mechanism of action of capreomycin is not well understood. Mycobacterial species that have become resistant to other agents are usually still sensitive to the action of capreomycin. However, significant cross-resistance with viomycin, kanamycin, and neomycin occurs.

Pharmacodynamics/Kinetics

Absorption: Oral: Poor absorption necessitates parenteral administration

Half-life: Dependent upon renal function and varies with creatinine clearance; 4-6 hours

Time to peak serum concentration: I.M.: Within 1 hour

Elimination: Essentially excreted unchanged in the urine; no significant accumulation after ≥30 day of 1 g/day dosing in patients with normal renal function

Usual Dosage I.M.:

Infants and Children: 15-20 mg/kg/day, up to 1 g/day maximum

Adults: 15-30 mg/kg/day up to 1 g/day for 60-120 days, followed by 1 g 2-3 times/week

Dosing interval in renal impairment: Cl_{cr} <10 mL/minute: Decrease dose to ~33% of usual and administer every 48 hours; consult manufacturer's guidelines for specific dosing recommendations

Test Interactions ↓ potassium (S), ↑ BUN, leukocytosis ↓ platelets

Patient Information Report any hearing loss to physician immediately; do not discontinue without notifying physician

Nursing Implications The solution for injection may acquire a pale straw color and darken with time; this is not associated with a loss of potency or development of toxicity

Dosage Forms Injection, as sulfate: 100 mg/mL (10 mL)

Capreomycin Sulfate *see* Capreomycin *on previous page*

Capsaicin (kap SAY sin)

Brand Names Capsin® [OTC]; Capzasin-P® [OTC]; Dolorac® [OTC]; No Pain-HP® [OTC]; R-Gel® [OTC]; Zostrix® [OTC]; Zostrix-® HP [OTC]

Therapeutic Category Analgesic, Topical; Topical Skin Product

Use FDA approved for the topical treatment of pain associated with postherpetic neuralgia, rheumatoid arthritis, osteoarthritis, diabetic neuropathy, and postsurgical pain.

Unlabeled uses: Treatment of pain associated with psoriasis, chronic neuralgias unresponsive to other forms of therapy, and intractable pruritus

Pregnancy Risk Factor C

Contraindications Hypersensitivity to capsaicin or components

Warnings/Precautions Avoid contact with eyes, mucous membrane, or with damaged or irritated skin

Adverse Reactions

>10%: Local: ≥30%: Transient burning on application which usually diminishes with repeated use

1% to 10%:

Dermatologic: Itching, stinging sensation, erythema

Respiratory: Cough

Mechanism of Action Induces release of substance P, the principal chemomediator of pain impulses from the periphery to the CNS, from peripheral sensory neurons; after repeated application, capsaicin depletes the neuron of substance P and prevents reaccumulation

Pharmacodynamics/Kinetics Data following the use of topical capsaicin in humans are lacking

Onset of action: Pain relief is usually seen within 14-28 days of regular topical application; maximal response may require 4-6 weeks of continuous therapy

Duration: Several hours

Usual Dosage Children ≥2 years and Adults: Topical: Apply to affected area at least 3-4 times/day; application frequency less than 3-4 times/day prevents the total depletion, inhibition of synthesis, and transport of substance P resulting in decreased clinical efficacy and increased local discomfort

Patient Information For external use only. Avoid washing treated areas for 30 minutes after application; should not be applied to wounds or damaged skin; avoid eye and mucous membrane exposure; discontinue if severe burning or itching occurs; if symptoms persist longer than 14-28 days, contact physician

Dosage Forms

Cream:

Capzasin-P®, Zostrix®: 0.025% (45 g, 90 g)

Dolorac®: 0.25% (28 g)

Zostrix-® HP: 0.075% (30 g, 60 g)

Gel (R-Gel®): 0.025% (15 g, 30 g)

Lotion (Capsin®): 0.025% (59 mL); 0.075% (59 mL)

Roll-on (No Pain-HP®): 0.075% (60 mL)

Capsin® [OTC] *see* Capsaicin *on this page*

Captopril (KAP toe pril)

Related Information

Angiotensin-Converting Enzyme Inhibitors Comparison *on page 1386*

Antacid Drug Interactions *on page 1388*

Heart Failure: Management of Patients With Left-Ventricular Systolic Dysfunction *on page 1533*

Therapy of Hypertension *on page 1540*

Brand Names Capoten®

Canadian/Mexican Brand Names Apo-Capto® (Canada); Novo-Captopril® (Canada); Nu-Capto® (Canada); Syn-Captopril® (Canada); Capotena® (Mexico); Capitral® (Mexico); Cardipril® (Mexico); Cryopril® (Mexico); Ecapresan® (Mexico); Ecaten® (Mexico); Kenolan® (Mexico); Lenpryl® (Mexico); Precaptil® (Mexico)

Synonyms ACE

Therapeutic Category Angiotensin-Converting Enzyme (ACE) Inhibitors; Antihypertensive

Use Management of hypertension and treatment of congestive heart failure; believed to prolong survival in heart failure

(Continued)

Captopril *(Continued)*

Unlabeled use: Hypertensive crisis, diabetic nephropathy, rheumatoid arthritis, diagnosis of anatomic renal artery stenosis, hypertension secondary to scleroderma renal crisis, diagnosis of aldosteronism, idiopathic edema, Bartter's syndrome, postmyocardial infarction for prevention of ventricular failure; increase circulation in Raynaud's phenomenon

Pregnancy Risk Factor C (first trimester); D (second and third trimester)

Pregnancy/Breast-Feeding Implications

Clinical effects on the fetus: No data available on crossing the placenta. Cranial defects, hypocalvaria/acalvaria, oligohydramnios, persistent anuria following delivery, hypotension, renal defects, renal dysgenesis/dysplasia, renal failure, pulmonary hypoplasia, limb contractures secondary to oligohydramnios and still-birth reported. ACE inhibitors should be avoided during pregnancy.

Breast-feeding/lactation: Crosses into breast milk. American Academy of Pediatrics considers COMPATIBLE with breast-feeding.

Contraindications Hypersensitivity to captopril, other ACE inhibitors, or any component

Warnings/Precautions Use with caution and modify dosage in patients with renal impairment (decrease dosage) (especially renal artery stenosis), severe congestive heart failure, or with coadministered diuretic therapy; experience in children is limited. Severe hypotension may occur in patients who are sodium and/or volume depleted, initiate lower doses and monitor closely when starting therapy in these patients; ACE inhibitors may be preferred agents in elderly patients with congestive heart failure and diabetes mellitus (diabetic proteinuria is reduced, minimal CNS effects, and enhanced insulin sensitivity); however due to decreased renal function, tolerance must be carefully monitored.

Adverse Reactions

1% to 10%:

Cardiovascular: Tachycardia, chest pain, palpitations
Central nervous system: Insomnia, headache, dizziness, fatigue, malaise
Dermatologic: Rash, pruritus, alopecia
Gastrointestinal: Abdominal pain, vomiting, nausea, diarrhea, anorexia, constipation, abnormal taste
Neuromuscular & skeletal: Paresthesias
Renal: Oliguria
Respiratory: Transient cough

<1%:

Cardiovascular: Hypotension
Dermatologic: Angioedema
Endocrine & metabolic: Hyperkalemia
Hematologic: Neutropenia, agranulocytosis
Renal: Proteinuria, increased BUN/serum creatinine

Overdosage/Toxicology Mild hypotension has been the only toxic effect seen with acute overdose. Bradycardia may also occur; hyperkalemia occurs even with therapeutic doses, especially in patients with renal insufficiency and those taking NSAIDs.

Following initiation of essential overdose management, toxic symptom treatment and supportive treatment should be initiated. Hypotension usually responds to I.V. fluids or Trendelenburg positioning.

Drug-Drug Interactions With ACEIs

Precipitant Drug	Drug (Category) and Effect	Description
Antacids	ACE Inhibitors: decreased	Decreased bioavailability of ACEIs. May be more likely with captopril. Separate administration times by 1-2 hours.
NSAIDs (indomethacin)	ACEIs: decreased	Reduced hypotensive effects of ACEIs. More prominent in low renin or volume dependent hypertensive patients.
Phenothiazines	ACEIs: increased	Pharmacologic effects of ACEIs may be increased.
ACEIs	Allopurinol: increased	Higher risk of hypersensitivity reaction possible when given concurrently. Three case reports of Stevens-Johnson syndrome with captopril.
ACEIs	Digoxin: increased	Increased plasma digoxin levels.
ACEIs	Lithium: increased	Increased serum lithium levels and symptoms of toxicity may occur.
ACEIs	Potassium preps/ potassium sparing diuretics increased	Coadministration may result in elevated potassium levels.

Drug Interactions

Increased toxicity:

Probenecid increases blood levels of captopril

Captopril and diuretics have additive hypotensive effects; see table.

Stability Unstable in aqueous solutions; to prepare solution for oral administration, mix prior to administration and use within 10 minutes

Mechanism of Action Competitive inhibitor of angiotensin-converting enzyme (ACE); prevents conversion of angiotensin I to angiotensin II, a potent vasoconstrictor; results in lower levels of angiotensin II which causes an increase in plasma renin activity and a reduction in aldosterone secretion

Pharmacodynamics/Kinetics

Onset of effect: Maximal decrease in blood pressure 1-1.5 hours after dose

Duration: Dose related, may require several weeks of therapy before full hypotensive effect is seen

Absorption: Oral: 60% to 75%; food decreases absorption of captopril 30% to 40%

Protein binding: 25% to 30%

Metabolism: 50%

Half-life (dependent upon renal and cardiac function):

Adults, normal: 1.9 hours

Congestive heart failure: 2.06 hours

Anuria: 20-40 hours

Time to peak: Within 1-2 hours

Elimination: 95% excreted in urine in 24 hours

Usual Dosage Note: Dosage must be titrated according to patient's response; use lowest effective dose. Oral:

Infants: Initial: 0.15-0.3 mg/kg/dose; titrate dose upward to maximum of 6 mg/kg/day in 1-4 divided doses; usual required dose: 2.5-6 mg/kg/day

Children: Initial: 0.5 mg/kg/dose; titrate upward to maximum of 6 mg/kg/day in 2-4 divided doses

Older Children: Initial: 6.25-12.5 mg/dose every 12-24 hours; titrate upward to maximum of 6 mg/kg/day

Adolescents: Initial: 12.5-25 mg/dose given every 8-12 hours; increase by 25 mg/dose to maximum of 450 mg/day

Adults:

Hypertension:

Initial dose: 12.5-25 mg 2-3 times/day; may increase by 12.5-25 mg/dose at 1- to 2-week intervals up to 50 mg 3 times/day; add diuretic before further dosage increases

Maximum dose: 150 mg 3 times/day

Congestive heart failure:

Initial dose: 6.25-12.5 mg 3 times/day in conjunction with cardiac glycoside and diuretic therapy; initial dose depends upon patient's fluid/electrolyte status

Target dose: 50 mg 3 times/day

Maximum dose: 100 mg 3 times/day

Dosing adjustment in renal impairment:

Cl_{cr} 10-50 mL/minute: Administer at 75% of normal dose

Cl_{cr} <10 mL/minute: Administer at 50% of normal dose

Note: Smaller dosages given every 8-12 hours are indicated in patients with renal dysfunction; renal function and leukocyte count should be carefully monitored during therapy

Hemodialysis: Moderately dialyzable (20% to 50%); administer dose postdialysis or administer 25% to 35% supplemental dose

Peritoneal dialysis: Supplemental dose is not necessary

Monitoring Parameters BUN, serum creatinine, urine dipstick for protein, complete leukocyte count, and blood pressure

Test Interactions ↑ BUN, creatinine, potassium, positive Coombs' [direct]; ↓ cholesterol (S); may cause false-positive results in urine acetone determinations using sodium nitroprusside reagent

Patient Information Take 1 hour before meals; do not stop therapy except under prescriber advice; notify physician if you develop sore throat, fever, swelling, rash, difficult breathing, irregular heartbeats, chest pains, or cough. May cause dizziness, fainting, and lightheadedness, especially in first week of therapy; sit and stand up slowly; do not add a salt substitute (potassium) without advice of physician.

Nursing Implications Watch for hypotensive effect within 1-3 hours of first dose or new higher dose

Additional Information A dosage ratio of 5:1 (captopril:lisinopril) was established and a regimen of 3 times/day vs 1 time/day (captopril vs lisinopril) was tolerated without an increased in adverse drug reactions

Dosage Forms Tablet: 12.5 mg, 25 mg, 50 mg, 100 mg

(Continued)

Captopril *(Continued)*

Extemporaneous Preparations Captopril has limited stability in aqueous preparations. The addition of an antioxidant (sodium ascorbate) has been shown to increase the stability of captopril in solution; captopril (1 mg/mL) in syrup with methylcellulose is stable for 7 days stored either at 4°C or 22°C; captopril (1 mg/mL) in distilled water (no additives) is stable for 14 days if stored at 4°C and 7 days if stored at 22°C; captopril (1 mg/mL) with sodium ascorbate (5 mg/mL) in distilled water is stable for 56 days at 4°C and 14 days at 22°C. Powder papers can also be made; powder papers are stable for 12 weeks when stored at room temperature.

Nahata MC, Morosco RS, and Hipple TF, "Stability of Captopril in Three Liquid Dosage Rorms", *Am J Hosp Pharm*, 1994, 51(1):95-96.

Taketomo CK, Chu SA, Cheng MH, et al, "Stability of Captopril in Powder Papers Under Three Storage Conditions", *Am J Hosp Pharm*, 1990;47(8):1799-1801.

Capzasin-P® [OTC] *see* Capsaicin *on page 197*

Carafate® *see* Sucralfate *on page 1168*

Carbachol (KAR ba kole)

Related Information

Glaucoma Drug Therapy Comparison *on page 1410*

Brand Names Carbastat® Ophthalmic; Carboptic® Ophthalmic; Isopto® Carbachol Ophthalmic; Miostat® Intraocular

Synonyms Carbacholine; Carbamylcholine Chloride

Therapeutic Category Cholinergic Agent, Ophthalmic; Ophthalmic Agent, Miotic

Use Lowers intraocular pressure in the treatment of glaucoma; cause miosis during surgery

Pregnancy Risk Factor C

Contraindications Acute iritis, acute inflammatory disease of the anterior chamber, hypersensitivity to carbachol or any component

Warnings/Precautions Use with caution in patients undergoing general anesthesia and in presence of corneal abrasion

Adverse Reactions

1% to 10%: Ocular: Blurred vision, eye pain

<1%:

Cardiovascular: Transient fall in blood pressure

Central nervous system: Headache

Gastrointestinal: Stomach cramps, diarrhea

Local: Ciliary spasm with temporary decrease of visual acuity

Ocular: Corneal clouding, persistent bullous keratopathy, postoperative keratitis, retinal detachment, transient ciliary and conjunctival injection

Respiratory: Asthma

Miscellaneous: Increased peristalsis

Overdosage/Toxicology Symptoms of overdose include miosis, flushing, vomiting, bradycardia, bronchospasm, involuntary urination

Atropine is the treatment of choice for intoxications manifesting with significant muscarinic symptoms. Atropine I.V. 2-4 mg every 3-60 minutes (or 0.04-0.08 mg I.V. every 5-60 minutes if needed for children) should be repeated to control symptoms and then continued as needed for 1-2 days following the acute ingestion. Epinephrine 0.1-1 mg S.C. may be useful in reversing severe cardiovascular or pulmonary sequel.

Stability

Intraocular: Store at room temperature of 15°C to 30°C/59°F to 86°F

Topical: Store at 8°C to 27°C/46°F to 80°F

Mechanism of Action Synthetic direct-acting cholinergic agent that causes miosis by stimulating muscarinic receptors in the eye

Pharmacodynamics/Kinetics

Ophthalmic instillation:

Onset of miosis: 10-20 minutes

Duration of reduction in intraocular pressure: 4-8 hours

Intraocular administration:

Onset of miosis: Within 2-5 minutes

Duration: 24 hours

Usual Dosage Adults:

Ophthalmic: Instill 1-2 drops up to 3 times/day

Intraocular: 0.5 mL instilled into anterior chamber before or after securing sutures

Patient Information May sting on instillation; may cause headache, altered distance vision, and decreased night vision

Nursing Implications Finger pressure should be applied on the lacrimal sac for 1-2 minutes following topical instillation; remove excess around the eye with a tissue. Instillation for miosis prior to eye surgery should be gentle and parallel to the iris face and tangential to the pupil border; discard unused portion.

Dosage Forms Solution:

Intraocular (Carbastat®, Miostat®): 0.01% (1.5 mL)

Topical, ophthalmic:

- Carboptic®: 3% (15 mL)
- Isopto® Carbachol: 0.75% (15 mL, 30 mL); 1.5% (15 mL, 30 mL); 2.25% (15 mL); 3% (15 mL, 30 mL)

Carbacholine *see* Carbachol *on previous page*

Carbamazepine (kar ba MAZ e peen)

Related Information

Anticonvulsants by Seizure Type *on page 1392*

Epilepsy Treatment *on page 1531*

Brand Names Epitol®; Tegretol®; Tegretol-XR®

Canadian/Mexican Brand Names Apo-Carbamazepine® (Canada); Mazepine® (Canada); Novo-Carbamaz® (Canada); Nu-Carbamazepine® (Canada); PMS-Carbamazepine (Canada); Carbazep® (Mexico); Carbazina® (Mexico); Neugeron® (Mexico)

Therapeutic Category Anticonvulsant

Use Prophylaxis of generalized tonic-clonic, partial (especially complex partial), and mixed partial or generalized seizure disorder; pain relief of trigeminal neuralgia

Unlabeled use: Treat bipolar disorders and other affective disorders; resistant schizophrenia, alcohol withdrawal, restless leg syndrome, and psychotic behavior associated with dementia

Pregnancy Risk Factor C

Pregnancy/Breast-Feeding Implications

Clinical effects on the fetus: Crosses the placenta. Dysmorphic facial features, cranial defects, cardiac defects, spina bifida, IUGR, and multiple other malformations reported. Epilepsy itself, number of medications, genetic factors, or a combination of these probably influence the teratogenicity of anticonvulsant therapy. Benefit:risk ratio usually favors continued use during pregnancy and breast-feeding.

Breast-feeding/lactation: Crosses into breast milk. American Academy of Pediatrics considers COMPATIBLE with breast-feeding.

Contraindications Hypersensitivity to carbamazepine or any component; **may have cross-sensitivity with tricyclic antidepressants**; should not be used in any patient with bone marrow suppression, MAO inhibitor use

Warnings/Precautions MAO inhibitors should be discontinued for a minimum of 14 days before carbamazepine is begun; administer with caution to patients with history of cardiac damage or hepatic disease; potentially fatal blood cell abnormalities have been reported following treatment; early detection of hematologic change is important; advise patients of early signs and symptoms including fever, sore throat, mouth ulcers, infections, easy bruising, petechial or purpuric hemorrhage; carbamazepine is not effective in absence, myoclonic or akinetic seizures; exacerbation of certain seizure types have been seen after initiation of carbamazepine therapy in children with mixed seizure disorders. Elderly may have increased risk of SIADH-like syndrome.

Adverse Reactions

Dermatologic: Rash; but does not necessarily mean the drug should not be stopped

>10%:

- Central nervous system: Sedation, dizziness, fatigue, slurred speech, ataxia, confusion
- Gastrointestinal: Nausea, vomiting
- Ocular: Blurred vision, nystagmus

1% to 10%:

- Dermatologic: Stevens-Johnson syndrome, toxic epidermal necrolysis
- Endocrine & metabolic: Hyponatremia, SIADH
- Gastrointestinal: Diarrhea
- Miscellaneous: Diaphoresis

<1%:

- Cardiovascular: Edema, congestive heart failure, syncope, bradycardia, hypertension or hypotension, A-V block, arrhythmias
- Central nervous system: Slurred speech, mental depression
- Endocrine & metabolic: Hypocalcemia, hyponatremia
- Genitourinary: Urinary retention, sexual problems in males
- Hematologic: Neutropenia (can be transient), aplastic anemia, agranulocytosis, eosinophilia, leukopenia, pancytopenia, thrombocytopenia, bone marrow suppression
- Hepatic: Hepatitis

(Continued)

Carbamazepine *(Continued)*

Neuromuscular & skeletal: Peripheral neuritis
Ocular: Diplopia
Miscellaneous: Swollen glands, hypersensitivity

Overdosage/Toxicology Symptoms of overdose include dizziness ataxia, drowsiness, nausea, vomiting, tremor, agitation, nystagmus, urinary retention, dysrhythmias, coma, seizures, twitches, respiratory depression, neuromuscular disturbances

Provide general supportive care. Activated charcoal is effective at binding certain chemicals and this is especially true for carbamazepine; other treatment is supportive/symptomatic. Treatment consists of inducing emesis or gastric lavage. EKG should also be monitored to detect cardiac dysfunction. Monitor blood pressure, body temperature, pupillary reflexes, bladder function for several days following ingestion.

Drug Interactions

Inducer of cytochrome P-450 3A enzymes
Cytochrome P-450 2C enzyme substrate

Decreased effect: Carbamazepine may induce the metabolism of warfarin, cyclosporine, doxycycline, oral contraceptives, phenytoin, theophylline, benzodiazepines, ethosuximide, valproic acid, corticosteroids, and thyroid hormones

Increased toxicity: Erythromycin, isoniazid, propoxyphene, verapamil, danazol, isoniazid, diltiazem, and cimetidine may inhibit hepatic metabolism of carbamazepine with resultant increase of carbamazepine serum concentrations and toxicity

Mechanism of Action In addition to anticonvulsant effects, carbamazepine has anticholinergic, antineuralgic, antidiuretic, muscle relaxant and antiarrhythmic properties; may depress activity in the nucleus ventralis of the thalamus or decrease synaptic transmission or decrease summation of temporal stimulation leading to neural discharge by limiting influx of sodium ions across cell membrane or other unknown mechanisms; stimulates the release of ADH and potentiates its action in promoting reabsorption of water; chemically related to tricyclic antidepressants

Pharmacodynamics/Kinetics

Absorption: Slowly absorbed from GI tract
Distribution: V_d:
- Neonates: 1.5 L/kg
- Children: 1.9 L/kg
- Adults: 0.59-2 L/kg

Protein binding: 75% to 90%; may be decreased in newborns
Metabolism: In the liver to active epoxide metabolite; induces liver enzymes to increase metabolism and shorten half-life over time
Bioavailability, oral: 85%
Half-life:
- Initial: 18-55 hours
- Multiple dosing:
  - Children: 8-14 hours
  - Adults: 12-17 hours

Time to peak serum concentration: Unpredictable, within 4-8 hours
Elimination: 1% to 3% excreted unchanged in urine

Usual Dosage Oral (dosage must be adjusted according to patient's response and serum concentrations):

Children:
- <6 years: Initial: 5 mg/kg/day; dosage may be increased every 5-7 days to 10 mg/kg/day; then up to 20 mg/kg/day if necessary; administer in 2-4 divided doses/day
- 6-12 years: Initial: 100 mg twice daily or 10 mg/kg/day in 2 divided doses; increase by 100 mg/day at weekly intervals depending upon response; usual maintenance: 20-30 mg/kg/day in 2-4 divided doses/day; maximum dose: 1000 mg/day

Children >12 years and Adults: 200 mg twice daily to start, increase by 200 mg/day at weekly intervals until therapeutic levels achieved; usual dose: 800-1200 mg/day in 3-4 divided doses; some patients have required up to 1.6-2.4 g/day

Dosing adjustment in renal impairment: Cl_{cr} <10 mL/minute: Administer 75% of dose

Dietary Considerations

Food: Drug may cause GI upset, take with large amount of water or food to decrease GI upset. May need to split doses to avoid GI upset.
Sodium: SIADH and water intoxication; monitor fluid status; may need to restrict fluid

Reference Range

Timing of serum samples: Absorption is slow, peak levels occur 6-8 hours after ingestion of the first dose; the half-life ranges from 8-60 hours, therefore, steady-state is achieved in 2-5 days

Therapeutic levels: 6-12 µg/mL (SI: 25-51 µmol/L)

Toxic concentration: >15 µg/mL; patients who require higher levels of 8-12 µg/mL (SI: 34-51 µmol/L) should be watched closely. Side effects including CNS effects occur commonly at higher dosage levels. If other anticonvulsants are given therapeutic range is 4-8 µg/mL.

Test Interactions ↑ BUN, AST, ALT, bilirubin, alkaline phosphatase (S); ↓ calcium, T_3, T_4, sodium (S)

Patient Information Take with food, may cause drowsiness, periodic blood test monitoring required; notify physician if you observe bleeding, bruising, jaundice, abdominal pain, pale stools, mental disturbances, fever, chills, sore throat, or mouth ulcers

Nursing Implications Observe patient for excessive sedation; suspension dosage form must be given on a 3-4 times/day schedule versus tablets which can be given 2-4 times/day

Dosage Forms

Suspension, oral (citrus-vanilla flavor): 100 mg/5 mL (450 mL)

Tablet: 200 mg

Tablet, chewable: 100 mg

Tablet, extended release: 100 mg, 200 mg, 400 mg

Extemporaneous Preparations A more concentrated oral suspension can be prepared with 24-hour carbamazepine 200 mg tablets to provide a final concentration of 200 mg/5 mL when mixed with 120 mL of simple syrup. The resultant suspension is stable for 90 days when refrigerated; "shake well" label and "refrigerate" label should be included.

Carbamide *see* Urea *on page 1280*

Carbamide Peroxide (KAR ba mide per OKS ide)

Brand Names Auro® Ear Drops [OTC]; Debrox® Otic [OTC]; E•R•O Ear [OTC]; Gly-Oxide® Oral [OTC]; Mollifene® Ear Wax Removing Formula [OTC]; Murine® Ear Drops [OTC]; Orajel® Perioseptic [OTC]; Proxigel® Oral [OTC]

Canadian/Mexican Brand Names Clamurid® (Canada)

Synonyms Urea Peroxide

Therapeutic Category Otic Agent, Cerumenolytic

Use Relief of minor inflammation of gums, oral mucosal surfaces and lips including canker sores and dental irritation; emulsify and disperse ear wax

Pregnancy Risk Factor C

Contraindications Otic preparation should not be used in patients with a perforated tympanic membrane; ear drainage, ear pain or rash in the ear; do not use in the eye; do not use otic preparation longer than 4 days; oral preparation should not be used in children <3 years

Warnings/Precautions

Oral: With prolonged use of oral carbamide peroxide, there is a potential for overgrowth of opportunistic organisms; damage to periodontal tissues; delayed wound healing; should not be used for longer than 7 days

Otic: Do not use if ear drainage or discharge, ear pain, irritation, or rash in ear; should not be used for longer than 4 days

Adverse Reactions 1% to 10%:

Dermatologic: Rash

Local: Irritation, redness

Miscellaneous: Superinfections

Stability Store in tight, light-resistant containers; oral gel should be stored under refrigeration

Mechanism of Action Carbamide peroxide releases hydrogen peroxide which serves as a source of nascent oxygen upon contact with catalase; deodorant action is probably due to inhibition of odor-causing bacteria; softens impacted cerumen due to its foaming action

Usual Dosage Children and Adults:

Gel: Gently massage on affected area 4 times/day; do not drink or rinse mouth for 5 minutes after use

Oral solution (should not be used for >7 days): Apply several drops undiluted on affected area 4 times/day after meals and at bedtime for up to 7 days; expectorate after 2-3 minutes **OR** as an adjunct to oral hygiene after brushing, place 10 drops onto tongue, mix with saliva, swish for several minutes, expectorate

Otic:

Children <12 years: Tilt head sideways and individualize the dose according to patient size; 3 drops (range: 1-5 drops) twice daily for up to 4 days, tip of applicator should not enter ear canal; keep drops in ear for several minutes by keeping head tilted and placing cotton in ear

(Continued)

Carbamide Peroxide *(Continued)*

Children ≥12 years and Adults: Tilt head sideways and instill 5-10 drops twice daily up to 4 days, tip of applicator should not enter ear canal; keep drops in ear for several minutes by keeping head tilted and placing cotton in ear

Patient Information Contact physician if dizziness or otic redness, rash, irritation, tenderness, pain, drainage, or discharge develop; do not drink or rinse mouth for 5 minutes after oral use of gel

Nursing Implications Patient may complain of foaming

Dosage Forms

Gel, oral (Proxigel®): 11% (36 g)

Solution:

Oral:

Gly-Oxide®: 10% in glycerin (15 mL, 60 mL)

Orajel® Perioseptic: 15% in glycerin (13.3 mL)

Otic: (Auro® Ear Drops, Debrox®, Mollifene® Ear Wax Removing, Murine® Ear Drops): 6.5% in glycerin (15 mL, 30 mL)

Carbamylcholine Chloride *see* Carbachol *on page 200*

Carbastat® Ophthalmic *see* Carbachol *on page 200*

Carbidopa (kar bi DOE pa)

Brand Names Lodosyn®

Therapeutic Category Anti-Parkinson's Agent

Use Given with levodopa in the treatment of parkinsonism to enable a lower dosage of levodopa to be used and a more rapid response to be obtained and to decrease side-effects; for details of administration and dosage, see Levodopa

Has no effect without levodopa

Pregnancy Risk Factor C

Contraindications Hypersensitivity to carbidopa or levodopa

Adverse Reactions Adverse reactions are associated with concomitant administration with levodopa

>10%: Central nervous system: Anxiety, confusion, nervousness, mental depression

1% to 10%:

Cardiovascular: Orthostatic hypotension, palpitations, cardiac arrhythmias

Central nervous system: Memory loss, nervousness, insomnia, fatigue, hallucinations, ataxia, dystonic movements

Gastrointestinal: Nausea, vomiting, GI bleeding

Ocular: Blurred vision

<1%:

Cardiovascular: Hypertension

Gastrointestinal: Duodenal ulcer

Hematologic: Hemolytic anemia

Drug Interactions Increased toxicity: Tricyclic antidepressant → hypertensive reactions and dyskinesia

Mechanism of Action Carbidopa is a peripheral decarboxylase inhibitor with little or no pharmacological activity when given alone in usual doses. It inhibits the peripheral decarboxylation of levodopa to dopamine; and as it does not cross the blood-brain barrier, unlike levodopa, effective brain concentrations of dopamine are produced with lower doses of levodopa. At the same time, reduced peripheral formation of dopamine reduces peripheral side-effects, notably nausea and vomiting, and cardiac arrhythmias, although the dyskinesias and adverse mental effects associated with levodopa therapy tend to develop earlier.

Pharmacodynamics/Kinetics

Absorption: Rapid but incomplete from GI tract

Distribution: Does not cross the blood-brain barrier; in rats, it has been reported to cross the placenta and to be excreted in milk

Elimination: Rapidly excreted in urine both unchanged and in the form of metabolites

Usual Dosage Adults: Oral: 70-100 mg/day; maximum daily dose: 200 mg

Administration Administer with meals to decrease GI upset

Patient Information Can take with food to prevent GI upset, do not stop taking this drug even if you do not think it is working; dizziness, lightheadedness, fainting may occur when getting up from a sitting or lying position

Dosage Forms Tablet: 25 mg

Carbidopa and Levodopa *see* Levodopa and Carbidopa *on page 715*

Carbinoxamine and Pseudoephedrine

(kar bi NOKS a meen & soo doe e FED rin)

Related Information

Pseudoephedrine *on page 1074*

Brand Names Biohist-LA®; Carbiset® Tablet; Carbiset-TR® Tablet; Carbodec® Syrup; Carbodec® Tablet; Carbodec TR® Tablet; Cardec-S® Syrup; Rondec® Drops; Rondec® Filmtab®; Rondec® Syrup; Rondec-TR®

Therapeutic Category Adrenergic Agonist Agent; Antihistamine, H_1 Blocker; Decongestant

Use Temporary relief of nasal congestion, running nose, sneezing, itching of nose or throat, and itchy, watery eyes due to the common cold, hay fever, or other respiratory allergies

Pregnancy Risk Factor C

Contraindications Hypersensitivity to carbinoxamine or pseudoephedrine or any component; severe hypertension or coronary artery disease, MAO inhibitor therapy, GI or GU obstruction, narrow-angle glaucoma; avoid use in premature or term infants due to a possible association with SIDS

Warnings/Precautions Narrow-angle glaucoma, bladder neck obstruction, symptomatic prostatic hypertrophy, asthmatic attack, and stenosing peptic ulcer

Adverse Reactions

>10%:
- Central nervous system: Slight to moderate drowsiness
- Respiratory: Thickening of bronchial secretions

1% to 10%:
- Central nervous system: Headache, fatigue, nervousness, dizziness
- Gastrointestinal: Appetite increase, weight gain, nausea, diarrhea, abdominal pain, xerostomia
- Neuromuscular & skeletal: Arthralgia
- Respiratory: Pharyngitis

<1%:
- Cardiovascular: Edema, palpitations
- Central nervous system: Depression
- Dermatologic: Angioedema, photosensitivity, rash
- Hepatic: Hepatitis
- Neuromuscular & skeletal: Myalgia, paresthesia
- Respiratory: Bronchospasm, epistaxis

Overdosage/Toxicology Symptoms of overdose include dry mouth, flushed skin, dilated pupils, CNS depression

There is no specific treatment for an antihistamine overdose, however, most of its clinical toxicity is due to anticholinergic effects. Anticholinesterase inhibitors including physostigmine, neostigmine, pyridostigmine, and edrophonium may be useful by reducing acetylcholinesterase; for anticholinergic overdose with severe life-threatening symptoms, physostigmine 1-2 mg (0.5 or 0.02 mg/kg for children) I.V., slowly may be given to reverse these effects.

Drug Interactions Increased toxicity: Barbiturates, TCAs, MAO inhibitors, ethanolamine antihistamines

Mechanism of Action Carbinoxamine competes with histamine for H_1-receptor sites on effector cells in the gastrointestinal tract, blood vessels, and respiratory tract

Usual Dosage Oral:

Children:
- Drops: 1-18 months: 0.25-1 mL 4 times/day
- Syrup:
  - 18 months to 6 years: 2.5 mL 3-4 times/day
  - >6 years: 5 mL 2-4 times/day

Adults:
- Liquid: 5 mL 4 times/day
- Tablets: 1 tablet 4 times/day

Patient Information May cause drowsiness, impaired coordination, or judgment; may cause blurred vision; may also cause CNS excitation and difficulty sleeping

Nursing Implications Raise bed rails; institute safety measures; assist with ambulation

Dosage Forms

Drops: Carbinoxamine maleate 2 mg and pseudoephedrine hydrochloride 25 mg per mL (30 mL with dropper)

Syrup: Carbinoxamine maleate 4 mg and pseudoephedrine hydrochloride 60 mg per 5 mL (120 mL, 480 mL)

Tablet:
- Film-coated: Carbinoxamine maleate 4 mg and pseudoephedrine hydrochloride 60 mg
- Sustained release: Carbinoxamine maleate 8 mg and pseudoephedrine hydrochloride 120 mg

Carbiset® Tablet *see* Carbinoxamine and Pseudoephedrine *on previous page*

Carbiset-TR® Tablet *see* Carbinoxamine and Pseudoephedrine *on previous page*

Carbocaine® *see* Mepivacaine *on page 783*

Carbodec® Syrup *see* Carbinoxamine and Pseudoephedrine *on previous page*

Carbodec® Tablet *see* Carbinoxamine and Pseudoephedrine *on page 204*
Carbodec TR® Tablet *see* Carbinoxamine and Pseudoephedrine *on page 204*

Carboplatin (KAR boe pla tin)

Related Information

Antiemetics for Chemotherapy Induced Nausea and Vomiting *on page 1348*
Cancer Chemotherapy Regimens *on page 1351*
Toxicities of Chemotherapeutic Agents *on page 1382*

Brand Names Paraplatin®

Synonyms CBDCA

Therapeutic Category Antineoplastic Agent, Alkylating Agent; Antineoplastic Agent, Irritant

Use Ovarian carcinoma, cervical, small cell lung carcinoma, esophageal, testicular, bladder cancer, mesothelioma, pediatric brain tumors, sarcoma, neuroblastoma, osteosarcoma

Pregnancy Risk Factor D

Contraindications Hypersensitivity to carboplatin or any component (anaphylactic-like reactions may occur), severe bone marrow suppression, or excessive bleeding

Warnings/Precautions The U.S. Food and Drug Administration (FDA) currently recommends that procedures for proper handling and disposal of antineoplastic agents be considered. High doses have resulted in severe abnormalities of liver function tests. Bone marrow suppression, which may be severe, and vomiting are dose related; reduce dosage in patients with bone marrow suppression and impaired renal function.

Adverse Reactions

>10%:
- Endocrine & metabolic: Electrolyte abnormalities such as hypocalcemia and hypomagnesemia, hyponatremia, hypokalemia
- Gastrointestinal: Nausea, vomiting, stomatitis
  - Emetic potential: Moderate
  - Time course for nausea and vomiting: Onset: 2-6 hours; Duration: 1-48 hours
- Hematologic: Neutropenia, leukopenia, thrombocytopenia, anemia
- Myelosuppressive: Dose-limiting toxicity
  - WBC: Severe (dose-dependent)
  - Platelets: Severe
  - Nadir: 21-24 days
  - Recovery: 28-35 days
- Hepatic: Abnormal liver function tests
- Local: Pain at injection site
- Neuromuscular & skeletal: Weakness

1% to 10%:
- Dermatologic: Alopecia
- Gastrointestinal: Diarrhea, anorexia
- Hematologic: Hemorrhagic complications
- Neuromuscular & skeletal: Peripheral neuropathy
- Otic: Ototoxicity in 1% of patients

<1%:
- Central nervous system: Neurotoxicity has only been noted in patients previously treated with cisplatin
- Dermatologic: Urticaria, rash, alopecia
- Ocular: Blurred vision
- Renal: Nephrotoxicity (uncommon)

Overdosage/Toxicology Symptoms of overdose include bone marrow suppression, hepatic toxicity

Drug Interactions Increased toxicity: Nephrotoxic drugs; aminoglycosides increase risk of ototoxicity

Stability

Store intact vials at room temperature (15°C to 30°C/59°F to 86°F) and protect from light; reconstitute powder to yield a final concentration of 10 mg/mL which is stable for 5 days at room temperature (25°C)

Aluminum needles should not be used for administration due to binding with the platinum ion

Compatible with etoposide

Standard I.V. dilution:
- Dose/250-1000 mL D_5W
  - Further dilution to a concentration as low as 0.5 mg/mL is stable at room temperature (25°C) or under refrigeration for 8 days in D_5W

Mechanism of Action Analogue of cisplatin which covalently binds to DNA; possible cross-linking and interference with the function of DNA

Pharmacodynamics/Kinetics Possible cross-linking and interference with the function of DNA

Distribution: V_d: 16 L/kg; distributes into liver, kidney, skin, and tumor tissue
Metabolism: To aquated and hydroxylated compounds
Protein binding: 0%; however, platinum is 30% irreversibly bound
Half-life: Terminal: 22-40 hours; 2.5-5.9 hours in patients with Cl_{cr} >60 mL/minute
Elimination: ~60% to 90% is excreted renally in the first 24 hours

Usual Dosage IVPB, I.V. infusion, Intraperitoneal (refer to individual protocols):

Children: Solid tumor: 600 mg/m² once every 4 weeks

Adults:

Ovarian cancer: Usual doses range from 360 mg/m² I.V. every 3 weeks single agent therapy to 300 mg/m² every 4 weeks as combination therapy

In general, however, single intermittent courses of carboplatin should not be repeated until the neutrophil count is at least 2000 and the platelet count is at least 100,000

The dose adjustments in the table are modified from a controlled trial in previously treated patients with ovarian carcinoma. Blood counts were done weekly, and the recommendations are based on the lowest post-treatment platelet or neutrophil value.

Carboplatin Dosage Adjustment based on Pretreatment Platelet Counts

Platelets (cells/mm³)	Neutrophils (cells/mm³)	Adjusted Dose (From Prior Course)
>100,000	>2,000	125%
50-100,000	500-2,000	No adjustment
<50,000	<500	75%

Carboplatin dosage adjustment based on the Egorin formula (based on platelet counts):

Previously untreated patients:

$$\text{dosage (mg/m}^2) = (0.091)\frac{(Cl_{cr})}{(BSA)}\frac{(\text{Pretreat Plt count - Plt nadir count desired x 100})}{(\text{Pretreatment Plt count})} + 86$$

Previously treated patients with heavily myelosuppressive agents:

$$\text{dosage (mg/m}^2) = (0.091)\frac{(Cl_{cr})}{(BSA)}\left[\frac{(\text{Pretreat Plt count - Plt nadir count desired x 100}) - 17}{(\text{Pretreatment Plt count})}\right] + 86$$

Autologous BMT: I.V.: 1600 mg/m² (total dose) divided over 4 days REQUIRES BMT

Dosing adjustment in renal impairment: These dosing recommendations apply to the initial course of treatment. Subsequent dosages should be adjusted according to the patient's tolerance based on the degree of bone marrow suppression.

Cl_{cr} <60 mL/minute: Increased risk of severe bone marrow suppression. In renally impaired patients who received single agent carboplatin therapy, the incidence of severe leukopenia, neutropenia, or thrombocytopenia has been about 25% when the following dosage modifications have been used:

Cl_{cr} 41-59 mL/minute: Recommended dose on day 1 is 250 mg/m²

Cl_{cr} 16-40 mL/minute: Recommended dose on day 1 is 200 mg/m²

Cl_{cr} <15 mL/minute: The data available for patients with severely impaired kidney function are too limited to permit a recommendation for treatment

or

Dosage adjustment in renal impairment: CALVERT FORMULA

Total dose (mg) = Target AUC x (GFR + 25)

Note: The dose of carboplatin calculated is **total mg dose** not mg/m². AUC is the area under the concentration versus time curve.

Target AUC value will vary depending upon:

Number of agents in the regimen

Treatment status (ie, previously untreated or treated)

Single Agent Carboplatin/No Prior Chemotherapy	Total dose (mg): 6-8 (GFR + 25)
Single Agent Carboplatin/Prior Chemotherapy	Total dose (mg): 4-6 (GFR + 25)
Combination Chemotherapy/No Prior Chemotherapy	Total dose (mg): 4.5-6 (GFR + 25)
Combination Chemotherapy/Prior Chemotherapy	A reasonable approach for these patients would be to use a target AUC value <5 for the initial cycle

(Continued)

Carboplatin *(Continued)*

Intraperitoneal: 200-650 mg/m^2 in 2 L of dialysis fluid have been administered into the peritoneum of ovarian cancer patients

Administration

Do not use needles or I.V. administration sets containing aluminum parts that may come in contact with carboplatin (aluminum can react causing precipitate formation and loss of potency)

Administer as IVPB over 15 minutes up to a CIV over 24 hours; may also be administered intraperitoneally

Monitoring Parameters CBC (with differential and platelet count), serum electrolytes, urinalysis, creatinine clearance, liver function tests

Patient Information Report any loss of hearing, numbness, or tingling in the extremities to the physician

Dosage Forms Powder for injection, lyophilized: 50 mg, 150 mg, 450 mg

Carboprost Tromethamine (KAR boe prost tro METH a meen)

Replaces Prostin/15M®

Brand Names Hemabate™

Therapeutic Category Abortifacient; Prostaglandin

Use Termination of pregnancy and refractory postpartum uterine bleeding

Investigational: Hemorrhagic cystitis

Pregnancy Risk Factor X

Contraindications Hypersensitivity to carboprost tromethamine or any component; acute pelvic inflammatory disease

Warnings/Precautions Use with caution in patients with history of asthma, hypotension or hypertension, cardiovascular, adrenal, renal or hepatic disease, anemia, jaundice, diabetes, epilepsy or compromised uteri

Adverse Reactions

>10%: Gastrointestinal: Nausea

1% to 10%: Cardiovascular: Flushing

<1%:

- Cardiovascular: Hypertension, hypotension
- Central nervous system: Drowsiness, vertigo, nervousness, fever, headache, dystonia, vasovagal syndrome
- Endocrine & metabolic: Breast tenderness
- Gastrointestinal: Xerostomia, vomiting, diarrhea, hematemesis, abnormal taste
- Genitourinary: Bladder spasms
- Neuromuscular & skeletal: Myalgia
- Ocular: Blurred vision
- Respiratory: Coughing, asthma, respiratory distress
- Miscellaneous: Septic shock, hiccups

Drug Interactions Increased toxicity: Oxytocic agents

Stability Refrigerate ampuls

Bladder irrigation: Dilute immediately prior to administration in NS; stability unknown

Mechanism of Action Carboprost tromethamine is a prostaglandin similar to prostaglandin F_2 alpha (dinoprost) except for the addition of a methyl group at the C-15 position. This substitution produces longer duration of activity than dinoprost; carboprost stimulates uterine contractility which usually results in expulsion of the products of conception and is used to induce abortion between 13-20 weeks of pregnancy. Hemostasis at the placentation site is achieved through the myometrial contractions produced by carboprost.

Usual Dosage Adults: I.M.:

Abortion: 250 mcg to start, 250 mcg at 1½-hour to 3½-hour intervals depending on uterine response; a 500 mcg dose may be given if uterine response is not adequate after several 250 mcg doses; do not exceed 12 mg total dose

Refractory postpartum uterine bleeding: Initial: 250 mcg; may repeat at 15- to 90-minute intervals to a total dose of 2 mg

Bladder irrigation for hemorrhagic cystitis (refer to individual protocols): [0.4-1.0 mg/dL as solution] 50 mL instilled into bladder 4 times/day for 1 hour

Administration Do not inject I.V.; may result in bronchospasm, hypertension, vomiting, and anaphylaxis

Dosage Forms Injection: Carboprost 250 mcg and tromethamine 83 mcg per mL (1 mL)

Carboptic® Ophthalmic *see* Carbachol *on page 200*

Cardec-S® Syrup *see* Carbinoxamine and Pseudoephedrine *on page 204*

Cardene® *see* Nicardipine *on page 898*

Cardene® SR *see* Nicardipine *on page 898*

Cardilate® *see* Erythrityl Tetranitrate *on page 460*

Cardioquin® *see* Quinidine *on page 1087*
Cardiovascular Agents Comparison *see page 1405*
Cardizem® CD *see* Diltiazem *on page 393*
Cardizem® Injectable *see* Diltiazem *on page 393*
Cardizem® Lyo-Ject™ *see* Diltiazem *on page 393*
Cardizem® SR *see* Diltiazem *on page 393*
Cardizem® Tablet *see* Diltiazem *on page 393*
Cardura® *see* Doxazosin *on page 423*
Carisoprodate *see* Carisoprodol *on this page*

Carisoprodol (kar i soe PROE dole)

Brand Names Rela®; Sodol®; Soma®; Soma® Compound; Soprodol®; Soridol®

Canadian/Mexican Brand Names Dolaren® (Carisoprodol with Diclofenac) (Mexico); Naxodol® (Carisoprodol with Naproxen) (Mexico)

Synonyms Carisoprodate; Isobamate

Therapeutic Category Skeletal Muscle Relaxant

Use Skeletal muscle relaxant

Pregnancy Risk Factor C

Contraindications Acute intermittent porphyria, hypersensitivity to carisoprodol, meprobamate or any component

Warnings/Precautions Use with caution in renal and hepatic dysfunction

Adverse Reactions

>10%: Central nervous system: Drowsiness

1% to 10%:

- Cardiovascular: Tachycardia, tightness in chest, flushing of face, syncope
- Central nervous system: Mental depression, allergic fever, dizziness, lightheadedness, headache, paradoxical CNS stimulation
- Dermatologic: Angioedema
- Gastrointestinal: Nausea, vomiting, stomach cramps
- Neuromuscular & skeletal: Trembling
- Ocular: Burning eyes
- Respiratory: Shortness of breath
- Miscellaneous: Hiccups

<1%:

- Central nervous system: Ataxia
- Dermatologic: Rash, urticaria, erythema multiforme
- Hematologic: Aplastic anemia, leukopenia, eosinophilia
- Ocular: Blurred vision

Overdosage/Toxicology Symptoms of overdose include CNS depression, stupor, coma, shock, respiratory depression

Treatment is supportive following attempts to enhance drug elimination. Hypotension should be treated with I.V. fluids and/or Trendelenburg positioning.

Drug Interactions Increased toxicity: Alcohol, CNS depressants, phenothiazines, clindamycin, MAO inhibitors

Mechanism of Action Precise mechanism is not yet clear, but many effects have been ascribed to its central depressant actions

Pharmacodynamics/Kinetics

Onset of action: Within 30 minutes

Duration: 4-6 hours

Distribution: Crosses the placenta; appears in high concentrations in breast milk

- Metabolism: By the liver
- Half-life: 8 hours
- Elimination: By the kidneys

Usual Dosage Adults: Oral: 350 mg 3-4 times/day; take last dose at bedtime; compound: 1-2 tablets 4 times/day

Dietary Considerations Alcohol: Additive CNS effects, avoid use

Monitoring Parameters Look for relief of pain and/or muscle spasm and avoid excessive drowsiness

Patient Information May cause drowsiness or dizziness; avoid alcohol and other CNS depressants

Nursing Implications Raise bed rails; institute safety measures; assist with ambulation

Dosage Forms Tablet: 350 mg

Extemporaneous Preparations A suspension can be prepared by triturating 60 carisoprodol 350 mg tablets, a small amount of water or glycerin, then mixing with a sufficient quantity of cherry syrup to bring the final volume to 60 mL; when refrigerated, the suspension is stable for 14 days; shake well before administration

Carmol® [OTC] *see* Urea *on page 1280*

Carmustine (kar MUS teen)

Related Information

Antiemetics for Chemotherapy Induced Nausea and Vomiting *on page 1348*
Cancer Chemotherapy Regimens *on page 1351*
Toxicities of Chemotherapeutic Agents *on page 1382*

Brand Names BiCNU®

Synonyms BCNU

Therapeutic Category Antineoplastic Agent, Alkylating Agent (Nitrosourea); Antineoplastic Agent, Vesicant; Vesicant

Use Treatment of brain tumors, multiple myeloma, Hodgkin's disease and non-Hodgkin's lymphomas, melanoma, lung cancer, colon cancer

Pregnancy Risk Factor D

Contraindications Hypersensitivity to carmustine or any component, myelosuppression from previous chemotherapy or other causes

Warnings/Precautions The U.S. Food and Drug Administration (FDA) currently recommends that procedures for proper handling and disposal of antineoplastic agents be considered. Administer with caution to patients with depressed platelet, leukocyte or erythrocyte counts, renal or hepatic impairment. Bone marrow suppression, notably thrombocytopenia and leukopenia, may lead to bleeding and overwhelming infections in an already compromised patient; will last for at least 6 weeks after a dose, **do not administer courses more frequently than every 6 weeks because the toxicity is cumulative.** Baseline pulmonary function tests are recommended.

Adverse Reactions

>10%:

- Cardiovascular: Hypotension is associated with HIGH-DOSE administration secondary to the high alcohol content of the diluent
- Central nervous system: Dizziness and ataxia
- Dermatologic: Hyperpigmentation of skin
- Gastrointestinal: Nausea and vomiting occur within 2-4 hours after drug injection; dose-related
  - Emetic potential:
  - <200 mg: Moderately high (60% to 90%)
  - ≥200 mg: High (>90%)
  - Time course of nausea/vomiting: Onset: 2-6 hours; Duration: 4-6 hours
- Hematologic: Myelosuppressive: Delayed, occurs 4-6 weeks after administration and is dose-related; usually persists for 1-2 weeks; thrombocytopenia is usually more severe than leukopenia. Myelofibrosis and preleukemic syndromes have been reported.
  - WBC: Moderate
  - Platelets: Severe
  - Onset (days): 14
  - Nadir (days): 21-35
  - Recovery (days): 42-50
- Local: Burning at injection site
  - **Irritant chemotherapy:** Pain at injection site
- Ocular: Ocular toxicity, and retinal hemorrhages

1% to 10%:

- Dermatologic: Facial flushing is probably due to the ethanol used in reconstitution, alopecia
- Gastrointestinal: Stomatitis, diarrhea, anorexia
- Hematologic: Anemia

<1%:

- Dermatologic: Hyperpigmentation, dermatitis
- Hepatic: Reversible toxicity, increased LFTs in 20%
- Respiratory: Fibrosis occurs mostly in patients treated with prolonged total doses >1400 mg/m^2 or with bone marrow transplantation doses; risk factors include a history of lung disease, concomitant bleomycin, or radiation therapy; PFTs should be conducted prior to therapy and monitored; patients with predicted FVC or DL_{co} <70% are at a higher risk
- Renal: Azotemia, decrease in kidney size

Overdosage/Toxicology Symptoms of overdose include nausea, vomiting, thrombocytopenia, leukopenia

There are no known antidotes and treatment is primarily symptomatic and supportive

Drug Interactions

Increased toxicity:

- Cimetidine: Reported to cause bone marrow suppression
- Etoposide: Reported to cause severe hepatic dysfunction with hyperbilirubinemia, ascites, and thrombocytopenia

Stability

Store intact vials under refrigeration: vials are stable for 7 days at room temperature

Initially dilute with 3 mL of absolute alcohol diluent. Further dilute with 27 mL SWI to result in a concentration of 3.3 mg/mL with 10% ethanol. Initial solutions are stable for 8 hours at room temperature (25°C) and 24 hours at refrigeration (2°C to 8°C) and protected from light.

Further dilution in D_5W or NS is stable for 8 hours at room temperature (25°C) and 48 hours at refrigeration (4°C) in glass or Excel® protected from light

Incompatible with sodium bicarbonate; **compatible** with cisplatin

Standard I.V. dilution:

Dose/150-500 mL D_5W or NS

Must use glass or Excel® containers for administration

PROTECT FROM LIGHT

Stable for 8 hours at room temperature (25°C) and 48 hours under refrigeration (4°C)

Mechanism of Action Interferes with the normal function of DNA by alkylation and cross-linking the strands of DNA, and by possible protein modification

Pharmacodynamics/Kinetics

Absorption: Highly lipid soluble

Distribution: Readily crosses the blood-brain barrier producing CSF levels equal to 15% to 70% of blood plasma levels; distributes into breast milk

Metabolism: Rapid

Half-life (biphasic):

Initial: 1.4 minutes

Secondary: 20 minutes (active metabolites may persist for days and have a plasma half-life of 67 hours)

Elimination: ~60% to 70% excreted in the urine within 96 hours and 6% to 10% excreted as CO_2 by the lungs

Usual Dosage I.V. (refer to individual protocols):

Children: 200-250 mg/m^2 every 4-6 weeks as a single dose

Adults: 150-200 mg/m^2 every 6 weeks as a single dose or divided into daily injections on 2 successive days; next dose is to be determined based on hematologic response to the previous dose. See table.

Suggested Carmustine Dose Following Initial Dose

Nadir After Prior Dose		% of Prior Dose to Be Given
Leukocytes/mm^3	Platelets/mm^3	
>4000	>100,000	100
3000-3999	75,000-99,999	100
2000-2999	25,000-74,999	70
<2000	<25,000	50

Primary brain cancer: 150-200 mg/m^2 every 6-8 weeks

Autologous BMT: ALL OF THE FOLLOWING DOSES ARE FATAL WITHOUT BMT

Combination therapy: Up to 300-900 mg/m^2

Single agent therapy: Up to 1200 mg/m^2 (fatal necrosis is associated with doses >2 g/m^2)

Hemodialysis: Supplemental dosing is not required

Dosing adjustment in hepatic impairment: Dosage adjustment may be necessary; however, no specific guidelines are available

Administration

Significant absorption to PVC containers - should be administered in either glass or Excel® container

Infuse I.V. infusion over ≥15-45 minutes is recommended to minimize severe burning/vein irritation; longer infusion times (1-2 hours) can alleviate venous pain/irritation

High-dose carmustine: Maximum rate of infusion of ≤3 mg/m^2/minute to avoid excessive flushing, agitation, and hypotension; infusions should run over at least 2 hours; some investigational protocols dictate shorter infusions.

Monitoring Parameters CBC with differential and platelet count, pulmonary function, liver function, and renal function tests; monitor blood pressure during administration

Patient Information Contraceptive measures are recommended during therapy

Dosage Forms Powder for injection: 100 mg/vial packaged with 3 mL of absolute alcohol for use as a sterile diluent

Carteolol (KAR tee oh lole)

Related Information

Beta-Blockers Comparison *on page 1398*

Glaucoma Drug Therapy Comparison *on page 1410*

Brand Names Cartrol®; Ocupress®

Synonyms Carteolol Hydrochloride

Therapeutic Category Beta-Adrenergic Blocker; Beta-Adrenergic Blocker, Ophthalmic

Use Management of hypertension; treatment of chronic open-angle glaucoma and intraocular hypertension

Pregnancy Risk Factor C

Contraindications Bronchial asthma, sinus bradycardia, second and third degree A-V block, cardiac failure (unless a functioning pacemaker present), cardiogenic shock, hypersensitivity to betaxolol or any component

Warnings/Precautions Some products contain sulfites which can cause allergic reactions; diminished response over time; may increase muscle weaknesses; use with a miotic in angle-closure glaucoma; use with caution in patients with decreased renal or hepatic function (dosage adjustment required) or patients with a history of asthma, congestive heart failure, or bradycardia; severe CNS, cardiovascular, and respiratory adverse effects have been seen following ophthalmic use

Adverse Reactions

1% to 10%:

Cardiovascular: Congestive heart failure, arrhythmia

Central nervous system: Mental depression, headache, dizziness

Neuromuscular & skeletal: Back pain, arthralgia

<1%:

Cardiovascular: Bradycardia, chest pain, mesenteric arterial thrombosis, A-V block, persistent bradycardia, hypotension, edema, Raynaud's phenomenon

Central nervous system: Fatigue, insomnia, lethargy, nightmares, confusion

Dermatologic: Purpura

Endocrine & metabolic: Hyperglycemia

Gastrointestinal: Ischemic colitis, constipation, nausea, diarrhea

Genitourinary: Impotence

Hematologic: Thrombocytopenia

Respiratory: Bronchospasm

Miscellaneous: Cold extremities

Overdosage/Toxicology Symptoms of intoxication include cardiac disturbances, CNS toxicity, bronchospasm, hypoglycemia, and hyperkalemia. The most common cardiac symptoms include hypotension and bradycardia; atrioventricular block, intraventricular conduction disturbances, cardiogenic shock, and systole may occur with severe overdose, especially with membrane-depressant drugs (eg, propranolol); CNS effects include convulsions, coma, and respiratory arrest (commonly seen with propranolol and other membrane-depressant and lipid-soluble drugs)

Treatment includes symptomatic treatment of seizures, hypotension, hyperkalemia, and hypoglycemia; bradycardia and hypotension resistant to atropine, isoproterenol, or pacing may respond to glucagon; wide QRS defects caused by the membrane-depressant poisoning may respond to hypertonic sodium bicarbonate; repeat-dose charcoal, hemoperfusion, or hemodialysis may be helpful in removal of only those beta-blockers with a small V_d, long half-life, or low intrinsic clearance (acebutolol, atenolol, nadolol, sotalol).

Drug Interactions

Decreased effect of beta-blockers with aluminum salts, barbiturates, calcium salts, cholestyramine, colestipol, NSAIDs, penicillins (ampicillin), rifampin, salicylates, and sulfinpyrazone due to decreased bioavailability and plasma levels

Beta-blockers may decrease the effect of sulfonylureas

Increased effect/toxicity of beta-blockers with calcium blockers (diltiazem, felodipine, nicardipine), contraceptives, flecainide, haloperidol (propranolol, hypotensive effects), H_2-antagonists (metoprolol, propranolol only by cimetidine, possibly ranitidine), hydralazine (metoprolol, propranolol), loop diuretics (propranolol, not atenolol), MAO inhibitors (metoprolol, nadolol, bradycardia), phenothiazines (propranolol), propafenone (metoprolol, propranolol), quinidine (in extensive metabolizers), ciprofloxacin, thyroid hormones (metoprolol, propranolol, when hypothyroid patient is converted to euthyroid state)

Beta-blockers may increase the effect/toxicity of flecainide, haloperidol (hypotensive effects), hydralazine, phenothiazines, acetaminophen, anticoagulants (propranolol, warfarin), benzodiazepines (not atenolol), clonidine (hypertensive crisis after or during withdrawal of either agent), epinephrine (initial hypertensive episode followed by bradycardia), nifedipine and verapamil lidocaine, ergots (peripheral ischemia), prazosin (postural hypotension)

Beta-blockers may affect the action or levels of ethanol, disopyramide, nondepolarizing muscle relaxants and theophylline although the effects are difficult to predict

Mechanism of Action Blocks both $beta_1$- and $beta_2$-receptors and has mild intrinsic sympathomimetic activity; has negative inotropic and chronotropic effects and can significantly slow A-V nodal conduction

Pharmacodynamics/Kinetics

Onset of effect: Oral: 1-1.5 hours

Peak effect: 2 hours

Duration: 12 hours

Absorption: Oral: 80%

Protein binding: 23% to 30%

Metabolism: 30% to 50%

Half-life: 6 hours

Elimination: Renally excreted metabolites

Usual Dosage Adults:

Oral: 2.5 mg as a single daily dose, with a maintenance dose normally 2.5-5 mg once daily; maximum daily dose: 10 mg; doses >10 mg do not increase response and may in fact decrease effect

Ophthalmic: Instill 1 drop in affected eye(s) twice daily

Dosing interval in renal impairment:

Cl_{cr} >60 mL/minute/1.73 m^2: Administer every 24 hours

Cl_{cr} 20-60 mL/minute/1.73 m^2: Administer every 48 hours

Cl_{cr} <20 mL/minute/1.73 m^2: Administer every 72 hours

Monitoring Parameters Ophthalmic: Intraocular pressure; Systemic: Blood pressure, pulse, CNS status

Patient Information Intended for twice daily dosing; keep eye open and do not blink for 30 seconds after instillation; wear sunglasses to avoid photophobic discomfort; apply gentle pressure to lacrimal sac during and immediately following instillation (1 minute); do not discontinue medication abruptly, sudden stopping of medication may precipitate or cause angina; consult pharmacist or physician before taking with other adrenergic drugs (eg, cold medications); notify physician if any systemic side effects occur; use with caution while driving or performing tasks requiring alertness; may mask signs of hypoglycemia in diabetics; may be taken without regard to meals

Nursing Implications Advise against abrupt withdrawal; monitor orthostatic blood pressures, apical and peripheral pulse, and mental status changes (ie, confusion, depression)

Dosage Forms

Solution, ophthalmic, as hydrochloride (Ocupress®): 1% (5 mL, 10 mL)

Tablet, as hydrochloride (Cartrol®): 2.5 mg, 5 mg

Carteolol Hydrochloride *see* Carteolol *on previous page*

Carter's Little Pills® [OTC] *see* Bisacodyl *on page 153*

Cartrol® *see* Carteolol *on previous page*

Carvedilol (KAR ve dil ole)

Brand Names Coreg®

Therapeutic Category Beta-Adrenergic Blocker

Use Management of hypertension; can be used alone or in combination with other agents, especially thiazide-type diuretics

An FDA advisory panel has recommended approval for the treatment of CHF since, in trials, it retarded disease progression, lowered hospitalization rates, increased the heart's inotropic action and improved physician and patient assessment of patients' well-being

Pregnancy Risk Factor C

Pregnancy/Breast-Feeding Implications Use during pregnancy only if the potential benefit justifies the risk; possible excretion in breast milk; avoid administration in lactating women, if possible

Contraindications Uncompensated congestive heart failure (NYHA Class IV), asthma or bronchospastic disease (status asthmaticus may result), cardiogenic shock, severe bradycardia or second or third degree heart block, and symptomatic hepatic disease; hypersensitivity to any component

Warnings/Precautions Use with caution in patients with congestive heart failure treated with digitalis, diuretic, or ACE inhibitor since A-V conduction may be slowed; discontinue therapy if any evidence of liver injury occurs; use caution in patients with peripheral vascular disease, those undergoing anesthesia, in hyperthyroidism and diabetes mellitus. If no other antihypertensive is tolerated, very small doses may be cautiously used in patients with bronchospastic disease. Abrupt withdrawal of the drug should be avoided, drug should be discontinued over 1-2 weeks; do not use in pregnant or nursing women; may potentiate

(Continued)

Carvedilol *(Continued)*

hypoglycemia in a diabetic patient and mask signs and symptoms; safety and efficacy in children have not been established.

Adverse Reactions

1% to 10%:

- Cardiovascular: Bradycardia, postural hypotension, edema
- Central nervous system: Dizziness, somnolence, insomnia, fatigue
- Gastrointestinal: Diarrhea, abdominal pain
- Neuromuscular & skeletal: Back pain
- Respiratory: Rhinitis, pharyngitis, dyspnea

<1%:

- Cardiovascular: A-V block, extrasystoles, hypertension, hypotension, palpitations, peripheral ischemia, syncope
- Central nervous system: Ataxia, vertigo, depression, nervousness, malaise
- Dermatologic: Pruritus, rash
- Endocrine & metabolic: Decreased male libido, hypercholesterolemia, hyperglycemia, hyperuricemia
- Gastrointestinal: Constipation, flatulence, xerostomia
- Genitourinary: Impotence
- Hematologic: Anemia, leukopenia
- Hepatic: Hyperbilirubinemia, increased LFTs
- Neuromuscular & skeletal: Paresthesia, myalgia, weakness
- Ocular: Abnormal vision
- Otic: Tinnitus
- Respiratory: Asthma, cough
- Miscellaneous: Diaphoresis (increased)

Overdosage/Toxicology Symptoms of intoxication include cardiac disturbances, CNS toxicity, bronchospasm, hypoglycemia, and hyperkalemia. The most common cardiac symptoms include hypotension and bradycardia; atrioventricular block, intraventricular conduction disturbances, cardiogenic shock, and systole may occur with severe overdose, especially with membrane-depressant drugs (eg, propranolol); CNS effects include convulsions, coma, and respiratory arrest which are commonly seen with propranolol and other membrane-depressant and lipid-soluble drugs.

Treatment includes symptomatic treatment of seizures, hypotension, hyperkalemia, and hypoglycemia; bradycardia and hypotension resistant to atropine, isoproterenol, or pacing may respond to glucagon; wide QRS defects caused by the membrane-depressant poisoning may respond to hypertonic sodium bicarbonate; repeat-dose charcoal, hemoperfusion, or hemodialysis may be helpful in removal of only those beta-blockers with a small V_d, long half-life, or low intrinsic clearance (acebutolol, atenolol, nadolol, sotalol)

Drug Interactions

Decreased effect: Rifampin may reduce the plasma concentration of carvedilol by up to 70%; decreased effect of beta-blockers has also occurred with aluminum salts, barbiturates, calcium salts, cholestyramine, colestipol, NSAIDs, penicillins (ampicillin), salicylates, and sulfinpyrazone due to decreased bioavailability and plasma levels; beta-blockers may decrease the effect of sulfonylureas

Increased effect: Carvedilol may enhance the action of antidiabetic agents, calcium channel blockers, digoxin; clonidine and cimetidine increase the effect and AUC of carvedilol, respectively

Increased effect/toxicity of beta-blockers with contraceptives, flecainide, haloperidol (propranolol, hypotensive effects), hydralazine, phenothiazines, acetaminophen, anticoagulants (propranolol, warfarin), benzodiazepines (not atenolol), epinephrine (initial hypertensive episode followed by bradycardia), lidocaine, ergots (peripheral ischemia), and prazocin (postural hypotension)

Mechanism of Action As a racemic mixture, carvedilol has nonselective beta-adrenoreceptor and alpha-adrenergic blocking activity at equal potency. No intrinsic sympathomimetic activity has been documented. Associated effects include reduction of cardiac output, exercise- or beta agonist-induced tachycardia, reduction of reflex orthostatic tachycardia, vasodilation, decreased peripheral vascular resistance (especially in standing position), decreased renal vascular resistance, reduced plasma renin activity, and increased levels of atrial natriuretic peptide.

Pharmacodynamics/Kinetics

Absorption: Rapid; food decreases the rate but not the extent of absorption; administration with food minimizes risks of orthostatic hypotension

Metabolism: First-pass metabolism; extensively metabolized primarily by aromatic ring oxidation and glucuronidation (2% excreted unchanged); three active metabolites (4-hydroxphenyl metabolite is 13 times more potent than parent drug); plasma concentrations in the elderly and those with cirrhotic liver disease are 50% and 4-7 times higher, respectively

Bioavailability: 25% to 35%
Half-life: 7-10 hours
Elimination: Primarily via bile into feces

Usual Dosage Adults: Oral:

Hypertension: 6.25 mg twice daily; if tolerated, dose should be maintained for 1-2 weeks, then increased to 12.5 mg twice daily; dosage may be increased to a maximum of 25 mg twice daily after 1-2 weeks; reduce dosage if heart rate drops <55 beats/minute
Congestive heart failure: 12.5-50 mg twice daily
Angina pectoris: 25-50 mg twice daily
Idiopathic cardiomyopathy: 6.25-25 mg twice daily

Dosing adjustment in renal impairment: None necessary

Dosing adjustment in hepatic impairment: Use is contraindicated in liver dysfunction

Monitoring Parameters Heart rate, blood pressure (base need for dosage increase on trough blood pressure measurements and for tolerance on standing systolic pressure 1 hour after dosing)

Patient Information Take with food to minimize the risk of hypotension; do not interrupt or discontinue using carvedilol without a physician's advice; use care to avoid standing abruptly or standing still for long periods; lie down if dizziness or faintness occurs and consult a physician for a reduced dosage; contact lens wearers may experience dry eyes

Nursing Implications Minimize risk of bradycardia with initiation of treatment with a low dose, slow upward titration, and administration with food; decrease dose if pulse rate drops <55 beats per minute

Dosage Forms Tablet: 6.25 mg, 12.5 mg, 25 mg

Cascara Sagrada (kas KAR a sah GRAH dah)

Related Information

Laxatives, Classification and Properties *on page 1412*

Therapeutic Category Laxative, Stimulant

Use Temporary relief of constipation; sometimes used with milk of magnesia ("black and white" mixture)

Pregnancy Risk Factor C

Contraindications Nausea, vomiting, abdominal pain, fecal impaction, intestinal obstruction, GI bleeding, appendicitis, congestive heart failure

Warnings/Precautions Excessive use can lead to electrolyte imbalance, fluid imbalance, vitamin deficiency, steatorrhea, osteomalacia, cathartic colon, and dependence; should be avoided during nursing because it may have a laxative effect on the infant

Adverse Reactions

1% to 10%:
- Central nervous system: Faintness
- Endocrine & metabolic: Electrolyte and fluid imbalance
- Gastrointestinal: Abdominal cramps, nausea, diarrhea
- Genitourinary: Discoloration of urine (reddish pink or brown)

Drug Interactions Decreased effect of oral anticoagulants

Stability Protect from light and heat

Mechanism of Action Direct chemical irritation of the intestinal mucosa resulting in an increased rate of colonic motility and change in fluid and electrolyte secretion

Pharmacodynamics/Kinetics

Onset of action: 6-10 hours
Absorption: Oral: Small amount absorbed from small intestine
Metabolism: In the liver

Usual Dosage Note: Cascara sagrada fluid extract is 5 times more potent than cascara sagrada aromatic fluid extract

Oral (aromatic fluid extract):
- Infants: 1.25 mL/day (range: 0.5-1.5 mL) as needed
- Children 2-11 years: 2.5 mL/day (range: 1-3 mL) as needed
- Children ≥12 years and Adults: 5 mL/day (range: 2-6 mL) as needed at bedtime (1 tablet as needed at bedtime)

Test Interactions ↓ calcium (S), ↓ potassium (S)

Patient Information Should not be used regularly for more than 1 week

Dosage Forms

Aromatic fluid extract: 120 mL, 473 mL
Tablet: 325 mg

Casodex® *see* Bicalutamide *on page 152*

Castor Oil (KAS tor oyl)

Related Information

Laxatives, Classification and Properties *on page 1412*

Brand Names Alphamul® [OTC]; Emulsoil® [OTC]; Fleet® Flavored Castor Oil [OTC]; Neoloid® [OTC]; Purge® [OTC]

Synonyms Oleum Ricini

Therapeutic Category Laxative, Stimulant

Use Preparation for rectal or bowel examination or surgery; rarely used to relieve constipation; also applied to skin as emollient and protectant

Pregnancy Risk Factor X

Contraindications Known hypersensitivity to castor oil; nausea, vomiting, abdominal pain, fecal impaction, GI bleeding, appendicitis, congestive heart failure, menstruation, dehydration

Warnings/Precautions Use only when a prompt and thorough catharsis is desired; use with caution during menstruation

Adverse Reactions

1% to 10%:

- Central nervous system: Dizziness
- Endocrine & metabolic: Electrolyte disturbance
- Gastrointestinal: Abdominal cramps, nausea, diarrhea

<1%: Genitourinary: Pelvic congestion

Stability Protect from heat (castor oil emulsion should be protected from freezing)

Mechanism of Action Acts primarily in the small intestine; hydrolyzed to ricinoleic acid which reduces net absorption of fluid and electrolytes and stimulates peristalsis

Pharmacodynamics/Kinetics Onset of action: Oral: 2-6 hours

Usual Dosage Oral:

Liquid:

- Infants <2 years: 1-5 mL or 15 mL/m²/dose as a single dose
- Children 2-11 years: 5-15 mL as a single dose
- Children ≥12 years and Adults: 15-60 mL as a single dose

Emulsified:

- 36.4%:
  - Infants: 2.5-7.5 mL/dose
  - Children <2 years: 5-15 mL/dose
  - Children 2-11 years: 7.5-30 mL/dose
  - Children ≥12 years and Adults: 30-60 mL/dose
- 60% to 67%:
  - Children <2 years: 1.25-5 mL
  - Children 2-12 years: 5-15 mL
  - Adults: 15-45 mL
- 95%, mix with ½ to 1 full glass liquid:
  - Children: 5-10 mL
  - Adults: 15-60 mL

Administration Do not administer at bedtime because of rapid onset of action

Patient Information Chill or take with juice or carbonated beverage to improve taste

Dosage Forms

Emulsion, oral:

- Alphamul®: 60% (90 mL, 3780 mL)
- Emulsoil®: 95% (63 mL)
- Fleet® Flavored Castor Oil: 67% (45 mL, 90 mL)
- Neoloid®: 36.4% (118 mL)

Liquid, oral:

- 100% (60 mL, 120 mL, 480 mL)
- Purge®: 95% (30 mL, 60 mL)

Cataflam® *see* Diclofenac *on page 373*

Catapres® *see* Clonidine *on page 299*

Catapres-TTS® *see* Clonidine *on page 299*

Caverject® Injection *see* Alprostadil *on page 51*

CBDCA *see* Carboplatin *on page 206*

CCNU *see* Lomustine *on page 738*

C-Crystals® [OTC] *see* Ascorbic Acid *on page 102*

2-CdA *see* Cladribine *on page 285*

CDDP *see* Cisplatin *on page 282*

Cebid® Timecelles® [OTC] *see* Ascorbic Acid *on page 102*

Ceclor® *see* Cefaclor *on next page*

Ceclor CD® *see* Cefaclor *on next page*

Cecon® [OTC] *see* Ascorbic Acid *on page 102*

Cedax® *see* Ceftibuten *on page 233*

CeeNU® *see* Lomustine *on page 738*

Cefaclor (SEF a klor)

Related Information

Antimicrobial Drugs of Choice *on page 1468*
Cephalosporins by Generation *on page 1447*

Brand Names Ceclor®; Ceclor CD®

Therapeutic Category Antibiotic, Cephalosporin (Second Generation)

Use Infections caused by susceptible organisms including *Staphylococcus aureus* and *H. influenzae*; treatment of otitis media, sinusitis, and infections involving the respiratory tract, skin and skin structure, bone and joint, and urinary tract

Pregnancy Risk Factor B

Contraindications Hypersensitivity to cefaclor, any component, or cephalosporins

Warnings/Precautions Modify dosage in patients with severe renal impairment; prolonged use may result in superinfection; a low incidence of cross-hypersensitivity to penicillins exists

Adverse Reactions

1% to 10%: Gastrointestinal: Pseudomembranous colitis, diarrhea

<1%:

- Dermatologic: Rash, urticaria, pruritus, Stevens-Johnson syndrome
- Gastrointestinal: Nausea, vomiting
- Hematologic: Eosinophilia, hemolytic anemia, neutropenia, positive Coombs' test
- Hepatic: Cholestatic jaundice, slight elevation of AST, ALT
- Neuromuscular & skeletal: Arthralgia

Overdosage/Toxicology Symptoms of overdose include neuromuscular hypersensitivity, convulsions

Hemodialysis may be helpful to aid in the removal of the drug from the blood, otherwise most treatment is supportive or symptom directed

Drug Interactions

Increased effect: Probenecid may decrease cephalosporin elimination

Increased toxicity: Furosemide, aminoglycosides may be a possible additive to nephrotoxicity

Stability Refrigerate suspension after reconstitution; discard after 14 days; do not freeze

Mechanism of Action Inhibits bacterial cell wall synthesis by binding to one or more of the penicillin-binding proteins (PBPs) which in turn inhibits the final transpeptidation step of peptidoglycan synthesis in bacterial cell walls, thus inhibiting cell wall biosynthesis. Bacteria eventually lyse due to ongoing activity of cell wall autolytic enzymes (autolysins and murein hydrolases) while cell wall assembly is arrested.

Pharmacodynamics/Kinetics

Peak serum levels:

- Capsule: 60 minutes
- Suspension: 45 minutes

Absorption: Oral: Well absorbed, acid stable

Distribution: Crosses the placenta; appears in breast milk

Protein binding: 25%

Metabolism: Partially

Half-life: 0.5-1 hour, prolonged with renal impairment

Elimination: 80% excreted unchanged in urine

Usual Dosage Oral:

Children >1 month: 20-40 mg/kg/day divided every 8-12 hours; maximum dose: 2 g/day (total daily dose may be divided into two doses for treatment of otitis media or pharyngitis)

Adults: 250-500 mg every 8 hours

- Extended release tablets: 500 mg every 12 hours for 7 days for acute bacterial exacerbations of or secondary infections with chronic bronchitis or 375 mg every 12 hour for 10 days for pharyngitis or tonsillitis or for uncomplicated skin and skin structure infections

Dosing adjustment in renal impairment: Cl_{cr} <50 mL/minute: Administer 50% of dose

Hemodialysis: Moderately dialyzable (20% to 50%)

Administration Administer around-the-clock rather than 3 times/day to promote less variation in peak and trough serum levels

Monitoring Parameters Assess patient at beginning and throughout therapy for infection

Test Interactions Positive Coombs' [direct], false-positive urine glucose (Clinitest®)

Patient Information Chilling of the oral suspension improves flavor (do not freeze); report persistent diarrhea; entire course of medication (10-14 days)
(Continued)

Cefaclor *(Continued)*

should be taken to ensure eradication of organism; should be taken in equal intervals around-the-clock to maintain adequate blood levels; may interfere with oral contraceptives; females should report symptoms of vaginitis

Dosage Forms

Capsule: 250 mg, 500 mg

Powder for oral suspension (strawberry flavor): 125 mg/5 mL (75 mL, 150 mL); 187 mg/5 mL (50 mL, 100 mL); 250 mg/5 mL (75 mL, 150 mL); 375 mg/5 mL (50 mL, 100 mL)

Tablet, extended release: 375 mg, 500 mg

Cefadroxil (sef a DROKS il)

Related Information

Cephalosporins by Generation *on page 1447*

Brand Names Duricef®; Ultracef®

Canadian/Mexican Brand Names Cefamox® (Mexico); Duracef® (Mexico)

Synonyms Cefadroxil Monohydrate

Therapeutic Category Antibiotic, Cephalosporin (First Generation)

Use Treatment of susceptible bacterial infections, including those caused by group A beta-hemolytic *Streptococcus*

Pregnancy Risk Factor B

Contraindications Hypersensitivity to cefadroxil or other cephalosporins

Warnings/Precautions Modify dosage in patients with severe renal impairment; prolonged use may result in superinfection; a low incidence of cross-hypersensitivity to penicillins exists

Adverse Reactions

1% to 10%: Gastrointestinal: Diarrhea

<1%:

- Central nervous system: Fatigue, chills
- Dermatologic: Maculopapular and erythematous rash
- Gastrointestinal: Dyspepsia, pseudomembranous colitis, nausea, vomiting, heartburn, gastritis, bloating
- Hematologic: Neutropenia
- Miscellaneous: Superinfections

Overdosage/Toxicology Symptoms of overdose include neuromuscular hypersensitivity, convulsions

Hemodialysis may be helpful to aid in the removal of the drug from the blood, otherwise most treatment is supportive or symptom directed

Drug Interactions

Increased effect: Probenecid may decrease cephalosporin elimination

Increased toxicity: Furosemide, aminoglycosides may be a possible additive to nephrotoxicity

Stability Refrigerate suspension after reconstitution; discard after 14 days

Mechanism of Action Inhibits bacterial cell wall synthesis by binding to one or more of the penicillin-binding proteins (PBPs) which in turn inhibits the final transpeptidation step of peptidoglycan synthesis in bacterial cell walls, thus inhibiting cell wall biosynthesis. Bacteria eventually lyse due to ongoing activity of cell wall autolytic enzymes (autolysins and murein hydrolases) while cell wall assembly is arrested.

Pharmacodynamics/Kinetics

Absorption: Oral: Rapid and well absorbed from GI tract

Distribution: V_d: 0.31 L/kg; crosses the placenta; appears in breast milk

Protein binding: 20%

Half-life: 1-2 hours; 20-24 hours in renal failure

Time to peak serum concentration: Within 70-90 minutes

Elimination: >90% of dose excreted unchanged in urine within 8 hours

Usual Dosage Oral:

Children: 30 mg/kg/day divided twice daily up to a maximum of 2 g/day

Adults: 1-2 g/day in 2 divided doses

Dosing interval in renal impairment:

Cl_{cr} 10-25 mL/minute: Administer every 24 hours

Cl_{cr} <10 mL/minute: Administer every 36 hours

Administration Administer around-the-clock to promote less variation in peak and trough serum levels

Test Interactions Positive Coombs' [direct], glucose, protein; ↓ glucose

Patient Information Report persistent diarrhea; entire course of medication (10-14 days) should be taken to ensure eradication of organism; should be taken in equal intervals around-the-clock to maintain adequate blood levels; may interfere with oral contraceptives; females should report symptoms of vaginitis

Dosage Forms

Capsule, as monohydrate: 500 mg

Suspension, oral, as monohydrate: 125 mg/5 mL, 250 mg/5 mL, 500 mg/5 mL (50 mL, 100 mL)

Tablet, as monohydrate: 1 g

Cefadroxil Monohydrate *see* Cefadroxil *on previous page*

Cefadyl® *see* Cephapirin *on page 242*

Cefamandole (sef a MAN dole)

Related Information

Cephalosporins by Generation *on page 1447*

Brand Names Mandol®

Synonyms Cefamandole Nafate

Therapeutic Category Antibiotic, Cephalosporin (Second Generation)

Use Treatment of susceptible bacterial infection; mainly respiratory tract, skin and skin structure, bone and joint, urinary tract and gynecologic, as well as, septicemia

Pregnancy Risk Factor B

Contraindications Hypersensitivity to cefamandole nafate, any component, or cephalosporins

Warnings/Precautions Modify dosage in patients with severe renal impairment; prolonged use may result in superinfection; a low incidence of cross-hypersensitivity to penicillins exists

Adverse Reactions

1% to 10%: Gastrointestinal: Diarrhea

<1%:

- Central nervous system: CNS irritation, seizures, fever
- Dermatologic: Rash, urticaria
- Gastrointestinal: Abdominal cramps, pseudomembraneous colitis
- Hematologic: Eosinophilia, hypoprothrombinemia, leukopenia, thrombocytopenia
- Hepatic: Transient elevation of liver enzymes, cholestatic jaundice
- Local: Pain at injection site
- Miscellaneous: Superinfections

Overdosage/Toxicology Symptoms of overdose include neuromuscular hypersensitivity, convulsions

Hemodialysis may be helpful to aid in the removal of the drug from the blood, otherwise most treatment is supportive or symptom directed

Drug Interactions

Disulfiram-like reaction has been reported when taken within 72 hours of alcohol consumption

Increased cefamandole plasma levels: Probenecid

Increased nephrotoxicity: Aminoglycosides, furosemide

Hypoprothrombinemic effect increased: Warfarin and heparin

Stability After reconstitution, CO_2 gas is liberated which allows solution to be withdrawn without injecting air; solution is stable for 24 hours at room temperature and 96 hours when refrigerated; for I.V., infusion in NS and D_5W is stable for 24 hours at room temperature, 1 week when refrigerated, or 26 weeks when frozen

Mechanism of Action Inhibits bacterial cell wall synthesis by binding to one or more of the penicillin-binding proteins (PBPs) which in turn inhibits the final transpeptidation step of peptidoglycan synthesis in bacterial cell walls, thus inhibiting cell wall biosynthesis. Bacteria eventually lyse due to ongoing activity of cell wall autolytic enzymes (autolysins and murein hydrolases) while cell wall assembly is arrested.

Pharmacodynamics/Kinetics

Time to peak serum concentration:

- I.M.: Within 1-2 hours
- I.V.: Within 10 minutes

Distribution: Distributes well throughout body, except CSF; poor penetration even with inflamed meninges; extensive enterohepatic circulation; high concentrations in the bile

Protein binding: 56% to 78%

Half-life: 30-60 minutes

Elimination: Extensive enterohepatic circulation; high concentrations in bile; majority of drug excreted unchanged in urine

Usual Dosage I.M., I.V.:

Children: 100-150 mg/kg/day in divided doses every 4-6 hours

Adults: 4-12 g/24 hours divided every 4-6 hours or 500-1000 mg every 4-8 hours; maximum: 2 g/dose

Dosing interval in renal impairment:

- Cl_{cr} 25-50 mL/minute: 1-2 g every 8 hours
- Cl_{cr} 10-25 mL/minute: 1 g every 8 hours

(Continued)

Cefamandole *(Continued)*

Cl_{cr} <10 mL/minute: 1 g every 12 hours

Hemodialysis: Moderately dialyzable (20% to 50%)

Administration Administer around-the-clock to promote less variation in peak and trough serum levels

Monitoring Parameters Monitor for signs of bruising or bleeding

Test Interactions ↑ alkaline phosphatase, AST, ALT, BUN, creatinine, prothrombin time (S), glucose, protein; ↓ glucose; positive Coombs' [direct]

Additional Information Sodium content of 1 g: 3.3 mEq

Dosage Forms Powder for injection, as nafate: 500 mg (10 mL); 1 g (10 mL, 100 mL); 2 g (20 mL, 100 mL); 10 g (100 mL)

Cefamandole Nafate *see* Cefamandole *on previous page*

Cefazolin (sef A zoe lin)

Related Information

Animal and Human Bites Guidelines *on page 1463*

Antibiotic Treatment of Adults With Infectious Endocarditis *on page 1465*

Antimicrobial Prophylaxis *on page 1445*

Cephalosporins by Generation *on page 1447*

Brand Names Ancef®; Kefzol®; Zolicef®

Canadian/Mexican Brand Names Cefamezin® (Mexico)

Synonyms Cefazolin Sodium

Therapeutic Category Antibiotic, Cephalosporin (First Generation)

Use Treatment of gram-positive bacilli and cocci (except enterococcus); some gram-negative bacilli including *E. coli*, *Proteus*, and *Klebsiella* may be susceptible

Pregnancy Risk Factor B

Contraindications Hypersensitivity to cefazolin sodium, any component, or cephalosporins

Warnings/Precautions Modify dosage in patients with severe renal impairment; prolonged use may result in superinfection; a low incidence of cross-hypersensitivity to penicillins exists

Adverse Reactions

1% to 10%: Gastrointestinal: Diarrhea

<1%:

Central nervous system: CNS irritation, seizures, confusion, fever

Dermatologic: Rash, urticaria

Hematologic: Leukopenia, thrombocytopenia, neutropenia

Hepatic: Transient elevation of liver enzymes, cholestatic jaundice

Miscellaneous: Superinfections

Overdosage/Toxicology Symptoms of overdose include neuromuscular hypersensitivity, convulsions; many beta-lactam containing antibiotics have the potential to cause neuromuscular hyperirritability or convulsive seizures

Hemodialysis may be helpful to aid in the removal of the drug from the blood, otherwise most treatment is supportive or symptom directed.

Drug Interactions

Increased effect: High-dose probenecid decreases clearance

Increased toxicity: Aminoglycosides increase nephrotoxic potential

Stability

Store intact vials at room temperature and protect from temperatures exceeding 40°C

Reconstituted solutions of cefazolin are light yellow to yellow

Protection from light is recommended for the powder and for the reconstituted solutions

Reconstituted solutions are stable for 24 hours at room temperature and 10 days under refrigeration

Stability of parenteral admixture at room temperature (25°C): 48 hours

Stability of parenteral admixture at refrigeration temperature (4°C): 14 days

Standard diluent: 1 g/50 mL D_5W; 2 g/50 mL D_5W

Mechanism of Action Inhibits bacterial cell wall synthesis by binding to one or more of the penicillin-binding proteins (PBPs) which in turn inhibits the final transpeptidation step of peptidoglycan synthesis in bacterial cell walls, thus inhibiting cell wall biosynthesis. Bacteria eventually lyse due to ongoing activity of cell wall autolytic enzymes (autolysins and murein hydrolases) while cell wall assembly is arrested.

Pharmacodynamics/Kinetics

Time to peak serum concentration:

I.M.: Within 0.5-2 hours

I.V.: Within 5 minutes

Distribution: Crosses the placenta; small amounts appear in breast milk; CSF penetration is poor

Protein binding: 74% to 86%
Metabolism: Hepatic is minimal
Half-life: 90-150 minutes (prolonged with renal impairment)
End stage renal disease: 40-70 hours
Elimination: 80% to 100% is excreted unchanged in urine

Usual Dosage I.M., I.V.:
Children >1 month: 50-100 mg/kg/day divided every 8 hours; maximum: 6 g/day
Adults: 1-2 g every 8 hours, depending on severity of infection; maximum dose: 12 g/day

Dosing adjustment in renal impairment:
Cl_{cr} 10-30 mL/minute: Administer every 12 hours
Cl_{cr} <10 mL/minute: Administer every 24 hours
Hemodialysis: Moderately dialyzable (20% to 50%); administer dose postdialysis or administer supplemental dose of 0.5-1 g after dialysis
Peritoneal dialysis: Administer 0.5 g every 12 hours
Continuous arterio-venous or veno-venous hemofiltration (CAVH/CAVHD): Removes 30 mg of cefazolin per liter of filtrate per day

Administration Administer around-the-clock rather than 3 times/day to promote less variation in peak and trough serum levels

Monitoring Parameters Renal function periodically when used in combination with other nephrotoxic drugs, hepatic function tests, CBC

Test Interactions False-positive urine glucose using Clinitest®, positive Coombs' [direct], false increase serum or urine creatinine

Additional Information Sodium content of 1 g: 47 mg (2 mEq)

Dosage Forms
Infusion, premixed, as sodium, in D_5W (frozen) (Ancef®): 500 mg (50 mL); 1 g (50 mL)
Injection, as sodium (Kefzol®): 500 mg, 1 g
Powder for injection, as sodium (Ancef®, Zolicef®): 250 mg, 500 mg, 1 g, 5 g, 10 g, 20 g

Cefazolin Sodium *see* Cefazolin *on previous page*

Cefepime (SEF e pim)

Related Information
Cephalosporins by Generation *on page 1447*

Brand Names Maxipime®

Synonyms Cefepime Hydrochloride

Therapeutic Category Antibiotic, Cephalosporin (Fourth Generation)

Use Treatment of respiratory tract infections (including bronchitis and pneumonia), cellulitis and other skin and soft tissue infections, and urinary tract infections; considered a fourth generation cephalosporin because it has good gram-negative coverage similar to third generation cephalosporins, but better gram-positive coverage

Pregnancy Risk Factor C

Contraindications Hypersensitivity to cefepime or its components, or other cephalosporins

Warnings/Precautions Modify dosage in patients with severe renal impairment; prolonged use may result in superinfection; a low incidence of cross-hypersensitivity to penicillins exists

Adverse Reactions
1% to 10%:
Central nervous system: Headache, lightheadedness
Gastrointestinal: Dyspepsia, antibiotic-associated diarrhea
Hepatic: Transient elevations in LFTs
Local: Phlebitis
Ocular: Blurred vision

Overdosage/Toxicology Symptoms of overdose include neuromuscular hypersensitivity, convulsions; hemodialysis may be helpful to aid in the removal of the drug from the blood; however, most often treatment is supportive and symptom directed

Drug Interactions
Increased effect: High-dose probenecid decreases clearance
Increased toxicity: Aminoglycosides increase nephrotoxic potential

Mechanism of Action Inhibits bacterial cell wall synthesis by binding to one or more of the penicillin-binding proteins (PBPs) which in turn inhibits the final transpeptidation step of peptidoglycan synthesis in bacterial cell walls, thus inhibiting cell wall biosynthesis. Bacterial eventually lyse due to ongoing activity of cell wall autolytic enzymes (autolysis and murein hydrolases) while cell wall assembly is arrested.

Pharmacodynamics/Kinetics
Absorption: I.M.: Rapid and complete; T_{max}: 0.5-1.5 hours
(Continued)

Cefepime *(Continued)*

Distribution: V_d: Adults: 14-20 L; penetrates into inflammatory fluid at concentrations ~80% of serum levels and into bronchial mucosa at levels ~60% of those reached in the plasma
Protein binding, plasma: 16% to 19%
Metabolism: Very little
Half-life: 2 hours
Elimination: Nearly completely eliminated as unchanged drug in urine

Usual Dosage I.V.:
Children: **Unlabeled**: 50 mg/kg every 8 hours; maximum dose: 2 g
Adults:
Most infections: 1-2 g every 12 hours for 5-10 days; higher doses or more frequent administration may be required in pseudomonal infections
Urinary tract infections, uncomplicated: 500 mg every 12 hours

Dosing adjustment in renal impairment:
Cl_{cr} 10-30 mL/minute: Administer 500 mg every 24 hours
Cl_{cr} <10 mL/minute: Administer 250 mg every 24 hours
Hemodialysis: Removed by dialysis; administer supplemental dose of 250 mg after each dialysis session
Peritoneal dialysis: Removed to a lesser extent than hemodialysis; administer 250 mg every 48 hours

Monitoring Parameters Obtain specimen for culture and sensitivity prior to the first dose

Test Interactions As with other cephalosporins; false-positive Coombs' test; may falsely elevate creatinine values when Jaffé reaction is used; may cause false-positive results in urine glucose tests when using cupric sulfate (Benedict's solution, Clinitest®), false-positive urinary proteins and steroids

Patient Information Report side effects such as diarrhea, dyspepsia, headache, blurred vision, and lightheadedness to your physician

Nursing Implications Do not admix with aminoglycosides in the same bottle/bag; observe for signs and symptoms of bacterial infection, including defervescence; observe for anaphylaxis during first dose

Dosage Forms Powder for injection, as hydrochloride: 500 mg, 1 g, 2 g

Cefepime Hydrochloride *see* Cefepime *on previous page*

Cefixime (sef IKS eem)

Related Information
Antimicrobial Drugs of Choice *on page 1468*
Cephalosporins by Generation *on page 1447*

Brand Names Suprax®

Therapeutic Category Antibiotic, Cephalosporin (Third Generation)

Use Treatment of urinary tract infections caused by *E. coli* and *P. mirabilis*, otitis media due to *H. influenzae (beta-lactamase (+) and (-) strains), M. catarrhalis and S. pyogenes*, pharyngitis, and tonsillitis due to *S. pyogenes*, acute bronchitis and acute exacerbations of chronic bronchitis due to *S. pneumoniae* and *H. influenzae* and uncomplicated cervical/urethral gonorrhea due to *N. gonorrhea* (penicillinase and nonpenicillinase producing); advantages include outpatient therapy of serious soft tissue or skeletal infections due to susceptible organisms and single-dose oral treatment of uncomplicated gonorrhea; has been used in treatment of shigellosis in areas with a high rate of resistance to TMP-SMX

Pregnancy Risk Factor B

Contraindications Hypersensitivity to cefixime or cephalosporins

Warnings/Precautions Prolonged use may result in superinfection

Adverse Reactions
Central nervous system: Fever, headache, dizziness, malaise, somnolence
Dermatologic: Skin rash
Gastrointestinal: Nausea, diarrhea, abdominal pain, flatulence, dyspepsia, pseudomembranous colitis
Hematologic: Transient thrombocytopenia, leukopenia, eosinophilia, and decreased hemoglobin and hematocrit
Hepatic: Transient elevation of liver enzymes
Renal: Transient elevation of BUN or creatinine

Drug Interactions Probenecid (increases cefixime concentration)

Stability After reconstitution, suspension may be stored for 14 days at room temperature

Mechanism of Action Inhibits bacterial cell wall synthesis by binding to one or more of the penicillin-binding proteins; inhibits the final transpeptidation step of peptidoglycan synthesis resulting in cell wall death

Pharmacodynamics/Kinetics
Absorption: Oral: 40% to 50%
Distribution: Into bile, sputum, middle ear discharge; crosses the placenta

Protein binding: 65%
Half-life:
Normal renal function: 3-4 hours
Renal failure: Up to 11.5 hours
Time to peak serum concentrations: Within 2-6 hours; peak serum concentrations are 15% to 50% higher for the oral suspension versus tablets; presence of food delays the time to reach peak concentrations
Elimination: 50% of absorbed dose excreted as active drug in urine and 10% in bile
10% removed by hemodialysis

Usual Dosage Oral:
Children: 8 mg/kg/day divided every 12-24 hours; maximum dose: 400 mg/day
Adolescents and Adults: 400 mg/day divided every 12-24 hours
Uncomplicated cervical/urethral gonorrhea due to *N. gonorrhoeae*: 400 mg as a single dose
For *S. pyogenes* infections, treat for 10 days; use suspension for otitis media due to increased peak serum levels as compared to tablet form

Dosing adjustment in renal impairment:
Cl_{cr} 21-60 mL/minute or with renal hemodialysis: Administer 75% of the standard dose
Cl_{cr} <20 mL/minute or with CAPD: Administer 50% of the standard dose

Administration Oral: May be administered with or without food; administer with food to decrease GI distress

Monitoring Parameters With prolonged therapy, monitor renal and hepatic function periodically

Test Interactions False-positive reaction for urine glucose using Clinitest®; false-positive urine ketones using tests with nitroprusside

Patient Information Report problems with diarrhea

Additional Information Otitis media should be treated with the suspension since it results in higher peak blood levels than the tablet

Dosage Forms
Powder for oral suspension (strawberry flavor): 100 mg/5 mL (50 mL, 100 mL)
Tablet, film coated: 200 mg, 400 mg

Cefizox® *see* Ceftizoxime *on page 235*

Cefmetazole (sef MET a zole)

Related Information
Antimicrobial Drugs of Choice *on page 1468*
Cephalosporins by Generation *on page 1447*

Brand Names Zefazone®

Synonyms Cefmetazole Sodium

Therapeutic Category Antibiotic, Cephalosporin (Second Generation)

Use Second generation cephalosporin with an antibacterial spectrum similar to cefoxitin, useful on many aerobic and anaerobic gram-positive and gram-negative bacteria

Pregnancy Risk Factor B

Contraindications Hypersensitivity to cefmetazole or any component or cephalosporins

Warnings/Precautions Modify dosage in patients with severe renal impairment; prolonged use may result in superinfection; a low incidence of cross-hypersensitivity to penicillins exists

Adverse Reactions
1% to 10%:
Dermatologic: Rash
Gastrointestinal: Diarrhea, nausea
<1%:
Cardiovascular: Shock, hypotension
Central nervous system: Headache, fever
Endocrine & metabolic: Hot flashes
Gastrointestinal: Epigastric pain, pseudomembraneous colitis
Genitourinary: Vaginitis
Hematologic: Hypoprothrombinemia, anemia
Local: Pain at injection site, phlebitis
Respiratory: Respiratory distress, dyspnea, epistaxis
Miscellaneous: Alteration of color, candidiasis

Overdosage/Toxicology Symptoms of overdose include neuromuscular hypersensitivity, convulsions; many beta-lactam containing antibiotics have the potential to cause neuromuscular hyperirritability or convulsive seizures

Hemodialysis may be helpful to aid in the removal of the drug from the blood, otherwise most treatment is supportive or symptom directed.
(Continued)

Cefmetazole *(Continued)*

Drug Interactions

Increased effect: Probenecid may decrease cephalosporin elimination

Increased toxicity: Furosemide, aminoglycosides may be a possible additive to nephrotoxicity

Stability Reconstituted solution and I.V. infusion in NS or D_5W solution are stable for 24 hours at room temperature, 7 days when refrigerated, or 6 weeks when frozen; after freezing, thawed solution is stable for 24 hours at room temperature or 7 days when refrigerated

Mechanism of Action Inhibits bacterial cell wall synthesis by binding to one or more of the penicillin-binding proteins (PBPs) which in turn inhibits the final transpeptidation step of peptidoglycan synthesis in bacterial cell walls, thus inhibiting cell wall biosynthesis. Bacteria eventually lyse due to ongoing activity of cell wall autolytic enzymes (autolysins and murein hydrolases) while cell wall assembly is arrested.

Pharmacodynamics/Kinetics

Protein binding: 65%

Metabolism: <15%

Half-life: 72 minutes

Elimination: Renal

Usual Dosage Adults: I.V.:

Infections: 2 g every 6-12 hours for 5-14 days

Prophylaxis: 2 g 30-90 minutes before surgery **or** 1 g 30-90 minutes before surgery; repeat 8 and 16 hours later

Dosing interval in renal impairment:

Cl_{cr} 50-90 mL/minute: Administer every 12 hours

Cl_{cr} 10-50 mL/minute: Administer every 16-24 hours

Cl_{cr} <10 mL/minute: Administer every 48 hours

Administration Administer around-the-clock rather than 2 times/day to promote less variation in peak and trough serum levels

Monitoring Parameters Monitor prothrombin times

Patient Information Do not drink alcohol for at least 24 hours after receiving dose; report persistent diarrhea; may interfere with oral contraceptives, females should report symptoms of vaginitis

Nursing Implications Do not admix with aminoglycosides in same bottle/bag

Additional Information Sodium content of 1 g: 2 mEq

Dosage Forms Powder for injection, as sodium: 1 g, 2 g

Cefmetazole Sodium *see* Cefmetazole *on previous page*

Cefobid® *see* Cefoperazone *on next page*

Cefol® Filmtab® *see* Vitamins, Multiple *on page 1310*

Cefonicid (se FON i sid)

Related Information

Cephalosporins by Generation *on page 1447*

Brand Names Monocid®

Canadian/Mexican Brand Names Monocidur® (Mexico)

Synonyms Cefonicid Sodium

Therapeutic Category Antibiotic, Cephalosporin (Second Generation)

Use Treatment of susceptible bacterial infection; mainly respiratory tract, skin and skin structure, bone and joint, urinary tract and gynecologic, as well as, septicemia; second generation cephalosporin

Pregnancy Risk Factor B

Contraindications Hypersensitivity to cefonicid sodium, any component, or cephalosporins

Warnings/Precautions Modify dosage in patients with severe renal impairment; prolonged use may result in superinfection; a low incidence of cross-hypersensitivity to penicillins exists

Adverse Reactions

1% to 10%:

Local: Pain at injection site

Hematologic: Increased platelets and eosinophils

Hepatic: Liver function alterations

<1%:

Central nervous system: Fever, headache

Dermatologic: Rash

Gastrointestinal: Nausea, diarrhea, abdominal pain, pseudomembranous colitis

Hematologic: Increased platelets and eosinophils

Hepatic: Transient elevation in liver enzymes

Renal: Transient elevation of BUN/creatinine

Overdosage/Toxicology Symptoms of overdose include neuromuscular hypersensitivity, convulsions

Hemodialysis may be helpful to aid in the removal of the drug from the blood, otherwise most treatment is supportive or symptom directed

Drug Interactions

Increased effect: Probenecid may decrease cephalosporin elimination

Increased toxicity: Furosemide, aminoglycosides may be a possible additive to nephrotoxicity

Stability Reconstituted solution and I.V. infusion in NS or D_5W solution are stable for 24 hours at room temperature or 72 hours if refrigerated

Mechanism of Action Inhibits bacterial cell wall synthesis by binding to one or more of the penicillin-binding proteins (PBPs) which in turn inhibits the final transpeptidation step of peptidoglycan synthesis in bacterial cell walls, thus inhibiting cell wall biosynthesis. Bacteria eventually lyse due to ongoing activity of cell wall autolytic enzymes (autolysins and murein hydrolases) while cell wall assembly is arrested.

Pharmacodynamics/Kinetics

Protein binding: 98%

Metabolism: None

Half-life: 6-7 hours

Elimination: Renal

Usual Dosage Adults: I.M., I.V.: 0.5-2 g every 24 hours

Prophylaxis: Preop: 1 g/hour

Dosing interval in renal impairment: See table.

Cefonicid Sodium

Cl_{cr} (mL/min/1.73 m^2)	Dose (mg/kg) for each dosing interval
60-79	10-24 q24h
40-59	8-20 q24h
20-39	4-15 q24h
10-19	4-15 q48h
5-9	4-15 q3-5d
<5	3-4 q3-5d

Administration Administer around-the-clock rather than 3 times/day to promote less variation in peak and trough serum levels

Additional Information Sodium content of 1 g: 3.7 mEq

Dosage Forms Powder for injection, as sodium: 500 mg, 1 g, 10 g

Cefonicid Sodium *see* Cefonicid *on previous page*

Cefoperazone (sef oh PER a zone)

Related Information

Cephalosporins by Generation *on page 1447*

Brand Names Cefobid®

Synonyms Cefoperazone Sodium

Therapeutic Category Antibiotic, Cephalosporin (Third Generation)

Use Treatment of susceptible bacterial infection; mainly respiratory tract, skin and skin structure, bone and joint, urinary tract and gynecologic, as well as, septicemia

Pregnancy Risk Factor B

Contraindications Hypersensitivity to cefoperazone or any component or cephalosporins

Warnings/Precautions Modify dosage in patients with severe renal impairment; prolonged use may result in superinfection; a low incidence of cross-hypersensitivity to penicillins exists

Adverse Reactions

1% to 10%: Gastrointestinal: Diarrhea

<1%:

- Dermatologic: Maculopapular and erythematous rash
- Gastrointestinal: Dyspepsia, pseudomembranous colitis, nausea, vomiting
- Hematologic: Hypoprothrombinemia
- Local: Pain and induration at injection site

Overdosage/Toxicology Symptoms of overdose include neuromuscular hypersensitivity, convulsions

Hemodialysis may be helpful to aid in the removal of the drug from the blood, otherwise most treatment is supportive or symptom directed

Stability Reconstituted solution and I.V. infusion in NS or D_5W solution are stable for 24 hours at room temperature, 5 days when refrigerated or 3 weeks, when

(Continued)

Cefoperazone *(Continued)*

frozen; after freezing, thawed solution is stable for 48 hours at room temperature or 10 days when refrigerated

Mechanism of Action Inhibits bacterial cell wall synthesis by binding to one or more of the penicillin-binding proteins (PBPs) which in turn inhibits the final transpeptidation step of peptidoglycan synthesis in bacterial cell walls, thus inhibiting cell wall biosynthesis. Bacteria eventually lyse due to ongoing activity of cell wall autolytic enzymes (autolysins and murein hydrolases) while cell wall assembly is arrested.

Pharmacodynamics/Kinetics

Distribution: Widely distributed in most body tissues and fluids; highest concentrations in bile; low penetration in CSF; variable when meninges are inflamed; crosses placenta; small amounts into breast milk

Half-life: 2 hours, higher with hepatic disease or biliary obstruction

Time to peak serum concentration:

I.M.: Within 1-2 hours

I.V.: Within 15-20 minutes (serum levels 2-3 times the serum levels following I.M. administration)

Elimination: Principally in bile (70% to 75%); 20% to 30% recovered unchanged in urine within 6-12 hours

Usual Dosage I.M., I.V.:

Children: 100-150 mg/kg/day divided every 8-12 hours; up to 12 g/day

Adults: 2-4 g/day in divided doses every 12 hours; up to 12 g/day

Dosing adjustment in hepatic impairment: Reduce dose 50% in patients with advanced liver cirrhosis; maximum daily dose: 4 g

Administration Administer around-the-clock to promote less variation in peak and trough serum levels

Monitoring Parameters Monitor for coagulation abnormalities and diarrhea; observe for signs and symptoms of anaphylaxis during first dose

Test Interactions Prothrombin time (S), glucose, protein; ↓ positive Coombs' [direct]

Nursing Implications Do not admix with aminoglycosides in same bottle/bag

Additional Information Sodium content of 1 g: 34.5 mg (1.5 mEq); contains the n-methylthiotetrazole side chain

Dosage Forms

Injection, as sodium, premixed (frozen): 1 g (50 mL); 2 g (50 mL)

Powder for injection, as sodium: 1 g, 2 g

Cefoperazone Sodium *see* Cefoperazone *on previous page*

Cefotan® *see* Cefotetan *on next page*

Cefotaxime (sef oh TAKS eem)

Related Information

Antibiotic Treatment of Adults With Infectious Endocarditis *on page 1465*

Antimicrobial Drugs of Choice *on page 1468*

Bacterial Meningitis Practical Guidelines for Management *on page 1475*

Cephalosporins by Generation *on page 1447*

Treatment of Sexually Transmitted Diseases *on page 1485*

Brand Names Claforan®

Canadian/Mexican Brand Names Alfotax® (Mexico); Benaxima® (Mexico); Biosint® (Mexico); Cefaxim® (Mexico); Cefoclin® (Mexico); Fotexina® (Mexico); Taporin® (Mexico); Viken® (Mexico)

Synonyms Cefotaxime Sodium

Therapeutic Category Antibiotic, Cephalosporin (Third Generation)

Use Treatment of susceptible infection in respiratory tract, skin and skin structure, bone and joint, urinary tract, gynecologic as well as septicemia, and documented or suspected meningitis

Pregnancy Risk Factor B

Contraindications Hypersensitivity to cefotaxime, any component, or cephalosporins

Warnings/Precautions Modify dosage in patients with severe renal impairment; prolonged use may result in superinfection; a low incidence of cross-hypersensitivity to penicillins exists

Adverse Reactions

1% to 10%:

Central nervous system: Fever

Dermatologic: Rash, pruritus

Gastrointestinal: Colitis, diarrhea, nausea, vomiting

Hematologic: Eosinophilia

Local: Pain at injection site

<1%:

Central nervous system: Headache

Gastrointestinal: Pseudomembranous colitis
Hematologic: Transient neutropenia, thrombocytopenia
Hepatic: Transient elevation of liver enzymes
Local: Phlebitis
Renal: Transient elevation of BUN/creatinine

Overdosage/Toxicology Symptoms of overdose include neuromuscular hypersensitivity, convulsions

Hemodialysis may be helpful to aid in the removal of the drug from the blood, otherwise most treatment is supportive or symptom directed

Drug Interactions

Increased effect: Probenecid may decrease cephalosporin elimination

Increased toxicity: Furosemide, aminoglycosides may be a possible additive to nephrotoxicity

Stability Reconstituted solution is stable for 24 hours at room temperature and 10 days when refrigerated; for I.V. infusion in NS or D_5W solution is stable for 24 hours at room temperature, 5 days when refrigerated, or 13 weeks when frozen; after freezing, thawed solution is stable for 24 hours at room temperature or 10 days when refrigerated

Mechanism of Action Inhibits bacterial cell wall synthesis by binding to one or more of the penicillin-binding proteins (PBPs) which in turn inhibits the final transpeptidation step of peptidoglycan synthesis in bacterial cell walls, thus inhibiting cell wall biosynthesis. Bacteria eventually lyse due to ongoing activity of cell wall autolytic enzymes (autolysins and murein hydrolases) while cell wall assembly is arrested.

Pharmacodynamics/Kinetics

Distribution: Widely distributed to body tissues and fluids including aqueous humor, ascitic and prostatic fluids, and bone; penetrates CSF when meninges are inflamed; crosses the placenta and appears in breast milk

Metabolism: Partially in the liver to active metabolite, desacetylcefotaxime

Half-life:
- Cefotaxime:
  - Premature neonates <1 week: 5-6 hours
  - Full-term neonates <1 week: 2-3.4 hours
  - Adults: 1-1.5 hours (prolonged with renal and/or hepatic impairment)
- Desacetylcefotaxime: 1.5-1.9 hours (prolonged with renal impairment)

Time to peak serum concentration: I.M.: Within 30 minutes

Elimination: Renal excretion of parent drug and metabolites

Usual Dosage I.M., I.V.:

Infants and Children 1 month to 12 years:
- <50 kg: 100-150 mg/kg/day in divided doses every 6-8 hours
- Meningitis: 200 mg/kg/day in divided doses every 6 hours
- >50 kg: Moderate to severe infection: 1-2 g every 6-8 hours; life-threatening infection: 2 g/dose every 4 hours; maximum dose: 12 g/day

Children >12 years and Adults: 1-2 g every 6-8 hours (up to 12 g/day)

Dosing interval in renal impairment:
- Cl_{cr} 10-50 mL/minute: Administer every 8-12 hours
- Cl_{cr} <10 mL/minute: Administer every 24 hours

Hemodialysis: Moderately dialyzable (20% to 50%)

Dosing adjustment in hepatic impairment: Moderate dosage reduction is recommended in severe liver disease

Administration Can be administered IVP over 3-5 minutes or I.V. retrograde or I.V. intermittent infusion over 15-30 minutes; do not admix with aminoglycosides in same bottle/bag

Monitoring Parameters Observe for signs and symptoms of anaphylaxis during first dose

Test Interactions False-positive Coombs' test, false-positive reaction for urine glucose tests using Clinitest® or Benedict's solution, false elevation of creatinine using Jaffé test

Additional Information Sodium content of 1 g: 2.2 mEq

Dosage Forms

Infusion, as sodium, premixed, in D_5W (frozen): 1 g (50 mL); 2 g (50 mL)

Powder for injection, as sodium: 500 mg, 1 g, 2 g, 10 g

Cefotaxime Sodium *see* Cefotaxime *on previous page*

Cefotetan (SEF oh tee tan)

Related Information

Animal and Human Bites Guidelines *on page 1463*
Antimicrobial Drugs of Choice *on page 1468*
Cephalosporins by Generation *on page 1447*
Treatment of Sexually Transmitted Diseases *on page 1485*

Brand Names Cefotan®

(Continued)

Cefotetan *(Continued)*

Synonyms Cefotetan Disodium

Therapeutic Category Antibiotic, Cephalosporin (Second Generation)

Use Treatment of susceptible bacterial infection; mainly respiratory tract, skin and skin structure, bone and joint, urinary tract and gynecologic, as well as, septicemia, similar spectrum to cefoxitin

Pregnancy Risk Factor B

Contraindications Hypersensitivity to cefotetan, any component, or cephalosporins

Warnings/Precautions Modify dosage in patients with severe renal impairment; prolonged use may result in superinfection; a low incidence of cross-hypersensitivity to penicillins exists

Adverse Reactions

1% to 10%:

- Gastrointestinal: Diarrhea
- Hepatic: Hepatic enzyme elevation
- Miscellaneous: Hypersensitivity reactions

<1%:

- Central nervous system: Fever
- Dermatologic: Rash, pruritus
- Gastrointestinal: Nausea, vomiting, antibiotic-associated colitis
- Hematologic: Prolongation of bleeding time or prothrombin time, neutropenia, thrombocytopenia
- Local: Phlebitis

Overdosage/Toxicology Symptoms of overdose include neuromuscular hypersensitivity, convulsions

Hemodialysis may be helpful to aid in the removal of the drug from the blood, otherwise most treatment is supportive or symptom directed

Drug Interactions

Increased effect: Probenecid may decrease cephalosporin elimination

Increased toxicity: Furosemide, aminoglycosides may be a possible additive to nephrotoxicity

May cause disulfiram-like reaction with concomitant alcohol use

Stability Reconstituted solution is stable for 24 hours at room temperature and 96 hours when refrigerated; for I.V. infusion in NS or D_5W solution and after freezing, thawed solution is stable for 24 hours at room temperature or 96 hours when refrigerated; frozen solution is stable for 12 weeks

Mechanism of Action Inhibits bacterial cell wall synthesis by binding to one or more of the penicillin-binding proteins (PBPs) which in turn inhibits the final transpeptidation step of peptidoglycan synthesis in bacterial cell walls, thus inhibiting cell wall biosynthesis. Bacteria eventually lyse due to ongoing activity of cell wall autolytic enzymes (autolysins and murein hydrolases) while cell wall assembly is arrested.

Pharmacodynamics/Kinetics

Distribution: Widely distributed to body tissues and fluids including bile, sputum, prostatic and peritoneal fluids; low concentrations enter CSF; crosses the placenta and appears in breast milk

Protein binding: 76% to 90%

Half-life: 1.5-3 hours

Time to peak serum concentration: I.M.: Within 1.5-3 hours

Elimination: Primarily excreted unchanged in urine with 20% excreted in bile

Usual Dosage I.M., I.V.:

Children: 20-40 mg/kg/dose every 12 hours

Adults: 1-6 g/day in divided doses every 12 hours, 1-2 g may be given every 24 hours for urinary tract infection

Dosing interval in renal impairment:

Cl_{cr} 10-30 mL/minute: Administer every 24 hours

Cl_{cr} <10 mL/minute: Administer every 48 hours

Hemodialysis: Slightly dialyzable (5% to 20%)

Administration Administer around-the-clock to promote less variation in peak and trough serum levels

Monitoring Parameters Monitor for unusual bleeding or bruising; observe for signs and symptoms of anaphylaxis during first dose

Test Interactions ↑ alkaline phosphatase, AST, ALT, BUN, creatinine, glucose, protein; decreased glucose; positive Coombs' test

Nursing Implications Do not admix with aminoglycosides in same bottle/bag

Additional Information Sodium content of 1 g: 34.5 mg (1.5 mEq); contains the n-methylthiotetrazole side chain

Dosage Forms Powder for injection, as disodium: 1 g (10 mL, 100 mL); 2 g (20 mL, 100 mL); 10 g (100 mL)

Cefotetan Disodium *see* Cefotetan *on previous page*

Cefoxitin (se FOKS i tin)

Related Information

Antimicrobial Drugs of Choice *on page 1468*
Cephalosporins by Generation *on page 1447*
Treatment of Sexually Transmitted Diseases *on page 1485*

Brand Names Mefoxin®

Synonyms Cefoxitin Sodium

Therapeutic Category Antibiotic, Cephalosporin (Second Generation)

Use Less active against staphylococci and streptococci than first generation cephalosporins, but active against anaerobes including *Bacteroides fragilis*; active against gram-negative enteric bacilli including *E. coli*, *Klebsiella*, and *Proteus*; used predominantly for respiratory tract, skin and skin structure, bone and joint, urinary tract and gynecologic as well as septicemia; surgical prophylaxis; intra-abdominal infections and other mixed infections; indicated for bacterial *Eikenella corrodeas* infections

Pregnancy Risk Factor B

Contraindications Hypersensitivity to cefoxitin, any component, or cephalosporins

Warnings/Precautions Use with caution in patients with history of colitis; cefoxitin may increase resistance of organisms by inducing beta-lactamase; modify dosage in patients with severe renal impairment; prolonged use may result in superinfection; a low incidence of cross-hypersensitivity to penicillins exists

Adverse Reactions

1% to 10%: Gastrointestinal: Diarrhea

<1%:

- Cardiovascular: Hypotension
- Central nervous system: Fever
- Dermatologic: Rash, exfoliative dermatitis
- Gastrointestinal: Nausea, vomiting, pseudomembranous colitis
- Hematologic: Transient leukopenia, thrombocytopenia, anemia, eosinophilia
- Hepatic: Elevation in serum AST concentration
- Local: Thrombophlebitis
- Renal: Elevations in serum creatinine and/or BUN
- Respiratory: Dyspnea

Overdosage/Toxicology Symptoms of overdose include neuromuscular hypersensitivity, convulsions

Hemodialysis may be helpful to aid in the removal of the drug from the blood, otherwise most treatment is supportive or symptom directed

Drug Interactions

Increased effect: Probenecid may decrease cephalosporin elimination

Increased toxicity: Furosemide, aminoglycosides may be a possible additive to nephrotoxicity

Stability Reconstituted solution is stable for 24 hours at room temperature and 48 hours when refrigerated; I.V. infusion in NS or D_5W solution is stable for 24 hours at room temperature, 1 week when refrigerated, or 26 weeks when frozen; after freezing, thawed solution is stable for 24 hours at room temperature or 5 days when refrigerated

Mechanism of Action Inhibits bacterial cell wall synthesis by binding to one or more of the penicillin-binding proteins (PBPs) which in turn inhibits the final transpeptidation step of peptidoglycan synthesis in bacterial cell walls, thus inhibiting cell wall biosynthesis. Bacteria eventually lyse due to ongoing activity of cell wall autolytic enzymes (autolysins and murein hydrolases) while cell wall assembly is arrested.

Pharmacodynamics/Kinetics

Distribution: Widely distributed to body tissues and fluids including pleural, synovial, ascitic fluid, and bile; poorly penetrates into CSF even with inflammation of the meninges; crosses the placenta and small amounts appear in breast milk

Protein binding: 65% to 79%

Half-life: 45-60 minutes, increases significantly with renal insufficiency

Time to peak serum concentration:

- I.M.: Within 20-30 minutes
- I.V.: Within 5 minutes

Elimination: Rapidly excreted as unchanged drug (85%) in urine

Usual Dosage I.M., I.V.:

Infants >3 months and Children:

- Mild-moderate infection: 80-100 mg/kg/day in divided doses every 4-6 hours
- Severe infection: 100-160 mg/kg/day in divided doses every 4-6 hours
- Maximum dose: 12 g/day

Adults: 1-2 g every 6-8 hours (I.M. injection is painful); up to 12 g/day

Dosing interval in renal impairment:

Cl_{cr} 30-50 mL/minute: Administer every 8-12 hours

(Continued)

Cefoxitin *(Continued)*

Cl_{cr} 10-30 mL/minute: Administer every 12-24 hours
Cl_{cr} <10 mL/minute: Administer every 24-48 hours
Hemodialysis: Moderately dialyzable (20% to 50%)

Administration Administer around-the-clock rather than 4 times/day to promote less variation in peak and trough serum levels

Monitoring Parameters Monitor renal function periodically when used in combination with other nephrotoxic drugs

Test Interactions Positive Coombs' [direct]; false-positive urine glucose (Clinitest®), false increase in serum or urine creatinine with the Jaffé method

Additional Information Sodium content of 1 g: 53 mg (2.3 mEq)

Dosage Forms

Infusion, as sodium, premixed, in D_5W (frozen): 1 g (50 mL); 2 g (50 mL)
Powder for injection, as sodium: 1 g, 2 g, 10 g

Cefoxitin Sodium *see* Cefoxitin *on previous page*

Cefpodoxime (sef pode OKS eem)

Related Information

Cephalosporins by Generation *on page 1447*

Brand Names Vantin®

Synonyms Cefpodoxime Proxetil

Therapeutic Category Antibiotic, Cephalosporin (Second Generation)

Use Treatment of susceptible acute, community-acquired pneumonia caused by *S. pneumoniae* or nonbeta-lactamase producing *H. influenzae*; acute uncomplicated gonorrhea caused by *N. gonorrhoeae*; uncomplicated skin and skin structure infections caused by *S. aureus* or *S. pyogenes*; acute otitis media caused by *S. pneumoniae, H. influenzae*, or *M. catarrhalis*; pharyngitis or tonsillitis; and uncomplicated urinary tract infections caused by *E. coli*, *Klebsiella*, and *Proteus*

Pregnancy Risk Factor B

Contraindications Hypersensitivity to cefpodoxime or cephalosporins

Warnings/Precautions Modify dosage in patients with severe renal impairment; prolonged use may result in superinfection; a low incidence of cross-hypersensitivity to penicillins exists

Adverse Reactions

1% to 10%: Gastrointestinal: Diarrhea

<1%:

Central nervous system: Headache
Dermatologic: Diaper rash
Gastrointestinal: Nausea, vomiting, abdominal pain, pseudomembranous colitis
Genitourinary: Vaginal fungal infections

Overdosage/Toxicology Symptoms of overdose include neuromuscular hypersensitivity, convulsions

Hemodialysis may be helpful to aid in the removal of the drug from the blood, otherwise most treatment is supportive or symptom directed

Drug Interactions

Decreased effect: Antacids and H_2-receptor antagonists (reduce absorption and serum concentration of cefpodoxime)
Increased effect: Probenecid may decrease cephalosporin elimination
Increased toxicity: Furosemide, aminoglycosides may be a possible additive to nephrotoxicity

Stability After mixing, keep suspension in refrigerator, shake well before using; discard unused portion after 14 days

Mechanism of Action Inhibits bacterial cell wall synthesis by binding to one or more of the penicillin-binding proteins (PBPs) which in turn inhibits the final transpeptidation step of peptidoglycan synthesis in bacterial cell walls, thus inhibiting cell wall biosynthesis. Bacteria eventually lyse due to ongoing activity of cell wall autolytic enzymes (autolysins and murein hydrolases) while cell wall assembly is arrested.

Pharmacodynamics/Kinetics

Absorption: Oral: Rapidly and well absorbed (50%), acid stable; enhanced in the presence of food or low gastric pH
Distribution: Good tissue penetration, including lung and tonsils; penetrates into pleural fluid
Protein binding: 18% to 23%
Metabolism: Oral: De-esterified in the GI tract to the active metabolite, cefpodoxime
Half-life: 2.2 hours (prolonged with renal impairment)
Time to peak: Within 1 hour (oral)
Elimination: Plasma clearance: ~200-300 mL/minute; primarily eliminated by the kidney with 80% of dose excreted unchanged in urine in 24 hours

Usual Dosage Oral:

Children >5 months to 12 years:

Acute otitis media: 10 mg/kg/day as a single dose or divided every 12 hours (400 mg/day)

Pharyngitis/tonsillitis: 10 mg/kg/day in 2 divided doses (maximum: 200 mg/day)

Children ≥13 years and Adults:

Acute community-acquired pneumonia and bacterial exacerbations of chronic bronchitis: 200 mg every 12 hours for 14 days and 10 days, respectively

Skin and skin structure: 400 mg every 12 hours for 7-14 days

Uncomplicated gonorrhea (male and female) and rectal gonococcal infections (female): 200 mg as a single dose

Pharyngitis/tonsillitis: 100 mg every 12 hours for 10 days

Uncomplicated urinary tract infection: 100 mg every 12 hours for 7 days

Dosing adjustment in renal impairment: Cl_{cr} <30 mL/minute: Administer every 24 hours

Administration Administer around-the-clock to promote less variation in peak and trough serum levels

Monitoring Parameters Assess patient at beginning and throughout therapy for infection

Test Interactions Positive Coombs' [direct]

Patient Information Take with food; chilling improves flavor (do not freeze); report persistent diarrhea; entire course of medication (10-14 days) should be taken to ensure eradication of organism; should be taken in equal intervals around-the-clock to maintain adequate blood levels; may interfere with oral contraceptives; females should report symptoms of vaginitis

Additional Information Dose adjustment is not necessary in patients with cirrhosis

Dosage Forms

Granules for oral suspension, as proxetil (lemon creme flavor): 50 mg/5 mL (100 mL); 100 mg/5 mL (100 mL)

Tablet, film coated, as proxetil: 100 mg, 200 mg

Cefpodoxime Proxetil *see* Cefpodoxime *on previous page*

Cefprozil (sef PROE zil)

Related Information

Cephalosporins by Generation *on page 1447*

Brand Names Cefzil®

Therapeutic Category Antibiotic, Cephalosporin (Second Generation)

Use Infections causes by susceptible organisms including *S. pneumoniae, S. aureus, S. pyogenes*; treatment of otitis media and infections involving the respiratory tract and skin and skin structure; also indicated for the treatment of acute sinusitis caused by *S. pneumoniae, S. aureas, H. influenzae* and *M. catarrhalis.*

Pregnancy Risk Factor B

Contraindications Hypersensitivity to cefprozil or any component or cephalosporins

Warnings/Precautions Modify dosage in patients with severe renal impairment; prolonged use may result in superinfection; a low incidence of cross-hypersensitivity to penicillins exists

Adverse Reactions

1% to 10%:

Central nervous system: Dizziness

Dermatologic: Diaper rash

Gastrointestinal: Diarrhea, nausea, vomiting, abdominal pain

Genitourinary: Vaginitis, genital pruritus

Hematologic: Eosinophilia

Hepatic: Elevation of AST, ALT and alkaline phosphatase

Miscellaneous: Superinfection

<1%:

Central nervous system: Headache, insomnia, confusion

Dermatologic: Rash, urticaria

Hematologic: Prolonged PT

Hepatic: Cholestatic jaundice

Neuromuscular & skeletal: Arthralgia

Renal: Elevated BUN/serum creatinine

Overdosage/Toxicology Symptoms of overdose include neuromuscular hypersensitivity, convulsions

Hemodialysis may be helpful to aid in the removal of the drug from the blood, otherwise most treatment is supportive or symptom directed

Drug Interactions

Increased effect: Probenecid may decrease cephalosporin elimination

(Continued)

Cefprozil *(Continued)*

Increased toxicity: Furosemide, aminoglycosides may be a possible additive to nephrotoxicity

Mechanism of Action Inhibits bacterial cell wall synthesis by binding to one or more of the penicillin-binding proteins (PBPs) which in turn inhibits the final transpeptidation step of peptidoglycan synthesis in bacterial cell walls, thus inhibiting cell wall biosynthesis. Bacteria eventually lyse due to ongoing activity of cell wall autolytic enzymes (autolysins and murein hydrolases) while cell wall assembly is arrested.

Pharmacodynamics/Kinetics

Absorption: Oral: Well absorbed (94%)

Distribution: Low distribution into breast milk

Protein binding: 35% to 45%

Half-life, elimination: 1.3 hours (normal renal function)

Peak serum levels: 1.5 hours (fasting state)

Elimination: 61% excreted unchanged in urine

Usual Dosage Oral:

Infants and Children >6 months to 12 years: Otitis media: 15 mg/kg every 12 hours for 10 days

Pharyngitis/tonsillitis:

- Children 2-12 years: 7.5 -15 mg/kg/day divided every 12 hours for 10 days (administer for >10 days if due to *S. pyogenes*); maximum: 1 g/day
- Children >13 years and Adults: 500 mg every 24 hours for 10 days

Uncomplicated skin and skin structure infections:

- Children 2-12 years: 20 mg/kg every 24 hours for 10 days; maximum: 1 g/day
- Children >13 years and Adults: 250 mg every 12 hours, or 500 mg every 12-24 hours for 10 days

Secondary bacterial infection of acute bronchitis or acute bacterial exacerbation of chronic bronchitis: 500 mg every 12 hours for 10 days

Dosing adjustment in renal impairment: Cl_{cr} <30 mL/minute: Reduce dose by 50%

Hemodialysis: Reduced by hemodialysis; administer dose after the completion of hemodialysis

Administration Administer around-the-clock to promote less variation in peak and trough serum levels

Monitoring Parameters Assess patient at beginning and throughout therapy for infection

Test Interactions Positive Coombs' [direct]; may produce false-positive reaction for urine glucose with Clinitest®

Patient Information Chilling improves flavor (do not freeze); report persistent diarrhea; entire course of medication (10-14 days) should be taken to ensure eradication of organism; should be taken in equal intervals around-the-clock to maintain adequate blood levels; may interfere with oral contraceptives; females should report symptoms of vaginitis

Dosage Forms

Powder for oral suspension, as anhydrous: 125 mg/5 mL (50 mL, 75 mL, 100 mL); 250 mg/5 mL (50 mL, 75 mL, 100 mL)

Tablet, as anhydrous: 250 mg, 500 mg

Ceftazidime (SEF tay zi deem)

Related Information

Antimicrobial Drugs of Choice *on page 1468*

Bacterial Meningitis Practical Guidelines for Management *on page 1475*

Cephalosporins by Generation *on page 1447*

Brand Names Ceptaz™; Fortaz®; Tazicef®; Tazidime®

Canadian/Mexican Brand Names Ceptaz™ (Canada); Ceftazim® (Mexico); Fortum® (Mexico); Tagal® (Mexico); Taloken® (Mexico); Waytrax® (Mexico)

Therapeutic Category Antibiotic, Cephalosporin (Third Generation)

Use Treatment of documented susceptible *Pseudomonas aeruginosa* infection; *Pseudomonas* infection in patients at risk of developing aminoglycoside-induced nephrotoxicity and/or ototoxicity; empiric therapy of febrile, granulocytopenic patients

Pregnancy Risk Factor B

Contraindications Hypersensitivity to ceftazidime, any component, or cephalosporins

Warnings/Precautions Modify dosage in patients with severe renal impairment; prolonged use may result in superinfection; a low incidence of cross-hypersensitivity to penicillins exists

Adverse Reactions

1% to 10%:

Gastrointestinal: Diarrhea

Local: Pain at injection site

<1%:

Central nervous system: Fever, headache, dizziness
Dermatologic: Rash, angioedema
Gastrointestinal: Nausea, vomiting, pseudomembranous colitis
Hematologic: Eosinophilia, thrombocytosis, transient leukopenia, hemolytic anemia
Hepatic: Transient elevation in liver enzymes
Local: Phlebitis
Neuromuscular & skeletal: Paresthesia
Renal: Transient elevation of BUN/creatinine
Miscellaneous: Candidiasis

Overdosage/Toxicology Symptoms of overdose include neuromuscular hypersensitivity, convulsions

Hemodialysis may be helpful to aid in the removal of the drug from the blood, otherwise most treatment is supportive or symptom directed

Drug Interactions

Increased effect: Probenecid may decrease cephalosporin elimination; aminoglycosides: *in vitro* studies indicate additive or synergistic effect against some strains of Enterobacteriaceae and *Pseudomonas aeruginosa*

Increased toxicity: Furosemide, aminoglycosides may be a possible additive to nephrotoxicity

Stability Reconstituted solution and I.V. infusion in NS or D_5W solution are stable for 24 hours at room temperature, 10 days when refrigerated, or 12 weeks when frozen; after freezing, thawed solution is stable for 24 hours at room temperature or 4 days when refrigerated; 96 hours under refrigeration, after mixing

Mechanism of Action Inhibits bacterial cell wall synthesis by binding to one or more of the penicillin-binding proteins (PBPs) which in turn inhibits the final transpeptidation step of peptidoglycan synthesis in bacterial cell walls, thus inhibiting cell wall biosynthesis. Bacteria eventually lyse due to ongoing activity of cell wall autolytic enzymes (autolysins and murein hydrolases) while cell wall assembly is arrested.

Pharmacodynamics/Kinetics

Distribution: Widely distributes throughout the body including bone, bile, skin, CSF (diffuses into CSF with higher concentrations when the meninges are inflamed), endometrium, heart, pleural and lymphatic fluids

Protein binding: 17%

Half-life: 1-2 hours (prolonged with renal impairment)
Neonates <23 days: 2.2-4.7 hours

Time to peak serum concentration: I.M.: Within 1 hour

Elimination: By glomerular filtration with 80% to 90% of the dose excreted as unchanged drug within 24 hours

Usual Dosage I.M., I.V.:

Infants and Children 1 month to 12 years: 30-50 mg/kg/dose every 8 hours; maximum dose: 6 g/day

Adults: 1-2 g every 8-12 hours
Urinary tract infections: 250-500 mg every 12 hours

Dosing interval in renal impairment:

Cl_{cr} 30-50 mL/minute: Administer every 12 hours
Cl_{cr} 10-30 mL/minute: Administer every 24 hours
Cl_{cr} <10 mL/minute: Administer every 48-72 hours

Hemodialysis: Dialyzable (50% to 100%)

Administration Any carbon dioxide bubbles that may be present in the withdrawn solution should be expelled prior to injection; administer around-the-clock to promote less variation in peak and trough serum levels; ceftazidime can be administered IVP over 3-5 minutes, or I.V. retrograde or I.V. intermittent infusion over 15-30 minutes; do not admix with aminoglycosides in same bottle/bag; final concentration for I.V. administration should not exceed 100 mg/mL

Monitoring Parameters Observe for signs and symptoms of anaphylaxis during first dose

Test Interactions Positive Coombs' [direct], false-positive urine glucose (Clinitest®)

Additional Information Sodium content of 1 g: 2.3 mEq

Dosage Forms

Infusion, premixed (frozen) (Fortaz®): 1 g (50 mL); 2 g (50 mL)
Powder for injection: 500 mg, 1 g, 2 g, 6 g

Ceftibuten (sef TYE byoo ten)

Brand Names Cedax®

Therapeutic Category Antibiotic, Cephalosporin (Third Generation)

Use Oral cephalosporin for bronchitis, otitis media, and pharyngitis/tonsillitis due to *H. influenzae* (highly sensitive) and *M. catarrhalis* (moderately sensitive), both (Continued)

Ceftibuten *(Continued)*

beta-lactamase-producing and nonproducing strains, as well as *S. pneumoniae* (weak) and *S. pyogenes*. **Note:** Documented sensitivity of *S. pneumoniae* to ceftibuten should be present before use, since resistance is known to penicillin-resistant strains (up to 25% of strains in the U.S.). It is highly active against group A streptococci, *N. gonorrhoeae* and *N. meningitidis*, as well. It has the broadest gram-negative spectrum of any oral cephalosporin, active against most strains of Enterobacteriaceae, including *E. coli*, *Salmonella*, *Shigella*, and *Yersinia*. Although ceftibuten may eradicate *S. pyogenes* from the oropharynx, proof of efficacy for prophylaxis of rheumatic fever is not available.

Pregnancy Risk Factor B

Pregnancy/Breast-Feeding Implications Cephalosporins cross the placenta, use only when potential benefits outweigh risk to the fetus; avoid breast-feeding in women needing to take this medication due to modification of bowel flora and interference with interpretation of culture result if a fever work-up is needed in the infant

Warnings/Precautions Modify dosage in patients with severe renal impairment, prolonged use may result in superinfection; a low incidence of cross-hypersensitivity to penicillins exist

Adverse Reactions

1% to 10%: Gastrointestinal: Diarrhea

<1%:

Central nervous system: Dizziness, fatigue, headache
Dermatologic: Rash
Gastrointestinal: Nausea, vomiting, pseudomembranous colitis
Hematologic: Transient neutropenia, anemia
Hepatic: Transient elevation in LFTs

Overdosage/Toxicology As with other cephalosporins, symptoms of overdose include neuromuscular hypersensitivity, convulsions

Hemodialysis may be helpful to aid in the removal of the drug from the blood; otherwise most treatment is supportive or symptom directed

Drug Interactions

Increased effect: High-dose probenecid decreases clearance
Increased toxicity: Aminoglycosides increase nephrotoxic potential

Stability Reconstituted suspension is stable for 14 days in the refrigerator

Mechanism of Action Inhibits bacterial cell wall synthesis by binding to one or more of the penicillin-binding proteins (PBPs) which in turn inhibits the final transpeptidation step of peptidoglycan synthesis in bacterial cell walls, thus inhibiting cell wall biosynthesis. Bacteria eventually lyse due to ongoing activity of cell wall autolytic enzymes (autolysins and murein hydrolases) while cell wall assembly is arrested.

Pharmacodynamics/Kinetics

Absorption: Rapid (T_{max}: 2-3 hours); food decreases peak concentrations, delays T_{max} and lowers the AUC (total amount of drug absorbed)
Half-life: 2 hours
Elimination: In urine

Usual Dosage Oral:

Children <12 years: 9 mg/kg/day for 10 days; maximum daily dose: 400 mg
Children ≥12 years and Adults: 400 mg once daily for 10 days; maximum: 400 mg

Dosage adjustment in renal impairment:

Cl_{cr} 30-49 mL//minute: Administer 4.5 mg/kg or 200 mg every 24 hours
Cl_{cr} 29 mL/minute: Administer 2.25 mg/kg or 100 mg every 24 hours

Monitoring Parameters Observe for signs and symptoms of anaphylaxis during first dose; with prolonged therapy, monitor renal, hepatic, and hematologic function periodically

Test Interactions False-positive Coombs' test; may falsely elevate creatinine values when Jaffé reaction is used; may cause false-positive results in urine glucose tests using cupric sulfate (Benedict's solution, Clinitest®)

Patient Information Must be administered at least 2 hours before meals or 1 hour after a meal; shake suspension well before use; suspension may be kept for 14 days if stored in refrigerator; discard any unused portion after 14 days; report prolonged diarrhea; entire course of medication should be taken to ensure eradication of organism; take at the same time each day to maintain adequate blood levels; may interfere with oral contraceptive; females should report symptoms of vaginitis

Nursing Implications Administer at the same time each day to maintain adequate blood levels; obtain specimens for culture and sensitivity testing prior to the first dose, if possible

Additional Information In clinical trials, ceftibuten once or twice daily was at least as effective as cefaclor or ciprofloxacin for treatment of acute bacterial exacerbations of bronchitis, as effective as amoxicillin/clavulanic acid or cefaclor for otitis media, as effective as penicillin for pharyngitis, and as effective as trimethoprim-sulfamethoxazole for urinary tract infections

Dosage Forms

Capsule: 400 mg

Powder for oral suspension (cherry flavor): 90 mg/5 mL (30 mL, 60 mL, 120 mL); 180 mg/5 mL (30 mL, 60 mL, 120 mL)

Ceftin® *see* Cefuroxime *on page 238*

Ceftizoxime (sef ti ZOKS eem)

Related Information

Antimicrobial Drugs of Choice *on page 1468*
Antimicrobial Prophylaxis *on page 1445*
Cephalosporins by Generation *on page 1447*
Treatment of Sexually Transmitted Diseases *on page 1485*

Brand Names Cefizox®

Canadian/Mexican Brand Names Ultracef® (Mexico)

Synonyms Ceftizoxime Sodium

Therapeutic Category Antibiotic, Cephalosporin (Third Generation)

Use Treatment of susceptible nonpseudomonal gram-negative rod infections or mixed gram-negative and anaerobic infections; predominantly respiratory tract, skin and skin structure, bone and joint, urinary tract and gynecologic, as well as septicemia

Pregnancy Risk Factor B

Contraindications Hypersensitivity to ceftizoxime, any component, or cephalosporins

Warnings/Precautions Modify dosage in patients with severe renal impairment; prolonged use may result in superinfection; a low incidence of cross-hypersensitivity to penicillins exists

Adverse Reactions

1% to 10%:

- Central nervous system: Fever
- Dermatologic: Rash, pruritus
- Hematologic: Eosinophilia, thrombocytosis
- Hepatic: Transient elevation of AST, ALT, and alkaline phosphatase
- Local: Pain, burning at injection site

<1%:

- Genitourinary: Vaginitis
- Hematologic: Anemia, leukopenia, neutropenia, thrombocytopenia
- Hepatic: Elevation of bilirubin
- Neuromuscular & skeletal: Numbness
- Renal: Transient elevations of BUN/creatinine

Overdosage/Toxicology Symptoms of overdose include neuromuscular hypersensitivity, convulsions

Hemodialysis may be helpful to aid in the removal of the drug from the blood, otherwise most treatment is supportive or symptom directed

Drug Interactions

Increased effect: Probenecid may decrease cephalosporin elimination

Increased toxicity: Furosemide, aminoglycosides may be a possible additive to nephrotoxicity

Stability Reconstituted solution is stable for 24 hours at room temperature and 96 hours when refrigerated; for I.V. infusion in NS or D_5W solution is stable for 24 hours at room temperature, 96 hours when refrigerated or 12 weeks when frozen; after freezing, thawed solution is stable for 24 hours at room temperature or 10 days when refrigerated

Mechanism of Action Inhibits bacterial cell wall synthesis by binding to one or more of the penicillin-binding proteins (PBPs) which in turn inhibits the final transpeptidation step of peptidoglycan synthesis in bacterial cell walls, thus inhibiting cell wall biosynthesis. Bacteria eventually lyse due to ongoing activity of cell wall autolytic enzymes (autolysins and murein hydrolases) while cell wall assembly is arrested.

Pharmacodynamics/Kinetics

Distribution: V_d: 0.35-0.5 L/kg; widely distributed into most body tissues and fluids including gallbladder, liver, kidneys, bone, sputum, bile, and pleural and synovial fluids; has good CSF penetration; crosses placenta; small amounts excreted in breast milk

Protein binding: 30%

Half-life: 1.6 hours, increases to 25 hours when Cl_{cr} falls to <10 mL/minute

Time to peak serum concentration: I.M.: Within 0.5-1 hour

Elimination: Excreted unchanged in urine

(Continued)

Ceftizoxime *(Continued)*

Usual Dosage I.M., I.V.:

Children ≥6 months: 150-200 mg/kg/day divided every 6-8 hours (maximum of 12 g/24 hours)

Adults: 1-2 g every 8-12 hours, up to 2 g every 4 hours or 4 g every 8 hours for life-threatening infections

Dosing interval in renal impairment:

Cl_{cr} 10-50 mL/minute: Administer every 24-48 hours

Cl_{cr} <10 mL/minute: Administer every 48-72 hours

Hemodialysis: Moderately dialyzable (20% to 50%)

Monitoring Parameters Observe for signs and symptoms of anaphylaxis during first dose

Test Interactions False-positive Coombs' test, may falsely elevate creatinine values when Jaffé reaction is used, may cause false-positive results in urine glucose tests using cupric sulfate (Benedict's solution, Clinitest®)

Nursing Implications Do not admix with aminoglycosides in same bottle/bag

Additional Information Sodium content of 1 g: 60 mg (2.6 mEq)

Dosage Forms

Injection, as sodium, in D_5W (frozen): 1 g (50 mL); 2 g (50 mL)

Powder for injection, as sodium: 500 mg, 1 g, 2 g, 10 g

Ceftizoxime Sodium *see* Ceftizoxime *on previous page*

Ceftriaxone (sef trye AKS one)

Related Information

Animal and Human Bites Guidelines *on page 1463*

Antibiotic Treatment of Adults With Infectious Endocarditis *on page 1465*

Antimicrobial Drugs of Choice *on page 1468*

Bacterial Meningitis Practical Guidelines for Management *on page 1475*

Cephalosporins by Generation *on page 1447*

Treatment of Sexually Transmitted Diseases *on page 1485*

Brand Names Rocephin®

Canadian/Mexican Brand Names Benaxona® (Mexico); Cefaxona® (Mexico); Tacex® (Mexico); Triaken® (Mexico)

Synonyms Ceftriaxone Sodium

Therapeutic Category Antibiotic, Cephalosporin (Third Generation)

Use Treatment of lower respiratory tract infections, skin and skin structure infections, bone and joint infections, intra-abdominal and urinary tract infections, sepsis and meningitis due to susceptible organisms; documented or suspected infection due to susceptible organisms in home care patients and patients without I.V. line access; treatment of documented or suspected gonococcal infection or chancroid; emergency room management of patients at high risk for bacteremia, periorbital or buccal cellulitis, salmonellosis or shigellosis, and pneumonia of unestablished etiology (<5 years of age); treatment of Lyme disease, depends on the stage of the disease (used in Stage II and Stage III, but not stage I); doxycycline is the drug of choice for Stage I

Pregnancy Risk Factor B

Contraindications Hypersensitivity to ceftriaxone sodium, any component, or cephalosporins; **do not use in hyperbilirubinemic neonates**, particularly those who are premature since ceftriaxone is reported to displace bilirubin from albumin binding sites

Warnings/Precautions Modify dosage in patients with severe renal impairment; prolonged use may result in superinfection with yeasts, enterococci, *B. fragilis*, or *P. aeruginosa*; a low incidence of cross-hypersensitivity to penicillins exists

Adverse Reactions

1% to 10%:

Dermatologic: Rash

Gastrointestinal: Diarrhea

Hematologic: Eosinophilia, thrombocytosis, leukopenia

Hepatic: Elevations of SGOT [AST], SGPT [ALT]

Local: Pain at injection site

Renal: Elevations of BUN

<1%:

Cardiovascular: Flushing

Central nervous system: Fever, chills, headache, dizziness

Dermatologic: Pruritus

Gastrointestinal: Nausea, vomiting, abnormal taste

Genitourinary: Presence of casts in urine, vaginitis

Hematologic: Anemia, hemolytic anemia, neutropenia, lymphopenia, thrombocytopenia

Hepatic: Elevations of alkaline phosphatase and bilirubin

Local: Phlebitis

Renal: Elevation of creatinine
Miscellaneous: Moniliasis, diaphoresis

Overdosage/Toxicology Symptoms of overdose include neuromuscular hypersensitivity, convulsions

Hemodialysis may be helpful to aid in the removal of the drug from the blood, otherwise most treatment is supportive or symptom directed

Drug Interactions

Increased effect:
- Aminoglycosides may result in synergistic antibacterial activity
- High-dose probenecid decreases clearance

Increased toxicity: Aminoglycosides increase nephrotoxic potential

Stability Reconstituted solution (100 mg/mL) is stable for 3 days at room temperature and 3 days when refrigerated; for I.V. infusion in NS or D_5W solution is stable for 3 days at room temperature, 10 days when refrigerated, or 26 weeks when frozen; after freezing, thawed solution is stable for 3 days at room temperature or 10 days when refrigerated

Mechanism of Action Inhibits bacterial cell wall synthesis by binding to one or more of the penicillin-binding proteins (PBPs) which in turn inhibits the final transpeptidation step of peptidoglycan synthesis in bacterial cell walls, thus inhibiting cell wall biosynthesis. Bacteria eventually lyse due to ongoing activity of cell wall autolytic enzymes (autolysins and murein hydrolases) while cell wall assembly is arrested.

Pharmacodynamics/Kinetics

Distribution: Widely distributes throughout the body including gallbladder, lungs, bone, bile, CSF (diffuses into the CSF at higher concentrations when the meninges are inflamed)

Protein binding: 85% to 95%

Half-life: Normal renal and hepatic function: 5-9 hours
- Neonates: Postnatal:
  - 1-4 days: 16 hours
  - 9-30 days: 9 hours

Time to peak serum concentration:
- I.M.: Within 1-2 hours
- I.V.: Within minutes

Elimination: Excreted unchanged in urine (33% to 65%) by glomerular filtration and in feces

Usual Dosage I.M., I.V.:

Neonates:
- Postnatal age ≤7 days: 50 mg/kg/day given every 24 hours
- Postnatal age >7 days:
  - ≤2000 g: 50 mg/kg/day given every 24 hours
  - >2000 g: 50-75 mg/kg/day given every 24 hours
- Gonococcal prophylaxis: 25-50 mg/kg as a single dose (dose not to exceed 125 mg)
- Gonococcal infection: 25-50 mg/kg/day (maximum dose: 125 mg) given every 24 hours for 10-14 days

Infants and Children: 50-75 mg/kg/day in 1-2 divided doses every 12-24 hours; maximum: 2 g/24 hours
- Meningitis: 100 mg/kg/day divided every 12-24 hours, up to a maximum of 4 g/24 hours; loading dose of 75 mg/kg/dose may be given at start of therapy
- Otitis media: Single I.M. injection
- Uncomplicated gonococcal infections, sexual assault, and STD prophylaxis: I.M.: 125 mg as a single dose
- Complicated gonococcal infections:
  - <45 kg: 50 mg/kg/day once daily; maximum: 1 g/day; for ophthalmia, peritonitis, arthritis, or bacteremia: 50-100 mg/kg/day divided every 12-24 hours; maximum: 2 g/day for meningitis or endocarditis
  - >45 kg: 1 g/day once daily for disseminated gonococcal infections; 1-2 g dose every 12 hours for meningitis or endocarditis
- Acute epididymitis: I.M.: 250 mg in a single dose

Adults: 1-2 g every 12-24 hours (depending on the type and severity of infection); maximum dose: 2 g every 12 hours for treatment of meningitis
- Uncomplicated gonorrhea: I.M.: 250 mg as a single dose

Dosing adjustment in renal or hepatic impairment: No change necessary

Hemodialysis: Not dialyzable (0% to 5%); administer dose postdialysis

Peritoneal dialysis: Administer 750 mg every 12 hours

Continuous arterio-venous or veno-venous hemofiltration (CAVH/CAVHD): Removes 10 mg of ceftriaxone of liter of filtrate per day

Monitoring Parameters Assess patient at beginning and throughout therapy for infection; observe for signs and symptoms of anaphylaxis

Test Interactions False-positive urine glucose with Clinitest®

(Continued)

Ceftriaxone *(Continued)*

Nursing Implications Obtain specimens for culture and sensitivity before the first dose

Additional Information Sodium content of 1 g: 2.6 mEq

Dosage Forms

Infusion, as sodium, premixed (frozen): 1 g in $D_{3.8}W$ (50 mL); 2 g in $D_{2.4}W$ (50 mL)

Injection, as sodium: 350 mg/mL

Powder for injection, as sodium: 250 mg, 500 mg, 1 g, 2 g, 10 g

Ceftriaxone Sodium *see* Ceftriaxone *on page 236*

Cefuroxime (se fyoor OKS eem)

Related Information

Antimicrobial Drugs of Choice *on page 1468*
Cephalosporins by Generation *on page 1447*

Brand Names Ceftin®; Kefurox®; Zinacef®

Canadian/Mexican Brand Names Froxal® (Mexico); Zinnat® (Mexico)

Synonyms Cefuroxime Axetil; Cefuroxime Sodium

Therapeutic Category Antibiotic, Cephalosporin (Second Generation)

Use Treatment of infections caused by staphylococci, group B streptococci, *H. influenzae* (type A and B), *E. coli*, *Enterobacter*, *Salmonella*, and *Klebsiella*; treatment of susceptible infections of the lower respiratory tract, otitis media, urinary tract, skin and soft tissue, bone and joint, sepsis and gonorrhea

Pregnancy Risk Factor B

Contraindications Hypersensitivity to cefuroxime, any component, or cephalosporins

Warnings/Precautions Modify dosage in patients with severe renal impairment; prolonged use may result in superinfection; a low incidence of cross-hypersensitivity to penicillins exists

Adverse Reactions

1% to 10%:

Hematologic: Decreased hemoglobin and hematocrit, eosinophilia

Hepatic: Transient rise in SGOT [AST]/SGPT [ALT] and alkaline phosphatase

Local: Thrombophlebitis

<1%:

Central nervous system: Dizziness, fever, headache

Dermatologic: Rash

Gastrointestinal: Nausea, vomiting, diarrhea, stomach cramps, colitis, GI bleeding

Genitourinary: Vaginitis

Hematologic: Transient neutropenia and leukopenia

Hepatic: Transient increase in liver enzymes

Local: Pain at the injection site

Renal: Increase in BUN/creatinine

Overdosage/Toxicology Symptoms of overdose include neuromuscular hypersensitivity, convulsions

Hemodialysis may be helpful to aid in the removal of the drug from the blood, otherwise most treatment is supportive or symptom directed

Drug Interactions

Increased effect: High-dose probenecid decreases clearance

Increased toxicity: Aminoglycosides increase nephrotoxic potential

Stability Reconstituted solution is stable for 24 hours at room temperature and 48 hours when refrigerated; I.V. infusion in NS or D_5W solution is stable for 24 hours at room temperature, 7 days when refrigerated, or 26 weeks when frozen; after freezing, thawed solution is stable for 24 hours at room temperature or 21 days when refrigerated

Mechanism of Action Inhibits bacterial cell wall synthesis by binding to one or more of the penicillin-binding proteins (PBPs) which in turn inhibits the final transpeptidation step of peptidoglycan synthesis in bacterial cell walls, thus inhibiting cell wall biosynthesis. Bacteria eventually lyse due to ongoing activity of cell wall autolytic enzymes (autolysins and murein hydrolases) while cell wall assembly is arrested.

Pharmacodynamics/Kinetics

Absorption: Increased when given with or shortly after food or infant formula

Distribution: Widely distributed to body tissues and fluids; crosses blood-brain barrier; therapeutic concentrations achieved in CSF even when meninges are not inflamed; crosses placenta and reaches breast milk

Protein binding: 33% to 50%

Bioavailability, axetil: Oral: 37% to 52%

Half-life:
- Neonates:
  - ≤3 days: 5.1-5.8 hours
  - 6-14 days: 2-4.2 hours
  - 3-4 weeks: 1-1.5 hours
- Adults: 1-2 hours (prolonged in renal impairment)
  - I.M.: Within 15-60 minutes
  - I.V.: 2-3 minutes

Elimination: Primarily excreted 66% to 100% as unchanged drug in urine by both glomerular filtration and tubular secretion

Usual Dosage

Children:
- Pharyngitis, tonsillitis: Oral:
  - Suspension: 20 mg/kg/day (maximum: 500 mg/day) in 2 divided doses
  - Tablet: 125 mg every 12 hours
- Acute otitis media, impetigo: Oral:
  - Suspension: 30 mg/kg/day (maximum: 1 g/day) in 2 divided doses
  - Tablet: 250 mg every 12 hours
- I.M., I.V.: 75-150 mg/kg/day divided every 8 hours; maximum dose: 6 g/day
  - Meningitis: Not recommended (doses of 200-240 mg/kg/day divided every 6-8 hours have been used); maximum dose: 9 g/day

Adults:
- Oral: 250-500 mg twice daily; uncomplicated urinary tract infection: 125-250 mg every 12 hours
- I.M., I.V.: 750 mg to 1.5 g/dose every 8 hours or 100-150 mg/kg/day in divided doses every 6-8 hours; maximum: 6 g/24 hours

Dosing adjustment in renal impairment:
- Cl_{cr} 10-20 mL/minute: Administer every 12 hours
- Cl_{cr} <10 mL/minute: Administer every 24 hours

Hemodialysis: Dialyzable (25%)

Note: Cefuroxime axetil film-coated tablets and oral suspension are not bioequivalent and are not substitutable on a mg/mg basis

Administration Administer around-the-clock to promote less variation in peak and trough serum levels

Monitoring Parameters Observe for signs and symptoms of anaphylaxis during first dose; with prolonged therapy, monitor renal, hepatic, and hematologic function periodically

Test Interactions False-positive Coombs' test; may falsely elevate creatinine values when Jaffé reaction is used; may cause false-positive results in urine glucose tests using cupric sulfate (Benedict's solution, Clinitest®)

Patient Information Report prolonged diarrhea; entire course of medication (10-14 days) should be taken to ensure eradication of organism; should be taken in equal intervals around-the-clock to maintain adequate blood levels; may interfere with oral contraceptives; females should report symptoms of vaginitis

Nursing Implications Do not admix with aminoglycosides in same bottle/bag; obtain specimens for culture and sensitivity prior to the first dose

Additional Information Sodium content of 1 g: 54.2 mg (2.4 mEq)

Dosage Forms
- Infusion, as sodium, premixed (frozen) (Zinacef®): 750 mg (50 mL); 1.5 g (50 mL)
- Powder for injection, as sodium: 750 mg, 1.5 g, 7.5 g
- Powder for injection, as sodium (Kefurox®, Zinacef®): 750 mg, 1.5 g, 7.5 g
- Powder for oral suspension, as axetil (tutti-frutti flavor) (Ceftin®): 125 mg/5 mL (50 mL, 100 mL, 200 mL)
- Tablet, as axetil (Ceftin®): 125 mg, 250 mg, 500 mg

Cefuroxime Axetil *see* Cefuroxime *on previous page*

Cefuroxime Sodium *see* Cefuroxime *on previous page*

Cefzil® *see* Cefprozil *on page 231*

Celestone® *see* Betamethasone *on page 147*

CellCept® *see* Mycophenolate *on page 865*

Celontin® *see* Methsuximide *on page 813*

Cel-U-Jec® *see* Betamethasone *on page 147*

Cenafed® [OTC] *see* Pseudoephedrine *on page 1074*

Cenafed® Plus Tablet [OTC] *see* Triprolidine and Pseudoephedrine *on page 1270*

Cena-K® *see* Potassium Chloride *on page 1024*

Cenolate® *see* Sodium Ascorbate *on page 1140*

Cephalexin (sef a LEKS in)

Related Information
- Animal and Human Bites Guidelines *on page 1463*
- Cephalosporins by Generation *on page 1447*

Brand Names Biocef; Keflex®; Keftab®

(Continued)

Cephalexin *(Continued)*

Canadian/Mexican Brand Names Apo-Cephalex® (Canada); Novo-Lexin® (Canada); Nu-Cephalex® (Canada); Ceporex® (Mexico)

Synonyms Cephalexin Hydrochloride; Cephalexin Monohydrate

Therapeutic Category Antibiotic, Cephalosporin (First Generation)

Use Treatment of susceptible bacterial infections, including those caused by group A beta-hemolytic *Streptococcus, Staphylococcus, Klebsiella pneumoniae, E. coli, Proteus mirabilis*, and *Shigella*; predominantly used for lower respiratory tract, urinary tract, skin and soft tissue, and bone and joint

Pregnancy Risk Factor B

Contraindications Hypersensitivity to cephalexin, any component, or cephalosporins

Warnings/Precautions Modify dosage in patients with severe renal impairment; prolonged use may result in superinfection; a low incidence of cross-hypersensitivity to penicillins exists

Adverse Reactions

1% to 10%: Gastrointestinal: Diarrhea

<1%:

- Central nervous system: Dizziness, fatigue, headache
- Dermatologic: Rash
- Gastrointestinal: Nausea, vomiting, pseudomembranous colitis
- Hematologic: Transient neutropenia, anemia
- Hepatic: Transient elevation in liver enzymes

Overdosage/Toxicology Symptoms of overdose include neuromuscular hypersensitivity, convulsions

Hemodialysis may be helpful to aid in the removal of the drug from the blood, otherwise most treatment is supportive or symptom directed

Drug Interactions

Increased effect: High-dose probenecid increases clearance

Increased toxicity: Aminoglycosides increase nephrotoxic potential

Stability Refrigerate suspension after reconstitution; discard after 14 days

Mechanism of Action Inhibits bacterial cell wall synthesis by binding to one or more of the penicillin-binding proteins (PBPs) which in turn inhibits the final transpeptidation step of peptidoglycan synthesis in bacterial cell walls, thus inhibiting cell wall biosynthesis. Bacteria eventually lyse due to ongoing activity of cell wall autolytic enzymes (autolysins and murein hydrolases) while cell wall assembly is arrested.

Pharmacodynamics/Kinetics

Absorption: Delayed in young children; may be decreased up to 50% in neonates

Distribution: Widely distributed into most body tissues and fluids, including gallbladder, liver, kidneys, bone, sputum, bile, and pleural and synovial fluids; CSF penetration is poor; crosses placenta; appears in breast milk

Protein binding: 6% to 15%

Half-life:

- Neonates: 5 hours
- Children 3-12 months: 2.5 hours
- Adults: 0.5-1.2 hours (prolonged with renal impairment)

Time to peak serum concentration: Oral: Within 1 hour

Elimination: 80% to 100% of dose excreted as unchanged drug in urine within 8 hours

Usual Dosage Oral:

Children: 25-50 mg/kg/day every 6 hours; severe infections: 50-100 mg/kg/day in divided doses every 6 hours; maximum: 3 g/24 hours

Adults: 250-1000 mg every 6 hours; maximum: 4 g/day

Dosing interval in renal impairment: Cl_{cr} <10 mL/minute: Administer every 8-12 hours

Hemodialysis: Moderately dialyzable (20% to 50%)

Dietary Considerations Food: Peak antibiotic serum concentration is lowered and delayed, but total drug absorbed is not affected; take on an empty stomach. If GI distress, take with food.

Administration Administer on an empty stomach (ie, 1 hour prior to, or 2 hours after meals) to increase total absorption; administer around-the-clock rather than 4 times/day to promote less variation in peak and trough serum levels

Monitoring Parameters With prolonged therapy monitor renal, hepatic, and hematologic function periodically

Test Interactions False-positive Coombs' test, may falsely elevate creatinine values when Jaffé reaction is used, may cause false-positive results in urine glucose tests using cupric sulfate (Benedict's solution, Clinitest®), false-positive urinary proteins and steroids

Patient Information Report prolonged diarrhea; entire course of medication (10-14 days) should be taken to ensure eradication of organism; should be taken in equal intervals around-the-clock to maintain adequate blood levels; may interfere with oral contraceptives; females should report symptoms of vaginitis

Nursing Implications Obtain specimens for culture and sensitivity prior to the first dose

Dosage Forms

Capsule, as monohydrate: 250 mg, 500 mg

Powder for oral suspension, as monohydrate: 125 mg/5 mL (5 mL unit dose, 60 mL, 100 mL, 200 mL); 250 mg/5 mL (5 mL unit dose, 100 mL, 200 mL)

Suspension, oral, as monohydrate, pediatric: 100 mg/mL [5 mg/drop] (10 mL)

Tablet, as monohydrate: 250 mg, 500 mg, 1 g

Tablet, as hydrochloride: 500 mg

Cephalexin Hydrochloride *see* Cephalexin *on page 239*

Cephalexin Monohydrate *see* Cephalexin *on page 239*

Cephalosporins by Generation *see page 1447*

Cephalothin (sef A loe thin)

Related Information

Cephalosporins by Generation *on page 1447*

Brand Names Keflin®

Canadian/Mexican Brand Names Ceporacin® (Canada); Ceftina® (Mexico)

Synonyms Cephalothin Sodium

Therapeutic Category Antibiotic, Cephalosporin (First Generation)

Use Treatment of susceptible bacterial infections, including those caused by group A beta-hemolytic *Streptococcus*; respiratory, genitourinary, gastrointestinal, skin and soft tissue, bone and joint infections; septicemia; cephalexin is the oral equivalent

Pregnancy Risk Factor B

Contraindications Hypersensitivity to cephalothin or cephalosporins

Warnings/Precautions Modify dosage in patients with severe renal impairment; prolonged use may result in superinfection; a low incidence of cross-hypersensitivity to penicillins exists

Adverse Reactions

1% to 10%: Gastrointestinal: Nausea, vomiting, diarrhea

<1%:

Dermatologic: Maculopapular and erythematous rash

Gastrointestinal: Dyspepsia, pseudomembranous colitis

Hematologic: Bleeding, thrombocytopenia

Local: Pain and induration at injection site

Overdosage/Toxicology Symptoms of overdose include neuromuscular hypersensitivity, convulsions

Hemodialysis may be helpful to aid in the removal of the drug from the blood, otherwise most treatment is supportive or symptom directed

Stability Reconstituted solution is stable for 12-24 hours at room temperature and 96 hours when refrigerated; for I.V. infusion in NS or D_5W solution is stable for 24 hours at room temperature, 96 hours when refrigerated or 12 weeks when frozen; after freezing, thawed solution is stable for 24 hours at room temperature or 96 hours when refrigerated

Mechanism of Action Inhibits bacterial cell wall synthesis by binding to one or more of the penicillin-binding proteins (PBPs) which in turn inhibits the final transpeptidation step of peptidoglycan synthesis in bacterial cell walls, thus inhibiting cell wall biosynthesis. Bacteria eventually lyse due to ongoing activity of cell wall autolytic enzymes (autolysins and murein hydrolases) while cell wall assembly is arrested.

Pharmacodynamics/Kinetics

Distribution: Does not penetrate the CSF unless the meninges are inflamed; crosses the placenta; small amounts appear in breast milk

Protein binding: 65% to 80%

Metabolism: Partially deacetylated in the liver and kidney

Half-life: 30-60 minutes

Time to peak serum concentration:

I.M.: Within 30 minutes

I.V.: Within 15 minutes

Elimination: 50% to 75% of a dose appearing as unchanged drug in urine

Usual Dosage

Children: I.M., I.V.: 75-125 mg/kg/day divided every 4-6 hours; maximum dose: 10 g in a 24-hour period

Adults: I.M., I.V.: 500 mg to 2 g every 4-6 hours

Dosing interval in renal impairment:

Cl_{cr} 10-50 mL/minute: Administer every 6-8 hours

Cl_{cr} <10 mL/minute: Administer every 12 hours

(Continued)

Cephalothin *(Continued)*

Administration Administer around-the-clock to promote less variation in peak and trough serum levels

Monitoring Parameters Observe for signs and symptoms of anaphylaxis during first dose; obtain specimen for culture and sensitivity prior to the first dose

Test Interactions False-positive Coombs' test, may falsely elevate creatinine values when Jaffé reaction is used; may cause false-positive results in urine glucose test using cupric sulfate (Benedict's solution, Clinitest®), false-positive urinary proteins and steroids

Nursing Implications Do not admix with aminoglycosides in same bottle/bag

Additional Information Sodium content of 1 g: 2.8 mEq

Dosage Forms

Infusion, as sodium, in D_5W (frozen): 1 g (50 mL); 2 g (50 mL)
Powder for injection, as sodium: 1 g, 2 g, 20 g

Cephalothin Sodium *see* Cephalothin *on previous page*

Cephapirin (sef a PYE rin)

Related Information

Cephalosporins by Generation *on page 1447*

Brand Names Cefadyl®

Synonyms Cephapirin Sodium

Therapeutic Category Antibiotic, Cephalosporin (First Generation)

Use Treatment of infections when caused by susceptible strains including group A beta-hemolytic *Streptococcus*; used in serious respiratory, genitourinary, gastrointestinal, skin and soft tissue, bone and joint infections; septicemia; endocarditis; identical to cephalothin

Pregnancy Risk Factor B

Contraindications Hypersensitivity to cephapirin sodium, any component, or cephalosporins

Warnings/Precautions Modify dosage in patients with severe renal impairment; prolonged use may result in superinfection; a low incidence of cross-hypersensitivity to penicillins exists

Adverse Reactions

1% to 10%: Gastrointestinal: Diarrhea

<1%:

- Central nervous system: CNS irritation, seizures, fever
- Dermatologic: Rash, urticaria
- Hematologic: Leukopenia, thrombocytopenia
- Hepatic: Transient elevation of liver enzymes

Overdosage/Toxicology Symptoms of overdose include neuromuscular hypersensitivity, convulsions

Hemodialysis may be helpful to aid in the removal of the drug from the blood, otherwise most treatment is supportive or symptom directed

Drug Interactions

Increased effect: High-dose probenecid decreases clearance
Increased toxicity: Aminoglycosides increase nephrotoxic potential

Stability Reconstituted solution is stable for 24 hours at room temperature and 10 days when refrigerated; for I.V. infusion in NS or D_5W solution is stable for 24 hours at room temperature, 10 days when refrigerated or 14 days when frozen; after freezing, thawed solution is stable for 12 hours at room temperature or 10 days when refrigerated

Mechanism of Action Inhibits bacterial cell wall synthesis by binding to one or more of the penicillin-binding proteins (PBPs) which in turn inhibits the final transpeptidation step of peptidoglycan synthesis in bacterial cell walls, thus inhibiting cell wall biosynthesis. Bacteria eventually lyse due to ongoing activity of cell wall autolytic enzymes (autolysins and murein hydrolases) while cell wall assembly is arrested.

Pharmacodynamics/Kinetics

Distribution: Widely distributed into most body tissues and fluids including gallbladder, liver, kidneys, bone, sputum, bile, and pleural and synovial fluids; CSF penetration is poor; crosses the placenta and small amounts appear in breast milk

Protein binding: 22% to 25%

Metabolism: Partially in the liver, kidney, and plasma to metabolites (50% active)

Half-life: 36-60 minutes

Time to peak serum concentration:

- I.M.: Within 30 minutes
- I.V.: Within 5 minutes

Elimination: 60% to 85% excreted as unchanged drug in urine

Usual Dosage I.M., I.V.:

Children: 10-20 mg/kg/dose every 6 hours up to 4 g/24 hours

Adults: 500 mg to 1 g every 6 hours up to 12 g/day

Dosing interval in renal impairment:

Cl_{cr} 10-50 mL/minute: Administer every 6-8 hours

Cl_{cr} <10 mL/minute: Administer every 12 hours

Administration Administer around-the-clock rather than 4 times/day to promote less variation in peak and trough serum levels

Monitoring Parameters Observe for signs and symptoms of anaphylaxis during first dose

Test Interactions False-positive Coombs' test, may falsely elevate creatinine values when Jaffé reaction is used, may cause false-positive results in urine glucose tests using cupric sulfate (Benedict's solution, Clinitest®), false-positive urinary proteins and steroids

Nursing Implications Do not admix with aminoglycosides in same bottle/bag; obtain specimens for culture and sensitivity prior to administration of first dose

Additional Information Sodium content of 1 g: 2.4 mEq

Dosage Forms Powder for injection, as sodium: 500 mg, 1 g, 2 g, 4 g, 20 g

Cephapirin Sodium *see* Cephapirin *on previous page*

Cephradine (SEF ra deen)

Related Information

Cephalosporins by Generation *on page 1447*

Brand Names Velosef®

Canadian/Mexican Brand Names Veracef® (Mexico)

Therapeutic Category Antibiotic, Cephalosporin (First Generation)

Use Treatment of susceptible bacterial infections, including those caused by group A beta-hemolytic *Streptococcus*; used in in respiratory, genitourinary, gastrointestinal, skin and soft tissue, bone and joint infections

Pregnancy Risk Factor B

Contraindications Hypersensitivity to cephradine, any component, or cephalosporins

Warnings/Precautions Prolonged use may result in superinfection; use with caution in patients with a history of colitis; reduce dose in patients with renal dysfunction; a low incidence of cross-hypersensitivity with penicillins exists

Adverse Reactions

1% to 10%: Gastrointestinal: Diarrhea

<1%:

Dermatologic: Rash

Gastrointestinal: Nausea, vomiting, pseudomembranous colitis

Renal: Increased BUN/creatinine

Overdosage/Toxicology Symptoms of overdose include neuromuscular hypersensitivity, convulsions

Hemodialysis may be helpful to aid in the removal of the drug from the blood, otherwise most treatment is supportive or symptom directed

Stability Reconstituted solution is stable for 2 hours at room temperature and 24 hours when refrigerated; for I.V. infusion in NS or D_5W solution is stable for 10 hours at room temperature, 48 hours when refrigerated or 6 weeks when frozen; after freezing, thawed solution is stable for 10 hours at room temperature or 48 hours when refrigerated

Mechanism of Action Inhibits bacterial cell wall synthesis by binding to one or more of the penicillin-binding proteins (PBPs) which in turn inhibits the final transpeptidation step of peptidoglycan synthesis in bacterial cell walls, thus inhibiting cell wall biosynthesis. Bacteria eventually lyse due to ongoing activity of cell wall autolytic enzymes (autolysins and murein hydrolases) while cell wall assembly is arrested.

Pharmacodynamics/Kinetics

Absorption: Oral is faster than I.M., but well absorbed from all routes

Distribution: Widely distributed into most body tissues and fluids including gallbladder, liver, kidneys, bone, sputum, bile, and pleural and synovial fluids; CSF penetration is poor; crosses the placenta and appears in breast milk

Protein binding: 18% to 20%

Half-life: 1-2 hours

Time to peak serum concentration: Oral, I.M.: Within 1-2 hours

Elimination: ~80% to 90% unchanged drug is recovered in urine within 6 hours

Usual Dosage Oral:

Children ≥9 months: 25-50 mg/kg/day in divided doses every 6 hours

Adults: 250-500 mg every 6-12 hours

Dosing adjustment in renal impairment:

Cl_{cr} 10-50 mL/minute: Administer 50% of dose

Cl_{cr} <10 mL/minute: Administer 25% of dose

or

(Continued)

Cephradine *(Continued)*

Cl_{cr} 25-50 mL/minute: Administer every 12 hours
Cl_{cr} 10-25 mL/minute: Administer every 24 hours
Cl_{cr} <10 mL/minute: Administer every 36 hours

Administration Administer around-the-clock to promote less variation in peak and trough serum levels

Monitoring Parameters Observe for signs and symptoms of anaphylaxis during first dose

Test Interactions False-positive Coombs' test, may falsely elevate creatinine values when Jaffé reaction is used, may cause false-positive results in urine glucose tests using cupric sulfate (Benedict's solution, Clinitest®), false-positive urinary proteins and steroids

Patient Information Take until gone, do not miss doses; report diarrhea promptly; entire course of medication (10-14 days) should be taken to ensure eradication of organism; should be taken in equal intervals around-the-clock to maintain adequate blood levels; may interfere with oral contraceptives; females should report symptoms of vaginitis

Nursing Implications Do not admix with aminoglycosides in same bottle/bag; obtain specimen for culture and sensitivity prior to the first dose

Dosage Forms

Capsule: 250 mg, 500 mg
Powder for oral suspension: 125 mg/5 mL (5 mL, 100 mL, 200 mL); 250 mg/5 mL (5 mL, 100 mL, 200 mL)

Cephulac® *see* Lactulose *on page 703*
Ceptaz™ *see* Ceftazidime *on page 232*
Ceredase® *see* Alglucerase *on page 47*
Cerezyme® *see* Alglucerase *on page 47*
Cerubidine® *see* Daunorubicin Hydrochloride *on page 345*
Cerumenex® *see* Triethanolamine Polypeptide Oleate-Condensate *on page 1261*
Cervidil® Vaginal Insert *see* Dinoprostone *on page 397*
C.E.S. *see* Estrogens, Conjugated *on page 471*
Cetacort® *see* Hydrocortisone *on page 623*
Cetamide® Ophthalmic *see* Sulfacetamide Sodium *on page 1171*
Cetapred® Ophthalmic *see* Sulfacetamide Sodium and Prednisolone *on page 1172*

Cetirizine (se TI ra zeen)

Brand Names Zyrtec™

Canadian/Mexican Brand Names Reactine™ (Canada)

Synonyms Cetirizine Hydrochloride; P-071; UCB-P071

Therapeutic Category Antihistamine

Use Perennial and seasonal allergic rhinitis and other allergic symptoms including urticaria

Pregnancy Risk Factor B

Contraindications Hypersensitivity to cetirizine, hydroxyzine, or any component

Warnings/Precautions Cetirizine should be used cautiously in patients with hepatic or renal dysfunction, the elderly and in nursing mothers. Doses >10 mg/day may cause significant drowsiness

Adverse Reactions

>10%: Central nervous system: Headache has been reported to occur in 10% to 12% of patients, drowsiness has been reported in as much as 26% of patients on high doses

1% to 10%:
Central nervous system: Somnolence, fatigue, dizziness
Gastrointestinal: Xerostomia

<1%: Central nervous system: Depression

Overdosage/Toxicology Symptoms of overdose include seizures, sedation, hypotension. There is no specific treatment for an antihistamine overdose, however, most of its clinical toxicity is due to anticholinergic effects

Anticholinesterase inhibitors may be useful by reducing acetylcholinesterase. For anticholinergic overdose with severe life-threatening symptoms, physostigmine 1-2 mg (0.5 or 0.02 mg/kg for children) I.V., slowly may be given to reverse these effects.

Drug Interactions Increased toxicity: CNS depressants, anticholinergics

Mechanism of Action Competes with histamine for H_1-receptor sites on effector cells in the gastrointestinal tract, blood vessels, and respiratory tract

Pharmacodynamics/Kinetics

Onset of effect: Within 15-30 minutes
Absorption: Oral: Rapid
Metabolism: Exact fate is unknown, limited hepatic metabolism
Half-life: 8-11 hours

Time to peak serum concentration: Within 30-60 minutes

Usual Dosage Children ≥6 years and Adults: Oral: 5-10 mg once daily, depending upon symptom severity

Dosing interval in renal/hepatic impairment:

Cl_{cr} ≤31 mL/minute: Administer 5 mg once daily

Monitoring Parameters Relief of symptoms, sedation and anticholinergic effects

Dosage Forms

Syrup, as hydrochloride: 5 mg/5 mL (120 mL)

Tablet, as hydrochloride: 5 mg, 10 mg

Cetirizine Hydrochloride *see* Cetirizine *on previous page*

Cevalin® [OTC] *see* Ascorbic Acid *on page 102*

Cevi-Bid® [OTC] *see* Ascorbic Acid *on page 102*

Ce-Vi-Sol® [OTC] *see* Ascorbic Acid *on page 102*

CG *see* Chorionic Gonadotropin *on page 272*

Charcoaid® [OTC] *see* Charcoal *on this page*

Charcoal (CHAR kole)

Brand Names Actidose-Aqua® [OTC]; Actidose® With Sorbitol [OTC]; Charcoaid® [OTC]; Charcocaps® [OTC]; Insta-Char® [OTC]; Liqui-Char® [OTC]; SuperChar® [OTC]

Canadian/Mexican Brand Names Charcodole® (Canada); Charcodole® AQ (Canada); Charcodole® TFS

Synonyms Activated Carbon; Activated Charcoal; Adsorbent Charcoal; Liquid Antidote; Medicinal Carbon; Medicinal Charcoal

Therapeutic Category Antidiarrheal; Antidote, Adsorbent; Antiflatulent

Use Emergency treatment in poisoning by drugs and chemicals; repetitive doses for gastric dialysis in uremia to adsorb various waste products, and repetitive doses have proven useful to enhance the elimination of certain drugs (eg, theophylline, phenobarbital, and aspirin)

Pregnancy Risk Factor C

Contraindications Not effective for cyanide, mineral acids, caustic alkalis, organic solvents, iron, ethanol, methanol poisoning, lithium; do not use charcoal with sorbitol in patients with fructose intolerance; charcoal with sorbitol is not recommended in children <1 year.

Warnings/Precautions When using ipecac with charcoal, induce vomiting with ipecac before administering activated charcoal since charcoal adsorbs ipecac syrup; charcoal may cause vomiting which is hazardous in petroleum distillate and caustic ingestions; if charcoal in sorbitol is administered, doses should be limited to prevent excessive fluid and electrolyte losses; do not mix charcoal with milk, ice cream, or sherbet

Adverse Reactions

>10%:

Gastrointestinal: Vomiting, diarrhea with sorbitol, constipation

Miscellaneous: Stools will turn black

<1%: Gastrointestinal: Swelling of abdomen

Drug Interactions Do not administer concomitantly with syrup of ipecac; do not mix with milk, ice cream, or sherbet

Stability Adsorbs gases from air, store in closed container

Mechanism of Action Adsorbs toxic substances or irritants, thus inhibiting GI absorption; adsorbs intestinal gas; the addition of sorbitol results in hyperosmotic laxative action causing catharsis

Pharmacodynamics/Kinetics

Absorption: Not absorbed from GI tract

Metabolism: Not metabolized

Elimination: As charcoal in feces

Usual Dosage Oral:

Acute poisoning:

Charcoal with sorbitol: Single-dose:

Children 1-12 years: 1-2 g/kg/dose or 15-30 g or approximately 5-10 times the weight of the ingested poison; 1 g adsorbs 100-1000 mg of poison; the use of repeat oral charcoal with sorbitol doses is not recommended. In young children, sorbitol should be repeated no more than 1-2 times/day.

Adults: 30-100 g

Charcoal in water:

Single-dose:

Infants <1 year: 1 g/kg

Children 1-12 years: 15-30 g or 1-2 g/kg

Adults: 30-100 g or 1-2 g/kg

Multiple-dose:

Infants <1 year: 0.5 g/kg every 4-6 hours

(Continued)

Charcoal *(Continued)*

Children 1-12 years: 20-60 g or 0.5-1 g/kg every 2-6 hours until clinical observations, serum drug concentration have returned to a subtherapeutic range, or charcoal stool apparent

Adults: 20-60 g or 0.5-1 g/kg every 2-6 hours

Gastric dialysis: Adults: 20-50 g every 6 hours for 1-2 days

Intestinal gas, diarrhea, GI distress: Adults: 520-975 mg after meals or at first sign of discomfort; repeat as needed to a maximum dose of 4.16 g/day

Administration Flavoring agents (eg, chocolate) and sorbitol can enhance charcoal's palatability; marmalade, milk, ice cream, and sherbet should be avoided since they can reduce charcoal's effectiveness

Patient Information Charcoal causes the stools to turn black; should not be used prior to calling a poison control center or a physician

Nursing Implications Too concentrated of slurries may clog airway; often given with a laxative or cathartic; check for presence of bowel sounds before administration

Dosage Forms

Capsule (Charcocaps®): 260 mg

Liquid, activated:

- Actidose-Aqua®: 12.5 g (60 mL); 25 g (120 mL)
- Liqui-Char®: 12.5 g (60 mL); 15 g (75 mL); 25 g (120 mL); 30 g (120 mL); 50 g (240 mL)
- SuperChar®: 30 g (240 mL)

Liquid, activated, with propylene glycol: 12.5 g (60 mL); 25 g (120 mL)

Liquid, activated, with sorbitol:

- Actidose® With Sorbitol: 25 g (120 mL); 50 g (240 mL)
- Charcoaid®: 30 g (150 mL)
- SuperChar®: 30 g (240 mL)

Powder for suspension, activated:

- 15 g, 30 g, 40 g, 120 g, 240 g
- SuperChar®: 30 g

Charcocaps® [OTC] *see* Charcoal *on previous page*

Chealamide® *see* Edetate Disodium *on page 438*

Chelated Manganese® [OTC] *see* Manganese *on page 757*

Chemet® *see* Succimer *on page 1165*

Chenix® *see* Chenodiol *on this page*

Chenodeoxycholic Acid *see* Chenodiol *on this page*

Chenodiol (kee noe DYE ole)

Brand Names Chenix®

Synonyms Chenodeoxycholic Acid

Therapeutic Category Bile Acid; Gallstone Dissolution Agent

Use Oral dissolution of cholesterol gallstones in selected patients

Pregnancy Risk Factor X

Contraindications Presence of known hepatocyte dysfunction or bile ductal abnormalities; a gallbladder confirmed as nonvisualizing after two consecutive single doses of dye; radiopaque stones; gallstone complications or compelling reasons for gallbladder surgery; inflammatory bowel disease or active gastric or duodenal ulcer; pregnancy

Warnings/Precautions Chenodiol is hepatotoxic in animal models including subhuman Primates; chenodiol should be discontinued if aminotransferases exceed 3 times the upper normal limit; chenodiol may contribute to colon cancer in otherwise susceptible individuals

Adverse Reactions

>10%:

- Gastrointestinal: Diarrhea (mild), biliary pain
- Miscellaneous: Aminotransferase increases

1% to 10%:

- Endocrine & metabolic: Increases in cholesterol and LDL cholesterol
- Gastrointestinal: Dyspepsia

<1%:

- Gastrointestinal: Diarrhea (severe), cramps, nausea, vomiting, flatulence, constipation
- Hematologic: Leukopenia
- Hepatic: Intrahepatic cholestasis, higher cholecystectomy rates

Overdosage/Toxicology Symptoms of overdose include diarrhea and a rise in liver function tests have been observed; no specific antidote, institute supportive therapy

Drug Interactions Decreased effect: Antacids, cholestyramine, colestipol, oral contraceptives

Mechanism of Action Chenodiol is a primary acid excreted into bile, normally constituting one-third of the total biliary bile acids. Synthesis of chenodiol is regulated by the relative composition and flux of cholesterol and bile acids through the hepatocyte by a negative feedback effect on the rate-limiting enzymes for synthesis of cholesterol (HMGCoA reductase) and bile acids (cholesterol 7 alpha-hydroxyl).

Usual Dosage Adults: Oral: 13-16 mg/kg/day in 2 divided doses, starting with 250 mg twice daily the first 2 weeks and increasing by 250 mg/day each week thereafter until the recommended or maximum tolerated dose is achieved

Dosing comments in hepatic impairment: Contraindicated for use in presence of known hepatocyte dysfunction or bile ductal abnormalities

Monitoring Parameters Oral cholecystograms and/or ultrasonograms should be used to monitor response; dissolutions of stones should be confirmed 1-3 months later

Test Interactions ↑ aminotransferases, ↑ cholesterol, ↑ LDL cholesterol, ↓ triglycerides, ↑ bilirubin (I)

Patient Information Periodic liver function tests and oral cholecystograms are required to monitor therapy; contact the physician immediately if nonspecific abdominal pain, right upper quadrant pain, nausea, and vomiting are severe

Dosage Forms Tablet, film coated: 250 mg

Cheracol® *see* Guaifenesin and Codeine *on page 590*

Cheracol® D [OTC] *see* Guaifenesin and Dextromethorphan *on page 591*

Chibroxin™ *see* Norfloxacin *on page 915*

Chicken Pox Vaccine *see* Varicella Virus Vaccine *on page 1290*

Chigger-Tox® [OTC] *see* Benzocaine *on page 138*

Children's Advil® Oral Suspension [OTC] *see* Ibuprofen *on page 639*

Children's Hold® [OTC] *see* Dextromethorphan *on page 366*

Children's Kaopectate® [OTC] *see* Attapulgite *on page 118*

Children's Motrin® Oral Suspension [OTC] *see* Ibuprofen *on page 639*

Children's Silfedrine® [OTC] *see* Pseudoephedrine *on page 1074*

Children's Vitamins *see* Vitamins, Multiple *on page 1310*

Chlo-Amine® [OTC] *see* Chlorpheniramine *on page 260*

Chloral *see* Chloral Hydrate *on this page*

Chloral Hydrate (KLOR al HYE drate)

Brand Names Aquachloral® Supprettes®

Canadian/Mexican Brand Names Novo-Chlorhydrate® (Canada); PMS-Chloral Hydrate (Canada)

Synonyms Chloral; Hydrated Chloral; Trichloroacetaldehyde Monohydrate

Therapeutic Category Hypnotic; Sedative

Use Short-term sedative and hypnotic (<2 weeks), sedative/hypnotic for dental and diagnostic procedures; sedative prior to EEG evaluations

Restrictions C-IV

Pregnancy Risk Factor C

Contraindications Hypersensitivity to chloral hydrate or any component; hepatic or renal impairment; gastritis or ulcers; severe cardiac disease

Warnings/Precautions Use with caution in patients with porphyria; use with caution in neonates, drug may accumulate with repeated use, prolonged use in neonates associated with hyperbilirubinemia; tolerance to hypnotic effect develops, therefore, not recommended for use >2 weeks; taper dosage to avoid withdrawal with prolonged use; trichloroethanol (TCE), a metabolite of chloral hydrate, is a carcinogen in mice; there is no data in humans. Chloral hydrate is considered a second line hypnotic agent in the elderly. Recent interpretive guidelines from the Health Care Financing Administration (HCFA) discourage the use of chloral hydrate in residents of long-term care facilities.

Adverse Reactions

>10%: Gastrointestinal: Gastric irritation, nausea, vomiting, diarrhea

1% to 10%:

- Central nervous system: Ataxia, hallucinations, drowsiness, "hangover" effect
- Dermatologic: Rash, urticaria

<1%:

- Central nervous system: Disorientation, sedation, ataxia, excitement (paradoxical), dizziness, fever, headache, confusion
- Gastrointestinal: Gastric irritation, flatulence
- Hematologic: Leukopenia, eosinophilia
- Miscellaneous: Physical and psychological dependence may occur with prolonged use of large doses

Overdosage/Toxicology Symptoms of overdose include hypotension, respiratory depression, coma, hypothermia, cardiac arrhythmias

(Continued)

Chloral Hydrate *(Continued)*

Treatment is supportive and symptomatic; lidocaine or propranolol may be used for ventricular dysrhythmias, while isoproterenol or atropine may be required for torsade de pointes; activated charcoal may prevent drug absorption

Drug Interactions Increased toxicity: May potentiate effects of warfarin, central nervous system depressants, alcohol; vasodilation reaction (flushing, tachycardia, etc) may occur with concurrent use of alcohol; concomitant use of furosemide (I.V.) may result in flushing, diaphoresis, and blood pressure changes

Stability Sensitive to light; exposure to air causes volatilization; store in light-resistant, airtight container

Mechanism of Action Central nervous system depressant effects are due to its active metabolite trichloroethanol, mechanism unknown

Pharmacodynamics/Kinetics

Peak effect: Within 0.5-1 hour

Duration: 4-8 hours

Absorption: Oral, rectal: Well absorbed

Distribution: Crosses the placenta; negligible amounts appear in breast milk

Metabolism: Rapidly to trichloroethanol (active metabolite); variable amounts metabolized in liver and kidney to trichloroacetic acid (inactive)

Half-life: Active metabolite: 8-11 hours

Elimination: Metabolites excreted in urine, small amounts excreted in feces via bile

Usual Dosage

Children:

Sedation, anxiety: Oral, rectal: 5-15 mg/kg/dose every 8 hours, maximum: 500 mg/dose

Prior to EEG: Oral, rectal: 20-25 mg/kg/dose, 30-60 minutes prior to EEG; may repeat in 30 minutes to maximum of 100 mg/kg or 2 g total

Hypnotic: Oral, rectal: 20-40 mg/kg/dose up to a maximum of 50 mg/kg/24 hours or 1 g/dose or 2 g/24 hours

Sedation, nonpainful procedure: Oral: 50-75 mg/kg/dose 30-60 minutes prior to procedure; may repeat 30 minutes after initial dose if needed, to a total maximum dose of 120 mg/kg or 1 g total

Adults: Oral, rectal:

Sedation, anxiety: 250 mg 3 times/day

Hypnotic: 500-1000 mg at bedtime or 30 minutes prior to procedure, not to exceed 2 g/24 hours

Dosing adjustment/comments in renal impairment: Cl_{cr} <50 mL/minute: Avoid use

Hemodialysis: Dialyzable (50% to 100%); supplemental dose is not necessary

Dosing adjustment/comments in hepatic impairment: Avoid use in patients with severe hepatic impairment

Dietary Considerations Alcohol: Additive CNS effects, avoid use

Administration Do not crush capsule, contains drug in liquid form

Monitoring Parameters Vital signs, O_2 saturation and blood pressure with doses used for conscious sedation

Test Interactions False-positive urine glucose using Clinitest® method; may interfere with fluorometric urine catecholamine and urinary 17-hydroxycorticosteroid tests

Patient Information Take a capsule with a full glass of water or fruit juice; swallow capsules whole, do not chew; avoid alcohol and other CNS depressants; avoid activities needing good psychomotor coordination until CNS effects are known; drug may cause physical or psychological dependence; avoid abrupt discontinuation after prolonged use; if taking at home prior to a diagnostic procedure, have someone else transport

Nursing Implications Gastric irritation may be minimized by diluting dose in water or other oral liquid

Dosage Forms

Capsule: 250 mg, 500 mg

Suppository, rectal: 324 mg, 500 mg, 648 mg

Syrup: 250 mg/5 mL (10 mL); 500 mg/5 mL (5 mL, 10 mL, 480 mL)

Chlorambucil (klor AM byoo sil)

Related Information

Antiemetics for Chemotherapy Induced Nausea and Vomiting *on page 1348*

Cancer Chemotherapy Regimens *on page 1351*

Toxicities of Chemotherapeutic Agents *on page 1382*

Brand Names Leukeran®

Therapeutic Category Antineoplastic Agent, Alkylating Agent

Use Management of chronic lymphocytic leukemia, Hodgkin's and non-Hodgkin's lymphoma; breast and ovarian carcinoma; Waldenström's macroglobulinemia, testicular carcinoma, thrombocythemia, choriocarcinoma

Pregnancy Risk Factor D

Pregnancy/Breast-Feeding Implications Carcinogenic and mutagenic in humans

Contraindications Previous resistance; hypersensitivity to chlorambucil or any component or other alkylating agents

Warnings/Precautions The U.S. Food and Drug Administration (FDA) currently recommends that procedures for proper handling and disposal of antineoplastic agents be considered. Use with caution in patients with seizure disorder and bone marrow suppression; reduce initial dosage if patient has received radiation therapy, myelosuppressive drugs or has a depressed baseline leukocyte or platelet count within the previous 4 weeks. Can severely suppress bone marrow function; affects human fertility; carcinogenic in humans and probably mutagenic and teratogenic as well; chromosomal damage has been documented; secondary AML may be associated with chronic therapy.

Adverse Reactions

>10%:

- Hematologic: Myelosuppressive: Use with caution when receiving radiation; bone marrow suppression frequently occurs and occasionally bone marrow failure has occurred; blood counts should be monitored closely while undergoing treatment; leukopenia, thrombocytopenia, anemia
  - WBC: Moderate
  - Platelets: Moderate
  - Onset (days): 7
  - Nadir (days): 10-14
  - Recovery (days): 28

1% to 10%:

- Dermatologic: Skin rashes
- Endocrine & metabolic: Hyperuricemia, menstrual changes
- Gastrointestinal: Nausea, vomiting, diarrhea, oral ulceration are all infrequent
  - Emetic potential: Low (<10%)

<1%:

- Central nervous system: Confusion, agitation, drug fever, ataxia, hallucination; rarely generalized or focal seizures
- Dermatologic: Rash
- Endocrine & metabolic: Fertility impairment: Has caused chromosomal damage in men, both reversible and permanent sterility have occurred in both sexes; can produce amenorrhea in females
- Gastrointestinal: Oral ulceration
- Genitourinary: Oligospermia
- Hepatic: Hepatotoxicity, hepatic necrosis
- Neuromuscular & skeletal: Weakness, tremors, muscular twitching, peripheral neuropathy
- Respiratory: Pulmonary fibrosis
- Miscellaneous: Secondary malignancies; Increased incidence of AML; skin hypersensitivity

Overdosage/Toxicology Symptoms of overdose include vomiting, ataxia, coma, seizures, pancytopenia

There are no known antidotes for chlorambucil intoxication, and treatment is mainly supportive, directed at decontaminating the GI tract and controlling symptoms; blood products may be used to treat the hematologic toxicity

Stability Store at room temperature

Mechanism of Action Interferes with DNA replication and RNA transcription by alkylation and cross-linking the strands of DNA

Pharmacodynamics/Kinetics

- Absorption/bioavailability: 70% to 80%; **food will interfere with absorption** resulting in a 10% to 20% decrease in bioavailability
- Distribution: V_d: 0.14-0.24 L/kg
- Protein binding: ~99% bound to albumin; extensive binding to tissues and plasma proteins
- Metabolism: In the liver to an active metabolite
- Half-life: 90 minutes to 2 hours
- Elimination: 60% excreted in urine within 24 hours, principally as metabolites

Usual Dosage Oral (refer to individual protocols):

Children:

- General short courses: 0.1-0.2 mg/kg/day **OR** 4.5 mg/m^2/day for 3-6 weeks for remission induction (usual: 4-10 mg/day); maintenance therapy: 0.03-0.1 mg/kg/day (usual: 2-4 mg/day)
- Nephrotic syndrome: 0.1-0.2 mg/kg/day every day for 5-15 weeks with low-dose prednisone

(Continued)

Chloramb**ucil** *(Continued)*

Chronic lymphocytic leukemia (CLL):

Biweekly regimen: Initial: 0.4 mg/kg/dose every 2 weeks; increase dose by 0.1 mg/kg every 2 weeks until a response occurs and/or myelosuppression occurs

Monthly regimen: Initial: 0.4 mg/kg, increase dose by 0.2 mg/kg every 4 weeks until a response occurs and/or myelosuppression occurs

Malignant lymphomas:

Non-Hodgkin's lymphoma: 0.1 mg/kg/day

Hodgkin's lymphoma: 0.2 mg/kg/day

Adults: 0.1-0.2 mg/kg/day **OR** 3-6 mg/m^2/day for 3-6 weeks, then adjust dose on basis of blood counts. Pulse dosing has been used in CLL as intermittent, biweekly, or monthly doses of 0.4 mg/kg and increased by 0.1 mg/kg until the disease is under control or toxicity ensues. An alternate regimen is 14 mg/m^2/day for 5 days, repeated every 21-28 days.

Hemodialysis: Supplemental dosing is not necessary

Peritoneal dialysis: Supplemental dosing is not necessary

Monitoring Parameters Liver function tests, CBC, leukocyte counts, platelets, serum uric acid

Patient Information Notify physician immediately if sore throat or bleeding occurs, contraceptive measures are recommended during therapy

Dosage Forms Tablet, sugar coated: 2 mg

Extemporaneous Preparations A 2 mg/mL suspension was stable for 7 days when refrigerated and compounded as follows: Pulverize sixty 2 mg tablets; levigate with a small amount of glycerin; add 20 mL Cologel® and levigate until a uniform mixture is obtained; add a 2:1 simple syrup/cherry syrup mixture to make a total volume of 60 mL

Handbook in Extemporaneous Formulations, Bethesda, MD: American Society of Hospital Pharmacists, 1987.

Chloramphenicol (klor am FEN i kole)

Related Information

Antimicrobial Drugs of Choice *on page 1468*

Bacterial Meningitis Practical Guidelines for Management *on page 1475*

Brand Names AK-Chlor®; Chloromycetin®; Chloroptic®

Canadian/Mexican Brand Names Diochloram® (Canada); Pentamycetin® (Canada); Sopamycetin® (Canada); Cetina® (Mexico); Clorafen® (Mexico); Paraxin® (Mexico); Quemicetina® (Mexico)

Therapeutic Category Antibiotic, Ophthalmic; Antibiotic, Otic; Antibiotic, Miscellaneous

Use Treatment of serious infections due to organisms resistant to other less toxic antibiotics or when its penetrability into the site of infection is clinically superior to other antibiotics to which the organism is sensitive; useful in infections caused by *Bacteroides, H. influenzae, Neisseria meningitidis, Salmonella*, and *Rickettsia*

Pregnancy Risk Factor C

Contraindications Hypersensitivity to chloramphenicol or any component

Warnings/Precautions Use with caution in patients with impaired renal or hepatic function and in neonates; reduce dose with impaired liver function; use with care in patients with glucose 6-phosphate dehydrogenase deficiency. Serious and fatal blood dyscrasias have occurred after both short-term and prolonged therapy; should not be used when less potentially toxic agents are effective; prolonged use may result in superinfection.

Adverse Reactions

<1%:

Central nervous system: Nightmares, headache

Dermatologic: Rash

Gastrointestinal: Diarrhea, stomatitis, enterocolitis, nausea, vomiting

Hematologic: Bone marrow suppression, aplastic anemia

Neuromuscular & skeletal: Peripheral neuropathy

Ocular: Optic neuritis

Miscellaneous: Gray baby syndrome

Three (3) major toxicities associated with chloramphenicol include:

Aplastic anemia, an idiosyncratic reaction which can occur with any route of administration; usually occurs 3 weeks to 12 months after initial exposure to chloramphenicol

Bone marrow suppression is thought to be dose-related with serum concentrations >25 µg/mL and reversible once chloramphenicol is discontinued; anemia and neutropenia may occur during the first week of therapy

Gray baby syndrome is characterized by circulatory collapse, cyanosis, acidosis, abdominal distention, myocardial depression, coma, and death;

reaction appears to be associated with serum levels ≥50 μg/mL; may result from drug accumulation in patients with impaired hepatic or renal function

Overdosage/Toxicology Symptoms of overdose include anemia, metabolic acidosis, hypotension, hypothermia; treatment is supportive following GI decontamination

Drug Interactions

Decreased effect: Phenobarbital and rifampin may decrease concentration of chloramphenicol

Increased toxicity: Chloramphenicol inhibits the metabolism of chlorpropamide, phenytoin, oral anticoagulants

Stability Refrigerate ophthalmic solution; constituted solutions remain stable for 30 days; use only clear solutions; frozen solutions remain stable for 6 months

Mechanism of Action Reversibly binds to 50S ribosomal subunits of susceptible organisms preventing amino acids from being transferred to growing peptide chains thus inhibiting protein synthesis

Pharmacodynamics/Kinetics

Absorption: Oral: 75% to 100%; in neonates, GI absorption of chloramphenicol palmitate is slow and erratic

Distribution: Readily crosses placenta; appears in breast milk; distributes to most tissues and body fluids

- Relative diffusion of antimicrobial agents from blood into cerebrospinal fluid (CSF): Adequate with or without inflammation (exceeds usual MICs)
- Ratio of CSF to blood level (%):
  - Normal meninges: 66
  - Inflamed meninges: 66+

Protein binding: 60%

Metabolism: Extensive in the liver (90%) to inactive metabolites, principally by glucuronidation, chloramphenicol palmitate is hydrolyzed by lipases in the GI tract to the active base; chloramphenicol sodium succinate is hydrolyzed by esterases to active base

Half-life: (Prolonged with markedly reduced liver function or combined liver/kidney dysfunction):

- Normal renal function: 1.6-3.3 hours
- End stage renal disease: 3-7 hours
- Cirrhosis: 10-12 hours
- Neonates: Postnatal:
  - 1-2 days: 24 hours
  - 10-16 days: 10 hours

Time to peak serum concentration: Oral: Within 0.5-3 hours

Elimination: 5% to 15% excreted as unchanged drug in the urine, 4% excreted in bile; in neonates, 6% to 80% may be excreted unchanged in urine

Usual Dosage

Meningitis: Oral, I.V.: Infants >30 days and Children: 75-100 mg/kg/day divided every 6 hours

Other infections: Oral, I.V.:

- Infants and Children: 50-75 mg/kg/day divided every 6 hours; maximum daily dose: 4 g/day
- Adults: 50-100 mg/kg/day in divided doses every 6 hours; maximum daily dose: 4 g/day

Ophthalmic: Children and Adults: Instill 1-2 drops or 1.25 cm (½" of ointment every 3-4 hours); increase interval between applications after 48 hours to 2-3 times/day

Otic solution: Instill 2-3 drops into ear 3 times/day

Topical: Gently rub into the affected area 1-4 times/day

Dosing adjustment/comments in hepatic impairment: Avoid use in severe liver impairment as increased toxicity may occur

Hemodialysis: Slightly dialyzable (5% to 20%) via hemo- and peritoneal dialysis; no supplemental doses needed in dialysis or continuous arterio-venous or veno-venous hemofiltration (CAVH/CAVHD)

Dietary Considerations Folic acid, iron salts, vitamin B_{12}: May decrease intestinal absorption of vitamin B_{12}; may have increased dietary need for riboflavin, pyridoxine, and vitamin B_{12}; monitor hematological status

Administration Administer around-the-clock rather than 4 times/day to promote less variation in peak and trough serum levels

Monitoring Parameters CBC with reticulocyte and platelet counts, periodic liver and renal function tests, serum drug concentration

Reference Range

Therapeutic levels: 15-20 μg/mL; Toxic concentration: >40 μg/mL; Trough: 5-10 μg/mL

Timing of serum samples: Draw levels 1.5 hours and 3 hours after completion of I.V. or oral dose; trough levels may be preferred; should be drawn ≤1 hour prior to dose

(Continued)

Chloramphenicol *(Continued)*

Test Interactions ↑ iron (B), prothrombin time (S); ↓ urea nitrogen (B)

Patient Information Take on empty stomach; take with food if GI upset occurs, at evenly spaced intervals (every 6 hours around-the-clock); notify physician if persistent sore throat, tiredness, or unusual bleeding or bruising

Additional Information Sodium content of 1 g (injection): 51.8 mg (2.25 mEq)

Dosage Forms

Capsule: 250 mg

Ointment, ophthalmic: 1% [10 mg/g] (3.5 g)

AK-Chlor®, Chloromycetin®, Chloroptic® S.O.P.: 1% [10 mg/g] (3.5 g)

Powder for injection, as sodium succinate: 1 g

Powder for ophthalmic solution (Chloromycetin®): 25 mg/vial (15 mL)

Solution: 0.5% [5 mg/mL] (7.5 mL, 15 mL)

Ophthalmic (AK-Chlor®, Chloroptic®): 0.5% [5 mg/mL] (2.5 mL, 7.5 mL, 15 mL)

Otic (Chloromycetin®): 0.5% (15 mL)

Chlorate® [OTC] *see* Chlorpheniramine *on page 260*

Chlordiazepoxide (klor dye az e POKS ide)

Related Information

Benzodiazepines Comparison *on page 1397*

Brand Names Libritabs®; Librium®; Mitran®; Reposans-10®

Canadian/Mexican Brand Names Apo-Chlordiazepoxide® (Canada); Corax® (Canada); Medilium® (Canada); Novo-Poxide® (Canada); Solium® (Canada)

Synonyms Methaminodiazepoxide Hydrochloride

Therapeutic Category Benzodiazepine; Hypnotic; Sedative

Use Approved for anxiety, may be useful for acute alcohol withdrawal symptoms

Restrictions C-IV

Pregnancy Risk Factor D

Contraindications Hypersensitivity to chlordiazepoxide or any component, pre-existing CNS depression, severe uncontrolled pain

Warnings/Precautions Use with caution in patients with respiratory depression, CNS impairment, liver dysfunction, or a history of drug dependence

Adverse Reactions

>10%:

Cardiovascular: Chest pain

Central nervous system: Drowsiness, fatigue, ataxia, lightheadedness, memory impairment, insomnia, anxiety, depression, headache

Dermatologic: Skin eruptions, rash

Endocrine & metabolic: Decreased libido

Gastrointestinal: Nausea, constipation, vomiting, diarrhea, xerostomia, increased or decreased appetite, decreased salivation

Neuromuscular & skeletal: Dysarthria

Ocular: Blurred vision

Miscellaneous: Diaphoresis

1% to 10%:

Cardiovascular: Hypotension, tachycardia, edema, syncope

Central nervous system: Ataxia, confusion, mental impairment, nervousness, dizziness, akathisia

Dermatologic: Dermatitis

Gastrointestinal: Weight gain or loss, increased salivation

Neuromuscular & skeletal: Rigidity, tremor, muscle cramps

Ocular: Blurred vision

Otic: Tinnitus

Respiratory: Nasal congestion, hyperventilation

<1%:

Endocrine & metabolic: Menstrual irregularities

Hematologic: Blood dyscrasias

Neuromuscular & skeletal: Depressed reflexes

Miscellaneous: Drug dependence

Overdosage/Toxicology Symptoms of overdose include hypotension, respiratory depression, coma, hypothermia, cardiac arrhythmias

Treatment for benzodiazepine overdose is supportive; rarely is mechanical ventilation required; flumazenil has been shown to selectively block the binding of benzodiazepines to CNS receptors, resulting in a reversal of benzodiazepine-induced CNS depression. Respiratory depression may not be reversed.

Drug Interactions Increased toxicity (CNS depression): Oral anticoagulants, alcohol, tricyclic antidepressants, sedative-hypnotics, MAO inhibitors

Stability Refrigerate injection; protect from light; **incompatible** when mixed with Ringer's solution, normal saline, ascorbic acid, benzquinamide, heparin, phenytoin, promethazine, secobarbital

Pharmacodynamics/Kinetics

Distribution: V_d: 3.3 L/kg; crosses the placenta; appears in breast milk
Protein binding: 90% to 98%
Metabolism: Extensive in the liver to desmethyldiazepam (active and long-acting)
Half-life: 6.6-25 hours
  End stage renal disease: 5-30 hours
  Cirrhosis: 30-63 hours
Time to peak serum concentration:
  Oral: Within 2 hours
  I.M.: Results in lower peak plasma levels than oral
Elimination: Very little excretion in urine as unchanged drug

Usual Dosage

Children:
  <6 years: Not recommended
  >6 years: Anxiety: Oral, I.M.: 0.5 mg/kg/24 hours divided every 6-8 hours

Adults:
  Anxiety:
    Oral: 15-100 mg divided 3-4 times/day
    I.M., I.V.: Initial: 50-100 mg followed by 25-50 mg 3-4 times/day as needed
  Preoperative anxiety: I.M.: 50-100 mg prior to surgery
  Alcohol withdrawal symptoms: Oral, I.V.: 50-100 mg to start, dose may be repeated in 2-4 hours as necessary to a maximum of 300 mg/24 hours

Dosing adjustment in renal impairment: Cl_{cr} <10 mL/minute: Administer 50% of dose

Hemodialysis: Not dialyzable (0% to 5%)

Dosing adjustment/comments in hepatic impairment: Avoid use

Dietary Considerations Alcohol: Additive CNS effects, avoid use

Administration Up to 300 mg may be given I.M. or I.V. during a 6-hour period, but not more than this in any 24-hour period; do not use diluent provided with parenteral form for I.V. administration; dissolve with normal saline instead; I.V. form is a powder and should be reconstituted with 5 mL of sterile water or saline prior to administration

Monitoring Parameters Respiratory and cardiovascular status, mental status, check for orthostasis

Reference Range Therapeutic: 0.1-3 μg/mL (SI: 0-10 μmol/L); Toxic: >23 μg/mL (SI: >77 μmol/L)

Test Interactions ↓ HDL, ↑ triglycerides (S)

Patient Information Avoid alcohol and other CNS depressants; avoid activities needing good psychomotor coordination until CNS effects are known; drug may cause physical or psychological dependence; avoid abrupt discontinuation after prolonged use, may cause drowsiness, poor balance

Nursing Implications Raise bed rails; initiate safety measures; aid with ambulation

Dosage Forms

Capsule, as hydrochloride: 5 mg, 10 mg, 25 mg
Powder for injection, as hydrochloride: 100 mg
Tablet: 5 mg, 10 mg, 25 mg

Chlorhexidine Gluconate (klor HEKS i deen GLOO koe nate)

Brand Names BactoShield® Topical [OTC]; Betasept® [OTC]; Dyna-Hex® Topical [OTC]; Exidine® Scrub [OTC]; Hibiclens® Topical [OTC]; Hibistat® Topical [OTC]; Peridex® Oral Rinse; PerioGard®

Therapeutic Category Antibacterial, Oral Rinse; Mouthwash

Use Skin cleanser for surgical scrub, cleanser for skin wounds, germicidal hand rinse, and as antibacterial dental rinse. Chlorhexidine is active against gram-positive and gram-negative organisms, facultative anaerobes, aerobes, and yeast.

Pregnancy Risk Factor B

Contraindications Known hypersensitivity to chlorhexidine gluconate

Warnings/Precautions Staining of oral surfaces, tooth restorations, and dorsum of tongue may occur; keep out of eyes and ears; for topical use only; there have been case reports of anaphylaxis following chlorhexidine disinfection

Adverse Reactions

>10%:
  Oral: Increase of tartar on teeth, changes in taste. Staining of oral surfaces (mucosa, teeth, dorsum of tongue) may be visible as soon as 1 week after therapy begins and is more pronounced when there is a heavy accumulation of unremoved plaque and when teeth fillings have rough surfaces. Stain does not have a clinically adverse effect but because removal may not be possible, patient with frontal restoration should be advised of the potential permanency of the stain.

(Continued)

Chlorhexidine Gluconate *(Continued)*

1% to 10%: Gastrointestinal: Tongue irritation, oral irritation

<1%:

Cardiovascular: Facial edema

Respiratory: Nasal congestion, shortness of breath

Overdosage/Toxicology Symptoms of oral overdose include gastric distress, nausea, or signs of alcohol intoxication

Mechanism of Action The bactericidal effect of chlorhexidine is a result of the binding of this cationic molecule to negatively charged bacterial cell walls and extramicrobial complexes. At low concentrations, this causes an alteration of bacterial cell osmotic equilibrium and leakage of potassium and phosphorous resulting in a bacteriostatic effect. At high concentrations of chlorhexidine, the cytoplasmic contents of the bacterial cell precipitate and result in cell death.

Pharmacodynamics/Kinetics

Absorption: ~30% of chlorhexidine is retained in the oral cavity following rinsing and is slowly released into the oral fluids; chlorhexidine is poorly absorbed from the GI tract

Serum concentrations: Detectable levels are not present in the plasma 12 hours after administration

Elimination: Primarily through the feces (approximately 90%); <1% excreted in the urine

Usual Dosage Adults: Oral rinse (Peridex®):

Precede use of solution by flossing and brushing teeth; completely rinse toothpaste from mouth. Swish 15 mL undiluted oral rinse around in mouth for 30 seconds, then expectorate. Caution patient not to swallow the medicine. Avoid eating for 2-3 hours after treatment. (The cap on bottle of oral rinse is a measure for 15 mL.)

When used as a treatment of gingivitis, the regimen begins with oral prophylaxis. Patient treats mouth with 15 mL chlorhexidine, swishes for 30 seconds, then expectorates. This is repeated twice daily (morning and evening). Patient should have a re-evaluation followed by a dental prophylaxis every 6 months.

Cleanser:

Surgical scrub: Scrub 3 minutes and rinse thoroughly, wash for an additional 3 minutes

Hand wash: Wash for 15 seconds and rinse

Hand rinse: Rub 15 seconds and rinse

Patient Information

Oral rinse: Do not swallow, do not rinse after use; may cause reduced taste perception which is reversible; may cause discoloration of teeth

Topical administration is for external use only

Dosage Forms

Foam, topical, with isopropyl alcohol 4% (BactoShield®): 4% (180 mL)

Liquid, topical, with isopropyl alcohol 4%:

Dyna-Hex® Skin Cleanser: 2% (120 mL, 240 mL, 480 mL, 960 mL, 4000 mL); 4% (120 mL, 240 mL, 480 mL, 4000 mL)

BactoShield® 2: 2% (960 mL)

BactoShield®, Betasept®, Exidine® Skin Cleanser, Hibiclens® Skin Cleanser: 4% (15 mL, 120 mL, 240 mL, 480 mL, 960 mL, 4000 mL)

Rinse:

Oral (mint flavor) (Peridex®, PerioGard®): 0.12% with alcohol 11.6% (480 mL)

Topical (Hibistat® Hand Rinse): 0.5% with isopropyl alcohol 70% (120 mL, 240 mL)

Sponge/Brush (Hibiclens®): 4% with isopropyl alcohol 4% (22 mL)

Wipes (Hibistat®): 0.5% (50s)

2-Chlorodeoxyadenosine *see* Cladribine *on page 285*

Chloromycetin® *see* Chloramphenicol *on page 250*

Chloroprocaine (klor oh PROE kane)

Brand Names Nesacaine®; Nesacaine®-MPF

Synonyms Chloroprocaine Hydrochloride

Therapeutic Category Local Anesthetic, Injectable

Use Infiltration anesthesia and peripheral and epidural anesthesia

Pregnancy Risk Factor C

Contraindications Known hypersensitivity to chloroprocaine, or other ester type anesthetics; myasthenia gravis; concurrent use of bupivacaine; do not use for subarachnoid administration

Warnings/Precautions Use with caution in patients with cardiac disease, renal disease, and hyperthyroidism; convulsions and cardiac arrest have been reported presumably due to intravascular injection

Adverse Reactions

<1%:

Cardiovascular: Myocardial depression, hypotension, bradycardia, cardiovascular collapse, edema
Central nervous system: Anxiety, restlessness, disorientation, confusion, seizures, drowsiness, unconsciousness, chills
Dermatologic: Urticaria
Gastrointestinal: Nausea, vomiting
Local: Transient stinging or burning at injection site
Neuromuscular & skeletal: Tremor
Ocular: Blurred vision
Otic: Tinnitus
Respiratory: Respiratory arrest
Miscellaneous: Anaphylactoid reactions, shivering

Overdosage/Toxicology Treatment is primarily symptomatic and supportive. Termination of anesthesia by pneumatic tourniquet inflation should be attempted when the agent is administered by infiltration or regional injection. Hypotension responds to I.V. fluids and Trendelenburg positioning. Other symptoms (seizures, bradyarrhythmias, metabolic acidosis, methemoglobinemia) respond to conventional treatments.

Mechanism of Action Chloroprocaine HCl is benzoic acid, 4-amino-2-chloro-2-(diethylamino) ethyl ester monohydrochloride. Chloroprocaine is an ester-type local anesthetic, which stabilizes the neuronal membranes and prevents initiation and transmission of nerve impulses thereby affecting local anesthetic actions. Local anesthetics including chloroprocaine, reversibly prevent generation and conduction of electrical impulses in neurons by decreasing the transient increase in permeability to sodium. The differential sensitivity generally depends on the size of the fiber; small fibers are more sensitive than larger fibers and require a longer period for recovery. Sensory pain fibers are usually blocked first, followed by fibers that transmit sensations of temperature, touch, and deep pressure. High concentrations block sympathetic somatic sensory and somatic motor fibers. The spread of anesthesia depends upon the distribution of the solution. This is primarily dependent on the volume of drug injected.

Usual Dosage Dosage varies with anesthetic procedure, the area to be anesthetized, the vascularity of the tissues, depth of anesthesia required, degree of muscle relaxation required, and duration of anesthesia; range: 1.5-25 mL of 2% to 3% solution; single adult dose should not exceed 800 mg

Infiltration and peripheral nerve block: 1% to 2%
Infiltration, peripheral and central nerve block, including caudal and epidural block: 2% to 3%, without preservatives

Administration Before injecting, withdraw syringe plunger to ensure injection is not into vein or artery

Nursing Implications Must have resuscitative equipment available

Dosage Forms Injection, as hydrochloride:

Preservative free (Nesacaine®-MPF): 2% (30 mL); 3% (30 mL)
With preservative (Nesacaine®): 1% (30 mL); 2% (30 mL)

Chloroprocaine Hydrochloride *see* Chloroprocaine *on previous page*
Chloroptic® *see* Chloramphenicol *on page 250*

Chloroquine and Primaquine (KLOR oh kwin & PRIM a kween)

Brand Names Aralen® Phosphate With Primaquine Phosphate

Synonyms Primaquine and Chloroquine

Therapeutic Category Antimalarial Agent

Use Prophylaxis of malaria, regardless of species, in all areas where the disease is endemic

Pregnancy Risk Factor C

Contraindications Retinal or visual field changes, known hypersensitivity to chloroquine or primaquine

Warnings/Precautions Use with caution in patients with psoriasis, porphyria, hepatic dysfunction, G-6-PD deficiency

Adverse Reactions

1% to 10%: Gastrointestinal: Diarrhea, nausea

<1%:

Cardiovascular: Hypotension, EKG changes
Central nervous system: Fatigue, personality changes, headache
Dermatologic: Pruritus, hair bleaching
Gastrointestinal: Anorexia, vomiting, stomatitis
Hematologic: Blood dyscrasias
Ocular: Retinopathy, blurred vision

Overdosage/Toxicology Symptoms of overdose include headache, visual changes, cardiovascular collapse, seizures, abdominal cramps, vomiting, cyanosis, methemoglobinemia, leukopenia, respiratory and cardiac arrest

(Continued)

Chloroquine and Primaquine *(Continued)*

Following initial measures (immediate GI decontamination), treatment is supportive and symptomatic

Drug Interactions

Decreased absorption if administered concomitantly with kaolin and magnesium trisilicate

Increased toxicity/levels with cimetidine

Mechanism of Action Chloroquine concentrates within parasite acid vesicles and raises internal pH resulting in inhibition of parasite growth; may involve aggregates of ferriprotoporphyrin IX acting as chloroquine receptors causing membrane damage; may also interfere with nucleoprotein synthesis. Primaquine eliminates the primary tissue exoerythrocytic forms of *P. falciparum*; disrupts mitochondria and binds to DNA.

Pharmacodynamics/Kinetics

Absorption: Oral: Both drugs are readily absorbed

Distribution: Concentrated in liver, spleen, kidney, heart, and brain

Protein binding: ~55%; binds strongly to melanin

Metabolism: 25% of chloroquine is metabolized

Elimination: Drug may remain in tissue for 3-5 days; up to 70% excreted unchanged

Usual Dosage Oral: Start at least 1 day before entering the endemic area; continue for 8 weeks after leaving the endemic area

Children: For suggested weekly dosage (based on body weight), see table:

Weight		Chloroquine Base (mg)	Primaquine Base (mg)	Dose* (mL)
lb	kg			
10-15	4.5-6.8	20	3	2.5
16-25	7.3-11.4	40	6	5
26-35	11.8-15.9	60	9	7.5
36-45	16.4-20.5	80	12	10
46-55	20.9-25	100	15	12.5
56-100	25.4-45.4	150	22.5	½ tablet
100+	>45.4	300	45	1 tablet

*Dose based on liquid containing approximately 40 mg of chloroquine base and 6 mg primaquine base per 5 mL, prepared from chloroquine phosphate with primaquine phosphate tablets.

Adults: 1 tablet/week on the same day each week

Monitoring Parameters Periodic CBC, examination for muscular weakness, and ophthalmologic examination in patients receiving prolonged therapy

Patient Information Take with meals; report any visual disturbances or difficulty in hearing or ringing in the ears; tablets are bitter tasting; may cause diarrhea, loss of appetite, nausea, stomach pain; notify physician if these become severe

Dosage Forms Tablet: Chloroquine phosphate 500 mg [base 300 mg] and primaquine phosphate 79 mg [base 45 mg]

Chloroquine Phosphate (KLOR oh kwin FOS fate)

Related Information

Prevention of Malaria *on page 1441*

Brand Names Aralen® Phosphate

Therapeutic Category Amebicide; Antimalarial Agent

Use Suppression or chemoprophylaxis of malaria; treatment of uncomplicated or mild-moderate malaria; extraintestinal amebiasis; rheumatoid arthritis; discoid lupus erythematosus, scleroderma, pemphigus

Pregnancy Risk Factor C

Contraindications Retinal or visual field changes; patients with psoriasis; known hypersensitivity to chloroquine

Warnings/Precautions Use with caution in patients with liver disease, G-6-PD deficiency, alcoholism or in conjunction with hepatotoxic drugs, psoriasis, porphyria

Adverse Reactions

1% to 10%: Gastrointestinal: Nausea, diarrhea

<1%:

Cardiovascular: Hypotension, EKG changes

Central nervous system: Fatigue, personality changes, headache

Dermatologic: Pruritus, hair bleaching

Gastrointestinal: Anorexia, vomiting, stomatitis

Hematologic: Blood dyscrasias

Ocular: Retinopathy, blurred vision

Overdosage/Toxicology Symptoms of overdose include headache, visual changes, cardiovascular collapse, seizures, abdominal cramps, vomiting, cyanosis, methemoglobinemia, leukopenia, respiratory and cardiac arrest

Following initial measures (immediate GI decontamination), treatment is supportive and symptomatic

Drug Interactions

Decreased absorption if administered concomitantly with kaolin and magnesium trisilicate

Increased toxicity/levels with cimetidine

Mechanism of Action Binds to and inhibits DNA and RNA polymerase; interferes with metabolism and hemoglobin utilization by parasites; inhibits prostaglandin effects; chloroquine concentrates within parasite acid vesicles and raises internal pH resulting in inhibition of parasite growth; may involve aggregates of ferriprotoporphyrin IX acting as chloroquine receptors causing membrane damage; may also interfere with nucleoprotein synthesis

Pharmacodynamics/Kinetics

Absorption: Oral: Rapid (~89%)

Distribution: Widely distributed in body tissues such as eyes, heart, kidneys, liver, and lungs where retention is prolonged; crosses the placenta; appears in breast milk

Metabolism: Partial hepatic metabolism occurs

Half-life: 3-5 days

Time to peak serum concentration: Within 1-2 hours

Elimination: ~70% excreted unchanged in urine; acidification of the urine increases elimination of drug; small amounts of drug may be present in urine months following discontinuation of therapy

Usual Dosage Oral (**dosage expressed in terms of mg of base**):

Suppression or prophylaxis of malaria:

- Children: Administer 5 mg base/kg/week on the same day each week (not to exceed 300 mg base/dose); begin 1-2 weeks prior to exposure; continue for 4-6 weeks after leaving endemic area; if suppressive therapy is not begun prior to exposure, double the initial loading dose to 10 mg base/kg and administer in 2 divided doses 6 hours apart, followed by the usual dosage regimen
- Adults: 300 mg/week (base) on the same day each week; begin 1-2 weeks prior to exposure; continue for 4-6 weeks after leaving endemic area; if suppressive therapy is not begun prior to exposure, double the initial loading dose to 600 mg base and administer in 2 divided doses 6 hours apart, followed by the usual dosage regimen

Acute attack:

- Children: 10 mg/kg on day 1, followed by 5 mg/kg 6 hours later and 5 mg/kg on days 2 and 3
- Adults: 600 mg on day 1, followed by 300 mg 6 hours later, followed by 300 mg on days 2 and 3

Extraintestinal amebiasis:

- Children: 10 mg/kg once daily for 2-3 weeks (up to 300 mg base/day)
- Adults: 600 mg base/day for 2 days followed by 300 mg base/day for at least 2-3 weeks

Dosing adjustment in renal impairment: Cl_{cr} <10 mL/minute: Administer 50% of dose

Hemodialysis: Minimally removed by hemodialysis

Monitoring Parameters Periodic CBC, examination for muscular weakness, and ophthalmologic examination in patients receiving prolonged therapy

Patient Information Take with meals; report any visual disturbances or difficulty in hearing or ringing in the ears; tablets are bitter tasting; may cause diarrhea, loss of appetite, nausea, stomach pain; notify physician if these become severe

Dosage Forms Tablet: 250 mg [150 mg base]; 500 mg [300 mg base]

Extemporaneous Preparations A 10 mg chloroquine base/mL suspension is made by pulverizing two Aralen® 500 mg phosphate = 300 mg base/tablet, levigating with sterile water, and adding by geometric proportion, a significant amount of the cherry syrup and levigating until a uniform mixture is obtained; qs ad to 60 mL with cherry syrup, stable for up to 4 weeks when stored in the refrigerator or at a temperature of 29°C

Mirochnick M, Barnett E, Clarke DF, et al, "Stability of Chloroquine in an Extemporaneously Prepared Suspension Stored at Three Temperatures," *Pediatr Infect Dis J*, 1994, 13(9):827-8.

Chlorothiazide (klor oh THYE a zide)

Related Information

Sulfonamide Derivatives *on page 1420*

Brand Names Diurigen®; Diuril®

(Continued)

Chlorothiazide *(Continued)*

Therapeutic Category Antihypertensive; Diuretic, Thiazide

Use Management of mild to moderate hypertension, or edema associated with congestive heart failure, pregnancy, or nephrotic syndrome in patients unable to take oral hydrochlorothiazide, when a thiazide is the diuretic of choice

Pregnancy Risk Factor D

Pregnancy/Breast-Feeding Implications

Clinical effects on the fetus: Crosses the placenta. Hypoglycemia, thrombocytopenia, hemolytic anemia, electrolyte disturbances reported. May exhibit a tocolytic effect. Generally, use of diuretics during pregnancy is avoided due to risk of decreased placental perfusion.

Breast-feeding/lactation: Crosses into breast milk

Clinical effects on the infant: May suppress lactation with high doses. American Academy of Pediatrics considers COMPATIBLE with breast-feeding.

Contraindications Hypersensitivity to chlorothiazide or any component; cross-sensitivity with other thiazides or sulfonamides; do not use in anuric patients.

Warnings/Precautions Injection must not be administered S.C. or I.M.; may cause hyperbilirubinemia, hypokalemia, alkalosis, hyperglycemia, hyperuricemia; chlorothiazide is minimally effective in patients with a Cl_{cr} <40 mL/minute; this may limit the usefulness of chlorothiazide in the elderly

Adverse Reactions

1% to 10%: Endocrine & metabolic: Hypokalemia, hyponatremia

<1%:

- Cardiovascular: Arrhythmia, weak pulse, orthostatic hypotension
- Central nervous system: Dizziness, vertigo, headache, fever
- Dermatologic: Rash, photosensitivity
- Endocrine & metabolic: Hypochloremic alkalosis, hyperglycemia, hyperlipidemia, hyperuricemia
- Hematologic: Rarely blood dyscrasias, leukopenia, agranulocytosis, aplastic anemia
- Neuromuscular & skeletal: Paresthesias
- Renal: Prerenal azotemia

Overdosage/Toxicology Symptoms of overdose include hypermotility, diuresis, lethargy, confusion, muscle weakness, coma; following GI decontamination, therapy is supportive with I.V. fluids, electrolytes, and I.V. pressors if needed

Drug Interactions

Decreased effect: NSAIDs + chlorothiazide → decreased antihypertensive effect; decreased absorption of thiazides with cholestyramine resins; chlorothiazide causes a decreased effect of oral hypoglycemics

Increased toxicity: Digitalis glycosides, lithium (decreased clearance), probenecid

Stability Reconstituted solution is stable for 24 hours at room temperature; precipitation will occur in <24 hours in pH <7.4

Mechanism of Action Inhibits sodium reabsorption in the distal tubules causing increased excretion of sodium and water as well as potassium and hydrogen ions, magnesium, phosphate, calcium

Pharmacodynamics/Kinetics

Absorption: Oral: Poor

Onset of diuresis: Oral: 2 hours

Duration of diuretic action:

- Oral: 6-12 hours
- I.V.: ~2 hours

Half-life: 1-2 hours

Time to peak serum concentration: Within 4 hours

Usual Dosage I.V. form not recommended for children and should only be used in adults if unable to take oral in emergency situations:

Infants <6 months:

- Oral: 20-40 mg/kg/day in 2 divided doses
- I.V.: 2-8 mg/kg/day in 2 divided doses

Infants >6 months and Children:

- Oral: 20 mg/kg/day in 2 divided doses
- I.V.: 4 mg/kg/day

Adults:

- Oral: 500 mg to 2 g/day divided in 1-2 doses
- I.V.: 100-500 mg/day

Elderly: Oral: 500 mg once daily **or** 1 g 3 times/week

Administration Injection must **not** be administered S.C. or I.M.

Monitoring Parameters Serum electrolytes, renal function, blood pressure; assess weight, I & O reports daily to determine fluid loss

Test Interactions ↑ creatine phosphokinase [CPK] (S), ammonia (B), amylase (S), calcium (S), chloride (S), cholesterol (S), glucose, ↑ acid (S), ↓ chloride (S), magnesium, potassium (S), sodium (S)

Patient Information Shake well; may be taken with food or milk; take early in day to avoid nocturia; take the last dose of multiple doses no later than 6 PM unless instructed otherwise; to avoid photosensitivity, use sun block SPF ≥15 on exposed skin areas

Nursing Implications Take blood pressure with patient lying down and standing; avoid extravasation of parenteral solution since it is extremely irritating to tissues

Additional Information Sodium content of injection, 500 mg: 57.5 mg (2 mEq)

Dosage Forms

Powder for injection, lyophilized, as sodium: 500 mg
Suspension, oral: 250 mg/5 mL (237 mL)
Tablet: 250 mg, 500 mg

Chlorotrianisene (klor oh trye AN i seen)

Brand Names TACE®

Therapeutic Category Estrogen Derivative, Oral

Use Treat inoperable prostatic cancer; management of atrophic vaginitis, female hypogonadism, vasomotor symptoms of menopause

Pregnancy Risk Factor X

Contraindications Thrombophlebitis, breast cancer, undiagnosed abnormal vaginal bleeding, known or suspected pregnancy

Warnings/Precautions Estrogens have been reported to increase the risk of endometrial carcinoma; do not use estrogens during pregnancy

Adverse Reactions

>10%:

- Cardiovascular: Peripheral edema
- Endocrine & metabolic: Enlargement of breasts (female and male), breast tenderness
- Gastrointestinal: Nausea, anorexia, bloating

1% to 10%:

- Central nervous system: Headache
- Endocrine & metabolic: Increased libido (female), decreased libido (male)
- Gastrointestinal: Vomiting, diarrhea

<1%:

- Cardiovascular: Hypertension, thromboembolism, myocardial infarction, edema
- Central nervous system: Depression, dizziness, anxiety, stroke
- Dermatologic: Chloasma, melasma, rash
- Endocrine & metabolic: Amenorrhea, alterations in frequency and flow of menses, decreased glucose tolerance, increased triglycerides and LDL
- Gastrointestinal: Nausea, GI distress
- Hepatic: Cholestatic jaundice
- Ocular: Intolerance to contact lenses
- Miscellaneous: Increased susceptibility to *Candida* infection, breast tumors

Overdosage/Toxicology Serious adverse effects have not been reported following ingestion of large doses of estrogen-containing oral contraceptives; overdosage of estrogen may cause nausea; withdrawal bleeding may occur in females

Mechanism of Action Diethylstilbestrol derivative with similar estrogenic actions

Pharmacodynamics/Kinetics

Onset of therapeutic effect: Commonly occurs within 14 days of therapy
Distribution: Stored in fat tissues and slowly released
Metabolism: In the liver to a more potent estrogen compound

Usual Dosage Adults: Oral:

- Atrophic vaginitis: 12-25 mg/day in 28-day cycles (21 days on and 7 days off)
- Female hypogonadism: 12-25 mg cyclically for 21 days. May be followed by I.M. progesterone 100 mg or 5 days of oral progestin; next course may begin on day 5 of induced uterine bleeding.
- Postpartum breast engorgement: 12 mg 4 times/day for 7 days or 50 mg every 6 hours for 6 doses; administer first dose within 8 hours after delivery
- Vasomotor symptoms associated with menopause: 12-25 mg cyclically for 30 days; one or more courses may be prescribed
- Prostatic cancer (inoperable/progressing): 12-25 mg/day

Patient Information Patients should inform their physicians if signs or symptoms of thromboembolic or thrombotic disorders including sudden severe headache or vomiting, disturbance of vision or speech, loss of vision, numbness or weakness in an extremity, sharp or crushing chest pain, calf pain, shortness of breath, severe abdominal pain or mass, mental depression or unusual bleeding.

Dosage Forms Capsule: 12 mg, 25 mg

Chlorphed® [OTC] *see* Brompheniramine *on page 166*

Chlorphed®-LA Nasal Solution [OTC] *see* Oxymetazoline *on page 940*

Chlorpheniramine (klor fen IR a meen)

Brand Names Aller-Chlor® [OTC]; AL-R® [OTC]; Chlo-Amine® [OTC]; Chlorate® [OTC]; Chlor-Pro® [OTC]; Chlor-Trimeton® [OTC]; Efidac® 24 [OTC]; Kloromin® [OTC]; Phenetron®; Telachlor®; Teldrin® [OTC]

Canadian/Mexican Brand Names Chlor-Tripolon® (Canada)

Synonyms Chlorpheniramine Maleate; CTM

Therapeutic Category Antihistamine, H_1 Blocker

Use Perennial and seasonal allergic rhinitis and other allergic symptoms including urticaria

Pregnancy Risk Factor B

Contraindications Hypersensitivity to chlorpheniramine maleate or any component; narrow-angle glaucoma, bladder neck obstruction, symptomatic prostate hypertrophy, during acute asthmatic attacks, stenosing peptic ulcer, pyloroduodenal obstruction. Avoid use in premature and term newborns due to possible association with SIDS.

Warnings/Precautions Do not administer to premature or full-term neonates; young children may be more susceptible to side effects and CNS stimulation; bladder neck obstruction, symptomatic prostate hypertrophy, asthmatic attacks, and stenosing peptic ulcer; swallow whole, do not crush or chew sustained release tablets. Anticholinergic action may cause significant confusional symptoms.

Adverse Reactions

Genitourinary: Urinary retention, polyuria

Ocular: Diplopia

>10%:

- Central nervous system: Slight to moderate drowsiness
- Respiratory: Thickening of bronchial secretions

1% to 10%:

- Central nervous system: Headache, excitability, fatigue, nervousness, dizziness
- Gastrointestinal: Nausea, xerostomia, diarrhea, abdominal pain, appetite increase, weight gain
- Neuromuscular & skeletal: Arthralgia, weakness
- Respiratory: Pharyngitis

<1%:

- Cardiovascular: Palpitations
- Central nervous system: Depression
- Dermatologic: Dermatitis, photosensitivity, angioedema
- Hepatic: Hepatitis
- Neuromuscular & skeletal: Myalgia, paresthesia
- Respiratory: Bronchospasm, epistaxis

Overdosage/Toxicology Symptoms of overdose include dry mouth, flushed skin, dilated pupils, CNS depression

There is no specific treatment for an antihistamine overdose, however, most of its clinical toxicity is due to anticholinergic effects. For anticholinergic overdose with severe life-threatening symptoms, physostigmine 1-2 mg (0.5 or 0.02 mg/kg for children) I.V., slowly may be given to reverse these effects.

Drug Interactions Increased toxicity (CNS depression): CNS depressants, MAO inhibitors, tricyclic antidepressants, phenothiazines

Stability Injectable form should be protected from light; **incompatible** when mixed in same syringe with calcium chloride, kanamycin, norepinephrine, pentobarbital

Mechanism of Action Competes with histamine for H_1-receptor sites on effector cells in the gastrointestinal tract, blood vessels, and respiratory tract

Pharmacodynamics/Kinetics

Protein binding: 69% to 72%

Metabolism: In the liver

Half-life: 20-24 hours

Elimination: Metabolites and parent drug (3% to 4%) excreted in urine, 35% of total within 48 hours

Usual Dosage

Children: Oral: 0.35 mg/kg/day in divided doses every 4-6 hours

- 2-6 years: 1 mg every 4-6 hours, not to exceed 6 mg in 24 hours
- 6-12 years: 2 mg every 4-6 hours, not to exceed 12 mg/day or sustained release 8 mg at bedtime

Children >12 years and Adults: Oral: 4 mg every 4-6 hours, not to exceed 24 mg/day or sustained release 8-12 mg every 8-12 hours, not to exceed 24 mg/day

Adults: Allergic reactions: I.M., I.V., S.C.: 10-20 mg as a single dose; maximum recommended dose: 40 mg/24 hours

Elderly: 4 mg once or twice daily. **Note:** Duration of action may be 36 hours or more when serum concentrations are low.

Hemodialysis: Supplemental dose is not necessary

Dietary Considerations Alcohol: Additive CNS effects, avoid use

Patient Information May cause drowsiness; swallow whole, do not crush or chew sustained release product; avoid alcohol, may impair coordination and judgment

Nursing Implications Do not crush sustained release drug product; raise bed rails, institute safety measures, assist with ambulation

Dosage Forms

Capsule, as maleate: 12 mg
Capsule, as maleate, timed release: 8 mg, 12 mg
Injection, as maleate: 10 mg/mL (1 mL, 30 mL); 100 mg/mL (2 mL)
Syrup, as maleate: 2 mg/5 mL (120 mL, 473 mL)
Tablet, as maleate: 4 mg, 8 mg, 12 mg
Tablet, as maleate:
  Chewable: 2 mg
  Timed release: 8 mg, 12 mg

Chlorpheniramine Maleate *see* Chlorpheniramine *on previous page*

Chlor-Pro® [OTC] *see* Chlorpheniramine *on previous page*

Chlorpromazine (klor PROE ma zeen)

Related Information

Antipsychotic Agents Comparison *on page 1396*
Drugs and Routes of Administration Not Recommended for Treatment of Cancer Pain *on page 1378*

Brand Names Ormazine; Thorazine®

Canadian/Mexican Brand Names Apo-Chlorpromazine® (Canada); Chlorprom® (Canada); Chlorpromanyl® (Canada); Largactil® (Canada); Novo-Chlorpromazine® (Canada)

Synonyms Chlorpromazine Hydrochloride

Therapeutic Category Antiemetic; Antipsychotic Agent; Phenothiazine Derivative

Use Treatment of nausea and vomiting; psychoses; Tourette's syndrome; mania; intractable hiccups (adults); behavioral problems (children)

Pregnancy Risk Factor C

Contraindications Hypersensitivity to chlorpromazine hydrochloride or any component; cross-sensitivity with other phenothiazines may exist; avoid use in patients with narrow-angle glaucoma

Warnings/Precautions Safety in children <6 months of age has not been established; use with caution in patients with seizures, bone marrow suppression, or severe liver disease

Significant hypotension may occur, especially when the drug is administered parenterally; injection contains benzyl alcohol; injection also contains sulfites which may cause allergic reaction

Tardive dyskinesia: Prevalence rate may be 40% in elderly; development of the syndrome and the irreversible nature are proportional to duration and total cumulative dose over time. May be reversible if diagnosed early in therapy.

Extrapyramidal reactions are more common in elderly with up to 50% developing these reactions after 60 years of age. Drug-induced **Parkinson's syndrome** occurs often. **Akathisia** is the most common extrapyramidal reaction in elderly.

Increased confusion, memory loss, psychotic behavior, and agitation frequently occur as a consequence of anticholinergic effects

Orthostatic hypotension is due to alpha-receptor blockade, the elderly are at greater risk for orthostatic hypotension

Antipsychotic associated sedation in nonpsychotic patients is extremely unpleasant due to feelings of depersonalization, derealization, and dysphoria

Life-threatening arrhythmias have occurred at therapeutic doses of antipsychotics

Adverse Reactions

>10%:

Cardiovascular: Hypotension (especially with I.V. use), tachycardia, arrhythmias, orthostatic hypotension
Central nervous system: Pseudoparkinsonism, akathisia, dystonias, tardive dyskinesia (persistent), dizziness
Gastrointestinal: Constipation
Ocular: Pigmentary retinopathy
Respiratory: Nasal congestion
Miscellaneous: Diaphoresis (decreased)

1% to 10%:

Dermatologic: Pruritus, rash, increased sensitivity to sun
Endocrine & metabolic: Amenorrhea, galactorrhea, gynecomastia, changes in libido, pain in breasts

(Continued)

Chlorpromazine *(Continued)*

Gastrointestinal: GI upset, nausea, vomiting, stomach pain, weight gain, xerostomia
Genitourinary: Dysuria, ejaculatory disturbances, urinary retention
Neuromuscular & skeletal: Trembling of fingers
Ocular: Blurred vision

<1%:

Central nervous system: Sedation, drowsiness, restlessness, anxiety, extrapyramidal reactions, seizures, altered central temperature regulation, lowering of seizures threshold, neuroleptic malignant syndrome (NMS)
Dermatologic: Discoloration of skin (blue-gray), photosensitivity
Endocrine & metabolic: Galactorrhea
Genitourinary: Priapism
Hematologic: Agranulocytosis (more often in women between 4th and 10th weeks of therapy), leukopenia (usually in patients with large doses for prolonged periods)
Hepatic: Cholestatic jaundice, hepatotoxicity
Ocular: Cornea and lens changes
Miscellaneous: Anaphylactoid reactions

Overdosage/Toxicology Symptoms of overdose include deep sleep, coma, extrapyramidal symptoms, abnormal involuntary muscle movements, hypotension

Following initiation of essential overdose management, toxic symptom treatment and supportive treatment should be initiated. Hypotension usually responds to I.V. fluids or Trendelenburg positioning. If unresponsive to these measures, the use of a parenteral inotrope may be required. Seizures commonly respond to diazepam (I.V. 5-10 mg bolus in adults every 15 minutes if needed up to a total of 30 mg; I.V. 0.25-0.4 mg/kg/dose up to a total of 10 mg in children) or to phenytoin or phenobarbital; critical cardiac arrhythmias often respond to I.V. phenytoin (15 mg/kg up to 1 g), while other antiarrhythmics can be used. Neuroleptics often cause extrapyramidal symptoms (eg, dystonic reactions) requiring management with benztropine mesylate I.V. 1-2 mg (adults) may be effective. These agents are generally effective within 2-5 minutes.

Drug Interactions Cytochrome P-450 2D6 enzyme substrate

Increased toxicity: Additive effects with other CNS-depressants; epinephrine (hypotension); may increase valproic acid serum concentrations

Stability Protect from light; a slightly yellowed solution does not indicate potency loss, but a markedly discolored solution should be discarded; diluted injection (1 mg/mL) with NS and stored in 5 mL vials remains stable for 30 days

Mechanism of Action Blocks postsynaptic mesolimbic dopaminergic receptors in the brain; exhibits a strong alpha-adrenergic blocking effect and depresses the release of hypothalamic and hypophyseal hormones; believed to depress the reticular-activating system, thus affecting basal metabolism, body temperature, wakefulness, vasomotor tone, and emesis

Pharmacodynamics/Kinetics

Distribution: Crosses the placenta; appears in breast milk
Metabolism: Extensively in the liver to active and inactive metabolites
Half-life, biphasic:
Initial: 2 hours
Terminal: 30 hours
Elimination: <1% excreted in urine as unchanged drug within 24 hours

Usual Dosage

Children >6 months:

Psychosis:

Oral: 0.5-1 mg/kg/dose every 4-6 hours; older children may require 200 mg/day or higher
I.M., I.V.: 0.5-1 mg/kg/dose every 6-8 hours; maximum dose for <5 years (22.7 kg): 40 mg/day; maximum for 5-12 years (22.7-45.5 kg): 75 mg/day

Nausea and vomiting:

Oral: 0.5-1 mg/kg/dose every 4-6 hours as needed
I.M., I.V.: 0.5-1 mg/kg/dose every 6-8 hours; maximum dose for <5 years (22.7 kg): 40 mg/day; maximum for 5-12 years (22.7-45.5 kg): 75 mg/day
Rectal: 1 mg/kg/dose every 6-8 hours as needed

Adults:

Psychosis:

Oral: Range: 30-800 mg/day in 1-4 divided doses, initiate at lower doses and titrate as needed; usual dose: 200 mg/day; some patients may require 1-2 g/day
I.M., I.V.: Initial: 25 mg, may repeat (25-50 mg) in 1-4 hours, gradually increase to a maximum of 400 mg/dose every 4-6 hours until patient is controlled; usual dose: 300-800 mg/day

Intractable hiccups: Oral, I.M.: 25-50 mg 3-4 times/day

Nausea and vomiting:

Oral: 10-25 mg every 4-6 hours

I.M., I.V.: 25-50 mg every 4-6 hours

Rectal: 50-100 mg every 6-8 hours

Elderly (nonpsychotic patient; dementia behavior): Initial: 10-25 mg 1-2 times/day; increase at 4- to 7-day intervals by 10-25 mg/day. Increase dose intervals (bid, tid, etc) as necessary to control behavior response or side effects; maximum daily dose: 800 mg; gradual increases (titration) may prevent some side effects or decrease their severity.

Hemodialysis: Not dialyzable (0% to 5%)

Dosing adjustment/comments in hepatic impairment: Avoid use in severe hepatic dysfunction

Dietary Considerations Alcohol: Additive CNS effects, avoid use

Administration Dilute oral concentrate solution in juice before administration

Monitoring Parameters Orthostatic blood pressures; tremors, gait changes, abnormal movement in trunk, neck, buccal area, or extremities; monitor target behaviors for which the agent is given; watch for hypotension when administering I.M. or I.V.

Reference Range

Therapeutic: 50-300 ng/mL (SI: 157-942 nmol/L)

Toxic: >750 ng/mL (SI: >2355 nmol/L); serum concentrations poorly correlate with expected response

Test Interactions False-positives for phenylketonuria, amylase, uroporphyrins, urobilinogen; may cause photosensitivity; avoid excessive sunlight; do not stop taking without consulting physician

Patient Information Do not stop taking unless informed by your physician; oral concentrate must be diluted in 2-4 oz of liquid (water, fruit juice, carbonated drinks, milk, or pudding); do not take antacid within 1 hour of taking drug; avoid alcohol; avoid excess sun exposure (use sun block); may cause drowsiness, rise slowly from recumbent position; use of supportive stockings may help prevent orthostatic hypotension

Nursing Implications Avoid contact of oral solution or injection with skin (contact dermatitis)

Dosage Forms

Capsule, as hydrochloride, sustained action: 30 mg, 75 mg, 150 mg, 200 mg, 300 mg

Concentrate, oral, as hydrochloride: 30 mg/mL (120 mL); 100 mg/mL (60 mL, 240 mL)

Injection, as hydrochloride: 25 mg/mL (1 mL, 2 mL, 10 mL)

Suppository, rectal, as base: 25 mg, 100 mg

Syrup, as hydrochloride: 10 mg/5 mL (120 mL)

Tablet, as hydrochloride: 10 mg, 25 mg, 50 mg, 100 mg, 200 mg

Chlorpromazine Hydrochloride *see* Chlorpromazine *on page 261*

Chlorpropamide (klor PROE pa mide)

Related Information

Hypoglycemic Drugs, Comparison of Oral Agents *on page 1411*

Sulfonamide Derivatives *on page 1420*

Brand Names Diabinese®

Canadian/Mexican Brand Names Apo-Chlorpropamide® (Canada); Novo-Propamide® (Canada); Deavynfar® (Mexico); Insogen® (Mexico)

Therapeutic Category Antidiabetic Agent, Oral; Antihyperglycemic Agent; Hypoglycemic Agent, Oral; Sulfonylurea Agent

Use Control blood sugar in adult onset, noninsulin-dependent diabetes (type II)

Unlabeled use: Neurogenic diabetes insipidus

Pregnancy Risk Factor D

Pregnancy/Breast-Feeding Implications

Clinical effects on the fetus: Crosses the placenta. Hypoglucemia; ear defects reported; other malformations reported but may have been secondary to poor maternal glucose control/diabetes. Insulin is the drug of choice for the control of diabetes mellitus during pregnancy.

Breast-feeding/lactation: Crosses into breast milk

Contraindications Cross-sensitivity may exist with other hypoglycemics or sulfonamides; do not use with type I diabetes or with severe renal, hepatic, thyroid, or other endocrine disease

Warnings/Precautions

Patients should be properly instructed in the early detection and treatment of hypoglycemia; long half-life may complicate recovery from excess effects

Because of chlorpropamide's long half-life, duration of action, and the increased risk for hypoglycemia, it is not considered a hypoglycemic agent of choice in the elderly; see Pharmacodynamics/Kinetics

(Continued)

Chlorpropamide *(Continued)*

Adverse Reactions

>10%:

Central nervous system: Headache, dizziness

Gastrointestinal: Anorexia, constipation, heartburn, epigastric fullness, nausea, vomiting, diarrhea

1% to 10%: Dermatologic: Skin rash, urticaria, photosensitivity

<1%:

Cardiovascular: Edema

Endocrine & metabolic: Hypoglycemia, hyponatremia, SIADH

Hematologic: Blood dyscrasias, aplastic anemia, hemolytic anemia, bone marrow suppression, thrombocytopenia, agranulocytosis

Hepatic: Cholestatic jaundice

Overdosage/Toxicology Symptoms of overdose include low blood glucose levels, tingling of lips and tongue, tachycardia, convulsions, stupor, coma

Antidote is glucose; intoxications with sulfonylureas can cause hypoglycemia and are best managed with glucose administration (oral for milder hypoglycemia or by injection in more severe forms); prolonged effects lasting up to 1 week may occur with this agent

Drug Interactions

Decreased effect: Thiazides and hydantoins (eg, phenytoin) ↓ chlorpropamide effectiveness may increase blood glucose

Increased toxicity:

Increases alcohol-associated disulfiram reactions

Increases oral anticoagulant effects

Salicylates → ↑ chlorpropamide effects → ↓ blood glucose

Sulfonamides → ↓ sulfonylureas clearance

Mechanism of Action Stimulates insulin release from the pancreatic beta cells; reduces glucose output from the liver; insulin sensitivity is increased at peripheral target sites

Pharmacodynamics/Kinetics

Peak effect: Oral: Within 6-8 hours

Distribution: V_d: 0.13-0.23 L/kg; appears in breast milk

Protein binding: 60% to 90%

Metabolism: Extensive (~80%) in the liver

Half-life: 30-42 hours; prolonged in the elderly or with renal disease

End stage renal disease: 50-200 hours

Time to peak serum concentration: Within 3-4 hours

Elimination: 10% to 30% excreted in the urine as unchanged drug

Usual Dosage Oral: The dosage of chlorpropamide is variable and should be individualized based upon the patient's response

Initial dose:

Adults: 250 mg/day in mild to moderate diabetes in middle-aged, stable diabetic

Elderly: 100 mg/day in older patients

Subsequent dosages may be increased or decreased by 50-125 mg/day at 3- to 5-day intervals

Maintenance dose: 100-250 mg/day; severe diabetics may require 500 mg/day; avoid doses >750 mg/day

Dosing adjustment/comments in renal impairment:

Cl_{cr} <50 mL/minute: Avoid use

Hemodialysis: Removed with hemoperfusion

Peritoneal dialysis: Supplemental dose is not necessary

Dosing adjustment in hepatic impairment: Dosage reduction is recommended

Dietary Considerations

Alcohol: A disulfiram-like reaction characterized by flushing, headache, nausea, vomiting, sweating or tachycardia; avoid use. Inform patient of chlorpropamide-alcohol flush (facial reddening and an increase in facial temperature).

Food: Chlorpropamide may cause GI upset; take with food. Take at the same time each day; eat regularly and do not skip meals.

Glucose: Decreases blood glucose concentration; hypoglycemia may occur. Educate patients how to detect and treat hypoglycemia. Monitor for signs and symptoms of hypoglycemia. Administer glucose if necessary. Evaluate patient's diet and exercise regimen. May need to decrease or discontinue dose of sulfonylurea.

Sodium: Reports of hyponatremia and SIADH. Those at increased risk include patients on medications or who have medical conditions that predispose them to hyponatremia. Monitor sodium serum concentration and fluid status. May need to restrict water intake.

Monitoring Parameters Fasting blood glucose, normal Hgb A_{1c} or fructosamine levels; monitor for signs and symptoms of hypoglycemia, (fatigue, sweating, numbness of extremities); monitor urine for glucose and ketones

Reference Range Target range: Adults:

Fasting blood glucose: <120 mg/dL

Glycosylated hemoglobin: <7%

Patient Information Avoid alcohol; take at the same time each day; avoid hypoglycemia, eat regularly, do not skip meals; carry a quick source of sugar

Dosage Forms Tablet: 100 mg, 250 mg

Chlortetracycline (klor tet ra SYE kleen)

Brand Names Aureomycin®

Canadian/Mexican Brand Names Aureomicina® (Mexico)

Synonyms Chlortetracycline Hydrochloride

Therapeutic Category Antibiotic, Ophthalmic; Antibiotic, Tetracycline Derivative; Antibiotic, Topical

Use

Ophthalmic: Treatment of superficial ocular infections involving the conjunctiva or cornea due to strains of susceptible microorganisms

Topical: Treatment of superficial infections of the skin due to susceptible organisms, also infection prophylaxis in minor skin abrasions

Pregnancy Risk Factor D

Contraindications Hypersensitivity to tetracycline or any component; do not use topical formulation in eyes

Warnings/Precautions Prolonged use may cause superinfection; ophthalmic ointments may retard corneal epithelial healing

Adverse Reactions

1% to 10%: Dermatologic: Faint yellowing of skin

<1%:

- Cardiovascular: Edema
- Dermatologic: Reddening of skin, photosensitivity
- Local: Irritation

Mechanism of Action Inhibits bacterial protein synthesis by binding with the 30S and possibly the 50S ribosomal subunit(s) of susceptible bacteria; may also cause alterations in the cytoplasmic membrane; usually bacteriostatic, may be bactericidal

Usual Dosage

Ophthalmic:

- Acute infections: Instill ½" (1.25 cm) every 3-4 hours until improvement
- Mild to moderate infections: Instill ½" (1.25 cm) 2-3 times/day

Topical: Apply 1-4 times/day, cover with sterile bandage if needed

Patient Information

For ophthalmic use, tilt head back, place medication in conjunctival sac and close eye, apply light finger pressure on lacrimal sac following instillation

Topical is for external use only, contact physician if rash or irritation develops, may stain clothing

Nursing Implications Cleanse affected area of skin prior to application unless otherwise directed

Dosage Forms Ointment, as hydrochloride:

Ophthalmic: 1% [10 mg/g] (3.5 g)

Topical: 3% (14.2 g, 30 g)

Chlortetracycline Hydrochloride *see* Chlortetracycline *on this page*

Chlorthalidone (klor THAL i done)

Related Information

Heart Failure: Management of Patients With Left-Ventricular Systolic Dysfunction *on page 1533*

Sulfonamide Derivatives *on page 1420*

Brand Names Hygroton®; Thalitone®

Canadian/Mexican Brand Names Apo-Chlorthalidone® (Canada); Novo-Thalidone® (Canada); Uridon® (Canada); Higroton® 50 (Mexico)

Therapeutic Category Antihypertensive; Diuretic, Miscellaneous

Use Management of mild to moderate hypertension, used alone or in combination with other agents; treatment of edema associated with congestive heart failure, nephrotic syndrome, or pregnancy. Recent studies have found chlorthalidone effective in the treatment of isolated systolic hypertension in the elderly.

Pregnancy Risk Factor D

Contraindications Hypersensitivity to chlorthalidone or any component, cross-sensitivity with other thiazides or sulfonamides; do not use in anuric patients

Warnings/Precautions Use with caution in patients with hypokalemia, renal disease, hepatic disease, gout, lupus erythematosus, diabetes mellitus; use with caution in severe renal diseases

(Continued)

Chlorthalidone *(Continued)*

Adverse Reactions

1% to 10%: Endocrine & metabolic: Hypokalemia

<1%:

Cardiovascular: Hypotension

Dermatologic: Photosensitivity

Endocrine & metabolic: Fluid and electrolyte imbalances (hypocalcemia, hypomagnesemia, hyponatremia), hyperglycemia

Hematologic: Rarely blood dyscrasias

Renal: Prerenal azotemia

Overdosage/Toxicology Symptoms of overdose include hypermotility, diuresis, lethargy, confusion, muscle weakness, coma; following GI decontamination, therapy is supportive with I.V. fluids, electrolytes, and I.V. pressors if needed

Drug Interactions

Decreased effect: NSAIDs + chlorothiazide → decreased antihypertensive effect; decreased absorption of thiazides with cholestyramine resins; chlorothiazide causes a decreased effect of oral hypoglycemics

Increased toxicity: Digitalis glycosides, lithium (decreased clearance), probenecid

Increased effect: Furosemide and other loop diuretics

Mechanism of Action Sulfonamide-derived diuretic that inhibits sodium and chloride reabsorption in the cortical-diluting segment of the ascending loop of Henle

Pharmacodynamics/Kinetics

Peak effect: 2-6 hours

Absorption: Oral: 65%

Distribution: Crosses placenta; appears in breast milk

Metabolism: In the liver

Half-life: 35-55 hours; may be prolonged with renal impairment, with anuria: 81 hours

Elimination: ~50% to 65% excreted unchanged in urine

Usual Dosage Oral:

Children: 2 mg/kg/dose 3 times/week or 1-2 mg/kg/day

Adults: 25-100 mg/day or 100 mg 3 times/week

Elderly: Initial: 12.5-25 mg/day or every other day; there is little advantage to using doses >25 mg/day

Dosing interval in renal impairment: Cl_{cr} <10 mL/minute: Administer every 48 hours

Monitoring Parameters Assess weight, I & O records daily to determine fluid loss; blood pressure, serum electrolytes, renal function

Test Interactions ↑ creatine phosphokinase [CPK] (S), ammonia (B), amylase (S), calcium (S), chloride (S), cholesterol (S), glucose, ↑ acid (S), ↓ chloride (S), magnesium, potassium (S), sodium (S)

Patient Information May be taken with food or milk; take early in day to avoid nocturia; take the last dose of multiple doses no later than 6 PM unless instructed otherwise; to avoid photosensitivity, use sun block SPF ≥15 on exposed skin areas

Nursing Implications Take blood pressure with patient lying down and standing

Dosage Forms

Tablet: 25 mg, 50 mg, 100 mg

Hygroton®: 25 mg, 50 mg, 100 mg

Thalitone®: 15 mg, 25 mg

Chlor-Trimeton® [OTC] *see* Chlorpheniramine *on page 260*

Chlorzoxazone (klor ZOKS a zone)

Brand Names Flexaphen®; Mus-Lax®; Paraflex®; Parafon Forte™ DSC

Synonyms Chlorzoxazone with Acetaminophen

Therapeutic Category Centrally Acting Muscle Relaxant; Skeletal Muscle Relaxant

Use Symptomatic treatment of muscle spasm and pain associated with acute musculoskeletal conditions

Pregnancy Risk Factor C

Contraindications Known hypersensitivity to chlorzoxazone; impaired liver function

Adverse Reactions

>10%: Central nervous system: Drowsiness

1% to 10%:

Cardiovascular: Tachycardia, tightness in chest, flushing of face, syncope

Central nervous system: Mental depression, allergic fever, dizziness, lightheadedness, headache, paradoxical stimulation

Dermatologic: Angioedema

Gastrointestinal: Nausea, vomiting, stomach cramps
Neuromuscular & skeletal: Trembling
Ocular: Burning of eyes
Respiratory: Shortness of breath
Miscellaneous: Hiccups

<1%:

Central nervous system: Ataxia
Dermatologic: Rash, urticaria, erythema multiforme
Hematologic: Aplastic anemia, leukopenia, eosinophilia
Ocular: Blurred vision

Overdosage/Toxicology Symptoms of overdose include nausea, vomiting, diarrhea, drowsiness, dizziness, headache, absent tendon reflexes, hypotension

Treatment is supportive following attempts to enhance drug elimination. Hypotension should be treated with I.V. fluids and/or Trendelenburg positioning. Dialysis and hemoperfusion and osmotic diuresis have all been useful in reducing serum drug concentrations; patient should be observed for possible relapses due to incomplete gastric emptying.

Drug Interactions Increased effect/toxicity: Alcohol, CNS depressants

Mechanism of Action Acts on the spinal cord and subcortical levels by depressing polysynaptic reflexes

Pharmacodynamics/Kinetics

Onset of action: Within 1 hour
Absorption: Oral: Readily absorbed
Metabolism: Extensively in the liver by glucuronidation
Elimination: Excretion in urine as conjugates

Usual Dosage Oral:

Children: 20 mg/kg/day or 600 mg/m^2/day in 3-4 divided doses
Adults: 250-500 mg 3-4 times/day up to 750 mg 3-4 times/day

Dietary Considerations Alcohol: Additive CNS effects, avoid use

Monitoring Parameters Periodic liver functions tests

Patient Information May cause drowsiness or dizziness; avoid alcohol and other CNS depressants

Nursing Implications Raise bed rails; institute safety measures; assist with ambulation

Dosage Forms

Caplet (Parafon Forte™ DSC): 500 mg
Capsule (Flexaphen®, Mus-Lax®): 250 mg with acetaminophen 300 mg
Tablet: Paraflex®: 250 mg

Chlorzoxazone with Acetaminophen *see* Chlorzoxazone *on previous page*
Cholac® *see* Lactulose *on page 703*
Choledyl® *see* Theophylline Salts *on page 1207*

Cholera Vaccine (KOL er a vak SEEN)

Related Information

Recommendations for Travelers *on page 1442*

Therapeutic Category Vaccine, Inactivated Bacteria

Use The World Health Organization no longer recommends cholera vaccination for travel to or from cholera-endemic areas. Some countries may still require evidence of a complete primary series or a booster dose given within 6 months of arrival. Vaccination should not be considered as an alternative to continued careful selection of foods and water. Ideally, cholera and yellow fever vaccines should be administered at least 3 weeks apart.

Pregnancy Risk Factor C

Contraindications Presence of any acute illness, history of severe systemic reaction, or allergic response following a prior dose of cholera vaccine

Warnings/Precautions There is no data on the safety of cholera vaccination during pregnancy. Use in pregnancy should reflect actual increased risk. Persons who have had severe local or systemic reactions to a previous dose should not be revaccinated. Have epinephrine (1:1000) available for immediate use.

Adverse Reactions

>10%:

Central nervous system: Malaise, fever, headache
Local: Pain, edema, tenderness, erythema, and induration at injection site

Drug Interactions Decreased effect with yellow fever vaccine; data suggests that giving both vaccines within 3 weeks of each other may decrease the response to both

Stability Refrigerate, avoid freezing

Mechanism of Action Inactivated vaccine producing active immunization

(Continued)

Cholera Vaccine *(Continued)*

Usual Dosage

Children:

6 months to 4 years: Two 0.2 mL doses I.M./S.C. 1 week to 1 month apart; booster doses (0.2 mL I.M./S.C.) every 6 months

5-10 years: Two 0.3 mL doses I.M./S.C. or two 0.2 mL intradermal doses 1 week to 1 month apart; booster doses (0.3 mL I.M./S.C. or 0.2 mL I.D.) every 6 months

Children ≥10 years and Adults: Two 0.5 mL doses given I.M./S.C. or two 0.2 mL doses I.D. 1 week to 1 month apart; booster doses (0.5 mL I.M. or S.C. or 0.2 mL I.D.) every 6 months

Administration Do not administer I.V.

Patient Information Local reactions can occur up to 7 days after injection

Nursing Implications Defer immunization in individuals with moderate or severe febrile illness

Additional Information Inactivated bacteria vaccine

Dosage Forms Injection: Suspension of killed *Vibrio cholerae* (Inaba and Ogawa types) 8 units of each serotype per mL (1.5 mL, 20 mL)

Cholestyramine Resin (koe LES tir a meen REZ in)

Related Information

Lipid-Lowering Agents *on page 1413*

Brand Names Questran®; Questran® Light

Canadian/Mexican Brand Names PMS-Cholestyramine (Canada)

Therapeutic Category Antilipemic Agent

Use Adjunct in the management of primary hypercholesterolemia; pruritus associated with elevated levels of bile acids; diarrhea associated with excess fecal bile acids; binding toxicologic agents; pseudomembraneous colitis

Pregnancy Risk Factor C

Contraindications Avoid using in complete biliary obstruction; hypersensitive to cholestyramine or any component; hypolipoproteinemia types III, IV, V

Warnings/Precautions Use with caution in patients with constipation (GI dysfunction); caution patients with phenylketonuria (Questran® Light contains aspartame); overdose may result in GI obstruction

Adverse Reactions

1% to 10%: Gastrointestinal: Constipation

<1%:

Dermatologic: Rash, irritation of perianal area, or skin

Endocrine & metabolic: Hyperchloremic acidosis

Gastrointestinal: Nausea, vomiting, abdominal distention and pain, malabsorption of fat-soluble vitamins, intestinal obstruction, steatorrhea, tongue irritation

Hematologic: Hypoprothrombinemia (secondary to vitamin K deficiency)

Renal: Increased urinary calcium excretion

Overdosage/Toxicology Symptoms of overdose include GI obstruction; treatment is supportive

Drug Interactions Decreased effect: Decreased absorption (oral) of digitalis glycosides, warfarin, thyroid hormones, valproic acid, thiazide diuretics, propranolol, phenobarbital, amiodarone, methotrexate, NSAIDs, and other drugs by binding to the drug in the intestine

Mechanism of Action Forms a nonabsorbable complex with bile acids in the intestine, releasing chloride ions in the process; inhibits enterohepatic reuptake of intestinal bile salts and thereby increases the fecal loss of bile salt-bound low density lipoprotein cholesterol

Pharmacodynamics/Kinetics

Peak effect: 21 days

Absorption: Not absorbed from the GI tract

Elimination: In feces as an insoluble complex with bile acids

Usual Dosage Oral (dosages are expressed in terms of anhydrous resin):

Powder:

Children: 240 mg/kg/day in 3 divided doses; need to titrate dose depending on indication

Adults: 4 g 1-6 times/day to a maximum of 16-32 g/day

Tablet: Adults: Initial: 4 g once or twice daily; maintenance: 8-16 g/day in 2 divided doses

Dialysis: Not removed by hemo- or peritoneal dialysis; supplemental doses not necessary with dialysis or continuous arterio-venous or veno-venous hemofiltration effects

Test Interactions ↑ prothrombin time (S); ↓ cholesterol (S), iron (B)

Patient Information Do not administer the powder in its dry form, mix with fluid or with applesauce; chew bars thoroughly; drink plenty of fluids; take other medications 1 hour before or 4-6 hours after binding resin; GI adverse reactions may decrease over time with continued use; do not take with meals; adhere to prescribed diet

Nursing Implications Administer warfarin and other drugs at least 1-2 hours prior to, or 6 hours after cholestyramine because cholestyramine may bind to them, decreasing their total absorption. (**Note:** Cholestyramine itself may cause hypoprothrombinemia in patients with impaired enterohepatic circulation.)

Dosage Forms

Powder: 4 g of resin/9 g of powder (9 g, 378 g)

Powder, for oral suspension, with aspartame: 4 g of resin/5 g of powder (5 g, 210 g)

Powder, for oral suspension, with phenylalanine: 4 g of resin/5.5 g of powder (60s)

Choline Magnesium Trisalicylate

(KOE leen mag NEE zhum trye sa LIS i late)

Related Information

Dosing Data for Acetaminophen and NSAIDs *on page 1377*

Brand Names Tricosal®; Trilisate®

Therapeutic Category Analgesic, Salicylate; Anti-inflammatory Agent; Nonsteroidal Anti-inflammatory Agent (NSAID), Oral; Salicylate

Use Management of osteoarthritis, rheumatoid arthritis, and other arthritis; salicylate salts may not inhibit platelet aggregation and, therefore, should not be substituted for aspirin in the prophylaxis of thrombosis

Pregnancy Risk Factor C

Contraindications Bleeding disorders; hypersensitivity to salicylates or other nonacetylated salicylates or other NSAIDs; tartrazine dye hypersensitivity, asthma

Warnings/Precautions Use with caution in patients with impaired renal function, erosive gastritis, or peptic ulcer; avoid use in patients with suspected varicella or influenza (salicylates have been associated with Reye's syndrome in children <16 years of age when used to treat symptoms of chickenpox or the flu). Tinnitus or impaired hearing may indicate toxicity; discontinue use 1 week prior to surgical procedures.

Elderly are a high-risk population for adverse effects from nonsteroidal anti-inflammatory agents. As much as 60% of elderly can develop peptic ulceration and/or hemorrhage asymptomatically. Use lowest effective dose for shortest period possible. Tinnitus may be a difficult and unreliable indication of toxicity due to age-related hearing loss or eighth cranial nerve damage. CNS adverse effects may be observed in the elderly at lower doses than younger adults.

Adverse Reactions

>10%: Gastrointestinal: Nausea, heartburn, stomach pains, dyspepsia, epigastric discomfort

1% to 10%:

- Central nervous system: Fatigue
- Dermatologic: Rash
- Gastrointestinal: Gastrointestinal ulceration
- Hematologic: Hemolytic anemia
- Neuromuscular & skeletal: Weakness
- Respiratory: Dyspnea
- Miscellaneous: Anaphylactic shock

<1%:

- Central nervous system: Insomnia, nervousness, jitters
- Hematologic: Occult bleeding, prolongation of bleeding time, leukopenia, thrombocytopenia, iron deficiency anemia
- Hepatic: Hepatotoxicity
- Renal: Impaired renal function
- Respiratory: Bronchospasm

Overdosage/Toxicology Symptoms of overdose include tinnitus, vomiting, acute renal failure, hyperthermia, irritability, seizures, coma, metabolic acidosis

For acute ingestions, determine serum salicylate levels 6 hours after ingestion; the "Done" nomogram may be helpful for estimating the severity of aspirin poisoning and directing treatment using serum salicylate levels. Treatment can also be based upon symptomatology.

(Continued)

Salicylates

Toxic Symptoms	Treatment
Overdose	Induce emesis with ipecac, and/or lavage with saline, followed with activated charcoal
Dehydration	I.V. fluids with KCl (no D_5W only)
Metabolic acidosis (must be treated)	Sodium bicarbonate
Hyperthermia	Cooling blankets or sponge baths
Coagulopathy/hemorrhage	Vitamin K I.V.
Hypoglycemia (with coma, seizures, or change in mental status)	Dextrose 25 g I.V.
Seizures	Diazepam 5-10 mg I.V.

Drug Interactions

Decreased effect: Antacids + Trilisate® may decrease salicylate concentration

Increased toxicity: Warfarin + Trilisate® may possibly increase hypoprothrombinemic effect

Mechanism of Action Inhibits prostaglandin synthesis; acts on the hypothalamus heat-regulating center to reduce fever; blocks the generation of pain impulses

Pharmacodynamics/Kinetics

Absorption: Absorbed from the stomach and small intestine

Distribution: Readily distributes into most body fluids and tissues; crosses the placenta; appears in breast milk

Half-life: Dose-dependent ranging from 2-3 hours at low doses to 30 hours at high doses

Time to peak serum concentration: ~2 hours

Usual Dosage Oral (based on total salicylate content):

Children <37 kg: 50 mg/kg/day given in 2 divided doses

Adults: 500 mg to 1.5 g 2-3 times/day; usual maintenance dose: 1-4.5 g/day

Dosing adjustment/comments in renal impairment: Avoid use in severe renal impairment

Dietary Considerations

Alcohol: Combination causes GI irritation, possible bleeding; avoid or limit alcohol. Patients at increased risk include those prone to hypoprothrombinemia, vitamin K deficiency, thrombocytopenia, thrombotic thrombocytopenia purpura, severe hepatic impairment, and those receiving anticoagulants.

Food: May decrease the rate but not the extent of oral absorption. Drug may cause GI upset, bleeding, ulceration, perforation. Take with food or or large volume of water or milk to minimize GI upset.

Folic acid: Hyperexcretion of folate; folic acid deficiency may result, leading to macrocytic anemia. Supplement with folic acid if necessary.

Iron: With chronic use and at doses of 3-4 g/day, iron deficiency anemia may result; supplement with iron if necessary

Magnesium: Hypermagnesemia resulting from magnesium salicylate; avoid or use with caution in renal insufficiency

Sodium: Hypernatremia resulting from buffered aspirin solutions or sodium salicylate containing high sodium content. Avoid or use with caution in CHF or any condition where hypernatremia would be detrimental.

Curry powder, paprika, licorice, Benedictine liqueur, prunes, raisins, tea and gherkins: Potential salicylate salicylate accumulation. These foods contain 6 mg salicylate/100 g. An ordinary American diet contains 10-200 mg/day of salicylate. Foods containing salicylates may contribute to aspirin hypersensitivity. Patients at greatest risk for aspirin hypersensitivity include those with asthma, nasal polyposis, or chronic urticaria.

Monitoring Parameters Serum magnesium with high dose therapy or in patients with impaired renal function; serum salicylate levels, renal function, hearing changes or tinnitus, abnormal bruising, weight gain and response (ie, pain)

Reference Range Salicylate blood levels for anti-inflammatory effect: 150-300 µg/mL; analgesia and antipyretic effect: 30-50 µg/mL

Test Interactions False-negative results for glucose oxidase urinary glucose tests (Clinistix®); false-positives using the cupric sulfate method (Clinitest®); also, interferes with Gerhardt test (urinary ketone analysis), VMA determination; 5-HIAA, xylose tolerance test, and T_3 and T_4; increased PBI; increased uric acid

Brand Name	Dosage Form	Total Salicylate	Choline Salicylate	Magnesium Salicylate
Trilisate®	Liquid	500 mg/5 mL	293 mg/5 mL	362 mg/5 mL
Trilisate 500®	Tablet	500 mg	293 mg	362 mg
Trilisate 750®	Tablet	750 mg	440 mg	544 mg
Trilisate 1000®	Tablet	1000 mg	587 mg	725 mg

Patient Information Take with food; do not take with antacids; watch for bleeding gums or any signs of GI bleeding; take with food or milk to minimize GI distress, notify physician if ringing in ears or persistent GI pain occurs

Nursing Implications Liquid may be mixed with fruit juice just before drinking; do not administer with antacids

Dosage Forms See table.

Choline Salicylate (KOE leen sa LIS i late)

Related Information

Dosing Data for Acetaminophen and NSAIDs *on page 1377*

Brand Names Arthropan® [OTC]

Canadian/Mexican Brand Names Teejel® (Canada)

Therapeutic Category Analgesic, Salicylate; Anti-inflammatory Agent; Nonsteroidal Anti-inflammatory Agent (NSAID), Oral; Salicylate

Use Temporary relief of pain of rheumatoid arthritis, rheumatic fever, osteoarthritis, and other conditions for which oral salicylates are recommended; useful in patients in which there is difficulty in administering doses in a tablet or capsule dosage form, because of the liquid dosage form

Pregnancy Risk Factor C

Contraindications Hypersensitivity to salicylates or any component or other nonacetylated salicylates

Warnings/Precautions Use with caution in patients with impaired renal function, erosive gastritis, or peptic ulcer; avoid use in patients with suspected varicella or influenza (salicylates have been associated with Reye's syndrome in children <16 years of age when used to treat symptoms of chickenpox or the flu)

Adverse Reactions

>10%: Gastrointestinal: Nausea, heartburn, stomach pains, dyspepsia, epigastric discomfort

1% to 10%:

- Central nervous system: Fatigue
- Dermatologic: Rash
- Gastrointestinal: Gastrointestinal ulceration
- Hematologic: Hemolytic anemia
- Neuromuscular & skeletal: Weakness
- Respiratory: Dyspnea
- Miscellaneous: Anaphylactic shock

<1%:

- Central nervous system: Insomnia, nervousness, jitters
- Hematologic: Occult bleeding, prolongation of bleeding time, leukopenia, thrombocytopenia, iron deficiency anemia
- Hepatic: Hepatotoxicity
- Renal: Impaired renal function
- Respiratory: Bronchospasm

Overdosage/Toxicology Symptoms of overdose include tinnitus, vomiting, acute renal failure, hyperthermia, irritability, seizures, coma, metabolic acidosis

For acute ingestions, determine serum salicylate levels 6 hours after ingestion; the "Done" nomogram may be helpful for estimating the severity of aspirin poisoning and directing treatment using serum salicylate levels. Treatment can also be based upon symptomatology.

Salicylates

Toxic Symptoms	Treatment
Overdose	Induce emesis with ipecac, and/or lavage with saline, followed with activated charcoal
Dehydration	I.V. fluids with KCl (no D_5W only)
Metabolic acidosis (must be treated)	Sodium bicarbonate
Hyperthermia	Cooling blankets or sponge baths
Coagulopathy/hemorrhage	Vitamin K I.V.
Hypoglycemia (with coma, seizures, or change in mental status)	Dextrose 25 g I.V.
Seizures	Diazepam 5-10 mg I.V.

Drug Interactions

Decreased effect with antacids

Increased effect of warfarin

Mechanism of Action Inhibits prostaglandin synthesis; acts on the hypothalamus heat-regulating center to reduce fever; blocks the generation of pain impulses

Pharmacodynamics/Kinetics

Absorption: From the stomach and small intestine within ~2 hours

(Continued)

Choline Salicylate *(Continued)*

Distribution: Readily distributes into most body fluids and tissues; crosses the placenta; appears in breast milk
Protein binding: 75% to 90%
Metabolism: Hydrolyzed to salicylate in the liver
Half-life: Dose-dependent ranging from 2-3 hours at low doses to 30 hours at high doses
Time to peak serum concentration: 1-2 hours
Elimination: In urine

Usual Dosage
Children >12 years and Adults: Oral: 5 mL (870 mg) every 3-4 hours, if necessary, but not more than 6 doses in 24 hours
Rheumatoid arthritis: 870-1740 mg (5-10 mL) up to 4 times/day

Dosing adjustment/comments in renal impairment: Avoid use in severe renal impairment

Test Interactions False-negative results for Clinistix® urine test; false-positive results with Clinitest®; ↑ bleeding time

Patient Information Take with food; do not take with antacids; watch for bleeding gums or any signs of GI bleeding; take with food or milk to minimize GI distress, notify physician if ringing in ears or persistent GI pain occurs

Nursing Implications Liquid may be mixed with fruit juice just before drinking; do not administer with antacids

Dosage Forms Liquid (mint flavor): 870 mg/5 mL (240 mL, 480 mL)

Choline Theophyllinate *see* Theophylline Salts *on page 1207*

Choloxin® *see* Dextrothyroxine *on page 367*

Chondroitin Sulfate-Sodium Hyaluronate

(kon DROY tin SUL fate-SOW de um hye a loo ROE nate)

Brand Names Viscoat®

Synonyms Sodium Hyaluronate-Chrondroitin Sulfate

Therapeutic Category Ophthalmic Agent, Viscoelastic

Use Surgical aid in anterior segment procedures, protects corneal endothelium and coats intraocular lens thus protecting it

Pregnancy Risk Factor C

Contraindications Hypersensitivity to hyaluronate

Warnings/Precautions Product is extracted from avian tissues and contains minute amounts of protein, potential risks of hypersensitivity may exist. Intraocular pressure may be elevated as a result of pre-existing glaucoma, compromised outflow and by operative procedures and sequelae, including coma, compromised outflow and by operative procedures and sequelae, including enzymatic zonulysis, absence of an iridectomy, trauma to filtration structures and by blood and lenticular remnants in the anterior chamber. Monitor IOP, especially during the immediate postoperative period.

Adverse Reactions 1% to 10%: Ocular: Increased intraocular pressure

Stability Store at 2°C to 8°C/36°F to 46°F; do not freeze

Mechanism of Action Functions as a tissue lubricant and is thought to play an important role in modulating the interactions between adjacent tissues

Pharmacodynamics/Kinetics
Absorption: Following intravitreous injection, diffusion occurs slowly
Elimination: By way of the Canal of Schlemm

Usual Dosage Carefully introduce (using a 27-gauge needle or cannula) into anterior chamber after thoroughly cleaning the chamber with a balanced salt solution

Administration May inject prior to or following delivery of the crystalline lens. Instillation prior to lens delivery provides additional protection to corneal endothelium, protecting it from possible damage arising from surgical instrumentation. May also be used to coat intraocular lens and tips of surgical instruments prior to implantation surgery. May inject additional solution during anterior segment surgery to fully maintain the solution lost during surgery. At the end of surgery, remove solution by thoroughly irrigating with a balanced salt solution.

Test Interactions False-negative results for Clinistix® urine test; false-positive results with Clinitest®

Dosage Forms Solution: Sodium chondroitin 40 mg and sodium hyaluronate 30 mg (0.25 mL, 0.5 mL)

Chooz® [OTC] *see* Calcium Carbonate *on page 185*

Chorex® *see* Chorionic Gonadotropin *on this page*

Chorionic Gonadotropin (kor ee ON ik goe NAD oh troe pin)

Brand Names A.P.L.®; Chorex®; Choron®; Follutein®; Glukor®; Gonic®; Pregnyl®; Profasi® HP

Synonyms CG; hCG

Therapeutic Category Ovulation Stimulator

Use Induces ovulation and pregnancy in anovulatory, infertile females; treatment of hypogonadotropic hypogonadism, prepubertal cryptorchidism

Pregnancy Risk Factor C

Contraindications Hypersensitivity to chorionic gonadotropin or any component; precocious puberty, prostatic carcinoma or similar neoplasms

Warnings/Precautions Use with caution in asthma, seizure disorders, migraine, cardiac or renal disease; **not** effective in the treatment of obesity

Adverse Reactions

1% to 10%:

- Central nervous system: Mental depression, fatigue
- Endocrine & metabolic: Pelvic pain, ovarian cysts, enlargement of breasts, precocious puberty
- Local: Pain at the injection site
- Neuromuscular & skeletal: Premature closure of epiphyses

<1%:

- Cardiovascular: Peripheral edema
- Central nervous system: Irritability, restlessness, headache
- Endocrine & metabolic: Ovarian hyperstimulation syndrome, gynecomastia

Stability Following reconstitution with the provided diluent, solutions are stable for 30-90 days, depending on the specific preparation, when stored at 2°C to 15°C

Mechanism of Action Stimulates production of gonadal steroid hormones by causing production of androgen by the testis; as a substitute for luteinizing hormone (LH) to stimulate ovulation

Pharmacodynamics/Kinetics

Half-life, biphasic:

- Initial: 11 hours
- Terminal: 23 hours

Elimination: Excreted unchanged in urine within 3-4 days

Usual Dosage I.M.:

Children:

- Prepubertal cryptorchidism: 1000-2000 units/m^2/dose 3 times/week for 3 weeks **OR** 4000 units 3 times/week for 3 weeks **OR** 5000 units every second day for 4 injections **OR** 500 units 3 times/week for 4-6 weeks
- Hypogonadotropic hypogonadism: 500-1000 units 3 times/week for 3 weeks, followed by the same dose twice weekly for 3 weeks **OR** 1000-2000 units 3 times/week **OR** 4000 units 3 times/week for 6-9 months; reduce dosage to 2000 units 3 times/week for additional 3 months

Adults: Induction of ovulation: 5000-10,000 units one day following last dose of menotropins

Administration I.M. administration only

Reference Range Depends on application and methodology; <3 mIU/mL (SI: <3 units/L) usually normal (nonpregnant)

Patient Information Discontinue immediately if possibility of pregnancy

Dosage Forms Powder for injection (human origin): 200 units/mL (10 mL, 25 mL); 500 units/mL (10 mL); 1000 units/mL (10 mL); 2000 units/mL (10 mL)

Choron® *see* Chorionic Gonadotropin *on previous page*

Chromagen® OB [OTC] *see* Vitamins, Multiple *on page 1310*

Chronulac® *see* Lactulose *on page 703*

Cibacalcin® Injection *see* Calcitonin *on page 181*

Ciclopirox (sye kloe PEER oks)

Brand Names Loprox®

Synonyms Ciclopirox Olamine

Therapeutic Category Antifungal Agent, Topical

Use Treatment of tinea pedis (athlete's foot), tinea cruris (jock itch), tinea corporis (ringworm), cutaneous candidiasis, and tinea versicolor (pityriasis)

Pregnancy Risk Factor B

Contraindications Known hypersensitivity to ciclopirox

Warnings/Precautions For external use only; avoid contact with eyes

Adverse Reactions

1% to 10%:

- Central nervous system: Pain
- Local: Irritation, redness, or burning; worsening of clinical condition

Mechanism of Action Inhibiting transport of essential elements in the fungal cell causing problems in synthesis of DNA, RNA, and protein

Pharmacodynamics/Kinetics

Absorption: <2% absorbed through intact skin

Protein binding: 94% to 98%

Half-life: 1.7 hours

(Continued)

Ciclopirox *(Continued)*

Elimination: Of the small amounts of systemically absorbed drug, majority excreted by the kidney with small amounts excreted in feces

Usual Dosage Children >10 years and Adults: Apply twice daily, gently massage into affected areas; if no improvement after 4 weeks of treatment, re-evaluate the diagnosis

Patient Information Avoid contact with eyes; if sensitivity or irritation occurs, discontinue use

Dosage Forms

Cream, topical, as olamine: 1% (15 g, 30 g, 90 g)

Lotion, as olamine: 1% (30 mL)

Ciclopirox Olamine *see* Ciclopirox *on previous page*

Cidofovir (si DOF o veer)

Brand Names Vistide®

Therapeutic Category Antiviral Agent, Parenteral

Use Treatment of cytomegalovirus (CMV) retinitis in patients with acquired immunodeficiency syndrome (AIDS); currently under Phase I and II trials for systemic treatment of AIDS. **Note:** Should be administered with probenecid

Pregnancy Risk Factor C

Pregnancy/Breast-Feeding Implications Although studies are inconclusive, adenocarcinomas have occurred in animal studies with cidofovir; use during pregnancy only if the potential benefit justifies the potential risk to the fetus. Excretion of cidofovir into breast milk is unknown, however, the US Public Health Service recommends HIV-infected women **not** breast-feed to avoid potential transmission to infants.

Contraindications Patients with hypersensitivity to cidofovir and in patients with a history of clinically severe hypersensitivity to probenecid or other sulfa-containing medications; direct intraocular injection of cidofovir is contraindicated

Warnings/Precautions Dose-dependent nephrotoxicity requires dose adjustment or discontinuation if changes in renal function occur during therapy (eg, proteinuria, glycosuria, decreased serum phosphate, uric acid or bicarbonate, and elevated Cr); avoid use in patients with Cr >1.5 mg/dL; Cl_{cr} <55 mL/minute; use great caution with elderly patients; neutropenia and ocular hypotony have also occurred; safety and efficacy have not been established in children; administration must be accompanied by oral probenecid and intravenous saline prehydration

Adverse Reactions

>10%:

Central nervous system: Infection, chills, fever, headache, amnesia, anxiety, confusion, seizures, insomnia

Dermatologic: Alopecia, rash, acne, skin discoloration

Gastrointestinal: Nausea, vomiting, diarrhea, anorexia, abdominal pain, constipation, dyspepsia, gastritis

Hematologic: Thrombocytopenia, neutropenia, anemia

Neuromuscular & skeletal: Weakness, paresthesia

Ocular: Amblyopia, conjunctivitis, ocular hypotony

Renal: Tubular damage, proteinuria, Cr elevations

Respiratory: Asthma, bronchitis, coughing, dyspnea, pharyngitis

1% to 10%:

Cardiovascular: Hypotension, pallor, syncope, tachycardia

Central nervous system: Dizziness, hallucinations, depression, somnolence, malaise

Dermatologic: Pruritus, urticaria

Endocrine & metabolic: Hyperglycemia, hyperlipidemia, hypocalcemia, hypokalemia, dehydration

Gastrointestinal: Abnormal taste, stomatitis

Genitourinary: Glycosuria, urinary incontinence, urinary tract infections

Neuromuscular & skeletal: Skeletal pain

Ocular: Retinal detachment, iritis, uveitis, abnormal vision

Renal: Hematuria

Respiratory: Pneumonia, rhinitis, sinusitis

Miscellaneous: Diaphoresis, allergic reactions

Overdosage/Toxicology No reports of acute toxicity have been reported, however, hemodialysis and hydration may reduce drug plasma concentrations; probenecid may assist in decreasing active tubular secretion

Drug Interactions Increased effect/toxicity: Drugs with nephrotoxic potential (eg, amphotericin B, aminoglycosides, foscarnet, and I.V. pentamidine) should be avoided during cidofovir therapy

Stability Store admixtures under refrigeration for ≤24 hours; prepare admixtures in a class two laminar flow hood, wearing protective gear; dispose of cidofovir as directed; wash and flush skin thoroughly with water if contact with skin

Mechanism of Action As a nucleotide analog, cidofovir suppresses CMV replication by selective prevention of viral DNA synthesis through inhibition of CMV DNA polymerase; the active form is the intracellular metabolite, cidofovir diphosphate; cross-resistance to ganciclovir but not foscarnet has been demonstrated *in vitro*

Pharmacodynamics/Kinetics The following pharmacokinetic data is based on a combination of cidofovir administered with probenecid:

Distribution: V_d: 0.54 L/kg; does not cross significantly into the CSF

Protein binding: <6%

Metabolism: Minimal; phosphorylation occurs intracellularly

Half-life, plasma: ~2.6 hours

Elimination: Renal tubular secretion and glomerular filtration

Usual Dosage

Induction: 5 mg/kg I.V. over 1 hour once weekly for 2 consecutive weeks

Maintenance: 5 mg/kg over 1 hour once every other week

Administer with probenecid - 2 g orally 3 hours prior to the cidofovir dose and 1 g at 2 and 8 hours after completion of the infusion (total: 4 g)

Hydrate with 1 L of 0.9% NS I.V. prior to cidofovir infusion; a second liter may be administered over a 1- to 3-hour period immediately following infusion, if tolerated

Dosing adjustment in renal impairment:

Cl_{cr} 41-55 mL/minute: 2 mg/kg

Cl_{cr} 30-40 mL/minute: 1.5 mg/kg

Cl_{cr} 20-29 mL/minute: 1 mg/kg

Cl_{cr} <19 mL/minute: 0.5 mg/kg

If the Cr increases by 0.3-0.4 mg/dL, reduce the cidofovir dose to 3 mg/kg; DC therapy for increases ≥0.5 mg/dL or development of ≥3+ proteinuria

Monitoring Parameters Renal function (Cr, BUN, UAs), LFTs, WBCs, intraocular pressure and visual acuity

Patient Information Cidofovir is not a cure for CMV retinitis; regular follow-up ophthalmologic exams and careful monitoring of renal function are necessary; probenecid must be administered concurrently with cidofovir; report rash immediately to your physician; avoid use during pregnancy; use contraception during and for 3 months following treatment

Nursing Implications Zidovudine (AZT) doses should be decreased or discontinued during cidofovir therapy since probenecid decreases its elimination; administration of probenecid with a meal may decrease associated nausea; acetaminophen and antihistamines may ameliorate hypersensitivity reactions; dilute in 100 mL 0.9% saline; administer probenecid and I.V. saline before each infusion; allow the admixture to come to room temperature before administration

Dosage Forms Injection: 75 mg/mL (5 mL)

Ciloxan™ Ophthalmic *see* Ciprofloxacin *on page 277*

Cimetidine (sye MET i deen)

Related Information

Antacid Drug Interactions *on page 1388*

Brand Names Tagamet®; Tagamet-HB® [OTC]

Canadian/Mexican Brand Names Apo-Cimetidine® (Canada); Novo-Cimetidine® (Canada); Nu-Cimet® (Canada); Peptol® (Canada); Blocan® (Mexico); Cimetase® (Mexico); Cimetigal® (Mexico); Columina® (Mexico); Ulcedine® (Mexico); Zymerol® (Mexico)

Therapeutic Category Antihistamine, H_2 Blocker; Histamine-2 Antagonist

Use Short-term treatment of active duodenal ulcers and benign gastric ulcers; long-term prophylaxis of duodenal ulcer; gastric hypersecretory states; gastroesophageal reflux; prevention of upper GI bleeding in critically ill patients.

Pregnancy Risk Factor B

Contraindications Hypersensitivity to cimetidine, other component, or other H_2-antagonists

Warnings/Precautions Adjust dosages in renal/hepatic impairment or patients receiving drugs metabolized through the P-450 system

Adverse Reactions

1% to 10%:

Central nervous system: Dizziness, agitation, headache, drowsiness

Gastrointestinal: Diarrhea, nausea, vomiting

<1%:

Cardiovascular: Bradycardia, hypotension, tachycardia

Central nervous system: Confusion, fever

Dermatologic: Rash

Endocrine & metabolic: Gynecomastia, edema of the breasts, decreased sexual ability

Hematologic: Neutropenia, agranulocytosis, thrombocytopenia

(Continued)

Cimetidine *(Continued)*

Hepatic: Elevated AST and ALT
Neuromuscular & skeletal: Myalgia
Renal: Elevated creatinine

Overdosage/Toxicology Treatment is primarily symptomatic and supportive. No experience with intentional overdose; reported ingestions of 20 g have had transient side effects seen with recommended doses; animal data have shown respiratory failure, tachycardia, muscle tremors, vomiting, restlessness, hypotension, salivation, emesis, and diarrhea.

Drug Interactions

Increased toxicity: Decreased elimination of lidocaine, theophylline, phenytoin, metronidazole, triamterene, procainamide, quinidine, and propranolol

Inhibition of warfarin metabolism, tricyclic antidepressant metabolism, diazepam elimination and cyclosporine elimination

Stability

Intact vials of cimetidine should be stored at room temperature and protected from light; cimetidine may precipitate from solution upon exposure to cold but can be redissolved by warming without degradation

Stability at room temperature:

Prepared bags: 7 days

Premixed bags: Manufacturer expiration dating and out of overwrap stability: 15 days

Stable in parenteral nutrition solutions for up to 7 days when protected from light

Physically incompatible with barbiturates, amphotericin B, and cephalosporins

Mechanism of Action Competitive inhibition of histamine at H_2-receptors of the gastric parietal cells resulting in reduced gastric acid secretion, gastric volume and hydrogen ion concentration reduced

Pharmacodynamics/Kinetics

Distribution: Crosses the placenta; appears in breast milk

Protein binding: 20%

Bioavailability: 60% to 70%

Half-life:

Neonates: 3.6 hours

Children: 1.4 hours

Adults (with normal renal function): 2 hours

Time to peak serum concentration: Oral: Within 1-2 hours

Elimination: Principally as unchanged drug by the kidney; some excretion in bile and feces

Usual Dosage

Children: Oral, I.M., I.V.: 20-40 mg/kg/day in divided doses every 4 hours

Adults: Short-term treatment of active ulcers:

Oral: 300 mg 4 times/day or 800 mg at bedtime or 400 mg twice daily for up to 8 weeks

I.M., I.V.: 300 mg every 6 hours or 37.5 mg/hour by continuous infusion; I.V. dosage should be adjusted to maintain an intragastric pH ≥5

Patients with an active bleed: Administer cimetidine as a continuous infusion (see above)

Duodenal ulcer prophylaxis: Oral: 400-800 mg at bedtime

Gastric hypersecretory conditions: Oral, I.M., I.V.: 300-600 mg every 6 hours; dosage not to exceed 2.4 g/day

Dosing adjustment/interval in renal impairment: Children and Adults:

Cl_{cr} 20-40 mL/minute: Administer every 8 hours or 75% of normal dose

Cl_{cr} 0-20 mL/minute: Administer every 12 hours or 50% of normal dose

Hemodialysis: Slightly dialyzable (5% to 20%)

Dosing adjustment/comments in hepatic impairment: Usual dose is safe in mild liver disease but use with caution and in reduced dosage in severe liver disease; increased risk of CNS toxicity in cirrhosis suggested by enhanced penetration of CNS

Dietary Considerations Alcohol: Additive CNS effects, avoid or limit use

Administration Administer with meals so that the drug's peak effect occurs at the proper time (peak inhibition of gastric acid secretion occurs at 1 and 3 hours after dosing in fasting subjects and approximately 2 hours in nonfasting subjects; this correlates well with the time food is no longer in the stomach offering a buffering effect)

Monitoring Parameters Blood pressure with I.V. push administration, CBC, gastric pH, signs and symptoms of peptic ulcer disease, occult blood with GI bleeding, monitor renal function to correct dose; monitor for side effects

Test Interactions ↑ creatinine, AST, ALT, creatinine (S)

Patient Information Take with or immediately after meals; take 1 hour before or 2 hours after antacids; may cause drowsiness, impaired judgment, or coordination; avoid excessive alcohol

Dosage Forms
Infusion, as hydrochloride, in NS: 300 mg (50 mL)
Injection, as hydrochloride: 150 mg/mL (2 mL, 8 mL)
Liquid, oral, as hydrochloride (mint-peach flavor): 300 mg/5 mL with alcohol 2.8% (5 mL, 240 mL)
Tablet: 200 mg, 300 mg, 400 mg, 800 mg

Cinobac® Pulvules® *see* Cinoxacin *on this page*

Cinoxacin (sin OKS a sin)

Brand Names Cinobac® Pulvules®
Canadian/Mexican Brand Names Gugecin® (Mexico)
Therapeutic Category Antibiotic, Quinolone
Use Treatment of urinary tract infections
Pregnancy Risk Factor B
Contraindications History of convulsive disorders, hypersensitivity to cinoxacin or any component or other quinolones
Warnings/Precautions CNS stimulation may occur (tremor, restlessness, confusion, and very rarely hallucinations or seizures). Use with caution in patients with known or suspected CNS disorders or renal impairment. Not recommended in children <18 years of age, ciprofloxacin (a related compound), has caused a transient arthropathy in children; prolonged use may result in superinfection; modify dosage in patients with renal impairment.
Adverse Reactions
1% to 10%:
Central nervous system: Headache, dizziness
Gastrointestinal: Heartburn, abdominal pain, GI bleeding, belching, flatulence, anorexia, nausea
<1%:
Central nervous system: Insomnia, confusion
Gastrointestinal: Diarrhea
Hematologic: Thrombocytopenia
Ocular: Photophobia
Otic: Tinnitus
Overdosage/Toxicology Symptoms of overdose include acute renal failure, seizures; GI decontamination and supportive care; not removed by peritoneal or hemodialysis
Drug Interactions
Decreased effect: Decreased urine levels with probenecid; decreased absorption with aluminum-, magnesium-, calcium-containing antacids
Increased serum levels: Probenecid
Mechanism of Action Inhibits microbial synthesis of DNA with resultant inhibition of protein synthesis
Pharmacodynamics/Kinetics
Absorption: Oral: Rapid and complete; food decreases peak levels by 30% but not total amount absorbed
Distribution: Crosses the placenta; concentrates in prostate tissue
Protein binding: 60% to 80%
Half-life: 1.5 hours, prolonged in renal impairment
Time to peak serum concentration: Oral: Within 2-3 hours
Elimination: ~60% excreted as unchanged drug in urine
Usual Dosage Children >12 years and Adults: 1 g/day in 2-4 doses for 7-14 days
Dosing interval in renal impairment:
Cl_{cr} 20-50 mL/minute: 250 mg twice daily
Cl_{cr} <20 mL/minute: 250 mg/day
Administration Administer around-the-clock to promote less variation in peak and trough serum levels
Patient Information May be taken with food to minimize upset stomach; avoid antacid use; drink fluid liberally; may cause dizziness; use caution when driving or performing other tasks requiring alertness
Nursing Implications Hold antacids for 3-4 hours after giving
Dosage Forms Capsule: 250 mg, 500 mg

Cipro™ *see* Ciprofloxacin *on this page*

Ciprofloxacin (sip roe FLOKS a sin)

Related Information
Antimicrobial Drugs of Choice *on page 1468*
Bacterial Meningitis Practical Guidelines for Management *on page 1475*
Desensitization Protocols *on page 1496*
Guidelines for the Prevention of Opportunistic Infections in Persons with HIV *on page 1457*
Brand Names Ciloxan™ Ophthalmic; Cipro™; Cipro® I.V.
(Continued)

Ciprofloxacin *(Continued)*

Canadian/Mexican Brand Names Cimogal® (Mexico); Ciproflox® (Mexico); Ciproflur® (Mexico); Ciproxina® (Mexico); Eni® (Mexico); Italnik® (Mexico); Kenzoflex® (Mexico); Microrgan® (Mexico); Mitroken® (Mexico); Nivoflox® (Mexico); Sophixin® Ofteno (Mexico)

Synonyms Ciprofloxacin Hydrochloride

Therapeutic Category Antibiotic, Ophthalmic; Antibiotic, Quinolone

Use Treatment of documented or suspected infections of the lower respiratory tract, skin and skin structure, bone/joints, and urinary tract due to susceptible bacterial strains; especially indicated for *Pseudomonal* infections (eg, home care patients) and those due to multidrug resistant gram-negative organisms, chronic bacterial prostatitis, infectious diarrhea, complicated gram (-) and anaerobic intra-abdominal infections (with metronidazole) due to *E. coli* (enteropathic strains), *B. fragilis, P. mirabilis, K. pneumoniae, P. aeruginosa, Campylobacter jejuni* or *Shigella*; also used to treat typhoid fever due to *Salmonella typhi* (although eradication of the chronic typhoid carrier state has not been proven), osteomyelitis when parenteral therapy is not feasible, and sexually transmitted diseases such as uncomplicated cervical and urethral gonorrhea due to *Neisseria gonorrhoeae.* **Note:** Resistance is developing, (avoid use in Asian or Wester Pacific travelers); used ophthalmologically for superficial ocular infections (corneal ulcers, conjunctivitis) due to susceptible strains; the I.V. form has been used for nosocomial pneumonia due to *H. influenzae* or *K. pneumoniae.*

Pregnancy Risk Factor C

Contraindications Hypersensitivity to ciprofloxacin, any component or other quinolones

Warnings/Precautions Not recommended in children <18 years of age; has caused transient arthropathy in children; CNS stimulation may occur (tremor, restlessness, confusion, and very rarely hallucinations or seizures); use with caution in patients with known or suspected CNS disorder; green discoloration of teeth in newborns has been reported; prolonged use may result in superinfection; may rarely cause inflamed or ruptured tendons (discontinue use immediately with signs of inflammation or tendon pain)

Adverse Reactions

1% to 10%:

- Central nervous system: Headache, restlessness
- Gastrointestinal: Nausea, diarrhea, vomiting, abdominal pain
- Dermatologic: Rash

<1%:

- Central nervous system: Dizziness, confusion, seizures
- Hematologic: Anemia
- Hepatic: Increased liver enzymes
- Neuromuscular & skeletal: Tremor, arthralgia, ruptured tendons
- Renal: Acute renal failure

Overdosage/Toxicology Symptoms of overdose include acute renal failure, seizures; GI decontamination and supportive care; not removed by peritoneal or hemodialysis

Drug Interactions Inhibitor of cytochrome P-450 1A2 enzymes

Decreased effect:

Enteral feedings may ↓ plasma concentrations of ciprofloxacin probably by >30% inhibition of absorption. Ciprofloxacin should not be administered with enteral feedings. The feeding would need to be discontinued for 1-2 hours prior to and after ciprofloxacin administration. Nasogastric administration produces a greater loss of ciprofloxacin bioavailability than does nasoduodenal administration.

Aluminum/magnesium products may decrease absorption of ciprofloxacin by ≥ 90% if administered concurrently

RECOMMENDATION: Administer ciprofloxacin 2 hours before dose OR administer ciprofloxacin at least 4 hours and preferably 6 hours after the dose of aluminum/magnesium OR change to an H_2-antagonist or omeprazole

Calcium products may decrease absorption of ciprofloxacin by 50% if administered concurrently

RECOMMENDATION: Administer ciprofloxacin 2 hours before dose OR administer ciprofloxacin at least 2 hours after the dose of calcium product

Didanosine may decrease absorption of ciprofloxacin by >90% if administered concurrently

RECOMMENDATION: Administer ciprofloxacin 2 hours before dose OR administer ciprofloxacin at least 4 hours after the dose of didanosine

Iron products may decrease absorption of ciprofloxacin 40% to 90% if administered concurrently

RECOMMENDATION: Administer ciprofloxacin 2 hours before dose OR administer ciprofloxacin at least 2 hours after the dose of iron product.

Multivitamins with minerals and/or zinc may decrease absorption of ciprofloxacin by 20% to 50% if administered concomitantly

RECOMMENDATION: Administer ciprofloxacin 2 hours before dose OR administer ciprofloxacin at least 2 hours after the dose of product

Sucralfate may decrease absorption of ciprofloxacin by >90% if administered concurrently

RECOMMENDATION: Administer ciprofloxacin 2 hours before dose OR administer ciprofloxacin at least 4 hours after the dose of sucralfate OR change to an H_2-antagonist or omeprazole

Zinc products may decrease absorption of ciprofloxacin by 20% to 50% if administered concurrently

RECOMMENDATION: Administer ciprofloxacin 2 hours before dose OR administer ciprofloxacin at least 2 hours after the dose of zinc product

Increased toxicity:

Caffeine and theophylline → CNS stimulation when concurrent with ciprofloxacin

Cyclosporine may increase serum creatinine levels

Stability Refrigeration and room temperature: Prepared bags: 14 days; Premixed bags: Manufacturer expiration dating

Mechanism of Action Inhibits DNA-gyrase in susceptible organisms; inhibits relaxation of supercoiled DNA and promotes breakage of double-stranded DNA

Pharmacodynamics/Kinetics

Absorption: Oral: Rapid from GI tract (~50% to 85%)

Distribution: Crosses the placenta; appears in breast milk; distributes widely throughout body; tissue concentrations often exceed serum concentrations especially in the kidneys, gallbladder, liver, lungs, gynecological tissue, and prostatic tissue; CSF concentrations reach 10% with noninflamed meninges and 14% to 37% with inflamed meninges

Protein binding: 16% to 43%

Metabolism: Partially metabolized in the liver

Bioavailability: Oral: T_{max}: 0.5-2 hours

Half-life:

Children: 2.5 hours

Adults with normal renal function: 3-5 hours

Elimination: 30% to 50% excreted as unchanged drug in urine; 20% to 40% of dose excreted in feces primarily from biliary excretion

Usual Dosage

Children (see Warnings):

Oral: 20-30 mg/kg/day in 2 divided doses; maximum: 1.5 g/day

Cystic fibrosis: 20-40 mg/kg/day divided every 12 hours

I.V.: 15-20 mg/kg/day divided every 12 hours

Cystic fibrosis: 15-30 mg/kg/day divided every 8-12 hours

Adults: Oral:

Urinary tract infection: 250-500 mg every 12 hours for 7-10 days, depending on severity of infection and susceptibility; (3 investigations (n=975) indicate the minimum effective dose for women with acute, uncomplicated urinary tract infection may be 100 mg twice daily for 3 days)

Lower respiratory tract, skin/skin structure infections: 500-750 mg twice daily for 7-14 days depending on severity and susceptibility

Bone/joint infections: 500-750 mg twice daily for 4-6 weeks, depending on severity and susceptibility

Infectious diarrhea: 500 mg every 12 hours for 5-7 days

Typhoid fever: 500 mg every 12 hours for 10 days

Urethral/cervical gonococcal infections: 250-500 mg as a single dose (CDC recommends concomitant doxycycline or azithromycin due to developing resistance; avoid use in Asian or Wester Pacific travelers)

Disseminated gonococcal infection: 500 mg twice daily to complete 7 days of therapy (initial treatment with ceftriaxone 1 g I.M./I.V. daily for 24-48 hours after improvement begins)

Chancroid: 500 mg twice daily for 3 days

Adults: I.V.

Urinary tract infection: 200-400 mg every 12 hours for 7-10 days

Lower respiratory tract, skin/skin structure infection (mild-moderate): 400 mg every 12 hours for 7-14 days

Ophthalmic: Instill 1-2 drops in eye(s) every 2 hours while awake for 2 days and 1-2 drops every 4 hours while awake for the next 5 days

Dosing adjustment in renal impairment:

Cl_{cr} <30 mL/minute: Administer every 18 hours (oral) and every 18-24 hours (I.V.)

Dialysis: Only small amounts of ciprofloxacin are removed by hemo- or peritoneal dialysis (<10%); usual dose: 250-500 mg every 24 hours following dialysis

(Continued)

Ciprofloxacin *(Continued)*

Dietary Considerations

Food: Decreases rate, but not extent, of absorption. Drug may cause GI upset; take without regard to meals (manufacturer prefers that drug is taken 2 hours after meals)

Dairy products, oral multivitamins, and mineral supplements: Absorption decreased by divalent and trivalent cations. These cations bind to and form insoluble complexes with quinolones. Avoid taking these substrates with ciprofloxacin. The manufacturer states that the usual dietary intake of calcium has not been shown to interfere with ciprofloxacin absorption.

Caffeine: Possible exaggerated or prolonged effects of caffeine. Ciprofloxacin reduces total body clearance of caffeine. Patients consuming regular large quantities of caffeinated beverages may need to restrict caffeine intake if excessive cardiac or CNS stimulation occurs.

Administration

Oral: Administer 2 hours after a meal; may administer with food to minimize GI upset; avoid antacid use; drink plenty of fluids to maintain proper hydration and urine output

Parenteral: Administer by slow I.V. infusion over 60 minutes to reduce the risk of venous irritation (burning, pain, erythema, and swelling); final concentration for administration should not exceed 2 mg/mL

Monitoring Parameters Patients receiving concurrent ciprofloxacin, theophylline, or cyclosporine should have serum levels monitored

Reference Range Therapeutic: 2.6-3 µg/mL; Toxic: >5 µg/mL

Patient Information May be taken with food to minimize upset stomach; avoid antacids containing magnesium or aluminum, or products containing zinc or iron within 4 hours before or 2 hours after dosing; may cause dizziness or drowsiness; drink fluid liberally; consult your physician immediately if inflammation or tendon pain develop

Nursing Implications Hold antacids for 2 hours after giving

Dosage Forms

Infusion, as hydrochloride, in D_5W: 400 mg (200 mL)
Infusion, as hydrochloride, in NS or D_5W: 200 mg (100 mL)
Injection, as hydrochloride: 200 mg (20 mL); 400 mg (40 mL)
Solution, ophthalmic, as hydrochloride: 3.5 mg/mL (2.5 mL, 5 mL)
Tablet, as hydrochloride: 100 mg, 250 mg, 500 mg, 750 mg

Ciprofloxacin Hydrochloride *see* Ciprofloxacin *on page 277*

Cipro® I.V. *see* Ciprofloxacin *on page 277*

Cisapride (SIS a pride)

Brand Names Propulsid®

Canadian/Mexican Brand Names Prepulsid® (Canada); Enteropride® (Mexico); Kinestase® (Mexico); Unamol® (Mexico)

Therapeutic Category Antiemetic; Cholinergic Agent

Use Treatment of nocturnal symptoms of gastroesophageal reflux disease (GERD), also demonstrated effectiveness for gastroparesis, refractory constipation, and nonulcer dyspepsia

Pregnancy Risk Factor C

Contraindications Hypersensitivity to cisapride or any of its components; GI hemorrhage, mechanical obstruction, GI perforation, or other situations when GI motility stimulation is dangerous

Warnings/Precautions Pregnancy, lactation and when stimulation of GI motility may be dangerous (eg, obstruction, perforation, hemorrhage)

Adverse Reactions

>5%:

Central nervous system: Headache
Dermatologic: Rash
Gastrointestinal: Diarrhea, GI cramping, dyspepsia, flatulence, nausea, xerostomia
Respiratory: Rhinitis

<5%:

Cardiovascular: Tachycardia
Central nervous system: Extrapyramidal effects, somnolence, fatigue, seizures, insomnia, anxiety
Hematologic: Thrombocytopenia, increased LFTs, pancytopenia, leukopenia, granulocytopenia, aplastic anemia
Respiratory: Sinusitis, coughing, upper respiratory tract infection, increased incidence of viral infection

Drug Interactions

Decreased effect: Atropine, digoxin

Increased toxicity: Warfarin, diazepam increased levels, cimetidine, and ranitidine, CNS depressants; erythromycin and other macrolides and the triazole antifungal agents such as ketoconazole or miconazole have increased cisapride levels, which has been associated with prolonged Q-T intervals and the potential for torsade de pointes

Mechanism of Action Enhances the release of acetylcholine at the myenteric plexus. *In vitro* studies have shown cisapride to have serotonin-4 receptor agonistic properties which may increase gastrointestinal motility and cardiac rate; increases lower esophageal sphincter pressure and lower esophageal peristalsis; accelerates gastric emptying of both liquids and solids.

Pharmacodynamics/Kinetics

Onset of effect: 0.5-1 hour

Bioavailability: 35% to 40%

Protein binding: 97.5% to 98%

Metabolism: Extensively to norcisapride, which is eliminated in urine and feces

Half-life: 6-12 hours

Elimination: <10% of dose excreted into feces and urine

Usual Dosage Oral:

Children: 0.15-0.3 mg/kg/dose 3-4 times/day; maximum: 10 mg/dose

Adults: Initial: 10 mg 4 times/day at least 15 minutes before meals and at bedtime; in some patients the dosage will need to be increased to 20 mg to obtain a satisfactory result

Additional Information Safety and effectiveness in children have not been established

Dosage Forms

Suspension, oral (cherry cream flavor): 1 mg/mL (450 mL)

Tablet, scored: 10 mg, 20 mg

Cisatracurium (sis a tra KYOO ree um)

Related Information

Neuromuscular Blocking Agents Comparison *on page 1417*

Brand Names Nimbex®

Synonyms Cisatracurium Besylate

Therapeutic Category Neuromuscular Blocker Agent, Nondepolarizing; Skeletal Muscle Relaxant

Use Drug for neuromuscular blockade in patients with renal and/or hepatic failure; eases endotracheal intubation as an adjunct to general anesthesia and relaxes skeletal muscle during surgery or mechanical ventilation; does not relieve pain

Pregnancy Risk Factor C

Contraindications Hypersensitivity to cisatracurium besylate or any component

Warnings/Precautions Not recommended for rapid sequence intubation; may produce profound effects in patients with neuromuscular disorders (myasthenia gravis); patients with severe burns may develop resistance; maintenance of an adequate airway and respiratory support is critical

Adverse Reactions

<1%:

- Cardiovascular: Effects are minimal and transient, bradycardia and hypotension, flushing
- Dermatologic: Rash
- Respiratory: Bronchospasm

Overdosage/Toxicology Symptoms of overdose include respiratory depression, cardiovascular collapse

Neostigmine 1-3 mg slow I.V. push in adults (0.5 mg in children) antagonizes the neuromuscular blockade, and should be administered with or immediately after atropine 1-1.5 mg I.V. push (adults). This may be especially useful in the presence of bradycardia.

Drug Interactions

Prolonged neuromuscular blockade:

- Inhaled anesthetics:
  - Halothane has only a marginal effect, enflurane and isoflurane increase the potency and prolong duration of neuromuscular blockade induced by cisatracurium
  - Dosage should be reduced by 30% to 40% in patients receiving isoflurane or enflurane
  - Local anesthetics
  - Lithium
  - Magnesium salts
  - Antiarrhythmics (eg, quinidine or procainamide)
  - Antibiotics (eg, aminoglycosides, tetracyclines, vancomycin, clindamycin)

Resistance to neuromuscular blockade:

- Chronic phenytoin or carbamazepine

(Continued)

Cisatracurium *(Continued)*

Stability Refrigerate (do not freeze); unstable in alkaline solutions; **compatible** with D_5W, D_5NS, and NS; do not dilute in lactated Ringers

Mechanism of Action Blocks neural transmission at the myoneural junction by binding with cholinergic receptor sites

Pharmacodynamics/Kinetics

Onset of action: I.V.: 2-3 minutes

Peak effect: Within 3-5 minutes

Duration: Recovery begins in 20-35 minutes when anesthesia is balanced; recovery is attained in 90% of patients in 25-93 minutes

Metabolism: Some metabolites are active; undergoes rapid nonenzymatic degradation in the blood stream, additional metabolism occurs via ester hydrolysis

Half-life: 22 minutes

Usual Dosage I.V. (not to be used I.M.):

Children 2 to 12 years: Initial: 0.10 mg/kg followed by maintenance doses of 1-5 mcg/kg/minute as needed to maintain neuromuscular blockade

Cisatracurium Besylate Infusion Chart

Drug Delivery Rate (mcg/kg/min)	Infusion Rate (mL/min) 0.1 mg/mL (10 mg/100 mL)	Infusion Rate (mL/min) 0.4 mg/mL (40 mg/100 mL)
1.0	42	10.5
1.5	63	15.8
2.0	84	21.0
3.0	126	31.5
5.0	210	52.5

Infusions (requires use of an infusion pump): 0.1 mg/mL or 0.4 mg/mL in D_5W or NS, see table.

Dosage adjustment in renal or hepatic: None necessary

Administration Administer undiluted as a bolus injection; not for I.M. inject, too much tissue irritation; continuous administration requires the use of an infusion pump

Monitoring Parameters Vital signs (heart rate, blood pressure, respiratory rate)

Patient Information May be difficult to talk because of head and neck muscle blockade

Additional Information Neuromuscular blocking potency is 3 times that of atracurium; maximum block is up to 2 minutes longer than for equipotent doses of atracurium

Dosage Forms Injection, as besylate: 2 mg/mL (5 mL, 10 mL); 10 mg/mL (20 mL)

Cisatracurium Besylate *see* Cisatracurium *on previous page*

Cisplatin (SIS pla tin)

Related Information

Antiemetics for Chemotherapy Induced Nausea and Vomiting *on page 1348*

Cancer Chemotherapy Regimens *on page 1351*

Toxicities of Chemotherapeutic Agents *on page 1382*

Brand Names Platinol®; Platinol®-AQ

Synonyms CDDP

Therapeutic Category Antineoplastic Agent, Alkylating Agent; Antineoplastic Agent, Vesicant; Vesicant

Use Treatment of head and neck, breast, testicular, and ovarian cancer; Hodgkin's and non-Hodgkin's lymphoma; neuroblastoma; sarcomas, bladder, gastric, lung, esophageal, cervical, and prostate cancer; myeloma, melanoma, mesothelioma, small cell lung cancer, and osteosarcoma

Pregnancy Risk Factor D

Contraindications Hypersensitivity to cisplatin or any other platinum-containing compounds or any component, anaphylactic-like reactions have been reported; pre-existing renal insufficiency, myelosuppression, hearing impairment

Warnings/Precautions The U.S. Food and Drug Administration (FDA) currently recommends that procedures for proper handling and disposal of antineoplastic agents be considered. All patients should receive adequate hydration prior to and for 24 hours after cisplatin administration, with or without mannitol and/or furosemide, to ensure good urine output and decrease the chance of nephrotoxicity; reduce dosage in renal impairment. Cumulative renal toxicity may be severe; dose-related toxicities include myelosuppression, nausea, and vomiting; cumulative ototoxicity, especially pronounced in children, is manifested by tinnitus or loss of high frequency hearing and occasionally, deafness. **Serum magnesium,**

as well as other electrolytes, should be monitored both before and within 48 hours after cisplatin therapy. Patients who are magnesium depleted should receive replacement therapy before the cisplatin is administered.

Adverse Reactions

>10%:

Endocrine & metabolic: Hyperuricemia

Gastrointestinal: Cisplatin is one of the most emetogenic agents used in cancer chemotherapy; nausea and vomiting occur in 76% to 100% of patients and is dose related. **Prophylactic antiemetics should always be prescribed**; nausea and vomiting may last up to 1 week after therapy. Antiemetics should be included in discharge medications.

Emetic potential:

<75 mg: Moderately high (60% to 90%)

≥75 mg: High (>90%)

Time course of nausea/vomiting: Onset: 1-4 hours; Duration: 12-96 hours

Hematologic: Myelosuppressive: Mild with moderate doses, mild to moderate with high-dose therapy

WBC: Mild

Platelets: Mild

Onset (days): 10

Nadir (days): 14-23

Recovery (days): 21-39

Anemia: Can be chronic, when high dose cisplatin is given for multiple cycles which is responsive to epoetin alfa. Cisplatin has also been associated with Coombs' + hemolytic anemia.

Neuromuscular & skeletal: Neurotoxicity: Peripheral neuropathy is dose- and duration-dependent. The mechanism is through axonal degeneration with subsequent damage to the long sensory nerves. Toxicity can first be noted at doses of 200 mg/m^2, with measurable toxicity at doses >350 mg/m^2. This process is irreversible and progressive with continued therapy. Ototoxicity occurs in 10% to 30%, and is manifested as high frequency hearing loss. Baseline audiography should be performed.

Otic: Ototoxicity (especially pronounced in children)

Renal: Nephrotoxicity: Related to elimination, protein binding, and uptake of cisplatin; two types of nephrotoxicity: acute renal failure and chronic renal insufficiency

Acute renal failure and azotemia is a dose-dependent process and can be minimized with proper administration and prophylaxis. Damage to the proximal tubules by the aquation products of cisplatin is suspected to cause the toxicity. Proper preplatinum hydration with a chloride containing intravenous fluid is believed to minimize the production of the more nephrotoxic aqua products. It is manifested as increased BUN and creatinine, oliguria, protein wasting, and potassium, calcium, and magnesium wasting.

Chronic renal dysfunction can develop in patients receiving multiple courses of cisplatin. This occurs with slow release of the platinum ion from tissues, which then accumulates in the distal tubules. Manifestations of this toxicity are varied, and can include sodium and water wasting, nephropathy, decreased Cl_{cr}, and magnesium wasting.

Recommendations for minimizing nephrotoxicity include:

Prepare cisplatin in saline-containing vehicles

Vigorous hydration with saline-containing intravenous fluids (125-150 mL/hour) before, during, and after cisplatin administration

Simultaneous administration of either mannitol or furosemide

Avoid other nephrotoxic agents (aminoglycosides, amphotericin, etc)

Miscellaneous: Anaphylactic reaction occurs within minutes after administration and can be controlled with epinephrine, antihistamines, and steroids

1% to 10%:

Extravasation: May cause thrombophlebitis and tissue damage if infiltrated; may use sodium thiosulfate as antidote, but consult UCH extravasation policy for guidelines

Irritant chemotherapy

<1%:

Cardiovascular: Bradycardia, arrhythmias

Dermatologic: Mild alopecia

Endocrine & Metabolic: SIADH, hypomagnesemia, hypocalcemia, hypokalemia, hypophosphatemia

Gastrointestinal: Mouth sores, elevation of liver enzymes

Local: Phlebitis

Ocular: Optic neuritis, blurred vision, papilledema

Overdosage/Toxicology Symptoms of overdose include severe myelosuppression, intractable nausea and vomiting, kidney and liver failure, deafness, ocular toxicity, and neuritis

(Continued)

Cisplatin *(Continued)*

No known antidote; hemodialysis appears to have little effect; treatment is supportive therapy

Drug Interactions

Decreased toxicity: Sodium thiosulfate theoretically inactivates drug systemically; has been used clinically to reduce systemic toxicity with intraperitoneal administration of cisplatin

Increased toxicity:

Ethacrynic acid has resulted in severe ototoxicity in animals

Bleomycin resulted in delayed bleomycin elimination

Stability Store intact vials at room temperature (15°C to 25°C/59°F to 77°F); protect from light; do not refrigerate solution - a precipitate may form. If inadvertently refrigerated, the precipitate will slowly dissolve within hours to days, when placed at room temperature. The precipitate may be dissolved without loss of potency by warming solution to 37°C/98.6°F.

Multidose (preservative-free) vials: After initial entry into the vial, solution is stable for 28 days protected from light or for at least 7 days under fluorescent room light at room temperature. Further dilution stability is dependent on the chloride ion concentration and should be mixed in solutions of NS (at least 0.3% NaCl). Further dilution in NS, D_5/0.45% NaCl or D_5/NS to a concentration of 0.05-2 mg/mL are stable for 72 hours at 4°C to 25°C in combination with mannitol; may administer 12.5-50 g mannitol/L

Incompatible with D_5W and other chloride-lacking solutions due to nephrotoxicity; **incompatible** with sodium bicarbonate

Aluminum-containing I.V. infusion sets and needles should NOT be used due to binding with the platinum

Standard I.V. dilution:

Dose/250-1000 mL NS, D_5/NS or D_5/0.45% NaCl

Stable for 72 hours at 4°C to 25°C (in combination with mannitol)

Mechanism of Action Inhibits DNA synthesis by the formation of DNA cross-links; denatures the double helix; covalently binds to DNA bases and disrupts DNA function; may also bind to proteins; the *cis*-isomer is 14 times more cytotoxic than the *trans*-isomer; both forms cross-link DNA but cis-platinum is less easily recognized by cell enzymes and, therefore, not repaired. Cisplatin can also bind two adjacent guanines on the same strand of DNA producing intrastrand cross-linking and breakage

Pharmacodynamics/Kinetics

Distribution: I.V.: Rapidly distributes into tissue; found in high concentrations in the kidneys, liver, ovaries, uterus, and lungs

Protein binding: >90%

Half-life:

Initial: 20-30 minutes

Beta: 60 minutes

Terminal: ~24 hours

Secondary half-life: 44-73 hours

Metabolism: Undergoes nonenzymatic metabolism; the drug is inactivated (in both the cell and the bloodstream) by sulfhydryl groups; cisplatin covalently binds to glutathione and to thiosulfate

Elimination: >90% excreted in the urine and 10% in bile

Usual Dosage I.V. (refer to individual protocols):

An estimated Cl_{cr} should be on all cisplatin chemotherapy orders along with other patient parameters (ie, patient's height, weight, and body surface area). Pharmacy and nursing staff should check the Cl_{cr} on the order and determine the appropriateness of cisplatin dosing.

The manufacturer recommends that subsequent cycles should only be given when serum creatinine <1.5 mg%, WBC ≥4,000/mm^3, platelets ≥ 100,000/mm^3, and BUN <25.

It is recommended that a 24-hour urine creatinine clearance be checked prior to a patient's first dose of cisplatin and periodically thereafter (ie, after every 2-3 cycles of cisplatin)

Pretreatment hydration with 1-2 L of chloride-containing fluid is recommended prior to cisplatin administration; adequate hydration and urinary output (>100 mL/hour) should be maintained for 24 hours after administration

If the dose prescribed is a reduced dose, then this should be indicated on the chemotherapy order

Children: Various dosage schedules range from 30-100 mg/m^2 once every 2-3 weeks; may also dose similar to adult dosing

Recurrent brain tumors: 60 mg/m^2 once daily for 2 consecutive days every 3-4 weeks

Adults:

Advanced bladder cancer: 50-70 mg/m^2 every 3-4 weeks

Head and neck cancer: 100-120 mg/m^2 every 3-4 weeks

Testicular cancer: 10-20 mg/m^2/day for 5 days repeated every 3-4 weeks

Metastatic ovarian cancer: 75-100 mg/m^2 every 3 weeks

Intraperitoneal: cisplatin has been administered intraperitoneal with systemic sodium thiosulfate for ovarian cancer; doses up to 90-270 mg/m^2 have been administered and retained for 4 hours before draining

Dosing adjustment in renal impairment:

Cl_{cr} 10-50 mL/minute: Administer 50% of normal dose

Cl_{cr} <10 mL/minute: Do not administer

Hemodialysis: Partially cleared by hemodialysis; administer dose posthemodialysis

CAPD effects: Unknown

CAVH effects: Unknown

Administration

I.V.: Rate of administration has varied from a 15- to 120-minute infusion, 1 mg/minute infusion, 6- to 8-hour infusion, 24-hour infusion, or per protocol

Maximum rate of infusion of 1 mg/minute in patients with CHF

Pretreatment hydration with 1-2 Liters of fluid is recommended prior to cisplatin administration; adequate hydration and urinary output (>100 mL/hour) should be maintained for 24 hours after administration

Needles, syringes, catheters, or I.V. administration sets that contain aluminum parts should not be used for administration of drug

Monitoring Parameters Renal function tests (serum creatinine, BUN, Cl_{cr}), electrolytes (particularly magnesium, calcium, potassium); hearing test, neurologic exam (with high dose), liver function tests periodically, CBC with differential and platelet count; urine output, urinalysis

Patient Information Drink plenty of fluids to maintain urine output, be prepared for severe nausea and vomiting following drug administration which can be delayed up to 48 hours; notify physician of numbness or tingling in extremities or hearing loss

Nursing Implications Perform pretreatment hydration (see Usual Dosage); monitor for possible anaphylactoid reaction; monitor renal, hematologic, otic, and neurologic function frequently

Management of extravasation:

Large extravasations (>20 mL) of concentrated solutions (>0.5 mg/mL) produce tissue necrosis. **Treatment is not recommended unless a large amount of highly concentrated solution is extravasated.**

Mix 4 mL of 10% sodium thiosulfate with 6 mL sterile water for injection: Inject 1-4 mL through existing I.V. line cannula. Administer 1 mL for each mL extravasated; inject S.C. if needle is removed.

Additional Information

Sodium content: 9 mg/mL (equivalent to 0.9% sodium chloride solution)

Osmolality of Platinol®-AQ = 285-286 mOsm

Dosage Forms

Injection, aqueous: 1 mg/mL (50 mL, 100 mL)

Powder for injection: 10 mg, 50 mg

13-*cis*-Retinoic Acid *see* Isotretinoin *on page 686*

Citracal® [OTC] *see* Calcium Citrate *on page 188*

Citrate of Magnesia *see* Magnesium Citrate *on page 751*

Citrovorum Factor *see* Leucovorin *on page 708*

CI-719 *see* Gemfibrozil *on page 569*

Cla *see* Clarithromycin *on page 287*

Cladribine (KLA dri been)

Related Information

Antiemetics for Chemotherapy Induced Nausea and Vomiting *on page 1348*

Cancer Chemotherapy Regimens *on page 1351*

Toxicities of Chemotherapeutic Agents *on page 1382*

Brand Names Leustatin™

Synonyms 2-CdA; 2-Chlorodeoxyadenosine

Therapeutic Category Antineoplastic Agent, Antimetabolite (Purine)

Use Treatment of hairy cell leukemia (HCL) and chronic lymphocytic leukemias

Pregnancy Risk Factor D

Contraindications Patients with a prior history of hypersensitivity to cladribine

Warnings/Precautions The U.S. Food and Drug Administration (FDA) currently recommends that procedures for proper handling and disposal of antineoplastic agents be considered. Because of its myelosuppressive properties, cladribine

(Continued)

Cladribine *(Continued)*

should be used with caution in patients with pre-existing hematologic or immunologic abnormalities; prophylactic administration of allopurinol should be considered in patients receiving cladribine because of the potential for hyperuricemia secondary to tumor lysis; appropriate antibiotic therapy should be administered promptly in patients exhibiting signs and symptoms of neutropenia and infection.

Adverse Reactions

>10%:

Bone marrow suppression: Commonly observed in patients treated with cladribine, especially at high doses; at the initiation of treatment, however, most patients in clinical studies had hematologic impairment as a result of HCL. During the first 2 weeks after treatment initiation, mean platelet counts decline and subsequently increased with normalization of mean counts by day 12. Absolute neutrophil counts and hemoglobin declined and subsequently increased with normalization of mean counts by week 5 and week 6. CD_4 counts nadir at approximately 270, 4-6 months after treatments. Mean CD_4 counts after 15 months were <500/mm^3. Patients should be considered immunosuppressed for up to one year after cladribine therapy.

Central nervous system: Fatigue, headache

Fever: Temperature ≥101°F has been associated with the use of cladribine in approximately 66% of patients in the first month of therapy. Although 69% of patients developed fevers, less than 33% of febrile events were associated with documented infection.

Dermatologic: Rash

Gastrointestinal: Nausea and vomiting are not severe with cladribine at any dose level. Most cases of nausea were mild, not accompanied by vomiting and did not require treatment with antiemetics. In patients requiring antiemetics, nausea was easily controlled most often by chlorpromazine.

Local: Injection site reactions

1% to 10%:

Cardiovascular: Edema, tachycardia

Central nervous system: Dizziness, insomnia, pain, chills, malaise

Dermatologic: Pruritus, erythema

Gastrointestinal: Constipation, abdominal pain

Neuromuscular & skeletal: Myalgia, arthralgia, weakness

Miscellaneous: Diaphoresis, trunk pain

Stability Store intact vials under refrigeration (2°C to 8°C). Further dilution in 100-1000 mL NS is stable for 72 hours. Stable in PVC containers for 24 hours at room temperature and 7 days in Pharmacia Deltec® medication cassettes at room temperature. For 7-day infusion, dilute with bacteriostatic NS and filter through 0.22 μ filter prior to addition into infusion reservoir.

Incompatible with D_5W

Standard I.V. 24-hour infusion dilution:

24-hour dose/500 mL NS

24-hour infusion solution is stable for 24 hours at room temperature

Standard I.V. 7-day infusion dilution:

7-day dose/q.s. to 100 mL with bacteriostatic NS

7-day infusion solution is stable for 7 days at room temperature

Mechanism of Action A purine nucleoside analogue; prodrug which is activated via phosphorylation by deoxycytidine kinase to a 5'-triphosphate derivative. This active form incorporates into susceptible cells and into DNA to result in the breakage of DNA strand and shutdown of DNA synthesis. This also results in a depletion of nicotinamide adenine dinucleotide and adenosine triphosphate (ATP). The induction of strand breaks results in a drop in the cofactor nicotinamide adenine dinucleotide and disruption of cell metabolism. ATP is depleted to deprive cells of an important source of energy. Cladribine effectively kills resting as well as dividing cells.

Pharmacodynamics/Kinetics

Distribution: V_d: 4.52±2.82 L/kg

Protein binding: 20% to plasma proteins

Half-life: Biphasic:

Alpha: 25 minutes

Beta: 6.7 hours

Terminal, mean (normal renal function): 5.4 hours

Elimination: Mean: 978±422 mL/hour/kg; estimated systemic clearance: 640 mL/hour/kg

Usual Dosage I.V.:

Children:

Acute leukemia:

The safety and effectiveness of cladribine in children have not been established; in a phase I study involving patients 1-21 years of age with relapsed acute leukemia, cladribine was administered by CIV at doses ranging from 3-10.7 mg/m²/day for 5 days (0.5-2 times the dose recommended in HCL). Investigators reported beneficial responses in this study; the dose-limiting toxicity was severe myelosuppression with profound neutropenia and thrombocytopenia.

CIV: 15-18 mg/m²/day for 5 days

Adults:

Hairy cell leukemia:

CIV: 0.09-0.1 mg/kg/day continuous infusion for 7 consecutive days

CIV: 4 mg/m²/day for 7 days

Non-Hodgkin's lymphoma: CIV: 0.1 mg/kg/day for 7 days

Administration Single daily infusion: Administer diluted in an infusion bag containing 500 mL of 0.9% sodium chloride and repeated for a total of 7 consecutive days

7-day infusion: Prepare with bacteriostatic 0.9% sodium chloride. Both cladribine and diluent should be passed through a sterile 0.22 micron hydrophilic filter as it is being introduced into the infusion reservoir. The calculated dose of cladribine (7 days x 0.09 mg/kg) should first be added to the infusion reservoir through a filter then the bacteriostatic 0.9% sodium chloride should be added to the reservoir to obtain a total volume of 100 mL.

Dosage Forms Injection, preservative free: 1 mg/mL (10 mL)

Claforan® *see* Cefotaxime *on page 226*

Clarithromycin (kla RITH roe mye sin)

Related Information

Antimicrobial Drugs of Choice *on page 1468*

Guidelines for the Prevention of Opportunistic Infections in Persons with HIV *on page 1457*

Helicobacter pylori Treatment *on page 1534*

Brand Names Biaxin™

Canadian/Mexican Brand Names Klaricid® (Mexico)

Synonyms Cla

Therapeutic Category Antibiotic, Macrolide

Use

In adults, for treatment of pharyngitis/tonsillitis, acute maxillary sinusitis, acute exacerbation of chronic bronchitis, pneumonia, uncomplicated skin/skin structure infections due to (eg, *S. pyogenes, S. pneumoniae, S. agalactiae,* viridans *Streptococcus, M. catarrhalis, C. trachomatis, Legionella* sp, *Mycoplasma pneumoniae,S. aureus, H. influenzae*) (MICs ≤0.25 mcg/mL); has activity against *M. avium* and *M. intracellulare* infection and is indicated for treatment of and prevention of disseminated mycobacterial infections due to *M. avium* complex disease (eg, patients with advanced HIV infection); indicated for the treatment of duodenal ulcer disease due to *H. pylori*in regimens with other drugs including omeprazole, ranitidine bismuth citrate, bismuth subsalicylate, tetracycline and/or an H_2-antagonist (see index).

In children, for treatment of pharyngitis/tonsillitis, acute maxillary sinusitis, acute otitis media, uncomplicated skin/skin structure infections due to the above organisms; also for treatment of and prevention of disseminated mycobacterial infections due to *M. avium* complex disease (eg, patients with advanced HIV infection)

Exhibits the same spectrum of *in vitro* activity as erythromycin, but with significantly increased potency against those organisms

Pregnancy Risk Factor C

Contraindications Hypersensitivity to clarithromycin, erythromycin, or any macrolide antibiotic; use with pimozide

Warnings/Precautions In presence of severe renal impairment with or without coexisting hepatic impairment, decreased dosage or prolonged dosing interval may be appropriate; antibiotic associated colitis has been reported with use of clarithromycin; elderly patients have experienced increased incidents of adverse effects due to known age-related decreases in renal function

Adverse Reactions

1% to 10%:

Central nervous system: Headache

Gastrointestinal: Diarrhea, nausea, abnormal taste, dyspepsia, abdominal pain

<1%:

Cardiovascular: Ventricular tachycardia, torsade de pointes

Hematologic: Decreased white blood count, elevated prothrombin time

Hepatic: Elevated AST, alkaline phosphatase, and bilirubin

Renal: Elevated BUN/serum creatinine

Overdosage/Toxicology Symptoms of overdose include nausea, vomiting, diarrhea, prostration, reversible pancreatitis, hearing loss with or without tinnitus or vertigo; treatment includes symptomatic and supportive care

(Continued)

Clarithromycin *(Continued)*

Drug Interactions

Increased levels: Clarithromycin increases serum theophylline levels by as much as 20%; significantly increases carbamazepine levels and those of cyclosporine, digoxin, ergot alkaloid, tacrolimus, omeprazole and triazolam; peak levels (but not AUC) of zidovudine are often increased; terfenadine and astemizole should be avoided with use of clarithromycin since plasma levels may be increased by >3 times; serious arrhythmias have occurred with cisapride and other drugs which inhibit cytochrome P-450 IIIA4 (eg, clarithromycin); fluconazole increases clarithromycin levels and AUC by ~25%

Note: While other drug interactions (bromocriptine, disopyramide, lovastatin, phenytoin, pimozide and valproate) known to occur with erythromycin have not been reported in clinical trials with clarithromycin, concurrent use of these drugs should be monitored closely

Mechanism of Action Exerts its antibacterial action by binding to 50S ribosomal subunit resulting in inhibition of protein synthesis. The 14-OH metabolite of clarithromycin is twice as active as the parent compound.

Pharmacodynamics/Kinetics

Absorption: Highly stable in the presence of gastric acid (unlike erythromycin)

Distribution: Widely distributes into most body tissues with the exception of the CNS

Metabolism: Partially converted to the microbiologically active metabolite, 14-OH clarithromycin

Bioavailability: 50%; food delays but does not affect extent of bioavailability; T_{max}: 2-4 hours

Half-life: 5-7 hours

Elimination: Primarily renal excretion; clearance approximates normal GFR

Usual Dosage Safe use in children has not been established

Children ≥6 months: 15 mg/kg/day divided every 12 hours; dosages of 7.5 mg/kg twice daily up to 500 mg twice daily children with AIDS and disseminated MAC infection

Adults: Oral: Usual dose: 250-500 mg every 12 hours for 7-14 days

Upper respiratory tract: 250-500 mg every 12 hours for 10-14 days

Pharyngitis/tonsillitis: 250 mg every 12 hours for 10 days

Acute maxillary sinusitis: 500 mg every 12 hours for 14 days

Lower respiratory tract: 250-500 mg every 12 hours for 7-14 days

Acute exacerbation of chronic bronchitis due to:

M. catarrhalis and *S. pneumoniae*: 250 mg every 12 hours for 7-14 days

H. influenzae: 500 mg every 12 hours for 7-14 days

Pneumonia due to *M. pneumoniae* and *S. pneumoniae*: 250 mg every 12 hours for 7-14 days

Mycobacterial infection (prevention and treatment): 500 mg twice daily (use with other antimycobacterial drugs, eg, ethambutol, clofazimine, or rifampin)

Uncomplicated skin and skin structure: 250 mg every 12 hours for 7-14 days

Helicobacter pylori: In combination regimen with bismuth subsalicylate, tetracycline, and an H_2-receptor antagonist; or in combination with omeprazole (and possibly metronidazole or amoxicillin) or ranitidine bismuth citrate (Tritec) (and possibly tetracycline or amoxicillin): 250 mg twice daily to 500 mg 3 times/day (for first 2 weeks only of regimen with Tritec or omeprazole)

Dosing adjustment in severe renal impairment: Decreased doses or prolonged dosing intervals are recommended

Dietary Considerations Food: Slight decrease in onset of absorption; extent of absorption is increased or unaffected; take without regard to meals

Patient Information May be taken with meals; finish all medication; do not skip doses

Nursing Implications Administer every 12 hours rather than twice daily to avoid peak and trough variation

Dosage Forms

Granules for oral suspension: 125 mg/5 mL (100 mL, 200 mL); 250 mg/5 mL (100 mL, 200 mL)

Tablet, film coated: 250 mg, 500 mg

Claritin® *see* Loratadine *on page 741*

Clear Away® Disc [OTC] *see* Salicylic Acid *on page 1120*

Clear By Design® Gel [OTC] *see* Benzoyl Peroxide *on page 140*

Clear Eyes® [OTC] *see* Naphazoline *on page 879*

Clearsil® Maximum Strength [OTC] *see* Benzoyl Peroxide *on page 140*

Clear Tussin® 30 *see* Guaifenesin and Dextromethorphan *on page 591*

Clemastine (KLEM as teen)

Brand Names Antihist-1® [OTC]; Tavist®; Tavist®-1 [OTC]

Synonyms Clemastine Fumarate

Therapeutic Category Antihistamine, H_1 Blocker

Use Perennial and seasonal allergic rhinitis and other allergic symptoms including urticaria

Pregnancy Risk Factor C

Contraindications Narrow-angle glaucoma, hypersensitivity to clemastine or any component

Warnings/Precautions Safety and efficacy have not been established in children <6 years of age; bladder neck obstruction, symptomatic prostate hypertrophy, asthmatic attacks, and stenosing peptic ulcer

Adverse Reactions

>10%:
- Central nervous system: Slight to moderate drowsiness
- Respiratory: Thickening of bronchial secretions

1% to 10%:
- Central nervous system: Headache, fatigue, nervousness, increased dizziness
- Gastrointestinal: Appetite increase, weight gain, nausea, diarrhea, abdominal pain, xerostomia
- Neuromuscular & skeletal: Arthralgia
- Respiratory: Pharyngitis

<1%:
- Cardiovascular: Edema, palpitations
- Central nervous system: Depression
- Dermatologic: Angioedema, photosensitivity, rash
- Hepatic: Hepatitis
- Neuromuscular & skeletal: Myalgia, paresthesia
- Respiratory: Bronchospasm, epistaxis

Overdosage/Toxicology Symptoms of overdose include anemia, metabolic acidosis, hypotension, hypothermia

There is no specific treatment for an antihistamine overdose, however, most of its clinical toxicity is due to anticholinergic effects. For anticholinergic overdose with severe life-threatening symptoms, physostigmine 1-2 mg (0.5 or 0.02 mg/kg for children) I.V., slowly may be given to reverse these effects.

Drug Interactions Increased toxicity (CNS depression): CNS depressants, MAO inhibitors, tricyclic antidepressants, phenothiazines

Mechanism of Action Competes with histamine for H_1-receptor sites on effector cells in the gastrointestinal tract, blood vessels, and respiratory tract

Pharmacodynamics/Kinetics
- Peak therapeutic effect: Within 5-7 hours
- Absorption: Almost 100% from GI tract
- Metabolism: In the liver
- Elimination: In urine

Usual Dosage Oral:
- Children: <12 years: 0.4-1 mg twice daily
- Children >12 years and Adults: 1.34 mg twice daily to 2.68 mg 3 times/day; do not exceed 8.04 mg/day; lower doses should be considered in patients >60 years

Dietary Considerations Alcohol: Additive CNS effects, avoid use

Monitoring Parameters Look for a reduction of rhinitis, urticaria, eczema, pruritus, or other allergic symptoms

Patient Information Avoid alcohol; may cause drowsiness, may impair coordination or judgment

Nursing Implications Raise bed rails, institute safety measures, assist with ambulation

Dosage Forms
- Syrup, as fumarate (citrus flavor): 0.67 mg/5 mL with alcohol 5.5% (120 mL)
- Tablet, as fumarate: 1.34 mg, 2.68 mg

Clemastine Fumarate *see* Clemastine *on this page*

Cleocin HCl® *see* Clindamycin *on this page*

Cleocin Pediatric® *see* Clindamycin *on this page*

Cleocin Phosphate® *see* Clindamycin *on this page*

Cleocin T® *see* Clindamycin *on this page*

Climara® Transdermal *see* Estradiol *on page 468*

Clinda-Derm® Topical Solution *see* Clindamycin *on this page*

Clindamycin (klin da MYE sin)

Related Information

Animal and Human Bites Guidelines *on page 1463*

(Continued)

Clindamycin *(Continued)*

Antimicrobial Drugs of Choice *on page 1468*
Antimicrobial Prophylaxis *on page 1445*
Guidelines for the Prevention of Opportunistic Infections in Persons with HIV *on page 1457*
Prevention of Bacterial Endocarditis *on page 1449*
Treatment of Sexually Transmitted Diseases *on page 1485*

Brand Names Cleocin HCl®; Cleocin Pediatric®; Cleocin Phosphate®; Cleocin T®; Clinda-Derm® Topical Solution; C/T/S® Topical Solution

Canadian/Mexican Brand Names Dalacin® C [Hydrochloride] (Canada); Dalacin® C (Mexico); Galecin® (Mexico); Klyndaken® (Mexico)

Synonyms Clindamycin Hydrochloride; Clindamycin Phosphate

Therapeutic Category Acne Products; Antibiotic, Anaerobic; Antibiotic, Topical

Use Treatment against aerobic and anaerobic streptococci (except enterococci), most staphylococci, *Bacteroides* sp and *Actinomyces*; used topically in treatment of severe acne, vaginally for *Gardnerella vaginalis*, alternate treatment for toxoplasmosis, PCP

Pregnancy Risk Factor B

Contraindications Hypersensitivity to clindamycin or any component; previous pseudomembranous colitis, hepatic impairment

Warnings/Precautions Dosage adjustment may be necessary in patients with severe hepatic dysfunction; no change necessary with renal insufficiency; can cause severe and possibly fatal colitis; use with caution in patients with a history of pseudomembranous colitis; discontinue drug if significant diarrhea, abdominal cramps, or passage of blood and mucus occurs

Adverse Reactions

>10%: Gastrointestinal: Diarrhea

1% to 10%:
- Dermatologic: Rashes
- Gastrointestinal: Pseudomembranous colitis, nausea, vomiting

<1%:
- Cardiovascular: Hypotension
- Dermatologic: Urticaria, Stevens-Johnson syndrome
- Hematologic: Eosinophilia, neutropenia, granulocytopenia, thrombocytopenia
- Hepatic: Elevation of liver enzymes
- Local: Thrombophlebitis, sterile abscess at I.M. injection site
- Neuromuscular & skeletal: Polyarthritis
- Renal: Rare renal dysfunction

Overdosage/Toxicology Symptoms of overdose include diarrhea, nausea, vomiting; following GI decontamination, treatment is supportive

Drug Interactions Increased duration of neuromuscular blockade from tubocurarine, pancuronium

Stability Do **not** refrigerate reconstituted oral solution because it will thicken; oral solution is stable for 2 weeks at room temperature following reconstitution; I.V. infusion solution in NS or D_5W solution is stable for 24 hours at room temperature

Mechanism of Action Reversibly binds to 50S ribosomal subunits preventing peptide bond formation thus inhibiting bacterial protein synthesis; bacteriostatic or bactericidal depending on drug concentration, infection site, and organism

Pharmacodynamics/Kinetics

Absorption: ~10% of topically applied drug is absorbed systemically; 90% absorbed rapidly from GI tract following oral administration

Distribution: No significant levels are seen in CSF, even with inflamed meninges; crosses the placenta; distributes into breast milk; high concentrations in bone, bile, and urine

Metabolism: Hepatic

Half-life:
- Neonates:
- Premature: 8.7 hours
- Full-term: 3.6 hours
- Adults: 1.6-5.3 hours, average: 2-3 hours

Time to peak serum concentration:
- Oral: Within 60 minutes
- I.M.: Within 1-3 hours

Elimination: Most of drug eliminated by hepatic metabolism

Usual Dosage Avoid in neonates (contains benzyl alcohol)

Infants and Children:
- Oral: 10-30 mg/kg/day in 3-4 divided doses
- I.M., I.V.: 25-40 mg/kg/day in 3-4 divided doses

Children and Adults: Topical: Apply a thin film twice daily

Adults:
- Oral: 150-450 mg/dose every 6-8 hours; maximum dose: 1.8 g/day
- I.M., I.V.: 1.2-1.8 g/day in 2-4 divided doses; maximum dose: 4.8 g/day

Pneumocystis carinii pneumonia:
Oral: 300-450 mg 4 times/day with primaquine
I.M., I.V.: 1200-2400 mg/day with pyrimethamine
I.V.: 600 mg 4 times/day with primaquine
Vaginal: One full applicator (100 mg) inserted intravaginally once daily before bedtime for seven consecutive days

Dosing adjustment in hepatic impairment: Adjustment recommended in patients with severe hepatic disease

Dietary Considerations Food: Peak serum concentration delayed but the extent of absorption is not changed; take with food or a full glass of water to avoid esophageal irritation

Administration Administer oral dosage form with a full glass of water to minimize esophageal ulceration; administer around-the-clock to promote less variation in peak and trough serum levels

Monitoring Parameters Observe for changes in bowel frequency, monitor for colitis and resolution of symptoms; during prolonged therapy monitor CBC, liver and renal function tests periodically

Patient Information Report any severe diarrhea immediately and do not take antidiarrheal medication; take each oral dose with a full glass of water; finish all medication; do not skip doses; should not engage in sexual intercourse during treatment with vaginal product; avoid contact of topical gel/solution with eyes, abraded skin, or mucous membranes

Dosage Forms
Capsule, as hydrochloride: 75 mg, 150 mg, 300 mg
Cream, vaginal: 2% (40 g)
Gel, topical, as phosphate: 1% [10 mg/g] (7.5 g, 30 g)
Granules for oral solution, as palmitate: 75 mg/5 mL (100 mL)
Infusion, as phosphate, in D_5W: 300 mg (50 mL); 600 mg (50 mL)
Injection, as phosphate: 150 mg/mL (2 mL, 4 mL, 6 mL, 50 mL, 60 mL)
Lotion: 1% [10 mg/mL] (60 mL)
Solution, topical, as phosphate: 1% [10 mg/mL] (30 mL, 60 mL, 480 mL)

Clindamycin Hydrochloride *see* Clindamycin *on page 289*
Clindamycin Phosphate *see* Clindamycin *on page 289*
Clinoril® *see* Sulindac *on page 1181*

Clioquinol (klye oh KWIN ole)

Brand Names Vioform® [OTC]

Canadian/Mexican Brand Names Clioquinol® (Canada)

Synonyms Iodochlorhydroxyquin

Therapeutic Category Antifungal Agent, Topical

Use Topically in the treatment of tinea pedis, tinea cruris, and skin infections caused by dermatophytic fungi (ring worm)

Pregnancy Risk Factor C

Contraindications Not effective in the treatment of scalp or nail fungal infections; children <2 years of age, hypersensitivity to any component

Warnings/Precautions May irritate sensitized skin; topical application poses a potential risk of toxicity to infants and children; known to cause serious and irreversible optic atrophy and peripheral neuropathy with muscular weakness, sensory loss, spastic paraparesis, and blindness; use with caution in patients with iodine intolerance

Adverse Reactions
1% to 10%:
Dermatologic: Skin irritation, rash
Neuromuscular & skeletal: Peripheral neuropathy
Ocular: Optic atrophy

Mechanism of Action Chelates bacterial surface and trace metals needed for bacterial growth

Pharmacodynamics/Kinetics
Absorption: With an occlusive dressing, up to 40% of dose can be absorbed systemically during a 12-hour period; absorption is enhanced when applied under diapers
Half-life: 11-14 hours
Elimination: Conjugated and excreted in urine

Usual Dosage Children and Adults: Topical: Apply 2-3 times/day; do not use for longer than 7 days

Test Interactions Thyroid function tests (decreased ^{131}I uptake); false-positive ferric chloride test for phenylketonuria

Patient Information Cleanse affected area before application; can stain skin and fabrics; for external use only; avoid contact with eyes and mucous membranes

Nursing Implications Watch affected area for increased irritation
(Continued)

Clioquinol *(Continued)*

Dosage Forms

Cream: 3% (30 g)

Ointment, topical: 3% (30 g)

Clobetasol (kloe BAY ta sol)

Related Information

Corticosteroids Comparison *on page 1407*

Brand Names Temovate®

Canadian/Mexican Brand Names Dermasone® (Canada); Dermovate® (Canada); Gen-Clobetasol® (Canada); Novo-Clobetasol® (Canada); Dermatovate® (Mexico)

Synonyms Clobetasol Propionate

Therapeutic Category Corticosteroid, Topical (Low Potency); Corticosteroid, Topical (Very High Potency)

Use **Short-term** relief of inflammation of moderate to severe corticosteroid-responsive dermatosis (very high potency topical corticosteroid)

Pregnancy Risk Factor C

Contraindications Known hypersensitivity to clobetasol; viral, fungal, or tubercular skin lesions

Warnings/Precautions Adrenal suppression can occur if used for >14 days

Adverse Reactions

1% to 10%:

Dermatologic: Itching, erythema

Local: Burning, dryness, irritation, papular rashes

<1%:

Dermatologic: Hypertrichosis, acneiform eruptions, maceration of skin, skin atrophy, striae, hypopigmentation, perioral dermatitis

Endocrine & metabolic: Miliaria

Mechanism of Action Stimulates the synthesis of enzymes needed to decrease inflammation, suppress mitotic activity, and cause vasoconstriction

Pharmacodynamics/Kinetics

Absorption: Percutaneous absorption variable and dependent upon many factors including vehicle used, integrity of epidermis, dose, and use of occlusive dressings

Metabolism: Remains to be defined

Elimination: In urine and bile

Usual Dosage Adults: Topical: Apply twice daily for up to 2 weeks with no more than 50 g/week

Patient Information A thin film of cream or ointment is effective; do not overuse; do not use tight-fitting diapers or plastic pants on children being treated in the diaper area; use only as prescribed and for no longer than the period prescribed; apply sparingly in light film; rub in lightly; avoid contact with eyes; notify physician if condition being treated persists or worsens

Nursing Implications For external use only; do not use on open wounds; apply sparingly to occlusive dressings; should not be used in the presence of open or weeping lesions

Dosage Forms

Cream, as propionate: 0.05% (15 g, 30 g, 45 g)

Cream, as propionate, in emollient base: 0.05% (15 g, 30 g, 60 g)

Gel, as propionate: 0.05% (15 g, 30 g, 45 g)

Ointment, topical, as propionate: 0.05% (15 g, 30 g, 45 g)

Scalp application, as propionate: 0.05% (25 mL, 50 mL)

Clobetasol Propionate *see* Clobetasol *on this page*

Clocort® Maximum Strength *see* Hydrocortisone *on page 623*

Clocortolone (kloe KOR toe lone)

Related Information

Corticosteroids Comparison *on page 1407*

Brand Names Cloderm®

Synonyms Clocortolone Pivalate

Therapeutic Category Corticosteroid, Topical (Medium Potency)

Use Inflammation of corticosteroid-responsive dermatoses (medium potency topical corticosteroid)

Pregnancy Risk Factor C

Contraindications Known hypersensitivity to clocortolone; viral, fungal, or tubercular skin lesions

Warnings/Precautions Adrenal suppression can occur if used for >14 days

Adverse Reactions

1% to 10%:

Dermatologic: Itching, erythema

Local: Burning, dryness, irritation, papular rashes

<1%:

Dermatologic: Hypertrichosis, acneiform eruptions, maceration of skin, skin atrophy, striae

Local: Hypopigmentation, perioral dermatitis, miliaria

Mechanism of Action Stimulates the synthesis of enzymes needed to decrease inflammation, suppress mitotic activity, and cause vasoconstriction

Pharmacodynamics/Kinetics

Absorption: Percutaneous absorption is variable and dependent upon many factors including vehicle used, integrity of epidermis, dose, and use of occlusive dressings;

Distribution: Small amounts enter systemic circulation mostly throughout skin

Metabolism: Remains to be defined (largely in liver)

Elimination: In urine and bile

Usual Dosage Adults: Apply sparingly and gently; rub into affected area from 1-4 times/day

Patient Information A thin film of cream or ointment is effective; do not overuse; do not use tight-fitting diapers or plastic pants on children being treated in the diaper area; use only as prescribed, and for no longer than the period prescribed; apply sparingly in light film; rub in lightly; avoid contact with eyes; notify physician if condition being treated persists or worsens

Nursing Implications For external use only; do not use on open wounds; apply sparingly to occlusive dressings; should not be used in the presence of open or weeping lesions

Dosage Forms Cream, as pivalate: 0.1% (15 g, 45 g)

Clocortolone Pivalate *see* Clocortolone *on previous page*

Cloderm® *see* Clocortolone *on previous page*

Clofazimine (kloe FA zi meen)

Related Information

Antimicrobial Drugs of Choice *on page 1468*

Brand Names Lamprene®

Synonyms Clofazimine Palmitate

Therapeutic Category Antibiotic, Miscellaneous; Leprostatic Agent

Use Treatment of dapsone-resistant leprosy; multibacillary dapsone-sensitive leprosy; erythema nodosum leprosum; *Mycobacterium avium-intracellulare* (MAI) infections

Pregnancy Risk Factor C

Contraindications Hypersensitivity to clofazimine or any component

Warnings/Precautions Use with caution in patients with GI problems; dosages >100 mg/day should be used for as short a duration as possible; skin discoloration may lead to depression

Adverse Reactions

>10%:

Dermatologic: Dry skin

Gastrointestinal: Abdominal pain, nausea, vomiting, diarrhea

Miscellaneous: Pink to brownish-black discoloration of the skin and conjunctiva

1% to 10%:

Dermatologic: Rash, pruritus

Endocrine & metabolic: Elevated blood sugar

Gastrointestinal: Fecal discoloration

Genitourinary: Discoloration of urine

Ocular: Irritation of the eyes

Miscellaneous: Discoloration of sputum, sweat

<1%:

Cardiovascular: Edema, vascular pain

Central nervous system: Dizziness, drowsiness, fatigue, headache, giddiness, taste disorder, fever

Dermatologic: Erythroderma, acneiform eruptions, monilial cheilosis, phototoxicity

Endocrine & metabolic: Hypokalemia

Gastrointestinal: Bowel obstruction, GI bleeding, anorexia, constipation, weight loss, eosinophilic enteritis

Genitourinary: Cystitis

Hematologic: Eosinophilia, anemia

Hepatic: Hepatitis, jaundice, enlarged liver, elevated albumin, serum bilirubin and AST

Neuromuscular & skeletal: Bone pain, neuralgia

Ocular: Diminished vision

Miscellaneous: Lymphadenopathy

Overdosage/Toxicology Following GI decontamination, treatment is supportive

Drug Interactions Decreased effect with dapsone (unconfirmed)

(Continued)

Clofazimine *(Continued)*

Mechanism of Action Binds preferentially to mycobacterial DNA to inhibit mycobacterial growth; also has some anti-inflammatory activity through an unknown mechanism

Pharmacodynamics/Kinetics

Absorption: Oral: 45% to 70% absorbed slowly

Distribution: Remains in tissues for prolonged periods; appears in breast milk; highly lipophilic; deposited primarily in fatty tissue and cells of the reticuloendothelial system; taken up by macrophages throughout the body; also distributed to breast milk, mesenteric lymph nodes, adrenal glands, subcutaneous fat, liver, bile, gallbladder, spleen, small intestine, muscles, bones, and skin; does not appear to cross blood-brain barrier

Metabolism: Partially in the liver to two metabolites

Half-life:

Terminal: 8 days

Tissue: 70 days

Time to peak serum concentration: 1-6 hours with chronic therapy

Elimination: Mainly in feces; negligible amounts excreted unchanged in urine; small amounts excreted in sputum, saliva, and sweat

Usual Dosage Oral:

Children: Leprosy: 1 mg/kg/day every 24 hours in combination with dapsone and rifampin

Adults:

Dapsone-resistant leprosy: 100 mg/day in combination with one or more antileprosy drugs for 3 years; then alone 100 mg/day

Dapsone-sensitive multibacillary leprosy: 100 mg/day in combination with two or more antileprosy drugs for at least 2 years and continue until negative skin smears are obtained, then institute single drug therapy with appropriate agent

Erythema nodosum leprosum: 100-200 mg/day for up to 3 months or longer then taper dose to 100 mg/day when possible

Pyoderma gangrenosum: 300-400 mg/day for up to 12 months

Dosing adjustment in hepatic impairment: Should be considered in severe hepatic dysfunction

Monitoring Parameters GI complaints

Test Interactions ↑ ESR, ↑ glucose (S), ↑ albumin, ↑ bilirubin, ↑ AST

Patient Information Drug may cause a pink to brownish-black discoloration of the skin, conjunctiva, tears, sweat, urine, feces, and nasal secretions; although reversible, may take months to years to disappear after therapy is complete; take with meals

Dosage Forms Capsule, as palmatate: 50 mg, 100 mg

Clofazimine Palmitate *see* Clofazimine *on previous page*

Clofibrate (kloe FYE brate)

Related Information

Lipid-Lowering Agents *on page 1413*

Brand Names Atromid-S®

Canadian/Mexican Brand Names Abitrate® (Canada); Claripex® (Canada); Novo-Fibrate® (Canada)

Therapeutic Category Antilipemic Agent

Use Adjunct to dietary therapy in the management of hyperlipidemias associated with high triglyceride levels (types III, IV, V); primarily lowers triglycerides and very low density lipoprotein

Pregnancy Risk Factor C

Contraindications Hypersensitivity to clofibrate or any component, severe hepatic or renal impairment, primary biliary cirrhosis

Warnings/Precautions Clofibrate has been shown to be tumorigenic in animal studies; increased risk of cholelithiasis, cholecystitis; discontinue if lipid response is not obtained; no evidence substantiates a beneficial effect on cardiovascular mortality

Adverse Reactions

>10%: Gastrointestinal: Nausea

1% to 10%: Gastrointestinal: Diarrhea, vomiting, dyspepsia, flatulence, abdominal distress

<1%:

Cardiovascular: Angina, cardiac arrhythmias

Central nervous system: Headache, dizziness, fatigue

Dermatologic: Rash, urticaria, pruritus, alopecia

Gastrointestinal: Gallstones

Genitourinary: Impotence

Hematologic: Leukopenia, anemia, eosinophilia, agranulocytosis

Hepatic: Increased liver function test
Neuromuscular & skeletal: Muscle cramping, aching, weakness, myalgia
Renal: Renal toxicity, rhabdomyolysis-induced renal failure
Miscellaneous: Dry, brittle hair

Overdosage/Toxicology Symptoms of overdose include nausea, vomiting, diarrhea, GI distress; following GI decontamination, treatment is supportive

Drug Interactions
Increased effect: Effects of warfarin, insulin, and sulfonylureas may be increased
Increased toxicity/levels: Clofibrate's levels may be increased with probenecid

Mechanism of Action Mechanism is unclear but thought to reduce cholesterol synthesis and triglyceride hepatic-vascular transference

Pharmacodynamics/Kinetics
Absorption: Occurs completely; intestinal transformation is required to activate the drug
Distribution: V_d: 5.5 L/kg; crosses the placenta
Protein binding: 95%
Metabolism: In the liver to an inactive glucuronide ester
Half-life: 6-24 hours, increases significantly with reduced renal function; with anuria: 110 hours
Time to peak serum concentration: Within 3-6 hours
Elimination: 40% to 70% excreted in urine

Usual Dosage Adults: Oral: 500 mg 4 times/day; some patients may respond to lower doses

Dosing interval in renal impairment:
Cl_{cr} >50 mL/minute: Administer every 6-12 hours
Cl_{cr} 10-50 mL/minute: Administer every 12-18 hours
Cl_{cr} <10 mL/minute: Avoid use
Hemodialysis: Elimination is not enhanced via hemodialysis; supplemental dose is not necessary

Monitoring Parameters Serum lipids, cholesterol and triglycerides, LFTs, CBC

Test Interactions ↑ creatine phosphokinase [CPK] (S); ↓ alkaline phosphatase (S), cholesterol (S), glucose, uric acid (S)

Patient Information If GI upset occurs, may be taken with food; notify physician of chest pain, shortness of breath, irregular heartbeat, severe stomach pain with nausea and vomiting, persistent fever, sore throat, or unusual bleeding or bruising; adhere to prescribed diet

Dosage Forms Capsule: 500 mg

Clomid® *see* Clomiphene *on this page*

Clomiphene (KLOE mi feen)

Brand Names Clomid®; Milophene®; Serophene®

Canadian/Mexican Brand Names Omifin® (Mexico)

Synonyms Clomiphene Citrate

Therapeutic Category Ovulation Stimulator

Use Treatment of ovulatory failure in patients desiring pregnancy

Unlabeled use: Male infertility

Pregnancy Risk Factor X

Contraindications Liver disease, abnormal uterine bleeding, suspected pregnancy, enlargement or development of ovarian cyst, uncontrolled thyroid or adrenal dysfunction

Warnings/Precautions Patients unusually sensitive to pituitary gonadotropins (eg, polycystic ovary disease); multiple pregnancies, blurring or other visual symptoms can occur

Adverse Reactions
>10%: Endocrine & metabolic: Hot flashes, ovarian enlargement
1% to 10%:
Cardiovascular: Thromboembolism
Central nervous system: Mental depression, headache
Endocrine & metabolic: Breast enlargement (males), abnormal menstrual flow
Gastrointestinal: Distention, bloating, nausea, vomiting, hepatotoxicity
Ocular: Blurring of vision, diplopia, floaters, after-images, phosphenes, photophobia
<1%:
Central nervous system: Insomnia, fatigue
Dermatologic: Alopecia (reversible)
Gastrointestinal: Weight gain
Genitourinary: Polyuria

Stability Protect from light

Mechanism of Action Induces ovulation by stimulating the release of pituitary gonadotropins

(Continued)

Clomiphene *(Continued)*

Pharmacodynamics/Kinetics

Half-life: 5-7 days

Elimination: Enterohepatically circulated; excreted primarily in feces with small amounts appearing in urine

Usual Dosage Adults: Oral:

Male (infertility): 25 mg/day for 25 days with 5 days rest, or 100 mg every Monday, Wednesday, Friday

Female (ovulatory failure): 50 mg/day for 5 days (first course); start the regimen on or about the fifth day of cycle; if ovulation occurs do not increase dosage; if not, increase next course to 100 mg/day for 5 days. Three courses of therapy are an adequate therapeutic trial. Further treatment is not recommended in patients who do not exhibit ovulation.

Reference Range FSH and LH are expected to peak 5-9 days after completing clomiphene; ovulation assessed by basal body temperature or serum progesterone 2 weeks after last clomiphene dose

Test Interactions Clomiphene may increase levels of serum thyroxine and thyroxine-binding globulin (TBG)

Patient Information May cause visual disturbances, dizziness, lightheadedness; if possibility of pregnancy, stop the drug and consult your physician

Dosage Forms Tablet, as citrate: 50 mg

Clomiphene Citrate *see* Clomiphene *on previous page*

Clomipramine (kloe MI pra meen)

Related Information

Antidepressant Agents Comparison *on page 1393*

Brand Names Anafranil®

Canadian/Mexican Brand Names Apo-Clomipramine® (Canada)

Synonyms Clomipramine Hydrochloride

Therapeutic Category Antidepressant, Tricyclic

Use Treatment of obsessive-compulsive disorder (OCD); may also relieve depression, panic attacks, and chronic pain

Pregnancy Risk Factor C

Contraindications Patients in acute recovery stage of recent myocardial infarction; not to be used within 14 days of MAO inhibitors

Warnings/Precautions Seizures are likely and are dose-related; can be additive when coadministered with other drugs that can lower the seizure threshold; use with caution in patients with asthma, bladder outlet destruction, narrow-angle glaucoma

Adverse Reactions

>10%:

- Central nervous system: Dizziness, drowsiness, headache
- Gastrointestinal: Xerostomia, constipation, increased appetite, nausea, unpleasant taste, weight gain
- Neuromuscular & skeletal: Weakness

1% to 10%:

- Cardiovascular: Arrhythmias, hypotension
- Central nervous system: Confusion, delirium, hallucinations, nervousness, restlessness, parkinsonian syndrome, insomnia
- Gastrointestinal: Diarrhea, heartburn
- Genitourinary: Dysuria, sexual dysfunction
- Neuromuscular & skeletal: Fine muscle tremors
- Ocular: Blurred vision, eye pain
- Miscellaneous: Diaphoresis (excessive)

<1%:

- Central nervous system: Anxiety, seizures
- Dermatologic: Alopecia, photosensitivity
- Endocrine & metabolic: Breast enlargement, galactorrhea, SIADH
- Gastrointestinal: Trouble with gums, decreased lower esophageal sphincter tone may cause GE reflux
- Genitourinary: Testicular edema
- Hematologic: Agranulocytosis, leukopenia, eosinophilia
- Hepatic: Cholestatic jaundice, increased liver enzymes
- Ocular: Increased intraocular pressure
- Otic: Tinnitus
- Miscellaneous: Allergic reactions

Overdosage/Toxicology Symptoms of overdose include agitation, confusion, hallucinations, urinary retention, hypothermia, hypotension, tachycardia, ventricular tachycardia, seizures, coma

Following initiation of essential overdose management, toxic symptoms should be treated. Sodium bicarbonate is indicated when QRS interval is >0.10 seconds or QT_c >0.42 seconds. Ventricular arrhythmias and EKG abnormalities (eg, QRS widening) often respond to systemic alkalinization (sodium bicarbonate 0.5-2 mEq/kg I.V.) and/or phenytoin 15-20 mg/kg (adults). Arrhythmias unresponsive to this therapy may respond to lidocaine 1 mg/kg I.V. followed by a titrated infusion. Physostigmine (1-2 mg I.V. slowly for adults or 0.5 mg I.V. slowly for children) may be indicated in reversing cardiac arrhythmias that are life-threatening. Seizures usually respond to diazepam I.V. boluses (5-10 mg for adults up to 30 mg or 0.25-0.4 mg/kg/dose for children up to 10 mg/dose). If seizures are unresponsive or recur, phenytoin or phenobarbital may be required.

Drug Interactions

Decreased effect with barbiturates, carbamazepine, phenytoin

Increased effect of alcohol, CNS depressants, anticholinergics, sympathomimetics

Increased toxicity: MAO inhibitors (increase temperature, seizures, coma, and death)

Mechanism of Action Clomipramine appears to affect serotonin uptake while its active metabolite, desmethylclomipramine, affects norepinephrine uptake

Pharmacodynamics/Kinetics

Absorption: Oral: Rapid

Metabolism: Extensive first-pass metabolism; metabolized to desmethylclomipramine (active) in the liver

Half-life: 20-30 hours

Usual Dosage Oral: Initial:

Children: 25 mg/day and gradually increase, as tolerated, to a maximum of 3 mg/kg/day or 200 mg/day, whichever is smaller

Adults: 25 mg/day and gradually increase, as tolerated, to 100 mg/day the first 2 weeks, may then be increased to a total of 250 mg/day maximum

Test Interactions ↑ glucose

Patient Information May cause seizures; caution should be used in activities that require alertness like driving, operating machinery, or swimming; effect of drug may take several weeks to appear

Dosage Forms Capsule, as hydrochloride: 25 mg, 50 mg, 75 mg

Clomipramine Hydrochloride *see* Clomipramine *on previous page*

Clonazepam (kloe NA ze pam)

Related Information

Anticonvulsants by Seizure Type *on page 1392*

Benzodiazepines Comparison *on page 1397*

Epilepsy Treatment *on page 1531*

Brand Names Klonopin™

Canadian/Mexican Brand Names PMS-Clonazepam (Canada); Rivotril® (Canada); Rivotril® (Mexico)

Therapeutic Category Anticonvulsant

Use Prophylaxis of petit mal, petit mal variant (Lennox-Gastaut), akinetic, and myoclonic seizures

Unlabeled use: Restless legs syndrome, neuralgia, multifocal tic disorder, parkinsonian dysarthria, acute manic episodes, and adjunct therapy for schizophrenia

Restrictions C-IV

Pregnancy Risk Factor C

Pregnancy/Breast-Feeding Implications

Clinical effects on the fetus: Crosses into breast milk. Two reports of cardiac defects; respiratory depression, lethargy, hypotonia may be observed in newborns exposed near time of delivery. Epilepsy itself, number of medications, genetic factors, or a combination of these probably influence the teratogenicity of anticonvulsant therapy. Benefit:risk ratio usually favors continued use during pregnancy and breast-feeding.

Breast-feeding/lactation: Crosses into breast milk

Clinical effects on the infant: CNS depression, respiratory depression reported. No recommendation from the American Academy of Pediatrics.

Contraindications Hypersensitivity to clonazepam, any component, or other benzodiazepines; severe liver disease, acute narrow-angle glaucoma

Warnings/Precautions Use with caution in patients with chronic respiratory disease or impaired renal function; abrupt discontinuance may precipitate withdrawal symptoms, status epilepticus or seizures, in patients with a history of substance abuse; clonazepam-induced behavioral disturbances may be more frequent in mentally handicapped patients

Adverse Reactions

>10%:

Cardiovascular: Tachycardia, chest pain

Central nervous system: Drowsiness, fatigue, ataxia, lightheadedness, memory impairment, insomnia, anxiety, depression, headache

(Continued)

Clonazepam *(Continued)*

Dermatologic: Rash
Endocrine & metabolic: Decreased libido
Gastrointestinal: Xerostomia, constipation, diarrhea, nausea, increased or decreased appetite, vomiting, decreased salivation
Neuromuscular & skeletal: Dysarthria
Ocular: Blurred vision
Miscellaneous: Diaphoresis

1% to 10%:
Cardiovascular: Syncope, hypotension
Central nervous system: Confusion, nervousness, dizziness, akathisia
Dermatologic: Dermatitis
Gastrointestinal: Weight gain or loss, increased salivation
Neuromuscular & skeletal: Rigidity, tremor, muscle cramps
Otic: Tinnitus
Respiratory: Nasal congestion, hyperventilation

<1%:
Endocrine & metabolic: Menstrual irregularities
Hematologic: Blood dyscrasias
Neuromuscular & skeletal: Reflex slowing
Miscellaneous: Drug dependence

Overdosage/Toxicology May produce somnolence, confusion, ataxia, diminished reflexes, or coma

Treatment for benzodiazepine overdose is supportive. Rarely is mechanical ventilation required. Flumazenil has been shown to selectively block the binding of benzodiazepines to CNS receptors, resulting in a reversal of benzodiazepine-induced CNS depression, but not respiratory depression

Drug Interactions
Decreased effect: Phenytoin, barbiturates may increase clonazepam clearance
Increased toxicity: CNS depressants may increase sedation

Mechanism of Action Suppresses the spike-and-wave discharge in absence seizures by depressing nerve transmission in the motor cortex

Pharmacodynamics/Kinetics
Onset of effect: 20-60 minutes
Duration: Up to 6-8 hours in infants and young children, up to 12 hours in adults
Absorption: Oral: Well absorbed
Distribution: Adults: V_d: 1.5-4.4 L/kg
Protein binding: 85%
Metabolism: Extensive; glucuronide and sulfate conjugation
Half-life:
Children: 22-33 hours
Adults: 19-50 hours
Time to peak serum concentration: Oral: 1-3 hours
Steady-state: 5-7 days
Elimination: <2% excreted unchanged in urine; metabolites excreted as glucuronide or sulfate conjugates

Usual Dosage Oral:
Children <10 years or 30 kg:
Initial daily dose: 0.01-0.03 mg/kg/day (maximum: 0.05 mg/kg/day) given in 2-3 divided doses; increase by no more than 0.5 mg every third day until seizures are controlled or adverse effects seen
Usual maintenance dose: 0.1-0.2 mg/kg/day divided 3 times/day; not to exceed 0.2 mg/kg/day

Adults:
Initial daily dose not to exceed 1.5 mg given in 3 divided doses; may increase by 0.5-1 mg every third day until seizures are controlled or adverse effects seen
Usual maintenance dose: 0.05-0.2 mg/kg; do not exceed 20 mg/day

Hemodialysis: Supplemental dose is not necessary

Dietary Considerations Alcohol: Additive CNS depression has been reported with benzodiazepines; avoid or limit alcohol

Reference Range Relationship between serum concentration and seizure control is not well established
Timing of serum samples: Peak serum levels occur 1-3 hours after oral ingestion; the half-life is 20-40 hours; therefore, steady-state occurs in 5-7 days
Therapeutic levels: 20-80 ng/mL; Toxic concentration: >80 ng/mL

Patient Information Avoid alcohol and other CNS depressants; avoid activities needing good psychomotor coordination until CNS effects are known; drug may cause physical or psychological dependence; avoid abrupt discontinuation after prolonged use

Nursing Implications Observe patient for excess sedation, respiratory depression; raise bed rails, initiate safety measures, assist with ambulation

Dosage Forms Tablet: 0.5 mg, 1 mg, 2 mg

Extemporaneous Preparations A 0.1 mg/mL oral suspension has been made using five 2 mg tablets, purified water USP (10 mL) and methylcellulose 1% (qsad 100 mL); the expected stability of this preparation is 2 weeks if stored under refrigeration; shake well before use

Nahata MC and Hipple TF, *Pediatric Drug Formulations*, 2nd ed, Cincinnati, OH: Harvey Whitney Books Co, 1992.

Clonidine (KLOE ni deen)

Related Information

Therapy of Hypertension *on page 1540*

Brand Names Catapres®; Catapres-TTS®

Canadian/Mexican Brand Names Apo-Clonidine® (Canada); Dixarit® (Canada); Novo-Clonidine® (Canada); Nu-Clonidine® (Canada); Catapresan-100® (Mexico)

Synonyms Clonidine Hydrochloride

Therapeutic Category Alpha$_2$-Adrenergic Agonist Agent; Antihypertensive

Use Management of mild to moderate hypertension; either used alone or in combination with other antihypertensives; not recommended for first-line therapy for hypertension; as a second-line agent for decreasing heroin or nicotine withdrawal symptoms in patients with severe symptoms; indicated by the epidural route, in combination with opiates, for treatment of severe pain in refractory cancer patients (most effective in patients with neuropathic pain); other uses may include prophylaxis of migraines, glaucoma, and diabetes-associated diarrhea

Pregnancy Risk Factor C

Pregnancy/Breast-Feeding Implications

Clinical effects on the fetus: Crosses the placenta. Caution should be used with this drug due to the potential of rebound hypertension with abrupt discontinuation.

Breast-feeding/lactation: Crosses into breast milk. American Academy of Pediatrics has NO RECOMMENDATION.

Contraindications Hypersensitivity to clonidine hydrochloride or any component

Warnings/Precautions Use with caution in cerebrovascular disease, coronary insufficiency, renal impairment, sinus node dysfunction; do not abruptly discontinue (rapid increase in blood pressure, and symptoms of sympathetic overactivity, ie, increased heart rate, tremor, agitation, anxiety, insomnia, sweating, palpitations) may occur; **if need to discontinue, taper dose gradually over 1 week or more (2-4 days with epidural product)**; adjust dosage in patients with renal dysfunction (especially the elderly); not recommended for obstetrical, postpartum or perioperative pain management or in those with severe hemodynamic instability due to unacceptable risk of hypotension and bradycardia; clonidine injection should be administered via a continuous epidural infusion device

Adverse Reactions

>10%:

- Central nervous system: Drowsiness, dizziness, confusion, anxiety
- Cardiovascular: Orthostatic hypotension (especially with epidural route), rebound hypertension, bradycardia
- Gastrointestinal: Xerostomia, constipation, nausea
- Genitourinary: Urinary tract infection

1% to 10%:

- Central nervous system: Mental depression, headache, fatigue, hyperaesthesia, pain
- Dermatologic: Rash, skin ulcer
- Respiratory: Dyspnea, hypoventilation
- Cardiovascular: Chest pain
- Endocrine & metabolic: Decreased sexual activity, loss of libido
- Gastrointestinal: vomiting, constipation
- Genitourinary: Nocturia, impotence
- Hepatic: Abnormal liver function tests
- Neuromuscular & skeletal: Weakness
- Otic: Tinnitus

<1%:

- Cardiovascular: Palpitations, tachycardia, Raynaud's phenomenon, congestive heart failure
- Central nervous system: Insomnia, vivid dreams, delirium, fever
- Dermatologic: Pruritus, urticaria, alopecia
- Endocrine & metabolic: Gynecomastia
- Gastrointestinal: Weight gain
- Genitourinary: Urinary retention, dysuria
- Ocular: Burning eyes, blurred vision

(Continued)

Clonidine *(Continued)*

Overdosage/Toxicology Symptoms of overdose include bradycardia, CNS depression, hypothermia, diarrhea, respiratory depression, apnea

Treatment is primarily supportive and symptomatic. Hypotension usually responds to I.V. fluids or Trendelenburg positioning. Naloxone may be utilized in treating CNS depression and/or apnea and should be given I.V. 0.4-2 mg, with repeated doses as needed or as an infusion.

Drug Interactions

Decreased effect: Tricyclic antidepressants antagonize hypotensive effects of clonidine

Increased toxicity: Beta-blockers may potentiate bradycardia in patients receiving clonidine and may increase the rebound hypertension of withdrawal; discontinue beta-blocker several days before clonidine is tapered; narcotic analgesics may potentiate hypotensive effects of clonidine; alcohol and barbiturates may increase the CNS-depression; epidural clonidine may prolong the sensory and motor blockade of local anesthetics

Mechanism of Action Stimulates $alpha_2$-adrenoceptors in the brain stem, thus activating an inhibitory neuron, resulting in reduced sympathetic outflow, producing a decrease in vasomotor tone and heart rate; epidural clonidine may produce pain relief at spinal presynaptic and postjunctional $alpha_2$-adrenoceptors by preventing pain signal transmission; pain relief occurs only for the body regions innervated by the spinal segments where analgesic concentrations of clonidine exist

Pharmacodynamics/Kinetics

Onset of effect: Oral: 0.5-1 hour; T_{max}: 2-4 hours

Duration: 6-10 hours

Distribution: V_d: 2.1 L/kg (adults); highly lipid soluble; distributes readily into extravascular sites; protein binding: 20% to 40%

Metabolism: Hepatic (enterohepatic recirculation); extensively metabolized to inactive metabolites

Bioavailability: 75% to 95%

Half-life: Adults:

- Normal renal function: 6-20 hours
- Renal impairment: 18-41 hours

Elimination: 65% excreted in urine, 32% unchanged, and 22% excreted in feces; not removed significantly by hemodialysis

Usual Dosage

Oral:

- Children: Initial: 5-10 mcg/kg/day in divided doses every 8-12 hours; increase gradually at 5- to 7-day intervals to 25 mcg/kg/day in divided doses every 6 hours; maximum: 0.9 mg/day
  - Clonidine tolerance test (test of growth hormone release from pituitary): 0.15 mg/m² or 4 mcg/kg as single dose
- Adults: Initial dose: 0.1 mg twice daily, usual maintenance dose: 0.2-1.2 mg/day in 2-4 divided doses; maximum recommended dose: 2.4 mg/day
  - Nicotine withdrawal symptoms: 0.1 mg twice daily to maximum of 0.4 mg/day for 3-4 weeks
- Elderly: Initial: 0.1 mg once daily at bedtime, increase gradually as needed

Transdermal: Apply once every 7 days; for initial therapy start with 0.1 mg and increase by 0.1 mg at 1- to 2-week intervals; dosages >0.6 mg do not improve efficacy

Epidural infusion: Starting dose: 30 mcg/hour; titrate as required for relief of pain or presence of side effects; minimal experience with doses >40 mcg/hour; should be considered an adjunct to intraspinal opiate therapy

Dosing adjustment in renal impairment:

Cl_{cr} <10 mL/minute: Administer 50% to 75% of normal dose initially

Dialysis: Not dialyzable (0% to 5%) via hemo- or peritoneal dialysis; supplemental dose not necessary

Monitoring Parameters Blood pressure, standing and sitting/supine, respiratory rate and depth, pain relief, mental status, heart rate (bradycardia may be treated with atropine)

Reference Range Therapeutic: 1-2 ng/mL (SI: 4.4-8.7 nmol/L)

Test Interactions ↑ sodium (S); ↓ catecholamines (U)

Patient Information Do not discontinue drug except on instruction of physician; check daily to be sure patch is present; may cause drowsiness, impaired coordination, and judgment; use extreme caution while driving or operating machines

Nursing Implications Patches should be applied weekly at bedtime to a clean, hairless area of the upper outer arm or chest; rotate patch sites weekly; redness under patch may be reduced if a topical corticosteroid spray is applied to the area before placement of the patch; if needed, gradually reduce dose over 2-4 days to avoid rebound hypertension; during epidural administration, monitor cardiovascular and respiratory status carefully

Dosage Forms

Injection, preservative free, as hydrochloride: 100 mcg/mL (10 mL)

Patch, transdermal, as hydrochloride: 1, 2, and 3 (0.1, 0.2, 0.3 mg/day, 7-day duration)

Tablet, as hydrochloride: 0.1 mg, 0.2 mg, 0.3 mg

Clonidine Hydrochloride *see* Clonidine *on page 299*

Clopra® *see* Metoclopramide *on page 824*

Clorazepate (klor AZ e pate)

Related Information

Benzodiazepines Comparison *on page 1397*

Epilepsy Treatment *on page 1531*

Brand Names Gen-XENE®; Tranxene®

Canadian/Mexican Brand Names Apo-Clorazepate® (Canada); Novo-Clopate® (Canada)

Synonyms Clorazepate Dipotassium

Therapeutic Category Anticonvulsant; Benzodiazepine; Sedative

Use Treatment of generalized anxiety and panic disorders; management of alcohol withdrawal; adjunct anticonvulsant in management of partial seizures

Restrictions C-IV

Pregnancy Risk Factor D

Contraindications Hypersensitivity to clorazepate dipotassium or any component; cross-sensitivity with other benzodiazepines may exist; avoid using in patients with pre-existing CNS depression, severe uncontrolled pain, or narrow-angle glaucoma

Warnings/Precautions Use with caution in patients with hepatic or renal disease; abrupt discontinuation may cause withdrawal symptoms or seizures

Adverse Reactions

>10%:

- Cardiovascular: Tachycardia, chest pain
- Central nervous system: Drowsiness, fatigue, ataxia, lightheadedness, memory impairment, insomnia, anxiety, headache, depression
- Dermatologic: Rash
- Endocrine & metabolic: Decreased libido
- Gastrointestinal: Xerostomia, constipation, diarrhea, decreased salivation, nausea, vomiting, increased or decreased appetite
- Neuromuscular & skeletal: Dysarthria
- Ocular: Blurred vision
- Miscellaneous: Diaphoresis

1% to 10%:

- Cardiovascular: Syncope, hypotension
- Central nervous system: Confusion, nervousness, dizziness, akathisia
- Dermatologic: Dermatitis
- Gastrointestinal: Nausea, increased salivation, weight gain or loss
- Neuromuscular & skeletal: Rigidity, tremor, muscle cramps
- Otic: Tinnitus
- Respiratory: Nasal congestion, hyperventilation

<1%:

- Endocrine & metabolic: Menstrual irregularities
- Hematologic: Blood dyscrasias
- Neuromuscular & skeletal: Reflex slowing
- Miscellaneous: Drug dependence; long-term use may also be associated with renal or hepatic injury and reduced hematocrit

Overdosage/Toxicology May produce somnolence, confusion, ataxia, diminished reflexes, coma

Treatment for benzodiazepine overdose is supportive; rarely is mechanical ventilation required; flumazenil has been shown to selectively block the binding of benzodiazepines to CNS receptors, resulting in a reversal of benzodiazepine-induced CNS depression, but not respiratory depression.

Drug Interactions Increased effect: Cimetidine, CNS depressants, alcohol

Stability Unstable in water

Mechanism of Action Facilitates gamma aminobutyric acid (GABA)-mediated transmission inhibitory neurotransmitter action, depresses subcortical levels of CNS

Pharmacodynamics/Kinetics

Distribution: Crosses the placenta; appears in urine

Metabolism: Rapidly decarboxylated to desmethyldiazepam (active) in acidic stomach prior to absorption; metabolized in the liver to oxazepam (active)

Half-life: Adults:

- Desmethyldiazepam: 48-96 hours
- Oxazepam: 6-8 hours

Time to peak serum concentration: Oral: Within 1 hour

(Continued)

Clorazepate *(Continued)*

Elimination: Primarily in urine

Usual Dosage Oral:

Children 9-12 years: Anticonvulsant: Initial: 3.75-7.5 mg/dose twice daily; increase dose by 3.75 mg at weekly intervals, not to exceed 60 mg/day in 2-3 divided doses

Children >12 years and Adults: Anticonvulsant: Initial: Up to 7.5 mg/dose 2-3 times/day; increase dose by 7.5 mg at weekly intervals; not to exceed 90 mg/day

Adults:

Anxiety: 7.5-15 mg 2-4 times/day, or given as single dose of 11.25 or 22.5 mg at bedtime

Alcohol withdrawal: Initial: 30 mg, then 15 mg 2-4 times/day on first day; maximum daily dose: 90 mg; gradually decrease dose over subsequent days

Dietary Considerations Alcohol: Additive CNS effects, avoid use

Monitoring Parameters Respiratory and cardiovascular status, excess CNS depression

Reference Range Therapeutic: 0.12-1 μg/mL (SI: 0.36-3.01 μmol/L)

Test Interactions ↓ hematocrit, abnormal liver and renal function tests

Patient Information Avoid alcohol and other CNS depressants; avoid activities needing good psychomotor coordination until CNS effects are known; drug may cause physical or psychological dependence; avoid abrupt discontinuation after prolonged use

Nursing Implications Observe patient for excess sedation, respiratory depression; raise bed rails, initiate safety measures, assist with ambulation

Dosage Forms

Capsule, as dipotassium: 3.75 mg, 7.5 mg, 15 mg

Tablet, as dipotassium: 3.75 mg, 7.5 mg, 15 mg

Tablet, as dipotassium, single dose: 11.25 mg, 22.5 mg

Clorazepate Dipotassium *see* Clorazepate *on previous page*

Clotrimazole (kloe TRIM a zole)

Related Information

Guidelines for the Prevention of Opportunistic Infections in Persons with HIV *on page 1457*

Treatment of Sexually Transmitted Diseases *on page 1485*

Brand Names Femizole-7® [OTC]; Gyne-Lotrimin® [OTC]; Lotrimin®; Lotrimin® AF Cream [OTC]; Lotrimin® AF Lotion [OTC]; Lotrimin® AF Solution [OTC]; Mycelex®; Mycelex®-7; Mycelex®-G

Therapeutic Category Antifungal Agent, Oral Nonabsorbed; Antifungal Agent, Topical; Antifungal Agent, Vaginal

Use Treatment of susceptible fungi infections, including oropharyngeal, candidiasis, dermatophytoses, superficial mycoses, and cutaneous candidiasis, as well as vulvovaginal candidiasis; limited data suggest that clotrimazole troches may be effective for prophylaxis against oropharyngeal candidiasis in neutropenic patients

Pregnancy Risk Factor B/C (oral)

Contraindications Hypersensitivity to clotrimazole or any component

Warnings/Precautions Clotrimazole should not be used for treatment of systemic fungal infection; safety and effectiveness of clotrimazole lozenges (troches) in children <3 years of age have not been established

Adverse Reactions

>10%: Hepatic: Abnormal liver function tests

1% to 10%:

Gastrointestinal: Nausea and vomiting may occur in patients on clotrimazole troches

Local: Mild burning, irritation, stinging to skin or vaginal area

Mechanism of Action Binds to phospholipids in the fungal cell membrane altering cell wall permeability resulting in loss of essential intracellular elements

Pharmacodynamics/Kinetics

Absorption: Topical: Negligible through intact skin

Time to peak serum concentration:

Oral topical administration: Salivary levels occur within 3 hours following 30 minutes of dissolution time in the mouth

Vaginal cream: High vaginal levels occur within 8-24 hours

Vaginal tablet: High vaginal levels occur within 1-2 days

Elimination: As metabolites via bile

Usual Dosage

Children >3 years and Adults:

Oral:

Prophylaxis: 10 mg troche dissolved 3 times/day for the duration of chemotherapy or until steroids are reduced to maintenance levels

Treatment: 10 mg troche dissolved slowly 5 times/day for 14 consecutive days

Topical: Apply twice daily; if no improvement occurs after 4 weeks of therapy, re-evaluate diagnosis

Children >12 years and Adults:

Vaginal:

Cream: Insert 1 applicatorful of 1% vaginal cream daily (preferably at bedtime) for 7 consecutive days

Tablet: Insert 100 mg/day for 7 days or 500 mg single dose

Topical: Apply to affected area twice daily (morning and evening) for 7 consecutive days

Monitoring Parameters Periodic liver function tests during oral therapy with clotrimazole lozenges

Patient Information May cause irritation to the skin; avoid contact with eyes; lozenge (troche) must be dissolved slowly in the mouth

Dosage Forms

Combination pack (Mycelex-7®): Vaginal tablet 100 mg (7's) and vaginal cream 1% (7 g)

Cream:

Topical (Lotrimin®, Lotrimin® AF, Mycelex®, Mycelex® OTC) : 1% (15 g, 30 g, 45 g, 90 g)

Vaginal (Femizole-7®, Gyne-Lotrimin®, Mycelex®-G): 1% (45 g, 90 g)

Lotion (Lotrimin®): 1% (30 mL)

Solution, topical (Lotrimin®, Lotrimin® AF, Mycelex®, Mycelex® OTC): 1% (10 mL, 30 mL)

Tablet, vaginal (Gyne-Lotrimin®, Mycelex®-G): 100 mg (7s); 500 mg (1s)

Troche (Mycelex®): 10 mg

Twin pack (Mycelex®): Vaginal tablet 500 mg (1's) and vaginal cream 1% (7 g)

Cloxacillin (kloks a SIL in)

Brand Names Cloxapen®; Tegopen®

Canadian/Mexican Brand Names Apo-Cloxi® (Canada); Novo-Cloxin® (Canada); Nu-Cloxi® (Canada); Orbenin® (Canada); Taro-Cloxacillin® (Canada)

Synonyms Cloxacillin Sodium

Therapeutic Category Antibiotic, Penicillin

Use Treatment of susceptible bacterial infections, notably penicillinase-producing staphylococci causing respiratory tract, skin and skin structure, bone and joint, urinary tract infections, endocarditis, septicemia, and meningitis

Pregnancy Risk Factor B

Contraindications Hypersensitivity to cloxacillin or any component, or penicillins

Warnings/Precautions Monitor PT if patient concurrently on warfarin, elimination of drug is slow in renally impaired; use with caution in patients allergic to cephalosporins due to a low incidence of cross-hypersensitivity

Adverse Reactions

1% to 10%: Gastrointestinal: Nausea, diarrhea

<1%:

Central nervous system: Fever

Dermatologic: Rash

Gastrointestinal: Vomiting

Hematologic: Eosinophilia, leukopenia, neutropenia, thrombocytopenia, agranulocytosis

Hepatic: Hepatotoxicity

Renal: Hematuria

Miscellaneous: Serum sickness-like reactions

Overdosage/Toxicology Symptoms of penicillin overdose include neuromuscular hypersensitivity (agitation, hallucinations, asterixis, encephalopathy, confusion, and seizures) and electrolyte imbalance with potassium or sodium salts, especially in renal failure

Hemodialysis may be helpful to aid in the removal of the drug from the blood, otherwise most treatment is supportive or symptom directed

Drug Interactions

Decreased effect: Efficacy of oral contraceptives may be reduced

Increased effect: Disulfiram, probenecid may increase penicillin levels, increased effect of anticoagulants

Stability Refrigerate oral solution after reconstitution; discard after 14 days; stable for 3 days at room temperature

(Continued)

Cloxacillin *(Continued)*

Mechanism of Action Inhibits bacterial cell wall synthesis by binding to one or more of the penicillin-binding proteins (PBPs) which in turn inhibits the final transpeptidation step of peptidoglycan synthesis in bacterial cell walls, thus inhibiting cell wall biosynthesis. Bacteria eventually lyse due to ongoing activity of cell wall autolytic enzymes (autolysins and murein hydrolases) while cell wall assembly is arrested.

Pharmacodynamics/Kinetics

Absorption: Oral: ~50%

Distribution: Crosses the placenta; appears in breast milk; distributed widely to most body fluids and bone; penetration into cells, into the eye, and across normal meninges is poor; inflammation increased amount that crosses the blood-brain barrier

Protein binding: 90% to 98%

Metabolism: Significant in the liver to active and inactive metabolites

Half-life: 0.5-1.5 hours (prolonged with renal impairment and in neonates)

Time to peak serum concentration: Oral: Within 0.5-2 hours

Elimination: In urine and through bile

Usual Dosage Oral:

Children >1 month (<20 kg): 50-100 mg/kg/day in divided doses every 6 hours; up to a maximum of 4 g/day

Children (>20 kg) and Adults: 250-500 mg every 6 hours

Hemodialysis: Not dialyzable (0% to 5%)

Administration Administer around-the-clock to lessen peak and tough concentrations

Test Interactions May interfere with urinary glucose tests using cupric sulfate (Benedict's solution, Clinitest®); may inactivate aminoglycosides *in vitro*; false-positive urine and serum proteins; false-positive in uric acid, urinary steroids

Patient Information Take 1 hour before or 2 hours after meals; finish all medication; do not skip doses

Dosage Forms

Capsule, as sodium: 250 mg, 500 mg

Powder for oral suspension, as sodium: 125 mg/5 mL (100 mL, 200 mL)

Cloxacillin Sodium *see* Cloxacillin *on previous page*

Cloxapen® *see* Cloxacillin *on previous page*

Clozapine (KLOE za peen)

Related Information

Antipsychotic Agents Comparison *on page 1396*

Brand Names Clozaril®

Canadian/Mexican Brand Names Leponex® (Mexico)

Therapeutic Category Antipsychotic Agent

Use Management of schizophrenic patients

Pregnancy Risk Factor B

Contraindications In patients with WBC ≤3500 cells/mm³ before therapy; if WBC falls to <3000 cells/mm³ during therapy the drug should be withheld until signs and symptoms of infection disappear and WBC rises to >3000 cells/mm³

Warnings/Precautions Medication should not be stopped abruptly; taper off over 1-2 weeks; WBC testing should occur weekly for the duration of therapy; significant risk of agranulocytosis, potentially life-threatening; use with caution in patients receiving other marrow suppressive agents

Adverse Reactions

>10%:

- Cardiovascular: Tachycardia, hypotension, orthostatic hypotension
- Central nervous system: Fever, headache, drowsiness
- Gastrointestinal: Constipation, nausea, vomiting, unusual weight gain

1% to 10%:

- Cardiovascular: EKG changes, hypertension
- Central nervous system: Agitation, akathisia
- Gastrointestinal: Abdominal discomfort, heartburn, xerostomia
- Ocular: Blurred vision
- Miscellaneous: Diaphoresis (increased)

<1%:

- Central nervous system: Insomnia, seizures, tardive dyskinesia, neuroleptic malignant syndrome
- Genitourinary: Dysuria, impotence
- Hematologic: Agranulocytosis, eosinophilia, granulocytopenia, leukopenia, thrombocytopenia
- Neuromuscular & skeletal: Rigidity, tremor

Overdosage/Toxicology Symptoms of overdose include altered states of consciousness, tachycardia, hypotension, hypersalivation, respiratory depression

Following initiation of essential overdose management, toxic symptom treatment and supportive treatment should be initiated. Hypotension usually responds to I.V. fluids or Trendelenburg positioning. If unresponsive to these measures, the use of a parenteral inotrope may be required. Seizures commonly respond to diazepam (I.V. 5-10 mg bolus in adults every 15 minutes if needed up to a total of 30 mg; I.V. 0.25-0.4 mg/kg/dose up to a total of 10 mg in children) or to phenytoin or phenobarbital; critical cardiac arrhythmias often respond to I.V. phenytoin (15 mg/kg up to 1 g), while other antiarrhythmics can be used. Neuroleptics often cause extrapyramidal symptoms (eg, dystonic reactions) requiring management with benztropine mesylate I.V. 1-2 mg (adults) may be effective. These agents are generally effective within 2-5 minutes.

Drug Interactions

Decreased effect of epinephrine; decreased effect with phenytoin

Increased effect of CNS depressants, guanabenz, anticholinergics

Increased toxicity with cimetidine, MAO inhibitors, neuroleptics, TCAs

Mechanism of Action Clozapine is a weak dopamine$_1$ and dopamine$_2$ receptor blocker; in addition, it blocks the serotonin$_2$, alpha-adrenergic, and histamine H_1 central nervous system receptors

Pharmacodynamics/Kinetics

Metabolism: Undergoes extensive metabolism primarily to unconjugated forms

Elimination: In urine

Usual Dosage Adults: Oral: 25 mg once or twice daily initially and increased, as tolerated to a target dose of 300-450 mg/day after 2 weeks, but may require doses as high as 600-900 mg/day

Patient Information Report any lethargy, fever, sore throat, flu-like symptoms, or any other signs or symptoms of infection; may cause drowsiness; frequent blood samples must be taken; do not stop taking even if you think it is not working

Nursing Implications Benign, self-limiting temperature elevations sometimes occur during the first 3 weeks of treatment, weekly CBC mandatory

Dosage Forms Tablet: 25 mg, 100 mg

Clozaril® *see* Clozapine *on previous page*

Clysodrast® *see* Bisacodyl *on page 153*

CMV-IGIV *see* Cytomegalovirus Immune Globulin (Intravenous-Human) *on page 335*

Coagulant Complex Inhibitor *see* Anti-Inhibitor Coagulant Complex *on page 96*

Cobex® *see* Cyanocobalamin *on page 319*

Cocaine (koe KANE)

Synonyms Cocaine Hydrochloride

Therapeutic Category Local Anesthetic, Ester Type; Local Anesthetic, Topical

Use Topical anesthesia (ester derivative) for mucous membranes

Restrictions C-II

Pregnancy Risk Factor C (X if nonmedicinal use)

Contraindications Systemic use, hypersensitivity to cocaine or any component

Warnings/Precautions Use with caution in patients with hypertension, severe cardiovascular disease, or thyrotoxicosis; use with caution in patients with severely traumatized mucosa and sepsis in the region of intended application. Repeated topical application can result in psychic dependence and tolerance. May cause cornea to become clouded or pitted, therefore, normal saline should be used to irrigate and protect cornea during surgery; not for injection.

Adverse Reactions

>10%:

- Central nervous system: CNS stimulation
- Gastrointestinal: Loss of taste perception
- Respiratory: Chronic rhinitis, nasal congestion
- Miscellaneous: Loss of smell

1% to 10%:

- Cardiovascular: Decreased heart rate with low doses, increased heart rate with moderate doses, hypertension, tachycardia, cardiac arrhythmias
- Central nervous system: Nervousness, restlessness, euphoria, excitement, hallucination, seizures
- Gastrointestinal: Vomiting
- Neuromuscular & skeletal: Tremors and clonic-tonic reactions
- Ocular: Sloughing of the corneal epithelium, ulceration of the cornea
- Respiratory: Tachypnea, respiratory failure

Overdosage/Toxicology Symptoms of overdose include anxiety, excitement, confusion, nausea, vomiting, headache, rapid pulse, irregular respiration,

(Continued)

Cocaine *(Continued)*

delirium, fever, seizures, respiratory arrest, hallucinations, dilated pupils, muscle spasms, sensory aberrations, cardiac arrhythmias

Fatal dose: Oral: 500 mg to 1.2 g; severe toxic effects have occurred with doses as low as 20 mg

Since no specific antidote for cocaine exists, serious toxic effects are treated symptomatically. Maintain airway and respiration. Attempt delay of absorption (if ingested) with activated charcoal, gastric lavage or emesis. Seizures are treated with diazepam while propranolol or labetalol may be useful for life-threatening arrhythmias, agitation, and/or hypertension.

Drug Interactions Increased toxicity: MAO inhibitors

Stability Store in well closed, light-resistant containers

Mechanism of Action Ester local anesthetic blocks both the initiation and conduction of nerve impulses by decreasing the neuronal membrane's permeability to sodium ions, which results in inhibition of depolarization with resultant blockade of conduction; interferes with the uptake of norepinephrine by adrenergic nerve terminals producing vasoconstriction

Pharmacodynamics/Kinetics Following topical administration to mucosa:

Onset of action: Within 1 minute

Peak action: Within 5 minutes

Duration: ≥30 minutes, depending on dosage administered

Absorption: Well absorbed through mucous membranes; limited by drug-induced vasoconstriction; enhanced by inflammation

Distribution: Appears in breast milk

Metabolism: In the liver; major metabolites are ecgonine methyl ester and benzoyl ecgonine

Half-life: 75 minutes

Elimination: Primarily in urine as metabolites and unchanged drug (<10%); cocaine metabolites may appear in the urine of neonates for up to 5 days after birth due to maternal cocaine use shortly before birth

Usual Dosage Dosage depends on the area to be anesthetized, tissue vascularity, technique of anesthesia, and individual patient tolerance; use the lowest dose necessary to produce adequate anesthesia should be used, not to exceed 1 mg/kg. Use reduced dosages for children, elderly, or debilitated patients.

Topical application (ear, nose, throat, bronchoscopy): Concentrations of 1% to 4% are used; concentrations >4% are not recommended because of potential for increased incidence and severity of systemic toxic reactions

Monitoring Parameters Vital signs

Reference Range Therapeutic: 100-500 ng/mL (SI: 330 nmol/L); Toxic: >1000 ng/mL (SI: >3300 nmol/L)

Nursing Implications Use only on mucous membranes of the oral, laryngeal, and nasal cavities, do not use on extensive areas of broken skin

Dosage Forms

Powder, as hydrochloride: 5 g, 25 g

Solution, topical:

As hydrochloride: 4% [40 mg/mL] (2 mL, 4 mL, 10 mL); 10% [100 mg/mL] (4 mL, 10 mL)

Viscous, as hydrochloride: 4% [40 mg/mL] (4 mL, 10 mL); 10% [100 mg/mL] (4 mL, 10 mL)

Tablet, soluble, for topical solution, as hydrochloride: 135 mg

Cocaine Hydrochloride *see* Cocaine *on previous page*

Codeine (KOE deen)

Related Information

Narcotic Agonists Comparison *on page 1414*

Dose Equivalents for Opioid Analgesics in Opioid-Naive Adults <50 kg *on page 1376*

Dose Equivalents for Opioid Analgesics in Opioid-Naive Adults ≥50 kg *on page 1375*

Canadian/Mexican Brand Names Codeine Conhn® (Canada); Linctus Codeine Blac (Canada); Linctus With Codeine Phosphate (Canada); Paveral Stanley Syrup With Codeine Phosphate (Canada)

Synonyms Codeine Phosphate; Codeine Sulfate; Methylmorphine

Therapeutic Category Analgesic, Narcotic; Antitussive

Use Treatment of mild to moderate pain; antitussive in lower doses; dextromethorphan has equivalent antitussive activity but has much lower toxicity in accidental overdose

Restrictions C-II

Pregnancy Risk Factor C (D if used for prolonged periods or in high doses at term)

Contraindications Hypersensitivity to codeine or any component

Warnings/Precautions Use with caution in patients with hypersensitivity reactions to other phenanthrene derivative opioid agonists (morphine, hydrocodone, hydromorphone, levorphanol, oxycodone, oxymorphone); respiratory diseases including asthma, emphysema, COPD, or severe liver or renal insufficiency; some preparations contain sulfites which may cause allergic reactions; may be habit-forming

Not recommended for use for cough control in patients with a productive cough; not recommended as an antitussive for children <2 years of age; the elderly may be particularly susceptible to the CNS depressant and confusion as well as constipating effects of narcotics

Adverse Reactions

>10%:

- Central nervous system: Drowsiness
- Gastrointestinal: Constipation

1% to 10%:

- Cardiovascular: Tachycardia or bradycardia, hypotension
- Central nervous system: Dizziness, lightheadedness, false feeling of well being, malaise, headache, restlessness, paradoxical CNS stimulation, confusion
- Dermatologic: Rash, urticaria
- Gastrointestinal: Xerostomia, anorexia, nausea, vomiting
- Genitourinary: Decreased urination, ureteral spasm
- Local: Burning at injection site
- Ocular: Blurred vision
- Neuromuscular & skeletal: Weakness
- Respiratory: Shortness of breath, dyspnea
- Miscellaneous: Histamine release

<1%:

- Central nervous system: Convulsions, hallucinations, mental depression, nightmares, insomnia
- Gastrointestinal: Paralytic ileus, biliary spasm, stomach cramps
- Neuromuscular & skeletal: Muscle rigidity, trembling

Overdosage/Toxicology Symptoms of overdose include CNS and respiratory depression, gastrointestinal cramping, constipation

Naloxone 2 mg I.V. (0.01 mg/kg for children) with repeat administration as necessary up to a total of 10 mg

Drug Interactions Cytochrome P-450 2D6 enzyme substrate and minor cytochrome P-450 3A enzyme substrate

Decreased effect with cigarette smoking

Increased toxicity: CNS depressants, phenothiazines, TCAs, other narcotic analgesics, guanabenz, MAO inhibitors, neuromuscular blockers

Stability Store injection between 15°C to 30°C, avoid freezing; do not use if injection is discolored or contains a precipitate; protect injection from light

Mechanism of Action Binds to opiate receptors in the CNS, causing inhibition of ascending pain pathways, altering the perception of and response to pain; causes cough supression by direct central action in the medulla; produces generalized CNS depression

Pharmacodynamics/Kinetics

Onset of action:

- Oral: 0.5-1 hour
- I.M.: 10-30 minutes

Peak action:

- Oral: 1-1.5 hours
- I.M.: 0.5-1 hour

Duration of action: 4-6 hours

Absorption: Oral: Adequate

Distribution: Crosses the placenta; appears in breast milk

Protein binding: 7%

Metabolism: Hepatic to morphine (active)

Half-life: 2.5-3.5 hours

Elimination: 3% to 16% excreted in urine as unchanged drug, norcodeine, and free and conjugated morphine

Usual Dosage Doses should be titrated to appropriate analgesic effect; when changing routes of administration, note that oral dose is $^2/_3$ as effective as parenteral dose

Analgesic:

- Children: Oral, I.M., S.C.: 0.5-1 mg/kg/dose every 4-6 hours as needed; maximum: 60 mg/dose
- Adults: Oral, I.M., I.V., S.C.: 30 mg/dose; range: 15-60 mg every 4-6 hours as needed; maximum: 360 mg/24 hours

(Continued)

Codeine *(Continued)*

Antitussive: Oral (for nonproductive cough):
Children: 1-1.5 mg/kg/day in divided doses every 4-6 hours as needed: Alternative dose according to age:
2-6 years: 2.5-5 mg every 4-6 hours as needed; maximum: 30 mg/day
6-12 years: 5-10 mg every 4-6 hours as needed; maximum: 60 mg/day
Adults: 10-20 mg/dose every 4-6 hours as needed; maximum: 120 mg/day

Dosing adjustment in renal impairment:
Cl_{cr} 10-50 mL/minute: Administer 75% of dose
Cl_{cr} <10 mL/minute: Administer 50% of dose

Dosing adjustment in hepatic impairment: Probably necessary in hepatic insufficiency

Dietary Considerations
Alcohol: Additive CNS effects, avoid or limit alcohol; watch for sedation
Food: Glucose may cause hyperglycemia; monitor blood glucose concentrations

Monitoring Parameters Pain relief, respiratory and mental status, blood pressure, heart rate

Reference Range Therapeutic: Not established; Toxic: >1.1 μg/mL

Test Interactions ↑ aminotransferase [ALT (SGPT)/AST (SGOT)] (S)

Patient Information Avoid alcohol, may cause drowsiness, impaired judgment, or coordination; may cause physical and psychological dependence with prolonged use

Nursing Implications Observe patient for excessive sedation, respiratory depression, implement safety measures, assist with ambulation

Dosage Forms
Injection, as phosphate: 30 mg (1 mL, 2 mL); 60 mg (1 mL, 2 mL)
Solution, oral: 15 mg/5 mL
Tablet, as sulfate: 15 mg, 30 mg, 60 mg
Tablet, as phosphate, soluble: 30 mg, 60 mg
Tablet, as sulfate, soluble: 15 mg, 30 mg, 60 mg

Codeine and Acetaminophen *see* Acetaminophen and Codeine *on page 21*
Codeine and Aspirin *see* Aspirin and Codeine *on page 109*
Codeine and Guaifenesin *see* Guaifenesin and Codeine *on page 590*
Codeine Phosphate *see* Codeine *on page 306*
Codeine Sulfate *see* Codeine *on page 306*
Codimal-A® *see* Brompheniramine *on page 166*
Codoxy® *see* Oxycodone and Aspirin *on page 939*
Codroxomin® *see* Hydroxocobalamin *on page 629*
Cogentin® *see* Benztropine *on page 142*
Co-Gesic® *see* Hydrocodone and Acetaminophen *on page 620*
Cognex® *see* Tacrine *on page 1185*
Colace® [OTC] *see* Docusate *on page 415*

Colchicine (KOL chi seen)

Canadian/Mexican Brand Names Colchiquim® (Mexico); Colchiquim-30® (Mexico)

Therapeutic Category Anti-inflammatory Agent; Uricosuric Agent

Use Treat acute gouty arthritis attacks and prevent recurrences of such attacks, management of familial Mediterranean fever

Pregnancy Risk Factor C (oral)/D (parenteral)

Contraindications Hypersensitivity to colchicine or any component; serious renal, gastrointestinal, hepatic, or cardiac disorders; blood dyscrasias

Warnings/Precautions Severe local irritation can occur following S.C. or I.M. administration; use with caution in debilitated patients or elderly patients or patients with severe GI, renal, or liver disease

Adverse Reactions
>10%: Gastrointestinal: Nausea, vomiting, diarrhea, abdominal pain
1% to 10%:
Dermatologic: Alopecia
Gastrointestinal: Anorexia
<1%:
Dermatologic: Rash
Genitourinary: Azoospermia
Hematologic: Agranulocytosis, aplastic anemia, bone marrow suppression
Hepatic: Hepatotoxicity
Neuromuscular & skeletal: Myopathy, peripheral neuritis

Overdosage/Toxicology Symptoms of overdose include nausea, vomiting, abdominal pain, shock, kidney damage, muscle weakness, burning in throat, watery to bloody diarrhea, hypotension, anuria, cardiovascular collapse, delirium, convulsions

Treatment includes gastric lavage and measures to prevent shock, hemodialysis or peritoneal dialysis; atropine and morphine may relieve abdominal pain

Drug Interactions

Decreased effect: Vitamin B_{12} absorption may be decreased
Increased toxicity:
Sympathomimetic agents
CNS depressant effects are enhanced

Stability Protect tablets from light; I.V. colchicine is **incompatible** with I.V. solutions with preservatives; **incompatible** with dextrose

Mechanism of Action Decreases leukocyte motility, decreases phagocytosis in joints and lactic acid production, thereby reducing the deposition of urate crystals that perpetuates the inflammatory response

Pharmacodynamics/Kinetics

Onset of effect:
Oral: Relief of pain and inflammation occurs after 24-48 hours
I.V.: 6-12 hours
Distribution: Concentrates in leukocytes, kidney, spleen, and liver; does not distribute in heart, skeletal muscle, and brain
Protein binding: 10% to 31%
Metabolism: Partially deacetylated in the liver
Half-life: 12-30 minutes
End stage renal disease: 45 minutes
Time to peak serum concentration: Oral: Within 0.5-2 hours declining for the next 2 hours before increasing again due to enterohepatic recycling
Elimination: Primarily in the feces via bile; 10% to 20% excreted in the urine

Usual Dosage

Prophylaxis of familial Mediterranean fever: Oral:
Children:
≤5 years: 0.5 mg/day
>5 years: 1-1.5 mg/day in 2-3 divided doses
Adults: 1-2 mg/day in 2-3 divided doses

Gouty arthritis, acute attacks: Adults:
Oral: Initial: 0.5-1.2 mg, then 0.5-0.6 mg every 1-2 hours or 1-1.2 mg every 2 hours until relief or GI side effects (nausea, vomiting, or diarrhea) occur to a maximum total dose of 8 mg; wait 3 days before initiating another course of therapy
I.V.: Initial: 1-3 mg, then 0.5 mg every 6 hours until response, not to exceed 4 mg/day; if pain recurs, it may be necessary to administer a daily dose of 1-2 mg for several days, however, do not administer more colchicine by any route for at least 7 days after a full course of I.V. therapy (4 mg), transfer to oral colchicine in a dose similar to that being given I.V.

Gouty arthritis, prophylaxis of recurrent attacks: Adults: Oral: 0.5-0.6 mg/day or every other day

Dosing adjustment in renal impairment:
Cl_{cr} <50 mL/minute: Avoid chronic use or administration
Cl_{cr} <10 mL/minute: Decrease dose by 50% for treatment of acute attacks

Hemodialysis: Not dialyzable (0% to 5%); supplemental dose is not necessary
Peritoneal dialysis: Supplemental dose is not necessary

Dietary Considerations

Alcohol: Avoid use
Food: Cyanocobalamin (Vitamin B_{12}): Malabsorption of the substrate. May result in macrocytic anemia or neurologic dysfunction. May need to supplement with Vitamin B_{12}.

Administration Injection should be made over 2-5 minutes into tubing of free-flowing I.V. with compatible fluid; do not administer I.M. or S.C.

Monitoring Parameters CBC and renal function test

Test Interactions May cause false-positive results in urine tests for erythrocytes or hemoglobin

Patient Information Avoid alcohol; discontinue if nausea or vomiting occurs; if taking for acute attack, discontinue as soon as pain resolves or if nausea, vomiting, or diarrhea occurs

Dosage Forms

Injection: 0.5 mg/mL (2 mL)
Tablet: 0.5 mg, 0.6 mg

Colestid® *see* Colestipol *on this page*

Colestipol (koe LES ti pole)

Related Information

Lipid-Lowering Agents *on page 1413*
(Continued)

Colestipol *(Continued)*

Brand Names Colestid®

Synonyms Colestipol Hydrochloride

Therapeutic Category Antilipemic Agent

Use Adjunct in management of primary hypercholesterolemia; regression of arteriolosclerosis; relief of pruritus associated with elevated levels of bile acids; possibly used to decrease plasma half-life of digoxin in toxicity

Pregnancy Risk Factor C

Contraindications Hypersensitivity to colestipol or any component; avoid using in complete biliary obstruction

Warnings/Precautions Avoid in patients with high triglycerides, GI dysfunction (constipation); may be associated with increased bleeding tendency as a result of hypothrombinemia secondary to vitamin K deficiency; may cause depletion of vitamins A, D, E

Adverse Reactions

>10%: Gastrointestinal: Constipation

1% to 10%: Gastrointestinal: Abdominal pain and distention, belching, flatulence, nausea, vomiting, diarrhea

<1%:

Central nervous system: Headache, dizziness, anxiety, vertigo, drowsiness, fatigue

Dermatologic: Dermatitis, urticaria

Gastrointestinal: Peptic ulceration, GI irritation and bleeding, anorexia

Hepatic: Cholelithiasis, cholecystitis

Neuromuscular & skeletal: Arthralgia, arthritis, weakness

Respiratory: Shortness of breath

Miscellaneous: Increased serum phosphorous and chloride with decrease of sodium and potassium

Overdosage/Toxicology Symptoms of overdose include GI obstruction, nausea, GI distress; treatment is supportive

Drug Interactions Decreased absorption of tetracycline, penicillin G, vitamins A, D, E and K, digitalis glycosides, warfarin, thyroid hormones, thiazide diuretics, propranolol, phenobarbital, amiodarone, methotrexate, NSAIDs, and other drugs by binding to the drug in the intestine

Mechanism of Action Binds with bile acids to form an insoluble complex that is eliminated in feces; it thereby increases the fecal loss of bile acid-bound low density lipoprotein cholesterol

Pharmacodynamics/Kinetics Absorption: Oral: Not absorbed

Usual Dosage Adults: Oral: 5-30 g/day in divided doses 2-4 times/day

Administration Dry powder should be added to at least 90 mL of liquid and stirred until completely mixed; other drugs should be administered at least 1 hour before or 4 hours after colestipol

Test Interactions ↑ prothrombin time (S); ↓ cholesterol (S)

Patient Information Take in water or fruit juice (~90 mL) or sprinkled on food; other drugs should not be taken at least 1 hour before or 4 hours after colestipol; rinse glass with small amount of liquid to ensure full dose is taken

Dosage Forms

Granules, as hydrochloride: 5 g packet, 300 g, 500 g

Tablet, as hydrochloride: 1 g

Colestipol Hydrochloride *see* Colestipol *on previous page*

Colfosceril Palmitate (kole FOS er il PALM i tate)

Brand Names Exosurf® Neonatal

Synonyms Dipalmitoylphosphatidylcholine; DPPC; Synthetic Lung Surfactant

Therapeutic Category Lung Surfactant

Use Neonatal respiratory distress syndrome:

Prophylactic therapy: Body weight <1350 g in infants at risk for developing RDS; body weight >1350 g in infants with evidence of pulmonary immaturity

Rescue therapy: Treatment of infants with RDS based on respiratory distress not attributable to any other causes and chest radiographic findings consistent with RDS

Warnings/Precautions Pulmonary hemorrhaging may occur especially in infants <700 g. Mucous plugs may have formed in the endotracheal tube in those infants whose ventilation was markedly impaired during or shortly after dosing. If chest expansion improves substantially, the ventilator PIP setting should be reduced immediately. Hyperoxia and hypocarbia (hypocarbia can decrease blood flow to the brain) may occur requiring appropriate ventilator adjustments.

Adverse Reactions

1% to 10%: Respiratory: Pulmonary hemorrhage, apnea, mucous plugging, decrease in transcutaneous O_2 of >20%

Stability Reconstituted suspension should be used immediately and unused portion discarded; store at room temperature of 15°C to 30°C (59°F to 86°F); do not refrigerate

Mechanism of Action Replaces deficient or ineffective endogenous lung surfactant in neonates with respiratory distress syndrome (RDS) or in neonates at risk of developing RDS; reduces surface tension and stabilizes the alveoli from collapsing

Pharmacodynamics/Kinetics

Absorption: Intratracheal: Absorbed from the alveolus

Metabolism: Catabolized and reutilized for further synthesis and secretion in lung tissue

Usual Dosage For intratracheal use only. Neonates:

Prophylactic treatment: Administer 5 mL/kg (as two 2.5 mL/kg half-doses) as soon as possible; the second and third doses should be administered at 12 and 24 hours later to those infants remaining on ventilators

Rescue treatment: Administer 5 mL/kg (as two 2.5 mL/kg half-doses) as soon as the diagnosis of RDS is made; the second 5 mL/kg (as two 2.5 mL/kg half-doses) dose should be administered 12 hours later

Administration For intratracheal administration only. Suction infant prior to administration; inspect solution to verify complete mixing of the suspension. Administer via sideport on the special ETT adapter without interrupting mechanical ventilation. Administer the dose in two 2.5 mL/kg aliquots. Each half-dose is instilled slowly over 1-2 minutes in small bursts with each inspiration. After the first 2.5 mL/kg dose, turn the infant's head and torso 45° to the right for 30 seconds, then return to the midline position and administer the second dose as above. Following the second dose, turn the infant's head and torso 45° to the left for 30 seconds and return the infant to the midline position.

Monitoring Parameters Continuous EKG and transcutaneous O_2 saturation should be monitored during administration; frequent ABG sampling is necessary to prevent post-dosing hyperoxia and hypocarbia

Dosage Forms Powder for injection, lyophilized: 108 mg (10 mL)

Collagen *see* Microfibrillar Collagen Hemostat *on page 836*

Collagenase (KOL la je nase)

Brand Names Biozyme-C®; Santyl®

Therapeutic Category Enzyme, Topical Debridement

Use Promotes debridement of necrotic tissue in dermal ulcers and severe burns

Pregnancy Risk Factor C

Contraindications Known hypersensitivity to collagenase

Warnings/Precautions For external use only; avoid contact with eyes; monitor debilitated patients for systemic bacterial infections because debriding enzymes may increase the risk of bacteremia

Adverse Reactions

1% to 10%: Local: Irritation

<1%: Local: Pain and burning may occur at site of application

Overdosage/Toxicology Action of enzyme may be stopped by applying Burow's solution

Drug Interactions Decreased effect: Enzymatic activity is inhibited by detergents, benzalkonium chloride, hexachlorophene, nitrofurazone, tincture of iodine, and heavy metal ions (silver and mercury)

Mechanism of Action Collagenase is an enzyme derived from the fermentation of *Clostridium histolyticum* and differs from other proteolytic enzymes in that its enzymatic action has a high specificity for native and denatured collagen. Collagenase will not attack collagen in healthy tissue or newly formed granulation tissue. In addition, it does not act on fat, fibrin, keratin, or muscle.

Usual Dosage Topical: Apply once daily (or more frequently if the dressing becomes soiled)

Nursing Implications Do not introduce into major body cavities; monitor debilitated patients for systemic bacterial infections

Dosage Forms Ointment, topical: 250 units/g (15 g, 30 g)

Collyrium Fresh® [OTC] *see* Tetrahydrozoline *on page 1205*

Colovage® *see* Polyethylene Glycol-Electrolyte Solution *on page 1017*

CoLyte® *see* Polyethylene Glycol-Electrolyte Solution *on page 1017*

Comfort® [OTC] *see* Naphazoline *on page 879*

Comparative Pharmacokinetic Properties of Antiarrhythmic Agents *see page 1391*

Compazine® *see* Prochlorperazine *on page 1051*

Compound E *see* Cortisone Acetate *on next page*

Compound F *see* Hydrocortisone *on page 623*

Compound S *see* Zidovudine *on page 1320*

Compound W® [OTC] *see* Salicylic Acid *on page 1120*
Compoz® Gel Caps [OTC] *see* Diphenhydramine *on page 399*
Compoz® Nighttime Sleep Aid [OTC] *see* Diphenhydramine *on page 399*
Constant-T® *see* Theophylline Salts *on page 1207*
Constilac® *see* Lactulose *on page 703*
Constulose® *see* Lactulose *on page 703*
Contac® Cough Formula Liquid [OTC] *see* Guaifenesin and Dextromethorphan *on page 591*
Control® [OTC] *see* Phenylpropanolamine *on page 991*
Convulsive Status Epilepticus *see page 1528*
Copaxone® *see* Glatiramer Acetate *on page 574*
Cophene-B® *see* Brompheniramine *on page 166*
Copolymer-1 *see* Glatiramer Acetate *on page 574*
Cordarone® *see* Amiodarone *on page 67*
Cordran® *see* Flurandrenolide *on page 545*
Cordran® SP *see* Flurandrenolide *on page 545*
Coreg® *see* Carvedilol *on page 213*
Corgard® *see* Nadolol *on page 868*
CortaGel® [OTC] *see* Hydrocortisone *on page 623*
Cortaid® Maximum Strength [OTC] *see* Hydrocortisone *on page 623*
Cortaid® with Aloe [OTC] *see* Hydrocortisone *on page 623*
Cortatrigen® Otic *see* Neomycin, Polymyxin B, and Hydrocortisone *on page 890*
Cort-Dome® *see* Hydrocortisone *on page 623*
Cortef® *see* Hydrocortisone *on page 623*
Cortef® Feminine Itch [OTC] *see* Hydrocortisone *on page 623*
Cortenema® *see* Hydrocortisone *on page 623*
Corticaine® [OTC] *see* Hydrocortisone *on page 623*
Corticosteroids Comparison *see page 1407*
Cortisol *see* Hydrocortisone *on page 623*

Cortisone Acetate (KOR ti sone AS e tate)

Related Information
Corticosteroids Comparison *on page 1407*

Brand Names Cortone® Acetate

Synonyms Compound E

Therapeutic Category Anti-inflammatory Agent; Corticosteroid; Corticosteroid, Adrenal; Corticosteroid, Systemic; Diagnostic Agent, Adrenocortical Insufficiency; Glucocorticoid; Mineralocorticoid

Use Management of adrenocortical insufficiency

Pregnancy Risk Factor D

Contraindications Serious infections, except septic shock or tuberculous meningitis, idiopathic thrombocytopenia purpura (I.M. use), administration of live virus vaccines

Warnings/Precautions Use with caution in patients with hypothyroidism, cirrhosis, hypertension, congestive heart failure, ulcerative colitis, thromboembolic disorders, osteoporosis, convulsive disorders, peptic ulcer, diabetes mellitus, myasthenia gravis; prolonged therapy (>5 days) of pharmacologic doses of corticosteroids may lead to hypothalamic-pituitary-adrenal suppression, the degree of adrenal suppression varies with the degree and duration of glucocorticoid therapy; this must be taken into consideration when taking patients off steroids

Adverse Reactions

>10%:
- Central nervous system: Insomnia, nervousness
- Gastrointestinal: Increased appetite, indigestion

1% to 10%:
- Dermatologic: Hirsutism
- Endocrine & metabolic: Diabetes mellitus
- Neuromuscular & skeletal: Arthralgia
- Ocular: Cataracts, glaucoma
- Respiratory: Epistaxis

<1%:
- Cardiovascular: Edema, hypertension
- Central nervous system: Vertigo, seizures, headache, psychoses, pseudotumor cerebri, mood swings, delirium, hallucinations, euphoria
- Dermatologic: Acne, skin atrophy, bruising, hyperpigmentation
- Endocrine & metabolic: Cushing's syndrome, pituitary-adrenal axis suppression, growth suppression, glucose intolerance, hypokalemia, alkalosis, amenorrhea, sodium and water retention, hyperglycemia

Gastrointestinal: Peptic ulcer, nausea, vomiting, abdominal distention, ulcerative esophagitis, pancreatitis

Neuromuscular & skeletal: Myalgia, osteoporosis, fractures, muscle wasting

Miscellaneous: Hypersensitivity reactions

Overdosage/Toxicology When consumed in excessive quantities for prolonged periods, systemic hypercorticism and adrenal suppression may occur; in those cases, discontinuation and withdrawal of the corticosteroid should be done judiciously. Cushingoid changes from continued administration of large doses results in moonface, central obesity, striae, hirsutism, acne, ecchymoses, hypertension, osteoporosis, myopathy, sexual dysfunction, diabetes, hyperlipidemia, peptic ulcer, increased susceptibility to infection and electrolyte and fluid imbalance.

Drug Interactions

Inducer of cytochrome P-450 enzymes

Cytochrome P-450 3A enzyme substrate

Decreased effect:

- Barbiturates, phenytoin, rifampin may decrease cortisone effects
- Live virus vaccines, diuretics (potassium depleting)
- Anticholinesterase agents may decrease effect
- Cortisone may decrease warfarin effects
- Cortisone may decrease effects of salicylates

Increased effect:

- Estrogens (increase cortisone effects)

Increased toxicity:

- Cortisone + NSAIDs may increase ulcerogenic potential
- Cortisone may increase potassium deletion due to diuretics

Mechanism of Action Decreases inflammation by suppression of migration of polymorphonuclear leukocytes and reversal of increased capillary permeability

Pharmacodynamics/Kinetics

Peak effect:

- Oral: Within 2 hours
- I.M.: Within 20-48 hours

Duration of action: 30-36 hours

Absorption: Slow rate of absorption

Distribution: Crosses the placenta; appears in breast milk; distributes to muscles, liver, skin, intestines, and kidneys

Metabolism: In the liver to inactive metabolites

Half-life: 30 minutes to 2 hours

- End stage renal disease: 3.5 hours

Elimination: In bile and urine

Note: Insoluble in water; supplemental doses may be warranted during times of stress in the course of withdrawing therapy

Usual Dosage If possible, administer glucocorticoids before 9 AM to minimize adrenocortical suppression; dosing depends upon the condition being treated and the response of the patient; supplemental doses may be warranted during times of stress in the course of withdrawing therapy

Children:

- Anti-inflammatory or immunosuppressive:
  - Oral: 2.5-10 mg/kg/day **OR** 20-300 mg/m ^{2}/day in divided doses every 6-8 hours
  - I.M.: 1-5 mg/kg/day **OR** 14-375 mg/m^2/day in divided doses every 12-24 hours
- Physiologic replacement:
  - Oral: 0.5-0.75 mg/kg/day **OR** 20-25 mg/m^2/day in divided doses every 8 hours
  - I.M.: 0.25-0.35 mg/kg/day once daily **OR** 12.5 mg/m^2/day
- Stress coverage for surgery: I.M.: 1 and 2 days before preanesthesia, and 1-3 days after surgery: 50-62.5 mg/m^2/day; 4 days after surgery: 31-50 mg/m^2/day; 5 days after surgery, resume presurgical corticosteroid dose.

Adults: Oral, I.M.: 25-300 mg/day in divided doses every 12-24 hours

Hemodialysis: Supplemental dose is not necessary

Peritoneal dialysis: Supplemental dose is not necessary

Administration Administer I.M. daily dose before 9 AM to minimize adrenocortical suppression

Patient Information Take with meals or take with food or milk; do not discontinue drug without notifying physician

Nursing Implications I.M. use only; shake vial before measuring out dose; withdraw gradually following long-term therapy

Additional Information Insoluble in water

Dosage Forms

Injection: 50 mg/mL (10 mL)

Tablet: 5 mg, 10 mg, 25 mg

Cortisporin® Ophthalmic Ointment *see* Bacitracin, Neomycin, Polymyxin B, and Hydrocortisone *on page 130*

Cortisporin® Ophthalmic Suspension *see* Neomycin, Polymyxin B, and Hydrocortisone *on page 890*

Cortisporin® Otic *see* Neomycin, Polymyxin B, and Hydrocortisone *on page 890*

Cortisporin® Topical Cream *see* Neomycin, Polymyxin B, and Hydrocortisone *on page 890*

Cortisporin® Topical Ointment *see* Bacitracin, Neomycin, Polymyxin B, and Hydrocortisone *on page 130*

Cortizone®-5 [OTC] *see* Hydrocortisone *on page 623*

Cortizone®-10 [OTC] *see* Hydrocortisone *on page 623*

Cortone® Acetate *see* Cortisone Acetate *on page 312*

Cortrosyn® *see* Cosyntropin *on this page*

Corvert® *see* Ibutilide *on page 641*

Cosmegen® *see* Dactinomycin *on page 337*

Cosyntropin (koe sin TROE pin)

Brand Names Cortrosyn®

Synonyms Synacthen; Tetracosactide

Therapeutic Category Diagnostic Agent, Adrenocortical Insufficiency

Use Diagnostic test to differentiate primary adrenal from secondary (pituitary) adrenocortical insufficiency

Pregnancy Risk Factor C

Contraindications Known hypersensitivity to cosyntropin

Warnings/Precautions Use with caution in patients with pre-existing allergic disease or a history of allergic reactions to corticotropin

Adverse Reactions

1% to 10%:

- Cardiovascular: Flushing
- Central nervous system: Mild fever
- Dermatologic: Pruritus
- Gastrointestinal: Chronic pancreatitis

<1%: Miscellaneous: Hypersensitivity reactions

Stability Reconstitute with NS

Stability of parenteral admixture at room temperature (25°C): 24 hours

Stability of parenteral admixture at refrigeration temperature (4°C): 21 days

I.V. infusion in NS or D_5W is stable 12 hours at room temperature

Mechanism of Action Stimulates the adrenal cortex to secrete adrenal steroids (including hydrocortisone, cortisone), androgenic substances, and a small amount of aldosterone

Pharmacodynamics/Kinetics

Distribution: Crosses the placenta

Metabolism: Unknown

Time to peak serum concentration: Within 1 hour (plasma cortisol levels rise in healthy individuals within 5 minutes of administration I.M. or I.V. push)

Usual Dosage

Adrenocortical insufficiency: I.M., I.V. (over 2 minutes): Peak plasma cortisol concentrations usually occur 45-60 minutes after cosyntropin administration

- Children <2 years: 0.125 mg
- Children >2 years and Adults: 0.25 mg
- When greater cortisol stimulation is needed, an I.V. infusion may be used:
  - Children >2 years and Adults: 0.25 mg administered at 0.04 mg/hour over 6 hours

Congenital adrenal hyperplasia evaluation: 1 mg/m^2/dose up to a maximum of 1 mg

Reference Range Normal baseline cortisol; increase in serum cortisol after cosyntropin injection of >7 mcg/dL or peak response >18 mcg/dL; plasma cortisol concentrations should be measured immediately before and exactly 30 minutes after a dose

Test Interactions Decreased effect: Spironolactone, hydrocortisone, cortisone

Nursing Implications Patient should not receive corticosteroids or spironolactone the day prior and the day of the test

Additional Information Each 0.25 mg of cosyntropin is equivalent to 25 units of corticotropin

Dosage Forms Powder for injection: 0.25 mg

Cotazym® *see* Pancrelipase *on page 949*

Cotazym-S® *see* Pancrelipase *on page 949*

Cotrim® *see* Co-Trimoxazole *on next page*

Cotrim® DS *see* Co-Trimoxazole *on next page*

Co-Trimoxazole (koe trye MOKS a zole)

Related Information

Animal and Human Bites Guidelines *on page 1463*
Antimicrobial Drugs of Choice *on page 1468*
Bacterial Meningitis Practical Guidelines for Management *on page 1475*
Guidelines for the Prevention of Opportunistic Infections in Persons with HIV *on page 1457*

Brand Names Bactrim™; Bactrim™ DS; Cotrim®; Cotrim® DS; Septra®; Septra® DS; Sulfatrim®

Canadian/Mexican Brand Names Apo-Sulfatrim® (Canada); Novo-Trimel® (Canada); Nu-Cotrimox® (Canada); Pro-Trin® (Canada); Roubac® (Canada); Trisulfa® (Canada); Trisulfa-S® (Canada); Anitrim® (Mexico); Bactelan® (Mexico); Batrizol® (Mexico); Ectaprim® (Mexico); Ectaprim-F® (Mexico); Enterobacticel® (Mexico); Esteprim® (Mexico); Isobac® (Mexico); Kelfiprim® (Mexico); Metoxiprim® (Mexico); Syraprim® (Mexico); Trimesuxol® (Mexico); Trimetoger® (Mexico); Trimetox® (Mexico); Trimzol® (Mexico)

Synonyms SMX-TMP; SMZ-TMP; Sulfamethoxazole and Trimethoprim; TMP-SMX; TMP-SMZ; Trimethoprim and Sulfamethoxazole

Therapeutic Category Antibiotic, Sulfonamide Derivative

Use

Oral treatment of urinary tract infections due to *E. coli, Klebsiella* and *Enterobacter sp, M. morganii, P. mirabilis* and *P, vulgaris*; acute otitis media in children and acute exacerbations of chronic bronchitis in adults due to susceptible strains of *H. influenzae* or *S. pneumoniae*; prophylaxis of *Pneumocystis carinii* pneumonitis (PCP), traveler's diarrhea due to enterotoxigenic *E. coli* or *Cyclospora*

I.V. treatment or severe or complicated infections when oral therapy is not feasible, for documented PCP, empiric treatment of PCP in immune compromised patients; treatment of documented or suspected shigellosis, typhoid fever, *Nocardia asteroides* infection, or other infections caused by susceptible bacteria

Unlabeled use: Cholera and salmonella-type infections and nocardiosis; chronic prostatitis; as prophylaxis in neutropenic patients with *P. carinii* infections, in leukemics, and in patients following renal transplantation, to decrease incidence of g(-) rod infections

Pregnancy Risk Factor C

Contraindications Hypersensitivity to any sulfa drug or any component; porphyria; megaloblastic anemia due to folate deficiency; infants <2 months of age

Warnings/Precautions Use with caution in patients with G-6-PD deficiency, impaired renal or hepatic function; adjust dosage in patients with renal impairment; injection vehicle contains benzyl alcohol and sodium metabisulfite; fatalities associated with severe reactions including Stevens-Johnson syndrome, toxic epidermal necrolysis, hepatic necrosis, agranulocytosis, aplastic anemia and other blood dyscrasias; discontinue use at first sign of rash; elderly patients appear at greater risk for more severe adverse reactions

Adverse Reactions

>10%:
- Dermatologic: Allergic skin reactions including rashes and urticaria, photosensitivity
- Gastrointestinal: Nausea, vomiting, anorexia

1% to 10%:
- Dermatologic: Stevens-Johnson syndrome, toxic epidermal necrolysis
- Hematologic: Blood dyscrasias
- Hepatic: Hepatitis

<1%:
- Central nervous system: Confusion, depression, hallucinations, seizures, fever, ataxia, kernicterus in neonates
- Dermatologic: Erythema multiforme
- Gastrointestinal: Stomatitis, diarrhea, pseudomembranous colitis
- Hematologic: Thrombocytopenia, megaloblastic anemia, granulocytopenia, aplastic anemia, hemolysis (with G-6-PD deficiency)
- Hepatic: Hepatitis
- Renal: Interstitial nephritis
- Miscellaneous: Serum sickness

Overdosage/Toxicology Symptoms of overdose include nausea, vomiting, GI distress, hematuria, crystalluria

Following GI decontamination, treatment is supportive; adequate fluid intake is essential; peritoneal dialysis is not effective and hemodialysis only moderately effective in removing co-trimoxazole

Drug Interactions Co-trimoxazole causes:

Decreased effect: Cyclosporines

(Continued)

Co-Trimoxazole *(Continued)*

Increased effect: Sulfonylureas and oral anticoagulants

Increased toxicity: Phenytoin, cyclosporines (nephrotoxicity), methotrexate (displaced from binding sites)

Stability Do not refrigerate injection; is less soluble in more alkaline pH; protect from light; do not use NS as a diluent; injection vehicle contains benzyl alcohol and sodium metabisulfite

Stability of parenteral admixture at room temperature (25°C):

5 mL/125 mL D_5W = 6 hours
5 mL/100 mL D_5W = 4 hours
5 mL/75 mL D_5W = 2 hours

Mechanism of Action Sulfamethoxazole interferes with bacterial folic acid synthesis and growth via inhibition of dihydrofolic acid formation from para-aminobenzoic acid; trimethoprim inhibits dihydrofolic acid reduction to tetrahydrofolate resulting in sequential inhibition of enzymes of the folic acid pathway

Pharmacodynamics/Kinetics

Absorption: Oral: 90% to 100%

Distribution: Crosses the placenta; distributes into breast milk

Protein binding:

SMX: 68%
TMP: 68%

Metabolism:

SMX is N-acetylated and glucuronidated
TMP is metabolized to oxide and hydroxylated metabolites

Half-life:

SMX: 9 hours
TMP: 6-17 hours, both are prolonged in renal failure

Time to peak serum concentration: Within 1-4 hours

Elimination: In urine as metabolites and unchanged drug

Usual Dosage Dosage recommendations are based on the trimethoprim component

Children >2 months:

Mild to moderate infections: Oral, I.V.: 8 mg TMP/kg/day in divided doses every 12 hours

Serious infection/*Pneumocystis*: I.V.: 20 mg TMP/kg/day in divided doses every 6 hours

Urinary tract infection prophylaxis: Oral: 2 mg TMP/kg/dose daily

Prophylaxis of *Pneumocystis*: Oral, I.V.: 10 mg TMP/kg/day or 150 mg TMP/m^2/day in divided doses every 12 hours for 3 days/week; dose should not exceed 320 mg trimethoprim and 1600 mg sulfamethoxazole 3 days/week

Adults:

Urinary tract infection/chronic bronchitis: Oral: 1 double strength tablet every 12 hours for 10-14 days

Sepsis: I.V.: 20 TMP/kg/day divided every 6 hours

Pneumocystis carinii:

Prophylaxis: Oral, I.V.: 10 mg TMP/kg/day divided every 12 hours for 3 days/week

Treatment: I.V.: 20 mg TMP/kg/day divided every 6 hours

Dosing interval/adjustment in renal impairment:

Cl_{cr} 30-50 mL/minute: Administer every 12-18 hours or reduce dose by 25%
Cl_{cr} 15-30 mL/minute: Administer every 18-24 hours or reduce dose by 50%
Cl_{cr} <15 mL/minute: Not recommended

Administration Infuse over 60-90 minutes, must dilute well before giving; may be given less diluted in a central line; not for I.M. injection; maintain adequate fluid intake to prevent crystalluria; administer around-the-clock every 6-12 hours

Test Interactions ↑ creatinine (Jaffé alkaline picrate reaction); increased serum methotrexate by dihydrofolate reductase method; does not interfere with RAI method

Patient Information Take oral medication with 8 oz of water on an empty stomach (1 hour before or 2 hours after meals) for best absorption; report any skin rashes immediately; finish all medication, do not skip doses

Dosage Forms The 5:1 ratio (SMX to TMP) remains constant in all dosage forms:

Injection: Sulfamethoxazole 80 mg and trimethoprim 16 mg per mL (5 mL, 10 mL, 20 mL, 30 mL, 50 mL)

Suspension, oral: Sulfamethoxazole 200 mg and trimethoprim 40 mg per 5 mL (20 mL, 100 mL, 150 mL, 200 mL, 480 mL)

Tablet: Sulfamethoxazole 400 mg and trimethoprim 80 mg

Tablet, double strength: Sulfamethoxazole 800 mg and trimethoprim 160 mg

Coumadin® *see* Warfarin *on page 1312*

Covera-HS® *see* Verapamil *on page 1297*

Cozaar® *see* Losartan *on page 744*

CPM *see* Cyclophosphamide *on page 323*

CPT-11 *see* Irinotecan *on page 673*

Creon 10® *see* Pancrelipase *on page 949*

Creon 20® *see* Pancrelipase *on page 949*

Crixivan® *see* Indinavir *on page 655*

Crolom® Ophthalmic Solution *see* Cromolyn Sodium *on this page*

Cromoglycic Acid *see* Cromolyn Sodium *on this page*

Cromolyn Sodium (KROE moe lin SOW dee um)

Related Information

Asthma, Guidelines for the Diagnosis and Management of *on page 1518*

Estimated Clinical Comparability of Doses for Inhaled Corticosteroids *on page 1522*

Brand Names Crolom® Ophthalmic Solution; Gastrocrom® Oral; Intal® Inhalation Capsule; Intal® Nebulizer Solution; Intal® Oral Inhaler; Nasalcrom® Nasal Solution [OTC]

Canadian/Mexican Brand Names Novo-Cromolyn® (Canada); Opticrom® (Canada); PMS-Sodium Cromoglycate (Canada); Rynacrom® (Canada)

Synonyms Cromoglycic Acid; Disodium Cromoglycate; DSCG

Therapeutic Category Antiallergic, Inhalation; Antiallergic, Ophthalmic

Use Adjunct in the prophylaxis of allergic disorders, including rhinitis, giant papillary conjunctivitis, and asthma; inhalation product may be used for prevention of exercise-induced bronchospasm; systemic mastocytosis, food allergy, and treatment of inflammatory bowel disease; **cromolyn is a prophylactic drug with no benefit for acute situations**

Pregnancy Risk Factor B

Pregnancy/Breast-Feeding Implications

Clinical effects on the fetus: No data on whether cromolyn crosses the placenta or clinical effects on the fetus. Available evidence suggests safe use during pregnancy.

Breast-feeding/lactation: No data on whether cromolyn crosses into breast milk or clinical effects on the infant

Contraindications Hypersensitivity to cromolyn or any component; acute asthma attacks

Warnings/Precautions Severe anaphylactic reactions may occur rarely; cromolyn is a prophylactic drug with no benefit for acute situations; do not use in patients with severe renal or hepatic impairment; caution should be used when withdrawing the drug or tapering the dose as symptoms may reoccur; use with caution in patients with a history of cardiac arrhythmias

Adverse Reactions

>10%:

- Gastrointestinal: Unpleasant taste (inhalation aerosol)
- Respiratory: Hoarseness, coughing

1% to 10%:

- Dermatologic: Angioedema
- Gastrointestinal: Xerostomia
- Genitourinary: Dysuria
- Respiratory: Sneezing, nasal congestion

<1%:

- Central nervous system: Dizziness, headache
- Dermatologic: Rash, urticaria
- Gastrointestinal: Nausea, vomiting, diarrhea
- Neuromuscular & skeletal: Arthralgia
- Ocular: Ocular stinging, lacrimation
- Respiratory: Wheezing, throat irritation, eosinophilic pneumonia, pulmonary infiltrates, nasal burning
- Miscellaneous: Anaphylactic reactions

Overdosage/Toxicology Symptoms of overdose include bronchospasm, laryngeal edema, dysuria

Stability Nebulizer solution is **compatible** with metaproterenol sulfate, isoproterenol hydrochloride, 0.25% isoetharine hydrochloride, epinephrine hydrochloride, terbutaline sulfate, and 20% acetylcysteine solution for at least 1 hour after their admixture; store nebulizer solution protected from direct light

Mechanism of Action Prevents the mast cell release of histamine, leukotrienes and slow-reacting substance of anaphylaxis by inhibiting degranulation after contact with antigens

Pharmacodynamics/Kinetics

Absorption:

- Inhalation: ~8% of dose reaches the lungs upon inhalation of the powder and is well absorbed
- Oral: Only 0.5% to 2% of dose absorbed

Half-life: 80-90 minutes

(Continued)

Cromolyn Sodium *(Continued)*

Time to peak serum concentration: Inhalation: Within 15 minutes

Elimination: Absorbed cromolyn is equally excreted unchanged in the urine and the feces (via bile); small amounts are exhaled

Usual Dosage Not effective for immediate relief of symptoms in acute asthmatic attacks; must be used at regular intervals for 2-4 weeks to be effective

Children:

Inhalation (taper frequency to the lowest effective dose, ie, qid → tid → bid):

Initial dose: Metered spray: >5 years: 2 inhalations 4 times/day by metered spray

Initial dose: Nebulization solution: >2 years: 20 mg 4 times/day

Prevention of exercise-induced bronchospasm: Metered spray: >5 years: Single dose of 2 inhalations (aerosol) just prior to (10 minutes to 1 hour) exercise

Nasal: >6 years: Instill 1 spray in each nostril 3-4 times/day

Infants ≤2 years: Oral: 20 mg/kg/day in 4 divided doses, not to exceed 30 mg/kg/day

Children 2-12 years: Oral: 100 mg 4 times/day 15-20 minutes before meals, not to exceed 40 mg/kg/day

Children >12 years and Adults: Oral: 200 mg 4 times/day 15-20 minutes before meal, up to 400 mg 4 times/day

Adults:

Inhalation: Metered spray: 2 inhalations 4 times/day

Nasal: Instill 1 spray in each nostril 3-4 times/day

Ophthalmic: Instill 1-2 drops 4-6 times/day into each eye

Monitoring Parameters Periodic pulmonary function tests

Patient Information Do not discontinue abruptly; not effective for acute relief of symptoms; must be taken on a regularly scheduled basis; do not mix oral capsule with fruit juice, milk, or foods

Nursing Implications Advise patient to clear as much mucus as possible before inhalation treatments

Dosage Forms

Capsule, oral (Gastrocrom®): 100 mg

Inhalation, oral (Intal®): 800 mcg/spray (8.1 g)

Solution, for nebulization:

10 mg/mL (2 mL)

Intal®: 10 mg/mL (2 mL)

Solution, nasal (Nasalcrom®): 40 mg/mL (13 mL)

Solution, ophthalmic (Crolom®): 4% (2.5 mL, 10 mL)

Crotamiton (kroe TAM i tonn)

Brand Names Eurax®

Therapeutic Category Scabicidal Agent

Use Treatment of scabies (*Sarcoptes scabiei*) and symptomatic treatment of pruritus

Pregnancy Risk Factor C

Contraindications Hypersensitivity to crotamiton or other components; patients who manifest a primary irritation response to topical medications

Warnings/Precautions Avoid contact with face, eyes, mucous membranes, and urethral meatus; do not apply to acutely inflamed or raw skin; for external use only

Adverse Reactions <1%:

Local: Irritation

Dermatologic: Pruritus, contact dermatitis, warm sensation

Overdosage/Toxicology Symptoms of ingestion include burning sensation in mouth, irritation of the buccal, esophageal and gastric mucosa, nausea, vomiting and abdominal pain

There is no specific antidote; general measures to eliminate the drug and reduce its absorption, combined with symptomatic treatment, are recommended

Mechanism of Action Crotamiton has scabicidal activity against *Sarcoptes scabiei*; mechanism of action unknown

Usual Dosage Topical:

Scabicide: Children and Adults: Wash thoroughly and scrub away loose scales, then towel dry; apply a thin layer and massage drug onto skin of the entire body from the neck to the toes (with special attention to skin folds, creases, and interdigital spaces). Repeat application in 24 hours. Take a cleansing bath 48 hours after the final application. Treatment may be repeated after 7-10 days if live mites are still present.

Pruritus: Massage into affected areas until medication is completely absorbed; repeat as necessary

Patient Information For topical use only; all contaminated clothing and bed linen should be washed to avoid reinfestation

Nursing Implications Lotion: Shake well before using; avoid contact with face, eyes, mucous membranes, and urethral meatus

Dosage Forms

Cream: 10% (60 g)

Lotion: 10% (60 mL, 454 mL)

Crystalline Penicillin *see* Penicillin G, Parenteral, Aqueous *on page 962*

Crystamine® *see* Cyanocobalamin *on this page*

Crysticillin® A.S. *see* Penicillin G Procaine *on page 964*

Crystodigin® *see* Digitoxin *on page 384*

CsA *see* Cyclosporine *on page 327*

CTM *see* Chlorpheniramine *on page 260*

C/T/S® Topical Solution *see* Clindamycin *on page 289*

CTX *see* Cyclophosphamide *on page 323*

Cuprid® *see* Trientine *on page 1260*

Cuprimine® *see* Penicillamine *on page 959*

Curretab® *see* Medroxyprogesterone Acetate *on page 771*

Cutivate™ *see* Fluticasone *on page 549*

CyA *see* Cyclosporine *on page 327*

Cyanocobalamin (sye an oh koe BAL a min)

Brand Names Berubigen®; Cobex®; Crystamine®; Cyanoject®; Cyomin®; Ener-B® [OTC]; Kaybovite-1000®; Redisol®; Rubramin-PC®; Sytobex®

Canadian/Mexican Brand Names Rubramin® (Canada)

Synonyms Vitamin B_{12}

Therapeutic Category Vitamin, Water Soluble

Use Treatment of pernicious anemia; vitamin B_{12} deficiency; increased B_{12} requirements due to pregnancy, thyrotoxicosis, hemorrhage, malignancy, liver or kidney disease

Pregnancy Risk Factor A (C if dose exceeds RDA recommendation)

Contraindications Hypersensitivity to cyanocobalamin or any component, cobalt; patients with hereditary optic nerve atrophy

Warnings/Precautions I.M. route used to treat pernicious anemia; vitamin B_{12} deficiency for >3 months results in irreversible degenerative CNS lesions; treatment of vitamin B_{12} megaloblastic anemia may result in severe hypokalemia, sometimes, fatal, when anemia corrects due to cellular potassium requirements. B_{12} deficiency masks signs of polycythemia vera; vegetarian diets may result in B_{12} deficiency; pernicious anemia occurs more often in gastric carcinoma than in general population.

Adverse Reactions

1% to 10%:

- Dermatologic: Itching
- Gastrointestinal: Diarrhea

<1%:

- Cardiovascular: Peripheral vascular thrombosis
- Dermatologic: Urticaria
- Miscellaneous: Anaphylaxis

Stability Clear pink to red solutions are stable at room temperature; protect from light; **incompatible** with chlorpromazine, phytonadione, prochlorperazine, warfarin, ascorbic acid, dextrose, heavy metals, oxidizing or reducing agents

Mechanism of Action Coenzyme for various metabolic functions, including fat and carbohydrate metabolism and protein synthesis, used in cell replication and hematopoiesis

Pharmacodynamics/Kinetics

Absorption: Absorbed from the terminal ileum in the presence of calcium; for absorption to occur gastric "intrinsic factor" must be present to transfer the compound across the intestinal mucosa

Distribution: Principally stored in the liver, also stored in the kidneys and adrenals

Protein binding: Bound to transcobalamin II

Metabolism: Converted in the tissues to active coenzymes methylcobalamin and deoxyadenosylcobalamin

Usual Dosage I.M. or deep S.C. (oral is not generally recommended due to poor absorption and I.V. is not recommended due to more rapid elimination):

Recommended daily allowance (RDA):

- Children: 0.3-2 mcg
- Adults: 2 mcg

Pernicious anemia, congenital (if evidence of neurologic involvement): 1000 mcg/day for at least 2 weeks; maintenance: 50 mcg/month

(Continued)

Cyanocobalamin *(Continued)*

Children: 30-50 mcg/day for 2 or more weeks (to a total dose of 1000-5000 mcg), then follow with 100 mcg/month as maintenance dosage

Adults: 100 mcg/day for 6-7 days; if improvement, administer same dose on alternate days for 7 doses; then every 3-4 days for 2-3 weeks; once hematologic values have returned to normal, maintenance dosage: 100 mcg/month. **Note:** Use only parenteral therapy as oral therapy is not dependable.

Vitamin B_{12} deficiency:

Children: 100 mcg/day for 10-15 days (total dose of 1-1.5 mg), then once or twice weekly for several months; may taper to 60 mcg every month

Adults: Initial: 30 mcg/day for 5-10 days; maintenance: 100-200 mcg/month

Administration I.M. or deep S.C. are preferred routes of administration

Monitoring Parameters Serum potassium, erythrocyte and reticulocyte count, hemoglobin, hematocrit

Reference Range Normal range of serum B_{12} is 150-750 pg/mL; this represents 0.1% of total body content. Metabolic requirements are 2-5 μg/day; years of deficiency required before hematologic and neurologic signs and symptoms are seen. Occasional patients with significant neuropsychiatric abnormalities may have no hematologic abnormalities and normal serum cobalamin levels, 200 pg/mL (SI: >150 pmol/L), or more commonly between 100-200 pg/mL (SI: 75-150 pmol/L). There exists evidence that people, particularly elderly whose serum cobalamin concentrations <300 pg/mL, should receive replacement parenteral therapy; this recommendation is based upon neuropsychiatric disorders and cardiovascular disorders associated with lower sodium cobalamin concentrations.

Test Interactions Methotrexate, pyrimethamine, and most antibiotics invalidate folic acid and vitamin B_{12} diagnostic microbiological blood assays

Patient Information Pernicious anemia will require monthly injections for life

Nursing Implications Oral therapy is markedly inferior to parenteral therapy; monitor potassium concentrations during early therapy

Dosage Forms

Gel, nasal (Ener-B®): 400 mcg/0.1 mL

Injection: 30 mcg/mL (30 mL); 100 mcg/mL (1 mL, 10 mL, 30 mL); 1000 mcg/mL (1 mL, 10 mL, 30 mL)

Tablet [OTC]: 25 mcg, 50 mcg, 100 mcg, 250 mcg, 500 mcg, 1000 mcg

Cyanoject® *see* Cyanocobalamin *on previous page*

Cyclan® *see* Cyclandelate *on this page*

Cyclandelate (sye KLAN de late)

Brand Names Cyclan®; Cyclospasmol®

Therapeutic Category Vasodilator, Peripheral

Use Considered as "possibly effective" for adjunctive therapy in peripheral vascular disease and possibly senility due to cerebrovascular disease or multi-infarct dementia; migraine prophylaxis, vertigo, tinnitus, and visual disturbances secondary to cerebrovascular insufficiency and diabetic peripheral polyneuropathy

Pregnancy Risk Factor C

Contraindications Hypersensitivity to cyclandelate or any component

Warnings/Precautions Use with caution in patients with severe obliterative coronary artery or cerebral vascular disease, in patients with active bleeding or a bleeding tendency, and patients with glaucoma

Adverse Reactions

<1%:

Cardiovascular: Flushing of face, tachycardia

Central nervous system: Headache, pain, dizziness; paresthesia in face, fingers, or toes

Gastrointestinal: Belching, heartburn

Neuromuscular & skeletal: Weakness

Overdosage/Toxicology Symptoms of overdose include drowsiness, weakness, respiratory depression, hypotension; treatment following decontamination is supportive; fluids followed by vasopressors are most helpful

Mechanism of Action Cyclandelate, 3,3,5-trimethylcyclohexyl mandelate is a vasodilator that exerts a direct, papaverine-like action on smooth muscles, particularly that found within the blood vessels. Animal data indicate that cyclandelate also has antispasmodic properties; exhibits no adrenergic stimulation or blocking action; action exceeds that of papaverine; mild calcium channel blocking agent, may benefit in mild hypercalcemia; calcium channel blocking activity may explain some of its pharmacologic effects (enhanced blood flow) and inhibition of platelet aggregation

Usual Dosage Adults: Oral: Initial: 1.2-1.6 g/day in divided doses before meals and at bedtime until response; maintenance therapy: 400-800 mg/day in 2-4

divided doses; start with lowest dose in elderly due to hypotensive potential; decrease dose by 200 mg decrements to achieve minimal maintenance dose; improvement can usually be seen over weeks of therapy and prolonged use; short courses of therapy are usually ineffective and not recommended

Administration Administer with meals

Patient Information Take medication with meals or antacids to decrease gastrointestinal side effects. **Note:** Use of antacids not recommended with reduced renal function (Cl_{cr} <30 mL/minute) or when bowel function may be adversely affected (eg, elderly).

Nursing Implications Observe for orthostatic hypotension

Dosage Forms

Capsule: 200 mg, 400 mg
Tablet: 200 mg, 400 mg

Cyclizine (SYE kli zeen)

Brand Names Marezine® [OTC]

Synonyms Cyclizine Hydrochloride; Cyclizine Lactate

Therapeutic Category Antiemetic; Antihistamine, H_1 Blocker

Use Prevention and treatment of nausea, vomiting, and vertigo associated with motion sickness; control of postoperative nausea and vomiting

Pregnancy Risk Factor B

Contraindications Hypersensitivity to cyclizine or any component

Warnings/Precautions Do not administer to premature or full-term neonates; young children may be more susceptible to side effects and CNS stimulation; bladder neck obstruction, symptomatic prostate hypertrophy, asthmatic attacks, and stenosing peptic ulcer

Adverse Reactions

>10%:
- Central nervous system: Drowsiness
- Gastrointestinal: Xerostomia

1% to 10%:
- Central nervous system: Headache
- Dermatologic: Dermatitis
- Gastrointestinal: Nausea
- Genitourinary: Urinary retention, polyuria
- Ocular: Diplopia

Overdosage/Toxicology Symptoms of overdose include dry mouth, flushed skin, dilated pupils, CNS depression

There is no specific treatment for an antihistamine overdose, however, most of its clinical toxicity is due to anticholinergic effects. For anticholinergic overdose with severe life-threatening symptoms, physostigmine 1-2 mg (0.5 or 0.02 mg/kg for children) I.V., slowly may be given to reverse these effects.

Drug Interactions Increased effect/toxicity with CNS depressants, alcohol

Stability I.M. formulation is **incompatible** when mixed in the same syringe with tetracyclines, methohexital, penicillin, pentobarbital, phenobarbital, secobarbital, thiopental

Mechanism of Action Cyclizine is a piperazine derivative with properties of histamines. The precise mechanism of action in inhibiting the symptoms of motion sickness is not known. It may have effects directly on the labyrinthine apparatus and central actions on the labyrinthine apparatus and on the chemoreceptor trigger zone. Cyclizine exerts a central anticholinergic action.

Usual Dosage

Children 6-12 years:
- Oral: 25 mg up to 3 times/day
- I.M.: Not recommended

Adults:
- Oral: 50 mg taken 30 minutes before departure, may repeat in 4-6 hours if needed, up to 200 mg/day
- I.M.: 50 mg every 4-6 hours as needed

Dietary Considerations Alcohol: Additive CNS effects, avoid use

Monitoring Parameters CNS effects or unusual movements

Patient Information May cause drowsiness, may impair judgment and coordination; avoid alcohol; drink plenty of fluids for dry mouth and to prevent constipation

Nursing Implications Raise bed rails, institute safety measures, assist with ambulation

Dosage Forms

Injection, as lactate: 50 mg/mL (1 mL)
Tablet, as hydrochloride: 50 mg

Cyclizine Hydrochloride *see* Cyclizine *on this page*

Cyclizine Lactate *see* Cyclizine *on this page*

Cyclobenzaprine (sye kloe BEN za preen)

Brand Names Flexeril®

Canadian/Mexican Brand Names Novo-Cycloprine® (Canada)

Synonyms Cyclobenzaprine Hydrochloride

Therapeutic Category Skeletal Muscle Relaxant

Use Treatment of muscle spasm associated with acute painful musculoskeletal conditions; supportive therapy in tetanus

Pregnancy Risk Factor B

Contraindications Hypersensitivity to cyclobenzaprine or any component; do not use concomitantly or within 14 days of MAO inhibitors; hyperthyroidism, congestive heart failure, arrhythmias

Warnings/Precautions Cyclobenzaprine shares the toxic potentials of the tricyclic antidepressants and the usual precautions of tricyclic antidepressant therapy should be observed; use with caution in patients with urinary hesitancy or angle-closure glaucoma

Adverse Reactions

>10%:

- Central nervous system: Drowsiness, dizziness, lightheadedness
- Gastrointestinal: Xerostomia

1% to 10%:

- Cardiovascular: Edema of the face/lips, syncope
- Gastrointestinal: Bloated feeling
- Genitourinary: Problems in urinating, polyuria
- Hepatic: Hepatitis
- Neuromuscular & skeletal: Problems in speaking, muscle weakness
- Ocular: Blurred vision
- Otic: Tinnitus

<1%:

- Cardiovascular: Tachycardia, hypotension, arrhythmia
- Central nervous system: Headache, fatigue, nervousness, confusion, ataxia
- Dermatologic: Rash, dermatitis
- Gastrointestinal: Dyspepsia, nausea, constipation, stomach cramps, unpleasant taste

Overdosage/Toxicology Symptoms of overdose include troubled breathing, drowsiness, syncope, seizures, tachycardia, hallucinations, vomiting

Following initiation of essential overdose management, toxic symptoms should be treated. Ventricular arrhythmias often respond to systemic alkalinization (sodium bicarbonate 0.5-2 mEq/kg I.V.) and/or phenytoin 15-20 mg/kg (adults). Arrhythmias unresponsive to this therapy may respond to lidocaine 1 mg/kg I.V. followed by a titrated infusion. Physostigmine (1-2 mg I.V. slowly for adults or 0.5 mg I.V. slowly for children) may be indicated in reversing cardiac arrhythmias that are life-threatening. Seizures usually respond to diazepam I.V. boluses (5-10 mg for adults up to 30 mg or 0.25-0.4 mg/kg/dose for children up to 10 mg/dose). If seizures are unresponsive or recur, phenytoin or phenobarbital may be required.

Drug Interactions Cytochrome P-450 1A2 enzyme substrate and cytochrome P-450 3A enzyme substrate

Increased toxicity:

- Do not use concomitantly or within 14 days after MAO inhibitors
- Because of similarities to the tricyclic antidepressants, may have additive toxicities
- Anticholinergics: Because of cyclobenzaprine's anticholinergic action, use with caution in patients receiving these agents
- Alcohol, barbiturates, and other CNS depressants: Effects may be enhanced by cyclobenzaprine

Mechanism of Action Centrally acting skeletal muscle relaxant pharmacologically related to tricyclic antidepressants; reduces tonic somatic motor activity influencing both alpha and gamma motor neurons

Pharmacodynamics/Kinetics

- Onset of action: Commonly occurs within 1 hour
- Absorption: Oral: Completely
- Metabolism: Hepatic; may undergo enterohepatic recycling
- Time to peak serum concentration: Within 3-8 hours
- Elimination: Renally as inactive metabolites and in feces (via bile) as unchanged drug

Usual Dosage Oral: **Note:** Do not use longer than 2-3 weeks

- Children: Dosage has not been established
- Adults: 20-40 mg/day in 2-4 divided doses; maximum dose: 60 mg/day

Patient Information Drug may impair ability to perform hazardous activities requiring mental alertness or physical coordination, such as operating machinery or driving a motor vehicle

Nursing Implications Raise bed rails, institute safety measures, assist with ambulation

Dosage Forms Tablet, as hydrochloride: 10 mg

Cyclobenzaprine Hydrochloride *see* Cyclobenzaprine *on previous page*

Cyclocort® *see* Amcinonide *on page 58*

Cyclogyl® *see* Cyclopentolate *on this page*

Cyclopentolate (sye kloe PEN toe late)

Related Information

Cycloplegic Mydriatics Comparison *on page 1409*

Brand Names AK-Pentolate®; Cyclogyl®; I-Pentolate®; Ocu-Pentolate®

Synonyms Cyclopentolate Hydrochloride

Therapeutic Category Anticholinergic Agent, Ophthalmic; Ophthalmic Agent, Mydriatic

Use Diagnostic procedures requiring mydriasis and cycloplegia

Pregnancy Risk Factor C

Contraindications Narrow-angle glaucoma, known hypersensitivity to drug

Warnings/Precautions 2% solution may result in psychotic reactions and behavioral disturbances in children, usually occurring approximately 30-45 minutes after instillation; use with caution in elderly patients and other patients who may be predisposed to increased intraocular pressure

Adverse Reactions

1% to 10%:

- Cardiovascular: Tachycardia
- Central nervous system: Restlessness, hallucinations, psychosis, hyperactivity, seizures, incoherent speech, ataxia
- Dermatologic: Burning sensation
- Ocular: Increase in intraocular pressure, loss of visual accommodation
- Miscellaneous: Allergic reaction

Overdosage/Toxicology Antidote, if needed, is pilocarpine

Drug Interactions Decreased effect of carbachol, cholinesterase inhibitors

Stability Store in tight containers

Mechanism of Action Prevents the muscle of the ciliary body and the sphincter muscle of the iris from responding to cholinergic stimulation, causing mydriasis and cycloplegia

Pharmacodynamics/Kinetics

Peak effect:

- Cycloplegia: 25-75 minutes
- Mydriasis: 30-60 minutes

Duration: Recovery takes up to 24 hours

Usual Dosage

Infants: Instill 1 drop of 0.5% into each eye 5-10 minutes before examination

Children: Instill 1 drop of 0.5%, 1%, or 2% in eye followed by 1 drop of 0.5% or 1% in 5 minutes, if necessary

Adults: Instill 1 drop of 1% followed by another drop in 5 minutes; 2% solution in heavily pigmented iris

Patient Information May cause blurred vision and increased sensitivity to light

Nursing Implications Finger pressure should be applied to lacrimal sac for 1-2 minutes after instillation to decrease risk of absorption and systemic reactions

Dosage Forms Solution, ophthalmic, as hydrochloride: 0.5% (2 mL, 5 mL, 15 mL); 1% (2 mL, 5 mL, 15 mL); 2% (2 mL, 5 mL, 15 mL)

Cyclopentolate Hydrochloride *see* Cyclopentolate *on this page*

Cyclophosphamide (sye kloe FOS fa mide)

Related Information

Antiemetics for Chemotherapy Induced Nausea and Vomiting *on page 1348*

Cancer Chemotherapy Regimens *on page 1351*

Toxicities of Chemotherapeutic Agents *on page 1382*

Brand Names Cytoxan®; Neosar®

Canadian/Mexican Brand Names Procytox® (Canada); Genoxal® (Mexico); Ledoxina® (Mexico)

Synonyms CPM; CTX; CYT

Therapeutic Category Antineoplastic Agent, Alkylating Agent

Use Treatment of Hodgkin's and non-Hodgkin's lymphoma, Burkitt's lymphoma, chronic lymphocytic leukemia, chronic granulocytic leukemia, AML, ALL, mycosis fungoides, breast cancer, multiple myeloma, neuroblastoma, retinoblastoma, rhabdomyosarcoma, Ewing's sarcoma; testicular, endometrium and ovarian, and lung cancer, and as a conditioning regimen for BMT; prophylaxis of rejection for kidney, heart, liver, and BMT transplants, severe rheumatoid disorders, nephrotic syndrome, Wegener's granulomatosis, idiopathic pulmonary hemosideroses, myasthenia gravis, multiple sclerosis, systemic lupus erythematosus, lupus nephritis, autoimmune hemolytic anemia, idiopathic thrombocytic purpura, macroglobulinemia, and antibody-induced pure red cell aplasia

(Continued)

Cyclophosphamide *(Continued)*

Pregnancy Risk Factor D

Contraindications Hypersensitivity to cyclophosphamide or any component

Warnings/Precautions The U.S. Food and Drug Administration (FDA) currently recommends that procedures for proper handling and disposal of antineoplastic agents be considered. Possible dosage adjustment needed for renal or hepatic failure; use with caution in patients with bone marrow suppression.

Adverse Reactions

>10%:

Dermatologic: Alopecia is frequent, but hair will regrow although it may be of a different color or texture; alopecia usually occurs 3 weeks after therapy

Endocrine & metabolic: Fertility: May cause sterility; interferes with oogenesis and spermatogenesis; may be irreversible in some patients; gonadal suppression (amenorrhea)

Gastrointestinal: Nausea and vomiting occur more frequently with larger doses, usually beginning 6-10 hours after administration; also seen are anorexia, diarrhea, stomatitis; mucositis

Emetic potential:

Oral: Low (<10%)

<1 g: Moderate (30% to 60%)

≥1 g: High (>90%)

Time course of nausea/vomiting: Onset: 6-8 hours; Duration: 8-24 hours

Hepatic: Jaundice seen occasionally

1% to 10%:

Central nervous system: Headache

Dermatologic: Skin rash, facial flushing

Hematologic: Myelosuppressive: Thrombocytopenia occurs less frequently than with mechlorethamine, anemia

WBC: Moderate

Platelets: Moderate

Onset (days): 7

Nadir (days): 10-14

Recovery (days): 21

<1%:

Cardiovascular: High-dose therapy may cause cardiac dysfunction manifested as congestive heart failure; cardiac necrosis or hemorrhagic myocarditis has occurred rarely, but is fatal. Cyclophosphamide may also potentiate the cardiac toxicity of anthracyclines.

Central nervous system: Dizziness

Dermatologic: Darkening of skin/fingernails

Endocrine & metabolic: Hyperglycemia, hypokalemia, distortion, hyperuricemia, SIADH has occurred with I.V. doses >50 mg/kg

Gastrointestinal: Stomatitis

Genitourinary: Acute hemorrhagic cystitis is believed to be a result of chemical irritation of the bladder by acrolein, a cyclophosphamide metabolite. Acute hemorrhagic cystitis occurs in 7% to 12% of patients, and has been reported in up to 40% of patients. Hemorrhagic cystitis can be severe and even fatal. Patients should be encouraged to drink plenty of fluids (3-4 L/day) during therapy, void frequently, and avoid taking the drug at nighttime. If large I.V. doses are being administered, I.V. hydration should be given during therapy. The administration of mesna or continuous bladder irrigation may also be warranted.

Hepatic: Hepatic toxicity

Renal: Renal tubular necrosis has occurred, but usually resolves after the discontinuation of therapy

Respiratory: Nasal congestion: Occurs when given in large I.V. doses via 30-60 minute infusion; patients experience runny eyes, nasal burning, rhinorrhea, sinus congestion, and sneezing during or immediately after the infusion; interstitial pulmonary fibrosis with prolonged high dosage has occurred

Miscellaneous: Secondary malignancy: Has developed with cyclophosphamide alone or in combination with other antineoplastics; both bladder carcinoma and acute leukemia are well documented; rare instances of anaphylaxis have been reported

Overdosage/Toxicology Symptoms of overdose include myelosuppression, alopecia, nausea, vomiting; treatment is supportive

Drug Interactions Cytochrome P-450 2B6 enzyme substrate and cytochrome P-450 2C enzyme substrate

Decreased effect: Digoxin: Cyclophosphamide may ↓ digoxin serum levels

Increased toxicity:

Allopurinol may cause ↑ in bone marrow suppression and may result in significant elevations of cyclophosphamide cytotoxic metabolites

Anesthetic agents: Cyclophosphamide reduces serum pseudocholinesterase concentrations and may prolong the neuromuscular blocking activity of succinylcholine; use with caution with halothane, nitrous oxide, and succinylcholine

Chloramphenicol results in prolonged cyclophosphamide half-life to ↑ toxicity

Cimetidine inhibits hepatic metabolism of drugs and may ↓ or ↑ the activation of cyclophosphamide

Doxorubicin: Cyclophosphamide may enhance cardiac toxicity of anthracyclines

Phenobarbital and phenytoin induce hepatic enzymes and cause a more rapid production of cyclophosphamide metabolites with a concurrent ↓ in the serum half-life of the parent compound

Tetrahydrocannabinol results in enhanced immunosuppression in animal studies

Thiazide diuretics: Leukopenia may be prolonged

Stability

Store intact vials of powder at room temperature (25°C to 35°C)

Reconstitute vials with SWI to a concentration of 20 mg/mL as follows below; reconstituted solutions are stable for 24 hours at room temperature (25°C) and 6 days at refrigeration (5°C)

100 mg vial = 5 mL
200 mg vial = 10 mL
500 mg vial = 25 mL
1 g vial = 50 mL
2 g vial = 100 mL

Further dilutions in D_5W or NS are stable for 24 hours at room temperature (25°C) and 6 days at refrigeration (5°C)

Maximum concentration of cyclophosphamide is **limited** to 20 mg/mL due to solubility of cyclophosphamide

Standard I.V. push dilution:

Dose up to 500 mg/30 mL syringe

Maximum syringe size for IVP is a 30 mL syringe syringe should be ≤75% full

Standard IVPB dilution:

May further dilute in D_5W or NS after initial reconstitution with SWI

Doses up to 2 g/250 mL volume

Doses up to 4 g/500 mL volume

Mechanism of Action Interferes with the normal function of DNA by alkylation and cross-linking the strands of DNA, and by possible protein modification; cyclophosphamide also possesses potent immunosuppressive activity; note that cyclophosphamide must be metabolized to its active form in the liver

Pharmacodynamics/Kinetics

Absorption: Completely from the GI tract (>75%)

Distribution: V_d: 0.48-0.71 L/kg; well distributed; crosses the placenta; appears in breast milk; does cross into the CSF, but not in concentrations high enough to treat meningeal leukemia

Protein binding: 10% to 56%

Metabolism: In the liver into its active components, one of which is 4-HC

Bioavailability: >75%

Half-life: 4-6.5 hours

Time to peak serum concentration: Oral: Within 1 hour

Elimination: In the urine as unchanged drug (<10%) and as metabolites (85% to 90%); most of which are inactive

Usual Dosage Refer to individual protocols

Patients with compromised bone marrow function may require a 33% to 50% reduction in initial loading dose

Children:

SLE: I.V.: 500-750 mg/m^2 every month; maximum dose: 1 g/m^2

JRA/vasculitis: I.V.: 10 mg/kg every 2 weeks

Children and Adults:

Oral: 50-100 mg/m^2/day as continuous therapy or 400-1000 mg/m^2 in divided doses over 4-5 days as intermittent therapy

I.V.:

Single Doses: 400-1800 mg/m^2 (30-50 mg/kg) per treatment course (1-5 days) which can be repeated at 2-4 week intervals

MAXIMUM SINGLE DOSE WITHOUT BMT is 7 g/m^2 (190 mg/kg) SINGLE AGENT THERAPY

Continuous daily doses: 60-120 mg/m^2 (1-2.5 mg/kg) per day

Autologous BMT: IVPB: 50 mg/kg/dose x 4 days or 60 mg/kg/dose for 2 days; total dose is usually divided over 2-4 days

Nephrotic syndrome: Oral: 2-3 mg/kg/day every day for up to 12 weeks when corticosteroids are unsuccessful

(Continued)

Cyclophosphamide *(Continued)*

Dosing adjustment in renal impairment: A large fraction of cyclophosphamide is eliminated by hepatic metabolism

Some authors recommend no dose adjustment unless severe renal insufficiency (Cl_{cr} <20 mL/minute)

Cl_{cr} >10 mL/minute: Administer 100% of normal dose

Cl_{cr} <10 mL/minute: Administer 75% of normal dose

Hemodialysis: Moderately dialyzable (20% to 50%); administer dose posthemodialysis or administer supplemental 50% dose

CAPD effects: Unknown

CAVH effects: Unknown

Dosing adjustment in hepatic impairment: Some authors recommend dosage reductions (of up to 30%); however, the pharmacokinetics of cyclophosphamide are not significantly altered in the presence of hepatic insufficiency. Cyclophosphamide undergoes hepatic transformation in the liver to its 4-hydroxycyclophosphamide, which breaks down to its active form, phosphoramide mustard.

Administration

May be administered I.M., I.P., intrapleurally, IVPB, or CIV

I.V. infusions may be administered over 1-2 hours

Doses >500 mg to approximately 1 g may be administered over 20-30 minutes

May also be administered slow IVP in lower doses

Force fluids up to 2 L/day to minimize bladder toxicity; high-dose regimens should be accompanied by vigorous hydration ± MESNA therapy

Monitoring Parameters CBC with differential and platelet count, BUN, UA, serum electrolytes, serum creatinine

Patient Information Drink plenty of fluids before and after doses; report any blood in urine

Nursing Implications Encourage adequate hydration and frequent voiding to help prevent hemorrhagic cystitis

Dosage Forms

Powder for injection: 100 mg, 200 mg, 500 mg, 1 g, 2 g

Powder for injection, lyophilized: 100 mg, 200 mg, 500 mg, 1 g, 2 g

Tablet: 25 mg, 50 mg

Cycloplegic Mydriatics Comparison *see page 1409*

Cycloserine (sye kloe SER een)

Related Information

Antimicrobial Drugs of Choice *on page 1468*

Brand Names Seromycin® Pulvules®

Therapeutic Category Antibiotic, Miscellaneous; Antitubercular Agent

Use Adjunctive treatment in pulmonary or extrapulmonary tuberculosis; treatment of acute urinary tract infections caused by *E. coli* or *Enterobacter* sp when less toxic conventional therapy has failed or is contraindicated

Pregnancy Risk Factor C

Contraindications Known hypersensitivity to cycloserine

Warnings/Precautions Epilepsy, depression, severe anxiety, psychosis, severe renal insufficiency, chronic alcoholism

Adverse Reactions

1% to 10%: Central nervous system: Drowsiness, headache

<1%:

Cardiovascular: Cardiac arrhythmias

Central nervous system: Dizziness, vertigo, seizures, confusion, psychosis, paresis, coma

Dermatologic: Rash

Hematologic: Folate deficiency

Hepatic: Elevated liver enzymes

Neuromuscular & skeletal: Tremor

Miscellaneous: Vitamin B_{12} deficiency

Overdosage/Toxicology Symptoms of overdose include confusion, CNS depression, psychosis, coma, seizures

Decontaminate with activated charcoal; can be hemodialyzed; management is supportive; administer 100-300 mg/day of pyridoxine to reduce neurotoxic effects; acute toxicity can occur with ingestions >1 g

Drug Interactions Increased toxicity: Alcohol, isoniazid, ethionamide increase toxicity of cycloserine; cycloserine inhibits the hepatic metabolism of phenytoin

Mechanism of Action Inhibits bacterial cell wall synthesis by competing with amino acid (D-alanine) for incorporation into the bacterial cell wall; bacteriostatic or bactericidal

Pharmacodynamics/Kinetics

Absorption: Oral: ~70% to 90% from the GI tract

Distribution: Crosses the placenta; appears in breast milk; distributed widely to most body fluids and tissues including CSF, breast milk, bile, sputum, lymph tissue, lungs, and ascitic, pleural, and synovial fluids

Half-life: 10 hours in patients with normal renal function

Metabolism: Extensive in liver

Time to peak serum concentration: Oral: Within 3-4 hours

Elimination: 60% to 70% of oral dose excreted unchanged in urine by glomerular filtration within 72 hours, small amounts excreted in feces, remainder is metabolized

Usual Dosage Some of the neurotoxic effects may be relieved or prevented by the concomitant administration of pyridoxine

Tuberculosis: Oral:

Children: 10-20 mg/kg/day in 2 divided doses up to 1000 mg/day for 18-24 months

Adults: Initial: 250 mg every 12 hours for 14 days, then administer 500 mg to 1 g/day in 2 divided doses for 18-24 months (maximum daily dose: 1 g)

Dosing interval in renal impairment:

Cl_{cr} 10-50 mL/minute: Administer every 12-24 hours

Cl_{cr} <10 mL/minute: Administer every 24 hours

Monitoring Parameters Periodic renal, hepatic, hematological tests, and plasma cycloserine concentrations

Reference Range Toxicity is greatly increased at levels >30 μg/mL

Patient Information May cause drowsiness; notify physician if skin rash, mental confusion, dizziness, headache, or tremors occur; do not skip doses; do not drink excessive amounts of alcoholic beverages

Dosage Forms Capsule: 250 mg

Cyclospasmol® *see* Cyclandelate *on page 320*

Cyclosporin A *see* Cyclosporine *on this page*

Cyclosporine (SYE kloe spor een)

Brand Names Neoral®; Sandimmune®

Canadian/Mexican Brand Names Consupren® (Mexico); Sandimmun® Neoral (Mexico)

Synonyms CsA; CyA; Cyclosporin A

Therapeutic Category Immunosuppressant Agent

Use Immunosuppressant which may be used with azathioprine and/or corticosteroids to prolong organ and patient survival in kidney, liver, heart, and bone marrow transplants; also used in some cases of severe autoimmune disease that are resistant to corticosteroids and other therapy.

Pregnancy Risk Factor C

Pregnancy/Breast-Feeding Implications Based on small numbers of patients, the use of cyclosporine during pregnancy apparently does not pose a major risk to the fetus

Contraindications Hypersensitivity to cyclosporine, Cremephor EL® (I.V. solution), or any other I.V. component (ie, polyoxyl 35 castor oil is an ingredient of the parenteral formulation and polyoxyl 40 hydrogenated castor oil is an ingredient of the cyclosporine capsules and solution for microemulsion)

Warnings/Precautions Infection and possible development of lymphoma may result. Make dose adjustments to avoid toxicity or possible organ rejection using cyclosporine blood levels because absorption is erratic and elimination is highly variable. Adjustment of dose should only be made under the direct supervision of an experienced physician; reserve the use of I.V. for use only in patients who cannot take oral; adequate airway and other supportive measures and agents for treating anaphylaxis should be present when I.V. drug is given. Nephrotoxic, if possible avoid concomitant use of other potentially nephrotoxic drugs (eg, acyclovir, aminoglycoside antibiotics, amphotericin B, ciprofloxacin).

Adverse Reactions

>10%:

Cardiovascular: Hypertension

Dermatologic: Hirsutism

Gastrointestinal: Gingival hypertrophy

Neuromuscular & skeletal: Tremor

Renal: Nephrotoxicity

1% to 10%:

Central nervous system: Seizure, headache

Dermatologic: Acne

Gastrointestinal: Abdominal discomfort, nausea, vomiting

Neuromuscular & skeletal: Leg cramps

(Continued)

Cyclosporine *(Continued)*

<1%:

Cardiovascular: Hypotension, tachycardia, warmth, flushing

Endocrine & metabolic: Hyperkalemia, hypomagnesemia, hyperuricemia

Gastrointestinal: Pancreatitis

Hepatic: Hepatotoxicity

Neuromuscular & skeletal: Myositis, paresthesias

Respiratory: Respiratory distress, sinusitis

Miscellaneous: Anaphylaxis, increased susceptibility to infection, and sensitivity to temperature extremes

Overdosage/Toxicology Symptoms of overdose include hepatotoxicity, nephrotoxicity, nausea, vomiting, tremor. CNS secondary to direct action of the drug may not be reflected in serum concentrations, may be more predictable by renal magnesium loss.

Drug Interactions Cytochrome P-450 3A enzyme substrate

Decreased effect: Drugs that decrease cyclosporine concentrations: Carbamazepine, phenobarbital, phenytoin, rifampin, isoniazid

Increased toxicity:

Drugs that increase cyclosporine concentrations: Azithromycin, clarithromycin, diltiazem, erythromycin, fluconazole, itraconazole, ketoconazole, nicardipine, verapamil, grapefruit juice

Drugs that enhance nephrotoxicity of cyclosporine: Aminoglycosides, amphotericin B, acyclovir

Lovastatin - myositis, myalgias, rhabdomyolysis, acute renal failure

Nifedipine - increases risk of gingival hyperplasia

Stability

Cyclosporine injection is a clear, faintly brown-yellow solution which should be stored at <30°C and protected from light

Cyclosporine concentrate for injection should be further diluted [1 mL (50 mg) of concentrate in 20-100 mL of D_5W or or NS] for administration by intravenous infusion. Light protection is not required for intravenous admixtures of cyclosporine.

Stability of injection of parenteral admixture at room temperature (25°C): 6 hours in PVC; 24 hours in Excel, PAB containers, or glass

Polyoxyethylated castor oil (Cremophor EL®) surfactant in cyclosporin injection may leach phthalate from PVC containers such as bags and tubing. The actual amount of diethylhexyl phthalate (DEHP) plasticizer leached from PVC containers and administration sets may vary in clinical situations, depending on surfactant concentration, bag size, and contact time.

Doses <250 mg should be prepared in 100 mL of D_5W or NS

Doses >250 mg should be prepared in 250 mL of D_5W or NS

Minimum volume: 100 mL D_5W or NS

Do not refrigerate oral or I.V. solution

Oral solution: Use the contents of the oral solution within two months after opening; should be mixed in glass containers

Mechanism of Action Inhibition of production and release of interleukin II and inhibits interleukin II-induced activation of resting T-lymphocytes

Pharmacodynamics/Kinetics

Absorption: Oral:

Solution or soft gelatin capsule (Sandimmune®): Erratically and incompletely absorbed; dependent on the presence of food, bile acids, and GI motility; larger oral doses of cyclosporine are needed in pediatric patients versus adults due to a shorter bowel length resulting in limited intestinal absorption

Solution in microemulsion or soft gelatin capsule in a microemulsion are bioequivalent (Neoral®): Erratically and incompletely absorbed; increased absorption, up to 30% when compared to Sandimmune®; absorption is less dependent on food intake, bile, or GI motility when compared to Sandimmune®

Distribution: Widely distributed in tissues and body fluids including the liver, pancreas, and lungs; crosses the placenta; excreted into breast milk

V_{dss}: 4-6 L/kg in renal, liver, and marrow transplant recipients (slightly lower values in cardiac transplant patients; children <10 years of age have higher values)

Protein binding: 90% of dose binds to blood proteins

Metabolism: Undergoes extensive first-pass metabolism following oral administration; extensively metabolized by the cytochrome P-450 system in the liver

Bioavailability:

Solution or soft gelatin capsule (Sandimmune®): Dependent on patient population and transplant type (<10% in adult liver transplant patients and as high as 89% in renal patients)

Children: 28% (range: 17% to 42%); with gut dysfunction commonly seen in BMT patients, oral bioavailability is further reduced

Solution or soft gelatin capsule in a microemulsion (Neoral®):

Children: 43% (range: 30& to 68%)

Adults: 23% greater than with Sandimmune® in renal transplant patients. 50% greater in liver transplant patients

Half-life:

Solution or soft gelatin capsule (Sandimmune®): Biphasic, alpha phase: 1.4 hours and terminal phase 6-24 hours (prolonged in patients with hepatic dysfunction)

Solution or soft gelatin capsule in a microemulsion (Neoral®): 8.4 hours, lower in pediatric patients versus adults due to the higher metabolism rate

Time to peak serum concentration:

Oral solution or capsule (Sandimmune®): 2-6 hours; some patients have a second peak at 5-6 hours

Oral solution or capsule in a microemulsion (Neoral®): 1.5-2 hours (in renal transplant patients)

Elimination: Primarily in the bile; clearance is more rapid in pediatric patients than in adults; clearance is decreased in patients with liver disease; 6% of dose excreted in the urine as unchanged drug (0.1%) and metabolites

Usual Dosage Children and Adults (oral dosage is ~3 times the I.V. dosage); dosage should be based on ideal body weight:

I.V.:

Initial: 5-6 mg/kg/day beginning 4-12 hours prior to organ transplantation; patients should be switched to oral cyclosporine as soon as possible; dose should be infused over 2-24 hours

Maintenance: 2-10 mg/kg/day in divided doses every 8-12 hours; dose should be adjusted to maintain whole blood FPIA trough concentrations in the reference range

Oral: **Solution or soft gelatin capsule (Sandimmune®):**

Initial: 14-18 mg/kg/day, beginning 4-12 hours prior to organ transplantation

Maintenance: 5-15 mg/kg/day divided every 12-24 hours; maintenance dose is usually tapered to 3-10 mg/kg/day

Focal segmental glomerulosclerosis: Initial: 3 mg/kg/day divided every 12 hours

Autoimmune diseases: 1-3 mg/kg/day

Dosing considerations of cyclosporine, see table.

Cyclosporine

Condition	Cyclosporine
Switch from I.V. to oral therapy	Threefold increase in dose
T-tube clamping	Decrease dose; increase availability of bile facilitates absorption of CsA
Pediatric patients	About 2-3 times higher dose compared to adults
Liver dysfunction	Decrease I.V. dose; increase oral dose
Renal dysfunction	Decrease dose to decrease levels if renal dysfunction is related to the drug
Dialysis	Not removed
Inhibitors of hepatic metabolism	Decrease dose
Inducers of hepatic metabolism	Monitor drug level; may need to increase dose

Oral: **Solution or soft gelatin capsule in a microemulsion (Neoral®):** Based on the organ transplant population:

Initial: Same as the initial dose for solution or soft gelatin capsule (listed above) **or**

Renal: 9 mg/kg/day (range: 6-12 mg/kg/day)

Liver: 8 mg/kg/day (range: 4-12 mg/kg/day)

Heart: 7 mg/kg/day (range: 4-10 mg/kg/day)

Note: A 1:1 ratio conversion from Sandimmune® to Neoral® has been recommended initially; however, lower doses of Neoral® may be required after conversion to prevent overdose. Total daily doses should be adjusted based on the cyclosporine trough blood concentration and clinical assessment of organ rejection. CsA blood trough levels should be determined prior to conversion. After conversion to Neoral®, CsA trough levels should be monitored every 4-7 days. **Neoral® and Sandimmune® are not bioequivalent and cannot be used interchangeably.**

Hemodialysis: Supplemental dose is not necessary

Peritoneal dialysis: Supplemental dose is not necessary

(Continued)

Cyclosporine *(Continued)*

Dosing adjustment in hepatic impairment: Probably necessary, monitor levels closely

Monitoring Parameters Cyclosporine trough levels, serum electrolytes, renal function, hepatic function, blood pressure, serum cholesterol

Reference Range Reference ranges are method dependent and specimen dependent; use the same analytical method consistently; trough levels should be obtained immediately prior to next dose

Method-dependent and specimen-dependent

Trough levels should be obtained:

Oral: 12-18 hours after dose (chronic usage)

I.V.: 12 hours after dose **or** immediately prior to next dose

Therapeutic range: Not absolutely defined, dependent on organ transplanted, time after transplant, organ function and CsA toxicity

General range of 100-400 ng/mL

Toxic level: Not well defined, nephrotoxicity may occur at any level

Test Interactions Cyclosporine adsorbs to silicone; specific whole blood assay for cyclosporine may be falsely elevated if sample is drawn from the same line through which dose was administered (even if flush has been administered and/or dose was given hours before)

Patient Information Use glass droppers or glass to hold dose; rinse container to get full dose; mix with milk, chocolate milk, or orange juice preferably at room temperature, improves palatability; stir well and drink at once. Take dose at same time each day.

Nursing Implications Do not administer liquid from plastic or styrofoam cup; mixing with milk, chocolate milk, or orange juice preferably at room temperature, improves palatability; stir well; do not allow to stand before drinking; rinse with more diluent to ensure that the total dose is taken; after use, dry outside of pipette; do not rinse with water or other cleaning agents; may cause inflamed gums

Dosage Forms

Capsule, microemulsion (Neoral®): 25 mg; 100 mg

Capsule, soft gelatin (Sandimmune®): 25 mg; 50 mg; 100 mg

Injection: 50 mg/mL (5 mL)

Solution, oral (Sandimmune®): 100 mg/mL (50 mL)

Solution, oral, microemulsion (Neoral®): 100 mg/mL (50 mL)

Cycrin® *see* Medroxyprogesterone Acetate *on page 771*

Cyklokapron® *see* Tranexamic Acid *on page 1248*

Cylert® *see* Pemoline *on page 958*

Cylex® [OTC] *see* Benzocaine *on page 138*

Cyomin® *see* Cyanocobalamin *on page 319*

Cyproheptadine (si proe HEP ta deen)

Brand Names Periactin®

Canadian/Mexican Brand Names PMS-Cyproheptadine (Canada)

Synonyms Cyproheptadine Hydrochloride

Therapeutic Category Antihistamine, H_1 Blocker

Use Perennial and seasonal allergic rhinitis and other allergic symptoms including urticaria; its off-labeled uses have included appetite stimulation, blepharospasm, cluster headaches, migraine headaches, Nelson's syndrome, pruritus, schizophrenia, spinal cord damage associated spasticity, and tardive dyskinesia

Pregnancy Risk Factor B

Contraindications Hypersensitivity to cyproheptadine or any component; narrow-angle glaucoma, bladder neck obstruction, acute asthmatic attack, stenosing peptic ulcer, GI tract obstruction, those on MAO inhibitors; avoid use in premature and term newborns due to potential association with SIDS

Warnings/Precautions Do not use in neonates, safety and efficacy have not been established in children <2 years of age; symptomatic prostate hypertrophy; antihistamines are more likely to cause dizziness, excessive sedation, syncope, toxic confusion states, and hypotension in the elderly. In case reports, cyproheptadine has promoted weight gain in anorexic adults, though it has not been specifically studied in the elderly. All cases of weight loss or decreased appetite should be adequately assessed.

Adverse Reactions

>10%:

Central nervous system: Slight to moderate drowsiness

Respiratory: Thickening of bronchial secretions

1% to 10%:

Central nervous system: Headache, fatigue, nervousness, dizziness

Gastrointestinal: Appetite stimulation, nausea, diarrhea, abdominal pain, xerostomia

Neuromuscular & skeletal: Arthralgia
Respiratory: Pharyngitis
<1%:
Cardiovascular: Tachycardia, palpitations, edema
Central nervous system: Sedation, CNS stimulation, seizures, depression
Dermatologic: Photosensitivity, rash, angioedema
Hematologic: Hemolytic anemia, leukopenia, thrombocytopenia
Hepatic: Hepatitis
Neuromuscular & skeletal: Myalgia, paresthesia
Respiratory: Bronchospasm, epistaxis
Miscellaneous: Allergic reactions

Overdosage/Toxicology Symptoms of overdose include CNS depression or stimulation, dry mouth, flushed skin, fixed and dilated pupils, apnea

There is no specific treatment for an antihistamine overdose, however, most of its clinical toxicity is due to anticholinergic effects. Anticholinesterase inhibitors may be useful by reducing acetylcholinesterase. Anticholinesterase inhibitors include physostigmine, neostigmine, pyridostigmine, and edrophonium. For anticholinergic overdose with severe life-threatening symptoms, physostigmine 1-2 mg (0.5 or 0.02 mg/kg for children) I.V., slowly may be given to reverse these effects.

Drug Interactions Increased toxicity: MAO inhibitors → hallucinations

Mechanism of Action A potent antihistamine and serotonin antagonist, competes with histamine for H_1-receptor sites on effector cells in the gastrointestinal tract, blood vessels, and respiratory tract

Pharmacodynamics/Kinetics
Metabolism: Almost completely
Elimination: >50% excreted in urine (primarily as metabolites); ~25% excreted in feces

Usual Dosage Oral:
Children: 0.25 mg/kg/day in 2-3 divided doses or 8 mg/m^2/day in 2-3 divided doses
2-6 years: 2 mg every 8-12 hours (not to exceed 12 mg/day)
7-14 years: 4 mg every 8-12 hours (not to exceed 16 mg/day)
Adults: 4-20 mg/day divided every 8 hours (not to exceed 0.5 mg/kg/day)

Dosing adjustment in hepatic impairment: Dosage should be reduced in patients with significant hepatic dysfunction

Dietary Considerations Alcohol: Additive CNS effects, avoid use

Test Interactions Diagnostic antigen skin tests, ↑ amylases (S), ↓ fasting glucose (S)

Patient Information May cause drowsiness; may stimulate appetite; avoid alcohol and other CNS depressants; may impair judgment and coordination

Nursing Implications Raise bed rails, institute safety measures, assist with ambulation

Dosage Forms
Syrup, as hydrochloride: 2 mg/5 mL with alcohol 5% (473 mL)
Tablet, as hydrochloride: 4 mg

Cyproheptadine Hydrochloride *see* Cyproheptadine *on previous page*

Cystagon® *see* Cysteamine *on this page*

Cysteamine (sis TEE a meen)

Brand Names Cystagon®

Synonyms Cysteamine Bitartrate

Therapeutic Category Anticystine Agent; Urinary Tract Product

Use Management of nephropathic cystinosis; approved as orphan drug 8/15/94

Pregnancy Risk Factor C

Pregnancy/Breast-Feeding Implications Use only when the potential benefits outweigh the potential hazards to the fetus; in animal studies, cysteamine reduced the fertility of rats and offspring survival at very large doses; it is unknown whether cysteamine is excreted in breast milk; discontinue nursing or discontinue drug during lactation

Contraindications Hypersensitivity to cysteamine or penicillamine

Warnings/Precautions Withhold cysteamine if a mild rash develops; restart at a lower dose and titrate to therapeutic dose; adjust cysteamine dose if CNS symptoms due to the drug develop, rather than the disease; adjust cysteamine dose downward if severe GI symptoms develop (most common during initiation of therapy)

Adverse Reactions
5% to 10%:
Gastrointestinal: Vomiting, anorexia, diarrhea
Central nervous system: Fever, lethargy
Dermatologic: Rash

(Continued)

Cysteamine *(Continued)*

<5%:

Cardiovascular: Hypertension

Central nervous system: Somnolence, encephalopathy, headache, seizures, ataxia, confusion, dizziness, jitteriness, nervousness, impaired cognition, emotional changes, hallucinations, nightmares

Dermatologic: Urticaria

Endocrine & metabolic: Dehydration

Gastrointestinal: Bad breath, abdominal pain, dyspepsia, constipation, gastroenteritis, duodenitis, duodenal ulceration

Hematologic: Anemia, leukopenia

Hepatic: Abnormal LFTs

Neuromuscular & skeletal: Tremor, hyperkinesia

Otic: Decreased hearing

Overdosage/Toxicology Symptoms may include vomiting, reduction of motor activity, GI or renal hemorrhage; treatment is generally supportive; hemodialysis may be appropriate

Mechanism of Action Reacts with cystine in the lysosome to convert it to cysteine and to a cysteine-cysteamine mixed disulfide, both of which can then exit the lysosome in patients with cystinosis, an inherited defect of lysosomal transport

Usual Dosage Initiate therapy with $^1/_4$ to $^1/_8$ of maintenance dose; titrate slowly upward over 4-6 weeks

Children <12 years: Oral: Maintenance: 1.3 $g/m^2/day$ divided into 4 doses

Children >12 years and Adults (>110 lbs): 2 g/day in 4 divided doses; dosage may be increased to 1.95 $g/m^2/day$ if cystine levels are <1 nmol/$^1/_2$ cystine/mg protein, although intolerance and incidence of adverse events may be increased

Administration Sprinkle capsule contents over food for children <6 years of age

Monitoring Parameters Blood counts and LFTs during therapy; monitor leukocyte cystine measurements every 3 months to determine adequate dosage and compliance (measure 5-6 hours after administration); monitor more frequently when switching salt forms

Reference Range Leukocyte cystine: <1 nmol/$^1/_2$ cystine/mg protein

Patient Information Following initiation of therapy, do not engage in hazardous tasks until the effects of the drug on mental performance are known

Dosage Forms Capsule, as bitartrate: 50 mg, 150 mg

Cysteamine Bitartrate *see* Cysteamine *on previous page*

Cystospaz® *see* Hyoscyamine *on page 635*

Cystospaz-M® *see* Hyoscyamine *on page 635*

CYT *see* Cyclophosphamide *on page 323*

Cytadren® *see* Aminoglutethimide *on page 65*

Cytarabine (sye TARE a been)

Related Information

Antiemetics for Chemotherapy Induced Nausea and Vomiting *on page 1348*

Cancer Chemotherapy Regimens *on page 1351*

Toxicities of Chemotherapeutic Agents *on page 1382*

Brand Names Cytosar-U®

Synonyms Arabinosylcytosine; Ara-C; Cytarabine Hydrochloride; Cytosine Arabinosine Hydrochloride

Therapeutic Category Antineoplastic Agent, Antimetabolite (Purine)

Use Ara-C is one of the most active agents in leukemia; also active against lymphoma, meningeal leukemia, and meningeal lymphoma; has little use in the treatment of solid tumors

Pregnancy Risk Factor D

Contraindications Hypersensitivity to cytarabine or any component

Warnings/Precautions The U.S. Food and Drug Administration (FDA) currently recommends that procedures for proper handling and disposal of antineoplastic agents be considered. Use with caution in pregnant women or women of child-bearing age and in infants; must monitor drug tolerance, protect and maintain a patient compromised by drug toxicity that includes bone marrow suppression with leukopenia, thrombocytopenia and anemia along with nausea, vomiting, diarrhea, abdominal pain, oral ulceration and hepatic impairment; marked bone marrow suppression necessitates dosage reduction by a decrease in the number of days of administration.

Adverse Reactions

>10%:

High-dose therapy toxicities: Cerebellar toxicity, conjunctivitis (make sure the patient is on steroid eye drops during therapy), corneal keratitis, hyperbilirubinemia, pulmonary edema, pericarditis, and tamponade

Central nervous system: Has produced seizures when given I.T.; cerebellar syndrome (or cerebellar toxicity), manifested as ataxia, dysarthria, and dysdiadochokinesia, has been reported to be dose-related. This may or may not be reversible.

Dermatologic: Oral/anal ulceration, rash

Gastrointestinal: Nausea, vomiting, diarrhea, and mucositis which subside quickly after discontinuing the drug; GI effects may be more pronounced with divided I.V. bolus doses than with continuous infusion

Emetic potential:

<500 mg: Moderately low (10% to 30%)

500 mg to 1500 mg: Moderately high (60% to 90%)

>1-1.5 g: High (>90%)

Time course of nausea/vomiting: Onset: 1-3 hours; Duration: 3-8 hours

Hematologic: Bleeding

Myelosuppressive: Occurs within the first week of treatment and lasts for 10-14 days; primarily manifested as granulocytopenia, but anemia can also occur

WBC: Severe

Platelets: Severe

Onset (days): 4-7

Nadir (days): 14-18

Recovery (days): 21-28

Hepatic: Hepatic dysfunction, mild jaundice and acute increase in transaminases can be produced

Local: Thrombophlebitis

1% to 10%:

Cardiovascular: Cardiomegaly

Central nervous system: Dizziness, headache, somnolence, confusion, neuritis, malaise

Dermatologic: Skin freckling, itching, alopecia, cellulitis at injection site

Genitourinary: Urinary retention

Neuromuscular & skeletal: Myalgia, bone pain, peripheral neuropathy

Respiratory: Syndrome of sudden respiratory distress progressing to pulmonary edema, pneumonia

Miscellaneous: Sepsis

Overdosage/Toxicology Symptoms of overdose include myelosuppression, megaloblastosis, nausea, vomiting, respiratory distress, pulmonary edema. A syndrome of sudden respiratory distress progressing to pulmonary edema and cardiomegaly has been reported following high doses.

Drug Interactions

Decreased effect of gentamicin, flucytosine; ↓ digoxin oral tablet absorption

Increased toxicity: Alkylating agents and radiation; purine analogs; methotrexate

Stability

Store intact vials of powder at room temperature 15°C to 30°C (59°F to 86°F)

WARNING: Bacteriostatic diluent should not be used for the preparation of either high-doses or intrathecal doses of cytarabine

Reconstitute with SWI, D_5W or NS; dilute to a concentration of 100 mg/mL as follows; reconstituted solutions are stable for 48 hours at 15°C to 30°C

100 mg vial = 1 mL

500 mg vial = 5 mL

1 g vial = 10 mL

2 g vial = 20 mL

Further dilution in D_5W or NS is stable for 8 days at room temperature (25°C)

Standard I.V. dilution:

I.V. push: Dose/syringe (concentration: 100 mg/mL)

Maximum syringe size for IVP is 30 mL syringe and syringe should be ≤75% full

IVPB: Dose/100 mL D_5W or NS

CIV: Dose/250-1000 mL D_5W or NS

Compatible with vincristine, potassium chloride, calcium, magnesium, and idarubicin

Incompatible with 5-FU, gentamicin, heparin, insulin, methylprednisolone, nafcillin, oxacillin, penicillin G sodium

Intrathecal solutions in 3-20 mL lactated Ringers are stable for 7 days at room temperature (30°C); however, should be used within 24 hours due to sterility concerns

Standard intrathecal dilutions:

Dose/3-5 mL lactated Ringers ± methotrexate (12 mg) ± hydrocortisone (15-50 mg)

Compatible with methotrexate and hydrocortisone in lactated Ringers or NS for 24 hours at room temperature (25°C)

Mechanism of Action Inhibition of DNA synthesis; cell cycle-specific for the S phase of cell division; cytosine gains entry into cells by a carrier process, and

(Continued)

Cytarabine *(Continued)*

then must be converted to its active compound; cytosine acts as an analog and is incorporated into DNA; however, the primary action is inhibition of DNA polymerase resulting in decreased DNA synthesis and repair; degree of its cytotoxicity correlates linearly with its incorporation into DNA; therefore, incorporation into the DNA is responsible for drug activity and toxicity

Pharmacodynamics/Kinetics

Absorption: Because high concentrations of cytidine deaminase are in the GI mucosa and liver, 3-10 fold higher doses than I.V. would need to be given orally; therefore, the oral route is not used

Distribution: V_d = total body water. Widely and rapidly distributed since it enters the cells readily; crosses the blood-brain barrier, and CSF levels of 40% to 50% of the plasma level are reached

Metabolism: Primarily in the liver; Ara-C must be metabolized to Ara-CTP to be active

Half-life:

Initial: 7-20 minutes

Terminal: 0.5-2.6 hours

Elimination: ~80% of dose excreted in the urine as metabolites within 36 hours

Usual Dosage I.V. bolus, IVPB, and CIV doses of cytarabine are very different. Bolus doses are relatively well tolerated since the drug is rapidly metabolized; bolus doses are associated with greater gastrointestinal and neurotoxicity; continuous infusion uniformly results in myelosuppression. Refer to individual protocols.

Children and Adults:

Induction remission:

I.V.: 200 mg/m²/day for 5 days at 2-week intervals

100-200 mg/m²/day for 5- to 10-day therapy course or every day until remission

I.T.: 5-75 mg/m² every 4 days until CNS findings normalize

or

<1 year: 20 mg

1-2 years: 30 mg

2-3 years: 50 mg

>3 years: 70 mg

Maintenance remission:

I.V.: 70-200 mg/m²/day for 2-5 days at monthly intervals

I.M., S.C.: 1-1.5 mg/kg single dose for maintenance at 1- to 4-week intervals

High-dose therapies:

Doses as high as 1-3 g/m² have been used for refractory or secondary leukemias or refractory non-Hodgkin's lymphoma

Doses of 3 g/m² every 12 hours for up to 12 doses have been used

Bone marrow transplant: 1.5 g/m² continuous infusion over 48 hours

Dosage adjustment of high-dose therapy in patients with renal insufficiency: In one study, 76% of patients with a Cl_{cr} <60 mL/minute experienced neurotoxicity; dosage adjustment should be considered in these patients

Dose may need to be adjusted in patients with liver failure since cytarabine is partially detoxified in the liver

Hemodialysis: Supplemental dose is not necessary

Peritoneal dialysis: Supplemental dose is not necessary

Administration Can be administered I.M., IVP, I.V. infusion, I.T., or S.C. at a concentration not to exceed 100 mg/mL; I.V. may be administered either as a bolus, IVPB (high-doses of > 500 mg/m²) or continuous intravenous infusion (doses of 100-200 mg/m²)

I.V. doses of >200 mg/m² may produce conjunctivitis which can be ameliorated with prophylactic use of corticosteroid (0.1% dexamethasone) eye drops. Dexamethasone eye drops should be administered at 1-2 drops every 6 hours for 2-7 days after cytarabine is done.

Monitoring Parameters Liver function tests, CBC with differential and platelet count, serum creatinine, BUN, serum uric acid

Patient Information Notify physician of any fever, sore throat, bleeding, or bruising

Additional Information Supplied with diluent containing benzyl alcohol, which should not be used when preparing either high-dose or I.T. doses

Dosage Forms

Powder for injection, as hydrochloride: 100 mg, 500 mg, 1 g, 2 g

Powder for injection, as hydrochloride (Cytosar-U®): 100 mg, 500 mg, 1 g, 2 g

Cytarabine Hydrochloride *see* Cytarabine *on page 332*

Cytochrome P-450 and Drug Interactions *see page 1572*

CytoGam™ *see* Cytomegalovirus Immune Globulin (Intravenous-Human) *on this page*

Cytomegalovirus Immune Globulin (Intravenous-Human)

(sye toe meg a low VYE rus i MYUN GLOB yoo lin in tra VEE nus HYU man)

Brand Names CytoGam™

Synonyms CMV-IGIV

Therapeutic Category Immune Globulin

Use Attenuation of primary CMV disease associated with kidney transplantation

Contraindications Hypersensitivity to any component, patients with selective immunoglobulin A deficiency (↑ potential for anaphylaxis)

Warnings/Precautions Studies indicate that product carries little or no risk for transmission of HIV

Adverse Reactions

1% to 10%:

- Cardiovascular: Flushing of the face
- Gastrointestinal: Nausea, vomiting
- Neuromuscular & skeletal: Muscle cramps, back pain
- Respiratory: Wheezing
- Miscellaneous: Diaphoresis

<1%:

- Cardiovascular: Tightness in the chest
- Central nervous system: Dizziness, fever, headache, chills
- Miscellaneous: Hypersensitivity reactions

Drug Interactions May inactivate live virus vaccines (eg, measles, mumps, rubella)

Stability Use reconstituted product within 6 hours

Mechanism of Action CMV-IGIV is a preparation of immunoglobulin G derived from pooled healthy blood donors with a high titer of CMV antibodies; administration provides a passive source of antibodies against cytomegalovirus

Usual Dosage I.V.:

Dosing schedule:

- Initial dose (within 72 hours after transplant): 150 mg/kg/dose
- 2 weeks after transplant: 100 mg/kg/dose
- 4, 6, 8 weeks after transplant: 100 mg/kg/dose
- 12 and 16 weeks after transplant: 50 mg/kg/dose

Administration rate: Administer at 15 mg/kg/hour initially, then increase to 30 mg/kg/hour after 30 minutes if no untoward reactions, then increase to 60 mg/kg/hour after another 30 minutes; volume not to exceed 75 mL/hour

Administration I.V. use only; administer as separate infusion; infuse beginning at 15 mg/kg/hour; may titrate up to 60 mg/kg/hour; do not administer faster than 75 mL/hour

Dosage Forms Powder for injection, lyophilized, detergent treated: 2500 mg ± 250 mg (50 mL)

Cytomel® *see* Liothyronine *on page 729*

Cytosar-U® *see* Cytarabine *on page 332*

Cytosine Arabinosine Hydrochloride *see* Cytarabine *on page 332*

Cytotec® *see* Misoprostol *on page 845*

Cytovene® *see* Ganciclovir *on page 566*

Cytoxan® *see* Cyclophosphamide *on page 323*

D-3-Mercaptovaline *see* Penicillamine *on page 959*

d4T *see* Stavudine *on page 1158*

Dacarbazine (da KAR ba zeen)

Related Information

Antiemetics for Chemotherapy Induced Nausea and Vomiting *on page 1348*
Cancer Chemotherapy Regimens *on page 1351*

Brand Names DTIC-Dome®

Synonyms DIC; Dimethyl Triazeno Imidazol Carboxamide; Imidazole Carboxamide

Therapeutic Category Antineoplastic Agent, Vesicant; Antineoplastic Agent, Miscellaneous; Vesicant

Use Treatment of malignant melanoma, Hodgkin's disease, soft-tissue sarcomas, fibrosarcomas, rhabdomyosarcoma, islet cell carcinoma, medullary carcinoma of the thyroid, and neuroblastoma

Pregnancy Risk Factor C

Contraindications Hypersensitivity to dacarbazine or any component

Warnings/Precautions The U.S. Food and Drug Administration (FDA) currently recommends that procedures for proper handling and disposal of antineoplastic

(Continued)

Dacarbazine *(Continued)*

agents be considered. Use with caution in patients with bone marrow suppression; in patients with renal and/or hepatic impairment since dosage reduction may be necessary; avoid extravasation of the drug.

Adverse Reactions

>10%:

Extravasation: Dacarbazine is an irritant; may cause tissue necrosis after extravasation; apply ice and consult extravasation policy if this occurs

Irritant chemotherapy: Pain and burning at infusion site

Gastrointestinal: Moderate to severe nausea and vomiting in 90% of patients and lasting up to 12 hours after administration; nausea and vomiting are dose-related and occur more frequently when given as a one-time dose, as opposed to a less intensive 5-day course; diarrhea may also occur

Emetic potential:

<500 mg: Moderately high (60% to 90%)

≥500 mg: High (>90%)

Time course of nausea/vomiting: Onset: 1-2 hours; Duration: 2-4 hours

1% to 10%:

Cardiovascular: Facial flushing

Central nervous system: Headache

Dermatologic: Alopecia, rash

Flu-like effects: Fever, malaise, headache, myalgia, and sinus congestion may last up to several days after administration

Gastrointestinal: Anorexia, metallic taste

Hematologic: Myelosuppressive: Mild to moderate is common and dose-related; leukopenia and thrombocytopenia may be delayed 2-3 weeks and may be the dose-limiting toxicity

WBC: Mild (primarily leukocytes)

Platelets: Mild

Onset (days): 7

Nadir (days): 21-25

Recovery (days): 21-28

Neuromuscular & skeletal: Paresthesias

Respiratory: Sinus congestion

Miscellaneous: Anaphylactic reactions, hypocalcemia with high-dose DTIC

<1%:

Cardiovascular: Orthostatic hypotension

Central nervous system: Polyneuropathy, headache, and seizures have been reported

Dermatologic: Photosensitivity reactions, alopecia

Gastrointestinal: Stomatitis, diarrhea

Hepatic: Elevated LFTs, hepatic vein thrombosis and hepatocellular necrosis

Neuromuscular & skeletal: Weakness

Ocular: Blurred vision

Miscellaneous: Anaphylaxis

Overdosage/Toxicology Symptoms of overdose include myelosuppression, diarrhea; there are no known antidotes and treatment is primarily symptomatic and supportive

Stability

Store intact vials under refrigeration (2°C to 8°C) and protect from light; vials are stable for 4 weeks at room temperature

Reconstitute with a minimum of 2 mL (100 mg vial) or 4 mL (200 mg vial) of SWI, D_5W, or NS; dilute to a concentration of 10 mg/mL as follows; reconstituted solution is stable for 24 hours at room temperature (20°C) and 96 hours under refrigeration (4°C)

100 mg vial = 9.9 mL

200 mg vial = 19.7 mL

500 mg vial = 49.5 mL

Further dilution in 200-500 mL of D_5W or NS is stable for 24 hours at room temperature and protected from light

Decomposed drug turns pink

Standard I.V. dilution:

Dose/250-500 mL D_5W or NS

Stable for 24 hours at room temperature and refrigeration (4°C) when protected from light

Mechanism of Action Alkylating agent which forms methylcarbonium ions that attack nucleophilic groups in DNA; cross-links strands of DNA resulting in the inhibition of DNA, RNA, and protein synthesis, but the exact mechanism of action is still unclear; originally developed as a purine antimetabolite, but it does not interfere with purine synthesis; metabolism by the host is necessary for activation of dacarbazine, then the methylated species acts by alkylation of nucleic acids; dacarbazine is active in all phases of the cell cycle

Pharmacodynamics/Kinetics

Onset of action: I.V.: 18-24 days

Absorption: Oral administration demonstrates slow and variable absorption; preferable to administer by I.V. route

Distribution: V_d: 0.6 L/kg, exceeding total body water and suggesting binding to some tissue (probably the liver)

Protein binding: Minimal (5%)

Metabolism: Extensive in the liver, and hepatobiliary excretion is probably of some importance; metabolites may also have an antineoplastic effect

Half-life (biphasic):

Initial: 20-40 minutes

Terminal: 5 hours

Elimination: Hepatobiliary; ~30% to 50% of dose excreted unchanged in the urine by tubular secretion

Usual Dosage I.V. (refer to individual protocols):

Children:

Pediatric solid tumors: 200-470 mg/m²/day over 5 days every 21-28 days

Pediatric neuroblastoma: 800-900 mg/m² as a single dose on day 1 of therapy every 3-4 weeks in combination therapy

Hodgkin's disease: 375 mg/m² on days 1 and 15 of treatment course, repeat every 28 days

Adults:

Malignant melanoma: 2-4.5 mg/kg/day for 10 days, repeat in 4 weeks **OR** may use 250 mg/m²/day for 5 days, repeat in 3 weeks

Hodgkin's disease: 150 mg/m²/day for 5 days, repeat every 4 weeks **OR** 375 mg/m² on day 1, repeat in 15 days of each 28-day cycle in combination with other agents **OR** 375 mg/m² repeated in 15 days of each 28-day cycle

Dosing adjustment in renal impairment: Adjustment is warranted

Dosing adjustment/comments in hepatic impairment: Monitor closely for signs of toxicity

Monitoring Parameters CBC (with differential, erythrocyte, and platelet count), liver function tests

Patient Information Report any persistent fever, sore throat, or malaise or fatigue

Nursing Implications

Extravasation management: Local pain, burning sensation, and irritation at the injection site may be relieved by local application of hot packs; if extravasation occurs, apply cold packs; protect exposed tissue from light following extravasation

Dosage Forms Injection: 100 mg (10 mL, 20 mL); 200 mg (20 mL, 30 mL); 500 mg (50 mL)

Dacodyl® [OTC] *see* Bisacodyl *on page 153*

Dactinomycin (dak ti noe MYE sin)

Related Information

Antiemetics for Chemotherapy Induced Nausea and Vomiting *on page 1348*

Cancer Chemotherapy Regimens *on page 1351*

Toxicities of Chemotherapeutic Agents *on page 1382*

Brand Names Cosmegen®

Synonyms ACT; Actinomycin D

Therapeutic Category Antineoplastic Agent, Antibiotic; Antineoplastic Agent, Vesicant; Vesicant

Use Treatment of testicular tumors, melanoma, choriocarcinoma, Wilms' tumor, neuroblastoma, retinoblastoma, rhabdomyosarcoma, uterine sarcomas, Ewing's sarcoma, Kaposi's sarcoma, and soft tissue sarcoma

Pregnancy Risk Factor C

Contraindications Hypersensitivity to dactinomycin or any component; patients with chickenpox or herpes zoster; avoid in infants <6 months of age

Warnings/Precautions The U.S. Food and Drug Administration (FDA) currently recommends that procedures for proper handling and disposal of antineoplastic agents be considered. Drug is extremely irritating to tissues and must be administered I.V.; if extravasation occurs during I.V. use, severe damage to soft tissues will occur; use with caution in patients who have received radiation therapy or in the presence of hepatobiliary dysfunction; reduce dosage in patients who are receiving radiation therapy simultaneously.

Adverse Reactions

>10%:

Central nervous system: Unusual fatigue, malaise, fever

Dermatologic: Alopecia (reversible), skin eruptions, acne, increased pigmentation of previously irradiated skin

(Continued)

Dactinomycin *(Continued)*

Extravasation: An irritant and should be administered through a rapidly running I.V. line; extravasation can lead to tissue necrosis, pain, and ulceration

Vesicant chemotherapy

Endocrine & metabolic: Hypocalcemia

Gastrointestinal: **Highly emetogenic**

Severe nausea and vomiting occurs in most patients and persists for up to 24 hours; stomatitis, anorexia, abdominal pain, esophagitis, diarrhea

Time course of nausea/vomiting: Onset: 2-5 hours; Duration: 4-24 hours

Hematologic: Myelosuppressive: Dose-limiting toxicity; anemia, aplastic anemia, agranulocytosis, pancytopenia

WBC: Moderate

Platelets: Moderate

Onset (days): 7

Nadir (days): 14-21

Recovery (days): 21-28

1% to 10%: Gastrointestinal: Diarrhea, mucositis

<1%:

Endocrine & metabolic: Hyperuricemia

Hepatic: Hepatitis, liver function tests abnormalities

Miscellaneous: Anaphylactoid reaction

Overdosage/Toxicology Symptoms of overdose include myelosuppression, nausea, vomiting, glossitis, oral ulceration; there are no known antidotes and treatment is primarily symptomatic and supportive

Drug Interactions

Increased toxicity: Dactinomycin potentiates the effects of radiation therapy: Radiation may cause skin erythema which may become severe and is also associated with ↑ incidence of GI toxicity

Stability

Store intact vials at room temperature (30°C) and protect from light; storage at high temperatures (up to 50°C) for up to 2 weeks is permissible

Dilute with 1.1 mL of preservative-free SWI to yield a final concentration of 500 mcg/mL; do not use preservative diluent as precipitation may occur. Solution is chemically stable for 24 hours at room temperature (25°C). Significant binding of the drug occurs with micrometer nitrocellulose filter materials.

Compatible with D_5W or NS

Standard I.V. dilution:

I.V. push: Dose/syringe (500 mcg/mL)

IVPB: Dose/50 mL D_5W or NS

Stable for 24 hours at room temperature

Mechanism of Action Binds to the guanine portion of DNA intercalating between guanine and cytosine base pairs inhibiting DNA and RNA synthesis and protein synthesis; product of *Streptomyces parvullus* (a yeast species)

Pharmacodynamics/Kinetics

Distribution: Poor penetration into CSF; crosses placenta; high concentrations found in bone marrow and tumor cells, submaxillary gland, liver, and kidney

Metabolism: Minimal

Half-life: 36 hours

Time to peak serum concentration: I.V.: Within 2-5 minutes

Elimination: ~10% of dose excreted as unchanged drug in the urine, 14% excreted in feces, while 50% appears in the bile

Usual Dosage Refer to individual protocols

Calculation of the dosage for obese or edematous patients should be on the basis of surface area in an effort to relate dosage to lean body mass

Children >6 months and Adults: I.V.:

15 mcg/kg/day **or** 400-600 mcg/m²/day (maximum: 500 mcg) for 5 days, may repeat every 3-6 weeks **or**

2.5 mg/m² given in divided doses over 1-week period and repeated at 2-week intervals **or**

0.75-2 mg/m² as a single dose given at intervals of 1-4 weeks have been used

Dosing in renal impairment: No adjustment necessary

Administration

Administer slow I.V. push over 10-15 minutes

An in-line cellulose membrane filter should not be used during administration of dactinomycin solutions; do not administer I.M. or S.C.

Avoid extravasation: Extremely damaging to soft tissue and will cause a severe local reaction if extravasation occurs

Monitoring Parameters CBC with differential and platelet count, liver function tests, and renal function tests

Patient Information Notify physician if fever, persistent sore throat, bleeding, bruising, fatigue, or malaise occurs

Nursing Implications Care should be taken to avoid extravasation of the drug; an in-line cellulose membrane filter should not be used during administration of dactinomycin solutions; do not administer I.M. or S.C.

Management of extravasation: Apply ice immediately for 30-60 minutes; then alternate off/on every 15 minutes for one day. Data is not currently available regarding potential antidotes for dactinomycin.

Dosage Forms Powder for injection, lyophilized: 0.5 mg

Dakin's Solution *see* Sodium Hypochlorite Solution *on page 1145*

Dalalone L.A.® *see* Dexamethasone *on page 356*

Dalgan® *see* Dezocine *on page 368*

Dalmane® *see* Flurazepam *on page 546*

***d*-Alpha Tocopherol** *see* Vitamin E *on page 1309*

Dalteparin (dal TE pa rin)

Brand Names Fragmin®

Therapeutic Category Anticoagulant

Use Prevention of deep vein thrombosis which may lead to pulmonary embolism, in patients requiring abdominal surgery who are at risk for thromboembolism complications (ie, patients >40 years of age, obese, patients with malignancy, history of deep vein thrombosis or pulmonary embolism, and surgical procedures requiring general anesthesia and lasting longer than 30 minutes)

Contraindications Hypersensitivity to dalteparin or other low-molecular weight heparins; cerebrovascular disease or other active hemorrhage; cerebral aneurysm; severe uncontrolled hypertension

Warnings/Precautions Use with caution in patients with pre-existing thrombocytopenia, recent childbirth, subacute bacterial endocarditis, peptic ulcer disease, pericarditis or pericardial effusion, liver or renal function impairment, recent lumbar puncture, vasculitis, concurrent use of aspirin (increased bleeding risk), previous hypersensitivity to heparin, heparin-associated thrombocytopenia

Adverse Reactions

1% to 10%:

Central nervous system: Allergic fever

Dermatologic: Pruritus, rash, bullous eruption, skin necrosis

Hematologic: Bleeding, thrombocytopenia, wound hematoma

Local: Pain at injection site, injection site hematoma, injection site reactions

Miscellaneous: Anaphylactoid reactions, allergic reactions

Drug Interactions Increased toxicity: Caution should be used when using aspirin, other platelet inhibitors, and oral anticoagulants in combination with dalteparin due to an increased risk of bleeding

Stability Store at temperatures ≤25°C

Mechanism of Action Low molecular weight heparin analog with a molecular weight of 4000-6000 daltons; the commercial product contains 3% to 15% heparin with a molecular weight <3000 daltons, 65% to 78% with a molecular weight of 3000-8000 daltons and 14% to 26% with a molecular weight >8000 daltons; while dalteparin has been shown to inhibit both factor Xa and factor IIa (thrombin), the antithrombotic effect of dalteparin is characterized by a higher ratio of antifactor Xa to antifactor IIa activity (ratio = 4)

Usual Dosage Adults: S.C.:

Low-moderate risk patients: 2500 units 1-2 hours prior to surgery, then once daily for 5-10 days postoperatively

High risk patients: 5000 units 1-2 hours prior to surgery and then once daily for 5-10 days postoperatively

Monitoring Parameters Periodic CBC including platelet count; stool occult blood tests; monitoring of PT and PTT is not necessary

Dosage Forms Injection: Prefilled syringe: Anti-Factor Xa 2500 units per 0.2 mL; anti-Factor Xa 5000 units per 0.2 mL

Damason-P® *see* Hydrocodone and Aspirin *on page 621*

Danaparoid (da NAP a roid)

Brand Names Orgaran®

Synonyms Danaparoid Sodium

Therapeutic Category Anticoagulant

Use Prevention of postoperative deep vein thrombosis following elective hip replacement surgery

Pregnancy Risk Factor B

Contraindications Patients with severe hemorrhagic diathesis including active major bleeding, hemorrhagic stroke in the acute phase, hemophilia and idiopathic thrombocytopenic purpura; type II thrombocytopenia associated with a

(Continued)

Danaparoid *(Continued)*

positive *in vitro* test for antiplatelet antibody in the presence of danaparoid, hypersensitivity to danaparoid or known hypersensitivity to pork products

Warnings/Precautions Do not administer intramuscularly; use with extreme caution in patients with a history of bacterial endocarditis, hemorrhagic stroke, recent CNS or ophthalmological surgery, bleeding diathesis, uncontrolled arterial hypertension, or a history of recent gastrointestinal ulceration and hemorrhage. Danaparoid shows a low cross-sensitivity with antiplatelet antibodies in individuals with type II heparin-induced thrombocytopenia. This product contains sodium sulfite which may cause allergic-type reactions, including anaphylactic symptoms and life-threatening asthmatic episodes in susceptible people; this is seen more frequently in asthmatics.

Adverse Reactions

1% to 10%:

Cardiovascular: Peripheral edema, generalized edema
Central nervous system: Fever, insomnia, headache, dizziness
Dermatologic: Rash, pruritus
Gastrointestinal: Nausea, constipation, vomiting
Genitourinary: Urinary tract infections, urinary retention
Hematologic: Anemia, hemorrhage, hematoma
Local: Injection site pain
Neuromuscular & skeletal: Joint disorder, weakness

Overdosage/Toxicology Symptoms of overdose include hemorrhage; protamine zinc has been used to reverse effects

Drug Interactions Increased toxicity with oral anticoagulants, platelet inhibitors

Pharmacodynamics/Kinetics

Onset of effect: Maximum anti-factor Xa and antithrombin (anti-factor IIa) activities occur 2-5 hours after S.C. administration
Half-life, plasma: Mean terminal half-life: ~24 hours
Elimination: Primarily by the kidneys

Usual Dosage S.C.:

Children: Safety and effectiveness have not been established
Adults: 750 anti-Xa units twice daily; beginning 1-4 hours before surgery and then not sooner than 2 hours after surgery and every 12 hours until the risk of DVT has diminished, the average duration of therapy is 7-10 days

Dosing adjustment in renal impairment: Adjustment may be necessary in elderly and patients with severe renal impairment; patients with serum creatinine levels ≥2.0 mg/dL should be carefully monitored

Monitoring Parameters Platelets, occult blood, and anti-Xa activity, if available; the monitoring of PT and/or PTT is not necessary

Dosage Forms Injection, as sodium: 750 anti-Xa units/0.6 mL

Danaparoid Sodium *see* Danaparoid *on previous page*

Danazol (DA na zole)

Brand Names Danocrine®

Canadian/Mexican Brand Names Cyclomen® (Canada); Ladogal® (Mexico); Zoldan-A® (Mexico)

Therapeutic Category Androgen; Antigonadotropic Agent

Use Treatment of endometriosis, fibrocystic breast disease, and hereditary angioedema

Pregnancy Risk Factor X

Contraindications Undiagnosed genital bleeding, hypersensitivity to danazol or any component

Warnings/Precautions Use with caution in patients with seizure disorders, migraine, or conditions influenced by edema; impaired hepatic, renal, or cardiac disease, pregnancy, lactation

Adverse Reactions

>10%:

Cardiovascular: Edema
Dermatologic: Oily skin, acne, hirsutism
Endocrine & metabolic: Fluid retention, breakthrough bleeding, irregular menstrual periods, decreased breast size
Gastrointestinal: Weight gain
Hepatic: Hepatic impairment
Miscellaneous: Voice deepening

1% to 10%:

Endocrine & metabolic: Virilization, androgenic effects, amenorrhea, hypoestrogenism
Neuromuscular & skeletal: Weakness

<1%:

Cardiovascular: Benign intracranial hypertension

Central nervous system: Dizziness, headache
Dermatologic: Skin rashes, photosensitivity
Gastrointestinal: Pancreatitis, bleeding gums
Genitourinary: Monilial vaginitism, testicular atrophy, enlarged clitoris
Hepatic: Cholestatic jaundice
Neuromuscular & skeletal: Carpal tunnel syndrome

Drug Interactions
Increased toxicity:
↓ insulin requirements
Warfarin → ↑ anticoagulant effects

Mechanism of Action Suppresses pituitary output of follicle-stimulating hormone and luteinizing hormone that causes regression and atrophy of normal and ectopic endometrial tissue; decreases rate of growth of abnormal breast tissue; reduces attacks associated with hereditary angioedema by increasing levels of C4 component of complement

Pharmacodynamics/Kinetics
Onset of therapeutic effect: Within 4 weeks following daily doses
Metabolism: Extensive hepatic metabolism, primarily to 2-hydroxymethylethisterone
Half-life: 4.5 hours (variable)
Time to peak serum concentration: Within 2 hours
Elimination: In urine

Usual Dosage Adults: Oral:
Endometriosis: 100-400 mg twice daily for 3-6 months (may extend to 9 months)
Fibrocystic breast disease: 50-200 mg twice daily for 2-6 months
Hereditary angioedema: 400-600 mg/day in 2-3 divided doses

Patient Information Notify physician if masculinity effects occur; virilization may occur in female patients; report menstrual irregularities; male patients report persistent penile erections; all patients should report persistent GI distress, diarrhea, or jaundice

Dosage Forms Capsule: 50 mg, 100 mg, 200 mg

Danocrine® *see* Danazol *on previous page*

Dantrium® *see* Dantrolene *on this page*

Dantrolene (DAN troe leen)

Brand Names Dantrium®

Synonyms Dantrolene Sodium

Therapeutic Category Antidote, Malignant Hyperthermia; Hyperthermia, Treatment; Skeletal Muscle Relaxant

Use Treatment of spasticity associated with spinal cord injury, stroke, cerebral palsy, or multiple sclerosis; also used as treatment of malignant hyperthermia

Pregnancy Risk Factor C

Contraindications Active hepatic disease; should not be used where spasticity is used to maintain posture or balance

Warnings/Precautions Use with caution in patients with impaired cardiac function or impaired pulmonary function; has potential for hepatotoxicity; overt hepatitis has been most frequently observed between the third and twelfth month of therapy; hepatic injury appears to be greater in females and in patients >35 years of age

Adverse Reactions
>10%:
Central nervous system: Drowsiness, dizziness, lightheadedness, fatigue
Dermatologic: Rash
Gastrointestinal: Diarrhea (mild), nausea, vomiting
Neuromuscular & skeletal: Muscle weakness
1% to 10%:
Cardiovascular: Pleural effusion with pericarditis
Central nervous system: Chills, fever, headache, insomnia, nervousness, mental depression
Gastrointestinal: Diarrhea (severe), constipation, anorexia, stomach cramps
Ocular: Blurred vision
Respiratory: Respiratory depression
<1%:
Central nervous system: Seizures, confusion
Hepatic: Hepatitis

Overdosage/Toxicology Symptoms of overdose include CNS depression, hypotension, nausea, vomiting

For decontamination, lavage/activated charcoal with cathartic; do not use ipecac; hypotension can be treated with isotonic I.V. fluids with the patient placed in the Trendelenburg position; dopamine or norepinephrine can be given if hypotension is refractory to above therapy
(Continued)

Dantrolene *(Continued)*

Drug Interactions Increased toxicity: Estrogens (hepatotoxicity), CNS depressants (sedation), MAO inhibitors, phenothiazines, clindamycin (increased neuromuscular blockade), verapamil (hyperkalemia and cardiac depression), warfarin, clofibrate and tolbutamide

Stability Reconstitute vial by adding 60 mL of sterile water for injection USP (**not bacteriostatic water for injection**); protect from light; use within 6 hours; avoid glass bottles for I.V. infusion

Mechanism of Action Acts directly on skeletal muscle by interfering with release of calcium ion from the sarcoplasmic reticulum; prevents or reduces the increase in myoplasmic calcium ion concentration that activates the acute catabolic processes associated with malignant hyperthermia

Pharmacodynamics/Kinetics

Absorption: Slow and incomplete from GI tract

Metabolism: Slowly in liver

Half-life: 8.7 hours

Elimination: 25% excreted in urine as metabolites and unchanged drug, 45% to 50% excreted in feces via bile

Usual Dosage

Spasticity: Oral:

Children: Initial: 0.5 mg/kg/dose twice daily, increase frequency to 3-4 times/day at 4- to 7-day intervals, then increase dose by 0.5 mg/kg to a maximum of 3 mg/kg/dose 2-4 times/day up to 400 mg/day

Adults: 25 mg/day to start, increase frequency to 2-4 times/day, then increase dose by 25 mg every 4-7 days to a maximum of 100 mg 2-4 times/day or 400 mg/day

Malignant hyperthermia: Children and Adults:

Oral: 4-8 mg/kg/day in 4 divided doses

Preoperative prophylaxis: Begin 1-2 days prior to surgery with last dose 3-4 hours prior to surgery

I.V.: 1 mg/kg; may repeat dose up to cumulative dose of 10 mg/kg (mean effective dose is 2.5 mg/kg), then switch to oral dosage

Preoperative: 2.5 mg/kg ~1¼ hours prior to anesthesia and infused over 1 hour with additional doses as needed and individualized

Dietary Considerations Alcohol: Additive CNS effects, avoid use

Monitoring Parameters Motor performance should be monitored for therapeutic outcomes; nausea, vomiting, and liver function tests should be monitored for potential hepatotoxicity; intravenous administration requires cardiac monitor and blood pressure monitor

Test Interactions ↑ serum AST (SGOT), ALT (SGPT), alkaline phosphatase, LDH, BUN, and total serum bilirubin

Patient Information Avoid unnecessary exposure to sunlight (or use sunscreen, protective clothing); avoid alcohol and other CNS depressants; patients should use caution while driving or performing other tasks requiring alertness

Nursing Implications 36 vials needed for adequate hyperthermia therapy; exercise caution at meals on the day of administration because difficulty swallowing and choking has been reported; avoid extravasation as is a tissue irritant

Dosage Forms

Capsule, as sodium: 25 mg, 50 mg, 100 mg

Powder for injection, as sodium: 20 mg

Extemporaneous Preparations A 5 mg/mL suspension may be made by adding five 100 mg capsules to a citric acid solution (150 mg citric acid powder in 10 mL water) and then adding syrup to a total volume of 100 mL; stable 2 days in refrigerator

Nahata MC and Hipple TF, *Pediatric Drug Formulations*, 1st ed, Cincinnati, OH: Harvey Whitney Books Co, 1990.

Dantrolene Sodium *see* Dantrolene *on previous page*

Dapa® [OTC] *see* Acetaminophen *on page 19*

Dapiprazole (DA pi pray zole)

Brand Names Rēv-Eyes™

Synonyms Dapiprazole Hydrochloride

Therapeutic Category Alpha-Adrenergic Blocking Agent, Ophthalmic

Use Reverse dilation due to drugs (adrenergic or parasympathomimetic) after eye exams

Pregnancy Risk Factor B

Contraindications Contraindicated in the presence of conditions where miosis is unacceptable, such as acute iritis and in patients with a history of hypersensitivity to any component of the formulation

Warnings/Precautions For ophthalmic use only

Adverse Reactions

>10%:

Central nervous system: Headache

Ocular: Conjunctival injection, burning and itching eyes, lid edema, ptosis, lid erythema, chemosis, punctate keratitis, corneal edema, photophobia

1% to 10%: Ocular: Dry eyes, blurring of vision, tearing of eye

Stability After reconstitution, drops are stable at room temperature for 21 days. Store at room temperature (15°C to 30°C/59°F to 86°F)

Mechanism of Action Dapiprazole is a selective alpha-adrenergic blocking agent, exerting effects primarily on alpha$_1$-adrenoceptors. It induces miosis via relaxation of the smooth dilator (radial) muscle of the iris, which causes pupillary constriction. It is devoid of cholinergic effects. Dapiprazole also partially reverses the cycloplegia induced with parasympatholytic agents such as tropicamide. Although the drug has no significant effect on the ciliary muscle *per se*, it may increase accommodative amplitude, therefore relieving the symptoms of paralysis of accommodation.

Usual Dosage Adults: Administer 2 drops followed 5 minutes later by an additional 2 drops applied to the conjunctiva of each eye; should not be used more frequently than once a week in the same patient

Administration Shake container for several minutes to ensure mixing. Instill 2 drops into the conjunctiva of each eye followed 5 minutes later by an additional 2 drops. Administer after the ophthalmic examination to reverse the diagnostic mydriasis.

Patient Information May still be sensitive to sunlight and sensitivity may return in 2 or more hours: exercise caution when driving at night or performing other activities in poor illumination. To avoid contamination, do not touch tip of container to any surface.

Nursing Implications Finger pressure should be applied to lacrimal sac for 1-2 minutes after instillation to decrease risk of absorption and systemic reactions

Dosage Forms Powder, lyophilized, as hydrochloride: 25 mg [0.5% solution when mixed with supplied diluent]

Dapiprazole Hydrochloride *see* Dapiprazole *on previous page*

Dapsone (DAP sone)

Related Information

Antimicrobial Drugs of Choice *on page 1468*

Guidelines for the Prevention of Opportunistic Infections in Persons with HIV *on page 1457*

Brand Names Avlosulfon®

Synonyms Diaminodiphenylsulfone

Therapeutic Category Antibiotic, Sulfone; Leprostatic Agent

Use Treatment of leprosy and dermatitis herpetiformis (infections caused by *Mycobacterium leprae*), alternative agent for *Pneumocystis carinii* pneumonia prophylaxis (given alone) and treatment (given with trimethoprim)

Pregnancy Risk Factor C

Contraindications Hypersensitivity to dapsone or any component

Warnings/Precautions Use with caution in patients with severe anemia, G-6-PD deficiency; hypersensitivity to other sulfonamides

Adverse Reactions

1% to 10%:

Central nervous system: Reactional states

Hematologic: Dose-related hemolysis, methemoglobinemia with cyanosis

<1%:

Central nervous system: Insomnia, headache

Dermatologic: Exfoliative dermatitis

Gastrointestinal: Nausea, vomiting

Hematologic: Hemolytic anemia, methemoglobinemia, leukopenia, agranulocytosis

Hepatic: Hepatitis, cholestatic jaundice

Neuromuscular & skeletal: Peripheral neuropathy

Ocular: Blurred vision

Otic: Tinnitus

Overdosage/Toxicology Symptoms of overdose include nausea, vomiting, hyperexcitability, methemoglobin-induced depression, seizures, cyanosis, hemolysis

Following decontamination, methylene blue 1-2 mg/kg I.V. is treatment of choice

Drug Interactions Cytochrome P-450 3A enzyme substrate

Decreased effect/levels: Para-aminobenzoic acid and rifampin

Increased toxicity: Folic acid antagonists

Stability Protect from light

Mechanism of Action Dapsone is a sulfone antimicrobial. The mechanism of action of the sulfones is similar to that of the sulfonamides. Sulfonamides are

(Continued)

Dapsone *(Continued)*

competitive antagonists of para-aminobenzoic acid (PABA) and prevent normal bacterial utilization of PABA for the synthesis of folic acid.

Pharmacodynamics/Kinetics

Absorption: Oral: Well absorbed

Distribution: V_d: 1.5 L/kg; throughout total body water and present in all tissues, especially liver and kidney

Metabolism: In the liver

Half-life, elimination: 30 hours (range: 10-50 hours)

Elimination: In urine

Usual Dosage Oral:

Leprosy:

Children: 1-2 mg/kg/24 hours, up to a maximum of 100 mg/day

Adults: 50-100 mg/day for 3-10 years

Dermatitis herpetiformis: Adults: Start at 50 mg/day, increase to 300 mg/day, or higher to achieve full control, reduce dosage to minimum level as soon as possible

Prophylaxis of *Pneumocystis carinii* pneumonia: Children >1 month: 1 mg/kg/day; maximum: 100 mg

Treatment of *Pneumocystis carinii* pneumonia: Adults: 100 mg/day in combination with trimethoprim (20 mg/kg/day) for 21 days

Dosing in renal impairment: Adjustment is necessary, but no specific guidelines are available

Monitoring Parameters Monitor patient for signs of jaundice and hemolysis

Patient Information Frequent blood tests are required during early therapy; discontinue if rash develops and contact physician if persistent sore throat, fever, malaise, or fatigue occurs; may cause photosensitivity

Dosage Forms Tablet: 25 mg, 100 mg

Extemporaneous Preparations One report indicated that dapsone may not be well absorbed when administered to children as suspensions made from pulverized tablets

Mirochnick M, Clarke D, Brenn A, et al, "Low Serum Dapsone Concentrations in Children Receiving an Extemporaneously Prepared Oral Formulation," [Abstract Th B 365], APS-SPR, Baltimore, MD: 1992.

Jacobus Pharmaceutical Company (609) 921-7447 makes a 2 mg/mL proprietary liquid formulation available under an IND for the prophylaxis of *Pneumocystis carinii* pneumonia

Daraprim® *see* Pyrimethamine *on page 1082*

Darvocet-N® *see* Propoxyphene and Acetaminophen *on page 1067*

Darvocet-N® 100 *see* Propoxyphene and Acetaminophen *on page 1067*

Darvon® *see* Propoxyphene *on page 1065*

Darvon-N® *see* Propoxyphene *on page 1065*

Datril® [OTC] *see* Acetaminophen *on page 19*

Daunomycin *see* Daunorubicin Hydrochloride *on next page*

Daunorubicin Citrate (Liposomal)

(daw noe ROO bi sin SI trate lip po SOE mal)

Related Information

Daunorubicin Hydrochloride *on next page*

Brand Names DaunoXome®

Therapeutic Category Antineoplastic Agent, Anthracycline; Antineoplastic Agent, Antibiotic

Use Advanced HIV-associated Kaposi's sarcoma; first-line cytotoxic therapy for advanced HIV-associated Kaposi's sarcoma

Pregnancy Risk Factor D

Contraindications Hypersensitivity to previous doses or any constituents of the product

Warnings/Precautions

The U.S. Food and Drug Administration (FDA) currently recommends that procedures for proper handling and disposal of antineoplastic agents be considered.

The primary toxicity is myelosuppression, especially off the granulocytic series, which may be severe, with much less marked effects on platelets and erythroid series. Potential cardiac toxicity, particularly in patients who have received prior anthracyclines or who have pre-existing cardiac disease, may occur. Refer to Daunorubicin monograph.

Although grade 3-4 injection site inflammation has been reported in patients treated with the liposomal daunorubicin, no instances of local tissue necrosis were observed with extravasation. However, refer to daunorubicin monograph and avoid extravasation.

Reduce dosage in patients with impaired hepatic function. Hyperuricemia can be induced secondary to rapid lysis of leukemic cells. As a precaution, administer allopurinol prior to initiating antileukemic therapy.

Adverse Reactions

>10%:

- Central nervous system: Fatigue, headache
- Gastrointestinal: Abdominal pain, anorexia, diarrhea, nausea, vomiting
- Hematologic: Neutropenia
- Neuromuscular & skeletal: Neuropathy
- Respiratory: Cough, dyspnea, rhinitis
- Miscellaneous: Infection

5% to 10%:

- Cardiovascular: Hypertension, palpitations, syncope, tachycardia, chest pain, edema
- Central nervous system: Depression, dizziness, insomnia, malaise
- Dermatologic: Alopecia, pruritus
- Endocrine & metabolic: Hot flashes
- Gastrointestinal: Constipation, stomatitis, tenesmus
- Neuromuscular & skeletal: Arthralgia, myalgia
- Ocular: Abnormal vision
- Respiratory: Sinusitis

Overdosage/Toxicology Symptoms of acute overdose are increased severities of the observed dose-limiting toxicities of therapeutic doses, myelosuppression (especially granulocytopenia), fatigue, nausea, vomiting; treatment is symptomatic

Stability Store intact vials under refrigeration (2°C to 8°C/36°F to 46°F). Reconstitute liposomal daunorubicin 1:1 with 5% dextrose injection before administration. Store reconstituted solution for a maximum of 6 hours. Do not freeze and protect from light. Do not use an in-line filter for intravenous infusion.

Mechanism of Action Liposomal daunorubicin contains an aqueous solution of the citrate salt of daunorubicin encapsulated with lipid vesicles (liposomes) composed of a lipid bilayer of distearoylphosphatidylcholine and cholesterol (2:1 molar ratio). This liposomal daunorubicin is formulated to maximum the selectivity of daunorubicin for solid tumors *in situ*; refer to Daunorubicin monograph.

Pharmacodynamics/Kinetics

Distribution: V_d: 6.4 L

Half-life: 4.4 hours

Elimination: Plasma clearance: 17.3 mL/minute

Usual Dosage Adults: I.V.: 40 mg/m^2 over 1 hour; repeat every 2 weeks; continue treatment until there is evidence of progressive disease

Dosing adjustment in renal/hepatic impairment:

Serum Bilirubin	Serum Creatinine	Recommended Dose
1.2-3 mg/dL		3/4 normal dose
>3 mg/dL	>3 mg/dL	1/2 normal dose

Administration Administer intravenously over 1 hour; avoid extravasation; refer to Daunorubicin monograph

Monitoring Parameters Observe patient closely and monitor chemical and laboratory tests extensively. Evaluate cardiac, renal, and hepatic function prior to each course of treatment. Repeat blood counts prior to each dose and withhold if the absolute granulocyte count is <750 cells/mm^3. Monitor serum uric acid levels.

Dosage Forms Injection: 2 mg/mL (equivalent to 50 mg daunorubicin base) (1 mL, 4 mL, 10 mL unit packs)

Daunorubicin Hydrochloride

(daw noe ROO bi sin hye droe KLOR ide)

Related Information

Antiemetics for Chemotherapy Induced Nausea and Vomiting *on page 1348*

Cancer Chemotherapy Regimens *on page 1351*

Extravasation Management of Chemotherapeutic Agents *on page 1379*

Brand Names Cerubidine®

Synonyms Daunomycin; DNR; Rubidomycin Hydrochloride

Therapeutic Category Antineoplastic Agent, Anthracycline; Antineoplastic Agent, Antibiotic; Antineoplastic Agent, Vesicant; Vesicant

Use Treatment of ANLL and myeloblastic leukemia; lymphoma

Pregnancy Risk Factor D

Contraindications Congestive heart failure, cardiopathy or arrhythmias; hypersensitivity to daunorubicin or any component

Warnings/Precautions The U.S. Food and Drug Administration (FDA) currently recommends that procedures for proper handling and disposal of antineoplastic agents be considered. I.V. use only, severe local tissue necrosis will result if

(Continued)

Daunorubicin Hydrochloride *(Continued)*

extravasation occurs; reduce dose in patients with impaired hepatic, renal, or biliary function; severe myelosuppression is possible when used in therapeutic doses. Total cumulative dose should take into account previous or concomitant treatment with cardiotoxic agents or irradiation of chest.

Irreversible myocardial toxicity may occur as total dosage approaches:

- 550 mg/m^2 in adults
- 400 mg/m^2 in patients receiving chest radiation
- 300 mg/m^2 in children >2 years of age or
- 10 mg/kg in children <2 years; this may occur during therapy or several months after therapy

Adverse Reactions

>10%:

- Dermatologic: Alopecia (reversible)
- Gastrointestinal: Mild nausea or vomiting occurs in 50% of patients within the first 24 hours; stomatitis may occur 3-7 days after administration, but is not as severe as that caused by doxorubicin
  - Time course for nausea/vomiting: Onset: 1-3 hours; Duration 4-24 hours
- Genitourinary: Discoloration of urine (red)

1% to 10%:

- Cardiovascular: Congestive heart failure; maximum lifetime dose: Refer to Warnings/Precautions
- Extravasation: Daunorubicin is a vesicant; infiltration can cause severe inflammation, tissue necrosis, and ulceration; if the drug is infiltrated, consult institutional policy, apply ice to the area, and elevate the limb
  - **Vesicant chemotherapy**
- Endocrine & metabolic: Hyperuricemia
- Gastrointestinal: GI ulceration, diarrhea
- Hematologic: Myelosuppressive: Dose-limiting toxicity; occurs in all patients; leukopenia is more significant than thrombocytopenia
  - WBC: Severe
  - Platelets: Severe
  - Onset (days): 7
  - Nadir (days): 14
  - Recovery (days): 21-28

<1%:

- Cardiovascular: Pericarditis, myocarditis
- Central nervous system: Chills
- Dermatologic: Skin rash, pigmentation of nail beds, urticaria
- Hepatic: Elevation in serum bilirubin, AST, and alkaline phosphatase
- Miscellaneous: Fertility impairment

Overdosage/Toxicology Symptoms of overdose include myelosuppression, nausea, vomiting, stomatitis; there are no known antidotes; treatment is primarily symptomatic and supportive

Stability

Store intact vials at room temperature and protect from light

Dilute vials with 4 mL SWI for a final concentration of 5 mg/mL; reconstituted solution is stable for 4 days at 15°C to 25°C

- Protect from fluorescent light to decrease photo-inactivation after storage in solution for several days; protect from direct sunlight
  - Decomposed drug turns purple
- For I.V. push administration, desired dose is withdrawn into a syringe containing 10-15 mL NS
- Further dilution in D_5W, LR, or NS is stable for 24 hours at room temperature (25°C) and up to 4 weeks if protected from light
- **Incompatible** with heparin, sodium bicarbonate, 5-FU, and dexamethasone

Standard I.V. dilution:

- I.V. push: Dose/syringe (initial concentration is 5 mg/mL; however, qs to 10-15 mL with NS)
  - Maximum syringe size for IVP is a 30 mL syringe and syringe should be <75% full
- IVPB: Dose/50-100 mL NS or D_5W
- Stable for 24 hours at room temperature (25°C)

Mechanism of Action Inhibition of DNA and RNA synthesis, by intercalating between DNA base pairs and by steric obstruction; is not cell cycle-specific for the S phase of cell division; daunomycin is preferred over doxorubicin for the treatment of ANLL because of its dose-limiting toxicity (myelosuppression) is not of concern in the therapy of this disease; has less mucositis associated with its use

Pharmacodynamics/Kinetics

Distribution: V_d: 40 L/kg; crosses the placenta; distributed to many body tissues, particularly the liver, kidneys, lung, spleen, and heart; does not distribute into the CNS

Metabolism: Primarily in the liver to daunorubicinol (active), which circulates

Half-life:

- Distribution: 2 minutes
- Elimination: 14-20 hours
- Terminal: 18.5 hours
- Daunorubicinol plasma half-life: 24-48 hours

Elimination: 40% of dose excreted in the bile; ~25% is excreted in the urine as metabolite and unchanged drug; can turn the urine red during first 24-48 hours after treatment

Usual Dosage I.V. (refer to individual protocols):

Children:

- ALL combination therapy: Remission induction: 25-45 mg/m^2 on day 1 every week for 4 cycles **or** 30-45 mg/m^2/day for 3 days
- In children <2 years or <0.5 m^2, daunorubicin should be based on weight (mg/kg): 1 mg/kg per protocol with frequency dependent on regimen employed
- Cumulative dose should not exceed 300 mg/m^2 in children >2 years or 10 mg/kg in children <2 years

Adults:

- 30-60 mg/m^2/day for 3-5 days, repeat dose in 3-4 weeks
- Single agent induction for AML: 60 mg/m^2/day for 3 days; repeat every 3-4 weeks
- Combination therapy induction for AML: 45 mg/m^2/day for 3 days of the first course of induction therapy; subsequent courses: Every day for 2 days
- ALL combination therapy: 45 mg/m^2/day for 3 days
  - Cumulative dose should not exceed 400-600 mg/m^2

Dosing adjustment in renal impairment:

- Cl_{cr} <10 mL/minute: Administer 75% of normal dose
- Serum creatine >3 mg/dL: Administer 50% of normal dose

Dosing adjustment in hepatic impairment:

- Serum bilirubin 1.2-3 mg/dL or AST 60-180 IU: Reduce dose to 75%
- Serum bilirubin 3.1-5 mg/dL or AST >180 IU: Reduce dose to 50%
- Serum bilirubin >5 mg/dL: Omit use

Administration

Administer IVP over 1-5 minutes into the tubing of a rapidly infusing I.V. solution of D_5W or NS; daunorubicin has also been diluted in 100 mL of D_5W or NS and infused over 15-30 minutes

Avoid extravasation, can cause severe tissue damage; flush with 5-10 mL of I.V. solution before and after drug administration

Monitoring Parameters CBC with differential and platelet count, liver function test, EKG, ventricular ejection fraction, renal function test

Patient Information Discoloration of urine (red) may occur transiently; immediately report any change in sensation (eg, stinging) at injection site during infusion (may be an early sign of infiltration)

Nursing Implications

Daunorubicin is a vesicant and should never be administered I.M. or S.C.

Extravasation management:

- Apply ice immediately for 30-60 minutes; then alternate off/on every 15 minutes for one day
- Topical cooling may be achieved using ice packs or cooling pad with circulating ice water; cooling of site for 24 hours as tolerated by the patient. Elevate and rest extremity 24-48 hours, then resume normal activity as tolerated. Application of cold inhibits vesicant's cytotoxicity.
- Application of heat or sodium bicarbonate can be harmful and is contraindicated
- If pain, erythema, and/or swelling persist beyond 48 hours, refer patient immediately to plastic surgeon for consultation and possible debridement

Dosage Forms Powder for injection, lyophilized: 20 mg

DaunoXome® *see* Daunorubicin Citrate (Liposomal) *on page 344*

Daypro™ *see* Oxaprozin *on page 932*

DC 240® Softgels® [OTC] *see* Docusate *on page 415*

DCF *see* Pentostatin *on page 973*

DDAVP® *see* Desmopressin Acetate *on page 353*

ddC *see* Zalcitabine *on page 1318*

ddI *see* Didanosine *on page 377*

1-Deamino-8-D-Arginine Vasopressin *see* Desmopressin Acetate *on page 353*

Debrisan® [OTC] *see* Dextranomer *on page 364*

Debrox® Otic [OTC] *see* Carbamide Peroxide *on page 203*

Decaderm® *see* Dexamethasone *on page 356*

Decadron® *see* Dexamethasone *on page 356*

Decadron®-LA *see* Dexamethasone *on page 356*

Decadron® Turbinaire® *see* Dexamethasone *on page 356*

Deca-Durabolin® *see* Nandrolone *on page 878*

Decaject-L.A.® *see* Dexamethasone *on page 356*

Decaspray® *see* Dexamethasone *on page 356*

Declomycin® *see* Demeclocycline *on page 350*

Decofed® Syrup [OTC] *see* Pseudoephedrine *on page 1074*

Deferoxamine (de fer OKS a meen)

Brand Names Desferal® Mesylate

Synonyms Deferoxamine Mesylate

Therapeutic Category Antidote, Aluminum Toxicity; Antidote, Iron Toxicity

Use Acute iron intoxication; chronic iron overload secondary to multiple transfusions; diagnostic test for iron overload; iron overload secondary to congenital anemias; hemochromatosis; removal of corneal rust rings following surgical removal of foreign bodies

Investigational: Treatment of aluminum accumulation in renal failure

Pregnancy Risk Factor C

Contraindications Patients with anuria, primary hemochromatosis

Warnings/Precautions Use with caution in patients with severe renal disease, pyelonephritis; may increase susceptibility to *Yersinia enterocolitica*

Adverse Reactions

1% to 10%: Local: Pain and induration at injection site

<1%:

Cardiovascular: Flushing, hypotension, tachycardia, shock, edema
Central nervous system: Fever
Dermatologic: Erythema, urticaria, pruritus, rash, cutaneous wheal formation
Gastrointestinal: Abdominal discomfort, diarrhea
Neuromuscular & skeletal: Leg cramps
Ocular: Blurred vision, cataracts
Otic: Hearing loss
Miscellaneous: Anaphylaxis

Overdosage/Toxicology Symptoms of overdose include hypotension, blurring of vision, diarrhea, leg cramps, tachycardia; treatment is symptomatic and supportive

Stability Protect from light; reconstituted solutions (sterile water) may be stored at room temperature for 7 days

Mechanism of Action Complexes with trivalent ions (ferric ions) to form ferrioxamine, which are removed by the kidneys

Pharmacodynamics/Kinetics

Absorption: Oral: <15%
Metabolism: In the liver to ferrioxamine
Half-life:
Parent drug: 6.1 hours
Ferrioxamine: 5.8 hours
Elimination: Renal excretion of the metabolite and unchanged drug

Usual Dosage

Children:

Acute iron intoxication (I.M. is preferred route for patients not in shock). Treat until urine is no longer pink salmon colored:
I.M.: 50 mg/kg/dose every 6 hours to a maximum of 6 g/day
I.V.: 15 mg/kg/hour; maximum: 6 g/day

Chronic iron overload:
I.M., I.V.: 50 mg/kg/dose to a maximum of 6 g/24 hours or 2 g/dose; do not exceed 15 mg/kg/hour I.V.
S.C.: 20-40 mg/kg/day over 8-12 hours (via a portable, controlled infusion device)

Aluminum-induced bone disease: 20-40 mg/kg every hemodialysis treatment, frequency dependent on clinical status of the patient

Adults:

Acute iron intoxication: (I.M. is preferred route for patients not in shock). Treat until urine is no longer pink salmon colored:
I.M., I.V.: 1 g stat, then 0.5 g every 4 hours for two doses, then 0.5 g every 4-12 hours up to 6 g/day; do not exceed 15 mg/kg/hour I.V.

Chronic iron overload:
I.M.: 0.5-1 g every day
I.V.: 2 g after each unit of blood infusion at 15 mg/kg/hour
S.C.: 1-2 g every day over 8-24 hours

Dosing adjustment in renal impairment: Cl_{cr} <10 mL/minute: Administer 50% of dose

Has been used investigationally as a single 40 mg/kg I.V. dose over 2 hours, to promote mobilization of aluminum from tissue stores as an aid in the diagnosis of aluminum-associated osteodystrophy

Administration I.M. is preferred route; maximum I.V. rate is 15 mg/kg/hour. Urticaria, hypotension, and shock have occurred following rapid I.V. administration; administer I.M., slow S.C., or I.V. infusion. Add 2 mL sterile water to 500 mg vial; for I.M. or S.C. administration, no further dilution is required; for I.V. infusion, dilute in dextrose, normal saline, or lactated Ringer's; 10 mg/mL (maximum: 25 mg/mL); maximum rate of infusion: 15 mg/kg/hour.

Monitoring Parameters Serum iron, total iron binding capacity; ophthalmologic exam and audiometry with chronic therapy

Patient Information May turn urine pink; blood and urine tests are necessary to follow therapy

Nursing Implications Iron chelate colors urine salmon pink

Dosage Forms Powder for injection, as mesylate: 500 mg

Deferoxamine Mesylate *see* Deferoxamine *on previous page*

Deficol® [OTC] *see* Bisacodyl *on page 153*

Degas® [OTC] *see* Simethicone *on page 1136*

Degest® 2 [OTC] *see* Naphazoline *on page 879*

Dehist® *see* Brompheniramine *on page 166*

Dekasol-L.A.® *see* Dexamethasone *on page 356*

Del Aqua-5® Gel *see* Benzoyl Peroxide *on page 140*

Del Aqua-10® Gel *see* Benzoyl Peroxide *on page 140*

Delatest® Injection *see* Testosterone *on page 1198*

Delatestryl® Injection *see* Testosterone *on page 1198*

Delaxin® *see* Methocarbamol *on page 805*

Delcort® *see* Hydrocortisone *on page 623*

Delestrogen® Injection *see* Estradiol *on page 468*

Delsym® [OTC] *see* Dextromethorphan *on page 366*

Delta-Cortef® *see* Prednisolone *on page 1037*

Deltacortisone *see* Prednisone *on page 1039*

Deltadehydrocortisone *see* Prednisone *on page 1039*

Deltahydrocortisone *see* Prednisolone *on page 1037*

Deltasone® *see* Prednisone *on page 1039*

Delta-Tritex® *see* Triamcinolone *on page 1255*

Del-Vi-A® *see* Vitamin A *on page 1307*

Demadex® *see* Torsemide *on page 1246*

Demecarium (dem e KARE ee um)

Related Information

Glaucoma Drug Therapy Comparison *on page 1410*

Brand Names Humorsol®

Synonyms Demecarium Bromide

Therapeutic Category Cholinergic Agent, Ophthalmic; Ophthalmic Agent, Miotic

Use Management of chronic simple glaucoma, chronic and acute angle-closure glaucoma; strabismus

Pregnancy Risk Factor C

Pregnancy/Breast-Feeding Implications Although there are no reports of use in pregnancy, demecarium is an ophthalmic medication and transplacental passage in significant amounts would not be expected

Contraindications Hypersensitivity to demecarium or any component, acute inflammatory disease of anterior chamber; pregnancy

Adverse Reactions

1% to 10%: Ocular: Stinging, burning eyes, myopia, visual blurring

<1%:

- Cardiovascular: Bradycardia, hypotension, flushing
- Gastrointestinal: Nausea, vomiting, diarrhea
- Neuromuscular & skeletal: Muscle weakness
- Ocular: Retinal detachment, miosis, twitching eyelids, watering eyes
- Respiratory: Dyspnea
- Miscellaneous: Diaphoresis

Overdosage/Toxicology Antidote: Atropine sulfate: Adults: 0.4-0.6 mg (1/150-1/100 grain) or more parenterally

Stability Do not freeze; protect from heat

Mechanism of Action Cholinesterase inhibitor (anticholinesterase) which causes acetylcholine to accumulate at cholinergic receptor sites and produces

(Continued)

Demecarium *(Continued)*

effects equivalent to excessive stimulation of cholinergic receptors. Demecarium mainly acts by inhibiting true (erythrocyte) cholinesterase and causes a reduction in intraocular pressure due to facilitation of outflow of aqueous humor; the reduction is likely to be particularly marked in eyes in which the pressure is elevated.

Usual Dosage Children/Adults: Ophthalmic:

Glaucoma: Instill 1 drop into eyes twice weekly to a maximum dosage of 1 or 2 drops twice daily for up to 4 months

Strabismus:

Diagnosis: Instill 1 drop daily for 2 weeks, then 1 drop every 2 days for 2-3 weeks. If eyes become straighter, an accommodative factor is demonstrated.

Therapy: Instill not more than 1 drop at a time in both eyes every day for 2-3 weeks. Then reduce dosage to 1 drop every other day for 3-4 weeks and re-evaluate. Continue at 1 drop every 2 days to 1 drop twice a week and evaluate the patient's condition every 4-12 weeks. If improvement continues, reduce dose to 1 drop once a week and eventually off of medication. Discontinue therapy after 4 months if control of the condition still requires 1 drop every 2 days.

Patient Information For the eye; do not touch dropper to eye; transient burning or stinging may occur; do not use more often than directed

Nursing Implications Finger pressure should be applied to lacrimal sac for 1-2 minutes after instillation to decrease risk of absorption and systemic reactions; patient must be under supervision and tonometric examinations performed every 3-4 hours following initiation of therapy

Dosage Forms Solution, ophthalmic, as bromide: 0.125% (5 mL); 0.25% (5 mL)

Demecarium Bromide *see* Demecarium *on previous page*

Demeclocycline (dem e kloe SYE kleen)

Brand Names Declomycin®

Canadian/Mexican Brand Names Ledermicina® (Mexico)

Synonyms Demeclocycline Hydrochloride; Demethylchlortetracycline

Therapeutic Category Antibiotic, Tetracycline Derivative

Use Treatment of susceptible bacterial infections (acne, gonorrhea, pertussis and urinary tract infections) caused by both gram-negative and gram-positive organisms; used when penicillin is contraindicated (other agents are preferred); treatment of chronic syndrome of inappropriate secretion of antidiuretic hormone (SIADH)

Pregnancy Risk Factor D

Contraindications Hypersensitivity to demeclocycline, tetracyclines, or any component

Warnings/Precautions Do not administer to children <9 years of age; photosensitivity reactions occur frequently with this drug, avoid prolonged exposure to sunlight, do not use tanning equipment

Adverse Reactions

1% to 10%:

Dermatologic: Photosensitivity

Gastrointestinal: Nausea, diarrhea

<1%:

Cardiovascular: Pericarditis

Central nervous system: Increased intracranial pressure, bulging fontanels in infants

Dermatologic: Dermatologic effects, pruritus, exfoliative dermatitis

Endocrine & metabolic: Diabetes insipidus syndrome

Gastrointestinal: Vomiting, esophagitis, anorexia, abdominal cramps

Neuromuscular & skeletal: Paresthesia

Renal: Acute renal failure, azotemia

Miscellaneous: Superinfections, anaphylaxis, pigmentation of nails

Overdosage/Toxicology Symptoms of overdose include diabetes insipidus, nausea, anorexia, diarrhea; following GI decontamination, treatment is supportive

Drug Interactions

Decreased effect with antacids (aluminum, calcium, zinc, or magnesium), bismuth salts, sodium bicarbonate, barbiturates, carbamazepine, hydantoins

Decreased effect of oral contraceptives

Increased effect of warfarin

Mechanism of Action Inhibits protein synthesis by binding with the 30S and possibly the 50S ribosomal subunit(s) of susceptible bacteria; may also cause alterations in the cytoplasmic membrane

Pharmacodynamics/Kinetics

Onset of action for diuresis in SIADH: Several days

Absorption: ~50% to 80% from GI tract; food and dairy products reduce absorption

Protein binding: 41% to 50%

Metabolism: Small amounts metabolized in the liver to inactive metabolites; enterohepatically recycled

Half-life: Reduced renal function: 10-17 hours

Time to peak serum concentration: Oral: Within 3-6 hours

Elimination: As unchanged drug (42% to 50%) in urine

Usual Dosage Oral:

Children ≥8 years: 8-12 mg/kg/day divided every 6-12 hours

Adults: 150 mg 4 times/day or 300 mg twice daily

Uncomplicated gonorrhea (penicillin sensitive): 600 mg stat, 300 mg every 12 hours for 4 days (3 g total)

SIADH: 900-1200 mg/day or 13-15 mg/kg/day divided every 6-8 hours initially, then decrease to 0.6-0.9 g/day

Dosing adjustment/comments in renal/hepatic impairment: Should be avoided in patients with renal/hepatic dysfunction

Administration Administer 1 hour before or 2 hours after food or milk with plenty of fluid

Monitoring Parameters CBC, renal and hepatic function

Test Interactions May interfere with tests for urinary glucose (false-negative urine glucose using Clinistix®, Tes-Tape®)

Patient Information Avoid prolonged exposure to sunlight or sunlamps; avoid taking antacids before tetracyclines

Dosage Forms

Capsule, as hydrochloride: 150 mg

Tablet, as hydrochloride: 150 mg, 300 mg

Demeclocycline Hydrochloride *see* Demeclocycline *on previous page*

Demerol® *see* Meperidine *on page 780*

4-demethoxydaunorubicin *see* Idarubicin *on page 642*

Demethylchlortetracycline *see* Demeclocycline *on previous page*

Demser® *see* Metyrosine *on page 831*

Demulen® *see* Ethinyl Estradiol and Ethynodiol Diacetate *on page 482*

Denavir® *see* Penciclovir *on page 959*

Deodorized Opium Tincture *see* Opium Tincture *on page 928*

Deoxycoformycin *see* Pentostatin *on page 973*

2′-deoxycoformycin *see* Pentostatin *on page 973*

Depakene® *see* Valproic Acid and Derivatives *on page 1285*

Depakote® *see* Valproic Acid and Derivatives *on page 1285*

depAndro® Injection *see* Testosterone *on page 1198*

Depen® *see* Penicillamine *on page 959*

depGynogen® Injection *see* Estradiol *on page 468*

depMedalone® *see* Methylprednisolone *on page 819*

Depo®-Estradiol Injection *see* Estradiol *on page 468*

Depogen® Injection *see* Estradiol *on page 468*

Depoject® *see* Methylprednisolone *on page 819*

Depo-Medrol® *see* Methylprednisolone *on page 819*

Deponit® *see* Nitroglycerin *on page 909*

Depopred® *see* Methylprednisolone *on page 819*

Depo-Provera® *see* Medroxyprogesterone Acetate *on page 771*

Depotest® Injection *see* Testosterone *on page 1198*

Depo®-Testosterone Injection *see* Testosterone *on page 1198*

Deprenyl *see* Selegiline *on page 1130*

Dermacort® *see* Hydrocortisone *on page 623*

Dermaflex® Gel *see* Lidocaine *on page 723*

Dermarest Dricort® *see* Hydrocortisone *on page 623*

Derma-Smoothe/FS® *see* Fluocinolone *on page 533*

Dermatop® *see* Prednicarbate *on page 1037*

DermiCort® *see* Hydrocortisone *on page 623*

Dermolate® [OTC] *see* Hydrocortisone *on page 623*

Dermoplast® [OTC] *see* Benzocaine *on page 138*

Dermoxyl® Gel [OTC] *see* Benzoyl Peroxide *on page 140*

Dermtex® HC with Aloe *see* Hydrocortisone *on page 623*

DES *see* Diethylstilbestrol *on page 381*

Desensitization Protocols *see page 1496*

Desferal® Mesylate *see* Deferoxamine *on page 348*

Desiccated Thyroid *see* Thyroid *on page 1223*

Desipramine (des IP ra meen)

Related Information

Antidepressant Agents Comparison *on page 1393*

Brand Names Norpramin®; Pertofrane®

Canadian/Mexican Brand Names PMS-Desipramine (Canada)

Synonyms Desipramine Hydrochloride; Desmethylimipramine Hydrochloride

Therapeutic Category Antidepressant, Tricyclic

Use Treatment of various forms of depression, often in conjunction with psychotherapy; analgesic adjunct in chronic pain, peripheral neuropathies

Pregnancy Risk Factor C

Contraindications Hypersensitivity to desipramine (cross-sensitivity with other tricyclic antidepressants may occur); patients receiving MAO inhibitors within past 14 days; narrow-angle glaucoma

Warnings/Precautions Use with caution in patients with cardiovascular disease, conduction disturbances, urinary retention, seizure disorders, hyperthyroidism or those receiving thyroid replacement; some formulations contain tartrazine which may cause allergic reaction; do not discontinue abruptly in patients receiving long-term high-dose therapy

Adverse Reactions

>10%:

Central nervous system: Dizziness, drowsiness, headache

Gastrointestinal: Xerostomia, constipation, increased appetite, nausea, unpleasant taste, weight gain

Neuromuscular & skeletal: Weakness

1% to 10%:

Cardiovascular: Arrhythmias, hypotension

Central nervous system: Confusion, delirium, hallucinations, nervousness, restlessness, parkinsonian syndrome, insomnia

Gastrointestinal: Diarrhea, heartburn

Genitourinary: Dysuria, sexual dysfunction

Neuromuscular & skeletal: Fine muscle tremors

Ocular: Blurred vision, eye pain

Miscellaneous: Diaphoresis (excessive)

<1%:

Central nervous system: Anxiety, seizures

Dermatologic: Alopecia, photosensitivity

Endocrine & metabolic: Breast enlargement, galactorrhea, SIADH

Gastrointestinal: Trouble with gums, decreased lower esophageal sphincter tone may cause GE reflux

Genitourinary: Testicular edema

Hematologic: Agranulocytosis, leukopenia, eosinophilia

Hepatic: Cholestatic jaundice, increased liver enzymes

Ocular: Increased intraocular pressure

Otic: Tinnitus

Miscellaneous: Allergic reactions

Overdosage/Toxicology Symptoms of overdose include agitation, confusion, hallucinations, hyperthermia, urinary retention, CNS depression, cyanosis, dry mucous membranes, cardiac arrhythmias, seizures

Following GI decontamination, treatment is supportive. Sodium bicarbonate is indicated when QRS interval is >0.10 seconds or QT_c >0.42 seconds. Ventricular arrhythmias and EKG changes (eg, QRS widening) often respond with concurrent systemic alkalinization (sodium bicarbonate 0.5-2 mEq/kg I.V.). Arrhythmias unresponsive to phenytoin 15-20 mg/kg (adults) may respond to lidocaine 1 mg/kg I.V. followed by a titrated infusion. Physostigmine (1-2 mg I.V. slowly for adults or 0.5 mg I.V. slowly for children) may be indicated in reversing cardiac arrhythmias that are life-threatening. Seizures usually respond to diazepam I.V. boluses (5-10 mg for adults up to 30 mg or 0.25-0.4 mg/kg/dose for children up to 10 mg/dose). If seizures are unresponsive or recur, phenytoin or phenobarbital may be required.

Drug Interactions Cytochrome P-450 2D6 enzyme substrate

Decreased effects: Guanethidine, clonidine; decreased effect with barbiturates, carbamazepine, phenytoin

Increased effects: Sympathomimetics, benzodiazepines

Increased toxicity: Anticholinergics; increased toxicity with MAO inhibitors (hyperpyrexia, tachycardia, hypertension, seizures, and death may occur), alcohol, CNS depressants, cimetidine

Mechanism of Action Traditionally believed to increase the synaptic concentration of norepinephrine in the central nervous system by inhibition of its reuptake by the presynaptic neuronal membrane. However, additional receptor effects have been found including desensitization of adenyl cyclase, down regulation of beta-adrenergic receptors, and down regulation of serotonin receptors.

Pharmacodynamics/Kinetics
Onset of action: 1-3 weeks (maximum antidepressant effects: after >2 weeks)
Absorption: Well absorbed (90%) from GI tract
Metabolism: In the liver
Half-life: Adults: 12-57 hours
Elimination: 70% excreted in urine

Usual Dosage Oral:
Children 6-12 years: 10-30 mg/day or 1-5 mg/kg/day in divided doses; do not exceed 5 mg/kg/day
Adolescents: Initial: 25-50 mg/day; gradually increase to 100 mg/day in single or divided doses; maximum: 150 mg/day
Adults: Initial: 75 mg/day in divided doses; increase gradually to 150-200 mg/day in divided or single dose; maximum: 300 mg/day
Elderly: Initial dose: 10-25 mg/day; increase by 10-25 mg every 3 days for inpatients and every week for outpatients if tolerated; usual maintenance dose: 75-100 mg/day, but doses up to 300 mg/day may be necessary
Hemodialysis/peritoneal dialysis: Supplemental dose is not necessary

Dietary Considerations Alcohol: Additive CNS effects, avoid use

Monitoring Parameters Monitor blood pressure and pulse rate prior to and during initial therapy; evaluate mental status; monitor weight

Reference Range
Plasma levels do not always correlate with clinical effectiveness
Timing of serum samples: Draw trough just before next dose
Therapeutic: 100-300 ng/mL
In elderly patients the response rate is greatest with steady-state plasma concentrations >115 ng/mL
Possible toxicity: >300 ng/mL
Toxic: >1000 ng/mL

Test Interactions ↑ glucose

Patient Information Avoid alcohol ingestion; do not discontinue medication abruptly; may cause urine to turn blue-green; may cause drowsiness; avoid unnecessary exposure to sunlight; sugarless hard candy or gum can help with dry mouth; full effect may not occur for 3-4 weeks

Nursing Implications May increase appetite

Dosage Forms
Capsule, as hydrochloride (Pertofrane®): 25 mg, 50 mg
Tablet, as hydrochloride (Norpramin®): 10 mg, 25 mg, 50 mg, 75 mg, 100 mg, 150 mg

Desipramine Hydrochloride *see* Desipramine *on previous page*
Desitin® [OTC] *see* Zinc Oxide, Cod Liver Oil, and Talc *on page 1324*
Desmethylimipramine Hydrochloride *see* Desipramine *on previous page*

Desmopressin Acetate (des moe PRES in AS e tate)

Brand Names DDAVP®; Stimate™

Canadian/Mexican Brand Names Octostim® (Canada)

Synonyms 1-Deamino-8-D-Arginine Vasopressin

Therapeutic Category Antihemophilic Agent; Hemostatic Agent; Vasopressin Analog, Synthetic

Use Treatment of diabetes insipidus and controlling bleeding in mild hemophilia, von Willebrand's disease, and thrombocytopenia (eg, uremia)

Pregnancy Risk Factor B

Contraindications Hypersensitivity to desmopressin or any component; avoid using in patients with type IIB or platelet-type von Willebrand's disease, patients with <5% factor VIII activity level

Warnings/Precautions Avoid overhydration especially when drug is used for its hemostatic effect

Adverse Reactions
1% to 10%:
Cardiovascular: Facial flushing
Central nervous system: Headache, dizziness
Gastrointestinal: Nausea, abdominal cramps
Genitourinary: Vulval pain
Local: Pain at the injection site
Respiratory: Nasal congestion
<1%:
Cardiovascular: Increase in blood pressure
Endocrine & metabolic: Hyponatremia, water intoxication

Overdosage/Toxicology Symptoms of overdose include drowsiness, headache, confusion, anuria, water intoxication

Drug Interactions
Decreased effect: Demeclocycline, lithium → ↓ ADH effects
(Continued)

Desmopressin Acetate *(Continued)*

Increased effect: Chlorpropamide, fludrocortisone → ↑ ADH response

Stability Keep in refrigerator, avoid freezing; discard discolored solutions; nasal solution stable for 3 weeks at room temperature; injection stable for 2 weeks at room temperature

Mechanism of Action Enhances reabsorption of water in the kidneys by increasing cellular permeability of the collecting ducts; possibly causes smooth muscle constriction with resultant vasoconstriction; raises plasma levels of von Willebrand factor and factor VIII

Pharmacodynamics/Kinetics

Intranasal administration:

- Onset of ADH effects: Within 1 hour
- Peak effect: Within 1-5 hours
- Duration: 5-21 hours

I.V. infusion:

- Onset of increased factor VIII activity: Within 15-30 minutes
- Peak effect: 90 minutes to 3 hours

Absorption: Nasal: Slow; 10% to 20%

Metabolism: Unknown

Half-life: Elimination (terminal): 75 minutes

Usual Dosage Dilute I.V. dose in 50 mL 0.9% sodium chloride and infuse over 15-30 minutes

Children:

Diabetes insipidus: 3 months to 12 years: Intranasal: Initial: 5 mcg/day divided 1-2 times/day; range: 5-30 mcg/day divided 1-2 times/day

Von Willebrand disease, thrombocytopathies, hemophilia: >3 months:

Intranasal: 2-4 mcg/kg/dose

I.V.: 0.3 mcg/kg by slow infusion over 15-30 minutes; usually tachyphylaxis occurs after 2-3 doses in 24 hours, recovery of response may take 48-72 hours

Nocturnal enuresis: ≥6 years: Intranasal: Initial: 20 mcg at bedtime; range: 10-40 mcg

Adults:

Diabetes insipidus: I.V., S.C.: 2-4 mcg/day in 2 divided doses or $^1/_{10}$ of the maintenance intranasal dose; intranasal: 5-40 mcg/day 1-3 times/day

Von Willebrand disease, thrombocytopathies, hemophilia:

Intranasal: 2-4 mcg/kg/dose

I.V.: 0.3 mcg/kg by slow infusion over 15-30 minutes; usually tachyphylaxis occurs after 2-3 doses in 24 hours; recovery of responsiveness may take 48-72 hours

Oral: Begin therapy 12 hours after the last intranasal dose for patients previously on intranasal therapy

Children: Initial: 0.05 mg; fluid restrictions are required in children to prevent hyponatremia and water intoxication

Adults: 0.05 mg twice daily; adjust individually to optimal therapeutic dose. Total daily dose should be increased or decreased (range: 0.1-1.2 mg divided 2-3 times/day) as needed to obtain adequate antidiuresis.

Administration For I.V. administration, dilute in 10-50 mL 0.9% sodium chloride and infuse over 15-30 minutes

Monitoring Parameters Blood pressure and pulse should be monitored during I.V. infusion

Diabetes insipidus: Fluid intake, urine volume, specific gravity, plasma and urine osmolality, serum electrolytes

Hemophilia: Factor VIII antigen levels, APTT, bleeding time (for von Willebrand's disease and thrombocytopathies)

Patient Information Avoid overhydration; notify physician if headache, shortness of breath, heartburn, nausea, abdominal cramps, or vulval pain occur

Dosage Forms

Injection (DDAVP®): 4 mcg/mL (1 mL)

Solution, nasal:

- DDAVP®: 100 mcg/mL (2.5 mL, 5 mL)
- Stimate™: 1.5 mg/mL (2.5 mL)

Tablet (DDAVP®): 0.1 mg, 0.2 mg

Desonide (DES oh nide)

Related Information

Corticosteroids Comparison *on page 1407*

Brand Names DesOwen®; Tridesilon®

Canadian/Mexican Brand Names Desocort® (Canada)

Therapeutic Category Corticosteroid, Topical (Low Potency); Corticosteroid, Topical (Medium Potency)

Use Adjunctive therapy for inflammation in acute and chronic corticosteroid responsive dermatosis (low potency corticosteroid)

Pregnancy Risk Factor C

Contraindications Known hypersensitivity to desonide, fungal infections, tuberculosis of skin, herpes simplex

Warnings/Precautions Use with caution in patients with impaired circulation, skin infections

Adverse Reactions

<1%:

Dermatologic: Itching, dry skin, folliculitis, hypertrichosis, acneiform eruptions, hypopigmentation, perioral dermatitis, allergic contact dermatitis, skin maceration, skin atrophy, striae

Local: Burning, irritation, miliaria

Miscellaneous: Secondary infection

Overdosage/Toxicology Symptoms of overdose include moon face, central obesity, hypertension, diabetes, hyperlipidemia, peptic ulcer, increased susceptibility to infection, electrolyte and fluid imbalance, psychosis, hallucinations. When consumed in excessive quantities, systemic hypercorticism and adrenal suppression may occur; in those cases discontinuation and withdrawal of the corticosteroid should be done judiciously.

Mechanism of Action Stimulates the synthesis of enzymes needed to decrease inflammation, suppress mitotic activity, and cause vasoconstriction

Pharmacodynamics/Kinetics

Onset of effect: Commonly noted within 7 days of continued therapy

Absorption: Topical absorption extensive from the scalp, face, axilla and scrotum; adequate through epidermis on appendages; absorption can be increased with occlusion or the addition of penetrants (eg, urea, DMSO)

Metabolism: By the liver

Elimination: Primarily in urine

Usual Dosage Children and Adults: Topical: Apply 2-4 times/day sparingly

Patient Information A thin film of cream or ointment is effective, do not overuse; rub in lightly; do not use tight-fitting diapers or plastic pants on children being treated in the diaper area; use only as prescribed and for no longer than the period prescribed; avoid contact with eyes; notify physician if condition being treated persists or worsens

Nursing Implications For external use only; do not use on open wounds; apply sparingly to occlusive dressings; should not be used in the presence of open or weeping lesions

Dosage Forms

Cream, topical: 0.05% (15 g, 60 g)

Lotion: 0.05% (60 mL, 120 mL)

Ointment, topical: 0.05% (15 g, 60 g)

DesOwen® *see* Desonide *on previous page*

Desoximetasone (des oks i MET a sone)

Related Information

Corticosteroids Comparison *on page 1407*

Brand Names Topicort®; Topicort®-LP

Therapeutic Category Corticosteroid, Topical (Medium Potency); Corticosteroid, Topical (High Potency)

Use Relieves inflammation and pruritic symptoms of corticosteroid-responsive dermatosis [medium to high potency topical corticosteroid]

Pregnancy Risk Factor C

Contraindications Known hypersensitivity to desoximetasone, topical fungal infections, tuberculosis of skin herpes simplex

Warnings/Precautions Use with caution in patients with impaired circulation; skin infections

Adverse Reactions

<1%:

Dermatologic: Itching, dry skin, folliculitis, hypertrichosis, acneiform eruptions, allergic contact dermatitis, skin maceration, skin atrophy, striae, perioral dermatitis, hypopigmentation

Local: Burning, irritation, miliaria

Miscellaneous: Secondary infection

Overdosage/Toxicology Symptoms of overdose include moon face, central obesity, hypertension, diabetes, hyperlipidemia, peptic ulcer, increased susceptibility to infection, electrolyte and fluid imbalance, psychosis, hallucinations. When consumed in excessive quantities, systemic hypercorticism and adrenal suppression may occur; in those cases discontinuation and withdrawal of the corticosteroid should be done judiciously.

Mechanism of Action Stimulates the synthesis of enzymes needed to decrease inflammation, suppress mitotic activity, and cause vasoconstriction

(Continued)

Desoximetasone *(Continued)*

Pharmacodynamics/Kinetics Topical:

Absorption: Extensive from the scalp, face, axilla, and scrotum and adequate through epidermis on appendages; absorption can be increased with occlusion or the addition of penetrants

Distribution: Only small amounts reach the systemic circulation or dermal layers

Usual Dosage Topical:

Children: Apply sparingly in a very thin film to affected area 1-2 times/day

Adults: Apply sparingly in a thin film twice daily

Patient Information A thin film of cream or ointment is effective, do not overuse; rub in lightly; do not use tight-fitting diapers or plastic pants on children being treated in the diaper area; use only as prescribed and for no longer than the period prescribed; avoid contact with eyes; notify physician if condition being treated persists or worsens

Nursing Implications For external use only; apply sparingly to occlusive dressings; should not be used in the presence of open or weeping lesions

Dosage Forms Topical:

Cream:

Topicort®: 0.25% (15 g, 60 g, 120 g)

Topicort®-LP: 0.05% (15 g, 60 g)

Gel, topical: 0.05% (15 g, 60 g)

Ointment (Topicort®): 0.25% (15 g, 60 g)

Desoxyephedrine Hydrochloride *see* Methamphetamine *on page 800*

Desoxyn® *see* Methamphetamine *on page 800*

Desoxyphenobarbital *see* Primidone *on page 1042*

Desquam-E® Gel *see* Benzoyl Peroxide *on page 140*

Desquam-X® Gel *see* Benzoyl Peroxide *on page 140*

Desquam-X® Wash *see* Benzoyl Peroxide *on page 140*

Desyrel® *see* Trazodone *on page 1250*

Devrom® [OTC] *see* Bismuth *on page 154*

Dexacidin® *see* Neomycin, Polymyxin B, and Dexamethasone *on page 889*

Dex-A-Diet® [OTC] *see* Phenylpropanolamine *on page 991*

Dexair® *see* Dexamethasone *on this page*

Dexamethasone (deks a METH a sone)

Related Information

Cancer Chemotherapy Regimens *on page 1351*

Corticosteroids Comparison *on page 1407*

Toxicities of Chemotherapeutic Agents *on page 1382*

Brand Names Aeroseb-Dex®; AK-Dex®; Alba-Dex®; Baldex®; Dalalone L.A.®; Decaderm®; Decadron®; Decadron®-LA; Decadron® Turbinaire®; Decaject-L.A.®; Decaspray®; Dekasol-L.A.®; Dexair®; Dexasone L.A.®; Dexone ®; Dexone L.A.®; Dezone®; Hexadrol®; I-Methasone®; Maxidex®; Ocu-Dex®; Solurex L.A.®

Canadian/Mexican Brand Names Alin® (Mexico); Alin® Depot (Mexico); Decadronal® (Mexico); Decorex® (Mexico); Dibasona® (Mexico)

Synonyms Dexamethasone Acetate; Dexamethasone Sodium Phosphate

Therapeutic Category Antiemetic; Anti-inflammatory Agent, Inhalant; Anti-inflammatory Agent, Ophthalmic; Corticosteroid, Inhalant; Corticosteroid, Ophthalmic; Corticosteroid, Systemic; Corticosteroid, Topical (Low Potency); Glucocorticoid

Use Systemically and locally for chronic inflammation, allergic, hematologic, neoplastic, and autoimmune diseases; may be used in management of cerebral edema, septic shock, as a diagnostic agent, antiemetic

Pregnancy Risk Factor C

Pregnancy/Breast-Feeding Implications

Dexamethasone has been used in patients with premature labor (26-34 weeks gestation) to stimulate fetal lung maturation

Effects on the fetus: Crosses the placenta; transient leukocytosis reported. Available evidence suggests safe use during pregnancy

Breast-feeding/lactation: No data on crossing into breast milk or effects on the infant

Contraindications Active untreated infections; use in ophthalmic viral, fungal, or tuberculosis diseases of the eye

Warnings/Precautions Fatalities have occurred due to adrenal insufficiency in asthmatic patients during and after transfer from systemic corticosteroids to aerosol steroids; aerosol steroids do **not** provide the systemic steroid needed to treat patients having trauma, surgery, or infections; use with caution in patients with hypothyroidism, cirrhosis, hypertension, congestive heart failure, ulcerative colitis, thromboembolic disorders. Because of the risk of adverse effects, systemic corticosteroids should be used cautiously in the elderly in the smallest possible dose and for the shortest possible time.

Adverse Reactions

Systemic:

>10%:

Central nervous system: Insomnia, nervousness

Gastrointestinal: Increased appetite, indigestion

1% to 10%:

Dermatologic: Hirsutism

Endocrine & metabolic: Diabetes mellitus

Neuromuscular & skeletal: Arthralgia

Ocular: Cataracts

Respiratory: Epistaxis

<1%:

Central nervous system: Seizures, mood swings, headache, delirium, hallucinations, euphoria

Dermatologic: Skin atrophy, bruising, hyperpigmentation, acne

Endocrine & metabolic: Amenorrhea, sodium and water retention, Cushing's syndrome, hyperglycemia, bone growth suppression

Gastrointestinal: Abdominal distention, ulcerative esophagitis, pancreatitis

Neuromuscular & skeletal: Muscle wasting

Miscellaneous: Hypersensitivity reactions

Topical:

<1%:

Dermatologic: Itching, dryness, folliculitis, hypertrichosis, acneiform eruptions, hypopigmentation, perioral dermatitis, allergic contact dermatitis, skin maceration, skin atrophy, striae

Endocrine & metabolic: Miliaria

Local: Burning, irritation

Miscellaneous: Secondary infection

Overdosage/Toxicology Symptoms of overdose include moon face, central obesity, hypertension, psychosis, hallucinations, diabetes, hyperlipidemia, peptic ulcer, increased susceptibility to infection, electrolyte and fluid imbalance. When consumed in excessive quantities, systemic hypercorticism and adrenal suppression may occur; in those cases, discontinuation and withdrawal of the corticosteroid should be done judiciously.

Drug Interactions Cytochrome P-450 3A enzyme substrate

Decreased effect:

Barbiturates, phenytoin, rifampin → ↓ dexamethasone effects

Dexamethasone decreases effect of salicylates, vaccines, toxoids

Stability

Dexamethasone 4 mg/mL injection solution is clear and colorless and dexamethasone 24 mg/mL injection solution is clear and colorless to light yellow. Injection solution should be protected from light and freezing.

Stability of injection of parenteral admixture at room temperature (25°C): 24 hours

Stability of injection of parenteral admixture at refrigeration temperature (4°C): 2 days; protect from light and freezing

Standard diluent: 4 mg/50 mL D_5W; 10 mg/50 mL D_5W

Minimum volume: 50 mL D_5W

Mechanism of Action Decreases inflammation by suppression of migration of polymorphonuclear leukocytes and reversal of increased capillary permeability; suppresses normal immune response

Pharmacodynamics/Kinetics

Duration of metabolic effect: Can last for 72 hours; acetate is a long-acting repository preparation with a prompt onset of action

Metabolism: In the liver

Half-life:

Normal renal function: 1.8-3.5 hours

Biological half-life: 36-54 hours

Time to peak serum concentration:

Oral: Within 1-2 hours

I.M.: Within 8 hours

Elimination: In the urine and bile

Usual Dosage

Neonates:

Airway edema or extubation: I.V.: Usual: 0.25 mg/kg/dose given 4 hours prior to scheduled extubation and then every 8 hours for 3 doses total; range: 0.25-1 mg/kg/dose for 1-3 doses; maximum dose: 1 mg/kg/day. **Note:** A longer duration of therapy may be needed with more severe cases

Bronchopulmonary dysplasia (to facilitate ventilator weaning): Oral:, I.V.: Numerous dosing schedules have been proposed; range: 0.5-0.6 mg/kg/day

(Continued)

Dexamethasone *(Continued)*

given in divided doses every 12 hours for 3-7 days, then taper over 1-6 weeks

Children:

Antiemetic (prior to chemotherapy): I.V. (should be given as sodium phosphate): 10 mg/m²/dose (maximum: 20 mg) for first dose then 5 mg/m²/dose every 6 hours as needed

Anti-inflammatory immunosuppressant: Oral, I.M., I.V. (injections should be given as sodium phosphate): 0.08-0.3 mg/kg/day **or** 2.5-10 mg/m²/day in divided doses every 6-12 hours

Extubation or airway edema: Oral, I.M., I.V. (injections should be given as sodium phosphate): 0.5-2 mg/kg/day in divided doses every 6 hours beginning 24 hours prior to extubation and continuing for 4-6 doses afterwards

Cerebral edema: I.V. (should be given as sodium phosphate): Loading dose: 1-2 mg/kg/dose as a single dose; maintenance: 1-1.5 mg/kg/day (maximum: 16 mg/day) in divided doses every 4-6 hours for 5 days then taper for 5 days, then discontinue

Bacterial meningitis in infants and children >2 months: I.V. (should be given as sodium phosphate): 0.6 mg/kg/day in 4 divided doses every 6 hours for the first 4 days of antibiotic treatment; start dexamethasone at the time of the first dose of antibiotic

Physiologic replacement: Oral, I.M., I.V.: 0.03-0.15 mg/kg/day or 0.6-0.75 mg/m²/day in divided doses every 6-12 hours

Adults:

Acute nonlymphoblastic leukemia (ANLL) protocol: I.V.: 2 mg/m²/dose every 8 hours for 12 doses

Antiemetic (prior to chemotherapy): Oral/I.V. (should be given as sodium phosphate): 10 mg/m²/dose (usually 20 mg) for first dose then 5 mg/m²/dose every 6 hours as needed

Anti-inflammatory:

Oral, I.M., I.V. (injections should be given as sodium phosphate): 0.75-9 mg/day in divided doses every 6-12 hours

I.M. (as acetate): 8-16 mg; may repeat in 1-3 weeks

Intralesional (as acetate): 0.8-1.6 mg

Intra-articular/soft tissue (as acetate): 4-16 mg; may repeat in 1-3 weeks

Intra-articular, intralesional, or soft tissue (as sodium phosphate): 0.4-6 mg/day

Cerebral edema: I.V. 10 mg stat, 4 mg I.M./I.V. (should be given as sodium phosphate) every 6 hours until response is maximized, then switch to oral regimen, then taper off if appropriate; dosage may be reduced after 24 days and gradually discontinued over 5-7 days

Diagnosis for Cushing's syndrome: Oral: 1 mg at 11 PM, draw blood at 8 AM the following day for plasma cortisol determination

Physiological replacement: Oral, I.M., I.V. (should be given as sodium phosphate): 0.03-0.15 mg/kg/day **OR** 0.6-0.75 mg/m²/day in divided doses every 6-12 hours

Shock therapy:

Addisonian crisis/shock (ie, adrenal insufficiency/responsive to steroid therapy): I.V. (given as sodium phosphate): 4-10 mg as a single dose, which may be repeated if necessary

Unresponsive shock (ie, unresponsive to steroid therapy): I.V. (given as sodium phosphate): 1-6 mg/kg as a single I.V. dose or up to 40 mg initially followed by repeat doses every 2-6 hours while shock persists

Hemodialysis: Supplemental dose is not necessary
Peritoneal dialysis: Supplemental dose is not necessary

Ophthalmic:

Ointment: Apply thin coating into conjunctival sac 3-4 times/day; gradually taper dose to discontinue

Suspension: Instill 2 drops into conjunctival sac every hour during the day and every other hour during the night; gradually reduce dose to every 3-4 hours, then to 3-4 times/day

Topical: Apply 1-4 times/day

Administration Administer oral formulation with meals to decrease GI upset

Monitoring Parameters Hemoglobin, occult blood loss, serum potassium, and glucose

Reference Range Dexamethasone suppression test, overnight: 8 AM cortisol <6 μg/100 mL (dexamethasone 1 mg); plasma cortisol determination should be made on the day after giving dose

Patient Information Notify physician of any signs of infection or injuries during therapy; inform physician or dentist before surgery if you are taking a corticosteroid; may cause GI upset, take with food; do not overuse; use only as prescribed and for no longer than the period prescribed; notify physician if condition being treated persists or worsens

Topical: Thin film of cream or ointment is effective, do not overuse; do not use tight-fitting diapers or plastic pants on children being treated in the diaper area; use only as prescribed, and for no longer than the period prescribed; rub in lightly; avoid contact with eyes; notify physician if condition being treated persists or worsens

Nursing Implications Topical formation is for external use, do not use on open wounds; apply sparingly to occlusive dressings; should not be used in the presence of open or weeping lesions; **acetate injection is not for I.V. use**

Dosage Forms

Aerosol:
- Oral, as sodium phosphate: 84 mcg dexamethasone per activation (12.6 g)
- Nasal, as sodium phosphate: 84 mcg dexamethasone/spray (12.6 g)

Cream, as sodium phosphate: 0.1% (15 g, 30 g)
Elixir: 0.5 mg/5 mL (5 mL, 20 mL, 100 mL, 120 mL, 237 mL, 240 mL, 500 mL)
Injection, as acetate suspension: 8 mg/mL (1 mL, 5 mL); 16 mg/mL (1 mL, 5 mL)
Injection, as sodium phosphate: 4 mg/mL (1 mL, 5 mL, 10 mL, 25 mL, 30 mL); 10 mg/mL (1 mL, 10 mL); 20 mg/mL (5 mL); 24 mg/mL (5 mL, 10 mL)
Ointment, ophthalmic, as sodium phosphate: 0.05% (3.5 g)
Solution, oral:
- Concentrate: 0.5 mg/0.5 mL (30 mL) (30% alcohol)
- Oral: 0.5 mg/5 mL (5 mL, 20 mL, 500 mL)

Suspension, ophthalmic, as sodium phosphate: 0.1% with methylcellulose 0.5% (5 mL, 15 mL)
Tablet: 0.25 mg, 0.5 mg, 0.75 mg, 1 mg, 1.5 mg, 2 mg, 4 mg, 6 mg
Tablet, therapeutic pack: 6 x 1.5 mg; 8 x 0.75 mg
Topical: 0.01% (58 g); 0.04% (25 g)

Dexamethasone Acetate *see* Dexamethasone *on page 356*

Dexamethasone and Tobramycin *see* Tobramycin and Dexamethasone *on page 1236*

Dexamethasone Sodium Phosphate *see* Dexamethasone *on page 356*

Dexasone L.A.® *see* Dexamethasone *on page 356*

Dexasporin® *see* Neomycin, Polymyxin B, and Dexamethasone *on page 889*

Dexatrim® [OTC] *see* Phenylpropanolamine *on page 991*

Dexchlor® *see* Dexchlorpheniramine *on this page*

Dexchlorpheniramine (deks klor fen EER a meen)

Brand Names Dexchlor®; Poladex®; Polaramine®

Synonyms Dexchlorpheniramine Maleate

Therapeutic Category Antihistamine, H_1 Blocker

Use Perennial and seasonal allergic rhinitis and other allergic symptoms including urticaria

Pregnancy Risk Factor B

Contraindications Narrow-angle glaucoma, hypersensitivity to dexchlorpheniramine or any component

Warnings/Precautions Bladder neck obstruction, symptomatic prostatic hypertrophy, asthmatic attack, and stenosing peptic ulcer

Adverse Reactions

>10%:
- Central nervous system: Slight to moderate drowsiness
- Respiratory: Thickening of bronchial secretions

1% to 10%:
- Central nervous system: Headache, fatigue, nervousness, dizziness
- Gastrointestinal: Appetite increase, weight gain, nausea, diarrhea, abdominal pain, xerostomia
- Neuromuscular & skeletal: Arthralgia
- Respiratory: Pharyngitis

<1%:
- Cardiovascular: Edema, palpitations
- Central nervous system: Depression
- Dermatologic: Angioedema, photosensitivity, rash
- Hepatic: Hepatitis
- Neuromuscular & skeletal: Myalgia, paresthesia
- Respiratory: Bronchospasm, epistaxis

Overdosage/Toxicology Symptoms of overdose include dry mouth, flushed skin, dilated pupils, CNS depression
(Continued)

Dexchlorpheniramine *(Continued)*

There is no specific treatment for an antihistamine overdose, however, most of its clinical toxicity is due to anticholinergic effects. For anticholinergic overdose with severe life-threatening symptoms, physostigmine 1-2 mg (0.5 or 0.02 mg/kg for children) I.V., slowly may be given to reverse these effects.

Drug Interactions Increased effect/toxicity: CNS depressants, MAO inhibitors, TCAs, phenothiazines, guanabenz

Mechanism of Action Competes with histamine for H_1-receptor sites on effector cells in the gastrointestinal tract, blood vessels, and respiratory tract

Pharmacodynamics/Kinetics

Peak effect: Oral: Within 3 hours
Duration: 3-6 hours
Absorption: Well absorbed from GI tract
Distribution: Small amounts appear in breast milk
Metabolism: In the liver
Elimination: In urine within 24 hours as inactive metabolites

Usual Dosage Oral:

Children:
- 2-5 years: 0.5 mg every 4-6 hours (do not use timed release)
- 6-11 years: 1 mg every 4-6 hours or 4 mg timed release at bedtime

Adults: 2 mg every 4-6 hours or 4-6 mg timed release at bedtime or every 8-10 hours

Dietary Considerations Alcohol: Additive CNS effects, avoid use

Test Interactions May interfere with a methacholine bronchial challenge

Patient Information May cause drowsiness; swallow whole, do not crush or chew sustained release product; avoid alcohol, may impair coordination and judgment

Nursing Implications Raise bed rails, institute safety measures, assist with ambulation

Dosage Forms

Syrup, as maleate (orange flavor): 2 mg/5 mL with alcohol 6% (480 mL)
Tablet, as maleate: 2 mg
Tablet, as maleate, sustained action: 4 mg, 6 mg

Dexchlorpheniramine Maleate *see* Dexchlorpheniramine *on previous page*
Dexedrine® *see* Dextroamphetamine *on page 365*

Dexfenfluramine (deks fen FLURE a meen)

Brand Names Redux®

Synonyms Dexfenfluramine Hydrochloride; S5614

Therapeutic Category Anorexiant

Use Management of obesity (initial body mass [BMI] >30 kg/m^2 or >27 kg/m^2 with other risk factors such as hypertension, diabetes, or hyperlipidemia); given as an adjunct to dietary restriction

Restrictions C-IV

Pregnancy Risk Factor C

Pregnancy/Breast-Feeding Implications Spontaneous abortions in 1st trimester has been described

Contraindications Hypersensitivity to dexfenfluramine or fenfluramine, glaucoma, pulmonary hypertension or use of monoamine oxidase inhibitors within 2 weeks of dexfenfluramine; children, pregnancy, or nursing women

Warnings/Precautions Use with caution in patients with cardiac disease, renal or hepatic insufficiency, porphyria, drug abuse, psychiatric disorder, or organic causes for obesity

Adverse Reactions

>10%:
- Central nervous system: Headache, insomnia
- Gastrointestinal: Xerostomia, diarrhea
- Neuromuscular & skeletal: Weakness

1% to 10%:
- Cardiovascular: Hypertension, angina, palpitations
- Central nervous system: Chills, somnolence, dizziness, depression, vertigo, emotional lability, headache, abnormal dreams, abnormal thoughts
- Dermatologic: Rash
- Endocrine & metabolic: Increased libido, decreased libido
- Gastrointestinal: Vomiting, abdominal pain, constipation, nausea, dyspepsia, increased appetite, gastritis, flatulence
- Genitourinary: Polyuria
- Neuromuscular & skeletal: Peripheral neuritis, arthralgia, myalgia
- Respiratory: Pharyngitis, rhinitis, cough, bronchitis
- Miscellaneous: Thirst

<1%:

Cardiovascular: Pulmonary hypertension (18 cases per 1 million users per year), heart block

Overdosage/Toxicology Three deaths have occurred as a result of overdoses; symptoms include agitation, drowsiness, mydriasis, diaphoresis, shivering, nausea, and vomiting

There is no specific antidote; the bulk of the treatment is supportive; effectiveness of dialysis is unknown. Hyperactivity and agitation usually respond to reduced sensory input; however, with extreme agitation, haloperidol (2-5 mg I.M. for adults) may be required. Hyperthermia is best treated with external cooling measures; when severe or unresponsive, muscle paralysis with pancuronium may be needed. Hypertension is usually transient and generally does not require treatment unless severe. For diastolic blood pressures >110 mm Hg, a nitroprusside infusion should be initiated. Seizures usually respond to diazepam IVP and/or phenytoin maintenance regimens.

Drug Interactions Increased toxicity: Serotonin reuptake inhibitors and monoamine oxidase inhibitors may cause rigidity, hyperthermia, tremor, seizures, and delirium

Mechanism of Action Can cause elevation of serotonin in the brain which suppresses appetite for carbohydrates (but not protein-rich foods); dexflenfluramine (d-fenfluramine) is the dextrostereoisomer of fenfluramine (dl-fenfluramine Pondimin®). In contrast to fenfluramine, dexfenfluramine is a relatively pure serotonin agonist, with minimal to no sympathomimetic activity or effects on the dopaminergic system. Studies in animal models have indicated that dexfenfluramine stimulates the release and inhibits reuptake of serotonin, leading to increased serotonin levels in the hypothalamic centers for feeding behavior. By increasing the levels of serotonin in these brain synapses, dexfenfluramine is thought to selectively suppress food intake.

Pharmacodynamics/Kinetics

Peak serum levels: 2-4 hours

Metabolism: Hepatic to d-norfenfluramine (active metabolite)

Half-life:

18 hours (dexfenfluramine)

30 hours (d-norfenfluramine)

Usual Dosage Oral: Adults: 15 mg twice daily with meals; doses >30 mg/day are not recommended

Monitoring Parameters Monitor weight, eating habits, cardiopulmonary function including cardiac insufficiency, palpitations, exertional dyspnea, and/or chest pain; blood should also be monitored

Reference Range After a 20 mg oral dose, peak serum level: ~16 µg/L; peak serum metabolite d-norfenfluramine is 6 µg/L

Test Interactions False-positive urine drug tests for amphetamine by ELISA have been observed for up to 24 hours after a dose

Nursing Implications Monitor CNS and pulmonary function for signs of drug toxicity

Additional Information BMI = (kg) weight divided by $[H + (m)]^2$

Dosage Forms Capsule, as hydrochloride: 15 mg

Dexfenfluramine Hydrochloride *see* Dexfenfluramine *on previous page*

Dexferrum® *see* Iron Dextran Complex *on page 676*

Dexone ® *see* Dexamethasone *on page 356*

Dexone L.A.® *see* Dexamethasone *on page 356*

Dexpanthenol (deks PAN the nole)

Brand Names Ilopan®; Ilopan-Choline®; Panthoderm® [OTC]

Synonyms Pantothenyl Alcohol

Therapeutic Category Gastrointestinal Agent, Stimulant

Use Prophylactic use to minimize paralytic ileus, treatment of postoperative distention

Pregnancy Risk Factor C

Contraindications Hemophilia; mechanical obstruction of ileus

Warnings/Precautions If hypersensitivity occurs, discontinue the drug; if ileus is secondary to mechanical obstruction, therapy must be directed at the obstruction

Adverse Reactions

<1%:

Cardiovascular: Slight drop in blood pressure

Dermatologic: Dermatitis, urticaria

Gastrointestinal: Vomiting, diarrhea, hyperperistalsis

Hematologic: Prolonged bleeding time

Local: Irritation

Neuromuscular & skeletal: Paresthesia

Respiratory: Dyspnea

(Continued)

Dexpanthenol *(Continued)*

Overdosage/Toxicology May cause diarrhea or intestinal upset

Drug Interactions Increased/prolonged effect of succinylcholine (do not administer within 1 hour)

Mechanism of Action A pantothenic acid B vitamin analog that is converted to coenzyme A internally; coenzyme A is essential to normal fatty acid synthesis, amino acid synthesis and acetylation of choline in the production of the neurotransmitter, acetylcholine

Pharmacodynamics/Kinetics

Absorption: Well absorbed

Elimination: As pantothenic acid principally in urine with small amounts in bile

Usual Dosage

Children and Adults: Relief of itching and aid in skin healing: Topical: Apply to affected area 1-2 times/day

Adults:

- Relief of gas retention: Oral: 2-3 tablets 3 times/day
- Prevention of postoperative ileus: I.M.: 250-500 mg stat, repeat in 2 hours, followed by doses every 6 hours until danger passes
- Paralyzed ileus: I.M.: 500 mg stat, repeat in 2 hours, followed by doses every 6 hours, if needed

Administration Not for direct I.V. administration; must be diluted

Dosage Forms

Cream: 2% (30 g, 60 g)

Injection (Ilopan®): 250 mg/mL (2 mL, 10 mL, 30 mL)

Tablet (Ilopan-Choline®): 50 mg with choline bitartrate 25 mg

Dexrazoxane (deks ray ZOKS ane)

Brand Names Zinecard®

Therapeutic Category Cardioprotective Agent

Use Reduction of the incidence and severity of cardiomyopathy associated with doxorubicin administration in women with metastatic breast cancer who have received a cumulative doxorubicin dose of 300 mg/m^2 and who would benefit from continuing therapy with doxorubicin. It is not recommended for use with the initiation of doxorubicin therapy.

Pregnancy Risk Factor C

Pregnancy/Breast-Feeding Implications Avoid use in pregnant women unless the potential benefit justifies the potential risk to the fetus; discontinue nursing during dexrazoxane therapy

Contraindications Do not use with chemotherapy regimens that do not contain an anthracycline

Warnings/Precautions Dexrazoxane may add to the myelosuppression caused by chemotherapeutic agents. There is some evidence that the use of dexrazoxane concurrently with the initiation of fluorouracil, doxorubicin, and cyclophosphamide (FAC) therapy interferes with the antitumor efficacy of the regimen, and this use is not recommended. Dexrazoxane should only be used in those patients who have received a cumulative doxorubicin dose of 300 mg/m^2 and are continuing with doxorubicin therapy. Dexrazoxane does not eliminate the potential for anthracycline-induced cardiac toxicity. Carefully monitor cardiac function.

Adverse Reactions The adverse experiences are likely attributable to the FAC regimen, with the exception of pain on injection that was observed mainly with dexrazoxane. Patients receiving FAC with dexrazoxane experienced more severe leukopenia, granulocytopenia, and thrombocytopenia at nadir than patients receiving FAC without dexrazoxane; but recovery counts were similar for the two groups.

1% to 2%: Dermatologic: Urticaria, recall skin reaction, extravasation

Overdosage/Toxicology Management includes good supportive care until resolution of myelosuppression, and related conditions, is complete. Management of overdose should include treatment of infections, fluid regulation, and management of nutritional requirements. Retention of a significant dose fraction of the unchanged drug in the plasma pool, minimal tissue partitioning or binding and availability of >90% of the systemic drug levels in the unbound form suggest that dexrazoxane could be removed using conventional peritoneal or hemodialysis.

Drug Interactions Decreased effect: There is some evidence that the use of dexrazoxane concurrently with the initiation of FAC therapy interferes with the antitumor efficacy of the regimen, and this use is not recommended

Stability

Store intact vials at controlled room temperature, (15°C to 30°C/59°F to 86°F). Reconstituted and diluted solutions are stable for 6 hours at controlled room temperature or under refrigeration (2°C to 8°C/36°F to 46°F).

Must be reconstituted with 0.167 Molar (M/6) sodium lactate injection to a concentration of 10 mg dexrazoxane/mL sodium lactate. Reconstituted dexrazoxane solution may be diluted with either 0.9% sodium chloride injection or 5% dextrose injection to a concentration of 1.3-5 mg/mL in intravenous infusion bags.

Caution should be exercised in the handling and preparation of the reconstituted solution; the use of gloves is recommended. If dexrazoxane powder or solutions contact the skin or mucosae, immediately wash with soap and water.

Mechanism of Action Derivative of EDTA and potent intracellular chelating agent. The mechanism of cardioprotectant activity is not fully understood. Appears to be converted intracellularly to a ring-opened chelating agent that interferes with iron-mediated free radical generation thought to be responsible, in part, for anthracycline-induced cardiomyopathy.

Pharmacodynamics/Kinetics

Distribution: V_d: 22-22.4 L/m^2; not bound to plasma proteins

Half-life: 2.1-2.5 hours

Elimination: 42% of dose excreted in the urine; renal clearance: 3.35 L/hour/m^2; plasma clearance: 6.25-7.88 L/hour/m^2

Usual Dosage Adults: I.V.: The recommended dosage ratio of dexrazoxane:doxorubicin is 10:1 (eg, 500 mg/m^2 dexrazoxane:50 mg/m^2 doxorubicin). Administer the reconstituted solution by slow I.V. push or rapid I.V. infusion from a bag. After completing the infusion, and prior to a total elapsed time of 30 minutes (from the beginning of the dexrazoxane infusion), administer the I.V. injection of doxorubicin.

Administration Doxorubicin should not be given prior to the I.V. injection of dexrazoxane. Administer dexrazoxane by slow I.V. push or rapid drip I.V. infusion from a bag. Administer doxorubicin within 30 minutes after beginning the infusion with dexrazoxane.

Monitoring Parameters Since dexrazoxane will always be used with cytotoxic drugs, and since it may add to the myelosuppressive effects of cytotoxic drugs, frequent complete blood counts are recommended

Nursing Implications Observe for signs and symptoms of cardiac toxicity, infection, and anemia

Additional Information Reimbursement Guarantee Program: 1-800-808-9111

Dosage Forms Powder for injection, lyophilized: 250 mg, 500 mg (10 mg/mL when reconstituted)

Dextran (DEKS tran)

Brand Names Gentran®; LMD®; Macrodex®; Rheomacrodex®

Synonyms Dextran 40; Dextran 70; Dextran, High Molecular Weight; Dextran, Low Molecular Weight

Therapeutic Category Plasma Volume Expander, Colloid

Use Blood volume expander used in treatment of shock or impending shock when blood or blood products are not available

Pregnancy Risk Factor C

Contraindications Hypersensitivity to dextrans or components (see Dextran 1)

Warnings/Precautions Use caution in patients with CHF, renal insufficiency, thrombocytopenia, or active hemorrhage; **observe patients closely during the first minute of infusion and have other means of maintaining circulation and epinephrine and diphenhydramine available should dextran therapy result in an anaphylactoid reaction;** patients should be well hydrated at the start of therapy; discontinue dextran if urine specific gravity is low and/or if oliguria or anuria occurs or if there is a precipitous rise in central venous pressure and signs of circulatory overload

Adverse Reactions

<1%:

- Cardiovascular: Mild hypotension, tightness of chest
- Central nervous system: Fever
- Dermatologic: Urticaria
- Gastrointestinal: Nausea, vomiting
- Neuromuscular & skeletal: Arthralgia
- Respiratory: Nasal congestion, wheezing
- Miscellaneous: Anaphylaxis

Overdosage/Toxicology Symptoms include fluid overload, pulmonary edema, increased bleeding time, decreased platelet function; treatment is supportive, blood products containing clotting factors may be necessary

Stability Store at room temperature; discard partially used containers

Mechanism of Action Produces plasma volume expansion by virtue of its highly colloidal starch structure, similar to albumin

Pharmacodynamics/Kinetics

Onset of action: I.V.: Within minutes to 1 hour (depending upon the molecular weight polysaccharide administered), infusion volume expansion occurs

(Continued)

Dextran *(Continued)*

Elimination: ~75% excreted in urine within 24 hours

Usual Dosage I.V.: (requires an infusion pump):

Children: Total dose should not be >20 mL/kg during first 24 hours

Adults: 500-1000 mL at rate of 20-40 mL/minute; if therapy continues beyond 24 hours, total daily dosage should not exceed 10 mL/kg and therapy should not continue beyond 5 days

Dosing in renal and/or hepatic impairment: Use with extreme caution

Administration I.V. infusion only (use an infusion pump)

Monitoring Parameters Observe patient for signs of circulatory overload and/or monitor central venous pressure; observe patients closely during the first minute of infusion and have other means of maintaining circulation should dextran therapy result in an anaphylactoid reaction

Nursing Implications Patients should be well hydrated at the start of therapy; discontinue dextran if urine specific gravity is low, and/or if oliguria or anuria occurs, or if there is a precipitous rise in central venous pressure or sign of circulatory overloading

Dosage Forms Injection:

High molecular weight:

- 6% dextran 75 in dextrose 5% (500 mL)
- Gentran®: 6% dextran 75 in sodium chloride 0.9% (500 mL)
- Gentran®, Macrodex®: 6% dextran 70 in sodium chloride 0.9% (500 mL)
- Macrodex®: 6% dextran 70 in dextrose 5% (500 mL)

Low molecular weight: Gentran®, LMD®, Rheomacrodex®:

- 10% dextran 40 in dextrose 5% (500 mL)
- 10% dextran 40 in sodium chloride 0.9% (500 mL)

Dextran 1 (DEKS tran won)

Brand Names Promit®

Therapeutic Category Dextran Adjunct; Plasma Volume Expander, Colloid

Use Prophylaxis of serious anaphylactic reactions to I.V. infusion of dextran

Pregnancy Risk Factor C

Contraindications Known hypersensitivity to dextrans or any component

Warnings/Precautions If immune adverse reactions occur, do not administer large volumes of dextran solutions for clinical use

Adverse Reactions

<1%:

- Cardiovascular: Mild hypotension, tightness of chest
- Central nervous system: Fever
- Dermatologic: Urticaria
- Gastrointestinal: Nausea, vomiting
- Local: Cutaneous reactions
- Neuromuscular & skeletal: Arthralgia
- Respiratory: Nasal congestion, wheezing

Stability Protect from freezing

Mechanism of Action Binds to dextran-reactive immunoglobulin without bridge formation and no formation of large immune complexes

Usual Dosage I.V. (time between dextran 1 and dextran solution should not exceed 15 minutes):

Children: 0.3 mL/kg 1-2 minutes before I.V. infusion of dextran

Adults: 20 mL 1-2 minutes before I.V. infusion of dextran

Nursing Implications Do not dilute or admix with dextrans

Dosage Forms Injection: 150 mg/mL (20 mL)

Dextran 40 *see* Dextran *on previous page*

Dextran 70 *see* Dextran *on previous page*

Dextran, High Molecular Weight *see* Dextran *on previous page*

Dextran, Low Molecular Weight *see* Dextran *on previous page*

Dextranomer (deks TRAN oh mer)

Brand Names Debrisan® [OTC]

Therapeutic Category Topical Skin Product

Use Clean exudative ulcers and wounds such as venous stasis ulcers, decubitus ulcers, and infected traumatic and surgical wounds; no controlled studies have found dextranomer to be more effective than conventional therapy

Pregnancy Risk Factor C

Contraindications Deep fistulas, sinus tracts, hypersensitivity to any component

Warnings/Precautions Do not use in deep fistulas or any area where complete removal is not assured; do not use on dry wounds (ineffective); avoid contact with eyes

Adverse Reactions 1% to 10%:

Local: Transitory pain, blistering

Dermatologic: Maceration may occur, erythema

Hematologic: Bleeding

Mechanism of Action Dextranomer is a network of dextran-sucrose beads possessing a great many exposed hydroxy groups; when this network is applied to an exudative wound surface, the exudate is drawn by capillary forces generated by the swelling of the beads, with vacuum forces producing an upward flow of exudate into the network

Usual Dosage Debride and clean wound prior to application; apply to affected area once or twice daily in a 1/4" layer; apply a dressing and seal on all four sides; removal should be done by irrigation

Patient Information For external use only; avoid contact with eyes; contact physician if condition worsens or persists beyond 14-21 days

Nursing Implications Sprinkle beads into ulcer (or apply paste) to 1/4" thickness; change dressings 1-4 times/day depending on drainage; change dressing before it is completely dry to facilitate removal

Dosage Forms

Beads: 4 g, 25 g, 60 g, 120 g

Paste: 10 g foil packets

Dextroamphetamine (deks troe am FET a meen)

Brand Names Dexedrine®; Ferndex; Oxydess® II; Spancap® No. 1

Synonyms Dextroamphetamine Sulfate

Therapeutic Category Amphetamine; Anorexiant; Central Nervous System Stimulant, Amphetamine

Use Narcolepsy, exogenous obesity, abnormal behavioral syndrome in children (minimal brain dysfunction), attention deficit hyperactive disorder (ADHD)

Restrictions C-II

Pregnancy Risk Factor C

Contraindications Hypersensitivity to dextroamphetamine or any component; advanced arteriosclerosis, hypertension, hyperthyroidism, glaucoma, MAO inhibitors

Warnings/Precautions Use with caution in patients with psychopathic personalities, cardiovascular disease, HTN, angina, and glaucoma; has high potential for abuse; use in weight reduction programs only when alternative therapy has been ineffective; prolonged administration may lead to drug dependence

Adverse Reactions

>10%:

- Cardiovascular: Arrhythmia
- Central nervous system: False feeling of well being, nervousness, restlessness, insomnia

1% to 10%:

- Cardiovascular: Hypertension
- Central nervous system: Mood or mental changes, dizziness, lightheadedness, headache
- Endocrine & metabolic: Changes in libido
- Gastrointestinal: Diarrhea, nausea, vomiting, stomach cramps, constipation, anorexia, weight loss, xerostomia
- Ocular: Blurred vision
- Miscellaneous: Diaphoresis (increased)

<1%:

- Cardiovascular: Chest pain
- Central nervous system: CNS stimulation (severe), Tourette's syndrome, hyperthermia, seizures, paranoia
- Dermatologic: Rash, urticaria
- Miscellaneous: Tolerance and withdrawal with prolonged use

Overdosage/Toxicology Symptoms of overdose include restlessness, tremor, confusion, hallucinations, panic, dysrhythmias, nausea, vomiting

There is no specific antidote for dextroamphetamine intoxication and the bulk of the treatment is supportive. Hyperactivity and agitation usually respond to reduced sensory input; however, with extreme agitation, haloperidol (2-5 mg I.M. for adults) may be required.

Hyperthermia is best treated with external cooling measures, or when severe or unresponsive, muscle paralysis with pancuronium may be needed

Hypertension is usually transient and generally does not require treatment unless severe. For diastolic blood pressures >110 mm Hg, a nitroprusside infusion should be initiated.

Seizures usually respond to diazepam I.V. and/or phenytoin maintenance regimens

(Continued)

Dextroamphetamine *(Continued)*

Drug Interactions

Decreased effect: Methyldopa decreased antihypertensive efficacy; ethosuximide; decreased effect with acidifiers, psychotropics

Increased toxicity: May precipitate hypertensive crisis in patients receiving MAO inhibitors and arrhythmias in patients receiving general anesthetics

Increased effect/toxicity of TCAs, phenytoin, phenobarbital, propoxyphene, norepinephrine and meperidine

Stability Protect from light

Mechanism of Action Blocks reuptake of dopamine and norepinephrine from the synapse, thus increases the amount of circulating dopamine and norepinephrine in cerebral cortex to reticular activating system; inhibits the action of monoamine oxidase and causes catecholamines to be released

Pharmacodynamics/Kinetics

Onset of action: 1-1.5 hours

Metabolism: In the liver

Half-life: Adults: 34 hours (pH dependent)

Time to peak serum concentration: Oral: Within 3 hours

Elimination: In urine as unchanged drug and inactive metabolites after oral dose

Usual Dosage Oral:

Children:

- Narcolepsy: 6-12 years: Initial: 5 mg/day, may increase at 5 mg increments in weekly intervals until side effects appear; maximum dose: 60 mg/day
- Attention deficit disorder:
  - 3-5 years: Initial: 2.5 mg/day given every morning; increase by 2.5 mg/day in weekly intervals until optimal response is obtained, usual range: 0.1-0.5 mg/kg/dose every morning with maximum of 40 mg/day
  - ≥6 years: 5 mg once or twice daily; increase in increments of 5 mg/day at weekly intervals until optimal response is reached, usual range: 0.1-0.5 mg/kg/dose every morning (5-20 mg/day) with maximum of 40 mg/day

Children >12 years and Adults:

- Narcolepsy: Initial: 10 mg/day, may increase at 10 mg increments in weekly intervals until side effects appear; maximum: 60 mg/day
- Exogenous obesity: 5-30 mg/day in divided doses of 5-10 mg 30-60 minutes before meals

Administration Administer as single dose in morning or as divided doses with breakfast and lunch

Monitoring Parameters Growth in children and CNS activity in all

Patient Information Take during day to avoid insomnia; do not discontinue abruptly, may cause physical and psychological dependence with prolonged use

Nursing Implications Last daily dose should be given 6 hours before retiring; do not crush sustained release drug product

Dosage Forms

Capsule, as sulfate, sustained release: 5 mg, 10 mg, 15 mg

Elixir, as sulfate: 5 mg/5 mL (480 mL)

Tablet, as sulfate: 5 mg, 10 mg (5 mg tablets contain tartrazine)

Dextroamphetamine Sulfate *see* Dextroamphetamine *on previous page*

Dextromethorphan (deks troe meth OR fan)

Brand Names Benylin® DM [OTC]; Children's Hold® [OTC]; Delsym® [OTC]; Hold® DM [OTC]; Pertussin® CS [OTC]; Pertussin® ES [OTC]; Robitussin® Cough Calmers [OTC]; Robitussin® Pediatric [OTC]; Scot-Tussin DM® Cough Chasers [OTC]; St. Joseph® Cough Suppressant [OTC]; Sucrets® Cough Calmers [OTC]; Suppress® [OTC]; Trocal® [OTC]; Vicks Formula 44® [OTC]; Vicks Formula 44® Pediatric Formula [OTC]

Canadian/Mexican Brand Names Balminil-DM® (Canada)

Therapeutic Category Antitussive; Cough Preparation

Use Symptomatic relief of coughs caused by minor viral upper respiratory tract infections or inhaled irritants; most effective for a chronic nonproductive cough

Pregnancy Risk Factor C

Contraindications Hypersensitivity to dextromethorphan or any component

Warnings/Precautions Use in children <2 years of age has not been proven safe and effective

Adverse Reactions

<1%:

- Central nervous system: Drowsiness, dizziness, coma, respiratory depression
- Gastrointestinal: Nausea, GI upset, constipation, abdominal discomfort

Overdosage/Toxicology Symptoms of overdose include nausea, vomiting, drowsiness, blurred vision, nystagmus, urinary retention, stupor, hallucinations, ataxia, respiratory depression, convulsions

Treatment is supportive; naloxone 2 mg I.V. with repeat administration as necessary up to a total of 10 mg

Mechanism of Action Chemical relative of morphine lacking narcotic properties except in overdose; controls cough by depressing the medullary cough center

Pharmacodynamics/Kinetics

Onset of antitussive action: Within 15-30 minutes

Duration: Up to 6 hours

Metabolism: In the liver

Elimination: Principally in urine

Usual Dosage Oral:

Children:

<2 years: Use only as directed by a physician

2-6 years (syrup): 2.5-7.5 mg every 4-8 hours; extended release is 15 mg twice daily (maximum: 30 mg/24 hours)

6-12 years: 5-10 mg every 4 hours or 15 mg every 6-8 hours; extended release is 30 mg twice daily (maximum: 60 mg/24 hours)

Children >12 years and Adults: 10-20 mg every 4 hours or 30 mg every 6-8 hours; extended release: 60 mg twice daily; maximum: 120 mg/day

Patient Information Shake well; do not exceed recommended dosage; take with a large glass of water; if cough lasts more than 1 week or is accompanied by a rash, fever, or headache, notify physician

Nursing Implications Raise side rails, institute safety measures

Dosage Forms

Capsule (Drixoral® Cough Liquid Caps): 30 mg

Liquid:

Creo-Terpin®: 10 mg/15 mL (120 mL)

Pertussin® CS: 3.5 mg/5 mL (120 mL)

Robitussin® Pediatric, St. Joseph® Cough Suppressant: 7.5 mg/5 mL (60 mL, 120 mL, 240 mL)

Pertussin® ES, Vicks Formula 44®: 15 mg/5 mL (120 mL, 240 mL)

Liquid, sustained release, as polistirex (Delsym®): 30 mg/5 mL (89 mL)

Lozenges:

Scot-Tussin DM® Cough Chasers: 2.5 mg

Children's Hold®, Hold® DM, Robitussin® Cough Calmers, Sucrets® Cough Calmers: 5 mg

Suppress®, Trocal®: 7.5 mg

Syrup:

Benylin® Pediatric: 7.5 mg/mL (118 mL)

Benylin DM®, Silphen DM®: 10 mg/5 mL (120 mL, 3780 mL)

Vicks Formula 44® Pediatric Formula: 15 mg/15 mL (120 mL)

Dextromethorphan and Guaifenesin *see* Guaifenesin and Dextromethorphan *on page 591*

Dextropropoxyphene *see* Propoxyphene *on page 1065*

Dextrothyroxine (deks troe thye ROKS een)

Brand Names Choloxin®

Synonyms Dextrothyroxine Sodium

Therapeutic Category Antilipemic Agent

Use Reduction of elevated serum cholesterol

Pregnancy Risk Factor C

Contraindications Organic heart disease, congestive heart failure, advanced renal or hepatic disease

Warnings/Precautions Use with caution in patients with a history of angina pectoris, severe hypertension, or myocardial infarction; do not use for treatment of obesity; discontinue 2 weeks prior to elective surgery

Adverse Reactions

<1%:

Cardiovascular: Myocardial infarction, angina, arrhythmias

Central nervous system: Insomnia, headache

Dermatologic: Alopecia, rash

Gastrointestinal: Weight loss

Neuromuscular & skeletal: Tremor, paresthesia

Ocular: Visual disturbances

Otic: Tinnitus

Miscellaneous: Diaphoresis

Overdosage/Toxicology Symptoms of overdose include palpitations, diarrhea, abdominal cramps, sweating, heat intolerance, congestive heart failure, tachycardia, hypertension, cardiac arrhythmias, angina, restlessness, tremor, seizures

Propranolol can be used to treat adrenergic adverse effects, adults rarely have severe toxicity following a single overdose

(Continued)

Dextrothyroxine *(Continued)*

Drug Interactions

Decreased effect of beta-blockers, digitalis, hypoglycemics; decreased effect with cholestyramine

Increased effect of anticoagulants

Mechanism of Action Unclear mechanism, thought to increase the liver breakdown of cholesterol

Pharmacodynamics/Kinetics

Absorption: Poorly absorbed from GI tract (25%)

Distribution: Small amounts cross the placenta; appears in breast milk

Metabolism: In the liver

Half-life: 18 hours

Elimination: In urine and bile in approximately equal amounts as unchanged drug and metabolites

Usual Dosage Oral:

Children: 0.05 mg/kg/day, increase at 1-month intervals by 0.05 mg/kg/day to a maximum of 0.4 mg/kg/day or 4 mg/day

Adults: 1-2 mg/day, increase at 1-2 mg at intervals of 4 weeks, up to a maximum of 8 mg/day

Patient Information If chest pain, palpitations, sweating, diarrhea develop during therapy, discontinue drug

Dosage Forms Tablet, as sodium: 2 mg, 4 mg, 6 mg

Dextrothyroxine Sodium *see* Dextrothyroxine *on previous page*

Dey-Dose® Isoproterenol *see* Isoproterenol *on page 681*

Dey-Dose® Metaproterenol *see* Metaproterenol *on page 793*

Dey-Lute® Isoetharine *see* Isoetharine *on page 678*

Dezocine (DEZ oh seen)

Related Information

Narcotic Agonists Comparison *on page 1414*

Brand Names Dalgan®

Therapeutic Category Analgesic, Narcotic

Use Relief of moderate to severe postoperative, acute renal and ureteral colic, and cancer pain

Pregnancy Risk Factor C

Contraindications Patients experiencing immediate type hypersensitivity reactions (anaphylaxis) to dezocine or structurally related compounds should not receive this drug. Use of other central nervous system depressants concurrently to dezocine is contraindicated.

Warnings/Precautions Use with caution in patients with head injuries or increased intracranial pressure, respiratory depression, asthma, emphysema, COPD, renal or hepatic disease, labor and delivery, biliary surgery, or in patients with a history of drug abuse; abuse potential is apparent; may be better tolerated than other opioid agonist-antagonist; does not affect cardiac performance; contains bisulfites, avoid use in those sensitive to bisulfites

Adverse Reactions

1% to 10%:

- Central nervous system: Sedation, dizziness, vertigo
- Gastrointestinal: Nausea, vomiting
- Local: Injection site reactions

<1%:

- Cardiovascular: Hypotension, palpitations, bradycardia, peripheral vasodilation
- Central nervous system: Increased intracranial pressure, CNS depression, drowsiness
- Endocrine & metabolic: Antidiuretic hormone release
- Gastrointestinal: Constipation, biliary tract spasm
- Genitourinary: Urinary tract spasm
- Ocular: Miosis
- Respiratory: Respiratory depression
- Miscellaneous: Histamine release, physical and psychological dependence with prolonged use

Overdosage/Toxicology Symptoms of overdose include CNS and respiratory depression, gastrointestinal cramping, constipation

Naloxone 2 mg I.V. (0.01 mg/kg for children) with repeat administration as necessary up to a total of 10 mg

Drug Interactions Increased effect with CNS depressants

Stability Store at room temperature; protect from light

Mechanism of Action Binds to opiate receptors in the CNS, causing inhibition of ascending pain pathways, altering the perception of and response to pain; produces generalized CNS depression; it is a mixed agonist-antagonist that appears to bind selectively to CNS μ and Δ opiate receptors

Pharmacodynamics/Kinetics

Onset of analgesia: Within 15-30 minutes

Peak effect: 1 hour

Duration of analgesia: 4-6 hours

Half-life: 2.6-2.8 hours

Metabolism: Glucuronidated in liver

Elimination: Excretion of inactive metabolites and unchanged drug in the urine

Usual Dosage Adults (not recommended for patients <18 years):

I.M.: Initial: 5-20 mg; may be repeated every 3-6 hours as needed; maximum: 120 mg/day and 20 mg/dose

I.V.: Initial: 2.5-10 mg; may be repeated every 2-4 hours as needed

Dosing adjustment in renal impairment: Should be used cautiously at reduced doses

Monitoring Parameters Monitor blood pressure and heart rate during adjustment of dose

Patient Information Avoid driving or operating machinery until the effect of drug wears off; may cause physical and psychological dependence with prolonged use

Nursing Implications Watch closely for respiratory depression; induced respiratory depression is greater than that seen with morphine during the first hour after administration

Dosage Forms Injection, single-dose vial: 5 mg/mL (2 mL); 10 mg/mL (2 mL); 15 mg/mL (2 mL)

Dezone® *see* Dexamethasone *on page 356*

DFMO *see* Eflornithine *on page 441*

DFP *see* Isoflurophate *on page 679*

DHAD *see* Mitoxantrone *on page 849*

DHC Plus® *see* Dihydrocodeine Compound *on page 390*

D.H.E. 45® *see* Dihydroergotamine *on page 390*

DHPG Sodium *see* Ganciclovir *on page 566*

DHT™ *see* Dihydrotachysterol *on page 391*

Diaβeta® *see* Glyburide *on page 578*

Diabetes Mellitus Treatment *see page 1530*

Diabetic Tussin EX® [OTC] *see* Guaifenesin *on page 589*

Diabinese® *see* Chlorpropamide *on page 263*

Dialose® [OTC] *see* Docusate *on page 415*

Dialume® [OTC] *see* Aluminum Hydroxide *on page 55*

Diamine T.D.® [OTC] *see* Brompheniramine *on page 166*

Diaminodiphenylsulfone *see* Dapsone *on page 343*

Diamox® *see* Acetazolamide *on page 22*

Diamox Sequels® *see* Acetazolamide *on page 22*

Diapid® *see* Lypressin *on page 750*

Diar-aid® [OTC] *see* Loperamide *on page 739*

Diasorb® [OTC] *see* Attapulgite *on page 118*

Diazepam (dye AZ e pam)

Related Information

Adult ACLS Algorithm, Electrical Conversion *on page 1515*

Anticonvulsants by Seizure Type *on page 1392*

Benzodiazepines Comparison *on page 1397*

Convulsive Status Epilepticus *on page 1528*

Febrile Seizures *on page 1532*

Brand Names Dizac® Injection; Valium®

Canadian/Mexican Brand Names Apo-Diazepam® (Canada); Diazemuls® (Canada); E Pam® (Canada); Meval® (Canada); Novo-Dipam® (Canada); PMS-Diazepam (Canada); Vivol® (Canada)

Therapeutic Category Antianxiety Agent; Anticonvulsant; Benzodiazepine; Sedative

Use Management of general anxiety disorders, panic disorders, and provide preoperative sedation, light anesthesia, and amnesia; treatment of status epilepticus, alcohol withdrawal symptoms; used as a skeletal muscle relaxant

Restrictions C-IV

Pregnancy Risk Factor D

Pregnancy/Breast-Feeding Implications

Clinical effects on the fetus: Crosses the placenta. Oral clefts reported, however, more recent data does not support an association between drug and oral clefts; inguinal hernia, cardiac defects, spina bifida, dysmorphic facial features, skeletal defects, multiple other malformations reported; hypotonia and withdrawal symptoms reported following use near time of delivery

(Continued)

Diazepam *(Continued)*

Breast-feeding/lactation: Crosses into breast milk

Clinical effects on the infant: Sedation; American Academy of Pediatrics reports that USE MAY BE OF CONCERN.

Contraindications Hypersensitivity to diazepam or any component; there may be a cross-sensitivity with other benzodiazepines; do not use in a comatose patient, in those with pre-existing CNS depression, respiratory depression, narrow-angle glaucoma, or severe uncontrolled pain; do not use in pregnant women

Warnings/Precautions Use with caution in patients receiving other CNS depressants, patients with low albumin, hepatic dysfunction, and in the elderly and young infants. Due to its long-acting metabolite, diazepam is not considered a drug of choice in the elderly; long-acting benzodiazepines have been associated with falls in the elderly.

Adverse Reactions

>10%:

- Cardiovascular: Cardiac arrest, hypotension, bradycardia, cardiovascular collapse, tachycardia, chest pain
- Central nervous system: Drowsiness, ataxia, amnesia, slurred speech, paradoxical excitement or rage, fatigue, lightheadedness, insomnia, memory impairment, headache, anxiety, depression
- Dermatologic: Rash
- Endocrine & metabolic: Decreased libido
- Gastrointestinal: Xerostomia, changes in salivation, constipation, nausea, vomiting, diarrhea, increased or decreased appetite
- Local: Phlebitis, pain with injection
- Neuromuscular & skeletal: Dysarthria
- Ocular: Blurred vision, diplopia
- Respiratory: Decrease in respiratory rate, apnea, laryngospasm
- Miscellaneous: Diaphoresis

1% to 10%:

- Cardiovascular: Syncope, hypotension
- Central nervous system: Confusion, nervousness, dizziness, akathisia
- Dermatologic: Dermatitis
- Gastrointestinal: Weight gain or loss
- Neuromuscular & skeletal: Rigidity, tremor, muscle cramps
- Otic: Tinnitus
- Respiratory: Nasal congestion, hyperventilation
- Miscellaneous: Hiccups

<1%:

- Endocrine & metabolic: Menstrual irregularities
- Hematologic: Blood dyscrasias
- Neuromuscular & skeletal: Reflex slowing
- Miscellaneous: Physical and psychological dependence with prolonged use

Overdosage/Toxicology Symptoms of overdose include somnolence, confusion, coma, hypoactive reflexes, dyspnea, hypotension, slurred speech, impaired coordination

Treatment for benzodiazepine overdose is supportive. Rarely is mechanical ventilation required. Flumazenil has been shown to selectively block the binding of benzodiazepines to CNS receptors, resulting in a reversal of benzodiazepine-induced CNS depression, but not respiratory depression.

Drug Interactions Diazepam and desmethyldiazepam are cytochrome P-450 2C enzyme substrates

Decreased effect: Enzyme inducers may increase the metabolism of diazepam

Increased toxicity: CNS depressants (alcohol, barbiturates, opioids) may enhance sedation and respiratory depression; cimetidine may decrease the metabolism of diazepam; cisapride can significantly increase diazepam levels; valproic acid may displace diazepam from binding sites which may result in an increase in sedative effects; selective serotonin reuptake inhibitors (eg, fluoxetine, sertraline, paroxetine) have greatly increased diazepam levels by altering its clearance

Stability Protect parenteral dosage form from light; potency is retained for up to 3 months when kept at room temperature; most stable at pH 4-8, hydrolysis occurs at pH <3; do not mix I.V. product with other medications

Mechanism of Action Depresses all levels of the CNS, including the limbic and reticular formation, probably through the increased action of gamma-aminobutyric acid (GABA), which is a major inhibitory neurotransmitter in the brain

Pharmacodynamics/Kinetics

I.V. for status epilepticus:

- Onset of action: Almost immediate
- Duration: Short, 20-30 minutes

Absorption: Oral: 85% to 100%, more reliable than I.M.

Protein binding: 98%
Metabolism: In the liver
Half-life:
Parent drug: Adults: 20-50 hours, increased half-life in neonates, elderly, and those with severe hepatic disorders
Active major metabolite (desmethyldiazepam): 50-100 hours, can be prolonged in neonates

Usual Dosage **Oral absorption is more reliable than I.M.**
Children:
Conscious sedation for procedures: Oral: 0.2-0.3 mg/kg (maximum: 10 mg) 45-60 minutes prior to procedure
Sedation or muscle relaxation or anxiety:
Oral: 0.12-0.8 mg/kg/day in divided doses every 6-8 hours
I.M., I.V.: 0.04-0.3 mg/kg/dose every 2-4 hours to a maximum of 0.6 mg/kg within an 8-hour period if needed
Status epilepticus:
Infants 30 days to 5 years: I.V.: 0.05-0.3 mg/kg/dose given over 2-3 minutes, every 15-30 minutes to a maximum total dose of 5 mg; repeat in 2-4 hours as needed **or** 0.2-0.5 mg/dose every 2-5 minutes to a maximum total dose of 5 mg
>5 years: I.V.: 0.05-0.3 mg/kg/dose given over 2-3 minutes every 15-30 minutes to a maximum total dose of 10 mg; repeat in 2-4 hours as needed **or** 1 mg/dose given over 2-3 minutes, every 2-5 minutes to a maximum total dose of 10 mg
Rectal: 0.5 mg/kg, then 0.25 mg/kg in 10 minutes if needed

Adolescents: Conscious sedation for procedures:
Oral: 10 mg
I.V.: 5 mg, may repeat with ½ dose if needed

Adults:
Anxiety/sedation/skeletal muscle relaxation:
Oral: 2-10 mg 2-4 times/day
I.M., I.V.: 2-10 mg, may repeat in 3-4 hours if needed
Status epilepticus: I.V.: 5-10 mg every 10-20 minutes, up to 30 mg in an 8-hour period; may repeat in 2-4 hours if necessary

Elderly: Oral: Initial:
Anxiety: 1-2 mg 1-2 times/day; increase gradually as needed, rarely need to use >10 mg/day
Skeletal muscle relaxant: 2-5 mg 2-4 times/day

Hemodialysis: Not dialyzable (0% to 5%); supplemental dose is not necessary

Dosing adjustment in hepatic impairment: Reduce dose by 50% in cirrhosis and avoid in severe/acute liver disease

Dietary Considerations Alcohol: Additive CNS depression has been reported with benzodiazepines; avoid or limit alcohol

Administration In children, do not exceed 1-2 mg/minute IVP; adults 5 mg/minute

Monitoring Parameters Respiratory rate, heart rate, blood pressure with I.V. use

Reference Range Therapeutic: Diazepam: 0.2-1.5 μg/mL (SI: 0.7-5.3 μmol/L); N-desmethyldiazepam (nordiazepam): 0.1-0.5 μg/mL (SI: 0.35-1.8 μmol/L)

Test Interactions False-negative urinary glucose determinations when using Clinistix® or Diastix®

Patient Information Avoid alcohol and other CNS depressants; avoid activities needing good psychomotor coordination until CNS effects are known; drug may cause physical or psychological dependence; avoid abrupt discontinuation after prolonged use

Nursing Implications Provide safety measures (ie, side rails, night light, and call button); supervise ambulation

Dosage Forms
Injection: 5 mg/mL (1 mL, 2 mL, 5 mL, 10 mL)
Injection, emulsified (Dizac®): 5 mg/mL (3 mL)
Solution, oral (wintergreen-spice flavor): 5 mg/5 mL (5 mL, 10 mL, 500 mL)
Solution, oral concentrate: 5 mg/mL (30 mL)
Tablet: 2 mg, 5 mg, 10 mg

Diazoxide (dye az OKS ide)

Related Information
Therapy of Hypertension *on page 1540*

Brand Names Hyperstat® I.V.; Proglycem®

Canadian/Mexican Brand Names Sefulken® (Mexico)

Therapeutic Category Antihypoglycemic Agent; Hypoglycemic Agent, Oral

(Continued)

Diazoxide *(Continued)*

Use

Oral: Hypoglycemia related to islet cell adenoma, carcinoma, hyperplasia, or adenomatosis, nesidioblastosis, leucine sensitivity, or extrapancreatic malignancy

I.V.: Emergency lowering of blood pressure

Pregnancy Risk Factor C

Contraindications Hypersensitivity to diazoxide, thiazides, or other sulfonamide derivatives; aortic coarctation, arteriovenous shunts, dissecting aortic aneurysm

Warnings/Precautions Diabetes mellitus, renal or liver disease, coronary artery disease, or cerebral vascular insufficiency; patients may require a diuretic with repeated I.V. doses

Adverse Reactions

1% to 10%:

- Cardiovascular: Hypotension
- Central nervous system: Dizziness
- Gastrointestinal: Nausea, vomiting
- Neuromuscular & skeletal: Weakness

<1%:

- Cardiovascular: Tachycardia, flushing
- Central nervous system: Seizures, headache, extrapyramidal symptoms and development of abnormal facies with chronic oral use
- Dermatologic: Rash, hirsutism, cellulitis
- Endocrine & metabolic: Hyperglycemia, ketoacidosis, sodium and water retention, hyperuricemia, inhibition of labor
- Gastrointestinal: Anorexia, constipation
- Hematologic: Leukopenia, thrombocytopenia
- Local: Pain, burning, phlebitis upon extravasation

Overdosage/Toxicology Symptoms of overdose include hyperglycemia, ketoacidosis, hypotension

Treatment: Insulin, fluid, and electrolyte restoration; I.V. pressors may be needed to support blood pressure

Drug Interactions

Decreased effect: Diazoxide may increase phenytoin metabolism or free fraction

Increased toxicity:

- Diuretics and hypotensive agents may potentiate diazoxide adverse effects
- Diazoxide may decrease warfarin protein binding

Stability Protect from light, heat, and freezing; avoid using darkened solutions

Mechanism of Action Inhibits insulin release from the pancreas; produces direct smooth muscle relaxation of the peripheral arterioles which results in decrease in blood pressure and reflex increase in heart rate and cardiac output

Pharmacodynamics/Kinetics

Hyperglycemic effect: Oral:

- Onset of action: Within 1 hour
- Duration (normal renal function): 8 hours

Hypotensive effect: I.V.:

- Peak: Within 5 minutes
- Duration: Usually 3-12 hours

Protein binding: 90%

Half-life:

- Children: 9-24 hours
- Adults: 20-36 hours
- End stage renal disease: >30 hours

Elimination: 50% excreted unchanged in urine

Usual Dosage

Hypertension: Children and Adults: I.V.: 1-3 mg/kg up to a maximum of 150 mg in a single injection; repeat dose in 5-15 minutes until blood pressure adequately reduced; repeat administration at intervals of 4-24 hours; monitor the blood pressure closely; do not use longer than 10 days

Hyperinsulinemic hypoglycemia: Oral: **Note:** Use lower dose listed as initial dose

- Newborns and Infants: 8-15 mg/kg/day in divided doses every 8-12 hours
- Children and Adults: 3-8 mg/kg/day in divided doses every 8-12 hours

Dosing adjustment in renal impairment: None

Dialysis: Elimination is not enhanced via hemo- or peritoneal dialysis; supplemental dose is not necessary

Administration I.V. diazoxide is given undiluted by rapid I.V. injection over a period of 30 seconds or less but may also be given by continuous infusion

Monitoring Parameters Blood pressure, blood glucose, serum uric acid; intravenous administration requires cardiac monitor and blood pressure monitor

Test Interactions False-negative insulin response to glucagon

Patient Information Check blood glucose carefully, monitor urine glucose/ketones; shake suspension well before using

Nursing Implications Extravasation can be treated with warm compresses; monitor blood glucose daily in patients receiving I.V. therapy

Dosage Forms

Capsule (Proglycem®): 50 mg
Injection (Hyperstat®): 15 mg/mL (1 mL, 20 mL)
Suspension, oral (chocolate-mint flavor) (Proglycem®): 50 mg/mL (30 mL)

Dibent® Injection *see* Dicyclomine *on page 376*
Dibenzyline® *see* Phenoxybenzamine *on page 986*

Dibucaine (DYE byoo kane)

Brand Names Nupercainal® [OTC]

Therapeutic Category Local Anesthetic, Amide Derivative; Local Anesthetic, Rectal; Local Anesthetic, Topical

Use Fast, temporary relief of pain and itching due to hemorrhoids, minor burns, or other minor skin conditions [amide derivative local anesthetic]

Pregnancy Risk Factor C

Contraindications Known hypersensitivity to amide-type anesthetics, ophthalmic use

Adverse Reactions

1% to 10%:
- Dermatologic: Angioedema, contact dermatitis
- Local: Burning

<1%:
- Cardiovascular: Edema
- Dermatologic: Urticaria
- Genitourinary: Urethritis
- Local: Tenderness, irritation, inflammation, cutaneous lesions

Overdosage/Toxicology Symptoms of overdose are due to high plasma levels and include convulsions or hypotension

Treatment is supportive; maintain an airway and support ventilation; methemoglobinemia may be treated with methylene blue

Mechanism of Action Blocks both the initiation and conduction of nerve impulses by decreasing the neuronal membrane's permeability to sodium ions, which results in inhibition of depolarization with resultant blockade of conduction

Pharmacodynamics/Kinetics

Onset of action: Within 15 minutes
Duration: 2-4 hours
Absorption: Poorly through intact skin, but well absorbed through mucous membranes and excoriated skin

Usual Dosage Children and Adults:

Rectal: Hemorrhoids: Insert ointment into rectum using a rectal applicator; administer each morning, evening, and after each bowel movement

Topical: Apply gently to the affected areas; no more than 30 g for adults or 7.5 g for children should be used in any 24-hour period

Patient Information If condition worsens or if symptoms persist for >7 days, stop using the ointment and consult a physician; wash hands after use to avoid getting ointment in eyes

Nursing Implications Do not use near the eyes or over denuded surfaces or blistered areas

Dosage Forms

Cream, topical: 0.5% (45 g)
Ointment, topical: 1% (30 g, 60 g, 454 g)

DIC *see* Dacarbazine *on page 335*
Dicarbosil® [OTC] *see* Calcium Carbonate *on page 185*
Dichysterol *see* Dihydrotachysterol *on page 391*

Diclofenac (dye KLOE fen ak)

Related Information

Nonsteroidal Anti-Inflammatory Agents Comparison *on page 1419*

Brand Names Cataflam®; Voltaren®; Voltaren-XR®

Canadian/Mexican Brand Names Apo-Diclo® (Canada); Novo-Difenac® (Canada); Novo-Difenac-SR® (Canada); Nu-Diclo® (Canada); Voltaren Rapide® (Canada); Artrenac® (Mexico); Clonodifen® (Mexico); Dolo Pangavit D® (Mexico); Fustaren® Retard (Mexico); Galedol® (Mexico); Liroken® (Mexico)

Synonyms Diclofenac Potassium; Diclofenac Sodium

Therapeutic Category Analgesic, Nonsteroidal Anti-inflammatory Drug; Anti-inflammatory Agent; Anti-Inflammatory Agent, Ophthalmic; Nonsteroidal Anti-Inflammatory Agent (NSAID), Ophthalmic; Nonsteroidal Anti-inflammatory Agent (NSAID), Oral

(Continued)

Diclofenac *(Continued)*

Use Acute treatment of mild to moderate pain; acute and chronic treatment of rheumatoid arthritis, ankylosing spondylitis, and osteoarthritis; used for juvenile rheumatoid arthritis, gout, dysmenorrhea; ophthalmic solution for postoperative inflammation after cataract extraction

Pregnancy Risk Factor B

Contraindications Known hypersensitivity to diclofenac, any component, aspirin or other nonsteroidal anti-inflammatory drugs (NSAIDs); porphyria

Warnings/Precautions Use with caution in patients with congestive heart failure, hypertension, decreased renal or hepatic function, history of GI disease, or those receiving anticoagulants

Adverse Reactions

>10%:

- Dermatologic: Rash
- Gastrointestinal: Abdominal cramps, heartburn, indigestion, nausea

1% to 10%:

- Cardiovascular: Angina pectoris, arrhythmias
- Central nervous system: Dizziness, nervousness
- Dermatologic: Itching
- Gastrointestinal: GI ulceration, vomiting
- Genitourinary: Vaginal bleeding
- Otic: Tinnitus

<1%:

- Cardiovascular: Chest pain, congestive heart failure, hypertension, tachycardia
- Central nervous system: Convulsions, forgetfulness, mental depression, drowsiness, insomnia
- Dermatologic: Urticaria, exfoliative dermatitis, erythema multiforme, Stevens-Johnson syndrome, angioedema
- Gastrointestinal: Stomatitis
- Genitourinary: Cystitis
- Hematologic: Agranulocytosis, anemia, pancytopenia, leukopenia, thrombocytopenia
- Hepatic: Hepatitis
- Neuromuscular & skeletal: Peripheral neuropathy, trembling, weakness
- Ocular: Blurred vision, change in vision
- Otic: Decreased hearing
- Renal: Interstitial nephritis, nephrotic syndrome, renal impairment
- Respiratory: Wheezing, laryngeal edema, shortness of breath, epistaxis
- Miscellaneous: Anaphylaxis, diaphoresis (increased)

Overdosage/Toxicology Symptoms of overdose include acute renal failure, vomiting, drowsiness, leukocytosis

Management of a nonsteroidal anti-inflammatory drug (NSAID) intoxication is primarily supportive and symptomatic. Fluid therapy is commonly effective in managing the hypotension that may occur following an acute NSAID overdose, except when this is due to an acute blood loss.

Drug Interactions

- Decreased effect with aspirin; decreased effect of thiazides, furosemide
- Increased toxicity of digoxin, methotrexate, cyclosporine, lithium, insulin, sulfonylureas, potassium-sparing diuretics, aspirin

Mechanism of Action Inhibits prostaglandin synthesis by decreasing the activity of the enzyme, cyclo-oxygenase, which results in decreased formation of prostaglandin precursors

Pharmacodynamics/Kinetics

- Onset of action: Cataflam® has a more rapid onset of action than does the sodium salt (Voltaren®), because it is absorbed in the stomach instead of the duodenum
- Protein binding: 99%
- Metabolism: In the liver to inactive metabolites
- Half-life: 2 hours
- Time to peak serum concentration:
  - Cataflam®: Within 1 hour
  - Voltaren®: Within 2 hours
- Elimination: Primarily in urine

Usual Dosage Adults:

Oral:

- Analgesia (Cataflam®): Starting dose: 50 mg 3 times/day
- Rheumatoid arthritis: 150-200 mg/day in 2-4 divided doses (100 mg/day of sustained release product)
- Osteoarthritis: 100-150 mg/day in 2-3 divided doses (100-200 mg/day of sustained release product)
- Ankylosing spondylitis: 100-125 mg/day in 4-5 divided doses

Ophthalmic: Instill 1 drop into affected eye 4 times/day beginning 24 hours after cataract surgery and continuing for 2 weeks

Monitoring Parameters Monitor CBC, liver enzymes; monitor urine output and BUN/serum creatinine in patients receiving diuretics; occult blood loss

Patient Information Do not crush tablets; take with food, milk, or water; report any signs of blood in stool

Nursing Implications Do not crush tablets

Additional Information

Diclofenac potassium = Cataflam®; potassium content: 5.8 mg (0.15 mEq) per 50 mg tablet

Diclofenac sodium = Voltaren®

Diclofenac sodium = Voltaren-XR®

Dosage Forms

Solution, ophthalmic, as sodium (Voltaren®): 0.1% (2.5 mL, 5 mL)

Tablet, enteric coated, as sodium: 25 mg, 50 mg, 75 mg

Voltaren®: 25 mg, 50 mg, 75 mg

Tablet, extended release, as sodium (Voltaren-XR®): 100 mg

Tablet, as potassium (Cataflam®): 50 mg

Diclofenac Potassium *see* Diclofenac *on page 373*

Diclofenac Sodium *see* Diclofenac *on page 373*

Dicloxacillin (dye kloks a SIL in)

Related Information

Animal and Human Bites Guidelines *on page 1463*

Brand Names Dycill®; Dynapen®; Pathocil®

Canadian/Mexican Brand Names Brispen® (Mexico); Posipen® (Mexico)

Synonyms Dicloxacillin Sodium

Therapeutic Category Antibiotic, Penicillin

Use Treatment of systemic infections such as pneumonia, skin and soft tissue infections, and osteomyelitis caused by penicillinase-producing staphylococci

Pregnancy Risk Factor B

Contraindications Known hypersensitivity to dicloxacillin, penicillin, or any components

Warnings/Precautions Monitor PT if patient concurrently on warfarin; elimination of drug is slow in neonates; use with caution in patients allergic to cephalosporins; bad taste of suspension may make compliance difficult

Adverse Reactions

1% to 10%: Gastrointestinal: Diarrhea

<1%:

Central nervous system: Fever

Dermatologic: Rash

Gastrointestinal: Nausea, vomiting

Hematologic: Eosinophilia, neutropenia, leukopenia, thrombocytopenia

Hepatic: Elevated liver enzymes

Miscellaneous: Sickness-like reaction

Overdosage/Toxicology Symptoms of penicillin overdose include neuromuscular hypersensitivity (agitation, hallucinations, asterixis, encephalopathy, confusion, and seizures) and electrolyte imbalance with potassium or sodium salts, especially in renal failure

Hemodialysis may be helpful to aid in the removal of the drug from the blood, otherwise most treatment is supportive or symptom directed

Drug Interactions

Decreased effect: Efficacy of oral contraceptives may be reduced

Increased effect: Disulfiram, probenecid may increase penicillin levels; increased effect of anticoagulants

Stability Refrigerate suspension after reconstitution; discard after 14 days if refrigerated or 7 days if kept at room temperature; unit dose antibiotic oral syringes are stable for 48 hours

Mechanism of Action Interferes with bacterial cell wall synthesis during active multiplication, causing cell wall death and resultant bactericidal activity against susceptible bacteria

Pharmacodynamics/Kinetics

Absorption: 35% to 76% from GI tract; food decreases rate and extent of absorption

Distribution: Crosses the placenta; distributes into breast milk

Protein binding: 96%

Half-life: 0.6-0.8 hours, slightly prolonged in patients with renal impairment

Time to peak serum concentration: Within 0.5-2 hours

Elimination: Prolonged in neonates; partially eliminated by the liver and excreted in bile, 56% to 70% is eliminated in urine as unchanged drug

(Continued)

Dicloxacillin *(Continued)*

Usual Dosage Oral:

Children <40 kg: 12.5-50 mg/kg/day divided every 6 hours; doses of 50-100 mg/kg/day in divided doses every 6 hours have been used for therapy of osteomyelitis

Children >40 kg and Adults: 125-500 mg every 6 hours

Dosage adjustment in renal impairment: Not necessary

Hemodialysis: Not dialyzable (0% to 5%); supplemental dosage not necessary

Peritoneal dialysis: Supplemental dosage not necessary

Continuous arterio-venous or veno-venous hemofiltration (CAVH/CAVHD): Supplemental dosage not necessary

Dietary Considerations Food: Decreases drug absorption rate; decreases drug serum concentration. Administer on an empty stomach 1 hour before or 2 hours after meals.

Administration Administer around-the-clock rather than 4 times/day to promote less variation in peak and trough serum levels

Monitoring Parameters Monitor prothrombin time if patient concurrently on warfarin

Test Interactions Positive Coombs' test [direct]

Patient Information Take until all medication used; take 1 hour before or 2 hours after meals, do not skip doses

Additional Information

Sodium content of 250 mg capsule: 13 mg (0.6 mEq)

Sodium content of suspension 65 mg/5 mL: 27 mg (1.2 mEq)

Dosage Forms

Capsule, as sodium: 125 mg, 250 mg, 500 mg

Powder for oral suspension, as sodium: 62.5 mg/5 mL (80 mL, 100 mL, 200 mL)

Dicloxacillin Sodium *see* Dicloxacillin *on previous page*

Dicyclomine (dye SYE kloe meen)

Brand Names Antispas® Injection; Bentyl® Hydrochloride Injection; Bentyl® Hydrochloride Oral; Byclomine® Injection; Dibent® Injection; Dilomine® Injection; Di-Spaz® Injection; Di-Spaz® Oral; Or-Tyl® Injection; Spasmoject® Injection

Canadian/Mexican Brand Names Bentylol® (Canada); Formulex® (Canada)

Synonyms Dicyclomine Hydrochloride; Dicycloverine Hydrochloride

Therapeutic Category Antispasmodic Agent, Gastrointestinal

Use Treatment of functional disturbances of GI motility such as irritable bowel syndrome

Unlabeled use: Urinary incontinence

Pregnancy Risk Factor B

Contraindications Hypersensitivity to any anticholinergic drug; narrow-angle glaucoma, myasthenia gravis; should not be used in infants <6 months of age

Warnings/Precautions Use with caution in patients with hepatic or renal disease, ulcerative colitis, hyperthyroidism, cardiovascular disease, hypertension, tachycardia, GI obstruction, obstruction of the urinary tract. The elderly are at increased risk for anticholinergic effects, confusion and hallucinations.

Adverse Reactions

>10%:

- Dermatologic: Dry skin
- Gastrointestinal: Constipation, dry throat, xerostomia
- Local: Injection site reactions
- Respiratory: Dry nose
- Miscellaneous: Diaphoresis (decreased)

1% to 10%:

- Dermatologic: Increased sensitivity to light
- Endocrine & metabolic: Decreased flow of breast milk
- Gastrointestinal: Dysphagia
- Ocular: Blurred vision

<1%:

- Cardiovascular: Orthostatic hypotension, tachycardia, palpitations
- Central nervous system: Confusion, drowsiness, headache, lightheadedness, loss of memory, fatigue, seizures, coma, nervousness, excitement, insomnia
- Dermatologic: Rash
- Gastrointestinal: Bloated feeling, nausea, vomiting
- Genitourinary: Dysuria, urinary retention
- Neuromuscular & skeletal: Muscular hypotonia, weakness
- Ocular: Increased intraocular pain
- Respiratory: Asphyxia, respiratory distress

Overdosage/Toxicology Symptoms of overdose include CNS stimulation followed by depression, confusion, delusions, nonreactive pupils, tachycardia, hypertension

Anticholinergic toxicity is caused by strong binding of the drug to cholinergic receptors. For anticholinergic overdose with severe life-threatening symptoms, physostigmine 1-2 mg (0.5 or 0.02 mg/kg for children) S.C. or I.V., slowly may be given to reverse these effects.

Drug Interactions

Decreased effect: Phenothiazines, anti-Parkinson's drugs, haloperidol, sustained release dosage forms; decreased effect with antacids

Increased toxicity: Anticholinergics, amantadine, narcotic analgesics, type I antiarrhythmics, antihistamines, phenothiazines, TCAs

Mechanism of Action Blocks the action of acetylcholine at parasympathetic sites in smooth muscle, secretory glands and the CNS

Pharmacodynamics/Kinetics

Onset of effect: 1-2 hours

Duration: Up to 4 hours

Absorption: Oral: Well absorbed

Metabolism: Extensive

Half-life:

- Initial phase: 1.8 hours
- Terminal phase: 9-10 hours

Elimination: In urine with only a small amount excreted as unchanged drug

Usual Dosage

Oral:

- Infants >6 months: 5 mg/dose 3-4 times/day
- Children: 10 mg/dose 3-4 times/day
- Adults: Begin with 80 mg/day in 4 equally divided doses, then increase up to 160 mg/day

I.M. **(should not be used I.V.)**: Adults: 80 mg/day in 4 divided doses (20 mg/dose)

Dietary Considerations Alcohol: Additive CNS effects, avoid use

Administration Do not administer I.V.

Monitoring Parameters Pulse, anticholinergic effect, urinary output, GI symptoms

Patient Information May cause drowsiness; avoid alcohol; may impair coordination and judgment; may cause blurred vision or dizziness; take 30-60 minutes before a meal; may cause dry mouth, difficult urination, or constipation

Nursing Implications Raise bed rails, institute safety measures

Dosage Forms

Capsule, as hydrochloride: 10 mg, 20 mg

Injection, as hydrochloride: 10 mg/mL (2 mL, 10 mL)

Syrup, as hydrochloride: 10 mg/5 mL (118 mL, 473 mL, 946 mL)

Tablet, as hydrochloride: 20 mg

Dicyclomine Hydrochloride *see* Dicyclomine *on previous page*

Dicycloverine Hydrochloride *see* Dicyclomine *on previous page*

Didanosine (dye DAN oh seen)

Brand Names Videx®

Synonyms ddI

Therapeutic Category Antiretroviral Agent; Antiviral Agent, Oral; Reverse Transcriptase Inhibitor

Use May be used as initial treatment in AIDS patients with no prior history of antiretroviral drug use; often used for treatment of advanced HIV infection in patients who are intolerant of zidovudine therapy or who have demonstrated significant clinical or immunologic deterioration during zidovudine therapy; may be used as monotherapy when antiretroviral therapy is warranted although often used in combination with zidovudine and possibly a protease inhibitor ("triple therapy"); combination with zalcitabine should be avoided due to possible toxicity or resistance

Pregnancy Risk Factor B

Pregnancy/Breast-Feeding Implications

Administer during pregnancy only if benefits to mother outweigh risks to the fetus

HIV-infected mothers are discouraged from breast-feeding to decrease potential transmission of HIV

Contraindications Hypersensitivity to any component

Warnings/Precautions Didanosine is indicated for treatment of HIV infection only in patients intolerant of zidovudine or who have failed zidovudine. Patients receiving didanosine may still develop opportunistic infections. Peripheral neuropathy occurs in ~35% of patients receiving the drug; pancreatitis (sometimes fatal) occurs in ~9%; risk factors for developing pancreatitis include a previous history of the condition, concurrent cytomegalovirus or *Mycobacterium avium-intracellulare* infection, and concomitant use of pentamidine or co-trimoxazole; discontinue didanosine if clinical signs of pancreatitis occur. Didanosine may cause retinal depigmentation in children receiving doses >300 mg/m²/day. (Continued)

Didanosine *(Continued)*

Patients should undergo retinal examination every 6-12 months. Use with caution in patients with decreased renal or hepatic function, phenylketonuria, sodium-restricted diets, or with edema, congestive heart failure or hyperuricemia; in high concentrations, didanosine is mutagenic.

Adverse Reactions

>10%:

Central nervous system: Anxiety, headache, irritability, insomnia, restlessness
Gastrointestinal: Abdominal pain, nausea, diarrhea
Neuromuscular & skeletal: Peripheral neuropathy

1% to 10%:

Central nervous system: Depression
Dermatologic: Rash, pruritus
Gastrointestinal: Pancreatitis

<1%:

Central nervous system: Seizures
Hematologic: Anemia, granulocytopenia, leukopenia, thrombocytopenia
Hepatic: Hepatitis
Ocular: Retinal depigmentation
Renal: Renal impairment
Miscellaneous: Hypersensitivity

Overdosage/Toxicology Chronic overdose may cause pancreatitis, peripheral neuropathy, diarrhea, hyperuricemia, and hepatic impairment; there is no known antidote for didanosine overdose; treatment is asymptomatic

Drug Interactions Drugs whose absorption depends on the level of acidity in the stomach such as ketoconazole, itraconazole, and dapsone should be administered at least 2 hours prior to didanosine

Decreased effect: Didanosine may decrease absorption of quinolones or tetracyclines, didanosine should be held during PCP treatment with pentamidine

Increased toxicity: Concomitant administration of other drugs which have the potential to cause peripheral neuropathy or pancreatitis may increase the risk of these toxicities

Stability Tablets should be stored in tightly closed bottles at 15°C to 30°C; undergoes rapid degradation when exposed to an acidic environment; tablets dispersed in water are stable for 1 hour at room temperature; reconstituted buffered solution is stable for 4 hours at room temperature; reconstituted pediatric solution is stable for 30 days if refrigerated; unbuffered powder for oral solution must be reconstituted and mixed with an equal volume of antacid at time of preparation

Mechanism of Action Didanosine, a purine nucleoside analogue and the deamination product of dideoxyadenosine (ddA), inhibits HIV replication *in vitro* in both T cells and monocytes. Didanosine is converted within the cell to the mono-, di-, and triphosphates of ddA. These ddA triphosphates act as substrate and inhibitor of HIV reverse transcriptase substrate and inhibitor of HIV reverse transcriptase thereby blocking viral DNA synthesis and suppressing HIV replication.

Pharmacodynamics/Kinetics

Absorption: Subject to degradation by the acidic pH of the stomach; buffered to resist the acidic pH; as much as 50% reduction in the peak plasma concentration is observed in the presence of food

Distribution: V_d: 54 L; children: 35.6 L/m^2

Protein binding: <5%

Metabolism: Has not been evaluated in man; studies conducted in dogs, shows didanosine extensively metabolized with allantoin, hypoxanthine, xanthine, and uric acid being the major metabolites found in the urine

Bioavailability: 21% (range: 2% to 89%)

Half-life:

Children and Adolescents: 0.8 hour

Adults:

Normal renal function: 1.5 hours; however, its active metabolite ddATP has an intracellular half-life >12 hours *in vitro*; this permits the drug to be dosed at 12-hour intervals; total body clearance averages 800 mL/minute

Impaired renal function: Half-life is increased, with values ranging from 2.5-5 hours

Elimination: ~55% of drug is eliminated unchanged in urine

Usual Dosage Oral (administer on an empty stomach):

Children: 180 mg/m^2/day divided every 12 hours **or** dosing is based on body surface area (m^2): See table.

Adults: Dosing is based on patient weight: See table.

Didanosine — Pediatric Dosing

Body Surface Area (m^2)	Dosing (Tablets) (mg bid)
≤0.4	25
0.5-0.7	50
0.8-1	75
1.1-1.4	100

Didanosine — Adult Dosing

Patient Weight (kg)	Dosing (Tablets) (mg bid)
35-49	125
50-74	200
≥75	300

Note: Children >1 year and Adults should receive 2 tablets per dose and children <1 year should receive 1 tablet per dose for adequate buffering and absorption; tablets should be chewed

Dosing adjustment in renal impairment: Patients with severe renal dysfunction should receive appropriate dose based on patient's weight on a once-a-day dosing schedule instead of twice daily dosing

Cl_{cr} 10-<60 mL/minute: Adjustment should be considered

Cl_{cr} <10 mL/minute: Administer every 24 hours

Hemodialysis: Removed by hemodialysis (40% to 60%)

Dosing adjustment in hepatic impairment: Should be considered

Patient Information Thoroughly chew tablets or manually crush or disperse 2 tablets in 1 oz of water prior to taking; for powder, open packet and pour contents into 4 oz of liquid; do not mix with fruit juice or other acid-containing liquid; stir until dissolved, drink immediately; do not take with meals

Nursing Implications Administer liquified powder immediately after dissolving; avoid creating dust if powder spilled, use wet mop or damp sponge

Additional Information A recent study (n=245) indicated that a change from AZT to ddI in clinically stable HIV-infected patients with CD4 cell counts of 200-500, resulted in a slowed disease progression rate, a sustained increase in CD4 counts, and a decreased probability of developing a high level of resistance to AZT

Dosage Forms

Powder for oral solution:

Buffered (single dose packet): 100 mg, 167 mg, 250 mg, 375 mg

Pediatric: 2 g, 4 g

Tablet, buffered, chewable (mint flavor): 25 mg, 50 mg, 100 mg, 150 mg

Dideoxycytidine *see* Zalcitabine *on page 1318*

Didronel® *see* Etidronate Disodium *on page 493*

Dienestrol (dye en ES trole)

Brand Names DV® Cream; Ortho® Dienestrol

Therapeutic Category Estrogen Derivative, Vaginal

Use Symptomatic management of atrophic vaginitis or kraurosis vulvae in postmenopausal women

Pregnancy Risk Factor X

Contraindications Pregnancy; should not be used during lactation or undiagnosed vaginal bleeding

Warnings/Precautions Use with caution in patients with a history of thromboembolism, stroke, myocardial infarction (especially age >40 who smoke), liver tumor, hypertension, cardiac, renal or hepatic insufficiency

Adverse Reactions

1% to 10%:

Cardiovascular: Peripheral edema

Endocrine & metabolic: Breast tenderness, breast enlargement

Gastrointestinal: Anorexia, abdominal cramping

<1%:

Cardiovascular: Hypertension, thromboembolism, myocardial infarction

Central nervous system: Stroke, migraine, dizziness, anxiety, depression, headache

Dermatologic: Chloasma, melasma, rash

Endocrine & metabolic: Decreased glucose tolerance, alterations in frequency and flow of menses, breast tenderness or enlargement, increased triglycerides and LDL

Gastrointestinal: Nausea, GI distress

Hepatic: Cholestatic jaundice

(Continued)

Dienestrol *(Continued)*

Miscellaneous: Increased susceptibility to *Candida* infection

Mechanism of Action Increases the synthesis of DNA, RNA, and various proteins in target tissues; reduces the release of gonadotropin-releasing hormone from the hypothalamus; reduces FSH and LH release from the pituitary

Pharmacodynamics/Kinetics

Time to peak serum concentration: Topical: Within 3-4 hours

Metabolism: In the liver

Usual Dosage Adults: Vaginal: Insert 1 applicatorful once or twice daily for 1-2 weeks and then 1/2 of that dose for 1-2 weeks; maintenance dose: 1 applicatorful 1-3 times/week for 3-6 months

Patient Information Insert applicator high into vagina. Patients should inform their physician if signs or symptoms of any of the following occur: Thromboembolic or thrombotic disorders including sudden severe headache or vomiting, disturbance of vision or speech, loss of vision, numbness or weakness in an extremity, sharp or crushing chest pain, calf pain, shortness of breath, severe abdominal pain or mass, mental depression, or unusual bleeding. Patients should discontinue taking the medication if they suspect they are pregnant or become pregnant.

Dosage Forms Cream, vaginal: 0.01% (30 g with applicator; 78 g with applicator)

Diethylpropion (dye eth il PROE pee on)

Brand Names Tenuate®; Tenuate® Dospan®; Tepanil®

Canadian/Mexican Brand Names Nobesine® (Canada)

Synonyms Amfepramone; Diethylpropion Hydrochloride

Therapeutic Category Anorexiant

Use Short-term adjunct in exogenous obesity

Restrictions C-IV

Pregnancy Risk Factor B

Contraindications Known hypersensitivity to diethylpropion

Warnings/Precautions Prolonged administration may lead to dependence; use with caution in patients with mental illness or diabetes mellitus, cardiovascular disease, nephritis, angina pectoris, hypertension, glaucoma, and patients with a history of drug abuse

Adverse Reactions

>10%:

Cardiovascular: Hypertension

Central nervous system: Euphoria, nervousness, insomnia

1% to 10%:

Central nervous system: Confusion, mental depression

Endocrine & metabolic: Changes in libido

Gastrointestinal: Nausea, vomiting, restlessness, constipation

Hematologic: Blood dyscrasias

Neuromuscular & skeletal: Tremor

Ocular: Blurred vision

<1%:

Cardiovascular: Tachycardia, arrhythmias

Central nervous system: Depression, headache

Dermatologic: Alopecia

Gastrointestinal: Diarrhea, abdominal cramps

Genitourinary: Dysuria, polyuria

Neuromuscular & skeletal: Myalgia, tremor

Respiratory: Dyspnea

Miscellaneous: Diaphoresis (increased)

Overdosage/Toxicology There is no specific antidote for amphetamine intoxication and the bulk of the treatment is supportive. Hyperactivity and agitation usually respond to reduced sensory input; however, with extreme agitation, haloperidol (2-5 mg I.M. for adults) may be required. Hyperthermia is best treated with external cooling measures, or when severe or unresponsive, muscle paralysis with pancuronium may be needed. Hypertension is usually transient and generally does not require treatment unless severe. For diastolic blood pressures >110 mm Hg, a nitroprusside infusion should be initiated. Seizures usually respond to diazepam I.V. and/or phenytoin maintenance regimens.

Drug Interactions

Decreased effect of guanethidine; decreased effect with phenothiazines

Increased effect/toxicity with MAO inhibitors (hypertensive crisis), CNS depressants, general anesthetics (arrhythmias), sympathomimetics

Mechanism of Action Diethylpropion is used as an anorexiant agent possessing pharmacological and chemical properties similar to those of amphetamines. The mechanism of action of diethylpropion in reducing appetite appears to be secondary to CNS effects, specifically stimulation of the hypothalamus to release catecholamines into the central nervous system; anorexiant effects are mediated via norepinephrine and dopamine metabolism. An increase in physical activity and metabolic effects (inhibition of lipogenesis and enhancement of lipolysis) may also contribute to weight loss.

Usual Dosage Adults: Oral:

Tablet: 25 mg 3 times/day before meals or food

Tablet, controlled release: 75 mg at midmorning

Dietary Considerations Alcohol: Avoid use

Monitoring Parameters Monitor CNS

Patient Information Avoid alcoholic beverages; take during day to avoid insomnia; do not discontinue abruptly, may cause physical and psychological dependence with prolonged use

Nursing Implications Do not crush 75 mg controlled release tablets; dose should not be given in evening or at bedtime

Dosage Forms

Tablet, as hydrochloride: 25 mg

Tablet, as hydrochloride, controlled release: 75 mg

Diethylpropion Hydrochloride *see* Diethylpropion *on previous page*

Diethylstilbestrol (dye eth il stil BES trole)

Brand Names Stilphostrol®

Canadian/Mexican Brand Names Honvol® (Canada)

Synonyms DES; Diethylstilbestrol Diphosphate Sodium; Stilbestrol

Therapeutic Category Estrogen Derivative; Estrogen Derivative, Oral; Estrogen Derivative, Parenteral

Use Palliative treatment of inoperable metastatic prostatic carcinoma and post-menopausal inoperable, progressing breast cancer

Pregnancy Risk Factor X

Contraindications Undiagnosed vaginal bleeding, during pregnancy; breast cancer except in select patients with metastatic disease

Warnings/Precautions Use with caution in patients with a history of thromboembolism, stroke, myocardial infarction (especially >40 of age who smoke), liver tumor, hypertension, cardiac, renal or hepatic insufficiency; estrogens have been reported to increase the risk of endometrial carcinoma; do not use estrogens during pregnancy

Adverse Reactions

>10%:

- Cardiovascular: Peripheral edema
- Endocrine & metabolic: Enlargement of breasts (female and male), breast tenderness
- Gastrointestinal: Nausea, anorexia, bloating

1% to 10%:

- Central nervous system: Headache
- Endocrine & metabolic: Increased libido (female), decreased libido (male)
- Gastrointestinal: Vomiting, diarrhea

<1%:

- Cardiovascular: Hypertension, thromboembolism, myocardial infarction, edema
- Central nervous system: Stroke, depression, dizziness, anxiety
- Dermatologic: Chloasma, melasma, rash
- Endocrine & metabolic: Amenorrhea, alterations in frequency and flow of menses, increased triglycerides
- Gastrointestinal: Nausea, GI distress
- Hepatic: Increased LDL, cholestatic jaundice
- Ocular: Intolerance to contact lenses
- Miscellaneous: Decreased glucose tolerance, increased susceptibility to *Candida* infection, breast tumors

Overdosage/Toxicology Symptoms of overdose include nausea

Stability Intravenous solution should be stored at room temperature and away from direct light; solution is stable for 3 days as long as cloudiness or precipitation has not occurred

Mechanism of Action Competes with estrogenic and androgenic compounds for binding onto tumor cells and thereby inhibits their effects on tumor growth

Pharmacodynamics/Kinetics

Metabolism: In the liver

Elimination: In urine and feces

Usual Dosage Adults:

Male:

- Prostate carcinoma (inoperable, progressing): Oral: 1-3 mg/day
- Diphosphate: (inoperable, progressing): Oral: 50 mg 3 times/day; increase up to 200 mg or more 3 times/day; maximum daily dose: 1 g
- I.V.: Administer 0.5 g, dissolved in 250 mL of saline or D_5W, administer slowly the first 10-15 minutes then adjust rate so that the entire amount is given in 1

(Continued)

Diethylstilbestrol *(Continued)*

hour; repeat for ≥5 days depending on patient response, then repeat 0.25-0.5 g 1-2 times for one week or change to oral therapy

Female: Postmenopausal (inoperable, progressing) breast carcinoma: Oral: 15 mg/day

Test Interactions

Increased prothrombin and factors VII, VIII, IX, X
Decreased antithrombin III
Increased platelet aggregability
Increased thyroid binding globulin
Increased total thyroid hormone (T_4)
Decreased serum folate concentration
Increased serum triglycerides/phospholipids

Patient Information Patients should inform their physicians if signs or symptoms of thromboembolic or thrombotic disorders including sudden severe headache or vomiting, disturbance of vision or speech, loss of vision, numbness or weakness in an extremity, sharp or crushing chest pain, calf pain, shortness of breath, severe abdominal pain or mass, mental depression or unusual bleeding.

Dosage Forms

Injection, as diphosphate sodium (Stilphostrol®): 0.25 g (5 mL)
Tablet: 1 mg, 2.5 mg, 5 mg
Tablet (Stilphostrol®): 50 mg

Diethylstilbestrol Diphosphate Sodium *see* Diethylstilbestrol *on previous page*

Differin™ *see* Adapalene *on page 32*

Diflorasone (dye FLOR a sone)

Related Information

Corticosteroids Comparison *on page 1407*

Brand Names Florone®; Florone E®; Maxiflor®; Psorcon™

Synonyms Diflorasone Diacetate

Therapeutic Category Corticosteroid, Topical (High Potency); Corticosteroid, Topical (Very High Potency)

Use Relieves inflammation and pruritic symptoms of corticosteroid-responsive dermatosis (high to very high potency topical corticosteroid)

Maxiflor™: High potency topical corticosteroid
Psorcon™: Very high potency topical corticosteroid

Pregnancy Risk Factor C

Contraindications Known hypersensitivity to diflorasone

Warnings/Precautions Use with caution in patients with impaired circulation; skin infections

Adverse Reactions

<1%:

Dermatologic: Itching, folliculitis, maceration
Local: Burning, dryness
Neuromuscular & skeletal: Muscle atrophy, arthralgia
Miscellaneous: Secondary infection

Overdosage/Toxicology Symptoms of overdose include moon face, central obesity, hypertension, diabetes, hyperlipidemia, peptic ulcer, increased susceptibility to infection, electrolyte and fluid imbalance, psychosis, hallucinations. When consumed in excessive quantities, systemic hypercorticism and adrenal suppression may occur; in those cases discontinuation and withdrawal of the corticosteroid should be done judiciously.

Mechanism of Action Decreases inflammation by suppression of migration of polymorphonuclear leukocytes and reversal of increased capillary permeability

Pharmacodynamics/Kinetics

Absorption: Topical: Negligible, around 1% reaches dermal layers or systemic circulation; occlusive dressings increase absorption percutaneously
Metabolism: Primarily in the liver

Usual Dosage Topical: Apply ointment sparingly 1-3 times/day; apply cream sparingly 2-4 times/day

Patient Information A thin film of cream or ointment is effective; do not overuse; do not use tight-fitting diapers or plastic pants on children being treated in the diaper area; use only as prescribed, and for no longer than the period prescribed; apply sparingly in light film; rub in lightly; avoid contact with eyes; notify physician if condition being treated persists or worsens

Nursing Implications For external use only; do not use on open wounds; apply sparingly to occlusive dressings; should not be used in the presence of open or weeping lesions

Dosage Forms

Cream, as diacetate: 0.05% (15 g, 30 g, 60 g)
Ointment, topical, as diacetate: 0.05% (15 g, 30 g, 60 g)

Diflorasone Diacetate *see* Diflorasone *on previous page*
Diflucan® *see* Fluconazole *on page 524*

Diflunisal (dye FLOO ni sal)

Related Information
Dosing Data for Acetaminophen and NSAIDs *on page 1377*

Brand Names Dolobid®

Canadian/Mexican Brand Names Apo-Diflunisal® (Canada); Novo-Diflunisal® (Canada); Nu-Diflunisal® (Canada)

Therapeutic Category Analgesic, Nonsteroidal Anti-inflammatory Drug; Anti-inflammatory Agent; Nonsteroidal Anti-inflammatory Agent (NSAID), Oral

Use Management of inflammatory disorders usually including rheumatoid arthritis and osteoarthritis; can be used as an analgesic for treatment of mild to moderate pain

Pregnancy Risk Factor C (D if used in the 3rd trimester)

Contraindications Hypersensitivity to diflunisal or any component, may be a cross-sensitivity with other nonsteroidal anti-inflammatory agents including aspirin; should not be used in patients with active GI bleeding

Warnings/Precautions Peptic ulceration and GI bleeding have been reported; platelet function and bleeding time are inhibited; ophthalmologic effects; impaired renal function, use lower dosage; peripheral edema; possibility of Reye's syndrome; elevation in liver tests

Adverse Reactions

>10%:
- Central nervous system: Headache
- Endocrine & metabolic: Fluid retention

1% to 10%:
- Cardiovascular: Angina pectoris, arrhythmias
- Central nervous system: Dizziness
- Dermatologic: Rash, itching
- Gastrointestinal: GI ulceration
- Genitourinary: Vaginal bleeding
- Otic: Tinnitus

<1%:
- Cardiovascular: Chest pain, vasculitis, tachycardia
- Central nervous system: Convulsions, hallucinations, mental depression, drowsiness, nervousness, insomnia
- Dermatologic: Toxic epidermal necrolysis, urticaria, exfoliative dermatitis, itching, erythema multiforme, Stevens-Johnson syndrome, angioedema
- Gastrointestinal: Stomatitis, esophagitis or gastritis
- Genitourinary: Cystitis
- Hematologic: Hemolytic anemia, agranulocytosis, thrombocytopenia
- Hepatic: Hepatitis
- Neuromuscular & skeletal: Peripheral neuropathy, trembling, weakness
- Ocular: Blurred vision, change in vision
- Otic: Decreased hearing
- Renal: Interstitial nephritis, nephrotic syndrome, renal impairment
- Respiratory: Wheezing, shortness of breath
- Miscellaneous: Anaphylaxis, diaphoresis (increased)

Overdosage/Toxicology Symptoms of overdose include drowsiness, nausea, vomiting, hyperventilation, tachycardia, tinnitus, stupor, coma, renal failure, leukocytosis

Management of a nonsteroidal anti-inflammatory drug (NSAID) intoxication is primarily supportive and symptomatic. Fluid therapy is commonly effective in managing the hypotension that may occur following an acute NSAID overdose, except when this is due to an acute blood loss.

Drug Interactions

Decreased effect with antacids

Increased effect/toxicity of digoxin, methotrexate, anticoagulants, phenytoin, sulfonylureas, sulfonamides, lithium, indomethacin, hydrochlorothiazide, acetaminophen (levels)

Mechanism of Action Inhibits prostaglandin synthesis by decreasing the activity of the enzyme, cyclo-oxygenase, which results in decreased formation of prostaglandin precursors

Pharmacodynamics/Kinetics
- Onset of analgesia: Within 1 hour
- Duration of action: 8-12 hours
- Absorption: Well absorbed from GI tract
- Distribution: Appears in breast milk
- Metabolism: Extensively in the liver
- Half-life: 8-12 hours, prolonged with renal impairment
- Time to peak serum concentration: Oral: Within 2-3 hours

(Continued)

Diflunisal *(Continued)*

Elimination: In urine within 72-96 hours, ~3% as unchanged drug and 90% as glucuronide conjugates

Usual Dosage Adults: Oral:

Pain: Initial: 500-1000 mg followed by 250-500 mg every 8-12 hours; maximum daily dose: 1.5 g

Inflammatory condition: 500-1000 mg/day in 2 divided doses; maximum daily dose: 1.5 g

Dosing adjustment in renal impairment: Cl_{cr} <50 mL/minute: Administer 50% of normal dose

Test Interactions ↑ chloride (S), glucose, ketone (U), uric acid (S), sodium (S); ↓ uric acid (S), catecholamines (U), glucose, potassium (S), prothrombin time (S), uric acid (S), ↑ bleeding time

Patient Information May cause GI upset, take with water, milk, or meals; do not take aspirin with diflunisal, swallow tablets whole, do not crush or chew

Dosage Forms Tablet: 250 mg, 500 mg

Digibind® *see* Digoxin Immune Fab *on page 389*

Digitoxin (di ji TOKS in)

Brand Names Crystodigin®

Canadian/Mexican Brand Names Digitaline® (Canada)

Therapeutic Category Antiarrhythmic Agent, Miscellaneous; Cardiac Glycoside

Use Treatment of congestive heart failure, atrial fibrillation, atrial flutter, paroxysmal atrial tachycardia, and cardiogenic shock

Pregnancy Risk Factor C

Contraindications Hypersensitivity to digitoxin or any component (rare); digitalis toxicity, beriberi heart disease, A-V block, idiopathic hypertrophic subaortic stenosis, constrictive pericarditis, ventricular fibrillation, or tachycardia

Warnings/Precautions Use with caution in patients with hypoxia, hypothyroidism, acute myocarditis,; do not use to treat obesity; patients with incomplete A-V block (Stokes-Adams attack) may progress to complete block with digitalis drug administration; use with caution in patients with acute myocardial infarction, severe pulmonary disease, advanced heart failure, idiopathic hypertrophic subaortic stenosis, Wolff-Parkinson-White syndrome, sick-sinus syndrome (bradyarrhythmias), amyloid heart disease, and constrictive cardiomyopathies; adjust dose with renal or hepatic impairment and aged patients; elderly may develop exaggerated serum/tissue concentrations due to decreased lean body mass, total body water, and age-related reduction in renal/hepatic function; exercise will reduce serum concentrations of digoxin due to increased skeletal muscle uptake

Adverse Reactions

1% to 10%: Gastrointestinal: Anorexia, nausea, vomiting

<1%:

- Cardiovascular: Sinus bradycardia, A-V block, S-A block, atrial or nodal ectopic beats, ventricular arrhythmias, bigeminy, trigeminy, atrial tachycardia with A-V block
- Central nervous system: Drowsiness, headache, fatigue, lethargy, vertigo, disorientation
- Endocrine & metabolic: Hyperkalemia with acute toxicity
- Gastrointestinal: Feeding intolerance, abdominal pain, diarrhea
- Neuromuscular & skeletal: Neuralgia
- Ocular: Blurred vision, halos, yellow or green vision, diplopia, photophobia, flashing lights

Overdosage/Toxicology Antidote: Life-threatening digitoxin toxicity is treated with Digibind®; discontinue digitalis preparation; administer potassium 40-80 mEq in divided doses in D_5W at 20 mEq/hour I.V.; do not administer potassium with complete heart block secondary to digitalis product or in cases of renal failure; digitalis-induced arrhythmias not responsive to potassium may be treated with phenytoin (0.5 mg/kg I.V. at 50 mg/minute), lidocaine (1 mg/kg over 5 minutes); cholestyramine, colestipol, activated charcoal may decrease absorption; other agents to consider, based on EKG and clinical assessment are atropine, quinidine, procainamide, and propranolol. **Note:** Other antiarrhythmics appear more dangerous to use in toxicity.

Drug Interactions

Decreased effect/levels of digoxin: Antacids (magnesium, aluminum)•, penicillamine•, dietary bran fiber•, radiotherapy⁺, antineoplastic drugs⁺, sucralfate⁺, sulfasalazine⁺, thiazide and loop diuretics⁺, aminosalicylic acid⁺, neomycin••, phenytoin••, cholestyramine/colestipol/kaolin-pectin••, aminoglutethimide••

Decreased effect/levels of digitoxin: Antacids (magnesium, aluminum)•, phenylbutazone••, phenobarbital••, phenytoin••, cholestyramine••, aminoglutethimide••, rifampin⁺⁺

Increased effect/toxicity/levels of digoxin: Diltiazem•, spironolactone/triamterene•, ibuprofen•, cimetidine•, omeprazole•, flecainide⁺, acetylsalicylic acid⁺, indomethacin⁺, benzodiazepines⁺, bepridil••, reserpine••, amphotericin B••, erythromycin••, quinine sulfate••, tetracycline••, cyclosporin••, amiodarone⁺⁺, propafenone⁺⁺, quinidine⁺⁺, verapamil⁺⁺, calcium preparations⁺⁺, itraconazole⁺⁺

Increased effect/toxicity/levels of digitoxin: Diltiazem•, spironolactone•, amphotericin B••, quinidine⁺⁺, calcium preparations⁺⁺

Note:

• = improbable clinical importance

⁺ = uncertain clinical significance

•• = interaction proven needing monitoring for possible dosage adjustments

⁺⁺ important interaction needing monitoring, dosage adjustments are likely

Mechanism of Action Digitalis binds to and inhibits magnesium and adenosine triphosphate dependent sodium and potassium ATPase thereby increasing the influx of calcium ions, from extracellular to intracellular cytoplasm due to the inhibition of sodium and potassium ion movement across the myocardial membranes; this increase in calcium ions results in a potentiation of the activity of the contractile heart muscle fibers and an increase in the force of myocardial contraction (positive inotropic effect); digitalis may also increase intracellular entry of calcium via slow calcium channel influx; stimulates release and blocks re-uptake of norepinephrine; decreases conduction through the S-A and A-V nodes

Pharmacodynamics/Kinetics

Absorption: 90% to 100%

Distribution: V_d: 7 L/kg

Protein binding: 90% to 97%

Metabolism: Hepatic, 50% to 70%

Time to peak: 8-12 hours

Half-life: 7-8 days

Elimination: 30% to 50% excreted unchanged in urine/feces

Usual Dosage Oral:

Children: Doses are very individualized; **when recommended**, digitalizing dose is as follows:

- <1 year: 0.045 mg/kg
- 1-2 years: 0.04 mg/kg
- >2 years: 0.03 mg/kg which is equivalent to 0.75 mg/m^2
- Maintenance: Approximately $^1/_{10}$ of the digitalizing dose

Adults: Oral:

- Rapid loading dose: Initial: 0.6 mg followed by 0.4 mg and then 0.2 mg at intervals of 4-6 hours
- Slow loading dose: 0.2 mg twice daily for a period of 4 days followed by a maintenance dose
- Maintenance: 0.05-0.3 mg/day
- Most common dose: 0.15 mg/day

Dosing adjustment in renal impairment:

Cl_{cr} <10 mL/minute: Administer 50% to 75% of normal dose

Hemodialysis: Not dialyzable (0% to 5%)

Dosing adjustment in hepatic impairment:

Dosage reduction is necessary in severe liver disease

Reference Range Therapeutic: 20-35 ng/mL; Toxic: >45 ng/mL

Patient Information Do not discontinue medication without physician's advice; instruct patients to notify physician if they suffer loss of appetite, visual changes, nausea, vomiting, weakness, drowsiness, headache, confusion, or depression

Nursing Implications Observe patients for noncardiac signs of toxicity: anorexia, vision changes (blurred), confusion, and depression

Dosage Forms Tablet: 0.1 mg, 0.2 mg

Digoxin (di JOKS in)

Related Information

Adult ACLS Algorithm, Hypotension, Shock *on page 1516*

Adult ACLS Algorithm, Tachycardia *on page 1512*

Antacid Drug Interactions *on page 1388*

Antiarrhythmic Drugs *on page 1389*

Heart Failure: Management of Patients With Left-Ventricular Systolic Dysfunction *on page 1533*

Brand Names Lanoxicaps®; Lanoxin®

Canadian/Mexican Brand Names Novo-Digoxin® (Canada); Mapluxin® (Mexico)

Therapeutic Category Antiarrhythmic Agent, Miscellaneous; Cardiac Glycoside

Use Treatment of congestive heart failure and to slow the ventricular rate in tachyarrhythmias such as atrial fibrillation, atrial flutter, and supraventricular tachycardia (paroxysmal atrial tachycardia); cardiogenic shock; may not slow

(Continued)

Digoxin *(Continued)*

progression of heart failure or affect survival but proven to relieve signs and symptoms of heart failure.

Pregnancy Risk Factor C

Contraindications Hypersensitivity to digoxin or any component; A-V block, idiopathic hypertrophic subaortic stenosis, or constrictive pericarditis

Warnings/Precautions Use with caution in patients with hypoxia, myxedema, hypothyroidism, acute myocarditis; patients with incomplete A-V block (Stokes-Adams attack) may progress to complete block with digitalis drug administration; use with caution in patients with acute myocardial infarction, severe pulmonary disease, advanced heart failure, idiopathic hypertrophic subaortic stenosis, Wolff-Parkinson-White syndrome, sick-sinus syndrome (bradyarrhythmias), amyloid heart disease, and constrictive cardiomyopathies; adjust dose with renal impairment; elderly and neonates may develop exaggerated serum/tissue concentrations due to age-related alterations in clearance and pharmacodynamic differences; exercise will reduce serum concentrations of digoxin due to increased skeletal muscle uptake; recent studies indicate photopsia, chromatopsia and decreased visual acuity may occur even with therapeutic serum drug levels

Adverse Reactions

1% to 10%: Gastrointestinal: Anorexia, nausea, vomiting

<1%:

- Cardiovascular: Sinus bradycardia, A-V block, S-A block, atrial or nodal ectopic beats, ventricular arrhythmias, bigeminy, trigeminy, atrial tachycardia with A-V block
- Central nervous system: Drowsiness, headache, fatigue, lethargy, vertigo, disorientation
- Endocrine & metabolic: Hyperkalemia with acute toxicity
- Gastrointestinal: Feeding intolerance, abdominal pain, diarrhea
- Neuromuscular & skeletal: Neuralgia
- Ocular: Blurred vision, halos, yellow or green vision, diplopia, photophobia, flashing lights

Overdosage/Toxicology Manifested by a wide variety of signs and symptoms difficult to distinguish from effects associated with cardiac disease; nausea and vomiting are common early signs of toxicity and may precede or follow evidence of cardiotoxicity; anorexia, diarrhea, abdominal discomfort, headache, weakness, drowsiness, visual disturbances, mental depression, confusion, restlessness, disorientation, seizures, hallucinations; cardiac abnormalities include ventricular tachycardia, unifocal or multifocal PVCs (bigeminal, trigeminal); paroxysmal nodal rhythms, A-V dissociation; excessive slowing of the pulse, A-V block of varying degree; P-R prolongation, S-T depression; occasional arterial fibrillation; ventricular fibrillation is common cause of death (alterations in cardiac rate and rhythm can result in any type of known arrhythmia)

Antidote: Life-threatening digoxin toxicity is treated with Digibind®; administer potassium except in cases of complete heart block or renal failure; digitalis-induced arrhythmias not responsive to potassium may be treated with phenytoin lidocaine; cholestyramine, and colestipol may decrease absorption; other agents to consider, based on EKG and clinical assessment are atropine, quinidine, procainamide, and propranolol. **Note:** Other antiarrhythmics appear more dangerous to use in toxicity.

Drug Interactions

Decreased effect/levels of digoxin: Antacids (magnesium, aluminum)•, penicillamine•, dietary bran fiber•, radiotherapy⁺, antineoplastic drugs⁺, sucralfate⁺, sulfasalazine⁺, thiazide and loop diuretics⁺, aminosalicylic acid⁺, neomycin••, phenytoin••, cholestyramine/colestipol/kaolin-pectin••, aminoglutethimide••

Decreased effect/levels of digitoxin: Antacids (magnesium, aluminum)•, phenylbutazone••, phenobarbital••, phenytoin••, cholestyramine••, aminoglutethimide••, rifampin⁺⁺

Increased effect/toxicity/levels of digoxin: Diltiazem•, spironolactone/triamterene•, ibuprofen•, cimetidine•, omeprazole•, flecainide⁺, acetylsalicylic acid⁺, indomethacin ⁺, benzodiazepines⁺, bepridil••, reserpine••, amphotericin B••, erythromycin••, clarithromycin, quinine sulfate••, tetracycline••, nefazodone, cyclosporin••, amiodarone⁺⁺, propafenone⁺⁺, quinidine⁺⁺, verapamil⁺⁺, calcium preparations⁺⁺, itraconazole ⁺⁺

Increased effect/toxicity/levels of digitoxin: diltiazem•, spironolactone•, amphotericin B••, quinidine⁺⁺, calcium preparations⁺⁺

Note:

- • = improbable clinical importance
- ⁺ = uncertain clinical significance
- •• = interaction proven needing monitoring for possible dosage adjustments
- ⁺⁺ important interaction needing monitoring, dosage adjustments are likely

Stability Protect elixir and injection from light; solution **compatibility**: D_5W, $D_{10}W$, NS, sterile water for injection (when diluted fourfold or greater)

Mechanism of Action

Congestive heart failure: Inhibition of the sodium/potassium ATPase pump which acts to increase the intracellular sodium-calcium exchange to increase intracellular calcium leading to increased contractility

Supraventricular arrhythmias: Direct suppression of the A-V node conduction to increase effective refractory period and decrease conduction velocity - positive inotropic effect, enhanced vagal tone, and decreased ventricular rate to fast atrial arrhythmias. Atrial fibrillation may decrease sensitivity and increase tolerance to higher serum digoxin concentrations.

Pharmacodynamics/Kinetics

Onset of action:
- Oral: 1-2 hours
- I.V.: 5-30 minutes

Peak effect:
- Oral: 2-8 hours
- I.V.: 1-4 hours

Duration: Adults: 3-4 days both forms

Absorption: By passive nonsaturable diffusion in the upper small intestine; food may delay, but does not affect extent of digoxin absorption

Distribution:
- Normal renal function: 6-7 L/kg
- V_d: Extensive to peripheral tissues, with a distinct distribution phase which lasts 6-8 hours; concentrates in heart, liver, kidney, skeletal muscle and intestines. Heart/serum concentration is 70:1. Pharmacologic effects are delayed and do not correlate well with serum concentrations during distribution phase.
- Hyperthyroidism: Increased V_d
- Hyperkalemia, hyponatremia: Decreased digoxin distribution to heart and muscle
- Hypokalemia: Increased digoxin distribution to heart and muscles
- Concomitant quinidine therapy: Decreased V_d
- Chronic renal failure: 4-6 L/kg
- Decreased sodium/potassium ATPase activity - decreased tissue binding
- Neonates, full term: 7.5-10 L/kg
- Children: 16 L/kg
- Adults: 7 L/kg, decreased with renal disease

Protein binding: 30% (in uremic patients, digoxin is displaced from plasma protein binding sites)

Metabolism: By sequential sugar hydrolysis in the stomach or by reduction of lactone ring by intestinal bacteria (in ~10% of population, gut bacteria may metabolize up to 40% of digoxin dose); metabolites may contribute to therapeutic and toxic effects of digoxin; metabolism is reduced in patients with CHF

Bioavailability: Oral (dependent upon formulation):
- Elixir: 75% to 85%
- Tablets: 70% to 80%

Half-life: Dependent upon age, renal and cardiac function:
- Neonates:
  - Premature: 61-170 hours
  - Full-term: 35-45 hours
- Infants: 18-25 hours
- Children: 35 hours
- Adults: 38-48 hours
- Adults, anephric: 4-6 days

Half-life:
- Parent drug: 38 hours
- Metabolites:
  - Digoxigenin: 4 hours
  - Monodigitoxoside: 3-12 hours

Time to peak serum concentration: Oral: Within 1 hour

Elimination: 50% to 70% excreted unchanged in urine

Usual Dosage When changing from oral (tablets or liquid) or I.M. to I.V. therapy, dosage should be reduced by 20% to 25%. See table.

Dosing adjustment/interval in renal impairment:
- Cl_{cr} 10-50 mL/minute: Administer 25% to 75% of dose or every 36 hours
- Cl_{cr} <10 mL/minute: Administer 10% to 25% of dose or every 48 hours
- Reduce loading dose by 50% in ESRD

Hemodialysis: Not dialyzable (0% to 5%)

(Continued)

Digoxin *(Continued)*

Age	Total Digitalizing Dose† (mcg/kg)*		Daily Maintenance Dose‡ (mcg/kg*)	
	P.O.	I.V. or I.M.	P.O.	I.V. or I.M.
Preterm infant*	20-30	15-25	5-7.5	4-6
Full-term infant*	25-35	20-30	6-10	5-8
1 mo - 2 y*	35-60	30-50	10-15	7.5-12
2-5 y*	30-40	25-35	7.5-10	6-9
5-10 y*	20-35	15-30	5-10	4-8
>10 y*	10-15	8-12	2.5-5	2-3
Adults	0.75-1.5 mg	0.5-1 mg	0.125-0.5 mg	0.1-0.4 mg

†Give one-half of the total digitalizing dose (TDD) in the initial dose, then give one-quarter of the TDD in each of two subsequent doses at 8- to 12-hour intervals. Obtain EKG 6 hours after each dose to assess potential toxicity.

*Based on lean body weight and normal renal function for age. Decrease dose in patients with ↓ renal function; digitalizing dose often not recommended in infants and children.

‡Divided every 12 hours in infants and children <10 years of age. Given once daily to children >10 years of age and adults.

Monitoring Parameters

When to draw serum digoxin concentrations: Digoxin serum concentrations are monitored because digoxin possesses a narrow therapeutic serum range; the therapeutic endpoint is difficult to quantify and digoxin toxicity may be life threatening. Digoxin serum levels should be drawn **at least 4 hours after an intravenous dose** and **at least 6 hours after an oral dose (optimally 12-24 hours after a dose).**

Initiation of therapy:

If a loading dose is given: Digoxin serum concentration may be drawn within 12-24 hours after the initial loading dose administration. Levels drawn this early may confirm the relationship of digoxin plasma levels and response but are of little value in determining maintenance doses.

If a loading dose is not given: Digoxin serum concentration should be obtained after 3-5 days of therapy

Maintenance therapy:

Trough concentrations should be followed just prior to the next dose or at a minimum of 4 hours after an I.V. dose and at least 6 hours after an oral dose

Digoxin serum concentrations should be obtained within 5-7 days (approximate time to steady-state) after any dosage changes. Continue to obtain digoxin serum concentrations 7-14 days after any change in maintenance dose. **Note:** In patients with end stage renal disease, it may take 15-20 days to reach steady-state.

Additionally, patients who are receiving potassium-depleting medications such as diuretics, should be monitored for potassium, magnesium, and calcium levels

Digoxin serum concentrations should be obtained whenever any of the following conditions occur:

Questionable patient compliance or to evaluate clinical deterioration following an initial good response

Changing renal function

Suspected digoxin toxicity

Initiation or discontinuation of therapy with drugs (amiodarone, quinidine, verapamil) which potentially interact with digoxin; if quinidine therapy is started; digoxin levels should be drawn within the first 24 hours after starting quinidine therapy, then 7-14 days later or empirically skip one day's digoxin dose and decrease the daily dose by 50%

Any disease changes (hypothyroidism)

Heart rate and rhythm should be monitored along with periodic EKGs to assess both desired effects and signs of toxicity

Follow closely (especially in patients receiving diuretics or amphotericin) for decreased serum potassium and magnesium or increased calcium, all of which predispose to digoxin toxicity

Assess renal function

Be aware of drug interactions

Reference Range

Digoxin therapeutic serum concentrations:

Congestive heart failure: 0.8-2 ng/mL

Arrhythmias: 1.5-2.5 ng/mL

Adults: <0.5 ng/mL; probably indicates underdigitalization unless there are special circumstances

Toxic: >2.5 ng/mL; tachyarrhythmias commonly require levels >2 ng/mL

Digoxin-like immunoreactive substance (DLIS) may crossreact with digoxin immunoassay. DLIS has been found in patients with renal and liver disease, congestive heart failure, neonates, and pregnant women (third trimester).

Patient Information Do not discontinue medication without checking with physician; notify physician if loss of appetite or visual changes occur

Nursing Implications Observe patients for noncardiac signs of toxicity, ie, anorexia, vision changes (blurred), confusion, and depression

Dosage Forms

Capsule: 50 mcg, 100 mcg, 200 mcg

Elixir, pediatric (lime flavor): 50 mcg/mL with alcohol 10% (60 mL)

Injection: 250 mcg/mL (1 mL, 2 mL)

Injection, pediatric: 100 mcg/mL (1 mL)

Tablet: 125 mcg, 250 mcg, 500 mcg

Digoxin Immune Fab (di JOKS in i MYUN fab)

Brand Names Digibind®

Synonyms Antidigoxin Fab Fragments

Therapeutic Category Antidote, Digoxin

Use Digoxin immune Fab are specific antibodies for the treatment of digitalis intoxication in carefully selected patients; use in life-threatening ventricular arrhythmias secondary to digoxin, acute digoxin ingestion (ie, >10 mg in adults or >4 mg in children), hyperkalemia (serum potassium >5 mEq/L) in the setting of digoxin toxicity

Pregnancy Risk Factor C

Contraindications Hypersensitivity to sheep products

Warnings/Precautions Use with caution in renal or cardiac failure; allergic reactions possible (sheep product)-skin testing not routinely recommended; epinephrine should be immediately available, Fab fragments may be eliminated more slowly in patients with renal failure, heart failure may be exacerbated as digoxin level is reduced; total serum digoxin concentration may rise precipitously following administration of Digibind®, but this will be almost entirely bound to the Fab fragment and not able to react with receptors in the body; Digibind® will interfere with digitalis immunoassay measurements - this will result in clinically misleading serum digoxin concentrations until the Fab fragment is eliminated from the body (several days to >1 week after Digibind® administration). Hypokalemia has been reported to occur following reversal of digitalis intoxication as has exacerbation of underlying heart failure; Serum digoxin levels drawn prior to therapy may be difficult to evaluate if 6-8 hours have not elapsed after the last dose of digoxin (time to equilibration between serum and tissue); redigitalization should not be initiated until Fab fragments have been eliminated from the body, which may occur over several days or greater than a week in patients with impaired renal function.

Adverse Reactions

<1%:

Cardiovascular: Worsening of low cardiac output or congestive heart failure, rapid ventricular response in patients with atrial fibrillation as digoxin is withdrawn, facial edema and redness

Endocrine & metabolic: Hypokalemia

Dermatologic: Urticarial rash

Miscellaneous: Allergic reactions

Overdosage/Toxicology Symptoms of overdose include delayed serum sickness

Treatment of serum sickness includes acetaminophen, $histamine_1$ and possibly $histamine_2$ blockers and corticosteroids

Stability Should be refrigerated (2°C to 8°C); reconstituted solutions should be used within 4 hours if refrigerated

Mechanism of Action Binds with molecules of digoxin or digitoxin and then is excreted by the kidneys and removed from the body

Pharmacodynamics/Kinetics

Onset of action: I.V.: Improvement in signs and symptoms occur within 2-30 minutes

Half-life: 15-20 hours; prolonged in patients with renal impairment

Elimination: Renally with levels declining to undetectable amounts within 5-7 days

Usual Dosage Each vial of Digibind® will bind approximately 0.6 mg of digoxin or digitoxin

I.V.: To determine the dose of digoxin immune Fab, first determine the total body load of digoxin (TBL using either an approximation of the amount ingested or a postdistribution serum digoxin concentration). If neither ingestion amount or serum level is known: Adult dosage is 20 vials (800 mg) I.V. infusion.

Administration Continuous I.V. infusion over 15-30 minutes is preferred; digoxin immune Fab is reconstituted by adding 4 mL sterile water, resulting in 10 mg/mL for I.V. infusion, the reconstituted solution may be further diluted with NS to a convenient volume (eg, 1 mg/mL)

(Continued)

Digoxin Immune Fab *(Continued)*

Monitoring Parameters Serum potassium, serum digoxin concentration prior to first dose of digoxin immune Fab; **digoxin levels will greatly increase with Digibind® use and are not an accurate determination of body stores**

Dosage Forms Powder for injection, lyophilized: 40 mg

Dihydrex® Injection *see* Diphenhydramine *on page 399*

Dihydrocodeine Compound (dye hye droe KOE deen KOM pound)

Brand Names DHC Plus®; Synalgos®-DC

Therapeutic Category Analgesic, Narcotic

Use Management of mild to moderate pain that requires relaxation

Restrictions C-III

Pregnancy Risk Factor B (D if used for prolonged periods or in high doses at term)

Contraindications Hypersensitivity to dihydrocodeine or any component

Warnings/Precautions Use with caution in patients with hypersensitivity reactions to other phenanthrene derivative opioid agonists (morphine, hydrocodone, hydromorphone, levorphanol, oxycodone, oxymorphone); respiratory diseases including asthma, emphysema, COPD, or severe liver or renal insufficiency; some preparations contain sulfites which may cause allergic reactions; may be habit-forming; dextromethorphan has equivalent antitussive activity but has much lower toxicity in accidental overdose

Adverse Reactions

>10%:

- Central nervous system: Lightheadedness, dizziness, drowsiness, sedation
- Dermatologic: Pruritus, skin reactions
- Gastrointestinal: Nausea, vomiting, constipation

1% to 10%:

- Cardiovascular: Hypotension, palpitations, bradycardia, peripheral vasodilation
- Central nervous system: Increased intracranial pressure
- Endocrine & metabolic: Antidiuretic hormone release
- Gastrointestinal: Biliary tract spasm
- Genitourinary: Urinary tract spasm
- Ocular: Miosis
- Respiratory: Respiratory depression
- Miscellaneous: Histamine release, physical and psychological dependence with prolonged use

Overdosage/Toxicology Naloxone 2 mg I.V. (0.01 mg/kg for children) with repeat administration as necessary up to a total of 10 mg; see Aspirin toxicology

Drug Interactions Increased toxicity: MAO inhibitors may increase adverse symptoms

Mechanism of Action Binds to opiate receptors in the CNS, causing inhibition of ascending pain pathways, altering the perception of and response to pain; causes cough suppression by direct central action in the medulla; produces generalized CNS depression

Usual Dosage Adults: Oral: 1-2 capsules every 4-6 hours as needed for pain

Dietary Considerations Alcohol: Additive CNS effects, avoid use

Patient Information Avoid alcohol, may cause drowsiness, impaired judgment or coordination; may cause physical and psychological dependence with prolonged use

Nursing Implications Observe patient for excessive sedation, respiratory depression; implement safety measures, assist with ambulation

Dosage Forms Capsule:

- DHC Plus®: Dihydrocodeine bitartrate 16 mg, acetaminophen 356.4 mg, and caffeine 30 mg
- Synalgos®-DC: Dihydrocodeine bitartrate 16 mg, aspirin 356.4 mg, and caffeine 30 mg

Dihydroergotamine (dye hye droe er GOT a meen)

Brand Names D.H.E. 45®

Synonyms Dihydroergotamine Mesylate

Therapeutic Category Ergot Alkaloid and Derivative

Use Aborts or prevents vascular headaches; also as an adjunct for DVT prophylaxis for hip surgery, for orthostatic hypotension, xerostomia secondary to antidepressant use, and pelvic congestion with pain

Pregnancy Risk Factor X

Contraindications High-dose aspirin therapy, hypersensitivity to dihydroergotamine or any component

Warnings/Precautions Use with caution in hypertension, angina, peripheral vascular disease, impaired renal or hepatic function; avoid pregnancy

Adverse Reactions

>10%:

Cardiovascular: Localized edema, peripheral vascular effects (numbness and tingling of fingers and toes)

Central nervous system: Drowsiness, dizziness

Gastrointestinal: Xerostomia, diarrhea, nausea, vomiting

1% to 10%:

Cardiovascular: Precordial distress and pain, transient tachycardia or bradycardia

Neuromuscular & skeletal: Muscle pain in the extremities, weakness in the legs

Overdosage/Toxicology Symptoms of overdose include peripheral ischemia, paresthesia, headache, nausea, vomiting

Activated charcoal is effective at binding certain chemicals; this is especially true for ergot alkaloids

Drug Interactions

Increased effect of heparin

Increased toxicity with erythromycin, clarithromycin, nitroglycerin, propranolol, troleandomycin

Stability Store in refrigerator

Mechanism of Action Ergot alkaloid alpha-adrenergic blocker directly stimulates vascular smooth muscle to vasoconstrict peripheral and cerebral vessels; also has effects on serotonin receptors

Pharmacodynamics/Kinetics

Onset of action: Within 15-30 minutes

Duration: 3-4 hours

Distribution: V_d: 14.5 L/kg

Protein binding: 90%

Metabolism: Extensively in the liver

Half-life: 1.3-3.9 hours

Time to peak serum concentration: I.M.: Within 15-30 minutes

Elimination: Predominately into bile and feces and 10% excreted in urine, mostly as metabolites

Usual Dosage Adults:

I.M.: 1 mg at first sign of headache; repeat hourly to a maximum dose of 3 mg total

I.V.: Up to 2 mg maximum dose for faster effects; maximum dose: 6 mg/week

Dosing adjustment in hepatic impairment: Dosage reductions are probably necessary but specific guidelines are not available

Reference Range Minimum concentration for vasoconstriction is reportedly 0.06 ng/mL

Patient Information Rare feelings of numbness or tingling of fingers, toes, or face may occur; avoid using this medication if you are pregnant, have heart disease, hypertension, liver disease, infection, itching

Dosage Forms Injection, as mesylate: 1 mg/mL (1 mL)

Dihydroergotamine Mesylate *see* Dihydroergotamine *on previous page*

Dihydroergotoxine *see* Ergoloid Mesylates *on page 457*

Dihydrogenated Ergot Alkaloids *see* Ergoloid Mesylates *on page 457*

Dihydrohydroxycodeinone *see* Oxycodone *on page 936*

Dihydromorphinone *see* Hydromorphone *on page 627*

Dihydrotachysterol (dye hye droe tak IS ter ole)

Brand Names DHT™; Hytakerol®

Synonyms Dichysterol

Therapeutic Category Vitamin, Fat Soluble

Use Treatment of hypocalcemia associated with hypoparathyroidism; prophylaxis of hypocalcemic tetany following thyroid surgery

Pregnancy Risk Factor A (D if used in doses above the recommended daily allowance)

Contraindications Hypercalcemia, known hypersensitivity to dihydrotachysterol

Warnings/Precautions Calcium-phosphate product (serum calcium and phosphorus) must not exceed 70; avoid hypercalcemia; use with caution in coronary artery disease, decreased renal function (especially with secondary hyperparathyroidism), renal stones, and elderly

Adverse Reactions

>10%:

Endocrine & metabolic: Hypercalcemia

Renal: Elevated serum creatinine, hypercalciuria

<1%:

Central nervous system: Convulsions

Endocrine & metabolic: Polydipsia

Gastrointestinal: Nausea, vomiting, anorexia, weight loss

(Continued)

Dihydrotachysterol *(Continued)*

Genitourinary: Polyuria
Hematologic: Anemia
Neuromuscular & skeletal: Weakness, metastatic calcification
Renal: Renal damage

Overdosage/Toxicology Symptoms of overdose include hypercalcemia, anorexia, nausea, weakness, constipation, diarrhea, vague aches, mental confusion, tinnitus, ataxia, depression, hallucinations, syncope, coma; polyuria, polydypsia, nocturia, hypercalciuria, irreversible renal insufficiency or proteinuria, azotemia; will spread tissue calcifications, hypertension

Following withdrawal of the drug, treatment consists of bed rest, liberal intake of fluids, reduced calcium intake, and cathartic administration. Severe hypercalcemia requires I.V. hydration and forced diuresis. Urine output should be monitored and maintained at >3 mL/kg/hour. I.V. saline can quickly and significantly increase excretion of calcium into the urine. Calcitonin, cholestyramine, prednisone, sodium EDTA and mithramycin have all been used successfully to treat the more resistant cases of vitamin D-induced hypercalcemia.

Drug Interactions

Decreased effect/levels of vitamin D: Cholestyramine, colestipol, mineral oil; phenytoin and phenobarbital may inhibit activation may decrease effectiveness
Increased toxicity: Thiazide diuretics increase calcium

Stability Protect from light

Mechanism of Action Synthetic analogue of vitamin D with a faster onset of action; stimulates calcium and phosphate absorption from the small intestine, promotes secretion of calcium from bone to blood; promotes renal tubule resorption of phosphate

Pharmacodynamics/Kinetics

Peak hypercalcemic effect: Within 2-4 weeks
Duration: Can be as long as 9 weeks
Absorption: Well absorbed from the GI tract
Elimination: In bile and feces; stored in liver, fat, skin, muscle, and bone

Usual Dosage Oral:

Hypoparathyroidism:
Infants and young Children: Initial: 1-5 mg/day for 4 days, then 0.1-0.5 mg/day
Older Children and Adults: Initial: 0.8-2.4 mg/day for several days followed by maintenance doses of 0.2-1 mg/day
Nutritional rickets: 0.5 mg as a single dose or 13-50 mcg/day until healing occurs
Renal osteodystrophy: Maintenance: 0.25-0.6 mg/24 hours adjusted as necessary to achieve normal serum calcium levels and promote bone healing

Monitoring Parameters Monitor renal function, serum calcium, and phosphate concentrations; if hypercalcemia is encountered, discontinue agent until serum calcium returns to normal

Reference Range Calcium (serum): 9-10 mg/dL (4.5-5 mEq/L)

Patient Information Do not take more than the recommended amount. While taking this medication, your physician may want you to follow a special diet or take a calcium supplement; follow this diet closely. Avoid taking magnesium supplements or magnesium-containing antacids. Early symptoms of hypercalcemia include weakness, fatigue, headache, metallic taste, stomach upset, muscle or bone pain, and irritability.

Nursing Implications Monitor symptoms of hypercalcemia (weakness, fatigue, somnolence, headache, anorexia, dry mouth, metallic taste, nausea, vomiting, cramps, diarrhea, muscle pain, bone pain, and irritability)

Dosage Forms

Capsule (Hytakerol®): 0.125 mg
Solution:
Oral Concentrate (DHT™): 0.2 mg/mL (30 mL)
Oral, in oil (Hytakerol®): 0.25 mg/mL (15 mL)
Tablet (DHT™): 0.125 mg, 0.2 mg, 0.4 mg

1,25 Dihydroxycholecalciferol *see* Calcitriol *on page 183*

Diiodohydroxyquin *see* Iodoquinol *on page 670*

Diisopropyl Fluorophosphate *see* Isoflurophate *on page 679*

Dilacor™ XR *see* Diltiazem *on next page*

Dilantin® *see* Phenytoin *on page 992*

Dilatrate®-SR *see* Isosorbide Dinitrate *on page 684*

Dilaudid® *see* Hydromorphone *on page 627*

Dilaudid-5® *see* Hydromorphone *on page 627*

Dilaudid-HP® *see* Hydromorphone *on page 627*

Dilocaine® *see* Lidocaine *on page 723*

Dilomine® Injection *see* Dicyclomine *on page 376*

Diltiazem (dil TYE a zem)

Related Information

Adult ACLS Algorithm, Tachycardia *on page 1512*
Antiarrhythmic Drugs *on page 1389*
Calcium Channel Blockers Comparative Actions *on page 1401*
Calcium Channel Blockers Comparative Pharmacokinetics *on page 1402*
Calcium Channel Blockers FDA-Approved Indications *on page 1403*
Comparative Pharmacokinetic Properties of Antiarrhythmic Agents *on page 1391*
Therapy of Hypertension *on page 1540*

Brand Names Cardizem® CD; Cardizem® Injectable; Cardizem® Lyo-Ject™; Cardizem® SR; Cardizem® Tablet; Dilacor™ XR; Tiazac®

Canadian/Mexican Brand Names Apo-Diltiaz® (Canada); Novo-Diltazem® (Canada); Nu-Diltiaz® (Canada); Syn-Diltiazem® (Canada); Angiotrofen® (Mexico); Angiotrofen A.P.® (Mexico); Angiotrofen® Retard (Mexico); Presoken® (Mexico); Presoquim® (Mexico); Tilazem® (Mexico)

Therapeutic Category Antianginal Agent; Antihypertensive; Calcium Channel Blocker

Use

Capsule: Essential hypertension (alone or in combination) - sustained release only; chronic stable angina or angina from coronary artery spasm

Injection: Atrial fibrillation or atrial flutter; paroxysmal supraventricular tachycardia (PSVT)

Pregnancy Risk Factor C

Pregnancy/Breast-Feeding Implications

Teratogenic and embryotoxic effects have been demonstrated in small animals

Clinical effects on the fetus: No data on crossing the placenta. 2 reports of cardiac defects.

Breast milk/Lactation: Freely diffuses into breast milk; however, the American Academy of Pediatrics considers diltiazem to be COMPATIBLE with breast-feeding. Available evidence suggest safe use during breast-feeding.

Contraindications Severe hypotension or second and third degree heart block; hypersensitivity to other calcium channel blockers, adenosine; atrial and ventricular arrhythmias, acute myocardial infarction, and pulmonary congestion

Warnings/Precautions Use with caution and titrate dosages for patients with impaired renal or hepatic function; use caution when treating patients with congestive heart failure, sick-sinus syndrome, severe left ventricular dysfunction, hypertrophic cardiomyopathy (especially obstructive), concomitant therapy with beta-blockers or digoxin, edema, or increased intracranial pressure with cranial tumors; do not abruptly withdraw (may cause chest pain); elderly may experience hypotension and constipation more readily.

Adverse Reactions

>10%: Central nervous system: Headache

1% to 10%:

- Cardiovascular: Bradycardia, A-V block (first degree), edema, EKG abnormality
- Central nervous system: Dizziness
- Gastrointestinal: Nausea, vomiting
- Neuromuscular & skeletal: Weakness

<1%:

- Cardiovascular: A-V block (second degree), angina
- Central nervous system: Abnormal dreams, amnesia, depression, gait abnormality, insomnia, nervousness
- Dermatologic: Urticaria, photosensitivity, alopecia, purpura
- Gastrointestinal: Anorexia, constipation, diarrhea, abnormal taste, dyspepsia
- Hematologic: Hemolytic anemia, leukopenia, thrombocytopenia
- Neuromuscular & skeletal: Paresthesia, tremor
- Ocular: Amblyopia, retinopathy
- Respiratory: Pharyngitis, cough increase
- Miscellaneous: Flu syndrome

Overdosage/Toxicology The primary cardiac symptoms of calcium blocker overdose includes hypotension and bradycardia. The hypotension is caused by peripheral vasodilation, myocardial depression, and bradycardia. Bradycardia results from sinus bradycardia, second- or third-degree atrioventricular block, or sinus arrest with junctional rhythm. Intraventricular conduction is usually not affected so QRS duration is normal (verapamil does prolong the P-R interval and bepridil prolongs the Q-T and may cause ventricular arrhythmias, including torsade de pointes).

The noncardiac symptoms include confusion, stupor, nausea, vomiting, metabolic acidosis and hyperglycemia. Following initial gastric decontamination, if possible, repeated calcium administration may promptly reverse the depressed cardiac contractility (but not sinus node depression or peripheral vasodilation);

(Continued)

Diltiazem *(Continued)*

glucagon, epinephrine, and amrinone may treat refractory hypotension; glucagon and epinephrine also increase the heart rate (outside the U.S., 4-aminopyridine may be available as an antidote); dialysis and hemoperfusion are not effective in enhancing elimination although repeat-dose activated charcoal may serve as an adjunct with sustained-release preparations.

Drug Interactions

Inhibitor of cytochrome P-450 3A enzymes
Cytochrome P-450 3A enzyme substrate

Decreased effect:

- Diltiazem and carbamazepine may cause decreased diltiazem effectiveness due to enhanced metabolism

Increased toxicity:

- Diltiazem and rifampin may cause increased diltiazem effectiveness due to enhanced metabolism
- Diltiazem and amiodarone may cause increased bradycardia and decreased cardiac output
- Verapamil and aspirin may cause bruising
- Diltiazem and H_2 blockers may cause increased bioavailability of diltiazem secondary to increased gastric pH
- Diltiazem and encainide may increase may increase encainide effects effects on A-V conduction, severe hypotension
- Diltiazem and cyclosporine may cause increased cyclosporine levels and subsequent renal toxicity
- Diltiazem and digoxin may cause increased digoxin levels
- Diltiazem and imipramine may cause increased imipramine levels
- Diltiazem and nitroprusside may cause increased nitroprusside levels
- Diltiazem and propranolol or metoprolol may cause increased cardiac depressant
- Diltiazem and vecuronium may cause increased vecuronium levels

Mechanism of Action Inhibits calcium ion from entering the "slow channels" or select voltage-sensitive areas of vascular smooth muscle and myocardium during depolarization, producing a relaxation of coronary vascular smooth muscle and coronary vasodilation; increases myocardial oxygen delivery in patients with vasospastic angina

Pharmacodynamics/Kinetics

Onset of action: Oral: 30-60 minutes (including sustained release)
Absorption: 80% to 90%
Time to peak serum concentration:
- Short-acting tablets: Within 2-3 hours
- Sustained release: 6-11 hours

Distribution: V_d: 1.7 L/kg; appears in breast milk
Protein binding: 77% to 85%
Metabolism: Extensive first-pass metabolism; metabolized in the liver; following single I.V. injection, plasma concentrations of N-monodesmethyldiltiazem and desacetyldiltiazem are typically undetectable; however, these metabolites accumulate to detectable concentrations following 24-hour constant rate infusion. N-monodesmethyldiltiazem appears to have 20% of the potency of diltiazem; desacetyldiltiazem is about 50% as potent as the parent compound.
Bioavailability: ~40% to 60% due to significant first-pass effect
Half-life: 4-6 hours, may increase with renal impairment; 5-7 hours with sustained release
Elimination: In urine and bile mostly as metabolites

Usual Dosage Adults:

Oral: 30-120 mg 3-4 times/day; dosage should be increased gradually, at 1- to 2-day intervals until optimum response is obtained; usual maintenance dose: 240-360 mg/day

Sustained-release capsules:

- **Cardizem SR®**: Initial: 60-12 mg twice daily; adjust to maximum antihypertensive effect (usually within 14 days); usual range: 240-360 mg/day
- **Cardizem® CD, Tiazac®:** Hypertension: Total daily dose of short-acting administered once daily or initially 180 or 240 mg once daily; adjust to maximum effect (usually within 14 days); maximum: 360 mg/day; usual range: 240-360 mg/day
- **Cardizem® CD:** Angina: Initial: 120-180 mg once daily; maximum: 480 mg once/day
- **Dilacor XR®:**
  - Hypertension: 180-240 mg once daily; maximum: 540 mg/day; usual range: 180-480 mg/day; use lower dose in elderly
  - Angina: Initial: 120 mg/day; titrate slowly over 7-14 days up to 480 mg/day, as needed

Note: Hypertensive or anginal patients treated with other formulations of diltiazem sustained release can be safely switched to Dilacor XR® at the nearest equivalent total daily dose; subsequent titration may be needed

I.V. (requires an infusion pump): See table.

Diltiazem — I.V. Dosage and Administration

Initial Bolus Dose	0.25 mg/kg actual body weight over 2 min (average adult dose: 20 mg)
Repeat Bolus Dose may be administered after 15 min if the response is inadequate	0.35 mg/kg actual body weight over 2 min (average adult dose: 25 mg)
Continuous Infusion Infusions >24 h or infusion rates >15 mg/h are not recommended due to potential accumulation of metabolites and increased toxicity	Initial infusion rate of 10 mg/h; rate may be increased in 5 mg/h increments up to 15 mg/h as needed; some patients may respond to an initial rate of 5 mg/h

If Cardizem® injectable is administered by continuous infusion for >24 hours, the possibility of decreased diltiazem clearance, prolonged elimination half-life, and increased diltiazem and/or diltiazem metabolite plasma concentrations should be considered

Conversion from I.V. diltiazem to oral diltiazem: Start oral approximately 3 hours after bolus dose

Oral dose (mg/day) is approximately equal to [rate (mg/hour) x 3 + 3] x 10

3 mg/hour = 120 mg/day
5 mg/hour = 180 mg/day
7 mg/hour = 240 mg/day
11 mg/hour = 360 mg/day (maximum recommended dose)

Dosing comments in renal/hepatic impairment: Use with caution as extensively metabolized by the liver and excreted in the kidneys and bile

Dialysis: Not removed by hemo- or peritoneal dialysis; supplemental dose is not necessary

Dietary Considerations Alcohol: Avoid use

Patient Information Sustained release products should be taken in the morning on an empty stomach, if possible and not crushed or chewed; limit caffeine intake; avoid alcohol; notify physician if angina pain is not reduced when taking this drug, irregular heartbeat, shortness of breath, swelling, dizziness, constipation, nausea, or hypotension occurs; do not stop therapy without advice of physician

Nursing Implications Do not crush sustained release capsules

Additional Information Although there is some initial data which may show increased risk of myocardial infarction with the treatment of hypertension with calcium antagonists, controlled trial (eg, ALL-HAT) are ongoing to examine the long-term effects of not only these agents but other antihypertensives in preventing heart disease. Until these studies are completed, patients taking calcium antagonists should be encouraged to continue with the prescribed antihypertensive regimens although a switch from high-dose short-acting products to sustained release agents may be warranted. It is also generally agreed that calcium antagonist should be avoided as primary treatment for hypertension unless diuretics or beta-blockers are contraindicated and as primary therapy of angina after acute myocardial infarction

An investigation (n=121) found diltiazem superior to nitroglycerin infusion in decreasing cardiac ischemia events at 48 hours

Dosage Forms

Capsule, sustained release:
- Cardizem® CD: 120 mg, 180 mg, 240 mg, 300 mg
- Cardizem® SR: 60 mg, 90 mg, 120 mg
- Dilacor™ XR: 180 mg, 240 mg
- Tiazac®: 120 mg, 180 mg, 240 mg, 300 mg, 360 mg

Injection: 5 mg/mL (5 mL, 10 mL)
- Cardizem®: 5 mg/mL (5 mL, 10 mL)

Tablet (Cardizem®): 30 mg, 60 mg, 90 mg, 120 mg

Tablet, extended release (Tiamate®): 120 mg, 180 mg, 240 mg

Dimenhydrinate (dye men HYE dri nate)

Brand Names Calm-X® Oral [OTC]; Dimetabs® Oral; Dinate® Injection; Dramamine® Oral [OTC]; Dramilin® Injection; Dramoject® Injection; Dymenate® Injection; Hydrate® Injection; Marmine® Injection; Marmine® Oral [OTC]; Tega-Vert® Oral; TripTone® Caplets® [OTC]

Canadian/Mexican Brand Names Apo-Dimenhydrinate® (Canada); Gravol® (Canada); PMS-Dimenhydrinate (Canada); Travel Aid® (Canada); Travel Tabs (Canada); Vomisen® (Mexico)

(Continued)

Dimenhydrinate *(Continued)*

Therapeutic Category Antiemetic; Antihistamine, H_1 Blocker

Use Treatment and prevention of nausea, vertigo, and vomiting associated with motion sickness

Pregnancy Risk Factor B

Contraindications Hypersensitivity to dimenhydrinate or any component

Warnings/Precautions Use with caution with prostatic hypertrophy, peptic ulcer, narrow-angle glaucoma, bronchial asthma, and cardiac arrhythmias

Adverse Reactions

>10%:
- Central nervous system: Slight to moderate drowsiness
- Respiratory: Thickening of bronchial secretions

1% to 10%:
- Central nervous system: Headache, fatigue, nervousness, dizziness
- Gastrointestinal: Appetite increase, weight gain, nausea, diarrhea, abdominal pain, xerostomia
- Neuromuscular & skeletal: Arthralgia
- Respiratory: Pharyngitis

<1%:
- Cardiovascular: Edema, palpitations, hypotension
- Central nervous system: Depression, drowsiness, paradoxical CNS stimulation
- Dermatologic: Angioedema, photosensitivity, rash
- Gastrointestinal: Anorexia
- Genitourinary: Polyuria
- Hepatic: Hepatitis
- Local: Pain at the injection site
- Neuromuscular & skeletal: Myalgia, paresthesia
- Ocular: Blurred vision
- Otic: Tinnitus
- Respiratory: Bronchospasm, epistaxis

Overdosage/Toxicology Toxicity may resemble atropine overdosage; CNS depression or stimulation; there is no specific treatment for an antihistamine overdose, however, most of its clinical toxicity is due to anticholinergic effects. For anticholinergic overdose with severe life-threatening symptoms, physostigmine 1-2 mg (0.5 or 0.02 mg/kg for children) I.V., slowly may be given to reverse these effects.

Drug Interactions

Increased effect/toxicity with CNS depressants, anticholinergics, TCAs, MAO inhibitors

Increased toxicity of antibiotics, especially aminoglycosides (ototoxicity)

Stability When mixed in the same syringe, drugs reported to be **incompatible** include aminophylline, barbiturates, butorphanol, chlorpromazine, glycopyrrolate, heparin, hydrocortisone, hydroxyzine, midazolam, phenytoin, prednisolone, prochlorperazine, promethazine, tetracycline, trifluoperazine

Mechanism of Action Competes with histamine for H_1-receptor sites on effector cells in the gastrointestinal tract, blood vessels, and respiratory tract; blocks chemoreceptor trigger zone, diminishes vestibular stimulation, and depresses labyrinthine function through its central anticholinergic activity

Pharmacodynamics/Kinetics

Onset of action: Oral: Within 15-30 minutes

Absorption: Well absorbed from GI tract

Distribution: Small amounts appear in breast milk

Metabolism: Extensively in the liver

Usual Dosage

Children:
- Oral:
  - 2-5 years: 12.5-25 mg every 6-8 hours, maximum: 75 mg/day
  - 6-12 years: 25-50 mg every 6-8 hours, maximum: 150 mg/day
- I.M.: 1.25 mg/kg or 37.5 mg/m^2 4 times/day, not to exceed 300 mg/day

Adults: Oral, I.M., I.V.: 50-100 mg every 4-6 hours, not to exceed 400 mg/day

Dietary Considerations Alcohol: Additive CNS effects, avoid use

Administration I.V. injection must be diluted to 10 mL with NS and given at 25 mg/minute

Patient Information May cause drowsiness, may impair judgment and coordination; avoid alcohol; drink plenty of fluids for dry mouth and to prevent constipation

Nursing Implications Raise bed rails, institute safety measures, assist with ambulation

Dosage Forms

Capsule: 50 mg

Injection: 50 mg/mL (1 mL, 5 mL, 10 mL)

Liquid: 12.5 mg/4 mL (90 mL, 473 mL); 16.62 mg/5 mL (480 mL)

Tablet: 50 mg
Tablet, chewable: 50 mg

Dimercaprol (dye mer KAP role)

Brand Names BAL in Oil®

Synonyms BAL; British Anti-Lewisite; Dithioglycerol

Therapeutic Category Antidote, Arsenic Toxicity; Antidote, Gold Toxicity; Antidote, Lead Toxicity; Antidote, Mercury Toxicity

Use Antidote to gold, arsenic, and mercury poisoning; adjunct to edetate calcium disodium in lead poisoning

Pregnancy Risk Factor C

Contraindications Hepatic insufficiency (unless due to arsenic poisoning); do not use on iron, cadmium, or selenium poisoning

Warnings/Precautions Potentially a nephrotoxic drug, use with caution in patients with oliguria or glucose 6-phosphate dehydrogenase deficiency; keep urine alkaline to protect kidneys; administer all injections deep I.M. at different sites

Adverse Reactions

>10%:
- Cardiovascular: Hypertension, tachycardia
- Central nervous system: Convulsions

1% to 10%: Gastrointestinal: Nausea, vomiting

<1%:
- Central nervous system: Nervousness, fever, headache
- Gastrointestinal: Salivation
- Hematologic: Transient neutropenia
- Local: Pain at the injection site
- Ocular: Blepharospasm, burning eyes
- Renal: Nephrotoxicity
- Miscellaneous: Burning sensation of the lips, mouth, throat, and penis

Drug Interactions Toxic complexes with iron, cadmium, selenium, or uranium

Mechanism of Action Sulfhydryl group combines with ions of various heavy metals to form relatively stable, nontoxic, soluble chelates which are excreted in urine

Pharmacodynamics/Kinetics

Distribution: Distributes to all tissues including the brain
Metabolism: Rapidly to inactive products
Time to peak serum concentration: 0.5-1 hour
Elimination: In urine

Usual Dosage Children and Adults: Deep I.M.:

Mild arsenic and gold poisoning: 2.5 mg/kg/dose every 6 hours for 2 days, then every 12 hours on the third day, and once daily thereafter for 10 days

Severe arsenic and gold poisoning: 3 mg/kg/dose every 4 hours for 2 days then every 6 hours on the third day, then every 12 hours thereafter for 10 days

Mercury poisoning: Initial: 5 mg/kg followed by 2.5 mg/kg/dose 1-2 times/day for 10 days

Lead poisoning (use with edetate calcium disodium):
- Mild: 3 mg/kg/dose every 4 hours for 5-7 days
- Severe and acute encephalopathy: 4 mg/kg/dose initially alone then every 4 hours in combination of edetate calcium disodium

Dosing adjustment in hepatic impairment: Necessary in acute hepatic insufficiency

Administration Administer deep I.M. only

Test Interactions Iodine ^{131}I thyroidal uptake values may be decreased

Patient Information Frequent blood and urine tests may be required

Nursing Implications Urine should be kept alkaline because chelate dissociates in acid media

Dosage Forms Injection: 100 mg/mL (3 mL)

Dimetabs® Oral *see* Dimenhydrinate *on page 395*

Dimetane® [OTC] *see* Brompheniramine *on page 166*

Dimethoxyphenyl Penicillin Sodium *see* Methicillin *on page 803*

β,β-Dimethylcysteine *see* Penicillamine *on page 959*

Dimethyl Triazeno Imidazol Carboxamide *see* Dacarbazine *on page 335*

Dinate® Injection *see* Dimenhydrinate *on page 395*

Dinoprostone (dye noe PROST one)

Brand Names Cervidil® Vaginal Insert; Prepidil® Vaginal Gel; Prostin E_2® Vaginal Suppository

Synonyms PGE_2; Prostaglandin E_2

Therapeutic Category Abortifacient; Prostaglandin

(Continued)

Dinoprostone *(Continued)*

Use

Gel: Promote cervical ripening prior to labor induction; usage for gel include any patient undergoing induction of labor with an unripe cervix, most commonly for pre-eclampsia, eclampsia, postdates, diabetes, intrauterine growth retardation, and chronic hypertension

Suppositories: Terminate pregnancy from 12th through 28th week of gestation; evacuate uterus in cases of missed abortion or intrauterine fetal death; manage benign hydatidiform mole

Pregnancy Risk Factor X

Contraindications

Gel: Hypersensitivity to prostaglandins or any constituents of the cervical gel, history of asthma, contracted pelvis, malpresentation of the fetus

Gel: The following are "relative" contraindications and should only be considered by the physician under these circumstances: Patients in whom vaginal delivery is not indicated (ie, herpes genitalia with a lesion at the time of delivery), prior uterine surgery, breech presentation, multiple gestation, polyhydramnios, premature rupture of membranes

Suppository: Known hypersensitivity to dinoprostone, acute pelvic inflammatory disease, uterine fibroids, cervical stenosis

Warnings/Precautions Dinoprostone should be used only by medically trained personnel in a hospital; caution in patients with cervicitis, infected endocervical lesions, acute vaginitis, compromised (scarred) uterus or history of asthma, hypertension or hypotension, epilepsy, diabetes mellitus, anemia, jaundice, or cardiovascular, renal, or hepatic disease. Oxytocin should not be used simultaneously with Prepidil™ (>6 hours of the last dose of Prepidil™).

Adverse Reactions

>10%:
- Central nervous system: Headache
- Gastrointestinal: Vomiting, diarrhea, nausea

1% to 10%:
- Cardiovascular: Bradycardia
- Central nervous system: Fever
- Neuromuscular & skeletal: Back pain

<1%:
- Cardiovascular: Hypotension, cardiac arrhythmias, syncope, flushing, tightness of the chest
- Central nervous system: Vasomotor and vasovagal reactions, dizziness, chills, pain
- Endocrine & metabolic: Hot flashes
- Respiratory: Wheezing, dyspnea, coughing, bronchospasm
- Miscellaneous: Shivering

Overdosage/Toxicology Symptoms of overdose include vomiting, bronchospasm, hypotension, chest pain, abdominal cramps, uterine contractions; treatment is symptomatic

Drug Interactions Increased effect of oxytocics

Stability Suppositories must be kept frozen, store in freezer not above -20°F (-4°C); bring to room temperature just prior to use; cervical gel should be stored under refrigeration 2°C to 8°C (36°F to 46°F)

Mechanism of Action A synthetic prostaglandin E_2 abortifacient that stimulates uterine contractions similar to those seen during natural labor

Pharmacodynamics/Kinetics

Onset of effect (uterine contractions): Within 10 minutes
Duration: Up to 2-3 hours
Absorption: Vaginal: Slow following administration
Metabolism: In many tissues including the kidney, lungs, and spleen
Elimination: Primarily in urine with small amounts excreted in feces

Usual Dosage

Abortifacient: Insert 1 suppository high in vagina, repeat at 3- to 5-hour intervals until abortion occurs up to 240 mg (maximum dose); continued administration for longer than 2 days is not advisable

Cervical ripening:
- Gel:
  - Intracervical: 0.25-1 mg
  - Intravaginal: 2.5 mg
- Suppositories: Intracervical: 2-3 mg

Administration Intracervically: For cervical ripening, patient should be supine in the dorsal position

Nursing Implications Bring suppository to room temperature just prior to use; patient should remain supine for 10 minutes following insertion; commercially available suppositories should not be used for extemporaneous preparation of any other dosage form of drug

Dosage Forms
Insert, vaginal (Cervidil®): 10 mg
Gel, endocervical: 0.5 mg in 3 g syringes [each package contains a 10-mm and 20-mm shielded catheter]
Suppository, vaginal: 20 mg

Diocto® [OTC] *see* Docusate *on page 415*

Diocto-K® [OTC] *see* Docusate *on page 415*

Dioctyl Calcium Sulfosuccinate *see* Docusate *on page 415*

Dioctyl Potassium Sulfosuccinate *see* Docusate *on page 415*

Dioctyl Sodium Sulfosuccinate *see* Docusate *on page 415*

Dioeze® [OTC] *see* Docusate *on page 415*

Dioval® Injection *see* Estradiol *on page 468*

Diovan® *see* Valsartan *on page 1287*

Dipalmitoylphosphatidylcholine *see* Colfosceril Palmitate *on page 310*

Dipentum® *see* Olsalazine *on page 924*

Diphenacen-50® Injection *see* Diphenhydramine *on this page*

Diphen® Cough [OTC] *see* Diphenhydramine *on this page*

Diphenhist [OTC] *see* Diphenhydramine *on this page*

Diphenhydramine (dye fen HYE dra meen)

Related Information
Desensitization Protocols *on page 1496*

Brand Names AllerMax® Oral [OTC]; Banophen® Oral [OTC]; Belix® Oral [OTC]; Benadryl® Injection; Benadryl® Oral [OTC]; Benadryl® Topical; Ben-Allergin-50® Injection; Benylin® Cough Syrup [OTC]; Bydramine® Cough Syrup [OTC]; Compoz® Gel Caps [OTC]; Compoz® Nighttime Sleep Aid [OTC]; Dihydrex® Injection; Diphenacen-50® Injection; Diphen® Cough [OTC]; Diphenhist [OTC]; Dormarex® 2 Oral [OTC]; Dormin® Oral [OTC]; Genahist® Oral; Hydramyn® Syrup [OTC]; Hyrexin-50® Injection; Maximum Strength Nytol® [OTC]; Miles Nervine® Caplets [OTC]; Nidryl® Oral [OTC]; Nordryl® Injection; Nordryl® Oral; Nytol® Oral [OTC]; Phendry® Oral [OTC]; Siladryl® Oral [OTC]; Silphen® Cough [OTC]; Sleep-eze 3® Oral [OTC]; Sleepinal® [OTC]; Sleepwell 2-nite® [OTC]; Sominex® Oral [OTC]; Tusstat® Syrup; Twilite® Oral [OTC]; Uni-Bent® Cough Syrup; 40 Winks® [OTC]

Canadian/Mexican Brand Names Allerdryl® (Canada); Allernix® (Canada); Nytol® Extra Strength

Synonyms Diphenhydramine Hydrochloride

Therapeutic Category Antidote, Hypersensitivity Reactions; Antihistamine, H_1 Blocker; Sedative

Use Symptomatic relief of allergic symptoms caused by histamine release which include nasal allergies and allergic dermatosis; can be used for mild nighttime sedation; prevention of motion sickness and as an antitussive; has antinauseant and topical anesthetic properties; treatment of phenothiazine-induced dystonic reactions

Pregnancy Risk Factor C

Contraindications Hypersensitivity to diphenhydramine or any component; should not be used in acute attacks of asthma

Warnings/Precautions Use with caution in patients with angle-closure glaucoma, peptic ulcer, urinary tract obstruction, hyperthyroidism; some preparations contain sodium bisulfite; syrup contains alcohol; diphenhydramine has high sedative and anticholinergic properties, so it may not be considered the antihistamine of choice for prolonged use in the elderly

Adverse Reactions
>10%:
Central nervous system: Slight to moderate drowsiness
Respiratory: Thickening of bronchial secretions
1% to 10%:
Central nervous system: Headache, fatigue, nervousness
Gastrointestinal: Nausea, vomiting, diarrhea, abdominal pain, xerostomia, appetite increase, weight gain, dry mucous membranes
Neuromuscular & skeletal: Arthralgia
Respiratory: Pharyngitis
<1%:
Cardiovascular: Hypotension, palpitations, edema
Central nervous system: Sedation, dizziness, paradoxical excitement, insomnia, depression
Dermatologic: Photosensitivity, rash, angioedema
Genitourinary: Urinary retention
Hepatic: Hepatitis
Neuromuscular & skeletal: Myalgia, paresthesia, tremor
Ocular: Blurred vision

(Continued)

Diphenhydramine *(Continued)*

Respiratory: Bronchospasm, epistaxis

Overdosage/Toxicology Symptoms of overdose include CNS stimulation or depression; overdose may result in death in infants and children

There is no specific treatment for an antihistamine overdose, however, most of its clinical toxicity is due to anticholinergic effects. Anticholinesterase inhibitors (eg, physostigmine, neostigmine, pyridostigmine, or edrophonium) may be useful by reducing acetylcholinesterase. For anticholinergic overdose with severe life-threatening symptoms, physostigmine 1-2 mg (0.5 or 0.02 mg/kg for children) I.V., slowly may be given to reverse these effects.

Drug Interactions Cytochrome P-450 2D6 enzyme substrate

Increased toxicity: CNS depressants worsens CNS and respiratory depression, monoamine oxidase inhibitors may increase anticholinergic effects; syrup should not be given to patients taking drugs that can cause disulfiram reactions (ie, metronidazole, chlorpropamide) due to high alcohol content

Stability Protect from light; the following drugs are **incompatible** with diphenhydramine when mixed in the same syringe: Amobarbital, amphotericin B, cephalothin, diatrizoate, foscarnet, heparin, hydrocortisone, hydroxyzine, pentobarbital, phenobarbital, phenytoin, prochlorperazine, promazine, promethazine, tetracycline, thiopental

Mechanism of Action Competes with histamine for H_1-receptor sites on effector cells in the gastrointestinal tract, blood vessels, and respiratory tract

Pharmacodynamics/Kinetics

Maximum sedative effect: 1-3 hours

Duration of action: 4-7 hours

Absorption: Oral: 40% to 60% reaches systemic circulation due to first-pass metabolism

Metabolism: Extensive in the liver and, to smaller degrees, in the lung and kidney

Half-life: 2-8 hours; elderly: 13.5 hours

Protein binding: 78%

Time to peak serum concentration: 2-4 hours

Usual Dosage

Children:

Oral: (>10 kg): 12.5-25 mg 3-4 times/day; maximum daily dose: 300 mg

I.M., I.V.: 5 mg/kg/day or 150 mg/m²/day in divided doses every 6-8 hours, not to exceed 300 mg/day

Adults:

Oral: 25-50 mg every 6-8 hours

Nighttime sleep aid: 50 mg at bedtime

I.M., I.V.: 10-50 mg in a single dose every 2-4 hours, not to exceed 400 mg/day

Topical: For external application, not longer than 7 days

Dietary Considerations Alcohol: Additive CNS effects, avoid use

Reference Range

Antihistamine effects at levels >25 ng/mL

Drowsiness at levels 30-40 ng/mL

Mental impairment at levels >60 ng/mL

Therapeutic: Not established

Toxic: >0.1 µg/mL

Test Interactions May suppress the wheal and flare reactions to skin test antigens

Patient Information May cause drowsiness; swallow whole, do not crush or chew sustained release product; avoid alcohol, may impair coordination and judgment

Nursing Implications Raise bed rails, institute safety measures, assist with ambulation

Dosage Forms

Capsule, as hydrochloride: 25 mg, 50 mg

Cream, as hydrochloride: 1%, 2%

Elixir, as hydrochloride: 12.5 mg/5 mL (5 mL, 10 mL, 20 mL, 120 mL, 480 mL, 3780 mL)

Injection, as hydrochloride: 10 mg/mL (10 mL, 30 mL); 50 mg/mL (1 mL, 10 mL)

Lotion, as hydrochloride: 1% (75 mL)

Solution, topical spray, as hydrochloride: 1% (60 mL)

Syrup, as hydrochloride: 12.5 mg/5 mL (5 mL, 120 mL, 240 mL, 480 mL, 3780 mL)

Tablet, as hydrochloride: 25 mg, 50 mg

Diphenhydramine Hydrochloride *see* Diphenhydramine *on previous page*

Diphenoxylate and Atropine (dye fen OKS i late & A troe peen)

Brand Names Lofene®; Logen®; Lomanate®; Lomodix®; Lomotil®; Lonox®; Low-Quel®

Synonyms Atropine and Diphenoxylate

Therapeutic Category Antidiarrheal

Use Treatment of diarrhea

Restrictions C-V

Pregnancy Risk Factor C

Contraindications Hypersensitivity to diphenoxylate, atropine or any component; severe liver disease, jaundice, dehydrated patient, and narrow-angle glaucoma; it should not be used for children <2 years of age

Warnings/Precautions High doses may cause physical and psychological dependence with prolonged use; use with caution in patients with ulcerative colitis, dehydration, and hepatic dysfunction; reduction of intestinal motility may be deleterious in diarrhea resulting from *Shigella*, *Salmonella*, toxigenic strains of *E. coli*, and from pseudomembranous enterocolitis associated with broad spectrum antibiotics; children may develop signs of atropinism (dryness of skin and mucous membranes, thirst, hyperthermia, tachycardia, urinary retention, flushing) even at the recommended dosages; if there is no response with 48 hours, the drug is unlikely to be effective and should be discontinued; if chronic diarrhea is not improved symptomatically within 10 days at maximum dosage of 20 mg/day, control is unlikely with further use.

Adverse Reactions

1% to 10%:

Central nervous system: Nervousness, restlessness, dizziness, drowsiness, headache, mental depression

Gastrointestinal: Paralytic ileus, xerostomia

Genitourinary: Urinary retention and dysuria

Ocular: Blurred vision

Respiratory: Respiratory depression

<1%:

Cardiovascular: Tachycardia

Central nervous system: Sedation, euphoria, hyperthermia

Dermatologic: Pruritus, urticaria

Gastrointestinal: Nausea, vomiting, abdominal discomfort, pancreatitis, stomach cramps

Neuromuscular & skeletal: Muscle cramps, weakness

Miscellaneous: Diaphoresis (increased)

Overdosage/Toxicology Symptoms of overdose include drowsiness, hypotension, blurred vision, flushing, dry mouth, miosis

Administration of activated charcoal will reduce bioavailability of diphenoxylate; naloxone 2 mg I.V. (0.01 mg/kg for children) with repeat administration as necessary up to a total of 10 mg; for anticholinergic overdose with severe life-threatening symptoms, physostigmine 1-2 mg (0.5 or 0.02 mg/kg for children) S.C. or I.V., slowly may be given to reverse these effects

Drug Interactions Increased toxicity: MAO inhibitors (hypertensive crisis), CNS depressants, antimuscarinics (paralytic ileus); may prolong half-life of drugs metabolized in liver

Stability Protect from light

Mechanism of Action Diphenoxylate inhibits excessive GI motility and GI propulsion; commercial preparations contain a subtherapeutic amount of atropine to discourage abuse

Pharmacodynamics/Kinetics

Onset of action: Within 45-60 minutes

Peak effect: Within 2 hours

Duration: 3-4 hours

Absorption: Oral: Well absorbed

Metabolism: Extensively in the liver to diphenoxylic acid (active)

Half-life: Diphenoxylate: 2.5 hours

Time to peak serum concentration: 2 hours

Elimination: Primarily in feces (via bile); ~14% excreted in urine; <1% excreted unchanged in urine

Usual Dosage Oral:

Children (use with caution in young children due to variable responses): Liquid: 0.3-0.4 mg of diphenoxylate/kg/day in 2-4 divided doses **or**

<2 years: Not recommended

2-5 years: 2 mg of diphenoxylate 3 times/day

5-8 years: 2 mg of diphenoxylate 4 times/day

8-12 years: 2 mg of diphenoxylate 5 times/day

Adults: 15-20 mg/day of diphenoxylate in 3-4 divided doses; maintenance: 5-15 mg/day in 2-3 divided doses

Dietary Considerations Alcohol: Additive CNS effects, avoid use

(Continued)

Diphenoxylate and Atropine *(Continued)*

Monitoring Parameters Watch for signs of atropinism (dryness of skin and mucous membranes, tachycardia, thirst, flushing); monitor number and consistency of stools; observe for signs of toxicity, fluid and electrolyte loss, hypotension, and respiratory depression

Patient Information Drowsiness, dizziness, dry mouth; use caution while driving or performing hazardous tasks; avoid alcohol or other CNS depressants; do not exceed prescribed dose; report persistent diarrhea, fever, or palpitations to physician

Nursing Implications Raise bed rails, institute safety measures

Dosage Forms

Solution, oral: Diphenoxylate hydrochloride 2.5 mg and atropine sulfate 0.025 mg per 5 mL (4 mL, 10 mL, 60 mL)

Tablet: Diphenoxylate hydrochloride 2.5 mg and atropine sulfate 0.025 mg

Diphenylan Sodium® *see* Phenytoin *on page 992*

Diphenylhydantoin *see* Phenytoin *on page 992*

Diphtheria and Tetanus Toxoid

(dif THEER ee a & TET a nus TOKS oyd)

Related Information

Adverse Events and Vaccination *on page 1439*

Immunization Guidelines *on page 1421*

Recommendations for Travelers *on page 1442*

Recommendations of the Advisory Committee on Immunization Practices (ACIP) *on page 1424*

Skin Tests *on page 1501*

Synonyms DT; Td; Tetanus and Diphtheria Toxoid

Therapeutic Category Toxoid

Use Active immunity against diphtheria and tetanus when pertussis vaccine is contraindicated

DT: Infants and children through 6 years of age

Td: Children and adults ≥7 years of age

Note: Since protective tetanus and diphtheria antibodies decline with age, only 28% of persons >70 years of age in the U.S. are believed to be immune to tetanus, and most of the tetanus-induced deaths occur in people >60 years of age, it is advisable to offer Td especially to the elderly concurrent with their influenza and other immunization programs if history of vaccination is unclear; boosters should be given at 10-year intervals; earlier for wounds

Pregnancy Risk Factor C

Pregnancy/Breast-Feeding Implications Td and T vaccines are not known to cause special problems for pregnant women or their unborn babies. While physicians do not usually recommend giving any drugs or vaccines to pregnant women, a pregnant women who needs Td vaccine should get it; wait until 2nd trimester if possible.

Contraindications Patients receiving immunosuppressive agents, prior anaphylactic, allergic, or systemic reactions; hypersensitivity to diphtheria and tetanus toxoid or any component; acute respiratory infection or other active infection

Warnings/Precautions History of a neurologic reaction or immediate hypersensitivity reaction following a previous dose. History of severe local reaction (Arthus-type) following previous dose (such individuals should not be given further routine or emergency doses of tetanus and diphtheria toxoids for 10 years). Do not confuse pediatric DT with adult diphtheria and tetanus toxoid (Td), absorbed (Td) is used in patients >7 years of age; primary immunization should be postponed until the second year of life due to possibility of CNS damage or convulsion; have epinephrine 1:1000 available.

Adverse Reactions Severe adverse reactions must be reported to the FDA

>10%: Central nervous system: Fretfulness, drowsiness

1% to 10%:

Central nervous system: Persistent crying

Gastrointestinal: Anorexia, vomiting

<1%:

Cardiovascular: Tachycardia, hypotension, edema

Central nervous system: Convulsions (rarely), pain

Dermatologic: Redness, urticaria, pruritus

Local: Tenderness

Miscellaneous: Arthus-type hypersensitivity reactions, transient fever

Drug Interactions Decreased effect with immunosuppressive agents, immunoglobulins if given within 1 month (eg, concomitant administration with tetanus immune globulin decreased the immune response to Td, especially in the elderly or other individuals with low prevaccination antibody titers (n=119))

Stability Refrigerate

Usual Dosage I.M.:

Infants and Children (DT):

6 weeks to 1 year: Three 0.5 mL doses at least 4 weeks apart; administer a reinforcing dose 6-12 months after the third injection

1-6 years: Two 0.5 mL doses at least 4 weeks apart; reinforcing dose 6-12 months after second injection; if final dose is given after seventh birthday, use adult preparation

4-6 years (booster immunization): 0.5 mL; not necessary if all 4 doses were given after fourth birthday - routinely administer booster doses at 10-year intervals with the adult preparation

Children >7 years and Adults: Should receive Td; 2 primary doses of 0.5 mL each, given at an interval of 4-6 weeks; third (reinforcing) dose of 0.5 mL 6-12 months later; boosters every 10 years

Tetanus Prophylaxis in Wound Management

Number of Prior Tetanus Toxoid Doses	Clean, Minor Wounds		All Other Wounds	
	Td*	TIG†	Td*	TIG†
Unknown or <3	Yes	No	Yes	Yes
≥3‡	No#	No	No¶	No

*Adult tetanus and diphtheria toxoids; use pediatric preparations (DT or DTP) if the patient is <7 years old.

†Tetanus immune globulin.

‡If only three doses of fluid tetanus toxoid have been received, a fourth dose of toxoid, preferably an adsorbed toxoid, should be given.

#Yes, if >10 years since last dose.

¶Yes, if >5 years since last dose.

Adapted from Report of the Committee on Infectious Diseases, American Academy of Pediatrics, Elk Grove Village, IL: American Academy of Pediatrics, 1986.

Administration Administer only I.M.; do not inject the same site more than once

Patient Information DT, Td and T vaccines cause few problems (mild fever or soreness, swelling, and redness/knot at the injection site); these problems usually last 1-2 days, but this does not happen nearly as often as with DTP vaccine

Nursing Implications Shake well before giving

Additional Information Pediatric dosage form should only be used in patients ≤6 years of age. Federal law requires that the date of administration, the vaccine manufacturer, lot number of vaccine, and the administering person's name, title, and address be entered into the patient's permanent medical record.

Dosage Forms Injection:

Pediatric use:

Diphtheria 6.6 Lf units and tetanus 5 Lf units per 0.5 mL (5 mL)

Diphtheria 10 Lf units and tetanus 5 Lf units per 0.5 mL (0.5 mL, 5 mL)

Diphtheria 12.5 Lf units and tetanus 5 Lf units per 0.5 mL (5 mL)

Diphtheria 15 Lf units and tetanus 10 Lf units per 0.5 mL (5 mL)

Adult use:

Diphtheria 1.5 Lf units and tetanus 5 Lf units per 0.5 mL (0.5 mL, 5 mL)

Diphtheria 2 Lf units and tetanus 5 Lf units per 0.5 mL (5 mL)

Diphtheria 2 Lf units and tetanus 10 Lf units per 0.5 mL (5 mL)

Diphtheria CRM_{197} Protein Conjugate *see Haemophilus* b Conjugate Vaccine *on page 595*

Diphtheria, Tetanus Toxoids, and Acellular Pertussis Vaccine

(dif THEER ee a, TET a nus TOKS oyds & ay CEL yoo lar per TUS sis vak SEEN)

Related Information

Adverse Events and Vaccination *on page 1439*

Guidelines for the Prevention of Opportunistic Infections in Persons with HIV *on page 1457*

Immunization Guidelines *on page 1421*

Miscellaneous Vaccination Information *on page 1437*

Prophylaxis for Patients Exposed to Common Communicable Diseases *on page 1452*

Recommendations of the Advisory Committee on Immunization Practices (ACIP) *on page 1424*

Recommended Childhood Immunization Schedule - US - January-December, 1997 *on page 1423*

Brand Names Acel-Imune®; Infanrix®; Tripedia®

Synonyms DTaP

Therapeutic Category Toxoid; Vaccine

(Continued)

Diphtheria, Tetanus Toxoids, and Acellular Pertussis Vaccine *(Continued)*

Use Approved for the primary immunization of children 2 months to 5 years of age, ideally beginning at the age of 2-3 months or at 6-week check-up. Administer 0.5 mL I.M. on 3 occasions at ~2-month intervals (eg, 2, 4 and 6 months), followed by a fourth 0.5 mL dose at approximately 15 months of age (at least prior to seventh birthday)

Pregnancy Risk Factor B

Pregnancy/Breast-Feeding Implications Effects on the fetus: Animal reproduction studies have not been conducted. It is not known whether the vaccine can cause fetal harm when administered to a pregnant woman or can affect reproductive capacity. Tripedia® vaccine is NOT recommended for use in a pregnant woman.

Contraindications Patients >7 years of age, patients with cancer, immunodeficiencies, an acute respiratory infection, or any other active infection; children with a history of neurologic disorders should not receive the pertussis or any component; history of any of the following effects from previous administration of pertussis vaccine precludes further use: >103°F fever (39.4°C), convulsions, focal neurologic signs, screaming episodes, shock, collapse, sleepiness or encephalopathy; known hypersensitivity to diphtheria and tetanus toxoids or pertussis vaccine; do not use for treatment of actual tetanus, diphtheria, or whooping cough infections

Warnings/Precautions DTaP should not be used in children <15 months of age and should not be used in children who have received fewer than 3 doses of DTP

Adverse Reactions All serious adverse reactions must be reported to the FDA

<1%:

Cardiovascular: Edema

Central nervous system: Convulsions, screaming episodes, malaise, sleepiness, focal neurological signs, shock, collapse, fever, chills

Dermatologic: Erythema, induration, rash, urticaria

Local: Tenderness

Neuromuscular & skeletal: Arthralgias

Drug Interactions Decreased effect with immunosuppressive agents, corticosteroids within 1 month

Stability Refrigerate at 2°C to 8°C (35°F to 46°F); do not freeze

Usual Dosage The primary immunization for children 2 months to 5 years of age, ideally beginning at the age of 2-3 months or at 6-week check-up: Administer 0.5 mL I.M. on 3 occasions at ~2-month intervals, followed by a fourth 0.5 mL dose at ~15 months of age

Administration Administer only I.M. in anterolateral aspect of thigh or deltoid muscle of upper arm

Patient Information A nodule may be palpable at the injection site for a few weeks

Nursing Implications Acetaminophen 10-15 mg/kg before and every 4 hours to 12-24 hours may reduce or prevent fever; shake well before administering; the child's medical record should document that the small risk of postvaccination seizure and the benefits of the pertussis vaccination were discussed with the patient

Additional Information This preparation contains less endotoxin relative to DTP and, although immunogenic, it apparently is less reactogenic than DTP. Federal law requires that the date of administration, the vaccine manufacturer, lot number of vaccine, and the administering person's name, title, and address be entered into the patient's permanent medical record.

Dosage Forms Injection:

Acel-Immune®: Diphtheria 7.5 Lf units, tetanus 5 Lf units, and acellular pertussis vaccine 40 mcg per 0.5 mL (7.5 mL)

Tripedia®: Diphtheria 6.7 Lf units, tetanus 5 Lf units, and acellular pertussis vaccine 46.8 mcg per 0.5 mL (7.5 mL)

Infanrix®: Diphtheria 25 Lf units, tetanus 10 Lf units, and acellular pertussis vaccine 25 mcg per 0.5 mL (0.5 mL)

Diphtheria, Tetanus Toxoids, Whole-Cell Pertussis, and *Haemophilus Influenzae* Type b Conjugate Vaccines

(dif THEER ee a, TET a nus TOKS oyds, hole-sel per TUS sis vak SEEN, & hem OF fil us bee KON joo gate vak SEEN)

Related Information

Adverse Events and Vaccination *on page 1439*

Immunization Guidelines *on page 1421*

Recommended Childhood Immunization Schedule - US - January-December, 1997 *on page 1423*

Brand Names Tetramune®; Tripedia/ActHIB

Synonyms DTwP-HIB

Therapeutic Category Toxoid

Use Active immunization of infants and children through 5 years of age (between 2 months and the sixth birthday) against diphtheria, tetanus, and pertussis and *Haemophilus* b disease when indications for immunization with DTP vaccine and HIB vaccine coincide

Pregnancy Risk Factor B

Contraindications Children with any febrile illness or active infection, known hypersensitivity to *Haemophilus* b polysaccharide vaccine (thimerosal), children who are immunosuppressed or receiving immunosuppressive therapy; patients >7 years of age, patients with cancer, immunodeficiencies, an acute respiratory infection, or any other active infection; children with a history of neurologic disorders should not receive the pertussis any component; history of any of the following effects from previous administration of pertussis vaccine precludes further use: fever >103°F (39.4°C), convulsions, focal neurologic signs, screaming episodes, shock, collapse, sleepiness or encephalopathy; known hypersensitivity to diphtheria and tetanus toxoids or pertussis vaccine; do not use DTP for treatment of actual tetanus, diphtheria or whooping cough infections

Warnings/Precautions If adverse reactions occurred with previous doses, immunization should be completed with diphtheria and tetanus toxoid absorbed (pediatric); any febrile illness or active infection is reason for delaying use of *Haemophilus* b conjugate vaccine

Adverse Reactions All serious adverse reactions must be reported to the US Department of Health and Human Services (DHHS) Vaccine Adverse Event Reporting System (VAERS). Reporting forms and information about reporting requirements or completion of the form can be obtained from VAERS through a toll-free number 1-800-822-7967.

>10%:
- Central nervous system: Fever, chills, irritability, restlessness, drowsiness
- Local: Erythema, edema, induration, pain and warmth at injection site

1% to 10%:
- Dermatologic: Rash
- Gastrointestinal: Vomiting, diarrhea, loss of appetite

<1%:
- Central nervous system: Convulsions, screaming episodes, malaise, sleepiness, focal neurological signs, shock, collapse, chills
- Dermatologic: Urticaria
- Local: Local tenderness
- Neuromuscular & skeletal: Arthralgia
- Miscellaneous: Increased risk of *Haemophilus* b infections in the week after vaccination, rarely allergic or anaphylactic reactions

Drug Interactions Decreased effect: Immunosuppressive agents; may interfere with antigen detection tests

Stability Keep in refrigerator, may be frozen (not diluent) without affecting potency; unopened vials are stable for up to 24 hours at <70°C

Usual Dosage The primary immunization for children 2 months to 5 years of age, ideally beginning at the age of 2-3 months or at 6-week check-up. Administer 0.5 mL I.M. on 3 occasions at ~2-month intervals, followed by a fourth 0.5 mL dose at ~15 months of age.

Administration Administer I.M. only

Patient Information A nodule may be palpable at the injection site for a few weeks

Nursing Implications
- Acetaminophen 10-15 mg/kg before and every 4 hours to 12-24 hours may reduce or prevent fever
- Shake well before administering
- The child's medical record should document that the small risk of past vaccination seizure and the benefits of the pertussis vaccination were discussed with the patient

Additional Information Inactivated bacterial vaccine; Federal law requires that the date of administration, the vaccine manufacturer, lot number of vaccine and the administering person's name, title, and address be entered into the patient's permanent medical record. **Note:** Diphtheria and Tetanus Toxoids, and Acellular Pertussis and *Haemophilus Influenzae Type B* Conjugate Vaccine is Tripedia/Act HIB®

Dosage Forms Injection: Diphtheria toxoid 12.5 Lf units, tetanus toxoid 5 Lf units, and whole-cell pertussis vaccine 4 units, and *Haemophilus influenzae* type b oligosaccharide 10 mcg per 0.5 mL (5 mL)

Diphtheria Toxoid Conjugate *see* *Haemophilus* b Conjugate Vaccine *on page 595*

Dipivalyl Epinephrine *see* Dipivefrin *on next page*

Dipivefrin (dye PI ve frin)

Related Information

Glaucoma Drug Therapy Comparison *on page 1410*

Brand Names AKPro® Ophthalmic; Propine® Ophthalmic

Canadian/Mexican Brand Names DPE™ (Canada); Ophtho-Dipivefrin™ (Canada)

Synonyms Dipivalyl Epinephrine; Dipivefrin Hydrochloride; DPE

Therapeutic Category Adrenergic Agonist Agent, Ophthalmic; Ophthalmic Agent, Vasoconstrictor

Use Reduces elevated intraocular pressure in chronic open-angle glaucoma; also used to treat ocular hypertension, low tension, and secondary glaucomas

Pregnancy Risk Factor B

Contraindications Hypersensitivity to dipivefrin, ingredients in the formulation, or epinephrine; contraindicated in patients with angle-closure glaucoma

Warnings/Precautions Use with caution in patients with vascular hypertension or cardiac disorders and in aphakic patients; contains sodium metabisulfite

Adverse Reactions

1% to 10%:
- Central nervous system: Headache
- Local: Burning, stinging
- Ocular: Ocular congestion, photophobia, mydriasis, blurred vision, ocular pain, bulbar conjunctival follicles, blepharoconjunctivitis, cystoid macular edema

<1%: Cardiovascular: Arrhythmias, hypertension

Drug Interactions Increased or synergistic effect when used with other agents to lower intraocular pressure

Stability Avoid exposure to light and air; discolored or darkened solutions indicate loss of potency

Mechanism of Action Dipivefrin is a prodrug of epinephrine which is the active agent that stimulates alpha- and/or beta-adrenergic receptors increasing aqueous humor outflow

Pharmacodynamics/Kinetics

Ocular pressure effect:
- Onset of action: Within 30 minutes
- Duration: ≥12 hours

Mydriasis:
- Onset of action: May occur within 30 minutes
- Duration: Several hours

Absorption: Rapid into the aqueous humor

Metabolism: Converted to epinephrine

Usual Dosage Adults: Ophthalmic: Instill 1 drop every 12 hours into the eyes

Patient Information Discolored solutions should be discarded; may cause transient burning or stinging

Nursing Implications Finger pressure should be applied to lacrimal sac for 1-2 minutes after instillation to decrease risk of absorption and systemic reactions

Dosage Forms Solution, ophthalmic, as hydrochloride: 0.1% (5 mL, 10 mL, 15 mL)

Dipivefrin Hydrochloride *see* Dipivefrin *on this page*

Diprivan® *see* Propofol *on page 1063*

Diprolene® *see* Betamethasone *on page 147*

Diprolene® AF *see* Betamethasone *on page 147*

Dipropylacetic Acid *see* Valproic Acid and Derivatives *on page 1285*

Diprosone® *see* Betamethasone *on page 147*

Dipyridamole (dye peer ID a mole)

Brand Names Persantine®

Canadian/Mexican Brand Names Apo-Dipyridamole® FC (Canada); Apo-Dipyridamole® SC (Canada); Novo-Dipiradol® (Canada); Dirinol® (Mexico); Lodimol® (Mexico); Trompersantin® (Mexico)

Therapeutic Category Antiplatelet Agent; Vasodilator, Coronary

Use Maintains patency after surgical grafting procedures including coronary artery bypass; used with warfarin to decrease thrombosis in patients after artificial heart valve replacement; used with aspirin to prevent coronary artery thrombosis; in combination with aspirin or warfarin to prevent other thromboembolic disorders. Dipyridamole may also be given 2 days prior to open heart surgery to prevent platelet activation by extracorporeal bypass pump and as a diagnostic agent in CAD; also approved as an alternative to exercise during Thallium myocardial perfusion imaging for the evaluation of coronary artery disease in patients who cannot exercise adequately

Pregnancy Risk Factor C

Contraindications Hypersensitivity to dipyridamole or any component

Warnings/Precautions Safety and effectiveness in children <12 years of age have not been established; may further decrease blood pressure in patients with hypotension due to peripheral vasodilation; use with caution in patients taking other drugs which affect platelet function or coagulation and in patients with hemostatic defects. Since evidence suggests that clinically used doses are ineffective for prevention of platelet aggregation, consideration for low-dose aspirin (81-325 mg/day) alone may be necessary; this will decrease cost as well as inconvenience.

Adverse Reactions

>10%:
- Cardiovascular: Exacerbation of angina pectoris
- Central nervous system: Dizziness

1% to 10%:
- Cardiovascular: Hypotension, hypertension, tachycardia
- Central nervous system: Headache
- Dermatologic: Rash
- Gastrointestinal: Abdominal distress
- Respiratory: Dyspnea

<1%:
- Cardiovascular: Vasodilatation, flushing, syncope, edema
- Central nervous system: Migraine
- Neuromuscular & skeletal: Weakness, hypertonia
- Respiratory: Rhinitis, hyperventilation
- Miscellaneous: Allergic reaction, pleural pain

Overdosage/Toxicology Symptoms of overdose include hypotension, peripheral vasodilation; dialysis is not effective

Treatment includes fluids and vasopressors although hypotension is often transient

Drug Interactions

Increased toxicity: Heparin may increase anticoagulation

Decreased hypotensive effect (I.V.): Theophylline

Stability Do not freeze, protect I.V. preparation from light

Mechanism of Action Inhibits the activity of adenosine deaminase and phosphodiesterase, which causes an accumulation of adenosine, adenine nucleotides, and cyclic AMP; these mediators then inhibit platelet aggregation and may cause vasodilation; may also stimulate release of prostacyclin or PGD_2; causes coronary vasodilation

Pharmacodynamics/Kinetics

Absorption: Readily absorbed from GI tract but variable

Distribution: V_d: 2-3 L/kg in adults

Protein binding: 91% to 99%

Metabolism: Concentrated and metabolized in the liver

Half-life, terminal: 10-12 hours

Time to peak serum concentration: 2-2.5 hours

Elimination: In feces via bile as glucuronide conjugates and unchanged drug

Usual Dosage

Oral:
- Children: 3-6 mg/kg/day in 3 divided doses
  - Doses of 4-10 mg/kg/day have been used investigationally to treat proteinuria in pediatric renal disease
- Adults: 75-400 mg/day in 3-4 divided doses

I.V.: 0.14 mg/kg/minute for 4 minutes; maximum dose: 60 mg

Patient Information Notify physician or pharmacist if taking other medications that affect bleeding, such as NSAIDs or warfarin

Dosage Forms

Injection: 10 mg/2 mL

Tablet: 25 mg, 50 mg, 75 mg

Extemporaneous Preparations A 10 mg/mL oral suspension has been made using four 25 mg tablets and purified water USP qs ad to 10 mL; expected stability is 3 days

Nahata MC and Hipple TF, *Pediatric Drug Formulations*, 2nd ed, Cincinnati, OH: Harvey Whitney Books Co, 1992.

Dirithromycin (dye RITH roe mye sin)

Brand Names Dynabac®

Therapeutic Category Antibiotic, Macrolide

Use Treatment of mild to moderate upper and lower respiratory tract infections due to *Moraxella catarrhalis, Streptococcus pneumoniae, Legionella pneumophila*, or *S. pyogenes* (ie, acute exacerbation of chronic bronchitis, secondary bacterial infection of acute bronchitis, community-acquired pneumonia, pharyngitis/tonsillitis, not proven to be effective in prevention of potentially subsequent rheumatic

(Continued)

Dirithromycin *(Continued)*

fever), and uncomplicated infections of the skin and skin structure due to *Staphylococcus aureus*

Note: Serum levels of dirithromycin are not adequate to treat bacteremias due to other sensitive strains; **empiric** treatment of acute bacterial exacerbations of chronic or secondary bronchitis is not recommended since resistance of the frequently causative agent, *H. influenzae*, occurs

Pregnancy Risk Factor C

Pregnancy/Breast-Feeding Implications Animal studies indicate the use of dirithromycin during pregnancy should be avoided if possible; use caution when administering to nursing women

Contraindications Hypersensitivity to any macrolide or component of dirithromycin; use with pimozide

Warnings/Precautions Contrary to potential serious consequences with other macrolides (eg, cardiac arrhythmias), the combination of terfenadine and dirithromycin has not shown alteration of terfenadine metabolism; however, caution should be taken during coadministration of dirithromycin and terfenadine; pseudomembranous colitis has been reported and should be considered in patients presenting with diarrhea subsequent to therapy with dirithromycin

Adverse Reactions

1% to 10%:

Central nervous system: Headache, dizziness, vertigo, insomnia
Dermatologic: Rash, pruritus, urticaria
Endocrine & metabolic: Hyperkalemia, increased CPK
Gastrointestinal: Abdominal pain, nausea, diarrhea, vomiting, dyspepsia, flatulence
Hematologic: Thrombocytosis, eosinophilia, segmented neutrophils
Neuromuscular & skeletal: Weakness, pain
Respiratory: Increased cough, dyspnea

<1%:

Cardiovascular: Palpitations, vasodilation, syncope, edema
Central nervous system: Anxiety, depression, somnolence, fever, malaise
Endocrine & metabolic: Dysmenorrhea, hypochloremia, hypophosphatemia, increased uric acid, dehydration
Gastrointestinal: Abnormal stools, anorexia, gastritis, constipation, abnormal taste, xerostomia, abdominal pain, mouth ulceration
Genitourinary: Polyuria, vaginitis
Hematologic: Neutropenia, thrombocytopenia, decreased hemoglobin/hematocrit; increased alkaline phosphatase, bands, basophils; leukocytosis, monocytosis
Hepatic: Increased ALT, AST, GGT; hyperbilirubinemia
Neuromuscular & skeletal: Paresthesia, tremor, myalgia
Ocular: Amblyopia
Otic: Tinnitus
Renal: Increased creatinine, phosphorus
Respiratory: Epistaxis, hemoptysis, hyperventilation
Miscellaneous: Hypoalbuminemia, flu-like syndrome, diaphoresis, thirst

Overdosage/Toxicology Symptoms of overdose include nausea, vomiting, abdominal pain, diarrhea; treatment is supportive; dialysis has not been found effective

Drug Interactions

Increased effect: Absorption of dirithromycin is slightly enhanced with concomitant antacids and H_2-antagonists; dirithromycin may, like erythromycin, increase the effect of alfentanil, anticoagulants, bromocriptine, carbamazepine, cyclosporine, digoxin, disopyramide, ergots, methylprednisolone, and triazolam

Note: Interactions with nonsedating antihistamines (eg, terfenadine) and theophylline are not known to occur, however, caution is advised with coadministration

Mechanism of Action After being converted during intestinal absorption to its active form, erythromycylamine, dirithromycin inhibits protein synthesis by binding to the 50S ribosomal subunits of susceptible microorganisms

Pharmacodynamics/Kinetics

Absorption: Rapidly absorbed and nonenzymatically hydrolyzed to erythromycylamine; T_{max}: 4 hours
Distribution: V_d: 800 L; rapidly and widely distributed (higher levels in tissues than plasma)
Protein binding: 14% to 30%
Metabolism: Minimal hepatic metabolism
Bioavailability: 10%
Half-life: 8 hours (range: 2-36 hours)
Elimination: Via bile (81% to 97% of dose)

Usual Dosage Adults: Oral: 500 mg once daily for 7-14 days (14 days required for treatment of community-acquired pneumonia due to *Legionella*, *Mycoplasma*, or *S. pneumoniae*; 10 days is recommended for treatment of *S. pyogenes* pharyngitis/tonsillitis)

Dosing adjustment in renal impairment: None necessary

Dosing adjustment in hepatic impairment: None needed in mild dysfunction; not studied in moderate to severe dysfunction

Administration Administer with food or within an hour following a meal; administer at the same time each day to promote less variation in peak and trough serum levels

Monitoring Parameters Temperature, CBC

Patient Information Take with food or within an hour following a meal; do not cut, chew, or crush tablets; entire course of medication should be taken to ensure eradication of organism

Nursing Implications Do not alter enteric coated dosage form

Dosage Forms Tablet, enteric coated: 250 mg

Disalcid® *see* Salsalate *on page 1122*

Disalicylic Acid *see* Salsalate *on page 1122*

Disodium Cromoglycate *see* Cromolyn Sodium *on page 317*

d-Isoephedrine Hydrochloride *see* Pseudoephedrine *on page 1074*

Disonate® [OTC] *see* Docusate *on page 415*

Disopyramide (dye soe PEER a mide)

Related Information

Antiarrhythmic Drugs *on page 1389*

Comparative Pharmacokinetic Properties of Antiarrhythmic Agents *on page 1391*

Brand Names Norpace®

Canadian/Mexican Brand Names Dimodan® (Mexico)

Synonyms Disopyramide Phosphate

Therapeutic Category Antiarrhythmic Agent, Class I-A

Use Suppression and prevention of unifocal and multifocal premature, ventricular premature complexes, coupled ventricular tachycardia; effective in the conversion of atrial fibrillation, atrial flutter, and paroxysmal atrial tachycardia to normal sinus rhythm and prevention of the reoccurrence of these arrhythmias after conversion by other methods

Pregnancy Risk Factor C

Contraindications Pre-existing second or third degree A-V block, cardiogenic shock, or known hypersensitivity to the drug

Warnings/Precautions Pre-existing urinary retention, family history, or existing angle-closure glaucoma, myasthenia gravis, hypotension during initiation of therapy, congestive heart failure unless caused by an arrhythmias, widening of QRS complex during therapy or Q-T interval (>25% to 50% of baseline QRS complex or Q-T interval), sick-sinus syndrome or WPW, renal or hepatic impairment require decrease in dosage; disopyramide ineffective in hypokalemia and potentially toxic with hyperkalemia. Due to changes in total clearance (decreased) in elderly, monitor closely; the anticholinergic action may be intolerable and require discontinuation.

Adverse Reactions

>10%: Genitourinary: Urinary retention/hesitancy

1% to 10%:

- Cardiovascular: Chest pains, congestive heart failure, hypotension
- Endocrine & metabolic: Hypokalemia
- Gastrointestinal: Stomach pain, bloating, xerostomia
- Neuromuscular & skeletal: Muscle weakness
- Ocular: Blurred vision

<1%:

- Cardiovascular: Syncope and conduction disturbances including A-V block, widening QRS complex and lengthening of Q-T interval
- Central nervous system: Fatigue, malaise, nervousness, acute psychosis, depression, dizziness, headache, pain
- Dermatologic: Generalized rashes
- Endocrine & metabolic: Hypoglycemia, may initiate contractions of pregnant uterus, hyperkalemia may enhance toxicities, increased cholesterol and triglycerides
- Gastrointestinal: Constipation, nausea, vomiting, diarrhea, flatulence, anorexia, weight gain, dry throat
- Hepatic: Hepatic cholestasis, elevated liver enzymes
- Ocular: Dry eyes
- Respiratory: Dyspnea, dry nose

(Continued)

Disopyramide *(Continued)*

Overdosage/Toxicology Has a low toxic therapeutic ratio and may easily produce fatal intoxication (acute toxic dose: 1 g in adults); symptoms of overdose include sinus bradycardia, sinus node arrest or asystole, P-R, QRS or Q-T interval prolongation, torsade de pointes (polymorphous ventricular tachycardia) and depressed myocardial contractility, which along with alpha-adrenergic or ganglionic blockade, may result in hypotension and pulmonary edema; other effects are anticholinergic (dry mouth, dilated pupils, and delirium) as well as seizures, coma and respiratory arrest.

Treatment is primarily symptomatic and effects usually respond to conventional therapies (fluids, positioning, vasopressors, anticonvulsants, antiarrhythmics). **Note:** Do not use other type Ia or Ic antiarrhythmic agents to treat ventricular tachycardia; sodium bicarbonate may treat wide QRS intervals or hypotension; markedly impaired conduction or high degree A-V block, unresponsive to bicarbonate, indicates consideration of a pacemaker.

Drug Interactions

Decreased effect with hepatic microsomal enzyme-inducing agents (ie, phenytoin, phenobarbital, rifampin)

Increased effect/levels/toxicity with erythromycin; increased levels of digoxin

Mechanism of Action Class IA antiarrhythmic: Decreases myocardial excitability and conduction velocity; reduces disparity in refractory between normal and infarcted myocardium; possesses anticholinergic, peripheral vasoconstrictive, and negative inotropic effects

Pharmacodynamics/Kinetics

Onset of action: 0.5-3.5 hours

Duration of effect: 1.5-8.5 hours

Absorption: 60% to 83%

Protein binding: Concentration dependent, ranges from 20% to 60%

Metabolism: In the liver to inactive metabolites

Half-life: Adults: 4-10 hours, increased half-life with hepatic or renal disease

Elimination: 40% to 60% excreted unchanged in urine and 10% to 15% in feces

Usual Dosage Oral:

Children:

- <1 year: 10-30 mg/kg/24 hours in 4 divided doses
- 1-4 years: 10-20 mg/kg/24 hours in 4 divided doses
- 4-12 years: 10-15 mg/kg/24 hours in 4 divided doses
- 12-18 years: 6-15 mg/kg/24 hours in 4 divided doses

Adults:

- <50 kg: 100 mg every 6 hours or 200 mg every 12 hours (controlled release)
- >50 kg: 150 mg every 6 hours or 300 mg every 12 hours (controlled release); if no response, may increase to 200 mg every 6 hours; maximum dose required for patients with severe refractory ventricular tachycardia is 400 mg every 6 hours

Dosing adjustment in renal impairment: 100 mg (nonsustained release) given at the following intervals: See table.

Creatinine Clearance (mL/min)	Dosage Interval
30-40	q8h
15-30	q12h
<15	q24h

or alter the dose as follows:

- Cl_{cr} 30-<40 mL/minute: Reduce dose 50%
- Cl_{cr} 15-30 mL/minute: Reduce dose 75%

Dialysis: Not dialyzable (0% to 5%) by hemo- or peritoneal methods; supplemental dose not necessary

Dosing interval in hepatic impairment: 100 mg every 6 hours or 200 mg every 12 hours (controlled release)

Administration Administer around-the-clock rather than 4 times/day (ie, 12-6-12-6, not 9-1-5-9) to promote less variation in peak and trough serum levels

Monitoring Parameters EKG, blood pressure, disopyramide drug level, urinary retention, CNS anticholinergic effects (confusion, agitation, hallucinations, etc)

Reference Range

Therapeutic concentration:

- Atrial arrhythmias: 2.8-3.2 μg/mL
- Ventricular arrhythmias 3.3-7.5 μg/mL

Toxic concentration: >7 μg/mL

Patient Information Notify physician if urinary retention or worsening CHF; do not break or chew sustained release capsules

Nursing Implications Do not crush controlled release capsules

Dosage Forms

Capsule, as phosphate: 100 mg, 150 mg

Capsule, sustained action, as phosphate: 100 mg, 150 mg

Extemporaneous Preparations Extemporaneous suspensions in cherry syrup (1 mg/mL and 10 mg/mL) are stable for 4 weeks in amber glass bottles stored at 5°C, 30°C, or at room temperature; shake well before use; do not use extended release capsules for this suspension

Mathur LK, Lai PK, and Shively CD, "Stability of Disopyramide Phosphate in Cherry Syrup," *J Hosp Pharm*, 1982, 39(2):309-10.

Disopyramide Phosphate *see* Disopyramide *on page 409*

Disotate® *see* Edetate Disodium *on page 438*

Di-Spaz® Injection *see* Dicyclomine *on page 376*

Di-Spaz® Oral *see* Dicyclomine *on page 376*

Dispos-a-Med® Isoproterenol *see* Isoproterenol *on page 681*

Disulfiram (dye SUL fi ram)

Brand Names Antabuse®

Therapeutic Category Aldehyde Dehydrogenase Inhibitor Agent; Antialcoholic Agent

Use Management of chronic alcoholism

Pregnancy Risk Factor C

Contraindications Severe myocardial disease and coronary occlusion, hypersensitivity to disulfiram or any component, patient receiving alcohol, paraldehyde, alcohol-containing preparations like cough syrup or tonics

Warnings/Precautions Use with caution in patients with diabetes, hypothyroidism, seizure disorders, hepatic cirrhosis, or insufficiency; should never be administered to a patient when he/she is in a state of alcohol intoxication, or without his/her knowledge

Adverse Reactions

>10%: Central nervous system: Drowsiness

1% to 10%:

- Central nervous system: Headache, fatigue, mood changes, neurotoxicity
- Dermatologic: Rash
- Gastrointestinal: Metallic or garlic-like aftertaste
- Genitourinary: Impotence

<1%:

- Central nervous system: Encephalopathy
- Hepatic: Hepatitis
- **Disulfiram reaction with alcohol**: Flushing, diaphoresis, cardiovascular collapse, myocardial infarction, vertigo, seizures, headache, nausea, vomiting, dyspnea, chest pain, death

Overdosage/Toxicology Management of disulfiram reaction: Institute support measures to restore blood pressure (pressors and fluids); monitor for hypokalemia

Drug Interactions

Increased effect: Diazepam, chlordiazepoxide

Increased toxicity:

- Alcohol and disulfiram: Antabuse® reaction
- Tricyclic antidepressants, metronidazole, isoniazid: Encephalopathy
- Phenytoin may increase serum levels and toxicity
- Warfarin may increase prothrombin time

Mechanism of Action Disulfiram is a thiuram derivative which interferes with aldehyde dehydrogenase. When taken concomitantly with alcohol, there is an increase in serum acetaldehyde levels. High acetaldehyde causes uncomfortable symptoms including flushing, nausea, thirst, palpitations, chest pain, vertigo, and hypotension. This reaction is the basis for disulfiram use in postwithdrawal long-term care of alcoholism.

Pharmacodynamics/Kinetics

Absorption: Rapid from GI tract

Full effect: 12 hours

Metabolism: To diethylthiocarbamate

Duration: May persist for 1-2 weeks after last dose

Usual Dosage Adults: Oral: Do not administer until the patient has abstained from alcohol for at least 12 hours

Initial: 500 mg/day as a single dose for 1-2 weeks; maximum daily dose is 500 mg

Average maintenance dose: 250 mg/day; range: 125-500 mg; duration of therapy is to continue until the patient is fully recovered socially and a basis for permanent self control has been established; maintenance therapy may be required for months or even years

(Continued)

Disulfiram *(Continued)*

Dietary Considerations Alcohol: Avoid use, including alcohol-containing products

Patient Information Do not drink any alcohol, including products containing alcohol (cough and cold syrups), or use alcohol-containing skin products for at least 3 days and preferably 14 days after stopping this medication or while taking this medication; not for treatment of alcohol intoxication; may cause drowsiness; tablets can be crushed or mixed with water

Nursing Implications Administration of any medications containing alcohol including topicals is contraindicated

Dosage Forms Tablet: 250 mg, 500 mg

Dithioglycerol *see* Dimercaprol *on page 397*
Ditropan® *see* Oxybutynin *on page 935*
Diucardin® *see* Hydroflumethiazide *on page 626*
Diurigen® *see* Chlorothiazide *on page 257*
Diuril® *see* Chlorothiazide *on page 257*
Divalproex Sodium *see* Valproic Acid and Derivatives *on page 1285*
Dizac® Injection *see* Diazepam *on page 369*
Dizmiss® [OTC] *see* Meclizine *on page 769*
***dl*-Alpha Tocopherol** *see* Vitamin E *on page 1309*
***dl*-Norephedrine Hydrochloride** *see* Phenylpropanolamine *on page 991*
***D*-Mannitol** *see* Mannitol *on page 758*
4-dmdr *see* Idarubicin *on page 642*
DNase *see* Dornase Alfa *on page 419*
DNR *see* Daunorubicin Hydrochloride *on page 345*

Dobutamine (doe BYOO ta meen)

Related Information

Adrenergic Agonists, Cardiovascular Comparison *on page 1385*
Adult ACLS Algorithm, Hypotension, Shock *on page 1516*
Cardiovascular Agents Comparison *on page 1405*
Extravasation Treatment of Other Drugs *on page 1381*

Brand Names Dobutrex®

Canadian/Mexican Brand Names Dobuject® (Mexico); Oxiken® (Mexico)

Synonyms Dobutamine Hydrochloride

Therapeutic Category Adrenergic Agonist Agent; Sympathomimetic

Use Short-term management of patients with cardiac decompensation

Pregnancy Risk Factor C

Contraindications Hypersensitivity to sulfites (commercial preparation contains sodium bisulfite); patients with idiopathic hypertrophic subaortic stenosis, atrial fibrillation or atrial flutter

Warnings/Precautions Hypovolemia should be corrected prior to use; infiltration causes local inflammatory changes, extravasation may cause dermal necrosis; use with extreme caution following myocardial infarction; potent drug, must be diluted prior to use

Adverse Reactions

>10%: Cardiovascular: Ectopic heartbeats, increased heart rate, chest pain, angina, palpitations, elevation in blood pressure; in higher doses ventricular tachycardia or arrhythmias may be seen; patients with atrial fibrillation or flutter are at risk of developing a rapid ventricular response

1% to 10%:
- Cardiovascular: Premature ventricular beats, chest pain, angina, palpitations
- Central nervous system: Headache
- Gastrointestinal: Nausea, vomiting
- Neuromuscular & skeletal: Mild leg cramps, paresthesia
- Respiratory: Dyspnea, shortness of breath

Overdosage/Toxicology Symptoms of overdose include fatigue, nervousness, tachycardia, hypertension, arrhythmias; reduce rate of administration or discontinue infusion until condition stabilizes

Drug Interactions

Decreased effect: Beta-adrenergic blockers (increased peripheral resistance)

Increased toxicity: General anesthetics (ie, halothane or cyclopropane) and usual doses of dobutamine have resulted in ventricular arrhythmias in animals

Stability Remix solution every 24 hours; store reconstituted solution under refrigeration for 48 hours or 6 hours at room temperature; pink discoloration of solution indicates slight oxidation but **no** significant loss of potency.

Stability of parenteral admixture at room temperature (25°C): 48 hours; at refrigeration (4°C): 7 days

Standard adult diluent: 250 mg/500 mL D_5W; 500 mg/500 mL D_5W

Incompatible with heparin, sodium bicarbonate, cefazolin, penicillin; **incompatible** in alkaline solutions (sodium bicarbonate)

Compatible with dopamine, epinephrine, isoproterenol, lidocaine

Mechanism of Action Stimulates $beta_1$-adrenergic receptors, causing increased contractility and heart rate, with little effect on $beta_2$- or alpha-receptors

Pharmacodynamics/Kinetics

Onset of action: I.V.: 1-10 minutes

Peak effect: Within 10-20 minutes

Metabolism: In tissues and the liver to inactive metabolites

Half-life: 2 minutes

Elimination: Metabolites are excreted in urine

Usual Dosage I.V. infusion:

Children: 2.5-15 mcg/kg/minute, titrate to desired response

Adults: 2.5-15 mcg/kg/minute; maximum: 40 mcg/kg/minute, titrate to desired response

Infusion Rates of Various Dilutions of Dobutamine

Desired Delivery Rate (mcg/kg/min)	Infusion Rate (mL/kg/min)	
	500 mcg/mL*	1000 mcg/mL†
2.5	0.005	0.0025
5.0	0.01	0.005
7.5	0.015	0.0075
10.0	0.02	0.01
12.5	0.025	0.0125
15.0	0.03	0.015

*500 mg per liter or 250 mg per 500 mL of diluent.

†1000 mg per liter or 250 mg per 250 mL of diluent.

Administration Use infusion device to control rate of flow; administer into large vein

To prepare for infusion:

$$\frac{6 \times \text{weight (kg)} \times \text{desired dose (mcg/kg/min)}}{\text{I.V. infusion rate (mL/h)}} = \text{mg of drug to be added to 100 mL of I.V. fluid}$$

Do not administer through same I.V. line as heparin, hydrocortisone sodium succinate, cefazolin, or penicillin

Monitoring Parameters Blood pressure, EKG, heart rate, CVP, RAP, MAP, urine output; if pulmonary artery catheter is in place, monitor CI, PCWP, and SVR; also monitor serum potassium

Patient Information May affect serum assay of chloramphenicol

Nursing Implications **Management of extravasation:** Phentolamine: Mix 5 mg with 9 mL of NS; inject a small amount of this dilution into extravasation area; blanching should reverse immediately. Monitor site; if blanching should recur, additional injections of phentolamine may be needed.

Dosage Forms Injection, as hydrochloride: 12.5 mg/mL (20 mL)

Dobutamine Hydrochloride *see* Dobutamine *on previous page*

Dobutrex® *see* Dobutamine *on previous page*

Docetaxel (doe se TAKS el)

Brand Names Taxotere®

Therapeutic Category Antineoplastic Agent, Antimicrotubular

Use FDA-approved: Treatment of patients with locally advanced or metastatic breast cancer who have progressed during anthracycline-based therapy or have relapsed during anthracycline-based adjuvant therapy

Investigational: Treatment of nonsmall cell lung cancer, gastric, pancreatic, head and neck, ovarian, soft tissue sarcoma, and melanoma

Pregnancy Risk Factor D

Contraindications History of hypersensitivity to any component

Warnings/Precautions

Early studies reported severe hypersensitivity reactions characterized by hypotension, bronchospasms, or minor reactions characterized by generalized rash/erythema. The overall incidence was 25% in patients who did not receive premedication.

Fluid retention syndrome characterized by pleural effusions, ascites, edema and weight gain (2-15 kg) has also been reported. It has not been associated with cardiac, pulmonary, renal, hepatic, or endocrine dysfunction. The incidence

(Continued)

Docetaxel *(Continued)*

and severity of the syndrome increase sharply at cumulative doses ≥400 mg/m^2.

Premedication to reduce fluid retention and hypersensitivity reactions: Oral dexamethasone 16 mg/day for 3 days starting on one day prior to docetaxel exposure

Neutropenia was the dose-limiting toxicity; however this rarely resulted in treatment delays and prophylactic colony stimulating factors have not been routinely used. Patients with increased liver function tests experienced more episodes of neutropenia with a greater number of severe infections. Patients with an absolute neutrophil count <1500 cells/mm^3 should not receive docetaxel.

Adverse Reactions

Irritant chemotherapy

>10%:

Central nervous system: Fever
Dermatologic: Alopecia
Gastrointestinal: Nausea, vomiting, diarrhea, stomatitis
Hematologic: Neutropenia, leukopenia, thrombocytopenia, anemia
Neuromuscular & skeletal: Myalgia

1% to 10%: Cardiovascular: Severe fluid retention: poorly tolerated peripheral edema, generalized edema, pleural effusion requiring urgent drainage, dyspnea at rest, cardiac tamponade or pronounced abdominal distention (due to ascites)

>1%: Miscellaneous: Hypersensitivity reactions

Drug Interactions Cytochrome P-450 substrate

Increased toxicity: Possibility of an inhibition of metabolism in patients treated with ketoconazole, erythromycin, terfenadine, and cyclosporine

Stability Docetaxel is available in 20 mg and 80 mg vials prepackaged with a special diluent and formulated in polysorbate 80. Docetaxel is diluted with 13% (w/w) ethanol in water giving a final concentration of 10 mg/mL. Docetaxel is slightly more water soluble than paclitaxel. Intact vials should stored under refrigeration (2°C to 8°C/36°F to 46°F) and protected from light. Vials should be stored at room temperature for approximately 5 minutes before using.

Docetaxel is **compatible** with 0.9% sodium chloride or 5% dextrose in water and should be diluted to a final concentration of 0.3-0.9 mg/mL. Diluted solutions are stable for 8 hours at either room temperature (15°C to 25°C/59°F to 77°F) or refrigeration (2°C to 8°C/36°F to 46°F). Solutions must be prepared in a glass bottle, polypropylene, or polyolefin plastic bag to prevent leaching of plasticizers. Nonpolyvinylchloride tubing should be used.

Mechanism of Action Semisynthetic agent prepared from a noncytotoxic precursor which is extracted from the needles of the European Yew *Taxus baccatta*. Docetaxel differs structurally from the prototype taxoid, paclitaxel, by substitutions at the C-10 and C-5 positions. It is an antimicrotubule agent, but exhibits a unique mechanism of action. Unlike other antimicrotubule agents that induce microtubule disassembly (eg, vinca alkaloids and colchicine), docetaxel promotes the assembly of microtubules from tubulin dimers, and inhibits the depolymerization of tubulin which leads to bundles of microtubules in the cell.

Pharmacodynamics/Kinetics Administered by I.V. infusion and exhibits linear pharmacokinetics at the recommended dosage range

Distribution: Exhibits a triphasic decline in plasma concentrations. Initial rapid decline represents distribution to the peripheral compartment and the terminal phase reflects a relatively slow efflux of docetaxel from the peripheral compartment. mean steady state: 36.6-95.6 L/m^2, indicating extensive extravascular distribution and/or tissue binding. Mean steady state volume of distribution is 113 Liters.

Protein binding: 94% mainly to alpha$_1$-acid glycoprotein, albumin, and lipoproteins

Metabolism: Oxidative metabolism by the liver. Isoenzymes of cytochrome P-450 (CYA3A) are involved in the metabolism

Half-lifes; α, β, and γ phases are 4 minutes, 36 minutes, and 11.1 hours, respectively

Elimination: Following oxidative metabolism, docetaxel is eliminated in both urine (6%) and feces (75%) with approximately 80% eliminated in the first 48 hours

Mean values for total body clearance 21 L/hour/m^2

Usual Dosage Corticosteroids (oral dexamethasone 8 mg twice daily for 3 days starting 1 day prior to docetaxel administration) are necessary to reduce the potential for hypersensitivity and severe fluid retention.

Adults: I.V. infusion: Refer to individual protocol

Locally advanced or metastatic carcinoma of the breast: 60-100 mg/m^2 over 1 hour every 3 weeks

Dosage adjustment in patients who are initially started at 100 mg/m² (>1 week), cumulative cutaneous reactions, or severe peripheral neuropathy: 75 mg/m².

Note: If the patient continues to experience these adverse reactions, the dosage should be reduced to 55 mg/m² or therapy should be discontinued.

Dosage adjustment in hepatic impairment:

Total bilirubin ≥ the upper limit of normal (ULN), or SGOT/SGPT >1.5 times the ULN concomitant with alkaline phosphatase >2.5 times the ULN: Docetaxel **should not be administered** secondary to increased incidence of treatment-related mortality

Administration

Anaphylactoid-like reactions have been reported: Premedication with dexamethasone (8 mg orally twice daily for 5 days starting one day prior to administration of docetaxel)

Administer I.V. infusion over 1-hour

Monitoring Parameters Monitor for hypersensitivity reactions and fluid retention

Patient Information Alopecia occurs in almost all patients

Dosage Forms Injection: 10 mg/mL (2 mL, 8 mL)

Docusate (DOK yoo sate)

Related Information

Laxatives, Classification and Properties *on page 1412*

Brand Names Colace® [OTC]; DC 240® Softgels® [OTC]; Dialose® [OTC]; Diocto® [OTC]; Diocto-K® [OTC]; Dioeze® [OTC]; Disonate® [OTC]; DOK® [OTC]; DOS® Softgel® [OTC]; D-S-S® [OTC]; Kasof® [OTC]; Modane® Soft [OTC]; Pro-Cal-Sof® [OTC]; Regulax SS® [OTC]; Sulfalax® [OTC]; Surfak® [OTC]

Canadian/Mexican Brand Names Albert® Docusate (Canada); Colax-C® (Canada); PMS-Docusate Calcium (Canada); Regulex® (Canada); Selax® (Canada); SoFlax® (Canada)

Synonyms Dioctyl Calcium Sulfosuccinate; Dioctyl Potassium Sulfosuccinate; Dioctyl Sodium Sulfosuccinate; Docusate Calcium; Docusate Potassium; Docusate Sodium; DOSS; DSS

Therapeutic Category Laxative, Surfactant; Stool Softener

Use Stool softener in patients who should avoid straining during defecation and constipation associated with hard, dry stools; prophylaxis for straining (valsalva) following myocardial infarction. A safe agent to be used in elderly; some evidence that doses <200 mg are ineffective; stool softeners are unnecessary if stool is well hydrated or "mushy" and soft; shown to be ineffective used long-term.

Pregnancy Risk Factor C

Contraindications Concomitant use of mineral oil; intestinal obstruction, acute abdominal pain, nausea, vomiting; hypersensitivity to docusate or any component

Warnings/Precautions Prolonged, frequent or excessive use may result in dependence or electrolyte imbalance

Adverse Reactions

1% to 10%:

Gastrointestinal: Intestinal obstruction, diarrhea, abdominal cramping

Miscellaneous: Throat irritation

Overdosage/Toxicology Symptoms of overdose include abdominal cramps, diarrhea, fluid loss, hypokalemia; treatment is symptomatic

Drug Interactions

Decreased effect of Coumadin® with high doses of docusate

Increased toxicity with mineral oil, phenolphthalein

Mechanism of Action Reduces surface tension of the oil-water interface of the stool resulting in enhanced incorporation of water and fat allowing for stool softening

Pharmacodynamics/Kinetics Onset of action: 12-72 hours

Usual Dosage Docusate salts are interchangeable; the amount of sodium, calcium, or potassium per dosage unit is clinically insignificant

Infants and Children <3 years: Oral: 10-40 mg/day in 1-4 divided doses

Children: Oral:

3-6 years: 20-60 mg/day in 1-4 divided doses

6-12 years: 40-150 mg/day in 1-4 divided doses

Adolescents and Adults: Oral: 50-500 mg/day in 1-4 divided doses

Older Children and Adults: Rectal: Add 50-100 mg of docusate liquid to enema fluid (saline or water); administer as retention or flushing enema

Test Interactions ↓ potassium (S), ↓ chloride (S)

Patient Information Adults: Docusate should be taken with a full glass of water; do not use if abdominal pain, nausea, or vomiting are present; laxative use should be used for a short period of time (<1 week); prolonged use may result in

(Continued)

Docusate *(Continued)*

abuse, dependence, as well as fluid and electrolyte loss; notify physician if bleeding occurs or if constipation is not relieved

Nursing Implications Docusate liquid should be given with milk, fruit juice, or infant formula to mask the bitter taste

Dosage Forms

Capsule, as calcium:
- DC 240® Softgels®, Pro-Cal-Sof®, Sulfalax®: 240 mg
- Surfak®: 50 mg, 240 mg

Capsule, as potassium:
- Diocto-K®: 100 mg
- Kasof®: 240 mg

Capsule, as sodium:
- Colace®: 50 mg, 100 mg
- Dioeze®: 250 mg
- Disonate®: 100 mg, 240 mg
- DOK®: 100 mg, 250 mg
- DOS® Softgel®: 100 mg, 250 mg
- D-S-S®: 100 mg
- Modane® Soft: 100 mg
- Regulax SS®: 100 mg, 250 mg

Liquid, as sodium (Diocto®, Colace®, Disonate®, DOK®): 150 mg/15 mL (30 mL, 60 mL, 480 mL)

Solution, oral, as sodium (Doxinate®): 50 mg/mL with alcohol 5% (60 mL, 3780 mL)

Syrup, as sodium:
- 50 mg/15 mL (15 mL, 30 mL)
- Colace®, Diocto®, Disonate®, DOK®: 60 mg/15 mL (240 mL, 480 mL, 3780 mL)

Tablet, as sodium (Dialose®): 100 mg

Docusate Calcium *see* Docusate *on previous page*
Docusate Potassium *see* Docusate *on previous page*
Docusate Sodium *see* Docusate *on previous page*
DOK® [OTC] *see* Docusate *on previous page*
Doktors® Nasal Solution [OTC] *see* Phenylephrine *on page 989*
Dolacet® *see* Hydrocodone and Acetaminophen *on page 620*
Dolene® *see* Propoxyphene *on page 1065*
Dolobid® *see* Diflunisal *on page 383*
Dolophine® *see* Methadone *on page 798*
Dolorac® [OTC] *see* Capsaicin *on page 197*
Dome Paste Bandage *see* Zinc Gelatin *on page 1323*

Donepezil (don EH pa zil)

Brand Names Aricept®

Synonyms E2020

Therapeutic Category Cholinergic Agent

Use Treatment of mild to moderate dementia of the Alzheimer's type

Pregnancy Risk Factor C

Contraindications Patients who are hypersensitive to donepezil or piperidine derivatives

Warnings/Precautions Use with caution in patients with sick sinus syndrome or other supraventricular cardiac conduction abnormalities, in patients with seizures or asthma; avoid use in nursing mothers

Adverse Reactions

>10%:
- Central nervous system: Headache
- Gastrointestinal: Nausea, diarrhea

1% to 10%:
- Cardiovascular: Syncope, chest pain
- Central nervous system: Fatigue, insomnia, dizziness, depression, abnormal dreams, somnolence
- Dermatologic: Bruising
- Gastrointestinal: Anorexia, vomiting, weight loss
- Genitourinary: Polyuria
- Neuromuscular & skeletal: Muscle cramps, arthritis, body pain

Overdosage/Toxicology General supportive measures; can cause a cholinergic crisis characterized by severe nausea, vomiting, salivation, sweating, bradycardia, hypotension, collapse, and convulsions; increased muscle weakness is a possibility and may result in death if respiratory muscles are involved

Tertiary anticholinergics, such as atropine, may be used as an antidote for overdosage. I.V. atropine sulfate titrated to effect is recommended; initial dose of

1-2 mg I.V. with subsequent doses based upon clinical response. Atypical increases in blood pressure and heart rate have been reported with other cholinomimetics when coadministered with quaternary anticholinergics such as glycopyrrolate.

Drug Interactions Increased effects of succinylcholine, cholinesterase inhibitors, or cholinergic agonists (bethanechol). Concomitant NSAIDs may increase the risk of gastrointestinal bleeding.

Usual Dosage Adults: Initial: 5 mg/day at bedtime; may increase to 10 mg/day at bedtime after 4-6 weeks

Dosage Forms Tablet: 5 mg, 10 mg

Donnamar® *see* Hyoscyamine *on page 635*

Donnapine® *see* Hyoscyamine, Atropine, Scopolamine, and Phenobarbital *on page 637*

Donna-Sed® *see* Hyoscyamine, Atropine, Scopolamine, and Phenobarbital *on page 637*

Donnatal® *see* Hyoscyamine, Atropine, Scopolamine, and Phenobarbital *on page 637*

Donphen® *see* Hyoscyamine, Atropine, Scopolamine, and Phenobarbital *on page 637*

Dopamine (DOE pa meen)

Related Information

Adrenergic Agonists, Cardiovascular Comparison *on page 1385*
Adult ACLS Algorithm, Bradycardia *on page 1514*
Adult ACLS Algorithm, Hypotension, Shock *on page 1516*
Cardiovascular Agents Comparison *on page 1405*
Extravasation Treatment of Other Drugs *on page 1381*

Brand Names Intropin®

Synonyms Dopamine Hydrochloride

Therapeutic Category Adrenergic Agonist Agent; Sympathomimetic; Vesicant

Use Adjunct in the treatment of shock which persists after adequate fluid volume replacement

Pregnancy Risk Factor C

Contraindications Hypersensitivity to sulfites (commercial preparation contains sodium bisulfite); pheochromocytoma or ventricular fibrillation

Warnings/Precautions Safety in children has not been established; hypovolemia should be corrected by appropriate plasma volume expanders before administration; extravasation may cause tissue necrosis; potent drug, must be diluted prior to use; patient's hemodynamic status should be monitored; use with caution in patients with cardiovascular disease or cardiac arrhythmias or patients with occlusive vascular disease

Adverse Reactions

>10%:

- Cardiovascular: Ectopic heartbeats, tachycardia, vasoconstriction, hypotension, cardiac conduction abnormalities, widened QRS complex, ventricular arrhythmias
- Central nervous system: Headache
- Gastrointestinal: Nausea, vomiting
- Respiratory: Dyspnea

1% to 10%: Cardiovascular: Bradycardia, hypertension, gangrene of the extremities

<1%:

- Cardiovascular: Vasoconstriction
- Central nervous system: Anxiety
- Neuromuscular & skeletal: Piloerection
- Renal: Azotemia, decreased urine output

Overdosage/Toxicology Symptoms of overdose include severe hypertension, cardiac arrhythmias, acute renal failure

Important: Antidote for peripheral ischemia: To prevent sloughing and necrosis in ischemic areas, the area should be infiltrated as soon as possible with 10-15 mL of saline solution containing from 5-10 mg of Regitine® (brand of phentolamine), an adrenergic blocking agent. A syringe with a fine hypodermic needle should be used, and the solution liberally infiltrated throughout the ischemic area. Sympathetic blockade with phentolamine causes immediate and conspicuous local hyperemic changes if the area is infiltrated within 12 hours. Therefore, phentolamine should be given as soon as possible after the extravasation is noted.

Drug Interactions Increased effect: Dopamine's effects are prolonged and intensified by MAO inhibitors, alpha- and beta-adrenergic blockers, general anesthetics, phenytoin

(Continued)

Dopamine *(Continued)*

Stability Protect from light; solutions that are darker than slightly yellow should not be used; **incompatible** with alkaline solutions or iron salts; **compatible** when coadministered with dobutamine, epinephrine, isoproterenol, and lidocaine

Mechanism of Action Stimulates both adrenergic and dopaminergic receptors, lower doses are mainly dopaminergic stimulating and produce renal and mesenteric vasodilation, higher doses also are both dopaminergic and beta$_1$-adrenergic stimulating and produce cardiac stimulation and renal vasodilation; large doses stimulate alpha-adrenergic receptors

Pharmacodynamics/Kinetics

Children: With medication changes, may not achieve steady-state for ~1 hour rather than 20 minutes

Adults:

Onset of action: 5 minutes

Duration: <10 minutes

Metabolism: In the plasma, kidneys, and liver 75% to inactive metabolites by monoamine oxidase and 25% to norepinephrine (active)

Half-life: 2 minutes

Elimination: Metabolites are excreted in urine; neonatal clearance varies and appears to be age related; clearance is more prolonged with combined hepatic and renal dysfunction

Dopamine has exhibited nonlinear kinetics in children

Usual Dosage I.V. infusion:

Children: 1-20 mcg/kg/minute, maximum: 50 mcg/kg/minute continuous infusion, titrate to desired response

Adults: 1-5 mcg/kg/minute up to 50 mcg/kg/minute, titrate to desired response; infusion may be increased by 1-4 mcg/kg/minute at 10- to 30-minute intervals until optimal response is obtained

If dosages >20-30 mcg/kg/minute are needed, a more direct-acting pressor may be more beneficial (ie, epinephrine, norepinephrine)

The hemodynamic effects of dopamine are dose-dependent:

Low-dose: 1-5 mcg/kg/minute, increased renal blood flow and urine output

Intermediate-dose: 5-15 mcg/kg/minute, increased renal blood flow, heart rate, cardiac contractility, and cardiac output

High-dose: >15 mcg/kg/minute, alpha-adrenergic effects begin to predominate, vasoconstriction, increased blood pressure

Administration

Administer into large vein to prevent the possibility of extravasation; monitor continuously for free flow; use infusion device to control rate of flow; administration into an umbilical arterial catheter is not recommended; central line administration

To prepare for infusion:

$$\frac{6 \times \text{weight (kg)} \times \text{desired dose (mcg/kg/min)}}{\text{I.V. infusion rate (mL/h)}} = \text{mg of drug to be added to 100 mL of I.V. fluid}$$

Monitoring Parameters Blood pressure, EKG, heart rate, CVP, RAP, MAP, urine output; if pulmonary artery catheter is in place, monitor CI, PCWP, SVR, and PVR

Nursing Implications Extravasation: Due to short half-life, withdrawal of drug is often only necessary treatment. Use phentolamine as antidote; mix 5 mg with 9 mL of NS; inject a small amount of this dilution into extravasated area; blanching should reverse immediately. Monitor site; if blanching should recur, additional injections of phentolamine may be needed.

Dosage Forms

Infusion, as hydrochloride, in D_5W: 0.8 mg/mL (250 mL, 500 mL); 1.6 mg/mL (250 mL, 500 mL); 3.2 mg/mL (250 mL, 500 mL)

Injection, as hydrochloride: 40 mg/mL (5 mL, 10 mL, 20 mL); 80 mg/mL (5 mL, 20 mL); 160 mg/mL (5 mL)

Dopamine Hydrochloride *see* Dopamine *on previous page*

Dopar® *see* Levodopa *on page 714*

Dopram® *see* Doxapram *on page 422*

Doral® *see* Quazepam *on page 1083*

Dorcol® [OTC] *see* Acetaminophen *on page 19*

Dormarex® 2 Oral [OTC] *see* Diphenhydramine *on page 399*

Dormin® Oral [OTC] *see* Diphenhydramine *on page 399*

Dornase Alfa (DOOR nase AL fa)

Brand Names Pulmozyme®

Synonyms DNase; Recombinant Human Deoxyribonuclease

Therapeutic Category Enzyme

Use Management of cystic fibrosis patients to reduce the frequency of respiratory infections that require parenteral antibiotics, and to improve pulmonary function; has also demonstrated value in the treatment of chronic bronchitis

Pregnancy Risk Factor B

Contraindications Contraindicated in patients with known hypersensitivity to dornase alfa, Chinese hamster ovary cell products (eg, epoetin alfa), or any component

Warnings/Precautions No clinical trials have been conducted to demonstrate safety and effectiveness of dornase in children <5 years of age, in patients with pulmonary function <40% of normal, or in patients for longer treatment periods >12 months; no data exists regarding safety during lactation

Adverse Reactions

>10%:

- Respiratory: Pharyngitis
- Miscellaneous: Voice alteration

1% to 10%:

- Cardiovascular: Chest pain
- Dermatologic: Rash
- Ocular: Conjunctivitis
- Respiratory: Laryngitis, cough, dyspnea, hemoptysis, rhinitis, hoarse throat, wheezing

Stability Must be stored in the refrigerator at 2°C to 8°C (36°F to 46°F) and protected from strong light; should not be exposed to room temperature for a total of 24 hours

Mechanism of Action The hallmark of cystic fibrosis lung disease is the presence of abundant, purulent airway secretions composed primarily of highly polymerized DNA. The principal source of this DNA is the nuclei of degenerating neutrophils, which is present in large concentrations in infected lung secretions. The presence of this DNA produces a viscous mucous that may contribute to the decreased mucocilliary transport and persistent infections that are commonly seen in this population. Dornase alfa is a deoxyribonuclease (DNA) enzyme produced by recombinant gene technology. Dornase selectively cleaves DNA, thus reducing mucous viscosity and as a result, airflow in the lung is improved and the risk of bacterial infection may be decreased.

Pharmacodynamics/Kinetics Following nebulization, enzyme levels are measurable in the sputum within 15 minutes and decline rapidly thereafter

Usual Dosage Children >5 years and Adults: Inhalation: 2.5 mg once daily through selected nebulizers in conjunction with a Pulmo-Aide® or a Pari-Proneb® compressor

Nursing Implications Should not be diluted or mixed with any other drugs in the nebulizer, this may inactivate the drug

Dosage Forms Solution, inhalation: 1 mg/mL (2.5 mL)

Doryx® Oral *see* Doxycycline *on page 430*

Dorzolamide (dor ZOLE a mide)

Related Information

Glaucoma Drug Therapy Comparison *on page 1410*

Brand Names Trusopt®

Synonyms Dorzolamide Hydrochloride

Therapeutic Category Carbonic Anhydrase Inhibitor

Use Lowers intraocular pressure to treat glaucoma in patients with ocular hypertension or open-angle glaucoma

Pregnancy Risk Factor C

Contraindications Hypersensitivity to any component of the product; contains benzalkonium chloride as a preservative

Warnings/Precautions

Although administered topically, systemic absorption occurs. Same types of adverse reactions attributed to sulfonamides may occur with topical administration.

Because dorzolamide and its metabolite are excreted predominantly by the kidney, it is not recommended for use in patients with severe renal impairment (Cl_{cr} <30 mL/minute); use with caution in patients with hepatic impairment

Local ocular adverse effects (conjunctivitis and lid reactions) were reported with chronic administration. Many resolved with discontinuation of drug therapy. If such reactions occur, discontinue dorzolamide.

(Continued)

Dorzolamide *(Continued)*

There is a potential for an additive effect in patients receiving an oral carbonic anhydrase inhibitor and dorzolamide. The concomitant administration of dorzolamide and oral carbonic anhydrase inhibitors is not recommended.

Benzalkonium chloride is the preservative in dorzolamide which may be absorbed by soft contact lenses. Dorzolamide should not be administered while wearing soft contact lenses.

Adverse Reactions

>10%:

Gastrointestinal: Bitter taste following administration (25%)

Ocular: Burning, stinging or discomfort immediately following administration (33%); superficial punctate keratitis (10% to 15%); signs and symptoms of ocular allergic reaction (10%)

5% to 10% Ocular: Blurred vision, tearing, dryness, photophobia

<1%:

Central nervous system: Headache, fatigue

Dermatologic: Rashes

Gastrointestinal: Nausea

Genitourinary: Urolithiasis

Neuromuscular & skeletal: Weakness

Ocular: Iridocyclitis

Overdosage/Toxicology Symptoms of overdose include electrolyte imbalance, development of an acidotic state and possible CNS effects; treatment is symptomatic

Drug Interactions Increased toxicity: Salicylates use may result in carbonic anhydrase inhibitor accumulation and toxicity including CNS depression and metabolic acidosis

Stability Store at room temperature (25°C)

Mechanism of Action Reversible inhibition of the enzyme carbonic anhydrase resulting in reduction of hydrogen ion secretion at renal tubule and an increased renal excretion of sodium, potassium, bicarbonate, and water to decrease production of aqueous humor; also inhibits carbonic anhydrase in central nervous system to retard abnormal and excessive discharge from CNS neurons

Pharmacodynamics/Kinetics

Peak effect: 2 hours

Duration: 8-12 hours

Absorption: Topical: Reaches the systemic circulation where it accumulates in RBCs during chronic dosing as a result of binding to CA-11

Distribution: Accumulates in RBCs during chronic administration

Protein binding: 33%

Half-life: Terminal RBC half-life of 147 days

Metabolism: Metabolized to N-desethyl metabolite that also inhibits carbonic anhydrase less potently than the parent drug

Elimination: Dorzolamide and its metabolite (N-desethyl) are excreted in the urine. After dosing is stopped, dorzolamide washes out of RBCs nonlinearly, resulting in a rapid decline of drug concentration initially, followed by a slower elimination phase with a half-life of about 4 months.

Usual Dosage Adults: Glaucoma: Instill 1 drop in the affected eye(s) 3 times/day

Administration If more than one topical ophthalmic drug is being used, administer the drugs at least 10 minutes apart. Instruct patients to avoid allowing the tip of the dispensing container to contact the eye or surrounding structures. Ocular solutions can become contaminated by common bacteria known to cause ocular infections. Serious damage to the eye and subsequent loss of vision may occur from using contaminated solutions.

Monitoring Parameters Monitor serum electrolyte levels (potassium) and blood pH levels; Ophthalmic exams and IOP periodically

Patient Information

If serious or unusual reactions or signs of hypersensitivity occur, discontinue use of the product

If any ocular reactions, particularly conjunctivitis and lid reactions, discontinue use and seek physician's advice. If an intercurrent ocular condition (eg, trauma, ocular surgery, infection) occur, immediately seek your physician's advice concerning the continued use of the present multidose container.

Avoid allowing the tip of the dispensing container to contact the eye or surround structures

Dosage Forms Solution, ophthalmic, as hydrochloride: 2%

Dorzolamide Hydrochloride *see* Dorzolamide *on previous page*

Dose Equivalents for Opioid Analgesics in Opioid-Naive Adults <50 kg *see page 1376*

Dose Equivalents for Opioid Analgesics in Opioid-Naive Adults ≥50 kg *see page 1375*

Dosing Data for Acetaminophen and NSAIDs *see page 1377*

DOSS *see* Docusate *on page 415*

DOS® Softgel® [OTC] *see* Docusate *on page 415*

Dovonex® *see* Calcipotriene *on page 181*

Doxacurium (doks a KYOO ri um)

Related Information

Neuromuscular Blocking Agents Comparison *on page 1417*

Brand Names Nuromax® Injection

Synonyms Doxacurium Chloride

Therapeutic Category Neuromuscular Blocker Agent, Nondepolarizing; Skeletal Muscle Relaxant

Use Adjunct to general anesthesia; provides skeletal muscle relaxation during surgery. Doxacurium is a long-acting nondepolarizing neuromuscular blocker with virtually no cardiovascular side effects. The characteristics of this agent make it especially useful in procedures requiring careful maintenance of hemodynamic stability for prolonged periods.

Pregnancy Risk Factor C

Contraindications Hypersensitivity to doxacurium or any component

Warnings/Precautions Use with caution in the elderly, effects and duration are more variable; product contains benzoyl alcohol; use with caution in newborns; use with caution in patients with neuromuscular diseases such as myasthenia gravis; resistance may develop in burn patients; ensure proper electrolyte balance prior to use; use with caution in patients with renal or hepatic impairment

Adverse Reactions

<1%:

- Cardiovascular: Hypotension
- Central nervous system: Fever
- Dermatologic: Urticaria
- Neuromuscular & skeletal: Skeletal muscle weakness
- Ocular: Diplopia
- Respiratory: Respiratory insufficiency and apnea, wheezing
- Miscellaneous: **Produces little, if any, histamine release**

Overdosage/Toxicology Overdosage is manifested by prolonged neuromuscular blockage; treatment is supportive; reverse blockade with neostigmine, pyridostigmine, or edrophonium

Drug Interactions

Decreased effect: Phenytoin, carbamazepine (decreases neuromuscular blockade)

Increased effect: Magnesium, lithium

Prolonged neuromuscular blockade:

- Corticosteroids
- Inhaled anesthetics
- Local anesthetics
- Calcium channel blockers
- Antiarrhythmics (eg, quinidine or procainamide)
- Antibiotics (eg, aminoglycosides, tetracyclines, vancomycin, clindamycin)
- Immunosuppressants (eg, cyclosporine)

Mechanism of Action Doxacurium is a long-acting nondepolarizing skeletal muscle relaxant. The drug is a bis-quaternary benzylisoquinolinium diester, with a chemical structure similar to that of atracurium. Similar to other nondepolarizing neuromuscular blocking agents, doxacurium produces muscle relaxation by competing with acetylcholine for cholinergic receptor sites on the postjunctional membrane; significant presynaptic depressant activity is also observed.

Pharmacodynamics/Kinetics

Onset of effect: 5-11 minutes

Duration: 30 minutes (range: 12-54 minutes)

Protein binding: 30%

Elimination: Primarily as unchanged drug via the kidneys and biliary tract

Recovery time is longer in elderly patients

Usual Dosage I.V. (in obese patients, use ideal body weight to calculate dose):

Children >2 years: Initial: 0.03-0.05 mg/kg followed by maintenance doses of 0.005-0.01 mg/kg after 30-45 minutes

Adults: Surgery: 0.05 mg/kg with thiopental/narcotic or 0.025 mg/kg with succinylcholine; maintenance doses of 0.005-0.01 mg/kg after 60-100 minutes

Dosing adjustment in renal or hepatic impairment: Reduce initial dose and titrate carefully as duration may be prolonged

Monitoring Parameters Blockade is monitored with a peripheral nerve stimulator, should also evaluate EKG, blood pressure, and heart rate

Dosage Forms Injection, as chloride: 1 mg/mL (5 mL)

Doxacurium Chloride *see* Doxacurium *on this page*

Doxapram (DOKS a pram)

Brand Names Dopram®

Synonyms Doxapram Hydrochloride

Therapeutic Category Central Nervous System Stimulant, Nonamphetamine; Respiratory Stimulant

Use Respiratory and CNS stimulant; stimulates respiration in patients with drug-induced CNS depression or postanesthesia respiratory depression; in hospitalized patients with COPD associated with acute hypercapnia

Pregnancy Risk Factor B

Contraindications Hypersensitivity to doxapram or any component; epilepsy, cerebral edema, head injury, severe pulmonary disease, pheochromocytoma, cardiovascular disease, hypertension, hyperthyroidism

Warnings/Precautions Safety of doxapram in children <12 years of age has not been established; may cause severe CNS toxicity, seizures; should be used with caution in newborns as the U.S. product contains benzyl alcohol (0.9%); recommended doses of doxapram for neonates will deliver 5.4-27 mg/kg/day of benzyl alcohol; large amounts of benzyl alcohol (>100 mg/kg/day) have been associated with fatal toxicity (gasping syndrome); the use of doxapram in newborns should be reserved for neonates who are unresponsive to the treatment of apnea with therapeutic serum concentrations of theophylline or caffeine. Doxapram is neither a nonspecific CNS depressant antagonist nor an opiate antagonist.

Adverse Reactions

1% to 10%:

- Cardiovascular: Ectopic beats, hypotension, vasoconstriction, tachycardia, anginal pain, palpitations
- Central nervous system: Headache
- Gastrointestinal: Nausea, vomiting
- Respiratory: Dyspnea

<1%:

- Cardiovascular: Hypertension (dose related), arrhythmias, flushing
- Central nervous system: CNS stimulation, restlessness, lightheadedness, jitters, hallucinations, irritability, seizures, hyperpyrexia
- Gastrointestinal: Abdominal distension, retching
- Hematologic: Hemolysis
- Local: Phlebitis
- Neuromuscular & skeletal: Tremor, hyperreflexia
- Ocular: Mydriasis, lacrimation
- Respiratory: Coughing, laryngospasm
- Miscellaneous: Diaphoresis, feeling of warmth

Overdosage/Toxicology Symptoms of overdose include excessive increases in blood pressure, tachycardia, arrhythmias, muscle spasticity, dyspnea

Supportive care is the preferred treatment; seizures are unlikely and can be treated with benzodiazepines; **doxapram is not dialyzable**.

Drug Interactions Increased toxicity (elevated blood pressure): Sympathomimetics, MAO inhibitors

Halothane, cyclopropane, and enflurane may sensitize the myocardium to catecholamine and epinephrine which is released at the initiation of doxapram, hence, separate discontinuation of anesthetics and start of doxapram by at least 10 minutes

Stability **Incompatible** with aminophylline, thiopental, or sodium bicarbonate (alkali drugs)

Mechanism of Action Stimulates respiration through action on respiratory center in medulla or indirectly on peripheral carotid chemoreceptors

Pharmacodynamics/Kinetics

Onset of action (respiratory stimulation): I.V.: Within 20-40 seconds

Peak effect: Within 1-2 minutes

Duration: 5-12 minutes

Metabolism: In the liver

Half-life:

- Neonates, premature: ~7-10 hours
- Adults: 3.4 hours (mean half-life)

Elimination: In urine as metabolites within 24-48 hours

Usual Dosage Not for use in newborns since doxapram contains a significant amount of benzyl alcohol (0.9%)

Neonatal apnea (apnea of prematurity): I.V.:

- Initial: 1-1.5 mg/kg/hour
- Maintenance: 0.5-2.5 mg/kg/hour, titrated to the lowest rate at which apnea is controlled

Adults: Respiratory depression following anesthesia: I.V.:

- Initial: 0.5-1 mg/kg; may repeat at 5-minute intervals; maximum total dose: 2 mg/kg

I.V. infusion: Initial: 5 mg/minute until adequate response or adverse effects seen; decrease to 1-3 mg/minute; usual total dose: 0.5-4 mg/kg; maximum: 300 mg

Hemodialysis: Not dialyzable

Administration Dilute to 1 mg/mL in D_5W or NS for continuous infusion

Monitoring Parameters Heart rate, blood pressure, reflexes, CNS status, apnea episodes

Nursing Implications Avoid extravasation, rapid infusion may cause hemolysis; not for use in newborns since doxapram injection contains significant amount of benzyl alcohol (0.9%)

Dosage Forms Injection, as hydrochloride: 20 mg/mL (20 mL)

Doxapram Hydrochloride *see* Doxapram *on previous page*

Doxazosin (doks AYE zoe sin)

Brand Names Cardura®

Therapeutic Category Alpha-Adrenergic Blocking Agent, Oral; Antihypertensive

Use Treatment of hypertension alone or in conjunction with diuretics, cardiac glycosides, ACE inhibitors or calcium antagonists (particularly appropriate for those with hypertension and other cardiovascular risk factors such as hypercholesterolemia and diabetes mellitus); treatment of urinary outflow obstruction and/or obstructive and irritative symptoms associated with benign prostatic hyperplasia (particularly useful in patients with troublesome symptoms who are unable or unwilling to undergo invasive procedures, but who require rapid symptomatic relief)

Pregnancy Risk Factor B

Contraindications Hypersensitivity to doxazosin or any component

Warnings/Precautions Use with caution in patients with renal impairment. Can cause marked hypotension and syncope with sudden loss of consciousness with the first dose. Anticipate a similar effect if therapy is interrupted for a few days, if dosage is increased rapidly, or if another antihypertensive drug is introduced.

Adverse Reactions

>10%: Central nervous system: Dizziness

1% to 10%:

- Cardiovascular: Palpitations, arrhythmia
- Central nervous system: Vertigo, nervousness, somnolence, anxiety
- Endocrine & metabolic: Decreased libido
- Gastrointestinal: Nausea, vomiting, xerostomia, diarrhea, constipation
- Neuromuscular & skeletal: Shoulder, neck, back pain
- Ocular: Abnormal vision
- Respiratory: Rhinitis

<1%:

- Cardiovascular: Hypotension, tachycardia
- Central nervous system: Depression
- Gastrointestinal: Abdominal discomfort, flatulence
- Genitourinary: Incontinence, polyuria
- Ocular: Conjunctivitis
- Otic: Tinnitus
- Respiratory: Dyspnea, sinusitis, epistaxis

Overdosage/Toxicology Symptoms of overdose include severe hypotension, drowsiness, tachycardia

Hypotension usually responds to I.V. fluids, Trendelenburg positioning, or parenteral vasoconstrictor; treatment is primarily supportive and symptomatic.

Drug Interactions

Decreased effect with NSAIDs

Increased effect with diuretics and antihypertensive medications (especially beta-blockers)

Mechanism of Action Competitively inhibits postsynaptic alpha-adrenergic receptors which results in vasodilation of veins and arterioles and a decrease in total peripheral resistance and blood pressure; approximately 50% as potent on a weight by weight basis as prazosin

Usual Dosage Oral:

Adults: 1 mg once daily in morning or evening; may be increased to 2 mg once daily; thereafter titrate upwards, if needed, over several weeks, balancing therapeutic benefit with doxazosin-induced postural hypotension; maximum dose for hypertension: 16 mg/day, for BPH: 8 mg/day

Elderly: Initial: 0.5 mg once daily

Monitoring Parameters Blood pressure, standing and sitting/supine

Test Interactions Increased urinary VMA 17%, norepinephrine metabolite 42%

(Continued)

Doxazosin *(Continued)*

Patient Information Rise from sitting/lying position carefully; may cause dizziness; report to physician if painful persistent erection occurs; take the first dose at bedtime

Nursing Implications Syncope may occur usually within 90 minutes of the initial dose

Dosage Forms Tablet: 1 mg, 2 mg, 4 mg, 8 mg

Doxepin (DOKS e pin)

Related Information

Antidepressant Agents Comparison *on page 1393*

Brand Names Adapin® Oral; Sinequan® Oral; Zonalon® Topical Cream

Canadian/Mexican Brand Names Apo-Doxepin® (Canada); Novo-Doxepin® (Canada); Triadapin® (Canada)

Synonyms Doxepin Hydrochloride

Therapeutic Category Antianxiety Agent; Antidepressant, Tricyclic

Use

Oral: Treatment of various forms of depression, usually in conjunction with psychotherapy; treatment of anxiety disorders

Unlabeled use: Analgesic for certain chronic and neuropathic pain

Topical: Short-term (<8 days) management of moderate pruritus in adults with atopic dermatitis or lichen simplex chronicus

Pregnancy Risk Factor C

Contraindications Hypersensitivity to doxepin or any component (cross-sensitivity with other tricyclic antidepressants may occur); narrow-angle glaucoma

Warnings/Precautions Use with caution in patients with cardiovascular disease, conduction disturbances, seizure disorders, urinary retention, hyperthyroidism, or those receiving thyroid replacement; avoid use during lactation; use with caution in pregnancy; do not discontinue abruptly in patients receiving chronic high-dose therapy

Adverse Reactions

>10%:

- Central nervous system: Sedation, drowsiness, dizziness, headache
- Gastrointestinal: Xerostomia, constipation, increased appetite, nausea, unpleasant taste, weight gain
- Neuromuscular & skeletal: Weakness

1% to 10%:

- Cardiovascular: Hypotension, arrhythmias
- Central nervous system: Confusion, delirium, hallucinations, nervousness, restlessness, parkinsonian syndrome, insomnia
- Gastrointestinal: Diarrhea, heartburn
- Genitourinary: Sexual dysfunction, dysuria
- Neuromuscular & skeletal: Fine muscle tremors
- Ocular: Blurred vision, eye pain
- Miscellaneous: Diaphoresis (excessive)

<1%:

- Central nervous system: Anxiety, seizures
- Dermatologic: Alopecia, photosensitivity
- Endocrine & metabolic: Breast enlargement, galactorrhea, SIADH
- Gastrointestinal: Trouble with gums, decreased lower esophageal sphincter tone may cause GE reflux
- Genitourinary: Urinary retention, testicular edema
- Hematologic: Agranulocytosis, leukopenia, eosinophilia
- Hepatic: Hepatitis, cholestatic jaundice and increased liver enzymes
- Ocular: Increased intraocular pressure
- Otic: Tinnitus
- Miscellaneous: Allergic reactions

Overdosage/Toxicology Symptoms of overdose include confusion, hallucinations, seizures, urinary retention, hypothermia, hypotension, tachycardia, cyanosis

Following initiation of essential overdose management, toxic symptoms should be treated. Sodium bicarbonate is indicated when QRS interval is >0.10 seconds or QT_c >0.42 seconds. Ventricular arrhythmias often respond to systemic alkalinization with or without phenytoin 15-20 mg/kg (adults) (sodium bicarbonate 0.5-2 mEq/kg I.V.). Arrhythmias unresponsive to this therapy may respond to lidocaine 1 mg/kg I.V. followed by a titrated infusion. Physostigmine (1-2 mg I.V. slowly for adults or 0.5 mg I.V. slowly for children) may be indicated in reversing cardiac arrhythmias that are life-threatening. Seizures usually respond to diazepam I.V. boluses (5-10 mg for adults up to 30 mg or 0.25-0.4 mg/kg/dose for children up to 10 mg/dose). If seizures are unresponsive or recur, phenytoin or phenobarbital may be required.

Drug Interactions

Decreased effect of bretylium, guanethidine, clonidine, levodopa; decreased effect with ascorbic acid, cholestyramine

Increased effect/toxicity of carbamazepine, amphetamines, thyroid preparations, sympathomimetics

Increased toxicity with fluoxetine (seizures), thyroid preparations, MAO inhibitors, albuterol, CNS depressants (ie, benzodiazepines, opiate analgesics, phenothiazines, alcohol), anticholinergics, cimetidine

Stability Protect from light

Mechanism of Action Increases the synaptic concentration of serotonin and/or norepinephrine in the central nervous system by inhibition of their reuptake by the presynaptic neuronal membrane

Pharmacodynamics/Kinetics

Peak effect (antidepressant): Usually more than 2 weeks; anxiolytic effects may occur sooner

Distribution: Crosses the placenta; appears in breast milk

Protein binding: 80% to 85%

Metabolism: Hepatic; metabolites include desmethyldoxepin (active)

Half-life: Adults: 6-8 hours

Elimination: Renal

Usual Dosage

Oral (entire daily dose may be given at bedtime):

Adolescents: Initial: 25-50 mg/day in single or divided doses; gradually increase to 100 mg/day

Adults: Initial: 30-150 mg/day at bedtime or in 2-3 divided doses; may gradually increase up to 300 mg/day; single dose should not exceed 150 mg; select patients may respond to 25-50 mg/day

Dosing adjustment in hepatic impairment: Use a lower dose and adjust gradually

Topical: Adults: Apply a thin film 4 times/day with at least 3- to 4-hour interval between applications

Dietary Considerations Alcohol: Additive CNS effect, avoid use

Monitoring Parameters Monitor blood pressure and pulse rate prior to and during initial therapy; monitor mental status, weight

Reference Range Therapeutic: 30-150 ng/mL; Toxic: >500 ng/mL; utility of serum level monitoring is controversial

Test Interactions ↑ glucose

Patient Information Avoid unnecessary exposure to sunlight; avoid alcohol ingestion; do not discontinue medication abruptly; may cause urine to turn blue-green; may cause drowsiness; can use sugarless gum or hard candy for dry mouth; full effect may not occur for 4-6 weeks

Nursing Implications May increase appetite; may cause drowsiness, raise bed rails, institute safety precautions

Dosage Forms

Capsule, as hydrochloride: 10 mg, 25 mg, 50 mg, 75 mg, 100 mg, 150 mg

Concentrate, oral, as hydrochloride: 10 mg/mL (120 mL)

Cream: 5% (30 g)

Doxepin Hydrochloride *see* Doxepin *on previous page*

Doxil™ *see* Doxorubicin (Liposomal) *on page 428*

Doxorubicin (doks oh ROO bi sin)

Related Information

Antiemetics for Chemotherapy Induced Nausea and Vomiting *on page 1348*

Cancer Chemotherapy Regimens *on page 1351*

Extravasation Management of Chemotherapeutic Agents *on page 1379*

Toxicities of Chemotherapeutic Agents *on page 1382*

Brand Names Adriamycin PFS™; Adriamycin RDF™; Rubex®

Synonyms ADR; Doxorubicin Hydrochloride; Hydroxydaunomycin Hydrochloride

Therapeutic Category Antineoplastic Agent, Anthracycline; Antineoplastic Agent, Antibiotic; Vesicant

Use Treatment of leukemias, lymphomas, multiple myeloma, osseous and nonosseous sarcomas, mesotheliomas, germ cell tumors of the ovary or testis, and carcinomas of the head and neck, thyroid, lung, Wilms' tumor, breast, stomach, pancreas, liver, ovary, bladder, prostate, and uterus, neuroblastoma

Pregnancy Risk Factor D

Contraindications Hypersensitivity to doxorubicin or any component, severe congestive heart failure, cardiomyopathy, pre-existing myelosuppression, patients with impaired cardiac function, patients who received previous treatment with complete cumulative doses of doxorubicin, idarubicin, and/or daunorubicin

Warnings/Precautions The U.S. Food and Drug Administration (FDA) currently recommends that procedures for proper handling and disposal of antineoplastic

(Continued)

Doxorubicin *(Continued)*

agents be considered. Total dose should not exceed 550 mg/m^2 or 400 mg/m^2 in patients with previous or concomitant treatment (with daunorubicin, cyclophosphamide, or irradiation of the cardiac region); irreversible myocardial toxicity may occur as total dosage approaches 550 mg/m^2. A baseline cardiac evaluation (EKG, LVEF, +/- ECHO) is recommended, especially in patients with risk factors for increased cardiac toxicity. I.V. use only, severe local tissue necrosis will result if extravasation occurs; reduce dose in patients with impaired hepatic function; severe myelosuppression is also possible.

Adverse Reactions

>10%:

Dermatologic: Alopecia

Extravasation: Doxorubicin is one of the most notorious vesicants. Infiltration can cause severe inflammation, tissue necrosis, and ulceration. If the drug is infiltrated, consult institutional policy, apply ice to the area, and elevate the limb. Can have ongoing tissue destruction secondary to propagation of free radicals; may require debridement.

Vesicant chemotherapy

Gastrointestinal: Acute nausea and vomiting may be seen in 21% to 55% of patients; mucositis, ulceration, and necrosis of the colon, anorexia, and diarrhea, stomatitis, esophagitis

Emetic potential:

≤20 mg: Moderately low (10% to 30%)

>20 mg or < 60 mg: Moderate (30% to 60%)

≥60 mg: Moderately high (60% to 90%)

Time course for nausea/vomiting: Onset: 1-3 hours; Duration 4-24 hours

Genitourinary: Discoloration of urine (red)

Hematologic: Myelosuppressive: 60% to 80% of patients will have leukopenia; dose-limiting toxicity

WBC: Moderate

Platelets: Moderate

Onset (days): 7

Nadir (days): 10-14

Recovery (days): 21-28

1% to 10%:

Cardiac toxicity: Dose-limiting and related to cumulative dose; usually a maximum total lifetime dose of 450-550 mg/m^2 is administered; although, it has been demonstrated that if given by continuous infusion in breast cancer patients, higher doses may be tolerated. Patients may present with acute toxicity (arrhythmias, heart block, pericarditis-myocarditis) which may be fatal. More commonly, chronic toxicity is seen, in which patients present with signs of congestive heart failure. Treatment includes aggressive management of CHF with digoxin, diuretics and peripheral vasodilators. Several methods of monitoring cardiac toxicity have been utilized, including myocardial biopsy (expensive and hazardous procedure).

Cardiovascular: Facial flushing

Dermatologic: Hyperpigmentation of nail beds, erythematous streaking along the vein if administered too rapidly

Endocrine & metabolic: Hyperuricemia

<1%:

Central nervous system: Fever, chills

Dermatologic: Urticaria

Ocular: Conjunctivitis

Radiation recall: Noticed in patients who have had prior irradiation; reactions include redness, warmth, erythema, and dermatitis in the radiation port. Can progress to severe desquamation and ulceration. Occurs 5-7 days after doxorubicin administration; local therapy with topical corticosteroids and cooling have given the best relief.

Miscellaneous: Allergic reaction, anaphylaxis

Overdosage/Toxicology Symptoms of overdose include myelosuppression, nausea, vomiting, myocardial toxicity

Drug Interactions

Decreased effect:

Doxorubicin may decrease digoxin plasma levels and renal excretion

Phenobarbital increases elimination of doxorubicin

Phenytoin levels decreased by doxorubicin

Increased toxicity:

Cyclosporine may induce coma or seizures

Cyclophosphamide enhances the cardiac toxicity of doxorubicin by producing additional myocardial cell damage

Mercaptopurine increases toxicities

Streptozocin greatly enhances leukopenia and thrombocytopenia by inhibiting doxorubicin metabolism

Verapamil alters the cellular distribution of doxorubicin; may result in ↑ cell toxicity by inhibition of the P-glycoprotein pump

Stability

Store intact vials of solution under refrigeration (2°C to 8°C) and protected from light; store intact vials of lyophilized powder at room temperature (15°C to 30°C)

Reconstitute lyophilized powder with SWI or NS to a final concentration of 2 mg/mL as follows. Reconstituted solution is stable for 7 days at room temperature (25°C) and 15 days under refrigeration (5°C) when protected from light.

10 mg vial = 5 mL

20 mg vial = 10 mL

50 mg vial = 25 mL

Further dilution in D_5W or NS is stable for 48 hours at room temperature (25°C) when protected from light

Unstable in solutions with a pH <3 or >7; avoid aluminum needles and bacteriostatic diluents as precipitation occurs; decomposing drug turns purple; protect from direct sunlight

Incompatible with hydrocortisone, fluorouracil, sodium bicarbonate, aminophylline, heparin, cephalothin, dexamethasone, furosemide, dexamethasone, diazepam

Y-site compatible with vincristine, cyclophosphamide, dacarbazine, bleomycin, vinblastine

Standard I.V. dilution:

I.V. push: Dose/syringe (concentration: 2 mg/mL)

Maximum syringe size for IVP is a 30 mL syringe and syringe should be ≤75% full

Syringes are stable for 7 days at room temperature (25°C) and 15 days under refrigeration (5°C) when protected from light

IVPB: Dose/50-100 mL D_5W or NS

IVPB solutions are stable for 48 hours at room temperature (25°C) when protected from light

Mechanism of Action Doxorubicin works through inhibition of topoisomerase-II at the point of DNA cleavage. A second mechanism of action is the production of free radicals (the hydroxy radical OH) by doxorubicin, which in turn can destroy DNA and cancerous cells. Doxorubicin is also a very powerful iron chelator, equal to deferoxamine. The iron-doxorubicin complex can bind DNA and cell membranes rapidly and produce free radicals that immediately cleave the DNA and cell membranes. Inhibits DNA and RNA synthesis by intercalating between DNA base pairs and by steric obstruction; active throughout entire cell cycle.

Pharmacodynamics/Kinetics

Absorption: Oral: Poor, <50%

Distribution: V_d: 25 L/kg; rapidly distributed into the liver, spleen, kidney, lung and heart, also distributes into breast milk

Protein binding: 70% bound to plasma proteins

Metabolism: In both the liver and in plasma to both active and inactive metabolites

Half-life, triphasic:

Primary: 30 minutes

Secondary: 3-3.5 hours for metabolites

Terminal: 17-30 hours for doxorubicin and its metabolites

Elimination, triphasic: 80% eventually excreted in bile and feces

Usual Dosage Refer to individual protocols

I.V. (patient's ideal weight should be used to calculate body surface area):

Children: 35-75 mg/m^2 as a single dose, repeat every 21 days; **or** 20-30 mg/m^2 once weekly; **or** 60-90 mg/m^2 given as a continuous infusion over 96 hours every 3-4 weeks

Adults: 60-75 mg/m^2 as a single dose, repeat every 21 days **or** other dosage regimens like 20-30 mg/m^2/day for 2-3 days, repeat in 4 weeks **or** 20 mg/m^2 once weekly

The lower dose regimen should be given to patients with decreased bone marrow reserve, prior therapy or marrow infiltration with malignant cells

Currently the maximum cumulative dose is 550 mg/m^2 or 450 mg/m^2 in patients who have received RT to the mediastinal areas; a baseline MUGA should be performed prior to initiating treatment. If the LVEF is <30% to 40%, therapy should not be instituted; LVEF should be monitored during therapy.

Doxorubicin has also been administered intraperitoneal (phase I in refractory ovarian cancer patients) and intra-arterially.

Dosing adjustment in renal impairment: Adjustments not required in mild to moderate renal failure

Cl_{cr} <10 mL/minute: Reduce dose to 75% of normal dose in severe renal failure

Hemodialysis: Supplemental dose is not necessary

(Continued)

Doxorubicin *(Continued)*

Dosing adjustment in hepatic impairment:

Bilirubin 1.2-3 mg/dL or AST 60-180 IU: Administer 50% of dose
Bilirubin 3.1-5 mg/dL or AST >180 IU: Administer 25% of dose
Bilirubin >5 mg/dL: Avoid use

Administration

Administer I.V. push over 1-2 minutes or IVPB; may be further diluted in either NS of D_5W for I.V. administration. Continuous infusions must be administered via central line.

Avoid extravasation, associated with severe ulceration and soft tissue necrosis; flush with 5-10 mL of I.V. solution before and after drug administration

Monitoring Parameters CBC with differential and platelet count, echocardiogram, liver function tests

Patient Information Discolors urine red/orange; immediately report any change in sensation (eg, stinging) at injection site during infusion (may be an early sign of infiltration)

Nursing Implications

Local erythematous streaking along the vein and/or facial flushing may indicate too rapid a rate of administration

Extravasation management:

Apply ice immediately for 30-60 minutes; then alternate off/on every 15 minutes for one day

Topical cooling may be achieved using ice packs or cooling pad with circulating ice water. Cooling of site for 24 hours as tolerated by the patient. Elevate and rest extremity 24-48 hours, then resume normal activity as tolerated. Application of cold inhibits vesicant's cytotoxicity.

Application of heat or sodium bicarbonate can be harmful and is contraindicated

If pain, erythema, and/or swelling persist beyond 48 hours, refer patient immediately to plastic surgeon for consultation and possible debridement

Dosage Forms

Injection, as hydrochloride:
Aqueous, with NS: 2 mg/mL (5 mL, 10 mL, 25 mL)
Preservative free: 2 mg/mL (5 mL, 10 mL, 25 mL, 100 mL)
Powder for injection, as hydrochloride, lyophilized: 10 mg, 20 mg, 50 mg, 100 mg
Powder for injection, as hydrochloride, lyophilized, rapid dissolution formula: 10 mg, 20 mg, 50 mg, 150 mg

Doxorubicin Hydrochloride *see* Doxorubicin *on page 425*

Doxorubicin Hydrochloride (Liposomal) *see* Doxorubicin (Liposomal) *on this page*

Doxorubicin (Liposomal) (doks oh ROO bi sin lip pah SOW mal)

Brand Names Doxil™

Synonyms Doxorubicin Hydrochloride (Liposomal)

Therapeutic Category Antineoplastic Agent, Anthracycline; Antineoplastic Agent, Antibiotic

Use Treatment of AIDS-related Kaposi's sarcoma in patients with disease that has progressed on prior combination chemotherapy or in patients who are intolerant to such therapy

Off-label use: Breast cancer, ovarian cancer, and solid tumors

Pregnancy Risk Factor D

Contraindications Hypersensitivity to doxorubicin or the components of Doxil®

Warnings/Precautions The U.S. Food and Drug Administration (FDA) currently recommends that procedures for proper handling and disposal of antineoplastic agents be considered. Total dose should not exceed 550 mg/m^2 or 400 mg/m^2 in patients with previous or concomitant treatment (with daunorubicin, cyclophosphamide, or irradiation of the cardiac region); irreversible myocardial toxicity may occur as total dosage approaches 550 mg/m^2. I.V. use only, severe local tissue necrosis will result if extravasation occurs; reduce dose in patients with impaired hepatic function; severe myelosuppression is also possible.

Adverse Reactions Information on adverse events is based on the experience reported in 753 patients with AIDS-related Kaposi's sarcoma enrolled in four studies

>10%:

Extravasation: Doxorubicin is one of the most notorious vesicants. Infiltration can cause severe inflammation, tissue necrosis, and ulceration. If the drug is infiltrated, consult institutional policy, apply ice to the area, and elevate the limb. Can have ongoing tissue destruction secondary to propagation of free radicals; may require debridement.

Irritant chemotherapy

Gastrointestinal: Nausea; emetic potential:
- ≤20 mg: Moderately low (10% to 30%)
- >20 mg or <75 mg: Moderate (30% to 60%)
- ≥75 mg: Moderately high (49%)

Hematologic: Myelosuppressive: 60% to 80% of patients will have leukopenia; dose-limiting toxicity
- WBC: Moderate
- Platelets: Moderate
- Onset (days): 7
- Nadir (days): 10-14
- Recovery (days): 21-28

1% to 10%:
- Cardiovascular: Cardiac toxicity (9.7%): Cardiomyopathy, congestive heart failure, arrhythmia, pericardial effusion, tachycardia, facial flushing
- Dermatologic: Hyperpigmentation of nail beds, erythematous streaking along the vein if administered too rapidly
- Endocrine & metabolic: Hyperuricemia

<1%:
- Hypersensitivity: Allergic reaction, anaphylaxis, fever, chills, urticaria
- Ocular: Conjunctivitis

Overdosage/Toxicology Symptoms of overdose include increases in mucositis, leukopenia, and thrombocytopenia

Treatment of acute overdosage consists of treatment of the severely myelosuppressed patient with hospitalization, antibiotics, platelet and granulocyte transfusions and symptomatic treatment of mucositis

Drug Interactions

No formal drug interaction studies have been conducted with doxorubicin hydrochloride liposome injection, however, may interact with drugs known to interact with the conventional formulation of doxorubicin hydrochloride

Decreased effect: Doxorubicin may decrease digoxin plasma levels and renal excretion

Increased effect: Allopurinol may enhance the antitumor activity of doxorubicin (animal data only)

Increased toxicity:
- Cyclophosphamide enhances the cardiac toxicity of doxorubicin by producing additional myocardial cell damage
- Mercaptopurine enhances toxicities
- Streptozocin greatly enhances leukopenia and thrombocytopenia
- Verapamil alters the cellular distribution of doxorubicin; may result in increased cell toxicity by inhibition of the P-glycoprotein pump

Stability Store intact vials of solution under refrigeration (2°C to 8°C) and avoid freezing. Prolonged freezing may adversely affect liposomal drug products, however, short-term freezing (<1 month) does not appear to have a deleterious effect.

The appropriate dose (up to a maximum of 90 mg) must be diluted in 250 mL of dextrose 5% in water prior to administration. Diluted doxorubicin hydrochloride liposome injection should be refrigerated at 2°C to 8°C and administered within 24 hours. **Do not use with in-line filters.**

Mechanism of Action Doxil® is doxorubicin hydrochloride encapsulated in long-circulating STEALTH® liposomes. Liposomes are microscopic vesicles composed of a phospholipid bilayer that are capable of encapsulating active drugs. Doxorubicin works through inhibition of topoisomerase-II at the point of DNA cleavage. A second mechanism of action is the production of free radicals (the hydroxy radical OH) by doxorubicin, which in turn can destroy DNA and cancerous cells. Doxorubicin is also a very powerful iron chelator, equal to deferoxamine. The iron-doxorubicin complex can bind DNA and cell membranes rapidly and produce free radicals that immediately cleave the DNA and cell membranes. Inhibits DNA and RNA synthesis by intercalating between DNA base pairs and by steric obstruction; active throughout entire cell cycle.

Pharmacodynamics/Kinetics

Distribution: V_d: Steady state volume of distribution is confined mostly to the vascular fluid volume

Protein binding (doxorubicin): 70% bound to plasma proteins

Metabolism: In both the liver and in plasma to both active and inactive metabolites

Elimination: Mean clearance value of 0.041 L/hour/m^2

Usual Dosage Refer to individual protocols

I.V. (patient's ideal weight should be used to calculate body surface area): 20 mg/m^2 over 30 minutes, once every 3 weeks, for as long as patients respond satisfactorily and tolerate treatment.

Breast cancer: I.V.: 20-80 mg/m^2/dose has been studied in a limited number of phase I/II trials

(Continued)

Doxorubicin (Liposomal) *(Continued)*

Ovarian cancer: I.V.: 50 mg/m²/dose repeated every 3 weeks has been studied in a limited number of phase I/II trials

Solid tumors: I.V.: 50-60 mg/m²dose repeated every 3-4 weeks has been studied in a limited number of phase I/II trials

Dosing adjustment in hepatic impairment:

Bilirubin 1.2-3 mg/dL or AST 60-180 units: Administer 50% of dose

Bilirubin >3 mg/dL: Administer 25% of dose

Administration

Administer IVPB over 30 minutes; further dilute in D_5W; do not administer as a bolus injection or undiluted solution

Do not administer intramuscular or subcutaneous

Avoid extravasation, associated with severe ulceration and soft tissue necrosis; flush with 5-10 mL of D_5W solution before and after drug administration

Monitoring Parameters CBC with differential and platelet count, echocardiogram, liver function tests

Patient Information Discolors urine red/orange; immediately report any change in sensation (eg, stinging) at injection site during infusion (may be an early sign of infiltration)

Nursing Implications

Local erythematous streaking along the vein and/or facial flushing may indicate too rapid a rate of administration

Extravasation management:

Apply ice immediately for 30-60 minutes; then alternate off/on every 15 minutes for one day

Topical cooling may be achieved using ice packs or cooling pad with circulating ice water. Cooling of site for 24 hours as tolerated by the patient. Elevate and rest extremity 24-48 hours, then resume normal activity as tolerated. Application of cold inhibits vesicant's cytotoxicity.

Application of heat or sodium bicarbonate can be harmful and is contraindicated

If pain, erythema, and/or swelling persist beyond 48 hours, refer patient immediately to plastic surgeon for consultation and possible debridement

Dosage Forms Injection, as hydrochloride: 2 mg/mL (10 mL)

Doxychel® Injection *see* Doxycycline *on this page*

Doxychel® Oral *see* Doxycycline *on this page*

Doxycycline (doks i SYE kleen)

Related Information

Animal and Human Bites Guidelines *on page 1463*

Antimicrobial Drugs of Choice *on page 1468*

Antimicrobial Prophylaxis *on page 1445*

Prevention of Malaria *on page 1441*

Treatment of Sexually Transmitted Diseases *on page 1485*

Brand Names Bio-Tab® Oral; Doryx® Oral; Doxychel® Injection; Doxychel® Oral; Doxy® Oral; Monodox® Oral; Vibramycin® Injection; Vibramycin® Oral; Vibra-Tabs®

Canadian/Mexican Brand Names Apo-Doxy® (Canada); Apo-Doxy® Tabs (Canada); Doxycin® (Canada); Doxytec® (Canada); Novo-Doxylin® (Canada); Nu-Doxycycline® (Canada); Vibramicina® (Mexico)

Synonyms Doxycycline Hyclate; Doxycycline Monohydrate

Therapeutic Category Antibiotic, Tetracycline Derivative

Use Principally in the treatment of infections caused by susceptible *Rickettsia*, *Chlamydia*, and *Mycoplasma* along with uncommon susceptible gram-negative and gram-positive organisms; alternative to mefloquine for malaria prophylaxis; treatment of Lyme disease (Stage I)

Unapproved use: Treatment for syphilis in penicillin-allergic patients; sclerosing agent for pleural effusions

Pregnancy Risk Factor D

Contraindications Hypersensitivity to doxycycline, tetracycline or any component; children <8 years of age; severe hepatic dysfunction

Warnings/Precautions Use of tetracyclines during tooth development may cause permanent discoloration of the teeth and enamel hypoplasia; prolonged use may result in superinfection; photosensitivity reaction may occur with this drug; avoid prolonged exposure to sunlight or tanning equipment

Adverse Reactions

>10%: Miscellaneous: Discoloration of teeth in children

1% to 10%: Gastrointestinal: Esophagitis

<1%:

Central nervous system: Increased intracranial pressure, bulging fontanels in infants

Dermatologic: Rash, photosensitivity
Gastrointestinal: Nausea, diarrhea
Hematologic: Neutropenia, eosinophilia
Hepatic: Hepatotoxicity
Local: Phlebitis

Overdosage/Toxicology Symptoms of overdose include nausea, anorexia, diarrhea

Following GI decontamination, supportive care only; fluid support may be required for hypotension

Drug Interactions

Decreased effect with antacids containing aluminum, calcium, or magnesium
Iron and bismuth subsalicylate may decrease doxycycline bioavailability
Barbiturates, phenytoin, and carbamazepine decrease doxycycline's half-life
Increased effect of warfarin

Mechanism of Action Inhibits protein synthesis by binding with the 30S and possibly the 50S ribosomal subunit(s) of susceptible bacteria; may also cause alterations in the cytoplasmic membrane

Pharmacodynamics/Kinetics

Absorption: Almost completely from the GI tract; absorption can be reduced by food or milk by 20%
Distribution: Appears in breast milk
Protein binding: 90%
Metabolism: Not metabolized in the liver, instead is partially inactivated in the GI tract by chelate formation
Half-life: 12-15 hours (usually increases to 22-24 hours with multiple dosing)
End stage renal disease: 18-25 hours
Time to peak serum concentration: Within 1.5-4 hours
Elimination: In urine (23%) and feces (30%)

Usual Dosage Oral, I.V.:

Children ≥8 years (<45 kg): 2-5 mg/kg/day in 1-2 divided doses, not to exceed 200 mg/day
Children >8 years (>45 kg) and Adults: 100-200 mg/day in 1-2 divided doses
Sclerosing agent for pleural effusion injection: 500 mg as a single dose in 30-50 mL of NS or SWI

Dosing adjustment in renal impairment: No change is necessary

Dialysis: Not dialyzable; 0% to 5% by hemo- and peritoneal methods or by continuous arterio-venous or veno-venous hemofiltration (CAVH/CAVHD); no supplemental dosage necessary

Administration Infuse I.V. doxycycline over 1 hour; may administer with meals to decrease GI upset

Test Interactions False-negative urine glucose using Clinistix®, Tes-Tape®

Patient Information Avoid unnecessary exposure to sunlight; finish all medication; do not skip doses

Nursing Implications Avoid extravasation

Dosage Forms

Capsule, as hyclate:
Doxychel®, Vibramycin®: 50 mg
Doxy®, Doxychel®, Vibramycin®: 100 mg
Capsule, as monohydrate (Monodox®): 50 mg, 100 mg
Capsule, coated pellets, as hyclate (Doryx®): 100 mg
Powder for injection, as hyclate (Doxy®, Doxychel®, Vibramycin® IV): 100 mg, 200 mg
Powder for oral suspension, as monohydrate (raspberry flavor) (Vibramycin®): 25 mg/5 mL (60 mL)
Syrup, as calcium (raspberry-apple flavor) (Vibramycin®): 50 mg/5 mL (30 mL, 473 mL)
Tablet, as hyclate
Doxychel®: 50 mg
Bio-Tab®, Doxychel®, Vibra-Tabs®: 100 mg

Doxycycline Hyclate *see* Doxycycline *on previous page*

Doxycycline Monohydrate *see* Doxycycline *on previous page*

Doxy® Oral *see* Doxycycline *on previous page*

DPA *see* Valproic Acid and Derivatives *on page 1285*

DPE *see* Dipivefrin *on page 406*

D-Penicillamine *see* Penicillamine *on page 959*

DPH *see* Phenytoin *on page 992*

DPPC *see* Colfosceril Palmitate *on page 310*

Dramamine® II [OTC] *see* Meclizine *on page 769*

Dramamine® Oral [OTC] *see* Dimenhydrinate *on page 395*

Dramilin® Injection *see* Dimenhydrinate *on page 395*

Dramoject® Injection *see* Dimenhydrinate *on page 395*
Drisdol® *see* Ergocalciferol *on page 456*
Dristan® Long Lasting Nasal Solution [OTC] *see* Oxymetazoline *on page 940*
Dristan® Saline Spray [OTC] *see* Sodium Chloride *on page 1142*
Drithocreme® *see* Anthralin *on page 93*
Drithocreme® HP 1% *see* Anthralin *on page 93*
Dritho-Scalp® *see* Anthralin *on page 93*
Drixoral® Non-Drowsy [OTC] *see* Pseudoephedrine *on page 1074*

Dronabinol (droe NAB i nol)

Brand Names Marinol®

Synonyms Tetrahydrocannabinol; THC

Therapeutic Category Antiemetic

Use When conventional antiemetics fail to relieve the nausea and vomiting associated with cancer chemotherapy, AIDS-related anorexia

Restrictions C-II

Pregnancy Risk Factor B

Contraindications Use only for cancer chemotherapy-induced nausea; should not be used in patients with a history of schizophrenia or in patients with known hypersensitivity to dronabinol or any component

Warnings/Precautions Use with caution in patients with heart disease, hepatic disease, or seizure disorders; reduce dosage in patients with severe hepatic impairment

Adverse Reactions

>10%: Central nervous system: Drowsiness, dizziness, detachment, anxiety, difficulty concentrating, mood change

1% to 10%:
- Cardiovascular: Orthostatic hypotension, tachycardia
- Central nervous system: Ataxia, depression, headache, vertigo, hallucinations, memory lapse
- Gastrointestinal: Xerostomia
- Neuromuscular & skeletal: Paresthesia, weakness

<1%:
- Cardiovascular: Syncope
- Central nervous system: Nightmares, speech difficulties
- Gastrointestinal: Diarrhea
- Neuromuscular & skeletal: Myalgia
- Otic: Tinnitus
- Miscellaneous: Diaphoresis

Overdosage/Toxicology Symptoms of overdose include tachycardia, hypertension, and hypotension

Drug Interactions Increased toxicity (drowsiness) with alcohol, barbiturates, benzodiazepines

Stability Store in a cool place

Mechanism of Action Not well defined, probably inhibits the vomiting center in the medulla oblongata

Pharmacodynamics/Kinetics
- Absorption: Oral: Erratic
- Protein binding: 97% to 99%
- Metabolism: Extensive first-pass metabolism; metabolized in the liver to several metabolites, some of which are active
- Half-life: 19-24 hours
- Time to peak serum concentration: Within 2-3 hours
- Elimination: In feces and urine

Usual Dosage Oral:

Children: NCI protocol recommends 5 mg/m² starting 6-8 hours before chemotherapy and every 4-6 hours after to be continued for 12 hours after chemotherapy is discontinued

Adults: 5 mg/m² 1-3 hours before chemotherapy, then administer 5 mg/m²/dose every 2-4 hours after chemotherapy for a total of 4-6 doses/day; dose may be increased up to a maximum of 15 mg/m²/dose if needed (dosage may be increased by 2.5 mg/m² increments)

Appetite stimulant (AIDS-related): Initial: 2.5 mg twice daily (before lunch and dinner); titrate up to a maximum of 20 mg/day

Dietary Considerations Alcohol: Additive CNS effect, avoid use

Monitoring Parameters CNS effects, heart rate, blood pressure

Reference Range Antinauseant effects: 5-10 ng/mL

Test Interactions ↓ FSH, ↓ LH, ↓ growth hormone, ↓ testosterone

Patient Information Avoid activities such as driving which require motor coordination, avoid alcohol and other CNS depressants; may impair coordination and judgment

Nursing Implications Raise bed rails, institute safety measures, assist with ambulation

Dosage Forms Capsule: 2.5 mg, 5 mg, 10 mg

Droperidol (droe PER i dole)

Brand Names Inapsine®

Canadian/Mexican Brand Names Dehydrobenzperidol® (Mexico)

Therapeutic Category Antiemetic; Antipsychotic Agent

Use Tranquilizer and antiemetic in surgical and diagnostic procedures; antiemetic for cancer chemotherapy; preoperative medication; has good antiemetic effect as well as sedative and antianxiety effects

Pregnancy Risk Factor C

Pregnancy/Breast-Feeding Implications

Clinical effects on the fetus: Crosses the placenta

Breast-feeding/lactation: No data available

Contraindications Hypersensitivity to droperidol or any component

Warnings/Precautions Safety in children <6 months of age has not been established; use with caution in patients with seizures, bone marrow suppression, or severe liver disease

Significant hypotension may occur, especially when the drug is administered parenterally; injection contains benzyl alcohol; injection also contains sulfites which may cause allergic reaction

Tardive dyskinesia: Prevalence rate may be 40% in elderly; development of the syndrome and the irreversible nature are proportional to duration and total cumulative dose over time. May be reversible if diagnosed early in therapy.

Extrapyramidal reactions are more common in elderly with up to 50% developing these reactions after 60 years of age. Drug-induced **Parkinson's syndrome** occurs often. **Akathisia** is the most common extrapyramidal reaction in elderly.

Increased confusion, memory loss, psychotic behavior, and agitation frequently occur as a consequence of anticholinergic effects

Orthostatic hypotension is due to alpha-receptor blockade, the elderly are at greater risk for orthostatic hypotension

Antipsychotic associated sedation in nonpsychotic patients is extremely unpleasant due to feelings of depersonalization, derealization, and dysphoria

Life-threatening arrhythmias have occurred at therapeutic doses of antipsychotics

Adverse Reactions

>10%:

- Cardiovascular: Mild to moderate hypotension, tachycardia
- Central nervous system: Postoperative drowsiness

1% to 10%:

- Cardiovascular: Hypertension
- Central nervous system: Extrapyramidal reactions
- Respiratory: Respiratory depression

<1%:

- Central nervous system: Dizziness, chills, postoperative hallucinations
- Respiratory: Laryngospasm, bronchospasm
- Miscellaneous: Shivering

Overdosage/Toxicology Symptoms of overdose include hypotension, tachycardia, hallucinations, extrapyramidal symptoms

Following initiation of essential overdose management, toxic symptom treatment and supportive treatment should be initiated. Hypotension usually responds to I.V. fluids or Trendelenburg positioning. If unresponsive to these measures, the use of a parenteral inotrope may be required (eg, norepinephrine 0.1-0.2 mcg/kg/minute titrated to response). Seizures commonly respond to diazepam (I.V. 5-10 mg bolus in adults every 15 minutes if needed up to a total of 30 mg; I.V. 0.25-0.4 mg/kg/dose up to a total of 10 mg in children) or to phenytoin or phenobarbital. Critical cardiac arrhythmias often respond to I.V. phenytoin (15 mg/kg up to 1 g), while other antiarrhythmics can be used. Neuroleptics often cause extrapyramidal symptoms (eg, dystonic reactions) requiring management with diphenhydramine 1-2 mg/kg (adults) up to a maximum of 50 mg I.M. or I.V. slow push followed by a maintenance dose for 48-72 hours. When these reactions are unresponsive to diphenhydramine, benztropine mesylate I.V. 1-2 mg (adults) may be effective. These agents are generally effective within 2-5 minutes.

Drug Interactions Increased toxicity: CNS depressants, fentanyl and other analgesics increased blood pressure; conduction anesthesia decreased blood pressure; epinephrine decreased blood pressure; atropine, lithium

Stability

Droperidol ampuls/vials should be stored at room temperature and protected from light

Stability of parenteral admixture at room temperature (25°C): 7 days

Standard diluent: 2.5 mg/50 mL D_5W

(Continued)

Droperidol *(Continued)*

Incompatible with barbiturates

Mechanism of Action Alters the action of dopamine in the CNS, at subcortical levels, to produce sedation; reduces emesis by blocking dopamine stimulation of the chemotrigger zone

Pharmacodynamics/Kinetics

Following parenteral administration:

Peak effect: Within 30 minutes

Duration: 2-4 hours, may extend to 12 hours

Metabolism: In the liver

Half-life: Adults: 2.3 hours

Elimination: In urine (75%) and feces (22%)

Usual Dosage Titrate carefully to desired effect

Children 2-12 years:

Premedication: I.M.: 0.1-0.15 mg/kg; smaller doses may be sufficient for control of nausea or vomiting

Adjunct to general anesthesia: I.V. induction: 0.088-0.165 mg/kg

Nausea and vomiting: I.M., I.V.: 0.05-0.06 mg/kg/dose every 4-6 hours as needed

Adults:

Premedication: I.M.: 2.5-10 mg 30 minutes to 1 hour preoperatively

Adjunct to general anesthesia: I.V. induction: 0.22-0.275 mg/kg; maintenance: 1.25-2.5 mg/dose

Alone in diagnostic procedures: I.M.: Initial: 2.5-10 mg 30 minutes to 1 hour before; then 1.25-2.5 mg if needed

Nausea and vomiting: I.M., I.V.: 2.5-5 mg/dose every 3-4 hours as needed

Administration Administer I.M. or I.V.; I.V. should be administered slow IVP (over 2-5 minutes) or IVPB

Monitoring Parameters Blood pressure, heart rate, respiratory rate; observe for dystonias, extrapyramidal side effects, and temperature changes

Dosage Forms Injection: 2.5 mg/mL (1 mL, 2 mL, 5 mL, 10 mL)

Drotic® Otic *see* Neomycin, Polymyxin B, and Hydrocortisone *on page 890*

Dr Scholl's Athlete's Foot [OTC] *see* Tolnaftate *on page 1243*

Dr Scholl's® Cracked Heel Relief Cream [OTC] *see* Lidocaine *on page 723*

Dr Scholl's® Disk [OTC] *see* Salicylic Acid *on page 1120*

Dr Scholl's Maximum Strength Tritin [OTC] *see* Tolnaftate *on page 1243*

Dr Scholl's® Wart Remover [OTC] *see* Salicylic Acid *on page 1120*

Drugs and Routes of Administration Not Recommended for Treatment of Cancer Pain *see page 1378*

Dryox® Gel [OTC] *see* Benzoyl Peroxide *on page 140*

Dryox® Wash [OTC] *see* Benzoyl Peroxide *on page 140*

DSCG *see* Cromolyn Sodium *on page 317*

DSS *see* Docusate *on page 415*

D-S-S® [OTC] *see* Docusate *on page 415*

DT *see* Diphtheria and Tetanus Toxoid *on page 402*

DTaP *see* Diphtheria, Tetanus Toxoids, and Acellular Pertussis Vaccine *on page 403*

DTIC-Dome® *see* Dacarbazine *on page 335*

DTO *see* Opium Tincture *on page 928*

***d*-Tubocurarine Chloride** *see* Tubocurarine *on page 1277*

DTwP-HIB *see* Diphtheria, Tetanus Toxoids, Whole-Cell Pertussis, and *Haemophilus Influenzae* Type b Conjugate Vaccines *on page 404*

Dulcolax® [OTC] *see* Bisacodyl *on page 153*

Dull-C® [OTC] *see* Ascorbic Acid *on page 102*

DuoCet™ *see* Hydrocodone and Acetaminophen *on page 620*

DuoFilm® [OTC] *see* Salicylic Acid *on page 1120*

DuoPlant® Gel [OTC] *see* Salicylic Acid *on page 1120*

Duo-Trach® *see* Lidocaine *on page 723*

Duotrate® *see* Pentaerythritol Tetranitrate *on page 967*

DuP 753 *see* Losartan *on page 744*

Duphalac® *see* Lactulose *on page 703*

Durabolin® *see* Nandrolone *on page 878*

Duradyne DHC® *see* Hydrocodone and Acetaminophen *on page 620*

Dura-Estrin® Injection *see* Estradiol *on page 468*

Duragen® Injection *see* Estradiol *on page 468*

Duragesic™ *see* Fentanyl *on page 510*

Duralone® *see* Methylprednisolone *on page 819*

Duramist Plus® [OTC] *see* Oxymetazoline *on page 940*

Duramorph® *see* Morphine Sulfate *on page 858*
Duranest® *see* Etidocaine *on page 493*
Duraphyl™ *see* Theophylline Salts *on page 1207*
Duratest® Injection *see* Testosterone *on page 1198*
Durathate® Injection *see* Testosterone *on page 1198*
Duration® Nasal Solution [OTC] *see* Oxymetazoline *on page 940*
Duricef® *see* Cefadroxil *on page 218*
Durrax® *see* Hydroxyzine *on page 634*
Duvoid® *see* Bethanechol *on page 150*
DV® Cream *see* Dienestrol *on page 379*
Dyazide® *see* Hydrochlorothiazide and Triamterene *on page 618*
Dycill® *see* Dicloxacillin *on page 375*
Dyclone® *see* Dyclonine *on this page*

Dyclonine (DYE kloe neen)

Brand Names Dyclone®

Synonyms Dyclonine Hydrochloride

Therapeutic Category Local Anesthetic, Mucous Membrane; Local Anesthetic, Oral

Use Local anesthetic prior to laryngoscopy, bronchoscopy, or endotracheal intubation; use topically for temporary relief of pain associated with oral mucosa or anogenital lesions

Pregnancy Risk Factor C

Contraindications Contraindicated in patients allergic to chlorobutanol (preservative used in dyclonine) or dyclonine

Warnings/Precautions Use with caution in patients with sepsis or traumatized mucosa in the area of application to avoid rapid systemic absorption; may impair swallowing and enhance the danger of aspiration; use with caution in patients with shock or heart block; resuscitative equipment, oxygen, and resuscitative drugs should be immediately available when dyclonine topical solution is administered to mucous membranes; **not for injection or ophthalmic use**

Adverse Reactions <1%:

Cardiovascular: Hypotension, bradycardia, respiratory arrest, cardiac arrest

Central nervous system: Excitation, drowsiness, nervousness, dizziness, seizures

Local: Slight irritation and stinging may occur when applied

Ocular: Blurred vision

Sensitivity reactions: Allergic reactions

Overdosage/Toxicology Symptoms of overdose are primarily CNS (seizures, excitation) and cardiovascular (hypotension, myocardial depression)

Treatment is supportive with fluids and pressors (particularly those that stimulate the myocardium); diazepam 0.1 mg/kg can be used to control seizures

Stability Store in tight, light-resistant containers

Mechanism of Action Blocks impulses at peripheral nerve endings in skin and mucous membranes by altering cell membrane permeability to ionic transfer

Pharmacodynamics/Kinetics

Onset of local anesthesia: 2-10 minutes

Duration: 30-60 minutes

Usual Dosage Use the lowest dose needed to provide effective anesthesia

Children and Adults: Topical solution:

Mouth sores: 5-10 mL of 0.5% or 1% to oral mucosa (swab or swish and then spit) 3-4 times/day as needed; maximum single dose: 200 mg (40 mL of 0.5% solution or 20 mL of 1% solution)

Bronchoscopy: Use 2 mL of the 1% solution or 4 mL of the 0.5% solution sprayed onto the larynx and trachea every 5 minutes until the reflex has been abolished

Patient Information Food should not be ingested for 60 minutes following application in the mouth or throat area; numbness of the tongue and buccal mucosa may result in increased risk of biting trauma; may impair swallowing; not for use in small infants or children

Dosage Forms

Lozenges, as hydrochloride: 1.2 mg, 3 mg

Solution, topical, as hydrochloride: 0.5% (30 mL); 1% (30 mL)

Dyclonine Hydrochloride *see* Dyclonine *on this page*
Dyflos *see* Isoflurophate *on page 679*
Dymelor® *see* Acetohexamide *on page 25*
Dymenate® Injection *see* Dimenhydrinate *on page 395*
Dynabac® *see* Dirithromycin *on page 407*
Dynacin® Oral *see* Minocycline *on page 842*
DynaCirc® *see* Isradipine *on page 688*

Dyna-Hex® Topical [OTC] *see* Chlorhexidine Gluconate *on page 253*
Dynapen® *see* Dicloxacillin *on page 375*
Dyrenium® *see* Triamterene *on page 1257*
7E3 *see* Abciximab *on page 14*
E2020 *see* Donepezil *on page 416*
Ear-Eze® Otic *see* Neomycin, Polymyxin B, and Hydrocortisone *on page 890*
Easprin® *see* Aspirin *on page 106*

Echothiophate Iodide (ek oh THYE oh fate EYE oh dide)

Related Information

Glaucoma Drug Therapy Comparison *on page 1410*

Brand Names Phospholine Iodide®

Synonyms Ecostigmine Iodide

Therapeutic Category Ophthalmic Agent, Miotic

Use Reverse toxic CNS effects caused by anticholinergic drugs; used as miotic in treatment of open-angle glaucoma; may be useful in specific case of narrow-angle glaucoma; accommodative esotropia

Pregnancy Risk Factor C

Contraindications Hypersensitivity to echothiophate or any component; most cases of angle-closure glaucoma; active uveal inflammation or any inflammatory disease of the iris or ciliary body, glaucoma associated with iridocyclitis

Warnings/Precautions Tolerance may develop after prolonged use; a rest period restores response to the drug

Adverse Reactions

1% to 10%: Ocular: Stinging, burning eyes, myopia, visual blurring

<1%:

- Cardiovascular: Bradycardia, hypotension, flushing
- Gastrointestinal: Nausea, vomiting, diarrhea
- Neuromuscular & skeletal: Muscle weakness
- Ocular: Retinal detachment, diaphoresis, browache, miosis, twitching eyelids, watering eyes
- Respiratory: Dyspnea

Overdosage/Toxicology Symptoms of overdose include excessive salivation, urinary incontinence, dyspnea, diarrhea, profuse sweating

If systemic effects occur, administer parenteral atropine; for severe muscle weakness, pralidoxime may be used in addition to atropine

Drug Interactions Increased toxicity: Carbamate or organophosphate insecticides and pesticides; succinylcholine; systemic acetylcholinesterases may increase neuromuscular effects

Stability Store undiluted vials at room temperature (15°C to 30°C/59°F to 86°F); reconstituted solutions remain stable for 30 days at room temperature or 6 months when refrigerated

Mechanism of Action Produces miosis and changes in accommodation by inhibiting cholinesterase, thereby preventing the breakdown of acetylcholine; acetylcholine is, therefore, allowed to continuously stimulate the iris and ciliary muscles of the eye

Pharmacodynamics/Kinetics

Onset of action:
- Miosis: 10-30 minutes
- Intraocular pressure decrease: 4-8 hours

Peak intraocular pressure decrease: 24 hours

Duration: Up to 1-4 weeks

Usual Dosage Adults:

Ophthalmic: Glaucoma: Instill 1 drop twice daily into eyes with 1 dose just prior to bedtime; some patients have been treated with 1 dose daily or every other day

Accommodative esotropia:
- Diagnosis: Instill 1 drop of 0.125% once daily into both eyes at bedtime for 2-3 weeks
- Treatment: Use lowest concentration and frequency which gives satisfactory response, with a maximum dose of 0.125% once daily, although more intensive therapy may be used for short periods of time

Patient Information Be sure of solution expiration date; local irritation and headache may occur; notify physician if abdominal cramps, diarrhea, or salivation occurs; use caution if driving at night or performing hazardous tasks; do not touch dropper to eye; report any change in vision to physician

Nursing Implications Keep refrigerated; do not touch dropper to eye

Dosage Forms Powder for reconstitution, ophthalmic: 1.5 mg [0.03%] (5 mL); 3 mg [0.06%] (5 mL); 6.25 mg [0.125%] (5 mL); 12.5 mg [0.25%] (5 mL)

E-Complex-600® [OTC] *see* Vitamin E *on page 1309*

Econazole (e KONE a zole)

Brand Names Spectazole™

Canadian/Mexican Brand Names Ecostatin® (Canada); Micostyl® (Mexico)

Synonyms Econazole Nitrate

Therapeutic Category Antifungal Agent, Topical

Use Topical treatment of tinea pedis (athlete's foot), tinea cruris (jock itch), tinea corporis (ringworm), tinea versicolor, and cutaneous candidiasis

Pregnancy Risk Factor C

Pregnancy/Breast-Feeding Implications Do not use during the first trimester of pregnancy, unless essential to a patient's welfare; use during the second and third trimesters only if clearly needed

Contraindications Known hypersensitivity to econazole or any component

Warnings/Precautions Discontinue drug if sensitivity or chemical irritation occurs; not for ophthalmic or intravaginal use

Adverse Reactions 1% to 10%:

Dermatologic: Pruritus, erythema

Local: Burning, stinging

Mechanism of Action Alters fungal cell wall membrane permeability; may interfere with RNA and protein synthesis, and lipid metabolism

Pharmacodynamics/Kinetics

Absorption: Topical: <10%

Metabolism: In the liver to >20 metabolites

Elimination: <1% of applied dose recovered in urine or feces

Usual Dosage Children and Adults: Topical:

Tinea pedis, tinea cruris, tinea corporis, tinea versicolor: Apply sufficient amount to cover affected areas once daily

Cutaneous candidiasis: Apply sufficient quantity twice daily (morning and evening)

Duration of treatment: Candidal infections and tinea cruris, versicolor, and corporis should be treated for 2 weeks and tinea pedis for 1 month; occasionally, longer treatment periods may be required

Patient Information For external use only; avoid eye contact; if condition worsens or persists, or irritation occurs, notify physician

Dosage Forms Cream, as nitrate: 1% (15 g, 30 g, 85 g)

Econazole Nitrate *see* Econazole *on this page*

Econopred® *see* Prednisolone *on page 1037*

Econopred® Plus *see* Prednisolone *on page 1037*

Ecostigmine Iodide *see* Echothiophate Iodide *on previous page*

Ecotrin® [OTC] *see* Aspirin *on page 106*

Ectasule® *see* Ephedrine *on page 446*

Edathamil Disodium *see* Edetate Disodium *on next page*

Edecrin® *see* Ethacrynic Acid *on page 476*

Edetate Calcium Disodium

(ED e tate KAL see um dye SOW dee um)

Brand Names Calcium Disodium Versenate®

Synonyms Calcium Disodium Edetate; Calcium EDTA

Therapeutic Category Antidote, Lead Toxicity

Use Treatment of acute and chronic lead poisoning; used as an aid in the diagnosis of lead poisoning

Pregnancy Risk Factor C

Contraindications Severe renal disease, anuria

Warnings/Precautions Potentially nephrotoxic; renal tubular acidosis and fatal nephrosis may occur, especially with high doses; EKG changes may occur during therapy; do not exceed recommended daily dose; avoid rapid I.V. infusion in the management of lead encephalopathy, may increase intracranial pressure to lethal levels. If anuria, increasing proteinuria, or hematuria occurs during therapy, discontinue calcium EDTA.

Adverse Reactions

1% to 10%: Renal: Renal tubular necrosis

<1%:

Cardiovascular: Hypotension, arrhythmias

Central nervous system: Fever, headache, chills

Dermatologic: Skin lesions

Endocrine & metabolic: Hypercalcemia

Gastrointestinal: Nausea, vomiting

Hematologic: Transient marrow suppression

Local: Pain at injection site following I.M. injection, thrombophlebitis following I.V. infusion (when concentration >0.5%)

Neuromuscular & skeletal: Numbness, paresthesia

(Continued)

Edetate Calcium Disodium *(Continued)*

Ocular: Lacrimation
Renal: Proteinuria, microscopic hematuria
Respiratory: Sneezing, nasal congestion

Drug Interactions Decreased effect: Do not use simultaneously with zinc insulin preparations; do not mix in the same syringe with dimercaprol

Stability Dilute with 0.9% sodium chloride or D_5W; physically **incompatible** with $D_{10}W$, LR, Ringer's

Mechanism of Action Calcium is displaced by divalent and trivalent heavy metals, forming a nonionizing soluble complex that is excreted in urine

Pharmacodynamics/Kinetics

Absorption: I.M., S.C.: Well absorbed
Distribution: Into extracellular fluid; minimal CSF penetration
Half-life, plasma:
I.M.: 1.5 hours
I.V.: 20 minutes
Elimination: Rapidly excreted in urine as metal chelates or unchanged drug, decreased GFR decreases elimination; when administered I.V., urinary excretion of chelated lead begins in 1 hour and peak excretion of chelated lead occurs within 24-48 hours

Usual Dosage

Children: I.M. (preferred route of administration as rapid I.V. infusion may be lethal), I.V., S.C.:

Asymptomatic lead poisoning: (Blood lead concentration >55 mcg/dL or blood lead concentrations of 25-55 mcg/dL with blood erythrocyte protoporphyrin concentrations ≥35 mcg/dL and positive mobilization test) or **symptomatic lead poisoning without encephalopathy** with lead level <100 mcg/dL: 1 g/m²/day I.M./I.V. in divided doses every 8-12 hours for 3-5 days (usually 5 days) with dimercaprol; maximum: 1 g/24 hours or 50 mg/kg/day

Symptomatic lead poisoning with encephalopathy with lead level >100 mcg/dL (treatment with calcium EDTA and dimercaprol is preferred): 250 mg/m² I.M. or intermittent I.V. infusion 4 hours after dimercaprol, then at 4-hour intervals thereafter for 5 days (1.5 g/m²/day); dose (1.5 g/m²/day) can also be given as a single I.V. continuous infusion over 12-24 hours/day for 5 days; maximum: 1 g/24 hours or 75 mg/kg/day

Note: Course of therapy may be repeated in 2-3 weeks until blood lead level is normal

Adults: Treatment: I.M., I.V.: 2-4 g/day or 1.5 g/m²/day in divided doses every 12-24 hours for 5 days; may repeat course one time after at least 2 days (usually after 2 weeks) not more than 2 courses of therapy are recommended

Dosing adjustment/comments in renal impairment: Calcium disodium EDTA is almost exclusively eliminated in urine and should not be administered during periods of anuria

Administration For intermittent I.V. infusion, administer the dose I.V. over at least 1 hour in asymptomatic patients, 2 hours in symptomatic patients; for I.V. continuous infusion, dilute to 2-4 mg/mL in D_5W or NS and infuse over at least 8 hours, usually over 12-24 hours; for I.M. injection, 1 mL of 1% procaine hydrochloride may be added to each mL of EDTA calcium to minimize pain at injection site

Monitoring Parameters BUN, creatinine, urinalysis, I & O, and EKG during therapy; intravenous administration requires a cardiac monitor

Test Interactions If calcium EDTA is given as a continuous I.V. infusion, stop the infusion for at least 1 hour before blood is drawn for lead concentration to avoid a falsely elevated value

Dosage Forms Injection: 200 mg/mL (5 mL)

Edetate Disodium (ED e tate dye SOW dee um)

Brand Names Chealamide®; Disotate®; Endrate®

Synonyms Edathamil Disodium; EDTA; Sodium Edetate

Therapeutic Category Antidote, Hypercalcemia; Chelating Agent, Parenteral

Use Emergency treatment of hypercalcemia; control digitalis-induced cardiac dysrhythmias (ventricular arrhythmias)

Pregnancy Risk Factor C

Contraindications Severe renal failure or anuria

Warnings/Precautions Use of this drug is recommended only when the severity of the clinical condition justifies the aggressive measures associated with this type of therapy; use with caution in patients with renal dysfunction, intracranial lesions, seizure disorders, coronary or peripheral vascular disease

Adverse Reactions

Rapid I.V. administration or excessive doses may cause a sudden drop in serum calcium concentration which may lead to hypocalcemic tetany, seizures, arrhythmias, and death from respiratory arrest. Do **not** exceed recommended dosage and rate of administration.

1% to 10%: Gastrointestinal: Nausea, vomiting, abdominal cramps, diarrhea

<1%:

Cardiovascular: Arrhythmias, transient hypotension, acute tubular necrosis
Central nervous system: Seizures, fever, headache, tetany, chills
Dermatologic: Eruptions, dermatologic lesions
Endocrine & metabolic: Hypomagnesemia, hypokalemia
Hematologic: Anemia
Local: Thrombophlebitis, pain at the site of injection
Neuromuscular & skeletal: Paresthesia may occur, back pain, muscle cramps
Renal: Nephrotoxicity
Respiratory: Death from respiratory arrest

Overdosage/Toxicology Symptoms of overdose include hypotension, dysrhythmias, tetany, seizures

Treatment includes immediate I.V. calcium salts for hypocalcemia related adverse reactions; replace calcium cautiously in patients on digitalis

Drug Interactions Increased effect of insulin (edetate disodium may decrease blood glucose concentrations and reduce insulin requirements in diabetic patients treated with insulin)

Mechanism of Action Chelates with divalent or trivalent metals to form a soluble complex that is then eliminated in urine

Pharmacodynamics/Kinetics

Metabolism: Not metabolized
Half-life: 20-60 minutes
Elimination: Following chelation, 95% excreted in urine as chelates within 24-48 hours

Usual Dosage Hypercalcemia: I.V.:

Children: 40-70 mg/kg/day slow infusion over 3-4 hours or more to a maximum of 3 g/24 hours; administer for 5 days and allow 5 days between courses of therapy

Adults: 50 mg/kg/day over 3 or more hours to a maximum of 3 g/24 hours; a suggested regimen of 5 days followed by 2 days without drug and repeated courses up to 15 total doses

Administration Must be diluted before use in 500 mL D_5W or NS to <30 mg/mL

Monitoring Parameters Cardiac function (EKG monitoring); blood pressure during infusion; renal function should be assessed before and during therapy; monitor calcium, magnesium, and potassium levels; cardiac monitor required

Nursing Implications Avoid extravasation; patient should remain supine for a short period after infusion; infuse over 3-4 hours

Additional Information Sodium content of 1 g: 5.4 mEq

Dosage Forms Injection: 150 mg/mL (20 mL)

Edrophonium (ed roe FOE nee um)

Brand Names Enlon®; Reversol®; Tensilon®

Synonyms Edrophonium Chloride

Therapeutic Category Antidote, Neuromuscular Blocking Agent; Cholinergic Agent; Diagnostic Agent, Myasthenia Gravis

Use Diagnosis of myasthenia gravis; differentiation of cholinergic crises from myasthenia crises; reversal of nondepolarizing neuromuscular blockers; treatment of paroxysmal atrial tachycardia

Pregnancy Risk Factor C

Contraindications Hypersensitivity to edrophonium or any component, GI or GU obstruction, hypersensitivity to sulfite agents

Warnings/Precautions Use with caution in patients with bronchial asthma and those receiving a cardiac glycoside; atropine sulfate should always be readily available as an antagonist. Overdosage can cause cholinergic crisis which may be fatal. I.V. atropine should be readily available for treatment of cholinergic reactions.

Adverse Reactions

>10%:

Gastrointestinal: Nausea, vomiting, diarrhea, excessive salivation, stomach cramps
Miscellaneous: Diaphoresis (increased)

1% to 10%:

Genitourinary: Polyuria
Ocular: Small pupils, lacrimation
Respiratory: Increased bronchial secretions

<1%:

Cardiovascular: Bradycardia, A-V block
Central nervous system: Seizures, headache, drowsiness, dysphoria
Neuromuscular & skeletal: Weakness, muscle cramps, muscle spasms

(Continued)

Edrophonium *(Continued)*

Local: Thrombophlebitis
Ocular: Diplopia, miosis
Respiratory: Laryngospasm, bronchospasm, respiratory paralysis
Miscellaneous: Hypersensitivity, hyper-reactive cholinergic responses

Overdosage/Toxicology Symptoms of overdose include muscle weakness, nausea, vomiting, miosis, bronchospasm, respiratory paralysis

Maintain adequate airway; antidote is atropine for muscarinic symptoms; pralidoxime (2-PAM) may also be needed to reverse severe muscle weakness or paralysis; skeletal muscle effects of edrophonium not alleviated by atropine.

Drug Interactions

Decreased effect: Atropine, nondepolarizing muscle relaxants, procainamide, quinidine
Increased effect: Succinylcholine, digoxin, I.V. acetazolamide, neostigmine, physostigmine

Mechanism of Action Inhibits destruction of acetylcholine by acetylcholinesterase. This facilitates transmission of impulses across myoneural junction and results in increased cholinergic responses such as miosis, increased tonus of intestinal and skeletal muscles, bronchial and ureteral constriction, bradycardia, and increased salivary and sweat gland secretions.

Pharmacodynamics/Kinetics

I.M.:
  Onset of effect: Within 2-10 minutes
  Duration: 5-30 minutes
I.V.:
  Onset of effect: Within 30-60 seconds
  Duration: 10 minutes
Distribution: V_d: 1.1 L/kg
Half-life: 1.8 hours

Usual Dosage Usually administered I.V., however, if not possible, I.M. or S.C. may be used:

Infants:
  I.M.: 0.5-1 mg
  I.V.: Initial: 0.1 mg, followed by 0.4 mg if no response; total dose = 0.5 mg

Children:
  Diagnosis: Initial: 0.04 mg/kg over 1 minute followed by 0.16 mg/kg if no response, to a maximum total dose of 5 mg for children <34 kg, or 10 mg for children >34 kg
  I.M.:
    <34 kg: 1 mg
    >34 kg: 5 mg
  Titration of oral anticholinesterase therapy: 0.04 mg/kg once given 1 hour after oral intake of the drug being used in treatment; if strength improves, an increase in neostigmine or pyridostigmine dose is indicated

Adults:
  Diagnosis:
    I.V.: 2 mg test dose administered over 15-30 seconds; 8 mg given 45 seconds later if no response is seen; test dose may be repeated after 30 minutes
    I.M.: Initial: 10 mg; if no cholinergic reaction occurs, administer 2 mg 30 minutes later to rule out false-negative reaction
  Titration of oral anticholinesterase therapy: 1-2 mg given 1 hour after oral dose of anticholinesterase; if strength improves, an increase in neostigmine or pyridostigmine dose is indicated
  Reversal of nondepolarizing neuromuscular blocking agents (neostigmine with atropine usually preferred): I.V.: 10 mg over 30-45 seconds; may repeat every 5-10 minutes up to 40 mg
  Termination of paroxysmal atrial tachycardia: I.V. rapid injection: 5-10 mg
  Differentiation of cholinergic from myasthenic crisis: I.V.: 1 mg; may repeat after 1 minute. **Note:** Intubation and controlled ventilation may be required if patient has cholinergic crisis

Dosing adjustment in renal impairment: Dose may need to be reduced in patients with chronic renal failure

Test Interactions ↑ aminotransferase [ALT (SGPT)/AST (SGOT)] (S), amylase (S)

Dosage Forms Injection, as chloride: 10 mg/mL (1 mL, 10 mL, 15 mL)

Edrophonium Chloride *see* Edrophonium *on previous page*
ED-SPAZ® *see* Hyoscyamine *on page 635*
EDTA *see* Edetate Disodium *on page 438*
E.E.S.® *see* Erythromycin *on page 461*

Efedron® *see* Ephedrine *on page 446*

Effer-K™ *see* Potassium Bicarbonate and Potassium Citrate, Effervescent *on page 1023*

Effer-Syllium® [OTC] *see* Psyllium *on page 1075*

Effexor® *see* Venlafaxine *on page 1295*

Efidac® 24 [OTC] *see* Chlorpheniramine *on page 260*

Efidac/24® [OTC] *see* Pseudoephedrine *on page 1074*

Eflornithine (ee FLOR ni theen)

Brand Names Ornidyl®

Synonyms DFMO; Eflornithine Hydrochloride

Therapeutic Category Antiprotozoal

Use Treatment of meningoencephalitic stage of *Trypanosoma brucei gambiense* infection (sleeping sickness)

Pregnancy Risk Factor C

Contraindications Hypersensitivity to eflornithine or any component

Warnings/Precautions Must be diluted before use; frequent monitoring for myelosuppression should be done; use with caution in patients with a history of seizures and in patients with renal impairment; serial audiograms should be obtained; due to the potential for relapse, patients should be followed up for at least 24 months

Adverse Reactions

>10%: Hematologic: Anemia, leukopenia, thrombocytopenia

1% to 10%:

- Central nervous system: Seizures, dizziness
- Dermatologic: Alopecia
- Gastrointestinal: Vomiting, diarrhea
- Hematologic: Eosinophilia
- Otic: Hearing impairment

<1%:

- Cardiovascular: Facial edema
- Central nervous system: Headache
- Gastrointestinal: Abdominal pain, anorexia
- Neuromuscular & skeletal: Weakness

Overdosage/Toxicology No known antidote; treatment is supportive

Stability Must be diluted before use and used within 24 hours of preparation

Mechanism of Action Eflornithine exerts antitumor and antiprotozoal effects through specific, irreversible ("suicide") inhibition of the enzyme ornithine decarboxylase (ODC). ODC is the rate-limiting enzyme in the biosynthesis of putrescine, spermine, and spermidine, the major polyamines in nucleated cells. Polyamines are necessary for the synthesis of DNA, RNA, and proteins and are, therefore, necessary for cell growth and differentiation. Although many microorganisms and higher plants are able to produce polyamines from alternate biochemical pathways, all mammalian cells depend on ornithine decarboxylase to produce polyamines. Eflornithine inhibits ODC and rapidly depletes animal cells of putrescine and spermidine; the concentration of spermine remains the same or may even increase. Rapidly dividing cells appear to most susceptible to the effects of eflornithine.

Usual Dosage Adults: I.V. infusion: 100 mg/kg/dose given every 6 hours (over at least 45 minutes) for 14 days

Dosing adjustment in renal impairment: Dose should be adjusted although no specific guidelines are available

Monitoring Parameters CBC with platelet counts

Patient Information Report any persistent or unusual fever, sore throat, fatigue, bleeding, or bruising; frequent blood tests are needed during therapy

Dosage Forms Injection, as hydrochloride: 200 mg/mL (100 mL)

Eflornithine Hydrochloride *see* Eflornithine *on this page*

Efodine® [OTC] *see* Povidone-Iodine *on page 1031*

Efudex® *see* Fluorouracil *on page 538*

EHDP *see* Etidronate Disodium *on page 493*

E-IPV *see* Polio Vaccines *on page 1015*

Elavil® *see* Amitriptyline *on page 69*

Eldecort® *see* Hydrocortisone *on page 623*

Eldepryl® *see* Selegiline *on page 1130*

Eldercaps® [OTC] *see* Vitamins, Multiple *on page 1310*

Eldopaque® [OTC] *see* Hydroquinone *on page 628*

Eldopaque Forte® *see* Hydroquinone *on page 628*

Eldoquin® [OTC] *see* Hydroquinone *on page 628*

Eldoquin® Forte® *see* Hydroquinone *on page 628*

Electrolyte Lavage Solution *see* Polyethylene Glycol-Electrolyte Solution *on page 1017*

Elimite™ *see* Permethrin *on page 978*

Elixophyllin® *see* Theophylline Salts *on page 1207*

Elixophyllin® SR *see* Theophylline Salts *on page 1207*

Elmiron® *see* Pentosan Polysulfate Sodium *on page 972*

Elocon® *see* Mometasone Furoate *on page 856*

Elspar® *see* Asparaginase *on page 103*

Eltroxin™ *see* Levothyroxine *on page 721*

Emcyt® *see* Estramustine *on page 470*

Eminase® *see* Anistreplase *on page 92*

EMLA® *see* Lidocaine and Prilocaine *on page 725*

Empirin® [OTC] *see* Aspirin *on page 106*

Empirin® With Codeine *see* Aspirin and Codeine *on page 109*

Emulsoil® [OTC] *see* Castor Oil *on page 216*

E-Mycin® *see* Erythromycin *on page 461*

Enalapril (e NAL a pril)

Related Information

Angiotensin-Converting Enzyme Inhibitors Comparison *on page 1386*

Heart Failure: Management of Patients With Left-Ventricular Systolic Dysfunction *on page 1533*

Brand Names Vasotec®; Vasotec® I.V.

Canadian/Mexican Brand Names Apo-Enalapril® (Canada); Enaladil® (Mexico); Glioten® (Mexico); Renitec® (Mexico)

Synonyms Enalaprilat; Enalapril Maleate

Therapeutic Category Angiotensin-Converting Enzyme (ACE) Inhibitors; Antihypertensive

Use Management of mild to severe hypertension and congestive heart failure; believed to prolong survival in heart failure

Unlabeled use: Hypertensive crisis, diabetic nephropathy, rheumatoid arthritis, diagnosis of anatomic renal artery stenosis, hypertension secondary to scleroderma renal crisis, diagnosis of aldosteronism, idiopathic edema, Bartter's syndrome, postmyocardial infarction for prevention of ventricular failure

Pregnancy Risk Factor C (first trimester); D (second and third trimester)

Pregnancy/Breast-Feeding Implications

Clinical effects on the fetus: No data available on crossing the placenta. Cranial defects, hypocalvaria/acalvaria, oligohydramnios, persistent anuria following delivery, hypotension, renal defects, renal dysgenesis/dysplasia, renal failure, pulmonary hypoplasia, limb contractures secondary to oligohydramnios and still-birth reported. ACE inhibitors should be avoided during pregnancy.

Breast-feeding/lactation: Crosses into breast milk. Detectable levels but appears clinically insignificant. American Academy of Pediatrics considers COMPATIBLE with breast-feeding.

Contraindications Hypersensitivity to enalapril, enalaprilat, other ACE inhibitors, or any component

Warnings/Precautions Use with caution and modify dosage in patients with renal impairment (especially renal artery stenosis), severe congestive heart failure, or with coadministered diuretic therapy, valvular stenosis, hyperkalemia (>5.7 mEq/L); experience in children is limited. Severe hypotension may occur in patients who are sodium and/or volume depleted; initiate lower doses and monitor closely when starting therapy in these patients.

Adverse Reactions

1% to 10%:

- Cardiovascular: Chest pain, palpitations, tachycardia, syncope
- Central nervous system: Insomnia, headache, dizziness, fatigue, malaise
- Dermatologic: Rash
- Gastrointestinal: Abnormal taste, abdominal pain, vomiting, nausea, diarrhea, anorexia, constipation
- Neuromuscular & skeletal: Paresthesia, weakness
- Respiratory: Bronchitis, cough, dyspnea

<1%:

- Cardiovascular: Angina pectoris, flushing
- Dermatologic: Alopecia, erythema multiforme, pruritus, Stevens-Johnson syndrome, urticaria, angioedema
- Endocrine & metabolic: Hypoglycemia, hyperkalemia
- Genitourinary: Impotence
- Hematologic: Agranulocytosis, neutropenia, anemia
- Neuromuscular & skeletal: Myalgia
- Ocular: Blurred vision
- Otic: Tinnitus

Renal: Oliguria
Respiratory: Asthma, bronchospasm
Miscellaneous: Diaphoresis

Overdosage/Toxicology Mild hypotension has been the only toxic effect seen with acute overdose. Bradycardia may also occur; hyperkalemia occurs even with therapeutic doses, especially in patients with renal insufficiency and those taking NSAIDs

Following initiation of essential overdose management, toxic symptom treatment and supportive treatment should be initiated. Hypotension usually responds to I.V. fluids or Trendelenburg positioning.

Drug Interactions See table.

Drug-Drug Interactions With ACEIs

Precipitant Drug	Drug (Category) and Effect	Description
Antacids	ACE Inhibitors: decreased	Decreased bioavailability of ACEIs. May be more likely with captopril. Separate administration times by 1-2 hours.
NSAIDs (indomethacin)	ACEIs: decreased	Reduced hypotensive effects of ACEIs. More prominent in low renin or volume dependent hypertensive patients.
Phenothiazines	ACEIs: increased	Pharmacologic effects of ACEIs may be increased.
ACEIs	Allopurinol: increased	Higher risk of hypersensitivity reaction possible when given concurrently. Three case reports of Stevens-Johnson syndrome with captopril.
ACEIs	Digoxin: increased	Increased plasma digoxin levels.
ACEIs	Lithium: increased	Increased serum lithium levels and symptoms of toxicity may occur.
ACEIs	Potassium preps/ potassium sparing diuretics increased	Coadministration may result in elevated potassium levels.

Stability Enalaprilat: Clear, colorless solution which should be stored at <30°C; I.V. is 24 hours at room temperature in D_5W or NS

Mechanism of Action Competitive inhibitor of angiotensin-converting enzyme (ACE); prevents conversion of angiotensin I to angiotensin II, a potent vasoconstrictor; results in lower levels of angiotensin II which causes an increase in plasma renin activity and a reduction in aldosterone secretion

Pharmacodynamics/Kinetics

Oral:
- Onset of action: ~1 hour
- Duration: 12-24 hours

Absorption: Oral: 55% to 75%
Protein binding: 50% to 60%
Metabolism: Enalapril is a prodrug and undergoes biotransformation to enalaprilat in the liver
Half-life:
- Enalapril: Adults:
  - Healthy: 2 hours
  - With congestive heart failure: 3.4-5.8 hours
- Enalaprilat:
  - Infants 6 weeks to 8 months: 6-10 hours
  - Adults: 35-38 hours

Time to peak serum concentration: Oral:
- Enalapril: Within 0.5-1.5 hours
- Enalaprilat (active): Within 3-4.5 hours

Elimination: Principally in urine (60% to 80%) with some fecal excretion

Usual Dosage Use lower listed initial dose in patients with hyponatremia, hypovolemia, severe congestive heart failure, decreased renal function, or in those receiving diuretics

Infants and Children:
- Investigational initial oral doses of **enalapril**: 0.1 mg/kg/day increasing as needed over 2 weeks to 0.5 mg/kg/day have been used to treat severe congestive heart failure in infants
- Investigational I.V. doses of **enalaprilat**: 5-10 mcg/kg/dose administered every 8-24 hours have been used for the treatment of neonatal hypertension; monitor patients carefully; select patients may require higher doses

Adults:
- Oral: **Enalapril**

(Continued)

Enalapril *(Continued)*

Hypertension: 2.5-5 mg/day then increase as required, usual therapeutic dose for hypertension: 10-40 mg/day in 1-2 divided doses; usual therapeutic dose for heart failure: 5-20 mg/day

Heart failure: As adjunct with diuretics and digitalis, initiate with 2.5 mg once or twice daily (usual range: 5-20 mg/day in 2 divided doses; maximum: 40 mg)

Asymptomatic left ventricular dysfunction: 2.5 mg twice daily, titrated as tolerated to 20 mg/day

I.V.: **Enalaprilat**

Hypertension: 1.25 mg/dose, given over 5 minutes every 6 hours; doses as high as 5 mg/dose every 6 hours have been tolerated for up to 36 hours. **Note:** If patients are concomitantly receiving diuretic therapy, begin with 0.625 mg I.V. over 5 minutes; if the effect is not adequate after 1 hour, repeat the dose and administer 1.25 mg at 6-hour intervals thereafter; if adequate, administer 0.625 mg I.V. every 6 hours

Conversion from I.V. to oral therapy if not concurrently on diuretics: 5 mg once daily; subsequent titration as needed; if concurrently receiving diuretics and responding to 0.625 mg I.V. every 6 hours, initiate with 2.5 mg/day

Dosing adjustment in renal impairment:

Oral: Enalapril:

Cl_{cr} 30-80 mL/minute: Administer 5 mg/day titrated upwards to maximum of 40 mg

Cl_{cr} <30 mL/minute: Administer 2.5 mg day; titrated upward until blood pressure is controlled

For heart failure patients with sodium <130 mEq/L or serum creatinine >$^{1}/_{6}$ mg/dL, initiate dosage with 2.5 mg/day, increasing to twice daily as needed; increase further in increments of 2.5 mg/dose at >4-day intervals to a maximum daily dose of 40 mg

I.V.: Enalaprilat:

Cl_{cr} >30 mL/minute: Initiate with 1.25 mg every 6 hours and increase dose based on response

Cl_{cr} <30 mL/minute: Initiate with 0.625 mg every 6 hours and increase dose based on response

Hemodialysis: Moderately dialyzable (20% to 50%); administer dose postdialysis (eg, 0.625 mg I.V. every 6 hours) or administer 20% to 25% supplemental dose following dialysis; Clearance: 62 mL/minute

Peritoneal dialysis: Supplemental dose is not necessary, although some removal of drug occurs

Dosing adjustment in hepatic impairment: Hydrolysis of enalapril to enalaprilat may be delayed and/or impaired in patients with sever hepatic impairment, but the pharmacodynamic effects of the drug do not appear to be significantly altered; no dosage adjustment

Administration Administer direct IVP over at least 5 minutes or dilute up to 50 mL and infuse

Monitoring Parameters Blood pressure, renal function, WBC, serum potassium; blood pressure monitor required during intravenous administration

Test Interactions Positive Coombs' [direct]; may cause false-positive results in urine acetone determinations using sodium nitroprusside reagent

Patient Information Notify physician if vomiting, diarrhea, excessive perspiration, or dehydration should occur; also if swelling of face, lips, tongue, or difficulty in breathing occurs or if persistent cough develops

Nursing Implications May cause depression in some patients; discontinue if angioedema of the face, extremities, lips, tongue, or glottis occurs; watch for hypotensive effects within 1-3 hours of first dose or new higher dose

Dosage Forms

Injection, as enalaprilat: 1.25 mg/mL (1 mL, 2 mL)

Tablet, as maleate: 2.5 mg, 5 mg, 10 mg, 20 mg

Extemporaneous Preparations An enalapril oral suspension (0.2 mg/mL) has been made using one 2.5 mg tablet and 12.5 mL sterile water; stability unknown; suspension should be used immediately and the remaining amount discarded

Young TE and Mangum OB, "Neofax®, '95: A Manual of Drugs Used in Neonatal Care," 8th ed, Columbus, OH: Ross Products Division, Abbott Laboratories, 1995, 85.

Enalaprilat *see* Enalapril *on page 442*

Enalapril Maleate *see* Enalapril *on page 442*

Endep® *see* Amitriptyline *on page 69*

End Lice® Liquid [OTC] *see* Pyrethrins *on page 1079*

Endolor® *see* Butalbital Compound *on page 176*

Endrate® *see* Edetate Disodium *on page 438*

Enduron® *see* Methyclothiazide *on page 813*

Ener-B® [OTC] *see* Cyanocobalamin *on page 319*

Engerix-B® *see* Hepatitis B Vaccine *on page 607*

Enhanced-potency Inactivated Poliovirus Vaccine *see* Polio Vaccines *on page 1015*

Enlon® *see* Edrophonium *on page 439*

Enovil® *see* Amitriptyline *on page 69*

Enoxacin (en OKS a sin)

Brand Names Penetrex™

Canadian/Mexican Brand Names Comprecin® (Mexico)

Therapeutic Category Antibiotic, Quinolone

Use Treatment of complicated and uncomplicated urinary tract infections caused by susceptible gram-negative and gram-positive bacteria

Pregnancy Risk Factor C

Contraindications Hypersensitivity to enoxacin, any component, or other quinolones

Warnings/Precautions Use with caution in patients with a history of convulsions or epilepsy, renal dysfunction, psychosis, elevated intracranial pressure, prepubertal children, and pregnancy; nalidixic acid and ciprofloxacin (related compounds) have been associated with erosions of the cartilage in weight-bearing joints and other signs of arthropathy in immature animals and children; similar precautions are advised for enoxacin although no data is available; has rarely caused ruptured tendons (discontinue immediately with signs of inflammation or tendon pain)

Adverse Reactions

1% to 10%: Gastrointestinal: Nausea, vomiting

<1%:

Central nervous system: Restlessness, dizziness, confusion, seizures, headache

Dermatologic: Rash

Gastrointestinal: Diarrhea, GI bleeding

Hematologic: Anemia

Hepatic: Increased liver enzymes

Neuromuscular & skeletal: Tremor, arthralgia, ruptured tendons

Renal: Increased serum creatinine/BUN, acute renal failure

Overdosage/Toxicology Symptoms of overdose include acute renal failure, seizures

GI decontamination and supportive care; diazepam for seizures; not removed by peritoneal or hemodialysis

Drug Interactions

Decreased effect with antacids (magnesium, aluminum), iron and zinc salts, sucralfate, bismuth salts

Increased toxicity/levels of warfarin, cyclosporine, digoxin, caffeine; increased levels with cimetidine

Mechanism of Action Exerts a broad spectrum antimicrobial effect. The primary target of the fluoroquinolones is DNA gyrase (topoisomerase II) an essential bacterial enzyme that maintains the superhelical structure of DNA. DNA gyrase is required for DNA replication and transcription, DNA repair, recombination, and transposition.

Pharmacodynamics/Kinetics

Absorption: 98%

Distribution: Penetrates well into tissues and body secretions

Bioavailability: Has essentially the same bioavailability as intravenous administration; administration with food does not affect the bioavailability of enoxacin

Half-life: 3-6 hours (average)

Elimination: Primarily in urine, however, significant drug concentrations are achieved in feces

Usual Dosage Adults: Oral: 400 mg twice daily

Dosing adjustment in renal impairment:

Cl_{cr} <50 mL/minute: Administer 50% of dose

Patient Information Take at least 1 hour before or 2 hours after a meal

Dosage Forms Tablet: 200 mg, 400 mg

Enoxaparin (e noks ah PAIR in)

Brand Names Lovenox®

Synonyms Enoxaparin Sodium

Therapeutic Category Anticoagulant

(Continued)

Enoxaparin *(Continued)*

Use Prevention of deep vein thrombosis following orthopedic or abdominal surgery; has demonstrated effectiveness in the treatment of existing deep vein thromboses and pulmonary embolus

Pregnancy Risk Factor B

Contraindications Patients with active major bleeding, thrombocytopenia associated with a positive *in vitro* test for antiplatelet antibody or enoxaparin-induced platelet aggregation, hypersensitivity to enoxaparin, known hypersensitivity to heparin or pork products

Warnings/Precautions Do not administer intramuscularly; use with extreme caution in patients with a history of heparin-induced thrombocytopenia; bacterial endocarditis, hemorrhagic stroke, recent CNS or ophthalmological surgery, bleeding diathesis, uncontrolled arterial hypertension, or a history of recent gastrointestinal ulceration and hemorrhage. Elderly and patients with renal insufficiency may show delayed elimination of enoxaparin; avoid use in lactation.

Adverse Reactions

1% to 10%:

- Central nervous system: Fever, confusion, pain
- Dermatologic: Erythema, bruising
- Gastrointestinal: Nausea
- Hematologic: Hemorrhage, thrombocytopenia, hypochromic anemia, hematoma
- Local: Irritation

At the recommended doses, single injections of enoxaparin do not significantly influence platelet aggregation or affect global clotting time (ie, prothrombin time or activated partial thromboplastin time)

Overdosage/Toxicology Symptoms of overdose include hemorrhage; protamine zinc has been used to reverse effects

Drug Interactions Increased toxicity with oral anticoagulants, platelet inhibitors

Pharmacodynamics/Kinetics

Onset of effect: Maximum antifactor Xa and antithrombin (antifactor IIa) activities occur 3-5 hours after S.C. administration

Duration: Following a 40 mg dose, significant antifactor Xa activity persists in plasma for ~12 hours

Protein binding: Low molecular weight heparins do not bind to heparin binding proteins

Half-life, plasma: Low molecular weight heparin is 2-4 times longer than standard heparin independent of the dose

Usual Dosage S.C.:

Children: In one dose-finding study, children >2 months of age required 1 mg/kg twice daily for treatment of thrombotic disease

Adults:

Prophylaxis: 30 mg twice daily; first dose within 12 hours after orthopedic surgery and every 12 hours for 3 days (including day of surgery); after 3 days, switch to adjusted dose heparin

A single daily dose of 40 mg has been found to be equally effective in patients undergoing orthopedic or gynecologic surgical procedures

Abdominal surgery: 40 mg once daily; first dose beginning 2 hours before surgery and continuing for a maximum of 12 days (usual: 10 days)

Treatment of DVT: 1 mg/kg twice daily

Dosing adjustment in renal impairment: Adjustment may be necessary in elderly and patients with severe renal impairment

Monitoring Parameters Platelets, occult blood, and anti-Xa activity, if available; the monitoring of PT and/or PTT is not necessary

Dosage Forms Injection, as sodium, preservative free: 30 mg/0.3 mL; 40 mg/0.4 mL

Enoxaparin Sodium *see* Enoxaparin *on previous page*

Enulose® *see* Lactulose *on page 703*

Ephedrine (e FED rin)

Brand Names Ectasule®; Efedron®; Ephedsol®; Vicks Vatronol®

Synonyms Ephedrine Sulfate

Therapeutic Category Adrenergic Agonist Agent; Bronchodilator; Sympathomimetic

Use Treatment of bronchial asthma, nasal congestion, acute bronchospasm, idiopathic orthostatic hypotension

Pregnancy Risk Factor C

Contraindications Hypersensitivity to ephedrine or any component, cardiac arrhythmias, angle-closure glaucoma, patients on other sympathomimetic agents

Warnings/Precautions Blood volume depletion should be corrected before ephedrine therapy is instituted; use caution in patients with unstable vasomotor symptoms, diabetes, hyperthyroidism, prostatic hypertrophy, or a history of seizures; also use caution in the elderly and those patients with cardiovascular disorders such as coronary artery disease, arrhythmias, and hypertension. Ephedrine may cause hypertension resulting in intracranial hemorrhage. Long-term use may cause anxiety and symptoms of paranoid schizophrenia. Avoid as a bronchodilator; generally not used as a bronchodilator since new $beta_2$ agents are less toxic. Use with caution in the elderly, since it crosses the blood-brain barrier and may cause confusion.

Adverse Reactions

>10%: Central nervous system: CNS stimulating effects, nervousness, anxiety, apprehension, fear, tension, agitation, excitation, restlessness, irritability, insomnia, hyperactivity

1% to 10%:

- Cardiovascular: Hypertension, tachycardia, palpitations, elevation or depression of blood pressure, unusual pallor
- Central nervous system: Dizziness, headache
- Gastrointestinal: Xerostomia, nausea, anorexia, GI upset, vomiting
- Genitourinary: Painful urination
- Neuromuscular & skeletal: Trembling, tremor (more common in the elderly), weakness
- Miscellaneous: Diaphoresis (increased)

<1%:

- Cardiovascular: Chest pain, arrhythmias
- Respiratory: Dyspnea

Overdosage/Toxicology Symptoms of overdose include dysrhythmias, CNS excitation, respiratory depression, vomiting, convulsions

There is no specific antidote for ephedrine intoxication and the bulk of the treatment is supportive. Hyperactivity and agitation usually respond to reduced sensory input; however, with extreme agitation, haloperidol (2-5 mg I.M. for adults) may be required. Hyperthermia is best treated with external cooling measures; or when severe or unresponsive, muscle paralysis with pancuronium may be needed. Hypertension is usually transient and generally does not require treatment unless severe. For diastolic blood pressures >110 mm Hg, a nitroprusside infusion should be initiated. Seizures usually respond to diazepam I.V. and/or phenytoin maintenance regimens.

Drug Interactions

Decreased effect: Alpha- and beta-adrenergic blocking agents decrease ephedrine vasopressor effects

Increased toxicity: Additive cardiostimulation with other sympathomimetic agents; theophylline → cardiostimulation; MAO inhibitors or atropine may increase blood pressure; cardiac glycosides or general anesthetics may increase cardiac stimulation

Stability Protect all dosage forms from light

Mechanism of Action Releases tissue stores of epinephrine and thereby produces an alpha- and beta-adrenergic stimulation; longer-acting and less potent than epinephrine

Pharmacodynamics/Kinetics

Oral:

- Onset of bronchodilation: Within 0.25-1 hour
- Duration of action: 3-6 hours

Distribution: Crosses the placenta; appears in breast milk

Metabolism: Little hepatic metabolism

Half-life: 2.5-3.6 hours

Elimination: 60% to 77% of dose excreted as unchanged drug in urine within 24 hours

Usual Dosage

Children:

- Oral, S.C.: 3 mg/kg/day or 25-100 mg/m^2/day in 4-6 divided doses every 4-6 hours
- I.M., slow I.V. push: 0.2-0.3 mg/kg/dose every 4-6 hours

Adults:

- Oral: 25-50 mg every 3-4 hours as needed
- I.M., S.C.: 25-50 mg, parenteral adult dose should not exceed 150 mg in 24 hours
- I.V.: 5-25 mg/dose slow I.V. push repeated after 5-10 minutes as needed, then every 3-4 hours not to exceed 150 mg/24 hours

Monitoring Parameters Blood pressure, pulse, urinary output, mental status; cardiac monitor and blood pressure monitor required

Test Interactions Can cause a false-positive amphetamine EMIT assay

Patient Information May cause wakefulness or nervousness; take last dose 4-6 hours before bedtime

Nursing Implications Do not administer unless solution is clear

(Continued)

Ephedrine *(Continued)*

Dosage Forms

Capsule, as sulfate: 25 mg, 50 mg
Injection, as sulfate: 25 mg/mL (1 mL); 50 mg/mL (1 mL, 10 mL)
Jelly, as sulfate (Kondon's Nasal®): 1% (20 g)
Spray, as sulfate (Pretz-D®): 0.25% (15 mL)

Ephedrine Sulfate *see* Ephedrine *on page 446*

Ephedsol® *see* Ephedrine *on page 446*

Epifrin® *see* Epinephrine *on this page*

Epilepsy Treatment *see page 1531*

Epinal® *see* Epinephrine *on this page*

Epinephrine (ep i NEF rin)

Related Information

Adrenergic Agonists, Cardiovascular Comparison *on page 1385*
Adult ACLS Algorithm, Asystole *on page 1511*
Adult ACLS Algorithm, Bradycardia *on page 1514*
Adult ACLS Algorithm, Pulseless Electrical Activity *on page 1510*
Adult ACLS Algorithm, V. Fib and Pulseless V. Tach *on page 1509*
Cardiovascular Agents Comparison *on page 1405*
Desensitization Protocols *on page 1496*
Extravasation Treatment of Other Drugs *on page 1381*
Glaucoma Drug Therapy Comparison *on page 1410*
Pediatric ALS Algorithm, Asystole and Pulseless Arrest *on page 1507*
Pediatric ALS Algorithm, Bradycardia *on page 1506*

Brand Names Adrenalin®; AsthmaHaler®; AsthmaNefrin® [OTC]; Bronitin®; Bronkaid® Mist [OTC]; Epifrin®; Epinal®; EpiPen® Auto-Injector; EpiPen® Jr Auto-Injector; Glaucon®; microNefrin®; Primatene® Mist [OTC]; Sus-Phrine®; Vaponefrin®

Canadian/Mexican Brand Names Epi E-Z Pen™ (Canada); Epi E-Z Pen™ Jr (Canada)

Synonyms Adrenaline; Epinephrine Bitartrate; Epinephrine Hydrochloride; Racemic Epinephrine

Therapeutic Category Adrenergic Agonist Agent; Antidote, Hypersensitivity Reactions; Bronchodilator; Sympathomimetic

Use Treatment of bronchospasms, anaphylactic reactions, cardiac arrest, management of open-angle (chronic simple) glaucoma

Pregnancy Risk Factor C

Pregnancy/Breast-Feeding Implications

Clinical effects on the fetus: Crosses the placenta. Reported association with malformations in 1 study; may be secondary to severe maternal disease.

Breast-feeding/lactation: No data on crossing into breast milk or clinical effects on the infant

Contraindications Hypersensitivity to epinephrine or any component; cardiac arrhythmias, angle-closure glaucoma

Warnings/Precautions Use with caution in elderly patients, patients with diabetes mellitus, cardiovascular diseases (angina, tachycardia, myocardial infarction), thyroid disease, or cerebral arteriosclerosis, Parkinson's; some products contain sulfites as preservatives. Rapid I.V. infusion may cause death from cerebrovascular hemorrhage or cardiac arrhythmias. Oral inhalation of epinephrine is **not** the preferred route of administration.

Adverse Reactions

>10%:
- Cardiovascular: Tachycardia (parenteral), pounding heartbeat
- Central nervous system: Nervousness, restlessness

1% to 10%:
- Cardiovascular: Flushing, hypertension, unusual pallor
- Central nervous system: Headache, dizziness, lightheadedness, insomnia
- Gastrointestinal: Nausea, vomiting
- Neuromuscular & skeletal: Weakness, trembling
- Miscellaneous: Diaphoresis (increased)

<1%:
- Cardiovascular: Pallor, tachycardia, hypertension, chest pain, increased myocardial oxygen consumption, cardiac arrhythmias, sudden death
- Central nervous system: Anxiety
- Gastrointestinal: Xerostomia, dry throat
- Genitourinary: Decreased renal and splanchnic blood flow, acute urinary retention in patients with bladder outflow obstruction
- Ocular: Precipitation of or exacerbation of narrow-angle glaucoma
- Respiratory: Wheezing

Overdosage/Toxicology Hypertension which may result in subarachnoid hemorrhage and hemiplegia; symptoms of overdose include arrhythmias, unusually large pupils, pulmonary edema, renal failure, metabolic acidosis

There is no specific antidote for epinephrine intoxication and the bulk of the treatment is supportive. Hyperactivity and agitation usually respond to reduced sensory input; however, with extreme agitation, haloperidol (2-5 mg I.M. for adults) may be required. Hyperthermia is best treated with external cooling measures; or when severe or unresponsive, muscle paralysis with pancuronium may be needed. Hypertension is usually transient and generally does not require treatment unless severe. For diastolic blood pressures >110 mm Hg, a nitroprusside infusion should be initiated. Seizures usually respond to diazepam I.V. and/or phenytoin maintenance regimens.

Drug Interactions Increased toxicity: Increased cardiac irritability if administered concurrently with halogenated inhalational anesthetics, beta-blocking agents, alpha-blocking agents

Stability

Epinephrine is sensitive to light and air; protection from light is recommended

Oxidation turns drug pink, then a brown color; **solutions should not be used if they are discolored or contain a precipitate**

Stability of injection of parenteral admixture at room temperature (25°C) or refrigeration (4°C): 24 hours

Standard diluent: 1 mg/250 mL NS

Compatible with dopamine, dobutamine, diltiazem

Incompatible with aminophylline, sodium bicarbonate or other alkaline solutions

Mechanism of Action Stimulates alpha-, beta$_1$-, and beta$_2$-adrenergic receptors resulting in relaxation of smooth muscle of the bronchial tree, cardiac stimulation, and dilation of skeletal muscle vasculature; small doses can cause vasodilation via beta$_2$-vascular receptors; large doses may produce constriction of skeletal and vascular smooth muscle; decreases production of aqueous humor and increases aqueous outflow; dilates the pupil by contracting the dilator muscle

Pharmacodynamics/Kinetics

Onset of bronchodilation:
- Subcutaneous: Within 5-10 minutes
- Inhalation: Within 1 minute

Conjunctival instillation:
- Onset of effect: Intraocular pressures fall within 1 hour
- Peak effect: Within 4-8 hours

Duration of ocular effect: 12-24 hours

Absorption: Orally ingested doses are rapidly metabolized in the GI tract and liver; pharmacologically active concentrations are not achieved

Distribution: Crosses the placenta; appears in breast milk

Metabolism: Following administration, drug is taken up into the adrenergic neuron and metabolized by monoamine oxidase and catechol-o-methyltransferase; circulating drug is metabolized in the liver

Elimination: Inactive metabolites (metanephrine and the sulfate and hydroxy derivatives of mandelic acid) and a small amount of unchanged drug is excreted in urine

Usual Dosage

Bronchodilator:
- Children: S.C.: 10 mcg/kg (0.01 mL/kg of 1:1000) (single doses not to exceed 0.5 mg); injection suspension (1:200): 0.005 mL/kg/dose (0.025 mg/kg/dose) to a maximum of 0.15 mL (0.75 mg for single dose) every 8-12 hours
- Adults:
  - I.M., S.C. (1:1000): 0.1-0.5 mg every 10-15 minutes to 4 hours
  - Suspension (1:200) S.C.: 0.1-0.3 mL (0.5-1.5 mg)
  - I.V.: 0.1-0.25 mg (single dose maximum: 1 mg)

Cardiac arrest:
- Infants and Children: Asystole or pulseless arrest:
  - I.V., intraosseous: First dose: 0.01 mg/kg (0.1 mL/kg of a 1:10,000 solution); subsequent doses: 0.1 mg/kg (0.1 mL/kg of a 1:1000 solution); doses as high as 0.2 mg/kg may be effective; repeat every 3-5 minutes
  - Intratracheal: 0.1 mg/kg (0.1 mL/kg of a 1:1000 solution); doses as high as 0.2 mg/kg may be effective
- Adults: Asystole:
  - I.V.: 1 mg every 3-5 minutes; if this approach fails, alternative regimens include: Intermediate: 2-5 mg every 3-5 minutes; Escalating: 1 mg, 3 mg, 5 mg at 3-minute intervals; High: 0.1 mg/kg every 3-5 minutes
  - Intratracheal: Although optimal dose is unknown, doses of 2-2.5 times the I.V. dose may be needed

Bradycardia: Children:
- I.V.: 0.01 mg/kg (0.1 mL/kg of 1:10,000 solution) every 3-5 minutes as needed (maximum: 1 mg/10 mL)

(Continued)

Epinephrine *(Continued)*

Intratracheal: 0.1 mg/kg (0.1 mL/kg of 1:1000 solution every 3-5 minutes); doses as high as 0.2 mg/kg may be effective

Refractory hypotension (refractory to dopamine/dobutamine): I.V. infusion administration requires the use of an infusion pump:

Children: Infusion rate 0.1-4 mcg/kg/minute

Adults: I.V. infusion: 1 mg in 250 mL NS/D_5W at 0.1-1 mcg/kg/minute; titrate to desired effect

Hypersensitivity reaction:

Children: S.C.: 0.01 mg/kg every 15 minutes for 2 doses then every 4 hours as needed (single doses not to exceed 0.5 mg)

Adults: I.M., S.C.: 0.2-0.5 mg every 20 minutes to 4 hours (single dose maximum: 1 mg)

Nebulization:

Children <2 years: 0.25 mL of 1:1000 diluted in 3 mL NS with treatments ordered individually

Children >2 years and Adolescents: 0.5 mL of 1:1000 concentration diluted in 3 mL NS

Children >2 years and Adults (racemic epinephrine):

<10 kg: 2 mL of 1:8 dilution over 15 minutes every 1-4 hours
10-15 kg: 2 mL of 1:6 dilution over 15 minutes every 1-4 hours
15-20 kg: 2 mL of 1:4 dilution over 15 minutes every 1-4 hours
>20 kg: 2 mL of 1:3 dilution over 15 minutes every 1-4 hours

Adults: Instill 8-15 drops into nebulizer reservoirs; administer 1-3 inhalations 4-6 times/day

Ophthalmic: Instill 1-2 drops in eye(s) once or twice daily

Intranasal: Children ≥6 years and Adults: Apply locally as drops or spray or with sterile swab

Administration Central line administration only; intravenous infusions require an infusion pump

Endotracheal: Doses (2-2.5 times the I.V. dose) should be diluted to 10 mL with NS or distilled water prior to administration

Epinephrine can be administered S.C., I.M., I.V., or intracardiac injection

I.M. administration into the buttocks should be avoided

Desired pediatric intravenous infusion solution preparation: "RULE OF 6"

Simplified equation: 0.6 x weight (kg) = amount (mg) of drug to be added to 100 mL of I.V. fluid

When infused at 1 mL/hour, then it will deliver the drug at a rate of 0.1 mcg/kg/minute

Complex equation: 0.6 x desired dose (mcg/kg/minute) x body weight (kg) divided by desired rate (mL/hour) is the mg added to make 100 mL of solution

Preparation of adult I.V. infusion: Dilute 1 mg in 250 mL of D_5W or NS (4 mcg/mL); administer at an initial rate of 1 mcg/minute and increase to desired effects; at 20 mcg/minute pure alpha effects occur

1 mcg/minute: 15 mL/hour
2 mcg/minute: 30 mL/hour
3 mcg/minute: 45 mL/hour, etc

Monitoring Parameters Pulmonary function, heart rate, blood pressure, site of infusion for blanching, extravasation; cardiac monitor and blood pressure monitor required

Reference Range Therapeutic: 31-95 pg/mL (SI: 170-520 pmol/L)

Test Interactions ↑ bilirubin (S), catecholamines (U), glucose, uric acid (S)

Nursing Implications Patients should be cautioned to avoid the use of over-the-counter epinephrine inhalation products; $beta_2$-adrenergic agents for inhalation are preferred

Management of extravasation: Use phentolamine as antidote; mix 5 mg with 9 mL of NS; inject a small amount of this dilution into extravasated area; blanching should reverse immediately. Monitor site; if blanching should recur, additional injections of phentolamine may be needed.

Additional Information

Epinephrine: Primatene® Mist, Bronkaid® Mist, Sus-Phrine®

Epinephrine bitartrate: AsthmaHaler®, Bronitin®, Epitrate®, Medihaler-Epi®; Primatene® Mist

Epinephrine hydrochloride: Adrenalin®, Epifrin®, EpiPen®, EpiPen® Jr

Racemic epinephrine: AsthmaHaler®, Breatheasy®, microNefrin®, Vaponefrin®

Epinephryl borate: Epinal®

Dosage Forms

Aerosol, oral:

Bitartrate (AsthmaHaler®, Bronitin®, Medihaler-Epi®, Primatene® Suspension): 0.3 mg/spray [epinephrine base 0.16 mg/spray] (10 mL, 15 mL, 22.5 mL)

Bronkaid®: 0.5% (10 mL, 15 mL, 22.5 mL)

Primatene®: 0.2 mg/spray (15 mL, 22.5 mL)

Auto-injector:

EpiPen®: Delivers 0.3 mg I.M. of epinephrine 1:1000 (2 mL)

EpiPen® Jr.: Delivers 0.15 mg I.M. of epinephrine 1:2000 (2 mL)

Solution:

Inhalation:

Adrenalin®: 1% [10 mg/mL, 1:100] (7.5 mL)

AsthmaNefrin®, microNefrin®, Nephron®, S-2®: Racepinephrine 2% [epinephrine base 1.125%] (7.5 mL, 15 mL, 30 mL)

Vaponefrin®: Racepinephrine 2% [epinephrine base 1%] (15 mL, 30 mL)

Injection:

Adrenalin®: 0.01 mg/mL [1:100,000] (5 mL); 0.1 mg/mL [1:10,000] (3 mL, 10 mL); 1 mg/mL [1:1000] (1 mL, 2 mL, 30 mL)

Suspension (Sus-Phrine®): 5 mg/mL [1:200] (0.3 mL, 5 mL)

Nasal (Adrenalin®): 0.1% [1 mg/mL, 1:1000] (30 mL)

Ophthalmic, as borate (Epinal®): 0.5% (7.5 mL); 1% (7.5 mL)

Ophthalmic, as hydrochloride (Epifrin®, Glaucon®): 0.1% (1 mL, 30 mL); 0.5% (15 mL); 1% (1 mL, 10 mL, 15 mL); 2% (10 mL, 15 mL)

Topical (Adrenalin®): 0.1% [1 mg/mL, 1:1000] (10 mL, 30 mL)

Epinephrine Bitartrate *see* Epinephrine *on page 448*

Epinephrine Hydrochloride *see* Epinephrine *on page 448*

EpiPen® Auto-Injector *see* Epinephrine *on page 448*

EpiPen® Jr Auto-Injector *see* Epinephrine *on page 448*

Epipodophyllotoxin *see* Etoposide *on page 496*

Epitol® *see* Carbamazepine *on page 201*

Epivir® *see* Lamivudine *on page 704*

EPO *see* Epoetin Alfa *on this page*

Epoetin Alfa (e POE e tin AL fa)

Brand Names Epogen®; ProCrit®

Synonyms EPO; Erythropoietin; *r*HuEPO-α

Therapeutic Category Colony Stimulating Factor; Growth Factor; Recombinant Human Erythropoietin

Use

Anemia associated with end stage renal disease (FDA-approved indication)

Anemia in cancer patients with nonmyeloid malignancies on chemotherapy (FDA-approved indication)

Anemia related to AIDS and therapy with AZT-treated in HIV-infected patients (FDA-approved indication)

Endogenous serum erythropoietin (EPO) level which are inappropriately low for hemoglobin level (eg, anemia of neoplasia); (FDA-approved indication)

Patients undergoing autologous blood donation prior to surgery - EPO may accelerate recovery of hemoglobin level and, in some cases, permit more units of blood to be donated

HuEPO is not beneficial in the acute treatment of anemia (onset of reticulocyte response does not appear until 7-10 days and hemoglobin rise appears over 2-6 weeks after starting therapy). Therefore, emergency/stat orders for the drug are not appropriate.

Pregnancy Risk Factor C

Pregnancy/Breast-Feeding Implications Epoetin alfa has been shown to have adverse effects in rats when given in doses 5X the human dose. There are no adequate and well-controlled studies in pregnant women. Epoetin alfa should be used only if potential benefit justifies the potential risk to the fetus.

Contraindications Known hypersensitivity to albumin (human) or mammalian cell-derived products; uncontrolled hypertension

Warnings/Precautions Use with caution in patients with porphyria, hypertension, or a history of seizures; prior to and during therapy, iron stores must be evaluated. It is recommended that the epoetin dose be decreased if the hematocrit increase exceeds 4 points in any 2-week period.

Pretherapy parameters:

Serum ferritin >300 ng/dL

Transferrin saturation (serum iron/iron binding capacity x 100) of 20% to 30%

Iron supplementation (usual oral dosing of 325 mg 2-3 times/day) should be given during therapy to provide for increased requirements during expansion of the red cell mass secondary to marrow stimulation by EPO unless iron stores are already in excess.

(Continued)

Epoetin Alfa *(Continued)*

For patients with endogenous serum EPO levels which are inappropriately low for hemoglobin level, documentation of the serum EPO level will help indicate which patients may benefit from EPO therapy. Serum EPO levels can be ordered routinely from Clinical Chemistry (red-top serum separator tube). Refer to "Reference Range" for information on interpretation of EPO levels.

See table:

Factors Limiting Response to Epoetin Alfa

Factor	Mechanism
Iron deficiency	Limits hemoglobin synthesis
Blood loss/hemolysis	Counteracts epoetin alfa-stimulated erythropoiesis
Infection/inflammation	Inhibits iron transfer from storage to bone marrow Suppresses erythropoiesis through activated macrophages
Aluminum overload	Inhibits iron incorporation into heme protein
Bone marrow replacement Hyperparathyroidsm Metastatic, neoplastic	Limits bone marrow volume
Folic acid/vitamin B_{12} deficiency	Limits hemoglobin synthesis
Patient compliance	Self-administered epoetin alfa or iron therapy

Increased mortality has occurred when aggressive dosing is used in CHF or anginal patients undergoing hemodialysis. An Amgen-funded study determined that when patients were targeted for a hematocrit of 42% versus a less aggressive 30%, mortality was higher (35% versus 29%)

Adverse Reactions

>10%:

Cardiovascular: Hypertension

Central nervous system: Fatigue, headache, fever

1% to 10%:

Cardiovascular: Edema, chest pain

Central nervous system: Dizziness, seizures

Gastrointestinal: Nausea, vomiting, diarrhea

Hematologic: Clotted access

Neuromuscular & skeletal: Arthralgia, weakness

<1%:

Cardiovascular: Myocardial infarction, CVA/TIA

Dermatologic: Rash

Miscellaneous: Hypersensitivity reactions

Overdosage/Toxicology Symptoms of overdose include erythrocytosis

Adequate airway and other supportive measures and agents for treating anaphylaxis should be present when I.V. drug is given

Stability

Vials should be stored at 2°C to 8°C (36°F to 46°F); **do not freeze or shake**; vials are stable 2 weeks at room temperature

Single-dose 1 mL vial contains no preservative: Use one dose per vial; do not re-enter vial; discard unused portions

Multidose 2 mL vial contains preservative; store at 2°C to 8°C after initial entry and between doses; discard 21 days after initial entry

For minimal dilution: Mix with bacteriostatic 0.9% sodium chloride, containing 20 mL of 0.9% sodium chloride and benzyl alcohol as the bacteriostatic agent; dilutions of 1:10 and 1:20 (1 part epoetin:19 parts sodium chloride) are stable for 18 hours at room temperature; results showed no loss of epoetin alfa after a 1:20 dilution; 250 mcg/mL albumin remaining after a 1:10 dilution of formulated epoetin alfa should be sufficient to prevent it from binding to commonly encountered containers

Mechanism of Action Induces erythropoiesis by stimulating the division and differentiation of committed erythroid progenitor cells; induces the release of reticulocytes from the bone marrow into the blood stream, where they mature to erythrocytes. There is a dose response relationship with this effect. This results in an increase in reticulocyte counts followed by a rise in hematocrit and hemoglobin levels.

Pharmacodynamics/Kinetics

Onset of action: Several days

Peak effect: 2-3 weeks

Distribution: V_d: 9 L; rapid in the plasma compartment; majority of drug is taken up by the liver, kidneys, and bone marrow

Metabolism: Some metabolic degradation does occur

Bioavailability: S.C.: ~21% to 31%; intraperitoneal epoetin in a few patients demonstrated a bioavailability of only 3%

Half-life: Circulating: 4-13 hours in patients with chronic renal failure; 20% shorter in patients with normal renal function

Time to peak serum concentrations: S.C.: 2-8 hours

Elimination: Small amounts recovered in the urine; majority hepatically eliminated; 10% excreted unchanged in the urine of normal volunteers

Usual Dosage

Individuals with anemia due to iron deficiency, sickle cell disease, autoimmune hemolytic anemia, and bleeding, generally have appropriate endogenous EPO levels to drive erythropoiesis and would not ordinarily be candidates for EPO therapy

Dosing recommendations:

Dosing schedules need to be individualized and careful monitoring of patients receiving the drug is mandatory

HuEPO may be ineffective if other factors such as iron or B_{12}/folate deficiency limit marrow response

Initial dose: I.V., S.C.: 50-150 units/kg 3 times/week

Dose should be reduced when the hematocrit reaches the target range of 30% to 36% or a hematocrit increase of >4 points over any 2-week period

Dose should be held if the hematocrit exceeds 36% and until the hematocrit decreases to the target range (30% to 36%)

Dose should be increased by 25-50 units/kg 3 times/week if the hematocrit does not increase by 5-6 points after 8 weeks of therapy and hematocrit is below the target range; further increases of 25 units/kg 3 times/week may be made at 4- to 6-week intervals until the desired response is obtained. Doses exceeding 300 units/kg 3 times/week are not recommended because a greater biological response is not usually observed.

Maintenance dose: Should be individualized to maintain the hematocrit within the 30% to 36% target range

Dosing adjustment/comments in renal impairment:

Dialysis patients: Usually administered as I.V. bolus 3 times/week; while administration is independent of the dialysis procedure, it may be administered into the venous line at the end of the dialysis procedure to obviate the need for additional venous access

Chronic renal failure patients not on dialysis: May be given either as an I.V. or S.C. injection

Hemodialysis: Supplemental dose is not necessary

Peritoneal dialysis: Supplemental dose is not necessary

Monitoring Parameters

Careful monitoring of blood pressure is indicated; problems with hypertension have been noted especially in renal failure patients treated with *r*HuEPO. Other patients are less likely to develop this complication.

See table.

Test	Initial Phase Frequency	Maintenance Phase Frequency
Hematocrit/hemoglobin	2 x/week	2-4 x/month
Blood pressure	3 x/week	3 x/week
Serum ferritin	Monthly	Quarterly
Transferrin saturation	Monthly	Quarterly
Serum chemistries including CBC with differential, creatinine, blood urea nitrogen, potassium, phosphorous	Regularly per routine	Regularly per routine

Hematocrit should be determined twice weekly until stabilization within the target range (30% to 36%), and twice weekly for at least 2 to 6 weeks after a dose increase

Reference Range Guidelines should be based on the following figure or published literature

Guidelines for estimating appropriateness of endogenous EPO levels for varying levels of anemia via the EIA assay method: See figure. The reference range for erythropoietin in serum, for subjects with normal hemoglobin and hematocrit, is 4.1-22.2 mIU/mL by the EIA method. Erythropoietin levels are typically inversely related to hemoglobin (and hematocrit) levels in anemias not attributed to impaired erythropoietin production.

Zidovudine-treated HIV patients: Available evidence indicates patients with endogenous serum erythropoietin levels >500 mIU/mL are unlikely to respond

Cancer chemotherapy patients: Treatment of patients with endogenous serum erythropoietin levels >200 mIU/mL is not recommended

(Continued)

Epoetin Alfa *(Continued)*

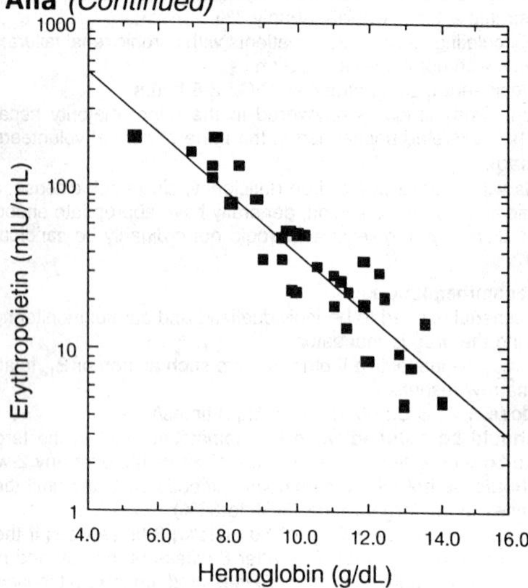

Patient Information

If necessary, the patient should be instructed as to the proper dosage and self-administration of epoetin alpha

Frequent blood tests are needed to determine the correct dose; notify physician if any severe headache develops

Additional Information

Reimbursement Hotline (Epogen®): 1-800-272-9376
Professional Services [Amgen]: 1-800-77-AMGEN
Reimbursement Hotline (Procrit®): 1-800-553-3851
Professional services [Ortho Biotech]: 1-800-325-7504

Dosage Forms

1 mL single-dose vials: Preservative-free solution
- 2000 units/mL
- 3000 units/mL
- 4000 units/mL
- 10,000 units/mL

2 mL multidose vials: Preserved solution: 10,000 units/mL

Epogen® *see* Epoetin Alfa *on page 451*

Epoprostenol (e poe PROST en ole)

Brand Names Flolan® Injection

Synonyms Epoprostenol Sodium; PGI_2; PGX; Prostacyclin

Therapeutic Category Plasma Volume Expander, Colloid; Prostaglandin

Use

Treatment of primary pulmonary hypertension in NYHA class III and IV patients

Other potential uses include pulmonary hypertension associated with ARDS, SLE, or CHF, neonatal pulmonary hypertension, cardiopulmonary bypass surgery, hemodialysis, atherosclerosis, peripheral vascular disorders, neonatal purpura fulminans, and refractory congestive heart failure

Pregnancy Risk Factor X

Contraindications Hyaline membrane disease or persistent fetal circulation and when a dominant left-to-right shunt is present, respiratory distress syndrome

Warnings/Precautions Abrupt interruptions or large sudden reductions in dosage may result in rebound pulmonary hypertension; some patients with primary pulmonary hypertension have developed pulmonary edema during dose ranging, which may be associated with pulmonary veno-occlusive disease; during chronic use, unless contraindicated, anticoagulants should be coadministered to reduce the risk of thromboembolism

Adverse Reactions

>10%:

Central nervous system: Fever, chills, anxiety, nervousness, dizziness, headache, hyperesthesia, pain

Cardiovascular: Flushing, tachycardia, shock, syncope, heart failure

Gastrointestinal: Diarrhea, nausea, vomiting

Neuromuscular & skeletal: Jaw pain, myalgia, tremor, paresthesia

Respiratory: Hypoxia

Miscellaneous: Sepsis, flu-like symptoms

1% to 10%:

Cardiovascular: Bradycardia, hypotension, tachycardia, angina pectoris, edema, arrhythmias, pallor, cyanosis, palpitations, cerebrovascular accident, myocardial ischemia, chest pain

Central nervous system: Seizures, confusion, depression, insomnia

Dermatologic: Pruritus, rash

Endocrine & metabolic: Hypokalemia, weight change

Gastrointestinal: Abdominal pain, anorexia, constipation

Hematologic: Hemorrhage

Hepatic: Ascites

Neuromuscular & skeletal: Arthralgias, bone pain, weakness

Hematologic: Disseminated intravascular coagulation

Ocular: Amblyopia

Respiratory: Cough increase, dyspnea, epistaxis, pleural effusion

Miscellaneous: Diaphoresis

Overdosage/Toxicology Symptoms of overdose include headache, hypotension, tachycardia, nausea, vomiting, diarrhea, and flushing

If any of these symptoms occur, the infusion rate should be reduced until the symptoms subside; if symptoms do not subside should then consider drug discontinuation; no fatal events have been reported following overdosage with epoprostenol

Drug Interactions Increased toxicity: The hypotensive effects of epoprostenol may be exacerbated by other vasodilators or by using acetate in dialysis fluids. Patients treated with anticoagulants and epoprostenol should be monitored for increased bleeding risk because of shared effects on platelet aggregation.

Stability Refrigerate ampuls; protect from freezing; prepare fresh solutions every 24 hours; **compatible** in D_5W, $D_{10}W$, and NS solutions

Mechanism of Action Epoprostenol is also known as prostacyclin and PG I2. It is a strong vasodilator of all vascular beds. In addition, it is a potent endogenous inhibitor of platelet aggregation. The reduction in platelet aggregation results from epoprostenol's activation of intracellular adenylate cyclase and the resultant increase in cyclic adenosine monophosphate concentrations within the platelets. Additionally, it is capable of decreasing thrombogenesis and platelet clumping in the lungs by inhibiting platelet aggregation.

Pharmacodynamics/Kinetics

Steady state levels are reached in about 15 minutes with continuous infusions

Metabolism: Rapidly hydrolyzed at neutral pH in blood and is subject to some enzymatic degradation to one active metabolite, and 13 inactive metabolites

Half-life: 2.7-6 minutes

Elimination: 12% excreted unchanged in urine

Usual Dosage I.V.: The drug is administered by continuous intravenous infusion via a central venous catheter using an ambulatory infusion pump; during dose ranging it may be administered peripherally

Acute dose ranging: The initial infusion rate should be 2 ng/kg/minute by continuous I.V. and increased in increments of 2 ng/kg/minute every 15 minutes or longer until dose-limiting effects are elicited (such as chest pain, anxiety, dizziness, changes in heart rate, dyspnea, nausea, vomiting, headache, hypotension and/or flushing)

Continuous chronic infusion: Initial: 4 ng/kg/minute **less** than the maximum-tolerated infusion rate determined during acute dose ranging.

If maximum-tolerated infusion rate is <5 ng/kg/minute the chronic infusion rate should be 1/2 the maximum-tolerated acute infusion rate

Preparation of Infusion

To make 100 mL of solution with concentration:	Directions:
3000 ng/mL	Dissolve one 0.5 mg vial with 6 mL supplied diluent, withdraw 3 mL and add to sufficient diluent to make a total of 100 mL
5000 ng/mL	Dissolve one 0.5 mg vial with 5 mL supplied diluent, withdraw entire vial contents and add a sufficient volume of diluent to make a total of 100 mL
10,000 ng/mL	Dissolve two 0.5 mg vials each with 5 mL supplied diluent, withdraw entire vial contents and add a sufficient volume of diluent to make a total of 100 mL
15,000 ng/mL	Dissolve one 1.5 mg vial with 5 mL supplied diluent, withdraw entire vial contents and add a sufficient volume of diluent to make a total of 100 mL

(Continued)

Epoprostenol *(Continued)*

Dosage adjustments: Dose adjustments in the chronic infusion rate should be based on persistence, recurrence or worsening of patient symptoms of pulmonary hypertension

If symptoms persist or recur after improving, the infusion rate should be increased by 1-2 ng/kg/minute increments, every 15 minutes or greater; following establishment of a new chronic infusion rate, the patient should be observed and vital signs monitored.

Monitoring Parameters Monitor for improvements in pulmonary function, decreased exertional dyspnea, fatigue, syncope and chest pain, pulmonary vascular resistance, pulmonary arterial pressure and quality of life. In addition, the pump device and catheters should be monitored frequently to avoid "system" related failure.

Patient Information Therapy with epoprostenol requires commitment to drug reconstitution, administration and care of the permanent central venous catheter; the decision to receive epoprostenol should be based upon the understanding that there is a high liklihood that therapy will be needed for prolonged periods, possibly for life, and that the care of the catheter and infusion pump will be required and should be carefully considered.

Nursing Implications Monitor arterial pressure; assess all vital functions; hypoxia, flushing and tachycardia may indicate overdose; epoprostenol must be reconstituted with manufacturer-supplied sterile diluent only and when given on an ongoing basis it must be infused through a permanent indwelling central venous catheter via a portable infusion pump

Additional Information All orders for epoprostenol are distributed only by Quantum Healthcare, Inc. To order the drug or to request reimbursement assistance, call 1-800-622-1820.

Dosage Forms Injection, as sodium: 0.5 mg/vial and 1.5 mg/vial, each supplied with 50 mL of sterile diluent

Epoprostenol Sodium *see* Epoprostenol *on page 454*

Epsom Salts *see* Magnesium Sulfate *on page 755*

EPT *see* Teniposide *on page 1191*

Equalactin® Chewable Tablet [OTC] *see* Calcium Polycarbophil *on page 195*

Equanil® *see* Meprobamate *on page 783*

Ercaf® *see* Ergotamine *on page 459*

Ergamisol® *see* Levamisole *on page 712*

Ergocalciferol (er goe kal SIF e role)

Brand Names Calciferol™; Drisdol®

Canadian/Mexican Brand Names Ostoforte®(Canada); Radiostol® (Canada)

Synonyms Activated Ergosterol; Viosterol; Vitamin D_2

Therapeutic Category Vitamin, Fat Soluble

Use Treatment of refractory rickets, hypophosphatemia, hypoparathyroidism

Pregnancy Risk Factor A (C if dose exceeds RDA recommendation)

Contraindications Hypercalcemia, hypersensitivity to ergocalciferol or any component; malabsorption syndrome; evidence of vitamin D toxicity

Warnings/Precautions Administer with extreme caution in patients with impaired renal function, heart disease, renal stones, or arteriosclerosis; must administer concomitant calcium supplementation; maintain adequate fluid intake; avoid hypercalcemia; renal function impairment with secondary hyperparathyroidism

Adverse Reactions

1% to 10%:

- Cardiovascular: Hypotension, cardiac arrhythmias, hypertension
- Central nervous system: Irritability, headache
- Gastrointestinal: Nausea, vomiting, anorexia, pancreatitis, metallic taste
- Genitourinary: Polyuria
- Dermatologic: Pruritus
- Endocrine & metabolic: Polydipsia
- Neuromuscular & skeletal: Bone pain, myalgia
- Ocular: Conjunctivitis, photophobia

<1%:

- Central nervous system: Overt psychosis
- Gastrointestinal: Weight loss

Overdosage/Toxicology Symptoms of chronic overdose include hypercalcemia, weakness, fatigue, lethargy, anorexia

Following withdrawal of the drug and oral decontamination, treatment consists of bedrest, liberal intake of fluids, reduced calcium intake, and cathartic administration. Severe hypercalcemia requires I.V. hydration and forced diuresis with I.V. furosemide. Urine output should be monitored and maintained at >3 mL/kg/hour.

I.V. saline can quickly and significantly increase excretion of calcium into urine. Calcitonin, mithramycin, and biphosphonates have all been used successfully to treat the more resistant cases of vitamin D-induced hypercalcemia.

Drug Interactions

Decreased effect: Cholestyramine, colestipol, mineral oil may decrease oral absorption

Increased effect: Thiazide diuretics may increase vitamin D effects

Increased toxicity: Cardiac glycosides may increase toxicity

Stability Protect from light

Mechanism of Action Stimulates calcium and phosphate absorption from the small intestine, promotes secretion of calcium from bone to blood; promotes renal tubule phosphate resorption

Pharmacodynamics/Kinetics

Peak effect: In ~1 month following daily doses

Absorption: Readily absorbed from GI tract; absorption requires intestinal presence of bile

Metabolism: Inactive until hydroxylated in the liver and the kidney to calcifediol and then to calcitriol (most active form)

Usual Dosage Oral dosing is preferred

Dietary supplementation (each mcg = 40 USP units):

- Premature infants: 10-20 mcg/day (400-800 units), up to 750 mcg/day (30,000 units)
- Infants and healthy Children: 10 mcg/day (400 units)
- Adults: 10 mcg/day (400 units)

Renal failure:

- Children: 100-1000 mcg/day (4000-40,000 units)
- Adults: 500 mcg/day (20,000 units)

Hypoparathyroidism:

- Children: 1.25-5 mg/day (50,000-200,000 units) and calcium supplements
- Adults: 625 mcg to 5 mg/day (25,000-200,000 units) and calcium supplements

Vitamin D-dependent rickets:

- Children: 75-125 mcg/day (3000-5000 units); maximum: 1500 mcg/day
- Adults: 250 mcg to 1.5 mg/day (10,000-60,000 units)

Nutritional rickets and osteomalacia:

- Children and Adults (with normal absorption): 25-125 mcg/day (1000-5000 units)
- Children with malabsorption: 250-625 mcg/day (10,000-25,000 units)
- Adults with malabsorption: 250-7500 mcg (10,000-300,000 units)

Vitamin D-resistant rickets:

- Children: Initial: 1000-2000 mcg/day (400,000-800,000 units) with phosphate supplements; daily dosage is increased at 3- to 4-month intervals in 250-500 mcg (10,000-20,000 units) increments
- Adults: 250-1500 mcg/day (10,000-60,000 units) with phosphate supplements

Administration Parenteral injection for I.M. use only

Monitoring Parameters Measure serum calcium, BUN, and phosphorus every 1-2 weeks

Reference Range Serum calcium times phosphorus should not exceed 70 mg/dL to avoid ectopic calcification; ergocalciferol levels: 10-60 ng/mL; serum calcium: 9-10 mg/dL, phosphorus: 2.5-5 mg/dL

Patient Information Early symptoms of hypercalcemia include weakness, fatigue, somnolence, headache, anorexia, dry mouth, metallic taste, nausea, vomiting, cramps, diarrhea, muscle pain, bone pain, and irritability. Your physician may place you on a special diet or have you take a calcium supplement. Follow this diet closely; do not take magnesium supplements or magnesium-containing antacids.

Nursing Implications Monitor serum calcium, phosphorus, and BUN every 2 weeks

Additional Information 1.25 mg ergocalciferol provides 50,000 units of vitamin D activity

Dosage Forms

Capsule (Drisdol®): 50,000 units [1.25 mg]

Injection (Calciferol™): 500,000 units/mL [12.5 mg/mL] (1 mL)

Liquid (Calciferol™, Drisdol®): 8000 units/mL [200 mcg/mL] (60 mL)

Tablet (Calciferol™): 50,000 units [1.25 mg]

Ergoloid Mesylates (ER goe loid MES i lates)

Brand Names Germinal®; Hydergine®; Hydergine® LC

Synonyms Dihydroergotoxine; Dihydrogenated Ergot Alkaloids

Therapeutic Category Ergot Alkaloid and Derivative

Use Treatment of cerebrovascular insufficiency in primary progressive dementia, Alzheimer's dementia, and senile onset

Pregnancy Risk Factor C

(Continued)

Ergoloid Mesylates *(Continued)*

Contraindications Acute or chronic psychosis, hypersensitivity to ergot or any component

Warnings/Precautions Exclude possibility that signs and symptoms of illness are from a potentially reversible and treatable condition

Adverse Reactions

1% to 10%:
- Gastrointestinal: Transient nausea
- Miscellaneous: Sublingual irritation

<1%:
- Cardiovascular: Bradycardia, orthostatic hypotension, flushing, syncope
- Central nervous system: Headache
- Dermatologic: Rash
- Gastrointestinal: Anorexia, nausea, vomiting, stomach cramps
- Ocular: Blurred vision
- Respiratory: Nasal congestion

Overdosage/Toxicology Symptoms of overdose include sinus bradycardia, blurred vision, headache, stomach cramps

Chronic overdose usually manifests as signs and symptoms of extremity or organ ischemia; nitroprusside has been shown to reverse the vasoconstriction associated with ergot toxicity

Drug Interactions Increased toxicity with dopamine

Mechanism of Action Ergot alkaloid alpha-adrenergic agonist directly stimulates vascular smooth muscle to vasoconstrict peripheral and cerebral vessels; may also have antagonist effects on serotonin

Pharmacodynamics/Kinetics

Absorption: Rapid yet incomplete
Metabolism: Significant first-pass metabolism
Half-life: 3.5 hours
Time to peak serum concentration: Within 1 hour

Usual Dosage Adults: Oral: 1 mg 3 times/day up to 4.5-12 mg/day; up to 6 months of therapy may be necessary

Monitoring Parameters Blood pressure, heart rate

Patient Information Do not chew or crush sublingual tablets, allow to dissolve under tongue

Dosage Forms

Capsule, liquid (Hydergine® LC): 1 mg
Liquid (Hydergine®): 1 mg/mL (100 mL)
Tablet:
- Oral:
  - 0.5 mg
  - Gerimal®, Hydergine®: 1 mg
- Sublingual:
  - Gerimal®, Hydergine®: 0.5 mg, 1 mg

Ergomar® *see* Ergotamine *on next page*

Ergometrine Maleate *see* Ergonovine *on this page*

Ergonovine (er goe NOE veen)

Brand Names Ergotrate® Maleate

Synonyms Ergometrine Maleate; Ergonovine Maleate

Therapeutic Category Ergot Alkaloid and Derivative

Use Prevention and treatment of postpartum and postabortion hemorrhage caused by uterine atony or subinvolution

Pregnancy Risk Factor X

Contraindications Induction of labor, threatened spontaneous abortion, hypersensitivity to ergonovine or any component

Warnings/Precautions Use with caution in patients with sepsis or with hepatic or renal impairment

Adverse Reactions

1% to 10%: Gastrointestinal: Nausea, vomiting

<1%:
- Cardiovascular: Palpitations, bradycardia, transient chest pain, hypertension, cerebrovascular accidents
- Central nervous system: Seizures, dizziness, headache
- Local: Thrombophlebitis
- Otic: Tinnitus
- Respiratory: Dyspnea
- Miscellaneous: Diaphoresis

Overdosage/Toxicology Symptoms of overdose include gangrene, seizures, chest pain, numbness in extremities, weak pulse, confusion, excitement, delirium, hallucinations

Treatment is supportive. Diazepam 0.1 mg/kg for seizures and excitement; haloperidol as needed for delirium or hallucinations; heparin for hypercoagulability; nitroprusside for arterial venospasm; nitroglycerin for coronary vasospasm.

Stability Refrigerate injection, protect from light; store intact ampuls in refrigerator, stable for 60-90 days; do not use if discoloration occurs

Mechanism of Action Ergot alkaloid alpha-adrenergic agonist directly stimulates vascular smooth muscle to vasoconstrict peripheral and cerebral vessels; may also have antagonist effects on serotonin

Pharmacodynamics/Kinetics

Onset of effect:

Oral: Within 5-15 minutes

I.M.: Within 2-5 minutes

Duration: Uterine effects persist for 3 hours, except when given I.V., then effects persist for ~45 minutes

Usual Dosage Adults:

Oral: 1-2 tablets (0.2-0.4 mg) every 6-12 hours for up to 48 hours

I.M., I.V. (I.V. should be reserved for emergency use only): 0.2 mg, repeat dose in 2-4 hours as needed

Administration I.V. doses should be administered over a period of not <1 minute; dilute in NS to 5 mL for I.V. administration

Patient Information May cause nausea, vomiting, dizziness, increased blood pressure, headache, ringing in the ears, chest pain, or shortness of breath

Nursing Implications I.V. use should be limited to patients with severe uterine bleeding or other life-threatening emergency situations

Dosage Forms Injection, as maleate: 0.2 mg/mL (1 mL)

Ergonovine Maleate *see* Ergonovine *on previous page*

Ergotamine (er GOT a meen)

Brand Names Cafatine®; Cafatine-PB®; Cafergot®; Cafetrate®; Ercaf®; Ergomar®; Phenerbel-S®; Wigraine®

Canadian/Mexican Brand Names Gynergen® (Canada); Megral® (Canada); Ergocaf® (Mexico); Sydolil® (Mexico)

Synonyms Ergotamine Tartrate; Ergotamine Tartrate and Caffeine

Therapeutic Category Adrenergic Blocking Agent; Ergot Alkaloid and Derivative

Use Abort or prevent vascular headaches, such as migraine or cluster

Pregnancy Risk Factor X

Contraindications Hypersensitivity to ergotamine, caffeine, or any component; peripheral vascular disease, hepatic or renal disease, hypertension, peptic ulcer disease, sepsis; avoid during pregnancy

Warnings/Precautions Avoid prolonged administration or excessive dosage because of the danger of ergotism and gangrene; patients who take ergotamine for extended periods of time may become dependent on it. May be harmful due to reduction in cerebral blood flow; may precipitate angina, myocardial infarction, or aggravate intermittent claudication; therefore, not considered a drug of choice in the elderly.

Adverse Reactions

>10%:

Cardiovascular: Tachycardia, bradycardia, arterial spasm, claudication and vasoconstriction; rebound headache may occur with sudden withdrawal of the drug in patients on prolonged therapy; localized edema, peripheral vascular effects (numbness and tingling of fingers and toes)

Central nervous system: Drowsiness, dizziness

Gastrointestinal: Nausea, vomiting, diarrhea, xerostomia

1% to 10%:

Cardiovascular: Transient tachycardia or bradycardia, precordial distress and pain

Neuromuscular & skeletal: Weakness in the legs, abdominal or muscle pain, muscle pains in the extremities, paresthesia

Overdosage/Toxicology Symptoms include vasospastic effects, nausea, vomiting, lassitude, impaired mental function, hypotension, hypertension, unconsciousness, seizures, shock, and death

Treatment includes general supportive therapy, gastric lavage, or induction of emesis, activated charcoal, saline cathartic; keep extremities warm. Activated charcoal is effective at binding certain chemicals, and this is especially true for ergot alkaloids; treatment is symptomatic with heparin, vasodilators (nitroprusside); vasodilators should be used with caution to avoid exaggerating any preexisting hypotension.

Drug Interactions Increased toxicity:

Propranolol: One case of severe vasoconstriction with pain and cyanosis has been reported

(Continued)

Ergotamine *(Continued)*

Erythromycin, troleandomycin and other macrolide antibiotics: Monitor for signs of ergot toxicity

Mechanism of Action Ergot alkaloid alpha-adrenergic blocker directly stimulates vascular smooth muscle to vasoconstrict peripheral and cerebral vessels; also has antagonist effects on serotonin

Pharmacodynamics/Kinetics

Absorption: Oral, rectal: Erratic; enhanced by caffeine coadministration

Metabolism: Extensively in the liver

Bioavailability: Poor overall (<5%)

Time to peak serum concentration: Within 0.5-3 hours following co-administration with caffeine

Elimination: In bile as metabolites (90%)

Usual Dosage Adults:

Oral:

Cafergot®: 2 tablets at onset of attack; then 1 tablet every 30 minutes as needed; maximum: 6 tablets per attack; do not exceed 10 tablets/week

Ergostat®: 1 tablet under tongue at first sign, then 1 tablet every 30 minutes, 3 tablets/24 hours, 5 tablets/week

Rectal (Cafergot® suppositories, Wigraine® suppositories, Cafatine® suppositories): 1 at first sign of an attack; follow with second dose after 1 hour, if needed; maximum dose: 2 per attack; do not exceed 5/week

Inhalation: Initial: 1 inhalation, followed by repeat inhalations 5 minutes apart to a maximum of 6 inhalations/24 hours or 15 inhalations/1 week

Patient Information Any symptoms such as nausea, vomiting, numbness or tingling, and chest, muscle, or abdominal pain should be reported to the physician. Initiate therapy at first sign of attack. Do **not** exceed recommended dosage.

Nursing Implications Do not crush sublingual drug product

Additional Information

Ergotamine tartrate: Ergostat®

Ergotamine tartrate and caffeine: Cafergot®

Dosage Forms

Suppository, rectal (Cafatine®, Cafergot®, Cafetrate®, Wigraine®): Ergotamine tartrate 2 mg and caffeine 100 mg (12s)

Tablet (Ercaf®, Wigraine®): Ergotamine tartrate 1 mg and caffeine 100 mg

Tablet, sublingual (Ergomar®): Ergotamine tartrate 2 mg

Ergotamine Tartrate *see* Ergotamine *on previous page*

Ergotamine Tartrate and Caffeine *see* Ergotamine *on previous page*

Ergotrate® Maleate *see* Ergonovine *on page 458*

E•R•O Ear [OTC] *see* Carbamide Peroxide *on page 203*

Erwiniar® *see* Asparaginase *on page 103*

Eryc® *see* Erythromycin *on next page*

EryPed® *see* Erythromycin *on next page*

Ery-Tab® *see* Erythromycin *on next page*

Erythrityl Tetranitrate (e RI thri til te tra NYE trate)

Brand Names Cardilate®

Therapeutic Category Antianginal Agent; Nitrate; Vasodilator, Coronary

Use Prophylaxis and long-term treatment of frequent or recurrent anginal pain and reduced exercise tolerance associated with angina pectoris

Unlabeled use: Reduce cardiac workload in CHF or following an MI; adjunct in treatment of Raynaud's disease

Pregnancy Risk Factor C

Contraindications Severe anemia, closed-angle glaucoma, postural hypotension, cerebral hemorrhage, head trauma, hypersensitivity to erythrityl tetranitrate or any component

Warnings/Precautions Use with caution in patients with hypertrophic cardiomyopathy, in patients with glaucoma, or volume depletion; tolerance may develop

Adverse Reactions

>10%: Central nervous system: Headache

1% to 10%: Cardiovascular: Tachycardia, hypotension, flushing

<1%:

Central nervous system: Restlessness, dizziness

Gastrointestinal: Nausea, vomiting, diarrhea

Hematologic: Methemoglobinemia

Neuromuscular & skeletal: Weakness

Overdosage/Toxicology Symptoms of overdose include hypotension, tachycardia, flushing, diaphoresis, dizziness, syncope, nausea, confusion, increased intracranial pressure, methemoglobinemia, cyanosis, metabolic acidosis, seizures

Following decontamination, keep patients recumbent, treat hypotension with fluids and pressors, treat methemoglobinemia with methylene-blue 1-2 mg/kg; epinephrine is ineffective in reversing hypotension.

Mechanism of Action Erythrityl tetranitrate, like other organic nitrates, induces vasodilation by dephosphorylation of the myosin light chain in smooth muscles. This is accomplished by activation of guanylate cyclase, which eventually stimulates a cyclic GMP-dependent protein kinase that alters the phosphorylation of the myosin. Venodilation causes peripheral blood pooling, which decreases venous return to the heart, central venous pressure, and pulmonary capillary wedge pressure. A reduction in pulmonary vascular resistance occurs secondary to pulmonary arteriolar dilation and afterload may be decreased by a lowering of systemic arterial pressure.

Usual Dosage Adults: Oral: 5 mg under the tongue or in the buccal pouch 3 times/day or 10 mg before meals or food, chewed 3 times/day, increasing in 2-3 days if needed; dosages of up to 100 mg/day are tolerated; some patients may need bedtime doses if they experience nocturnal symptoms

Monitoring Parameters Monitor blood pressure reduction for maximal effect and orthostatic hypotension

Test Interactions ↓ cholesterol (S)

Patient Information Do not change brands without consulting physician or pharmacist; notify physician if persistent headache, dizziness, or flushing occurs; seek medical help if chest pain is unresolved after 15 minutes; do not chew or swallow sublingual tablet; keep tablets in original container and keep container tightly closed; take sublingual and chewable tablets while sitting down

Nursing Implications Do not crush sublingual drug product

Dosage Forms Tablet, oral or sublingual: 10 mg

Erythrocin® *see* Erythromycin *on this page*

Erythromycin (er ith roe MYE sin)

Related Information

Animal and Human Bites Guidelines *on page 1463*
Antimicrobial Drugs of Choice *on page 1468*
Antimicrobial Prophylaxis *on page 1445*
Prevention of Bacterial Endocarditis *on page 1449*
Treatment of Sexually Transmitted Diseases *on page 1485*

Brand Names E.E.S.®; E-Mycin®; Eryc®; EryPed®; Ery-Tab®; Erythrocin®; Ilosone®; PCE®

Canadian/Mexican Brand Names Apo-Erythro® E-C (Canada); Diomycin® (Canada); Erybid® (Canada); Erythro-Base® (Canada); Novo-Rythro® Encap (Canada); PMS-Erythromycin (Canada); Eritroquim® (Mexico); Latotryd® (Mexico); Lauricin® (Mexico); Luritran® (Mexico); Lederpax® (Mexico); Pantomicina® (Mexico); Tromigal® (Mexico)

Synonyms Erythromycin Base; Erythromycin Estolate; Erythromycin Ethylsuccinate; Erythromycin Gluceptate; Erythromycin Lactobionate; Erythromycin Stearate

Therapeutic Category Antibiotic, Macrolide; Antibiotic, Ophthalmic

Use Treatment of susceptible bacterial infections including *M. pneumoniae, Legionella pneumophila*, diphtheria, pertussis, chancroid, *Chlamydia*, and *Campylobacter* gastroenteritis; used in conjunction with neomycin for decontaminating the bowel

Unlabeled use: Gastroparesis

Pregnancy Risk Factor B

Contraindications Hepatic impairment, known hypersensitivity to erythromycin or its components; concomitant use with pimozide or terfenadine

Warnings/Precautions Hepatic impairment with or without jaundice has occurred, it may be accompanied by malaise, nausea, vomiting, abdominal colic, and fever; discontinue use if these occur; avoid using erythromycin lactobionate in neonates since formulations may contain benzyl alcohol which is associated with toxicity in neonates

Adverse Reactions

>10%: Gastrointestinal: Abdominal pain, cramping, nausea, vomiting

1% to 10%:
- Gastrointestinal: Oral candidiasis
- Hepatic: Cholestatic jaundice
- Local: Phlebitis at the injection site
- Miscellaneous: Hypersensitivity reactions

<1%:
- Cardiovascular: Ventricular arrhythmias
- Central nervous system: Fever
- Dermatologic: Rash
- Gastrointestinal: Hypertrophic pyloric stenosis, diarrhea
- Hematologic: Eosinophilia

(Continued)

Erythromycin *(Continued)*

Local: Thrombophlebitis

Miscellaneous: Allergic reactions

Overdosage/Toxicology Symptoms of overdose include nausea, vomiting, diarrhea, prostration, reversible pancreatitis, hearing loss with or without tinnitus or vertigo; general and supportive care only

Drug Interactions Cytochrome P-450 IIIA enzyme inhibitor

Increased toxicity:

- Erythromycin decreases clearance of carbamazepine, cyclosporine, and triazolam
- Erythromycin may decrease theophylline clearance and increase theophylline's half-life by up to 60% (patients on high-dose theophylline and erythromycin or who have received erythromycin for >5 days may be at higher risk)
- Decreases metabolism of terfenadine resulting in an increase in Q-T interval and potential heart failure
- Inhibits felodipine (and other dihydropyridine calcium antagonist) metabolism in the liver resulting in a 2-fold increase in levels and consequent toxicity
- May potentiate anticoagulant effect of warfarin and decrease metabolism of vinblastine
- Concurrent use of erythromycin and lovastatin and simvastatin may result in significantly increased levels and rhabdomyolysis

Stability

Erythromycin lactobionate should be reconstituted with sterile water for injection without preservatives to avoid gel formation; the reconstituted solution is stable for 2 weeks when refrigerated for 24 hours at room temperature

Erythromycin I.V. infusion solution is stable at pH 6-8. Stability of lactobionate is pH dependent; I.V. form has the longest stability in 0.9% sodium chloride (NS) and should be prepared in this base solution whenever possible. Do not use D_5W as a diluent unless sodium bicarbonate is added to solution. If I.V. must be prepared in D_5W, 0.5 mL of the 8.4% sodium bicarbonate solution should be added per each 100 mL of D_5W.

Stability of parenteral admixture at room temperature (25°C) and at refrigeration temperature (4°C): 24 hours

Standard diluent: 500 mg/250 mL D_5W/NS; 750 mg/250 mL D_5W/NS; 1 g/250 mL D_5W/NS

Refrigerate oral suspension

Mechanism of Action Inhibits RNA-dependent protein synthesis at the chain elongation step; binds to the 50S ribosomal subunit resulting in blockage of transpeptidation

Pharmacodynamics/Kinetics

Absorption: Variable but better with salt forms than with base form; 18% to 45% absorbed orally, ethylsuccinate may be better absorbed with food

Distribution: Crosses the placenta; appears in breast milk

- Relative diffusion of antimicrobial agents from blood into cerebrospinal fluid (CSF): Minimal even with inflammation
- Ratio of CSF to blood level (%):
  - Normal meninges: 1-12
  - Inflamed meninges: 7-25

Protein binding: 75% to 90%

Metabolism: In the liver by demethylation

Half-life: 1.5-2 hours (peak)

- End stage renal disease: 5-6 hours

Time to peak serum concentration: 4 hours for the base, 30 minutes to 2.5 hours for the ethylsuccinate; delayed in the presence of food; due to differences in absorption, **200 mg erythromycin ethylsuccinate produces the same serum levels as 125 mg of erythromycin base**

Elimination: 2% to 15% excreted as unchanged drug in urine and major excretion in feces (via bile)

Usual Dosage Erythromycin has been used as a prokinetic agent to improve gastric emptying time and intestinal motility. In adults, 200 mg was infused I.V. initially followed by 250 mg orally 3 times/day 30 minutes before meals. In children, erythromycin 3 mg/kg I.V. has been infused over 60 minutes initially followed by 20 mg/kg/day orally in 3-4 divided doses before meals or before meals and at bedtime

Infants and Children:

- Oral: Do not exceed 2 g/day; base and ethylsuccinate: 30-50 mg/kg/day divided every 6-8 hours
- Endocarditis prophylaxis in penicillin-allergic patients: Oral: Base: 20 mg/kg/dose 2 hours before procedure and 10 mg/kg/dose 6 hours later
- Preop bowel preparation: 20 mg/kg erythromycin base at 1, 2, and 11 PM on the day before surgery combined with mechanical cleansing of the large intestine and oral neomycin

I.V.: Lactobionate: 20-40 mg/kg/day divided every 6 hours, not to exceed 4 g/day

Adults:

Oral:

Base: 250-500 mg every 6-12 hours

Ethylsuccinate: 400-800 mg every 6-12 hours

Endocarditis prophylaxis in penicillin-allergic patients: Oral: 1 g 2 hours before procedure and 500 mg 6 hours later

Preop bowel preparation: Oral: 1 g erythromycin base at 1, 2, and 11 PM on the day before surgery combined with mechanical cleansing of the large intestine and oral neomycin

I.V.: Lactobionate: 15-20 mg/kg/day divided every 6 hours or 500 mg to 1 g every 6 hours, or given as a continuous infusion over 24 hours (maximum: 4 g/24 hours)

Children and Adults: Ophthalmic: Instill ½" (1.25 cm) 2-8 times/day depending on the severity of the infection

Dialysis: Slightly dialyzable (5% to 20%); no supplemental dosage necessary in hemo or peritoneal dialysis or in continuous arterio-venous or veno-venous hemofiltration (CAVH/CAVHD)

Dietary Considerations Food: Increased drug absorption with meals. Drug may cause GI upset; may take with food.

Administration Administer around-the-clock rather than 4 times/day to promote less variation in peak and trough serum levels; can administer with food to decrease GI upset

Test Interactions False-positive urinary catecholamines

Patient Information Refrigerate after reconstitution, take until gone, do not skip doses; chewable tablets should not be swallowed whole; report to physician if persistent diarrhea occurs; discard any unused portion after 10 days; drug absorption unaffected by food

Nursing Implications Some formulations may contain benzyl alcohol as a preservative; use with extreme care in neonates; do not crush enteric coated drug product; GI upset, including diarrhea, is common; I.V. infusion may be very irritating to the vein; if phlebitis/pain occurs with used dilution, consider diluting further (eg, 1:5), if fluid status of the patient will tolerate, or consider administering in larger available vein

Dosage Forms

Erythromycin base:

Capsule, delayed release: 250 mg

Capsule, delayed release, enteric coated pellets (Eryc®): 250 mg

Tablet, delayed release: 333 mg

Tablet, enteric coated (E-Mycin®, Ery-Tab®, E-Base®): 250 mg, 333 mg, 500 mg

Tablet, film coated: 250 mg, 500 mg

Tablet, polymer coated particles (PCE®): 333 mg, 500 mg

Erythromycin estolate:

Capsule (Ilosone® Pulvules®): 250 mg

Suspension, oral (Ilosone®): 125 mg/5 mL (480 mL); 250 mg/5 mL (480 mL)

Tablet (Ilosone®): 500 mg

Erythromycin ethylsuccinate:

Granules for oral suspension (EryPed®): 400 mg/5 mL (60 mL, 100 mL, 200 mL)

Powder for oral suspension (E.E.S.®): 200 mg/5 mL (100 mL, 200 mL)

Suspension, oral (E.E.S.®, EryPed®): 200 mg/5 mL (5 mL, 100 mL, 200 mL, 480 mL); 400 mg/5 mL (5 mL, 60 mL, 100 mL, 200 mL, 480 mL)

Suspension, oral [drops] (EryPed®): 100 mg/2.5 mL (50 mL)

Tablet (E.E.S.®): 400 mg

Tablet, chewable (EryPed®): 200 mg

Erythromycin gluceptate:

Injection: 1000 mg (30 mL)

Erythromycin lactobionate:

Powder for injection: 500 mg, 1000 mg

Erythromycin stearate:

Tablet, film coated (Eramycin®, Erythrocin®): 250 mg, 500 mg

Erythromycin and Sulfisoxazole

(er ith roe MYE sin & sul fi SOKS a zole)

Brand Names Eryzole®; Pediazole®

Synonyms Sulfisoxazole and Erythromycin

Therapeutic Category Antibiotic, Macrolide; Antibiotic, Sulfonamide Derivative

(Continued)

Erythromycin and Sulfisoxazole *(Continued)*

Use Treatment of susceptible bacterial infections of the upper and lower respiratory tract, otitis media in children caused by susceptible strains of *Haemophilus influenzae*, and other infections in patients allergic to penicillin

Pregnancy Risk Factor C

Contraindications Hepatic dysfunction, known hypersensitivity to erythromycin or sulfonamides; infants <2 months of age (sulfas compete with bilirubin for binding sites); patients with porphyria; concurrent use with pimozide or terfenadine

Warnings/Precautions Use with caution in patients with impaired renal or hepatic function, G-6-PD deficiency (hemolysis may occur)

Adverse Reactions

>10%: Gastrointestinal: Abdominal pain, cramping, nausea, vomiting

1% to 10%:

- Gastrointestinal: Oral candidiasis
- Hepatic: Cholestatic jaundice
- Local: Phlebitis at the injection site
- Miscellaneous: Hypersensitivity reactions

<1%:

- Cardiovascular: Ventricular arrhythmias
- Central nervous system: Fever, headache
- Dermatologic: Rash, Stevens-Johnson syndrome, toxic epidermal necrolysis
- Gastrointestinal: Hypertrophic pyloric stenosis, diarrhea
- Genitourinary: Crystalluria
- Hematologic: Eosinophilia, agranulocytosis, aplastic anemia
- Hepatic: Hepatic necrosis
- Local: Thrombophlebitis
- Renal: Toxic nephrosis

Overdosage/Toxicology Symptoms of overdose include nausea, vomiting, diarrhea, prostration, reversible pancreatitis, hearing loss with or without tinnitus or vertigo; general and supportive care only; keep patient well hydrated

Drug Interactions Increased effect/toxicity/levels of alfentanil, anticoagulants, astemizole, terfenadine (resulting in potentially life-threatening prolonged QT interval) , bromocriptine, carbamazepine, cyclosporine, digoxin, disopyramide, theophylline, triazolam, and warfarin

Stability Reconstituted suspension is stable for 14 days when refrigerated

Mechanism of Action Erythromycin inhibits bacterial protein synthesis; sulfisoxazole competitively inhibits bacterial synthesis of folic acid from para-aminobenzoic acid

Pharmacodynamics/Kinetics

Erythromycin ethylsuccinate:

- Absorption: Well absorbed from GI tract
- Distribution: Crosses the placenta; appears in breast milk
- Protein binding: 75% to 90%
- Metabolism: In the liver
- Half-life: 1-1.5 hours
- Elimination: Unchanged drug is excreted and concentrated in bile

Sulfisoxazole acetyl: Hydrolyzed in the GI tract to sulfisoxazole which has the following characteristics:

- Absorption: Readily absorbed
- Distribution: Crosses the placenta; appears in breast milk
- Protein binding: 85%
- Half-life: 6 hours, prolonged in renal impairment
- Elimination: 50% excreted in urine as unchanged drug

Usual Dosage Oral (dosage recommendation is based on the product's erythromycin content):

Children ≥2 months: 50 mg/kg/day erythromycin and 150 mg/kg/day sulfisoxazole in divided doses every 6 hours; not to exceed 2 g erythromycin/day or 6 g sulfisoxazole/day for 10 days

Adults: 400 mg erythromycin and 1200 mg sulfisoxazole every 6 hours

Dosing adjustment in renal impairment (sulfisoxazole must be adjusted in renal impairment):

- Cl_{cr} 10-50 mL/minute: Administer every 8-12 hours
- Cl_{cr} <10 mL/minute: Administer every 12-24 hours

Monitoring Parameters CBC and periodic liver function test

Test Interactions False-positive urinary protein

Patient Information Maintain adequate fluid intake; avoid prolonged exposure to sunlight; discontinue if rash appears; take until gone, do not skip doses

Nursing Implications Shake well before use; refrigerate

Dosage Forms Suspension, oral: Erythromycin ethylsuccinate 200 mg and sulfisoxazole acetyl 600 mg per 5 mL (100 mL, 150 mL, 200 mL, 250 mL)

Erythromycin Base *see* Erythromycin *on page 461*
Erythromycin Estolate *see* Erythromycin *on page 461*
Erythromycin Ethylsuccinate *see* Erythromycin *on page 461*
Erythromycin Gluceptate *see* Erythromycin *on page 461*
Erythromycin Lactobionate *see* Erythromycin *on page 461*
Erythromycin Stearate *see* Erythromycin *on page 461*
Erythropoietin *see* Epoetin Alfa *on page 451*
Eryzole® *see* Erythromycin and Sulfisoxazole *on page 463*
Eserine Salicylate *see* Physostigmine *on page 997*
Esgic® *see* Butalbital Compound *on page 176*
Esidrix® *see* Hydrochlorothiazide *on page 617*
Eskalith® *see* Lithium *on page 735*

Esmolol (ES moe lol)

Related Information

Antiarrhythmic Drugs *on page 1389*
Beta-Blockers Comparison *on page 1398*
Comparative Pharmacokinetic Properties of Antiarrhythmic Agents *on page 1391*
Extravasation Treatment of Other Drugs *on page 1381*
Therapy of Hypertension *on page 1540*

Brand Names Brevibloc®

Synonyms Esmolol Hydrochloride

Therapeutic Category Antiarrhythmic Agent, Class II; Beta-Adrenergic Blocker

Use Treatment of supraventricular tachycardia, atrial fibrillation/flutter (primarily to control ventricular rate), and hypertension (especially perioperatively)

Pregnancy Risk Factor C

Contraindications Sinus bradycardia or heart block; uncompensated congestive heart failure; cardiogenic shock; hypersensitivity to esmolol, any component, or other beta-blockers

Warnings/Precautions Must be diluted for continuous I.V. infusion; use with extreme caution in patients with hyper-reactive airway disease; use lowest dose possible and discontinue infusion if bronchospasm occurs; use with caution in diabetes mellitus, hypoglycemia, renal failure; avoid extravasation; caution should be exercised when discontinuing esmolol infusions to avoid withdrawal effects; esmolol shares the toxic potentials of beta-adrenergic blocking agents and the usual precautions of these agents should be observed

Adverse Reactions

>10%:
- Cardiovascular: Asymptomatic and symptomatic hypotension
- Miscellaneous: Diaphoresis

1% to 10%:
- Cardiovascular: Peripheral ischemia
- Central nervous system: Dizziness, somnolence, confusion, headache, agitation, fatigue
- Gastrointestinal: Nausea, vomiting
- Local: Infusion site reactions

<1%:
- Cardiovascular: Pallor, flushing, bradycardia, chest pain, syncope, heart block, edema
- Central nervous system: Depression, abnormal thinking, anxiety, fever, lightheadedness, seizures
- Dermatologic: Erythema, skin discoloration
- Gastrointestinal: Anorexia, dyspepsia, constipation, xerostomia, abdominal discomfort
- Genitourinary: Urinary retention
- Local: Thrombophlebitis
- Neuromuscular & skeletal: Paresthesia, rigors, midcapsular pain, weakness
- Ocular: Abnormal vision
- Respiratory: Bronchospasm, wheezing, dyspnea, nasal congestion, pulmonary edema
- Miscellaneous: Speech disorder

Overdosage/Toxicology Symptoms of overdose include hypotension, bradycardia, heart block

Sympathomimetics (eg, epinephrine or dopamine), glucagon, or a pacemaker can be used to treat the toxic bradycardia, asystole, and/or hypotension; initially, fluids may be the best treatment for hypotension

Drug Interactions

Decreased effect of beta-blockers with aluminum salts, barbiturates, calcium salts, cholestyramine, colestipol, NSAIDs, penicillins (ampicillin), rifampin,

(Continued)

Esmolol *(Continued)*

salicylates and sulfinpyrazone due to decreased bioavailability and plasma levels

Beta-blockers may decrease the effect of sulfonylureas

Increased effect/toxicity of beta-blockers with calcium blockers (diltiazem, felodipine, nicardipine), contraceptives, flecainide, haloperidol (propranolol, hypotensive effects), H_2-antagonists (metoprolol, propranolol only by cimetidine, possibly ranitidine), hydralazine (metoprolol, propranolol), loop diuretics (propranolol, not atenolol), MAO inhibitors (metoprolol, nadolol, bradycardia), phenothiazines (propranolol), propafenone (metoprolol, propranolol), quinidine (in extensive metabolizers), ciprofloxacin, thyroid hormones (metoprolol, propranolol, when hypothyroid patient is converted to euthyroid state)

Beta-blockers may increase the effect/toxicity of flecainide, haloperidol (hypotensive effects), hydralazine, phenothiazines, acetaminophen, anticoagulants (propranolol, warfarin), benzodiazepines (not atenolol), clonidine (hypertensive crisis after or during withdrawal of either agent), epinephrine (initial hypertensive episode followed by bradycardia), nifedipine and verapamil lidocaine, ergots (peripheral ischemia), prazosin (postural hypotension)

Beta-blockers may affect the action or levels of ethanol, disopyramide, nondepolarizing muscle relaxants and theophylline although the effects are difficult to predict

Stability Clear, colorless to light yellow solution which should be stored at room temperature and protected from temperatures >40°C

Stability of parenteral admixture at room temperature (25°C) and at refrigeration temperature (4°C): 24 hours

Standard diluent: 5 g/500 mL NS

Mechanism of Action Class II antiarrhythmic: Competitively blocks response to $beta_1$- and $beta_2$-adrenergic stimulation

Pharmacodynamics/Kinetics

Onset of beta-blockade: I.V.: Within 2-10 minutes (onset of effect is quickest when loading doses are administered)

Duration of activity: Short, 10-30 minutes; prolonged following higher cumulative doses, extended duration of use

Protein binding: 55%

Metabolism: In blood by esterases

Half-life: Adults: 9 minutes

Elimination: ~69% of dose excreted in urine as metabolites and 2% as unchanged drug

Usual Dosage I.V. administration requires an infusion pump (must be adjusted to individual response and tolerance):

Children: An extremely limited amount of information regarding esmolol use in pediatric patients is currently available

Some centers have utilized doses of 100-500 mcg/kg given over 1 minute for control of supraventricular tachycardias

Loading doses of 500 mcg/kg/minute over 1 minute with maximal doses of 50-250 mcg/kg/minute (mean 173) have been used in addition to nitroprusside to treat postoperative hypertension after coarctation of aorta repair

Adults: Loading dose: 500 mcg/kg over 1 minute; follow with a 50 mcg/kg/minute infusion for 4 minutes; if response is inadequate, rebolus with another 500 mcg/kg loading dose over 1 minute, and increase the maintenance infusion to 100 mcg/kg/minute. Repeat this process until a therapeutic effect has been achieved or to a maximum recommended maintenance dose of 200 mcg/kg/minute. Usual dosage range: 50-200 mcg/kg/minute with average dose of 100 mcg/kg/minute.

Esmolol: Hemodynamic effects of beta-blockade return to baseline within 20-30 minutes after discontinuing esmolol infusions

Guidelines for withdrawal of therapy:

Transfer to alternative antiarrhythmic drug (propranolol, digoxin, verapamil)

Infusion should be reduced by 50% 30 minutes following the first dose of the alternative agent

Following the second dose of the alternative drug, patient's response should be monitored and if control is adequate for the first hours, esmolol may be discontinued

Dialysis: Not removed by hemo- or peritoneal dialysis; supplemental dose is not necessary

Administration The 250 mg/mL ampul is **not** for direct I.V. injection, but rather must first be diluted to a final concentration of 10 mg/mL (ie, 2.5 g in 250 mL or 5 g in 500 mL); decrease or discontinue infusion if hypotension, congenital heart failure occur

Monitoring Parameters Blood pressure, heart rate, MAP, EKG, respiratory rate, I.V. site; cardiac monitor and blood pressure monitor required

Test Interactions Increases cholesterol (S), glucose

Dosage Forms Injection, as hydrochloride: 10 mg/mL (10 mL); 250 mg/mL (10 mL)

Esmolol Hydrochloride *see* Esmolol *on page 465*

Esoterica® Facial [OTC] *see* Hydroquinone *on page 628*

Esoterica® Regular [OTC] *see* Hydroquinone *on page 628*

Esoterica® Sensitive Skin Formula [OTC] *see* Hydroquinone *on page 628*

Esoterica® Sunscreen [OTC] *see* Hydroquinone *on page 628*

Estazolam (es TA zoe lam)

Related Information

Benzodiazepines Comparison *on page 1397*

Brand Names ProSom™

Canadian/Mexican Brand Names Tasedan® (Mexico)

Therapeutic Category Benzodiazepine; Hypnotic; Sedative

Use Short-term management of insomnia; there has been little experience with this drug in the elderly, but because of its lack of active metabolites, it is a reasonable choice when a benzodiazepine hypnotic is indicated

Restrictions C-IV

Pregnancy Risk Factor X

Contraindications Hypersensitivity to estazolam, cross-sensitivity with other benzodiazepines may occur, pre-existing CNS depression, sleep apnea, pregnancy, narrow-angle glaucoma

Warnings/Precautions Abrupt discontinuance may precipitate withdrawal or rebound insomnia; use with caution in patients receiving other CNS depressants, patients with low albumin, hepatic dysfunction, and in the elderly; do not use in pregnant women; may cause drug dependency; safety and efficacy have not been established in children <15 years of age, not recommended in nursing mothers

Adverse Reactions

>10%:

- Cardiovascular: Tachycardia, chest pain
- Central nervous system: Drowsiness, fatigue, ataxia, lightheadedness, memory impairment, insomnia, anxiety, depression, headache
- Dermatologic: Rash
- Endocrine & metabolic: Decreased libido
- Gastrointestinal: Xerostomia, constipation, decreased salivation, nausea, vomiting, diarrhea, increased or decreased appetite
- Neuromuscular & skeletal: Dysarthria
- Ocular: Blurred vision
- Miscellaneous: Diaphoresis

1% to 10%:

- Cardiovascular: Syncope, hypotension
- Central nervous system: Confusion, nervousness, dizziness, akathisia
- Dermatologic: Dermatitis
- Gastrointestinal: Weight gain or loss, increased salivation
- Neuromuscular & skeletal: Rigidity, tremor, muscle cramps
- Otic: Tinnitus
- Respiratory: Nasal congestion, hyperventilation

<1%:

- Endocrine & metabolic: Menstrual irregularities
- Hematologic: Blood dyscrasias
- Neuromuscular & skeletal: Reflex slowing
- Miscellaneous: Drug dependence

Overdosage/Toxicology Symptoms of overdose include respiratory depression, hypoactive reflexes, unsteady gait, hypotension

Treatment for benzodiazepine overdose is supportive; rarely is mechanical ventilation required; flumazenil has been shown to selectively block the binding of benzodiazepines to CNS receptors, resulting in a reversal of benzodiazepine-induced CNS depression.

Drug Interactions

Decreased effect: Enzyme inducers may increase the metabolism of estazolam

Increased toxicity: CNS depressants may increase CNS adverse effects; cimetidine may decrease metabolism of estazolam

Mechanism of Action Benzodiazepines may exert their pharmacologic effect through potentiation of the inhibitory activity of GABA. Benzodiazepines do not alter the synthesis, release, reuptake, or enzymatic degradation of GABA.

Usual Dosage Adults: Oral: 1 mg at bedtime, some patients may require 2 mg; start at doses of 0.5 mg in debilitated or small elderly patients

Dosing adjustment in hepatic impairment: May be necessary

Dietary Considerations Alcohol: Additive CNS effect, avoid use

Monitoring Parameters Respiratory and cardiovascular status

(Continued)

Estazolam *(Continued)*

Patient Information May cause daytime drowsiness, avoid alcohol and drugs with CNS depressant effects; avoid activities needing good psychomotor coordination until CNS effects are known; drug may cause physical or psychological dependence; avoid abrupt discontinuation after prolonged use

Nursing Implications Provide safety measures (ie, side rails, night light, and call button); remove smoking materials from area; supervise ambulation; avoid abrupt discontinuance in patients with prolonged therapy or seizure disorders

Dosage Forms Tablet: 1 mg, 2 mg

Estimated Clinical Comparability of Doses for Inhaled Corticosteroids *see page 1522*

Estinyl® *see* Ethinyl Estradiol *on page 481*

Estivin® II [OTC] *see* Naphazoline *on page 879*

Estrace® Oral *see* Estradiol *on this page*

Estraderm® Transdermal *see* Estradiol *on this page*

Estra-D® Injection *see* Estradiol *on this page*

Estradiol (es tra DYE ole)

Brand Names Alora® Transdermal; Climara® Transdermal; Delestrogen® Injection; depGynogen® Injection; Depo®-Estradiol Injection; Depogen® Injection; Dioval® Injection; Dura-Estrin® Injection; Duragen® Injection; Estrace® Oral; Estraderm® Transdermal; Estra-D® Injection; Estra-L® Injection; Estring®; Estro-Cyp® Injection; Estroject-L.A.® Injection; Gynogen L.A.® Injection; Valergen® Injection; Vivelle™ Transdermal

Canadian/Mexican Brand Names Ginedisc® (Mexico); Oestrogel® (Mexico); Systen® (Mexico)

Synonyms Estradiol Cypionate; Estradiol Transdermal; Estradiol Valerate

Therapeutic Category Estrogen Derivative, Intramuscular; Estrogen Derivative, Oral; Estrogen Derivative, Topical; Estrogen Derivative, Vaginal

Use Treatment of atrophic vaginitis, atrophic dystrophy of vulva, menopausal symptoms, female hypogonadism, ovariectomy, primary ovarian failure, inoperable breast cancer, inoperable prostatic cancer, mild to severe vasomotor symptoms associated with menopause

Pregnancy Risk Factor X

Contraindications Known or suspected pregnancy, undiagnosed genital bleeding, carcinoma of the breast (except in patients treated for metastatic disease), estrogen-dependent tumors, history of thrombophlebitis, thrombosis, or thromboembolic disorders associated with estrogen use

Warnings/Precautions Use with caution in patients with renal or hepatic insufficiency; estrogens may cause premature closure of epiphyses in young individuals; in patients with a history of thromboembolism, stroke, myocardial infarction (especially >40 years of age who smoke), liver tumor, hypertension.

Estrogens have been reported to increase the risk of endometrial carcinoma; do not use estrogens during pregnancy. Before prescribing estrogen therapy to postmenopausal women, the risks and benefits must be weighed for each patient. Women should be informed of these risks and benefits, as well as possible side effects and the return of menstrual bleeding (when cycled with a progestin), and be involved in the decision to prescribe. Oral therapy may be more convenient for vaginal atrophy and stress incontinence.

Adverse Reactions

>10%:

- Cardiovascular: Peripheral edema
- Endocrine & metabolic: Enlargement of breasts (female and male), breast tenderness
- Gastrointestinal: Nausea, anorexia, bloating

1% to 10%:

- Central nervous system: Headache
- Endocrine & metabolic: Increased libido (female), decreased libido (male)
- Gastrointestinal: Vomiting, diarrhea

<1%:

- Cardiovascular: Increase in blood pressure, edema, thromboembolic disorders, myocardial infarction
- Central nervous system: Depression, dizziness, anxiety, stroke
- Dermatologic: Chloasma, melasma, rash
- Endocrine & metabolic: Hypercalcemia, folate deficiency, change in menstrual flow, breast tumors, amenorrhea, decreased glucose tolerance, increased triglycerides and LDL
- Gastrointestinal: Nausea, GI distress
- Hepatic: Cholestatic jaundice
- Local: Pain at injection site
- Ocular: Intolerance to contact lenses

Miscellaneous: Increased susceptibility to *Candida* infection

Overdosage/Toxicology Symptoms of overdose include fluid retention, jaundice, thrombophlebitis, nausea, vomiting

Toxicity is unlikely following single exposures of excessive doses, any treatment following emesis and charcoal administration should be supportive and symptomatic

Drug Interactions

Decreased effect: Rifampin ↓ estrogen serum concentrations

Increased toxicity: Hydrocortisone ↑ corticosteroid toxic potential; ↑ potential for thromboembolic events with anticoagulants

Mechanism of Action Increases the synthesis of DNA, RNA, and various proteins in target tissues; reduces the release of gonadotropin-releasing hormone from the hypothalamus; reduces FSH and LH release from the pituitary

Pharmacodynamics/Kinetics

Absorption: Readily absorbed through skin and GI tract; reabsorbed from bile in GI tract and enterohepatically recycled

Distribution: Crosses the placenta; appears in breast milk

Metabolism: Principally degraded in the liver

Protein binding: 80%

Half-life: 50-60 minutes

Elimination: In urine as conjugates; small amounts excreted in feces via bile, reabsorbed from the GI tract and enterohepatically recycled

Usual Dosage Adults (all dosage needs to be adjusted based upon the patient's response):

Male:

Prostate cancer: Valerate: I.M.: ≥30 mg or more every 1-2 weeks

Prostate cancer (androgen-dependent, inoperable, progressing): Oral: 10 mg 3 times/day for at least 3 months

Female:

Breast cancer (inoperable, progressing): Oral: 10 mg 3 times/day for at least 3 months

Osteoporosis prevention: Oral: 0.5 mg/day in a cyclic regimen (3 weeks on and 1 week off of drug)

Hypogonadism, moderate to severe vasomotor symptoms:

Oral: 1-2 mg/day in a cyclic regimen for 3 weeks on drug, then 1 week off drug

Moderate to severe vasomotor symptoms:

I.M.: Cypionate: 1-5 mg every 3-4 weeks

I.M.: Valerate: 10-20 mg every 4 weeks

Postpartum breast engorgement: I.M.: Valerate: 10-25 mg at end of first stage of labor

Transdermal: Apply 0.05 mg patch initially (titrate dosage to response) applied twice weekly in a cyclic regimen, for 3 weeks on drug and 1 week off drug in patients with an intact uterus and continuously in patients without a uterus

Atrophic vaginitis, kraurosis vulvae: Vaginal: Insert 2-4 g/day for 2 weeks then gradually reduce to 1/2 the initial dose for 2 weeks followed by a maintenance dose of 1 g 1-3 times/week

Administration Injection for intramuscular use only

Reference Range

Children: <10 pg/mL (SI: <37 pmol/L)

Male: 10-50 pg/mL (SI: 37-184 pmol/L)

Female:

Premenopausal: 30-400 pg/mL (SI: 110-1468 pmol/L)

Postmenopausal: 0-30 pg/mL (SI: 0-110 pmol/L)

Test Interactions

Decreased antithrombin III

Decreased serum folate concentration

Increased prothrombin and factors VII, VIII, IX, X

Increased platelet aggregability

Increased thyroid binding globulin

Increased total thyroid hormone (T_4)

Increased serum triglycerides/phospholipids

Patient Information Patients should inform their physicians if signs or symptoms of any of the following occur: Thromboembolic or thrombotic disorders including sudden severe headache or vomiting, disturbance of vision or speech, loss of vision, numbness or weakness in an extremity, sharp or crushing chest pain, calf pain, shortness of breath, severe abdominal pain or mass, mental depression, or unusual bleeding.

Patients should discontinue taking the medication if they suspect they are pregnant or become pregnant. Notify physician if area under dermal patch becomes irritated or a rash develops. Patient package insert is available with product; insert vaginal product high into the vagina.

(Continued)

Estradiol *(Continued)*

Nursing Implications Aerosol topical corticosteroids applied under the patch may reduce allergic reactions; do not apply transdermal system to breasts, but place on trunk of body (preferably abdomen); rotate application sites

Additional Information

Estradiol: Estraderm®, Estrace®

Estradiol cypionate: Depo®-Estradiol, depGynogen®, Depogen®, Dura-Estrin®, Estra-D®, Estro-Cyp®, Estroject-L.A.®

Estradiol valerate: Delestrogen®, Dioval®, Duragen®, Estra-L®Gynogen®, Valergen®

Dosage Forms

Cream, vaginal (Estrace®): 0.1 mg/g (42.5 g)

Injection, as cypionate (depGynogen®, Depo®-Estradiol, Depogen®, Dura-Estrin®, Estra-D®, Estro-Cyp®, Estroject-L.A.®): 5 mg/mL (5 mL, 10 mL)

Injection, as valerate:

- Delestrogen®, Valergen®: 10 mg/mL (5 mL, 10 mL); 20 mg/mL (1 mL, 5 mL, 10 mL); 40 mg/mL (5 mL, 10 mL)
- Dioval®, Duragen®, Estra-L®, Gynogen L.A.®: 20 mg/mL (10 mL); 40 mg/mL (10 mL)

Tablet, micronized (Estrace®): 1 mg, 2 mg

Transdermal system

- Alora®:
  - 0.05 mg/24 hours [18 cm^2], total estradiol 1.5 mg
  - 0.075 mg/24 hours [27 cm^2], total estradiol 2.3 mg
  - 0.1 mg/24 hours [36 cm^2], total estradiol 3 mg
- Climara®:
  - 0.05 mg/24 hours [12.5 cm^2], total estradiol 3.9 mg
  - 0.1 mg/24 hours [25 cm^2], total estradiol 7.8 mg
- Estraderm®:
  - 0.05 mg/24 hours [10 cm^2], total estradiol 4 mg
  - 0.1 mg/24 hours [20 cm^2], total estradiol 8 mg
- Vivelle®:
  - 0.0375 mg/day
  - 0.05 mg/day
  - 0.075 mg/day

Vaginal ring (Estring®): 2 mg gradually released over 90 days

Estradiol Cypionate *see* Estradiol *on page 468*

Estradiol Transdermal *see* Estradiol *on page 468*

Estradiol Valerate *see* Estradiol *on page 468*

Estra-L® Injection *see* Estradiol *on page 468*

Estramustine (es tra MUS teen)

Brand Names Emcyt®

Synonyms Estramustine Phosphate Sodium

Therapeutic Category Antineoplastic Agent, Alkylating Agent; Antineoplastic Agent, Hormone; Antineoplastic Agent, Nitrogen Mustard

Use Palliative treatment of prostatic carcinoma (progressive or metastatic)

Pregnancy Risk Factor C

Contraindications Active thrombophlebitis or thromboembolic disorders, hypersensitivity to estramustine or any component, estradiol or nitrogen mustard

Warnings/Precautions The U.S. Food and Drug Administration (FDA) currently recommends that procedures for proper handling and disposal of antineoplastic agents be considered. Glucose tolerance may be decreased; elevated blood pressure may occur; exacerbation of peripheral edema or congestive heart disease may occur; use with caution in patients with impaired liver function, renal insufficiency, or metabolic bone diseases.

Adverse Reactions

>10%:

- Cardiovascular: Edema
- Gastrointestinal: Diarrhea, nausea, mild increases in AST (SGOT) or LDH
- Endocrine & metabolic: Decreased libido, breast tenderness, breast enlargement
- Respiratory: Dyspnea

1% to 10%:

- Cardiovascular: Myocardial infarction
- Central nervous system: Insomnia, lethargy
- Gastrointestinal: Anorexia, flatulence
- Hematologic: Leukopenia
- Local: Thrombophlebitis
- Neuromuscular & skeletal: Leg cramps
- Respiratory: Pulmonary embolism

<1%:
- Cardiovascular: Cardiac arrest
- Central nervous system: Depression
- Dermatologic: Pigment changes
- Endocrine & metabolic: Hypercalcemia, hot flashes
- Otic: Tinnitus
- Miscellaneous: Night sweats

Overdosage/Toxicology Symptoms of overdose include nausea, vomiting, myelosuppression

There are no known antidotes, treatment is primarily symptomatic and supportive

Drug Interactions Decreased effect: Milk products and calcium-rich foods/drugs may impair the oral absorption of estramustine phosphate sodium

Stability Refrigerate at 2°C to 8°C (36°F to 46°F); capsules may be stored outside of refrigerator for up to 24-48 hours without affecting potency

Mechanism of Action Mechanism is not completely clear, thought to act as an alkylating agent and as estrogen

Pharmacodynamics/Kinetics
- Absorption: Oral: Well absorbed (75%)
- Metabolism: Dephosphorylated in the intestines and eventually oxidized and hydrolyzed to estramustine, estrone, estradiol, and nitrogen mustard
- Half-life: 20 hours
- Time to peak serum concentration: Within 2-3 hours
- Elimination: In feces via bile

Usual Dosage Adults: Oral: 14 mg/kg/day (range: 10-16 mg/kg/day) in 3-4 divided doses for 30-90 days; some patients have been maintained for >3 years on therapy

Patient Information Take on an empty stomach, particularly avoid taking with milk

Dosage Forms Capsule, as phosphate sodium: 140 mg

Estramustine Phosphate Sodium *see* Estramustine *on previous page*

Estratab® *see* Estrogens, Esterified *on page 473*

Estring® *see* Estradiol *on page 468*

Estro-Cyp® Injection *see* Estradiol *on page 468*

Estrogenic Substance Aqueous *see* Estrone *on page 474*

Estrogenic Substances, Conjugated *see* Estrogens, Conjugated *on this page*

Estrogens, Conjugated (ES troe jenz KON joo gate ed)

Brand Names Premarin®

Canadian/Mexican Brand Names C.E.S.® (Canada); Congest® (Canada)

Synonyms C.E.S.; Estrogenic Substances, Conjugated

Therapeutic Category Estrogen Derivative; Estrogen Derivative, Intramuscular; Estrogen Derivative, Oral; Estrogen Derivative, Parenteral; Estrogen Derivative, Vaginal

Use Atrophic vaginitis; hypogonadism; primary ovarian failure; vasomotor symptoms of menopause; prostatic carcinoma; osteoporosis prophylactic

Pregnancy Risk Factor X

Contraindications Undiagnosed vaginal bleeding; hypersensitivity to estrogens or any component; thrombophlebitis, liver disease, known or suspected pregnancy, carcinoma of the breast, estrogen dependent tumor

Warnings/Precautions Use with caution in patients with asthma, epilepsy, migraine, diabetes, cardiac or renal dysfunction; estrogens may cause premature closure of the epiphyses in young individuals; safety and efficacy in children have not been established; estrogens have been reported to increase the risk of endometrial carcinoma; do not use estrogens during pregnancy

Adverse Reactions

>10%:
- Cardiovascular: Peripheral edema
- Endocrine & metabolic: Breast tenderness, hypercalcemia, enlargement of breasts
- Gastrointestinal: Nausea, anorexia, bloating

1% to 10%:
- Central nervous system: Headache
- Endocrine & metabolic: Increased libido
- Gastrointestinal: Vomiting, diarrhea
- Local: Pain at injection site

<1%:
- Cardiovascular: Increase in blood pressure, edema, thromboembolic disorder, myocardial infarction, hypertension
- Central nervous system: Depression, dizziness, anxiety, stroke
- Dermatologic: Chloasma, melasma, rash

(Continued)

Estrogens, Conjugated *(Continued)*

Endocrine & metabolic: Breast tumors, amenorrhea, alterations in frequency and flow of menses, decreased glucose tolerance, increased triglycerides and LDL
Gastrointestinal: Vomiting, GI distress
Hepatic: Cholestatic jaundice
Ocular: Intolerance to contact lenses
Miscellaneous: Increased susceptibility to *Candida* infection

Overdosage/Toxicology Symptoms of overdose include fluid retention, jaundice, thrombophlebitis

Toxicity is unlikely following single exposures of excessive doses, any treatment following emesis and charcoal administration should be supportive and symptomatic

Drug Interactions Inducer of cytochrome P-450 1A2 enzymes
Decreased effect: Rifampin ↓ estrogen serum concentrations
Increased toxicity:
Hydrocortisone ↑ corticosteroid toxic potential
↑ potential for thromboembolic events with anticoagulants

Stability
Refrigerate injection; at room temperature, the injection is stable for 24 months
Reconstituted solution is stable for 60 days at refrigeration
Compatible with normal saline, dextrose, and inert sugar solution
Incompatible with proteins, ascorbic acid, or solutions with acidic pH

Mechanism of Action Increases the synthesis of DNA, RNA, and various proteins in target tissues; reduces the release of gonadotropin-releasing hormone from the hypothalamus; reduces FSH and LH release from the pituitary

Pharmacodynamics/Kinetics
Absorption: Readily absorbed from GI tract
Metabolism: To inactive compounds in the liver
Elimination: In bile and urine

Usual Dosage Adolescents and Adults:
Male: Prostate cancer: Oral: 1.25-2.5 mg 3 times/day
Female:
Dysfunctional uterine bleeding:
Stable hematocrit: Oral: 1.25 mg twice daily for 21 days; if bleeding persists after 48 hours, increase to 2.5 mg twice daily; if bleeding persists after 48 more hours, increase to 2.5 mg 4 times/day; some recommend starting at 2.5 mg 4 times/day (**Note:** Medroxyprogesterone acetate 10 mg/day is also given on days 17-21)
Unstable hematocrit: Oral: I.V.: 5 mg 2-4 times/day; if bleeding is profuse, 20-40 mg every 4 hours up to 24 hours may be used. **Note:** A progestational-weighted contraception pill should also be given (eg, Ovral® 2 tablets stat and 1 tablet 4 times/day or medroxyprogesterone acetate 5-10 mg 4 times/day)
Alternatively: I.V.: 25 mg every 6-12 hours until bleeding stops
Hypogonadism: Oral: 2.5-7.5 mg/day for 20 days, off 10 days and repeat until menses occur
Moderate to severe vasomotor symptoms: Oral: 0.625-1.25 mg/day
Postpartum breast engorgement: Oral: 3.75 mg every 4 hours for 5 doses, then 1.25 mg every 4 hours for 5 days
Atrophic vaginitis, kraurosis vulvae: Vaginal: 2-4 g instilled/day 3 weeks on and 1 week off

Male/Female: Uremic bleeding: I.V.: 0.6 mg/kg/dose daily for 5 days

Administration May also be administered intramuscularly; when administered I.V., drug should be administered slowly to avoid the occurrence of a flushing reaction

Reference Range
Children: <10 μg/24 hours (SI: <35 μmol/day) (values at Mayo Medical Laboratories)
Adults:
Male: 15-40 μg/24 hours (SI: 52-139 μmol/day)
Female:
Menstruating: 15-80 μg/24 hours (SI: 52-277 μmol/day)
Postmenopausal: <20 μg/24 hours (SI: <69 μmol/day)

Test Interactions
Decreased antithrombin III
Decreased serum folate concentration
Increased prothrombin and factors VII, VIII, IX, X
Increased platelet aggregability
Increased thyroid binding globulin
Increased total thyroid hormone (T_4)
Increased serum triglycerides/phospholipids

Patient Information Insert vaginal product high into vagina

Patient package insert available with product

Women should inform their physicians if signs or symptoms of any of the following occur: Thromboembolic or thrombotic disorders including sudden severe headache or vomiting, disturbance of vision or speech, loss of vision, numbness or weakness in an extremity, sharp or crushing chest pain, calf pain, shortness of breath, severe abdominal pain or mass, mental depression or unusual bleeding

Women should discontinue taking the medication if they suspect they are pregnant or become pregnant

Nursing Implications May also be administered intramuscularly; administer at bedtime to minimize occurrence of adverse effects; when administered I.V., drug should be administered slowly to avoid the occurrence of a flushing reaction

Additional Information Contains 50% to 65% sodium estrone sulfate and 20% to 35% sodium equilin sulfate

Dosage Forms

Cream, vaginal: 0.625 mg/g (42.5 g)

Injection: 25 mg (5 mL)

Tablet: 0.3 mg, 0.625 mg, 0.9 mg, 1.25 mg, 2.5 mg

Estrogens, Esterified (ES troe jenz, es TER i fied)

Brand Names Estratab®; Menest®

Canadian/Mexican Brand Names Neo-Estrone® (Canada)

Therapeutic Category Estrogen Derivative; Estrogen Derivative, Oral

Use Atrophic vaginitis; hypogonadism; primary ovarian failure; vasomotor symptoms of menopause; prostatic carcinoma; osteoporosis prophylactic

Pregnancy Risk Factor X

Contraindications Known or suspected cancer of the breast, except in appropriately selected patients being treated for metastatic disease; known or suspected estrogen-dependent neoplasia; known or suspected pregnancy; undiagnosed abnormal genital bleeding; active thrombophlebitis or thromboembolic disorders; past history of thrombophlebitis, thrombosis, or thromboembolic disorders associated with previous estrogen use except when used in the treatment of breast or prostatic malignancy

Warnings/Precautions Use with caution in patients with asthma, epilepsy, migraine, diabetes, cardiac or renal dysfunction; estrogens may cause premature closure of the epiphyses in young individuals; safety and efficacy in children have not been established; estrogens have been reported to increase the risk of endometrial carcinoma, do not use estrogens during pregnancy

Adverse Reactions

>10%:

- Cardiovascular: Peripheral edema
- Endocrine & metabolic: Enlargement of breasts, breast tenderness
- Gastrointestinal: Nausea, anorexia, bloating

1% to 10%:

- Central nervous system: Headache
- Endocrine & metabolic: Increased libido
- Gastrointestinal: Vomiting, diarrhea

<1%:

- Cardiovascular: Hypertension, thromboembolism, myocardial infarction, edema
- Central nervous system: Stroke, depression, dizziness, anxiety
- Dermatologic: Chloasma, melasma, rash
- Endocrine & metabolic: Amenorrhea, alterations in frequency and flow of menses, decreased glucose tolerance, increased triglycerides and LDL
- Gastrointestinal: GI distress
- Hepatic: Cholestatic jaundice
- Ocular: Intolerance to contact lenses
- Miscellaneous: Increased susceptibility to *Candida* infection, breast tumors

Overdosage/Toxicology Symptoms of overdose include fluid retention, jaundice, thrombophlebitis

Toxicity is unlikely following single exposures of excessive doses, any treatment following emesis and charcoal administration should be supportive and symptomatic

Drug Interactions

Decreased effect: Rifampin decreases estrogen serum concentrations

Increased toxicity:

- Hydrocortisone increases corticosteroid toxic potential
- Anticoagulants: Increases potential for thromboembolic events with anticoagulants
- Carbamazepine, tricyclic antidepressants, and corticosteroids; increased thromboembolic potential with oral anticoagulants

(Continued)

Estrogens, Esterified *(Continued)*

Mechanism of Action Primary effects on the interphase DNA-protein complex (chromatin) by binding to a receptor (usually located in the cytoplasm of a target cell) and initiating translocation of the hormone-receptor complex to the nucleus

Pharmacodynamics/Kinetics

Absorption: Readily absorbed from GI tract
Metabolism: Rapidly in the liver to less active metabolites
Elimination: In urine as unchanged compound and metabolites

Usual Dosage Adults: Oral:

Male: Prostate cancer (inoperable, progressing): 1.25-2.5 mg 3 times/day
Female:
- Hypogonadism: 2.5-7.5 mg/day for 20 days, off 10 days and repeat until menses occur
- Moderate to severe vasomotor symptoms: 0.3-1.25 mg/day
- Breast cancer (inoperable, progressing): 10 mg 3 times/day for at least 3 months

Test Interactions Endocrine function test may be altered

Decreased antithrombin III
Decreased serum folate concentration
Increased prothrombin and factors VII, VIII, IX, X
Increased platelet aggregability
Increased thyroid binding globulin
Increased total thyroid hormone (T_4)
Increased serum triglycerides/phospholipids

Patient Information Patients should inform their physicians if signs or symptoms of thromboembolic or thrombotic disorders occur including sudden severe headache or vomiting, disturbance of vision or speech, loss of vision, numbness or weakness in an extremity, sharp or crushing chest pain, calf pain, shortness of breath, severe abdominal pain or mass, mental depression or unusual bleeding; patients should discontinue taking the medication if they suspect they are pregnant or become pregnant.

Additional Information Esterified estrogens are a combination of the sodium salts of the sulfate esters of estrogenic substances; the principal component is estrone, with preparations containing 75% to 85% sodium estrone sulfate and 6% to 15% sodium equilin sulfate such that the total is not <90%

Dosage Forms Tablet: 0.3 mg, 0.625 mg, 1.25 mg, 2.5 mg

Estroject-L.A.® Injection *see* Estradiol *on page 468*

Estrone (ES trone)

Brand Names Aquest®; Kestrone®

Canadian/Mexican Brand Names Femogen® (Canada); Neo-Estrone® (Canada); Oestrillin® (Canada)

Synonyms Estrogenic Substance Aqueous

Therapeutic Category Estrogen Derivative; Estrogen Derivative, Intramuscular

Use Hypogonadism; primary ovarian failure; vasomotor symptoms of menopause; prostatic carcinoma; inoperable breast cancer, kraurosis vulvae, abnormal uterine bleeding due to hormone imbalance

Pregnancy Risk Factor X

Contraindications Thrombophlebitis, undiagnosed vaginal bleeding, hypersensitivity to estrogens or any component, pregnancy

Warnings/Precautions Use with caution in patients with asthma, epilepsy, migraine, diabetes, cardiac or renal dysfunction; estrogens may cause premature closure of the epiphyses in young individuals; safety and efficacy in children have not been established; estrogens have been reported to increase the risk of endometrial carcinoma, do not use estrogens during pregnancy

Adverse Reactions

>10%:
- Cardiovascular: Peripheral edema
- Endocrine & metabolic: Enlargement of breasts, breast tenderness
- Gastrointestinal: Nausea, anorexia, bloating

1% to 10%:
- Central nervous system: Headache
- Endocrine & metabolic: Increased libido
- Gastrointestinal: Vomiting, diarrhea

<1%:
- Cardiovascular: Hypertension, thromboembolism, myocardial infarction, edema
- Central nervous system: Stroke, depression, dizziness, anxiety
- Dermatologic: Chloasma, melasma, rash
- Endocrine & metabolic: Amenorrhea, alterations in frequency and flow of menses, decreased glucose tolerance, increased triglycerides and LDL
- Gastrointestinal: GI distress

Hepatic: cholestatic jaundice
Ocular: Intolerance to contact lenses
Miscellaneous: Increased susceptibility to *Candida* infection, breast tumors

Overdosage/Toxicology Symptoms of overdose include fluid retention, jaundice, thrombophlebitis

Toxicity is unlikely following single exposures of excessive doses, any treatment should be supportive and symptomatic

Drug Interactions
Decreased effect: Rifampin decreases estrogen serum concentrations
Increased toxicity:
Hydrocortisone increases corticosteroid toxic potential
Anticoagulants: Increases potential for thromboembolic events with anticoagulants
Carbamazepine, tricyclic antidepressants, and corticosteroids; increased thromboembolic potential with oral anticoagulants

Mechanism of Action Estrone is a natural ovarian estrogenic hormone that is available as an aqueous mixture of water insoluble estrone and water soluble estrone potassium sulfate; all estrogens, including estrone, act in a similar manner; there is no evidence that there are biological differences among various estrogen preparations other than their ability to bind to cellular receptors inside the target cells

Usual Dosage Adults: I.M.:
Male: Prostatic carcinoma: 2-4 mg 2-3 times/week
Female:
Senile vaginitis and kraurosis vulvae: 0.1-0.5 mg 2-3 times/week
Breast cancer (inoperable, progressing): 5 mg 3 or more times/week
Primary ovarian failure, hypogonadism: 0.1-1 mg/week, up to 2 mg/week in single or divided doses
Abnormal uterine bleeding: 2.5 mg/day for several days

Administration Intramuscular injection only

Test Interactions
Decreased antithrombin III
Decreased serum folate concentration
Increased prothrombin and factors VII, VIII, IX, X
Increased platelet aggregability
Increased thyroid binding globulin
Increased total thyroid hormone (T_4)
Increased serum triglycerides/phospholipids

Patient Information Patients should inform their physicians if signs or symptoms of any of the following occur: Thromboembolic or thrombotic disorders including sudden severe headache or vomiting, disturbance of vision or speech, loss of vision, numbness or weakness in an extremity, sharp or crushing chest pain, calf pain, shortness of breath, severe abdominal pain or mass, mental depression or unusual bleeding; patients should discontinue taking the medication if they suspect they are pregnant or become pregnant

Dosage Forms Injection: 2 mg/mL (10 mL, 30 mL); 5 mg/mL (10 mL)

Estropipate (ES troe pih pate)

Brand Names Ogen®; Ortho-Est®

Canadian/Mexican Brand Names Estrouis® (Canada)

Synonyms Piperazine Estrone Sulfate

Therapeutic Category Estrogen Derivative; Estrogen Derivative, Oral; Estrogen Derivative, Vaginal

Use Atrophic vaginitis; hypogonadism; primary ovarian failure; vasomotor symptoms of menopause; osteoporosis prophylactic

Pregnancy Risk Factor X

Contraindications Thrombophlebitis, undiagnosed vaginal bleeding, hypersensitivity to estrogens or any component

Warnings/Precautions Use with caution in patients with asthma, epilepsy, migraine, diabetes, cardiac or renal dysfunction; estrogens may cause premature closure of the epiphyses in young individuals; safety and efficacy in children have not been established; estrogens have been reported to increase the risk of endometrial carcinoma, do not use estrogens during pregnancy

Adverse Reactions
>10%:
Cardiovascular: Peripheral edema
Endocrine & metabolic: Enlargement of breasts, breast tenderness
Gastrointestinal: Nausea, anorexia, bloating
1% to 10%:
Central nervous system: Headache
Endocrine & metabolic: Increased libido
Gastrointestinal: Vomiting, diarrhea

(Continued)

Estropipate *(Continued)*

<1%:

Cardiovascular: Hypertension, thromboembolism, myocardial infarction, edema

Central nervous system: Stroke, depression, dizziness, anxiety

Dermatologic: Chloasma, melasma, rash

Endocrine & metabolic: Amenorrhea, alterations in frequency and flow of menses, decreased glucose tolerance, increased triglycerides and LDL

Gastrointestinal: GI distress

Hepatic: Cholestatic jaundice

Ocular: Intolerance to contact lenses

Miscellaneous: Increased susceptibility to *Candida* infection, breast tumors

Overdosage/Toxicology Symptoms of overdose include fluid retention, jaundice, thrombophlebitis

Toxicity is unlikely following single exposures of excessive doses, any treatment following emesis and charcoal administration should be supportive and symptomatic

Drug Interactions

Decreased effect: Rifampin decreases estrogen serum concentrations

Increased toxicity:

Hydrocortisone increases corticosteroid toxic potential

Anticoagulants: Increases potential for thromboembolic events with anticoagulants

Carbamazepine, tricyclic antidepressants, and corticosteroids; increased thromboembolic potential with oral anticoagulants

Mechanism of Action Crystalline estrone that has been solubilized as the sulfate and stabilized with piperazine. Primary effects on the interphase DNA-protein complex (chromatin) by binding to a receptor (usually located in the cytoplasm of a target cell) and initiating translocation of the hormone receptor complex to the nucleus.

Usual Dosage Adults: Female:

Moderate to severe vasomotor symptoms: Oral: 0.625-5 mg/day

Hypogonadism or primary ovarian failure: Oral: 1.25-7.5 mg/day for 3 weeks followed by an 8- to 10-day rest period

Osteoporosis prevention: Oral: 0.625 mg/day for 25 days of a 31-day cycle

Atrophic vaginitis or kraurosis vulvae: Vaginal: Instill 2-4 g/day 3 weeks on and 1 week off

Test Interactions

Decreased antithrombin III

Decreased serum folate concentration

Increased prothrombin and factors VII, VIII, IX, X

Increased platelet aggregability

Increased thyroid binding globulin

Increased total thyroid hormone (T_4)

Increased serum triglycerides/phospholipids

Patient Information Patients should inform their physicians if signs or symptoms of any of the following occur: Thromboembolic or thrombotic disorders including sudden severe headache or vomiting, disturbance of vision or speech, loss of vision, numbness or weakness in an extremity, sharp or crushing chest pain, calf pain, shortness of breath, severe abdominal pain or mass, mental depression or unusual bleeding; patients should discontinue taking the medication if they suspect they are pregnant or become pregnant. Patient package insert is available; insert product high into the vagina.

Dosage Forms

Cream, vaginal: 0.15% [estropipate 1.5 mg/g] (42.5 g tube)

Tablet: 0.625 mg [estropipate 0.75 mg]; 1.25 mg [estropipate 1.5 mg]; 2.5 mg [estropipate 3 mg]; 5 mg [estropipate 6 mg]

Ethacrynate Sodium *see* Ethacrynic Acid *on this page*

Ethacrynic Acid (eth a KRIN ik AS id)

Related Information

Heart Failure: Management of Patients With Left-Ventricular Systolic Dysfunction *on page 1533*

Brand Names Edecrin®

Synonyms Ethacrynate Sodium

Therapeutic Category Diuretic, Loop

Use Management of edema associated with congestive heart failure; hepatic cirrhosis or renal disease; short-term management of ascites due to malignancy, idiopathic edema, and lymphedema

Pregnancy Risk Factor B

Pregnancy/Breast-Feeding Implications

Clinical effects on the fetus: No data available. Generally, use of diuretics during pregnancy is avoided due to risk of decreased placental perfusion.

Breast-feeding/lactation: No data available

Contraindications Hypersensitivity to ethacrynic acid or any component; anuria, hypotension, dehydration with low serum sodium concentrations; metabolic alkalosis with hypokalemia, or history of severe, watery diarrhea from ethacrynic acid

Warnings/Precautions Use with caution in patients with advanced hepatic cirrhosis, diabetes mellitus, hypotension, dehydration, history of watery diarrhea from ethacrynic acid, hearing impairment; ototoxicity occurs more frequently than with other loop diuretics; safety and efficacy in infants have not been established

Adverse Reactions

>10%: Gastrointestinal: Diarrhea

1% to 10%:

- Cardiovascular: Orthostatic hypotension
- Central nervous system: Headache
- Endocrine & metabolic: Hyponatremia, hypochloremic alkalosis, hypokalemia
- Gastrointestinal: Loss of appetite
- Ocular: Blurred vision
- Otic: Ototoxicity

<1%:

- Central nervous system: Nervousness
- Dermatologic: Rash
- Endocrine & metabolic: Hyperuricemia, gout
- Gastrointestinal: GI bleeding, pancreatitis, stomach cramps
- Hepatic: Hepatic dysfunction, abnormal LFTs
- Hematologic: Leukopenia, agranulocytosis, thrombocytopenia
- Local: Irritation
- Renal: Renal injury, hematuria

Overdosage/Toxicology Symptoms of overdose include electrolyte depletion, volume depletion, dehydration, circulatory collapse

Following GI decontamination, treatment is supportive; hypotension responds to fluids and Trendelenburg position

Drug Interactions

Increased toxicity:

- Hypotensive agents → additive decreased blood pressure
- Drugs affected by or causing potassium depletion → additive decreased potassium
- Increased nephrotoxic potential with aminoglycosides
- Digoxin increases cardiotoxic potential → arrhythmias
- Increased warfarin anticoagulant effects; increased lithium levels

Decreased effect:

- Probenecid decreases diuretic effects
- Decreased effectiveness of antidiabetic agents

Mechanism of Action Inhibits reabsorption of sodium and chloride in the ascending loop of Henle and distal renal tubule, interfering with the chloride-binding cotransport system, thus causing increased excretion of water, sodium, chloride, magnesium, and calcium

Pharmacodynamics/Kinetics

Onset of diuretic effect:

- Oral: Within 30 minutes
- I.V.: 5 minutes

Peak effect:

- Oral: 2 hours
- I.V.: 30 minutes

Duration of action:

- Oral: 12 hours
- I.V.: 2 hours

Absorption: Oral: Rapid

Metabolism: In the liver to active cysteine conjugate (35% to 40%)

Protein binding: >90%

Half-life: Normal renal function: 2-4 hours

Elimination: 30% to 60% excreted unchanged in bile and urine

Usual Dosage I.V. formulation should be diluted in D_5W or NS (1 mg/mL) and infused over several minutes

Children:

- Oral: 1 mg/kg/dose once daily; increase at intervals of 2-3 days as needed, to a maximum of 3 mg/kg/day
- I.V.: 1 mg/kg/dose, (maximum: 50 mg/dose); repeat doses not routinely recommended; however, if indicated, repeat doses every 8-12 hours

(Continued)

Ethacrynic Acid *(Continued)*

Adults:

Oral: 50-100 mg/day in 1-2 divided doses; may increase in increments of 25-50 mg at intervals of several days to a maximum of 400 mg/24 hours

I.V.: 0.5-1 mg/kg/dose (maximum: 100 mg/dose); repeat doses not routinely recommended; however, if indicated, repeat doses every 8-12 hours

Dosing adjustment/comments in renal impairment: Cl_{cr} <10 mL/minute: Avoid use

Dialysis: Not removed by hemo- or peritoneal dialysis; supplemental dose is not necessary

Administration Injection should **not** be given S.C. or I.M. due to local pain and irritation; single I.V. doses should not exceed 100 mg; if a second dose is needed, use a new injection site to avoid possible thrombophlebitis

Monitoring Parameters Blood pressure, renal function, serum electrolytes, and fluid status closely, including weight and I & O daily; hearing

Patient Information May be taken with food or milk; get up slowly from a lying or sitting position to minimize dizziness, lightheadedness, or fainting; also use extra care when exercising, standing for long periods of time, and during hot weather. Take in morning, take last dose of multiple doses before 6 PM unless instructed otherwise.

Dosage Forms

Powder for injection, as ethacrynate sodium: 50 mg (50 mL)

Tablet: 25 mg, 50 mg

Extemporaneous Preparations To make a 1 mg/mL suspension: Dissolve 120 mg ethacrynic acid powder in a small amount of 10% alcohol. Add a small amount of 50% sorbitol solution and stir. Adjust pH to 7 with 0.1N sodium hydroxide solution. Add sufficient 50% sorbitol solution to make a final volume of 120 mL. (Methylparaben 6 mg and propylparaben 2.4 mg are added as preservatives.) Stable 220 days at room temperature.

Handbook on Extemporaneous Formulations, Bethesda, MD: American Society of Hospital Pharmacists, 1987.

Ethambutol (e THAM byoo tole)

Related Information

Antimicrobial Drugs of Choice *on page 1468*

Desensitization Protocols *on page 1496*

Recommendations for Prophylaxis Against Tuberculosis *on page 1455*

Recommendations of the Advisory Council on the Elimination of Tuberculosis *on page 1483*

Brand Names Myambutol®

Canadian/Mexican Brand Names Etibl® (Canada)

Synonyms Ethambutol Hydrochloride

Therapeutic Category Antitubercular Agent

Use Treatment of tuberculosis and other mycobacterial diseases in conjunction with other antituberculosis agents; only indicated when patients are from areas where drug-resistant *M. tuberculosis* is endemic, in HIV-infected elderly patients, and when drug-resistant *M. tuberculosis* is suspected

Pregnancy Risk Factor B

Contraindications Hypersensitivity to ethambutol or any component; optic neuritis

Warnings/Precautions Use only in children whose visual acuity can accurately be determined and monitored (not recommended for use in children <13 years of age); dosage modification required in patients with renal insufficiency

Adverse Reactions

1% to 10%:

Central nervous system: Headache, confusion, disorientation

Endocrine & metabolic: Acute gout or hyperuricemia

Gastrointestinal: Abdominal pain, anorexia, nausea, vomiting

<1%:

Central nervous system: Malaise, mental confusion, fever

Dermatologic: Rash, pruritus

Hepatic: Abnormal liver function tests

Neuromuscular & skeletal: Peripheral neuritis

Ocular: Optic neuritis

Miscellaneous: Anaphylaxis

Overdosage/Toxicology Symptoms of overdose include decrease in visual acuity, anorexia, joint pain, numbness of the extremities; following GI decontamination, treatment is supportive

Drug Interactions Decreased absorption with aluminum salts

Mechanism of Action Suppresses mycobacteria multiplication by interfering with RNA synthesis

Pharmacodynamics/Kinetics

Absorption: Oral: ~80%

Distribution: Well distributed throughout the body with high concentrations in kidneys, lungs, saliva, and red blood cells

Relative diffusion of antimicrobial agents from blood into CSF: Adequate with or without inflammation (exceeds usual MICs)

Ratio of CSF to blood level (%):

Normal meninges: 0

Inflamed meninges: 25

Protein binding: 20% to 30%

Metabolism: 20% metabolized by the liver to inactive metabolite

Half-life: 2.5-3.6 hours

End stage renal disease: 7-15 hours

Time to peak serum concentration: 2-4 hours

Elimination: ~50% excreted in the urine and 20% excreted in the feces as unchanged drug

Usual Dosage Oral:

Ethambutol is generally not recommended in children whose visual acuity cannot be monitored (<6 years of age). However, ethambutol should be considered for all children with organisms resistant to other drugs, when susceptibility to ethambutol has been demonstrated, or susceptibility is likely.

Note: A four-drug regimen (isoniazid, rifampin, pyrazinamide, and either streptomycin or ethambutol) is preferred for the initial, empiric treatment of TB. When the drug susceptibility results are available, the regimen should be altered as appropriate.

Patients with tuberculosis and without HIV infection:

OPTION 1: Isoniazid resistance rate <4%: Administer daily isoniazid, rifampin, and pyrazinamide for 8 weeks followed by isoniazid and rifampin daily or directly observed therapy (DOT) 2-3 times/week for 16 weeks. If isoniazid resistance rate is not documented, ethambutol or streptomycin should also be administered until susceptibility to isoniazid or rifampin is demonstrated. Continue treatment for at least 6 months or 3 months beyond culture conversion.

OPTION 2: Administer daily isoniazid, rifampin, pyrazinamide, and either streptomycin or ethambutol for 2 weeks followed by DOT 2 times/week administration of the same drugs for 6 weeks, and subsequently, with isoniazid and rifampin DOT 2 times/week administration for 16 weeks

OPTION 3: Administer isoniazid, rifampin, pyrazinamide, and either ethambutol or streptomycin by DOT 3 times/week for 6 months

Patients with TB and with HIV infection: Administer any of the above OPTIONS 1, 2 or 3; however, treatment should be continued for a total of 9 months and at least 6 months beyond culture conversion

Note: Some experts recommend that the duration of therapy should be extended to 9 months for patients with disseminated disease, miliary disease, disease involving the bones or joints, or tuberculosis lymphadenitis

Children (>6 years) and Adults:

Daily therapy: 15-25 mg/kg/day (maximum: 2.5 g/day)

Directly observed therapy (DOT): Twice weekly: 50 mg/kg (maximum: 2.5 g)

DOT: 3 times/week: 25-30 mg/kg (maximum: 2.5 g)

Dosing interval in renal impairment:

Cl_{cr} 10-50 mL/minute: Administer every 24-36 hours

Cl_{cr} <10 mL/minute: Administer every 48 hours

Hemodialysis: Slightly dialyzable (5% to 20%); Administer dose postdialysis

Peritoneal dialysis: Dose for Cl_{cr} <10 mL/minute

Continuous arterio-venous or veno-venous hemofiltration: Administer every 24-36 hours

Monitoring Parameters Periodic visual testing in patients receiving more than 15 mg/kg/day; periodic renal, hepatic, and hematopoietic tests

Test Interactions ↑ uric acid (S)

Patient Information Report any visual changes or rash to physician; may cause stomach upset, take with food; do not take within 2 hours of aluminum-containing antacids

Dosage Forms Tablet, as hydrochloride: 100 mg, 400 mg

Ethambutol Hydrochloride *see* Ethambutol *on previous page*

Ethamolin® *see* Ethanolamine Oleate *on this page*

Ethanoic Acid *see* Acetic Acid *on page 24*

Ethanolamine Oleate (ETH a nol a meen OH lee ate)

Brand Names Ethamolin®

Therapeutic Category Sclerosing Agent

Use Mild sclerosing agent used for bleeding esophageal varices

(Continued)

Ethanolamine Oleate *(Continued)*

Pregnancy Risk Factor C

Contraindications Hypersensitivity to agent or oleic acid

Warnings/Precautions Fatal anaphylactic shock has been reported following administration; use with caution in children class C patients

Adverse Reactions

1% to 10%:

Central nervous system: Pyrexia
Gastrointestinal: Esophageal ulcer, esophageal stricture
Respiratory: Pleural effusion, pneumonia
Miscellaneous: Retrosternal pain

<1%:

Local: Injection necrosis
Neuromuscular & skeletal: Retrosternal pain
Renal: Acute renal failure
Respiratory: Aspiration
Miscellaneous: Anaphylaxis

Overdosage/Toxicology Anaphylaxis after administration of larger than normal volumes, severe intramural necrosis

Treatment is supportive with epinephrine, corticosteroids, fluids, and pressors

Mechanism of Action Derived from oleic acid and similar in physical properties to sodium morrhuate; however, the exact mechanism of the hemostatic effect used in endoscopic injection sclerotherapy is not known. Intravenously injected ethanolamine oleate produces a sterile inflammatory response resulting in fibrosis and occlusion of the vein; a dose-related extravascular inflammatory reaction occurs when the drug diffuses through the venous wall. Autopsy results indicate that variceal obliteration occurs secondary to mural necrosis and fibrosis. Thrombosis appears to be a transient reaction.

Usual Dosage Adults: 1.5-5 mL per varix, up to 20 mL total or 0.4 mL/kg; patients with severe hepatic dysfunction should receive less than recommended maximum dose

Nursing Implications Have epinephrine and resuscitative equipment nearby

Dosage Forms Injection: 5% [50 mg/mL] (2 mL)

Ethchlorvynol (eth klor VI nole)

Brand Names Placidyl®

Therapeutic Category Hypnotic; Sedative

Use Short-term management of insomnia

Restrictions C-IV

Pregnancy Risk Factor C

Contraindications Porphyria, hypersensitivity to ethchlorvynol or any component

Warnings/Precautions Administer with caution to depressed or suicidal patients or to patients with a history of drug abuse; intoxication symptoms may appear with prolonged daily doses of as little as 1 g; withdrawal symptoms may be seen upon abrupt discontinuation; use with caution in the elderly and in patients with hepatic or renal dysfunction; use with caution in patients who have a history of paradoxical restlessness to barbiturates or alcohol; some products may contain tartrazine

Adverse Reactions

>10%:

Central nervous system: Dizziness
Gastrointestinal: Indigestion, nausea, stomach pain, unpleasant aftertaste
Neuromuscular & skeletal: Weakness
Ocular: Blurred vision

1% to 10%:

Central nervous system: Nervousness, excitement, ataxia, confusion, drowsiness (daytime)
Dermatologic: Rash

<1%:

Cardiovascular: Bradycardia
Central nervous system: Hyperthermia, slurred speech
Hepatic: Cholestatic jaundice
Neuromuscular & skeletal: Trembling, weakness (severe)
Respiratory: Shortness of breath

Overdosage/Toxicology Symptoms of overdose include prolonged deep coma, respiratory depression, hypothermia, bradycardia, hypotension, nystagmus

Treatment is supportive in nature; hemoperfusion may be helpful in enhancing elimination

Drug Interactions

Decreased effect of oral anticoagulants

Increased toxicity (CNS depression) with alcohol, CNS depressants, MAO inhibitors, TCAs (delirium)

Stability Capsules should not be crushed and should not be refrigerated

Mechanism of Action Causes nonspecific depression of the reticular activating system

Pharmacodynamics/Kinetics

Onset of action: 15-60 minutes
Duration: 5 hours
Absorption: Rapid from GI tract
Metabolism: In the liver
Half-life: 10-20 hours
Time to peak serum concentration: 2 hours

Usual Dosage Adults: Oral: 500-1000 mg at bedtime

Dosing adjustment in renal impairment: Cl_{cr} <50 mL/minute: Avoid use

Dietary Considerations Alcohol: Additive CNS effect, avoid use

Monitoring Parameters Cardiac and respiratory function and abuse potential

Reference Range Therapeutic: 2-9 µg/mL; Toxic: >20 µg/mL

Patient Information May cause drowsiness, can impair judgment and coordination; avoid alcohol and other CNS depressants; ataxia can be reduced if taken with food, do not crush or refrigerate capsules

Nursing Implications Raise bed rails, institute safety measures, assist with ambulation

Dosage Forms Capsule: 200 mg, 500 mg, 750 mg

Ethinyl Estradiol (ETH in il es tra DYE ole)

Brand Names Estinyl®

Therapeutic Category Estrogen Derivative; Estrogen Derivative, Oral

Use Hypogonadism; primary ovarian failure; vasomotor symptoms of menopause; prostatic carcinoma; breast cancer

Pregnancy Risk Factor X

Contraindications Thrombophlebitis, undiagnosed vaginal bleeding, hypersensitivity to ethinyl estradiol or any component, pregnancy, estrogen dependent neoplasia

Warnings/Precautions Use with caution in patients with asthma, seizure disorders, migraine, cardiac, renal or hepatic impairment, cerebrovascular disorders or history of breast cancer, past or present thromboembolic disease, smokers >35 years of age

Adverse Reactions

>10%:

Cardiovascular: Peripheral edema
Endocrine & metabolic: Enlargement of breasts, breast tenderness, bloating
Gastrointestinal: Nausea, anorexia

1% to 10%:

Central nervous system: Headache
Endocrine & metabolic: Increased libido
Gastrointestinal: Vomiting, diarrhea

<1%:

Cardiovascular: Hypertension, thromboembolism, myocardial infarction, edema
Central nervous system: Stroke, depression, dizziness, anxiety
Dermatologic: Chloasma, melasma, rash
Endocrine & metabolic: Breast tumors, amenorrhea, alterations in frequency and flow of menses, decreased glucose tolerance, increased triglycerides and LDL
Gastrointestinal: GI distress
Hepatic: Cholestatic jaundice
Ocular: Intolerance to contact lenses
Miscellaneous: Increased susceptibility to *Candida* infection

Overdosage/Toxicology Symptoms of overdose include fluid retention, jaundice, thrombophlebitis, nausea

Toxicity is unlikely following single exposures of excessive doses, any treatment following emesis and charcoal administration should be supportive and symptomatic

Drug Interactions Cytochrome P-450 3A enzyme substrate

Increased toxicity:

Carbamazepine, tricyclic antidepressants, and corticosteroids

Increased thromboembolic potential with oral anticoagulants

Mechanism of Action Increases the synthesis of DNA, RNA, and various proteins in target tissues; reduces the release of gonadotropin-releasing hormone from the hypothalamus; reduces FSH and LH release from the pituitary

Pharmacodynamics/Kinetics

Absorption: Absorbed well from GI tract

(Continued)

Ethinyl Estradiol *(Continued)*

Protein binding: 50% to 80%
Metabolism: Inactivated by liver
Elimination: By the kidneys

Usual Dosage Adults: Oral:
Male: Prostatic cancer (inoperable, progressing): 0.15-2 mg/day for palliation
Female:
Hypogonadism: 0.05 mg 1-3 times/day for 2 weeks of a theoretical menstrual cycle followed by progesterone for 3-6 months
Vasomotor symptoms: 0.02-0.05 mg for 21 days, off 7 days and repeat
Breast cancer (inoperable, progressing): 1 mg 3 times/day for palliation

Test Interactions
Decreased antithrombin III
Decreased serum folate concentration
Increased prothrombin and factors VII, VIII, IX, X
Increased platelet aggregability
Increased thyroid binding globulin
Increased total thyroid hormone (T_4)
Increased serum triglycerides/phospholipids

Patient Information Photosensitivity may occur
Women should inform their physicians if signs or symptoms of any of the following occur: Thromboembolic or thrombotic disorders including sudden severe headache or vomiting, disturbance of vision or speech, loss of vision, numbness or weakness in an extremity, sharp or crushing chest pain, calf pain, shortness of breath, severe abdominal pain or mass, mental depression or unusual bleeding
Women should discontinue taking the medication if they suspect they are pregnant or become pregnant

Nursing Implications Administer at bedtime to minimize occurrence of adverse effects

Dosage Forms Tablet: 0.02 mg, 0.05 mg, 0.5 mg

Ethinyl Estradiol and Ethynodiol Diacetate

(ETH in il es tra DYE ole & e thye noe DYE ole dye AS e tate)

Brand Names Demulen®; Zovia®

Synonyms Ethynodiol Diacetate and Ethinyl Estradiol

Therapeutic Category Contraceptive, Oral (Intermediate Potency Estrogen, Intermediate Potency Progestin); Contraceptive, Oral (Low Potency Estrogen, Intermediate Potency Progestin); Contraceptive, Oral (Monophasic); Estrogen Derivative, Oral; Progestin Derivative

Use Prevention of pregnancy; treatment of hypermenorrhea, endometriosis, female hypogonadism

Pregnancy Risk Factor X

Contraindications Known or suspected pregnancy, undiagnosed genital bleeding, carcinoma of the breast, estrogen-dependent tumor

Warnings/Precautions In patients with a history of thromboembolism, stroke, myocardial infarction (especially >40 years of age who smoke), liver tumor, hypertension, cardiac, renal or hepatic insufficiency; use of any progestin during the first 4 months of pregnancy is not recommended; risk of cardiovascular side effects increases in those women who smoke cigarettes and in women >35 years of age

Adverse Reactions
>10%:
Cardiovascular: Peripheral edema
Endocrine & metabolic: Enlargement of breasts, breast tenderness
Gastrointestinal: Nausea, anorexia, bloating
1% to 10%:
Central nervous system: Headache
Endocrine & metabolic: Increased libido
Gastrointestinal: Vomiting, diarrhea
<1%:
Cardiovascular: Hypertension, thromboembolism, stroke, myocardial infarction, edema
Central nervous system: Depression, dizziness, anxiety
Dermatologic: Chloasma, melasma, rash
Endocrine & metabolic: Decreased glucose tolerance, amenorrhea, alterations in frequency and flow of menses, increased triglycerides and LDL
Gastrointestinal: GI distress
Hepatic: Cholestatic jaundice
Ocular: Intolerance to contact lenses
Miscellaneous: Increased susceptibility to *Candida* infection, breast tumors
See tables.

Achieving Proper Hormonal Balance in an Oral Contraceptive

Estrogen		Progestin	
Excess	**Deficiency**	**Excess**	**Deficiency**
Nausea, bloating Cervical mucorrhea, polyposis Melasma Migraine headache Breast fullness or tenderness Edema Hypertension	Early or midcycle breakthrough bleeding Increased spotting Hypomenorrhea	Increased appetite Weight gain Tiredness, fatigue Hypomenorrhea Acne, oily scalp* Hair loss, hirsutism* Depression Monilial vaginitis Breast regression	Late breakthrough bleeding Amenorrhea Hypermenorrhea

*Result of androgenic activity of progestins.

Pharmacological Effects of Progestins Used in Oral Contraceptives

	Progestin	Estrogen	Antiestrogen	Androgen
Norgestrel/levonorgestrel	+++	0	++	+++
Ethynodiol diacetate	++	+*	+*	+
Norethindrone acetate	+	+	+++	+
Norethindrone	+	+*	+*	+
Norethynodrel	+	+++	0	0

*Has estrogenic effect at low doses; may have antiestrogenic effect at higher doses.

+++ = pronounced effect

++ = moderate effect

+ = slight effect

0 = moderate effect

Overdosage/Toxicology Toxicity is unlikely following single exposures of excessive doses; any treatment following emesis and charcoal administration should be supportive and symptomatic

Drug Interactions

Decreased effect of oral contraceptives with barbiturates, hydantoins - phenytoin, rifampin, antibiotics - penicillins, tetracyclines, griseofulvin

Increased toxicity of acetaminophen, anticoagulants, benzodiazepines, caffeine, corticosteroids, metoprolol, theophylline, tricyclic antidepressants

Mechanism of Action Combination oral contraceptives inhibit ovulation via a negative feedback mechanism on the hypothalamus, which alters the normal pattern of gonadotropin secretion of a follicle-stimulating hormone (FSH) and luteinizing hormone by the anterior pituitary. The follicular phase FSH and midcycle surge of gonadotropins are inhibited. In addition, oral contraceptives produce alterations in the genital tract, including changes in the cervical mucus, rendering it unfavorable for sperm penetration even if ovulation occurs. Changes in the endometrium may also occur, producing an unfavorable environment for nidation. Oral contraceptive drugs may alter the tubal transport of the ova through the fallopian tubes. Progestational agents may also alter sperm fertility.

Pharmacodynamics/Kinetics

Ethinyl estradiol:

- Absorption: Absorbed well from GI tract
- Protein binding: 50% to 80%
- Metabolism: Inactivated by liver
- Elimination: By the kidneys

Ethynodiol diacetate:

- Converted to norethindrone
- Metabolism: By conjugation in the liver
- Half-life, terminal: 5-14 hours

Usual Dosage Adults: Female: Oral:

For 21-tablet cycle packs, with 21 active tablets (28-day packs have 21 active tablets and 7 inert tablets): Take 1 tablet daily starting on the fifth day of menstrual cycle, with day 1 being the first day of menstruation; begin taking a new cycle pack on the eighth day after taking the last tablet from the previous pack

With 28-tablet packages, dosage is 1 tablet daily without interruption; extra tablets are placebos or contain iron. If next menstrual period does not begin on schedule, rule out pregnancy before starting new dosing cycle. If menstrual period begins, start new dosing cycle 7 days after last tablet was taken. If all doses have been taken on schedule and one menstrual period is missed, continue dosing cycle. If two consecutive menstrual periods are missed, pregnancy test is required before new dosing cycle is started.

(Continued)

Ethinyl Estradiol and Ethynodiol Diacetate *(Continued)*

One dose missed: Take as soon as remembered or take 2 tablets next day

Two doses missed: Take 2 tablets as soon as remembered or 2 tablets next 2 days

Three doses missed: Begin new compact of tablets starting on day 1 of next cycle

Test Interactions

Decreased antithrombin III

Decreased serum folate concentration

Increased prothrombin and factors VII, VIII, IX, X

Increased platelet aggregability

Increased thyroid binding globulin

Increased total thyroid hormone (T_4)

Increased serum triglycerides/phospholipids

Patient Information Photosensitivity may occur

Inform your physician if signs or symptoms of any of the following occur: Thromboembolic or thrombotic disorders including sudden severe headache or vomiting, disturbance of vision or speech, loss of vision, numbness or weakness in an extremity, sharp or crushing chest pain, calf pain, shortness of breath, severe abdominal pain or mass, mental depression or unusual bleeding.

If any doses are missed, alternative contraceptive methods should be used for the next 2 days or until 2 days into the new cycle

Discontinue taking the medication if you suspect you are pregnant or become pregnant

Additional Information Monophasic oral contraceptive

Dosage Forms Tablet:

1/35: Ethinyl estradiol 0.035 mg and ethynodiol diacetate 1 mg (21s, 28s)

1/50: Ethinyl estradiol 0.05 mg and ethynodiol diacetate 1 mg (21s, 28s)

Ethinyl Estradiol and Levonorgestrel

(ETH in il es tra DYE ole & LEE voe nor jes trel)

Brand Names Levlen®; Levora®; Nordette®; Tri-Levlen®; Triphasil®

Canadian/Mexican Brand Names Microgynon® (Mexico); Nordet® (Mexico); Nordiol® (Mexico)

Synonyms Levonorgestrel and Ethinyl Estradiol

Therapeutic Category Contraceptive, Oral (Low Potency Estrogen, Intermediate Potency Progestin); Contraceptive, Oral (Low Potency Estrogen, Low Potency Progestin); Contraceptive, Oral (Monophasic); Contraceptive, Oral (Triphasic); Estrogen Derivative, Oral; Progestin Derivative

Use Prevention of pregnancy; treatment of hypermenorrhea, endometriosis, female hypogonadism

Pregnancy Risk Factor X

Contraindications Thrombophlebitis, undiagnosed vaginal bleeding, hypersensitivity to ethinyl estradiol or any component, known or suspected pregnancy, carcinoma of the breast, estrogen-dependent tumor

Warnings/Precautions Use of any progestin during the first 4 months of pregnancy is not recommended; use with caution in patients with asthma, seizure disorders, migraine, cardiac, renal or hepatic impairment, cerebrovascular disorders or history of breast cancer, past and present thromboembolic disease, smokers >35 years of age

Adverse Reactions

>10%:

Cardiovascular: Peripheral edema

Endocrine & metabolic: Enlargement of breasts, breast tenderness

Gastrointestinal: Nausea, anorexia, bloating

1% to 10%:

Central nervous system: Headache

Endocrine & metabolic: Increased libido

Gastrointestinal: Vomiting, diarrhea

<1%:

Cardiovascular: Hypertension, thromboembolism, stroke, myocardial infarction, edema

Central nervous system: Depression, dizziness, anxiety

Dermatologic: Chloasma, melasma, rash

Endocrine & metabolic: Decreased glucose tolerance, amenorrhea, alterations in frequency and flow of menses, increased triglycerides and LDL

Gastrointestinal: GI distress

Hepatic: Cholestatic jaundice

Ocular: Intolerance to contact lenses

Miscellaneous: Increased susceptibility to *Candida* infection, breast tumors

See tables.

Achieving Proper Hormonal Balance in an Oral Contraceptive

Estrogen		Progestin	
Excess	**Deficiency**	**Excess**	**Deficiency**
Nausea, bloating Cervical mucorrhea, polyposis Melasma Migraine headache Breast fullness or tenderness Edema Hypertension	Early or midcycle breakthrough bleeding Increased spotting Hypomenorrhea	Increased appetite Weight gain Tiredness, fatigue Hypomenorrhea Acne, oily scalp* Hair loss, hirsutism* Depression Monilial vaginitis Breast regression	Late breakthrough bleeding Amenorrhea Hypermenorrhea

*Result of androgenic activity of progestins.

Pharmacological Effects of Progestins Used in Oral Contraceptives

	Progestin	Estrogen	Antiestrogen	Androgen
Norgestrel/levonorgestrel	+++	0	++	+++
Ethynodiol diacetate	++	+*	+*	+
Norethindrone acetate	+	+	+++	+
Norethindrone	+	+*	+*	+
Norethynodrel	+	+++	0	0

*Has estrogenic effect at low doses; may have antiestrogenic effect at higher doses.

+++ = pronounced effect

++ = moderate effect

+ = slight effect

0 = moderate effect

Overdosage/Toxicology Toxicity is unlikely following single exposures of excessive doses; any treatment following emesis and charcoal administration should be supportive and symptomatic

Drug Interactions

Decreased effect of oral contraceptives with barbiturates, hydantoins - phenytoin, rifampin, antibiotics - penicillins, tetracyclines, griseofulvin

Increased toxicity of acetaminophen, anticoagulants, benzodiazepines, caffeine, corticosteroids, metoprolol, theophylline, tricyclic antidepressants

Mechanism of Action Combination oral contraceptives inhibit ovulation via a negative feedback mechanism on the hypothalamus, which alters the normal pattern of gonadotropin secretion of a follicle-stimulating hormone (FSH) and luteinizing hormone by the anterior pituitary. The follicular phase FSH and midcycle surge of gonadotropins are inhibited. In addition, oral contraceptives produce alterations in the genital tract, including changes in the cervical mucus, rendering it unfavorable for sperm penetration even if ovulation occurs. Changes in the endometrium may also occur, producing an unfavorable environment for nidation. Oral contraceptive drugs may alter the tubal transport of the ova through the fallopian tubes. Progestational agents may also alter sperm fertility.

Pharmacodynamics/Kinetics

Ethinyl estradiol:

- Absorption: Absorbed well from GI tract
- Protein binding: 50% to 80%
- Metabolism: Inactivated by liver
- Elimination: By the kidneys

Levonorgestrel:

- Bioavailability: Completely
- Metabolism: Does not undergo first-pass effect; chiefly metabolized by reduction and conjugation
- Time to peak: 0.5-2 hours
- Half-life, terminal: 11-45 hours

Usual Dosage Adults: Female: Oral:

Contraception: 1 tablet daily, beginning on day 5 of menstrual cycle (first day of menstrual flow is day 1). With 20-tablet and 21-tablet packages, new dosing cycle begins 7 days after last tablet taken. With 28-tablet packages, dosage is 1 tablet daily without interruption; extra tablets are placebos or contain iron. If next menstrual period does not begin on schedule, rule out pregnancy before starting new dosing cycle. If menstrual period begins, start new dosing cycle 7 days after last tablet was taken. If all doses have been taken on schedule and one menstrual period is missed, continue dosing cycle. If two consecutive menstrual periods are missed, pregnancy test is required before new dosing cycle is started.

(Continued)

Ethinyl Estradiol and Levonorgestrel *(Continued)*

One dose missed: Take as soon as remembered or take 2 tablets next day
Two doses missed: Take 2 tablets as soon as remembered or 2 tablets next 2 days
Three doses missed: Begin new compact of tablets starting on day 1 of next cycle

Triphasic oral contraceptive (Tri-Levlen®, Triphasil®): 1 tablet/day in the sequence specified by the manufacturer

Test Interactions

Decreased antithrombin III
Decreased serum folate concentration
Increased prothrombin and factors VII, VIII, IX, X
Increased platelet aggregability
Increased thyroid binding globulin
Increased total thyroid hormone (T_4)
Increased serum triglycerides/phospholipids

Patient Information

Inform your physician if signs or symptoms of any of the following occur: Thromboembolic or thrombotic disorders including sudden severe headache or vomiting, disturbance of vision or speech, loss of vision, numbness or weakness in an extremity, sharp or crushing chest pain, calf pain, shortness of breath, severe abdominal pain or mass, mental depression or unusual bleeding

If any doses are missed, alternative contraceptive methods should be used for the next 2 days or until 2 days into the new cycle

Discontinue taking the medication if you suspect you are pregnant or become pregnant

Additional Information

Monophasic oral contraceptives: Levlen®, Levora®, Nordette®
Triphasic oral contraceptives: Tri-Levlen® and Triphasil®

Dosage Forms Tablet:

Levlen®, Levora®, Nordette®: Ethinyl estradiol 0.03 mg and levonorgestrel 0.15 mg (21s, 28s)

Tri-Levlen®, Triphasil®: Phase 1 (6 brown tablets): Ethinyl estradiol 0.03 mg and levonorgestrel 0.05 mg; Phase 2 (5 white tablets): Ethinyl estradiol 0.04 mg and levonorgestrel 0.075 mg; Phase 3 (10 yellow tablets): Ethinyl estradiol 0.03 mg and levonorgestrel 0.125 mg (21s, 28s)

Ethinyl Estradiol and Norethindrone

(ETH in il es tra DYE ole & nor eth IN drone)

Brand Names Brevicon®; Genora® 0.5/35; Genora® 1/35; Jenest-28™; Loestrin®; Modicon™; N.E.E.® 1/35; Nelova™ 0.5/35E; Nelova™ 10/11; Norethin™ 1/35E; Norinyl® 1+35; Ortho-Novum® 1/35; Ortho-Novum® 7/7/7; Ortho-Novum® 10/11; Ovcon® 35; Ovcon® 50; Tri-Norinyl®

Canadian/Mexican Brand Names Ortho®0.5/35 (Canada); Synphasic® (Canada); Trinovum® (Mexico)

Synonyms Norethindrone Acetate and Ethinyl Estradiol

Therapeutic Category Contraceptive, Oral (Biphasic); Contraceptive, Oral (Intermediate Potency Estrogen, Intermediate Potency Progestin); Contraceptive, Oral (Intermediate Potency Estrogen, Low Potency Progestin); Contraceptive, Oral (Low Potency Estrogen, Low Potency Progestin); Contraceptive, Oral (Monophasic); Contraceptive, Oral (Triphasic); Estrogen Derivative, Oral; Progestin Derivative

Use Prevention of pregnancy; treatment of hypermenorrhea, endometriosis, female hypogonadism

Pregnancy Risk Factor X

Contraindications Thrombophlebitis, cerebral vascular disease, coronary artery disease, known or suspected breast carcinoma, undiagnosed abnormal genital bleeding, hypersensitivity to any component

Warnings/Precautions Use of any progestin during the first 4 months of pregnancy is not recommended; in patients with a history of thromboembolism, stroke, myocardial infarction (especially >40 years of age who smoke), liver tumor, hypertension, cardiac, renal or hepatic insufficiency; risk of cardiovascular side effects increases in those women who smoke cigarettes and in women >35 years of age

Adverse Reactions

>10%:

Cardiovascular: Peripheral edema
Endocrine & metabolic: Enlargement of breasts, breast tenderness
Gastrointestinal: Nausea, anorexia, bloating

1% to 10%:

Central nervous system: Headache
Endocrine & metabolic: Increased libido

Gastrointestinal: Vomiting, diarrhea

<1%:

Cardiovascular: Hypertension, thromboembolism, stroke, myocardial infarction, edema

Central nervous system: Depression, dizziness, anxiety

Dermatologic: Chloasma, melasma, rash

Endocrine & metabolic: Decreased glucose tolerance, breast tumors, amenorrhea, alterations in frequency and flow of menses, increased triglycerides and LDL

Gastrointestinal: GI distress

Hepatic: Cholestatic jaundice

Ocular: Intolerance to contact lenses

Miscellaneous: Increased susceptibility to *Candida* infection

Minimize these effects by adjusting the estrogen/progestin balance or dosage. The table categorizes products by both their estrogenic and progestational potencies; because overall activity is influenced by the interaction of components, it is difficult to precisely classify products; placement in the table is only approximate. Differences between products within a group are probably not clinically significant. See tables.

Achieving Proper Hormonal Balance in an Oral Contraceptive

Estrogen		Progestin	
Excess	**Deficiency**	**Excess**	**Deficiency**
Nausea, bloating	Early or midcycle breakthrough bleeding	Increased appetite	Late breakthrough bleeding
Cervical mucorrhea, polyposis	Increased spotting	Weight gain	Amenorrhea
Melasma	Hypomenorrhea	Tiredness, fatigue	Hypermenorrhea
Migraine headache		Hypomenorrhea	
Breast fullness or tenderness		Acne, oily scalp*	
Edema		Hair loss, hirsutism*	
Hypertension		Depression	
		Monilial vaginitis	
		Breast regression	

*Result of androgenic activity of progestins.

Pharmacological Effects of Progestins Used in Oral Contraceptives

	Progestin	Estrogen	Antiestrogen	Androgen
Norgestrel/levonorgestrel	+++	0	++	+++
Ethynodiol diacetate	++	+*	+*	+
Norethindrone acetate	+	+	+++	+
Norethindrone	+	+*	+*	+
Norethynodrel	+	+++	0	0

*Has estrogenic effect at low doses; may have antiestrogenic effect at higher doses.

+++ = pronounced effect

++ = moderate effect

+ = slight effect

0 = moderate effect

Overdosage/Toxicology Toxicity is unlikely following single exposures of excessive doses; any treatment following emesis and charcoal administration should be supportive and symptomatic

Drug Interactions Ethinyl estradiol is a cytochrome P-450 3A enzyme substrate

Decreased effect:

Potential contraceptive failure with barbiturates, hydantoins, and rifampin

Concomitant penicillins or tetracyclines may lead to contraceptive failure

Increased toxicity:

Increased toxicity of carbamazepine, tricyclic antidepressants, and corticosteroids

Increased thromboembolic potential with oral anticoagulants

Mechanism of Action Combination oral contraceptives inhibit ovulation via a negative feedback mechanism on the hypothalamus, which alters the normal pattern of gonadotropin secretion of a follicle-stimulating hormone (FSH) and luteinizing hormone by the anterior pituitary. The follicular phase FSH and midcycle surge of gonadotropins are inhibited. In addition, oral contraceptives produce alterations in the genital tract, including changes in the cervical mucus, rendering it unfavorable for sperm penetration even if ovulation occurs. Changes in the endometrium may also occur, producing an unfavorable environment for nidation. Oral contraceptive drugs may alter the tubal transport of the ova through the fallopian tubes. Progestational agents may also alter sperm fortility, (Continued)

Ethinyl Estradiol and Norethindrone *(Continued)*

Pharmacodynamics/Kinetics

Ethinyl estradiol:

Absorption: Absorbed well from GI tract
Protein binding: 50% to 80%
Metabolism: Inactivated by liver
Elimination: By the kidneys

Norethindrone:

Time to peak: Oral: 0.5-4 hours
Bioavailability: Overall 65% with first-pass metabolism
Half-life, terminal: 5-14 hours

Usual Dosage Adults: Female: Oral:

For 21-tablet cycle packs, with 21 active tablets (28-day packs have 21 active tablets and 7 inert tablets): Take 1 tablet daily starting on the fifth day of menstrual cycle, with day 1 being the first day of menstruation; begin taking a new cycle pack on the eighth day after taking the last tablet from the previous pack

With 28-tablet packages, dosage is 1 tablet daily without interruption; extra tablets are placebos or contain iron. If next menstrual period does not begin on schedule, rule out pregnancy before starting new dosing cycle. If menstrual period begins, start new dosing cycle 7 days after last tablet was taken. If all doses have been taken on schedule and one menstrual period is missed, continue dosing cycle. If two consecutive menstrual periods are missed, pregnancy test is required before new dosing cycle is started.

One dose missed: Take as soon as remembered or take 2 tablets next day

Two doses missed: Take 2 tablets as soon as remembered or 2 tablets next 2 days

Three doses missed: Begin new compact of tablets starting on day 1 of next cycle

Biphasic oral contraceptive (Jenest™-28, Ortho-Novum™ 10/11, Nelova™ 10/11): 1 color tablet/day for 10 days, then next color tablet for 11 days

Triphasic oral contraceptive (Ortho-Novum™ 7/7/7, Tri-Norinyl®, Triphasil®): 1 tablet/day in the sequence specified by the manufacturer

Test Interactions

Decreased antithrombin III
Decreased serum folate concentration
Increased prothrombin and factors VII, VIII, IX, X
Increased platelet aggregability
Increased thyroid binding globulin
Increased total thyroid hormone (T_4)
Increased serum triglycerides/phospholipids

Patient Information Take exactly as directed; use additional method of birth control during first week of administration of first cycle; photosensitivity may occur. Women should inform their physicians if signs or symptoms of any of the following occur thromboembolic or thrombotic disorders including sudden severe headache or vomiting, disturbance of vision or speech, loss of vision, numbness or weakness in an extremity, sharp or crushing chest pain, calf pain, shortness of breath, severe abdominal pain or mass, mental depression, or unusual bleeding.

When any doses are missed, alternative contraceptive methods should be used for the next 2 days or until 2 days into the new cycle

Women should discontinue taking the medication if they suspect they are pregnant or become pregnant

Nursing Implications Administer at bedtime to minimize occurrence of adverse effects

Additional Information

Monophasic oral contraceptives: Ovcon®, Genora®, Loestrin®, N.E.E.®, Nelova®, Norethin®, Norinyl®, Ortho-Novum®

Biphasic oral contraceptives: Jenest®, Nelova™ 10/11, Ortho-Novum™ 10/11

Triphasic oral contraceptives: Tri-Norinyl®, Ortho-Novum™ 7/7/7

Dosage Forms Tablet:

Brevicon®, Genora® 0.5/35, Modicon™, Nelova® 0.5/35E: Ethinyl estradiol 0.035 mg and norethindrone 0.5 mg (21s, 28s)

Genora® 1/35, N.E.E.®1/35, Nelova® 1/35E, Norethin® 1/35E, Norinyl® 1 + 35, Ortho-Novum® 1/35: Ethinyl estradiol 0.035 mg and norethindrone 1 mg (21s, 28s)

Jenest™-28: Phase 1 (7 white tablets): Ethinyl estradiol 0.035 mg and norethindrone 0.5 mg; Phase 2 (14 peach tablets): Ethinyl estradiol 0.035 mg and norethindrone 1 mg (21s, 28s)

Loestrin® 1/20: Ethinyl estradiol 0.02 mg and norethindrone acetate 1 mg (21s, 28s)

Loestrin® 1.5/30: Ethinyl estradiol 0.03 mg and norethindrone acetate 1.5 mg (21s, 28s)

Loestrin® Fe 1.5/30: Ethinyl estradiol 0.03 mg and norethindrone acetate 1.5 mg with ferrous fumarate 75 mg in 7 inert tablets (28s)
Loestrin® 1/20: Ethinyl estradiol 0.02 mg and norethindrone acetate 1 mg (21s)
Loestrin® Fe 1/20: Ethinyl estradiol 0.02 mg and norethindrone acetate 1 mg with ferrous fumarate 75 mg in 7 inert tablets (28s)
Nelova™ 10/11: Phase 1 (10 light yellow tablets): Ethinyl estradiol 0.035 mg and norethindrone 0.5 mg; Phase 2 (11 dark yellow tablets): Ethinyl estradiol 0.035 mg and norethindrone 1 mg (21s, 28s)
Ortho-Novum™ 10/11: Phase 1 (10 white tablets): Ethinyl estradiol 0.035 mg and norethindrone 0.5 mg; Phase 2 (11 peach tablets): Ethinyl estradiol 0.035 mg and norethindrone 1 mg (21s, 28s)
Ortho-Novum™ 7/7/7: Phase 1 (7 white tablets): Ethinyl estradiol 0.035 mg and norethindrone 0.5 mg; Phase 2 (7 light peach tablets): Ethinyl estradiol 0.035 mg and norethindrone 0.75 mg; Phase 3 (7 peach tablets): Ethinyl estradiol 0.035 mg and norethindrone 1 mg (21s, 28s)
Ovcon®-35: Ethinyl estradiol 0.035 mg and norethindrone acetate 0.4 mg (21s)
Ovcon®-50: Ethinyl estradiol 0.05 mg and norethindrone acetate 1 mg (21s, 28s)
Tri-Norinyl®: Phase 1 (7 blue tablets): Ethinyl estradiol 0.035 mg and norethindrone 0.5 mg; Phase 2 (9 yellow-green tablets): Ethinyl estradiol 0.035 mg and norethindrone 1 mg; Phase 3 (5 blue tablets): Ethinyl estradiol 0.035 mg and norethindrone 0.5 mg (21s, 28s)

Ethinyl Estradiol and Norgestrel

(ETH in il es tra DYE ole & nor JES trel)

Brand Names Lo/Ovral®; Ovral®

Synonyms Morning After Pill; Norgestrel and Ethinyl Estradiol

Therapeutic Category Contraceptive, Oral (Intermediate Potency Estrogen, High Potency Progestin); Contraceptive, Oral (Low Potency Estrogen, Intermediate Potency Progestin); Contraceptive, Oral (Monophasic); Estrogen Derivative, Oral; Progestin Derivative

Use Prevention of pregnancy; oral: postcoital contraceptive or "morning after" pill; treatment of hypermenorrhea, endometriosis, female hypogonadism

Pregnancy Risk Factor X

Contraindications Thromboembolic disorders, cerebrovascular or coronary artery disease; known or suspected breast cancer; undiagnosed abnormal vaginal bleeding; women smokers >35 years of age; all women >40 years of age, hypersensitivity to drug or components

Warnings/Precautions Use of any progestin during the first 4 months of pregnancy is not recommended; in patients with a history of thromboembolism, stroke, myocardial infarction (especially >40 years of age who smoke), liver tumor, hypertension, cardiac, renal or hepatic insufficiency; risk of cardiovascular side effects increases in those women who smoke cigarettes and in women >35 years of age

Adverse Reactions Effects can be minimized by adjusting the estrogen/progestin balance or dosage. See tables in Ethinyl Estradiol and Norethindrone monograph.

>10%:
Cardiovascular: Peripheral edema
Endocrine & metabolic: Enlargement of breasts, breast tenderness
Gastrointestinal: Nausea, anorexia, bloating

1% to 10%:
Central nervous system: Headache
Endocrine & metabolic: Increased libido
Gastrointestinal: Vomiting, diarrhea

<1%:
Cardiovascular: Hypertension, thromboembolism, myocardial infarction, edema
Central nervous system: Depression, dizziness, anxiety, stroke
Dermatologic: Chloasma, melasma, rash
Endocrine & metabolic: Decreased glucose tolerance, breast tumors, amenorrhea, alterations in frequency and flow of menses, increased triglycerides and LDL
Gastrointestinal: GI distress
Hepatic: Cholestatic jaundice
Ocular: Intolerance to contact lenses
Miscellaneous: Increased susceptibility to *Candida* infection

Overdosage/Toxicology Toxicity is unlikely following single exposures of excessive doses; any treatment following emesis and charcoal administration should be supportive and symptomatic

Drug Interactions Ethinyl estradiol is a cytochrome P-450 3A enzyme substrate
Decreased effect:
Potential contraceptive failure with barbiturates, hydantoins, and rifampin
Concomitant penicillins or tetracyclines may lead to contraceptive failure
(Continued)

Ethinyl Estradiol and Norgestrel *(Continued)*

Increased toxicity:

Increased toxicity of carbamazepine, tricyclic antidepressants, and corticosteroids

Increased thromboembolic potential with oral anticoagulants

Mechanism of Action Combination oral contraceptives inhibit ovulation via a negative feedback mechanism on the hypothalamus, which alters the normal pattern of gonadotropin secretion of a follicle-stimulating hormone (FSH) and luteinizing hormone by the anterior pituitary. The follicular phase FSH and midcycle surge of gonadotropins are inhibited. In addition, oral contraceptives produce alterations in the genital tract, including changes in the cervical mucus, rendering it unfavorable for sperm penetration even if ovulation occurs. Changes in the endometrium may also occur, producing an unfavorable environment for nidation. Oral contraceptive drugs may alter the tubal transport of the ova through the fallopian tubes. Progestational agents may also alter sperm fertility.

Pharmacodynamics/Kinetics

Ethinyl estradiol:

Absorption: Absorbed well from GI tract

Protein binding: 50% to 80%

Metabolism: Inactivated by liver

Elimination: By the kidneys

Norgestrel:

Metabolism: Reduction and conjugation

Time to peak: 0.5-2 hours

Bioavailability: Complete with no first-pass effect

Half-life, terminal: 11-45 hours

Usual Dosage Female: Oral: Contraceptive: 1 tablet daily, beginning on day 5 of menstrual cycle (first day of menstrual flow is day 1). With 20-tablet and 21-tablet packages, new dosing cycle begins 7 days after last tablet taken; with 28-tablet packages, dosage is 1 tablet daily without interruption; extra tablets are placebos or contain iron. If next menstrual period does not begin on schedule, rule out pregnancy before starting new dosing cycle; if menstrual period begins, start new dosing cycle 7 days after last tablet was taken; if all doses have been taken on schedule and one menstrual period is missed, continue dosing cycle; if two consecutive menstrual periods are missed, pregnancy test is required before new dosing cycle is started.

One dose missed: Take as soon as remembered or take 2 tablets next day

Two doses missed: Take 2 tablets as soon as remembered or 2 tablets next 2 days

Three doses missed: Begin new compact of tablets starting on day 1 of next cycle

Postcoital contraception or "morning after" pill: Oral (50 mcg ethinyl estradiol and 0.5 mg norgestrel): 2 tablets at initial visit and 2 tablets 12 hours later

Test Interactions

Decreased antithrombin III

Decreased serum folate concentration

Increased prothrombin and factors VII, VIII, IX, X

Increased platelet aggregability

Increased thyroid binding globulin

Increased total thyroid hormone (T_4)

Increased serum triglycerides/phospholipids

Patient Information Take exactly as directed; use additional method of birth control during first week of administration of first cycle; photosensitivity may occur. Women should inform their physicians if signs or symptoms of any of the following occur: Thromboembolic or thrombotic disorders including sudden severe headache or vomiting, disturbance of vision or speech, loss of vision, numbness or weakness in an extremity, sharp or crushing chest pain, calf pain, shortness of breath, severe abdominal pain or mass, mental depression or unusual bleeding.

Women should be advised that when any doses are missed, alternative contraceptive methods should be used for the next 2 days or until 2 days into the new cycle

Women should discontinue taking the medication if they suspect they are pregnant or become pregnant

Nursing Implications Administer at bedtime to minimize occurrence of adverse effects

Additional Information Monophasic oral contraceptives

Dosage Forms Tablet:

Lo/Ovral®: Ethinyl estradiol 0.03 mg and norgestrel 0.3 mg (21s and 28s)

Ovral®: Ethinyl estradiol 0.05 mg and norgestrel 0.5 mg (21s and 28s)

Ethiofos *see* Amifostine *on page 59*

Ethionamide (e thye on AM ide)

Related Information

Antimicrobial Drugs of Choice *on page 1468*

Recommendations for Prophylaxis Against Tuberculosis *on page 1455*

Brand Names Trecator®-SC

Therapeutic Category Antitubercular Agent

Use Treatment of tuberculosis and other mycobacterial diseases, in conjunction with other antituberculosis agents, when first-line agents have failed or resistance has been demonstrated

Pregnancy Risk Factor C

Contraindications Contraindicated in patients with severe hepatic impairment or in patients who are sensitive to the drug

Warnings/Precautions Use with caution in patients receiving cycloserine or isoniazid, in diabetics

Adverse Reactions

>10%: Gastrointestinal: Anorexia, nausea, vomiting

1% to 10%:

- Cardiovascular: Postural hypotension
- Central nervous system: Psychiatric disturbances
- Gastrointestinal: Metallic taste
- Hepatic: Hepatitis, jaundice
- Neuromuscular & skeletal: Peripheral neuritis

<1%:

- Central nervous system: Drowsiness, dizziness, seizures, headache
- Dermatologic: Rash
- Endocrine & metabolic: Hypothyroidism or goiter, hypoglycemia, gynecomastia
- Gastrointestinal: Stomatitis, abdominal pain, diarrhea
- Hematologic: Thrombocytopenia
- Ocular: Optic neuritis

Overdosage/Toxicology Symptoms of overdose include peripheral neuropathy, anorexia, joint pain

Following GI decontamination, treatment is supportive; pyridoxine may be given to prevent peripheral neuropathy

Mechanism of Action Inhibits peptide synthesis

Pharmacodynamics/Kinetics

Distribution: Crosses the placenta

Protein binding: 10%

Bioavailability: 80%

Half-life: 2-3 hours

Time to peak serum concentration: Oral: Within 3 hours

Elimination: As metabolites (active and inactive) and parent drug in urine

Usual Dosage Oral:

Children: 15-20 mg/kg/day in 2 divided doses, not to exceed 1 g/day

Adults: 500-1000 mg/day in 1-3 divided doses

Dosing adjustment in renal impairment:

Cl_{cr} <50 mL/minute: Administer 50% of dose

Monitoring Parameters Initial and periodic serum ALT and AST

Test Interactions ↓ thyroxine (S)

Patient Information Take with meals; notify physician of persistent or severe stomach upset, loss of appetite, or metallic taste; frequent blood tests are needed for monitoring; increase dietary intake of pyridoxine

Nursing Implications Neurotoxic effects may be relieved by the administration of pyridoxine

Dosage Forms Tablet, sugar coated: 250 mg

Ethmozine® *see* Moricizine *on page 856*

Ethosuximide (eth oh SUKS i mide)

Related Information

Anticonvulsants by Seizure Type *on page 1392*

Epilepsy Treatment *on page 1531*

Brand Names Zarontin®

Therapeutic Category Anticonvulsant

Use Management of absence (petit mal) seizures, myoclonic seizures, and akinetic epilepsy; considered to be drug of choice for simple absence seizures

Pregnancy Risk Factor C

Pregnancy/Breast-Feeding Implications

Clinical effects on the fetus: No data on crossing the placenta. Dysmorphic facial features and patent ductus arteriosus reported. Epilepsy itself, number of medications, genetic factors, or a combination of these probably influence the teratogenicity of anticonvulsant therapy. Benefit:risk ratio usually favors continued use during pregnancy and breast-feeding.

(Continued)

Ethosuximide *(Continued)*

Breast-feeding/Lactation: Crosses into breast milk. American Academy of Pediatrics considers COMPATIBLE with breast-feeding.

Contraindications Known hypersensitivity to ethosuximide

Warnings/Precautions Use with caution in patients with hepatic or renal disease; abrupt withdrawal of the drug may precipitate absence status; ethosuximide may increase tonic-clonic seizures in patients with mixed seizure disorders; ethosuximide must be used in combination with other anticonvulsants in patients with both absence and tonic-clonic seizures

Adverse Reactions

>10%:

Central nervous system: Ataxia, drowsiness, sedation, dizziness, lethargy, euphoria, hallucinations, insomnia, agitation, behavioral changes, headache
Dermatologic: Stevens-Johnson syndrome
Gastrointestinal: Weight loss
Gastrointestinal: Nausea, vomiting, anorexia, abdominal pain
Miscellaneous: Hiccups, SLE syndrome

1% to 10%:

Central nervous system: Aggressiveness, mental depression, nightmares, fatigue
Neuromuscular & skeletal: Weakness

<1%:

Central nervous system: Paranoid psychosis
Dermatologic: Rashes, urticaria, exfoliative dermatitis
Hematologic: Leukopenia, aplastic anemia, thrombocytopenia, agranulocytosis, pancytopenia

Overdosage/Toxicology Acute overdosage can cause CNS depression, ataxia, stupor, coma, hypotension; chronic overdose can cause skin rash, confusion, ataxia, proteinuria, hepatic dysfunction, hematuria

Treatment is supportive; hemoperfusion and hemodialysis may be useful

Drug Interactions

Decreased effect: Phenytoin, carbamazepine, primidone, phenobarbital may increase the hepatic metabolism of ethosuximide

Increased toxicity: Isoniazid may inhibit hepatic metabolism with a resultant increase in ethosuximide serum concentrations

Mechanism of Action Increases the seizure threshold and suppresses paroxysmal spike-and-wave pattern in absence seizures; depresses nerve transmission in the motor cortex

Pharmacodynamics/Kinetics

Time to peak serum concentration:
Capsule: Within 2-4 hours
Syrup: <2-4 hours

Distribution: Adults: V_d: 0.62-0.72 L/kg

Metabolism: ~80% metabolized in the liver to three inactive metabolites

Half-life:
Children: 30 hours
Adults: 50-60 hours

Elimination: Slowly excreted in urine as metabolites (50%) and as unchanged drug (10% to 20%); small amounts excreted in feces

Usual Dosage Oral:

Children 3-6 years: Initial: 250 mg/day (or 15 mg/kg/day) in 2 divided doses; increase every 4-7 days; usual maintenance dose: 15-40 mg/kg/day in 2 divided doses

Children >6 years and Adults: Initial: 250 mg twice daily; increase by 250 mg as needed every 4-7 days up to 1.5 g/day in 2 divided doses; usual maintenance dose: 20-40 mg/kg/day in 2 divided doses

Dietary Considerations Alcohol: Additive CNS depression has been reported with succimides; avoid or limit alcohol

Monitoring Parameters Seizure frequency, trough serum concentrations; CBC, platelets, liver enzymes, urinalysis

Reference Range Therapeutic: 40-100 μg/mL (SI: 280-710 μmol/L); Toxic: >150 μg/mL (SI: >1062 μmol/L)

Test Interactions ↑ alkaline phosphatase (S); positive Coombs' [direct]; ↓ calcium (S)

Patient Information Take with food; do not discontinue abruptly; may cause drowsiness and impair judgment

Nursing Implications Observe patient for excess sedation

Dosage Forms

Capsule: 250 mg
Syrup (raspberry flavor): 250 mg/5 mL (473 mL)

Ethoxynaphthamido Penicillin Sodium *see* Nafcillin *on page 871*

Ethyl Aminobenzoate *see* Benzocaine *on page 138*

Ethylenediamine *see* Theophylline Salts *on page 1207*

Ethynodiol Diacetate and Ethinyl Estradiol *see* Ethinyl Estradiol and Ethynodiol Diacetate *on page 482*

Ethyol® *see* Amifostine *on page 59*

Etidocaine (e TI doe kane)

Brand Names Duranest®

Synonyms Etidocaine Hydrochloride

Therapeutic Category Local Anesthetic, Injectable

Use Infiltration anesthesia; peripheral nerve blocks; central neural blocks

Pregnancy Risk Factor B

Contraindications Heart block, severe hemorrhage, severe hypotension, known hypersensitivity to etidocaine or other amide local anesthetics

Warnings/Precautions Use with caution in patients with cardiac disease and hyperthyroidism; fetal bradycardia may occur up to 20% of the time; use with caution in areas of inflammation or sepsis, in debilitated or elderly patients, and those with severe cardiovascular disease or hepatic dysfunction; some products may contain sulfites

Adverse Reactions

<1%:

Cardiovascular: Myocardial depression, hypotension, bradycardia, cardiovascular collapse

Central nervous system: Anxiety, restlessness, disorientation, confusion, seizures, drowsiness, unconsciousness, chills

Dermatologic: Urticaria

Gastrointestinal: Nausea, vomiting

Local: Transient stinging or burning at injection site

Neuromuscular & skeletal: Tremor

Ocular: Blurred vision

Otic: Tinnitus

Respiratory: Respiratory arrest

Miscellaneous: Anaphylactoid reactions, shivering

Overdosage/Toxicology Symptoms of overdose include seizures, hypoventilation, apnea, hypotension, cardiac depression, arrhythmias, cardiac arrest

Treatment is supportive; seizures may be treated with diazepam; hypotension, circulatory collapse respond best to fluids and Trendelenburg position

Mechanism of Action Blocks nervous conduction through the stabilization of neuronal membranes. By preventing the transient increase in membrane permeability to sodium, the ionic fluxes necessary for initiation and transmission of electrical impulses are inhibited and local anesthesia is induced.

Pharmacodynamics/Kinetics

Onset of anesthesia: Within 2-5 minutes

Duration: ~4-10 hours

Absorption: Rapid

Distribution: Wide V_d allows wide distribution into neuronal tissues

Protein binding: High

Metabolism: Extensively in the liver

Elimination: Small amounts excreted in urine

Usual Dosage Varies with procedure; use 1% for peripheral nerve block, central nerve block, lumbar peridural caudal; use 1.5% for maxillary infiltration or inferior alveolar nerve block; use 1% or 1.5% for intra-abdominal or pelvic surgery, lower limb surgery, or caesarean section

Reference Range Toxic concentration: >0.1 µg/mL

Nursing Implications Before injecting withdraw syringe plunger to ensure injection is not into vein or artery; have resuscitative equipment nearby

Dosage Forms

Injection, as hydrochloride: 1% [10 mg/mL] (30 mL)

Injection, as hydrochloride, with epinephrine 1:200,000: 1% [10 mg/mL] (30 mL); 1.5% [15 mg/mL] (20 mL)

Etidocaine Hydrochloride *see* Etidocaine *on this page*

Etidronate Disodium (e ti DROE nate dye SOW dee um)

Brand Names Didronel®

Synonyms EHDP; Sodium Etidronate

Therapeutic Category Antidote, Hypercalcemia; Bisphosphonate Derivative

Use Symptomatic treatment of Paget's disease and heterotopic ossification due to spinal cord injury or after total hip replacement, hypercalcemia associated with malignancy

Pregnancy Risk Factor B (oral)/C (parenteral)

(Continued)

Etidronate Disodium *(Continued)*

Contraindications Patients with serum creatinine >5 mg/dL; hypersensitivity to biphosphonates

Warnings/Precautions Use with caution in patients with restricted calcium and vitamin D intake; dosage modification required in renal impairment; I.V. form may be nephrotoxic and should be used with caution, if at all, in patients with impaired renal function (serum creatinine: 2.5-4.9 mg/dL)

Adverse Reactions

1% to 10%:

- Central nervous system: Fever, convulsions
- Endocrine & metabolic: Hypophosphatemia, hypomagnesemia, fluid overload
- Neuromuscular & skeletal: Bone pain
- Respiratory: Dyspnea

<1%:

- Central nervous system: Pain
- Dermatologic: Angioedema, rash
- Gastrointestinal: Abnormal taste
- Hematologic: Occult blood in stools
- Neuromuscular & skeletal: Increased risk of fractures
- Renal: Nephrotoxicity
- Miscellaneous: Hypersensitivity reactions

Overdosage/Toxicology Symptoms of overdose include diarrhea, nausea, vomiting, paresthesias, tetany, coma; antidote is calcium

Stability Store ampuls at room temperature and avoid excess heat (>40°C/104°F); intravenous solution diluted in ≥250 mL normal saline is stable for 48 hours at room temperature or refrigerated

Mechanism of Action Decreases bone resorption by inhibiting osteocystic osteolysis; decreases mineral release and matrix or collagen breakdown in bone

Pharmacodynamics/Kinetics

Onset of therapeutic effect: Within 1-3 months of therapy

Duration: Can persist for 12 months without continuous therapy

Absorption: Dependent upon dose administered

Metabolism: Not metabolized

Elimination: As unchanged drug primarily in urine with unabsorbed drug being eliminated in feces

Usual Dosage Adults:

Paget's disease: Oral: 5 mg/kg/day given every day for no more than 6 months; may administer 10 mg/kg/day for up to 3 months; daily dose may be divided if adverse GI effects occur

Heterotopic ossification with spinal cord injury: 20 mg/kg/day for 2 weeks, then 10 mg/kg/day for 10 weeks (this dosage has been used in children, however, treatment >1 year has been associated with a rachitic syndrome)

Hypercalcemia associated with malignancy:

- I.V. (Dilute dose in at least 250 mL NS): 7.5 mg/kg/day for 3 days; there should be at least 7 days between courses of treatment
- Oral: Start 20 mg/kg/day on the last day of infusion and continue for 30-90 days

Dosing adjustment in renal impairment:

- S_{cr} 2.5-5 mg/dL: Use with caution
- S_{cr} >5 mg/dL: Do not use

Administration Administer intravenous dose over at least 2 hours; I.V. doses should be diluted in at least 250 mL 0.9% sodium chloride

Monitoring Parameters Serum calcium and phosphorous; serum creatinine and BUN

Reference Range Calcium (total): Adults: 9.0-11.0 mg/dL

Patient Information Maintain adequate intake of calcium and vitamin D; take medicine on an empty stomach 2 hours before meals

Nursing Implications Ensure adequate hydration

Dosage Forms

Injection: 50 mg/mL (6 mL)

Tablet: 200 mg, 400 mg

Etodolac (ee toe DOE lak)

Related Information

Dosing Data for Acetaminophen and NSAIDs *on page 1377*

Nonsteroidal Anti-Inflammatory Agents Comparison *on page 1419*

Brand Names Lodine®; Lodine® XL

Canadian/Mexican Brand Names Lodine® Retard (Mexico); Utradol™ (Canada)

Synonyms Etodolic Acid

Therapeutic Category Analgesic, Nonsteroidal Anti-inflammatory Drug; Anti-inflammatory Agent; Nonsteroidal Anti-inflammatory Agent (NSAID), Oral

Use Acute and long-term use in the management of signs and symptoms of osteoarthritis and management of pain

Unapproved use: Rheumatoid arthritis

Pregnancy Risk Factor C

Contraindications Hypersensitivity to etodolac, aspirin, or other NSAIDs

Warnings/Precautions Use with caution in patients with congestive heart failure, hypertension, decreased renal or hepatic function, history of GI disease, or those receiving anticoagulants

Adverse Reactions

>10%:
- Central nervous system: Dizziness
- Dermatologic: Rash
- Gastrointestinal: Abdominal cramps, heartburn, indigestion, nausea

1% to 10%:
- Central nervous system: Headache, nervousness
- Dermatologic: Itching
- Endocrine & metabolic: Fluid retention
- Gastrointestinal: Vomiting
- Otic: Tinnitus

<1%:
- Cardiovascular: Congestive heart failure, hypertension, arrhythmia, tachycardia
- Central nervous system: Confusion, hallucinations, aseptic meningitis, mental depression, drowsiness, insomnia
- Dermatologic: Urticaria, erythema multiforme, toxic epidermal necrolysis, Stevens-Johnson syndrome, angioedema
- Endocrine & metabolic: Polydipsia, hot flashes
- Gastrointestinal: Gastritis, GI ulceration
- Genitourinary: Cystitis, polyuria
- Hematologic: Agranulocytosis, anemia, hemolytic anemia, bone marrow suppression, leukopenia, thrombocytopenia
- Hepatic: Hepatitis
- Neuromuscular & skeletal: Peripheral neuropathy
- Ocular: Toxic amblyopia, blurred vision, conjunctivitis, dry eyes
- Otic: Decreased hearing
- Renal: Acute renal failure
- Respiratory: Allergic rhinitis, shortness of breath, epistaxis

Overdosage/Toxicology Symptoms of overdose include acute renal failure, vomiting, drowsiness, leukocytes

Management of a nonsteroidal anti-inflammatory drug (NSAID) intoxication is primarily supportive and symptomatic. Fluid therapy is commonly effective in managing the hypotension that may occur following an acute NSAID overdose, except when this is due to an acute blood loss.

Drug Interactions

Decreased effect with aspirin

Increased effect/toxicity with aspirin (GI irritation), probenecid; increased effect/ toxicity of lithium, methotrexate, digoxin, cyclosporin (nephrotoxicity), warfarin (bleeding)

Stability Protect from moisture

Mechanism of Action Inhibits prostaglandin synthesis by decreasing the activity of the enzyme, cyclo-oxygenase, which results in decreased formation of prostaglandin precursors

Pharmacodynamics/Kinetics

Absorption: Oral: Well absorbed

Distribution: V_d: 0.4 L/kg

Protein binding: High

Half-life: 7 hours

Time to peak serum concentration: 1 hour

Usual Dosage Single dose of 76-100 mg is comparable to the analgesic effect of aspirin 650 mg; in patients ≥65 years, no substantial differences in the pharmacokinetics or side-effects profile were seen compared with the general population

Adults: Oral:
- Acute pain: 200-400 mg every 6-8 hours, as needed, not to exceed total daily doses of 1200 mg; for patients weighing <60 kg, total daily dose should not exceed 20 mg/kg/day
- Osteoarthritis: Initial: 800-1200 mg/day given in divided doses: 400 mg 2 or 3 times/day; 300 mg 2, 3 or 4 times/day; 200 mg 3 or 4 times/day; total daily dose should not exceed 1200 mg; for patients weighing <60 kg, total daily dose should not exceed 20 mg/kg/day

Monitoring Parameters Monitor CBC, liver enzymes; in patients receiving diuretics, monitor urine output and BUN/serum creatinine

Test Interactions False-positive for urinary bilirubin and ketone ↑ bleeding time

(Continued)

Etodolac *(Continued)*

Patient Information Do not crush tablets; take with food, milk, or water; report any signs of blood in stool

Dosage Forms

Capsule (Lodine®): 200 mg, 300 mg
Tablet: 400 mg
Lodine®: 400 mg
Tablet, extended release (Lodine® XL): 400 mg, 600 mg

Etodolic Acid *see* Etodolac *on page 494*

Etomidate (e TOM i date)

Related Information

Adult ACLS Algorithm, Electrical Conversion *on page 1515*

Brand Names Amidate®

Therapeutic Category General Anesthetic

Use Induction of general anesthesia

Pregnancy Risk Factor C

Contraindications Known hypersensitivity to etomidate

Warnings/Precautions Consider exogenous corticosteroid replacement in patients undergoing severe stress

Adverse Reactions

>10%:
Gastrointestinal: Nausea, vomiting
Local: Pain at injection site
Neuromuscular & skeletal: Transient skeletal movements
Ocular: Uncontrolled eye movements
1% to 10%: Hiccups
<1%:
Cardiovascular: Hypertension, hypotension, tachycardia, bradycardia, arrhythmias
Respiratory: Hyperventilation, hypoventilation, apnea, laryngospasm

Overdosage/Toxicology Symptoms of overdose include respiratory arrest, coma; supportive treatment

Stability Store in refrigerator

Mechanism of Action Ultrashort-acting nonbarbiturate hypnotic used for the induction of anesthesia; chemically, it is a carboxylated imidazole and has been shown to produce a rapid induction of anesthesia with minimal cardiovascular and respiratory effects

Usual Dosage Children >10 years and Adults: I.V.: 0.2-0.6 mg/kg over a period of 30-60 seconds for induction of anesthesia

Dosage Forms Injection: 2 mg/mL (10 mL, 20 mL)

Etopophos® *see* Etoposide Phosphate *on page 499*

Etoposide (e toe POE side)

Related Information

Antiemetics for Chemotherapy Induced Nausea and Vomiting *on page 1348*
Cancer Chemotherapy Regimens *on page 1351*
Extravasation Management of Chemotherapeutic Agents *on page 1379*
Toxicities of Chemotherapeutic Agents *on page 1382*

Brand Names Toposar® Injection; VePesid® Injection; VePesid® Oral

Canadian/Mexican Brand Names Etopos® (Mexico); Medsaposide® (Mexico); Serozide® (Mexico)

Synonyms Epipodophyllotoxin; VP-16; VP-16-213

Therapeutic Category Antineoplastic Agent, Irritant; Antineoplastic Agent, Podophyllotoxin Derivative; Vesicant

Use Treatment of lymphomas, ANLL, lung, testicular, bladder, and prostate carcinoma, hepatoma, rhabdomyosarcoma, uterine carcinoma, neuroblastoma, mycosis fungoides, Kaposi's sarcoma, histiocytosis, gestational trophoblastic disease, Ewing's sarcoma, Wilm's tumor, and brain tumors

Pregnancy Risk Factor D

Contraindications Hypersensitivity to etoposide or any component; **I.T. administration is contraindicated**

Warnings/Precautions The U.S. Food and Drug Administration (FDA) currently recommends that procedures for proper handling and disposal of antineoplastic agents be considered. Severe myelosuppression with resulting infection or bleeding may occur.

Dosage should be adjusted in patients with hepatic or renal impairment

Adverse Reactions

>10%:
Dermatologic: Alopecia (reversible)

Gastrointestinal: Occasional diarrhea and infrequent nausea and vomiting at standard doses; severe mucositis occurs with high (BMT) doses, anorexia
Emetic potential: Moderately low (10% to 30%)

Hematologic: Myelosuppressive: Principal dose-limiting toxicity of VP-16. White blood cell count nadir is 5-15 days after administration and is more frequent than thrombocytopenia. Recovery is usually within 24-28 days and cumulative toxicity has not been noted with VP-16 as a single agent. No difference in toxicity is seen when VP-16 is administered over a 24-hour period or over 2 hours on 5 consecutive days.
WBC: Mild to severe
Platelets: Mild
Onset (days): 10
Nadir (days): granulocytes 7-14 days; platelets 9-16 days
Recovery (days): 21-28

1% to 10%:
Cardiovascular: Hypotension: Related to drug infusion time; may be related to vehicle used in the I.V. preparation (polysorbate 80 plus polyethylene glycol). Best to administer the drug over 1 hour.
Central nervous system: Unusual fatigue
Gastrointestinal: Stomatitis, diarrhea, abdominal pain, hepatitic dysfunction

<1%:
Cardiovascular: Tachycardia
Central nervous system: Neurotoxicity, somnolence, fever, headache
Irritant chemotherapy, thrombophlebitis has been reported
Hepatic: Toxic hepatitis (with high-dose therapy)
Hypersensitivity: Reports of flushing or bronchospasm, which did not reoccur in one report if patients were pretreated with corticosteroids and antihistamines
Neuromuscular & skeletal: Peripheral neuropathy

Overdosage/Toxicology Symptoms of overdose include bone marrow suppression, leukopenia, thrombocytopenia, nausea, vomiting; treatment is supportive

Drug Interactions Cytochrome P-450 3A enzyme substrate

Increased toxicity:
Warfarin may elevate prothrombin time with concurrent use
Methotrexate: Alteration of MTX transport has been found as a slow efflux of MTX and its polyglutamated form out of the cell, leading to intercellular accumulation of MTX
Calcium antagonists: Increases the rate of VP-16-induced DNA damage and cytotoxicity *in vitro*
Carmustine: Reports of frequent hepatic dysfunction with hyperbilirubinemia, ascites, and thrombocytopenia
Cyclosporine: Additive cytotoxic effects on tumor cells

Stability

Store intact vials of injection at room temperature and protected from light; injection solution contains polyethylene glycol vehicle with absolute alcohol; store oral capsules under refrigeration

VP-16 should be further diluted in D_5W or NS for administration; diluted solutions have CONCENTRATION-DEPENDENT stability: More concentrated solutions have shorter stability times

At room temperature in D_5W or NS in polyvinyl chloride, the concentration is stable as follows:
0.2 mg/mL: 96 hours
0.4 mg/mL: 48 hours
0.6 mg/mL: 8 hours
1 mg/mL: 2 hours
2 mg/mL: 1 hour
20 mg/mL (undiluted): 24 hours

Y-site compatible with carboplatin, cytarabine, mesna, daunorubicin

Standard I.V. dilution:

Lower dose regimens (<1 g/dose):
Doses may be diluted in 100-1000 mL of D_5W or NS
If the concentration is less than or equal to 0.6 mg/mL, the bag should be mixed with the appropriate expiration dating
If the concentration is >0.6 mg/mL, the concentration is highly unstable and a syringe of UNDILUTED etoposide accompanied with the appropriate volume of diluent will be sent to the nursing unit to be mixed by the nursing staff just prior to administration

High dose regimens (>1g/dose):
Total dose should be drawn into an empty viaflex container and the appropriate amount of diluent (for a final concentration of 1 mg/mL) will be sent
Use the **2-Channel Pump Method**: Instill all of the etoposide dose into one viaflex container (concentration = 20 mg/mL). Infuse this into one channel (Baxter Flow-Guard 6300 Dual Channel Volumetric Infusion Pump - or any 2-channel infusion pump that does not require a "hard" plastic cassette).

(Continued)

Etoposide *(Continued)*

Infuse the indicated diluent (ie, D_5W or NS) at a rate of at least 20 times the infusion rate of the etoposide to simulate a 1 mg/mL concentration in the line. The etoposide should be Y-sited into the port most proximal to the patient. A 0.22 micron filter should be attached to the line after the Y-site and before entry into the patient.

Mechanism of Action Inhibits mitotic activity; inhibits cells from entering prophase; inhibits DNA synthesis. Initially thought to be mitotic inhibitors similar to podophyllotoxin, but actually have no effect on microtubule assembly. However, later shown to induce DNA strand breakage and inhibition of topoisomerase II (an enzyme which breaks and repairs DNA); etoposide acts in late S or early G2 phases.

Pharmacodynamics/Kinetics

Absorption: Oral: 32% to 57%

Distribution: Poor penetration across blood-brain barrier, with concentrations in the CSF being <10% that of plasma

Average V_d: 3-36 L/m²

Protein binding: 94% to 97%

Metabolism: In the liver (with a biphasic decay)

Half-life: Terminal: 4-15 hours

Children: 6-8 hours with normal renal and hepatic function

Time to peak serum concentration: Oral: 1-1.5 hours

Elimination: Both unchanged drug and metabolites are excreted in the urine and a small amount (2% to 16%) excreted in feces; up to 55% of an I.V. dose is excreted unchanged in urine in children

Usual Dosage Refer to individual protocols

Oral: Twice the I.V. dose rounded to the nearest 50 mg given once daily if total dose ≤400 mg or in divided doses if >400 mg

Children: I.V.: 60-120 mg/m²/day for 3-5 days every 3-6 weeks

AML:

Remission induction: 150 mg/m²/day for 2-3 days for 2-3 cycles

Intensification or consolidation: 250 mg/m²/day for 3 days, courses 2-5

Conditioning regimen for allogenic BMT: 60 mg/kg/dose as a single dose

Adults:

Small cell lung cancer:

Oral: Twice the I.V. dose rounded to the nearest 50 mg given once daily if

I.V.: 35 mg/m²/day for 4 days or 50 mg/m²/day for 5 days every 3-4 weeks

total dose ≤400 mg/day or in divided doses if >400 mg/day

IVPB: 60-100 mg/m² /day for 3 days (with cisplatin)

CIV.: 500 mg/m² over 24 hours every 3 weeks

Testicular cancer:

IVPB: 50-100 mg/m²/day for 5 days repeated every 3-4 weeks

I.V.: 100 mg/m² every other day for 3 doses repeated every 3-4 weeks

BMT/relapsed leukemia:

I.V.: 2.4-3.5 g/m² or 25-70 mg/kg administered over 4-36 hours

Dosage adjustment in renal impairment:

Cl_{cr} 10-50 mL/minute: Administer 75% of normal dose

Cl_{cr} <10 mL minute: Administer 50% of normal dose

Hemodialysis: Supplemental dose is not necessary

Peritoneal dialysis: Supplemental dose is not necessary

CAPD effects: Unknown

CAVH effects: Unknown

Dosage adjustment in hepatic impairment:

Bilirubin 1.5-3 mg/dL or AST 60-180 units: Reduce dose by 50%

Bilirubin 3-5 mg/dL or AST >180 units: Reduce by 75%

Bilirubin >5 mg/dL: Do not administer

Administration

Administer lower doses IVPB over at least 30 minutes to minimize the risk of hypotensive reactions

Administer high-doses (>1 g/dose) via the 2-channel pump method.

An in-line 0.22 micron filter should be attached to ALL etoposide infusions due to the high potential for precipitation

Monitoring Parameters CBC with differential, platelet count, and hemoglobin, vital signs (blood pressure), bilirubin, and renal function tests

Patient Information Any signs of infection, easy bruising or bleeding, shortness of breath, or painful or burning urination should be brought to physician's attention. Nausea, vomiting, or hair loss sometimes occur. The drug may cause permanent sterility and may cause birth defects. The drug may be excreted in breast milk, therefore, an alternative form of feeding your baby should be used.

Nursing Implications

Extravasation treatment:

Inject 150-900 units of hyaluronidase S.C. clockwise into the infiltrated area using a 25-gauge needle; change the needle with each injection; apply heat immediately for 1 hour, repeat 4 times/day for 3-5 days

Application of cold or hydrocortisone is contraindicated.

If necessary, the injection may be used for oral administration; mix with orange juice, apple juice, or lemonade to a concentration of 0.4 mg/mL or less, and use within a 3-hour period

Dosage Forms

Capsule: 50 mg

Injection: 20 mg/mL (5 mL, 10 mL, 25 mL)

Etoposide Phosphate (e toe POE side FOS fate)

Brand Names Etopophos®

Canadian/Mexican Brand Names Etopos® (Mexico); Medsaposide® (Mexico); Serozide® (Mexico)

Therapeutic Category Antineoplastic Agent, Irritant; Antineoplastic Agent, Podophyllotoxin Derivative; Vesicant

Use Treatment of refractory testicular tumors and small cell lung cancer

Pregnancy Risk Factor D

Contraindications Hypersensitivity to etoposide, etoposide phosphate, or any component; **I.T. administration is contraindicated**

Warnings/Precautions The U.S. Food and Drug Administration (FDA) currently recommends that procedures for proper handling and disposal of antineoplastic agents be considered. Severe myelosuppression with resulting infection or bleeding may occur.

Dosage should be adjusted in patients with hepatic or renal impairment

Adverse Reactions

>10%:

Dermatologic: Alopecia (reversible)

Gastrointestinal: Occasional diarrhea and infrequent nausea and vomiting at standard doses; severe mucositis occurs with high (BMT) doses, anorexia

Emetic potential: Moderately low (10% to 30%)

Hematologic: Myelosuppressive: Principal dose-limiting toxicity of VP-16. White blood cell count nadir is 5-15 days after administration and is more frequent than thrombocytopenia. Recovery is usually within 24-28 days and cumulative toxicity has not been noted with VP-16 as a single agent. No difference in toxicity is seen when VP-16 is administered over a 24-hour period or over 2 hours on 5 consecutive days.

WBC: Mild to severe

Platelets: Mild

Onset (days): 10

Nadir (days): granulocytes 7-14 days; platelets 9-16 days

Recovery (days): 21-28

1% to 10%:

Cardiovascular: Hypotension: Related to drug infusion time; may be related to vehicle used in the I.V. preparation (polysorbate 80 plus polyethylene glycol). Best to administer the drug over 1 hour.

Central nervous system: Unusual fatigue

Gastrointestinal: Stomatitis, diarrhea, abdominal pain, hepatitic dysfunction

<1%:

Cardiovascular: Tachycardia

Central nervous system: Neurotoxicity, somnolence, fever, headache

Hepatic: Toxic hepatitis (with high-dose therapy)

Hypersensitivity: Reports of flushing or bronchospasm, which did not reoccur in one report if patients were pretreated with corticosteroids and antihistamines

Neuromuscular & skeletal: Peripheral neuropathy

Overdosage/Toxicology Symptoms of overdose include bone marrow suppression, leukopenia, thrombocytopenia, nausea, vomiting; treatment is supportive

Drug Interactions Cytochrome P-450 3A enzyme substrate

Increased toxicity:

Warfarin may elevate prothrombin time with concurrent use

Methotrexate: Alteration of MTX transport has been found as a slow efflux of MTX and its polyglutamated form out of the cell, leading to intercellular accumulation of MTX

Calcium antagonists: Increases the rate of VP-16-induced DNA damage and cytotoxicity *in vitro*

Carmustine: Reports of frequent hepatic dysfunction with hyperbilirubinemia, ascites, and thrombocytopenia

Cyclosporine: Additive cytotoxic effects on tumor cells

(Continued)

Etoposide Phosphate *(Continued)*

Stability

Store intact vials of injection under refrigeration 2°C to 8°C (36°F to 46°F); protect from light

Reconstituted vials with 5 mL or 10 mL SWI, D_5W, NS, bacteriostatic SWI, or bacteriostatic NS to a concentration of 20 mg/mL or 10 mg/mL etoposide (22.7 mg/mL or 11.4 mg/mL etoposide phosphate), respectively. These solutions may be administered without further dilution or may be further diluted to a concentration as low as 0.1 mg/mL etoposide with either D_5W or NS. Solutions are stable in glass or plastic containers at room temperature 20°C to 25°C (68°F to 77°F) or under refrigeration 2°C to 8°C (36°F to 47°F) for up to 24 hours.

Mechanism of Action Etoposide phosphate is converted *in vivo* to the active moiety, etoposide, by dephosphorylation. Etoposide inhibits mitotic activity; inhibits cells from entering prophase; inhibits DNA synthesis. Initially thought to be mitotic inhibitors similar to podophyllotoxin, but actually have no effect on microtubule assembly. However, later shown to induce DNA strand breakage and inhibition of topoisomerase II (an enzyme which breaks and repairs DNA); etoposide acts in late S or early G2 phases.

Pharmacodynamics/Kinetics

Distribution: Average V_d: 3-36 L/m^2; poor penetration across blood-brain barrier, with concentrations in the CSF being <10% that of plasma

Protein binding: 94% to 97%

Metabolism: In the liver (with a biphasic decay)

Half-life: Terminal: 4-15 hours

Children: 6-8 hours with normal renal and hepatic function

Elimination: Both unchanged drug and metabolites are excreted in the urine and a small amount (2% to 16%) excreted in feces; up to 55% of an I.V. dose is excreted unchanged in urine in children

Usual Dosage Refer to individual protocols

Adults:

Small cell lung cancer:

I.V. (in combination with other approved chemotherapeutic drugs): **Equivalent doses of etoposide phosphate to an etoposide dosage** range of 35 mg/m^2/day for 4 days to 50 mg/m^2/day for 5 days. Courses are repeated at 3- to 4-week intervals after adequate recovery from any toxicity.

Testicular cancer:

I.V. (in combination with other approved chemotherapeutic agents): **Equivalent dose of etoposide phosphate to etoposide dosage** range of 50-100 mg/m^2/day on days 1-5 to 100 mg/m^2/day on days 1, 3, and 5. Courses are repeated at 3- to 4-week intervals after adequate recovery from any toxicity.

Dosage adjustment in renal impairment:

Cl_{cr} 15-50 mL/minute: Administer 75% of normal dose

Cl_{cr} <15 mL minute: Data are not available and further dose reduction should be considered in these patients.

Hemodialysis: Supplemental dose is not necessary

Peritoneal dialysis: Supplemental dose is not necessary

CAPD effects: Unknown

CAVH effects: Unknown

Dosage adjustment in hepatic impairment:

Bilirubin 1.5-3 mg/dL or AST 60-180 units: Reduce dose by 50%

Bilirubin 3-5 mg/dL or AST >180 units: Reduce by 75%

Bilirubin >5 mg/dL: Do not administer

Administration Etoposide phosphate solutions may be administered at infusion rates from 5-210 minutes

Monitoring Parameters CBC with differential, platelet count, and hemoglobin, vital signs (blood pressure), bilirubin, and renal function tests

Patient Information Any signs of infection, easy bruising or bleeding, shortness of breath, or painful or burning urination should be brought to physician's attention. Nausea, vomiting, or hair loss sometimes occur. The drug may cause permanent sterility and may cause birth defects. The drug may be excreted in breast milk, therefore, an alternative form of feeding your baby should be used.

Dosage Forms Powder for injection, lyophilized: 119.3 mg (100 mg base)

Etretinate (e TRET i nate)

Brand Names Tegison®

Therapeutic Category Antipsoriatic Agent, Systemic

Use Treatment of severe recalcitrant psoriasis in patients intolerant of or unresponsive to standard therapies

Pregnancy Risk Factor X

Contraindications Pregnancy, known hypersensitivity to etretinate; because of the high likelihood of long lasting teratogenic effects, do not prescribe etretinate for women who are or who are likely to become pregnant while or after using the drug

Warnings/Precautions Not to be used in severe obesity or women of child-bearing potential unless woman is capable of complying with effective contraceptive measures; therapy is normally begun on the second or third day of next normal menstrual period; effective contraception must be used for at least 1 month before beginning therapy, during therapy, and for 1 month after discontinuation of therapy; pregnancy test must be performed prior to starting therapy

Adverse Reactions

>10%:

Central nervous system: Fatigue, headache, fever
Dermatologic: Chapped lips, alopecia
Endocrine & metabolic: Hypercholesterolemia, hypertriglyceridemia
Gastrointestinal: Nausea, appetite change, xerostomia, sore tongue
Neuromuscular & skeletal: Hyperostosis, bone pain, arthralgia
Ocular: Eye irritation
Respiratory: Epistaxis

1% to 10%:

Cardiovascular: Edema
Central nervous system: Dizziness, lethargy
Hepatic: Hepatitis
Neuromuscular & skeletal: Myalgia
Ocular: Blurred vision
Otic: Otitis externa
Respiratory: Dyspnea

<1%:

Cardiovascular: Syncope
Central nervous system: Amnesia, confusion, pseudotumor cerebri, depression
Dermatologic: Urticaria
Gastrointestinal: Mouth ulcers, diarrhea, constipation, flatulence, weight loss, gingival bleeding
Endocrine & metabolic: Gout
Genitourinary: Dysuria, polyuria
Local: Phlebitis
Neuromuscular & skeletal: Hyperkinesia, hypertonia
Ocular: Photophobia
Otic: Ear infection
Renal: Kidney stones
Respiratory: Rhinorrhea

Drug Interactions

Increased effect: Milk increases absorption of etretinate
Increased toxicity: Additive toxicity with vitamin A

Mechanism of Action Unknown; related to retinoic acid and retinol (vitamin A)

Pharmacodynamics/Kinetics

Absorption: Oral: Absorbed from small intestine; absorption enhanced when coadministered with whole milk or a high lipid meal (highly lipophilic)
Protein binding: 99%
Metabolism: Undergoes significant first-pass metabolism to form acitretin (active)
Half-life: 4-8 days (with multiple doses)
Elimination: By metabolism and by excretion in feces of unchanged drug and metabolites

Usual Dosage Adults: Oral: Individualized; Initial: 0.75-1 mg/kg/day in divided doses, increase by 0.25 mg/kg/day at weekly intervals up to 1.5 mg/kg/day; maintenance dose established after 8-10 weeks of therapy 0.5-0.75 mg/kg/day

Patient Information Do not become pregnant while taking this drug, use effective contraceptive measures; if severe persistent nausea, abdominal pain, or vomiting recur stop taking the drug; if persistent or severe headache or visual disturbance occur, stop taking the drug; take with food, do not take vitamin A supplements while taking this drug, may have decreased tolerance to contact lenses before and after therapy

Dosage Forms Capsule: 10 mg, 25 mg

Eulexin® *see* Flutamide *on page 548*
Eurax® *see* Crotamiton *on page 318*
Evac-Q-Mag® [OTC] *see* Magnesium Citrate *on page 751*
Evalose® *see* Lactulose *on page 703*
Everone® Injection *see* Testosterone *on page 1198*
E-Vista® *see* Hydroxyzine *on page 634*
E-Vitamin® [OTC] *see* Vitamin E *on page 1309*
Exact® Cream [OTC] *see* Benzoyl Peroxide *on page 140*
Excedrin® IB [OTC] *see* Ibuprofen *on page 639*

Exelderm® *see* Sulconazole *on page 1170*
Exidine® Scrub [OTC] *see* Chlorhexidine Gluconate *on page 253*
Exna® *see* Benzthiazide *on page 141*
Exosurf® Neonatal *see* Colfosceril Palmitate *on page 310*
Exsel® *see* Selenium Sulfide *on page 1132*
Extra Action Cough Syrup [OTC] *see* Guaifenesin and Dextromethorphan *on page 591*
Extravasation Management of Chemotherapeutic Agents *see page 1379*
Extravasation Treatment of Other Drugs *see page 1381*
Eye-Sed® [OTC] *see* Zinc Supplements *on page 1324*
Eye-Zine® [OTC] *see* Tetrahydrozoline *on page 1205*
Ezide® *see* Hydrochlorothiazide *on page 617*
F_3T *see* Trifluridine *on page 1263*

Factor IX Complex (Human) (FAK ter nyne KOM pleks HYU man)

Brand Names AlphaNine®; Konȳne® 80; Mononine®; Profilnine® Heat-Treated; Proplex® SX-T; Proplex® T

Therapeutic Category Antihemophilic Agent

Use Controls bleeding in patients with factor IX deficiency (Hemophilia B or Christmas disease); prevention/control of bleeding in hemophilia A patients with inhibitors to factor VIII

Pregnancy Risk Factor C

Contraindications Liver disease with signs of intravascular coagulation or fibrinolysis, not for use in factor VII deficiencies, patients undergoing elective surgery

Warnings/Precautions Use with caution in patients with liver dysfunction; risk of viral transmission is not totally eradicated, prepared from pooled human plasma

Adverse Reactions

1% to 10%: Following rapid administration: Transient fever
- Central nervous system: Fever, headache, chills
- Neuromuscular & skeletal: Paresthesia

<1%:
- Cardiovascular: Flushing, DIC, thrombosis following high dosages in hemophilia B patients, tightness in chest
- Central nervous system: Somnolence
- Dermatologic: Urticaria
- Gastrointestinal: Nausea, vomiting
- Respiratory: Tightness in neck

Overdosage/Toxicology Disseminated intravascular coagulation (DIC)

Drug Interactions Increased toxicity: Do not coadminister with aminocaproic acid may increase risk for thrombosis

Stability When stored at refrigerator temperature, 2°C to 8°C (36°F to 46°F), coagulation factor IX is stable for the period indicated by the expiration date on its label. Avoid freezing which may damage container for the diluent.

Stability of parenteral admixture at room temperature (25°C): 24 hours; do **not** refrigerate after reconstitution
Standard diluent: Dose in units/bag
Minimum volume: Use complete vial(s) for entire dose
Comments: Infusion rate should be 2 mL/minute

Mechanism of Action Replaces deficient clotting factor including factor X; hemophilia B, or Christmas disease, is an X-linked recessively inherited disorder of blood coagulation characterized by insufficient or abnormal synthesis of the clotting protein factor IX. Factor IX is a vitamin K-dependent coagulation factor which is synthesized in the liver. Factor IX is activated by factor XIa in the intrinsic coagulation pathway. Activated factor IX (IXa), in combination with factor VII:C activates factor X to Xa, resulting ultimately in the conversion of prothrombin to thrombin and the formation of a fibrin clot. The infusion of exogenous factor IX to replace the deficiency present in hemophilia B temporarily restores hemostasis.

Pharmacodynamics/Kinetics

Half-life:
- VII component: Cleared rapidly from the serum in two phases; initial: 4-6 hours; terminal: 22.5 hours
- IX component: 24 hours

Usual Dosage Children and Adults: Dosage is expressed in units of factor IX activity and must be individualized. I.V. only:

Factor VII deficiency: Highly individualized
0.5 unit/kg x body weight (kg) x desired increase (%)
For example, for a 70 kg adult to increase level by 25%:
0.5 unit/kg x 70 kg x 25 = 875 units

Factor IX deficiency: Highly individualized
1 unit/kg x body weight (in kg) x desired increase (%)

For example, to increase the level by 25% in a 70 kg adult:
1 unit x 70 kg x 25 = 1,750 units

Formula for units required to raise blood level %:
Total blood volume (mL blood/kg) = 70 mL/kg (adults), 80 mL/kg (children)
Plasma volume = total blood volume (mL) x [1 - Hct (in decimals)]
For example, for a 70 kg adult with a Hct = 40%: Plasma volume = [70 kg x 70 mL/kg] x [1 - 0.4] = 2940 mL
To calculate number of units needed to increase level to desired range (highly individualized and dependent on patient's condition):
Number of units = desired level increase [desired level - actual level] x plasma volume (in mL)
For example, for a 100% level in the above patient who has an actual level of 20%: Number of units needed = [1 (for a 100% level) - 0.2] x 2940 mL = 2,352 units
As a general rule, the level of factor IX required for treatment of different conditions is shown in the table.

	Minor Spontaneous Hemorrhage, Prophylaxis	Major Trauma or Surgery
Desired levels of factor IX for hemostasis	15%-25%	25%-50%
Initial loading dose to achieve desired level	<20-30 units/kg	<75 units/kg
Frequency of dosing	Once; repeated in 24 h if necessary	q18-30h, depending on half-life and measured factor IX levels
Duration of treatment	Once; repeated if necessary	Up to 10 days, depending upon nature of insult

Factor VIII inhibitor patients: 75 units/kg/dose; may be given every 6-12 hours
Anticoagulant overdosage: I.V.: 15 units/kg

Administration Solution should be infused at room temperature
I.V. administration only: Should be infused **slowly**: Start infusion at a rate of 2-3 mL/minute. If headache, flushing, changes in pulse rate or blood pressure appear, the infusion rate should be decreased. Initially, stop the infusion until the symptoms disappear, then resume the infusion at a slower rate. **Infuse at a rate not exceeding 3 mL/minute.**

Monitoring Parameters Levels of factors II, IX, and X; PT and PTT

Reference Range Average normal factor VII and factor IX levels are 50% to 150%; patients with severe hemophilia will have levels <1%, often undetectable. Moderate forms of the disease have levels of 1% to 10% while some mild cases may have 11% to 49% of normal factor IX.

Maintain factor IX plasma level at least 20% until hemostasis achieved after acute joint or muscle bleeding
In preparation for and following surgery:
Level to prevent spontaneous hemorrhage: 5%
Minimum level for hemostasis following trauma and surgery: 30% to 50%
Severe hemorrhage: >60%
Major surgery: >60% prior to procedure, 30% to 50% for several days after surgery, and >20% for 7-10 days thereafter

Dosage Forms Injection:
AlphaNine®: 500 units, 1000 units, 1500 units
Konÿne® 80: 10 mL, 20 mL
Mononine®: 250 units, 500 units, 1000 units
Profilnine® Heat-Treated: Single dose vial
Proplex® SX-T: Vial
Proplex® T: Vial

Factor VIII *see* Antihemophilic Factor (Human) *on page 94*
Factrel® *see* Gonadorelin *on page 583*

Famciclovir (fam SYE kloe veer)

Brand Names Famvir™

Therapeutic Category Antiviral Agent, Oral

Use Management of acute herpes zoster (shingles); treatment of recurrent herpes simplex in immunocompetent patients

Pregnancy Risk Factor B

Pregnancy/Breast-Feeding Implications Use only if the benefit to the patient clearly exceeds the potential risk to the fetus; due to potential for excretion of famciclovir in breast milk and for its associated tumorigenicity, discontinue nursing or discontinue the drug during lactation

Contraindications Hypersensitivity to famciclovir

(Continued)

Famciclovir *(Continued)*

Warnings/Precautions Has not been studied in immunocompromised patients or patients with ophthalmic or disseminated zoster; dosage adjustment is required in patients with renal insufficiency (Cl_{cr} <60 mL/minute) and in patients with noncompensated hepatic disease; safety and efficacy have not been established in children <18 years of age; animal studies indicated increases in incidence of carcinomas, mutagenic changes, and decreases in fertility with extremely large doses

Adverse Reactions

>10%:

Central nervous system: Headache

Gastrointestinal: Nausea

1% to 10%:

Central nervous system: Fatigue, fever, dizziness, somnolence

Gastrointestinal: Diarrhea, vomiting, constipation, anorexia, abdominal pain

Neuromuscular & skeletal: Rigors, paresthesia

Overdosage/Toxicology Supportive and symptomatic care is recommended; hemodialysis may enhance elimination

Drug Interactions Increased effect/toxicity:

Cimetidine: Penciclovir AUC may increase due to impaired metabolism

Digoxin: C_{max} of digoxin increases by ~19%

Probenecid: Penciclovir serum levels significantly increase

Theophylline: Penciclovir AUC/C_{max} may increase and renal clearance decrease, although not clinically significant

Mechanism of Action After undergoing rapid biotransformation to the active compound, penciclovir, famciclovir is phosphorylated by viral thymidine kinase in HSV-1, HSV-2, and VZV-infected cells to a monophosphate form; this is then converted to penciclovir triphosphate and competes with deoxyguanosine triphosphate to inhibit HSV-2 polymerase (ie, herpes viral DNA synthesis/replication is selectively inhibited)

Pharmacodynamics/Kinetics

Absorption: Food decreases the maximum peak concentration and delays the time to peak; AUC remains the same

Distribution: V_{dss}: 0.98-1.08 L/kg

Protein binding: 20%

Metabolism: Rapidly deacetylated and oxidized to penciclovir (not by cytochrome P-450)

Bioavailability: 77%; T_{max}: 0.9 hours

Half-life: Penciclovir: 2-3 hours (10, 20, and 7 hours in HSV-1, HSV-2, and VZV-infected cells); linearly decreased with reductions in renal failure

Elimination: >90% of penciclovir is eliminated unchanged in urine; C_{max} and T_{max} are decreased and prolonged, respectively in patients with noncompensated hepatic impairment

Usual Dosage Adults: Oral:

Acute herpes zoster: 500 mg every 8 hours for 7 days

Recurrent herpes simplex in immunocompetent patients: 125 mg twice daily for 5 days

Dosing interval in renal impairment:

Cl_{cr} ≥60 mL/minute: Administer 500 mg every 8 hours

Cl_{cr} 40-59 mL/minute: Administer 500 mg every 12 hours

Cl_{cr} 20-39 mL/minute: Administer 500 mg every 24 hours

Cl_{cr} <20 mL/minute: Unknown

Administration Initiate therapy as soon as herpes zoster is diagnosed

Patient Information May take medication with food or on an empty stomach

Additional Information Most effective if therapy is initiated within 72 hours of initial lesion

Dosage Forms Tablet: 125 mg, 250 mg, 500 mg

Famotidine (fa MOE ti deen)

Brand Names Pepcid®; Pepcid® AC Acid Controller [OTC]

Canadian/Mexican Brand Names Apo-Famotidine® (Canada); Novo-Famotidine® (Canada); Nu-Famotidine® (Canada); Durater® (Mexico); Famoxal® (Mexico); Farmotex® (Mexico); Pepcidine® (Mexico); Sigafam® (Mexico)

Therapeutic Category Antihistamine, H_2 Blocker; Histamine-2 Antagonist

Use

Pepcid®: Therapy and treatment of duodenal ulcer, gastric ulcer, control gastric pH in critically ill patients, symptomatic relief in gastritis, gastroesophageal reflux, active benign ulcer, and pathological hypersecretory conditions

Pepcid® AC Acid Controller: Relieves heartburn, acid indigestion and sour stomach

Pregnancy Risk Factor B

Pregnancy/Breast-Feeding Implications

Clinical effects on the fetus: Crosses the placenta. No data on effects on the fetus (insufficient data).

Breast-feeding/lactation: Crosses into breast milk. American Academy of Pediatrics has NO RECOMMENDATIONS.

Contraindications Hypersensitivity to famotidine or other H_2-antagonists

Warnings/Precautions Modify dose in patients with renal impairment

Adverse Reactions

1% to 10%:

Central nervous system: Dizziness, headache

Gastrointestinal: Constipation, diarrhea

<1%:

Cardiovascular: Bradycardia, tachycardia, palpitations, hypertension

Central nervous system: Fever, fatigue, seizures, insomnia, drowsiness

Dermatologic: Acne, pruritus, urticaria, dry skin

Gastrointestinal: Abdominal discomfort, flatulence, belching, anorexia

Hematologic: Agranulocytosis, neutropenia, thrombocytopenia

Hepatic: Increases in AST, ALT

Neuromuscular & skeletal: Paresthesia, weakness

Renal: Increases in BUN/creatinine, proteinuria

Respiratory: Bronchospasm

Miscellaneous: Allergic reaction

Overdosage/Toxicology Symptoms of overdose include hypotension, tachycardia, vomiting, drowsiness; treatment is primarily symptomatic and supportive

Drug Interactions Decreased effect of ketoconazole, itraconazole

Stability Reconstituted I.V. solution is stable for 48 hours at room temperature; I.V. infusion in NS or D_5W solution is stable for 48 hours at room temperature; reconstituted oral solution is stable for 30 days at room temperature

Mechanism of Action Competitive inhibition of histamine at H_2 receptors of the gastric parietal cells, which inhibits gastric acid secretion

Pharmacodynamics/Kinetics

Onset of GI effect: Oral: Within 1 hour

Duration: 10-12 hours

Protein binding: 15% to 20%

Bioavailability: Oral: 40% to 50%

Half-life: 2.5-3.5 hours; increases with renal impairment, oliguric patients: 20 hours

Time to peak serum concentration: Oral: Within 1-3 hours

Elimination: In urine as unchanged drug

Usual Dosage

Children: Oral, I.V.: Doses of 1-2 mg/kg/day have been used; maximum dose: 40 mg

Adults:

Oral:

Duodenal ulcer, gastric ulcer: 40 mg/day at bedtime for 4-8 weeks

Hypersecretory conditions: Initial: 20 mg every 6 hours, may increase up to 160 mg every 6 hours

GERD: 20 mg twice daily for 6 weeks

I.V.: 20 mg every 12 hours

Dosing adjustment in renal impairment:

Cl_{cr} 30-50 mL/minute: Administer every 24 hours or 50% of dose

Cl_{cr} <30 mL/minute: Administer every 36-48 hours or 25% of dose

Administration Administer over 15-30 minutes; may be given undiluted I.V. push

Dosage Forms

Infusion, premixed in NS: 20 mg (50 mL)

Injection: 10 mg/mL (2 mL, 4 mL)

Powder for oral suspension (cherry-banana-mint flavor): 40 mg/5 mL (50 mL)

Tablet, film coated: 20 mg, 40 mg

Pepcid® AC Acid Controller: 10 mg

Famvir™ *see* Famciclovir *on page 503*

Fansidar® *see* Sulfadoxine and Pyrimethamine *on page 1174*

Fastin® *see* Phentermine *on page 987*

Fat Emulsion (fat e MUL shun)

Brand Names Intralipid®; Liposyn®; Nutrilipid®; Soyacal®

Synonyms Intravenous Fat Emulsion

Therapeutic Category Caloric Agent

Use Source of calories and essential fatty acids for patients requiring parenteral nutrition of extended duration

Pregnancy Risk Factor B/C

(Continued)

Fat Emulsion *(Continued)*

Contraindications Pathologic hyperlipidemia, lipoid nephrosis, known hypersensitivity to fat emulsion and severe egg or legume (soybean) allergies, pancreatitis with hyperlipemia

Warnings/Precautions Use caution in patients with severe liver damage, pulmonary disease, anemia, or blood coagulation disorder; use with caution in jaundiced, premature, and low birth weight children

Adverse Reactions

>10%: Local: Thrombophlebitis

1% to 10%: Endocrine & metabolic: Hyperlipemia

<1%:

- Cardiovascular: Cyanosis, flushing, chest pain
- Gastrointestinal: Nausea, vomiting, diarrhea
- Hepatic: Hepatomegaly
- Respiratory: Dyspnea
- Miscellaneous: Sepsis

Overdosage/Toxicology Too rapid administration results in fluid or fat overloading to cause dilution of serum electrolytes, overhydration, pulmonary edema, impaired pulmonary diffusion capacity, metabolic acidosis; treatment is supportive

Stability May be stored at room temperature; do not store partly used bottles for later use; do not use if emulsion appears to be oiling out

Mechanism of Action Essential for normal structure and function of cell membranes

Pharmacodynamics/Kinetics

Metabolism: Undergoes lipolysis to free fatty acids, which are utilized by reticuloendothelial cells

Half-life: 0.5-1 hour

Usual Dosage Fat emulsion should not exceed 60% of the total daily calories

Infants, premature: Initial dose: 0.25-0.5 g/kg/day, increase by 0.25-0.5 g/kg/day to a maximum of 3-4 g/kg/day; maximum rate of infusion: 0.15 g/kg/hour (0.75 mL/kg/hour of 20% solution)

Infants and Children: Initial dose: 0.5-1 g/kg/day, increase by 0.5 g/kg/day to a maximum of 3-4 g/kg/day; maximum rate of infusion: 0.25 g/kg/hour (1.25 mL/kg/hour of 20% solution)

Adolescents and Adults: Initial dose: 1 g/kg/day, increase by 0.5-1 g/kg/day to a maximum of 2.5 g/kg/day of 10% and 3 g/kg/day of 20%; maximum rate of infusion: 0.25 g/kg/hour (1.25 mL/kg/hour of 20% solution); do not exceed 50 mL/hour (20%) or 100 mL/hour (10%)

Note: At the onset of therapy, the patient should be observed for any immediate allergic reactions such as dyspnea, cyanosis, and fever. Slower initial rates of infusion may be used for the first 10-15 minutes of the infusion (eg, 0.1 mL/minute of 10% or 0.05 mL/minute of 20% solution).

Prevention of fatty acid deficiency (8% to 10% of total caloric intake): 0.5-1 g/kg/24 hours

- Children: 5-10 mL/kg/day at 0.1 mL/minute then up to 100 mL/hour
- Adults: 500 mL twice weekly at rate of 1 mL/minute for 30 minutes, then increase to 500 mL over 4-6 hours

Can be used in both children and adults on a daily basis as a caloric source in TPN

Administration May be simultaneously infused with amino acid dextrose mixtures by means of Y-connector located near infusion site. The 10% isotonic solution which has 1.1 cal/mL (10%) and may be administered peripherally; the 20% (2 cal/mL) is not recommended for use in low birth weight infants.

Monitoring Parameters Serum triglycerides; before initiation of therapy and at least weekly during therapy

Dosage Forms Injection: 10% [100 mg/mL] (100 mL, 250 mL, 500 mL); 20% [200 mg/mL] (100 mL, 250 mL, 500 mL)

5-FC *see* Flucytosine *on page 526*

^{18}FDG *see* Fludeoxyglucose F 18 *on page 529*

Febrile Seizures *see page 1532*

Feiba VH Immuno® *see* Anti-Inhibitor Coagulant Complex *on page 96*

Feldene® *see* Piroxicam *on page 1009*

Felodipine (fe LOE di peen)

Related Information

Calcium Channel Blockers Comparative Actions *on page 1401*

Calcium Channel Blockers Comparative Pharmacokinetics *on page 1402*

Calcium Channel Blockers FDA-Approved Indications *on page 1403*

Brand Names Plendil®

Canadian/Mexican Brand Names Renedil® (Canada); Munobal® (Mexico)

Therapeutic Category Calcium Channel Blocker

Use Treatment of hypertension, congestive heart failure

Pregnancy Risk Factor C

Contraindications Hypersensitivity to felodipine or any component or other calcium channel blocker; severe hypotension or second and third degree heart block

Warnings/Precautions Use with caution and titrate dosages for patients with impaired renal or hepatic function; use caution when treating patients with congestive heart failure, sick-sinus syndrome, severe left ventricular dysfunction, hypertrophic cardiomyopathy (especially obstructive), concomitant therapy with beta-blockers or digoxin, edema, or increased intracranial pressure with cranial tumors; do not abruptly withdraw (may cause chest pain); elderly may experience hypotension and constipation more readily.

Adverse Reactions

>10%: Cardiovascular: Peripheral edema

1% to 10%:

- Cardiovascular: Chest pain, tachycardia
- Central nervous system: Dizziness, lightheadedness
- Dermatologic: Rash
- Gastrointestinal: Constipation, diarrhea

<1%:

- Cardiovascular: Hypotension, arrhythmia, bradycardia, palpitations
- Central nervous system: Mental depression, headache
- Gastrointestinal: Gingival hyperplasia, xerostomia, nausea
- Hepatic: Marked elevations in liver function tests
- Ocular: Blurred vision
- Respiratory: Shortness of breath

Overdosage/Toxicology The primary cardiac symptoms of calcium blocker overdose includes hypotension and bradycardia. The hypotension is caused by peripheral vasodilation, myocardial depression, and bradycardia. Bradycardia results from sinus bradycardia, second- or third-degree atrioventricular block, or sinus arrest with junctional rhythm. Intraventricular conduction is usually not affected so QRS duration is normal (verapamil does prolong the P-R interval and bepridil prolongs the Q-T and may cause ventricular arrhythmias, including torsade de pointes).

The noncardiac symptoms include confusion, stupor, nausea, vomiting, metabolic acidosis and hyperglycemia. Following initial gastric decontamination, if possible, repeated calcium administration may promptly reverse the depressed cardiac contractility (but not sinus node depression or peripheral vasodilation); glucagon, epinephrine, and amrinone may treat refractory hypotension; glucagon and epinephrine also increase the heart rate (outside the U.S., 4-aminopyridine may be available as an antidote); dialysis and hemoperfusion are not effective in enhancing elimination although repeat-dose activated charcoal may serve as an adjunct with sustained-release preparations.

Drug Interactions

Decreased effect:

- Felodipine and carbamazepine may decrease felodipine effect
- Felodipine and theophylline may decrease pharmacologic actions of theophylline

Increased toxicity/effect/levels:

- Felodipine and metoprolol may increase cardiac depressant effects on A-V conduction
- Felodipine and erythromycin inhibits felodipine (and other dihydropyridine calcium antagonist) metabolism resulting in a 2-fold increase in levels and consequent toxicity

Mechanism of Action Inhibits calcium ions from entering the "slow channels" or select voltage-sensitive areas of vascular smooth muscle and myocardium during depolarization, producing a relaxation of coronary vascular smooth muscle and coronary vasodilation; increases myocardial oxygen delivery in patients with vasospastic angina

Pharmacodynamics/Kinetics

- Onset of effect: 2-5 hours
- Duration: 16-24 hours
- Absorption: 100%; absolute: 20% due to first-pass effect
- Protein binding: >99%
- Metabolism: >99% in liver
- Half-life: 11-16 hours
- Elimination: In urine as metabolites

Usual Dosage Adults: Oral: 5-10 mg once daily; increase by 5 mg at 2-week intervals, as needed, to a maximum of 20 mg/day (Elderly: Begin with 2.5 mg/day)

(Continued)

Felodipine *(Continued)*

Dosing adjustment/comments in hepatic impairment: Begin with 2.5 mg/day; do not use doses >10 mg/day

Patient Information Do not crush or chew tablets; do not discontinue abruptly; report any dizziness, shortness of breath, palpitations or edema occurs

Additional Information Although there is some initial data which may show increased risk of myocardial infarction following treatment of hypertension with calcium antagonists, controlled trials (eg, ALL-HAT) are ongoing to examine the long-term effects of not only calcium antagonists but other antihypertensives in preventing heart disease. Until these studies are completed, patients taking calcium antagonists should be encouraged to continue with prescribed antihypertensive regimes, although a switch from high-dose, short-acting agents to sustained release products may be warranted. It is also generally agreed that calcium antagonists should be avoided as the primary treatment for hypertension unless diuretics or beta-blockers are contraindicated and for the primary treatment of angina following acute myocardial infarction.

Dosage Forms Tablet, extended release: 2.5 mg, 5 mg, 10 mg

Femcet® *see* Butalbital Compound *on page 176*

Femiron® [OTC] *see* Ferrous Fumarate *on page 513*

Femizole-7® [OTC] *see* Clotrimazole *on page 302*

Femizol-M® [OTC] *see* Miconazole *on page 834*

Femstat® *see* Butoconazole *on page 178*

Fenesin™ *see* Guaifenesin *on page 589*

Fenesin DM® *see* Guaifenesin and Dextromethorphan *on page 591*

Fenfluramine (fen FLURE a meen)

Related Information

Dexfenfluramine *on page 360*

Brand Names Pondimin®

Canadian/Mexican Brand Names Ponderal® (Canada)

Synonyms Fenfluramine Hydrochloride

Therapeutic Category Anorexiant; Sympathomimetic

Use Short-term adjunct in exogenous obesity

Restrictions C-IV

Pregnancy Risk Factor C

Contraindications Known hypersensitivity to fenfluramine

Warnings/Precautions Cardiovascular disease, nephritis, angina pectoris, hypertension, glaucoma, patients with a history of drug abuse, known hypersensitivity to amphetamine

Adverse Reactions

1% to 10%:

- Central nervous system: Confusion, mental depression, restlessness
- Endocrine & metabolic: Changes in libido
- Gastrointestinal: Nausea, vomiting, constipation
- Hematologic: Blood dyscrasias
- Neuromuscular & skeletal: Tremor
- Ocular: Blurred vision

<1%:

- Cardiovascular: Tachycardia, arrhythmias, pulmonary hypertension
- Central nervous system: Restlessness, depression, headache
- Dermatologic: Alopecia
- Gastrointestinal: Diarrhea, abdominal cramps
- Genitourinary: Dysuria, polyuria
- Neuromuscular & skeletal: Myalgia
- Respiratory: Dyspnea
- Miscellaneous: Diaphoresis (increased)

Overdosage/Toxicology Symptoms of overdose include agitation, drowsiness, confusion, flushing, tremor, fever, diaphoresis, abdominal pain, dilated nonreactive pupils

There is no specific antidote for amphetamine intoxication; the bulk of the treatment is supportive. Hyperactivity and agitation usually respond to reduced sensory input; however, with extreme agitation haloperidol (2-5 mg I.M. for adults) may be required. Hyperthermia is best treated with external cooling measures; when severe or unresponsive, muscle paralysis with pancuronium may be needed. Hypertension is usually transient and generally does not require treatment unless severe. For diastolic blood pressures >110 mm Hg, a nitroprusside infusion should be initiated. Seizures usually respond to diazepam IVP and/or phenytoin maintenance regimens.

Mechanism of Action Fenfluramine hydrochloride is a phenethylamine structurally related to amphetamine; central nervous system depression is more common than stimulation, which makes fenfluramine pharmacologically different from amphetamine. Fenfluramine's exact mechanism of action is not well understood; the drug's appetite suppressing action may be due to the stimulation of the hypothalamus; the anorectic effect may also be due to delayed gastric emptying.

Usual Dosage Adults: Oral: 20 mg 3 times/day before meals or food, up to 40 mg 3 times/day; maximum daily dose: 120 mg

Patient Information Take during day to avoid insomnia; do not discontinue abruptly, may cause physical and psychological dependence with prolonged use; due to its potential for serious and possibly life-threatening adverse reactions, it should only be used in patients with morbid obesity (>30% overweight or BMI >30) and only for the short-term

Nursing Implications Monitor CNS, dose should not be given in evening or at bedtime

Dosage Forms Tablet, as hydrochloride: 20 mg

Fenfluramine Hydrochloride *see* Fenfluramine *on previous page*

Fenoprofen (fen oh PROE fen)

Related Information

Dosing Data for Acetaminophen and NSAIDs *on page 1377*
Nonsteroidal Anti-Inflammatory Agents Comparison *on page 1419*

Brand Names Nalfon®

Synonyms Fenoprofen Calcium

Therapeutic Category Analgesic, Nonsteroidal Anti-inflammatory Drug; Anti-inflammatory Agent; Nonsteroidal Anti-inflammatory Agent (NSAID), Oral

Use Symptomatic treatment of acute and chronic rheumatoid arthritis and osteoarthritis; relief of mild to moderate pain

Pregnancy Risk Factor B (D if used in the 3rd trimester or near delivery)

Contraindications Known hypersensitivity to fenoprofen or other NSAIDs

Warnings/Precautions Use with caution in patients with congestive heart failure, hypertension, decreased renal or hepatic function, history of GI disease, or those receiving anticoagulants

Adverse Reactions

>10%:
- Central nervous system: Dizziness
- Dermatologic: Rash
- Gastrointestinal: Abdominal cramps, heartburn, indigestion, nausea

1% to 10%:
- Central nervous system: Headache, nervousness
- Dermatologic: Itching
- Endocrine & metabolic: Fluid retention
- Gastrointestinal: Vomiting
- Otic: Tinnitus

<1%:
- Cardiovascular: Congestive heart failure, hypertension, arrhythmias, tachycardia
- Central nervous system: Confusion, hallucinations, aseptic meningitis, mental depression, drowsiness, insomnia
- Dermatologic: Urticaria, erythema multiforme, toxic epidermal necrolysis, Stevens-Johnson syndrome, angioedema
- Endocrine & metabolic: Polydipsia, hot flashes
- Gastrointestinal: Gastritis, GI ulceration
- Genitourinary: Cystitis, polyuria
- Hematologic: Agranulocytosis, anemia, hemolytic anemia, bone marrow suppression, leukopenia, thrombocytopenia
- Hepatic: Hepatitis
- Neuromuscular & skeletal: Peripheral neuropathy
- Ocular: Toxic amblyopia, blurred vision, conjunctivitis, dry eyes
- Otic: Decreased hearing
- Renal: Acute renal failure
- Respiratory: Allergic rhinitis, shortness of breath, epistaxis

Overdosage/Toxicology Symptoms of overdose include acute renal failure, vomiting, drowsiness, leukocytosis

Management of a nonsteroidal anti-inflammatory drug (NSAID) intoxication is primarily supportive and symptomatic. Fluid therapy is commonly effective in managing the hypotension that may occur following an acute NSAID overdose, except when this is due to an acute blood loss.

Drug Interactions

Decreased effect with phenobarbital
Increased effect/toxicity of phenytoin, sulfonamides, sulfonylureas
Increased toxicity with salicylates, oral anticoagulants
(Continued)

Fenoprofen *(Continued)*

Mechanism of Action Inhibits prostaglandin synthesis by decreasing the activity of the enzyme, cyclo-oxygenase, which results in decreased formation of prostaglandin precursors

Pharmacodynamics/Kinetics

Absorption: Rapid (to 80%) from upper GI tract
Distribution: Does not cross the placenta
Protein binding: 99%
Metabolism: Extensively in the liver
Half-life: 2.5-3 hours
Time to peak serum concentration: Within 2 hours
Elimination: In urine 2% to 5% as unchanged drug; small amounts appear in feces

Usual Dosage Adults: Oral:

Rheumatoid arthritis: 300-600 mg 3-4 times/day up to 3.2 g/day
Mild to moderate pain: 200 mg every 4-6 hours as needed

Monitoring Parameters Monitor CBC, liver enzymes; monitor urine output and BUN/serum creatinine in patients receiving diuretics

Reference Range Therapeutic: 20-65 μg/mL (SI: 82-268 μmol/L)

Test Interactions ↑ chloride (S), ↑ sodium (S)

Patient Information Do not crush tablets; take with food, milk, or water; report any signs of blood in stool

Dosage Forms

Capsule, as calcium: 200 mg, 300 mg
Tablet, as calcium: 600 mg

Fenoprofen Calcium *see* Fenoprofen *on previous page*

Fentanyl (FEN ta nil)

Related Information

Adult ACLS Algorithm, Electrical Conversion *on page 1515*
Narcotic Agonists Comparison *on page 1414*

Brand Names Duragesic™; Fentanyl Oralet®; Sublimaze®

Canadian/Mexican Brand Names Durogesic® (Mexico); Fentanest® (Mexico)

Synonyms Fentanyl Citrate

Therapeutic Category Analgesic, Narcotic

Use Sedation, relief of pain, preoperative medication, adjunct to general or regional anesthesia, management of chronic pain (transdermal product)

Restrictions C-II

Pregnancy Risk Factor B (D if used for prolonged periods or in high doses at term)

Contraindications Hypersensitivity to fentanyl or any component; increased intracranial pressure; severe respiratory depression; severe liver or renal insufficiency

Transmucosal is contraindicated in unmonitored settings where a risk of unrecognized hypoventilation exists or in treating acute or chronic pain

Warnings/Precautions Fentanyl shares the toxic potentials of opiate agonists, and precautions of opiate agonist therapy should be observed; use with caution in patients with bradycardia; rapid I.V. infusion may result in skeletal muscle and chest wall rigidity → impaired ventilation → respiratory distress → apnea, bronchoconstriction, laryngospasm; inject slowly over 3-5 minutes; nondepolarizing skeletal muscle relaxant may be required.

Transmucosal fentanyl: Fentanyl Oralet® is not indicated for use in unmonitored settings where there is a risk of unrecognized hypoventilation or in treating acute or chronic pain. Patients should be monitored by direct visual observation and by some means of measuring respiratory function such as pulse oximetry until they are recovered. Facilities for the administration of fluids, opioid antagonists, oxygen and resuscitation equipment (including facilities for endotracheal intubation) should be readily available.

Topical patches: Serum fentanyl concentrations may increase approximately one-third for patients with a body temperature of 40°C secondary to a temperature-dependent increase in fentanyl release from the system and increased skin permeability. Patients who experience adverse reactions should be monitored for at least 12 hours after removal of the patch.

The elderly may be particularly susceptible to the CNS depressant and constipating effects of narcotics

Adverse Reactions

>10%:

Cardiovascular: Hypotension, bradycardia
Central nervous system: CNS depression, drowsiness, sedation
Gastrointestinal: Nausea, vomiting, constipation

Respiratory: Respiratory depression

1% to 10%:

Cardiovascular: Cardiac arrhythmias, orthostatic hypotension

Central nervous system: Confusion, CNS depression

Gastrointestinal: Biliary tract spasm

Ocular: Miosis

<1%:

Cardiovascular: Circulatory depression

Central nervous system: Convulsions, dysesthesia, paradoxical CNS excitation or delirium; cold, clammy skin; dizziness

Dermatologic: Erythema, pruritus, rash, urticaria, itching

Endocrine & metabolic: ADH release

Gastrointestinal: Biliary tract spasm

Genitourinary: Urinary tract spasm

Respiratory: Bronchospasm, laryngospasm

Miscellaneous: Physical and psychological dependence with prolonged use

Overdosage/Toxicology Symptoms of overdose include CNS depression, respiratory depression, miosis

Treatment of an overdose includes support of the patient's airway, establishment of an I.V. line, and administration of naloxone 2 mg I.V. (0.01 mg/kg for children) with repeat administration as necessary up to a total of 10 mg

Drug Interactions Increased toxicity: CNS depressants, phenothiazines, tricyclic antidepressants may potentiate fentanyl's adverse effects

Stability Protect from light; **incompatible** when mixed in the same syringe with pentobarbital

Transmucosal: Store at controlled room temperature of 15°C to 30°C (59°F to 86°F)

Mechanism of Action Binds with stereospecific receptors at many sites within the CNS, increases pain threshold, alters pain reception, inhibits ascending pain pathways

Pharmacodynamics/Kinetics Respiratory depressant effect may last longer than analgesic effect

I.M.:

Onset of analgesia: 7-15 minutes

Duration: 1-2 hours

I.V.:

Onset of analgesia: Almost immediate

Duration: 0.5-1 hour

Transmucosal:

Onset of effect: 5-15 minutes with a maximum reduction in activity/apprehension

Peak analgesia: Within 20-30 minutes

Duration: Related to blood level of the drug

Absorption: Transmucosal: Rapid, ~25% from the buccal mucosa; 75% swallowed with saliva and slowly absorbed from gastrointestinal tract

Distribution: Highly lipophilic, redistributes into muscle and fat

Metabolism: In the liver

Bioavailability: Transmucosal: ~50% (range: 36% to 71%)

Half-life: 2-4 hours

Transmucosal: 6.6 hours (range: 5-15 hours)

Elimination: In urine primarily as metabolites and 10% as unchanged drug

Usual Dosage Doses should be titrated to appropriate effects; wide range of doses, dependent upon desired degree of analgesia/anesthesia

Children 1-12 years:

Sedation for minor procedures/analgesia:

I.M., I.V.: 1-2 mcg/kg/dose; may repeat at 30- to 60-minute intervals. **Note:** Children 18-36 months of age may require 2-3 mcg/kg/dose

Transmucosal (dosage strength is based on patient weight): 5 mcg/kg if child is not fearful; fearful children and some younger children may require doses of 5-15 mcg/kg (which also carries an increased risk of hypoventilation); drug effect begins within 10 minutes, with sedation beginning shortly thereafter

Continuous sedation/analgesia: Initial I.V. bolus: 1-2 mcg/kg then 1 mcg/kg/hour; titrate upward; usual: 1-3 mcg/kg/hour

Pain control: Transdermal: Not recommended

Children >12 years and Adults:

Sedation for minor procedures/analgesia:

I.M., I.V.: 0.5-1 mcg/kg/dose; higher doses are used for major procedures

Transmucosal: 5 mcg/kg, suck on lozenge vigorously approximately 20-40 minutes before the start of procedure, drug effect begins within 10 minutes, with sedation beginning shortly thereafter; see table.

(Continued)

Fentanyl *(Continued)*

Dosage Recommendations for Transmucosal Fentanyl (Oralet®)

Patient Age/Weight	5-10 mcg/kg/dose	10-15 mcg/kg/dose
Children <2 years of age OR <15 kg	NOT RECOMMENDED	NOT RECOMMENDED
<15 kg	NOT AVAILABLE	200 mcg
20 kg	200 mcg	200-300 mcg
25 kg	200 mcg	300 mcg
30 kg	300 mcg	300-400 mcg
35 kg	300 mcg	400 mcg
> 40 kg	400 mcg	400 mcg
Adults	400 mcg	400 mcg

Preoperative sedation, adjunct to regional anesthesia, postoperative pain: I.M., I.V.: 50-100 mcg/dose

Adjunct to general anesthesia: I.M., I.V.: 2-50 mcg/kg

General anesthesia without additional anesthetic agents: I.V. 50-100 mcg/kg with O_2 and skeletal muscle relaxant

Pain control: Transdermal: Initial: 25 mcg/hour system; if currently receiving opiates, convert to fentanyl equivalent and administer equianalgesic dosage titrated to minimize the adverse effects and provide analgesia. To convert patients from oral or parenteral opioids to Duragesic™, the previous 24-hour analgesic requirement should be calculated. This analgesic requirement should be converted to the equianalgesic oral morphine dose. See tables.

Equianalgesic Doses of Opioid Agonists

Drug	Equianalgesic Dose (mg)	
	I.M.	P.O.
Codeine	130	200
Hydromorphone	1.5	7.5
Levorphanol	2	4
Meperidine	75	—
Methadone	10	20
Morphine	10	60
Oxycodone	15	30
Oxymorphone	1	10 (PR)

From *N Engl J Med*, 1985, 313:84-95.

Corresponding Doses of Oral/Intramuscular Morphine and Duragesic™

Oral 24-Hour Morphine (mg/d)	I.M. 24-Hour Morphine (mg/d)	Duragesic™ Dose (mcg/h)
45-134	8-22	25
135-224	28-37	50
225-314	38-52	75
315-404	53-67	100
405-494	68-82	125
495-584	83-97	150
585-674	98-112	175
675-764	113-127	200
765-854	128-142	225
855-944	143-157	250
945-1034	158-172	275
1035-1124	173-187	300

Product information, Duragesic™— Janssen Pharmaceutica, January, 1991.

The dosage should not be titrated more frequently than every 3 days after the initial dose or every 6 days thereafter. The majority of patients are controlled on every 72-hour administration, however, a small number of patients require every 48-hour administration.

Elderly >65 years: Transmucosal: Dose should be reduced to 2.5-5 mcg/kg; elderly have been found to be twice as sensitive as younger patients to the effects of fentanyl

Dosing adjustment in renal impairment:

Cl_{cr} 10-50 mL/minute: Administer at 75% of normal dose

Cl_{cr} <10 mL/minute: Administer at 50% of normal dose

Dietary Considerations

Alcohol: Additive CNS effects, avoid or limit alcohol; watch for sedation

Food: Glucose may cause hyperglycemia; monitor blood glucose concentrations

Administration Transmucosal product should begin 20-40 minutes prior to the anticipated start of surgery, diagnostic, or therapeutic procedure; foil overwrap should be removed just prior to administration; once removed, patient should place the unit in mouth and suck (not chew) it; unit should be removed after it is consumed or if patient has achieved an adequate sedation and anxiolytic level, and/or shows signs of respiratory depression

Monitoring Parameters Respiratory and cardiovascular status, blood pressure, heart rate

Nursing Implications

May cause rebound respiratory depression postoperatively

Patients with increased temperature may have increased fentanyl absorption transdermally, observe for adverse effects, dosage adjustment may be needed

Pharmacologic and adverse effects can be seen after discontinuation of transdermal system, observe patients for at least 12 hours after transdermal product removed; keep transdermal product (both used and unused) out of the reach of children

Do **not** use soap, alcohol, or other solvents to remove transdermal gel if it accidentally touches skin as they may increase transdermal absorption, use copious amounts of water For patients who have received transmucosal product within 6-12 hours, it is recommended that if other narcotics are required, they should be used at starting doses $^1/_4$ to $^1/_3$ those usually recommended.

Dosage Forms

Injection, as citrate: 0.05 mg/mL (2 mL, 5 mL, 10 mL, 20 mL, 50 mL)

Lozenge, oral transmucosal (raspberry flavored): 200 mcg, 300 mcg, 400 mcg

Transdermal system: 25 mcg/hour [10 cm^2]; 50 mcg/hour [20 cm^2]; 75 mcg/hour [30 cm^2]; 100 mcg/hour [40 cm^2] (all available in 5s)

Fentanyl Citrate *see* Fentanyl *on page 510*

Fentanyl Oralet® *see* Fentanyl *on page 510*

Feosol® [OTC] *see* Ferrous Sulfate *on page 516*

Feostat® [OTC] *see* Ferrous Fumarate *on this page*

Feratab® [OTC] *see* Ferrous Sulfate *on page 516*

Fergon® [OTC] *see* Ferrous Gluconate *on page 515*

Fer-In-Sol® [OTC] *see* Ferrous Sulfate *on page 516*

Fer-Iron® [OTC] *see* Ferrous Sulfate *on page 516*

Ferndex *see* Dextroamphetamine *on page 365*

Fero-Gradumet® [OTC] *see* Ferrous Sulfate *on page 516*

Ferospace® [OTC] *see* Ferrous Sulfate *on page 516*

Ferralet® [OTC] *see* Ferrous Gluconate *on page 515*

Ferralyn® Lanacaps® [OTC] *see* Ferrous Sulfate *on page 516*

Ferra-TD® [OTC] *see* Ferrous Sulfate *on page 516*

Ferro-Sequels® [OTC] *see* Ferrous Fumarate *on this page*

Ferrous Fumarate (FER us FYOO ma rate)

Brand Names Femiron® [OTC]; Feostat® [OTC]; Ferro-Sequels® [OTC]; Fumasorb® [OTC]; Fumerin® [OTC]; Hemocyte® [OTC]; Ircon® [OTC]; Nephro-Fer™ [OTC]; Span-FF® [OTC]

Canadian/Mexican Brand Names Palafer® (Canada); Ferval® Ferroso (Mexico)

Therapeutic Category Iron Salt

Use Prevention and treatment of iron deficiency anemias

Pregnancy Risk Factor A

Contraindications Hemochromatosis, hemolytic anemia, known hypersensitivity to iron salts

Warnings/Precautions Avoid in patients with peptic ulcer, enteritis, or ulcerative colitis. Administration of iron for >6 months should be avoided except in patients with continuous bleeding or menorrhagia. Anemia in the elderly is often caused by "anemia of chronic disease" or associated with inflammation rather than blood loss. Iron stores are usually normal or increased, with a serum ferritin >50 ng/mL and a decreased total iron binding capacity. Hence, the "anemia of chronic disease" is not secondary to iron deficiency but the inability of the reticuloendothelial system to roclaim available iron stores.

Adverse Reactions

>10%: Gastrointestinal: Stomach cramping, constipation, nausea, vomiting, dark stools

(Continued)

Ferrous Fumarate *(Continued)*

1% to 10%:

Gastrointestinal: Heartburn, diarrhea, staining of teeth

Genitourinary: Discoloration of urine

<1%: Ocular: Contact irritation

Overdosage/Toxicology Symptoms of overdose include acute GI irritation, erosion of GI mucosa, hepatic and renal impairment, coma, hematemesis, lethargy, acidosis, serum Fe level >300 mcg/mL requires treatment of overdose due to severe toxicity

Following treatment for fluid losses, metabolic acidosis, and shock, a severe iron overdose may be treated with deferoxamine. Deferoxamine may be administered I.V. (80 mg/kg over 24 hours) or I.M. (40-90 mg/kg every 8 hours). Usual toxic dose of elemental iron: ≥35 mg/kg.

Drug Interactions

Decreased effect: Absorption of oral preparation of iron and tetracyclines are decreased when both of these drugs are given together; concurrent administration of antacids may decrease iron absorption; iron may decrease absorption of penicillamine when given at the same time; response to iron therapy may be delayed in patients receiving chloramphenicol

Milk may decrease absorption of iron

Increased effect: Current administration ≥200 mg vitamin C per 30 mg elemental iron increases absorption of oral iron

Mechanism of Action Replaces iron found in hemoglobin, myoglobin, and enzymes; allows the transportation of oxygen via hemoglobin

Pharmacodynamics/Kinetics

Onset of hematologic response (essentially the same to either oral or parenteral iron salts): Red blood cell form and color changes within 3-10 days

Peak reticulocytosis: Within 5-10 days; hemoglobin values increase within 2-4 weeks

Absorption: Iron is absorbed in the duodenum and upper jejunum; in persons with normal iron stores 10% of an oral dose is absorbed, this is increased to 20% to 30% in persons with inadequate iron stores; food and achlorhydria will decrease absorption

Elimination: Iron is largely bound to serum transferrin and excreted in the urine, sweat, sloughing of intestinal mucosa, and by menses

Usual Dosage Oral **(dose expressed in terms of elemental iron):**

Children:

Severe iron deficiency anemia: 4-6 mg Fe/kg/day in 3 divided doses

Mild to moderate iron deficiency anemia: 3 mg Fe/kg/day in 1-2 divided doses

Prophylaxis: 1-2 mg Fe/kg/day

Adults:

Iron deficiency: 60-100 mg twice daily up to 60 mg 2 times/day

Prophylaxis: 60-100 mg/day

To avoid GI upset, start with a single daily dose and increase by 1 tablet/day each week or as tolerated until desired daily dose is achieved

Elderly: 200 mg 3-4 times/day

Reference Range

Serum iron:

Male: 75-175 μg/dL (SI: 13.4-31.3 μmol/L)

Female: 65-165 μg/dL (SI: 11.6-29.5 μmol/L)

Total iron binding capacity: 230-430 μg/dL

Transferrin: 204-360 mg/dL

Percent transferrin saturation: 20% to 50%

Iron levels >300 μg/dL can be considered toxic, should be treated as an overdose

Patient Information May color stool black, take between meals for maximum absorption; may take with food if GI upset occurs, do not take with milk or antacids; keep out of reach of children

Additional Information Elemental iron content of ferrous fumarate: 33%

Dosage Forms Amount of elemental iron is listed in brackets

Capsule, controlled release (Span-FF®): 325 mg [106 mg]

Drops (Feostat®): 45 mg/0.6 mL [15 mg/0.6 mL] (60 mL)

Suspension, oral (Feostat®): 100 mg/5 mL [33 mg/5 mL] (240 mL)

Tablet:

325 mg [106 mg]

Chewable (chocolate flavor) (Feostat®): 100 mg [33 mg]

Femiron®: 63 mg [20 mg]

Fumerin®: 195 mg [64 mg]

Fumasorb®, Ircon®: 200 mg [66 mg]

Hemocyte®: 324 mg [106 mg]

Nephro-Fer™: 350 mg [115 mg]

Timed release (Ferro-Sequels®): Ferrous fumarate 150 mg [50 mg] and docusate sodium 100 mg

Ferrous Gluconate (FER us GLOO koe nate)

Brand Names Fergon® [OTC]; Ferralet® [OTC]; Simron® [OTC]

Canadian/Mexican Brand Names Apo-Ferrous® Gluconate (Canada)

Therapeutic Category Iron Salt

Use Prevention and treatment of iron deficiency anemias

Pregnancy Risk Factor A

Contraindications Hemochromatosis, hemolytic anemia; known hypersensitivity to iron salts

Warnings/Precautions Administration of iron for >6 months should be avoided except in patients with continued bleeding, menorrhagia, or repeated pregnancies; avoid in patients with peptic ulcer, enteritis, or ulcerative colitis. Anemia in the elderly is often caused by "anemia of chronic disease" or associated with inflammation rather than blood loss. Iron stores are usually normal or increased, with a serum ferritin >50 ng/mL and a decreased total iron binding capacity. Hence, the "anemia of chronic disease" is not secondary to iron deficiency but the inability of the reticuloendothelial system to reclaim available iron stores.

Adverse Reactions

>10%: Gastrointestinal: Stomach cramping, constipation, nausea, vomiting, dark stools

1% to 10%:

- Gastrointestinal: Heartburn, diarrhea, staining of teeth
- Genitourinary: Discoloration of urine

<1%: Ocular: Contact irritation

Overdosage/Toxicology Symptoms of overdose include acute GI irritation; erosion of GI mucosa, hepatic and renal impairment, coma, hematemesis, lethargy, acidosis

Following treatment for fluid losses, metabolic acidosis, and shock, a severe iron overdose may be treated with deferoxamine. Deferoxamine may be administered I.V. (80 mg/kg over 24 hours) or I.M. (40-90 mg/kg every 8 hours). Usual toxic dose of elemental iron: ≥35 mg/kg.

Drug Interactions Absorption of oral preparation of iron and tetracyclines is decreased when both of these drugs are given together; concurrent administration of antacids may decrease iron absorption; iron may decrease absorption of penicillamine when given at the same time. Response to iron therapy may be delayed in patients receiving chloramphenicol. Concurrent administration ≥200 mg vitamin C/30 mg elemental iron increases absorption of oral iron; milk may decrease absorption of iron.

Mechanism of Action Replaces iron found in hemoglobin, myoglobin, and enzymes; allows the transportation of oxygen via hemoglobin

Pharmacodynamics/Kinetics Onset of hematologic response (essentially the same to either oral or parenteral iron salts): Red blood cells form and color changes within 3-10 days, peak reticulocytosis occurs in 5-10 days, and hemoglobin values increase within 2-4 weeks

Usual Dosage Oral **(dose expressed in terms of elemental iron):**

Children:

- Severe iron deficiency anemia: 4-6 mg Fe/kg/day in 3 divided doses
- Mild to moderate iron deficiency anemia: 3 mg Fe/kg/day in 1-2 divided doses
- Prophylaxis: 1-2 mg Fe/kg/day

Adults:

- Iron deficiency: 60 mg twice daily up to 60 mg 4 times/day
- Prophylaxis: 60 mg/day

Reference Range Therapeutic: Male: 75-175 µg/dL (SI: 13.4-31.3 µmol/L); Female: 65-165 µg/dL (SI: 11.6-29.5 µmol/L); serum iron level >300 µg/dL usually requires treatment of overdose due to severe toxicity

Test Interactions False-positive for blood in stool by the guaiac test

Patient Information May color stool black, take between meals for maximum absorption; may take with food if GI upset occurs, do not take with milk or antacids; keep out of reach of children

Additional Information Elemental iron content of gluconate: 12%

Dosage Forms Amount of elemental iron is listed in brackets

Capsule, soft gelatin (Simron®): 86 mg [10 mg]

Elixir (Fergon®): 300 mg/5 mL [34 mg/5 mL] with alcohol 7% (480 mL)

Tablet: 300 mg [34 mg]; 325 mg [38 mg]

- Fergon®, Ferralet®: 320 mg [37 mg]
- Sustained release (Ferralet® Slow Release): 320 mg [37 mg]

Ferrous Sulfate (FER us SUL fate)

Brand Names Feosol® [OTC]; Feratab® [OTC]; Fer-In-Sol® [OTC]; Fer-Iron® [OTC]; Fero-Gradumet® [OTC]; Ferospace® [OTC]; Ferralyn® Lanacaps® [OTC]; Ferra-TD® [OTC]; Mol-Iron® [OTC]; Slow FE® [OTC]

Canadian/Mexican Brand Names Apo-Ferrous® Sulfate (Canada); Ferodan® (Canada); PMS-Ferrous Sulfate (Canada); Hemobion® 200 (Mexico); Hemobion® 400 (Mexico); Orafer® (Mexico)

Synonyms $FeSO_4$

Therapeutic Category Iron Salt

Use Prevention and treatment of iron deficiency anemias

Pregnancy Risk Factor A

Contraindications Hemochromatosis, hemolytic anemia; known hypersensitivity to iron salts

Warnings/Precautions Administration of iron for >6 months should be avoided except in patients with continued bleeding, menorrhagia, or repeated pregnancies; avoid in patients with peptic ulcer, enteritis, or ulcerative colitis. Anemia in the elderly is often caused by "anemia of chronic disease" or associated with inflammation rather than blood loss. Iron stores are usually normal or increased, with a serum ferritin >50 ng/mL and a decreased total iron binding capacity. Hence, the "anemia of chronic disease" is not secondary to iron deficiency but the inability of the reticuloendothelial system to reclaim available iron stores.

Adverse Reactions

>10%: Gastrointestinal: GI irritation, epigastric pain, nausea, dark stool, vomiting, stomach cramping, constipation

1% to 10%:

- Gastrointestinal: Heartburn, diarrhea
- Genitourinary: Discoloration of urine
- Miscellaneous: Liquid preparations may temporarily stain the teeth

<1%: Ocular: Contact irritation

Overdosage/Toxicology Symptoms of overdose include acute GI irritation; erosion of GI mucosa, hepatic and renal impairment, coma, hematemesis, lethargy, acidosis

Following treatment for fluid losses, metabolic acidosis, and shock, a severe iron overdose may be treated with deferoxamine. Deferoxamine may be administered I.V. (80 mg/kg over 24 hours) or I.M. (40-90 mg/kg every 8 hours). Usual toxic dose of elemental iron: ≥35 mg/kg.

Drug Interactions

Decreased effect: Absorption of oral preparation of iron and tetracyclines are decreased when both of these drugs are given together; concurrent administration of antacids may decrease iron absorption; iron may decrease absorption of penicillamine when given at the same time; response to iron therapy may be delayed in patients receiving chloramphenicol; milk may decrease absorption of iron

Increased effect: Concurrent administration ≥200 mg vitamin C per 30 mg elemental Fe increases absorption of oral iron

Mechanism of Action Replaces iron, found in hemoglobin, myoglobin, and other enzymes; allows the transportation of oxygen via hemoglobin

Pharmacodynamics/Kinetics

Onset of hematologic response (essentially the same to either oral or parenteral iron salts): Red blood cell form and color changes within 3-10 days

Peak reticulocytosis: Occurs in 5-10 days, and hemoglobin values increase within 2-4 weeks

Absorption: Iron is absorbed in the duodenum and upper jejunum; in persons with normal serum iron stores, 10% of an oral dose is absorbed; this is increased to 20% to 30% in persons with inadequate iron stores. Food and achlorhydria will decrease absorption

Elimination: Iron is largely bound to serum transferrin and excreted in the urine, sweat, sloughing of the intestinal mucosa, and by menstrual bleeding

Usual Dosage Oral:

Children **(dose expressed in terms of elemental iron)**:

- Severe iron deficiency anemia: 4-6 mg Fe/kg/day in 3 divided doses
- Mild to moderate iron deficiency anemia: 3 mg Fe/kg/day in 1-2 divided doses
- Prophylaxis: 1-2 mg Fe/kg/day up to a maximum of 15 mg/day

Adults **(dose expressed in terms of ferrous sulfate)**:

- Iron deficiency: 300 mg twice daily up to 300 mg 4 times/day or 250 mg (extended release) 1-2 times/day
- Prophylaxis: 300 mg/day

Administration Administer ferrous sulfate 2 hours prior to, or 4 hours after antacids

Reference Range

Serum iron:

- Male: 75-175 µg/dL (SI: 13.4-31.3 µmol/L)

Female: 65-165 µg/dL (SI: 11.6-29.5 µmol/L)
Total iron binding capacity: 230-430 µg/dL
Transferrin: 204-360 mg/dL
Percent transferrin saturation: 20% to 50%

Test Interactions False-positive for blood in stool by the guaiac test

Patient Information May color stool black, take between meals for maximum absorption; may take with food if GI upset occurs, do not take with milk or antacids; keep out of reach of children

Additional Information Elemental iron content of iron salts in ferrous sulfate is 20% (ie, 300 mg ferrous sulfate is equivalent to 60 mg ferrous iron)

Dosage Forms Amount of elemental iron is listed in brackets

Capsule:
- Exsiccated (Fer-In-Sol®): 190 mg [60 mg]
- Exsiccated, timed release (Feosol®): 159 mg [50 mg]
- Exsiccated, timed release (Ferralyn® Lanacaps®, Ferra-TD®): 250 mg [50 mg]
- Ferospace®: 250 mg [50 mg]

Drops, oral:
- Fer-In-Sol®: 75 mg/0.6 mL [15 mg/0.6 mL] (50 mL)
- Fer-Iron®: 125 mg/mL [25 mg/mL] (50 mL)

Elixir (Feosol®): 220 mg/5 mL [44 mg/5 mL] with alcohol 5% (473 mL, 4000 mL)
Syrup (Fer-In-Sol®): 90 mg/5 mL [18 mg/5 mL] with alcohol 5% (480 mL)
Tablet: 324 mg [65 mg]
- Exsiccated (Feosol®) 200 mg [65 mg]
- Exsiccated, timed release (Slow FE®): 160 mg [50 mg]
- Feratab®: 300 mg [60 mg]
- Mol-Iron®: 195 mg [39 mg]

Timed release (Fero-Gradumet®): 525 mg [105 mg]

Fertinex® Injection *see* Urofollitropin *on page 1281*

$FeSO_4$ *see* Ferrous Sulfate *on previous page*

Feverall™ [OTC] *see* Acetaminophen *on page 19*

Fexofenadine (feks oh FEN a deen)

Brand Names Allegra®

Synonyms Fexofenadine Hydrochloride

Use Nonsedating antihistamine indicated for the relief of seasonal allergic rhinitis

Pregnancy Risk Factor C

Contraindications Individuals demonstrating hypersensitivity to fexofenadine or any components of its formulation

Warnings/Precautions Safety and effectiveness in pediatric patients <12 years of age has not been established. Fexofenadine is classified in FDA pregnancy category C and no data is yet available evaluating its use in breast-feeding women.

Adverse Reactions

1% to 10%:
- Central nervous system: Drowsiness (1.3%), fatigue (1.3%)
- Endocrine & metabolic: Dysmenorrhea (1.5%)
- Gastrointestinal: Nausea (1.5%), dyspepsia (1.3%)
- Miscellaneous: Viral infection (2.5%)

Drug Interactions Fexofenadine levels have increased with erythromycin (82% higher) and with ketoconazole (135% higher); this has not been associated with any increased incidence of side effects

In two separate studies, fexofenadine 120 mg twice daily (high doses) was coadministered with standard doses of erythromycin or ketoconazole to healthy volunteers and although fexofenadine peak plasma concentrations increased, no differences in adverse events or QTc intervals were observed. **It remains unknown if a similar interaction occurs with other azole antifungal agents (eg, itraconazole) or other macrolide antibiotics (eg, clarithromycin).**

Stability Capsules should be stored at controlled room temperature 20°C to 25°C and protected from excessive moisture

Mechanism of Action Fexofenadine is an active metabolite of terfenadine and like terfenadine it competes with histamine for H_1-receptor sites on effector cells in the gastrointestinal tract, blood vessels and respiratory tract; it appears that fexofenadine does not cross the blood brain barrier to any appreciable degree, resulting in a reduced potential for sedation

Pharmacodynamics/Kinetics

Onset of action: 60 minutes
Duration of antihistaminic effect: At least 12 hours
Metabolism: ~5% metabolized mostly by gut flora; only 0.5% to 1.5% metabolized by cytochrome P-450 enzymes
Half-life: 14.4 hours
Time to peak serum concentration: ~2.6 hours after oral administration
Elimination: Primarily in feces (~80%) and in urine (~11%) as unchanged drug

(Continued)

Fexofenadine *(Continued)*

Usual Dosage Oral:

Children <12 years: Not recommended

Children ≥12 years and Adults: 1 capsule (60 mg) twice daily

Dosing adjustment in renal impairment: Recommended initial doses of 60 mg once daily

Monitoring Parameters Relief of symptoms

Patient Information Although relatively uncommon (1.3%), fexofenadine may cause drowsiness; contact your physician or pharmacist if you experience drowsiness, upset stomach, increased pain or cramping during menstruation while taking this medication

Dosage Forms Capsule, as hydrochloride: 60 mg

Fiberall® Chewable Tablet [OTC] *see* Calcium Polycarbophil *on page 195*

Fiberall® Powder [OTC] *see* Psyllium *on page 1075*

Fiberall® Wafer [OTC] *see* Psyllium *on page 1075*

FiberCon® Tablet [OTC] *see* Calcium Polycarbophil *on page 195*

Fiber-Lax® Tablet [OTC] *see* Calcium Polycarbophil *on page 195*

Filgrastim (fil GRA stim)

Related Information

Cancer Chemotherapy Regimens *on page 1351*

Sargramostim *on page 1125*

Toxicities of Chemotherapeutic Agents *on page 1382*

Brand Names Neupogen®

Synonyms G-CSF; Granulocyte Colony Stimulating Factor

Therapeutic Category Colony Stimulating Factor

Use FDA approved: Patients with nonmyeloid malignancies receiving myelosuppressive anticancer drugs associated with a significant incidence of neutropenia; cancer patients receiving bone marrow transplant (BMT); patients with severe chronic neutropenia (SCN)

Chronic administration in symptomatic patients with congenital neutropenia, cyclic neutropenia, or idiopathic neutropenia; filgrastim should not be started until the diagnosis of SCN is confirmed, as it may interfere with diagnostic efforts

Patients undergoing Peripheral Blood Progenitor Cell (PBPC) collection

Safety and efficacy of G-CSF given simultaneously with cytotoxic chemotherapy have not been established; concurrent treatment may increase myelosuppression; G-CSF should be avoided in patients receiving concomitant chemotherapy and radiation therapy

Pregnancy Risk Factor C

Contraindications Patients with known hypersensitivity to *E. coli*-derived proteins or G-CSF

Warnings/Precautions Complete blood count and platelet count should be obtained prior to chemotherapy. Do not use G-CSF in the period 24 hours before to 24 hours after administration of cytotoxic chemotherapy because of the potential sensitivity of rapidly dividing myeloid cells to cytotoxic chemotherapy. Precaution should be exercised in the usage of G-CSF in any malignancy with myeloid characteristics. G-CSF can potentially act as a growth factor for any tumor type, particularly myeloid malignancies. Tumors of nonhematopoietic origin may have surface receptors for G-CSF.

Allergic-type reactions have occurred in patients receiving G-CSF with first, or later, doses. Reactions tended to occur more frequently with intravenous administration and within 30 minutes of infusion. Most cases resolved rapidly with antihistamines, steroids, bronchodilators, and/or epinephrine. Symptoms recurred in >50% of patients on rechallenge.

Adverse Reactions Effects are generally mild and dose related

>10%:

Central nervous system: Neutropenic fever, fever

Dermatologic: Alopecia

Gastrointestinal: Nausea, vomiting, diarrhea, mucositis,

Splenomegaly: This occurs more commonly in patients with cyclic neutropenia/congenital agranulocytosis who received S.C. injections for a prolonged (>14 days) period of time; ~33% of these patients experience subclinical splenomegaly (detected by MRI or CT scan); ~3% of these patients experience clinical splenomegaly

Neuromuscular & skeletal: Medullary bone pain (24% incidence): This occurs most commonly in lower back pain, posterior iliac crest, and sternum and is controlled with non-narcotic analgesics

1% to 10%:

Cardiovascular: Chest pain, fluid retention

Central nervous system: Headache

Dermatologic: Skin rash
Gastrointestinal: Anorexia, stomatitis, constipation
Hematologic: Leukocytosis
Local: Pain at injection site
Neuromuscular & skeletal: Weakness
Respiratory: Dyspnea, cough, sore throat

<1%:

Cardiovascular: Transient supraventricular arrhythmia, pericarditis
Local: Thrombophlebitis
Miscellaneous: Anaphylactic reaction

Overdosage/Toxicology No clinical adverse effects seen with high dose producing ANC >10,000/mm^3. Leukocytosis which was not associated with any clinical adverse effects. After discontinuing the drug there is a 50% decrease in circulating levels of neutrophils within 1-2 days, return to pretreatment levels within 1-7 days.

Stability

Filgrastim is a clear, colorless solution and should be stored under refrigeration at 2°C to 8°C (36°F to 46°F) and protected from direct sunlight. Filgrastim should be protected from freezing and temperatures >30°C to avoid aggregation.

The solution should not be shaken since bubbles and/or foam may form. If foaming occurs, the solution should be left undisturbed for a few minutes until bubbles dissipate.

Filgrastim is stable for 24 hours at 9°C to 30°C, however, the manufacturer recommends discarding after 6 hours because of microbiological concerns. The product is packaged as single-use vial without a preservative.

Undiluted filgrastim is stable for 24 hours at 15°C to 30°C and 7 days at 2°C to 8°C in tuberculin syringes. However, refrigeration and use within 24 hours are recommended because of concern for bacterial contamination.

Filgrastim may be diluted in dextrose 5% in water to a concentration of ≥15 mcg/mL for I.V. infusion administration

Minimum concentration is 15 mcg/mL

Concentrations <15 mcg/mL require addition of albumin (1 mL of 5%) to the bag to prevent absorption to plastics/PVC

This diluted solution is stable for 7 days under refrigeration or at room temperature

Standard diluent: ≥375 mcg/25 mL D_5W; filgrastim is **incompatible** with 0.9% sodium chloride (normal saline)

Mechanism of Action Stimulates the production, maturation, and activation of neutrophils, G-CSF activates neutrophils to increase both their migration and cytotoxicity

Pharmacodynamics/Kinetics

Onset of action: Rapid elevation in neutrophil counts within the first 24 hours, reaching a plateau in 3-5 days

Duration: ANC decreases by 50% within 2 days after discontinuing G-CSF; white counts return to the normal range in 4-7 days

Absorption: S.C.: 100% absorbed; peak plasma levels can be maintained for up to 12 hours

Distribution: V_d: 150 mL/kg; no evidence of drug accumulation over a 11- to 20-day period

Metabolism: Systemically metabolized

Bioavailability: Oral: Not bioavailable

Half-life: 1.8-3.5 hours

Time to peak serum concentration: S.C.: Within 2-6 hours

Usual Dosage Children and Adults:

Dosage should be based on actual body weight (even in morbidly obese patients)

Existing clinical data suggest that starting G-CSF between 24 and 72 hours subsequent to chemotherapy may provide optimal neutrophil recover; continue therapy until the occurrence of an absolute neutrophil count of 10,000/ µL after the neutrophil nadir

The available data suggest that rounding the dose to the nearest vial size may enhance patient convenience and reduce costs without clinical detriment

Myelosuppressive chemotherapy S.C. or I.V. infusion: 5 mcg/kg/day

Doses may be increased in increments of 5 mcg/kg for each chemotherapy cycle, according to the duration and severity of the absolute neutrophil count (ANC) nadir

Bone marrow transplant patients

Bone marrow transplant patients: 5-10 mcg/kg/day as an I.V. infusion of 4 or 24 hours or as continuous 24-hour S.C. infusion; administer first dose at least 24

(Continued)

Filgrastim *(Continued)*

hours after cytotoxic chemotherapy and at least 24 hours after bone marrow infusion

Filgrastim Dose Based on Neutrophil Response

Absolute Neutrophil Count	Filgrastim Dose Adjustment
When ANC >1000/mm³ for 3 consecutive days	Reduce to 5 mcg/kg/day
If ANC remains >1000/mm³ for 3 more consecutive days	Discontinue filgrastim
If ANC decreases to <1000/mm³	Resume at 5 mcg/kg/day

Peripheral Blood Progenitor Cell (PBPC) Collection: 10 mcg/kg/day either S.C. or a bolus or continuous I.V. infusion. It is recommended that G-CSF be given for at least 4 days before the first leukapheresis procedure and continued until the last leukapheresis; although the optimal duration of administration and leukapheresis schedule have not been established, administration of G-CSF for 6-7 days with leukaphereses on days 5,6 and 7 was found to be safe and effective; neutrophil counts should be monitored after 4 days of G-CSF, and G-CSF dose-modification should be considered for those patients who develop a white blood cell count >100,000/mm³

Severe chronic neutropenia: S.C.:
- Congenital neutropenia: 6 mcg/kg/dose twice daily
- Idiopathic/cyclic neutropenia: 5 mcg/kg/day

Chronic daily administration is required to maintain clinical benefit; adjust dose based on the patients' clinical course as well as ANC; in phase III studies, the target ANC was 1500-10,000/mm³. Reduce the dose of the ANC is persistently >10,000/mm³

Premature discontinuation of G-CSF therapy prior to the time of recovery from the expected neutrophil is generally not recommended; a transient increase in neutrophil counts is typically seen 1-2 days after initiation of therapy

Hemodialysis: Supplemental dose is not necessary
Peritoneal dialysis: Supplemental dose is not necessary

Administration May be administered undiluted by S.C. or by I.V. infusion over 15-60 minutes in D_5W; **incompatible** with sodium chloride solutions

Monitoring Parameters Complete blood cell count and platelet count should be obtained twice weekly after chemotherapy or three times weekly after transplant. Leukocytosis (white blood cell counts of ≥100,000/mm³) has been observed in ~2% of patients receiving G-CSF at doses above 5 mcg/kg/day. Monitor platelets and hematocrit regularly. Monitor patients with pre-existing cardiac conditions closely as cardiac events (myocardial infarctions, arrhythmias) have been reported in premarketing clinical studies.

Reference Range No clinical benefit seen with ANC >10,000/mm³

Patient Information Possible bone pain

Nursing Implications Do not mix with sodium chloride solutions

Additional Information
Reimbursement Hotline: 1-800-272-9376
Professional Services [AMGEN]: 1-800-77-AMGEN

Dosage Forms Injection, preservative free: 300 mcg/mL (1 mL, 1.6 mL)

Filibon® [OTC] *see* Vitamins, Multiple *on page 1310*

Finasteride (fi NAS teer ide)

Brand Names Proscar®

Therapeutic Category Antiandrogen; Antineoplastic Agent, Miscellaneous

Use Early data indicate that finasteride is useful in the treatment of symptomatic benign prostatic hyperplasia (BPH)

Unlabeled use: Adjuvant monotherapy after radical prostatectomy in the treatment of prostatic cancer

Pregnancy Risk Factor X

Contraindications History of hypersensitivity to drug, pregnancy, lactation, children

Warnings/Precautions A minimum of 6 months of treatment may be necessary to determine whether an individual will respond to finasteride. Use with caution in those patients with liver function abnormalities. Carefully monitor patients with a large residual urinary volume or severely diminished urinary flow for obstructive uropathy. These patients may not be candidates for finasteride therapy.

Adverse Reactions

1% to 10%:
Endocrine & metabolic: Decreased libido

Genitourinary: <4% incidence of impotence, decreased volume of ejaculate

Mechanism of Action Finasteride is a 4-azo analog of testosterone and is a competitive inhibitor of both tissue and hepatic 5-alpha reductase. This results in inhibition of the conversion of testosterone to dihydrotestosterone and markedly suppresses serum dihydrotestosterone levels; depending on dose and duration, serum testosterone concentrations may or may not increase. Testosterone-dependent processes such as fertility, muscle strength, potency, and libido are not affected by finasteride.

Pharmacodynamics/Kinetics

Onset of clinical effect: Within 12 weeks to 6 months of ongoing therapy

Duration of action:

After a single oral dose as small as 0.5 mg: 65% depression of plasma dihydrotestosterone levels persists 5-7 days

After 6 months of treatment with 5 mg/day: Circulating dihydrotestosterone levels are reduced to castrate levels without significant effects on circulating testosterone; levels return to normal within 14 days of discontinuation of treatment

Absorption: Oral: Extent may be reduced if administered with food

Bioavailability: Mean: 63%

Time to peak serum concentration: Oral: 2-6 hours

Metabolism: Unchanged finasteride is major circulating component; two active metabolites have been identified

Half-life, serum: Parent drug: ~5-17 hours (mean: 1.9 fasting, 4.2 with breakfast)

Half-life:

Elderly: 8 hours

Adults: 6 hours (3-16)

Protein binding: 90%

Elimination: As metabolites in urine and feces; elimination rate is decreased in the elderly, but no dosage adjustment is needed

Usual Dosage Adults: Male: Benign prostatic hyperplasia: Oral: 5 mg/day as a single dose; clinical responses occur within 12 weeks to 6 months of initiation of therapy; long-term administration is recommended for maximal response

Dosing adjustment in renal impairment: No dosage adjustment is necessary

Dietary Considerations Food: Administration with food may delay the rate and reduce the extent of oral absorption

Monitoring Parameters Objective and subjective signs of relief of benign prostatic hyperplasia, including improvement in urinary flow, reduction in symptoms of urgency, and relief of difficulty in micturition

Dosage Forms Tablet, film coated: 5 mg

Fiorgen PF® *see* Butalbital Compound *on page 176*

Fioricet® *see* Butalbital Compound *on page 176*

Fiorinal® *see* Butalbital Compound *on page 176*

Fisalamine *see* Mesalamine *on page 787*

FK506 *see* Tacrolimus *on page 1186*

Flagyl® *see* Metronidazole *on page 829*

Flarex® *see* Fluorometholone *on page 537*

Flatulex® [OTC] *see* Simethicone *on page 1136*

Flavorcee® [OTC] *see* Ascorbic Acid *on page 102*

Flavoxate (fla VOKS ate)

Brand Names Urispas®

Synonyms Flavoxate Hydrochloride

Therapeutic Category Antispasmodic Agent, Urinary

Use Antispasmodic to provide symptomatic relief of dysuria, nocturia, suprapubic pain, urgency, and incontinence due to detrusor instability and hyper-reflexia in elderly with cystitis, urethritis, urethrocystitis, urethrotrigonitis, and prostatitis

Pregnancy Risk Factor B

Contraindications Pyloric or duodenal obstruction, GI hemorrhage, GI obstruction; ileus; achalasia; obstructive uropathies of lower urinary tract (BPH)

Warnings/Precautions May cause drowsiness, vertigo, and ocular disturbances; administer cautiously in patients with suspected glaucoma

Adverse Reactions

>10%:

Central nervous system: Drowsiness

Gastrointestinal: Xerostomia, dry throat

1% to 10%:

Cardiovascular: Tachycardia, palpitations,

Central nervous system: Nervousness, fatigue, vertigo, headache, hyperpyrexia

Gastrointestinal: Constipation, nausea, vomiting

(Continued)

Flavoxate *(Continued)*

<1%:

Central nervous system: Confusion (especially in the elderly)
Dermatologic: Rash
Hematologic: Leukopenia
Ocular: Increased intraocular pressure

Overdosage/Toxicology Symptoms of overdose include clumsiness, dizziness, drowsiness, flushing, hallucinations, irritability; supportive care only

Mechanism of Action Synthetic antispasmotic with similar actions to that of propantheline; it exerts a direct relaxant effect on smooth muscles via phosphodiesterase inhibition, providing relief to a variety of smooth muscle spasms; it is especially useful for the treatment of bladder spasticity, whereby it produces an increase in urinary capacity

Pharmacodynamics/Kinetics

Onset of action: 55-60 minutes
Metabolism: To methyl; flavone carboxylic acid active
Elimination: 10% to 30% of dose excreted in urine within 6 hours

Usual Dosage Children >12 years and Adults: Oral: 100-200 mg 3-4 times/day; reduce the dose when symptoms improve

Monitoring Parameters Monitor I & O closely

Patient Information May cause drowsiness, dizziness, or visual disturbances; use with caution if performing tasks requiring coordination or mental alertness; avoid other substances that may cause similar effects (eg, alcohol); may cause dry mouth

Dosage Forms Tablet, film coated, as hydrochloride: 100 mg

Flavoxate Hydrochloride *see* Flavoxate *on previous page*

Flecainide (fle KAY nide)

Related Information

Antacid Drug Interactions *on page 1388*
Antiarrhythmic Drugs *on page 1389*
Comparative Pharmacokinetic Properties of Antiarrhythmic Agents *on page 1391*

Brand Names Tambocor™

Synonyms Flecainide Acetate

Therapeutic Category Antiarrhythmic Agent, Class I-C

Use Prevention and suppression of documented life-threatening ventricular arrhythmias (ie, sustained ventricular tachycardia); controlling symptomatic, disabling supraventricular tachycardias in patients without structural heart disease in whom other agents fail

Pregnancy Risk Factor C

Contraindications Pre-existing second or third degree A-V block; right bundle-branch block associated with left hemiblock (bifascicular block) or trifascicular block; cardiogenic shock, myocardial depression; known hypersensitivity to the drug

Warnings/Precautions Pre-existing sinus node dysfunction, sick-sinus syndrome, history of congestive heart failure or myocardial dysfunction; increases in P-R interval ≥300 MS, QRS ≥180 MS, Q-T_c interval increases, and/or new bundle-branch block; patients with pacemakers, renal impairment, and/or hepatic impairment.

The manufacturer and FDA recommend that this drug be reserved for life-threatening ventricular arrhythmias unresponsive to conventional therapy. Its use for symptomatic nonsustained ventricular tachycardia, frequent premature ventricular complexes (PVCs), uniform and multiform PVCs and/or coupled PVCs is no longer recommended. Flecainide can worsen or cause arrhythmias with an associated risk of death. Proarrhythmic effects range from an increased number of PVCs to more severe ventricular tachycardias (eg, tachycardias that are more sustained or more resistant to conversion to sinus rhythm).

Adverse Reactions

>10%:

Central nervous system: Dizziness
Ocular: Visual disturbances
Respiratory: Dyspnea

1% to 10%:

Cardiovascular: Palpitations, chest pain, edema, tachycardia
Central nervous system: Headache, fatigue, fever
Dermatologic: Rash
Gastrointestinal: Nausea, constipation, abdominal pain
Neuromuscular & skeletal: Tremor, weakness

<1%:

Cardiovascular: Bradycardia, heart block, increased P-R, QRS duration, worsening ventricular arrhythmias, congestive heart failure

Central nervous system: Nervousness, hypoesthesia

Dermatologic: Alopecia

Hematologic: Blood dyscrasias

Hepatic: Possible hepatic dysfunction

Neuromuscular & skeletal: Paresthesia

Overdosage/Toxicology Has a narrow therapeutic index and severe toxicity may occur slightly above the therapeutic range, especially if combined with other antiarrhythmic drugs. (Acute single ingestion of twice the daily therapeutic dose is life-threatening.) Symptoms of overdose include increases in P-R, QRS, Q-T intervals and amplitude of the T wave, A-V block, bradycardia, hypotension, ventricular arrhythmias (monomorphic or polymorphic ventricular tachycardia), and asystole; other symptoms include dizziness, blurred vision, headache, and GI upset.

Treatment is supportive, using conventional treatment (fluids, positioning, anticonvulsants, antiarrhythmics). **Note:** Type Ia antiarrhythmic agents should not be used to treat cardiotoxicity caused by type Ic drugs; sodium bicarbonate may reverse QRS prolongation, bradycardia and hypotension; ventricular pacing may be needed; hemodialysis only of possible benefit for tocainide or flecainide overdose in patients with renal failure.

Drug Interactions Cytochrome P-450 2D6 enzyme substrate

Increased toxicity:

Digoxin, amiodarone (increased plasma concentrations)

Beta-adrenergic blockers, disopyramide, verapamil (possible additive negative inotropic effects)

Alkalinizing agents (high dose antacids, cimetidine, carbonic anhydrase inhibitors or sodium bicarbonate) may decrease flecainide clearance

Decreased toxicity: Smoking and acid urine (increases flecainide clearance)

Mechanism of Action Class Ic antiarrhythmic; slows conduction in cardiac tissue by altering transport of ions across cell membranes; causes slight prolongation of refractory periods; decreases the rate of rise of the action potential without affecting its duration; increases electrical stimulation threshold of ventricle, HIS-Purkinje system; possesses local anesthetic and moderate negative inotropic effects

Pharmacodynamics/Kinetics

Absorption: Oral: Rapid

Distribution: Adults: V_d: 5-13.4 L/kg

Protein binding: 40% to 50% ($alpha_1$ glycoprotein)

Bioavailability: 85% to 90%

Metabolism: In the liver

Half-life:

Infants: 11-12 hours

Children: 8 hours

Adults: 7-22 hours, increased with congestive heart failure or renal dysfunction

End stage renal disease: 19-26 hours

Time to peak serum concentration: Within 1.5-3 hours

Elimination: 80% to 90% excreted in urine as unchanged drug and metabolites (10% to 50%)

Usual Dosage Oral:

Children:

Initial: 3 mg/kg/day or 50-100 mg/m^2/day in 3 divided doses

Usual: 3-6 mg/kg/day or 100-150 mg/m^2/day in 3 divided doses; up to 11 mg/kg/day or 200 mg/m^2/day for uncontrolled patients with subtherapeutic levels

Adults:

Life-threatening ventricular arrhythmias:

Initial: 100 mg every 12 hours

Increase by 50-100 mg/day (given in 2 doses/day) every 4 days; maximum: 400 mg/day

For patients receiving 400 mg/day who are not controlled and have trough concentrations <0.6 μg/mL, dosage may be increased to 600 mg/day

Prevention of paroxysmal supraventricular arrhythmias in patients with disabling symptoms but no structural heart disease:

Initial: 50 mg every 12 hours

Increase by 50 mg twice daily at 4-day intervals; maximum: 300 mg/day

Dosing adjustment in severe renal impairment: Cl_{cr} <10 mL/minute: Decrease usual dose by 25% to 50%

Dialysis: Not dialyzable (0% to 5%) via hemo- or peritoneal dialysis; no supplemental dose necessary

Dosing adjustment/comments in hepatic impairment: Monitoring of plasma levels is recommended because of significantly increased half-life

(Continued)

Flecainide *(Continued)*

When transferring from another antiarrhythmic agent, allow for 2-4 half-lives of the agent to pass before initiating flecainide therapy

Administration Administer around-the-clock to promote less variation in peak and trough serum levels

Monitoring Parameters EKG, blood pressure, pulse, periodic serum concentrations, especially in patients with renal or hepatic impairment

Reference Range Therapeutic: 0.2-1 µg/mL; pediatric patients may respond at the lower end of the recommended therapeutic range

Patient Information Notify physician if chest pain, faintness, or palpitations occurs; take only as prescribed

Dosage Forms Tablet, as acetate: 50 mg, 100 mg, 150 mg

Extemporaneous Preparations A 5 mg/mL suspension compounded from tablets and an oral flavored commercially available diluent (Roxane®) was stable for up to 45 days when stored at 5°C or 25°C in amber glass bottles

Wiest DB, Garner SS, and Pagacz LR, "Stability of Flecainide Acetate in an Extemporaneously Compounded Oral Suspension," *Am J Hosp Pharm*, 1992, 49(6):1467-70.

Flecainide Acetate *see* Flecainide *on page 522*

Fleet® Babylax® [OTC] *see* Glycerin *on page 580*

Fleet® Enema [OTC] *see* Sodium Phosphates *on page 1146*

Fleet® Flavored Castor Oil [OTC] *see* Castor Oil *on page 216*

Fleet® Laxative [OTC] *see* Bisacodyl *on page 153*

Fleet® Mineral Oil Enema [OTC] *see* Mineral Oil *on page 841*

Fleet® Pain Relief [OTC] *see* Pramoxine *on page 1033*

Fleet® Phospho®-Soda [OTC] *see* Sodium Phosphates *on page 1146*

Flexaphen® *see* Chlorzoxazone *on page 266*

Flexeril® *see* Cyclobenzaprine *on page 322*

Flolan® Injection *see* Epoprostenol *on page 454*

Flonase™ *see* Fluticasone *on page 549*

Florinef® Acetate *see* Fludrocortisone Acetate *on page 529*

Florone® *see* Diflorasone *on page 382*

Florone E® *see* Diflorasone *on page 382*

Floropryl® *see* Isoflurophate *on page 679*

Florvite® *see* Vitamins, Multiple *on page 1310*

Flovent™ *see* Fluticasone *on page 549*

Floxin® *see* Ofloxacin *on page 922*

Flubenisolone *see* Betamethasone *on page 147*

Fluconazole (floo KOE na zole)

Related Information

Antifungal Agents *on page 1395*

Guidelines for the Prevention of Opportunistic Infections in Persons with HIV *on page 1457*

Treatment of Sexually Transmitted Diseases *on page 1485*

Brand Names Diflucan®

Canadian/Mexican Brand Names Oxifungol® (Mexico); Zonal® (Mexico)

Therapeutic Category Antifungal Agent, Systemic

Use Oral fluconazole should be used in persons able to tolerate oral medications; parenteral fluconazole should be reserved for patients who are both unable to take oral medications and are unable to tolerate amphotericin B (eg, due to hypersensitivity or renal insufficiency)

Indications for use in adult patients:

Oral or vaginal candidiasis unresponsive to nystatin or clotrimazole

Nonlife-threatening *Candida* infections (eg, cystitis, esophagitis)

Treatment of hepatosplenic candidiasis

Treatment of other *Candida* infections in persons unable to tolerate amphotericin B

Treatment of cryptococcal infections

Secondary prophylaxis for cryptococcal meningitis in persons with AIDS

Antifungal prophylaxis in allogeneic bone marrow transplant recipients

Pregnancy Risk Factor C

Contraindications Known hypersensitivity to fluconazole or other azoles

Warnings/Precautions Should be used with caution in patients with renal and hepatic dysfunction or previous hepatotoxicity from other azole derivatives. Patients who develop abnormal liver function tests during fluconazole therapy should be monitored closely and discontinued if symptoms consistent with liver disease develop.

Adverse Reactions

1% to 10%:

Central nervous system: Headache

Dermatologic: Rash

Gastrointestinal: Nausea, vomiting, abdominal pain, diarrhea

<1%:

Cardiovascular: Pallor

Central nervous system: Dizziness

Endocrine & metabolic: Hypokalemia

Hepatic: Elevated AST, ALT, or alkaline phosphatase

Overdosage/Toxicology Symptoms of overdose include decreased lacrimation, salivation, respiration and motility, urinary incontinence, cyanosis

Treatment includes supportive measures, a 3-hour hemodialysis will remove 50%

Drug Interactions Cytochrome P-450 IIIA4 enzyme inhibitor and cytochrome P-450 IIC enzyme inhibitor

Decreased effect: Rifampin decreases concentrations of fluconazole; fluconazole may decrease the effect of oral contraceptives

Increased toxicity:

May increase cyclosporine levels when high doses used

May increase phenytoin serum concentration

Fluconazole may also inhibit warfarin metabolism

Stability Parenteral admixture at room temperature (25°C): Manufacturer expiration dating; do not refrigerate

Standard diluent: 200 mg/100 mL NS (premixed); 400 mg/200 mL NS (premixed)

Incompatible with ampicillin, calcium gluconate, ceftazidime, cefotaxime, cefuroxime, ceftriaxone, clindamycin, furosemide, imipenem, ticarcillin, and piperacillin

Mechanism of Action Interferes with cytochrome P-450 activity, decreasing ergosterol synthesis (principal sterol in fungal cell membrane) and inhibiting cell membrane formation

Pharmacodynamics/Kinetics

Distribution: Relative diffusion of antimicrobial agents from blood into CSF: Adequate with or without inflammation (exceeds usual MICs)

Ratio of CSF to blood level (%):

Normal meninges: 70-80

Inflamed meninges: >70-80

Protein binding, plasma: 11% to 12%

Bioavailability: Oral: >90%

Half-life: 25-30 hours with normal renal function

Time to peak serum concentration: Oral: Within 2-4 hours

Elimination: 80% of a dose excreted unchanged in the urine

Usual Dosage The daily dose of fluconazole is the same for oral and I.V. administration

Efficacy of fluconazole has not been established in children; a small number of patients from 3-13 years of age have been treated with fluconazole using doses of 3-6 mg/kg/day once daily. Doses as high as 12 mg/kg/day once daily have been used to treat candidiasis in immunocompromised children; 10-12 mg/kg/day has been used prophylactically against fungal infections in pediatric bone marrow transplant patients.

Adults: Oral, I.V.: See table for once daily dosing.

Indication	Day 1	Daily Therapy	Minimum Duration of Therapy
Oropharyngeal candidiasis	200 mg	100 mg	14 d
Esophageal candidiasis	200 mg	100 mg	21 d
Systemic candidiasis	400 mg	200 mg	28 d
Cryptococcal meningitis			10-12 wk after CSF culture becomes negative
acute	400 mg	200 mg	
relapse	200 mg	200 mg	

Dosing adjustment/interval in renal impairment:

Cl_{cr} 21-50 mL/minute: Administer 50% of recommended dose or administer every 48 hours

Cl_{cr} <20 mL/minute: Administer 25% of recommended dose or administer every 72 hours

Hemodialysis: 50% removed by hemodialysis

Administration Parenteral fluconazole must be administered by I.V. infusion over approximately 1-2 hours; do not exceed 200 mg/hour when giving I.V. infusion; maximum rate of infusion: 200 mg/hour

(Continued)

Fluconazole *(Continued)*

Monitoring Parameters Periodic liver function tests (AST, ALT, alkaline phosphatase) and renal function tests, potassium

Patient Information May take with food; complete full course of therapy; contact physician or pharmacist if side effects develop; consider using an alternative method of contraception if taking concurrently with birth control pills

Nursing Implications Do not use if cloudy or precipitated

Dosage Forms

Injection: 2 mg/mL (100 mL, 200 mL)
Powder for oral suspension: 10 mg/mL (35 mL); 40 mg/mL (35 mL)
Tablet: 50 mg, 100 mg, 150 mg, 200 mg

Flucytosine (floo SYE toe seen)

Related Information

Antifungal Agents *on page 1395*

Brand Names Ancobon®

Canadian/Mexican Brand Names Ancotil® (Canada)

Synonyms 5-FC; 5-Flurocytosine

Therapeutic Category Antifungal Agent, Systemic

Use Adjunctive treatment of susceptible fungal infections (usually *Candida* or *Cryptococcus*); in combination with amphotericin B, fluconazole, or itraconazole; synergy with amphotericin B for fungal infections (*Aspergillus*)

Pregnancy Risk Factor C

Contraindications Hypersensitivity to flucytosine or any component

Warnings/Precautions Use with extreme caution in patients with renal impairment or bone marrow suppression; dosage modification required in patients with impaired renal function

Adverse Reactions

1% to 10%:
- Dermatologic: Rash
- Gastrointestinal: Abdominal pain, diarrhea, loss of appetite, nausea, vomiting
- Hematologic: Anemia, leukopenia, thrombocytopenia
- Hepatic: Hepatitis, jaundice

<1%:
- Cardiovascular: Cardiac arrest
- Central nervous system: Confusion, hallucinations, dizziness, drowsiness, headache, parkinsonism, psychosis, ataxia
- Dermatologic: Photosensitivity
- Endocrine & metabolic: Temporary growth failure, hypoglycemia, hypokalemia
- Hematologic: Bone marrow suppression
- Hepatic: Elevated liver enzymes
- Neuromuscular & skeletal: Paresthesia
- Otic: Hearing loss
- Respiratory: Respiratory arrest

Overdosage/Toxicology Symptoms of overdose include nausea, vomiting, diarrhea, bone marrow suppression; treatment is supportive

Drug Interactions Increased effect/toxicity (enterocolitis) with concurrent amphotericin administration

Stability Protect from light

Mechanism of Action Penetrates fungal cells and is converted to fluorouracil which competes with uracil interfering with fungal RNA and protein synthesis

Pharmacodynamics/Kinetics

Absorption: Oral: 75% to 90%
Distribution: Into CSF and bronchial secretions
Metabolism: Minimal
Protein binding: 2% to 4%
Half-life: 3-8 hours
- Anuria: May be as long as 200 hours
- End stage renal disease: 75-200 hours

Time to peak serum concentration: Within 2-6 hours
Elimination: 75% to 90% excreted unchanged in the urine by glomerular filtration

Usual Dosage Children and Adults: Oral: 50-150 mg/kg/day in divided doses every 6 hours

Dosing interval in renal impairment:
- Cl_{cr} 10-<50 mL/minute: Administer every 12 hours
- Cl_{cr} <10 mL/minute: Administer every 24 hours

Hemodialysis: Dialyzable (50% to 100%); administer dose post hemodialysis
Peritoneal dialysis: Administer 0.5-1 g every 24 hours (adults) and during continuous arterio-venous or veno-venous hemofiltration

Administration Administer around-the-clock rather than 4 times/day to promote less variation in peak and trough serum levels

Monitoring Parameters Serum creatinine, BUN, alkaline phosphatase, AST, ALT, CBC; serum flucytosine concentrations

Reference Range

Therapeutic: 25-100 μg/mL (SI: 195-775 μmol/L); levels should not exceed 100-120 μg/mL to avoid toxic bone marrow depressive effects

Trough: Draw just prior to dose administration

Peak: Draw 2 hours after an oral dose administration

Test Interactions Flucytosine causes markedly false elevations in serum creatinine values when the Ektachem® analyzer is used

Patient Information Take capsules a few at a time with food over a 15-minute period to avoid nausea

Dosage Forms Capsule: 250 mg, 500 mg

Extemporaneous Preparations Flucytosine oral liquid has been prepared by using the contents of ten 500 mg capsules triturated in a mortar and pestle with a small amount of distilled water; the mixture was transferred to a 500 mL volumetric flask; the mortar was rinsed several times with a small amount of distilled water and the fluid added to the flask; sufficient distilled water was added to make a total volume of 500 mL of a 10 mg/mL liquid; oral liquid was stable for 70 days when stored in glass or plastic prescription bottles at 4°C or for up to 14 days at room temperature.

Wintermeyer SM and Nahata MC, "Stability of Flucytosine in an Extemporaneously Compounded Oral Liquid," *Am J Health-Syst Pharm*, 1996, 53:407-9.

Fludara® *see* Fludarabine *on this page*

Fludarabine (floo DARE a been)

Related Information

Antiemetics for Chemotherapy Induced Nausea and Vomiting *on page 1348*
Cancer Chemotherapy Regimens *on page 1351*
Toxicities of Chemotherapeutic Agents *on page 1382*

Brand Names Fludara®

Synonyms Fludarabine Phosphate

Therapeutic Category Antineoplastic Agent, Antimetabolite (Purine)

Use Treatment of chronic lymphocytic leukemia (B-cell) in patients who have not responded to other alkylating agent regimen

Pregnancy Risk Factor D

Contraindications Hypersensitivity of fludarabine; patients with severe infections

Warnings/Precautions The U.S. Food and Drug Administration (FDA) currently recommends that procedures for proper handling and disposal of antineoplastic agents be considered. Use with caution with renal insufficiency, patients with a fever, documented infection, or pre-existing hematological disorders (particularly granulocytopenia) or in patients with pre-existing central nervous system disorder (epilepsy), spasticity, or peripheral neuropathy. Use with caution in patients with pre-existing renal insufficiency. Life-threatening and sometimes fatal autoimmune hemolytic anemia have occurred.

Adverse Reactions

>10%:

- Cardiovascular: Edema
- Central nervous system: Fever, chills, fatigue, pain
- Dermatologic: Rash
- Gastrointestinal: Mild nausea, vomiting, diarrhea, stomatitis, GI bleeding
- Genitourinary: Urinary infection
- Hematologic: Myelosuppression: Dose-limiting toxicity; myelosuppression may not be related to cumulative dose
  - Granulocyte nadir: 13 days (3-25)
  - Platelet nadir: 16 days (2-32)
  - WBC nadir: 8 days
  - Recovery: 5-7 weeks
- Neuromuscular & skeletal: Paresthesia, myalgia, weakness
- Respiratory: Manifested as dyspnea and a nonproductive cough; lung biopsy has shown pneumonitis in some patients, pneumonia
- Miscellaneous: Infection

1% to 10%:

- Cardiovascular: Congestive heart failure
- Central nervous system: Malaise, headache
- Dermatologic: Alopecia
- Endocrine & metabolic: Hyperglycemia
- Gastrointestinal: Anorexia
- Otic: Hearing loss

(Continued)

Fludarabine *(Continued)*

<1%:

Central nervous system: Reported with higher dose levels; most patients shown to have CNS demyelination; somnolence, blindness, coma, and death also occurred; severe neurotoxicity

Dermatologic: Skin rash

Endocrine & metabolic: Metabolic acidosis

Gastrointestinal: Metallic taste

Hematologic: Life-threatening and sometimes fatal autoimmune hemolytic anemia; often recurs on rechallenge; steroid treatment may or may not be beneficial

Hepatic: Reversible hepatotoxicity

Renal: Renal failure, hematuria, increased serum creatinine

Respiratory: Interstitial pneumonitis

Miscellaneous: Tumor lysis syndrome

Overdosage/Toxicology There are clear dose-dependent toxic neurologic effects associated with fludarabine. Doses of 96 mg/m²/day for 5-7 days are associated with a syndrome characterized by delayed blindness, coma, and death. Symptoms appeared from 21-60 days following the last dose. The central nervous system toxicity has distinctive features of delayed onset and progressive encephalopathy resulting in fatal outcomes. It is reported at an incidence rate of 36% at high doses (≥96 mg/m²/day for 5-7 days) and <0.2% for low doses (≤125 mg/m²/course).

Drug Interactions Increased toxicity: Cytarabine when administered with or prior to a fludarabine dose competes for deoxycytidine kinase decreasing the metabolism of F-ara-A to the active F-ara-ATP (inhibits the antineoplastic effect of fludarabine); however, administering fludarabine prior to cytarabine may stimulate activation of cytarabine

Stability

Store intact vials under refrigeration (2°C to 8°C)

Reconstitute vials with 2 mL SWI to result in a concentration of 25 mg/mL; solution is stable for 16 days at room temperature (22°C to 25°C) and under refrigeration (2°C to 8°C)

Further dilution in 100 mL D_5W or NS is stable for 48 hours at room temperature or refrigeration

Standard I.V. dilution:

Dose/100 mL D_5W or NS

Stable for 48 hours at 4°C to 25°C

Mechanism of Action Fludarabine is analogous to that of Ara-C and Ara-A. Following systemic administration, FAMP is rapidly dephosphorylated to 2-fluoro-Ara-A. 2-Fluoro-Ara-A enters the cell by a carrier-mediated transport process, then is phosphorylated intracellularly by deoxycytidine kinase to form the active metabolite 2-fluoro-Ara-ATP. 2-Fluoro-Ara-ATP inhibits DNA synthesis by inhibition of DNA polymerase and ribonucleotide reductase.

Pharmacodynamics/Kinetics

Absorption: Oral preparation is under study

Bioavailability: 75%

Distribution: V_d: 38-96 L/m²; widely distributed with extensive tissue binding

Metabolism: I.V.: Fludarabine phosphate is rapidly dephosphorylated to 2-fluoro-vidarabine, which subsequently enters tumor cells and is phosphorylated to the active triphosphate derivative; rapidly dephosphorylated in the serum

Half-life, elimination: 2-fluoro-vidarabine: 9 hours

Elimination: 23% of a dose of fludarabine is recovered in urine as 2-fluoro-vidarabine

Usual Dosage I.V.:

Children:

Acute leukemia: 10 mg/m² bolus over 15 minutes followed by continuous infusion of 30.5 mg/m²/day over 5 days **or**

10.5 mg/m² bolus over 15 minutes followed by 30.5 mg/m²/day over 48 hours followed by cytarabine has been used in clinical trials

Solid tumors: 9 mg/m² bolus followed by 27 mg/m²/day continuous infusion over 5 days

Adults:

Chronic lymphocytic leukemia: 25 mg/m²/day over a 30-minute period for 5 days; 5-day courses are repeated every 28 days days

Non-Hodgkin's lymphoma: Loading dose: 20 mg/m² followed by 30 mg/m²/day for 48 hours

Dosing in renal impairment: Cl_{cr} <50 mL/minute: Monitor closely for toxicity; dose reduction is indicated in patients with renal failure. However, no specific guidelines are available

Administration Administer I.V. over 15-30 minutes or continuous infusion

Monitoring Parameters CBC with differential, platelet count, AST, ALT, creatinine, serum albumin, uric acid

Reference Range Peak plasma levels: 0.3-0.9 μg/mL following a short infusion of 25 mg/m^2

Dosage Forms Powder for injection, as phosphate, lyophilized: 50 mg (6 mL)

Fludarabine Phosphate *see* Fludarabine *on page 527*

Fludeoxyglucose F 18 (floo dee OKS i GLOO kose eff AY teen)

Brand Names ^{18}FDG

Therapeutic Category Radiopharmaceutical

Use Identification of regions of abnormal glucose metabolism associated with foci of epileptic seizures, stroke, myocardial infarction, malignant tumors, and (brain, liver, thyroid) through the use of positron emission tomography; also used in cerebral imaging

Mechanism of Action Portion of the fludeoxyglucose molecule is labeled with F-18, a positron-emitting radionucleide which provides the signal for tumor identification in Positron Emission Tomography (PET) scanners

Pharmacodynamics/Kinetics Half-life: 110 minutes

Administration For I.V. use only

Additional Information Activity >37 x 10^3 MBg (1 ci)/mmol

Dosage Forms Injection:

Fludrocortisone Acetate (floo droe KOR ti sone AS e tate)

Brand Names Florinef® Acetate

Synonyms Fluohydrisone Acetate; Fluohydrocortisone Acetate; 9α-Fluorohydrocortisone Acetate

Therapeutic Category Mineralocorticoid

Use Partial replacement therapy for primary and secondary adrenocortical insufficiency in Addison's disease; treatment of salt-losing adrenogenital syndrome

Pregnancy Risk Factor C

Contraindications Known hypersensitivity to fludrocortisone; systemic fungal infections

Warnings/Precautions Taper dose gradually when therapy is discontinued; use with caution with Addison's disease, sodium retention and potassium loss

Adverse Reactions

1% to 10%:

- Cardiovascular: Hypertension, edema, congestive heart failure
- Central nervous system: Convulsions, headache, dizziness
- Dermatologic: Acne, rash, bruising
- Endocrine & metabolic: Hypokalemic alkalosis, suppression of growth, hyperglycemia, HPA suppression
- Gastrointestinal: Peptic ulcer
- Neuromuscular & skeletal: Muscle weakness
- Ocular: Cataracts
- Miscellaneous: Diaphoresis

Overdosage/Toxicology Symptoms of overdose include hypertension, edema, hypokalemia, excessive weight gain. When consumed in excessive quantities, systemic hypercorticism and adrenal suppression may occur; in those cases, discontinuation and withdrawal of the corticosteroid should be done judiciously.

Drug Interactions **Decreased effect:**

Anticholinesterases effects are antagonized

Decreased corticosteroid effects by rifampin, barbiturates, and hydantoins

Decreased salicylate levels

Mechanism of Action Promotes increased reabsorption of sodium and loss of potassium from renal distal tubules

Pharmacodynamics/Kinetics

Absorption: Rapid and complete from GI tract, partially absorbed through skin

Protein binding: 42%

Metabolism: In the liver

Half-life:

- Plasma: 30-35 minutes
- Biological: 18-36 hours

Time to peak serum concentration: Within 1.7 hours

Usual Dosage Oral:

Infants and Children: 0.05-0.1 mg/day

Adults: 0.1-0.2 mg/day with ranges of 0.1 mg 3 times/week to 0.2 mg/day

Administration Administration in conjunction with a glucocorticoid is preferable

Monitoring Parameters Monitor blood pressure and signs of edema when patient is on chronic therapy; very potent mineralocorticoid with high glucocorticoid activity; monitor serum electrolytes, serum renin activity, and blood pressure; monitor for evidence of infection

(Continued)

Fludrocortisone Acetate *(Continued)*

Patient Information Notify physician if dizziness, severe or continuing headaches, swelling of feet or lower legs or unusual weight gain occur

Dosage Forms Tablet: 0.1 mg

Flu-Imune® *see* Influenza Virus Vaccine *on page 658*

Flumadine® *see* Rimantadine *on page 1110*

Flumazenil (FLO may ze nil)

Related Information

Toxicology Information *on page 1553*

Replaces Mazicon™

Brand Names Romazicon™

Canadian/Mexican Brand Names Anexate® (Canada); Lanexat® (Mexico)

Therapeutic Category Antidote, Benzodiazepine

Use Benzodiazepine antagonist - reverses sedative effects of benzodiazepines used in general anesthesia; for management of benzodiazepine overdose; flumazenil does **not** antagonize the CNS effects of other GABA agonists (such as ethanol, barbiturates, or general anesthetics), **does not** reverse narcotics

Pregnancy Risk Factor C

Contraindications Known hypersensitivity to flumazenil or benzodiazepines; patients given benzodiazepines for control of potentially life-threatening conditions (eg, control of intracranial pressure or status epilepticus); patients who are showing signs of serious cyclic-antidepressant overdosage

Warnings/Precautions

Risk of seizures = high-risk patients:

- Patients on benzodiazepines for long-term sedation
- Tricyclic antidepressant overdose patients
- Concurrent major sedative-hypnotic drug withdrawal
- Recent therapy with repeated doses of parenteral benzodiazepines
- Myoclonic jerking or seizure activity prior to flumazenil administration

Hypoventilation: Does not reverse respiratory depression/hypoventilation or cardiac depression

Resedation: Occurs more frequently in patients where a large single dose or cumulative dose of a benzodiazepine is administered along with a neuromuscular blocking agent and multiple anesthetic agents

Flumazenil should be used with caution in the intensive care unit because of increased risk of unrecognized benzodiazepine dependence in such settings.

Adverse Reactions

>10%:

- Central nervous system: Dizziness
- Gastrointestinal: Vomiting, nausea

1% to 10%:

- Central nervous system: Headache, malaise, anxiety, nervousness, insomnia, abnormal crying, euphoria, depression
- Endocrine & metabolic: Hot flashes
- Gastrointestinal: Xerostomia
- Local: Pain at injection site
- Neuromuscular & skeletal: Tremor, weakness
- Ocular: Abnormal vision
- Respiratory: Dyspnea, hyperventilation
- Miscellaneous: Diaphoresis (increased disorders)

<1%:

- Cardiovascular: Bradycardia, tachycardia, chest pain, hypertension, ventricular extrasystoles, altered blood pressure (increases and decreases)
- Central nervous system: Anxiety and sensation of coldness, generalized convulsions, somnolence
- Gastrointestinal: Thick tongue
- Otic: Abnormal hearing
- Miscellaneous: Hiccups, withdrawal syndrome, shivering

Drug Interactions

Increased toxicity:

- Use with caution in overdosage involving mixed drug overdose
- Toxic effects may emerge (especially with cyclic antidepressants) with the reversal of the benzodiazepine effect by flumazenil

Stability For I.V. use only; **compatible** with D_5W, lactated Ringer's, or normal saline; once drawn up in the syringe or mixed with solution use within 24 hours; discard any unused solution after 24 hours

Mechanism of Action Antagonizes the effect of benzodiazepines on the GABA/benzodiazepine receptor complex. Flumazenil is benzodiazepine specific and does not antagonize other nonbenzodiazepine GABA agonists (including ethanol, barbiturates, general anesthetics); flumazenil does not reverse the effects of opiates

Pharmacodynamics/Kinetics

Onset of action: 1-3 minutes; 80% response within 3 minutes

Peak effect: 6-10 minutes

Duration: Resedation occurs usually within 1 hour; duration is related to dose given and benzodiazepine plasma concentrations; reversal effects of flumazenil may wear off before effects of benzodiazepine

Distribution: 0.63-1.06 L/kg

Initial V_d: 0.5 L/kg

V_{dss} 0.77-1.6 L/kg

Protein binding: 40% to 50%

Half-life, adults:

Alpha: 7-15 minutes

Terminal: 41-79 minutes

Elimination: Clearance dependent upon hepatic blood flow; hepatically eliminated, 0.2% unchanged in urine

Usual Dosage See table.

Flumazenil

Pediatric Dosage Further studies are needed Pediatric dosage for **reversal of conscious sedation:** Intravenously through a freely running intravenous infusion into a large vein to minimize pain at the injection site	
Initial dose	0.01 mg/kg over 15 seconds (maximum dose of 0.2 mg)
Repeat doses	0.005-0.01 mg/kg (maximum dose of 0.2 mg) repeated at 1-minute intervals
Maximum total cumulative dose	1 mg
Pediatric dosage for **management of benzodiazepine overdose:** Intravenously through a freely running intravenous infusion into a large vein to minimize pain at the injection site	
Initial dose	0.01 mg/kg (maximum dose: 0.2 mg)
Repeat doses	0.01 mg/kg (maximum dose of 0.2 mg) repeated at 1-minute intervals
Maximum total cumulative dose	1 mg
In place of repeat bolus doses, follow-up continuous infusions of 0.005-0.01 mg/kg/h have been used; further studies are needed.	
Adult Dosage Adult dosage for **reversal of conscious sedation:** Intravenously through a freely running intravenous infusion into a large vein to minimize pain at the injection site	
Initial dose	0.2 mg intravenously over 15 seconds
Repeat doses	If desired level of consciousness is not obtained, 0.2 mg may be repeated at 1-minute intervals.
Maximum total cumulative dose	1 mg (usual dose 0.6-1 mg) **In the event of resedation:** Repeat doses may be given at 20-minute intervals with maximum of 1 mg/dose and 3 mg/h.
Adult dosage for **suspected benzodiazepine overdose:** Intravenously through a freely running intravenous infusion into a large vein to minimize pain at the injection site	
Initial dose	0.2 mg intravenously over 30 seconds
Repeat doses	0.5 mg over 30 seconds repeated at 1-minute intervals
Maximum total cumulative dose	3 mg (usual dose 1-3 mg) Patients with a partial response at 3 mg may require additional titration up to a total dose of 5 mg. If a patient has not responded 5 minutes after cumulative dose of 5 mg, the major cause of sedation is not likely due to benzodiazepines. **In the event of resedation:** May repeat doses at 20-minute intervals with maximum of 1 mg/dose and 3 mg/h.

Resedation: Repeated doses may be given at 20-minute intervals as needed; repeat treatment doses of 1 mg (at a rate of 0.5 mg/minute) should be given at any time and no more than 3 mg should be given in any hour. After intoxication with high doses of benzodiazepines, the duration of a single dose of flumazenil is not expected to exceed 1 hour; if desired, the period of wakefulness may be prolonged with repeated low intravenous doses of flumazenil, or by an infusion

(Continued)

Flumazenil *(Continued)*

of 0.1-0.4 mg/hour. Most patients with benzodiazepine overdose will respond to a cumulative dose of 1-3 mg and doses >3 mg do not reliably produce additional effects. Rarely, patients with a partial response at 3 mg may require additional titration up to a total dose of 5 mg. **If a patient has not responded 5 minutes after receiving a cumulative dose of 5 mg, the major cause of sedation is not likely to be due to benzodiazepines.**

Dosing in renal impairment: Not significantly affected by renal failure (Cl_{cr} <10 mL/minute) or hemodialysis beginning 1 hour after drug administration

Dosing in hepatic impairment: Initial dose of flumazenil used for initial reversal of benzodiazepine effects is not changed; however, subsequent doses in liver disease patients should be reduced in size or frequency

Monitoring Parameters Monitor patients for return of sedation or respiratory depression

Patient Information Flumazenil does not consistently reverse amnesia; do not engage in activities requiring alertness for 18-24 hours after discharge; resedation may occur in patients on long-acting benzodiazepines (such as diazepam)

Dosage Forms Injection: 0.1 mg/mL (5 mL, 10 mL)

Flunisolide (floo NIS oh lide)

Related Information

Asthma, Guidelines for the Diagnosis and Management of *on page 1518*

Estimated Clinical Comparability of Doses for Inhaled Corticosteroids *on page 1522*

Brand Names AeroBid®-M Oral Aerosol Inhaler; AeroBid® Oral Aerosol Inhaler; Nasalide® Nasal Aerosol; Nasarel® Nasal Spray

Canadian/Mexican Brand Names Bronalide® (Canada); Rhinalar® (Canada); Rhinaris-F® (Canada); Syn-Flunisolide® (Canada)

Therapeutic Category Anti-inflammatory Agent, Inhalant; Corticosteroid, Inhalant; Corticosteroid, Intranasal

Use Steroid-dependent asthma; nasal solution is used for seasonal or perennial rhinitis

Pregnancy Risk Factor C

Pregnancy/Breast-Feeding Implications

Clinical effects on the fetus: No data on crossing the placenta or effects on the fetus

Breast-feeding/lactation: No data on crossing into breast milk or effects on the infant

Contraindications Known hypersensitivity to flunisolide, acute status asthmaticus; viral, tuberculosis, fungal or bacterial respiratory infections, or infections of nasal mucosa

Warnings/Precautions Use with caution in patients with hypothyroidism, cirrhosis, hypertension, congestive heart failure, ulcerative colitis, thromboembolic disorders; do not stop medication abruptly if on prolonged therapy; fatalities have occurred due to adrenal insufficiency in asthmatic patients during and after transfer from systemic corticosteroids to aerosol steroids; several months may be required for recovery of this syndrome; during this period, aerosol steroids do **not** provide the systemic steroid needed to treat patients having trauma, surgery or infections. When consumed in excessive quantities, systemic hypercorticism and adrenal suppression may occur; withdrawal and discontinuation of the corticosteroid should be done carefully.

Adverse Reactions

>10%:

- Cardiovascular: Pounding heartbeat
- Central nervous system: Dizziness, headache, nervousness
- Dermatologic: Itching, rash
- Endocrine & metabolic: Adrenal suppression, menstrual problems
- Gastrointestinal: GI irritation, anorexia, sore throat, bitter taste
- Local: Nasal burning, *Candida* infections of the nose or pharynx, atrophic rhinitis
- Respiratory: Sneezing, coughing, upper respiratory tract infection, bronchitis, nasal congestion, nasal dryness
- Miscellaneous: Increased susceptibility to infections

1% to 10%:

- Central nervous system: Insomnia, psychic changes
- Dermatologic: Acne, urticaria
- Gastrointestinal: Increase in appetite, xerostomia, dry throat, loss of taste perception
- Ocular: Cataracts
- Respiratory: Epistaxis
- Miscellaneous: Diaphoresis, loss of smell

<1%:

Gastrointestinal: Abdominal fullness

Respiratory: Bronchospasm, shortness of breath

Overdosage/Toxicology When consumed in excessive quantities, systemic hypercorticism and adrenal suppression may occur; in those cases; discontinuation and withdrawal of the corticosteroid should be done judiciously

Drug Interactions Expected interactions similar to other corticosteroids

Mechanism of Action Decreases inflammation by suppression of migration of polymorphonuclear leukocytes and reversal of increased capillary permeability; does not depress hypothalamus

Pharmacodynamics/Kinetics

Absorption: Nasal inhalation: ~50%

Metabolism: Rapidly in the liver to active metabolites

Half-life: 1.8 hours

Elimination: Equally in urine and feces

Usual Dosage

Children >6 years:

Oral inhalation: 2 inhalations twice daily (morning and evening) up to 4 inhalations/day

Nasal: 1 spray each nostril twice daily (morning and evening), not to exceed 4 sprays/day each nostril

Adults:

Oral inhalation: 2 inhalations twice daily (morning and evening) up to 8 inhalations/day maximum

Nasal: 2 sprays each nostril twice daily (morning and evening); maximum dose: 8 sprays/day in each nostril

Patient Information Inhaler should be shaken well immediately prior to use; while activating inhaler, deep breathe for 3-5 seconds, hold breath for ~10 seconds and allow ≥1 minute between inhalations

Nursing Implications Shake well before giving; do not use Nasalide® orally; throw out product after it has been opened for 3 months

Additional Information Does not contain fluorocarbons; contains polyethylene glycol vehicle

Dosage Forms

Inhalant:

Nasal (Nasalide®): 25 mcg/actuation [200 sprays] (25 mL)

Oral:

AeroBid®: 250 mcg/actuation [100 metered doses] (7 g)

AeroBid-M® (menthol flavor): 250 mcg/actuation [100 metered doses] (7 g)

Solution, spray: 0.025% [200 actuations] (25 mL)

Fluocinolone (floo oh SIN oh lone)

Related Information

Corticosteroids Comparison *on page 1407*

Brand Names Derma-Smoothe/FS®; Fluonid®; Flurosyn®; FS Shampoo®; Synalar®; Synalar-HP®; Synemol®

Canadian/Mexican Brand Names Lidemol® (Canada); Cremisona® (Mexico); Synalar® Simple (Mexico)

Synonyms Fluocinolone Acetonide

Therapeutic Category Corticosteroid, Shampoo; Corticosteroid, Topical (Low Potency); Corticosteroid, Topical (Medium Potency); Corticosteroid, Topical (High Potency)

Use Relief of susceptible inflammatory dermatosis [low, medium, high potency topical corticosteroid]

Pregnancy Risk Factor C

Contraindications Fungal infection, hypersensitivity to fluocinolone or any component, TB of skin, herpes (including varicella)

Warnings/Precautions Adverse systemic effects may occur when used on large areas of the body, denuded areas, for prolonged periods of time, with an occlusive dressing, and/or in infants or small children. Infants and small children may be more susceptible to adrenal axis suppression from topical corticosteroid therapy.

Adverse Reactions

<1%:

Dermatologic: Acne, hypopigmentation, allergic dermatitis, maceration of the skin, skin atrophy, folliculitis, hypertrichosis, dry skin, itching

Endocrine & metabolic: HPA suppression, Cushing's syndrome, growth retardation

Local: Burning, irritation

Miscellaneous: Secondary infection

(Continued)

Fluocinolone *(Continued)*

Overdosage/Toxicology When consumed in excessive quantities, systemic hypercorticism and adrenal suppression may occur; in those cases, discontinuation and withdrawal of the corticosteroid should be done judiciously

Mechanism of Action A synthetic corticosteroid which differs structurally from triamcinolone acetonide in the presence of an additional fluorine atom in the 6-alpha position on the steroid nucleus. The mechanism of action for all topical corticosteroids is not well defined, however, is believed to be a combination of three important properties: anti-inflammatory activity, immunosuppressive properties, and antiproliferative actions.

Pharmacodynamics/Kinetics

Absorption: Dependent on strength of preparation, amount applied,and nature of skin at application site; ranges from ~1% in thick stratum corneum areas (palms, soles, elbows, etc) to 36% in areas of thinnest stratum corneum (face, eyelids, etc); increased absorption in areas of skin damage, inflammation, or occlusion

Distribution: Throughout the local skin; absorbed drug is distributed rapidly into muscle, liver, skin, intestines, and kidneys

Metabolism: Primarily in the skin; small amount absorbed into systemic circulation is metabolized primarily in the liver to inactive compounds

Elimination: By the kidneys primarily as glucuronides and sulfate, but also as unconjugated products; small amounts of metabolites are excreted in feces

Usual Dosage Children and Adults: Topical: Apply a thin layer to affected area 2-4 times/day

Patient Information A thin film of cream or ointment is effective; do not overuse; do not use tight-fitting diapers or plastic pants on children being treated in the diaper area; use only as prescribed, and for no longer than the period prescribed; apply sparingly in light film; rub in lightly; avoid contact with eyes; notify physician if condition being treated persists or worsens

Dosage Forms

Cream, as acetonide: 0.01% (15 g, 60 g); 0.025% (15 g, 60 g)
- Flurosyn®, Synalar®: 0.01% (15 g, 30 g, 60 g, 425 g)
- Flurosyn®, Synalar®, Synemol®: 0.025% (15 g, 60 g, 425 g)
- Synalar-HP®: 0.2% (12 g)

Ointment, topical, as acetonide: 0.025% (15 g, 60 g)
- Flurosyn®, Synalar®: 0.025% (15 g, 30 g, 60 g, 425 g)

Oil, as acetonide (Derma-Smoothe/FS®): 0.01% (120 mL)

Shampoo, as acetonide (FS Shampoo®): 0.01% (180 mL)

Solution, topical, as acetonide: 0.01% (20 mL, 60 mL)
- Fluonid®, Synalar®: 0.01% (20 mL, 60 mL)

Fluocinolone Acetonide *see* Fluocinolone *on previous page*

Fluocinonide (floo oh SIN oh nide)

Related Information

Corticosteroids Comparison *on page 1407*

Brand Names Fluonex®; Lidex®; Lidex-E®

Canadian/Mexican Brand Names Lyderm® (Canada); Topactin® (Canada); Topsyn® (Canada); Gelisyn® (Mexico)

Therapeutic Category Corticosteroid, Topical (High Potency)

Use Anti-inflammatory, antipruritic, relief of inflammatory and pruritic manifestations [high potency topical corticosteroid]

Pregnancy Risk Factor C

Contraindications Viral, fungal, or tubercular skin lesions, herpes simplex, known hypersensitivity to fluocinonide

Warnings/Precautions Adverse systemic effects may occur when used on large areas of the body, denuded areas, for prolonged periods of time, with an occlusive dressing, and/or in infants or small children

Adverse Reactions <1%:

Central nervous system: Intracranial hypertension

Dermatologic: Acne, hypopigmentation, allergic dermatitis, maceration of the skin, skin atrophy, dry skin, itching, folliculitis, hypertrichosis

Endocrine & metabolic: HPA suppression, Cushing's syndrome, growth retardation

Local: Burning, irritation

Miscellaneous: Secondary infection

Mechanism of Action Fluorinated topical corticosteroid considered to be of high potency. The mechanism of action for all topical corticosteroids is not well defined, however, is felt to be a combination of three important properties: anti-inflammatory activity, immunosuppressive properties, and antiproliferative actions.

Pharmacodynamics/Kinetics

Absorption: Dependent on amount applied and nature of skin at application site; ranges from ~1% in areas of thick stratum corneum (palms, soles, elbows, etc) to 36% in areas of thin stratum corneum (face, eyelids, etc); absorption is increased in areas of skin damage, inflammation, or occlusion

Distribution: Distributed throughout local skin; any absorbed drug is removed rapidly from the blood and distributed into muscle, liver, skin, intestines, and kidneys

Metabolism: Primarily in the skin; small amount absorbed into systemic circulation is metabolized primarily in the liver to inactive compounds

Elimination: By the kidneys primarily as glucuronides and sulfates, but also as unconjugated products; small amounts of metabolites are excreted in feces

Usual Dosage Children and Adults: Topical: Apply thin layer to affected area 2-4 times/day depending on the severity of the condition

Patient Information Do not use tight-fitting diapers or plastic pants on children being treated in the diaper area; use only as prescribed, and for no longer than the period prescribed; apply sparingly in a light film; rub in lightly; notify physician if condition being treated persists or worsens; avoid contact with eyes

Dosage Forms

Cream: 0.05% (15 g, 30 g, 60 g, 120 g)
- Anhydrous, emollient (Lidex®): 0.05% (15 g, 30 g, 60 g, 120 g)
- Aqueous, emollient (Lidex-E®): 0.05% (15 g, 30 g, 60 g, 120 g)

Gel, topical: 0.05% (15 g, 60 g)
- Lidex®: 0.05% (15 g, 30 g, 60 g, 120 g)

Ointment, topical: 0.05% (15 g, 30 g, 60 g)
- Lidex®: 0.05% (15 g, 30 g, 60 g, 120 g)

Solution, topical: 0.05% (20 mL, 60 mL)
- Lidex®: 0.05% (20 mL, 60 mL)

Fluogen® *see* Influenza Virus Vaccine *on page 658*

Fluohydrisone Acetate *see* Fludrocortisone Acetate *on page 529*

Fluohydrocortisone Acetate *see* Fludrocortisone Acetate *on page 529*

Fluonex® *see* Fluocinonide *on previous page*

Fluonid® *see* Fluocinolone *on page 533*

Fluoracaine® Ophthalmic *see* Proparacaine and Fluorescein *on page 1062*

Fluorescein Sodium (FLURE e seen SOW dee um)

Brand Names AK-Fluor; Fluorescite®; Fluorets®; Fluor-I-Strip®; Fluor-I-Strip-AT®; Fluress®; Ful-Glo®; Funduscein®; Ophthifluor®

Synonyms Soluble Fluorescein

Therapeutic Category Diagnostic Agent, Ophthalmic Dye

Use Demonstrates defects of corneal epithelium; diagnostic aid in ophthalmic angiography

Pregnancy Risk Factor C (topical); X (parenteral)

Contraindications Hypersensitivity to fluorescein or any other component of the product; do not use with soft contact lenses, as this will cause them to discolor

Warnings/Precautions Use with caution in patients with history of hypersensitivity, allergies, or asthma; avoid extravasation; should not be used in patients with soft contact lenses, will cause them to discolor

Adverse Reactions

1% to 10%:
- Dermatologic: Burning sensation
- Local: Temporary stinging

<1%:
- Cardiovascular: Syncope, hypotension, cardiac arrest, basilar artery ischemia, severe shock
- Central nervous system: Headache
- Gastrointestinal: Nausea, GI distress, vomiting
- Local: Thrombophlebitis

Mechanism of Action Yellow, water soluble, dibasic acid xanthine dye which penetrates any break in epithelial barrier to permit rapid penetration

Usual Dosage

Ophthalmic:
- Solution: Instill 1-2 drops of 2% solution and allow a few seconds for staining; wash out excess with sterile water or irrigating solution
- Strips: Moisten strip with sterile water. Place moistened strip at the fornix into the lower cul-de-sac close to the punctum. For best results, patient should close lid tightly over strip until desired amount of staining is obtained. Patient should blink several times after application.
- Removal of foreign bodies, sutures or tonometry (Fluress®): Instill 1 or 2 drops (single instillations) into each eye before operating
- Deep ophthalmic anesthesia (Fluress®): Instill 2 drops into each eye very 90 seconds up to 3 doses

(Continued)

Fluorescein Sodium *(Continued)*

Injection: Prior to use, perform intradermal skin test; have epinephrine 1:1000, an antihistamine, and oxygen available
Children: 3.5 mg/lb (7.5 mg/kg) injected rapidly into antecubital vein
Adults: 500-750 mg injected rapidly into antecubital vein

Patient Information Do not replace soft contact lenses for at least 1 hour, flush eye before replacing; skin discoloration may last 6-12 hours, urine 24-36 hours if given systemically

Nursing Implications Avoid extravasation, results in severe local tissue damage; have epinephrine 1:1000, an antihistamine, and oxygen available

Dosage Forms
Injection (AK-Fluor, Fluorescite®, Funduscein®, Ophthifluor®): 10% [100 mg/mL] (5 mL); 25% [250 mg/mL] (2 mL, 3 mL)
Ophthalmic:
Solution: 2% [20 mg/mL] (1 mL, 2 mL, 15 mL)
Fluress®: 0.25% [2.5 mg/mL] with benoxinate 0.4% (5 mL)
Strip:
Ful-Glo®: 0.6 mg
Fluorets®, Fluor-I-Strip-AT®: 1 mg
Fluor-I-Strip®: 9 mg

Fluorescite® *see* Fluorescein Sodium *on previous page*

Fluorets® *see* Fluorescein Sodium *on previous page*

Fluoride (FLOR ide)

Brand Names ACT® [OTC]; Fluorigard® [OTC]; Fluorinse®; Fluoritab®; Flura®; Flura-Drops®; Flura-Loz®; Gel Kam®; Gel-Tin® [OTC]; Karidium®; Karigel®; Karigel®-N; Listermint® with Fluoride [OTC]; Luride®; Luride® Lozi-Tab®; Luride®-SF Lozi-Tab®; Minute-Gel®; Pediaflor®; Pharmaflur®; Phos-Flur®; Point-Two®; PreviDent®; Stop® [OTC]; Thera-Flur®; Thera-Flur-N®

Synonyms Acidulated Phosphate Fluoride; Sodium Fluoride; Stannous Fluoride

Therapeutic Category Mineral, Oral; Mineral, Oral Topical

Use Prevention of dental caries

Pregnancy Risk Factor C

Contraindications Hypersensitivity to fluoride, tartrazine, or any component; when fluoride content of drinking water exceeds 0.7 ppm; low sodium or sodium-free diets; do not use 1 mg tablets in children <3 years of age or when drinking water fluoride content is ≥0.3 ppm; do not use 1 mg/5 mL rinse (as supplement) in children <6 years of age

Warnings/Precautions Prolonged ingestion with excessive doses may result in dental fluorosis and osseous changes; do **not** exceed recommended dosage; some products contain tartrazine

Adverse Reactions
<1%:
Dermatologic: Rash
Gastrointestinal: Nausea, vomiting, products containing stannous fluoride may stain the teeth

Overdosage/Toxicology Symptoms of overdose include hypersalivation, salty or soapy taste, epigastric pain, nausea, vomiting, diarrhea, rash muscle weakness, tremor, seizures, cardiac failure, respiratory arrest, shock, death

Fatal dose not known. Children: 500 mg; Adults: 7-140 mg/kg

Treatment of overdose: Gastric lavage with $CaCl_2$ or $Ca(OH)_2$ solution; administer large quantity of milk at frequent intervals; $Al(OH)_3$ may also bind the fluoride ion

Drug Interactions Decreased effect/absorption with magnesium-, aluminum-, and calcium-containing products

Stability Store in tight plastic containers (not glass)

Mechanism of Action Promotes remineralization of decalcified enamel; inhibits the cariogenic microbial process in dental plaque; increases tooth resistance to acid dissolution

Pharmacodynamics/Kinetics
Absorption: Absorbed in GI tract, lungs, and skin; calcium, iron, or magnesium may delay absorption
Distribution: 50% of fluoride is deposited in teeth and bone after ingestion; topical application works superficially on enamel and plaque; crosses placenta; appears in breast milk
Elimination: In urine and feces

Usual Dosage Oral:
Recommended daily fluoride supplement (2.2 mg of sodium fluoride is equivalent to 1 mg of fluoride ion): See table.

Fluoride Ion

Fluoride Content of Drinking Water	Daily Dose, Oral (mg)
<0.3 ppm	
Birth - 6 mo	0
6 mo to 3 y	0.25
3-6 y	0.5
6-16 y	1
0.3-06 ppm	
Birth - 3 y	0
3-6 y	0.25
6-16 y	0.5
>0.6 ppm	
All ages	0

Adapted from *AAP News*, 1995, 11(2):18.

Dental rinse or gel:
Children 6-12 years: 5-10 mL rinse or apply to teeth and spit daily after brushing
Adults: 10 mL rinse or apply to teeth and spit daily after brushing

Patient Information Take with food (but not milk) to eliminate GI upset; with dental rinse or dental gel do **not** swallow, do **not** eat or drink for 30 minutes after use

Nursing Implications Avoid giving with milk or dairy products

Dosage Forms Fluoride ion content listed in brackets
Drops, oral, as sodium:
Fluoritab®, Flura-Drops®: 0.55 mg/drop [0.25 mg/drop] (22.8 mL, 24 mL)
Karidium®, Luride®: 0.275 mg/drop [0.125 mg/drop] (30 mL, 60 mL)
Pediaflor®: 1.1 mg/mL [0.5 mg/mL] (50 mL)
Gel, topical:
Acidulated phosphate fluoride (Minute-Gel®): 1.23% (480 mL)
Sodium fluoride (Karigel®, Karigel®-N, PreviDent®): 1.1% [0.5%] (24 g, 30 g, 60 g, 120 g, 130 g, 250 g)
Stannous fluoride (Gel Kam®, Gel-Tin®, Stop®): 0.4% [0.1%] (60 g, 65 g, 105 g, 120 g)
Lozenge, as sodium (Flura-Loz®) (raspberry flavor): 2.2 mg [1 mg]
Rinse, topical, as sodium:
ACT®, Fluorigard®: 0.05% [0.02%] (90 mL, 180 mL, 300 mL, 360 mL, 480 mL)
Fluorinse®, Point-Two®: 0.2% [0.09%] (240 mL, 480 mL, 3780 mL)
Listermint® with Fluoride: 0.02% [0.01%] (180 mL, 300 mL, 360 mL, 480 mL, 540 mL, 720 mL, 960 mL, 1740 mL)
Solution, oral, as sodium (Phos-Flur®): 0.44 mg/mL [0.2 mg/mL] (250 mL, 500 mL, 3780 mL)
Tablet, as sodium:
Chewable:
Fluoritab®, Luride® Lozi-Tab®, Pharmaflur®: 1.1 mg [0.5 mg]
Fluoritab®, Karidium®, Luride® Lozi-Tab®, Luride®-SF Lozi-Tab®, Pharmaflur®: 2.2 mg [1 mg]
Oral: Flura®, Karidium®: 2.2 mg [1 mg]

Fluorigard® [OTC] *see* Fluoride *on previous page*

Fluorinse® *see* Fluoride *on previous page*

Fluor-I-Strip® *see* Fluorescein Sodium *on page 535*

Fluor-I-Strip-AT® *see* Fluorescein Sodium *on page 535*

Fluoritab® *see* Fluoride *on previous page*

9α-Fluorohydrocortisone Acetate *see* Fludrocortisone Acetate *on page 529*

Fluorometholone (flure oh METH oh lone)

Brand Names Flarex®; Fluor-Op®; FML®; FML® Forte

Therapeutic Category Corticosteroid, Ophthalmic; Corticosteroid, Topical (Low Potency)

Use Inflammatory conditions of the eye, including keratitis, iritis, cyclitis, and conjunctivitis

Pregnancy Risk Factor C

Contraindications Herpes simplex, keratitis, fungal diseases of ocular structures, most viral diseases, hypersensitivity to any component

Warnings/Precautions Not recommended in children <2 years of age, prolonged use may result in glaucoma, elevated intraocular pressure, or other ocular damage; some products contain sulfites

(Continued)

Fluorometholone *(Continued)*

Adverse Reactions

1% to 10%: Ocular: Blurred vision

<1%: Ocular: Stinging, burning eyes, increased intraocular pressure, open-angle glaucoma, defect in visual acuity and field of vision, cataracts

Overdosage/Toxicology When consumed in excessive quantities, systemic hypercorticism and adrenal suppression may occur; in those cases, discontinuation and withdrawal of the corticosteroid should be done judiciously

Mechanism of Action Decreases inflammation by suppression of migration of polymorphonuclear leukocytes and reversal of increased capillary permeability

Pharmacodynamics/Kinetics Absorption: Into aqueous humor with slight systemic absorption

Usual Dosage Children >2 years and Adults: Ophthalmic:

Ointment: May be applied every 4 hours in severe cases; 1-3 times/day in mild to moderate cases

Solution: Instill 1-2 drops into conjunctival sac every hour during day, every 2 hours at night until favorable response is obtained, then use 1 drop every 4 hours; for mild to moderate inflammation, instill 1-2 drops into conjunctival sac 2-4 times/day

Patient Information Do not discontinue use without consulting a physician; photosensitivity may occur; notify physician if improvement does not occur after 7-8 days

Nursing Implications Use a separate individual container for each patient

Dosage Forms Ophthalmic:

Ointment (FML®): 0.1% (3.5 g)

Suspension:

Flarex®, Fluor-Op®, FML®: 0.1% (2.5 mL, 5 mL, 10 mL)

FML® Forte: 0.25% (2 mL, 5 mL, 10 mL, 15 mL)

Fluor-Op® *see* Fluorometholone *on previous page*

Fluoroplex® *see* Fluorouracil *on this page*

Fluorouracil (flure oh YOOR a sil)

Related Information

Antiemetics for Chemotherapy Induced Nausea and Vomiting *on page 1348*

Cancer Chemotherapy Regimens *on page 1351*

Toxicities of Chemotherapeutic Agents *on page 1382*

Brand Names Adrucil®; Efudex®; Fluoroplex®

Synonyms 5-Fluorouracil; 5-FU

Therapeutic Category Antineoplastic Agent, Antimetabolite (Pyrimidine)

Use Treatment of carcinoma of stomach, colon, rectum, breast, and pancreas; also used topically for management of multiple actinic keratoses and superficial basal cell carcinomas

Pregnancy Risk Factor D (injection); X (topical)

Contraindications Hypersensitivity to fluorouracil or any component; patients with poor nutritional status, bone marrow suppression

Warnings/Precautions The U.S. Food and Drug Administration (FDA) currently recommends that procedures for proper handling and disposal of antineoplastic agents be considered. Use with caution in patients with impaired kidney or liver function. The drug should be discontinued if intractable vomiting or diarrhea, precipitous falls in leukocyte or platelet counts, stomatitis, hemorrhage, or myocardial ischemia occurs. Use with caution in patients who have had high-dose pelvic radiation or previous use of alkylating agents. Patient should be hospitalized during initial course of therapy.

Adverse Reactions Toxicity depends on route and duration of infusion

>10%:

Dermatologic: Dermatitis, pruritic maculopapular rash, alopecia

Irritant chemotherapy

Gastrointestinal (route and schedule dependent): Heartburn, nausea, vomiting, anorexia, stomatitis, esophagitis, anorexia, stomatitis, and diarrhea; bolus dosing produces milder GI problems, while continuous infusion tends to produce severe mucositis and diarrhea; vomiting is moderate, occurring in 30% to 60% of patients, and responds well to phenothiazines and dexamethasone

Emetic potential:

<1000 mg: Moderately low (10% to 30%)

≥1000 mg: Moderate (30% to 60%)

Hematologic: Myelosuppressive: Granulocytopenia occurs around 9-14 days after 5-FU and thrombocytopenia around 7-17 days. The marrow recovers after 22 days. Myelosuppression tends to be more pronounced in patients receiving bolus dosing of 5-FU.

WBC: Moderate

Platelets: Mild to moderate
Onset (days): 7-10
Nadir (days): 14
Recovery (days): 21

1% to 10%:
Dermatologic: Dry skin
Gastrointestinal: GI ulceration

<1%:
Cardiovascular: Hypotension, chest pain, EKG changes similar to ischemic changes, and possibly cardiac enzyme abnormalities. Usually occurs within the first two days of therapy, and may resolve with nitroglycerin and calcium channel blockers. May be due to coronary vessel vasospasm induced by 5-FU.
Central nervous system: Neurologic: Cerebellar ataxia, headache, somnolence, ataxia are seen primarily in intracarotid arterial infusions for head and neck tumors. This is believed to be caused by fluorocitrate, a neurotoxic metabolite of the parent compound.
Dermatologic: Pruritic maculopapular rash, alopecia, hyperpigmentation of nailbeds, face, hands, and veins used in infusion; photosensitization with UV light; palmar-plantar syndrome (hand-foot syndrome)
Hematologic: Coagulopathy
Hepatic: Hepatotoxicity
Ocular: Conjunctivitis, tear duct stenosis, excessive lacrimation, visual disturbances
Respiratory: Shortness of breath

Overdosage/Toxicology Symptoms of overdose include myelosuppression, nausea, vomiting, diarrhea, alopecia

No specific antidote exists; monitor hematologically for at least 4 weeks; supportive therapy

Drug Interactions

Methotrexate: This interaction is schedule dependent; **5-FU should be given following MTX, not prior to**

If MTX is given first: The cells exposed to MTX before 5-FU have a depleted reduced folate pool which inhibits the binding of the 5dUMP to TS. However, it does not interfere with FUTP incorporation into RNA. Polyglutamines, which accumulate in the presence of MTX may be substituted for the folates and allow binding of FdUMP to TS. MTX given prior to 5-FU may actually activate 5-FU due to MTX inhibition of purine synthesis.

If 5-FU is given first: 5-FU inhibits the TS binding and thus the reduced folate pool is not depleted, thereby negating the effect of MTX

Increased effect: Leucovorin: ↑ the folate pool and in certain tumors, may promote TS inhibition and ↑ 5-FU activity. Must be given before or with the 5-FU to prime the cells; it is not used as a rescue agent in this case.

Increased toxicity:
Allopurinol: Inhibits thymidine phosphorylase (an enzyme that activates 5-FU). The antitumor effect of 5-FU appears to be unaltered, but ↓ toxicity
Cimetidine: Results in increased plasma levels of 5-FU due to drug metabolism inhibition and reduction of liver blood flow induced by cimetidine

Stability Store intact vials at room temperature and protect from light; slight discoloration does not usually denote decomposition. Further dilution in D_5W or NS at concentrations of 0.5-10 mg/mL are stable for 72 hours at 4°C to 25°C.

Incompatible with cytarabine, diazepam, doxorubicin, methotrexate; concentrations of >25 mg/mL of fluorouracil and >2 mg/mL of leucovorin are **incompatible** (precipitation occurs)

Compatible with vincristine, methotrexate, potassium chloride, magnesium sulfate

Standard I.V. dilution:
I.V. push: Dose/syringe (concentration: 50 mg/mL)
Maximum syringe size for IVP is a 30 mL syringe and syringe should be <75% full
CIV/IVPB: Dose/50-1000 mL D_5W or NS
Syringe and solution are stable for 72 hours at 4°C to 25°C

Mechanism of Action A pyrimidine antimetabolite that interferes with DNA synthesis by blocking the methylation of deoxyuridylic acid; 5-FU rapidly enters the cell and is activated to the nucleotide level; there it inhibits thymidylate synthetase (TS), or is incorporated into RNA (most evident during the GI phase of the cell cycle). The reduced folate cofactor is required for tight binding to occur between the 5-FdUMP and TS.

Pharmacodynamics/Kinetics

Absorption: Oral: Erratic and rarely used

(Continued)

Fluorouracil *(Continued)*

Distribution: V_d: ~22% of total body water; penetrates the extracellular fluid, CSF, and third space fluids (such as pleural effusions and ascitic fluid)

Metabolism: 5-FU must be metabolized to be active. 90% metabolized; accomplished by a dehydrogenase enzyme primarily found in the liver; dose may need to be omitted in patients with liver failure (bilirubin >5 mg/dL)

Bioavailability: <75%, erratic and undependable

Half-life (biphasic): Initial: 6-20 minutes; doses of 400-600 mg/m² produce drug concentrations above the threshold for cytotoxicity for normal tissue and remain there for 6 hours; 2 metabolites, FdUMP and FUTP, have prolonged half-lives depending on the type of tissue; the clinical effect of these metabolites has not been determined

Elimination: 5% of dose excreted as unchanged drug in the urine in 6 hours, and a large amount excreted as CO_2 from the lung

Usual Dosage Refer to individual protocols

All dosages are based on the patient's actual weight. However, the estimated lean body mass (dry weight) is used if the patient is obese or if there has been a spurious weight gain due to edema, ascites or other forms of abnormal fluid retention.

Children and Adults:

I.V.: Initial: 400-500 mg/m²/day (12 mg/kg/day; maximum: 800 mg/day) for 4-5 days either as a single daily I.V. push or 4-day CIV

I.V.: Maintenance dose regimens:

200-250 mg/m² (6 mg/kg) every other day for 4 days repeated in 4 weeks

500-600 mg/m² (15 mg/kg) weekly as a CIV or I.V. push

I.V.: Concomitant with leucovorin:

370 mg/m²/day x 5 days

500-1000 mg/m² every 2 weeks

600 mg/m² weekly for 6 weeks

Although the manufacturer recommends no daily dose >800 mg, higher doses of up to 2 g/day are routinely administered by CIV; higher daily doses have been successfully used

Hemodialysis: Administer dose posthemodialysis

Dosing adjustment/comments in hepatic impairment: Bilirubin >5 mg/dL: Omit use

Topical:

Actinic or solar keratosis: Apply twice daily for 2-6 weeks

Superficial basal cell carcinomas: Apply 5% twice daily for at least 3-6 weeks and up to 10-12 weeks

Administration Direct I.V. push injection (50 mg/mL solution needs no further dilution) or by I.V. infusion; myelotoxicity may be reduced by giving the drug as a constant infusion. Bolus doses may be administered by slow IVP or IVPB; continuous infusions may be administered in D_5W or NS. Solution should be protected from direct sunlight; 5-FU may also be administered intra-arterially or intrahepatically (refer to specific protocols).

Monitoring Parameters CBC with differential and platelet count, renal function tests, liver function tests

Test Interactions Fecal discoloration

Patient Information Avoid unnecessary exposure to sunlight; any signs of infection, easy bruising or bleeding, shortness of breath, or painful or burning urination should be brought to physician's attention. Nausea, vomiting, or hair loss sometimes occur. The drug may cause permanent sterility and may cause birth defects. The drug may be excreted in breast milk, therefore, an alternative form of feeding your baby should be used.

Nursing Implications Cool to body temperature before using; after vial has been entered, any unused portion should be discarded within 1 hour; wash hands immediately after topical application of the 5% cream; I.V. formulation may be given orally mixed in water, grape juice, or carbonated beverage

Dosage Forms

Cream, topical:

Efudex®: 5% (25 g)

Fluoroplex®: 1% (30 g)

Injection (Adrucil®): 50 mg/mL (10 mL, 20 mL, 50 mL, 100 mL)

Solution, topical:

Efudex®: 2% (10 mL); 5% (10 mL)

Fluoroplex®: 1% (30 mL)

5-Fluorouracil *see* Fluorouracil *on page 538*

Fluostigmin *see* Isoflurophate *on page 679*

Fluoxetine (floo OKS e teen)

Related Information

Antidepressant Agents Comparison *on page 1393*

Brand Names Prozac®

Canadian/Mexican Brand Names Fluoxac® (Mexico)

Synonyms Fluoxetine Hydrochloride

Therapeutic Category Antidepressant, Serotonin Reuptake Inhibitor

Use Treatment of major depression; treatment of binge-eating and vomiting in patients with moderate-to-severe bulimia nervosa; obsessive-compulsive disorder

Pregnancy Risk Factor B

Contraindications Hypersensitivity to fluoxetine; patients receiving MAO inhibitors currently or in past 2 weeks

Warnings/Precautions Use with caution in patients with hepatic impairment, history of seizures; MAO inhibitors should be discontinued at least 14 days before initiating fluoxetine therapy; add or initiate other antidepressants with caution for up to 5 weeks after stopping fluoxetine

Adverse Reactions Predominant adverse effects are CNS and GI

>10%:

- Central nervous system: Headache, nervousness, insomnia, drowsiness
- Gastrointestinal: Nausea, diarrhea, xerostomia

1% to 10%:

- Central nervous system: Anxiety, dizziness, fatigue, sedation
- Dermatologic: Rash, pruritus
- Endocrine & metabolic: SIADH, hypoglycemia, hyponatremia (elderly or volume-depleted patients)
- Gastrointestinal: Anorexia, dyspepsia, constipation
- Neuromuscular & skeletal: Tremor
- Miscellaneous: Diaphoresis (excessive)

<1%:

- Central nervous system: Extrapyramidal reactions (rare)
- Ocular: Visual disturbances
- Miscellaneous: Anaphylactoid reactions, allergies, suicidal ideation

Overdosage/Toxicology Symptoms of overdose include ataxia, sedation, and coma; respiratory depression may occur, especially with coingestion of alcohol or other drugs; seizures very rarely occur

Drug Interactions

Inhibitor of cytochrome P-450 2D6 enzymes
Cytochrome P-450 2D6 enzyme substrate

Increased effect with tricyclics (2 times ↑ plasma level)
Increased/decreased effect of lithium (both increased and decreased level has been reported)
Increased toxicity of diazepam, trazodone via decreased clearance; increased toxicity with MAO inhibitors (hyperpyrexia, tremors, seizures, delirium, coma)
May displace highly protein bound drugs (warfarin)

Mechanism of Action Inhibits CNS neuron serotonin uptake; minimal or no effect on reuptake of norepinephrine or dopamine; does not significantly bind to alpha-adrenergic, histamine or cholinergic receptors; may therefore be useful in patients at risk from sedation, hypotension, and anticholinergic effects of tricyclic antidepressants

Pharmacodynamics/Kinetics

Peak antidepressant effect: After >4 weeks
Absorption: Oral: Well absorbed
Metabolism: To norfluoxetine (active)
Half-life: Adults: 2-3 days; due to long half-life, resolution of adverse reactions after discontinuation may be slow
Time to peak serum concentration: Within 4-8 hours
Elimination: In urine as fluoxetine (2.5% to 5%) and norfluoxetine (10%)

Usual Dosage Oral:

Children <18 years: Dose and safety not established; preliminary experience in children 6-14 years using initial doses of 20 mg/day have been reported

Adults: 20 mg/day in the morning; may increase after several weeks by 20 mg/day increments; maximum: 80 mg/day; doses >20 mg should be divided into morning and noon doses

Usual dosage range:

- 20-80 mg/day for depression and OCD
- 20-60 mg/day for obesity
- 60-80 mg/day for bulimia nervosa

Note: Lower doses of 5 mg/day have been used for initial treatment

Elderly: Some patients may require an initial dose of 10 mg/day with dosage increases of 10 and 20 mg every several weeks as tolerated; should not be taken at night unless patient experiences sedation

(Continued)

Fluoxetine *(Continued)*

Dosing adjustment in renal impairment:

Single dose studies: Pharmacokinetics of fluoxetine and norfluoxetine were similar among subjects with all levels of impaired renal function, including anephric patients on chronic hemodialysis

Chronic administration: Additional accumulation of fluoxetine or norfluoxetine may occur in patients with severely impaired renal function

Hemodialysis: Not removed by hemodialysis

Dosing adjustment in hepatic impairment: Elimination half-life of fluoxetine is prolonged in patients with hepatic impairment; a lower or less frequent dose of fluoxetine should be used in these patients

Cirrhosis patients: Administer a lower dose or less frequent dosing interval

Compensated cirrhosis without ascites: Administer 50% of normal dose

Dietary Considerations Alcohol: Avoid use

Reference Range Therapeutic levels have not been well established

Therapeutic: Fluoxetine: 100-800 ng/mL (SI: 289-2314 nmol/L); Norfluoxetine: 100-600 ng/mL (SI: 289-1735 nmol/L)

Toxic: Fluoxetine plus norfluoxetine: >2000 ng/mL

Test Interactions ↑ albumin in urine

Patient Information Avoid alcoholic beverages, take in morning to avoid insomnia; fluoxetine's potential stimulating and anorexic effects may be bothersome to some patients. Use sugarless hard candy for dry mouth; avoid alcoholic beverages, may cause drowsiness, improvement may take several weeks; rise slowly to prevent dizziness.

Nursing Implications Offer patient sugarless hard candy for dry mouth

Dosage Forms

Capsule, as hydrochloride: 10 mg, 20 mg

Liquid, as hydrochloride (mint flavor): 20 mg/5 mL (120 mL)

Extemporaneous Preparations A 20 mg capsule may be mixed with 4 oz of water, apple juice, or Gatorade® to provide a solution that is stable for 14 days under refrigeration

Fluoxetine Hydrochloride *see* Fluoxetine *on previous page*

Fluoxymesterone (floo oks i MES te rone)

Related Information

Cancer Chemotherapy Regimens *on page 1351*

Brand Names Halotestin®

Canadian/Mexican Brand Names Stenox® (Mexico)

Therapeutic Category Androgen

Use Replacement of endogenous testicular hormone; in females, used as palliative treatment of breast cancer; stimulation of erythropoiesis, angioneurotic edema, postpartum breast engorgement

Restrictions C-III

Pregnancy Risk Factor X

Contraindications Serious cardiac disease, liver or kidney disease, hypersensitivity to fluoxymesterone or any component

Warnings/Precautions May accelerate bone maturation without producing compensatory gain in linear growth in children; in prepubertal children perform radiographic examination of the hand and wrist every 6 months to determine the rate of bone maturation and to assess the effect of treatment on the epiphyseal centers

Adverse Reactions

>10%:

- Males: Priapism
- Females: Menstrual problems (amenorrhea), virilism, breast soreness
- Cardiovascular: Edema
- Dermatologic: Acne

1% to 10%:

- Males: Prostatic carcinoma, hirsutism (increase in pubic hair growth), impotence, testicular atrophy
- Cardiovascular: Edema
- Gastrointestinal: GI irritation, nausea, vomiting
- Genitourinary: Prostatic hypertrophy
- Hepatic: Hepatic dysfunction

<1%:

- Males: Gynecomastia
- Females: Amenorrhea
- Endocrine & metabolic: Hypercalcemia
- Hematologic: Leukopenia, polycythemia
- Hepatic: Hepatic necrosis, cholestatic hepatitis
- Miscellaneous: Hypersensitivity reactions

Overdosage/Toxicology Symptoms of overdose include abnormal liver function tests, water retention

Drug Interactions

Decreased effect:

Fluphenazine effectiveness with anticholinergics

Barbiturate levels and ↓ fluphenazine effectiveness when given together

Increased toxicity:

Anticoagulants: Fluoxymesterone may suppress clotting factors II, V, VII, and X; therefore, bleeding may occur in patients on anticoagulant therapy

Cyclosporine: May elevate cyclosporine serum levels

Insulin: May enhance hypoglycemic effect of insulin therapy

May decrease blood glucose concentrations and insulin requirements in patients with diabetes

With ethanol, effects of both drugs may increase

EPSEs and other CNS effects may increase when coadministered with lithium

May potentiate the effects of narcotics including respiratory depression

Stability Protect from light

Mechanism of Action Synthetic androgenic anabolic hormone responsible for the normal growth and development of male sex hormones and development of male sex organs and maintenance of secondary sex characteristics; synthetic testosterone derivative with significant androgen activity; stimulates RNA polymerase activity resulting in an increase in protein production; increases bone development

Pharmacodynamics/Kinetics

Absorption: Oral: Rapid

Protein binding: 98%

Metabolism: In the liver

Half-life: 10-100 minutes

Elimination: Enterohepatic circulation and urinary excretion (90%)

Halogenated derivative of testosterone with up to 5 times the activity of methyltestosterone

Usual Dosage Adults: Oral:

Male:

Hypogonadism: 5-20 mg/day

Delayed puberty: 2.5-20 mg/day for 4-6 months

Female:

Inoperable breast carcinoma: 10-40 mg/day in divided doses for 1-3 months

Breast engorgement: 2.5 mg after delivery, 5-10 mg/day in divided doses for 4-5 days

Monitoring Parameters In prepubertal children, perform radiographic examination of the head and wrist every 6 months

Test Interactions Decreased levels of thyroxine-binding globulin; decreased total T_4 serum levels; increased resin uptake of T_3 and T_4

Patient Information Men should report overly frequent or persistent penile erections; women should report menstrual irregularities; all patients should report persistent GI distress, diarrhea, or jaundice

Dosage Forms Tablet: 2 mg, 5 mg, 10 mg

Fluphenazine (floo FEN a zeen)

Related Information

Antipsychotic Agents Comparison *on page 1396*

Brand Names Permitil®; Prolixin®; Prolixin Decanoate®; Prolixin Enanthate®

Canadian/Mexican Brand Names Apo-Fluphenazine® [Hydrochloride] (Canada); Modecate® [Fluphenazine Decanoate] (Canada); Modecate Enanthate [Fluphenazine Enanthate] (Canada); Moditen® Hydrochloride (Canada); PMS-Fluphenazine [Hydrochloride] (Canada)

Synonyms Fluphenazine Decanoate; Fluphenazine Enanthate; Fluphenazine Hydrochloride

Therapeutic Category Antipsychotic Agent; Phenothiazine Derivative

Use Management of manifestations of psychotic disorders

Pregnancy Risk Factor C

Contraindications Hypersensitivity to fluphenazine or any component, cross-sensitivity with other phenothiazines may exist; avoid use in patients with narrow-angle glaucoma

Warnings/Precautions Safety in children <6 months of age has not been established; use with caution in patients with cardiovascular disease or seizures; benefits of therapy must be weighed against risks of therapy; adverse effects may be of longer duration with Depot® form; watch for hypotension when administering I.M. or I.V.; use with caution in patients with severe liver or renal disease

(Continued)

Fluphenazine *(Continued)*

Adverse Reactions

>10%:

Cardiovascular: Orthostatic hypotension, hypotension, tachycardia, arrhythmias

Central nervous system: Parkinsonian symptoms, akathisia, dystonias, tardive dyskinesia (persistent), dizziness

Gastrointestinal: Constipation

Ocular: Pigmentary retinopathy

Respiratory: Nasal congestion

Miscellaneous: Diaphoresis (decreased)

1% to 10%:

Dermatologic: Increased sensitivity to sun, rash

Endocrine & metabolic: Changes in menstrual cycle, breast pain, amenorrhea, galactorrhea, gynecomastia, changes in libido

Gastrointestinal: Weight gain, nausea, vomiting, stomach pain

Genitourinary: Dysuria, ejaculatory disturbances

Neuromuscular & skeletal: Trembling of fingers

<1%:

Central nervous system: Sedation, drowsiness, restlessness, anxiety, extrapyramidal reactions, pseudoparkinsonian signs and symptoms, seizures, altered central temperature regulation

Dermatologic: Photosensitivity, hyperpigmentation, pruritus, rash, discoloration of skin (blue-gray)

Endocrine & metabolic: Galactorrhea

Gastrointestinal: Xerostomia

Genitourinary: Priapism, urinary retention

Hematologic: Agranulocytosis (more often in women between 4th and 10th weeks of therapy), leukopenia (usually in patients with large doses for prolonged periods)

Hepatic: Cholestatic jaundice, hepatotoxicity

Ocular: Cornea and lens changes, blurred vision

Overdosage/Toxicology Symptoms of overdose include deep sleep, hypotension, hypertension, dystonia, seizures, extrapyramidal symptoms, respiratory failure

Following initiation of essential overdose management, toxic symptom treatment and supportive treatment should be initiated. Hypotension usually responds to I.V. fluids or Trendelenburg positioning. If unresponsive to these measures, the use of a parenteral inotrope may be required. Seizures commonly respond to diazepam (I.V. 5-10 mg bolus in adults every 15 minutes if needed up to a total of 30 mg; I.V. 0.25-0.4 mg/kg/dose up to a total of 10 mg in children) or to phenytoin or phenobarbital. Cardiac arrhythmias often respond to I.V. lidocaine while other antiarrhythmics can be used. Neuroleptics often cause extrapyramidal symptoms (eg, dystonic reactions) requiring management; benztropine mesylate I.V. 1-2 mg (adults) may be effective. These agents are generally effective within 2-5 minutes.

Drug Interactions

Decreased effect: Barbiturate levels and decreased fluphenazine effectiveness when given together

Increased toxicity: With ethanol, effects of both drugs may be increased; EPSEs and other CNS effects may be increased when coadministered with lithium; may potentiate the effects of narcotics including respiratory depression

Mechanism of Action Blocks postsynaptic mesolimbic dopaminergic D_1 and D_2 receptors in the brain; exhibits a strong alpha-adrenergic blocking and anticholinergic effect, depresses the release of hypothalamic and hypophyseal hormones; believed to depress the reticular activating system thus affecting basal metabolism, body temperature, wakefulness, vasomotor tone, and emesis

Pharmacodynamics/Kinetics

Following I.M. or S.C. administration (derivative dependent):

Decanoate (lasts the longest and requires more time for onset):

Onset of action: 24-72 hours

Peak neuroleptic effect: Within 48-96 hours

Hydrochloride salt (acts quickly and persists briefly):

Onset of activity: Within 1 hour

Duration: 6-8 hours

Distribution: Crosses the placenta; appears in breast milk

Metabolism: In the liver

Half-life: Derivative dependent:

Enanthate: 84-96 hours

Hydrochloride: 33 hours

Decanoate: 163-232 hours

Usual Dosage Adults:
Oral: 0.5-10 mg/day in divided doses at 6- to 8-hour intervals; some patients may require up to 40 mg/day
I.M.: 2.5-10 mg/day in divided doses at 6- to 8-hour intervals (parenteral dose is 1/3 to 1/2 the oral dose for the hydrochloride salts)
I.M., S.C. (decanoate): 12.5 mg every 3 weeks
Conversion from hydrochloride to decanoate I.M. 0.5 mL (12.5 mg) decanoate every 3 weeks is approximately equivalent to 10 mg hydrochloride/day
I.M., S.C. (enanthate): 12.5-25 mg every 3 weeks

Hemodialysis: Not dialyzable (0% to 5%)

Dietary Considerations Alcohol: Additive CNS effect, avoid use

Reference Range Therapeutic: 5-20 ng/mL; correlation of serum concentrations and efficacy is controversial; most often dosed to best response

Test Interactions ↑ cholesterol (S), ↑ glucose; ↓ uric acid (S)

Patient Information Avoid alcoholic beverages, may cause drowsiness, do not discontinue without consulting physician

Nursing Implications Avoid contact of oral solution or injection with skin (contact dermatitis); watch for hypotension when administering I.M. or I.V.; oral liquid to be diluted in the following **only**: water, saline, 7-UP®, homogenized milk, carbonated orange beverages, pineapple, apricot, prune, orange, V8® juice, tomato, and grapefruit juices

Dosage Forms
Concentrate, as hydrochloride:
Permitil®: 5 mg/mL with alcohol 1% (118 mL)
Prolixin®: 5 mg/mL with alcohol 14% (120 mL)
Elixir, as hydrochloride (Prolixin®): 2.5 mg/5 mL with alcohol 14% (60 mL, 473 mL)
Injection, as decanoate (Prolixin Decanoate®): 25 mg/mL (1 mL, 5 mL)
Injection, as enanthate (Prolixin Enanthate®): 25 mg/mL (5 mL)
Injection, as hydrochloride (Prolixin®): 2.5 mg/mL (10 mL)
Tablet, as hydrochloride
Permitil®: 2.5 mg, 5 mg, 10 mg
Prolixin®: 1 mg, 2.5 mg, 5 mg, 10 mg

Fluphenazine Decanoate *see* Fluphenazine *on page 543*
Fluphenazine Enanthate *see* Fluphenazine *on page 543*
Fluphenazine Hydrochloride *see* Fluphenazine *on page 543*
Flura® *see* Fluoride *on page 536*
Flura-Drops® *see* Fluoride *on page 536*
Flura-Loz® *see* Fluoride *on page 536*

Flurandrenolide (flure an DREN oh lide)

Related Information
Corticosteroids Comparison *on page 1407*

Brand Names Cordran®; Cordran® SP

Canadian/Mexican Brand Names Drenison® (Canada)

Synonyms Flurandrenolone

Therapeutic Category Corticosteroid, Topical (Low Potency); Corticosteroid, Topical (Medium Potency)

Use Inflammation of corticosteroid-responsive dermatoses [medium potency topical corticosteroid]

Pregnancy Risk Factor C

Contraindications Viral, fungal, or tubercular skin lesions, known hypersensitivity to flurandrenolide

Warnings/Precautions Adverse systemic effects may occur when used on large areas of the body, denuded areas, for prolonged periods of time, with an occlusive dressing, and/or in infants or small children

Adverse Reactions
<1%:
Dermatologic: Itching, dry skin, folliculitis, hypertrichosis, acneiform eruptions, hypopigmentation, perioral dermatitis, allergic contact dermatitis, skin atrophy, striae, miliaria, intracranial hypertension, acne, maceration of the skin
Endocrine & metabolic: HPA suppression, Cushing's syndrome, growth retardation
Local: Burning, irritation
Miscellaneous: Secondary infection

Overdosage/Toxicology When consumed in excessive quantities, systemic hypercorticism and adrenal suppression may occur; in those cases, discontinuation and withdrawal of the corticosteroid should be done judiciously

Mechanism of Action Decreases inflammation by suppression of migration of polymorphonuclear leukocytes and reversal of increased capillary permeability

(Continued)

Flurandrenolide *(Continued)*

Pharmacodynamics/Kinetics

Absorption: Adequate with intact skin

Metabolism: In the liver

Elimination: By the kidney with small amounts appearing in bile

Repeated applications lead to depot effects on skin, potentially resulting in enhanced percutaneous absorption

Usual Dosage Topical:

Children:

Ointment, cream: Apply sparingly 1-2 times/day

Tape: Apply once daily

Adults: Cream, lotion, ointment: Apply sparingly 2-3 times/day

Patient Information A thin film of cream or ointment is effective; do not overuse; do not use tight-fitting diapers or plastic pants on children being treated in the diaper area; use only as prescribed, and for no longer than the period prescribed; apply sparingly in light film; rub in lightly; avoid contact with eyes; notify physician if condition being treated persists or worsens

Dosage Forms

Cream, emulsified base (Cordran® SP): 0.025% (30 g, 60 g); 0.05% (15 g, 30 g, 60 g)

Lotion (Cordran®): 0.05% (15 mL, 60 mL)

Ointment, topical (Cordran®): 0.025% (30 g, 60 g); 0.05% (15 g, 30 g, 60 g)

Tape, topical (Cordran®): 4 mcg/cm^2 (7.5 cm x 60 cm, 7.5 cm x 200 cm rolls)

Flurandrenolone *see* Flurandrenolide *on previous page*

Flurazepam (flure AZ e pam)

Related Information

Benzodiazepines Comparison *on page 1397*

Brand Names Dalmane®

Canadian/Mexican Brand Names Apo-Flurazepam® (Canada); Novo-Flupam® (Canada); PMS-Flupam (Canada); Somnol® (Canada); Som Pam® (Canada)

Synonyms Flurazepam Hydrochloride

Therapeutic Category Benzodiazepine; Hypnotic; Sedative

Use Short-term treatment of insomnia

Restrictions C-IV

Pregnancy Risk Factor X

Contraindications Hypersensitivity to flurazepam or any component (there may be cross-sensitivity with other benzodiazepines); pregnancy, pre-existing CNS depression, respiratory depression, narrow-angle glaucoma

Warnings/Precautions Use with caution in patients receiving other CNS depressants, patients with low albumin, hepatic dysfunction, and in the elderly; do not use in pregnant women; may cause drug dependency; safety and efficacy have not been established in children <15 years of age

Adverse Reactions

>10%:

Cardiovascular: Tachycardia, chest pain

Central nervous system: Drowsiness, fatigue, ataxia, lightheadedness, memory impairment, insomnia, anxiety, depression, headache

Dermatologic: Rash

Endocrine & metabolic: Decreased libido

Gastrointestinal: Xerostomia, constipation, decreased salivation, nausea, vomiting, diarrhea, increased or decreased appetite

Neuromuscular & skeletal: Dysarthria

Ocular: Blurred vision

Miscellaneous: Diaphoresis

1% to 10%:

Cardiovascular: Syncope, hypotension

Central nervous system: Confusion, nervousness, dizziness, akathisia

Dermatologic: Dermatitis

Gastrointestinal: Weight gain or loss, increased salivation

Neuromuscular & skeletal: Rigidity, tremor, muscle cramps

Otic: Tinnitus

Respiratory: Hyperventilation, nasal congestion

<1%:

Endocrine & metabolic: Menstrual irregularities

Hematologic: Blood dyscrasias

Neuromuscular & skeletal: Reflex slowing

Miscellaneous: Drug dependence

Overdosage/Toxicology Symptoms of overdose include respiratory depression, hypoactive reflexes, unsteady gait, hypotension

Treatment for benzodiazepine overdose is supportive. Rarely is mechanical ventilation required. Flumazenil has been shown to selectively block the binding of benzodiazepines to CNS receptors, resulting in a reversal of benzodiazepine-induced CNS depression.

Drug Interactions

Decreased effect with enzyme inducers

Increased toxicity with other CNS depressants and cimetidine

Stability Store in light-resistant containers

Mechanism of Action Depresses all levels of the CNS, including the limbic and reticular formation, probably through the increased action of gamma-aminobutyric acid (GABA), which is a major inhibitory neurotransmitter in the brain

Pharmacodynamics/Kinetics

Onset of hypnotic effect: 15-20 minutes

Peak: 3-6 hours

Duration of action: 7-8 hours

Metabolism: In the liver to N-desalkylflurazepam (active)

Half-life: Adults: 40-114 hours

Usual Dosage Oral:

Children:

<15 years: Dose not established

>15 years: 15 mg at bedtime

Adults: 15-30 mg at bedtime

Dietary Considerations Alcohol: Additive CNS effect, avoid use

Monitoring Parameters Respiratory and cardiovascular status

Reference Range Therapeutic: 0-4 ng/mL (SI: 0-9 nmol/L); Metabolite N-desalkylflurazepam: 20-110 ng/mL (SI: 43-240 nmol/L); Toxic: >0.12 μg/mL

Patient Information Avoid alcohol and other CNS depressants; avoid activities needing good psychomotor coordination until CNS effects are known; drug may cause physical or psychological dependence; avoid abrupt discontinuation after prolonged use

Nursing Implications Provide safety measures (ie, side rails, night light, and call button); remove smoking materials from area; supervise ambulation; avoid abrupt discontinuance in patients with prolonged therapy or seizure disorders

Dosage Forms Capsule, as hydrochloride: 15 mg, 30 mg

Flurazepam Hydrochloride *see* Flurazepam *on previous page*

Flurbiprofen (flure BI proe fen)

Related Information

Nonsteroidal Anti-Inflammatory Agents Comparison *on page 1419*

Brand Names Ansaid®; Ocufen®

Canadian/Mexican Brand Names Apro-Flurbiprofen® (Canada); Froben® (Canada); Froben-SR® (Canada); Novo-Flurprofen® (Canada); Nu-Flurprofen® (Canada)

Synonyms Flurbiprofen Sodium

Therapeutic Category Analgesic, Nonsteroidal Anti-inflammatory Drug; Anti-inflammatory Agent; Nonsteroidal Anti-Inflammatory Agent (NSAID), Ophthalmic; Nonsteroidal Anti-inflammatory Agent (NSAID), Oral

Use Inhibition of intraoperative miosis; acute or long-term treatment of signs and symptoms of rheumatoid arthritis and osteoarthritis; prevention and management of postoperative ocular inflammation and postoperative cystoid macular edema remains to be determined

Pregnancy Risk Factor C

Contraindications Dendritic keratitis, hypersensitivity to flurbiprofen or any component

Warnings/Precautions Should be used with caution in patients with a history of herpes simplex, keratitis, and patients who might be affected by inhibition of platelet aggregation; slowing of corneal wound healing patients in whom asthma, rhinitis, or urticaria is precipitated by aspirin or other NSAIDs.

Adverse Reactions

Ophthalmic:

>10%: Ocular: Slowing of corneal wound healing, mild ocular stinging, itching and burning eyes, ocular irritation

1% to 10%: Ocular: Eye redness

Oral:

>10%:

Central nervous system: Dizziness

Dermatologic: Rash

Gastrointestinal: Abdominal cramps, heartburn, indigestion, nausea

1% to 10%:

Central nervous system: Headache, nervousness

Dermatologic: Itching

(Continued)

Flurbiprofen *(Continued)*

Endocrine & metabolic: Fluid retention
Gastrointestinal: Vomiting
Otic: Tinnitus

<1%:

Cardiovascular: Congestive heart failure, hypertension, arrhythmias, tachycardia
Central nervous system: Confusion, hallucinations, aseptic meningitis, mental depression, drowsiness, insomnia
Dermatologic: Urticaria, erythema multiforme, toxic epidermal necrolysis, Stevens-Johnson syndrome, angioedema
Endocrine & metabolic: Polydipsia, hot flashes
Gastrointestinal: Gastritis, GI ulceration
Genitourinary: Cystitis, polyuria
Hematologic: Agranulocytosis, anemia, hemolytic anemia, bone marrow suppression, leukopenia, thrombocytopenia
Hepatic: Hepatitis
Neuromuscular & skeletal: Peripheral neuropathy
Ocular: Toxic amblyopia, blurred vision, conjunctivitis, dry eyes
Otic: Decreased hearing
Renal: Acute renal failure
Respiratory: Shortness of breath, allergic rhinitis, epistaxis

Overdosage/Toxicology Symptoms include apnea, metabolic acidosis, coma, and nystagmus; leukocytosis, renal failure

Management of a nonsteroidal anti-inflammatory drug (NSAID) intoxication is primarily supportive and symptomatic. Fluid therapy is commonly effective in managing the hypotension that may occur following an acute NSAIDs overdose, except when this is due to an acute blood loss. Seizures tend to be very short-lived and often do not require drug treatment; although, recurrent seizures should be treated with I.V. diazepam. Since many of the NSAID undergo enterohepatic cycling, multiple doses of charcoal may be needed to reduce the potential for delayed toxicities.

Drug Interactions Decreased effect: When used concurrently with flurbiprofen, reports acetylcholine chloride and carbachol being ineffective

Mechanism of Action Inhibits prostaglandin synthesis by decreasing the activity of the enzyme, cyclo-oxygenase, which results in decreased formation of prostaglandin precursors

Pharmacodynamics/Kinetics Onset of effect: Within 1-2 hours

Usual Dosage

Oral: Rheumatoid arthritis and osteoarthritis: 200-300 mg/day in 2, 3, or 4 divided doses

Ophthalmic: Instill 1 drop every 30 minutes, 2 hours prior to surgery (total of 4 drops to each affected eye)

Patient Information Take the oral formulation with food to decrease any abdominal complaints. Eye drops may cause mild burning or stinging, notify physician if this becomes severe or persistent; do not touch dropper to eye, visual acuity may be decreased after administration.

Nursing Implications Care should be taken to avoid contamination of the solution container tip

Dosage Forms

Solution, ophthalmic, as sodium (Ocufen®): 0.03% (2.5 mL, 5 mL, 10 mL)
Tablet, as sodium (Ansaid®): 50 mg, 100 mg

Flurbiprofen Sodium *see* Flurbiprofen *on previous page*

Fluress® *see* Fluorescein Sodium *on page 535*

5-Flurocytosine *see* Flucytosine *on page 526*

Flurosyn® *see* Fluocinolone *on page 533*

Flutamide (FLOO ta mide)

Related Information

Cancer Chemotherapy Regimens *on page 1351*

Brand Names Eulexin®

Therapeutic Category Antiandrogen; Antineoplastic Agent, Miscellaneous

Use In combination therapy with LHRH agonist analogues in treatment of metastatic prostatic carcinoma. A study has shown that the addition of flutamide to leuprolide therapy in patients with advanced prostatic cancer increased median actuarial survival time to 34.9 months versus 27.9 months with leuprolide alone. To achieve benefit to combination therapy, both drugs need to be started simultaneously.

Pregnancy Risk Factor D

Contraindications Known hypersensitivity to flutamide

Warnings/Precautions The U.S. Food and Drug Administration (FDA) currently recommends that procedures for proper handling and disposal of antineoplastic agents be considered. Animal data (based on using doses higher than recommended for humans) produced testicular interstitial cell adenoma. Do not discontinue therapy without physician's advice.

Adverse Reactions

>10%:

Gastrointestinal: Nausea, vomiting, diarrhea

Genitourinary: Impotence

Endocrine & metabolic: Loss of libido, hot flashes

1% to 10%:

Endocrine & metabolic: Gynecomastia

Gastrointestinal: Anorexia

Neuromuscular & skeletal: Numbness in extremities

<1%:

Cardiovascular: Hypertension, edema

Central nervous system: Drowsiness, nervousness, confusion

Hepatic: Hepatitis

Overdosage/Toxicology Symptoms of overdose include hypoactivity, ataxia, anorexia, vomiting, slow respiration, lacrimation

Management is supportive, dialysis not of benefit; induce vomiting

Stability Store at room temperature

Mechanism of Action Nonsteroidal antiandrogen that inhibits androgen uptake or inhibits binding of androgen in target tissues

Pharmacodynamics/Kinetics

Absorption: Rapid and complete

Metabolism: Extensively to more than 10 metabolites

Half-life: 5-6 hours

Elimination: All metabolites excreted primarily in urine

Usual Dosage Adults: Oral: 2 capsules every 8 hours for a total daily dose of 750 mg

Administration Contents of capsule may be opened and mixed with applesauce, pudding, or other soft foods; mixing with a beverage is not recommended

Monitoring Parameters LFTs, tumor reduction, testosterone/estrogen, and phosphatase serum levels

Patient Information Flutamide and the drug used for medical castration should be administered concomitantly; do not interrupt or stop taking medication; frequent blood tests may be needed to monitor therapy

Dosage Forms Capsule: 125 mg

Flutex® *see* Triamcinolone *on page 1255*

Fluticasone (floo TIK a sone)

Related Information

Asthma, Guidelines for the Diagnosis and Management of *on page 1518*

Corticosteroids Comparison *on page 1407*

Estimated Clinical Comparability of Doses for Inhaled Corticosteroids *on page 1522*

Brand Names Cutivate™; Flonase™; Flovent™

Synonyms Fluticasone Propionate

Therapeutic Category Corticosteroid, Inhalant; Corticosteroid, Topical (Medium Potency)

Use

Inhalation: Maintenance treatment of asthma as prophylactic therapy. It is also indicated for patients requiring oral corticosteroid therapy for asthma to assist in total discontinuation or reduction of total oral dose. NOT indicated for the relief of acute bronchospasm.

Intranasal: Management of seasonal and perennial allergic rhinitis in patients ≥12 years of age

Topical: Relief of inflammation and pruritus associated with corticosteroid-responsive dermatoses [medium potency topical corticosteroid]

Pregnancy Risk Factor C

Contraindications Hypersensitivity to any component, bacterial infections, ophthalmic use

Warnings/Precautions Adverse systemic effects may occur when used on large areas of the body, denuded areas, for prolonged periods of time, with an occlusive dressing, and/or in infants or small children

Adverse Reactions

>10%: Oral inhalation:

Central nervous system: Headache

Respiratory: Respiratory infection, pharyngitis, nasal congestion

1% to 10%: Oral Inhalation:

Central nervous system: Dysphonia

(Continued)

Fluticasone *(Continued)*

Gastrointestinal: Oral candidiasis
Respiratory: Sinusitis

<1%:

Dermatologic: Acne, hypopigmentation, allergic dermatitis, maceration of the skin, skin atrophy, folliculitis, hypertrichosis, itching, dry skin
Endocrine & metabolic: HPA suppression, Cushing's syndrome, growth retardation
Local: Burning, irritation
Miscellaneous: Secondary infection

Overdosage/Toxicology When consumed in excessive quantities, systemic hypercorticism and adrenal suppression may occur; in those cases, discontinuation and withdrawal of the corticosteroid should be done judiciously

Mechanism of Action Fluticasone belongs to a new group of corticosteroids which utilizes a fluorocarbothioate ester linkage at the 17 carbon position; extremely potent vasoconstrictive and anti-inflammatory activity; has a weak hypothalamic -pituitary- adrenocortical axis (HPA) inhibitory potency when applied topically, which gives the drug a high therapeutic index. The mechanism of action for all topical corticosteroids is believed to be a combination of three important properties: anti-inflammatory activity, immunosuppressive properties, and antiproliferative actions.

Usual Dosage

Adolescents:

Topical: Apply sparingly in a thin film twice daily
Intranasal: Initially 1 spray (50 mcg/spray) per nostril once daily. Patients not adequately responding or patients with more severe symptoms may use 2 sprays (200 mcg) per nostril. Depending on response, dosage may be reduced to 100 mcg daily. Total daily dosage should not exceed 4 sprays (200 mcg)/day.

Adults:

Topical: Apply sparingly in a thin film twice daily
Inhalation, Oral:

Recommended Oral Inhalation Doses

Previous Therapy	Recommended Starting Dose	Highest Recommended Dose
Bronchodilator Alone	88 mcg twice daily	440 mcg twice daily
Inhaled Corticosteroids	88–220 mcg twice daily	440 mcg twice daily
Oral Corticosteroids	880 mcg twice daily	880 mcg twice daily

Intranasal: Initial: 2 sprays (50 mcg/spray) per nostril once daily; after the first few days, dosage may be reduced to 1 spray per nostril once daily for maintenance therapy; maximum total daily dose should not exceed 4 sprays (200 mcg)/day

Patient Information A thin film of cream or ointment is effective; do not overuse; do not use tight-fitting diapers or plastic pants on children being treated in the diaper area; use only as prescribed, and for no longer than the period prescribed; apply sparingly in light film; rub in lightly; avoid contact with eyes; notify physician if condition being treated persists or worsens

Dosage Forms

Spray, aerosol, oral inhalation (Flovent®): 44 mcg/actuation (7.9 g = 60 actuations or 13 g = 120 actuations), 110 mcg/actuation (13 g = 120 actuations); 220 mcg/actuation (13 g = 120 actuations)
Spray, intranasal (Flonase™): 50 mcg/actuation (9 g = 60 actuations, 16 g = 120 actuations)
Topical (Cutivate™):
Cream: 0.05% (15 g, 30 g, 60 g)
Ointment: 0.005% (15 g, 60 g)

Fluticasone Propionate *see* Fluticasone *on previous page*

Fluvastatin (FLOO va sta tin)

Related Information

Lipid-Lowering Agents *on page 1413*

Brand Names Lescol®

Therapeutic Category Antilipemic Agent; HMG-CoA Reductase Inhibitor

Use Adjunct to dietary therapy to decrease elevated serum total and LDL cholesterol concentrations in primary hypercholesterolemia

Pregnancy Risk Factor X

Pregnancy/Breast-Feeding Implications Skeletal malformations have occurred in animals following agents with similar structure; avoid use in women of childbearing age; discontinue if pregnancy occurs; avoid use in nursing mothers; avoid use in nursing mothers

Contraindications Myopathy or marked elevations of CPK

Warnings/Precautions Avoid combination of clofibrate and fluvastatin due to possible myopathy; consider temporarily withholding therapy in patients with risk of developing renal failure; avoid prolonged exposure to the sun or other ultraviolet light

Adverse Reactions

1% to 10%:

Central nervous system: Headache, dizziness, insomnia

Dermatologic: Rash

Gastrointestinal: Dyspepsia, diarrhea, nausea, vomiting, constipation, flatulence, abdominal pain

Neuromuscular & skeletal: Back pain, myalgia, arthropathy

Miscellaneous: Cold symptoms

Overdosage/Toxicology No symptomatology has been reported in cases of significant overdosage, however, supportive measure should be instituted, as required; dialyzability is not known

Drug Interactions

Anticoagulant effect of warfarin may be increased

Concurrent use of erythromycin and HMG-CoA reductase inhibitors may result in rhabdomyolysis

Mechanism of Action Acts by competitively inhibiting 3-hydroxyl-3-methylglutaryl-coenzyme A (HMG-CoA) reductase, the enzyme that catalyzes the reduction of HMG-CoA to mevalonate; this is an early rate-limiting step in cholesterol biosynthesis. HDL is increased while total, LDL and VLDL cholesterols, apolipoprotein B, and plasma triglycerides are decreased.

Pharmacodynamics/Kinetics

Protein binding: >98%

Metabolism: Undergoes extensive first pass hepatic extraction; metabolized to inactive and active metabolites although the active forms do not circulate systemically

Bioavailability: Absolute (24%); T_{max}: ≤1 hour

Half-life: 1.2 hours

Elimination: Urine (5%), feces (90%)

Usual Dosage Adults: Oral:

Initial dose: 20 mg at bedtime

Usual dose: 20-40 mg at bedtime

Note: Splitting the 40 mg dose into a twice/daily regimen may provide a modest improvement in LDL response; maximum response occurs within 4-6 weeks; decrease dose and monitor effects carefully in patients with hepatic insufficiency

Administration Place patient on a standard cholesterol-lowering diet before and during treatment; fluvastatin may be taken without regard to meals; adjust dosage as needed in response to periodic lipid determinations during the first 4 weeks after a dosage change; lipid-lowering effects are additive when fluvastatin is combined with a bile-acid binding resin or niacin, however, it must be administered at least 2 hours following these drugs.

Test Interactions Increased serum transaminases, CPK, alkaline phosphatase, and bilirubin and thyroid function tests

Patient Information Avoid prolonged exposure to the sun and other ultraviolet light; report unexplained muscle pain or weakness, especially if accompanied by fever or malaise

Dosage Forms Capsule: 20 mg, 40 mg

Fluvoxamine (floo VOKS ah meen)

Related Information

Antidepressant Agents Comparison *on page 1393*

Brand Names Luvox®

Therapeutic Category Antidepressant, Serotonin Reuptake Inhibitor

Use Approved for the treatment of obsessive-compulsive disorder (OCD); effective in the treatment of major depression; may be useful for the treatment of panic disorder

Pregnancy Risk Factor C

Contraindications Concomitant terfenadine or astemizole; during or within 14 days of MAO inhibitors; hypersensitivity to fluvoxamine or any congeners (eg, fluoxetine)

Warnings/Precautions Use with caution in patients with liver dysfunction, suicidal tendencies, history of seizures, mania, or drug abuse, ECT, cardiovascular disease, and the elderly

Adverse Reactions

>10%: Gastrointestinal: Nausea

(Continued)

Fluvoxamine *(Continued)*

1% to 10%:

Cardiovascular: Palpitations

Central nervous system: Somnolence, headache, insomnia, dizziness, nervousness, mania, hypomania, vertigo, abnormal thinking, agitation, anxiety, malaise, amnesia

Endocrine & metabolic: Decreased libido

Gastrointestinal: Xerostomia, abdominal pain, vomiting, dyspepsia, constipation, diarrhea, abnormal taste, anorexia

Neuromuscular & skeletal: Tremors, weakness

Miscellaneous: Diaphoresis

<1%:

Central nervous system: Seizures

Dermatologic: Toxic epidermal necrolysis

Hematologic: Thrombocytopenia

Hepatic: Hepatic dysfunction

Renal: Increases in serum creatinine

Miscellaneous: Extrapyramidal reactions

Overdosage/Toxicology Symptoms of overdose include drowsiness, nausea, vomiting, abdominal pain, tremors, sinus bradycardia, and seizures

Specific antidote does not exist; treatment is supportive. Although vomiting has not been extensive in overdose to date, patients should be monitored for fluid and electrolyte loss, and appropriate replacement therapy instituted when necessary.

Drug Interactions Because fluvoxamine inhibits cytochrome P-450 isozymes IA2, IIC9, IIIA4, and possibly IID6, it is associated with numerous significant drug interactions

Increased toxicity: Terfenadine and astemizole are both metabolized by the cytochrome P-450 IIIA4 isozyme, increased levels of these drugs have been associated with prolongation of the Q-T interval and potentially fatal, torsade de pointes ventricular arrhythmias. Since fluvoxamine inhibits the enzyme responsible for their clearance, the concomitant use of these agents is contraindicated.

Potentiates triazolam and alprazolam (dose should be reduced by at least 50%), hypertensive crisis with MAO inhibitors, theophylline (doses should be reduced by 1/3 and plasma levels monitored), warfarin (reduce its dose and monitor PT/INR), carbamazepine (monitor levels), tricyclic antidepressants (monitor effects and reduce doses accordingly), methadone, beta-blockers (reduce dose of propranolol or metoprolol), diltiazem. Caution with other benzodiazepines, phenytoin, lithium, clozapine, alcohol, other CNS drugs, quinidine, ketoconazole.

Mechanism of Action Inhibits CNS neuron serotonin uptake; minimal or no effect on reuptake of norepinephrine or dopamine; does not significantly bind to alpha-adrenergic, histamine or cholinergic receptors

Usual Dosage

Adults: Initial: 50 mg at bedtime; adjust in 50 mg increments at 4- to 7-day intervals; usual dose range: 100-300 mg/day; divide total daily dose into 2 doses; administer larger portion at bedtime

Elderly or hepatic impairment: Reduce dose, titrate slowly

Dietary Considerations Alcohol: Additive CNS effect, avoid use

Monitoring Parameters Signs and symptoms of depression, anxiety, weight gain or loss, nutritional intake, sleep

Patient Information Its favorable side effect profile makes it a useful alternative to the traditional agents; use sugarless hard candy for dry mouth; avoid alcoholic beverages, may cause drowsiness; improvement may take several weeks; rise slowly to prevent dizziness. As with all psychoactive drugs, fluvoxamine may impair judgment, thinking, or motor skills, so use caution when operating hazardous machinery, including automobiles, especially early on into therapy. Inform your physician of any concurrent medications you may be taking.

Dosage Forms Tablet: 50 mg, 100 mg

Fluzone® *see* Influenza Virus Vaccine *on page 658*

FML® *see* Fluorometholone *on page 537*

FML® Forte *see* Fluorometholone *on page 537*

Foille® [OTC] *see* Benzocaine *on page 138*

Foille Medicated First Aid® [OTC] *see* Benzocaine *on page 138*

Folacin *see* Folic Acid *on next page*

Folate *see* Folic Acid *on next page*

Folex® PFS *see* Methotrexate *on page 806*

Folic Acid (FOE lik AS id)

Brand Names Folvite®

Canadian/Mexican Brand Names Apo-Folic® (Canada); Flodine® (Canada); Novo-Folacid® (Canada); Dalisol® (Mexico); Folitab® (Mexico); A.F. Valdecasas® (Mexico)

Synonyms Folacin; Folate; Pteroylglutamic Acid

Therapeutic Category Vitamin, Water Soluble

Use Treatment of megaloblastic and macrocytic anemias due to folate deficiency; dietary supplement to prevent neural tube defects

Pregnancy Risk Factor A (C if dose exceeds RDA recommendation)

Contraindications Pernicious, aplastic, or normocytic anemias

Warnings/Precautions Doses <0.1 mg/day may obscure pernicious anemia with continuing irreversible nerve damage progression. Resistance to treatment may occur with depressed hematopoiesis, alcoholism, deficiencies of other vitamins. Injection contains benzyl alcohol (1.5%) as preservative (use care in administration to neonates).

Adverse Reactions

<1%:

Cardiovascular: Slight flushing
Central nervous system: General malaise
Dermatologic: Pruritus, rash
Respiratory: Bronchospasm
Miscellaneous: Allergic reaction

Drug Interactions

Decreased effect: In folate-deficient patients, folic acid therapy may increase **phenytoin** metabolism. **Phenytoin, primidone, para-aminosalicylic acid, and sulfasalazine** may decrease serum folate concentrations and cause deficiency. **Oral contraceptives** may also impair folate metabolism producing depletion, but the effect is unlikely to cause anemia or megaloblastic changes. Concurrent administration of **chloramphenicol** and folic acid may result in antagonism of the hematopoietic response to folic acid.

Stability Incompatible with oxidizing and reducing agents and heavy metal ions

Mechanism of Action Folic acid is necessary for formation of a number of coenzymes in many metabolic systems, particularly for purine and pyrimidine synthesis; required for nucleoprotein synthesis and maintenance in erythropoiesis; stimulates WBC and platelet production in folate deficiency anemia

Pharmacodynamics/Kinetics

Peak effect: Oral: Within 0.5-1 hour
Absorption: In the proximal part of the small intestine

Usual Dosage Oral, I.M., I.V., S.C.:

Infants: 0.1 mg/day

Children: Initial: 1 mg/day
- Deficiency: 0.5-1 mg/day
- Maintenance dose:
  - <4 years: Up to 0.3 mg/day
  - >4 years: 0.4 mg/day

Adults: Initial: 1 mg/day
- Deficiency: 1-3 mg/day
- Maintenance dose: 0.5 mg/day
- Women of childbearing age, pregnant, and lactating women: 0.8 mg/day

Administration Oral, but may also be administered by deep I.M., S.C., or I.V. injection; a diluted solution for oral or for parenteral administration may be prepared by diluting 1 mL of folic acid injection (5 mg/mL), with 49 mL sterile water for injection; resulting solution is 0.1 mg folic acid per 1 mL

Reference Range Therapeutic: 0.005-0.015 μg/mL

Test Interactions Falsely low serum concentrations may occur with the *Lactobacillus casei* assay method in patients on anti-infectives (eg, tetracycline)

Patient Information Take folic acid replacement only under recommendation of physician

Dosage Forms

Injection, as sodium folate: 5 mg/mL (10 mL); 10 mg/mL (10 mL)
- Folvite®: 5 mg/mL (10 mL)

Tablet: 0.1 mg, 0.4 mg, 0.8 mg, 1 mg
- Folvite®: 1 mg

Extemporaneous Preparations A 1 mg/mL folic acid solution may be prepared by crushing fifty 1 mg tablets. Dissolve in a small amount of distilled water, then add sufficient distilled water to make a final volume of 50 mL. Adjust the pH to 8 with sodium hydroxide. It is stable for 42 days at room temperature.

Nahata MC and Hipple TF, *Pediatric Drug Formulations*, Harvey Whitney Books Company, 1992.

Folinic Acid *see* Leucovorin *on page 708*

Follutein® *see* Chorionic Gonadotropin *on page 272*
Folvite® *see* Folic Acid *on previous page*
Formula Q® *see* Quinine *on page 1089*
5-Formyl Tetrahydrofolate *see* Leucovorin *on page 708*
Fortaz® *see* Ceftazidime *on page 232*
Fosamax™ *see* Alendronate *on page 44*

Foscarnet (fos KAR net)

Related Information

Guidelines for the Prevention of Opportunistic Infections in Persons with HIV *on page 1457*

Brand Names Foscavir®

Synonyms PFA; Phosphonoformate; Phosphonoformic Acid

Therapeutic Category Antiviral Agent, Parenteral

Use Approved indications in adult patients:

Herpesvirus infections suspected to be caused by acyclovir (HSV, VZV) or ganciclovir (CMV) resistant strains (this occurs almost exclusively in immunocompromised persons with immunocompromised (eg, advanced AIDS), who have received prolonged treatment for a herpesvirus infection)

CMV retinitis in persons with AIDS

Other CMV infections in persons unable to tolerate ganciclovir

Pregnancy Risk Factor C

Contraindications Hypersensitivity to foscarnet, Cl_{cr} <0.4 mL/minute/kg during therapy

Warnings/Precautions Renal impairment occurs to some degree in the majority of patients treated with foscarnet; renal impairment may occur at any time and is usually reversible within 1 week following dose adjustment or discontinuation of therapy, however, several patients have died with renal failure within 4 weeks of stopping foscarnet; therefore, renal function should be closely monitored. Foscarnet is deposited in teeth and bone of young, growing animals; it has adversely affected tooth enamel development in rats; safety and effectiveness in children have not been studied. Imbalance of serum electrolytes or minerals occurs in 6% to 18% of patients (hypocalcemia, low ionized calcium, hypo- or hyperphosphatemia, hypomagnesemia or hypokalemia). Patients with a low ionized calcium may experience perioral tingling, numbness, paresthesias, tetany, and seizures. Seizures have been experienced by up to 10% of AIDS patients. Risk factors for seizures include a low baseline absolute neutrophil count (ANC), impaired baseline renal function and low total serum calcium. Some patients who have experienced seizures have died, while others have been able to continue or resume foscarnet treatment after their mineral or electrolyte abnormality has been corrected, their underlying disease state treated, or their dose decreased. Foscarnet has been shown to be mutagenic *in vitro* and in mice at very high doses. Information on the use of foscarnet is lacking in the elderly; dose adjustments and proper monitoring must be performed because of the decreased renal function common in older patients.

Adverse Reactions

>10%:

- Central nervous system: Fever, headache, seizures
- Gastrointestinal: Nausea, diarrhea, vomiting
- Hematologic: Anemia
- Renal: Abnormal renal function, decreased creatinine clearance

1% to 10%:

- Central nervous system: Fatigue, malaise, dizziness, hypoesthesia, depression, confusion, anxiety
- Dermatologic: Rash
- Endocrine & metabolic: Electrolyte imbalance
- Gastrointestinal: Anorexia
- Hematologic: Granulocytopenia, leukopenia
- Local: Injection site pain
- Neuromuscular & skeletal: Paresthesia, involuntary muscle contractions, rigors, neuropathy (peripheral), weakness
- Ocular: Vision abnormalities
- Respiratory: Coughing, dyspnea
- Miscellaneous: Sepsis, diaphoresis (increased)

<1%:

- Cardiovascular: Cardiac failure, bradycardia, arrhythmias, cerebral edema, leg edema, peripheral edema, syncope, substernal chest pain
- Central nervous system: Hypothermia, abnormal crying, malignant hyperpyrexia, vertigo, coma, speech disorders
- Endocrine & metabolic: Gynecomastia, decreased gonadotropins
- Hepatic: Cholecystitis, cholelithiasis, hepatitis, hepatosplenomegaly, ascites
- Neuromuscular & skeletal: Abnormal gait, dyskinesia, hypertonia
- Ocular: Nystagmus

Miscellaneous: Vocal cord paralysis

Overdosage/Toxicology Symptoms of overdose include seizures, renal dysfunction, perioral or limb paresthesias, hypocalcemia; treatment is supportive; I.V. calcium salts for hypocalcemia

Drug Interactions Increased toxicity: Pentamidine increases hypocalcemia; concurrent use with ciprofloxacin increases seizure potential; acute renal failure (reversible) has been reported with cyclosporin due most likely to toxic synergistic effect

Stability

Foscarnet injection is a clear, colorless solution; it should be stored at room temperature and protected from temperatures >40°C and from freezing

Foscarnet should be diluted in D_5W or NS and transferred to PVC containers; stable for 24 hours at room temperature or refrigeration

For peripheral line administration, foscarnet **must** be diluted to 12 mg/mL with D_5W or NS

For central line administration, foscarnet may be administered undiluted

Incompatible with dextrose 30%, I.V. solutions containing calcium, magnesium, vancomycin, TPN

Mechanism of Action Pyrophosphate analogue which acts as a noncompetitive inhibitor of many viral RNA and DNA polymerases as well as HIV reverse transcriptase. Inhibitory effects occur at concentrations which do not affect host cellular DNA polymerases; however, some human cell growth suppression has been observed with high *in vitro* concentrations. Similar to ganciclovir, foscarnet is a virostatic agent. Foscarnet does not require activation by thymidine kinase.

Pharmacodynamics/Kinetics

Absorption: Oral: Poorly absorbed; I.V. therapy is needed for the treatment of viral infections in AIDS patients

Distribution: Up to 28% of cumulative I.V. dose may be deposited in bone

Metabolism: Biotransformation does not occur

Half-life: ~3 hours

Elimination: Up to 28% excreted unchanged in urine

Usual Dosage

Adolescents and Adults: I.V.:

CMV retinitis:

Induction treatment: 60 mg/kg/dose every 8 hours for 14-21 days

Dose Adjustment for Renal Impairment

The induction dose of foscarnet should be adjusted according to creatinine clearance as follows:

Creatinine Clearance (mL/min/kg)	Foscarnet Induction Dose (mg/kg)
1.6	60 q8h
1.5	57 q8h
1.4	53 q8h
1.3	49 q8h
1.2	46 q8h
1.1	42 q8h
1	39 q12h
0.9	35 q12h
0.8	32 q12h
0.7	28 q12h
0.6	25 q24h
0.5	21 q24h
0.4	18 q24h
<0.4	Not recommended

The maintenance dose of foscarnet should be adjusted according to creatinine clearance as follows:

Creatinine Clearance (mL/min/kg)	Foscarnet Maintenance Dose (mg/kg)
1.4	90-120 q24h
1.2-1.4	78-104 q24h
1-1.2	75-100 q24h
0.8-1	71-94 q24h
0.6-0.8	63-84 q48h
0.4-0.6	57-75 q48h
<0.4	Not recommended

(Continued)

Foscarnet *(Continued)*

Maintenance therapy: 90-120 mg/kg/day as a single infusion

Acyclovir-resistant HSV induction treatment: 40 mg/kg/dose every 8-12 hours for 14-21 days

See table.

Administration

Foscarnet is administered by intravenous infusion, using an infusion pump, at a rate not exceeding 1 mg/kg/minute

Adult induction doses of 60 mg/kg are administered over 1 hour

Adult maintenance doses of 90-120 mg/kg are infused over 2 hours

Undiluted (24 mg/mL) solution can be administered without further dilution when using a central venous catheter for infusion

For peripheral vein administration, the solution **must** be diluted to a final concentration **not to exceed** 12 mg/mL

The recommended dosage, frequency, and rate of infusion should not be exceeded

Patient Information Close monitoring is important and any symptom of electrolyte abnormalities should be reported immediately; maintain adequate fluid intake and hydration; regular ophthalmic examinations are necessary. Foscarnet is not a cure; disease progression may occur during or following treatment. Report any numbness in the extremities, paresthesias, or perioral tingling.

Dosage Forms Injection: 24 mg/mL (250 mL, 500 mL)

Foscavir® *see* Foscarnet *on page 554*

Fosfomycin (fos foe MYE sin)

Brand Names Monurol®

Synonyms Fosfomycin Tromethamine

Therapeutic Category Antibiotic, Miscellaneous

Use As a single oral dose in the treatment of uncomplicated urinary tract infections in women; multiple doses have been investigated for complicated UTIs in men; may have an advantage over other agents since it maintains high concentration in the urine for up to 48 hours

Pregnancy Risk Factor B

Pregnancy/Breast-Feeding Implications Milk concentration approximates 10% of plasma

Adverse Reactions

>1%:

- Central nervous system: Headache
- Dermatologic: Rash
- Gastrointestinal: Diarrhea (2% to 8%), nausea, vomiting, epigastric discomfort, anorexia

<1%:

- Central nervous system: Dizziness, drowsiness, fatigue
- Dermatologic: Pruritus

Drug Interactions Decreased effect: Food decreases absorption significantly; antacids or calcium salts may cause precipitate formation and decrease fosfomycin absorption

Mechanism of Action As a phosphonic acid derivative, fosfomycin inhibits bacterial wall synthesis (bactericidal) by inactivating the enzyme, pyruvyl transferase, which is critical in the synthesis of cell walls by bacteria; the tromethamine salt is preferable to the calcium salt due to its superior absorption; many gram-positive and gram-negative organisms are inhibited staphylococci, pneumococci, *E. coli, Salmonella, Shigella, H. influenzae, Neisseria* spp, and some strains of *P. aeruginosa*, indole-negative *Proteus*, and *Providencia*; *B. fragilis*, and anaerobic g (-) cocci are resistant; *in vitro* synergism occurs with penicillins, cephalosporins, aminoglycosides, erythromycin, and tetracyclines

Pharmacodynamics/Kinetics

Absorption: Well absorbed

Distribution: V_d: 2 L/kg; high concentrations in urine; distributed well into other tissues, crosses maximally into CSF with inflamed meninges

Protein binding: Minimal (<3%)

Metabolism: None

Bioavailability: 34% to 58%

Half-life: 4-8 hours; prolonged in renal failure (50 hours with Cl_{cr} <10 mL/minute)

Time to peak serum concentration: 2 hours

Elimination: High urinary levels persist for >48 hours (100 mcg/mL); excreted unchanged

Usual Dosage Adults: Urinary tract infections: Oral:

Female: Single dose of 3 g in 4 oz of water

Male: 3 g once daily for 2-3 days for complicated urinary tract infections

Dosing adjustment in renal impairment: Decrease dose; 80% removed by dialysis, repeat dose after dialysis

Dosing adjustment in hepatic impairment: No dosage decrease needed

Administration Always mix with water before ingesting; do not administer in its dry form; pour contents of envelope into 90-120 mL of water (not hot), stir to dissolve and take immediately

Monitoring Parameters Signs and symptoms of urinary tract infection

Patient Information May be taken with or without food; avoid use of antacids or calcium salts within 4 hours before or 2 hours after taking fosfomycin; contact your physician if signs of allergy develop; if symptoms do not improve after 2-3 days, contact your health care provider

Dosage Forms Powder, as tromethamine: 3 g, to be mixed in 4 oz of water

Fosfomycin Tromethamine *see* Fosfomycin *on previous page*

Fosinopril (foe SIN oh pril)

Related Information

Angiotensin-Converting Enzyme Inhibitors Comparison *on page 1386*

Heart Failure: Management of Patients With Left-Ventricular Systolic Dysfunction *on page 1533*

Brand Names Monopril®

Therapeutic Category Angiotensin-Converting Enzyme (ACE) Inhibitors; Antihypertensive

Use Treatment of hypertension, either alone or in combination with other antihypertensive agents; congestive heart failure; believed to prolong survival in heart failure

Pregnancy Risk Factor C (first trimester); D (second and third trimester)

Contraindications Renal impairment, collagen vascular disease, hypersensitivity to fosinopril, any component, or other angiotensin-converting enzyme inhibitors

Warnings/Precautions Use with caution and modify dosage in patients with renal impairment (decrease dosage) (especially renal artery stenosis), severe congestive heart failure or with coadministered diuretic therapy; experience in children is limited. Severe hypotension may occur in patients who are sodium and/or volume depleted; initiate lower doses and monitor closely when starting therapy in these patients.

Adverse Reactions

1% to 10%:

Cardiovascular: Orthostatic hypotension

Central nervous system: Headache, dizziness, fatigue

Endocrine & metabolic: Sexual dysfunction

Gastrointestinal: Diarrhea, nausea, vomiting

Respiratory: Cough

<1%:

Cardiovascular: Syncope

Central nervous system: Vertigo, insomnia

Dermatologic: Angioedema, rash

Endocrine & metabolic: Hypoglycemia, hyperkalemia

Gastrointestinal: Abnormal taste

Genitourinary: Impotence

Hematologic: Neutropenia, agranulocytosis, anemia

Neuromuscular & skeletal: Muscle cramps

Renal: Deterioration in renal function

Overdosage/Toxicology Mild hypotension has been the only toxic effect seen with acute overdose. Bradycardia may also occur; hyperkalemia occurs even with therapeutic doses, especially in patients with renal insufficiency and those taking NSAIDs

Following initiation of essential overdose management, toxic symptom treatment and supportive treatment should be initiated. Hypotension usually responds to I.V. fluids or Trendelenburg positioning.

Drug Interactions

Increased toxicity:

Probenecid increases blood levels of captopril

Captopril and diuretics have additive hypotensive effects; see table.

Mechanism of Action Competitive inhibitor of angiotensin-converting enzyme (ACE); prevents conversion of angiotensin I to angiotensin II, a potent vasoconstrictor; results in lower levels of angiotensin II which causes an increase in plasma renin activity and a reduction in aldosterone secretion; a CNS mechanism may also be involved in hypotensive effect as angiotensin II increases adrenergic outflow from CNS; vasoactive kallikreins may be decreased in conversion to active hormones by ACE inhibitors, thus reducing blood pressure

(Continued)

Fosinopril *(Continued)*

Drug-Drug Interactions With ACEIs

Precipitant Drug	Drug (Category) and Effect	Description
Antacids	ACE Inhibitors: decreased	Decreased bioavailability of ACEIs. May be more likely with captopril. Separate administration times by 1-2 hours.
NSAIDs (indomethacin)	ACEIs: decreased	Reduced hypotensive effects of ACEIs. More prominent in low renin or volume dependent hypertensive patients.
Phenothiazines	ACEIs: increased	Pharmacologic effects of ACEIs may be increased.
ACEIs	Allopurinol: increased	Higher risk of hypersensitivity reaction possible when given concurrently. Three case reports of Stevens-Johnson syndrome with captopril.
ACEIs	Digoxin: increased	Increased plasma digoxin levels.
ACEIs	Lithium: increased	Increased serum lithium levels and symptoms of toxicity may occur.
ACEIs	Potassium preps/ potassium sparing diuretics increased	Coadministration may result in elevated potassium levels.

Pharmacodynamics/Kinetics

Absorption: 36%

Metabolism: Fosinopril is a prodrug and is hydrolyzed to its active metabolite fosinoprilat by intestinal wall and hepatic esterases

Half-life, serum (fosinoprilat): 12 hours

Time to peak serum concentration: ~3 hours

Elimination: In the urine and bile as fosinoprilat and it conjugates in roughly equal proportions (45% to 50%)

Usual Dosage Adults: Oral:

Hypertension: Initial: 10 mg/day; increase to a maximum dose of 80 mg/day; most patients are maintained on 20-40 mg/day; may need to divide the dose into two if trough effect is inadequate; discontinue the diuretic, if possible 2-3 days before initiation of therapy; resume diuretic therapy carefully, if needed.

Heart failure: Initial: 10 mg/day (5 mg if renal dysfunction present) and increase, as needed, to a maximum of 40 mg once daily over several weeks; usual dose: 20-40 mg/day; if hypotension, orthostasis, or azotemia occur during titration, consider decreasing concomitant diuretic dose, if any

Dosing adjustment/comments in renal impairment: None needed since hepatobiliary elimination compensates adequately diminished renal elimination

Hemodialysis: Moderately dialyzable (20% to 50%)

Monitoring Parameters Blood pressure (supervise for at least 2 hours after the initial dose or any increase for significant orthostasis); serum potassium, calcium, creatinine, BUN, WBC

Test Interactions Positive Coombs' [direct]; may cause false-positive results in urine acetone determinations using sodium nitroprusside reagent

Patient Information Notify physician if vomiting, diarrhea, excessive perspiration, or dehydration should occur; also if swelling of face, lips, tongue, or difficulty in breathing occurs or if persistent cough develops; may be taken with meals; do not stop therapy or add a potassium salt replacement without physician's advice

Nursing Implications May cause depression in some patients; discontinue if angioedema of the face, extremities, lips, tongue, or glottis occurs; watch for hypotensive effects within 1-3 hours of first dose or new higher dose

Dosage Forms Tablet: 10 mg, 20 mg

Fosphenytoin (FOS fen i toyn)

Synonyms Fosphenytoin Sodium; 3-Phosphoryloxymethyl Phenytoin Disodium

Therapeutic Category Anticonvulsant, Hydantoin

Use Indicated for short-term parenteral administration when other means of phenytoin administration are unavailable, inappropriate or deemed less advantageous; the safety and effectiveness of fosphenytoin in this use has not been systematically evaluated for more than 5 days; may be used for the control of generalized convulsive status epilepticus and prevention and treatment of seizures occurring during neurosurgery

Pregnancy Risk Factor D

Pregnancy/Breast-Feeding Implications Distributes into breast milk; crosses placenta with fetal serum concentrations equal to those of mother; eye, cardiac, cleft palate, and skeletal malformations have been noted; fetal hydantoin syndrome associated with maternal ingestion of 100-800 mg/kg during 1st trimester

Contraindications Hypersensitivity to phenytoin or fosphenytoin; occurrence of any rash while on treatment; the drug should not be resumed if rash is exfoliative, purpuric, or bullous; not recommended for use in children <4 years of age

Warnings/Precautions Use with caution in patients with severe cardiovascular, hepatic, renal disease or diabetes mellitus; avoid abrupt discontinuation; dosing should be slowly reduced to avoid precipitation of seizures; increased toxicity with nephrotic syndrome patient; may increase frequency of petit mal seizures; use with caution in patients with porphyria, fever, or hypothyroidism

Adverse Reactions

Cardiovascular: Facial edema

Central nervous system: Slurred speech, dizziness, drowsiness, choreoathetosis, fever, visual hallucinations

Dermatologic: Rash, exfoliative dermatitis, erythema multiforme, acne

Endocrine & metabolic: Folic acid depletion, osteomalacia, hyperglycemia, reduced plasma testosterone, gynecomastia

Gastrointestinal: Nausea, vomiting, gingival hyperplasia

Genitourinary: Priapism

Hematologic: Lymphadenopathy, neutropenia, thrombocytopenia, anemia (megaloblastic)

Local: Pain on injection; due to the fact that fosphenytoin is water soluble and has a lower pH (8.8) than phenytoin (12), necrosis or irritation at injection site is reduced

Neuromuscular & skeletal: Sensory paresthesia (long-term treatment)

Ocular: Nystagmus, blurred vision, diplopia

Renal: Nephrotic syndrome

Overdosage/Toxicology Signs and symptoms of toxicity include unsteady gait, tremors, hyperglycemia, chorea (extrapyramidal), gingival hyperplasia, gynecomastia, myoglobinuria, nephrotic syndrome, slurred speech, mydriasis, myoclonus, confusion, encephalopathy, hyperthermia, drowsiness, nausea, hypothermia, fever, hypotension, respiratory depression, leukopenia; neutropenia; agranulocytosis; granulocytopenia; hyperreflexia, coma, systemic lupus erythematosus (SLE), ophthalmoplegia

Treatment is supportive for hypotension; treat with I.V. fluids and place patient in Trendelenburg position; seizures may be controlled with lorazepam or diazepam 5-10 mg (0.25-0.4 mg/kg in children); intravenous albumin (25 g every 6 hours has been used to increase bound fraction of drug). Multiple dosing of activated charcoal may be effective; peritoneal dialysis, diuresis, hemodialysis, hemoperfusion, and plasmapheresis is of little value

Drug Interactions No drug interaction noted with diazepam

Stability Refrigerated vials are stable for 2 years; at room temperature, stable for 3 months; I.V. solutions are stable for one day when refrigerated

Compatible with all diluents and does not require propylene glycol or ethanol for solubility

Mechanism of Action Diphosphate ester salt of phenytoin which acts as a water soluble pro-drug of phenytoin; after administration, plasma esterases convert fosphenytoin to phosphate, formaldehyde and phenytoin as the active moiety; phenytoin works by stabilizing neuronal membranes and decreasing seizure activity by increasing efflux or decreasing influx of sodium ions across cell membranes in the motor cortex during generation of nerve impulses

Usual Dosage The dose, concentration in solutions, and infusion rates for fosphenytoin are expressed as phenytoin sodium equivalents; fosphenytoin should always be prescribed and dispensed in phenytoin sodium equivalents

Status epilepticus: I.V.: Adults: Loading dose: Phenytoin equivalent: 15-20 mg/kg I.V. administered at 100-150 mg/minute

Nonemergent loading and maintenance dosing: I.V. or I.M.: Adults:

Loading dose: Phenytoin equivalent: 10-20 mg/kg I.V. or I.M. (maximum I.V. rate: 150 mg/minute)

Initial daily maintenance dose: Phenytoin equivalent: 4-6 mg/kg/day I.V. or I.M.

I.M. or I.V. substitution for oral phenytoin therapy: May be substituted for oral phenytoin sodium at the same total daily dose, however, Dilantin® capsules are ~90% bioavailable by the oral route; phenytoin, supplied as fosphenytoin, is 100% bioavailable by both the I.M. and I.V. routes; for this reason, plasma phenytoin concentrations may increase when I.M. or I.V. fosphenytoin is substituted for oral phenytoin sodium therapy; in clinical trials I.M. fosphenytoin was administered as a single daily dose utilizing either 1 or 2 injection sites; some patients may require more frequent dosing

Dosing adjustments in renal/hepatic impairment: Phenytoin clearance may be substantially reduced in cirrhosis and plasma level monitoring with dose adjustment advisable; free phenytoin levels should be monitored closely in patients with renal or hepatic disease or in those with hypoalbuminemia;

(Continued)

Fosphenytoin *(Continued)*

furthermore, fosphenytoin clearance to phenytoin may be increased without a similar increase in phenytoin in these patients leading to increase frequency and severity of adverse events

Administration Since there is no precipitation problem with fosphenytoin, no I.V. filter is required

Monitoring Parameters Blood pressure, vital signs (with I.V. use), plasma level monitoring, CBC, liver function tests

Reference Range

Therapeutic: 10-20 μg/mL (SI: 40-79 μmol/L); toxicity is measured clinically, and some patients require levels outside the suggested therapeutic range

Toxic: 30-50 μg/mL (SI: 120-200 μmol/L)

Lethal: >100 μg/mL (SI: >400 μmol/L)

Manifestations of toxicity:

Nystagmus: 20 μg/mL (SI: 79 μmol/L)

Ataxia: 30 μg/mL (SI: 118.9 μmol/L)

Decreased mental status: 40 μg/mL (SI: 159 μmol/L)

Coma: 50 μg/mL (SI: 200 μmol/L)

Peak serum phenytoin level after a 375 mg I.M. fosphenytoin dose in healthy males: 5.7 μg/mL

Peak serum fosphenytoin levels and phenytoin levels after a 1.2 g infusion (I.V.) in healthy subjects over 30 minutes were 129 μg/mL and 17.2 μg/mL respectively

Test Interactions Increases glucose, alkaline phosphatase (S); decreases thyroxine (S), calcium (S); serum sodium increases in overdose setting

Nursing Implications I.V. injections should be followed by normal saline flushes through the same needle or I.V. catheter to avoid local irritation of the vein; must be diluted to concentrations <6 mg/mL, in normal saline, for I.V. infusion

Additional Information 1.5 mg fosphenytoin is approximately equivalent to 1 mg phenytoin; equimolar fosphenytoin dose is 375 mg (75 mg/mL solution) to phenytoin 250 mg (50 mg/mL)

Water solubility: 142 mg/mL at pH of 9

Antiarrhythmic effects may be similar to phenytoin; parenteral product contains no propylene sterol; this should allow for rapid intravenous bolus dosing without cardiovascular complications; formaldehyde production is not expected to be clinically consequential (about 200 mg) if used for one week

Dosage Forms Injection, as sodium: 150 mg [equivalent to phenytoin sodium 100 mg] in 2 mL vials; 750 mg [equivalent to phenytoin sodium 500 mg] in 10 mL vials

Fosphenytoin Sodium *see* Fosphenytoin *on page 558*
Fostex® 10% BPO Gel [OTC] *see* Benzoyl Peroxide *on page 140*
Fostex® 10% Wash [OTC] *see* Benzoyl Peroxide *on page 140*
Fostex® Bar [OTC] *see* Benzoyl Peroxide *on page 140*
Fragmin® *see* Dalteparin *on page 339*
Freezone® Solution [OTC] *see* Salicylic Acid *on page 1120*
Frusemide *see* Furosemide *on next page*
FS Shampoo® *see* Fluocinolone *on page 533*
5-FU *see* Fluorouracil *on page 538*
Ful-Glo® *see* Fluorescein Sodium *on page 535*
Fulvicin® P/G *see* Griseofulvin *on page 587*
Fulvicin-U/F® *see* Griseofulvin *on page 587*
Fumasorb® [OTC] *see* Ferrous Fumarate *on page 513*
Fumerin® [OTC] *see* Ferrous Fumarate *on page 513*
Funduscein® *see* Fluorescein Sodium *on page 535*
Fungizone® *see* Amphotericin B *on page 81*
Fungoid® Creme *see* Miconazole *on page 834*
Fungoid® Tincture *see* Miconazole *on page 834*
Furacin® *see* Nitrofurazone *on page 908*
Furadantin® *see* Nitrofurantoin *on page 907*
Furalan® *see* Nitrofurantoin *on page 907*
Furan® *see* Nitrofurantoin *on page 907*
Furanite® *see* Nitrofurantoin *on page 907*

Furazolidone (fyoor a ZOE li done)

Brand Names Furoxone®

Canadian/Mexican Brand Names Furoxona® Gotas (Mexico); Furoxona® Tabletas (Mexico); Fuxol® (Mexico)

Therapeutic Category Antibiotic, Miscellaneous; Antidiarrheal; Antiprotozoal

Use Treatment of bacterial or protozoal diarrhea and enteritis caused by susceptible organisms *Giardia lamblia* and *Vibrio cholerae*

Pregnancy Risk Factor C

Contraindications Known hypersensitivity to furazolidone; concurrent use of alcohol; patients <1 month of age because of the possibility of producing hemolytic anemia

Warnings/Precautions Use caution in patients with G-6-PD deficiency when administering large doses for prolonged periods; furazolidone inhibits monoamine oxidase

Adverse Reactions

>10%: Genitourinary: Discoloration of urine (dark yellow to brown)

1% to 10%:

- Central nervous system: Headache
- Gastrointestinal: Abdominal pain, diarrhea, nausea, vomiting

<1%:

- Cardiovascular: Orthostatic hypotension
- Central nervous system: Fever, dizziness, drowsiness, malaise
- Dermatologic: Rash
- Endocrine & metabolic: Hypoglycemia, disulfiram-like reaction after alcohol ingestion, leukopenia
- Hematologic: Agranulocytosis, hemolysis in patients with G-6-PD deficiency
- Neuromuscular & skeletal: Arthralgia

Overdosage/Toxicology Symptoms of overdose include nausea, vomiting, serotonin crisis; treatment is supportive care only; serotonin crisis may require dantrolene/bromocriptine

Drug Interactions

Increased effect with sympathomimetic amines, tricyclic antidepressants, tyramine-containing foods, MAO inhibitors, meperidine, anorexiants, dextromethorphan, fluoxetine, paroxetine, sertraline, trazodone

Increased effect/toxicity of levodopa

Disulfiram-like reaction with alcohol

Mechanism of Action Inhibits several vital enzymatic reactions causing antibacterial and antiprotozoal action

Pharmacodynamics/Kinetics

Absorption: Oral: Poor

Elimination: Oral: ⅓ of dose is excreted in urine as active drug and metabolites

Usual Dosage Oral:

Children >1 month: 5-8 mg/kg/day in 4 divided doses for 7 days, not to exceed 400 mg/day or 8.8 mg/kg/day

Adults: 100 mg 4 times/day for 7 days

Dietary Considerations

Alcohol: Avoid use

Food: Avoid tyramine-containing foods

Test Interactions False-positive results for urine glucose with Clinitest®

Patient Information May discolor urine to a brown tint; avoid drinking alcohol during or for 4 days after therapy or eating tyramine-containing foods; consult with physician or pharmacist for a list of these foods. Do not take any prescription or nonprescription drugs without consulting the physician or pharmacist; if result not achieved at the end of treatment contact physician.

Dosage Forms

Liquid: 50 mg/15 mL (60 mL, 473 mL)

Tablet: 100 mg

Furazosin *see* Prazosin *on page 1036*

Furosemide (fyoor OH se mide)

Related Information

Adult ACLS Algorithm, Hypotension, Shock *on page 1516*

Cardiovascular Agents Comparison *on page 1405*

Heart Failure: Management of Patients With Left-Ventricular Systolic Dysfunction *on page 1533*

Sulfonamide Derivatives *on page 1420*

Brand Names Lasix®

Canadian/Mexican Brand Names Apo-Furosemide® (Canada); Furoside® (Canada); Novo-Semide® (Canada); Uritol® (Canada); Edenol® (Mexico); Henexal® (Mexico)

Synonyms Frusemide

Therapeutic Category Antihypertensive; Diuretic, Loop

Use Management of edema associated with congestive heart failure and hepatic or renal disease; used alone or in combination with antihypertensives in treatment of hypertension

Pregnancy Risk Factor C

(Continued)

Furosemide *(Continued)*

Pregnancy/Breast-Feeding Implications

Clinical effects on the fetus: Crosses the placenta. Increased fetal urine production, electrolyte disturbances reported. Generally, use of diuretics during pregnancy is avoided due to risk of decreased placental perfusion.

Breast-feeding/Lactation: Crosses into breast milk

Clinical effects on the infant: May suppress lactation. American Academy of Pediatrics has NO RECOMMENDATION.

Contraindications Hypersensitivity to furosemide, any component, or other sulfonamides

Warnings/Precautions Loop diuretics are potent diuretics; close medical supervision and dose evaluation is required to prevent fluid and electrolyte imbalance; use caution with other nephrotoxic or ototoxic drugs

Adverse Reactions

>10%:

- Cardiovascular: Orthostatic hypotension
- Central nervous system: Dizziness

1% to 10%:

- Central nervous system: Headache
- Dermatologic: Photosensitivity
- Endocrine & metabolic: Electrolyte imbalance (hypokalemia, hyponatremia, hypochloremia, hypercalciuria, hyperuricemia), alkalosis, dehydration
- Gastrointestinal: Diarrhea, loss of appetite, stomach cramps or pain
- Ocular: Blurred vision

<1%:

- Dermatologic: Rash
- Gastrointestinal: Pancreatitis, nausea
- Hepatic: Hepatic dysfunction
- Hematologic: Agranulocytosis, leukopenia, anemia, thrombocytopenia
- Local: Redness at injection site
- Neuromuscular & skeletal: Gout
- Ocular: Xanthopsia
- Otic: Ototoxicity
- Renal: Nephrocalcinosis, interstitial nephritis, prerenal azotemia

Overdosage/Toxicology Symptoms of overdose include electrolyte depletion, volume depletion, hypotension, dehydration, circulatory collapse

Following GI decontamination, treatment is supportive; hypotension responds to fluids and Trendelenburg position

Drug Interactions

Decreased effect:

- Furosemide interferes with hypoglycemic effect of antidiabetic agents; decreased furosemide concentrations with metformin have been observed
- Indomethacin may reduce natriuretic and hypotensive effects of furosemide

Increased effect: Effects of antihypertensive agents may be enhanced

Increased toxicity:

- Lithium → renal clearance decreased; furosemide may increase toxicity of metformin
- Concomitant use of furosemide with aminoglycoside antibiotics or other ototoxic drugs should be avoided

Stability

Furosemide injection should be stored at controlled room temperature and protected from light

Exposure to light may cause discoloration; do not use furosemide solutions if they have a yellow color

Refrigeration may result in precipitation or crystallization, however, resolubilization at room temperature or warming may be performed without affecting the drugs stability

Furosemide solutions are unstable in acidic media but very stable in basic media

I.V. infusion solution mixed in NS or D_5W solution is stable for 24 hours at room temperature

Mechanism of Action Inhibits reabsorption of sodium and chloride in the ascending loop of Henle and distal renal tubule, interfering with the chloride-binding cotransport system, thus causing increased excretion of water, sodium, chloride, magnesium, and calcium

Pharmacodynamics/Kinetics

Onset of diuresis:

- Oral: Within 30-60 minutes
- I.M.: 30 minutes
- I.V.: Within 5 minutes

Peak effect: Oral: Within 1-2 hours

Duration:

- Oral: 6-8 hours

I.V.: 2 hours

Absorption: Oral: 60% to 67%

Protein binding: >98%

Half-life:

Normal renal function: 0.5-1.1 hours

End stage renal disease: 9 hours

Elimination: 50% of an oral or 80% of an I.V. dose is excreted in the urine within 24 hours; the remainder is eliminated by other nonrenal pathways, including liver metabolism and excretion of unchanged drug in the feces

Usual Dosage

Infants and Children:

Oral: 1-2 mg/kg/dose increased in increments of 1 mg/kg/dose with each succeeding dose until a satisfactory effect is achieved to a maximum of 6 mg/kg/dose no more frequently than 6 hours

I.M., I.V.: 1 mg/kg/dose, increasing by each succeeding dose at 1 mg/kg/dose at intervals of 6-12 hours until a satisfactory response up to 6 mg/kg/dose

Adults:

Oral: 20-80 mg/dose initially increased in increments of 20-40 mg/dose at intervals of 6-8 hours; usual maintenance dose interval is twice daily or every day

I.M., I.V.: 20-40 mg/dose, may be repeated in 1-2 hours as needed and increased by 20 mg/dose with each succeeding dose up to 1000 mg/day; usual dosing interval: 6-12 hours

Continuous I.V. infusion: Initial I.V. bolus dose of 0.1 mg/kg followed by continuous I.V. infusion doses of 0.1 mg/kg/hour doubled every 2 hours to a maximum of 0.4 mg/kg/hour if urine output is <1 mL/kg/hour have been found to be effective and result in a lower daily requirement of furosemide than with intermittent dosing. Other studies have used 20-160 mg/hour continuous I.V. infusion

Elderly: Oral, I.M., I.V.: Initial: 20 mg/day; increase slowly to desired response

Dosing adjustment/comments in renal impairment: Acute renal failure: Doses up to 100 mg/day may be necessary to initiate desired response; avoid use in oliguric states

Dialysis: Not removed by hemo- or peritoneal dialysis; supplemental dose is not necessary

Dosing adjustment/comments in hepatic disease: Diminished natriuretic effect with increased sensitivity to hypokalemia and volume depletion in cirrhosis; monitor effects, particularly with high doses

Administration I.V. injections should be given slowly over 1-2 minutes; maximum rate of administration for IVPB or infusion: 4 mg/minute; replace parenteral therapy with oral therapy as soon as possible

Monitoring Parameters Monitor weight and I & O daily; blood pressure, serum electrolytes, renal function; in high doses, monitor hearing

Patient Information May be taken with food or milk; rise slowly from a lying or sitting position to minimize dizziness, lightheadedness, or fainting; also use extra care when exercising, standing for long periods of time, and during hot weather; take last dose of day early in the evening to prevent nocturia

Additional Information Sodium content of 1 mL (injection): 0.162 mEq

Dosage Forms

Injection: 10 mg/mL (2 mL, 4 mL, 5 mL, 6 mL, 8 mL, 10 mL, 12 mL)

Solution, oral: 10 mg/mL (60 mL, 120 mL); 40 mg/5 mL (5 mL, 10 mL, 500 mL)

Tablet: 20 mg, 40 mg, 80 mg

Furoxone® *see* Furazolidone *on page 560*

G-1® *see* Butalbital Compound *on page 176*

Gabapentin (GA ba pen tin)

Related Information

Anticonvulsants by Seizure Type *on page 1392*

Epilepsy Treatment *on page 1531*

Brand Names Neurontin®

Therapeutic Category Anticonvulsant

Use Adjunct for treatment of drug-refractory partial and secondarily generalized seizures in adults with epilepsy; not effective for absence seizures

Pregnancy Risk Factor C

Pregnancy/Breast-Feeding Implications

Clinical effects on the fetus: No data on crossing the placenta; 4 reports of normal pregnancy outcomes; 1 report of infant with respiratory distress, pyloric stenosis, inguinal hernia following 1st trimester exposure to gabapentin plus carbamazepine; epilepsy itself, number of medications, genetic factors, or a combination of these probably influence the teratogenicity of anticonvulsant therapy

Breast-feeding/lactation: No data available

(Continued)

Gabapentin *(Continued)*

Contraindications Hypersensitivity to the drug or its ingredients

Warnings/Precautions Avoid abrupt withdrawal, may precipitate seizures; may be associated with a slight incidence (0.6%) of status epilepticus and sudden deaths (0.0038 deaths/patient year); use cautiously in patients with severe renal dysfunction; rat studies demonstrated an association with pancreatic adenocarcinoma in male rats; clinical implication unknown

Adverse Reactions

>10%: Central nervous system: Somnolence, dizziness, ataxia, fatigue

1% to 10%:

- Cardiovascular: Peripheral edema
- Central nervous system: Nervousness, amnesia, depression, anxiety, abnormal coordination
- Dermatologic: Pruritus
- Gastrointestinal: Dyspepsia, dry throat, xerostomia, nausea, constipation, appetite stimulation (weight gain)
- Genitourinary: Impotence
- Hematologic: Leukopenia
- Neuromuscular & skeletal: Back pain, myalgia, dysarthria, tremor
- Ocular: Diplopia, blurred vision, nystagmus
- Respiratory: Rhinitis, bronchospasm
- Miscellaneous: Hiccups

Overdosage/Toxicology

Decontamination: Lavage/activated charcoal with cathartic

Enhancement of elimination: Multiple dosing of activated charcoal may be useful; hemodialysis will be useful

Drug Interactions

Gabapentin does not modify plasma concentrations of standard anticonvulsant medications (ie, valproic acid, carbamazepine, phenytoin, or phenobarbital)

Decreased effect: Antacids reduce the bioavailability of gabapentin by 20%

Increased toxicity: Cimetidine may decrease clearance of gabapentin; gabapentin may increase levels of norethindrone by 13%

Mechanism of Action Exact mechanism of action is not known, but does have properties in common with other anticonvulsants; although structurally related to GABA, it does not interact with GABA receptors

Pharmacodynamics/Kinetics

Absorption: Oral: 50% to 60%

Distribution: V_d: 0.6-0.8 L/kg

Protein binding: 0%

Half-life: 5-6 hours

Elimination: Renal, 56% to 80%

Usual Dosage If gabapentin is discontinued or if another anticonvulsant is added to therapy, it should be done slowly over a minimum of 1 week

Children >12 years and Adults: Oral:

- Initial: 300 mg on day 1 (at bedtime to minimize sedation), then 300 mg twice daily on day 2, and then 300 mg 3 times/day on day 3
- Total daily dosage range: 900-1800 mg/day administered in 3 divided doses at 8-hour intervals
- Pain: 300-1800 mg/day given in 3 divided doses has been the most common dosage range

Dosing adjustment in renal impairment:

- Cl_{cr} >60 mL/minute: Administer 1200 mg/day
- Cl_{cr} 30-60 mL/minute: Administer 600 mg/day
- Cl_{cr} 15-30 mL/minute: Administer 300 mg/day
- Cl_{cr} <15 mL/minute: Administer 150 mg/day

Hemodialysis: 200-300 mg after each 4-hour dialysis following a loading dose of 300-400 mg

Dietary Considerations

Food: Does not change rate or extent of absorption; take without regard to meals

Serum lipids: May see increases in total cholesterol, HDL cholesterol and triglycerides. Hyperlipidemia and hypercholesterolemia have been reported with gabapentin.

Administration Administer first dose on first day at bedtime to avoid somnolence and dizziness

Monitoring Parameters Monitor serum levels of concomitant anticonvulsant therapy; routine monitoring of gabapentin levels is not mandatory

Reference Range Minimum effective serum concentration may be 2 μg/mL; **routine monitoring of drug levels is not required**

Patient Information Take only as prescribed; may cause dizziness, somnolence, and other symptoms and signs of CNS depression; do not operate machinery or drive a car until you have experience with the drug; may be administered without regard to meals

Nursing Implications Dosage must be adjusted for renal function and elderly often have reduced renal function

Dosage Forms Capsule: 100 mg, 300 mg, 400 mg

Gallium Nitrate (GAL ee um NYE trate)

Brand Names Ganite™

Therapeutic Category Antidote, Hypercalcemia

Use Treatment of clearly symptomatic cancer-related hypercalcemia that has not responded to adequate hydration

Pregnancy Risk Factor C

Contraindications Should not be used in patients with a serum creatinine >2.5 mg/dL, hypersensitivity to any component

Warnings/Precautions Safety and efficacy in children have not been established. Concurrent use of gallium nitrate with other potentially nephrotoxic drugs may increase the risk for developing severe renal insufficiency in patients with cancer-related hypercalcemia; use with caution in patients with impaired renal function or dehydration

Adverse Reactions

>10%:

- Endocrine & metabolic: Hypophosphatemia
- Gastrointestinal: Nausea, vomiting, diarrhea, metallic taste
- Renal: Renal toxicity

1% to 10%: Endocrine & metabolic: Hypocalcemia

<1%:

- Hematologic: Anemia
- Ocular: Optic neuritis
- Otic: Hearing impairment

Overdosage/Toxicology Symptoms of overdose include nausea, vomiting, renal failure, hypocalcemia, tetany; supportive measures ensure adequate hydration, calcium salts

Drug Interactions Increased toxicity: Nephrotoxic drugs (eg, aminoglycosides, amphotericin B)

Stability Store at room temperature (15°C to 30°C/59°F to 86°F); when diluted in NS or D_5W, stable for 48 hours at room temperature or 7 days at refrigeration (2°C to 8°C/36°F to 46°F)

Mechanism of Action Primarily via inhibition of bone resorption with associated reduction in urinary calcium excretion. Gallium has increased the calcium content of newly mineralized bone following short-term treatment *in vitro*, and this effect combined with its ability to inhibit bone resorption has suggested the use of gallium for other disorders associated with increased bone loss.

Pharmacodynamics/Kinetics

Metabolism: Not metabolized by liver or kidneys

Half-life, elimination: Terminal: 25-111 hours

Elimination: Up to 70% of dose excreted by the kidneys

Usual Dosage Adults:

I.V. infusion (over 24 hours): 200 mg/m^2 for 5 consecutive days in 1 L of NS or D_5W

Mild hypercalcemia/few symptoms: 100 mg/m^2/day for 5 days in 1 L of NS or D_5W

Dosing adjustment/comments in renal impairment:

Cl_{cr} <30 mL/minute: Avoid use

Monitoring Parameters Serum creatinine, BUN, and calcium

Reference Range Steady-state gallium serum levels: Generally obtained within 2 days following initiation of continuous I.V. infusions of gallium nitrate

Nursing Implications Patients should have adequate I.V. hydration, serum creatinine levels should be monitored during gallium nitrate therapy

Dosage Forms Injection: 25 mg/mL (20 mL)

Gamastan® *see* Immune Globulin, Intramuscular *on page 650*

Gamimune® N *see* Immune Globulin, Intravenous *on page 651*

Gamma Benzene Hexachloride *see* Lindane *on page 728*

Gammagard® *see* Immune Globulin, Intravenous *on page 651*

Gammagard® S/D *see* Immune Globulin, Intravenous *on page 651*

Gamma Globulin *see* Immune Globulin, Intramuscular *on page 650*

Gammaphos *see* Amifostine *on page 59*

Gammar® *see* Immune Globulin, Intramuscular *on page 650*

Gammar-P® I.V. *see* Immune Globulin, Intravenous *on page 651*

Gamulin® Rh *see* Rh_o(D) Immune Globulin *on page 1101*

Ganciclovir (gan SYE kloe veer)

Related Information

Guidelines for the Prevention of Opportunistic Infections in Persons with HIV *on page 1457*

Brand Names Cytovene®; Vitrasert®

Canadian/Mexican Brand Names Cymevene® (Mexico)

Synonyms DHPG Sodium; GCV Sodium; Nordeoxyguanosine

Therapeutic Category Antiviral Agent, Parenteral

Use Oral treatment of CMV retinitis in immunocompromised individuals, including patients with acquired immunodeficiency syndrome; for treatment of CMV pneumonia in marrow transplant recipients and AIDS patients, and for prophylaxis and treatment in organ transplant recipients with CMV colitis, pneumonitis, and multiorgan involvement; bone marrow transplant patients when given in combination with IVIG or CMV hyperimmune globulin

Oral: Alternative to the I.V. formulation for maintenance treatment of CMV retinitis in immunocompromised patients, including patients with AIDS, in whom retinitis is stable following appropriate induction therapy and for whom the risk of more rapid progression is balanced by the benefit associated with avoiding daily I.V. infusions

Pregnancy Risk Factor C

Contraindications Absolute neutrophil count $<500/mm^3$; platelet count $<25,000/mm^3$; known hypersensitivity to ganciclovir or acyclovir

Warnings/Precautions Dosage adjustment or interruption of ganciclovir therapy may be necessary in patients with neutropenia and/or thrombocytopenia and patients with impaired renal function. Use with extreme caution in children since long-term safety has not been determined and due to ganciclovir's potential for long-term carcinogenic and adverse reproductive effects; ganciclovir may adversely affect spermatogenesis and fertility; due to its mutagenic potential, contraceptive precautions for female and male patients need to be followed during and for at least 90 days after therapy with the drug; take care to administer only into veins with good blood flow.

Adverse Reactions

>10%:
- Central nervous system: Headache
- Hematologic: Granulocytopenia, thrombocytopenia

1% to 10%:
- Central nervous system: Confusion, fever
- Dermatologic: Rash
- Hematologic: Anemia
- Hepatic: Abnormal liver function values
- Miscellaneous: Sepsis

<1%:
- Cardiovascular: Arrhythmia, hypertension, hypotension, edema
- Central nervous system: Ataxia, dizziness, nervousness, psychosis, malaise, coma
- Dermatologic: Alopecia, pruritus, urticaria
- Gastrointestinal: Nausea, vomiting, diarrhea, abdominal pain
- Hematologic: Eosinophilia, hemorrhage
- Local: Inflammation or pain at injection site
- Neuromuscular & skeletal: Paresthesia, tremor
- Ocular: Retinal detachment
- Respiratory: Dyspnea

Overdosage/Toxicology Symptoms of overdose include neutropenia, vomiting, hypersalivation, bloody diarrhea, cytopenia, testicular atrophy

Treatment is supportive; hemodialysis removes 50% of drug; hydration may be of some benefit

Drug Interactions

Decreased effect: Didanosine: A decrease in steady-state ganciclovir AUC may occur

Increased toxicity:
- Zidovudine, immunosuppressive agents may increase hematologic toxicity
- Imipenem/cilastatin may increase seizure potential
- Zidovudine: Oral ganciclovir increased the AUC of zidovudine. Since both drugs have the potential to cause neutropenia and anemia, some patients may not tolerate concomitant therapy with these drugs at full dosage.
- Probenecid: The renal clearance of ganciclovir is decreased in the presence of probenecid

Stability

Preparation should take place in a vertical laminar flow hood with the same precautions as antineoplastic agents

Intact vials should be stored at room temperature and protected from temperatures >40°C

Reconstitute powder with sterile water **not** bacteriostatic water because parabens may cause precipitation

Reconstituted solution is stable for 12 hours at room temperature, however, conflicting data indicates that reconstituted solution is stable for 60 days under refrigeration (4°C)

Drug product should be reconstituted immediately before use and any unused portion should be discarded

Stability of parenteral admixture at room temperature (25°C) and at refrigeration temperature (4°C): 5 days

An in-line filter of 0.22-5 micron is recommended during the infusion of all ganciclovir solutions

Mechanism of Action Ganciclovir is phosphorylated to a substrate which competitively inhibits the binding of deoxyguanosine triphosphate to DNA polymerase resulting in inhibition of viral DNA synthesis

Pharmacodynamics/Kinetics

Absorption: Oral: Absolute bioavailability under fasting conditions: 5% and following food: 6% to 9%; following fatty meal: 28% to 31%

Protein binding: 1% to 2%

Half-life: 1.7-5.8 hours; increases with impaired renal function

End stage renal disease: 3.6 hours

Elimination: Majority (94% to 99%) excreted as unchanged drug in the urine

Usual Dosage

Slow I.V. infusion (dosing is based on total body weight):

Children >3 months and Adults:

Induction therapy: 5 mg/kg/dose every 12 hours for 14-21 days followed by maintenance therapy

Maintenance therapy: 5 mg/kg/day as a single daily dose for 7 days/week or 6 mg/kg/day for 5 days/week

Oral: 1000 mg 3 times/day with food **or** 500 mg 6 times/day with food

Dosing adjustment in renal impairment:

I.V.:

Cl_{cr} 50-79 mL/minute: Administer 2.5 mg/kg/dose every 12 hours

Cl_{cr} 25-49 mL/minute: Administer 2.5 mg/kg/dose every 24 hours

Cl_{cr} <25 mL/minute: Administer 1.25 mg/kg/dose every 24 hours

Oral:

Cl_{cr} 50-69 mL/minute: Administer 1500 mg/day or 500 mg 3 times/day

Cl_{cr} 25-49 mL/minute: Administer 1000 mg/day or 500 mg twice daily

Cl_{cr} 10-24 mL/minute: Administer 500 mg/day

Cl_{cr} <10 mL/minute: Administer 500 mg 3 times/week following hemodialysis

Hemodialysis: Dialyzable (50%) following hemodialysis; administer dose postdialysis

Peritoneal dialysis: Dose as for Cl_{cr} <10 mL/minute; during continuous arteriovenous or veno-venous hemofiltration (CAVH/CAVHD), administer 2.5 mg/kg/dose every 24 hours

Administration The same precautions utilized with antineoplastic agents should be followed with ganciclovir administration. Ganciclovir should not be administered by I.M., S.C., or rapid IVP administration; administer by slow I.V. infusion over at least 1 hour at a final concentration for administration not to exceed 10 mg/mL. **An IN-LINE filter of 0.22-5 micron is recommended during the infusion of all ganciclovir solutions**. Oral ganciclovir should be administered with food

Monitoring Parameters CBC with differential and platelet count, serum creatinine, ophthalmologic exams

Patient Information Ganciclovir is not a cure for CMV retinitis; regular ophthalmologic examinations should be done; close monitoring of blood counts should be done while on therapy and dosage adjustments may need to be made; take with food to increase absorption

Nursing Implications Must be prepared in vertical flow hood; use chemotherapy precautions during administration; discard appropriately

Additional Information Sodium content of 500 mg vial: 46 mg

Dosage Forms

Capsule: 250 mg

Implant, intravitreal: 4.5 mg released gradually over 5-8 months

Powder for injection, lyophilized: 500 mg (10 mL)

Ganite™ *see* Gallium Nitrate *on page 565*

Gantanol® *see* Sulfamethoxazole *on page 1175*

Gantrisin® *see* Sulfisoxazole *on page 1179*

Garamycin® *see* Gentamicin *on page 570*

Gas Relief® [OTC] *see* Simethicone *on page 1136*

Gastrocrom® Oral *see* Cromolyn Sodium *on page 317*

Gastrosed™ *see* Hyoscyamine *on page 635*

Gas-X® [OTC] *see* Simethicone *on page 1136*
G-CSF *see* Filgrastim *on page 518*
GCV Sodium *see* Ganciclovir *on page 566*
Gee Gee® [OTC] *see* Guaifenesin *on page 589*
Gel Kam® *see* Fluoride *on page 536*
Gel-Tin® [OTC] *see* Fluoride *on page 536*
Gelucast® *see* Zinc Gelatin *on page 1323*

Gemcitabine (jem SIT a been)

Brand Names Gemzar®

Synonyms Gemcitabine Hydrochloride

Therapeutic Category Antineoplastic Agent, Antimetabolite

Use Adenocarcinoma of the pancreas; first-line therapy for patients with locally advanced (nonresectable stage II of stage III) or metastatic (stage IV) adenocarcinoma of the pancreas. Indicated for patients previously treated with 5-FU.

Pregnancy Risk Factor D

Contraindications Known hypersensitivity to gemcitabine

Warnings/Precautions The U.S. Food & Drug Administration (FDA) recommends that procedures for proper handling and disposal of antineoplastic agents be considered. Prolongation of the infusion time >60 minutes and more frequent than weekly dosing have been shown to increase toxicity. Gemcitabine can suppress bone marrow function manifested by leukopenia, thrombocytopenia and anemia, and myelosuppression is usually the dose-limiting ototoxicity. The incidence of fever is 41% and gemcitabine may cause fever in the absence of clinical infection. Rash has been reported in 30% of patients - typically a macular or finely granular maculopapular pruritic eruption of mild-moderate severity involving the trunk and extremities. Gemcitabine should be used with caution in patients with pre-existing renal impairment (mild proteinuria and hematuria were commonly reported; hemolytic uremic syndrome has been reported) and hepatic impairment (associated with transient elevations of serum transaminases in 2/3 of patients - but no evidence of increasing hepatic toxicity).

Adverse Reactions

>10%:

- Cardiovascular: Peripheral edema
- Central nervous system: Fever
- Dermatologic: Rash, alopecia
- Gastrointestinal: Nausea, vomiting, constipation, diarrhea, stomatitis
- Hematologic: Anemia, leukopenia, neutropenia, thrombocytopenia
- Hepatic: Elevated liver enzymes (ALT, AST, alkaline phosphatase) and bilirubin
- Neuromuscular & skeletal: Pain
- Renal: Proteinuria, hematuria, elevated BUN
- Respiratory: Dyspnea
- Miscellaneous: Infection

Overdosage/Toxicology Symptoms of overdose include myelosuppression, paresthesia, and severe rash - the principle toxicities seen when a single dose as high as 5,700 mg/m^2 was administered by I.V. infusion over 30 minutes every 2 weeks

Treatment: Monitor blood counts and administer supportive therapy as needed

Stability

Store intact vials at room temperature (20°C to 25°C/68°F to 77°F). Reconstitute gemcitabine with 0.9% sodium chloride (preservative-free). Dilute as follows:
200 mg vial - 5 mL
1 g vial - 25 mL

These dilutions yield a concentration of 40 mg/mL - maximum concentration for reconstitution is 40 mg/mL. Store at room temperature (20°C to 25°C/68°F to 77°F) for up to 24 hours. The appropriate dose should be further diluted with 0.9% sodium chloride injection to concentrations as low as 0.1 mg/mL. Store at room temperature for up to 24 hours. Do not refrigerate.

Mechanism of Action Nucleoside analogue that primarily kills cells undergoing DNA synthesis (S-phase) and blocks the progression of cells through the G1/S-phase boundary

Pharmacodynamics/Kinetics

Distribution: V_d: 50 mL/m^2 (short infusions); 370 L/m^2 (long infusions)
Metabolism: To inactive metabolite (dFdU)
Half-life: 42-94 minutes
Elimination: In urine

Usual Dosage Adults: I.V.:

1000 mg/m^2 once weekly for up to 7 weeks (or until toxicity necessitates reducing or holding a dose), followed by a week of rest from treatment. Subsequent cycles should consist of infusions once weekly for 3 consecutive weeks out of every 4 weeks.

Dosing reductions based on hematologic function:

Absolute Granulocyte Count		Platelet Count	% of Full Dose
≥1000	AND	≥100,000	100
500-999	OR	50,000-99,000	75
<500	OR	<50,000	Hold

Patients who complete an entire 7-week initial cycle of gemcitabine therapy or a subsequent 3-week cycle at a dose of 1000 mg/m² may have the dose for subsequent cycles increased by 25% (1250 mg/m²), provided that the absolute granulocyte count and platelet nadirs exceed 1500 x 10^6/L and 100,000 x 10^6/L, respectively and if nonhematologic toxicity has not been more than World Health Organization Grade 1.

Patients who tolerate the subsequent course, at a dose of 1250 mg/m², the dose for the next cycle can be increased to 1500 mg/m², provided again that the AGC and platelet nadirs exceed 1500 x 10^6/L and 100,000 x 10^6/L, respectively, and again, if nonhematologic toxicity has not been greater than WHO Grade 1.

Dosing adjustment in renal/hepatic impairment: Use with caution; gemcitabine has not been studied in patients with significant renal or hepatic dysfunction

Administration I.V. over 30 minutes

Monitoring Parameters Patients should be monitored prior to each dose with a complete blood count (CBC), including differential and platelet count; suspension or modification of therapy should be considered when marrow suppression is detected

Hepatic and renal function should be performed prior to initiation of therapy and periodically, thereafter

Dosage Forms Powder for injection, as hydrochloride, lyophilized: 20 mg/mL (10 mL, 50 mL)

Gemcitabine Hydrochloride *see* Gemcitabine *on previous page*

Gemcor® *see* Gemfibrozil *on this page*

Gemfibrozil (jem FI broe zil)

Related Information

Lipid-Lowering Agents *on page 1413*

Brand Names Gemcor®; Lopid®

Canadian/Mexican Brand Names Apo-Gemfibrozil® (Canada); Nu-Gemfibrozil® (Canada)

Synonyms CI-719

Therapeutic Category Antilipemic Agent

Use Treatment of hypertriglyceridemia in types IV and V hyperlipidemia for patients who are at greater risk for pancreatitis and who have not responded to dietary intervention; reduction of coronary heart disease in type IIB patients who have low HDL cholesterol, ↑ LDL cholesterol, and ↑ triglycerides

Pregnancy Risk Factor B

Contraindications Renal or hepatic dysfunction, gallbladder disease, hypersensitivity to gemfibrozil or any component

Warnings/Precautions Abnormal elevation of AST, ALT, LDH, bilirubin, and alkaline phosphatase has occurred; if no appreciable triglyceride or cholesterol lowering effect occurs after 3 months, the drug should be discontinued; not useful for type I hyperlipidemia; myositis may be more common in patients with poor renal function

Adverse Reactions

>10%:

- Gastrointestinal: Dyspepsia, abdominal pain
- Hepatic: Cholelithiasis

1% to 10%:

- Central nervous system: Fatigue, vertigo, headache
- Dermatologic: Eczema, rash
- Gastrointestinal: Diarrhea, nausea, vomiting, constipation, acute appendicitis

<1%:

- Cardiovascular: Atrial fibrillation
- Central nervous system: Hyperesthesia, dizziness, drowsiness, somnolence, mental depression
- Gastrointestinal: Flatulence
- Neuromuscular & skeletal: Paresthesia
- Ocular: Blurred vision

(Continued)

Gemfibrozil *(Continued)*

Overdosage/Toxicology Symptoms of overdose include abdominal pain, diarrhea, nausea, vomiting; following GI decontamination, treatment is supportive

Drug Interactions

Increased toxicity:

May potentiate the effects of warfarin

Manufacturer warns against the use of gemfibrozil with concomitant lovastatin therapy

Mechanism of Action The exact mechanism of action of gemfibrozil is unknown, however, several theories exist regarding the VLDL effect; it can inhibit lipolysis and decrease subsequent hepatic fatty acid uptake as well as inhibit hepatic secretion of VLDL; together these actions decrease serum VLDL levels; increases HDL cholesterol; the mechanism behind HDL elevation is currently unknown

Pharmacodynamics/Kinetics

Absorption: Well absorbed

Protein binding: 99%

Metabolism: In the liver by oxidation to two inactive metabolites

Half-life: 1.4 hours

Time to peak serum concentration: Within 1-2 hours

Elimination: A portion of the drug undergoes enterohepatic recycling; excreted in urine, primarily as unchanged drug (70%)

Usual Dosage Adults: Oral: 1200 mg/day in 2 divided doses, 30 minutes before breakfast and dinner

Hemodialysis: Not removed by hemodialysis; supplemental dose is not necessary

Monitoring Parameters Serum cholesterol, LFTs

Patient Information May cause dizziness or blurred vision, abdominal or epigastric pain, diarrhea, nausea, or vomiting; notify physician if these become pronounced

Dosage Forms

Capsule: 300 mg

Tablet, film coated: 600 mg

Gemzar® *see* Gemcitabine *on page 568*

Genabid® *see* Papaverine *on page 951*

Genac® Tablet [OTC] *see* Triprolidine and Pseudoephedrine *on page 1270*

Genagesic® *see* Propoxyphene and Acetaminophen *on page 1067*

Genahist® Oral *see* Diphenhydramine *on page 399*

Genapap® [OTC] *see* Acetaminophen *on page 19*

Genaspor® [OTC] *see* Tolnaftate *on page 1243*

Genatuss® [OTC] *see* Guaifenesin *on page 589*

Genatuss DM® [OTC] *see* Guaifenesin and Dextromethorphan *on page 591*

Gen-K® *see* Potassium Chloride *on page 1024*

Genoptic® *see* Gentamicin *on this page*

Genora® 0.5/35 *see* Ethinyl Estradiol and Norethindrone *on page 486*

Genora® 1/35 *see* Ethinyl Estradiol and Norethindrone *on page 486*

Genora® 1/50 *see* Mestranol and Norethindrone *on page 791*

Genotropin® Injection *see* Human Growth Hormone *on page 613*

Genpril® [OTC] *see* Ibuprofen *on page 639*

Gentacidin® *see* Gentamicin *on this page*

Gentafair® *see* Gentamicin *on this page*

Gentak® *see* Gentamicin *on this page*

Gentamicin (jen ta MYE sin)

Related Information

Antibiotic Treatment of Adults With Infectious Endocarditis *on page 1465*

Antimicrobial Drugs of Choice *on page 1468*

Antimicrobial Prophylaxis *on page 1445*

Bacterial Meningitis Practical Guidelines for Management *on page 1475*

Prevention of Bacterial Endocarditis *on page 1449*

Treatment of Sexually Transmitted Diseases *on page 1485*

Brand Names Garamycin®; Genoptic®; Gentacidin®; Gentafair®; Gentak®; Gentrasul®; I-Gent®; Jenamicin®; Ocumycin®

Canadian/Mexican Brand Names Garalen® (Mexico); Garamicina® (Mexico); Genenicina® (Mexico); Genkova® (Mexico); Genrex® (Mexico); Gentarim® (Mexico); Nozolon® (Mexico); Quilagen® (Mexico); Yectamicina® (Mexico)

Synonyms Gentamicin Sulfate

Therapeutic Category Antibiotic, Aminoglycoside; Antibiotic, Ophthalmic; Antibiotic, Topical

Use Treatment of susceptible bacterial infections, normally gram-negative organisms including *Pseudomonas*, *Proteus*, *Serratia*, and gram-positive *Staphylococcus*; treatment of bone infections, respiratory tract infections, skin and soft tissue infections, as well as abdominal and urinary tract infections, endocarditis, and septicemia; used topically to treat superficial infections of the skin or ophthalmic infections caused by susceptible bacteria

Pregnancy Risk Factor C

Contraindications Hypersensitivity to gentamicin or other aminoglycosides

Warnings/Precautions

Not intended for long-term therapy due to toxic hazards associated with extended administration; pre-existing renal insufficiency, vestibular or cochlear impairment, myasthenia gravis, hypocalcemia, conditions which depress neuromuscular transmission

Parenteral aminoglycosides have been associated with significant nephrotoxicity or ototoxicity; the ototoxicity may be directly proportional to the amount of drug given and the duration of treatment; tinnitus or vertigo are indications of vestibular injury and impending hearing loss; renal damage is usually reversible

Adverse Reactions

>10%:

- Central nervous system: Neurotoxicity (vertigo, ataxia)
- Neuromuscular & skeletal: Gait instability
- Otic: Ototoxicity (auditory), ototoxicity (vestibular)
- Renal: Nephrotoxicity, decreased creatinine clearance

1% to 10%:

- Cardiovascular: Edema
- Dermatologic: Skin itching, reddening of skin, rash

<1%:

- Central nervous system: Drowsiness, headache, pseudomotor cerebri
- Dermatologic: Photosensitivity, erythema
- Gastrointestinal: Anorexia, nausea, vomiting, weight loss, increased salivation, enterocolitis
- Hematologic: Granulocytopenia, agranulocytosis, thrombocytopenia
- Hepatic: Elevated LFTs
- Local: Burning, stinging
- Neuromuscular & skeletal: Tremors, muscle cramps, weakness
- Respiratory: Dyspnea

Overdosage/Toxicology Symptoms of overdose include ototoxicity, nephrotoxicity, and neuromuscular toxicity; serum level monitoring is recommended

The treatment of choice, following a single acute overdose, appears to be the maintenance of good urine output of at least 3 mL/kg/hour. Dialysis is of questionable value in the enhancement of aminoglycoside elimination. If required, hemodialysis is preferred over peritoneal dialysis in patients with normal renal function. Careful hydration may be all that is required to promote diuresis and therefore the enhancement of the drug's elimination. Chelation with penicillins is experimental.

Drug Interactions

Increased toxicity:

- Penicillins, cephalosporins, amphotericin B, loop diuretics may increase nephrotoxic potential
- Neuromuscular blocking agents may increase neuromuscular blockade

Stability

Gentamicin is a colorless to slightly yellow solution which should be stored between 2°C to 30°C, but refrigeration is not recommended

I.V. infusion solutions mixed in NS or D_5W solution are stable for 24 hours at room temperature and refrigeration

Premixed bag: Manufacturer expiration date

Out of overwrap stability: 30 days

Mechanism of Action Interferes with bacterial protein synthesis by binding to 30S and 50S ribosomal subunits resulting in a defective bacterial cell membrane

Pharmacodynamics/Kinetics

Absorption: Oral: Not absorbed

Distribution: Crosses the placenta

V_d: Increased by edema, ascites, fluid overload; decreased in patients with dehydration. See table.

- Neonates: 0.4-0.6 L/kg
- Children: 0.3-0.35 L/kg
- Adults: 0.2-0.3 L/kg

Relative diffusion of antimicrobial agents from blood into cerebrospinal fluid (CSF): Minimal even with inflammation

Ratio of CSF to blood level (%):

- Normal meninges: Nil
- Inflamed meninges: 10-30

(Continued)

Gentamicin *(Continued)*

Aminoglycoside Penetration Into Various Tissues

Site	Extent of Distribution
Eye	Poor
CNS	Poor (<25%)
Pleural	Excellent
Bronchial secretions	Poor
Sputum	Fair (10%-50%)
Pulmonary tissue	Excellent
Ascitic fluid	Variable (43%-132%)
Peritoneal fluid	Poor
Bile	Variable (25%-90%)
Bile with obstruction	Poor
Synovial fluid	Excellent
Bone	Poor
Prostate	Poor
Urine	Excellent
Renal tissue	Excellent

Protein binding: <30%

Half-life:

Infants:

<1 week: 3-11.5 hours

1 week to 6 months: 3-3.5 hours

Adults: 1.5-3 hours; end stage renal disease: 36-70 hours

Time to peak serum concentration:

I.M.: Within 30-90 minutes

I.V.: 30 minutes after a 30-minute infusion

Elimination: Clearance is directly related to renal function, eliminated almost completely by glomerular filtration of unchanged drug with excretion into the urine

Usual Dosage Individualization is critical because of the low therapeutic index

Use of ideal body weight (IBW) for determining the mg/kg/dose appears to be more accurate than dosing on the basis of total body weight (TBW).

In morbid obesity, dosage requirement may best be estimated using a dosing weight of IBW + 0.4 (TBW - IBW)

Initial and periodic peak and trough plasma drug levels should be determined, particularly in critically ill patients with serious infections or in disease states known to significantly alter aminoglycoside pharmacokinetics (eg, cystic fibrosis, burns, or major surgery)

Once daily dosing: Higher peak serum drug concentration to MIC ratios, demonstrated aminoglycoside postantibiotic effect, decreased renal cortex drug uptake, and improved cost-time efficiency are supportive reasons for the use of once daily dosing regimens for aminoglycosides. Current research indicates these regimens to be as effective for nonlife-threatening infections, with no higher incidence of nephrotoxicity, than those requiring multiple daily doses. Doses are determined by calculating the entire day's dose via usual multiple dose calculation techniques and administering this quantity as a single dose. Doses are then adjusted to maintain mean serum concentrations above the MIC(s) of the causative organism(s). (Example: 4.0-4.5 mg/kg as a single dose; expected Cp_{max}: 10-20 mcg/mL and Cp_{min}: <1 mcg/mL). Further research is needed for universal recommendation in all patient populations and gram-negative disease; exceptions may include those with known high clearance (eg, children, patients with cystic fibrosis, or burns who may require shorter dosage intervals) and patients with renal function impairment for whom longer than conventional dosage intervals are usually required.

Newborns: Intrathecal: 1 mg every day

Infants >3 months: Intrathecal: 1-2 mg/day

Infants and Children <5 years: I.M., I.V.: 2.5 mg/kg/dose every 8 hours*

Cystic fibrosis: 2.5 mg/kg/dose every 6 hours

Children >5 years: I.M., I.V.: 1.5-2.5 mg/kg/dose every 8 hours*

*Some patients may require larger or more frequent doses (eg, every 6 hours) if serum levels document the need (ie, cystic fibrosis or febrile granulocytopenic patients)

Adults: I.M., I.V.:

Severe life-threatening infections: 2-2.5 mg/kg/dose

Urinary tract infections: 1.5 mg/kg/dose

Synergy (for gram-positive infections): 1 mg/kg/dose

Children and Adults:
Intrathecal: 4-8 mg/day
Ophthalmic:
Ointment: Instill ½" (1.25 cm) 2-3 times/day to every 3-4 hours
Solution: Instill 1-2 drops every 2-4 hours, up to 2 drops every hour for severe infections
Topical: Apply 3-4 times/day to affected area

Dosing interval in renal impairment:
Cl_{cr} ≥60 mL/minute: Administer every 8 hours
Cl_{cr} 40-60 mL/minute: Administer every 12 hours
Cl_{cr} 20-40 mL/minute: Administer every 24 hours
Cl_{cr} 10-20 mL/minute: Administer every 48 hours
Cl_{cr} <10 mL/minute: Administer every 72 hours
Hemodialysis: Dialyzable; removal by hemodialysis: 30% removal of aminoglycosides occurs during 4 hours of HD; administer dose after dialysis and follow levels
Removal by continuous ambulatory peritoneal dialysis (CAPD):
Administration via CAPD fluid:
Gram-negative infection: 4-8 mg/L (4-8 mcg/mL) of CAPD fluid
Gram-positive infection (ie, synergy): 3-4 mg/L (3-4 mcg/mL) of CAPD fluid
Administration via I.V., I.M. route during CAPD: Dose as for Cl_{cr} <10 mL/minute and follow levels
Removal via continuous arterio-venous or veno-venous hemofiltration (CAVH/CAVHD): Dose as for Cl_{cr} 10-15 mL/minute and follow levels

Dosing adjustment/comments in hepatic disease: Monitor plasma concentrations

Dietary Considerations Calcium, magnesium, potassium: Renal wasting may cause hypocalcemia, hypomagnesemia, and/or hypokalemia

Monitoring Parameters Urinalysis, urine output, BUN, serum creatinine; hearing should be tested before, during, and after treatment; particularly in those at risk for ototoxicity or who will be receiving prolonged therapy (>2 weeks)

Reference Range
Timing of serum samples: Draw peak 30 minutes after 30-minute infusion has been completed or 1 hour after I.M. injection; draw trough immediately before next dose
Sample size: 0.5-2 mL blood (red top tube) or 0.1-1 mL serum (separated)
Therapeutic levels:
Peak:
Serious infections: 6-8 μg/mL (12-17 μmol/L)
Life-threatening infections: 8-10 μg/mL (17-21 μmol/L)
Urinary tract infections: 4-6 μg/mL
Synergy against gram-positive organisms: 3-5 μg/mL
Trough:
Serious infections: 0.5-1 μg/mL
Life-threatening infections: 1-2 μg/mL
Monitor serum creatinine and urine output; obtain drug levels after the third dose unless renal dysfunction/toxicity suspected

Test Interactions ↑ protein; ↓ magnesium; ↑ BUN, AST, GPT, alk phos, serum creatinine; ↓ potassium, sodium, calcium

Patient Information Report any dizziness or sensations of ringing or fullness in ears; do not touch ophthalmics to eye; use no other eye drops within 5-10 minutes of instilling ophthalmic

Nursing Implications Slower absorption and lower peak concentrations probably due to poor circulation in the atrophic muscle, may occur following I.M. injection in paralyzed patients (suggest I.V. route); aminoglycoside levels measured in blood taken from Silastic® central catheters can sometimes give falsely high readings (draw via separate lumen or peripheral site if possible, otherwise flush very well). Monitor serum creatinine and urine output; obtain drug levels after the third dose unless otherwise directed (eg, suspected toxicity or renal dysfunction). Peak levels are drawn 30 minutes after the end of a 30-minute infusion or 60 minutes following I.M. injection; trough levels are drawn within 30 minutes before the next dose; administer other antibiotic drugs at least 1 hour before or after gentamicin. Hearing should be tested before, during, and after treatment in patients at risk for ototoxicity.

Dosage Forms
Cream, topical, as sulfate (Garamycin®, G-myticin®): 0.1% (15 g)
Infusion, in D_5W, as sulfate: 60 mg, 80 mg, 100 mg
Infusion, in NS, as sulfate: 40 mg, 60 mg, 80 mg, 90 mg, 100 mg, 120 mg
Injection, as sulfate: 40 mg/mL (1 mL, 1.5 mL, 2 mL)
Pediatric, as sulfate: 10 mg/mL (2 mL)
Intrathecal, preservative free, as sulfate (Garamycin®): 2 mg/mL (2 mL)
(Continued)

Gentamicin *(Continued)*

Ointment, as sulfate:
Ophthalmic: 0.3% [3 mg/g] (3.5 g)
Garamycin®, Genoptic® S.O.P., Gentacidin®, Gentak®: 0.3% [3 mg/g] (3.5 g)
Topical, as sulfate (Garamycin®, G-myticin®): 0.1% (15 g)
Solution, ophthalmic, as sulfate: 0.3% (5 mL, 15 mL)
Garamycin®, Genoptic®, Gentacidin®, Gentak®: 0.3% (1 mL, 5 mL, 15 mL)

Gentamicin Sulfate *see* Gentamicin *on page 570*

Gentran® *see* Dextran *on page 363*

Gentrasul® *see* Gentamicin *on page 570*

Gen-XENE® *see* Clorazepate *on page 301*

German Measles Vaccine *see* Rubella Virus Vaccine, Live *on page 1119*

Germinal® *see* Ergoloid Mesylates *on page 457*

GG *see* Guaifenesin *on page 589*

GG-Cen® [OTC] *see* Guaifenesin *on page 589*

GI87084B *see* Remifentanil *on page 1097*

Glatiramer Acetate (gla TIR a mer AS e tate)

Brand Names Copaxone®

Synonyms Copolymer-1

Therapeutic Category Biological, Miscellaneous

Use Relapsing-remitting type multiple sclerosis; studies indicate that it reduces the frequency of attacks and the severity of disability; appears to be most effective for patients with minimal disability and has not demonstrated benefits in the chronic progressive form of multiple sclerosis

Contraindications Previous hypersensitivity to any component of the copolymer formulation

Adverse Reactions

>10%:
Dermatologic: Erythema
Local: Pain

1% to 10%:
Cardiovascular: Chest pain or tightness, flushing
Central nervous system: Anxiety
Hematologic: Transient eosinophilia
Respiratory: Dyspnea
Miscellaneous: Diaphoresis

Overdosage/Toxicology Well tolerated; no serious toxicities can be anticipated

Stability Reconstituted product contains no preservative, use immediately; store unreconstituted product in freezer at -20° to -10°C (-4° to 14°F); diluent may be stored at room temperature

Mechanism of Action Glatiramer is a mixture of random polymers of four amino acids; L-alanine, L-glutamic acid, L-lysine and L-tyrosine, the resulting mixture is antigenically similar to myelin basic protein, which is an important component of the myelin sheath of nerves; glatiramer is thought to suppress T-lymphocytes specific for a myelin antigen, it is also proposed that glatiramer interferes with the antigen-presenting function of certain immune cells opposing pathogenic T-cell function

Usual Dosage Adults: S.C.: 20 mg daily

Patient Information It is essential to provide the patient with proper handling and reconstitution instruction, since they will most likely have to self-administer the drug for an extended period

Dosage Forms

Injection: Single-use vials containing 20 mg of glatiramer and 40 mg mannitol; packaged in 2 mL vials along with 1 mL vial of diluent (sterile water for injection)

Glaucoma Drug Therapy Comparison *see page 1410*

Glaucon® *see* Epinephrine *on page 448*

GlaucTabs® *see* Methazolamide *on page 801*

Glibenclamide *see* Glyburide *on page 578*

Glimepiride (GLYE me pye ride)

Related Information

Hypoglycemic Drugs, Comparison of Oral Agents *on page 1411*

Brand Names Amaryl®

Therapeutic Category Antidiabetic Agent; Hypoglycemic Agent, Oral; Sulfonylurea Agent

Use

Management of noninsulin-dependent diabetes mellitus (type II) as an adjunct to diet and exercise to lower blood glucose

Use in combination with insulin to lower blood glucose in patients whose hyperglycemia cannot be controlled by diet and exercise in conjunction with an oral hypoglycemic agent

Pregnancy Risk Factor C

Contraindications Hypersensitivity to glimepiride or any component, other sulfonamides; diabetic ketoacidosis (with or without coma)

Warnings/Precautions

The administration of oral hypoglycemic drugs (ie, tolbutamide) has been reported to be associated with increased cardiovascular mortality as compared to treatment with diet alone or diet plus insulin

All sulfonylurea drugs are capable of producing severe hypoglycemia. Hypoglycemia is more likely to occur when caloric intake is deficient, after severe or prolonged exercise, when alcohol is ingested, or when more than one glucose-lowering drug is used.

Adverse Reactions

1% to 10%: Central nervous system: Headache

<1%:

- Cardiovascular: Edema
- Dermatologic: Rash, urticaria, photosensitivity
- Endocrine & metabolic: Hypoglycemia, hyponatremia
- Gastrointestinal: Anorexia, nausea, vomiting, diarrhea, epigastric fullness, constipation, heartburn
- Hematologic: Blood dyscrasias, aplastic anemia, hemolytic anemia, bone marrow suppression, thrombocytopenia, agranulocytosis
- Hepatic: Cholestatic jaundice
- Renal: Diuretic effect

Overdosage/Toxicology Symptoms of overdose include low blood sugar, tingling of lips and tongue, nausea, yawning, confusion, agitation, tachycardia, sweating, convulsions, stupor, and coma

Intoxications with sulfonylureas can cause hypoglycemia and are best managed with glucose administration (oral for milder hypoglycemia or by injection in more severe forms). Patients should be monitored for a minimum of 24-48 hours after ingestion.

Drug Interactions

Decreased effects: Beta-blockers, cholestyramine, hydantoins, rifampin, thiazide diuretics, urinary alkalines, charcoal

Increased effects: H_2-antagonists, anticoagulants, androgens, fluconazole, salicylates, gemfibrozil, sulfonamides, tricyclic antidepressants, probenecid, MAO inhibitors, methyldopa, digitalis glycosides, urinary acidifiers

Increased toxicity: Cimetidine may increase hypoglycemic effects

Mechanism of Action Stimulates insulin release from the pancreatic beta cells; reduces glucose output from the liver; insulin sensitivity is increased at peripheral target sites

Pharmacodynamics/Kinetics

Duration of action: 24 hours

Peak blood glucose reductions: Within 2-3 hours

Protein binding: >99.5%

Absorption: 100% absorbed; delayed when given with food

Metabolism: Completely in the liver

Half-life: 5-9 hours

Elimination: Metabolites excreted in urine and feces

Usual Dosage Oral (allow several days between dose titrations):

Adults: Initial: 1-2 mg once daily, administered with breakfast or the first main meal; usual maintenance dose: 1-4 mg once daily; after a dose of 2 mg once daily, increase in increments of 2 mg at 1- to 2-week intervals based upon the patient's blood glucose response to a maximum of 8 mg once daily

Elderly: Initial: 1 mg/day

Combination with insulin therapy (fasting glucose level for instituting combination therapy is in the range of >150 mg/dL in plasma or serum depending on the patient): 8 mg once daily with the first main meal

After starting with low-dose insulin, upward adjustments of insulin can be done approximately weekly as guided by frequent measurements of fasting blood glucose. Once stable, combination-therapy patients should monitor their capillary blood glucose on an ongoing basis, preferably daily.

Dosing adjustment/comments in renal impairment: Cl_{cr} <22 mL/minute: Initial starting dose should be 1 mg and dosage increments should be based on fasting blood glucose levels

Dosing adjustment in hepatic impairment: No data available

Administration May be taken with a meal/food

(Continued)

Glimepiride *(Continued)*

Monitoring Parameters Urine for glucose and ketones; monitor for signs and symptoms of hypoglycemia (fatigue, excessive hunger, profuse sweating, numbness of extremities), fasting blood glucose, hemoglobin A_{1c}, fructosamine

Reference Range Target range: Adults:
Fasting blood glucose: <120 mg/dL
Glycosylated hemoglobin: <7%

Patient Information Patients must be counseled by someone experienced in diabetes education, signs and symptoms of hyper- and hypoglycemia, exercise and diet, blood glucose monitoring, and other related topics; eat regularly, do not skip meals; carry quick source of sugar; medical alert bracelet

Nursing Implications Patients who are NPO may need to have their dose held to avoid hypoglycemia

Dosage Forms Tablet: 1 mg, 2 mg, 4 mg

Glipizide (GLIP i zide)

Related Information
Hypoglycemic Drugs, Comparison of Oral Agents *on page 1411*
Sulfonamide Derivatives *on page 1420*

Brand Names Glucotrol®; Glucotrol® XL

Canadian/Mexican Brand Names Minodiab® (Mexico)

Synonyms Glydiazinamide

Therapeutic Category Antidiabetic Agent, Oral; Antihyperglycemic Agent; Hypoglycemic Agent, Oral; Sulfonylurea Agent

Use Management of noninsulin-dependent diabetes mellitus (type II)

Pregnancy Risk Factor C

Pregnancy/Breast-Feeding Implications
Clinical effects on the fetus: Crosses the placenta. Insulin is the drug of choice for the control of diabetes mellitus during pregnancy.
Breast-feeding/lactation: No data available

Contraindications Hypersensitivity to glipizide or any component, other sulfonamides, type I diabetes mellitus

Warnings/Precautions Use with caution in patients with severe hepatic disease; a useful agent since few drug to drug interactions and not dependent upon renal elimination of active drug

Adverse Reactions
>10%:
- Central nervous system: Headache
- Gastrointestinal: Anorexia, nausea, vomiting, diarrhea, epigastric fullness, constipation, heartburn

1% to 10%: Dermatologic: Rash, urticaria, photosensitivity

<1%:
- Cardiovascular: Edema
- Endocrine & metabolic: Hypoglycemia, hyponatremia
- Hematologic: Blood dyscrasias, aplastic anemia, hemolytic anemia, bone marrow suppression, thrombocytopenia, agranulocytosis
- Hepatic: Cholestatic jaundice
- Renal: Diuretic effect

Overdosage/Toxicology Symptoms of overdose include low blood sugar, tingling of lips and tongue, nausea, yawning, confusion, agitation, tachycardia, sweating, convulsions, stupor, and coma

Intoxications with sulfonylureas can cause hypoglycemia and are best managed with glucose administration (oral for milder hypoglycemia or by injection in more severe forms)

Drug Interactions
Decreased effects: Beta-blockers, cholestyramine, hydantoins, rifampin, thiazide diuretics, urinary alkalines, charcoal
Increased effects: H_2-antagonists, anticoagulants, androgens, fluconazole, salicylates, gemfibrozil, sulfonamides, tricyclic antidepressants, probenecid, MAO inhibitors, methyldopa, digitalis glycosides, urinary acidifiers
Increased toxicity: Cimetidine may increase hypoglycemic effects

Mechanism of Action Stimulates insulin release from the pancreatic beta cells; reduces glucose output from the liver; insulin sensitivity is increased at peripheral target sites

Pharmacodynamics/Kinetics
Duration of action: 12-24 hours
Peak blood glucose reductions: Within 1.5-2 hours
Protein binding: 92% to 99%
Absorption: Delayed when given with food
Metabolism: In the liver with metabolites (91% to 97%)
Half-life: 2-4 hours

Elimination: Metabolites (91% to 97%) excreted in urine (60% to 80%) and feces (11%)

Usual Dosage Oral (allow several days between dose titrations):

Adults: 2.5-40 mg/day; doses >15-20 mg/day should be divided and given twice daily

Elderly: Initial: 2.5-5 mg/day; increase by 2.5-5 mg/day at 1- to 2-week intervals

Dosing adjustment/comments in renal impairment: Cl_{cr} <10 mL/minute: Some investigators recommend not using

Dosing adjustment in hepatic impairment: Initial dosage should be 2.5 mg/day

Dietary Considerations

Alcohol: A disulfiram-like reaction characterized by flushing, headache, nausea, vomiting, sweating, or tachycardia; avoid use

Food: Food delays absorption by 40%; take glipizide before meals

Glucose: Decreases blood glucose concentration. Hypoglycemia may occur. Educate patients how to detect and treat hypoglycemia. Monitor for signs and symptoms of hypoglycemia. Administer glucose if necessary. Evaluate patient's diet and exercise regimen. May need to decrease or discontinue dose of sulfonylurea.

Sodium: Reports of hyponatremia and SIADH. Those at increased risk include patients on medications or who have medical conditions that predispose them to hyponatremia. Monitor sodium serum concentration and fluid status. May need to restrict water intake.

Administration Administer 30 minutes before a meal to achieve greatest reduction in postprandial hyperglycemia

Monitoring Parameters Urine for glucose and ketones; monitor for signs and symptoms of hypoglycemia (fatigue, excessive hunger, profuse sweating, numbness of extremities), fasting blood glucose, hemoglobin A_{1c}, fructosamine

Reference Range Target range: Adults:

Fasting blood glucose: <120 mg/dL

Glycosylated hemoglobin: <7%

Patient Information Patients must be counseled by someone experienced in diabetes education, signs and symptoms of hyper- and hypoglycemia, exercise and diet, blood glucose monitoring, and other related topics; eat regularly, do not skip meals; carry quick source of sugar; medical alert bracelet

Nursing Implications Patients who are NPO may need to have their dose held to avoid hypoglycemia

Dosage Forms

Tablet: 5 mg, 10 mg

Tablet, extended release: 5 mg, 10 mg

Glucagon (GLOO ka gon)

Therapeutic Category Antidote, Hypoglycemia; Diagnostic Agent, Gastrointestinal

Use Management of hypoglycemia; diagnostic aid in the radiologic examination of GI tract when a hypnotic state is needed; used with some success as a cardiac stimulant in management of severe cases of beta-adrenergic blocking agent overdosage

Pregnancy Risk Factor B

Contraindications Hypersensitivity to glucagon or any component

Warnings/Precautions Use with caution in patients with a history of insulinoma and/or pheochromocytoma

Adverse Reactions 1% to 10%:

Cardiovascular: Hypotension

Dermatologic: Urticaria

Gastrointestinal: Nausea, vomiting

Respiratory: Respiratory distress

Overdosage/Toxicology Symptoms of overdose include hypokalemia, nausea, vomiting

Drug Interactions Increased toxicity: Oral anticoagulant - hypoprothrombinemic effects may be increased possibly with bleeding

Stability After reconstitution, use immediately; may be kept at 5°C for up to 48 hours if necessary

Mechanism of Action Stimulates adenylate cyclase to produce increased cyclic AMP, which promotes hepatic glycogenolysis and gluconeogenesis, causing a raise in blood glucose levels

Pharmacodynamics/Kinetics

Peak effect on blood glucose levels: Parenteral: Within 5-20 minutes

Duration of action: 60-90 minutes

Metabolism: In the liver with some inactivation occurring in the kidneys and plasma

(Continued)

Glucagon *(Continued)*

Half-life, plasma: 3-10 minutes

Usual Dosage

Hypoglycemia or insulin shock therapy: I.M., I.V., S.C.:

Children: 0.025-0.1 mg/kg/dose, not to exceed 1 mg/dose, repeated in 20 minutes as needed

Adults: 0.5-1 mg, may repeat in 20 minutes as needed

If patient fails to respond to glucagon, I.V. dextrose must be given

Diagnostic aid: Adults: I.M., I.V.: 0.25-2 mg 10 minutes prior to procedure

Administration Reconstitute powder for injection by adding 1 or 10 mL of sterile diluent to a vial containing 1 or 10 units of the drug, respectively, to provide solutions containing 1 mg of glucagon/mL; if dose to be administered is <2 mg of the drug → use only the diluent provided by the manufacturer; if >2 mg → use sterile water for injection; use immediately after reconstitution

Monitoring Parameters Blood pressure, blood glucose

Patient Information Instruct a close associate on how to prepare and administer as a treatment for insulin shock

Additional Information 1 unit = 1 mg

Dosage Forms Powder for injection, lyophilized: 1 mg [1 unit]; 10 mg [10 units]

Glucocerebrosidase *see* Alglucerase *on page 47*

Glucophage® *see* Metformin *on page 795*

Glucotrol® *see* Glipizide *on page 576*

Glucotrol® XL *see* Glipizide *on page 576*

Glukor® *see* Chorionic Gonadotropin *on page 272*

Glyate® [OTC] *see* Guaifenesin *on page 589*

Glybenclamide *see* Glyburide *on this page*

Glybenzcyclamide *see* Glyburide *on this page*

Glyburide (GLYE byoor ide)

Related Information

Hypoglycemic Drugs, Comparison of Oral Agents *on page 1411*

Sulfonamide Derivatives *on page 1420*

Brand Names Diaβeta®; Glynase™ PresTab™; Micronase®

Canadian/Mexican Brand Names Albert® Glyburide (Canada); Apo-Glyburide® (Canada); Euglucon® (Canada); Gen-Glybe® (Canada); Novo-Glyburide® (Canada); Nu-Glyburide® (Canada); Daonil® (Mexico); Euglucon® (Mexico); Glibenil® (Mexico); Glucal® (Mexico); Norboral® (Mexico)

Synonyms Glibenclamide; Glybenclamide; Glybenzcyclamide

Therapeutic Category Antidiabetic Agent, Oral; Antihyperglycemic Agent; Hypoglycemic Agent, Oral; Sulfonylurea Agent

Use Management of noninsulin-dependent diabetes mellitus (type II)

Pregnancy Risk Factor C

Pregnancy/Breast-Feeding Implications

Clinical effects on the fetus: Crosses the placenta. Hypoglycemia; ear defects reported; other malformations reported but may have been secondary to poor maternal glucose control/diabetes. Insulin is the drug of choice for the control of diabetes mellitus during pregnancy.

Breast-feeding/lactation: No data available

Contraindications Hypersensitivity to glyburide or any component, or other sulfonamides; type I diabetes mellitus

Warnings/Precautions Use with caution in patients with hepatic impairment. Elderly: Rapid and prolonged hypoglycemia (>12 hours) despite hypertonic glucose injections have been reported; age and hepatic and renal impairment are independent risk factors for hypoglycemia; dosage titration should be made at weekly intervals. Use with caution in patients with renal and hepatic impairment.

Adverse Reactions

>10%:

Central nervous system: Headache, dizziness

Gastrointestinal: Nausea, epigastric fullness, heartburn, constipation, diarrhea, anorexia

1% to 10%:

Dermatologic: Pruritus, rash, urticaria, photosensitivity reaction

<1%:

Endocrine & metabolic: Hypoglycemia

Genitourinary: Nocturia

Hematologic: Leukopenia, thrombocytopenia, hemolytic anemia, aplastic anemia, bone marrow suppression, agranulocytosis

Hepatic: Cholestatic jaundice

Neuromuscular & skeletal: Arthralgia, paresthesia

Renal: Diuretic effect

Overdosage/Toxicology Symptoms of overdose include severe hypoglycemia, seizures, cerebral damage, tingling of lips and tongue, nausea, yawning, confusion, agitation, tachycardia, sweating, convulsions, stupor, and coma

Intoxications with sulfonylureas can cause hypoglycemia and are best managed with glucose administration (oral for milder hypoglycemia or by injection in more severe forms)

Drug Interactions

Decreased effect: Thiazides and beta-blockers may decrease effectiveness of glyburide

Increased toxicity:

Since this agent is highly protein bound, the toxic potential is increased when given concomitantly with other highly protein bound drugs (ie, phenylbutazole, oral anticoagulants, hydantoins, salicylates, NSAIDs, sulfonamides) - increase hypoglycemic effect

Alcohol increases disulfiram reactions

Phenylbutazone can increase hypoglycemic effects

Mechanism of Action Stimulates insulin release from the pancreatic beta cells; reduces glucose output from the liver; insulin sensitivity is increased at peripheral target sites

Pharmacodynamics/Kinetics

Onset of action: Oral: Insulin levels in the serum begin to increase within 15-60 minutes after a single dose

Duration: Up to 24 hours

Metabolism: To one moderately active and several inactive metabolites

Plasma protein binding: High (>99%)

Half-life: 5-16 hours; may be prolonged with renal insufficiency or hepatic insufficiency

Time to peak serum concentration: Adults: Within 2-4 hours

Usual Dosage Oral:

Adults: 1.25-5 mg to start then increase at weekly intervals to 1.25-20 mg maintenance dose/day divided in 1-2 doses

Elderly: Initial: 1.25-2.5 mg/day, increase by 1.25-2.5 mg/day every 1-3 weeks

Glynase™ PresTab™: Initial: 0.75-3 mg/day, increase by 1.5 mg/day in weekly intervals, maximum: 12 mg/day

Dosing adjustment/comments in renal impairment:

Cl_{cr} 10-50 mL/minute: Use conservative initial and maintenance doses

Cl_{cr} <10 mL/minute: Avoid use

Hemodialysis: Supplemental dose is not necessary

Peritoneal dialysis: Supplemental dose is not necessary

Continuous arterio-venous or veno-venous hemofiltration effects: Supplemental dose is not necessary

Dosing adjustment in hepatic impairment: Use conservative initial and maintenance doses and avoid use in severe disease

Dietary Considerations

Alcohol: A disulfiram-like reaction characterized by flushing, headache, nausea, vomiting, sweating, or tachycardia; avoid use

Food: Food does not affect absorption; glyburide may be taken with food

Glucose: Decreases blood glucose concentration. Hypoglycemia may occur. Educate patients how to detect and treat hypoglycemia. Monitor for signs and symptoms of hypoglycemia. Administer glucose if necessary. Evaluate patient's diet and exercise regimen. May need to decrease or discontinue dose of sulfonylurea.

Sodium: Reports of hyponatremia and SIADH. Those at increased risk include patients on medications or who have medical conditions that predispose them to hyponatremia. Monitor sodium serum concentration and fluid status. May need to restrict water intake.

Monitoring Parameters Signs and symptoms of hypoglycemia, fasting blood glucose, hemoglobin A_{1c}, fructosamine

Reference Range Target range: Adults:

Fasting blood glucose: <120 mg/dL

Glycosylated hemoglobin: <7%

Patient Information Patients must be counseled by someone experienced in diabetes education, signs and symptoms of hyper- and hypoglycemia, exercise and diet, blood glucose monitoring, and other related topics; eat regularly, do not skip meals; carry quick source of sugar; medical alert bracelet

Nursing Implications Patients who are anorexic or NPO, may need to have their dose held to avoid hypoglycemia

Dosage Forms

Tablet (Diaβeta®, Micronase®): 1.25 mg, 2.5 mg, 5 mg

Tablet, micronized (Glynase™ PresTab™): 1.5 mg, 3 mg, 6 mg

Glycate® [OTC] *see* Calcium Carbonate *on page 185*

Glycerin (GLIS er in)

Related Information
Laxatives, Classification and Properties *on page 1412*

Brand Names Fleet® Babylax® [OTC]; Ophthalgan®; Osmoglyn®; Sani-Supp® [OTC]

Synonyms Glycerol

Therapeutic Category Cathartic, Stimulant; Diuretic, Osmotic; Laxative, Hyperosmolar; Rectal Drug, Locally Acting

Use Constipation; reduction of intraocular pressure; reduction of corneal edema; glycerin has been administered orally to reduce intracranial pressure

Pregnancy Risk Factor C

Contraindications Known hypersensitivity to glycerin or any ingredients, anuria, pulmonary edema, severe dehydration

Warnings/Precautions Safety and efficacy of ophthalmic solution in children have not been established. The primary use of glycerin in the elderly is as a laxative, although it is not recommended as a first-line treatment. Oral: Use cautiously in hypovolemia, confused mental state, congestive heart failure, elderly, senile, diabetic, and severely dehydrated patients.

Adverse Reactions

>10%:
- Central nervous system: Headache
- Gastrointestinal: Vomiting

1% to 10%:
- Central nervous system: Dizziness, confusion
- Endocrine & metabolic: Polydipsia
- Gastrointestinal: Diarrhea, nausea, tenesmus, xerostomia
- Miscellaneous: Thirst

<1%:
- Cardiovascular: Arrhythmias
- Central nervous system: Pain
- Endocrine & metabolic: Hyperglycemia
- Local: Rectal irritation, burning, cramping pain

Stability
Refrigerate suppositories; protect from heat; freezing should be avoided
Ophthalmic: Keep bottle tightly closed; store at room temperature; discard 6 months after dropper is first placed in the solution

Mechanism of Action Osmotic dehydrating agent which increases osmotic pressure; draws fluid into colon and thus stimulates evacuation

Pharmacodynamics/Kinetics
Absorption:
- Oral: Well absorbed
- Rectal: Poorly absorbed

Decrease in intraocular pressure: Oral:
- Onset of action: Within 10-30 minutes
- Peak effect: Within 60-90 minutes
- Duration: 4-8 hours

Reduction of intracranial pressure: Oral:
- Onset of action: Within 10-60 minutes
- Peak effect: Within 60-90 minutes
- Duration: ~2-3 hours

Constipation: Suppository: Onset of action: 15-30 minutes
Metabolism: Primarily in the liver with 20% metabolized in the kidney
Half-life: 30-45 minutes
Elimination: Only a small percentage of drug is excreted unchanged in the urine

Usual Dosage
Constipation: Rectal:
- Children <6 years: 1 infant suppository 1-2 times/day as needed or 2-5 mL as an enema
- Children >6 years and Adults: 1 adult suppository 1-2 times/day as needed or 5-15 mL as an enema

Children and Adults:
- Reduction of intraocular pressure: Oral: 1-1.8 g/kg 1-1½ hours preoperatively; additional doses may be administered at 5-hour intervals
- Reduction of intracranial pressure: Oral: 1.5 g/kg/day divided every 4 hours; 1 g/kg/dose every 6 hours has also been used
- Reduction of corneal edema: Ophthalmic solution: Instill 1-2 drops in eye(s) prior to examination OR for lubricant effect, instill 1-2 drops in eye(s) every 3-4 hours

Patient Information Do not use if experiencing abdominal pain, nausea, or vomiting

Nursing Implications Apply topical anesthetic before instilling ophthalmic drops. Use caution during insertion of suppository to avoid intestinal perforation, especially in neonates; suppository needs to melt to provide laxative effect; primary use of glycerin in the elderly is as a laxative, although it is not recommended as a first line treatment.

Dosage Forms

Solution:

Ophthalmic, sterile (Ophthalgan®): Glycerin with chlorobutanol 0.55% (7.5 mL)

Oral (lime flavor)(Osmoglyn®): 50% (220 mL)

Rectal (Fleet Babylax®): 4 mL/applicator (6s)

Suppository, rectal (Sani-Supp®): Glycerin with sodium stearate (infant and adult sizes)

Glycerol *see* Glycerin *on previous page*

Glycerol Guaiacolate *see* Guaifenesin *on page 589*

Glyceryl Trinitrate *see* Nitroglycerin *on page 909*

Glycopyrrolate (glye koe PYE roe late)

Brand Names Robinul®; Robinul® Forte

Synonyms Glycopyrronium Bromide

Therapeutic Category Anticholinergic Agent; Antispasmodic Agent, Gastrointestinal

Use Adjunct in treatment of peptic ulcer disease; inhibit salivation and excessive secretions of the respiratory tract preoperatively; reversal of neuromuscular blockade; control of upper airway secretions

Pregnancy Risk Factor B

Contraindications Narrow-angle glaucoma, acute hemorrhage, tachycardia, hypersensitivity to glycopyrrolate or any component; ulcerative colitis, obstructive uropathy, paralytic ileus, obstructive disease of GI tract

Warnings/Precautions Not recommended in children <12 years of age for the management of peptic ulcer; infants, patients with Down syndrome, and children with spastic paralysis or brain damage may be hypersensitive to antimuscarine effects. Use caution in elderly, patients with autonomic neuropathy, hepatic or renal disease, ulcerative colitis may predispose megacolon, hyperthyroidism, CAD, CHF, arrhythmias, tachycardia, BPH, hiatal hernia, with reflux.

Adverse Reactions

>10%:

Dermatologic: Dry skin

Gastrointestinal: Constipation, dry throat, xerostomia

Local: Irritation at injection site

Respiratory: Dry nose

Miscellaneous: Diaphoresis (decreased)

1% to 10%:

Dermatologic: Increased sensitivity to light

Endocrine & metabolic: Decreased flow of breast milk

Gastrointestinal: Dysphagia

<1%:

Cardiovascular: Orthostatic hypotension, ventricular fibrillation, tachycardia, palpitations

Central nervous system: Confusion, drowsiness, headache, loss of memory, fatigue, ataxia

Dermatologic: Rash

Gastrointestinal: Bloated feeling, nausea, vomiting

Genitourinary: Dysuria

Neuromuscular & skeletal: Weakness

Ocular: Increased intraocular pain, blurred vision

Overdosage/Toxicology Symptoms of overdose include blurred vision, urinary retention, tachycardia, absent bowel sounds

Anticholinergic toxicity is caused by strong binding of the drug to cholinergic receptors. For anticholinergic overdose with severe life-threatening symptoms, physostigmine 1-2 mg (0.5 or 0.02 mg/kg for children) S.C. or I.V., slowly may be given to reverse these effects.

Drug Interactions

Decreased effect of levodopa

Increased toxicity with amantadine, cyclopropane

Stability Unstable at pH >6; **incompatible** with secobarbital (immediate precipitation), sodium bicarbonate (gas evolves), thiopental (immediate precipitation)

Mechanism of Action Blocks the action of acetylcholine at parasympathetic sites in smooth muscle, secretory glands, and the CNS

Pharmacodynamics/Kinetics

Oral:

Onset of action: Within 50 minutes

Peak effect: Within 1 hour

(Continued)

Glycopyrrolate *(Continued)*

I.M.: Onset of action: 20-40 minutes
I.V.: Onset of action: 10-15 minutes
Absorption: Oral: Poor and erratic
Bioavailability: ~10%

Usual Dosage

Children:

Control of secretions:

Oral: 40-100 mcg/kg/dose 3-4 times/day

I.M., I.V.: 4-10 mcg/kg/dose every 3-4 hours; maximum: 0.2 mg/dose or 0.8 mg/24 hours

Intraoperative: I.V.: 4 mcg/kg not to exceed 0.1 mg; repeat at 2- to 3-minute intervals as needed

Preoperative: I.M.:

<2 years: 4.4-8.8 mcg/kg 30-60 minutes before procedure

>2 years: 4.4 mcg/kg 30-60 minutes before procedure

Children and Adults: Reverse neuromuscular blockade: I.V.: 0.2 mg for each 1 mg of neostigmine or 5 mg of pyridostigmine administered

Adults:

Intraoperative: I.V.: 0.1 mg repeated as needed at 2- to 3-minute intervals

Preoperative: I.M.: 4.4 mcg/kg 30-60 minutes before procedure

Peptic ulcer:

Oral: 1-2 mg 2-3 times/day

I.M., I.V.: 0.1-0.2 mg 3-4 times/day

Administration For I.V. administration, glycopyrrolate may also be administered via the tubing of a running I.V. infusion of a compatible solution

Patient Information Maintain good oral hygiene habits, because lack of saliva may increase chance of cavities. Observe caution while driving or performing other tasks requiring alertness, as may cause drowsiness, dizziness, or blurred vision. Notify physician if skin rash, flushing or eye pain occurs; or if difficulty in urinating, constipation, or sensitivity to light becomes severe or persists.

Dosage Forms

Injection, as bromide: 0.2 mg/mL (1 mL, 2 mL, 5 mL, 20 mL)

Robinul®: 0.2 mg/mL (1 mL, 2 mL, 5 mL, 20 mL)

Tablet, as bromide:

Robinul®: 1 mg

Robinul® Forte: 2 mg

Glycopyrronium Bromide *see* Glycopyrrolate *on previous page*
Glycotuss® [OTC] *see* Guaifenesin *on page 589*
Glycotuss-dM® [OTC] *see* Guaifenesin and Dextromethorphan *on page 591*
Glydiazinamide *see* Glipizide *on page 576*
Glynase™ PresTab™ *see* Glyburide *on page 578*
Gly-Oxide® Oral [OTC] *see* Carbamide Peroxide *on page 203*
Glytuss® [OTC] *see* Guaifenesin *on page 589*
GM-CSF *see* Sargramostim *on page 1125*
GnRH *see* Gonadorelin *on next page*

Gold Sodium Thiomalate (gold SOW dee um thye oh MAL ate)

Brand Names Aurolate®; Myochrysine®

Therapeutic Category Gold Compound

Use Treatment of progressive rheumatoid arthritis

Pregnancy Risk Factor C

Contraindications Hypersensitivity to gold compounds or any component; systemic lupus erythematosus; history of blood dyscrasias; congestive heart failure, exfoliative dermatitis, colitis

Warnings/Precautions Frequent monitoring of patients for signs and symptoms of toxicity will prevent serious adverse reactions; nonsteroidal anti-inflammatory drugs (NSAIDs) and corticosteroids may be discontinued after initiating gold therapy; must not be injected I.V.

Explain the possibility of adverse reactions before initiating therapy; signs of gold toxicity include decrease in hemoglobin, leukopenia, granulocytes and platelets; proteinuria, hematuria, pigmentation, pruritus, stomatitis or persistent diarrhea, rash, metallic taste; advise patient to report any symptoms of toxicity; use with caution in patients with liver or renal disease

Adverse Reactions

>10%:

Dermatologic: Itching, rash

Gastrointestinal: Stomatitis, gingivitis, glossitis

Ocular: Conjunctivitis

1% to 10%:
- Dermatologic: Urticaria, alopecia
- Hematologic: Eosinophilia, leukopenia, thrombocytopenia
- Renal: Proteinuria, hematuria

<1%:
- Dermatologic: Angioedema
- Gastrointestinal: Ulcerative enterocolitis, GI hemorrhage, dysphagia, metallic taste
- Hematologic: Agranulocytosis, anemia, aplastic anemia
- Hepatic: Hepatotoxicity
- Neuromuscular & skeletal: Peripheral neuropathy
- Respiratory: Interstitial pneumonitis

Overdosage/Toxicology Symptoms of overdose include hematuria, proteinuria, fever, nausea, vomiting, diarrhea

For mild gold poisoning, dimercaprol 2.5 mg/kg 4 times/day for 2 days or for more severe forms of gold intoxication, dimercaprol 3-5 mg/kg every 4 hours for 2 days should be initiated; then after 2 days, the initial dose should be repeated twice daily on the third day, and once daily thereafter for 10 days. Other chelating agents have been used with some success.

Drug Interactions Decreased effect with penicillamine, acetylcysteine

Stability Should not be used if solution is darker than pale yellow

Mechanism of Action Unknown, may decrease prostaglandin synthesis or may alter cellular mechanisms by inhibiting sulfhydryl systems

Pharmacodynamics/Kinetics
- Half-life: 5 days; may lengthen with multiple doses
- Time to peak serum concentration: Within 4-6 hours
- Elimination: Majority (60% to 90%) excreted in urine with smaller amounts (10% to 40%) excreted in feces (via bile)

Usual Dosage I.M.:
- Children: Initial: Test dose of 10 mg is recommended, followed by 1 mg/kg/week for 20 weeks; maintenance: 1 mg/kg/dose at 2- to 4-week intervals thereafter for as long as therapy is clinically beneficial and toxicity does not develop. Administration for 2-4 months is usually required before clinical improvement is observed.
- Adults: 10 mg first week; 25 mg second week; then 25-50 mg/week until 1 g cumulative dose has been given; if improvement occurs without adverse reactions, administer 25-50 mg every 2-3 weeks for 2-20 weeks, then every 3-4 weeks indefinitely

Dosing adjustment in renal impairment:
- Cl_{cr} 50-80 mL/minute: Administer 50% of normal dose
- Cl_{cr} <50 mL/minute: Avoid use

Administration Deep I.M. injection into the upper outer quadrant of the gluteal region addition of 0.1 mL of 1% lidocaine to each injection may reduce the discomfort associated with I.M. administration

Monitoring Parameters Signs and symptoms of gold toxicity, CBC with differential and platelet count, urinalysis

Reference Range Gold: Normal: 0-0.1 μg/mL (SI: 0-0.0064 μmol/L); Therapeutic: 1-3 μg/mL (SI: 0.06-0.18 μmol/L); Urine: <0.1 μg/24 hour

Patient Information Minimize exposure to sunlight; benefits from drug therapy may take as long as 3 months to appear; notify physician of pruritus, rash, sore mouth; metallic taste may occur

Nursing Implications Explain the possibility of adverse reactions before initiating therapy

Additional Information Approximately 50% gold

Dosage Forms Injection: 25 mg/mL (1 mL); 50 mg/mL (1 mL, 2 mL, 10 mL)

GoLYTELY® *see* Polyethylene Glycol-Electrolyte Solution *on page 1017*

Gonadorelin (goe nad oh REL in)

Brand Names Factrel®; Lutrepulse®

Synonyms GnRH; Gonadorelin Acetate; Gonadorelin Hydrochloride; Gonadotropin Releasing Hormone; LH-RH; LRH; Luteinizing Hormone Releasing Hormone

Therapeutic Category Diagnostic Agent, Gonadotrophic Hormone; Gonadotropin

Use Evaluation of the functional capacity and response of gonadotrophic hormones; evaluate abnormal gonadotropin regulation as in precocious puberty and delayed puberty. Lutrepulse®: Induction of ovulation in females with hypothalamic amenorrhea.

Pregnancy Risk Factor B

Contraindications Known hypersensitivity to gonadorelin, women with any condition that could be exacerbated by pregnancy; patients who have ovarian

(Continued)

Gonadorelin *(Continued)*

cysts or causes of anovulation other than those of hypothalamic origin; any condition that may worsened by reproductive hormones

Warnings/Precautions Hypersensitivity and anaphylactic reactions have occurred following multiple-dose administration; multiple pregnancy is a possibility; use with caution in women in whom pregnancy could worsen pre-existing conditions (eg, pituitary prolactinemia). Multiple pregnancy is a possibility with Lutrepulse®.

Adverse Reactions

1% to 10%: Local: Pain at injection site

<1%:

Cardiovascular: Flushing
Central nervous system: Lightheadedness, headache
Dermatologic: Rash
Gastrointestinal: Nausea, abdominal discomfort

Overdosage/Toxicology Symptoms of overdose include abdominal discomfort, nausea, headache, flushing; symptomatic treatment

Drug Interactions

Decreased levels/effect: Oral contraceptives, digoxin, phenothiazines, dopamine antagonists

Increased levels/effect: Androgens, estrogens, progestins, glucocorticoids, spironolactone, levodopa

Stability

Factrel®: Prepare immediately prior to use; after reconstitution, store at room temperature and use within 1 day; discard unused portion

Lutrepulse®: Store at room temperature; reconstitute with diluent immediately prior to use and transfer to plastic reservoir. The solution will supply 90 minute pulsatile doses for 7 consecutive days (Lutrepulse® pump).

Mechanism of Action Stimulates the release of luteinizing hormone (LH) from the anterior pituitary gland

Pharmacodynamics/Kinetics

Peak effect: Maximal LH release occurs within 20 minutes
Duration of action: 3-5 hours
Half-life: 4 minutes

Usual Dosage

Diagnostic test: Children >12 years and Adults (female): I.V., S.C. hydrochloride salt: 100 mcg administered in women during early phase of menstrual cycle (day 1-7)

Primary hypothalamic amenorrhea: Female adults: Acetate: I.V.: 5 mcg every 90 minutes via Lutrepulse® pump kit at treatment intervals of 21 days (pump will pulsate every 90 minutes for 7 days)

Administration

Factrel®: Dilute in 3 mL of normal saline; administer I.V. push over 30 seconds

Lutrepulse®: A presterilized reservoir bag with the infusion catheter set supplied with the kit should be filled with the reconstituted solution and administered I.V. using the Lutrepulse® pump. Set the pump to deliver 25-50 mL of solution, based upon the dose, over a pulse period of 1 minute and at a pulse frequency of 90 minutes.

Monitoring Parameters LH, FSH

Dosage Forms

Injection, as acetate (Lutrepulse®): 0.8 mg, 3.2 mg
Injection, as hydrochloride (Factrel®): 100 mcg, 500 mcg

Gonadorelin Acetate *see* Gonadorelin *on previous page*
Gonadorelin Hydrochloride *see* Gonadorelin *on previous page*
Gonadotropin Releasing Hormone *see* Gonadorelin *on previous page*
Gonic® *see* Chorionic Gonadotropin *on page 272*
Gordofilm® Liquid *see* Salicylic Acid *on page 1120*

Goserelin (GOE se rel in)

Related Information

Cancer Chemotherapy Regimens *on page 1351*

Brand Names Zoladex®

Synonyms Goserelin Acetate

Therapeutic Category Antineoplastic Agent, Miscellaneous; Gonadotropin Releasing Hormone Analog; Luteinizing Hormone-Releasing Hormone Analog

Use Prostate carcinoma: palliative treatment of advanced carcinoma of the prostate. An alternative treatment of prostatic cancer when orchiectomy or estrogen administration are either not indicated or unacceptable to the patient.

3.6 mg implant ONLY:

Endometriosis: management of endometriosis, including pain relief and reduction of endometriotic lesions for the duration of therapy.

Advanced breast cancer: palliative treatment of advanced breast cancer in pre- and perimenopausal women. Estrogen and progesterone receptor values may help to predict whether goserelin therapy is likely to be beneficial.

Note: The 10.8 mg implant is not indicated in women as the data are insufficient to support reliable suppression of serum estradiol

Pregnancy Risk Factor X

Contraindications In women who are or may become pregnant, patients who are hypersensitive to the drug

Warnings/Precautions Initially, goserelin, transiently increases serum levels of testosterone. Transient worsening of signs and symptoms, usually manifested by an increase in cancer-related pain which was managed symptomatically, may develop during the first few weeks of treatment. Isolated cases of ureteral obstruction and spinal cord compression have been reported; patient's symptoms may initially worsen temporarily during first few weeks of therapy, cancer-related pain can usually be controlled by analgesics

Adverse Reactions

General: Worsening of signs and symptoms may occur during the first few weeks of therapy and are usually manifested by an increase in bone pain, increased difficulty in urinating, hot flashes, injection site irritation, and weakness; this will subside, but patients should be aware

>10%:

- Endocrine & metabolic: Gynecomastia, postmenopausal symptoms, sexual dysfunction, loss of libido, hot flashes
- Genitourinary: Impotence, decreased erection

1% to 10%:

- Cardiovascular: Edema
- Central nervous system: Headache, spinal cord compression (possible result of tumor flare), lethargy, dizziness, insomnia
- Dermatologic: Rash
- Gastrointestinal: Nausea and vomiting, anorexia, diarrhea, weight gain
- Genitourinary: Vaginal spotting and breakthrough bleeding, breast tenderness/enlargement
- Local: Pain on injection
- Neuromuscular & skeletal: Bone loss, increased bone pain
- Miscellaneous: Diaphoresis

Overdosage/Toxicology Symptomatic management

Stability Zoladex® should be stored at room temperature not to exceed 25°C or 77°F; must be dispensed in an amber bag

Mechanism of Action LHRH synthetic analog of luteinizing hormone-releasing hormone also known as gonadotropin-releasing hormone (GnRH) incorporated into a biodegradable depot material which allows for continuous slow release over 28 days; mechanism of action is similar to leuprolide

Pharmacodynamics/Kinetics

Absorption:

- Oral: Inactive when administered orally
- S.C.: Rapid and can be detected in the serum in 10 minutes

Distribution: V_d: 13.7 L

Time to peak serum concentration: S.C.: 12-15 days

Half-life: Following a bolus S.C. dose: 5 hours

Elimination: By the kidney; elimination time: 4.2 hours (prolonged in impaired renal function - 12 hours)

Usual Dosage

Adults: S.C.:

- Monthly implant: 3.6 mg injected into upper abdomen every 28 days; do not try to aspirate with the goserelin syringe, if the needle is in a large vessel, blood will immediately appear in syringe chamber. While a delay of a few days is permissible, attempt to adhere to the 28-day schedule.
- 3-month implant: 10.8 mg injected into the upper abdominal wall every 12 weeks; do not try to aspirate with the goserelin syringe, if the needle is in a large vessel, blood will immediately appear in syringe chamber. While a delay of a few days is permissible, attempt to adhere to the 12 week schedule.

Prostate carcinoma: Intended for long-term administration

Endometriosis: Recommended duration is 6 months; retreatment is not recommended since safety data is not available; if symptoms recur after a course of therapy, and further treatment is contemplated, consider monitoring bone mineral density. Currently there are no clinical data on the effect of treatment of benign gynecological conditions with goserelin for periods >6 months.

Dosage adjustment in renal/hepatic impairment: No dosage adjustment necessary

Administration

Do not remove the sterile syringe until immediately before use.

(Continued)

Goserelin *(Continued)*

After cleaning with an alcohol swab, a local anesthetic may be used on an area of skin on the upper abdominal wall.

Stretch the patient's skin with one hand, and grip the needle with fingers around the barrel of the syringe. Insert the hypodermic needle into the SC fat. Do not aspirate. If the hypodermic needle penetrates a large vessel, blood will be seen instantly in the syringe chamber.

Change the direction of the needle so it parallels the abdominal wall. Push the needle in until the barrel hub touches the patient's skin. Withdraw the needle 1 cm to create a space to discharge the drug; fully depress the plunger to discharge.

Withdraw needle and bandage the site. Confirm discharge by ensuring tip of the plunger is visible within the tip of the needle.

Test Interactions Serum alkaline phosphatase, serum acid phosphatase, serum testosterone, serum LH and FSH, serum estradiol

Patient Information Females must use reliable contraception during therapy; symptoms may worsen temporarily during first weeks of therapy

Dosage Forms Injection: 3.6 mg single dose disposable syringe with 16-gauge hypodermic needle; 10.8 mg single dose disposable syringe with 14-gauge hypodermic needle

Goserelin Acetate *see* Goserelin *on page 584*

GR122311X *see* Ranitidine Bismuth Citrate *on page 1094*

Granisetron (gra NI se tron)

Brand Names Kytril®

Therapeutic Category Antiemetic

Use Prophylaxis and treatment of chemotherapy-related emesis; may be prescribed for patients who are refractory to or have severe adverse reactions to standard antiemetic therapy. Granisetron may be prescribed for young patients (ie, <45 years of age who are more likely to develop extrapyramidal reactions to high-dose metoclopramide) who are to receive highly emetogenic chemotherapeutic agents as listed:

Agents with high emetogenic potential (>90%) (dose/m^2):
- Carmustine ≥200 mg
- Cisplatin ≥75 mg
- Cyclophosphamide ≥1000 mg
- Cytarabine ≥1000 mg
- Dacarbazine ≥500 mg
- Ifosfamide ≥1000 mg
- Lomustine ≥60 mg
- Mechlorethamine
- Pentostatin
- Streptozocin

or two agents classified as having high or moderately high emetogenic potential as listed:

Agents with moderately high emetogenic potential (60% to 90%) (dose/m^2):
- Carmustine <200 mg
- Cisplatin <75 mg
- Cyclophosphamide 1000 mg
- Cytarabine 250-1000 mg
- Dacarbazine <500 mg
- Doxorubicin ≥75 mg
- Ifosfamide
- Lomustine <60 mg
- Methotrexate ≥250 mg
- Mitomycin
- Mitoxantrone
- Procarbazine

Granisetron should not be prescribed for chemotherapeutic agents with a low emetogenic potential (eg, bleomycin, busulfan, cyclophosphamide <1000 mg, etoposide, 5-fluorouracil, vinblastine, vincristine)

Contraindications Previous hypersensitivity to granisetron

Warnings/Precautions Use with caution in patients with liver disease or in pregnant patients

Adverse Reactions

>10%: Central nervous system: Headache

1% to 10%:
- Cardiovascular: Hyper/hypotension
- Central nervous system: Dizziness, insomnia, anxiety
- Gastrointestinal: Constipation, abdominal pain, diarrhea

Neuromuscular & skeletal: Weakness

<1%:

Cardiovascular: Arrhythmias

Central nervous system: Somnolence, agitation

Endocrine & metabolic: Hot flashes

Hepatic: Liver enzyme elevations

Stability I.V.: Stable when mixed in NS or D_5W for 24 hours at room temperature; protect from light; do not freeze vials

Mechanism of Action Selective 5-HT_3-receptor antagonist, blocking serotonin, both peripherally on vagal nerve terminals and centrally in the chemoreceptor trigger zone

Pharmacodynamics/Kinetics

Onset of action: Commonly controls emesis within 1-3 minutes of administration

Duration: Effects generally last no more than 24 hours maximum

Distribution: V_d: 2-3 L/kg; widely distributed throughout the body

Half-life:

Cancer patients: 10-12 hours

Healthy volunteers: 3-4 hours

Elimination: Primarily nonrenal, 8% to 15% of a dose is excreted unchanged in urine

Usual Dosage

I.V.: Children and Adults: 10 mcg/kg for 1-3 doses. Doses should be administered as a single IVPB over 5 minutes to 1 hour or by undiluted IV push over 30 seconds, given just prior to chemotherapy (15-60 minutes before); as intervention therapy for breakthrough nausea and vomiting, during the first 24 hours following chemotherapy, 2 or 3 repeat infusions (same dose) have been administered, separated by at least 10 minutes

Oral: Adults: 1 mg twice daily; the first 1 mg dose should be given up to 1 hour before chemotherapy, and the second tablet, 12 hours after the first

Note: Granisetron should only be given on the day(s) of chemotherapy

Dosing interval in renal impairment: Creatinine clearance values have no relationship to granisetron clearance

Dosing interval in hepatic impairment: Kinetic studies in patients with hepatic impairment showed that total clearance was approximately halved, however, standard doses were very well tolerated

Nursing Implications Doses should be given at least 15 minutes prior to initiation of chemotherapy

Dosage Forms

Injection: 1 mg/mL

Tablet: 1 mg (2s), (20s)

Extemporaneous Preparations A 0.2 mg/mL oral suspension may be prepared by crushing twelve (12) 1 mg tablets and mixing with 30 mL water and enough cherry syrup to provide a final volume of 60 mL; this preparation is stable for 14 days at room temperature or when refrigerated

Granulocyte Colony Stimulating Factor *see* Filgrastim *on page 518*

Granulocyte-Macrophage Colony Stimulating Factor *see* Sargramostim *on page 1125*

Grifulvin® V *see* Griseofulvin *on this page*

Grisactin® *see* Griseofulvin *on this page*

Grisactin® Ultra *see* Griseofulvin *on this page*

Griseofulvin (gri see oh FUL vin)

Related Information

Antifungal Agents *on page 1395*

Brand Names Fulvicin® P/G; Fulvicin-U/F®; Grifulvin® V; Grisactin®; Grisactin® Ultra; Gris-PEG®

Canadian/Mexican Brand Names Grisovin-FP® (Canada); Fulvina® P/G (Mexico); Grisovin-FP® (Mexico)

Synonyms Griseofulvin Microsize; Griseofulvin Ultramicrosize

Therapeutic Category Antifungal Agent, Systemic

Use Treatment of susceptible tinea infections of the skin, hair, and nails

Pregnancy Risk Factor C

Contraindications Hypersensitivity to griseofulvin or any component; severe liver disease, porphyria (interferes with porphyrin metabolism)

Warnings/Precautions Safe use in children <2 years of age has not been established; during long-term therapy, periodic assessment of hepatic, renal, and hematopoietic functions should be performed; may cause fetal harm when administered to pregnant women; avoid exposure to intense sunlight to prevent photosensitivity reactions; hypersensitivity cross reaction between penicillins and griseofulvin is possible

(Continued)

Griseofulvin *(Continued)*

Adverse Reactions

>10%: Dermatologic: Rash, urticaria

1% to 10%:

Central nervous system: Headache, fatigue, dizziness, insomnia, mental confusion
Dermatologic: Photosensitivity
Gastrointestinal: Nausea, vomiting, epigastric distress, diarrhea
Miscellaneous: Oral thrush

<1%:

Dermatologic: Angioneurotic edema
Endocrine & metabolic: Menstrual toxicity
Gastrointestinal: GI bleeding
Hematologic: Leukopenia
Hepatic: Hepatic toxicity
Renal: Proteinuria, nephrosis

Overdosage/Toxicology Symptoms of overdose include lethargy, vertigo, blurred vision, nausea, vomiting, diarrhea; following GI decontamination, treatment is supportive

Drug Interactions

Decreased effect:

Barbiturates may decrease levels
Decreased warfarin activity
Decreased oral contraceptive effectiveness

Increased toxicity: With alcohol → tachycardia and flushing

Mechanism of Action Inhibits fungal cell mitosis at metaphase; binds to human keratin making it resistant to fungal invasion

Pharmacodynamics/Kinetics

Absorption: Ultramicrosize griseofulvin absorption is almost complete; absorption of microsize griseofulvin is variable (25% to 70% of an oral dose); absorption is enhanced by ingestion of a fatty meal
Distribution: Crosses the placenta
Metabolism: Extensive in the liver
Half-life: 9-22 hours
Elimination: <1% excreted unchanged in urine; also excreted in feces and perspiration

Usual Dosage Oral:

Children:

Microsize: 10-15 mg/kg/day in single or divided doses
Ultramicrosize: >2 months: 5.5-7.3 mg/kg/day in single or divided doses

Adults:

Microsize: 500-1000 mg/day in single or divided doses
Ultramicrosize: 330-375 mg/day in single or divided doses; doses up to 750 mg/day have been used for infections more difficult to eradicate such as tinea unguium and tinea pedis

Duration of therapy depends on the site of infection:

Tinea corporis: 2-4 weeks
Tinea capitis: 4-6 weeks or longer
Tinea pedis: 4-8 weeks
Tinea unguium: 4-6 months

Monitoring Parameters Periodic renal, hepatic, and hematopoietic function tests

Test Interactions False-positive urinary VMA levels

Patient Information Avoid exposure to sunlight, take with fatty meal; if patient gets headache, it usually goes away with continued therapy; may cause dizziness, drowsiness, and impair judgment; do not take if pregnant; if you become pregnant, discontinue immediately

Additional Information

Microsize: Fulvicin-U/F®, Grifulvin® V, Grisactin®
Ultramicrosize: Fulvicin® P/G, Grisactin® Ultra, Gris-PEG®; GI absorption of ultramicrosize is ~1.5 times that of microsize

Dosage Forms

Microsize:

Capsule (Grisactin®): 125 mg, 250 mg
Suspension, oral (Grifulvin® V): 125 mg/5 mL with alcohol 0.2% (120 mL)
Tablet:

Fulvicin-U/F®, Grifulvin® V: 250 mg
Fulvicin-U/F®, Grifulvin® V, Grisactin-500®: 500 mg

Ultramicrosize:

Tablet:

Fulvicin® P/G: 165 mg, 330 mg
Fulvicin® P/G, Grisactin® Ultra, Gris-PEG®: 125 mg, 250 mg

Grisactin® Ultra: 330 mg

Griseofulvin Microsize *see* Griseofulvin *on page 587*

Griseofulvin Ultramicrosize *see* Griseofulvin *on page 587*

Gris-PEG® *see* Griseofulvin *on page 587*

Growth Hormone *see* Human Growth Hormone *on page 613*

Guaifenesin (gwye FEN e sin)

Brand Names Anti-Tuss® Expectorant [OTC]; Breonesin® [OTC]; Diabetic Tussin EX® [OTC]; Fenesin™; Gee Gee® [OTC]; Genatuss® [OTC]; GG-Cen® [OTC]; Glyate® [OTC]; Glycotuss® [OTC]; Glytuss® [OTC]; Guaifenex LA®; GuiaCough® Expectorant [OTC]; Guiatuss® [OTC]; Halotussin® [OTC]; Humibid® L.A.; Humibid® Sprinkle; Hytuss® [OTC]; Hytuss-2X® [OTC]; Liquibid®; Malotuss® [OTC]; Medi-Tuss® [OTC]; Muco-Fen-LA®; Mytussin® [OTC]; Naldecon® Senior EX [OTC]; Organidin® NR; Pneumomist®; Respa-GF®; Robitussin® [OTC]; Scot-Tussin® [OTC]; Siltussin® [OTC]; Sinumist®-SR Capsulets®; Touro Ex®; Tusibron® [OTC]; Uni-tussin® [OTC]

Canadian/Mexican Brand Names Balminil® Expectorant (Canada); Calmylin® Expectorant (Canada)

Synonyms GG; Glycerol Guaiacolate

Therapeutic Category Cough Preparation; Expectorant

Use Temporary control of cough due to minor throat and bronchial irritation

Pregnancy Risk Factor C

Contraindications Hypersensitivity to guaifenesin or any component

Warnings/Precautions Not for persistent cough such as occurs with smoking, asthma, or emphysema or cough accompanied by excessive secretions

Adverse Reactions

1% to 10%:

- Central nervous system: Drowsiness, headache
- Dermatologic: Rash
- Gastrointestinal: Nausea, vomiting, stomach pain

Overdosage/Toxicology Symptoms of overdose include vomiting, lethargy, coma, respiratory depression; treatment is supportive

Stability Protect from light

Mechanism of Action Thought to act as an expectorant by irritating the gastric mucosa and stimulating respiratory tract secretions, thereby increasing respiratory fluid volumes and decreasing phlegm viscosity

Pharmacodynamics/Kinetics

Absorption: Well absorbed from GI tract

Metabolism: Hepatic, 60%

Elimination: Renal excretion of changed and unchanged drug

Usual Dosage Oral:

Children:

- <2 years: 12 mg/kg/day in 6 divided doses
- 2-5 years: 50-100 mg every 4 hours, not to exceed 600 mg/day
- 6-11 years: 100-200 mg every 4 hours, not to exceed 1.2 g/day

Children >12 years and Adults: 200-400 mg every 4 hours to a maximum of 2.4 g/day

Test Interactions Possible color interference with determination of 5-HIAA and VMA

Patient Information Take with a large quantity of fluid to ensure proper action; if cough persists for more than 1 week or is accompanied by fever, rash, or persistent headache, physician should be consulted

Additional Information Syrup contains 3.5% alcohol

Dosage Forms

Caplet, sustained release (Touro Ex®): 600 mg

Capsule (Breonesin®, GG-Cen®, Hytuss-2X®): 200 mg

Capsule, sustained release (Humibid® Sprinkle): 300 mg

Liquid:

- Diabetic Tussin EX®, Organidin® NR, Tusibron®: 100 mg/5 mL (118 mL)
- Naldecon® Senior EX: 200 mg/5 mL (118 mL, 480 mL)

Syrup (Anti-Tuss® Expectorant, Genatuss®, Glyate®, GuiaCough® Expectorant, Guiatuss®, Halotussin®, Malotuss®, Medi-Tuss®, Mytussin®, Robitussin®, Scot-tussin®, Siltussin®, Tusibron®, Uni-Tussin®): 100 mg/5 mL with alcohol 3.5% (30 mL, 120 mL, 240 mL, 473 mL, 946 mL)

Tablet:

- Duratuss-G®: 1200 mg
- Gee Gee®, Glytuss®, Organidin® NR: 200 mg
- Glycotuss®, Hytuss®: 100 mg
- Sustained release:
  - Fenesin™, Guaifenex LA®, Humibid® L.A., Liquibid®, Monafed®, Muco-Fen-LA®, Pneumomist®, Respa-GF®, Sinumist®-SR Capsulets®: 600 mg

Guaifenesin and Codeine (gwye FEN e sin & KOE deen)

Brand Names Brontex® Liquid; Brontex® Tablet; Cheracol®; Guaituss AC®; Guiatussin® with Codeine; Mytussin® AC; Robafen® AC; Robitussin® A-C; Tussi-Organidin® NR

Synonyms Codeine and Guaifenesin

Therapeutic Category Antitussive; Cough Preparation; Expectorant

Use Temporary control of cough due to minor throat and bronchial irritation

Restrictions C-V

Pregnancy Risk Factor C

Contraindications Hypersensitivity to guaifenesin, codeine or any component

Warnings/Precautions Should not be used for chronic productive coughs

Adverse Reactions

Codeine:

>10%:

Central nervous system: Drowsiness

Gastrointestinal: Constipation

1% to 10%:

Cardiovascular: Hypotension, palpitations, tachycardia or bradycardia, peripheral vasodilation

Central nervous system: CNS depression, drowsiness, sedation, confusion, headache, increased intracranial pressure, dizziness, lightheadedness, false feeling of well being, restlessness, paradoxical CNS stimulation, malaise

Dermatologic: Rash, urticaria

Endocrine & metabolic: Antidiuretic hormone release

Gastrointestinal: Nausea, vomiting, anorexia, xerostomia, biliary tract spasm

Genitourinary: Decreased urination, urinary tract spasm

Neuromuscular & skeletal: Weakness

Ocular: Miosis, blurred vision

Respiratory: Respiratory depression, shortness of breath, dyspnea

Miscellaneous: Histamine release, physical and psychological dependence with prolonged use

<1%:

Central nervous system: Convulsions, hallucinations, mental depression, nightmares, insomnia

Gastrointestinal: Biliary tract spasm, stomach cramps, paralytic ileus

Neuromuscular & skeletal: Trembling, muscle rigidity

Guaifenesin:

1% to 10%:

Central nervous system: Drowsiness, headache

Dermatologic: Rash

Gastrointestinal: Nausea, vomiting, stomach pain

Drug Interactions Increased toxicity: CNS depressant medications produce additive sedative properties

Mechanism of Action Refer to individual monographs for Guaifenesin and Codeine

Pharmacodynamics/Kinetics Refer to individual monographs for Guaifenesin and Codeine

Usual Dosage Oral:

Children:

2-6 years: 1-1.5 mg/kg codeine/day divided into 4 doses administered every 4-6 hours (maximum: 30 mg/24 hours)

6-12 years: 5 mL every 4 hours, not to exceed 30 mL/24 hours

Children >12 years and Adults: 5-10 mL every 4-8 hours not to exceed 60 mL/24 hours

Dietary Considerations

Codeine:

Alcohol: Additive CNS effects, avoid or limit alcohol; watch for sedation

Food: Glucose may cause hyperglycemia; monitor blood glucose concentration

Patient Information Take with a large quantity of fluid to ensure proper action; if cough persists for more than 1 week or is accompanied by fever, rash, or persistent headache, physician should be consulted; avoid CNS depressants and alcohol; do not use for chronic or persistent coughs

Dosage Forms

Liquid (Brontex®): Guaifenesin 75 mg and codeine phosphate 2.5 mg per 5 mL

Syrup (Cheracol®, Guaituss AC®, Guiatussin® with Codeine, Mytussin® AC, Robafen® AC, Robitussin® A-C, Tussi-Organidin® NR): Guaifenesin 100 mg and codeine phosphate 10 mg per 5 mL (60 mL, 120 mL, 480 mL)

Tablet (Brontex®): Guaifenesin 300 mg and codeine phosphate 10 mg

Guaifenesin and Dextromethorphan

(gwye FEN e sin & deks troe meth OR fan)

Brand Names Benylin® Expectorant [OTC]; Cheracol® D [OTC]; Clear Tussin® 30; Contac® Cough Formula Liquid [OTC]; Extra Action Cough Syrup [OTC]; Fenesin DM®; Genatuss DM® [OTC]; Glycotuss-dM® [OTC]; Guaifenex DM®; GuiaCough® [OTC]; Guiatuss DM® [OTC]; Halotussin® DM [OTC]; Humibid® DM [OTC]; Iobid DM®; Kolephrin® GG/DM [OTC]; Mytussin® DM [OTC]; Naldecon® Senior DX [OTC]; Phanatuss® [OTC]; Queltuss® [OTC]; Respa-DM®; Rhinosyn-DMX® [OTC]; Robitussin®-DM [OTC]; Siltussin DM® [OTC]; Syracol-CF® [OTC]; Tolu-Sed® DM [OTC]; Tusibron-DM® [OTC]; Tuss-DM® [OTC]; Tussi-Organidin® DM NR; Uni-tussin® DM [OTC]; Vicks® Pediatric Formula 44E [OTC]

Synonyms Dextromethorphan and Guaifenesin

Therapeutic Category Antitussive; Cough Preparation; Expectorant

Use Temporary control of cough due to minor throat and bronchial irritation

Pregnancy Risk Factor C

Contraindications Hypersensitivity to guaifenesin, dextromethorphan or any component

Warnings/Precautions Should not be used for persistent or chronic cough such as that occurring with smoking, asthma, chronic bronchitis, or emphysema or for cough associated with excessive phlegm

Adverse Reactions

1% to 10%:

- Central nervous system: Drowsiness, headache
- Dermatologic: Rash
- Gastrointestinal: Nausea, vomiting

Pharmacodynamics/Kinetics Refer to Dextromethorphan and Guaifenesin monographs

Onset of action: Exerts its antitussive effect in 15-30 minutes after oral administration

Usual Dosage Oral:

Children: Dextromethorphan: 1-2 mg/kg/24 hours divided 3-4 times/day

Children >12 years and Adults: 5 mL every 4 hours or 10 mL every 6-8 hours not to exceed 40 mL/24 hours

Patient Information Take with a large quantity of fluid to ensure proper action; if cough persists for more than one week, is recumbent, or is accompanied by fever, rash or persistent headache, physician should be consulted

Dosage Forms

Syrup:

- Benylin® Expectorant: Guaifenesin 100 mg and dextromethorphan hydrobromide 5 mg per 5 mL (118 mL, 236 mL)
- Cheracol® D, Clear Tussin® 30, Genatuss DM®, Mytussin® DM, Robitussin®-DM, Siltussin DM®, Tolu-Sed® DM, Tussi-Organidin® DM NR: Guaifenesin 100 mg and dextromethorphan hydrobromide 10 mg per 5 mL (5 mL, 10 mL, 120 mL, 240 mL, 360 mL, 480 mL, 3780 mL)
- Contac® Cough Formula Liquid: Guaifenesin 67 mg and dextromethorphan hydrobromide 10 mg per 5 mL (120 mL)
- Extra Action Cough Syrup, GuiaCough®, Guiatuss DM®, Halotussin® DM, Rhinosyn-DMX®, Tusibron-DM®, Uni-tussin® DM: Guaifenesin 100 mg and dextromethorphan hydrobromide 15 mg per 5 mL (120 mL, 240 mL, 480 mL)
- Kolephrin® GG/DM: Guaifenesin 150 mg and dextromethorphan hydrobromide 10 mg per 5 mL (120 mL)
- Naldecon® Senior DX: Guaifenesin 200 mg and dextromethorphan hydrobromide 15 mg per 5 mL (118 mL, 480 mL)
- Phanatuss®: Guaifenesin 85 mg and dextromethorphan hydrobromide 10 mg per 5 mL
- Vicks® 44E: Guaifenesin 66.7 mg and dextromethorphan hydrobromide 6.7 mg per 5 mL

Tablet:

- Extended release
- Guaifenex DM®, Iobid DM®, Fenesin DM®, Humibid® DM, Respa-DM®: Guaifenesin 600 mg and dextromethorphan hydrobromide 30 mg
- Glycotuss-dM®: Guaifenesin 100 mg and dextromethorphan hydrobromide 10 mg
- Queltuss®: Guaifenesin 100 mg and dextromethorphan hydrobromide 15 mg
- Syracol-CF®: Guaifenesin 200 mg and dextromethorphan hydrobromide 15 mg
- Tuss-DM®: Guaifenesin 200 mg and dextromethorphan hydrobromide 10 mg

Guaifenex DM® *see* Guaifenesin and Dextromethorphan *on this page*

Guaifenex LA® *see* Guaifenesin *on page 589*

Guaituss AC® *see* Guaifenesin and Codeine *on previous page*

Guanabenz (GWAHN a benz)

Brand Names Wytensin®

Synonyms Guanabenz Acetate

Therapeutic Category Alpha$_2$-Adrenergic Agonist Agent; Antihypertensive

Use Management of hypertension

Pregnancy Risk Factor C

Contraindications Hypersensitivity to guanabenz or any component

Warnings/Precautions Use with caution in patients with severe coronary insufficiency, recent myocardial infarction, severe renal or hepatic impairment

Adverse Reactions

>10%:

Central nervous system: Drowsiness or sedation, dizziness
Gastrointestinal: Xerostomia
Neuromuscular & skeletal: Weakness

1% to 10%:

Cardiovascular: Chest pain, edema
Central nervous system: Headache
Endocrine & metabolic: Decreased sexual ability
Gastrointestinal: Nausea

<1%:

Cardiovascular: Arrhythmias, palpitations
Central nervous system: Anxiety, ataxia, depression, sleep disturbances
Dermatologic: Rash, pruritus
Endocrine & metabolic: Disturbances of sexual function, gynecomastia
Gastrointestinal: Diarrhea, vomiting, constipation
Genitourinary: Polyuria
Neuromuscular & skeletal: Myalgia
Ocular: Blurring of vision
Respiratory: Nasal congestion, dyspnea
Miscellaneous: Taste disorders

Overdosage/Toxicology Symptoms of overdose include CNS depression, hypothermia, apnea, lethargy, diarrhea, hypotension, bradycardia

Treatment is primarily supportive and symptomatic. Hypotension usually responds to I.V. fluids, Trendelenburg positioning, or vasoconstrictors. CNS depression and/or apnea may respond to naloxone I.V. 0.4-2 mg, with repeats as needed.

Drug Interactions

Decreased hypotensive effect of guanabenz with tricyclic antidepressants
Increased effect: Other hypotensive agents

Stability Protect from light

Mechanism of Action Stimulates alpha$_2$-adrenoreceptors in the brain stem, thus activating an inhibitory neuron, resulting in reduced sympathetic outflow, producing a decrease in vasomotor tone and heart rate

Pharmacodynamics/Kinetics

Onset of antihypertensive effect: Within 1 hour
Absorption: ~75%
Metabolism: Extensive
Half-life: 7-10 hours
Elimination: <1% of dose excreted as unchanged drug in urine

Usual Dosage Adults: Oral: Initial: 4 mg twice daily, increase in increments of 4-8 mg/day every 1-2 weeks to a maximum of 32 mg twice daily

Dosing adjustment in hepatic impairment: Probably necessary

Monitoring Parameters Blood pressure, standing and sitting/supine

Patient Information May cause drowsiness; rise from sitting/lying position carefully, may cause dizziness; do not discontinue without notifying physician

Dosage Forms Tablet, as acetate: 4 mg, 8 mg

Guanabenz Acetate *see* Guanabenz *on this page*

Guanadrel (GWAHN a drel)

Brand Names Hylorel®

Synonyms Guanadrel Sulfate

Therapeutic Category Adrenergic Blocking Agent, Peripherally Acting; Antihypertensive

Use Considered a second line agent in the treatment of hypertension, usually with a diuretic

Pregnancy Risk Factor B

Contraindications Known hypersensitivity to guanadrel, pheochromocytoma, patients taking MAO inhibitors

Warnings/Precautions Orthostatic hypotension can occur frequently; use with caution in patients with CHF, in patients with regional vascular disease, and in patients with asthma or active peptic ulcer

Adverse Reactions

>10%:

Cardiovascular: Palpitations, chest pain, peripheral edema

Central nervous system: Fatigue, headache, faintness, drowsiness, confusion

Gastrointestinal: Increased bowel movements, gas pain, constipation, anorexia, weight gain/loss

Genitourinary: Nocturia, polyuria, ejaculation disturbances

Neuromuscular & skeletal: Paresthesia, aching limbs, leg cramps, backache, arthralgia

Ocular: Visual disturbances

Respiratory: Shortness of breath, coughing

1% to 10%:

Cardiovascular: Orthostatic hypotension

Central nervous system: Psychological problems, depression, sleep disorders

Gastrointestinal: Increased bowel movements, glossitis, nausea, vomiting, xerostomia

Genitourinary: Impotence

Renal: Hematuria

<1%: Cardiovascular: Syncope, angina

Overdosage/Toxicology Symptoms of overdose include hypotension, blurred vision, dizziness, syncope

Treatment is primarily supportive and symptomatic; hypotension usually responds to I.V. fluids, Trendelenburg positioning or vasoconstrictors

Drug Interactions

Decreased effect with tricyclic antidepressants, indirect-acting amines (ephedrine, phenylpropanolamine), phenothiazines

Increased toxicity of direct-acting amines (epinephrine, norepinephrine)

Increased effect of beta-blockers, vasodilators

Mechanism of Action Acts as a false neurotransmitter that blocks the adrenergic actions of norepinephrine; it displaces norepinephrine from its presynaptic storage granules and thus exposes it to degradation; it thereby produces a reduction in total peripheral resistance and, therefore, blood pressure

Pharmacodynamics/Kinetics

Peak effect: Within 4-6 hours

Duration: 4-14 hours

Absorption: Oral: Rapid

Distribution: Crosses the placenta; hydrophilic, therefore, does not cross the blood-brain barrier

Protein binding: 20%

Half-life, biphasic:

Initial: 1-4 hours

Terminal: 5-45 hours

Time to peak serum concentration: Within 1.5-2 hour

Elimination: In urine, 40% as unchanged drug

Usual Dosage

Adults: Oral: Initial: 10 mg/day (5 mg twice daily); adjust dosage until blood pressure is controlled, usual dosage: 20-75 mg/day, given twice daily

Elderly: Initial: 5 mg once daily

Dosing interval in renal impairment:

Cl_{cr} 10-50 mL/minute: Administer every 12-24 hours

Cl_{cr} <10 mL/minute: Administer every 24-48 hours

Monitoring Parameters Blood pressure, standing and sitting/supine

Patient Information May cause orthostatic hypotension, rise slowly from sitting or lying; take no new prescription or OTC medication without contacting your physician or pharmacist

Nursing Implications Tablet may be crushed; assist patient with rising and ambulation; monitor for orthostasis

Dosage Forms Tablet, as sulfate: 10 mg, 25 mg

Guanadrel Sulfate *see* Guanadrel *on previous page*

Guanethidine (gwahn ETH i deen)

Brand Names Ismelin®

Canadian/Mexican Brand Names Apo-Guanethidine® (Canada)

Synonyms Guanethidine Monosulfate

Therapeutic Category $Alpha_2$-Adrenergic Agonist Agent; Antihypertensive

Use Treatment of moderate to severe hypertension

Pregnancy Risk Factor C

Contraindications Pheochromocytoma, patients taking MAO inhibitors, hypersensitivity to guanethidine or any component

Warnings/Precautions Orthostatic hypotension can occur frequently; use with caution in patients with CHF, in patients with regional vascular disease, and in

(Continued)

Guanethidine *(Continued)*

patients with asthma or active peptic ulcer; withdraw therapy 2 weeks prior to surgery to decrease chance of vascular collapse and cardiac arrest during anesthesia

Adverse Reactions

>10%:

Cardiovascular: Palpitations, chest pain, peripheral edema

Central nervous system: Fatigue, headache, faintness, drowsiness, confusion

Gastrointestinal: Increased bowel movements, gas pain, constipation, anorexia, weight gain/loss

Genitourinary: Nocturia, polyuria, impotence, ejaculation disturbances

Neuromuscular & skeletal: Paresthesia, aching limbs, leg cramps, backache, arthralgia

Ocular: Visual disturbances

Respiratory: Shortness of breath, coughing

1% to 10%:

Cardiovascular: Orthostatic hypotension

Central nervous system: Psychological problems, depression, sleep disorders

Gastrointestinal: Increased bowel movements, glossitis, nausea, vomiting, xerostomia

Renal: Hematuria

<1%: Cardiovascular: Syncope, angina

Overdosage/Toxicology Symptoms of overdose include hypotension, blurred vision, dizziness, syncope

Hypotension usually responds to I.V. fluids, Trendelenburg positioning or vasoconstrictors; treatment is primarily supportive and symptomatic

Drug Interactions

Decreased effect with tricyclic antidepressants, indirect-acting amines (ephedrine, phenylpropanolamine)

Increased toxicity of direct-acting amines (epinephrine, norepinephrine)

Mechanism of Action Acts as a false neurotransmitter that blocks the adrenergic actions of norepinephrine; it displaces norepinephrine from its presynaptic storage granules and thus exposes it to degradation; it thereby produces a reduction in total peripheral resistance and, therefore, blood pressure

Pharmacodynamics/Kinetics

Onset of effect: Within 0.5-2 hours

Peak antihypertensive effect: Within 6-8 hours

Duration: 24-48 hours

Absorption: Irregular (3% to 55%)

Metabolism: Hepatic; metabolites inactive

Half-life: 5-10 days

Elimination: 25% to 60% of dose excreted unchanged in urine; small amounts also appear in feces

Usual Dosage Oral:

Children: Initial: 0.2 mg/kg/day, increase by 0.2 mg/kg/day at 7- to 10-day intervals to a maximum of 3 mg/kg/day

Adults:

Ambulatory patients: Initial: 10 mg/day, increase at 5- to 7-day intervals to a maximum of 25-50 mg/day

Hospitalized patients: Initial: 25-50 mg/day, increase by 25-50 mg/day or every other day to desired therapeutic response

Elderly: Initial: 5 mg once daily

Dosing interval in renal impairment: Cl_{cr} <10 mL/minute: Administer every 24-36 hours

Monitoring Parameters Blood pressure, standing and sitting/supine; monitor for orthostasis

Patient Information May cause drowsiness; rise from sitting/lying carefully, may cause dizziness; do not take any OTC or prescription cough or cold medication without consulting physician

Nursing Implications Tablet may be crushed

Dosage Forms Tablet, as monosulfate: 10 mg, 25 mg

Guanethidine Monosulfate *see* Guanethidine *on previous page*

Guanfacine (GWAHN fa seen)

Brand Names Tenex®

Synonyms Guanfacine Hydrochloride

Therapeutic Category Alpha$_2$-Adrenergic Agonist Agent; Antihypertensive

Use Management of hypertension

Pregnancy Risk Factor B

Contraindications Hypersensitivity to guanfacine or any component

Warnings/Precautions Use with caution in patients with severe coronary insufficiency, recent myocardial infarction, severe renal or hepatic impairment

Adverse Reactions

>10%:

Central nervous system: Somnolence, dizziness
Gastrointestinal: Xerostomia, constipation

1% to 10%:

Central nervous system: Fatigue, headache, insomnia
Endocrine & metabolic: Decreased sexual ability
Gastrointestinal: Nausea, vomiting
Ocular: Conjunctivitis

<1%:

Cardiovascular: Bradycardia, palpitations, substernal pain
Central nervous system: Amnesia, confusion, depression, malaise
Dermatologic: Dermatitis, pruritus, purpura
Gastrointestinal: Abdominal pain, diarrhea, dyspepsia, dysphagia, taste perversion
Genitourinary: Testicular disorder, urinary incontinence
Neuromuscular & skeletal: Leg cramps, hypokinesia, paresthesia
Otic: Tinnitus
Respiratory: Rhinitis, dyspnea
Miscellaneous: Diaphoresis

Overdosage/Toxicology Symptoms of overdose include CNS depression, hypothermia, apnea, lethargy, diarrhea, hypotension, bradycardia

Treatment is primarily supportive and symptomatic. Hypotension usually responds to I.V. fluids, Trendelenburg positioning or vasoconstrictors. Naloxone may be utilized in treating CNS depression and/or apnea.

Drug Interactions

Increased effect: Other hypotensive agents
Decreased hypotensive effect of guanfacine with tricyclic antidepressants

Mechanism of Action Stimulates $alpha_2$-adrenoreceptors in the brain stem, thus activating an inhibitory neuron, resulting in reduced sympathetic outflow, producing a decrease in vasomotor tone and heart rate

Pharmacodynamics/Kinetics

Peak effect: Within 8-11 hours
Duration: 24 hours following a single dose
Protein binding: 20% to 30%
Metabolism: In the liver to glucuronide and sulfate metabolites
Bioavailability: 80% to 100%
Half-life: 17 hours
Time to peak serum concentration: Within 1-4 hours
Elimination: Renal excretion of changed and unchanged drug (30%)

Usual Dosage Adults: Oral: 1 mg usually at bedtime, may increase if needed at 3- to 4-week intervals to a maximum of 3 mg/day; 1 mg/day is most common dose

Monitoring Parameters Blood pressure, standing and sitting/supine

Patient Information May cause drowsiness, dizziness; do not discontinue this medication without consulting your physician; take at bedtime; do not abruptly quit taking this medication

Nursing Implications Administer dose at bedtime; observe for orthostasis

Dosage Forms Tablet, as hydrochloride: 1 mg

Guanfacine Hydrochloride *see* Guanfacine *on previous page*
GuiaCough® [OTC] *see* Guaifenesin and Dextromethorphan *on page 591*
GuiaCough® Expectorant [OTC] *see* Guaifenesin *on page 589*
Guiatuss® [OTC] *see* Guaifenesin *on page 589*
Guiatuss DM® [OTC] *see* Guaifenesin and Dextromethorphan *on page 591*
Guiatussin® with Codeine *see* Guaifenesin and Codeine *on page 590*
Guidelines for the Prevention of Opportunistic Infections in Persons with HIV *see page 1457*
G-well® *see* Lindane *on page 728*
Gynecort® [OTC] *see* Hydrocortisone *on page 623*
Gyne-Lotrimin® [OTC] *see* Clotrimazole *on page 302*
Gyne-Sulf® *see* Sulfabenzamide, Sulfacetamide, and Sulfathiazole *on page 1171*
Gynogen L.A.® Injection *see* Estradiol *on page 468*
Habitrol™ Patch *see* Nicotine *on page 900*

Haemophilus b Conjugate Vaccine

(hem OF fi lus bee KON joo gate vak SEEN)

Related Information

Guidelines for the Prevention of Opportunistic Infections in Persons with HIV *on page 1457*
Haemophilus influenzae Vaccination *on page 1435*

(Continued)

Haemophilus b Conjugate Vaccine *(Continued)*

Immunization Guidelines *on page 1421*
Recommendations of the Advisory Committee on Immunization Practices (ACIP) *on page 1424*

Brand Names ActHIB®; HibTITER®; OmniHIB®; PedvaxHIB™; ProHIBiT®

Synonyms Diphtheria CRM_{197} Protein Conjugate; Diphtheria Toxoid Conjugate; *Haemophilus* b Oligosaccharide Conjugate Vaccine; *Haemophilus* b Polysaccharide Vaccine; HbCV; Hib Polysaccharide Conjugate; PRP-D

Therapeutic Category Vaccine, Inactivated Bacteria

Use Routine immunization of children 2 months to 5 years of age against invasive disease caused by *H. influenzae*

Unimmunized children ≥5 years of age with a chronic illness known to be associated with increased risk of *Haemophilus influenzae* type b disease, specifically, persons with anatomic or functional asplenia or sickle cell anemia or those who have undergone splenectomy, should receive Hib vaccine.

Haemophilus b conjugate vaccines are not indicated for prevention of bronchitis or other infections due to *H. influenzae* in adults; adults with specific dysfunction or certain complement deficiencies who are at especially high risk of *H. influenzae* type b infection (HIV-infected adults); patients with Hodgkin's disease (vaccinated at least 2 weeks before the initiation of chemotherapy or 3 months after the end of chemotherapy)

Pregnancy Risk Factor C

Contraindications Children with any febrile illness or active infection, known hypersensitivity to *Haemophilus* b polysaccharide vaccine (thimerosal), children who are immunosuppressed or receiving immunosuppressive therapy

Warnings/Precautions Have epinephrine 1:1000 available; children in whom DTP or DT vaccination is deferred: The carrier proteins used in HbOC (but not PRP-OMP) are chemically and immunologically related to toxoids contained in DTP vaccine. Earlier or simultaneous vaccination with diphtheria or tetanus toxoids may be required to elicit an optimal anti-PRP antibody response to HbOC. In contrast, the immunogenicity of PRP-OMP is not affected by vaccination with DTP. In infants in whom DTP or DT vaccination is deferred, PRP-OMP may be advantageous for *Haemophilus influenzae* type b vaccination.

Children with immunologic impairment: Children with chronic illness associated with increased risk of *Haemophilus influenzae* type b disease may have impaired anti-PRP antibody responses to conjugate vaccination. Examples include those with HIV infection, immunoglobulin deficiency, anatomic or functional asplenia, and sickle cell disease, as well as recipients of bone marrow transplants and recipients of chemotherapy for malignancy. Some children with immunologic impairment may benefit from more doses of conjugate vaccine than normally indicated.

Adverse Reactions When administered during the same visit that DTP vaccine is given, the rates of systemic reactions do not differ from those observed only when DTP vaccine is administered

25%:
- Cardiovascular: Edema
- Dermatologic: Local erythema
- Local: Increased risk of *Haemophilus* b infections in the week after vaccination
- Miscellaneous: Warmth

>10%: Acute febrile reactions

1% to 10%:
- Central nervous system: Fever (up to 102.2°F), irritability, lethargy
- Gastrointestinal: Anorexia, diarrhea
- Local: Irritation at injection site

<1%:
- Cardiovascular: Edema of the eyes/face
- Central nervous system: Convulsions, fever >102.2° F, unusual fatigue
- Dermatologic: Urticaria, itching
- Gastrointestinal: Vomiting
- Neuromuscular & skeletal: Weakness
- Respiratory: Dyspnea

Drug Interactions Decreased effect with immunosuppressive agents, immunoglobulins within 1 month may decrease antibody production; may interfere with antigen detection tests

Stability Keep in refrigerator, may be frozen (not diluent) without affecting potency; reconstituted Hib-Imune® remains stable for only 8 hours, whereas HibVAX® remain stable for 30 days when refrigerated

Mechanism of Action Stimulates production of anticapsular antibodies and provides active immunity to *Haemophilus influenzae*; Hib conjugate vaccines use covalent binding of capsular polysaccharide of *Haemophilus influenzae* type b to diphtheria CRM 197 (HibTITER®) to produce an antigen which is postulated to convert a T-independent antigen into a T-dependent antigen to result in enhanced antibody response and on immunologic memory

Pharmacodynamics/Kinetics

The seroconversion following one dose of Hib vaccine for children 18 months or 24 months of age or older is 75% to 90% respectively

Onset of serum antibody responses: 1-2 weeks after vaccination

Duration: Immunity appears to last 1.5 years

Usual Dosage Children: I.M.: 0.5 mL as a single dose should be administered according to one of the following "brand-specific" schedules; do not inject I.V.

Vaccination Schedule for Haemophilus b Conjugate Vaccines

Age at 1st Dose (mo)	HibTITER®		PedvaxHIB®		ProHIBiT®	
	Primary Series	Booster	Primary Series	Booster	Primary Series	Booster
2-6*	3 doses, 2 months apart	15 mo†	2 doses, 2 months apart	12 mo†		
7-11	2 doses, 2 months apart	15 mo†	2 doses, 2 months apart	15 mo†		
12-14	1 dose	15 mo†	1 dose	15 mo†		
15-60	1 dose	—	1 dose	—	1 dose	—

*It is not currently recommended that the various Haemophilus b conjugate vaccines be interchanged (ie, the same brand should be used throughout the entire vaccination series). If the health care provider does not know which vaccine was previously used, it is prudent that an infant, 2-6 months of age, be given a primary series of three doses.

†At least 2 months after previous dose.

Test Interactions May interfere with interpretation of antigen detection tests

Patient Information May use acetaminophen for postdose fever

Nursing Implications Defer immunization if infection or febrile illness present. Do not administer I.V.

Additional Information Federal law requires that the date of administration, the vaccine manufacturer, lot number of vaccine, and the administering person's name, title, and address be entered into the patient's permanent medical record

Haemophilus Influenzae type b Conjugate Vaccines

Manufacturer	Abbreviation	Trade Name	Carrier Protein
Connaught Laboratories	PRP-D*	ProHiBit®	Diphtheria toxoid
Lederle Laboratories	HbOC	HibTITER®	CRM_{197} (a nontoxic mutant diphtheria toxin)
Merck and Company	PRP-OMP	PedvaxHIB	OMP (an outer membrane protein complex of *Neisseria meningitidis*)
Pasteur Merieux Vaccines (Distributed by Connaught Laboratories, Inc, and SmithKline Beecham)	PRP-T**	ActHIB OmniHIB	Tetanus toxoid

*PRP-D is recommended by the American Academy of Pediatrics for only infants ≥12 months of age. HbOC, PRP-OMP, and PRP-T are recommended for infants beginning at approximately 2 months of age.

**PRP-T may be reconstituted with DTP, manufactured by Connaught Laboratories. Other licensed formulations of DTP have not been approved by the FDA for reconstitution and may not be used for this purpose.

Dosage Forms Injection:

ActHIB®, HibTITER®, OmniHIB®: Capsular oligosaccharide 10 mcg and diphtheria CRM_{197} protein ~25 mcg per 0.5 mL (0.5 mL, 2.5 mL, 5 mL)

PedvaxHIB™: Purified capsular polysaccharide 15 mcg and *Neisseria meningitidis* OMPC 250 mcg per dose (0.5 mL)

ProHIBiT®: Purified capsular polysaccharide 25 mcg and conjugated diphtheria toxoid protein 18 mcg per dose (0.5 mL, 2.5 mL, 5 mL)

***Haemophilus* b Oligosaccharide Conjugate Vaccine** *see Haemophilus* b Conjugate Vaccine *on page 595*

***Haemophilus* b Polysaccharide Vaccine** *see Haemophilus* b Conjugate Vaccine *on page 595*

***Haemophilus Influenzae* Vaccination** *see page 1435*

Halcinonide (hal SIN oh nide)

Related Information

Corticosteroids Comparison *on page 1407*

Brand Names Halog®; Halog®-E

Canadian/Mexican Brand Names Dermalog® Simple (Mexico)

Therapeutic Category Corticosteroid, Topical (Medium Potency); Corticosteroid, Topical (High Potency)

Use Inflammation of corticosteroid-responsive dermatoses [high potency topical corticosteroid]

Pregnancy Risk Factor C

Contraindications Viral, fungal, or tubercular skin lesions, known hypersensitivity to halcinonide or any component

Warnings/Precautions Adverse systemic effects may occur when used on large areas of the body, denuded areas, for prolonged periods of time, with an occlusive dressing, and/or in infants or small children

Adverse Reactions <1%:

Dermatologic: Itching, dry skin, folliculitis, hypertrichosis, acneiform eruptions, hypopigmentation, perioral dermatitis, allergic contact dermatitis, skin maceration, skin atrophy, striae

Local: Burning, irritation, miliaria

Miscellaneous: Secondary infection

Overdosage/Toxicology When consumed in excessive quantities, systemic hypercorticism and adrenal suppression may occur; in those cases, discontinuation and withdrawal of the corticosteroid should be done judiciously

Mechanism of Action Decreases inflammation by suppression of migration of polymorphonuclear leukocytes and reversal of increased capillary permeability

Pharmacodynamics/Kinetics

Absorption: Percutaneous absorption varies by location of topical application and the use of occlusive dressings

Metabolism: Primarily in the liver

Elimination: By the kidneys

Usual Dosage Children and Adults: Topical: Apply sparingly 1-3 times/day, occlusive dressing may be used for severe or resistant dermatoses; a thin film of cream or ointment is effective; do not overuse

Patient Information A thin film of cream or ointment is effective; do not overuse; do not use tight-fitting diapers or plastic pants on children being treated in the diaper area; use only as prescribed, and for no longer than the period prescribed; apply sparingly in light film; rub in lightly; avoid contact with eyes; notify physician if condition being treated persists or worsens

Dosage Forms

Cream (Halog®): 0.025% (15 g, 60 g, 240 g); 0.1% (15 g, 30 g, 60 g, 240 g)

Cream, emollient base (Halog®-E) : 0.1% (15 g, 30 g, 60 g)

Ointment, topical (Halog®): 0.1% (15 g, 30 g, 60 g, 240 g)

Solution (Halog®): 0.1% (20 mL, 60 mL)

Halcion® *see* Triazolam *on page 1258*

Haldol® *see* Haloperidol *on page 600*

Haldol® Decanoate *see* Haloperidol *on page 600*

Halenol® [OTC] *see* Acetaminophen *on page 19*

Halfan® *see* Halofantrine *on next page*

Halobetasol (hal oh BAY ta sol)

Related Information

Corticosteroids Comparison *on page 1407*

Brand Names Ultravate™

Synonyms Halobetasol Propionate

Therapeutic Category Corticosteroid, Topical (Very High Potency)

Use Relief of inflammatory and pruritic manifestations of corticosteroid-response dermatoses [very high potency topical corticosteroid]

Pregnancy Risk Factor C

Contraindications Hypersensitivity to halobetasol or any component; viral, fungal, or tubercular skin lesions

Warnings/Precautions Not for ophthalmic use; may cause adrenal suppression or insufficiency; application to abraded or inflamed areas or too large of areas of the body may increase the risk of systemic absorption and the risk of adrenal suppression, as may prolonged use or the use of >50 g/week. Topical halobetasol should not be used for the treatment of rosacea or perioral dermatitis.

Adverse Reactions <1%:

Dermatologic: Itching, dry skin, folliculitis, hypertrichosis, acneiform eruptions, hypopigmentation, perioral dermatitis, allergic contact dermatitis, skin maceration, skin atrophy, striae

Local: Burning, irritation, miliaria
Miscellaneous: Secondary infection

Overdosage/Toxicology When consumed in excessive quantities, systemic hypercorticism and adrenal suppression may occur; in those cases, discontinuation and withdrawal of the corticosteroid should be done judiciously

Mechanism of Action Corticosteroids inhibit the initial manifestations of the inflammatory process (ie, capillary dilation and edema, fibrin deposition, and migration and diapedesis of leukocytes into the inflamed site) as well as later sequelae (angiogenesis, fibroblast proliferation)

Pharmacodynamics/Kinetics

Absorption: Percutaneous absorption varies by location of topical application and the use of occlusive dressings; ~3% of a topically applied dose of ointment enters the circulation within 96 hours
Metabolism: Primarily in the liver
Elimination: By the kidneys

Usual Dosage Children and Adults: Topical: Apply sparingly to skin twice daily, rub in gently and completely; treatment should not exceed 2 consecutive weeks and total dosage should not exceed 50 g/week

Patient Information A thin film of cream or ointment is effective; do not overuse; do not use tight-fitting diapers or plastic pants on children being treated in the diaper area; use only as prescribed, and for no longer than the period prescribed; apply sparingly in light film; rub in lightly; avoid contact with eyes; notify physician if condition being treated persists or worsens

Dosage Forms

Cream, as propionate: 0.05% (15 g, 45 g)
Ointment, topical, as propionate: 0.05% (15 g, 45 g)

Halobetasol Propionate *see* Halobetasol *on previous page*

Halofantrine (ha loe FAN trin)

Brand Names Halfan®

Synonyms Halofantrine Hydrochloride

Therapeutic Category Antimalarial Agent

Use Treatment of mild to moderate acute malaria caused by susceptible strains of *Plasmodium falciparum* and *Plasmodium vivax*

Pregnancy Risk Factor X

Contraindications Pregnancy

Warnings/Precautions Monitor closely for decreased hematocrit and hemoglobin, patients with chronic liver disease

Adverse Reactions

>10%: Dermatologic: Pruritus

1% to 10%:
- Cardiovascular: Edema
- Central nervous system: Malaise, headache
- Gastrointestinal: Nausea, vomiting
- Hematologic: Leukocytosis
- Hepatic: Elevated LFTs
- Local: Tenderness
- Neuromuscular & skeletal: Myalgia
- Respiratory: Cough
- Miscellaneous: Lymphadenopathy

<1%:
- Cardiovascular: Tachycardia, hypotension
- Dermatologic: Urticaria
- Endocrine & metabolic: Hypoglycemia
- Local: Sterile abscesses
- Respiratory: Asthma
- Miscellaneous: Anaphylactic shock

Mechanism of Action Similar to mefloquine; destruction of asexual blood forms, possible inhibition of proton pump

Pharmacodynamics/Kinetics

Mean time to parasite clearance: 40-84 hours
Absorption: Erratic and variable; serum levels are proportional to dose up to 1000 mg; doses greater than this should be divided; may be increased 60% with high fat meals
Distribution: V_d: 570 L/kg; widely distributed in most tissues
Metabolism: To active metabolite in liver
Half-life: 23 hours; metabolite: 82 hours; may be increased in active disease
Elimination: Essentially unchanged in urine

Usual Dosage Oral:

Children <40 kg: 8 mg/kg every 6 hours for 3 doses
Adults: 500 mg every 6 hours for 3 doses

Monitoring Parameters CBC, LFTs, parasite counts

(Continued)

Halofantrine *(Continued)*

Test Interactions Increased serum transaminases, bilirubin

Patient Information Take with food, avoid high fat meals; notify physician of persistent nausea, vomiting, abdominal pain, light stools, dark urine

Nursing Implications Monitor closely for jaundice, other signs of hepatotoxicity

Dosage Forms

Suspension, as hydrochloride: 100 mg/5 mL

Tablet, as hydrochloride: 250 mg

Halofantrine Hydrochloride *see* Halofantrine *on previous page*

Halog® *see* Halcinonide *on page 598*

Halog®-E *see* Halcinonide *on page 598*

Haloperidol (ha loe PER i dole)

Related Information

Antipsychotic Agents Comparison *on page 1396*

Brand Names Haldol®; Haldol® Decanoate

Canadian/Mexican Brand Names Haldol™ LA (Canada); Peridol (Canada); Haloperil® (Mexico)

Synonyms Haloperidol Decanoate; Haloperidol Lactate

Therapeutic Category Antipsychotic Agent; Sedative

Use Treatment of psychoses, Tourette's disorder, and severe behavioral problems in children; may be used for the emergency sedation of severely agitated or delirious patients

Pregnancy Risk Factor C

Contraindications Hypersensitivity to haloperidol or any component; narrow-angle glaucoma, bone marrow suppression, CNS depression, severe liver or cardiac disease, subcortical brain damage; circulatory collapse; severe hypotension or hypertension

Warnings/Precautions Safety and efficacy have not been established in children <3 years of age; watch for hypotension when administering I.M. or I.V.; use with caution in patients with cardiovascular disease or seizures; benefits of therapy must be weighed against risks of therapy; decanoate form should never be given I.V.; some tablets contain tartrazine which may cause allergic reactions; use caution with CNS depression and severe liver or cardiac disease

Adverse Reactions EKG changes, retinal pigmentation are more common than with chlorpromazine

>10%:

- Central nervous system: Restlessness, anxiety, extrapyramidal reactions, dystonic reactions, pseudoparkinsonian signs and symptoms, tardive dyskinesia, neuroleptic malignant syndrome (NMS), seizures, altered central temperature regulation, akathisia
- Endocrine & metabolic: Edema of the breasts
- Gastrointestinal: Weight gain, constipation

1% to 10%:

- Cardiovascular: Hypotension (especially orthostatic), tachycardia, arrhythmias, abnormal T waves with prolonged ventricular repolarization
- Central nervous system: Hallucinations, sedation, drowsiness, persistent tardive dyskinesia
- Gastrointestinal: Nausea, vomiting
- Genitourinary: Dysuria

<1%:

- Central nervous system: Tardive dystonia
- Dermatologic: Hyperpigmentation, pruritus, rash, contact dermatitis, alopecia, photosensitivity (rare)
- Endocrine & metabolic: Amenorrhea, galactorrhea, gynecomastia, sexual dysfunction
- Gastrointestinal: Adynamic ileus, nausea, vomiting, xerostomia (problem for denture user)
- Genitourinary: Urinary retention, overflow incontinence, priapism
- Hematologic: Agranulocytosis, leukopenia (usually inpatients with large doses for prolonged periods)
- Hepatic: Cholestatic jaundice, obstructive jaundice
- Ocular: Blurred vision, retinal pigmentation, decreased visual acuity (may be irreversible)
- Respiratory: Laryngospasm, respiratory depression
- Miscellaneous: Heat stroke

Overdosage/Toxicology Symptoms of overdose include deep sleep, dystonia, agitation, dysrhythmias, extrapyramidal symptoms

Following initiation of essential overdose management, toxic symptom treatment and supportive treatment should be initiated. Critical cardiac arrhythmias often respond to I.V. lidocaine, while other antiarrhythmics can be used. Neuroleptics often cause extrapyramidal symptoms (eg, dystonic reactions) requiring management with benztropine mesylate I.V. 1-2 mg (adult) may be effective. These agents are generally effective within 2-5 minutes.

Drug Interactions Cytochrome P-450 IID6 enzyme inhibitor

Decreased effect: Carbamazepine and phenobarbital may increase metabolism and decreased effectiveness of haloperidol

Increased toxicity: CNS depressants may increase adverse effects; epinephrine may cause hypotension; haloperidol and anticholinergic agents may increase intraocular pressure; concurrent use with lithium has occasionally caused acute encephalopathy-like syndrome

Stability

Protect oral dosage forms from light

Haloperidol lactate injection should be stored at controlled room temperature and protected from light, freezing and temperatures >40°C; exposure to light may cause discoloration and the development of a grayish-red precipitate over several weeks

Haloperidol lactate may be administered IVPB or I.V. infusion in D_5W solutions; NS solutions should not be used due to reports of decreased stability and incompatibility

Standardized dose: 0.5-100 mg/50-100 mL D_5W

Stability of standardized solutions is 38 days at room temperature (24°C)

Mechanism of Action Blocks postsynaptic mesolimbic dopaminergic D_1 and D_2 receptors in the brain; exhibits a strong alpha-adrenergic blocking and anticholinergic effect, depresses the release of hypothalamic and hypophyseal hormones; believed to depress the reticular activating system thus affecting basal metabolism, body temperature, wakefulness, vasomotor tone, and emesis

Pharmacodynamics/Kinetics

Onset of sedation: I.V.: Within 1 hour

Duration of action: ~3 weeks for decanoate form

Distribution: Crosses the placenta; appears in breast milk

Protein binding: 90%

Metabolism: In the liver to inactive compounds

Bioavailability: Oral: 60%

Half-life: 20 hours

Time to peak serum concentration: 20 minutes

Elimination: 33% to 40% excreted in urine within 5 days; an additional 15% excreted in feces

Usual Dosage

Children: 3-12 years (15-40 kg): Oral:
- Initial: 0.05 mg/kg/day or 0.25-0.5 mg/day given in 2-3 divided doses; increase by 0.25-0.5 mg every 5-7 days; maximum: 0.15 mg/kg/day
- Usual maintenance:
  - Agitation or hyperkinesia: 0.01-0.03 mg/kg/day once daily
  - Nonpsychotic disorders: 0.05-0.075 mg/kg/day in 2-3 divided doses
  - Psychotic disorders: 0.05-0.15 mg/kg/day in 2-3 divided doses

Children 6-12 years: I.M. (as lactate): 1-3 mg/dose every 4-8 hours to a maximum of 0.15 mg/kg/day; change over to oral therapy as soon as able

Adults:
- Oral: 0.5-5 mg 2-3 times/day; usual maximum: 30 mg/day; some patients may require up to 100 mg/day
- I.M. (as lactate): 2-5 mg every 4-8 hours as needed
- I.M. (as decanoate): Initial: 10-15 times the daily oral dose administered at 3- to 4-week intervals

Sedation in the Intensive Care Unit:
- I.M./IVP/IVPB: May repeat bolus doses after 30 minutes until calm achieved then administer 50% of the maximum dose every 6 hours
  - Mild agitation: 0.5-2 mg
  - Moderate agitation: 2-5 mg
  - Severe agitation: 10-20 mg
- Continuous intravenous infusion (100 mg/100 mL D_5W): Rates of 1-40 mg/hour have been used

Elderly (nonpsychotic patients, dementia behavior):
- Initial: Oral: 0.25-0.5 mg 1-2 times/day; increase dose at 4- to 7-day intervals by 0.25-0.5 mg/day; increase dosing intervals (twice daily, 3 times/day, etc) as necessary to control response or side effects
- Maximum daily dose: 50 mg; gradual increases (titration) may prevent side effects or decrease their severity

Hemodialysis/peritoneal dialysis: Supplemental dose is not necessary

Dietary Considerations Alcohol: Additive CNS effect, avoid use

Administration The decanoate injectable formulation should be administered I.M. only, **do not administer decanoate I.V.** Dilute the oral concentrate with water or juice before administration

(Continued)

Haloperidol *(Continued)*

Monitoring Parameters Monitor orthostatic blood pressures 3-5 days after initiation of therapy or a dose increase; observe for tremor and abnormal movement or posturing (extrapyramidal symptoms)

Reference Range

Therapeutic: 5-15 ng/mL (SI: 10-30 nmol/L) (psychotic disorders - less for Tourette's and mania)

Toxic: >42 ng/mL (SI: >84 nmol/L)

Test Interactions ↓ cholesterol (S)

Patient Information May cause drowsiness, restlessness, avoid alcohol and other CNS depressants, rise slowly from recumbent position; use of supportive stockings may help prevent orthostatic hypotension; do not alter dosage or discontinue without consulting physician; oral concentrate must be diluted in 2-4 oz of liquid (water, fruit juice, carbonated drinks, milk, or pudding)

Nursing Implications Avoid skin contact with oral suspension or solution; may cause contact dermatitis

Dosage Forms

Concentrate, oral, as lactate: 2 mg/mL (5 mL, 10 mL, 15 mL, 120 mL, 240 mL)
Injection, as decanoate: 50 mg/mL (1 mL, 5 mL); 100 mg/mL (1 mL, 5 mL)
Injection, as lactate: 5 mg/mL (1 mL, 2 mL, 2.5 mL, 10 mL)
Tablet: 0.5 mg, 1 mg, 2 mg, 5 mg, 10 mg, 20 mg

Haloperidol Decanoate *see* Haloperidol *on page 600*

Haloperidol Lactate *see* Haloperidol *on page 600*

Haloprogin (ha loe PROE jin)

Brand Names Halotex®

Therapeutic Category Antifungal Agent, Topical

Use Topical treatment of tinea pedis (athlete's foot), tinea cruris (jock itch), tinea corporis (ring worm), tinea manuum caused by *Trichophyton rubrum, Trichophyton tonsurans, Trichophyton mentagrophytes, Microsporum canis,* or *Epidermophyton floccosum*. Topical treatment of *Malassezia furfur.*

Pregnancy Risk Factor B

Contraindications Hypersensitivity to haloprogin or any component

Warnings/Precautions Safety and efficacy have not been established in children

Adverse Reactions <1%:

Dermatologic: Pruritus, folliculitis, vesicle formation, erythema
Local: Irritation, burning sensation

Mechanism of Action Interferes with fungal DNA replication to inhibit yeast cell respiration and disrupt its cell membrane

Pharmacodynamics/Kinetics

Absorption: Poorly through the skin (~11%)
Metabolism: To trichlorophenol
Elimination: In urine, 75% as unchanged drug

Usual Dosage Topical: Children and Adults: Apply liberally twice daily for 2-3 weeks; intertriginous areas may require up to 4 weeks of treatment

Patient Information Avoid contact with eyes; for external use only; improvement should occur within 4 weeks; discontinue use if sensitization or irritation occur

Dosage Forms

Cream: 1% (15 g, 30 g)
Solution, topical: 1% with alcohol 75% (10 mL, 30 mL)

Halotestin® *see* Fluoxymesterone *on page 542*

Halotex® *see* Haloprogin *on this page*

Halotussin® [OTC] *see* Guaifenesin *on page 589*

Halotussin® DM [OTC] *see* Guaifenesin and Dextromethorphan *on page 591*

Haltran® [OTC] *see* Ibuprofen *on page 639*

Havrix® *see* Hepatitis A Vaccine *on page 606*

HbCV *see Haemophilus* b Conjugate Vaccine *on page 595*

H-BIG® *see* Hepatitis B Immune Globulin *on page 607*

25-HCC *see* Calcifediol *on page 180*

hCG *see* Chorionic Gonadotropin *on page 272*

HCTZ *see* Hydrochlorothiazide *on page 617*

HDCV *see* Rabies Virus Vaccine *on page 1091*

Head & Shoulders® Intensive Treatment [OTC] *see* Selenium Sulfide *on page 1132*

Healon® *see* Sodium Hyaluronate *on page 1144*

Healon® GV *see* Sodium Hyaluronate *on page 1144*

Heart Failure: Management of Patients With Left-Ventricular Systolic Dysfunction *see page 1533*

Heavy Mineral Oil *see* Mineral Oil *on page 841*
***Helicobacter pylori* Treatment** *see page 1534*
Helidac® *see* Bismuth Subsalicylate, Metronidazole, and Tetracycline *on page 155*
Helistat® *see* Microfibrillar Collagen Hemostat *on page 836*
Hemabate™ *see* Carboprost Tromethamine *on page 208*
Hemocyte® [OTC] *see* Ferrous Fumarate *on page 513*
Hemofil® M *see* Antihemophilic Factor (Human) *on page 94*
Hemotene® *see* Microfibrillar Collagen Hemostat *on page 836*
Hemril-HC™ *see* Hydrocortisone *on page 623*

Heparin (HEP a rin)

Brand Names Hep-Lock®

Canadian/Mexican Brand Names Calcilean® (Canada); Hepalean® (Canada); Hepalean®-LOK (Canada); Hepalean® LCO (Canada)

Synonyms Heparin Calcium; Heparin Lock Flush; Heparin Sodium

Therapeutic Category Anticoagulant

Use Prophylaxis and treatment of thromboembolic disorders

Pregnancy Risk Factor C

Contraindications Hypersensitivity to heparin or any component; severe thrombocytopenia, subacute bacterial endocarditis, suspected intracranial hemorrhage, uncontrollable bleeding (unless secondary to disseminated intravascular coagulation)

Warnings/Precautions

Use with caution as hemorrhaging may occur; risk factors for hemorrhage include I.M. injections, peptic ulcer disease, increased capillary permeability, menstruation; severe renal, hepatic or biliary disease; use with caution in patients with shock, severe hypotension

Some preparations contain benzyl alcohol as a preservative. In neonates, large amounts of benzyl alcohol (>100 mg/kg/day) have been associated with fatal toxicity (gasping syndrome). The use of preservative-free heparin is, therefore, recommended in neonates. Some preparations contain sulfite which may cause allergic reactions.

Heparin does not possess fibrinolytic activity and, therefore, cannot lyse established thrombi; discontinue heparin if hemorrhage occurs; severe hemorrhage or overdosage may require protamine

Use caution with white clot syndrome (new thrombus associated with thrombocytopenia) and heparin resistance

Adverse Reactions

>10%:
- Dermatologic: Unexplained bruising
- Gastrointestinal: Constipation, vomiting of blood
- Hematologic: Hemorrhage, blood in urine, bleeding from gums

1% to 10%:
- Cardiovascular: Chest pain
- Genitourinary: Frequent or persistent erection
- Neuromuscular & skeletal: Peripheral neuropathy
- Miscellaneous: Allergic reactions

<1%:
- Central nervous system: Fever, headache, chills
- Dermatologic: Urticaria
- Gastrointestinal: Nausea, vomiting
- Hematologic: Thrombocytopenia (heparin-associated thrombocytopenia occurs in <1% of patients, immune thrombocytopenia occurs with progressive fall in platelet counts and, in some cases, thromboembolic complications; daily platelet counts for 5-7 days at initiation of therapy may help detect the onset of this complication)
- Hepatic: Elevated liver enzymes
- Local: Irritation, ulceration, cutaneous necrosis have been rarely reported with deep S.C. injections
- Neuromuscular & skeletal: Osteoporosis (chronic therapy effect)

Overdosage/Toxicology The primary symptom of overdose is bleeding

Antidote is protamine; dose 1 mg per 1 mg (100 units) of heparin. Discontinue all heparin if evidence of progressive immune thrombocytopenia occurs.

Drug Interactions

Decreased effect with digoxin, TCN, nicotine, antihistamine, I.V. NTG

Increased toxicity with NSAIDs, ASA, dipyridamole, dextran, hydroxychloroquine

Stability

Heparin solutions are colorless to slightly yellow; minor color variations do not affect therapeutic efficacy

Heparin should be stored at controlled room temperature and protected from freezing and temperatures >40°C

(Continued)

Heparin *(Continued)*

Stability at room temperature and refrigeration:
- Prepared bag: 24 hours
- Premixed bag: After seal is broken 4 days
- Out of overwrap stability: 30 days

Standard diluent: 25,000 units/500 mL D_5W (premixed)

Minimum volume: 250 mL D_5W

Mechanism of Action Potentiates the action of antithrombin III and thereby inactivates thrombin (as well as activated coagulation factors IX, X, XI, XII, and plasmin) and prevents the conversion of fibrinogen to fibrin; heparin also stimulates release of lipoprotein lipase (lipoprotein lipase hydrolyzes triglycerides to glycerol and free fatty acids)

Pharmacodynamics/Kinetics

Onset of anticoagulation:
- I.V.: Immediate with use
- S.C.: Within 20-30 minutes

Absorption: Oral, rectal, S.C., I.M.: Erratic

Distribution: Does not cross placenta; does not appear in breast milk

Metabolism: Hepatic; believed to be partially metabolized in the reticuloendothelial system

Half-life:
- Mean: 1.5 hours
- Range: 1-2 hours; affected by obesity, renal function, hepatic function, malignancy, presence of pulmonary embolism, and infections

Elimination: Renal excretion, small amount excreted unchanged in urine

Usual Dosage

Line flushing: When using daily flushes of heparin to maintain patency of single and double lumen central catheters, 10 units/mL is commonly used for younger infants (eg, <10 kg) while 100 units/mL is used for older infants, children, and adults. Capped PVC catheters and peripheral heparin locks require flushing more frequently (eg, every 6-8 hours). Volume of heparin flush is usually similar to volume of catheter (or slightly greater). Additional flushes should be given when stagnant blood is observed in catheter, after catheter is used for drug or blood administration, and after blood withdrawal from catheter.

Addition of heparin (0.5-1 unit/mL) to peripheral and central TPN has been shown to increase duration of line patency. The final concentration of heparin used for TPN solutions may need to be decreased to 0.5 units/mL in small infants receiving larger amounts of volume in order to avoid approaching therapeutic amounts. Arterial lines are heparinized with a final concentration of 1 unit/mL.

Children:
- Intermittent I.V.: Initial: 50-100 units/kg, then 50-100 units/kg every 4 hours
- I.V. infusion: Initial: 50 units/kg, then 15-25 units/kg/hour; increase dose by 2-4 units/kg/hour every 6-8 hours as required

Standard Heparin Solution
(25,000 units/500 mL D_5W)

To Administer a Dose of	Set Infusion Rate at
400 units/h	8 mL/h
500 units/h	10 mL/h
600 units/h	12 mL/h
700 units/h	14 mL/h
800 units/h	16 mL/h
900 units/h	18 mL/h
1000 units/h	20 mL/h
1100 units/h	22 mL/h
1200 units/h	24 mL/h
1300 units/h	26 mL/h
1400 units/h	28 mL/h
1500 units/h	30 mL/h
1600 units/h	32 mL/h
1700 units/h	34 mL/h
1800 units/h	36 mL/h
1900 units/h	38 mL/h
2000 units/h	40 mL/h

Adults:

Prophylaxis (low-dose heparin): S.C.: 5000 units every 8-12 hours

Intermittent I.V.: Initial: 10,000 units, then 50-70 units/kg (5000-10,000 units) every 4-6 hours

I.V. infusion: 50 units/kg to start, then 15-25 units/kg/hour as continuous infusion; increase dose by 5 units/kg/hour every 4 hours as required according to PTT results, usual range: 10-30 units/hour

Weight-based protocol: 80 units/kg I.V. push followed by continuous infusion of 18 units/kg/hour. See table.

Administration Do not administer I.M. due to pain, irritation, and hematoma formation; central venous catheters must be flushed with heparin solution when newly inserted, daily (at the time of tubing change), after blood withdrawal or transfusion, and after an intermittent infusion through an injectable cap. A volume of at least 10 mL of blood should be removed and discarded from a heparinized line before blood samples are sent for coagulation testing.

Monitoring Parameters Platelet counts, PTT, hemoglobin, hematocrit, signs of bleeding

For intermittent I.V. injections, PTT is measured 3.5-4 hours after I.V. injection

Note: Continuous I.V. infusion is preferred vs I.V. intermittent injections. For full-dose heparin (ie, nonlow-dose), the dose should be titrated according to PTT results. For anticoagulation, an APTT 1.5-2.5 times normal is usually desired. APTT is usually measured prior to heparin therapy, 6-8 hours after initiation of a continuous infusion (following a loading dose), and 6-8 hours after changes in the infusion rate; increase or decrease infusion by 2-4 units/kg/hour dependent on PTT. See table.

Heparin Infusion Dose Adjustment

APTT	Adjustment
>3 x control	↓ Infusion rate 50%
2-3 x control	↓ Infusion rate 25%
1.5-2 x control	No change
<1.5 x control	↑ Rate of infusion 25%; max 2500 units/h

Reference Range Heparin: 0.3-0.5 unit/mL; APTT: 1.5-2.5 times **the patient's baseline**

Test Interactions ↑ thyroxine (S) (competitive protein binding methods); ↑ PT, ↑ PTT, ↑ bleeding time

Dosage Forms

Heparin sodium:

Lock flush injection:

Beef lung source: 10 units/mL (1 mL, 2 mL, 2.5 mL, 3 mL, 5 mL, 10 mL, 30 mL); 100 units/mL (1 mL, 2 mL, 2.5 mL, 3 mL, 5 mL, 10 mL, 30 mL)

Porcine intestinal mucosa source: 10 units/mL (1 mL, 2 mL, 10 mL, 30 mL); 100 units/mL (1 mL, 2 mL, 10 mL, 30 mL)

Porcine intestinal mucosa source, preservative free: 10 units/mL (1 mL); 100 units/mL (1 mL)

Multiple-dose vial injection:

Beef lung source, with preservative: 1000 units/mL (5 mL, 10 mL, 30 mL); 5000 units/mL (10 mL); 10,000 units/mL (4 mL, 5 mL, 10 mL); 20,000 units/mL (2 mL, 5 mL, 10 mL); 40,000 units/mL (5 mL)

Porcine intestinal mucosa source, with preservative: 1000 units/mL (10 mL, 30 mL); 5000 units/mL (10 mL); 10,000 units/mL (4 mL); 20,000 units/mL (2 mL, 5 mL)

Single-dose vial injection:

Beef lung source: 1000 units/mL (1 mL); 5000 units/mL (1 mL); 10,000 units/mL (1 mL); 20,000 units/mL (1 mL); 40,000 units/mL (1 mL)

Porcine intestinal mucosa: 1000 units/mL (1 mL); 5000 units/mL (1 mL); 10,000 units/mL (1 mL); 20,000 units/mL (1 mL); 40,000 units/mL (1 mL)

Unit dose injection:

Porcine intestinal mucosa source, with preservative: 1000 units/dose (1 mL, 2 mL); 2500 units/dose (1 mL); 5000 units/dose (0.5 mL, 1 mL); 7500 units/dose (1 mL); 10,000 units/dose (1 mL); 15,000 units/dose (1 mL); 20,000 units/dose (1 mL)

Heparin sodium infusion, porcine intestinal mucosa source:

D_5W: 40 units/mL (500 mL); 50 units/mL (250 mL, 500 mL); 100 units/mL (100 mL, 250 mL)

NaCl 0.45%: 2 units/mL (500 mL, 1000 mL); 50 units/mL (250 mL); 100 units/mL (250 mL)

NaCl 0.9%: 2 units/mL (500 mL, 1000 mL); 5 units/mL (1000 mL); 50 units/mL (250 mL, 500 mL, 1000 mL)

(Continued)

Heparin *(Continued)*

Heparin calcium:

Unit dose injection, porcine intestinal mucosa, preservative free (Calciparine®): 5000 units/dose (0.2 mL); 12,500 units/dose (0.5 mL); 20,000 units/dose (0.8 mL)

Heparin Calcium *see* Heparin *on page 603*

Heparin Cofactor I *see* Antithrombin III *on page 97*

Heparin Lock Flush *see* Heparin *on page 603*

Heparin Sodium *see* Heparin *on page 603*

Hepatitis A Vaccine (hep a TYE tis aye vak SEEN)

Related Information

Immunization Guidelines *on page 1421*

Miscellaneous Vaccination Information *on page 1437*

Prevention of Hepatitis A Through Active or Passive Immunization *on page 1440*

Prophylaxis for Patients Exposed to Common Communicable Diseases *on page 1452*

Brand Names Havrix®; VAQTA®

Therapeutic Category Vaccine, Inactivated Virus

Use For populations desiring protection against hepatitis A or for populations at high risk of exposure to hepatitis A virus (travelers to developing countries, household and sexual contacts of persons infected with hepatitis A), child day care employees, illicit drug users, male homosexuals, institutional workers (eg, institutions for the mentally and physically handicapped persons, prisons, etc), and healthcare workers who may be exposed to hepatitis A virus (eg, laboratory employees); protection lasts for approximately 15 years

Pregnancy Risk Factor C

Contraindications Hypersensitivity to any component of hepatitis A vaccine

Warnings/Precautions Use caution in patients with serious active infection, cardiovascular disease, or pulmonary disorders; treatment for anaphylactic reactions should be immediately available

Adverse Reactions

Central nervous system: Headache, fatigue, fever (rare)

Hepatic: Transient liver function test abnormalities

Local: Cutaneous reactions at the injection site (pain, soreness, tenderness, edema, warmth, and redness)

Drug Interactions No interference of immunogenicity was reported when mixed with hepatitis B vaccine

Mechanism of Action As an inactivated virus vaccine, hepatitis A vaccine offers active immunization against hepatitis A virus infection at an effective immune response rate in up to 99% of subjects

Pharmacodynamics/Kinetics

Onset of action (protection): 3 weeks after a single dose

Duration: Neutralizing antibodies have persisted for >3 years; unconfirmed evidence indicates that antibody levels may persist for 5-10 years

Usual Dosage I.M.:

Havrix®:

Children 2-18 years: 720 ELISA units (administered as 2 injections of 360 ELISA units [0.5 mL]) 15-30 days prior to travel with a booster 6-12 months following primary immunization; the deltoid muscle should be used for I.M. injection

Adults: 1440 ELISA units(1 mL) 15-30 days prior to travel with a booster 6-12 months following primary immunization; injection should be in the deltoid

Administration Inject I.M. into the deltoid muscle, if possible

Monitoring Parameters Liver function tests

Reference Range Seroconversion for Havrix®: Antibody >20 milli-international units/mL

Additional Information Some investigators suggest simultaneous or sequential administration of inactivated hepatitis A vaccine and immune globulin for postexposure protection, especially for travelers requiring rapid immunization, although a slight decrease in vaccine immunogenicity may be observed with this technique

Dosage Forms

Injection: 360 ELISA units/0.5 mL (0.5 mL); 1440 ELISA units/mL (1 mL)

Injection, pediatric: 720 ELISA units/0.5 mL (0.5 mL)

Injection (VAQTA®): 50 units/mL (1 mL)

Hepatitis B Immune Globulin

(hep a TYE tis bee i MYUN GLOB yoo lin)

Related Information

Immunization Guidelines *on page 1421*

Miscellaneous Vaccination Information *on page 1437*

Brand Names H-BIG®; HyperHep®

Therapeutic Category Immune Globulin

Use Provide prophylactic passive immunity to hepatitis B infection to those individuals exposed; newborns of mothers known to be hepatitis B surface antigen positive; hepatitis B immune globulin is not indicated for treatment of active hepatitis B infections and is ineffective in the treatment of chronic active hepatitis B infection

Pregnancy Risk Factor C

Contraindications Hypersensitivity to hepatitis B immune globulin or any component; allergies to gamma globulin or anti-immunoglobulin antibodies; allergies to thimerosal; IgA deficiency; I.M. injections in patients with thrombocytopenia or coagulation disorders

Adverse Reactions

1% to 10%:

- Central nervous system: Dizziness, malaise
- Dermatologic: Urticaria, angioedema, rash, erythema
- Local: Pain and tenderness at injection site
- Neuromuscular & skeletal: Arthralgia

<1%: Miscellaneous: Anaphylaxis

Drug Interactions Increased toxicity: Live virus vaccines

Stability Refrigerate at 2°C to 8°C (36°F to 46°F); do not freeze

Mechanism of Action Hepatitis B immune globulin (HBIG) is a nonpyrogenic sterile solution containing 10% to 18% protein of which at least 80% is monomeric immunoglobulin G (IgG). HBIG differs from immune globulin in the amount of anti-HB_s. Immune globulin is prepared from plasma that is not preselected for anti-HB_s content. HBIG is prepared from plasma preselected for high titer anti-HB_s. In the U.S., HBIG has an anti-HB_s high titer >1:100,000 by IRA. There is no evidence that the causative agent of AIDS (HTLV-III/LAV) is transmitted by HBIG.

Pharmacodynamics/Kinetics

Absorption: Slow

Time to peak serum concentration: 1-6 days

Usual Dosage I.M.:

Newborns: Hepatitis B: 0.5 mL as soon after birth as possible (within 12 hours)

Adults: Postexposure prophylaxis: 0.06 mL/kg; usual dose: 3-5 mL; maximum dose: 5 mL as soon as possible after exposure (within 96 hours); repeat at 28-30 days after exposure

Administration I.M. injection only in gluteal or deltoid region; to prevent injury from injection, care should be taken when giving to patients with thrombocytopenia or bleeding disorders; **do not administer I.V.**

Dosage Forms Injection:

H-BIG®: 4 mL, 5 mL

Hep-B-Gammagee®: 5 mL

HyperHep®: 0.5 mL, 1 mL, 5 mL

Hepatitis B Inactivated Virus Vaccine (plasma derived) *see* Hepatitis B Vaccine *on this page*

Hepatitis B Inactivated Virus Vaccine (recombinant DNA) *see* Hepatitis B Vaccine *on this page*

Hepatitis B Vaccine (hep a TYE tis bee vak SEEN)

Related Information

Guidelines for the Prevention of Opportunistic Infections in Persons with HIV *on page 1457*

Immunization Guidelines *on page 1421*

Miscellaneous Vaccination Information *on page 1437*

Prophylaxis for Patients Exposed to Common Communicable Diseases *on page 1452*

Recommendations for Travelers *on page 1442*

Recommendations of the Advisory Committee on Immunization Practices (ACIP) *on page 1424*

Recommended Childhood Immunization Schedule - US - January-December, 1997 *on page 1423*

Brand Names Engerix-B®; Recombivax HB®

Synonyms Hepatitis B Inactivated Virus Vaccine (plasma derived); Hepatitis B Inactivated Virus Vaccine (recombinant DNA)

Therapeutic Category Vaccine, Inactivated Virus

(Continued)

Hepatitis B Vaccine *(Continued)*

Use Immunization against infection caused by all known subtypes of hepatitis B virus, in individuals considered at high risk of potential exposure to hepatitis B virus or HB_sAg-positive materials; see chart.

Pre-exposure Prophylaxis for Hepatitis B
Health care workers*
Special patient groups (eg, adolescents, infants born to HB_sAg–positive mothers, military personnel, etc)
Hemodialysis patients†
Recipients of certain blood products‡
Lifestyle factors
Homosexual and bisexual men
Intravenous drug abusers
Heterosexually active persons with multiple sexual partners or recently acquired sexually transmitted diseases
Environmental factors
Household and sexual contacts of HBV carriers
Prison inmates
Clients and staff of institutions for the mentally handicapped
Residents, immigrants and refugees from areas with endemic HBV infection
International travelers at increased risk of acquiring HBV infection

*The risk of hepatitis B virus (HBV) infection for health care workers varies both between hospitals and within hospitals. Hepatitis B vaccination is recommended for all health care workers with blood exposure.

†Hemodialysis patients often respond poorly to hepatitis B vaccination; higher vaccine doses or increased number of doses are required. A special formulation of one vaccine is now available for such persons (Recombivax HB®, 40 mcg/mL). The anti-Hb_s (antibody to hepatitis B surface antigen) response of such persons should be tested after they are vaccinated, and those who have not responded should be revaccinated with 1-3 additional doses

Patients with chronic renal disease should be vaccinated as early as possible, ideally before they require hemodialysis. In addition, their anti-HB_s levels should be monitored at 6-12 month intervals to assess the need for revaccination.

‡Patients with hemophilia should be immunized subcutaneously, not intramuscularly.

Pregnancy Risk Factor C

Contraindications Hypersensitivity to yeast, hypersensitivity to hepatitis B vaccine or any component

Adverse Reactions

>10%:
- Central nervous system: Fever, malaise, fatigue, headache
- Local: Mild local tenderness, local inflammatory reaction

1% to 10%:
- Gastrointestinal: Nausea, diarrhea
- Respiratory: Pharyngitis

<1%:
- Cardiovascular: Tachycardia, hypotension, sensation of warmth, flushing
- Central nervous system: Lightheadedness, chills, somnolence, insomnia, irritability, agitation
- Dermatologic: Pruritus, rash, erythema, urticaria
- Gastrointestinal: Vomiting, GI disturbances, constipation, abdominal cramps, dyspepsia, anorexia
- Genitourinary: Dysuria
- Neuromuscular & skeletal: Arthralgia, myalgia, stiffness in back/neck/arm or shoulder
- Otic: Earache
- Respiratory: Rhinitis, cough, epistaxis
- Miscellaneous: Diaphoresis

Drug Interactions Decreased effect: Immunosuppressive agents

Stability Refrigerate, do not freeze

Mechanism of Action Recombinant hepatitis B vaccine is a noninfectious subunit viral vaccine. The vaccine is derived from hepatitis B surface antigen (HB_sAg) produced through recombinant DNA techniques from yeast cells. The portion of the hepatitis B gene which codes for HB_sAg is cloned into yeast which is then cultured to produce hepatitis B vaccine.

Pharmacodynamics/Kinetics Duration of action: Following all 3 doses of hepatitis B vaccine, immunity will last approximately 5-7 years

Usual Dosage See tables.

Immunization Regimen of Three I.M. Hepatitis B Vaccine Doses

Age	Initial		1 mo		6 mo	
	Recombivax HB® (mL)	Engerix-B® (mL)	Recombivax HB® (mL)	Engerix-B® (mL)	Recombivax HB® (mL)	Engerix-B® (mL)
Birth* - 10 y	0.25	0.5	0.25	0.5	0.25	0.5
11-19 y	0.5	1	0.5	1	0.5	1
≥20 y	1	1	1	1	1	1
Dialysis or immunocompromised patients		2†		2†		2†

*Infants born of HB_sAg negative mothers.

†Two 1 mL doses given at different sites.

Recommended Dosage for Infants Born to HB_sAg Positive Mothers

Treatment	Birth	Within 7 d	1 mo	6 mo
Engerix-B® (pediatric dose 10 mcg/0.5 mL)	*	0.5 mL*	0.5 mL	0.5 mL
Recombivax HB® (pediatric dose 5 mcg/0.5 mL)	*	0.5 mL*	0.5 mL	0.5 mL
Hepatitis B immune globulin	0.5 mL	—	—	—

*The first dose may be given at birth at the same time as HBIG, but give in the opposite anterolateral thigh. This may better ensure vaccine absorption.

Administration I.M. injection only; in adults, the deltoid muscle is the preferred site; the anterolateral thigh is the recommended site in infants and young children

Patient Information Must complete full course of injections for adequate immunization

Nursing Implications Rare chance of anaphylactoid reaction; have epinephrine available

Additional Information Inactivated virus vaccine; federal law requires that the date of administration, the vaccine manufacturer, lot number of vaccine, and the administering person's name, title and address be entered into the patient's permanent medical record

Dosage Forms Injection:

Recombinant DNA (Engerix-B®): Hepatitis B surface antigen 20 mcg/mL (1 mL)

Pediatric, recombinant DNA (Engerix-B®): Hepatitis B surface antigen 10 mcg/0.5 mL (0.5 mL)

Recombinant DNA (Recombivax HB®): Hepatitis B surface antigen 10 mcg/mL (1 mL, 3 mL)

Dialysis formulation, recombinant DNA (Recombivax HB®): Hepatitis B surface antigen 40 mcg/mL (1 mL)

Hep-Lock® *see* Heparin *on page 603*

Heptalac® *see* Lactulose *on page 703*

Herplex® Ophthalmic *see* Idoxuridine *on page 644*

HES *see* Hetastarch *on this page*

Hespan® *see* Hetastarch *on this page*

Hetastarch (HET a starch)

Brand Names Hespan®

Synonyms HES; Hydroxyethyl Starch

Therapeutic Category Plasma Volume Expander, Colloid

Use Blood volume expander used in treatment of shock or impending shock when blood or blood products are not available; does not have oxygen-carrying capacity and is not a substitute for blood or plasma

Pregnancy Risk Factor C

Contraindications Severe bleeding disorders, renal failure with oliguria or anuria, or severe congestive heart failure

Warnings/Precautions Anaphylactoid reactions have occurred; use with caution in patients with thrombocytopenia (may interfere with platelet function); large volume may cause drops in hemoglobin concentrations; use with caution in patients at risk from overexpansion of blood volume, including the very young or aged patients, those with congestive heart failure or pulmonary edema; large volumes may interfere with platelet function and prolong PT and PTT times

Adverse Reactions

<1%:

Cardiovascular: Peripheral edema, heart failure, circulatory overload

Central nervous system: Fever, chills, headaches

Dermatologic: Itching, pruritus

Gastrointestinal: Vomiting

(Continued)

Hetastarch *(Continued)*

Hematologic: Bleeding, prolongation of PT, PTT, clotting time, and bleeding time
Neuromuscular & skeletal: Myalgia
Miscellaneous: Hypersensitivity

Overdosage/Toxicology Symptoms of overdose include heart failure, nausea, vomiting, circulatory overload, bleeding; treatment is supportive

Stability Do not use if crystalline precipitate forms or is turbid deep brown

Mechanism of Action Produces plasma volume expansion by virtue of its highly colloidal starch structure, similar to albumin

Pharmacodynamics/Kinetics

Onset of volume expansion: I.V.: Within 30 minutes
Duration: 24-36 hours
Metabolism: Molecules >50,000 daltons require enzymatic degradation by the reticuloendothelial system or amylases in the blood prior to urinary and fecal excretion
Elimination: Smaller molecular weight molecules are readily excreted in urine

Usual Dosage I.V. infusion (requires an infusion pump):

Children: Safety and efficacy have not been established
Adults: 500-1000 mL (up to 1500 mL/day) or 20 mL/kg/day (up to 1500 mL/day); larger volumes (15,000 mL/24 hours) have been used safely in small numbers of patients

Dosing adjustment in renal impairment: Cl_{cr} <10 mL/minute: Initial dose is the same but subsequent doses should be reduced by 20% to 50% of normal

Administration I.V. only; may administer up to 1.2 g/kg/hour (20 mL/kg/hour)

Nursing Implications Anaphylactoid reactions can occur, have epinephrine and resuscitative equipment available

Dosage Forms Infusion, in sodium chloride 0.9%: 6% (500 mL)

Hexachlorocyclohexane *see* Lindane *on page 728*

Hexachlorophene (heks a KLOR oh feen)

Brand Names pHisoHex®; Septisol®

Therapeutic Category Antibacterial, Topical; Soap

Use Surgical scrub and as a bacteriostatic skin cleanser; control an outbreak of gram-positive infection when other procedures have been unsuccessful

Pregnancy Risk Factor C

Contraindications Known hypersensitivity to halogenated phenol derivatives or hexachlorophene; use in premature infants; use on burned or denuded skin; occlusive dressing; application to mucous membranes

Warnings/Precautions Discontinue use if signs of cerebral irritability occur; exposure of preterm infants or patients with extensive burns has been associated with apnea, convulsions, agitation and coma; do not use for bathing infants, premature infants are particularly susceptible to hexachlorophene topical absorption

Adverse Reactions

<1%:

Central nervous system: CNS injury, seizures, irritability
Dermatologic: Photosensitivity, dermatitis, redness, dry skin

Overdosage/Toxicology Symptoms of overdose include anorexia, vomiting, abdominal cramps, diarrhea, dehydration, seizures, hypotension, shock; treatment is supportive

Stability Store in nonmetallic container (**incompatible** with many metals); prolonged direct exposure to strong light may cause brownish surface discoloration, but this does not affect its action

Mechanism of Action Bacteriostatic polychlorinated biphenyl which inhibits membrane-bound enzymes and disrupts the cell membrane

Pharmacodynamics/Kinetics

Absorption: Percutaneously through inflamed, excoriated, and intact skin
Distribution: Crosses the placenta
Half-life: Infants: 6.1-44.2 hours

Usual Dosage Children and Adults: Topical: Apply 5 mL cleanser and water to area to be cleansed; lather and rinse thoroughly under running water

Patient Information Do not leave on skin for prolonged contact; for external use only; discontinue product if condition persists or worsens and call physician; if suds enter eye, rinse out thoroughly with water

Dosage Forms

Foam (Septisol®): 0.23% with alcohol 56% (180 mL, 600 mL)
Liquid, topical (pHisoHex®): 3% (8 mL, 150 mL, 500 mL, 3840 mL)

Hexadrol® *see* Dexamethasone *on page 356*
Hexalen® *see* Altretamine *on page 54*

Hexamethylenetetramine *see* Methenamine *on page 802*

Hexamethylmelamine *see* Altretamine *on page 54*

Hexavitamin *see* Vitamins, Multiple *on page 1310*

Hibiclens® Topical [OTC] *see* Chlorhexidine Gluconate *on page 253*

Hibistat® Topical [OTC] *see* Chlorhexidine Gluconate *on page 253*

Hib Polysaccharide Conjugate *see Haemophilus* b Conjugate Vaccine *on page 595*

HibTITER® *see Haemophilus* b Conjugate Vaccine *on page 595*

Hi-Cor 1.0® *see* Hydrocortisone *on page 623*

Hi-Cor-2.5® *see* Hydrocortisone *on page 623*

Hiprex® *see* Methenamine *on page 802*

Hismanal® *see* Astemizole *on page 110*

Histaject® *see* Brompheniramine *on page 166*

Histerone® Injection *see* Testosterone *on page 1198*

Histrelin (his TREL in)

Brand Names Supprelin™

Therapeutic Category Gonadotropin Releasing Hormone Analog; Luteinizing Hormone-Releasing Hormone Analog

Use Treatment of central idiopathic precocious puberty; treatment of estrogen-associated gynecological disorders such as acute intermittent porphyria, endometriosis, leiomyomata uteri, and premenstrual syndrome

Pregnancy Risk Factor X

Contraindications Hypersensitivity to histrelin, pregnancy, breast-feeding

Warnings/Precautions The site of injection should be varied daily; the dose should be administered at the same time each day. In precocious puberty, changing the dosage schedule or noncompliance may result in inadequate control of the pubertal process.

Adverse Reactions

>10%:

- Cardiovascular: Vasodilation
- Central nervous system: Headache
- Gastrointestinal: Abdominal pain
- Genitourinary: Vaginal bleeding, vaginal dryness
- Local: Skin reaction at injection site

1% to 10%:

- Central nervous system: Mood swings, headache, pain
- Dermatologic: Rashes, urticaria
- Endocrine & metabolic: Breast tenderness, hot flashes
- Gastrointestinal: Nausea, vomiting
- Genitourinary: Increased urinary calcium excretion
- Neuromuscular & skeletal: Joint stiffness

Stability Refrigerate at 2°C to 8°C (36°F to 46°F) and protect from light; allow vial to reach room temperature before injecting contents

Mechanism of Action Histrelin is a synthetic long-acting gonadotropin-releasing hormone analog; with daily administration, it desensitizes the pituitary to endogenous gonadotropin-releasing hormone (ie, suppresses gonadotropin release by causing down regulation of the pituitary); this results in a decrease in gonadal sex steroid production which stops the secondary sexual development

Pharmacodynamics/Kinetics

Precocious puberty: Onset of hormonal responses: Within 3 months of initiation of therapy

Acute intermittent porphyria associated with menses: Amelioration of symptoms: After 1-2 months of therapy

Treatment of endometriosis or leiomyomata uteri: Onset of responses: After 3-6 months of treatment

Usual Dosage

Central idiopathic precocious puberty: S.C.: Usual dose is 10 mcg/kg/day given as a single daily dose at the same time each day

Acute intermittent porphyria in women: S.C.: 5 mcg/day

Endometriosis: S.C.: 100 mcg/day

Leiomyomata uteri: S.C.: 20-50 mcg/day or 4 mcg/kg/day

Administration Injection site should be varied daily; dose should be administered at the same time each day

Monitoring Parameters Precocious puberty: Prior to initiating therapy: Height and weight, hand and wrist x-rays, total sex steroid levels, beta-hCG level, adrenal steroid level, gonadotropin-releasing hormone stimulation test, pelvic/adrenal/testicular ultrasound/head CT; during therapy monitor 3 months after initiation and then every 6-12 months; serial levels of sex steroids and gonadotropin-releasing hormone testing; physical exam; secondary sexual development;

(Continued)

Histrelin *(Continued)*

histrelin may be discontinued when the patient reaches the appropriate age for puberty

Dosage Forms Injection: 7-day kits of single use: 120 mcg/0.6 mL; 300 mcg/0.6 mL; 600 mcg/0.6 mL

Hivid® *see* Zalcitabine *on page 1318*

HMS Liquifilm® *see* Medrysone *on page 772*

HN_2 *see* Mechlorethamine *on page 767*

Hold® DM [OTC] *see* Dextromethorphan *on page 366*

Homatropine (hoe MA troe peen)

Related Information

Cycloplegic Mydriatics Comparison *on page 1409*

Brand Names AK-Homatropine®; Isopto® Homatropine

Synonyms Homatropine Hydrobromide

Therapeutic Category Anticholinergic Agent, Ophthalmic; Ophthalmic Agent, Mydriatic

Use Producing cycloplegia and mydriasis for refraction; treatment of acute inflammatory conditions of the uveal tract

Pregnancy Risk Factor C

Contraindications Narrow-angle glaucoma, acute hemorrhage or hypersensitivity to the drug or any component in the formulation

Warnings/Precautions Use with caution in patients with hypertension, cardiac disease, or increased intraocular pressure; safety and efficacy not established in infants and young children, therefore, use with extreme caution due to susceptibility of systemic effects; use with caution in obstructive uropathy, paralytic ileus, ulcerative colitis, unstable cardiovascular status in acute hemorrhage

Adverse Reactions

>10%: Ocular: Blurred vision, photophobia

1% to 10%:
- Local: Stinging, local irritation
- Ocular: Increased intraocular pressure
- Respiratory: Congestion

<1%:
- Cardiovascular: Vascular congestion, edema
- Central nervous system: Drowsiness
- Dermatologic: Exudate, eczematoid dermatitis
- Ocular: Follicular conjunctivitis

Overdosage/Toxicology Symptoms of overdose include blurred vision, urinary retention, tachycardia

Anticholinergic toxicity is caused by strong binding of the drug to cholinergic receptors. For anticholinergic overdose with severe life-threatening symptoms, physostigmine 1-2 mg (0.5 or 0.02 mg/kg for children) S.C. or I.V., slowly may be given to reverse these effects.

Stability Protect from light

Mechanism of Action Blocks response of iris sphincter muscle and the accommodative muscle of the ciliary body to cholinergic stimulation resulting in dilation and loss of accommodation

Pharmacodynamics/Kinetics

Onset of accommodation and pupil effect: Ophthalmic:
- Maximum mydriatic effect: Within 10-30 minutes
- Maximum cycloplegic effect: Within 30-90 minutes

Duration:
- Mydriasis: 6 hours to 4 days
- Cycloplegia: 10-48 hours

Usual Dosage

Children:
- Mydriasis and cycloplegia for refraction: Instill 1 drop of 2% solution immediately before the procedure; repeat at 10-minute intervals as needed
- Uveitis: Instill 1 drop of 2% solution 2-3 times/day

Adults:
- Mydriasis and cycloplegia for refraction: Instill 1-2 drops of 2% solution or 1 drop of 5% solution before the procedure; repeat at 5- to 10-minute intervals as needed
- Uveitis: Instill 1-2 drops of 2% or 5% 2-3 times/day up to every 3-4 hours as needed

Patient Information May cause blurred vision; if irritation persists or increases, discontinue use

Nursing Implications Finger pressure should be applied to lacrimal sac for 1-2 minutes after instillation to decrease risk of absorption and systemic reactions

Dosage Forms Solution, ophthalmic, as hydrobromide:
- 2% (1 mL, 5 mL); 5% (1 mL, 2 mL, 5 mL)
- AK-Homatropine®: 5% (15 mL)
- Isopto® Homatropine 2% (5 mL, 15 mL); 5% (5 mL, 15 mL)

Homatropine and Hydrocodone *see* Hydrocodone and Homatropine *on page 622*

Homatropine Hydrobromide *see* Homatropine *on previous page*

Horse Anti-human Thymocyte Gamma Globulin *see* Lymphocyte Immune Globulin *on page 749*

Human Diploid Cell Cultures Rabies Vaccine *see* Rabies Virus Vaccine *on page 1091*

Human Diploid Cell Cultures Rabies Vaccine (Intradermal use) *see* Rabies Virus Vaccine *on page 1091*

Human Growth Hormone (HYU man grothe HOR mone)

Brand Names Genotropin® Injection; Humatrope® Injection; Norditropin® Injection; Nutropin® AQ Injection; Nutropin® Injection; Protropin® Injection

Synonyms Growth Hormone; Somatrem; Somatropin

Therapeutic Category Growth Hormone

Use
- Long-term treatment of growth failure from lack of adequate endogenous growth hormone secretion
- Nutropin®: Treatment of children who have growth failure associated with chronic renal insufficiency up until the time of renal transplantation

Pregnancy Risk Factor C

Contraindications Closed epiphyses, known hypersensitivity to drug, benzyl alcohol (somatrem), or M-cresol or glycerin (somatropin); progression of any underlying intracranial lesion or actively growing intracranial tumor

Warnings/Precautions Use with caution in patients with diabetes; when administering to newborns, reconstitute with sterile water for injection

Adverse Reactions S.C. administration can cause local lipoatrophy or lipodystrophy and may enhance the development of neutralizing antibodies

1% to 10%: Endocrine & metabolic: Hypothyroidism

<1%:
- Dermatologic: Rash, itching
- Endocrine & metabolic: Hypoglycemia
- Local: Pain at injection site
- Miscellaneous: Small risk for developing leukemia, pain in hip/knee

Overdosage/Toxicology Symptoms include hypoglycemia, hyperglycemia, acromegaly

Drug Interactions Decreased effect: Glucocorticoid therapy may inhibit growth-promoting effects.

Stability
- Somatrem (Protropin®): Store vials at 2°C to 8°C/36°F to 46°F; reconstitute each 5 mg vial with 1-5 mL of bacteriostatic water for injection; use reconstituted vials within 7 days; avoid freezing
- Somatropin (Humatrope®/Nutropin®): Store vials at 2°C to 8°C/36°C to 46°F; avoid freezing; reconstitute each 5 mg vial with 1-5 mL of bacteriostatic water for injection; use reconstituted vials within 14 days; avoid freezing

Mechanism of Action Somatropin and somatrem are purified polypeptide hormones of recombinant DNA origin; somatropin contains the identical sequence of amino acids found in human growth hormone while somatrem's amino acid sequence is identical plus an additional amino acid, methionine; human growth hormone stimulates growth of linear bone, skeletal muscle, and organs; stimulates erythropoietin which increases red blood cell mass; exerts both insulin-like and diabetogenic effects

Pharmacodynamics/Kinetics Somatrem and somatropin have equivalent pharmacokinetic properties
- Duration of action: Maintains supraphysiologic levels for 18-20 hours
- Absorption: I.M.: Well absorbed
- Metabolism: ~90% in the liver
- Half-life: 15-50 minutes
- Elimination: 0.1% excreted in urine unchanged

Usual Dosage Children (individualize dose):
- Somatrem (Protropin®): I.M., S.C.: Up to 0.1 mg (0.26 units)/kg/dose 3 times/week
- Somatropin (Humatrope®): I.M., S.C.: Up to 0.06 mg (0.16 units)/kg/dose 3 times/week
- Somatropin (Nutropin®): S.C.:
  - Growth hormone inadequacy: Weekly dosage of 0.3 mg/kg (0.78 units/kg) administered daily

(Continued)

Human Growth Hormone *(Continued)*

Chronic renal insufficiency: Weekly dosage of 0.35 mg/kg (0.91 units/kg) administered daily

Therapy should be discontinued when patient has reached satisfactory adult height, when epiphyses have fused, or when the patient ceases to respond

Growth of 5 cm/year or more is expected, if growth rate does not exceed 2.5 cm in a 6-month period, double the dose for the next 6 months, if there is still no satisfactory response, discontinue therapy

Administration Do not shake; administer S.C. or I.M.; refer to product labeling; when administering to newborns, reconstitute with sterile water for injection

Monitoring Parameters Growth curve, periodic thyroid function tests, bone age (annually), periodical urine testing for glucose, somatomedin C levels

Nursing Implications Watch for glucose intolerance

Dosage Forms Powder for injection (lyophilized):

Somatropin:

- Genotropin®: 1.5 mg ~4 units (5 mL); 5.8 mg ~15 units (5 mL)
- Humatrope®: 5 mg ~13 units (5 mL)
- Norditropin®: 4 mg ~12 units; 8 mg ~24 units
- Nutropin®: 5 mg ~13 units (5 mL); 10 mg ~26 units (10 mL)
- Nutropin® AQ: 10 mg ~30 units (2 mL)

Somatrem, Protropin®: 5 mg ~13 units (10 mL)

Humate-P® *see* Antihemophilic Factor (Human) *on page 94*
Humatin® *see* Paromomycin *on page 953*
Humatrope® Injection *see* Human Growth Hormone *on previous page*
Humegon™ *see* Menotropins *on page 779*
Humibid® DM [OTC] *see* Guaifenesin and Dextromethorphan *on page 591*
Humibid® L.A. *see* Guaifenesin *on page 589*
Humibid® Sprinkle *see* Guaifenesin *on page 589*
HuMist® Nasal Mist [OTC] *see* Sodium Chloride *on page 1142*
Humorsol® *see* Demecarium *on page 349*
Humulin® 50/50 *see* Insulin Preparations *on page 659*
Humulin® 70/30 *see* Insulin Preparations *on page 659*
Humulin® L *see* Insulin Preparations *on page 659*
Humulin® N *see* Insulin Preparations *on page 659*
Humulin® R *see* Insulin Preparations *on page 659*
Humulin® U *see* Insulin Preparations *on page 659*
Hurricaine® *see* Benzocaine *on page 138*
Hyaluronic Acid *see* Sodium Hyaluronate *on page 1144*

Hyaluronidase (hye al yoor ON i dase)

Related Information

Extravasation Treatment of Other Drugs *on page 1381*

Brand Names Wydase®

Therapeutic Category Antidote, Extravasation

Use Increases the dispersion and absorption of other drugs; increases rate of absorption of parenteral fluids given by hypodermoclysis; enhances diffusion of locally irritating or toxic drugs in the management of I.V. extravasation

Pregnancy Risk Factor C

Contraindications Hypersensitivity to hyaluronidase or any component; do not inject in or around infected, inflamed, or cancerous areas

Warnings/Precautions Drug infiltrates in which hyaluronidase is contraindicated: Dopamine, alpha-adrenergic agonists; an intradermal skin test for sensitivity should be performed before actual administration using 0.02 mL of a 150 units/mL of hyaluronidase solution

Adverse Reactions

<1%:

- Cardiovascular: Tachycardia, hypotension
- Central nervous system: Dizziness, chills
- Dermatologic: Urticaria, erythema
- Gastrointestinal: Nausea, vomiting

Overdosage/Toxicology Symptoms of overdose include local edema, urticaria, erythema, chills, nausea, vomiting, hypotension

Drug Interactions Decreased effect: Salicylates, cortisone, ACTH, estrogens, antihistamines

Stability Reconstituted hyaluronidase solution remains stable for only 24 hours when stored in the refrigerator; do not use discolored solutions

Mechanism of Action Modifies the permeability of connective tissue through hydrolysis of hyaluronic acid, one of the chief ingredients of tissue cement which offers resistance to diffusion of liquids through tissues

Pharmacodynamics/Kinetics

Onset of action: Immediate by the subcutaneous or intradermal routes for the treatment of extravasation

Duration: 24-48 hours

Usual Dosage

Infants and Children:

Management of I.V. extravasation: Reconstitute the 150 unit vial of lyophilized powder with 1 mL normal saline; take 0.1 mL of this solution and dilute with 0.9 mL normal saline to yield 15 units/mL; using a 25- or 26-gauge needle, five 0.2 mL injections are made subcutaneously or intradermally into the extravasation site at the leading edge, changing the needle after each injection

Hypodermoclysis:

S.C.: 1 mL (150 units) is added to 1000 mL of infusion fluid and 0.5 mL (75 units) in injected into each clysis site at the initiation of the infusion

I.V.: 15 units is added to each 100 mL of I.V. fluid to be administered

Children <3 years: Limit volume of single clysis to 200 mL

Premature Infants: Do not exceed 25 mL/kg/day and not >2 mL/minute

Adults: Absorption and dispersion of drugs: 150 units are added to the vehicle containing the drug

Administration Administer hyaluronidase within the first few minutes to 1 hour after the extravasation of a necrotizing agent is recognized; do not administer I.V.

Nursing Implications Appropriate drugs for the management of an acute hypersensitivity (epinephrine, corticosteroids, and antihistamines) should be readily available

Additional Information The USP hyaluronidase unit is equivalent to the turbidity-reducing (TR) unit and the International Unit; each unit is defined as being the activity contained in 100 mcg of the International Standard Preparation

Dosage Forms

Injection, stabilized solution: 150 units/mL (1 mL, 10 mL)

Powder for injection, lyophilized: 150 units, 1500 units

Hyate®:C *see* Antihemophilic Factor (Porcine) *on page 95*

Hybalamin® *see* Hydroxocobalamin *on page 629*

Hybolin™ Decanoate *see* Nandrolone *on page 878*

Hybolin™ Improved *see* Nandrolone *on page 878*

Hycamptamine *see* Topotecan *on page 1244*

Hycamtin® *see* Topotecan *on page 1244*

Hycodan® *see* Hydrocodone and Homatropine *on page 622*

Hycort® *see* Hydrocortisone *on page 623*

Hydeltrasol® *see* Prednisolone *on page 1037*

Hydeltra-T.B.A.® *see* Prednisolone *on page 1037*

Hydergine® *see* Ergoloid Mesylates *on page 457*

Hydergine® LC *see* Ergoloid Mesylates *on page 457*

Hydralazine (hye DRAL a zeen)

Related Information

Heart Failure: Management of Patients With Left-Ventricular Systolic Dysfunction *on page 1533*

Therapy of Hypertension *on page 1540*

Brand Names Apresoline®

Canadian/Mexican Brand Names Apo-Hydralazine® (Canada); Novo-Hylazin® (Canada); Nu-Hydral® (Canada); Apresolina® (Mexico)

Synonyms Hydralazine Hydrochloride

Therapeutic Category Antihypertensive; Vasodilator

Use Management of moderate to severe hypertension, congestive heart failure, hypertension secondary to pre-eclampsia/eclampsia; also used to treat primary pulmonary hypertension

Pregnancy Risk Factor C

Pregnancy/Breast-Feeding Implications

Clinical effects on the fetus: Crosses the placenta. One report of fetal arrhythmia; transient neonatal thrombocytopenia and fetal distress reported following late 3rd trimester use. A large amount of clinical experience with the use of these drugs for management of hypertension during pregnancy is available. Available evidence suggests safe use during pregnancy and breast-feeding.

Breast-feeding/lactation: Crosses into breast milk in extremely small amounts. American Academy of Pediatrics considers COMPATIBLE with breast-feeding.

Contraindications Hypersensitivity to hydralazine or any component, dissecting aortic aneurysm, mitral valve rheumatic heart disease

Warnings/Precautions Discontinue hydralazine in patients who develop SLE-like syndrome or positive ANA. Use with caution in patients with severe renal disease or cerebral vascular accidents or with known or suspected coronary

(Continued)

Hydralazine *(Continued)*

artery disease; monitor blood pressure closely with I.V. use; some formulations may contain tartrazines or sulfites. Slow acetylators, patients with decreased renal function, and patients receiving >200 mg/day (chronically) are at higher risk for SLE. Titrate dosage to patient's response. Usually administered with diuretic and a beta-blocker to counteract side effects of sodium and water retention and reflex tachycardia.

Adverse Reactions

>10%:

Cardiovascular: Palpitations, flushing, tachycardia, angina pectoris
Central nervous system: Headache
Gastrointestinal: Nausea, vomiting, diarrhea, anorexia

1% to 10%:

Cardiovascular: Hypotension, redness or flushing of face
Gastrointestinal: Constipation
Ocular: Lacrimation
Respiratory: Dyspnea, nasal congestion

<1%:

Central nervous system: Malaise, fever, dizziness
Dermatologic: Rash, edema
Neuromuscular & skeletal: Arthralgias, weakness, peripheral neuritis
Miscellaneous: Positive ANA, positive LE cells

Note: Because of blunted beta-receptor response, the elderly are less likely to experience reflex tachycardia; this puts them at greater risk for orthostatic hypotension

Overdosage/Toxicology Symptoms of overdose include hypotension, tachycardia, shock

Hypotension usually responds to I.V. fluid, Trendelenburg positioning or vasoconstrictors; treatment is primarily supportive and symptomatic

Drug Interactions Increased toxicity: MAO inhibitors → significant decrease in blood pressure; indomethacin may decrease hypotensive effects

Stability

Intact ampuls/vials of hydralazine should not be stored under refrigeration because of possible precipitation or crystallization

Hydralazine should be diluted in NS for IVPB administration due to decreased stability in D_5W

Stability of IVPB solution in NS: 4 days at room temperature

Mechanism of Action Direct vasodilation of arterioles (with little effect on veins) with decreased systemic resistance

Pharmacodynamics/Kinetics

Onset of action:
- Oral: 20-30 minutes
- I.V.: 5-20 minutes

Duration:
- Oral: 2-4 hours
- I.V.: 2-6 hours

Distribution: Crosses placenta; appears in breast milk
Metabolism: Large first-pass effect orally, acetylated in liver
Protein binding: 85% to 90%
Bioavailability: 30% to 50%; enhanced by concurrent administration with food
Half-life:
- Normal renal function: 2-8 hours
- End stage renal disease: 7-16 hours

Elimination: 14% excreted unchanged in urine

Usual Dosage

Children:
- Oral: Initial: 0.75-1 mg/kg/day in 2-4 divided doses, not to exceed 25 mg/dose; increase over 3-4 weeks to maximum of 7.5 mg/kg/day in 2-4 divided doses; maximum daily dose: 200 mg/day
- I.M., I.V.: 0.1-0.2 mg/kg/dose (not to exceed 20 mg) every 4-6 hours as needed, up to 1.7-3.5 mg/kg/day in 4-6 divided doses

Adults:
- Oral: Hypertension:
  - Initial dose: 10 mg 4 times/day
  - Increase by 10-25 mg/dose every 2-5 days
  - Maximum dose: 300 mg/day
- Oral: Congestive heart failure:
  - Initial dose: 10-25 mg 3 times/day
  - Target dose: 75 mg 3 times/day
  - Maximum dose: 100 mg 3 times/day

I.M., I.V.:

Hypertensive Initial: 10-20 mg/dose every 4-6 hours as needed, may increase to 40 mg/dose; change to oral therapy as soon as possible

Pre-eclampsia/eclampsia: 5 mg/dose then 5-10 mg every 20-30 minutes as needed

Elderly: Oral: Initial: 10 mg 2-3 times/day; increase by 10-25 mg/day every 2-5 days

Dosing interval in renal impairment:

Cl_{cr} 10-50 mL/minute: Administer every 8 hours

Cl_{cr} <10 mL/minute: Administer every 8-16 hours in fast acetylators and every 12-24 hours in slow acetylators

Hemodialysis: Supplemental dose is not necessary

Peritoneal dialysis: Supplemental dose is not necessary

Monitoring Parameters Blood pressure (monitor closely with I.V. use), standing and sitting/supine, heart rate, ANA titer

Patient Information Report flu-like symptoms, rise slowly from sitting/lying position; take with meals

Nursing Implications Aid with ambulation, rising may cause orthostasis

Dosage Forms

Injection, as hydrochloride: 20 mg/mL (1 mL)

Tablet, as hydrochloride: 10 mg, 25 mg, 50 mg, 100 mg

Extemporaneous Preparations An oral solution (20 mg/5 mL) has been made from 20 mL of the hydralazine injection (20 mg/mL), 8 mL of propylene glycol and purified water USP qsad 100 mL; expected stability: 30 days if refrigerated

A flavored syrup (1.25 mg/mL) has been made using seventy-five hydralazine hydrochloride 50 mg tablets, dissolved in 250 mL of distilled water with 2250 g of Lycasin® (75% w/w maltitol syrup vehicle); edetate disodium 3 g and sodium saccharin 3 g dissolved in 50 mL distilled water was added; solution was preserved with 30 mL of a solution containing methylparaben 10% (w/v) and propylparaben 2% (w/v) in propylene glycol; flavored with 3 mL orange flavoring; qsad to 3 L with distilled water and then pH adjusted to pH of 3.7 using glacial acetic acid; measured stability was 5 days at room temperature (25°C); less than 2% loss of hydralazine occurred at 2 weeks when syrup was stored at 5°C

Alexander KS, Pudipeddi M, and Parker GA, "Stability of Hydralazine Hydrochloride Syrup Compounded From Tablets," *Am J Hosp Pharm*, 1993, 50(4):683-6.

Nahata MC and Hipple TF, *Pediatric Drug Formulations*, 2nd ed, Cincinnati, OH: Harvey Whitney Books Co, 1992.

Hydralazine Hydrochloride *see* Hydralazine *on page 615*

Hydramyn® Syrup [OTC] *see* Diphenhydramine *on page 399*

Hydrated Chloral *see* Chloral Hydrate *on page 247*

Hydrate® Injection *see* Dimenhydrinate *on page 395*

Hydrea® *see* Hydroxyurea *on page 632*

Hydrex® *see* Benzthiazide *on page 141*

Hydrocet® *see* Hydrocodone and Acetaminophen *on page 620*

Hydrochlorothiazide (hye droe klor oh THYE a zide)

Related Information

Heart Failure: Management of Patients With Left-Ventricular Systolic Dysfunction *on page 1533*

Sulfonamide Derivatives *on page 1420*

Brand Names Esidrix®; Ezide®; HydroDIURIL®; Hydro-Par®; Microzide®; Oretic®

Canadian/Mexican Brand Names Apo-Hydro® (Canada); Diuchlor® (Canada); Neo-Codema® (Canada); Novo-Hydrazide® (Canada); Urozide® (Canada); Diclotride® (Mexico)

Synonyms HCTZ

Therapeutic Category Antihypertensive; Diuretic, Thiazide

Use Management of mild to moderate hypertension; treatment of edema in congestive heart failure and nephrotic syndrome

Pregnancy Risk Factor D

Contraindications Anuria, renal decompensation, hypersensitivity to hydrochlorothiazide or any component, cross-sensitivity with other thiazides and sulfonamide derivatives

Warnings/Precautions Use with caution in renal disease, hepatic disease, gout, lupus erythematosus, diabetes mellitus; some products may contain tartrazine. Hydrochlorothiazide is not effective in patients with a Cl_{cr} <30 mL/minute, therefore, it may not be a useful agent in many elderly patients.

Adverse Reactions

1% to 10%: Endocrine & metabolic: Hypokalemia

<1%:

Cardiovascular: Hypotension

(Continued)

Hydrochlorothiazide *(Continued)*

Dermatologic: Photosensitivity
Endocrine & metabolic: Fluid and electrolyte imbalances, hyperglycemia
Hematologic: Rarely blood dyscrasias
Renal: Prerenal azotemia

Overdosage/Toxicology Symptoms of overdose include hypermotility, diuresis, lethargy, confusion, muscle weakness

Following GI decontamination, therapy is supportive with I.V. fluids, electrolytes, and I.V. pressors if needed

Drug Interactions

Decreased effect: Decreased antidiabetic drug efficacy
Increased toxicity:
Hypotensive agents may increase hypotensive potential
Increased digoxin related arrhythmias
Increased lithium levels
Tetracyclines may increase uremia

Mechanism of Action Inhibits sodium reabsorption in the distal tubules causing increased excretion of sodium and water as well as potassium and hydrogen ions

Pharmacodynamics/Kinetics

Onset of diuretic action: Oral: Within 2 hours
Peak effect: 4 hours
Duration: 6-12 hours
Absorption: Oral: ~60% to 80%
Elimination: Excreted unchanged in urine

Usual Dosage Oral (effect of drug may be decreased when used every day):

Children (In pediatric patients, chlorothiazide may be preferred over hydrochlorothiazide as there are more dosage formulations (eg, suspension) available):
<6 months: 2-3 mg/kg/day in 2 divided doses
>6 months: 2 mg/kg/day in 2 divided doses
Adults: 25-100 mg/day in 1-2 doses
Maximum: 200 mg/day
Elderly: 12.5-25 mg once daily
Minimal increase in response and more electrolyte disturbances are seen with doses >50 mg/day

Dosing adjustment/comments in renal impairment: Cl_{cr} <50 mL/minute: Not effective

Monitoring Parameters Assess weight, I & O reports daily to determine fluid loss; blood pressure, serum electrolytes, BUN, creatinine

Test Interactions ↑ creatine phosphokinase [CPK] (S), ammonia (B), amylase (S), calcium (S), chloride (S), cholesterol (S), glucose, ↑ acid (S), ↓ chloride (S), magnesium, potassium (S), sodium (S); Tyramine and phentolamine tests, histamine tests for pheochromocytoma

Patient Information May be taken with food or milk; take early in day to avoid nocturia; take the last dose of multiple doses no later than 6 PM unless instructed otherwise. A few people who take this medication become more sensitive to sunlight and may experience skin rash, redness, itching, or severe sunburn, especially if sun block SPF ≥15 is not used on exposed skin areas. May increase blood glucose levels in diabetics.

Nursing Implications Take blood pressure with patient lying down and standing

Dosage Forms

Solution, oral (mint flavor): 50 mg/5 mL (50 mL)
Tablet: 25 mg, 50 mg, 100 mg

Hydrochlorothiazide and Triamterene

(hye droe klor oh THYE a zide & trye AM ter een)

Brand Names Dyazide®; Maxzide®

Canadian/Mexican Brand Names Apo-Triazide® (Canada); Novo-Triamzide® (Canada); Nu-Triazide® (Canada)

Therapeutic Category Antihypertensive; Diuretic, Potassium Sparing; Diuretic, Thiazide

Use Management of mild to moderate hypertension; treatment of edema in congestive heart failure and nephrotic syndrome

Pregnancy Risk Factor C

Pregnancy/Breast-Feeding Implications Clinical effects on the fetus: Generally, use of diuretics during pregnancy is avoided due to risk of decreased placental perfusion

Contraindications Anuria, hyperkalemia, renal or hepatic failure, hypersensitivity to hydrochlorothiazide, triamterene or any component; concurrent use of potassium supplements

Warnings/Precautions This fixed combination is not indicated for initial therapy of hypertension; therapy requires titration to the individual patient, if dosage so determined represents this fixed combination, its use may be more convenient; safety and efficacy in children have not been established; avoid interchanging brands of drug.

Serum potassium concentrations do not necessarily indicate the true body potassium concentration. A rise in plasma pH or an increase in the circulating levels of insulin or epinephrine may cause a decrease in plasma potassium concentration and an increase in the intracellular potassium concentration. The efficacy of hydrochlorothiazide is limited in patients with Cl_{cr} <30 mL/minute.

Adverse Reactions

1% to 10%: Gastrointestinal: Loss of appetite, nausea, vomiting, stomach cramps, diarrhea, upset stomach

<1%:

- Central nervous system: Dizziness, fatigue
- Dermatologic: Purpura
- Endocrine & metabolic: Electrolyte disturbances
- Gastrointestinal: Burning of tongue
- Hematologic: Aplastic anemia, agranulocytosis, hemolytic anemia, leukopenia, thrombocytopenia, megaloblastic anemia
- Neuromuscular & skeletal: Muscle cramps
- Ocular: Xanthopsia, transient blurred vision
- Respiratory: Allergic pneumonitis, pulmonary edema, respiratory distress
- Miscellaneous: Bright orange tongue, cracked corners of mouth

Overdosage/Toxicology

Triamterene: Symptoms of overdose include drowsiness, confusion, clinical signs of dehydration, electrolyte imbalance, and hypotension; ingestion of large amounts of potassium-sparing diuretics, may result in life-threatening hyperkalemia. This can be treated with I.V. glucose with concurrent regular insulin, I.V. sodium bicarbonate and, if needed, Kayexalate® oral or rectal solutions in sorbitol may also be used.

Hydrochlorothiazide: Symptoms of overdose include hypermotility, diuresis, lethargy, confusion, muscle weakness; following GI decontamination, therapy is supportive with I.V. fluids, electrolytes, and I.V. pressors if needed

Drug Interactions

Hydrochlorothiazide:

- Decreased effect of oral hypoglycemics; decreased absorption with cholestyramine and colestipol
- Increased effect with furosemide and other loop diuretics
- Increased toxicity/levels of lithium

Triamterene:

- Increased risk of hyperkalemia if given together with amiloride, spironolactone, angiotensin-converting enzyme (ACE) inhibitors
- Increased toxicity of amantadine (possibly by decreasing its renal excretion)

Usual Dosage Oral:

Adults: 1-2 capsules twice daily after meals

Elderly: Initial: 1 capsule/day or every other day

Monitoring Parameters Blood pressure, serum electrolytes, BUN, creatinine, liver function tests

Test Interactions Serum creatinine and BUN, bentiromide test, fluorescent measurement of quinidine

Patient Information May be taken with food or milk; take early in day to avoid nocturia; take the last dose of multiple doses no later than 6 PM unless instructed otherwise. A few people who take this medication become more sensitive to sunlight and may experience skin rash, redness, itching, or severe sunburn, especially if sun block SPF ≥15 is not used on exposed skin areas. May increase blood glucose levels in diabetics. Notify physician if weakness, headache, joint swelling, or nausea becomes severe or persistent; may increase blood glucose and may impart a blue fluorescent color to urine.

Nursing Implications Assess weight, I & O reports daily to determine fluid loss; take blood pressure with patient lying down and standing; observe for hyperkalemia; if ordered once daily, dose should be given in the morning

Additional Information Dyazide® and Maxzide® are not bioequivalent. *One product should not be substituted for the other.* Retitration and appropriate changes in dosage may be necessary if patients are to be transferred from one dosage form to the other.

Dosage Forms

Capsule (Dyazide®): Hydrochlorothiazide 25 mg and triamterene 37.5 mg

Tablet:

- Maxzide®-25: Hydrochlorothiazide 25 mg and triamterene 37.5 mg
- Maxzide®: Hydrochlorothiazide 50 mg and triamterene 75 mg

Hydrocil® [OTC] *see* Psyllium *on page 1075*
Hydro-Cobex® *see* Hydroxocobalamin *on page 629*

Hydrocodone and Acetaminophen

(hye droe KOE done & a seet a MIN oh fen)

Related Information

Narcotic Agonists Comparison *on page 1414*

Dose Equivalents for Opioid Analgesics in Opioid-Naive Adults <50 kg *on page 1376*

Dose Equivalents for Opioid Analgesics in Opioid-Naive Adults ≥50 kg *on page 1375*

Brand Names Anexsia®; Anodynos-DHC®; Bancap HC®; Co-Gesic®; Dolacet®; DuoCet™; Duradyne DHC®; Hydrocet®; Hydrogesic®; Hy-Phen®; Lorcet®; Lorcet®-HD; Lorcet® Plus; Lortab®; Margesic® H; Norcet®; Stagesic®; T-Gesic®; Vicodin®; Vicodin® ES; Zydone®

Canadian/Mexican Brand Names Vapocet® (Canada)

Synonyms Acetaminophen and Hydrocodone

Therapeutic Category Analgesic, Narcotic

Use Relief of moderate to severe pain; antitussive (hydrocodone)

Restrictions C-III

Pregnancy Risk Factor C

Contraindications CNS depression, hypersensitivity to hydrocodone, acetaminophen or any component; severe respiratory depression

Warnings/Precautions Use with caution in patients with hypersensitivity reactions to other phenanthrene derivative opioid agonists (morphine, hydrocodone, hydromorphone, levorphanol, oxycodone, oxymorphone); tablets contain metabisulfite which may cause allergic reactions

Adverse Reactions

>10%:
- Cardiovascular: Hypotension
- Central nervous system: Lightheadedness, dizziness, sedation, drowsiness, fatigue
- Neuromuscular & skeletal: Weakness

1% to 10%:
- Cardiovascular: Bradycardia
- Central nervous system: Confusion
- Gastrointestinal: Nausea, vomiting
- Genitourinary: Decreased urination
- Respiratory: Shortness of breath, dyspnea

<1%:
- Cardiovascular: Hypertension
- Central nervous system: Hallucinations
- Gastrointestinal: Xerostomia, anorexia, biliary tract spasm
- Genitourinary: Urinary tract spasm
- Ocular: Diplopia, miosis
- Miscellaneous: Histamine release, physical and psychological dependence with prolonged use

Overdosage/Toxicology Symptoms of overdose include hepatic necrosis, blood dyscrasias, respiratory depression

Acetylcysteine 140 mg/kg orally (loading) followed by 70 mg/kg every 4 hours for 17 doses. Therapy should be initiated based upon laboratory analysis suggesting high probability of hepatotoxic potential. Naloxone (2 mg I.V.) can also be used to reverse the toxic effects of the opiate. Activated charcoal is effective at binding certain chemicals, and this is especially true for acetaminophen.

Drug Interactions
- Decreased effect with phenothiazines
- Increased effect with dextroamphetamine
- Increased toxicity with CNS depressants, TCAs

Mechanism of Action See individual agents

Pharmacodynamics/Kinetics
- Onset of narcotic analgesia: Within 10-20 minutes
- Duration: 3-6 hours
- Distribution: Crosses the placenta
- Metabolism: In the liver
- Half-life: 3.8 hours
- Elimination: In urine

Usual Dosage Oral (doses should be titrated to appropriate analgesic effect):

Children:
- Antitussive (hydrocodone): 0.6 mg/kg/day in 3-4 divided doses
  - A single dose should not exceed 10 mg in children >12 years, 5 mg in children 2-12 years, and 1.25 mg in children <2 years of age
- Analgesic (acetaminophen): Refer to Acetaminophen monograph

Adults: Analgesic: 1-2 tablets or capsules every 4-6 hours or 5-10 mL solution every 4-6 hours as needed for pain

Monitoring Parameters Pain relief, respiratory and mental status, blood pressure

Patient Information May cause drowsiness; do not exceed recommended dose; do not take for more than 10 days without physician's advice

Nursing Implications Observe patient for excessive sedation, respiratory depression

Dosage Forms

Capsule:

Bancap HC®, Dolacet®, Hydrocet®, Hydrogesic®, Lorcet®-HD, Margesic® H, Medipain 5®, Norcet®, Stagesic®, T-Gesic®, Zydone®: Hydrocodone bitartrate 5 mg and acetaminophen 500 mg

Elixir (tropical fruit punch flavor) (Lortab®): Hydrocodone bitartrate 2.5 mg and acetaminophen 167 mg per 5 mL with alcohol 7% (480 mL)

Solution, oral (tropical fruit punch flavor) (Lortab®): Hydrocodone bitartrate 2.5 mg and acetaminophen 167 mg per 5 mL with alcohol 7% (480 mL)

Tablet:

Lortab® 2.5/500: Hydrocodone bitartrate 2.5 mg and acetaminophen 500 mg

Anexsia® 5/500, Anodynos-DHC®, Co-Gesic®, DuoCet™, Duradyne DHC®, Hy-Phen®, Lorcet®, Lortab®® 5/500, Vicodin®: Hydrocodone bitartrate 5 mg and acetaminophen 500 mg

Lortab® 7.5/500: Hydrocodone bitartrate 7.5 mg and acetaminophen 500 mg

Anexsia® 7.5/650, Lorcet® Plus: Hydrocodone bitartrate 7.5 mg and acetaminophen 650 mg

Vicodin® ES: Hydrocodone bitartrate 7.5 mg and acetaminophen 750 mg

Lortab® 10/500: Hydrocodone bitartrate 10 mg and acetaminophen 500 mg

Lortab® 10/650: Hydrocodone bitartrate 10 mg and acetaminophen 650 mg

Vicodin® HP: Hydrocodone bitartrate 10 mg and acetaminophen 660 mg

Hydrocodone and Aspirin (hye droe KOE done & AS pir in)

Related Information

Narcotic Agonists Comparison *on page 1414*

Dose Equivalents for Opioid Analgesics in Opioid-Naive Adults <50 kg *on page 1376*

Dose Equivalents for Opioid Analgesics in Opioid-Naive Adults ≥50 kg *on page 1375*

Brand Names Azdone®; Damason-P®; Lortab® ASA; Panasal® 5/500

Therapeutic Category Analgesic, Narcotic

Use Relief of moderate to moderately severe pain

Restrictions C-III

Pregnancy Risk Factor D

Warnings/Precautions Use with caution in patients with impaired renal function, erosive gastritis, or peptic ulcer disease; children and teenagers should not use for chickenpox or flu symptoms before a physician is consulted about Reye's syndrome

Adverse Reactions

>10%:

Cardiovascular: Hypotension

Central nervous system: Lightheadedness, dizziness, sedation, drowsiness, fatigue

Gastrointestinal: Nausea, heartburn, stomach pains, dyspepsia, epigastric discomfort

Neuromuscular & skeletal: Weakness

1% to 10%:

Cardiovascular: Bradycardia

Central nervous system: Confusion

Dermatologic: Rash

Gastrointestinal: Vomiting, gastrointestinal ulceration

Genitourinary: Decreased urination

Hematologic: Hemolytic anemia

Respiratory: Shortness of breath, dyspnea

Miscellaneous: Anaphylactic shock

<1%:

Cardiovascular: Hypertension

Central nervous system: Hallucinations, insomnia, nervousness, jitters

Gastrointestinal: Xerostomia, anorexia, biliary tract spasm

Genitourinary: Urinary tract spasm

Hematologic: Occult bleeding, prolonged bleeding time, leukopenia, thrombocytopenia, iron deficiency anemia

Hepatic: Hepatotoxicity

Ocular: Diplopia, miosis

Renal: Impaired renal function

Respiratory: Bronchospasm

(Continued)

Hydrocodone and Aspirin *(Continued)*

Miscellaneous: Histamine release, physical and psychological dependence with prolonged use

Overdosage/Toxicology Antidote is naloxone for codeine. Naloxone 2 mg I.V. (0.01 mg/kg for children) with repeat administration as necessary up to a total of 10 mg. The "Done" nomogram is very helpful for estimating the severity of aspirin poisoning and directing treatment using serum salicylate levels. Treatment can also be based upon symptomatology; see Aspirin.

Drug Interactions Increased toxicity with CNS depressants, warfarin (bleeding)

Mechanism of Action Refer to individual agents

Usual Dosage Adults: Oral: 1-2 tablets every 4-6 hours as needed for pain

Dietary Considerations Alcohol: Additive CNS effect, avoid use

Administration Administer with food or a full glass of water to minimize GI distress

Monitoring Parameters Observe patient for excessive sedation, respiratory depression

Test Interactions Urine glucose, urinary 5-HIAA, serum uric acid

Patient Information May cause drowsiness; avoid alcohol; watch for bleeding gums or any signs of GI bleeding; take with food or milk to minimize GI distress, notify physician if ringing in ears or persistent GI pain occurs

Dosage Forms Tablet: Hydrocodone bitartrate 5 mg and aspirin 500 mg

Hydrocodone and Homatropine

(hye droe KOE done & hoe MA troe peen)

Related Information

Narcotic Agonists Comparison *on page 1414*

Brand Names Hycodan®; Hydromet®; Hydropane®; Hydrotropine®; Tussigon®

Synonyms Homatropine and Hydrocodone

Therapeutic Category Antitussive; Cough Preparation

Use Symptomatic relief of cough

Restrictions C-III

Pregnancy Risk Factor C

Contraindications Increased intracranial pressure, narrow-angle glaucoma, depressed ventilation, hypersensitivity to hydrocodone, homatropine, or any component

Warnings/Precautions Use with caution in patients with hypersensitivity to other phenanthrene derivatives; use with caution in patients with respiratory diseases, or severe liver or renal failure; use with caution in children with spastic paralysis, in the elderly, and in patients with prostatic hypertrophy

Adverse Reactions

>10%:

Cardiovascular: Hypotension

Central nervous system: Lightheadedness, dizziness, sedation, drowsiness, fatigue

Neuromuscular & skeletal: Weakness

1% to 10%:

Cardiovascular: Bradycardia, tachycardia

Central nervous system: Confusion

Gastrointestinal: Nausea, vomiting

Genitourinary: Decreased urination

Respiratory: Shortness of breath, dyspnea

<1%:

Central nervous system: Hallucinations

Cardiovascular: Hypertension

Dermatologic: Dry hot skin

Gastrointestinal: Xerostomia, anorexia, impaired GI motility, biliary tract spasm

Genitourinary: Urinary tract spasm

Ocular: Diplopia, miosis, mydriasis, blurred vision

Miscellaneous: Histamine release, physical and psychological dependence with prolonged use

Overdosage/Toxicology Symptoms of overdose include CNS and respiratory depression; gastrointestinal cramping; dilated, unreactive pupils; blurred vision; hot, dry flushed skin; dryness of mucous membranes; difficulty in swallowing, foul breath, diminished or absent bowel sounds, urinary retention, tachycardia, hyperthermia, hypertension, increased respiratory rate

CNS depression is an extension of pharmacologic effect; treatment is supportive; naloxone 0.4 mg I.V. (0.01 mg/kg for children) with repeat administrations as necessary; anticholinergic toxicity is caused by strong binding of the drug to cholinergic receptors. For anticholinergic overdose with severe life-threatening symptoms, physostigmine 1-2 mg (0.5 or 0.02 mg/kg for children) S.C. or I.V., slowly may be given to reverse these effects.

Usual Dosage Oral (based on hydrocodone component):

Children: 0.6 mg/kg/day in 3-4 divided doses; do not administer more frequently than every 4 hours

A single dose should not exceed 1.25 mg in children <2 years of age, 5 mg in children 2-12 years, and 10 mg in children >12 years

Adults: 5-10 mg every 4-6 hours, a single dose should not exceed 15 mg; do not administer more frequently than every 4 hours

Dietary Considerations Alcohol: Additive CNS effect, avoid use

Test Interactions ↑ ALT, AST (S)

Patient Information Avoid alcohol; may cause drowsiness and impair judgment or coordination; may cause physical and psychological dependence with prolonged use; lack of saliva may enhance cavities; maintain good oral hygiene; use caution while driving; may cause blurred vision; notify physician if difficulty in urinating or constipation becomes severe

Nursing Implications Dispense in light-resistant container; observe patient for excessive sedation, respiratory depression, implement safety measures, assist with ambulation

Dosage Forms

Syrup (Hycodan®, Hydromet®, Hydropane®, Hydrotropine®): Hydrocodone bitartrate 5 mg and homatropine methylbromide 1.5 mg per 5 mL (120 mL, 480 mL, 4000 mL)

Tablet (Hycodan®, Tussigon®): Hydrocodone bitartrate 5 mg and homatropine methylbromide 1.5 mg

Hydrocort® *see* Hydrocortisone *on this page*

Hydrocortisone (hye droe KOR ti sone)

Related Information

Corticosteroids Comparison *on page 1407*

Desensitization Protocols *on page 1496*

Brand Names Acticort™; Aeroseb-HC®; A-HydroCort®; Ala-Cort®; Ala-Scalp™; Anucort-HC®; Anumed HC™; Anusol-HC® [OTC]; Bactine™ Maximum Strength [OTC]; Caldecort® [OTC]; Caldecort® Anti-Itch Spray [OTC]; Cetacort®; Clocort® Maximum Strength; CortaGel® [OTC]; Cortaid® Maximum Strength [OTC]; Cortaid® with Aloe [OTC]; Cort-Dome®; Cortef®; Cortef® Feminine Itch [OTC]; Cortenema®; Corticaine® [OTC]; Cortizone®-5 [OTC]; Cortizone®-10 [OTC]; Delcort®; Dermacort®; Dermarest Dricort®; DermiCort®; Dermolate® [OTC]; Dermtex® HC with Aloe; Eldecort®; Gynecort® [OTC]; Hemril-HC™; Hi-Cor 1.0®; Hi-Cor-2.5®; Hycort®; Hydrocort®; Hydrocortone® Acetate; Hydrocortone® Phosphate; HydroSKIN®; Hydro-Tex® [OTC]; Hytone®; LactiCare-HC®; Lanacort® [OTC]; Locoid®; Nutracort®; Orabase® HCA; Pandel®; Penecort®; Proctocort™; ProctoCream-HC™; Scalpicin®; Solu-Cortef®; S-T Cort®; Synacort®; Tegrin®-HC; Texacort™; U-Cort™ Cortifoam®; Westcort®

Canadian/Mexican Brand Names Flebocortid® [Sodium Succinate] (Mexico); Nositrol® [Sodium Succinate] (Mexico)

Synonyms Compound F; Cortisol; Hydrocortisone Acetate; Hydrocortisone Buteprate; Hydrocortisone Butyrate; Hydrocortisone Cypionate; Hydrocortisone Sodium Phosphate; Hydrocortisone Sodium Succinate; Hydrocortisone Valerate

Therapeutic Category Anti-inflammatory Agent; Anti-inflammatory Agent, Rectal; Corticosteroid; Corticosteroid, Rectal; Corticosteroid, Systemic; Corticosteroid, Topical (Low Potency); Corticosteroid, Topical (Medium Potency); Glucocorticoid; Mineralocorticoid

Use Management of adrenocortical insufficiency; relief of inflammation of corticosteroid-responsive dermatoses (low and medium potency topical corticosteroid); adjunctive treatment of ulcerative colitis

Pregnancy Risk Factor C

Contraindications Serious infections, except septic shock or tuberculous meningitis; known hypersensitivity to hydrocortisone; viral, fungal, or tubercular skin lesions

Warnings/Precautions

Use with caution in patients with hyperthyroidism, cirrhosis, nonspecific ulcerative colitis, hypertension, osteoporosis, thromboembolic tendencies, CHF, convulsive disorders, myasthenia gravis, thrombophlebitis, peptic ulcer, diabetes

Acute adrenal insufficiency may occur with abrupt withdrawal after long-term therapy or with stress; young pediatric patients may be more susceptible to adrenal axis suppression from topical therapy

Because of the risk of adverse effects, systemic corticosteroids should be used cautiously in the elderly, in the smallest possible dose, and for the shortest possible time

Adverse Reactions

>10%:

Central nervous system: Insomnia, nervousness

(Continued)

Hydrocortisone *(Continued)*

Gastrointestinal: Increased appetite, indigestion

1% to 10%:

- Dermatologic: Hirsutism
- Endocrine & metabolic: Diabetes mellitus
- Neuromuscular & skeletal: Arthralgia
- Ocular: Cataracts
- Respiratory: Epistaxis

<1%:

- Cardiovascular: Hypertension, edema
- Central nervous system: Euphoria, headache, delirium, hallucinations, seizures, mood swings
- Dermatologic: Acne, dermatitis, skin atrophy, bruising, hyperpigmentation
- Endocrine & metabolic: Hypokalemia, hyperglycemia, Cushing's syndrome, sodium and water retention, bone growth suppression, amenorrhea
- Gastrointestinal: Peptic ulcer, abdominal distention, ulcerative esophagitis, pancreatitis
- Neuromuscular & skeletal: Muscle wasting
- Miscellaneous: Hypersensitivity reactions, immunosuppression

Overdosage/Toxicology Symptoms of overdose include cushingoid appearance (systemic), muscle weakness (systemic), osteoporosis (systemic) all with long-term use only. When consumed in excessive quantities for prolonged periods, systemic hypercorticism and adrenal suppression may occur. In those cases, discontinuation and withdrawal of the corticosteroid should be done judiciously.

Drug Interactions

Inducer of cytochrome P-450 enzymes

Cytochrome P-450 3A enzyme substrate

Decreased effect:

- Insulin decreases hypoglycemic effect
- Phenytoin, phenobarbital, ephedrine, and rifampin increase metabolism of hydrocortisone and decrease steroid blood level

Increased toxicity:

- Oral anticoagulants change prothrombin time; potassium-depleting diuretics increase risk of hypokalemia
- Cardiac glucosides increase risk of arrhythmias or digitalis toxicity secondary to hypokalemia

Stability

Hydrocortisone sodium phosphate and hydrocortisone sodium succinate are clear, light yellow solutions which are heat labile

After initial reconstitution, hydrocortisone sodium succinate solutions are stable for 3 days at room temperature and refrigeration if protected from light

Stability of parenteral admixture (Solu-Cortef®) at room temperature (25°C) and at refrigeration temperature (4°C) is concentration dependent

Minimum volume: Concentration should not exceed 1 mg/mL

Stability of concentration ≤1 mg/mL: 24 hours

Stability of concentration >1 mg/mL to <25 mg/mL: Unpredictable, 4-6 hours

Stability of concentration ≥25 mg/mL: 3 days

Standard diluent (Solu-Cortef®): 50 mg/50 mL D_5W; 100 mg/100 mL D_5W

Comments: Should be administered in a 0.1-1 mg/mL concentration due to stability problems

Mechanism of Action Decreases inflammation by suppression of migration of polymorphonuclear leukocytes and reversal of increased capillary permeability

Pharmacodynamics/Kinetics

Absorption: Rapid by all routes, except rectally

Metabolism: In the liver

Half-life, biologic: 8-12 hours

Elimination: Renally, mainly as 17-hydroxysteroids and 17-ketosteroids

Hydrocortisone acetate salt has a slow onset but long duration of action when compared with more soluble preparations

Hydrocortisone sodium phosphate salt is a water soluble salt with a rapid onset but short duration of action

Hydrocortisone sodium succinate salt is a water soluble salt with is rapidly active

Usual Dosage Dose should be based on severity of disease and patient response

Acute adrenal insufficiency: I.M., I.V.:

- Infants and young Children: Succinate: 1-2 mg/kg/dose bolus, then 25-150 mg/day in divided doses every 6-8 hours
- Older Children: Succinate: 1-2 mg/kg bolus then 150-250 mg/day in divided doses every 6-8 hours
- Adults: Succinate: 100 mg I.V. bolus, then 300 mg/day in divided doses every 8 hours or as a continuous infusion for 48 hours; once patient is stable change

to oral, 50 mg every 8 hours for 6 doses, then taper to 30-50 mg/day in divided doses

Chronic adrenal corticoid insufficiency: Adults: Oral: 20-30 mg/day

Anti-inflammatory or immunosuppressive:
- Infants and Children:
  - Oral: 2.5-10 mg/kg/day **or** 75-300 mg/m²/day every 6-8 hours
  - I.M., I.V.: Succinate: 1-5 mg/kg/day **or** 30-150 mg/m²/day divided every 12-24 hours
- Adolescents and Adults: Oral, I.M., I.V.: Succinate: 15-240 mg every 12 hours

Congenital adrenal hyperplasia: Oral: Initial: 30-36 mg/m²/day with 1/3 of dose every morning and 2/3 every evening or 1/4 every morning and mid-day and 1/2 every evening; maintenance: 20-25 mg/m²/day in divided doses

Physiologic replacement: Children:
- Oral: 0.5-0.75 mg/kg/day **or** 20-25 mg/m²/day every 8 hours
- I.M.: Succinate: 0.25-0.35 mg/kg/day **or** 12-15 mg/m²/day once daily

Shock: I.M., I.V.: Succinate:
- Children: Initial: 50 mg/kg, then repeated in 4 hours and/or every 24 hours as needed
- Adolescents and Adults: 500 mg to 2 g every 2-6 hours

Status asthmaticus: Children and Adults: I.V.: Succinate: 1-2 mg/kg/dose every 6 hours for 24 hours, then maintenance of 0.5-1 mg/kg every 6 hours

Rheumatic diseases:
- Adults: Intralesional, intra-articular, soft tissue injection: Acetate:
  - Large joints: 25 mg (up to 37.5 mg)
  - Small joints: 10-25 mg
- Tendon sheaths: 5-12.5 mg
- Soft tissue infiltration: 25-50 mg (up to 75 mg)
- Bursae: 25-37.5 mg
- Ganglia: 12.5-25 mg

Dermatosis: Children >2 years and Adults: Topical: Apply to affected area 3-4 times/day (Buteprate: Apply once or twice daily)

Ulcerative colitis: Adults: Rectal: 10-100 mg 1-2 times/day for 2-3 weeks

Administration
- Oral: Administer with food or milk to decrease GI upset
- Parenteral: Hydrocortisone sodium succinate may be administered by I.M. or I.V. routes
  - I.V. bolus: Dilute to 50 mg/mL and administer over 30 seconds to several minutes (depending on the dose)
  - I.V. intermittent infusion: Dilute to 1 mg/mL and administer over 20-30 minutes
- Topical: Apply a thin film to clean, dry skin and rub in gently

Monitoring Parameters Blood pressure, weight, serum glucose, and electrolytes

Reference Range Therapeutic: AM: 5-25 μg/dL (SI: 138-690 nmol/L), PM: 2-9 μg/dL (SI: 55-248 nmol/L) depending on test, assay

Patient Information Notify surgeon or dentist before surgical repair; oral formulation may cause GI upset, take with food; notify physician if any sign of infection occurs; avoid abrupt withdrawal when on long-term therapy. Before applying, gently wash area to reduce risk of infection; apply a thin film to cleansed area and rub in gently and thoroughly until medication vanishes; avoid exposure to sunlight, severe sunburn may occur.

Additional Information
- Sodium content of 1 g (sodium succinate injection): 47.5 mg (2.07 mEq)
- Hydrocortisone base topical cream, lotion, and ointments in concentrations of 0.25%, 0.5%, and 1% may be OTC or prescription depending on the product labeling

Dosage Forms

Hydrocortisone acetate:
- Cream, topical: 0.5% (15 g, 22.5 g, 30 g); 1% (15 g, 30 g, 120 g)
- Ointment, topical: 0.5% (15 g, 30 g); 1% (15 g, 21 g, 30 g)
- Injection, suspension: 25 mg/mL (5 mL, 10 mL); 50 mg/mL (5 mL, 10 mL)
- Suppositories, rectal: 10 mg, 25 mg

Hydrocortisone base:
- Aerosol, topical: 0.5% (45 g, 58 g); 1% (45 mL)
- Cream, rectal: 1% (30 g); 2.5% (30 g)
- Cream, topical: 0.5% (15 g, 30 g, 60 g, 120 g, 454 g); 1% (15 g, 20 g, 30 g, 60 g, 90 g, 120 g, 240 g, 454 g); 2.5% (15 g, 20 g, 30 g, 60 g, 120 g, 240 g, 454 g)
- Gel, topical: 0.5% (15 g, 30 g); 1% (15 g, 30 g)
- Lotion, topical: 0.25% (120 mL); 0.5% (30 mL, 60 mL, 120 mL); 1% (60 mL, 118 mL, 120 mL); 2% (30 mL) ; 2.5% (60 mL, 120 mL)

(Continued)

Hydrocortisone *(Continued)*

Ointment, rectal: 1% (30 g)
Ointment, topical: 0.5% (30 g) ; 1% (15 g, 20 g, 28 g, 30 g, 60 g, 120 g, 240 g, 454 g); 2.5% (20 g, 30 g)
Suspension, rectal: 100 mg/60 mL (7s)
Tablet, oral: 5 mg, 10 mg, 20 mg

Hydrocortisone buteprate: Cream: 1% (15 g, 45 g)

Hydrocortisone butyrate:
Cream: 0.1% (15 g, 45 g)
Ointment, topical: 0.1% (15 g, 45 g)
Solution, topical: 0.1% (20 mL, 50 mL)

Hydrocortisone cypionate:
Suspension, oral: 10 mg/5 mL (120 mL)

Hydrocortisone sodium phosphate:
Injection, I.M./I.V./S.C.: 50 mg/mL (2 mL, 10 mL)

Hydrocortisone sodium succinate:
Injection, IM/I.V.: 100 mg, 250 mg, 500 mg, 1000 mg

Hydrocortisone valerate:
Cream, topical: 0.2% (15 g, 45 g, 60 g)
Ointment, topical: 0.2% (15 g, 45 g, 60 g, 120 g)

Hydrocortisone Acetate *see* Hydrocortisone *on page 623*
Hydrocortisone Buteprate *see* Hydrocortisone *on page 623*
Hydrocortisone Butyrate *see* Hydrocortisone *on page 623*
Hydrocortisone Cypionate *see* Hydrocortisone *on page 623*
Hydrocortisone Sodium Phosphate *see* Hydrocortisone *on page 623*
Hydrocortisone Sodium Succinate *see* Hydrocortisone *on page 623*
Hydrocortisone Valerate *see* Hydrocortisone *on page 623*
Hydrocortone® Acetate *see* Hydrocortisone *on page 623*
Hydrocortone® Phosphate *see* Hydrocortisone *on page 623*
Hydro-Crysti-12® *see* Hydroxocobalamin *on page 629*
HydroDIURIL® *see* Hydrochlorothiazide *on page 617*

Hydroflumethiazide (hye droe floo meth EYE a zide)

Related Information
Sulfonamide Derivatives *on page 1420*

Brand Names Diucardin®; Saluron®

Therapeutic Category Antihypertensive; Diuretic, Thiazide

Use Management of mild to moderate hypertension; treatment of edema in congestive heart failure and nephrotic syndrome

Pregnancy Risk Factor D

Contraindications Anuria, renal decompensation, hypersensitivity to hydrochlorothiazide or any component, cross-sensitivity with other thiazides and sulfonamide derivatives

Warnings/Precautions Use with caution in renal disease, hepatic disease, gout, lupus erythematosus, diabetes mellitus; some products may contain tartrazine

Adverse Reactions
1% to 10%: Endocrine & metabolic: Hypokalemia
<1%:
Cardiovascular: Hypotension
Central nervous system: Drowsiness
Dermatologic: Photosensitivity, rash
Endocrine & metabolic: Fluid and electrolyte imbalances (hypocalcemia, hypomagnesemia, hyponatremia), hyperglycemia
Gastrointestinal: Anorexia
Genitourinary: Polyuria
Hematologic: Aplastic anemia, hemolytic anemia, leukopenia, agranulocytosis, thrombocytopenia, rarely blood dyscrasias
Hepatic: Hepatitis
Neuromuscular & skeletal: Paresthesia
Renal: Prerenal azotemia, uremia

Overdosage/Toxicology Symptoms of overdose include hypermotility, diuresis, lethargy

Following GI decontamination, therapy is supportive with I.V. fluids, electrolytes, and I.V. pressors if needed

Drug Interactions
Decreased effect of oral hypoglycemics; decreased absorption with cholestyramine and colestipol
Increased effect with furosemide and other loop diuretics
Increased toxicity/levels of lithium

Mechanism of Action The diuretic mechanism of action is primarily inhibition of sodium, chloride, and water reabsorption in the renal distal tubules, thereby producing diuresis with a resultant reduction in plasma volume

Pharmacodynamics/Kinetics

Onset of diuretic effect: Within ~2 hours

Peak effect: Within ~4 hours

Duration of action: 12-24 hours

Usual Dosage Oral:

Children: 1 mg/kg/24 hours

Adults: 50-200 mg/day

Monitoring Parameters Assess weight, I & O reports daily to determine fluid loss; blood pressure, serum electrolytes, BUN, creatinine

Test Interactions ↑ ammonia (B), ↑ amylase (S), ↑ calcium (S), ↑ chloride (S), ↑ glucose, ↑ uric acid (S); ↓ chloride (S), ↓ magnesium, ↓ potassium (S), ↓ sodium (S)

Patient Information May be taken with food or milk; take early in day to avoid nocturia; take the last dose of multiple doses no later than 6 PM unless instructed otherwise. A few people who take this medication become more sensitive to sunlight and may experience skin rash, redness, itching or severe sunburn, especially if sun block SPF ≥15 is not used on exposed skin areas.

Nursing Implications Take blood pressure with patient lying down and standing

Dosage Forms Tablet: 50 mg

Hydrogesic® *see* Hydrocodone and Acetaminophen *on page 620*

Hydromet® *see* Hydrocodone and Homatropine *on page 622*

Hydromorphone (hye droe MOR fone)

Related Information

Narcotic Agonists Comparison *on page 1414*

Dose Equivalents for Opioid Analgesics in Opioid-Naive Adults <50 kg *on page 1376*

Dose Equivalents for Opioid Analgesics in Opioid-Naive Adults ≥50 kg *on page 1375*

Brand Names Dilaudid®; Dilaudid-5®; Dilaudid-HP®; HydroStat IR®

Canadian/Mexican Brand Names Hydromorph Contin® (Canada); PMS-Hydromorphone (Canada)

Synonyms Dihydromorphinone; Hydromorphone Hydrochloride

Therapeutic Category Analgesic, Narcotic; Antitussive

Use Management of moderate to severe pain; antitussive at lower doses

Restrictions C-II

Pregnancy Risk Factor B (D if used for prolonged periods or in high doses at term)

Contraindications Hypersensitivity to hydromorphone or any component or other phenanthrene derivative

Warnings/Precautions Tablet and cough syrup contain tartrazine which may cause allergic reactions; hydromorphone shares toxic potential of opiate agonists, and precaution of opiate agonist therapy should be observed; extreme caution should be taken to avoid confusing the highly concentrated injection with the less concentrated injectable product, injection contains benzyl alcohol; use with caution in patients with hypersensitivity to other phenanthrene opiates, in patients with respiratory disease, or severe liver or renal failure

Adverse Reactions

Endocrine & metabolic: Antidiuretic hormone release

Gastrointestinal: Biliary tract spasm

Genitourinary: Urinary tract spasm

Ocular: Miosis

Sensitivity reactions: Histamine release

Miscellaneous: Physical and psychological dependence

>10%:

- Cardiovascular: Palpitations, hypotension, peripheral vasodilation
- Central nervous system: Dizziness, lightheadedness, drowsiness
- Gastrointestinal: Anorexia

1% to 10%:

- Cardiovascular: Tachycardia, bradycardia, flushing of face
- Central nervous system: CNS depression, increased intracranial pressure, fatigue, headache, nervousness, restlessness
- Gastrointestinal: Nausea, vomiting, constipation, stomach cramps, xerostomia
- Genitourinary: Decreased urination, ureteral spasm
- Neuromuscular & skeletal: Trembling, weakness
- Respiratory: Respiratory depression, dyspnea, shortness of breath

<1%:

- Central nervous system: Hallucinations, mental depression
- Dermatologic: Pruritus, rash, urticaria

(Continued)

Hydromorphone *(Continued)*

Gastrointestinal: Paralytic ileus

Overdosage/Toxicology Symptoms of overdose include CNS depression, respiratory depression, miosis, apnea, pulmonary edema, convulsions

Maintain airway, establish I.V. line; naloxone 2 mg I.V. (0.01 mg/kg for children) with repeat administration as necessary up to a total of 10 mg.

Drug Interactions Increased toxicity: CNS depressants, phenothiazines, tricyclic antidepressants may potentiate the adverse effects of hydromorphone

Stability Protect tablets from light; do not store intact ampuls in refrigerator; a slightly yellowish discoloration has not been associated with a loss of potency; I.V. is **incompatible** when mixed with minocycline, prochlorperazine, sodium bicarbonate, tetracycline, thiopental

Mechanism of Action Binds to opiate receptors in the CNS, causing inhibition of ascending pain pathways, altering the perception of and response to pain; causes cough supression by direct central action in the medulla; produces generalized CNS depression

Pharmacodynamics/Kinetics

Onset of analgesic effect: Within 15-30 minutes
Peak effect: Within 0.5-1.5 hours
Duration: 4-5 hours
Metabolism: Primarily in the liver
Bioavailability: 62%
Half-life: 1-3 hours
Elimination: In urine, principally as glucuronide conjugates

Usual Dosage

Doses should be titrated to appropriate analgesic effects; when changing routes of administration, note that oral doses are less than half as effective as parenteral doses (may be only one-fifth as effective)

Pain: Older Children and Adults:
- Oral, I.M., I.V., S.C.: 1-4 mg/dose every 4-6 hours as needed; usual adult dose: 2 mg/dose
- Rectal: 3 mg every 6-8 hours

Antitussive: Oral:
- Children 6-12 years: 0.5 mg every 3-4 hours as needed
- Children >12 years and Adults: 1 mg every 3-4 hours as needed

Dosing adjustment in hepatic impairment: Should be considered

Dietary Considerations

Alcohol: Additive CNS effects, avoid or limit alcohol; watch for sedation
Food: Glucose may cause hyperglycemia; monitor blood glucose concentrations

Monitoring Parameters Pain relief, respiratory and mental status, blood pressure

Test Interactions ↑ aminotransferase [ALT (SGPT)/AST (SGOT)] (S)

Patient Information May cause drowsiness; avoid alcohol; take with food or milk to minimize GI distress

Nursing Implications Observe patient for oversedation, respiratory depression, implement safety measures

Additional Information Equianalgesic doses: Morphine 10 mg I.M. = hydromorphone 1.5 mg I.M.

Dosage Forms

Injection, as hydrochloride:
- Dilaudid®: 1 mg/mL (1 mL); 2 mg/mL (1 mL, 20 mL); 3 mg/mL (1 mL); 4 mg/mL (1 mL)
- Dilaudid-HP®: 10 mg/mL (1 mL, 2 mL, 5 mL)

Liquid, as hydrochloride: 5 mg/5 mL (480 mL)
Powder for injection, as hydrochloride: (Dilaudid-HP®): 250 mg
Suppository, rectal, as hydrochloride: 3 mg (6s)
Tablet, as hydrochloride: 1 mg, 2 mg, 3 mg, 4 mg, 8 mg

Hydromorphone Hydrochloride *see* Hydromorphone *on previous page*
Hydromox® *see* Quinethazone *on page 1086*
Hydropane® *see* Hydrocodone and Homatropine *on page 622*
Hydro-Par® *see* Hydrochlorothiazide *on page 617*
Hydroquinol *see* Hydroquinone *on this page*

Hydroquinone (HYE droe kwin one)

Brand Names Ambi® Skin Tone [OTC]; Eldopaque® [OTC]; Eldopaque Forte®; Eldoquin® [OTC]; Eldoquin® Forte®; Esoterica® Facial [OTC]; Esoterica® Regular [OTC]; Esoterica® Sensitive Skin Formula [OTC]; Esoterica® Sunscreen [OTC]; Melanex®; Melpaque HP®; Melquin HP®; Nuquin HP®; Porcelana® [OTC]; Porcelana® Sunscreen [OTC]; Solaquin® [OTC]; Solaquin Forte®

Canadian/Mexican Brand Names Neostrata® HQ (Canada); Ultraquin® (Canada); Crema Blanca Bustillos (Mexico)

Synonyms Hydroquinol; Quinol

Therapeutic Category Depigmenting Agent

Use Gradual bleaching of hyperpigmented skin conditions

Pregnancy Risk Factor C

Contraindications Sunburn, depilatory usage, known hypersensitivity to hydroquinone

Warnings/Precautions Limit application to area no larger than face and neck or hands and arms

Adverse Reactions 1% to 10%:

Dermatologic: Dermatitis, dryness, erythema, stinging, inflammatory reaction, sensitization

Local: Irritation

Mechanism of Action Produces reversible depigmentation of the skin by suppression of melanocyte metabolic processes, in particular the inhibition of the enzymatic oxidation of tyrosine to DOPA (3,4-dihydroxyphenylalanine); sun exposure reverses this effect and will cause repigmentation.

Pharmacodynamics/Kinetics Onset and duration of depigmentation produced by hydroquinone varies among individuals

Usual Dosage Children >12 years and Adults: Topical: Apply thin layer and rub in twice daily

Patient Information Use sunscreens or clothing; do not use on irritated or denuded skin; stop using if rash or irritation develops; for external use only, avoid eye contact

Dosage Forms

Cream, topical:

- Esoterica® Sensitive Skin Formula: 1.5% (85 g)
- Eldopaque®, Eldoquin®, Esoterica® Facial, Esoterica® Regular, Porcelana®: 2% (14.2 g, 28.4 g, 60 g, 85 g, 120 g)
- Eldopaque Forte®, Eldoquin® Forte®, Melquin HP®: 4% (14.2 g, 28.4 g)

Cream, topical, with sunscreen:

- Esoterica® Sunscreen, Porcelana®, Solaquin®: 2% (28.4 g, 120 g)
- Melpaque HP®, Nuquin HP®, Solaquin Forte®: 4% (14.2 g, 28.4 g)

Gel, topical, with sunscreen (Solaquin Forte®): 4% (14.2 g, 28.4 g)

Solution, topical (Melanex®): 3% (30 mL)

HydroSKIN® *see* Hydrocortisone *on page 623*

HydroStat IR® *see* Hydromorphone *on page 627*

Hydro-Tex® [OTC] *see* Hydrocortisone *on page 623*

Hydrotropine® *see* Hydrocodone and Homatropine *on page 622*

Hydroxocobalamin (hye droks oh koe BAL a min)

Brand Names Alphamin®; Codroxomin®; Hybalamin®; Hydro-Cobex®; Hydro-Crysti-12®; LA-12®

Canadian/Mexican Brand Names Acti-B_{12}® (Canada); Duradoce® (Mexico)

Synonyms Vitamin B_{12}

Therapeutic Category Vitamin, Water Soluble

Use Treatment of pernicious anemia, vitamin B_{12} deficiency, increased B_{12} requirements due to pregnancy, thyrotoxicosis, hemorrhage, malignancy, liver or kidney disease

Pregnancy Risk Factor C

Contraindications Hypersensitivity to cyanocobalamin or any component, cobalt; patients with hereditary optic nerve atrophy

Warnings/Precautions Some products contain benzoyl alcohol; avoid use in premature infants; an intradermal test dose should be performed for hypersensitivity; use only if oral supplementation not possible or when treating pernicious anemia

Adverse Reactions

1% to 10%:

- Dermatologic: Itching
- Gastrointestinal: Diarrhea

<1%:

- Cardiovascular: Peripheral vascular thrombosis
- Dermatologic: Urticaria
- Miscellaneous: Anaphylaxis

Mechanism of Action Coenzyme for various metabolic functions, including fat and carbohydrate metabolism and protein synthesis, used in cell replication and hematopoiesis

Usual Dosage Vitamin B_{12} deficiency: I.M.:

Children: 1-5 mg given in single doses of 100 mcg over 2 or more weeks, followed by 30-50 mcg/month

(Continued)

Hydroxocobalamin *(Continued)*

Adults: 30 mcg/day for 5-10 days, followed by 100-200 mcg/month

Administration Administer I.M. only; may require coadministration of folic acid

Patient Information Therapy is required throughout life; do not take folic acid instead of B_{12} to prevent anemia

Dosage Forms Injection: 1000 mcg/mL (10 mL, 30 mL)

Hydroxycarbamide *see* Hydroxyurea *on page 632*

Hydroxychloroquine (hye droks ee KLOR oh kwin)

Brand Names Plaquenil®

Synonyms Hydroxychloroquine Sulfate

Therapeutic Category Antimalarial Agent

Use Suppresses and treats acute attacks of malaria; treatment of systemic lupus erythematosus and rheumatoid arthritis

Pregnancy Risk Factor C

Contraindications Retinal or visual field changes attributable to 4-aminoquinolines; hypersensitivity to hydroxychloroquine, 4-aminoquinoline derivatives, or any component

Warnings/Precautions Use with caution in patients with hepatic disease, G-6-PD deficiency, psoriasis, and porphyria; long-term use in children is not recommended; perform baseline and periodic (6 months) ophthalmologic examinations; test periodically for muscle weakness

Adverse Reactions

>10%:

Central nervous system: Headache

Dermatologic: Itching

Gastrointestinal: Diarrhea, loss of appetite, nausea, stomach cramps, vomiting

Ocular: Ciliary muscle dysfunction

1% to 10%:

Central nervous system: Dizziness, lightheadedness, nervousness, restlessness

Dermatologic: Bleaching of hair, rash, discoloration of skin (black-blue)

Ocular: Ocular toxicity, keratopathy, retinopathy

<1%:

Central nervous system: Emotional changes, seizures

Hematologic: Agranulocytosis, aplastic anemia, neutropenia, thrombocytopenia

Neuromuscular & skeletal: Neuromyopathy

Otic: Ototoxicity

Overdosage/Toxicology Symptoms of overdose include headache, drowsiness, visual changes, cardiovascular collapse, and seizures followed by respiratory and cardiac arrest

Treatment is symptomatic; urinary alkalinization will enhance renal elimination

Mechanism of Action Interferes with digestive vacuole function within sensitive malarial parasites by increasing the pH and interfering with lysosomal degradation of hemoglobin; inhibits locomotion of neutrophils and chemotaxis of eosinophils; impairs complement-dependent antigen-antibody reactions

Pharmacodynamics/Kinetics

Absorption: Oral: Complete

Protein binding: 55%

Metabolism: In the liver

Elimination: Metabolites and unchanged drug slowly excreted in urine, may be enhanced by urinary acidification

Usual Dosage Oral:

Children:

Chemoprophylaxis of malaria: 5 mg/kg (base) once weekly; should not exceed the recommended adult dose; begin 2 weeks before exposure; continue for 4-6 weeks after leaving endemic area

Acute attack: 10 mg/kg (base) initial dose; followed by 5 mg/kg at 6, 24, and 48 hours

JRA or SLE: 3-5 mg/kg/day divided 1-2 times/day to a maximum of 400 mg/day; not to exceed 7 mg/kg/day

Adults:

Chemoprophylaxis of malaria: 2 tablets weekly on same day each week; begin 2 weeks before exposure; continue for 4-6 weeks after leaving endemic area

Acute attack: 4 tablets first dose day 1; 2 tablets in 6 hours day 1; 2 tablets in 1 dose day 2; and 2 tablets in 1 dose on day 3

Rheumatoid arthritis: 2-3 tablets/day to start taken with food or milk; increase dose until optimum response level is reached; usually after 4-12 weeks dose should be reduced by ½ and a maintenance dose of 1-2 tablets/day given

Lupus erythematosus: 2 tablets every day or twice daily for several weeks depending on response; 1-2 tablets/day for prolonged maintenance therapy

Administration Administer with food or milk

Monitoring Parameters Ophthalmologic exam, CBC

Patient Information Take with food or milk; complete full course of therapy; wear sunglasses in bright sunlight; notify physician if blurring or other vision changes, ringing in the ears, or hearing loss occurs

Nursing Implications Periodic blood counts and eye examinations are recommended when patient is on chronic therapy

Dosage Forms Tablet, as sulfate: 200 mg [base 155 mg]

Extemporaneous Preparations A 25 mg/mL hydroxychloroquine sulfate suspension is made by removing the coating off of fifteen 200 mg hydroxychloroquine sulfate tablets with a towel moistened with alcohol; tablets are ground to a fine powder and levigated to a paste with 15 mL of Ora-Plus® suspending agent; add an additional 45 mL of suspending agent and levigate until a uniform mixture is obtained; qs ad to 120 mL with sterile water for irrigation; a 30 day expiration date is recommended, although stability testing has not been performed

Pesko LJ, "Compounding: Hydroxychloroquine," *Am Druggist*, 1993, 207:57.

Hydroxychloroquine Sulfate *see* Hydroxychloroquine *on previous page*

25-Hydroxycholecalciferol *see* Calcifediol *on page 180*

Hydroxydaunomycin Hydrochloride *see* Doxorubicin *on page 425*

Hydroxyethyl Starch *see* Hetastarch *on page 609*

Hydroxyprogesterone Caproate

(hye droks ee proe JES te rone KAP roe ate)

Brand Names Hylutin® Injection; Hyprogest® 250 Injection

Canadian/Mexican Brand Names Primolut® Depot (Mexico)

Therapeutic Category Progestin Derivative

Use Treatment of amenorrhea, abnormal uterine bleeding, endometriosis, uterine carcinoma

Pregnancy Risk Factor D

Contraindications Thrombophlebitis, thromboembolic disorders, cerebral hemorrhage, liver impairment, carcinoma of the breast, hypersensitivity to hydroxyprogesterone or any component, undiagnosed vaginal bleeding

Warnings/Precautions Use with caution in patients with asthma, seizure disorders, migraine, cardiac or renal impairment, history of mental depression; use of any progestin during the first 4 months of pregnancy is not recommended; observe patients closely for signs and symptoms of thrombotic disorders

Adverse Reactions

>10%:

Cardiovascular: Edema

Endocrine & metabolic: Breakthrough bleeding, spotting, changes in menstrual flow, amenorrhea

Gastrointestinal: Anorexia

Local: Pain at injection site

Neuromuscular & skeletal: Weakness

1% to 10%:

Cardiovascular: Edema

Central nervous system: Mental depression, insomnia, fever

Dermatologic: Melasma or chloasma, allergic rash with or without pruritus

Gastrointestinal: Weight gain or loss

Genitourinary: Changes in cervical erosion and secretions, increased breast tenderness

Hepatic: Cholestatic jaundice

Overdosage/Toxicology Toxicity is unlikely following single exposures of excessive doses; supportive treatment is adequate in most cases

Drug Interactions Decreased effect: Rifampin may increase clearance of hydroxyprogesterone

Stability Store at <40°C (15°C to 30°C); avoid freezing

Mechanism of Action Natural steroid hormone that induces secretory changes in the endometrium, promotes mammary gland development, relaxes uterine smooth muscle, blocks follicular maturation and ovulation and maintains pregnancy

Pharmacodynamics/Kinetics

Metabolism: Hepatic

Peak serum concentration: I.M.: 3-7 days; concentrations are measurable for 3-4 weeks after injection

Elimination: Renal

Usual Dosage Adults: Female: I.M.:

Amenorrhea: 375 mg; if no bleeding, begin cyclic treatment with estradiol valerate

(Continued)

Hydroxyprogesterone Caproate *(Continued)*

Production of secretory endometrium and desquamation: (Medical D and C): 125-250 mg administered on day 10 of cycle; repeat every 7 days until supression is no longer desired.

Uterine carcinoma: 1 g one or more times/day (1-7 g/week) for up to 12 weeks

Administration Administer deep I.M. only

Test Interactions Thyroid function tests and liver function tests and endocrine function tests

Patient Information Take this medicine only as directed; do not exceed recommended dosage nor take it for a longer period of time; if you suspect you may have become pregnant, stop taking this medicine; take with food; patient package insert is available upon request; notify physician of pain in calves along with swelling and warmth, severe headache, visual disturbance

Nursing Implications Patients should receive a copy of the patient labeling for the drug

Dosage Forms Injection:

125 mg/mL (10 mL)

Hylutin®, Hyprogest®: 250 mg/mL (5 mL)

Hydroxyurea (hye droks ee yoor EE a)

Related Information

Cancer Chemotherapy Regimens *on page 1351*

Toxicities of Chemotherapeutic Agents *on page 1382*

Brand Names Hydrea®

Synonyms Hydroxycarbamide

Therapeutic Category Antineoplastic Agent, Antimetabolite (Ribonucleotide Reductase Inhibitor)

Use CML in chronic phase; radiosensitizing agent in the treatment of primary brain tumors; head and neck tumors; uterine cervix and nonsmall cell lung cancer; psoriasis; sickle cell anemia and other hemoglobinopathies; hematologic conditions such as essential thrombocythemia, polycythemia vera, hypereosinophilia, and hyperleukocytosis due to acute leukemia. Has shown activity against renal cell cancer, melanoma, ovarian cancer, head and neck cancer, and prostate cancer.

Pregnancy Risk Factor D

Contraindications Severe anemia, severe bone marrow suppression; WBC <2500/mm³ or platelet count <100,000/mm³; hypersensitivity to hydroxyurea

Warnings/Precautions The U.S. Food and Drug Administration (FDA) currently recommends that procedures for proper handling and disposal of antineoplastic agents be considered. Use with caution in patients with renal impairment, in patients who have received prior irradiation therapy, and in the elderly.

Adverse Reactions

>10%:

Central nervous system: Drowsiness

Gastrointestinal: Mild to moderate nausea and vomiting may occur, as well as diarrhea, constipation, mucositis, ulceration of the GI tract, anorexia, and stomatitis

Hematologic: Myelosuppression: Dose-limiting toxicity, causes a rapid drop in leukocyte count (seen in 4-5 days in nonhematologic malignancy and more rapidly in leukemia); thrombocytopenia and anemia occur less often; reversal of WBC count occurs rapidly, but the platelet count may take 7-10 days to recover

WBC: Moderate
Platelets: Moderate
Onset (days): 7
Nadir (days): 10
Recovery (days): 21

1% to 10%:

Dermatologic: Dermatologic changes (hyperpigmentation, erythema of the hands and face, maculopapular rash, or dry skin), alopecia

Hepatic: Abnormal LFTs and hepatitis

Renal: Increased creatinine and BUN due to impairment of renal tubular function

Miscellaneous: Carcinogenic potential

<1%:

Central nervous system: Neurotoxicity, dizziness, disorientation, hallucination, seizures, headache, fever

Dermatologic: Facial erythema

Endocrine & metabolic: Hyperuricemia

Genitourinary: Dysuria

Hepatic: Elevation of hepatic enzymes

Respiratory: Rarely, acute diffuse pulmonary infiltrates; dyspnea

Overdosage/Toxicology Symptoms of overdose include myelosuppression, facial swelling, hallucinations, disorientation; treatment is supportive

Drug Interactions

Increased effect: AZT, ddC, ddl: Synergy

Increased toxicity:

Fluorouracil: The potential for neurotoxicity may ↑ with concomitant administration

Cytarabine: Modulation of its metabolism and cytotoxicity → reduction of cytarabine dose is recommended

Stability Store capsules at room temperature; capsules may be opened and emptied into water (will not dissolve completely)

Mechanism of Action Thought to interfere (unsubstantiated hypothesis) with synthesis of DNA, during the S phase of cell division, without interfering with RNA synthesis; inhibits ribonucleoside diphosphate reductase, preventing conversion of ribonucleotides to deoxyribonucleotides; cell-cycle specific for the S phase and may hold other cells in the G_1 phase of the cell cycle.

Pharmacodynamics/Kinetics

Absorption: Readily absorbed from GI tract (≥80%)

Distribution: Readily crosses the blood-brain barrier; well distributed into intestine, brain, lung, kidney tissues, effusions and ascites; appears in breast milk

Metabolism: In the liver

Half-life: 3-4 hours

Time to peak serum concentration: Within 2 hours

Elimination: Renal excretion of urea (metabolite) and respiratory excretion of CO_2 (metabolic end product); 50% of the drug is excreted unchanged in urine

Usual Dosage All dosage should be based on ideal or actual body weight, whichever is less. Oral (refer to individual protocols):

Children:

No FDA-approved dosage regimens have been established; dosages of 1500-3000 mg/m^2 as a single dose in combination with other agents every 4-6 weeks have been used in the treatment of pediatric astrocytoma, medulloblastoma and primitive neuroectodermal tumors

CML: Initial: 10-20 mg/kg/day once daily; adjust dose according to hematologic response

Adults: Dose should always be titrated to patient response and WBC counts; usual oral doses range from 10-30 mg/kg/day or 500-3000 mg/day; if WBC count falls <2500 cells/mm^3, or the platelet count <100,000/mm^3, therapy should be stopped for at least 3 days and resumed when values rise toward normal

Solid tumors:

Intermittent therapy: 80 mg/kg as a single dose every third day

Continuous therapy: 20-30 mg/kg/day given as a single dose/day

Concomitant therapy with irradiation: 80 mg/kg as a single dose every third day starting at least 7 days before initiation of irradiation

Resistant chronic myelocytic leukemia: 20-30 mg/kg/day divided daily

Sickle cell anemia (moderate/severe disease): Hydroxyurea administration in adults (age range: 22-42 years) has produced beneficial effects in several small studies

Initial: 15 mg/kg/day, increased by 5 mg/kg every 12 weeks unless toxicity is observed or the maximum tolerated dose of 35 mg/kg/day is achieved

Monitor for toxicity every 2 weeks; if toxicity occurs, stop treatment until the bone marrow recovers; restart at 2.5 mg/kg/day less than the dose at which toxicity occurs; if no toxicity occurs over the next 12 weeks, then the subsequent dose should be increased by 2.5 mg/kg/day; reduced dosage of hydroxyurea alternating with erythropoietin may decrease myelotoxicity and increase levels of fetal hemoglobin in patients who have not been helped by hydroxyurea alone

Dosing adjustment in renal impairment:

Cl_{cr} 10-50 mL/minute: Administer 50% of normal dose

Cl_{cr} <10 mL/minute: Administer 20% of normal dose

Hemodialysis: Supplemental dose is not necessary

CAPD effects: Unknown

CAVH effects: Unknown

Monitoring Parameters CBC with differential, platelets, hemoglobin, renal function and liver function tests, serum uric acid

Patient Information Contents of capsule may be emptied into a glass of water if taken immediately; inform the physician if you develop fever, sore throat, bruising, or bleeding; may cause drowsiness, constipation, and loss of hair

Dosage Forms Capsule: 500 mg

25-Hydroxyvitamin D_3 *see* Calcifediol *on page 180*

Hydroxyzine (hye DROKS i zeen)

Brand Names Anxanil®; Atarax®; Atozine®; Durrax®; E-Vista®; Hy-Pam®; Hyzine-50®; Neucalm®; Quiess®; Rezine®; Vamate®; Vistacon-50®; Vistaquel®; Vistaril®; Vistazine®

Canadian/Mexican Brand Names Apo-Hydroxyzine® (Canada); Multipax® (Canada); Novo-Hydroxyzine® (Canada); PMS-Hydroxyzine (Canada)

Synonyms Hydroxyzine Hydrochloride; Hydroxyzine Pamoate

Therapeutic Category Antianxiety Agent; Antiemetic; Antihistamine, H_1 Blocker; Sedative

Use Treatment of anxiety, as a preoperative sedative, an antipruritic, an antiemetic, and in alcohol withdrawal symptoms

Pregnancy Risk Factor C

Contraindications Hypersensitivity to hydroxyzine or any component

Warnings/Precautions S.C., intra-arterial and I.V. administration **not** recommended since thrombosis and digital gangrene can occur; extravasation can result in sterile abscess and marked tissue induration; should be used with caution in patients with narrow-angle glaucoma, prostatic hypertrophy, and bladder neck obstruction; should also be used with caution in patients with asthma or COPD

Anticholinergic effects are not well tolerated in the elderly. Hydroxyzine may be useful as a short-term antipruritic, but it is not recommended for use as a sedative or anxiolytic in the elderly.

Adverse Reactions

>10%:

- Central nervous system: Slight to moderate drowsiness
- Respiratory: Thickening of bronchial secretions

1% to 10%:

- Central nervous system: Headache, fatigue, nervousness, dizziness
- Gastrointestinal: Appetite increase, weight gain, nausea, diarrhea, abdominal pain, xerostomia
- Neuromuscular & skeletal: Arthralgia
- Respiratory: Pharyngitis

<1%:

- Cardiovascular: Palpitations, hypotension, edema
- Central nervous system: Depression, sedation, paradoxical excitement, insomnia
- Dermatologic: Angioedema, photosensitivity, rash
- Genitourinary: Urinary retention
- Hepatic: Hepatitis
- Neuromuscular & skeletal: Myalgia, tremor, paresthesia
- Ocular: Blurred vision
- Respiratory: Bronchospasm, epistaxis

Overdosage/Toxicology Symptoms of overdose include seizures, sedation, hypotension

There is no specific treatment for an antihistamine overdose, however, most of its clinical toxicity is due to anticholinergic effects. Anticholinesterase inhibitors may be useful by reducing acetylcholinesterase. For anticholinergic overdose with severe life-threatening symptoms, physostigmine 1-2 mg (0.5 or 0.02 mg/kg for children) I.V., slowly may be given to reverse these effects.

Drug Interactions

- Decreased effect: Epinephrine decreased vasopressor effect
- Increased toxicity: CNS depressants, anticholinergics

Stability Protect from light; store at 15°C to 30°C and protected from freezing; I.V. is **incompatible** when mixed with aminophylline, amobarbital, chloramphenicol, dimenhydrinate, heparin, penicillin G, pentobarbital, phenobarbital, phenytoin, ranitidine, sulfisoxazole, vitamin B complex with C

Mechanism of Action Competes with histamine for H_1-receptor sites on effector cells in the gastrointestinal tract, blood vessels, and respiratory tract

Pharmacodynamics/Kinetics

- Onset of effect: Within 15-30 minutes
- Duration: 4-6 hours
- Absorption: Oral: Rapid
- Metabolism: Exact fate is unknown
- Half-life: 3-7 hours
- Time to peak serum concentration: Within 2 hours

Usual Dosage

Children:

- Oral: 0.6 mg/kg/dose every 6 hours
- I.M.: 0.5-1 mg/kg/dose every 4-6 hours as needed

Adults:

- Antiemetic: I.M.: 25-100 mg/dose every 4-6 hours as needed

Anxiety: Oral: 25-100 mg 4 times/day; maximum dose: 600 mg/day
Preoperative sedation:
Oral: 50-100 mg
I.M.: 25-100 mg
Management of pruritus: Oral: 25 mg 3-4 times/day

Dosing interval in hepatic impairment: Change dosing interval to every 24 hours in patients with primary biliary cirrhosis

Dietary Considerations Alcohol: Additive CNS effect, avoid use

Administration For I.M. administration in children, injections should be made into the midlateral muscles of the thigh; S.C., intra-arterial, and I.V. administration **not** recommended since thrombosis and digital gangrene can occur

Monitoring Parameters Relief of symptoms, mental status, blood pressure

Patient Information Will cause drowsiness, avoid alcohol and other CNS depressants, avoid driving and other hazardous tasks until the CNS effects are known

Nursing Implications Extravasation can result in sterile abscess and marked tissue induration; provide safety measures (ie, side rails, night light, and call button); remove smoking materials from area; supervise ambulation

Additional Information

Hydroxyzine hydrochloride: Anxanil®, Atarax®, E-Vista®, Hydroxacen®, Quiess®, Vistaril® injection, Vistazine®

Hydroxyzine pamoate: Hy-Pam®, Vistaril® capsule and suspension

Dosage Forms

Hydroxyzine hydrochloride:
Injection:
Vistaject-25®, Vistaril®: 25 mg/mL (1 mL, 2 mL, 10 mL)
E-Vista®, Hydroxacen®, Hyzine-50®, Neucalm®, Quiess®, Vistacon-50®, Vistaject-50®, Vistaquel®, Vistaril®, Vistazine®: 50 mg/mL (1 mL, 2 mL, 10 mL)
Syrup (Atarax®): 10 mg/5 mL (120 mL, 480 mL, 4000 mL)
Tablet:
Anxanil®: 25 mg
Atarax®: 10 mg, 25 mg, 50 mg, 100 mg
Atozine®: 10 mg, 25 mg, 50 mg
Durrax®: 10 mg, 25 mg

Hydroxyzine pamoate:
Capsule:
Hy-Pam®: 25 mg, 50 mg
Vamate®: 25 mg, 50 mg, 100 mg
Vistaril®: 25 mg, 50 mg, 100 mg
Suspension, oral (Vistaril®:) 25 mg/5 mL (120 mL, 480 mL)

Hydroxyzine Hydrochloride *see* Hydroxyzine *on previous page*

Hydroxyzine Pamoate *see* Hydroxyzine *on previous page*

Hygroton® *see* Chlorthalidone *on page 265*

Hylorel® *see* Guanadrel *on page 592*

Hylutin® Injection *see* Hydroxyprogesterone Caproate *on page 631*

Hyoscine *see* Scopolamine *on page 1127*

Hyoscyamine (hye oh SYE a meen)

Brand Names Anaspaz®; A-Spas® S/L; Cystospaz®; Cystospaz-M®; Donnamar®; ED-SPAZ®; Gastrosed™; Levbid®; Levsin®; Levsinex®; Levsin/SL®

Synonyms Hyoscyamine Sulfate; *l*-Hyoscyamine Sulfate

Therapeutic Category Anticholinergic Agent; Antispasmodic Agent, Gastrointestinal

Use Treatment of GI tract disorders caused by spasm, adjunctive therapy for peptic ulcers

Pregnancy Risk Factor C

Contraindications Narrow-angle glaucoma, obstructive uropathy, obstructive GI tract disease, myasthenia gravis, known hypersensitivity to belladonna alkaloids

Warnings/Precautions Use with caution in children with spastic paralysis; use with caution in elderly patients. Low doses cause a paradoxical decrease in heart rates. Some commercial products contain sodium metabisulfite, which can cause allergic-type reactions. May accumulate with multiple inhalational administration, particularly in the elderly. Heat prostration may occur in hot weather. Use with caution in patients with autonomic neuropathy, prostatic hypertrophy, hyperthyroidism, congestive heart failure, cardiac arrhythmias, chronic lung disease, biliary tract disease.

Adverse Reactions

>10%:
Dermatologic: Dry skin
Gastrointestinal: Dry throat, xerostomia

(Continued)

Hyoscyamine *(Continued)*

Local: Irritation at injection site
Respiratory: Dry nose
Miscellaneous: Diaphoresis (decreased)

1% to 10%:
Dermatologic: Photosensitivity
Gastrointestinal: Constipation, dysphagia
Ocular: Blurred vision, mydriasis

<1%:
Cardiovascular: Palpitations, orthostatic hypotension
Central nervous system: Headache, lightheadedness, memory loss, fatigue, delirium, restlessness, ataxia
Dermatologic: Rash
Genitourinary: Dysuria
Neuromuscular & skeletal: Tremor
Ocular: Increased intraocular pressure

Overdosage/Toxicology Symptoms of overdose include dilated, unreactive pupils; blurred vision; hot, dry flushed skin; dryness of mucous membranes; difficulty in swallowing, foul breath, diminished or absent bowel sounds, urinary retention, tachycardia, hyperthermia, hypertension, increased respiratory rate

Anticholinergic toxicity is caused by strong binding of the drug to cholinergic receptors. Anticholinesterase inhibitors reduce acetylcholinesterase, the enzyme that breaks down acetylcholine and thereby allows acetylcholine to accumulate and compete for receptor binding with the offending anticholinergic. For anticholinergic overdose with severe life-threatening symptoms, physostigmine 1-2 mg (0.5 or 0.02 mg/kg for children) S.C. or I.V., slowly may be given to reverse these effects.

Drug Interactions

Decreased effect with antacids
Increased toxicity with amantadine, antimuscarinics, haloperidol, phenothiazines, TCAs, MAO inhibitors

Mechanism of Action Blocks the action of acetylcholine at parasympathetic sites in smooth muscle, secretory glands and the CNS; increases cardiac output, dries secretions, antagonizes histamine and serotonin

Pharmacodynamics/Kinetics

Onset of effect: 2-3 minutes
Duration: 4-6 hours
Absorption: Oral: Absorbed well
Distribution: Crosses the placenta; small amounts appear in breast milk
Protein binding: 50%
Metabolism: In the liver
Half-life: 13% to 38%
Elimination: In urine

Usual Dosage

Children: Oral, S.L.: Dose as per table repeated every 4 hours as needed

Hyoscyamine

Weight (kg)	Dose (mcg)	Maximum 24-Hour Dose (mcg)
Children <2 y		
2.3	12.5	75
3.4	16.7	100
5	20.8	125
7	25	150
10	31.3-33.3	200
15	45.8	275
Children 2-10 y		
10	31.3-33.3	Do not exceed 0.75 mg
20	62.5	
40	93.8	
50	125	

Adults:
Oral or S.L.: 0.125-0.25 mg 3-4 times/day before meals or food and at bedtime
Oral: 0.375-0.75 mg (timed release) every 12 hours
I.M., I.V., S.C.: 0.25-0.5 mg every 6 hours

Patient Information Maintain good oral hygiene habits, because lack of saliva may increase chance of cavities. Observe caution while driving or performing other tasks requiring alertness, as may cause drowsiness, dizziness, or blurred vision. Notify physician if skin rash, flushing or eye pain occurs; or if difficulty in urinating, constipation or sensitivity to light becomes severe or persists.

Nursing Implications Observe for tachycardia if patient has cardiac problems.

Dosage Forms

Capsule, as sulfate, timed release (Cystospaz-M®, Levsinex®): 0.375 mg
Elixir, as sulfate (Levsin®): 0.125 mg/5 mL with alcohol 20% (480 mL)
Injection, as sulfate (Levsin®): 0.5 mg/mL (1 mL, 10 mL)
Solution, oral (Gastrosed™, Levsin®): 0.125 mg/mL (15 mL)
Tablet, as sulfate:
Anaspaz®, Gastrosed™, Levsin®, Neoquess®: 0.125 mg
Cystospaz®: 0.15 mg

Hyoscyamine, Atropine, Scopolamine, and Phenobarbital

(hye oh SYE a meen, A troe peen, skoe POL a meen & fee noe BAR bi tal)

Brand Names Barbidonna®; Barophen®; Donnapine®; Donna-Sed®; Donnatal®; Donphen®; Hyosophen®; Kinesed®; Malatal®; Relaxadon®; Spaslin®; Spasmolin®; Spasmophen®; Spasquid®; Susano®

Therapeutic Category Anticholinergic Agent; Antispasmodic Agent, Gastrointestinal

Use Adjunct in treatment of peptic ulcer disease, irritable bowel, spastic colitis, spastic bladder, and renal colic

Pregnancy Risk Factor C

Contraindications Hypersensitivity to hyoscyamine, atropine, scopolamine, phenobarbital, or any component; narrow-angle glaucoma, tachycardia, GI and GU obstruction, myasthenia gravis

Warnings/Precautions Use with caution in patients with hepatic or renal disease, hyperthyroidism, cardiovascular disease, hypertension, prostatic hypertrophy, autonomic neuropathy in the elderly; abrupt withdrawal may precipitate status epilepticus. Because of the anticholinergic effects of this product, it is not recommended for use in the elderly.

Adverse Reactions

>10%:
Dermatologic: Dry skin
Gastrointestinal: Constipation, dry throat, xerostomia
Local: Irritation at injection site
Respiratory: Dry nose
Miscellaneous: Diaphoresis (decreased)

1% to 10%:
Dermatologic: Increased sensitivity to light
Endocrine & metabolic: Decreased flow of breast milk
Gastrointestinal: Dysphagia

<1%:
Cardiovascular: Orthostatic hypotension, ventricular fibrillation, tachycardia, palpitations
Central nervous system: Confusion, drowsiness, headache, loss of memory, fatigue, ataxia
Dermatologic: Rash
Gastrointestinal: Bloated feeling, nausea, vomiting
Genitourinary: Dysuria
Ocular: Increased intraocular pain, blurred vision

Overdosage/Toxicology Symptoms of overdose include unsteady gait, slurred speech, confusion, hypotension, respiratory collapse, dilated unreactive pupils, hot or flushed skin, diminished bowel sounds, urinary retention

Anticholinergic toxicity is caused by strong binding of the drug to cholinergic receptors. Anticholinesterase inhibitors reduce acetylcholinesterase, the enzyme that breaks down acetylcholine and thereby allows acetylcholine to accumulate and compete for receptor binding with the offending anticholinergic. For anticholinergic overdose with severe life-threatening symptoms, physostigmine 1-2 mg (0.5 or 0.02 mg/kg for children) S.C. or I.V., slowly may be given to reverse these effects.

Drug Interactions Increased toxicity: CNS depressants, coumarin anticoagulants, amantadine, antihistamine, phenothiazides, antidiarrheal suspensions, corticosteroids, digitalis, griseofulvin, tetracyclines, anticonvulsants, MAO inhibitors, tricyclic antidepressants

Mechanism of Action Refer to individual agents

Pharmacodynamics/Kinetics Absorption: Well absorbed from GI tract

Usual Dosage Oral:

Children 2-12 years: Kinesed® dose: ½ to 1 tablet 3-4 times/day

Children: Donnatal® elixir: 0.1 mL/kg/dose every 4 hours; maximum dose: 5 mL **or** see table for alternative.

(Continued)

Hyoscyamine, Atropine, Scopolamine, and Phenobarbital *(Continued)*

Weight (kg)	Dose (mL)	
	q4h	q6h
4.5	0.5	0.75
10	1	1.5
14	1.5	2
23	2.5	3.8
34	3.8	5
≥45	5	7.5

Adults: 1-2 capsules or tablets 3-4 times/day; or 1 Donnatal® Extentab® in sustained release form every 12 hours; or 5-10 mL elixir 3-4 times/day or every 8 hours

Patient Information Maintain good oral hygiene habits, because lack of saliva may increase chance of cavities. Observe caution while driving or performing other tasks requiring alertness, as may cause drowsiness, dizziness, or blurred vision. Notify physician if skin rash, flushing or eye pain occurs; or if difficulty in urinating, constipation, or sensitivity to light becomes severe or persists. Do not attempt tasks requiring mental alertness or physical coordination until you know the effects of the drug. Swallow extended release tablet whole, do not crush or chew.

Dosage Forms

Capsule (Donnatal®, Spasmolin®): Hyoscyamine sulfate 0.1037 mg, atropine sulfate 0.0194 mg, scopolamine hydrobromide 0.0065 mg, and phenobarbital 16.2 mg

Elixir (Barophen®, Donna-Sed®, Donnatal®, Hyosophen®, Spasmophen®, Spasquid®, Susano®): Hyoscyamine sulfate 0.1037 mg, atropine sulfate 0.0194 mg, scopolamine hydrobromide 0.0065 mg, and phenobarbital 16.2 mg per 5 mL (120 mL, 480 mL, 4000 mL)

Tablet:

Barbidonna®: Hyoscyamine hydrobromide 0.1286 mg, atropine sulfate 0.025 mg, scopolamine hydrobromide 0.0074 mg, and phenobarbital 16 mg

Barbidonna® No. 2: Hyoscyamine hydrobromide 0.1286 mg, atropine sulfate 0.025 mg, scopolamine hydrobromide 0.0074 mg, and phenobarbital 32 mg

Chewable (Kinesed®): Hyoscyamine hydrobromide 0.12 mg, atropine sulfate 0.12 mg, scopolamine hydrobromide 0.007 mg, and phenobarbital 16 mg

Donnapine®, Donnatal®, Hyosophen®, Malatal®, Relaxadon®, Spaslin®, Susano®: Hyoscyamine sulfate 0.1037 mg, atropine sulfate 0.0194 mg, scopolamine hydrobromide 0.0065 mg, and phenobarbital 16.2 mg

Donnatal® No. 2: Hyoscyamine sulfate 0.1037 mg, atropine sulfate 0.0194 mg, scopolamine hydrobromide 0.0065 mg, and phenobarbital 32.4 mg

Donphen®: Hyoscyamine sulfate 0.1 mg, atropine sulfate 0.02 mg, scopolamine hydrobromide 0.006 mg, and phenobarbital 15 mg

Long-acting (Donnatal®): Hyoscyamine sulfate 0.3111 mg, atropine sulfate 0.0582 mg, scopolamine hydrobromide 0.0195 mg, and phenobarbital 48.6 mg

Spasmophen®: Hyoscyamine sulfate 0.1037 mg, atropine sulfate 0.0194 mg, scopolamine hydrobromide 0.0065 mg, and phenobarbital 15 mg

Hyoscyamine Sulfate *see* Hyoscyamine *on page 635*

Hyosophen® *see* Hyoscyamine, Atropine, Scopolamine, and Phenobarbital *on previous page*

Hy-Pam® *see* Hydroxyzine *on page 634*

Hyperab® *see* Rabies Immune Globulin (Human) *on page 1091*

HyperHep® *see* Hepatitis B Immune Globulin *on page 607*

Hyperstat® I.V. *see* Diazoxide *on page 371*

Hyper-Tet® *see* Tetanus Immune Globulin (Human) *on page 1200*

Hy-Phen® *see* Hydrocodone and Acetaminophen *on page 620*

Hypoglycemic Drugs, Comparison of Oral Agents *see page 1411*

HypRho®-D *see* $Rh_o(D)$ Immune Globulin *on page 1101*

HypRho®-D Mini-Dose *see* $Rh_o(D)$ Immune Globulin *on page 1101*

Hyprogest® 250 Injection *see* Hydroxyprogesterone Caproate *on page 631*

Hyrexin-50® Injection *see* Diphenhydramine *on page 399*

Hytakerol® *see* Dihydrotachysterol *on page 391*

Hytone® *see* Hydrocortisone *on page 623*

Hytrin® *see* Terazosin *on page 1193*

Hytuss® [OTC] *see* Guaifenesin *on page 589*

Hytuss-2X® [OTC] *see* Guaifenesin *on page 589*

Hyzine-50® *see* Hydroxyzine *on page 634*

Iberet-Folic-500® *see* Vitamins, Multiple *on page 1310*

Ibidomide Hydrochloride *see* Labetalol *on page 700*

Ibuprin® [OTC] *see* Ibuprofen *on this page*

Ibuprofen (eye byoo PROE fen)

Related Information

Dosing Data for Acetaminophen and NSAIDs *on page 1377*

Nonsteroidal Anti-Inflammatory Agents Comparison *on page 1419*

Brand Names Aches-N-Pain® [OTC]; Advil® [OTC]; Children's Advil® Oral Suspension [OTC]; Children's Motrin® Oral Suspension [OTC]; Excedrin® IB [OTC]; Genpril® [OTC]; Haltran® [OTC]; Ibuprin® [OTC]; Ibuprohm® [OTC]; Ibu-Tab®; Junior Strength Motrin® [OTC]; Medipren® [OTC]; Menadol® [OTC]; Midol® 200 [OTC]; Motrin®; Motrin® IB [OTC]; Nuprin® [OTC]; Pamprin IB® [OTC]; PediaProfen™; Rufen®; Saleto-200® [OTC]; Saleto-400®; Trendar® [OTC]; Uni-Pro® [OTC]

Canadian/Mexican Brand Names Actiprofen® (Canada); Apo-Ibuprofen® (Canada); Novo-Profen® (Canada); Nu-Ibuprofen® (Canada); Butacortelone® (Mexico); Dibufen® (Mexico); Kedvil® (Mexico); Proartinal® (Mexico); Quadrax® (Mexico); Tabalon® (Mexico)

Synonyms *p*-Isobutylhydratropic Acid

Therapeutic Category Analgesic, Nonsteroidal Anti-inflammatory Drug; Anti-inflammatory Agent; Antipyretic; Nonsteroidal Anti-inflammatory Agent (NSAID), Oral

Use Inflammatory diseases and rheumatoid disorders including juvenile rheumatoid arthritis, mild to moderate pain, fever, dysmenorrhea, gout, ankylosing spondylitis, acute migraine headache

Pregnancy Risk Factor B (D if used in the 3rd trimester)

Contraindications Hypersensitivity to ibuprofen, any component, aspirin, or other nonsteroidal anti-inflammatory drugs (NSAIDs)

Warnings/Precautions Do not exceed 3200 mg/day; use with caution in patients with congestive heart failure, hypertension, decreased renal or hepatic function, history of GI disease (bleeding or ulcers), or those receiving anticoagulants; safety and efficacy in children <6 months of age have not yet been established; elderly are a high-risk population for adverse effects from nonsteroidal anti-inflammatory agents. As much as 60% of elderly can develop peptic ulceration and/or hemorrhage asymptomatically.

Use lowest effective dose for shortest period possible. Use of NSAIDs can compromise existing renal function especially when Cl_{cr} is <30 mL/minute. CNS adverse effects such as confusion, agitation, and hallucination are generally seen in overdose or high dose situations; but elderly may demonstrate these adverse effects at lower doses than younger adults.

Adverse Reactions

>10%:

- Central nervous system: Dizziness, fatigue
- Dermatologic: Rash, urticaria
- Gastrointestinal: Abdominal cramps, heartburn, indigestion, nausea

1% to 10%:

- Central nervous system: Headache, nervousness
- Dermatologic: Itching
- Endocrine & metabolic: Fluid retention
- Gastrointestinal: Dyspepsia, vomiting, abdominal pain, peptic ulcer, GI bleed, GI perforation
- Otic: Tinnitus

<1%:

- Cardiovascular: Edema, congestive heart failure, arrhythmias, tachycardia, hypertension
- Central nervous system: Confusion, hallucinations, mental depression, drowsiness, insomnia, aseptic meningitis
- Dermatologic: Erythema multiforme, toxic epidermal necrolysis, Stevens-Johnson syndrome
- Endocrine & metabolic: Polydipsia, hot flashes
- Gastrointestinal: Gastritis, GI ulceration
- Genitourinary: Cystitis, polyuria
- Hematologic: Neutropenia, anemia, agranulocytosis, inhibition of platelet aggregation, hemolytic anemia, bone marrow suppression, leukopenia, thrombocytopenia
- Hepatic: Hepatitis
- Neuromuscular & skeletal: Peripheral neuropathy
- Ocular: Vision changes, blurred vision, conjunctivitis, dry eyes, toxic amblyopia
- Otic: Decreased hearing

(Continued)

Ibuprofen *(Continued)*

Renal: Acute renal failure

Respiratory: Allergic rhinitis, shortness of breath, epistaxis

Overdosage/Toxicology Symptoms include apnea, metabolic acidosis, coma, and nystagmus; leukocytosis, renal failure

Management of a nonsteroidal anti-inflammatory drug (NSAID) intoxication is primarily supportive and symptomatic. Fluid therapy is commonly effective in managing the hypotension that may occur following an acute NSAID overdose, except when this is due to an acute blood loss. Seizures tend to be very short-lived and often do not require drug treatment; although, recurrent seizures should be treated with I.V. diazepam. Since many of the NSAIDs undergo enterohepatic cycling, multiple doses of charcoal may be needed to reduce the potential for delayed toxicities.

Drug Interactions Cytochrome P-450 2C enzyme substrate

Decreased effect: Aspirin may decrease ibuprofen serum concentrations

Increased toxicity: May increase digoxin, methotrexate, and lithium serum concentrations; other nonsteroidal anti-inflammatories may increase adverse gastrointestinal effects

Mechanism of Action Inhibits prostaglandin synthesis by decreasing the activity of the enzyme, cyclo-oxygenase, which results in decreased formation of prostaglandin precursors

Pharmacodynamics/Kinetics

Onset of analgesia: 30-60 minutes
Duration: 4-6 hours
Onset of anti-inflammatory effect: Up to 7 days
Peak action: 1-2 weeks
Absorption: Oral: Rapid (85%)
Time to peak serum concentration: Within 1-2 hours
Protein binding: 90% to 99%
Metabolism: In the liver by oxidation
Half-life: 2-4 hours
End stage renal disease: Unchanged
Elimination: In urine (1% as free drug); some biliary excretion occurs

Usual Dosage Oral:

Children:

Antipyretic: 6 months to 12 years: Temperature <102.5°F (39°C): 5 mg/kg/dose; temperature >102.5°F: 10 mg/kg/dose given every 6-8 hours; maximum daily dose: 40 mg/kg/day

Juvenile rheumatoid arthritis: 30-70 mg/kg/24 hours divided every 6-8 hours
<20 kg: Maximum: 400 mg/day
20-30 kg: Maximum: 600 mg/day
30-40 kg: Maximum: 800 mg/day
>40 kg: Adult dosage

Start at lower end of dosing range and titrate upward; maximum: 2.4 g/day

Analgesic: 4-10 mg/kg/dose every 6-8 hours

Adults:

Inflammatory disease: 400-800 mg/dose 3-4 times/day; maximum dose: 3.2 g/day

Analgesia/pain/fever/dysmenorrhea: 200-400 mg/dose every 4-6 hours; maximum daily dose: 1.2 g (unless directed by physician)

Dosing adjustment/comments in severe hepatic impairment: Avoid use

Dietary Considerations Food: May decrease the rate but not the extent of oral absorption; drug may cause GI upset, bleeding, ulceration, perforation; take with food or milk to minimize GI upset

Administration Administer with food

Monitoring Parameters CBC; occult blood loss and periodic liver function tests; monitor response (pain, range of motion, grip strength, mobility, ADL function), inflammation; observe for weight gain, edema; monitor renal function (urine output, serum BUN and creatinine); observe for bleeding, bruising; evaluate gastrointestinal effects (abdominal pain, bleeding, dyspepsia); mental confusion, disorientation; with long-term therapy, periodic ophthalmic exams

Reference Range Plasma concentrations >200 µg/mL may be associated with severe toxicity

Test Interactions ↑ chloride (S), ↑ sodium (S), ↑ bleeding time

Patient Information Serious gastrointestinal bleeding can occur as well as ulceration and perforation. Pain may or may not be present. Avoid aspirin and aspirin-containing products while taking this medication. If gastric upset occurs, take with food, milk, or antacid. If gastric adverse effects persist, contact physician. May cause drowsiness, dizziness, blurred vision, and confusion. Use caution when performing tasks that require alertness (eg, driving). Do not take for more than 3 days for fever or 10 days for pain without physician's advice.

Nursing Implications Do not crush tablet

Additional Information Sucrose content of 5 mL (suspension): 2.5 g

Dosage Forms

Caplet: 100 mg
Drops, oral (berry flavor): 40 mg/mL (15 mL)
Suspension, oral: 100 mg/5 mL [OTC] (60 mL, 120 mL, 480 mL)
Suspension, oral, drops: 40 mg/mL [OTC]
Tablet: 100 mg [OTC], 200 mg [OTC], 300 mg, 400 mg, 600 mg, 800 mg
Tablet, chewable: 50 mg, 100 mg

Ibuprohm® [OTC] *see* Ibuprofen *on page 639*

Ibu-Tab® *see* Ibuprofen *on page 639*

Ibutilide (i BYOO ti lide)

Brand Names Corvert®

Synonyms Ibutilide Fumarate

Therapeutic Category Antiarrhythmic Agent, Class III

Use Acute termination of atrial fibrillation or flutter of recent onset; the effectiveness of ibutilide has not been determined in patients with arrhythmias of >90 days in duration

Pregnancy Risk Factor C

Pregnancy/Breast-Feeding Implications Teratogenic and embryocidal in rats; avoid use in pregnancy; avoid breast-feeding during therapy

Contraindications Hypersensitivity to the drug or any component

Warnings/Precautions Potentially fatal arrhythmias (eg, polymorphic ventricular tachycardia) can occur with ibutilide, **usually** in association with torsade de pointes (Q-T prolongation). Studies indicate a 1.7% incidence of arrhythmias in treated patients. The drug should be given in a setting of continuous EKG monitoring and by personnel trained in treating arrhythmias particularly polymorphic ventricular tachycardia. Patients with chronic atrial fibrillation may not be the best candidates for ibutilide since they often revert after conversion and the risks of treatment may not be justified when compared to alternative management. Dosing adjustments in patients with renal or hepatic dysfunction since a maximum of only two 10-minute infusions are indicated and drug distribution is one of the primary mechanisms responsible for termination of the pharmacologic effect; safety and efficacy in children have not been established.

Adverse Reactions

1% to 10%:

Cardiovascular: Sustained polymorphic ventricular tachycardia (ie, torsade de pointes) (1.7%), often requiring cardioversion, nonsustained polymorphic ventricular tachycardia (2.7%), nonsustained monomorphic ventricular extrasystoles (5.1%), nonsustained monomorphic VT (4.9%), tachycardia/supraventricular tachycardia, hypotension (2%), bundle branch block (1.9%), A-V block (1.5%), bradycardia, Q-T segment prolongation, hypertension (1.2%), palpitations (1%)
Central nervous system: Headache (3.6%)
Gastrointestinal: Nausea (>1%)

<1%:

Cardiovascular: Supraventricular extrasystoles (0.9%), nodal arrhythmia (0.7%), congestive heart failure (0.5%), syncope, idioventricular rhythm, sustained monomorphic VT (0.2%)
Renal: Renal failure: (0.3%)

Overdosage/Toxicology Symptoms include CNS depression, rapid gasping breathing, and convulsions; arrhythmias occur

Treatment is supportive and includes measures appropriate for the condition; antiarrhythmics are generally avoided; pharmacologic therapies may include magnesium sulfate, correction of other electrolyte abnormalities, overdrive cardiac pacing, electrical cardioversion, or defibrillation

Drug Interactions

Increased toxicity: Class Ia antiarrhythmic drugs (disopyramide, quinidine, and procainamide) and other class III drugs such as amiodarone and sotalol, should not be given concomitantly with ibutilide due to their potential to prolong refractoriness; the potential for prolongation of the Q-T interval may occur if ibutilide is given concurrently with phenothiazines, tricyclic and tetracyclic antidepressants, and the nonsedating antihistamines (terfenadine and astemizole); signs of digoxin toxicity may be masked when coadministered with ibutilide

Stability Admixtures are chemically and physically stable for 24 hours at room temperature and for 48 hours at refrigerated temperatures

Mechanism of Action Exact mechanism of action is unknown; prolongs the action potential in cardiac tissue

Pharmacodynamics/Kinetics

Absorption: Onset: Within 90 minutes after start of infusion (1/2 of conversions to sinus rhythm occur during infusion)

(Continued)

Ibutilide *(Continued)*

Metabolism: Extensively metabolized in the liver
Half-life: 2-12 hours (average: 6 hours)
Elimination: Parent and metabolite excreted predominantly in the urine

Usual Dosage I.V.: Initial:
<60 kg: 0.01 mg/kg over 10 minutes
≥60 kg: 1 mg over 10 minutes
If the arrhythmia does not terminate within 10 minutes after the end of the initial infusion, a second infusion of equal strength may be infused over a 10-minute period

Administration May be administered undiluted or diluted in 50 mL diluent (0.9% NS or D_5W)

Monitoring Parameters Observe patient with continuous EKG monitoring for at least 4 hours following infusion or until Q-T_c has returned to baseline; skilled personnel and proper equipment should be available during administration of ibutilide and subsequent monitoring of the patient

Nursing Implications See Monitoring Parameters; EKG, electrolytes

Dosage Forms Injection, as fumarate: 0.1 mg/mL (10 mL)

Ibutilide Fumarate *see* Ibutilide *on previous page*

Idamycin® *see* Idarubicin *on this page*

Idarubicin (eye da ROO bi sin)

Related Information
Antiemetics for Chemotherapy Induced Nausea and Vomiting *on page 1348*
Cancer Chemotherapy Regimens *on page 1351*
Extravasation Management of Chemotherapeutic Agents *on page 1379*
Toxicities of Chemotherapeutic Agents *on page 1382*

Brand Names Idamycin®

Synonyms 4-demethoxydaunorubicin; 4-dmdr; Idarubicin Hydrochloride

Therapeutic Category Antineoplastic Agent, Anthracycline; Antineoplastic Agent, Antibiotic; Vesicant

Use In combination treatment of acute myeloid leukemia (AML), this includes classifications M1 through M7 of the French-American-British (FAB) classification system; also used for the treatment of acute lymphocytic leukemia (ALL) in children

Pregnancy Risk Factor D

Contraindications Hypersensitivity to idarubicin, daunorubicin, or any component

Warnings/Precautions The U.S. Food and Drug Administration (FDA) currently recommends that procedures for proper handling and disposal of antineoplastic agents be considered. Administer I.V. slowly into a freely flowing I.V. infusion; do not administer I.M. or S.C., severe necrosis can result if extravasation occurs; can cause myocardial toxicity and is more common in patients who have previously received anthracyclines or have pre-existing cardiac disease; reduce dose in patients with impaired hepatic function; irreversible myocardial toxicity may occur as total dosage approaches 137.5 mg/m^2; severe myelosuppression is also possible.

Adverse Reactions
>10%:
- Central nervous system: Headache, fever
- Dermatologic: Alopecia, rash, urticaria
- Gastrointestinal: Mucositis, nausea, vomiting, diarrhea, stomatitis
- Genitourinary: Reddish urine
- Hematologic: Hemorrhage, anemia
  - Leukopenia (nadir: 8-29 days)
  - Thrombocytopenia (nadir: 10-15 days)
- Local: Tissue necrosis upon extravasation, erythematous streaking
  - **Vesicant chemotherapy**
- Miscellaneous: Infection

1% to 10%:
- Central nervous system: Seizures
- Neuromuscular & skeletal: Peripheral neuropathy
- Miscellaneous: Pulmonary allergy

<1%:
- Cardiovascular: Arrhythmias, EKG changes, cardiomyopathy, congestive heart failure, myocardial toxicity, acute life-threatening arrhythmias
- Endocrine & metabolic: Hyperuricemia
- Hepatic: Elevations in liver enzymes or bilirubin

Overdosage/Toxicology Symptoms of overdose include severe myelosuppression and increased GI toxicity

Treatment is supportive; it is unlikely that therapeutic efficacy or toxicity would be altered by conventional peritoneal or hemodialysis

Stability

Store intact vials of lyophilized powder at room temperature and protect from light

Dilute powder with NS to a concentration of 1 mg/mL as follows: Solution is stable for 72 hours at room temperature and 7 days under refrigeration

5 mg = 5 mL

10 mg = 10 mL

Further dilution in D_5W or NS is stable for 4 weeks at room temperature and protected from light

Incompatible with fluorouracil, etoposide, dexamethasone, heparin, hydrocortisone, methotrexate, vincristine

Standard I.V. dilution:

I.V. push: Dose/syringe (concentration is 1 mg/mL)

Maximum syringe size for IVP is 30 mL syringe and syringe should be ≤75% full

IVPB: Dose/100 mL D_5W or NS

Syringe and IVPB solutions are stable for 72 hours at room temperature and 7 days under refrigeration

Mechanism of Action Derivative of daunorubicin; the only structural difference between idarubicin and the parent compound, daunorubicin, is lack of the methoxyl group at the C4 position of the aglycone. Similar to daunorubicin, idarubicin exhibits inhibitory effects on DNA and RNA polymerase *in vitro*. Idarubicin has an affinity for DNA similar to the parent compound and somewhat higher efficacy than daunorubicin in stabilizing the DNA double helix against heat denaturation.

Pharmacodynamics/Kinetics

Absorption: Oral: Rapid but erratic (20% to 30%) from the GI tract

Distribution: Large V_d due to extensive tissue binding and distributes into CSF

Protein binding: 94% to 97%

Metabolism: In the liver to idarubicinol, which is pharmacologically active

Half-life, elimination:

Oral: 14-35 hours

I.V.: 12-27 hours

Time to peak serum concentration: Within 2-4 hours and varies considerably

Elimination: ~15% of an I.V. dose has been recovered in urine as idarubicin and idarubicinol; urinary recovery of idarubicin and idarubicinol is lower following oral doses; similar amounts are excreted via the bile

Usual Dosage I.V.:

Children:

Leukemia: 10-12 mg/m^2 once daily for 3 days and repeat every 3 weeks

Solid tumors: 5 mg/m^2 once daily for 3 days and repeat every 3 weeks

Adults: 12 mg/m^2/day for 3 days by slow I.V. injection (10-15 minutes) in combination with Ara-C. The Ara-C may be given as 100 mg/m^2/day by continuous infusion for 7 days or 25 mg/m^2 bolus followed by Ara-C 200 mg/m^2/day for 5 days continuous infusion

Dosing adjustment in renal impairment: Dose reduction is recommended

Serum creatinine ≥2 mg/dL: Reduce dose by 25%

Hemodialysis: Significant drug removal is unlikely based on physiochemical characteristics

Peritoneal dialysis: Significant drug removal is unlikely based on physiochemical characteristics

Dosing adjustment/comments in hepatic impairment:

Bilirubin 1.5-5.0 mg/dL or AST 60-180 units: Reduce dose 50%

Bilirubin >5 mg/dL or AST >180 units: Do not administer

Administration

Administer by intermittent infusion over 10-15 minutes into a free flowing I.V. solution of NS or D_5W

Avoid extravasation - potent vesicant

Monitoring Parameters CBC with differential, platelet count, ECHO, EKG, serum electrolytes, creatinine, uric acid, ALT, AST, bilirubin, signs of extravasation

Patient Information May cause hair loss; notify physician if pain, burning, or stinging around injection site occur

Nursing Implications

Local erythematous streaking along the vein may indicate too rapid a rate of administration; unless specific data available, do not mix with other drugs

Extravasation management:

Apply ice immediately for 30-60 minutes; then alternate off/on every 15 minutes for one day

Topical cooling may be achieved using ice packs or cooling pad with circulating ice water. Cooling of site for 24 hours as tolerated by the patient. Elevate and rest extremity 24-48 hours, then resume normal activity as tolerated. Application of cold inhibits vesicant's cytotoxicity.

(Continued)

Idarubicin *(Continued)*

Application of heat or sodium bicarbonate can be harmful and is contraindicated

If pain, erythema, and/or swelling persist beyond 48 hours, refer patient immediately to plastic surgeon for consultation and possible debridement

Dosage Forms Powder for injection, lyophilized, as hydrochloride: 5 mg, 10 mg

Idarubicin Hydrochloride *see* Idarubicin *on page 642*

Idoxuridine (eye doks YOOR i deen)

Brand Names Herplex® Ophthalmic

Synonyms IDU; IUDR

Therapeutic Category Antiviral Agent, Ophthalmic

Use Treatment of herpes simplex keratitis

Pregnancy Risk Factor C

Contraindications Hypersensitivity to idoxuridine or any component; concurrent use in patients receiving corticosteroids with superficial dendritic keratitis

Warnings/Precautions Use with caution in patients with corneal ulceration or patients receiving corticosteroid applications; if no response in epithelial infections within 14 days, consider a second form of therapy

Adverse Reactions

1% to 10%:

- Central nervous system: Pain
- Dermatologic: Pruritus, follicular conjunctivitis
- Local: Irritation, inflammation
- Ocular: Visual haze, corneal clouding, photophobia, small punctate defects on the corneal epithelium, mild edema of the eyelids and cornea

<1%: Ocular: Small punctate defects on the corneal epithelium

Overdosage/Toxicology Due to frequent dosing, small defects on the epithelium may result. Mutagenic and cytotoxic and should be considered as being potentially carcinogenic; no treatment is indicated for accidental ingestion

Drug Interactions Increased toxicity: Do not coadminister with boric acid-containing solutions

Stability Store in tight, light-resistant containers at 2°C to 8°C until dispensed; do not mix with other medications; solution must be refrigerated

Mechanism of Action Incorporated into viral DNA in place of thymidine resulting in mutations and inhibition of viral replication

Pharmacodynamics/Kinetics

Absorption: Ophthalmic: Poorly absorbed following instillation; tissue uptake is a function of cellular metabolism, which is inhibited by high concentrations of the drug (absorption decreases as the concentration of drug increases)

Distribution: Crosses the placenta

Metabolism: To iodouracil, uracil, and iodide

Elimination: Unchanged drug and metabolites excreted in the urine

Usual Dosage Adults: Ophthalmic:

Ointment: Instill 5 times/day (every 4 hours) in the conjunctival sac with last dose at bedtime; continue therapy for 5-7 days after healing appears complete

Solution: Instill 1 drop in eye(s) every hour during day and every 2 hours at night, continue until definite improvement is noted, then reduce daytime dose to 1 drop every 2 hours and every 4 hours at night; continue for 5-7 days after healing appears complete

Alternative dosing schedule: Instill 1 drop every minute for 5 minutes; repeat every 4 hours day and night

Patient Information May cause sensitivity to bright light; minimize by wearing sunglasses; notify physician if improvement is not seen in 7-8 days, if condition worsens, or if pain, decreased vision, itching, or swelling of the eye occur; do not exceed recommended dose

Nursing Implications Idoxuridine solution should not be mixed with other medications

Dosage Forms Solution, ophthalmic: 0.1% (15 mL)

IDU *see* Idoxuridine *on this page*

Ifex® *see* Ifosfamide *on this page*

IFLrA *see* Interferon Alfa-2a *on page 663*

IFN *see* Interferon Alfa-2a *on page 663*

Ifosfamide (eye FOSS fa mide)

Related Information

Antiemetics for Chemotherapy Induced Nausea and Vomiting *on page 1348*
Cancer Chemotherapy Regimens *on page 1351*
Toxicities of Chemotherapeutic Agents *on page 1382*

Brand Names Ifex®

Therapeutic Category Antineoplastic Agent, Alkylating Agent; Antineoplastic Agent, Nitrogen Mustard

Use In combination with certain other antineoplastics in treatment of lung cancer, Hodgkin's and non-Hodgkin's lymphoma, breast cancer, acute and chronic lymphocytic leukemia, ovarian cancer, testicular cancer, and sarcomas, pancreatic and gastric carcinoma, osteosarcoma

Pregnancy Risk Factor D

Contraindications Patients who have demonstrated a previous hypersensitivity to ifosfamide; patients with severely depressed bone marrow function

Warnings/Precautions The U.S. Food and Drug Administration (FDA) currently recommends that procedures for proper handling and disposal of antineoplastic agents be considered. May require therapy cessation if confusion or coma occurs; be aware of hemorrhagic cystitis and severe myelosuppression. Use with caution in patients with impaired renal function or those with compromised bone marrow reserve.

Adverse Reactions

>10%:

Central nervous system: Somnolence, confusion, hallucinations in 12% and coma (rare) have occurred and are usually reversible; usually occur with higher doses or in patients with reduced renal function; depressive psychoses, polyneuropathy

Dermatologic: Alopecia occurs in 50% to 83% of patients 2-4 weeks after initiation of therapy; may be as high as 100% in combination therapy

Gastrointestinal: Nausea and vomiting in 58% of patients is dose and schedule related (more common with higher doses and after bolus regimens); nausea and vomiting can persist up to 3 days after therapy; also anorexia, diarrhea, constipation, transient increase in LFTs and stomatitis noted.

Emetic potential: Moderate (58%)

Time course of nausea/vomiting: Onset: 2-3 hours; Duration: 12-72 hours

Genitourinary: Hemorrhagic cystitis has been frequently associated with the use of ifosfamide. A urinalysis prior to each dose should be obtained. **Ifosfamide should never be administered without a uroprotective agent (MESNA).** Hematuria has been reported in 6% to 92% of patients. Renal toxicity occurs in 6% of patients and is manifested as an increase in BUN or serum creatinine and is most likely related to tubular damage. Renal toxicity, including ARF, may occur more frequently with high-dose ifosfamide. Metabolic acidosis may occur in up to 31% of patients.

1% to 10%:

Dermatologic: Phlebitis, dermatitis, nail ridging, skin hyperpigmentation, impaired wound healing

Endocrine & metabolic: SIADH

Hematologic: Myelosuppression: Less of a problem than with cyclophosphamide if used alone. Leukopenia is mild to moderate, thrombocytopenia and anemia are rare. However, myelosuppression can be severe when used with other chemotherapeutic agents or with high-dose therapy. Be cautious with patients with compromised bone marrow reserve.

WBC: Moderate

Platelets: Mild

Onset (days): 7

Nadir (days): 10-14

Hepatic: Elevated liver enzymes

Respiratory: Nasal congestion, pulmonary fibrosis

Miscellaneous: Immunosuppression, sterility, possible secondary malignancy, allergic reactions

<1%:

Cardiovascular: Cardiotoxicity

Respiratory: Pulmonary toxicity

Overdosage/Toxicology Symptoms of overdose include myelosuppression, nausea, vomiting, diarrhea, alopecia; direct extension of the drug's pharmacologic effect; treatment is supportive

Drug Interactions Cytochrome P-450 2B6 enzyme substrate, cytochrome P-450 2C enzyme substrate, and cytochrome P-450 3A enzyme substrate

Because ifosfamide undergoes hepatic activation by microsomal enzymes, induction of these enzymes is potentially possible by pretreatment with various enzyme-inducers such as phenobarbital, phenytoin, and chloral hydrate

Stability

Store intact vials at room temperature or under refrigeration

Dilute powder with SWI or NS to a concentration of 50 mg/mL as follows. **Do not use bacteriostatic SWI or NS - incompatible**; solution is stable for 7 days at room temperature and 3 weeks under refrigeration

1 g vial = 20 mL

3 g vial = 60 mL

Further dilution in NS, D_5W or LR is stable for 7 days at room temperature

(Continued)

Ifosfamide *(Continued)*

Compatible with mesna in NS for up to 9 days at room temperature.

Standard I.V. dilution:

I.V. push: Dose/syringe (concentration = 50 mg/mL)

Maximum syringe size for IVP is a 30 mL syringe and syringe should be ≤75% full

IVPB: Dose/100-1000 mL D_5W or NS

Syringe and IVPB are stable for 7 days at room temperature and 6 weeks under refrigeration

Mechanism of Action Causes cross-linking of strands of DNA by binding with nucleic acids and other intracellular structures; inhibits protein synthesis and DNA synthesis; an analogue of cyclophosphamide, and like cyclophosphamide, it undergoes activation by microsomal enzymes in the liver. Ifosfamide is metabolized to active compounds, ifosfamide mustard, and acrolein

Pharmacodynamics/Kinetics Pharmacokinetics are dose-dependent

Absorption: Oral: Peak plasma levels occur within 1 hour

Bioavailability: Estimated at 100%

Distribution: V_d: Has been calculated to be 5.7-49 L; does penetrate CNS, but not in therapeutic levels

Protein binding: Not appreciably protein bound

Metabolism: In the liver to active species; requires biotransformation in the liver before it can act as an alkylating agent; the metabolite acrolein is the toxic agent implicated in the development of hemorrhagic cystitis

Half-life: Beta phase: 11-15 hours with high-dose (3800-5000 mg/m^2) or 4-7 hours with lower doses (1800 mg/m^2)

Elimination: 15% to 50% excreted unchanged in urine

Usual Dosage I.V. (refer to individual protocols):

Children: 1200-1800 mg/m^2/day for 3-5 days every 21-28 days

Adults:

Doses may be given as 50 mg/kg/day **or** 700-2000 mg/m^2/day for 5 days

Alternatives include 2400 mg/m^2/day for 3 days **or** 5000 mg/m^2 as a single dose

Doses of 700-900 mg/m^2/day for 5 days may be given IVP; courses may be repeated every 3-4 weeks

To prevent bladder toxicity, ifosfamide should be given with extensive hydration consisting of at least 2 L of oral or I.V. fluid per day. A protector, such as mesna, should also be used to prevent hemorrhagic cystitis. The dose-limiting toxicity is hemorrhagic cystitis and ifosfamide should be used in conjunction with a uroprotective agent.

Dosing adjustment in renal impairment:

S_{cr} >3.0 mg/dL: Withhold drug

S_{cr} 2.1-3.0 mg/dL: Reduce dose by 25% to 50%

Dosing adjustment in hepatic impairment: Although no specific guidelines are available, it is possible that higher doses are indicated in hepatic disease

Administration

Administer slow I.V. push, IVPB over 30 minutes or continuour I.V. over 5 days

Adequate hydration (at least 2 L/day) of the patient before and for 72 hours after therapy is recommended to minimize the risk of hemorrhagic cystitis

MESNA should be administered concomitantly (20% of the ifosfamide dose 15 minutes before, 4 hours after and 8 hours after ifosfamide administration)

Monitoring Parameters CBC with differential, hemoglobin, and platelet count, urine output, urinalysis, liver function, and renal function tests

Patient Information Drink plenty of fluids after dose; notify physician if persistent sore throat, fever, sores on mucous membranes, fatigue, or unusual bleeding or bruising occur

Nursing Implications Mesna to be used concomitantly for prophylaxis against hemorrhagic cystitis

Dosage Forms Powder for injection: 1 g, 3 g

IG *see* Immune Globulin, Intramuscular *on page 650*

I-Gent® *see* Gentamicin *on page 570*

IGIM *see* Immune Globulin, Intramuscular *on page 650*

IL-2 *see* Aldesleukin *on page 40*

Ilopan® *see* Dexpanthenol *on page 361*

Ilopan-Choline® *see* Dexpanthenol *on page 361*

Ilosone® *see* Erythromycin *on page 461*

Ilozyme® *see* Pancrelipase *on page 949*

IMDUR™ *see* Isosorbide Mononitrate *on page 685*

I-Methasone® *see* Dexamethasone *on page 356*

Imidazole Carboxamide *see* Dacarbazine *on page 335*

Imipemide *see* Imipenem and Cilastatin *on this page*

Imipenem and Cilastatin (i mi PEN em & sye la STAT in)

Related Information

Animal and Human Bites Guidelines *on page 1463*
Antimicrobial Drugs of Choice *on page 1468*
Bacterial Meningitis Practical Guidelines for Management *on page 1475*

Brand Names Primaxin®

Canadian/Mexican Brand Names Tienam® (Mexico)

Synonyms Imipemide

Therapeutic Category Antibiotic, Miscellaneous

Use Treatment of documented multidrug resistant gram-negative infection due to organisms proven or suspected to be susceptible to imipenem/cilastatin; treatment of multiple organism infection in which other agents have an insufficient spectrum of activity or are contraindicated due to toxic potential; Antibacterial activity includes resistant gram-negative bacilli (*Pseudomonas aeruginosa* and *Enterococcus* sp), gram-positive bacteria (methicillin-sensitive *Staphylococcus aureus* and *Enterococcus* sp) and anaerobes

Pregnancy Risk Factor C

Contraindications Hypersensitivity to imipenem/cilastatin or any component

Warnings/Precautions Dosage adjustment required in patients with impaired renal function; safety and efficacy in children <12 years of age have not yet been established; prolonged use may result in superinfection; use with caution in patients with a history of seizures or hypersensitivity to beta-lactams; elderly patients often require lower doses

Adverse Reactions

1% to 10%:
- Gastrointestinal: Nausea, diarrhea, vomiting
- Local: Phlebitis

<1%:
- Cardiovascular: Hypotension, palpitations
- Central nervous system: Seizures
- Dermatologic: Rash
- Gastrointestinal: Pseudomembranous colitis
- Hematologic: Neutropenia, eosinophilia
- Local: Pain at injection site
- Miscellaneous: Emergence of resistant strains of *P. aeruginosa*

Overdosage/Toxicology Symptoms of overdose include neuromuscular hypersensitivity, seizures

Hemodialysis may be helpful to aid in the removal of the drug from the blood; otherwise most treatment is supportive or symptom directed

Drug Interactions Increased toxicity: Beta-lactam antibiotics, probenecid may increase toxic potential

Stability

Imipenem/cilastatin powder for injection should be stored at <30°C

Reconstituted solutions are stable 10 hours at room temperature and 48 hours at refrigeration (4°C) with NS

If reconstituted with 5% or 10% dextrose injection, 5% dextrose and sodium bicarbonate, 5% dextrose and 0.9% sodium chloride, is stable for 4 hours at room temperature and 24 hours when refrigerated

Imipenem/cilastatin is most stable at a pH of 6.5-7.5; imipenem is inactivated at acidic or alkaline pH

Standard diluent: 500 mg/100 mL NS; 1 g/250 mL NS

Comments: All IVPB should be prepared fresh; do not use dextrose as a diluent due to limited stability

Mechanism of Action A carbapenem with broad-spectrum antibacterial activity including resistant gram-negative bacilli (*Pseudomonas aeruginosa* and *Enterococcus* sp), gram-positive bacteria (methicillin-sensitive *Staphylococcus aureus* and *Enterococcus* sp) and anaerobes

Inhibits cell wall synthesis by binding to penicillin-binding proteins on the bacterial outer membrane; cilastatin prevents renal metabolism of imipenem by competitive inhibition of dehydropeptidase along the brush border of the proximal renal tubules

Pharmacodynamics/Kinetics

Imipenem:
- Distribution: Appears in breast milk; crosses the placenta
- Metabolism: In the kidney by dehydropeptidase
- Half-life: 1 hour, extended with renal insufficiency
- Elimination: When given with cilastatin, urinary excretion of unchanged imipenem increases to 70%

Cilastatin:
- Metabolism: Partially in the kidneys

(Continued)

Imipenem and Cilastatin *(Continued)*

Half-life: 1 hour, extended with renal insufficiency
Elimination: 70% to 80% of dose excreted in urine as unchanged cilastatin

Usual Dosage I.M. and I.V. (dosing based on imipenem component):

Children: I.V.: 60-100 mg/kg/24 hours divided every 6 hours (maximum: 4 g/day)

Adults: I.V.: 500 mg every 6-8 hours (1 g every 6-8 hours for severe *Pseudomonas* infection); infuse each 250-500 mg dose over 20-30 minutes; infuse each 1 g dose over 40-60 minutes

Mild to moderate infection **only**: I.M.: 500-750 mg every 12 hours (**Note:** 750 mg is recommended for intra-abdominal and more severe respiratory, dermatologic, or gynecologic infections; total daily I.M. dosages >1500 mg are not recommended; deep I.M. injection should be carefully made into a large muscle mass only)

Dosing adjustment in renal impairment: See table.

CreatinineClearance mL/min/1.73 m²	Frequency	% Decrease in Daily Maximum Dose
30-70	q6-8h	50
20-30	q8-12h	63
5-20	q12h	75

Hemodialysis: Imipenem (**not cilastatin**) is moderately dialyzable (20% to 50%); administer dose postdialysis

Peritoneal dialysis: Dose as for Cl_{cr} <10 mL/minute

Continuous arterio-venous or veno-venous hemofiltration (CAVH/CAVHD): Removes 20 mg of imipenem/L of filtrate per day

Administration Not for direct infusion; vial contents must be transferred to 100 mL of infusion solution; final concentration should not exceed 5 mg/mL; infuse over 30-60 minutes; watch for convulsions. If nausea and/or vomiting occur during administration, decrease the rate of I.V. infusion; do not mix with or physically add to other antibiotics; however, may administer concomitantly

Monitoring Parameters Periodic renal, hepatic, and hematologic function tests

Test Interactions Interferes with urinary glucose determination using Clinitest®

Additional Information Sodium content of 1 g: 3.2 mEq

Dosage Forms Powder for injection:

I.M.:
Imipenem 500 mg and cilastatin 500 mg
Imipenem 750 mg and cilastatin 750 mg

I.V.:
Imipenem 250 mg and cilastatin 250 mg
Imipenem 500 mg and cilastatin 500 mg

Imipramine (im IP ra meen)

Related Information

Antidepressant Agents Comparison *on page 1393*

Brand Names Janimine®; Tofranil®; Tofranil-PM®

Canadian/Mexican Brand Names Apo-Imipramine® (Canada); Novo-Pramine® (Canada); PMS-Imipramine (Canada); Talpramin® (Mexico)

Synonyms Imipramine Hydrochloride; Imipramine Pamoate

Therapeutic Category Antidepressant, Tricyclic

Use Treatment of various forms of depression, often in conjunction with psychotherapy; enuresis in children; analgesic for certain chronic and neuropathic pain

Pregnancy Risk Factor D

Contraindications Hypersensitivity to imipramine (cross-sensitivity with other tricyclics may occur); patients receiving MAO inhibitors or fluoxetine within past 14 days; narrow-angle glaucoma

Warnings/Precautions Use with caution in patients with cardiovascular disease, conduction disturbances, seizure disorders, urinary retention, hyperthyroidism or those receiving thyroid replacement; do not discontinue abruptly in patients receiving long-term, high-dose therapy; some oral preparations contain tartrazine and injection contains sulfites, both of which can cause allergic reactions

Orthostatic hypotension is a concern with this agent, especially in patients taking other medications that may affect blood pressure; may precipitate arrhythmias in predisposed patients; may aggravate seizures; a less anticholinergic antidepressant may be a better choice

Adverse Reactions Less sedation and anticholinergic effects than amitriptyline

>10%:

Central nervous system: Dizziness, drowsiness, headache

Gastrointestinal: Increased appetite, nausea, unpleasant taste, weight gain, xerostomia, constipation

Genitourinary: Urinary retention

Neuromuscular & skeletal: Weakness

1% to 10%:

Cardiovascular: Postural hypotension, arrhythmias, tachycardia, sudden death

Central nervous system: Confusion, delirium, hallucinations, nervousness, restlessness, parkinsonian syndrome, insomnia

Endocrine & metabolic: Sexual dysfunction

Gastrointestinal: Diarrhea, heartburn

Genitourinary: Dysuria

Neuromuscular & skeletal: Fine muscle tremors

Ocular: Blurred vision, eye pain

Miscellaneous: Diaphoresis (excessive)

<1%:

Central nervous system: Anxiety, seizures

Dermatologic: Alopecia, photosensitivity

Endocrine & metabolic: Breast enlargement, galactorrhea, SIADH

Gastrointestinal: Trouble with gums, decreased lower esophageal sphincter tone may cause GE reflux

Genitourinary: Testicular edema

Hematologic: Leukopenia, eosinophilia, rarely agranulocytosis

Hepatic: Increased liver enzymes, cholestatic jaundice

Ocular: Increased intraocular pressure

Otic: Tinnitus

Miscellaneous: Allergic reactions, has been associated with falls

Overdosage/Toxicology Symptoms of overdose include confusion, hallucinations, constipation, cyanosis, tachycardia, urinary retention, ventricular tachycardia, seizures

Following initiation of essential overdose management, toxic symptoms should be treated. Sodium bicarbonate is indicated when QRS interval is >0.10 seconds or QT_c >0.42 seconds. Ventricular arrhythmias often respond to concurrent systemic alkalinization (sodium bicarbonate 0.5-2 mEq/kg I.V.). Arrhythmias unresponsive to this therapy may respond to lidocaine 1 mg/kg I.V. followed by a titrated infusion. Physostigmine (1-2 mg I.V. slowly for adults or 0.5 mg I.V. slowly for children) may be indicated in reversing cardiac arrhythmias that are life-threatening. Seizures usually respond to diazepam I.V. boluses (5-10 mg for adults up to 30 mg or 0.25-0.4 mg/kg/dose for children up to 10 mg/dose). If seizures are unresponsive or recur, phenytoin or phenobarbital may be required.

Drug Interactions Cytochrome P-450 1A2 enzyme substrate, cytochrome P-450 2D6 enzyme substrate, and cytochrome P-450 2C enzyme substrate (minor)

Decreased effect: Clonidine, blocks uptake of guanethidine and prevents its hypotensive effects

Increased toxicity: MAO inhibitors: Hyperpyrexia, hypertension, tachycardia, confusion, seizures, and death have been reported; may increase the prothrombin time in patients stabilized on warfarin; may potentiate the action of other CNS depressants; potentiates the pressor and cardiac effects of sympathomimetic agents such as isoproterenol, epinephrine, etc; additive anticholinergic effects seen with other anticholinergic agents; cimetidine reduces the hepatic metabolism of imipramine

Stability Solutions stable at a pH of 4-5; turns yellowish or reddish on exposure to light. Slight discoloration does not affect potency; marked discoloration is associated with loss of potency. Capsules stable for 3 years following date of manufacture.

Mechanism of Action Traditionally believed to increase the synaptic concentration of serotonin and/or norepinephrine in the central nervous system by inhibition of their reuptake by the presynaptic neuronal membrane. However, additional receptor effects have been found including desensitization of adenyl cyclase, down regulation of beta-adrenergic receptors, and down regulation of serotonin receptors.

Pharmacodynamics/Kinetics

Peak antidepressant effect: Usually after ≥2 weeks

Absorption: Oral: Well absorbed

Distribution: Crosses the placenta

Metabolism: In the liver by microsomal enzymes to desipramine (active) and other metabolites; significant first-pass metabolism

Half-life: 6-18 hours

Elimination: Almost all compounds following metabolism are excreted in urine

Usual Dosage Maximum antidepressant effect may not be seen for 2 or more weeks after initiation of therapy.

Children: Oral:

Depression: 1.5 mg/kg/day with dosage increments of 1 mg/kg every 3-4 days to a maximum dose of 5 mg/kg/day in 1-4 divided doses; monitor carefully especially with doses ≥3.5 mg/kg/day

(Continued)

Imipramine *(Continued)*

Enuresis: ≥6 years: Initial: 10-25 mg at bedtime, if inadequate response still seen after 1 week of therapy, increase by 25 mg/day; dose should not exceed 2.5 mg/kg/day or 50 mg at bedtime if 6-12 years of age or 75 mg at bedtime if ≥12 years of age

Adjunct in the treatment of cancer pain: Initial: 0.2-0.4 mg/kg at bedtime; dose may be increased by 50% every 2-3 days up to 1-3 mg/kg/dose at bedtime

Adolescents: Oral: Initial: 25-50 mg/day; increase gradually; maximum: 100 mg/day in single or divided doses

Adults:

Oral: Initial: 25 mg 3-4 times/day, increase dose gradually, total dose may be given at bedtime; maximum: 300 mg/day

I.M.: Initial: Up to 100 mg/day in divided doses; change to oral as soon as possible

Elderly: Initial: 10-25 mg at bedtime; increase by 10-25 mg every 3 days for inpatients and weekly for outpatients if tolerated; average daily dose to achieve a therapeutic concentration: 100 mg/day; range: 50-150 mg/day

Dietary Considerations Alcohol: Additive CNS effect, avoid use

Monitoring Parameters Monitor blood pressure and pulse rate prior to and during initial therapy; EKG, CBC; evaluate mental status

Reference Range Therapeutic: Imipramine and desipramine: 150-250 ng/mL (SI: 530-890 nmol/L); desipramine: 150-300 ng/mL (SI: 560-1125 nmol/L); Toxic: >500 ng/mL (SI: 446-893 nmol/L); utility of serum level monitoring controversial

Test Interactions ↑ glucose

Patient Information May require 2-4 weeks to achieve desired effect; avoid alcohol ingestion; do not discontinue medication abruptly; may cause urine to turn blue-green; may cause drowsiness, avoid alcohol and other CNS depressants; dry mouth may be helped by sips of water, sugarless gum, or hard candy; rise slowly to avoid dizziness

Nursing Implications Raise bed rails, institute safety measures

Additional Information

Imipramine hydrochloride: Tofranil®, Janimine®

Imipramine pamoate: Tofranil-PM®

Dosage Forms

Capsule, as pamoate (Tofranil-PM®): 75 mg, 100 mg, 125 mg, 150 mg

Injection, as hydrochloride (Tofranil®): 12.5 mg/mL (2 mL)

Tablet, as hydrochloride (Janimine®, Tofranil®): 10 mg, 25 mg, 50 mg

Imipramine Hydrochloride *see* Imipramine *on page 648*

Imipramine Pamoate *see* Imipramine *on page 648*

Imitrex® *see* Sumatriptan Succinate *on page 1183*

Immune Globulin, Intramuscular

(i MYUN GLOB yoo lin, IN tra MUS kyoo ler)

Related Information

Immunization Guidelines *on page 1421*

Miscellaneous Vaccination Information *on page 1437*

Prophylaxis for Patients Exposed to Common Communicable Diseases *on page 1452*

Brand Names Gamastan®; Gammar®

Canadian/Mexican Brand Names Gammabulin Immuno (Canada); Iveegam® (Canada)

Synonyms Gamma Globulin; IG; IGIM; Immune Serum Globulin; ISG

Therapeutic Category Immune Globulin

Use Household and sexual contacts of persons with hepatitis A, measles, varicella, and possibly rubella; travelers to high-risk areas outside tourist routes; staff, attendees, and patients of diapered attendees in day-care center outbreaks

For travelers, IG is not an alternative to careful selection of foods and water; immune globulin can interfere with the antibody response to parenterally administered live virus vaccines. Frequent travelers should be tested for hepatitis A antibody, immune hemolytic anemia, and neutropenia (with ITP, I.V. route is usually used).

Pregnancy Risk Factor C

Contraindications Thrombocytopenia, hypersensitivity to immune globulin, thimerosal, IgA deficiency

Warnings/Precautions Skin testing should not be performed as local irritation can occur and be misinterpreted as a positive reaction; do not administer I.V.; IG should **not** be used to control outbreaks of measles; epidemiologic and laboratory data indicate current IMIG products do not have a discernible risk of transmitting HIV

Adverse Reactions

>10%: Local: Pain, tenderness, muscle stiffness at I.M. site

1% to 10%:

Cardiovascular: Flushing

Central nervous system: Chills

Gastrointestinal: Nausea

<1%:

Central nervous system: Lethargy, fever

Dermatologic: Urticaria, angioedema, erythema

Gastrointestinal: Vomiting

Neuromuscular & skeletal: Myalgia

Miscellaneous: Hypersensitivity reactions

Drug Interactions Increased toxicity: Live virus, vaccines (measles, mumps, rubella); do not administer within 3 months after administration of these vaccines

Stability Keep in refrigerator; do not freeze

Mechanism of Action Provides passive immunity by increasing the antibody titer and antigen-antibody reaction potential

Pharmacodynamics/Kinetics

Duration of immune effect: Usually 3-4 weeks

Half-life: 23 days

Time to peak serum concentration: I.M.: Within 24-48 hours

Usual Dosage I.M.:

Hepatitis A:

Pre-exposure prophylaxis upon travel into endemic areas:

0.02 mL/kg for anticipated risk 1-3 months

0.06 mL/kg for anticipated risk >3 months

Repeat approximate dose every 4-6 months if exposure continues

Postexposure prophylaxis: 0.02 mL/kg given within 2 weeks of exposure

Measles:

Prophylaxis: 0.25 mL/kg/dose (maximum dose: 15 mL) given within 6 days of exposure followed by live attenuated measles vaccine in 3 months or at 15 months of age (whichever is later)

For patients with leukemia, lymphoma, immunodeficiency disorders, generalized malignancy, or receiving immunosuppressive therapy: 0.5 mL/kg (maximum dose: 15 mL)

Poliomyelitis: Prophylaxis: 0.3 mL/kg/dose as a single dose

Rubella: Prophylaxis: 0.55 mL/kg/dose within 72 hours of exposure

Varicella:: Prophylaxis: 0.6-1.2 mL/kg (varicella zoster immune globulin preferred) within 72 hours of exposure

IgG deficiency: 1.3 mL/kg, then 0.66 mL/kg in 3-4 weeks

Hepatitis B: Prophylaxis: 0.06 mL/kg/dose (HBIG preferred)

Administration Intramuscular injection only

Test Interactions Skin tests should **not** be done

Nursing Implications Do not mix with other medications; skin testing should not be performed as local irritation can occur and be misinterpreted as a positive reaction

Dosage Forms Injection: I.M.: 165±15 mg (of protein)/mL (2 mL, 10 mL)

Immune Globulin, Intravenous

(i MYUN GLOB yoo lin, IN tra VEE nus)

Related Information

Immunization Guidelines *on page 1421*

Brand Names Gamimune® N; Gammagard®; Gammagard® S/D; Gammar-P® I.V.; Polygam®; Polygam® S/D; Sandoglobulin®; Venoglobulin®-I; Venoglobulin®-S

Synonyms IVIG

Therapeutic Category Immune Globulin

Use Treatment of immunodeficiency sufficiency (hypogammaglobulinemia, agammaglobulinemia, IgG subclass deficiencies, severe combined immunodeficiency syndromes (SCIDS), Wiskott-Aldrich syndrome), idiopathic thrombocytopenic purpura; used in conjunction with appropriate anti-infective therapy *to prevent or modify acute bacterial or viral infections* in patients with iatrogenically-induced or disease-associated immunodepression; *chronic lymphocytic leukemia (CLL) - chronic prophylaxis autoimmune neutropenia, bone marrow transplantation patients, autoimmune hemolytic anemia or neutropenia, refractory dermatomyositis/polymyositis, autoimmune diseases* (myasthenia gravis, SLE, bullous pemphigoid, severe rheumatoid arthritis), *Kawasaki disease, Guillain-Barré syndrome.* Therapy should be guided by clinical observation and serial determination of serum IgG levels.

Pregnancy Risk Factor C

Contraindications Hypersensitivity to immune globulin or any component, IgA deficiency (except with the use of Gammagard®, Polygam®)

(Continued)

Immune Globulin, Intravenous *(Continued)*

Warnings/Precautions Anaphylactic hypersensitivity reactions can occur, especially in IgA-deficient patients; studies indicate that the currently available products have no discernible risk of transmitting HIV or hepatitis B

Adverse Reactions

1% to 10%:
- Cardiovascular: Flushing of the face, tachycardia
- Central nervous system: Chills
- Gastrointestinal: Nausea
- Respiratory: Dyspnea

<1%:
- Cardiovascular: Hypotension, tightness in the chest
- Central nervous system: Dizziness, fever, headache
- Miscellaneous: Diaphoresis, hypersensitivity reactions

Drug Interactions Increased toxicity: Live virus, vaccines (measles, mumps, rubella); do not administer within 3 months after administration of these vaccines

Stability Stability and dilution is dependent upon the manufacturer and brand; do not mix with other drugs

Mechanism of Action Replacement therapy for primary and secondary immunodeficiencies; interference with F_c receptors on the cells of the reticuloendothelial system for autoimmune cytopenias and ITP; possible role of contained antiviral-type antibodies

Pharmacodynamics/Kinetics I.V. provides immediate antibody levels

Half-life: 21-24 days

Usual Dosage Children and Adults: I.V.:

Dosages should be based on ideal body weight and not actual body weight in morbidly obese patients

Primary immunodeficiency disorders: 200-400 mg/kg every 4 weeks or as per monitored serum IgG concentrations

Chronic lymphocytic leukemia (CLL): 400 mg/kg/dose every 3 weeks

Idiopathic thrombocytopenic purpura (ITP): Maintenance dose:
- 400 mg/kg/day for 5 consecutive days
- 800 mg/kg/day for 2 consecutive days

Chronic ITP: 400-1000 mg/kg/dose every 7 or 14 days

Kawasaki disease:
- 400 mg/kg/day for 4 days within 10 days of onset of fever
- 800 mg/kg/day for 1-2 days within 10 days of onset of fever
- 2 g/kg for one dose only

Acquired immunodeficiency syndrome (patients must be symptomatic):
- 200-250 mg/kg/dose every 2 weeks
- 400-500 mg/kg/dose every month or every 4 weeks

Autoimmune hemolytic anemia and neutropenia: 1000 mg/kg/dose for 2-3 days

Autoimmune diseases: 400 mg/kg/day for 4 days

Post allogeneic bone marrow transplant: 500 mg/kg/week for 4 months post-transplant

Adjuvant to severe cytomegalovirus infections: 500 mg/kg/dose every other day for 7 doses

Severe systemic viral and bacterial infections: Children: 500-1000 mg/kg/week

Prevention of gastroenteritis: Infants and Children: Oral: 50 mg/kg/day divided every 6 hours

Guillain-Barré syndrome:
- 400 mg/kg/day for 4 days
- 1000 mg/kg/day for 2 days
- 2000 mg/kg/day for one day

Refractory dermatomyositis: 2 g/kg/dose every month x 3-4 doses

Refractory polymyositis: 1 g/kg/day x 2 days every month x 4 doses

Chronic inflammatory demyelinating polyneuropathy:
- 400 mg/kg/day for 5 doses once each month
- 800 mg/kg/day for 3 doses once each month
- 1000 mg/kg/day for 2 days once each month

Dosing adjustment/comments in renal impairment: Cl_{cr} <10 mL/minute: Avoid use

Administration I.V. use only; for initial treatment, a lower concentration and/or a slower rate of infusion should be used

Dosage Forms

Injection: Gamimune® N: 5% [50 mg/mL] (10 mL, 50 mL, 100 mL); 10% [100 mg/mL] (50 mL, 100 mL, 200 mL)

Powder for injection, lyophilized:
- Gammagard®, Polygam®: 0.5 g, 2.5 g, 5 g, 10 g
- Gammar-P®-IV: 1 g, 2.5 g, 5 g
- Polygam®: 0.5 g, 2.5 g, 5 g, 10 g
- Sandoglobulin®: 1 g, 3 g, 6 g

INTRAVENOUS IMMUNE GLOBULIN PRODUCT COMPARISON

	Gamimune® N	Gammagard®	Gammar® -IV	Iveegam®	Polygam®	Sandoglobulin®	Venoglobulin® -I
FDA indication	Primary immunodeficiency, ITP	Primary immunodeficiency, ITP, CLL prophylaxis	Primary immunodeficiency	Primary immunodeficiency, Kawasaki syndrome	Primary immunodeficiency, ITP, CLL	Primary immunodeficiency, ITP	Primary immunodeficiency, ITP
Contraindication	IgA deficiency	None (caution with IgA deficiency)	IgA deficiency	IgA deficiency	None (caution with IgA deficiency)	IgA deficiency	IgA deficiency
IgA content	270 mcg/mL	0.92-1.6 mcg/mL	<20 mcg/mL	10 mcg/mL	0.74±0.33 mcg/mL	720 mcg/mL	20-24 mcg/mL
Adverse reactions (%)	5.2	6	15	1	6	2.5-6.6	6
Plasma source	>2000 paid donors	4000-5000 paid donors	>8000 paid donors	>6000 paid donors	50,000 voluntary donors	8000-15,000 voluntary donors	6000-9000 paid donors
Half-life	21 d	24 d	21-24 d	26-29 d	21-25 d	21-23 d	29 d
IgG subclass (%)							
IgG_1 (60-70)	60	67 (66.8)[1]	69	64.1[2]	67	60.5 (55.3)[1]	62.3[2]
IgG_2 (19-31)	29.4	25 (25.4)	23	30.3	25	30.2 (35.7)	32.8
IgG_3 (5-8.4)	6.5	5 (7.4)	6	4	5	6.6 (6.3)	2.9
IgG_4 (0.7-4)	4.1	3 (0.3)	2	1.5	3	2.6 (2.6)	2
Monomers (%)	>95	>95	>98	93.8	>95	>92	>98
Gammaglobulin (%)	>98	>90	>98	100	>90	>96	>98
Storage	Refrigerate	Room temp	Room temp	Refrigerate	Room temp	Room temp	Room temp
Recommendations for **initial** infusion rate	0.01-0.02 mL/kg/min	0.5 mL/kg/h	0.01-0.02 mL/kg/min	1 mL/min	0.5 mL/kg/h	0.01-0.03 mL/kg/min	0.01-0.02 mL/kg/min
Maximum infusion rate	0.08 mL/kg/min	4 mL/kg/h	0.06 mL/kg/min	2 mL/min	4 mL/kg/h	2.5 mL/min	0.04 mL/kg/min
Maximum concentration for infusion (%)	10	5	5	5	10	12	10

[1] Skvaril F and Gardi A, 'Differences Among Available Immunoglobulin Preparations for Intravenous Use,' *Pediatr Infect Dis J*, 1988, 7:543-48.

[2] Roomer J, Morgenthaler JJ, Scherz R, et al, 'Characterization of Various Immunoglobulin Preparations for Intravenous Application', *Vox Sang*, 1982, 42:62-73.

[3] ASHP Commission on Therapeutics, ASHP Therapeutic Guidelines for Intravenous Immune Globulin, *Clin Pharm*, 1992, 11:117-36.

[4] Manufacturer's Product Information/Personal Communication.

Immune Globulin, Intravenous *(Continued)*

Venoglobulin®-I: 2.5 g, 5 g
Detergent treated:
Gammagard® S/D: 2.5 g, 5 g, 10 g
Polygam® S/D: 2.5 g, 5 g, 10 g
Venoglobulin®-S: 2.5 g, 5 g, 10 g

Immune Serum Globulin *see* Immune Globulin, Intramuscular *on page 650*
Immunization Guidelines *see page 1421*
Imodium® *see* Loperamide *on page 739*
Imodium® A-D [OTC] *see* Loperamide *on page 739*
Imogam® *see* Rabies Immune Globulin (Human) *on page 1091*
Imovax® Rabies I.D. Vaccine *see* Rabies Virus Vaccine *on page 1091*
Imovax® Rabies Vaccine *see* Rabies Virus Vaccine *on page 1091*
Imuran® *see* Azathioprine *on page 122*
I-Naphline® *see* Naphazoline *on page 879*
Inapsine® *see* Droperidol *on page 433*

Indapamide (in DAP a mide)

Related Information

Sulfonamide Derivatives *on page 1420*

Brand Names Lozol®

Canadian/Mexican Brand Names Lozide® (Canada)

Therapeutic Category Antihypertensive; Diuretic, Miscellaneous

Use Management of mild to moderate hypertension; treatment of edema in congestive heart failure and nephrotic syndrome

Pregnancy Risk Factor D

Contraindications Anuria, hypersensitivity to hydrochlorothiazide or any component, cross-sensitivity with other thiazides and sulfonamide derivatives

Warnings/Precautions Use with caution in patients with renal or hepatic disease, gout, lupus erythematosus, or diabetes mellitus

Adverse Reactions

1% to 10%: Endocrine & metabolic: Hypokalemia

<1%:

Cardiovascular: Arrhythmia, weak pulse, hypotension
Central nervous system: Mood changes
Dermatologic: Photosensitivity
Endocrine & metabolic: Fluid and electrolyte imbalances (hypocalcemia, hypomagnesemia, hyponatremia), hyperglycemia
Gastrointestinal: Xerostomia
Hematologic: Rarely blood dyscrasias
Neuromuscular & skeletal: Numbness or paresthesia in hands, feet or lips, muscle cramps or pain, unusual weakness
Renal: Prerenal azotemia
Respiratory: Shortness of breath
Miscellaneous: Increased thirst

Overdosage/Toxicology Symptoms of overdose include lethargy, diuresis, hypermotility, confusion, muscle weakness

Following GI decontamination, therapy is supportive with I.V. fluids, electrolytes, and I.V. pressors if needed

Drug Interactions

Decreased effect of oral hypoglycemics; decreased absorption with cholestyramine and colestipol

Increased effect with furosemide and other loop diuretics

Increased toxicity/levels of lithium; when given with digoxin, diuretic-induced hypokalemia increases the risk of digoxin toxicity

Mechanism of Action Diuretic effect is localized at the proximal segment of the distal tubule of the nephron; it does not appear to have significant effect on glomerular filtration rate nor renal blood flow; like other diuretics, it enhances sodium, chloride, and water excretion by interfering with the transport of sodium ions across the renal tubular epithelium

Pharmacodynamics/Kinetics

Absorption: Completely from GI tract
Plasma protein binding: 71% to 79%
Metabolism: Extensively in the liver
Half-life: 14-18 hours
Time to peak serum concentration: 2-2.5 hours
Elimination: ~60% of dose excreted in urine within 48 hours, ~16% to 23% excreted via bile in feces

Usual Dosage Adults: Oral: 2.5-5 mg/day. **Note:** There is little therapeutic benefit to increasing the dose >5 mg/day; there is, however, an increased risk of electrolyte disturbances.

Monitoring Parameters Blood pressure (both standing and sitting/supine), serum electrolytes, renal function, assess weight, I & O reports daily to determine fluid loss

Patient Information May be taken with food or milk; take early in day to avoid nocturia; take the last dose of multiple doses no later than 6 PM unless instructed otherwise. A few people who take this medication become more sensitive to sunlight and may experience skin rash, redness, itching, or severe sunburn, especially if sun block SPF ≥15 is not used on exposed skin areas.

Nursing Implications Take blood pressure with patient lying down and standing; may increase serum glucose in diabetic patients

Dosage Forms Tablet: 1.25 mg, 2.5 mg

Inderal® *see* Propranolol *on page 1067*

Inderal® LA *see* Propranolol *on page 1067*

Indinavir (in DIN a veer)

Related Information

Occupational Exposure to HIV *on page 1448*

Brand Names Crixivan®

Therapeutic Category Antiretroviral Agent; Antiviral Agent, Oral; Protease Inhibitor

Use Treatment of HIV infection, especially advanced disease; usually administered as part of a three-drug regimen (two nucleosides plus a protease inhibitor) or double therapy (one nucleoside plus a protease inhibitor)

Pregnancy Risk Factor C

Pregnancy/Breast-Feeding Implications

Administer during pregnancy only if benefits to mother outweigh risks to the fetus

HIV-infected mothers are discouraged from breast-feeding to decrease potential transmission of HIV

Contraindications Hypersensitivity to the drug or its components; avoid use with terfenadine, astemizole, cisapride, or benzodiazepines

Warnings/Precautions Use caution in patients with hepatic insufficiency; dosage reduction may be needed; nephrolithiasis may occur with use; if signs and symptoms of nephrolithiasis occur, interrupt therapy for 1-3 days; ensure adequate hydration

Adverse Reactions

1% to 10%:

Gastrointestinal: Mild elevation of indirect bilirubin (10%)

Renal: Kidney stones (2% to 3%)

Drug Interactions

Decreased effect: Concurrent use of rifampin and rifabutin may decrease the effectiveness of indinavir; dosage decreases of rifampin/rifabutin is recommended

Increased toxicity: Gastric pH is lowered and absorption may be decreased when didanosine and indinavir are taken <1 hour apart; a reduction of dose is often required when coadministered with ketoconazole; terfenadine, astemizole, cisapride, and benzodiazepines should be avoided with indinavir due to a potentially serious toxicity

Mechanism of Action Indinavir is a protease inhibitor which prevents cleavage of protein precursors essential for HIV infection of new cells and viral replication. Some patients with advanced HIV infection have significantly improved clinically with the use of a protease; resistant strains are cross-resistant to ritonavir and saquinavir.

Pharmacodynamics/Kinetics

Protein binding: 60% in the plasma

Metabolism: Hepatically metabolized to 7 metabolites

Bioavailability: Oral: Good; T_{max}: 0.8 ± 0.3 hour

Half-life: 1.8 ± 0.4 hour

Elimination: In feces and urine

Usual Dosage Adults: Oral: 800 mg every 8 hours

Dosage adjustment in hepatic impairment: 600 mg every 8 hours with mild/medium impairment due to cirrhosis or with ketoconazole coadministration

Monitoring Parameters Signs of infection

Patient Information Drink at least 48 oz of water daily; take the drug with water, 1 hour before or 2 hours after a meal

Nursing Implications Administer around-the-clock to avoid significant fluctuation in serum levels; administer with plenty of water

Additional Information One study of previously untreated patients with a mean CD4-cell count of 250 cell/mm³ found that indinavir plus zidovudine lowered serum HIV below detectable levels in 56% of 52 patients treated for 24 weeks.

(Continued)

Indinavir *(Continued)*

Other studies show similar results. Indinavir alone has suppressed serum HIV below detectable levels in 40% to 60% of patients treated up to 48 weeks.

Dosage Forms Capsule: 400 mg

Indochron E-R® *see* Indomethacin *on this page*

Indocin® *see* Indomethacin *on this page*

Indocin® I.V. *see* Indomethacin *on this page*

Indocin® SR *see* Indomethacin *on this page*

Indometacin *see* Indomethacin *on this page*

Indomethacin (in doe METH a sin)

Related Information

Antacid Drug Interactions *on page 1388*

Nonsteroidal Anti-Inflammatory Agents Comparison *on page 1419*

Brand Names Indochron E-R®; Indocin®; Indocin® I.V.; Indocin® SR

Canadian/Mexican Brand Names Apo-Indomethacin® (Canada); Indocid® (Canada); Indocid® PDA (Canada); Indocid®-SR (Canada); Rhodacine® (Canada); Novo-Methacin® (Canada); Nu-Indo® (Canada); Pro-Indo® (Canada); Antalgin® Dialicels (Mexico); Indocid® (Mexico); Malival® y Malival® AP (Mexico)

Synonyms Indometacin; Indomethacin Sodium Trihydrate

Therapeutic Category Analgesic, Nonsteroidal Anti-inflammatory Drug; Anti-inflammatory Agent; Antipyretic; Nonsteroidal Anti-inflammatory Agent (NSAID), Oral; Nonsteroidal Anti-Inflammatory Agent (NSAID), Parenteral

Use Management of inflammatory diseases and rheumatoid disorders; moderate pain; acute gouty arthritis; I.V. form used as alternative to surgery for closure of patent ductus arteriosus in neonates

Pregnancy Risk Factor B (D if used longer than 48 hours or after 34-week gestation)

Contraindications Hypersensitivity to indomethacin, any component, aspirin, or other nonsteroidal anti-inflammatory drugs (NSAIDs); active GI bleeding, ulcer disease; premature neonates with necrotizing enterocolitis, impaired renal function, active bleeding, thrombocytopenia

Warnings/Precautions Use with caution in patients with cardiac dysfunction, hypertension, renal or hepatic impairment, epilepsy, history of GI bleeding, patients receiving anticoagulants, and for treatment of JRA in children (fatal hepatitis has been reported); may have adverse effects on fetus; may affect platelet and renal function in neonates; elderly are a high-risk population for adverse effects from nonsteroidal anti-inflammatory agents. As much as 60% of elderly can develop peptic ulceration and/or hemorrhage asymptomatically.

Use lowest effective dose for shortest period possible. Use of NSAIDs can compromise existing renal function especially when Cl_{cr} is <30 mL/minute.

CNS adverse effects such as confusion, agitation, and hallucination are generally seen in overdose or high-dose situations; but elderly may demonstrate these adverse effects at lower doses than younger adults.

Adverse Reactions

>10%:

- Central nervous system: Dizziness
- Dermatologic: Rash
- Gastrointestinal: Nausea, epigastric pain, abdominal pain, anorexia, GI bleeding, ulcers, perforation, abdominal cramps, heartburn, indigestion

1% to 10%:

- Central nervous system: Headache, nervousness
- Dermatologic: Itching
- Endocrine & metabolic: Fluid retention
- Gastrointestinal: Vomiting
- Otic: Tinnitus

<1%:

- Cardiovascular: Hypertension, congestive heart failure, arrhythmias, tachycardia
- Central nervous system: Somnolence, fatigue, depression, confusion, drowsiness, hallucinations, aseptic meningitis
- Dermatologic: Urticaria, erythema multiforme, toxic epidermal necrolysis, Stevens-Johnson syndrome, angioedema
- Endocrine & metabolic: Hyperkalemia, dilutional hyponatremia (I.V.), hypoglycemia (I.V.), polydipsia, hot flashes
- Gastrointestinal: Gastritis, GI ulceration
- Genitourinary: Cystitis, polyuria
- Hematologic: Hemolytic anemia, bone marrow suppression, agranulocytosis, thrombocytopenia, inhibition of platelet aggregation, anemia, leukopenia
- Hepatic: Hepatitis
- Neuromuscular & skeletal: Peripheral neuropathy

Ocular: Corneal opacities, blurred vision, conjunctivitis, dry eyes, toxic amblyopia
Otic: Decreased hearing
Renal: Oliguria, renal failure
Respiratory: Shortness of breath, allergic rhinitis, epistaxis
Miscellaneous: Hypersensitivity reactions

Overdosage/Toxicology Symptoms of overdose include drowsiness, lethargy, nausea, vomiting, seizures, paresthesia, headache, dizziness, GI bleeding, cerebral edema, tinnitus, leukocytosis, renal failure

Management of a nonsteroidal anti-inflammatory drug (NSAID) intoxication is primarily supportive and symptomatic. Fluid therapy is commonly effective in managing the hypotension that may occur following an acute NSAID overdose, except when this is due to an acute blood loss. Seizures tend to be very short-lived and often do not require drug treatment. Although, recurrent seizures should be treated with I.V. diazepam.

Drug Interactions

Decreased effect: May decrease antihypertensive effects of beta-blockers, hydralazine and captopril; aspirin may decrease antihypertensive and diuretic effects of furosemide and thiazides

Increased toxicity: May increase serum potassium with potassium-sparing diuretics; probenecid may increase indomethacin serum concentrations; other NSAIDs may increase GI adverse effects; may increase nephrotoxicity of cyclosporin

Indomethacin may increase serum concentrations of digoxin, methotrexate, lithium, and aminoglycosides (reported with I.V. use in neonates)

Stability I.V.: Protect from light; not stable in alkaline solution; reconstitute just prior to administration; discard any unused portion; do not use preservative-containing diluents for reconstitution; suppositories do not require refrigeration

Mechanism of Action Inhibits prostaglandin synthesis by decreasing the activity of the enzyme, cyclo-oxygenase, which results in decreased formation of prostaglandin precursors

Pharmacodynamics/Kinetics

Onset of action: Within 30 minutes
Duration: 4-6 hours
Absorption: Prompt and extensive
Distribution: V_d: 0.34-1.57 L/kg; crosses the placenta; appears in breast milk
Protein binding: 90%
Metabolism: In the liver with significant enterohepatic cycling
Half-life: 4.5 hours, longer in neonates
Time to peak serum concentration: Oral: Within 3-4 hours
Elimination: Significant enterohepatic recycling; excreted in urine principally as glucuronide conjugates

Usual Dosage

Patent ductus arteriosus: Neonates: I.V.: Initial: 0.2 mg/kg; followed with: 2 doses of 0.1 mg/kg at 12- to 24-hour intervals if age <48 hours at time of first dose; 0.2 mg/kg 2 times if 2-7 days old at time of first dose; or 0.25 mg/kg 2 times if over 7 days at time of first dose; discontinue if significant adverse effects occur. Dose should be withheld if patient has anuria or oliguria.

Analgesia:

Children: Oral: Initial: 1-2 mg/kg/day in 2-4 divided doses; maximum: 4 mg/kg/day; not to exceed 150-200 mg/day

Adults: Oral, rectal: 25-50 mg/dose 2-3 times/day; maximum dose: 200 mg/day; extended release capsule should be given on a 1-2 times/day schedule

Dietary Considerations

Food: May decrease the rate but not the extent of oral absorption. Drug may cause GI upset, bleeding, ulceration, perforation; take with food or milk to minimize GI upset.

Potassium: Hyperkalemia has been reported. The elderly and those with renal insufficiency are at greatest risk. Monitor potassium serum concentration in those at greatest risk. Avoid salt substitutes.

Sodium: Hyponatremia from sodium retention. Suspect secondary to suppression of renal prostaglandin. Monitor serum concentration and fluid status. May need to restrict fluid.

Administration Administer orally with food, milk, or antacids to decrease GI adverse effects

I.V.: Administer over 20-30 minutes at a concentration of 0.5-1 mg/mL in preservative-free sterile water for injection or normal saline. Reconstitute I.V. formulation just prior to administration; discard any unused portion; avoid I.V. bolus administration or infusion via an umbilical catheter into vessels near the superior mesenteric artery as these may cause vasoconstriction and can compromise blood flow to the intestines. Do not administer intra-arterially.

Monitoring Parameters Monitor response (pain, range of motion, grip strength, mobility, ADL function), inflammation; observe for weight gain, edema; monitor

(Continued)

Indomethacin *(Continued)*

renal function (serum creatinine, BUN); observe for bleeding, bruising; evaluate gastrointestinal effects (abdominal pain, bleeding, dyspepsia); mental confusion, disorientation, CBC, liver function tests

Test Interactions Positive Coombs' [direct]; ↑ sodium, ↑ chloride, ↑ bleeding time

Patient Information Take with food, milk, or with antacids; extended release capsules must be swallowed whole/intact, can cause dizziness or drowsiness

Nursing Implications Extended release capsules must be swallowed intact

Dosage Forms

Capsule: 25 mg, 50 mg
  Indocin®: 25 mg, 50 mg
Capsule, sustained release (Indocin® SR): 75 mg
Powder for injection, as sodium trihydrate (Indocin® I.V.): 1 mg
Suppository, rectal (Indocin®): 50 mg
Suspension, oral (Indocin®): 25 mg/5 mL (5 mL, 10 mL, 237 mL, 500 mL)

Indomethacin Sodium Trihydrate *see* Indomethacin *on page 656*

INF *see* Interferon Alfa-2b *on page 665*

INF-alpha 2 *see* Interferon Alfa-2b *on page 665*

Infanrix® *see* Diphtheria, Tetanus Toxoids, and Acellular Pertussis Vaccine *on page 403*

InFed™ *see* Iron Dextran Complex *on page 676*

Inflamase® *see* Prednisolone *on page 1037*

Inflamase® Mild *see* Prednisolone *on page 1037*

Influenza Virus Vaccine (in floo EN za VYE rus vak SEEN)

Related Information

Guidelines for the Prevention of Opportunistic Infections in Persons with HIV *on page 1457*
Immunization Guidelines *on page 1421*
Miscellaneous Vaccination Information *on page 1437*

Brand Names Flu-Imune®; Fluogen®; Fluzone®

Canadian/Mexican Brand Names Fluviral® (Canada)

Synonyms Influenza Virus Vaccine (inactivated whole-virus); Influenza Virus Vaccine (split-virus) Influenza Virus Vaccine (purified surface antigen)

Therapeutic Category Vaccine, Inactivated Virus

Use Provide active immunity to influenza virus strains contained in the vaccine; for high risk persons, previous year vaccines should not be to prevent present year influenza

Those at risk for influenza injection:
- Persons ≥65 years of age
- Institutionalized patients
- Persons of any age with chronic disorders of pulmonary and/or cardiovascular system
- Persons who have required medical follow-up following hospitalization for other chronic diseases such as diabetes, renal disease, immunodepressive disorders, etc
- Travelers, especially those at risk (above)

Pregnancy Risk Factor C

Contraindications Persons with allergy history to eggs or egg products, chicken, chicken feathers or chicken dander, hypersensitivity to thimerosal, influenza virus vaccine or any component, presence of acute respiratory disease or other active infections or illnesses, delay immunization in a patient with an active neurological disorder

Warnings/Precautions Waiting until the second or third trimester to vaccinate the pregnant woman with a high-risk condition may be reasonable. Antigenic response may not be as great as expected in patients requiring immunosuppressive drug; hypersensitivity reactions may occur; because of potential for febrile reactions, risks and benefits must carefully be considered in patients with history of febrile convulsions; influenza vaccines from previous seasons must not be used; patients with sulfite sensitivity may be affected by this product.

Adverse Reactions

1% to 10%:
  Central nervous system: Fever, malaise
  Local: Tenderness, redness, or induration at the site of injection

<1%:
  Central nervous system: Guillain-Barré syndrome, fever
  Dermatologic: Urticaria, angioedema
  Neuromuscular & skeletal: Myalgia
  Respiratory: Asthma

Miscellaneous: Anaphylactoid reactions (most likely to residual egg protein), allergic reactions

Drug Interactions

Decreased effect with immunosuppressive agents; do not administer within 7 days after administration of diphtheria and tetanus toxoids and pertussis vaccine adsorbed (DTP)

Increased effect/toxicity of theophylline and warfarin

Stability Refrigerate

Usual Dosage I.M.:

Children:

6-35 months: 1-2 doses of 0.25 mL with ≥4 weeks between doses and the last dose administered before December

3-8 years: 1-2 doses of 0.5 mL (in anterolateral aspect of thigh) with ≥4 weeks between doses and the last dose administered before December

Note: The split virus or purified surface antigen is recommended for children ≤12 years of age; if the child has received at least one dose of the 1978-79 or later vaccine, one dose is sufficient

Children ≥9 years and Adults: 0.5 mL each year of appropriate vaccine for the year, one dose is all that is necessary; administer in late fall to allow maximum titers to develop by peak epidemic periods usually occurring in early December

Administration Inspect for particulate matter and discoloration prior to administration; for I.M. administration only

Additional Information Pharmacies will stock the formulations(s) standardized according to the USPHS requirements for the season. Influenza vaccines from previous seasons must not be used. Federal law requires that the date of administration, the vaccine manufacturer, lot number of vaccine, and the administering person's name, title and address be entered into the patient's permanent medical record.

Dosage Forms Injection:

Purified surface antigen (Flu-Imune®): 5 mL

Split-virus (Fluogen®, Fluzone®): 0.5 mL, 5 mL

Whole-virus (Fluzone®): 5 mL

Influenza Virus Vaccine (inactivated whole-virus) *see* Influenza Virus Vaccine *on previous page*

Influenza Virus Vaccine (split-virus) Influenza Virus Vaccine (purified surface antigen) *see* Influenza Virus Vaccine *on previous page*

Inocor® *see* Amrinone *on page 88*

Insta-Char® [OTC] *see* Charcoal *on page 245*

Insulin Preparations (IN su lin prep a RAY shuns)

Related Information

Desensitization Protocols *on page 1496*

Diabetes Mellitus Treatment *on page 1530*

Brand Names Humulin® 50/50; Humulin® 70/30; Humulin® L; Humulin® N; Humulin® R; Humulin® U; Lente® Iletin® I; Lente® Iletin® II; Lente® Insulin; Lente® L; Novolin® 70/30; Novolin® L; Novolin® N; Novolin® R; NPH Iletin® I; NPH Insulin; NPH-N; Pork NPH Iletin® II; Pork Regular Iletin® II; Regular (Concentrated) Iletin® II U-500; Regular Iletin® I; Regular Insulin; Regular Purified Pork Insulin; Velosulin® Human

Canadian/Mexican Brand Names Insulina Lenta® (Mexico); Insulina NPH® (Mexico); Insulina Regular® (Mexico)

Therapeutic Category Antidiabetic Agent, Parenteral; Antidote, Hyperglycemia; Antihyperglycemic Agent

Use Treatment of insulin-dependent diabetes mellitus, also noninsulin-dependent diabetes mellitus unresponsive to treatment with diet and/or oral hypoglycemics; to assure proper utilization of glucose and reduce glucosuria in nondiabetic patients receiving parenteral nutrition whose glucosuria cannot be adequately controlled with infusion rate adjustments or those who require assistance in achieving optimal caloric intakes; hyperkalemia (use with glucose to shift potassium into cells to lower serum potassium levels)

Pregnancy Risk Factor B

Pregnancy/Breast-Feeding Implications

Clinical effects on the fetus: Does not cross the placenta. Insulin is the drug of choice for the control of diabetes mellitus during pregnancy.

Breast-feeding/lactation: No data on crossing into breast milk

Warnings/Precautions Any change of insulin should be made cautiously; changing manufacturers, type and/or method of manufacture, may result in the need for a change of dosage; human insulin differs from animal-source insulin; regular insulin is the only insulin to be used I.V.; hypoglycemia may result from increased work or exercise without eating

(Continued)

Insulin Preparations *(Continued)*

Adverse Reactions

1% to 10%:

Cardiovascular: Palpitation, tachycardia, pallor

Central nervous system: Fatigue, mental confusion, loss of consciousness, headache, hypothermia

Dermatologic: Urticaria, redness

Endocrine & metabolic: Hypoglycemia

Gastrointestinal: Hunger, nausea, numbness of mouth

Local: Itching, edema, stinging, or warmth at injection site, atrophy or hypertrophy of S.C. fat tissue

Neuromuscular & skeletal: Muscle weakness, paresthesia, tremors

Ocular: Transient presbyopia or blurred vision, blurred vision

Miscellaneous: Diaphoresis, anaphylaxis

Overdosage/Toxicology Symptoms of overdose include tachycardia, anxiety, hunger, tremors, pallor, headache, motor dysfunction, speech disturbances, sweating, palpitations, coma, death

Antidote is glucose and glucagon, if necessary

Drug Interactions See table.

Drug Interactions With Insulin Injection

Decrease Hypoglycemic Effect of Insulin	Increase Hypoglycemic Effect of Insulin
Contraceptives, oral	Alcohol
Corticosteroids	Alpha blockers
Dextrothyroxine	Anabolic steroids
Diltiazem	Beta-blockers*
Dobutamine	Clofibrate
Epinephrine	Fenfluramine
Smoking	Guanethidine
Thiazide diuretics	MAO inhibitors
Thyroid hormone	Pentamidine
Niacin	Phenylbutazone
	Salicylates
	Sulfinpyrazone
	Tetracyclines

*Nonselective beta-blockers may delay recovery from hypoglycemic episodes and mask signs/symptoms of hypoglycemia. Cardioselective agents may be alternatives.

Stability

Newer neutral formulation of insulin is stable at room temperature up to one month (studies indicate up to 24-30 months)

Freezing causes more damage to insulin than room temperatures up to 100°F

Avoid direct sunlight; for compatibility, see table.

Insulin

Insulin Preparations	Compatible Mixed With
Rapid-Acting	
Insulin injection (regular)	All
Prompt insulin zinc suspension (Semilente®)	Lente®
Intermediate-Acting	
Isophane insulin suspension (NPH)	Regular
Insulin zinc suspension (Lente®)	Regular Semilente®
Long-Acting	
Protamine zinc insulin suspension* (PZI)	Regular
Extended insulin zinc suspension (Ultralente®)	Regular Semilente®

When mixing with NPH insulin in any proportion, the excess protamine may combine with regular insulin and may reduce or delay activity of regular insulin (does not appear to be clinically significant); phosphate-buffered regular insulins bind with Lente® insulins forming short-acting insulin; excess protamine in PZI combines with regular insulin and prolongs its action, therefore, should not be mixed; administer as a separate injection

Stability of parenteral admixture of regular insulin at room temperature (25°C) and at refrigeration temperature (4°C): 24 hours

Standard diluent: 100 units/100 mL NS

Comments: All bags should be prepared fresh; tubing should be flushed 30 minutes prior to administration to allow adsorption as time permits

Mechanism of Action The principal hormone required for proper glucose utilization in normal metabolic processes; it is obtained from beef or pork pancreas or a biosynthetic process converting pork insulin to human insulin; insulins are categorized into 3 groups related to promptness, duration, and intensity of action

Pharmacodynamics/Kinetics

Onset and duration of hypoglycemic effects depend upon preparation administered. See table.

Pharmacokinetics/Pharmacodynamics: Onset and Duration of Hypoglycemic Effects Depend Upon Preparation Administered

	Onset (h)	Peak (h)	Duration (h)
Insulin, regular (Novolin® R)	½-1	2-3	5-7
Prompt insulin zinc suspension (Semilente®)	0.5-1	4-7	18-24
Insulin zinc suspension (NPH) (Novolin® N)	1-1½	4-12	18-24
Isophane insulin suspension (Lente®)	1-2½	8-12	18-24
Isophane insulin suspension and regular insulin injection (Novolin® 70/30)	½ (½)	4-8 (2-12)	24 (24)
Prompt zinc insulin suspension (PZI)	4-8	14-24	36
Extended insulin zinc suspension (Ultralente®)	4-8	16-18	>36

Onset and duration: Biosynthetic NPH human insulin shows a more rapid onset and shorter duration of action than corresponding porcine insulins; human insulin and purified porcine regular insulin are similarly efficacious following S.C. administration. The duration of action of highly purified porcine insulins is shorter than that of conventional insulin equivalents. Duration depends on type of preparation and route of administration as well as patient related variables. In general, the larger the dose of insulin, the longer the duration of activity.

Absorption: Biosynthetic regular human insulin is absorbed from the S.C. injection site more rapidly than insulins of animal origin (60-90 minutes peak vs 120-150 minutes peak respectively) and lowers the initial blood glucose much faster. Human Ultralente® insulin is absorbed about twice as quickly as its bovine equivalent, and bioavailability is also improved. Human Lente® insulin preparations are also absorbed more quickly than their animal equivalents.

Bioavailability: Medium-acting S.C. Lente®-type human insulins did not differ from the corresponding porcine insulins

Usual Dosage Dose requires continuous medical supervision; may administer I.V. (regular), I.M., S.C.

Diabetes mellitus:

Children and Adults: 0.5-1 unit/kg/day in divided doses

Adolescents (growth spurts): 0.8-1.2 units/kg/day in divided doses

Adjust dose to maintain premeal and bedtime blood glucose of 80-140 mg/dL (children <5 years: 100-200 mg/dL)

Hyperkalemia: Administer calcium gluconate and $NaHCO_3$ first then 50% dextrose at 0.5-1 mL/kg and insulin 1 unit for every 4-5 g dextrose given

Diabetic ketoacidosis: Children and Adults: I.V. loading dose: 0.1 unit/kg, then maintenance continuous infusion: 0.1 unit/kg/hour (range: 0.05-0.2 units/kg/hour depending upon the rate of decrease of serum glucose - too rapid decrease of serum glucose may lead to cerebral edema).

Optimum rate of decrease (serum glucose): 80-100 mg/dL/hour

Note: Newly diagnosed patients with IDDM presenting in DKA and patients with blood sugars <800 mg/dL may be relatively "sensitive" to insulin and should receive loading and initial maintenance doses approximately ½ of those indicated above.

Dosing adjustment in renal impairment (regular):

Cl_{cr} 10-50 mL/minute: Administer at 75% of normal dose

Cl_{cr} <10 mL/minute: Administer at 25% to 50% of normal dose and monitor glucose closely

Hemodialysis: Because of a large molecular weight (6,000 daltons), insulin is not significantly removed by either peritoneal or hemodialysis

Supplemental dose is not necessary

Peritoneal dialysis: Supplemental dose is not necessary

(Continued)

Insulin Preparations *(Continued)*

Continuous arterio-venous or veno-venous hemofiltration effects: Supplemental dose is not necessary

Dietary Considerations

Alcohol: Increase in hypoglycemic effect of insulin; monitor blood glucose concentration; avoid or limit use

Food:

Potassium: Shifts potassium from extracellular to intracellular space. Decreases potassium serum concentration; monitor potassium serum concentration.

Sodium: SIADH; water retention and dilutional hyponatremia may occur. Patients at greatest risk are those with CHF or hepatic cirrhosis. Monitor sodium serum concentration and fluid status.

Administration

Regular insulin may be administered by S.C., I.M., or I.V. routes

S.C. administration is usually made into the thighs, arms, buttocks, or abdomen, with sites rotated

When mixing regular insulin with other preparations of insulin, regular insulin should be drawn into syringe first

I.V. administration (requires use of an infusion pump): **Only regular insulin** may be administered I.V.

I.V. infusions: To minimize adsorption problems to I.V. solution bag:

If new tubing is **not** needed: Wait a minimum of 30 minutes between the preparation of the solution and the initiation of the infusion

If new tubing is needed: After receiving the insulin drip solution, the administration set should be attached to the I.V. container and the line should be flushed with the insulin solution. The nurse should then wait 30 minutes, then flush the line again with the insulin solution prior to initiating the infusion

If insulin is required prior to the availability of the insulin drip, regular insulin should be administered by I.V. push injection

Because of adsorption, the actual amount of insulin being administered could be substantially less than the apparent amount. Therefore, adjustment of the insulin drip rate should be based on effect and not solely on the apparent insulin dose. Furthermore, the apparent dose should not be used as the basis for determining the subsequent insulin dose upon discontinuing the insulin drip. Dose requires continuous medical supervision.

To be ordered as units/hour

Example: Standard diluent of regular insulin only: 100 units/100 mL NS (can be given as a more diluted solution, ie, 100 units/250 mL NS)

Insulin rate of infusion (100 units regular/100 mL NS)

1 unit/hour: 1 mL/hour
2 units/hour: 2 mL/hour
3 units/hour: 3 mL/hour
4 units/hour: 4 mL/hour
5 units/hour: 5 mL/hour, etc

Monitoring Parameters Urine sugar and acetone, serum glucose, electrolytes

Reference Range

Therapeutic, serum insulin (fasting): 5-20 µIU/mL (SI: 35-145 pmol/L)

Glucose, fasting:

Newborns: 60-110 mg/dL
Adults: 60-110 mg/dL
Elderly: 100-180 mg/dL

Patient Information Do not change insulins without physician's approval; titrate vials to mix, do not shake; store in a cool place; when mixing insulins, draw up regular insulin into syringe first and use as soon as possible after mixing. Patients must be counseled by someone experienced in diabetes education, signs and symptoms of hyper- and hypoglycemia, exercise and diet, blood glucose monitoring, and other related topics.

Nursing Implications Patients using human insulin may be less likely to recognize hypoglycemia than if they use pork insulin, patients on pork insulin that have low blood sugar exhibit hunger and sweating; regular insulin is the only form for I.V. use. Patients who are unable to accurately draw up their dose will need assistance such as prefilled syringes.

Additional Information The term "purified" refers to insulin preparations containing no more than 10 ppm proinsulin (purified and human insulins are less immunogenic)

Dosage Forms All insulins are 100 units/mL (10 mL) except where indicated:

RAPID ACTING:

Insulin lispro rDNA origin: Humalog® [*Lilly*] (1.5 mL, 10 mL)

Insulin injection (Regular Insulin)

Beef and pork: Regular Iletin® I [*Lilly*]

Human:
rDNA: Humulin® R [*Lilly*], Novolin® R [*Novo Nordisk*]
Semisynthetic: Velosulin® Human [*Novo Nordisk*]
Pork: Regular Insulin [*Novo Nordisk*]
Purified pork:
Pork Regular Iletin® II [*Lilly*], Regular Purified Pork Insulin [*Novo Nordisk*]
Regular (concentrated) Iletin® II U-500 (*Lilly*): 500 units/mL

INTERMEDIATE-ACTING:
Insulin zinc suspension (Lente)
Beef and pork: Lente® Iletin® I [*Lilly*]
Human, rDNA: Humulin® L [*Lilly*], Novolin® L [*Novo Nordisk*]
Purified pork: Lente® Iletin® II [*Lilly*], Lente® L [*Novo Nordisk*]

Isophane insulin suspension (NPH)
Beef and pork: NPH Iletin® I [*Lilly*]
Human, rDNA: Humulin® N [*Lilly*], Novolin® N [*Novo Nordisk*]
Purified pork: Pork NPH Iletin® II [*Lilly*], NPH-N [*Novo Nordisk*]

LONG-ACTING:
Insulin zinc suspension, extended (Ultralente®)
Human, rDNA: Humulin® U [Lilly]

COMBINATIONS:
Isophane insulin suspension and insulin injection
Isophane insulin suspension (50%) and insulin injection (50%) human (rDNA): Humulin® 50/50 [*Lilly*]
Isophane insulin suspension (70%) and insulin injection (30%) human (rDNA): Humulin® 70/30 [*Lilly*], Novolin® 70/30 [*Novo Nordisk*]

Intal® Inhalation Capsule *see* Cromolyn Sodium *on page 317*
Intal® Nebulizer Solution *see* Cromolyn Sodium *on page 317*
Intal® Oral Inhaler *see* Cromolyn Sodium *on page 317*
α-2-interferon *see* Interferon Alfa-2b *on page 665*

Interferon Alfa-2a (in ter FEER on AL fa too aye)

Related Information
Toxicities of Chemotherapeutic Agents *on page 1382*

Brand Names Roferon-A®

Synonyms IFLrA; IFN; rIFN-A

Therapeutic Category Biological Response Modulator; Interferon

Use FDA approved: Patients >18 years of age: Hairy cell leukemia, AIDS-related Kaposi's sarcoma, chronic myelogenous leukemia (CML), Chronic Hepatitis C, adjuvant treatment to surgery for primary or recurrent malignant melanoma; multiple unlabeled uses; indications and dosage regimens are specific for a particular brand of interferon

Pregnancy Risk Factor C

Contraindications Hypersensitivity to alfa-2a interferon or any component of the product

Warnings/Precautions The U.S. Food and Drug Administration (FDA) currently recommends that procedures for proper handling and disposal of antineoplastic agents be considered. Use with caution in patients with seizure disorders, brain metastases, compromised CNS, multiple sclerosis, and patients with pre-existing cardiac disease, severe renal or hepatic impairment, or myelosuppression; safety and efficacy in children <18 years of age have not been established. Higher doses in the elderly or in malignancies other than hairy cell leukemia may result in severe obtundation.

Adverse Reactions
>10%:
Central nervous system: Dizziness, fatigue, malaise, fever (usually within 4-6 hours), chills
Dermatologic: Rash
Gastrointestinal: Xerostomia, nausea, vomiting, diarrhea, abdominal cramps, weight loss, metallic taste
Hematologic: Mildly myelosuppressive and well tolerated if used without adjunct antineoplastic agents; thrombocytosis has been reported, leukopenia (mainly neutropenia), anemia, thrombocytopenia, decreased hemoglobin, hematocrit, platelets
Myelosuppressive:
WBC: Mild
Platelets: Mild
Onset (days): 7-10
Nadir (days): 14
Recovery (days): 21
Neuromuscular & skeletal: Rigors, arthralgia
Miscellaneous: Flu-like syndrome, diaphoresis

(Continued)

Interferon Alfa-2a *(Continued)*

1% to 10%:
- Central nervous system: Headache, delirium, somnolence, neurotoxicity
- Dermatologic: Alopecia, dry skin
- Gastrointestinal: Anorexia, stomatitis
- Hepatic: Hepatotoxicity
- Neuromuscular & skeletal: Peripheral neuropathy, leg cramps
- Ocular: Blurred vision
- Miscellaneous: Diaphoresis

<1%:
- Cardiovascular: Tachycardia, arrhythmias, chest pain, hypotension, SVT, edema
- Central nervous system: Confusion, sensory neuropathy, psychiatric effects, EEG abnormalities, depression
- Endocrine & metabolic: Hypothyroidism, increased uric acid level
- Gastrointestinal: Change in taste
- Hepatic: Increased hepatic transaminase
- Neuromuscular & skeletal: Myalgia
- Ocular: Visual disturbances
- Renal: Proteinuria, increased BUN/creatinine
- Respiratory: Coughing, dyspnea, nasal congestion
- Miscellaneous: Neutralizing antibodies, local sensitivity to injection; usually patient can build up a tolerance to side effects

Overdosage/Toxicology Symptoms of overdose include CNS depression, obtundation, flu-like symptoms, myelosuppression; treatment is supportive

Drug Interactions

Increased effect:
- Cimetidine: May augment the antitumor effects of interferon in melanoma
- Theophylline: Clearance has been reported to be decreased in hepatitis patients receiving interferon

Increased toxicity: Vinblastine: Enhances interferon toxicity in several patients; increased incidence of paresthesia has also been noted

Stability Refrigerate (2°C to 8°C/36°F to 46°F); do not freeze; do not shake; after reconstitution, the solution is stable for 24 hours at room temperature and for 1 month when refrigerated

Pharmacodynamics/Kinetics

Absorption: Filtered and absorbed at the renal tubule

Distribution: The V_d of interferon is 31 L; but has been noted to be much greater (370-720 L) in leukemia patients receiving continuous infusion IFN; IFN does not penetrate the CSF

Metabolism: Majority of dose thought to be metabolized in the kidney

Bioavailability:
- I.M.: 83%
- S.C.: 90%

Half-life: Elimination:
- I.M., I.V.: 2 hours after administration
- S.C.: 3 hours

Time to peak serum concentration: I.M., S.C.: ~6-8 hours

Usual Dosage Refer to individual protocols

Infants and Children: Hemangiomas of infancy, pulmonary hemangiomatosis: S.C.: 1-3 million units/m²/day once daily

Adults >18 years: I.M., S.C.:
- Hairy cell leukemia:
  - Induction: 3 million units/day for 16-24 weeks.
  - Maintenance: 3 million units 3 times/week (may be treated for up to 20 consecutive weeks)
- AIDS-related Kaposi's sarcoma:
  - Induction: 36 million units/day for 10-12 weeks
  - Maintenance: 36 million units 3 times/week (may begin with dose escalation from 3-9-18 million units each day over 3 consecutive days followed by 36 million units/day for the remainder of the 10-12 weeks of induction)
  - If severe adverse reactions occur, modify dosage (50% reduction) or temporarily discontinue therapy until adverse reactions abate

Administration S.C. administration is suggested for those who are at risk for bleeding or are thrombocytopenic; rotate S.C. injection site; patient should be well hydrated

Monitoring Parameters Baseline chest x-ray, EKG, CBC with differential, liver function tests, electrolytes, platelets, weight; patients with pre-existing cardiac abnormalities, or in advanced stages of cancer should have EKGs taken before and during treatment

Patient Information Do not change brands as changes in dosage may result; possible mental status changes may occur while on therapy; report to physician any persistent or severe sore throat, fever, fatigue, unusual bleeding, or bruising; do not operate heavy machinery while on therapy since changes in mental status may occur

Nursing Implications Do not freeze or shake solution; a flu-like syndrome (fever, chills) occurs in the majority of patients 2-6 hours after a dose; pretreatment with nonsteroidal anti-inflammatory drug (NSAID) or acetaminophen can decrease fever and its severity and alleviate headache

Dosage Forms

Injection: 3 million units/mL (1 mL); 6 million units/mL (3 mL); 9 million units/mL (0.9 mL, 3 mL); 36 million units/mL (1 mL)

Powder for injection: 6 million units/mL when reconstituted

Interferon Alfa-2b (in ter FEER on AL fa too bee)

Related Information

Cancer Chemotherapy Regimens *on page 1351*
Toxicities of Chemotherapeutic Agents *on page 1382*

Brand Names Intron® A

Synonyms INF; INF-alpha 2; α-2-interferon; rLFN-α2

Therapeutic Category Biological Response Modulator; Interferon

Use FDA approved: Hairy-cell leukemia in patients >18 years, condylomata acuminata, AIDS-related Kaposi's sarcoma in patients >18 years, chronic non-A/non-B/C hepatitis in patients >18 years, chronic hepatitis B in patients >18 years (indications and dosage are specific for a particular brand of interferon)

Pregnancy Risk Factor C

Contraindications Known hypersensitivity to interferon alfa-2b or any components, patients with pre-existing thyroid disease uncontrolled by medication, coagulation disorders, diabetics prone to DKA, pulmonary disease

Warnings/Precautions The U.S. Food and Drug Administration (FDA) currently recommends that procedures for proper handling and disposal of antineoplastic agents be considered. Use with caution in patients with seizure disorders, brain metastases, compromised CNS, multiple sclerosis, and patients with pre-existing cardiac disease, severe renal or hepatic impairment, or myelosuppression; safety and efficacy in children <18 years has not been established. Higher doses in the elderly or in malignancies other than hairy cell leukemia may result in severe obtundation. A baseline ocular exam is recommended in patients with diabetes or hypertension.

Adverse Reactions

>10%:

- Central nervous system: Dizziness, fatigue, malaise, fever (usually within 4-6 hours), chills
- Dermatologic: Skin rash
- Gastrointestinal: Xerostomia, nausea, vomiting, diarrhea, dizziness, abdominal cramps, weight loss, metallic taste, anorexia
- Hematologic: Mildly myelosuppressive and well tolerated if used without adjunct antineoplastic agents; thrombocytosis has been reported, leukopenia (mainly neutropenia), anemia, thrombocytopenia, decreased hemoglobin, hematocrit, platelets
- Myelosuppressive:
  - WBC: Mild
  - Platelets: Mild
  - Onset (days): 7-10
  - Nadir (days): 14
  - Recovery (days): 21
- Neuromuscular & skeletal: Rigors, arthralgia
- Miscellaneous: Flu-like syndrome, diaphoresis

1% to 10%:

- Central nervous system: Neurotoxicity
- Dermatologic: Dry skin, alopecia
- Gastrointestinal: Stomatitis
- Hepatic: Hepatotoxicity
- Neuromuscular & skeletal: Peripheral neuropathy, leg cramps
- Ocular: Blurred vision
- Miscellaneous: Diaphoresis

<1%:

- Cardiovascular: Cardiotoxicity, tachycardia, arrhythmias, hypotension, SVT, arrhythmias, chest pain, edema
- Central nervous system: EEG abnormalities, confusion, sensory neuropathy, fever, headache, psychiatric effects, delirium, somnolence, chills
- Dermatologic: Partial alopecia, rash
- Endocrine & metabolic: Increased uric acid level, hypothyroidism
- Gastrointestinal: Change in taste
- Hematologic: Decreased hemoglobin, hematocrit, platelets
- Hepatic: Increased hepatic transaminase, increased ALT and AST

(Continued)

Interferon Alfa-2b *(Continued)*

Local: Sensitivity to injection
Neuromuscular & skeletal: Myalgia, rigors
Ocular: Visual disturbances, blurred vision
Renal: Proteinuria, increased creatinine, increased BUN
Respiratory: Coughing, dyspnea, nasal congestion
Miscellaneous: Neutralizing antibodies; usually patient can build up a tolerance to side effects

Overdosage/Toxicology Symptoms of overdose include CNS depression, obtundation, flu-like symptoms, myelosuppression; treatment is supportive

Drug Interactions

Increased effect: Cimetidine: May augment the antitumor effects of interferon in melanoma

Increased toxicity:

Theophylline: Clearance has been reported to be ↓ in hepatitis patients receiving interferon

Vinblastine: Enhances interferon toxicity in several patients; ↑ incidence of paresthesia has also been noted

Zidovudine: Increased myelosuppression

Stability

Store intact vials at refrigeration (2°C to 8°C)

Reconstitute vials with diluent; solution is stable for 30 days under refrigeration (2°C to 8°C)

Standard I.M./S.C. dilution:

Dose/syringe or dispense vial to floor

Solution is stable for 7 days at room temperature and 30 days under refrigeration (2°C to 8°C)

Mechanism of Action Alpha interferons are a family of proteins, produced by nucleated cells, that have antiviral, antiproliferative, and immune-regulating activity. There are 16 known subtypes of alpha interferons. Interferons interact with cells through high affinity cell surface receptors. Following activation, multiple effects can be detected including induction of gene transcription. Inhibits cellular growth, alters the state of cellular differentiation, interferes with oncogene expression, alters cell surface antigen expression, increases phagocytic activity of macrophages, and augments cytotoxicity of lymphocytes for target cells

Pharmacodynamics/Kinetics

Absorption: Filtered and absorbed at the renal tubule

Distribution: The V_d of interferon is 31 L; but has been noted to be much greater (370-720 L) in leukemia patients receiving continuous infusion IFN; IFN does not penetrate the CSF

Metabolism: Majority of dose thought to be metabolized in the kidney

Bioavailability:

I.M.: 83%

S.C.: 90%

Half-life: Elimination:

I.M., I.V.: 2 hours

S.C.: 3 hours

Time to peak serum concentration: I.M., S.C.: ~6-8 hours

Usual Dosage Adults (refer to individual protocols):

Hairy cell leukemia: I.M., S.C.: 2 million units/m² 3 times/week for 2 to ≥6 months of therapy

AIDS-related Kaposi's sarcoma: I.M., S.C. (use 50 million IU vial): 30 million units/m² 3 times/week

Condylomata acuminata: Intralesionally (use 10 million IU vial): 1 million units/lesion 3 times/week for 4-8 weeks; not to exceed 5 million units per treatment (maximum: 5 lesions at one time)

Chronic hepatitis C (non-A/non-B): I.M., S.C.: 3 million units 3 times/week for approximately a 6-month course

Chronic hepatitis B: I.M., S.C.: 5 million IU/day or 10 million IU 3 times/week for 16 weeks; if severe adverse reactions occur, reduce dosage 50% or temporarily discontinue therapy until adverse reactions abate; when platelet/granulocyte count returns to normal, reinstitute therapy

Hemodialysis: Supplemental dose is not necessary

Peritoneal dialysis: Supplemental dose is not necessary

Monitoring Parameters Baseline chest x-ray, EKG, CBC with differential, liver function tests, electrolytes, thyroid function tests, platelets, weight; patients with pre-existing cardiac abnormalities, or in advanced stages of cancer should have EKGs taken before and during treatment

Patient Information Do not change brands of interferon as changes in dosage may result; do not operate heavy machinery while on therapy since changes in mental status may occur; report to physician any persistent or severe sore throat, fever, fatigue, unusual bleeding, or bruising

Nursing Implications Use acetaminophen to prevent or partially alleviate headache and fever; do not use 3, 5, 18, and 25 million unit strengths intralesionally, solutions are hypertonic; 50 million unit strength is not for use in condylomata, hairy cell leukemia, or chronic hepatitis.

Dosage Forms Powder for injection, lyophilized: 3 million units, 5 million units, 10 million units, 18 million units, 25 million units, 50 million units

Interferon Alfa-n3 (in ter FEER on AL fa en three)

Related Information

Toxicities of Chemotherapeutic Agents *on page 1382*

Brand Names Alferon® N

Therapeutic Category Interferon

Use FDA approved (Patients ≥18 years of age): Condylomata acuminata, intralesional treatment of refractory or recurring genital or venereal warts; useful in patients who do not respond or are not candidates for usual treatments; indications and dosage regimens are specific for a particular brand of interferon

Pregnancy Risk Factor C

Contraindications Patients with known hypersensitivity to alpha interferon, mouse immunoglobulin, or any component of the product

Warnings/Precautions The U.S. Food and Drug Administration (FDA) currently recommends that procedures for proper handling and disposal of antineoplastic agents be considered. Use with caution in patients with seizure disorders, brain metastases, compromised CNS function, cardiac disease, severe renal or hepatic impairment, multiple sclerosis; safety and efficacy in children <18 years have not been established.

Adverse Reactions

>10%:

- Central nervous system: Fatigue, malaise, fever (usually within 4-6 hours), chills, dizziness
- Dermatologic: Rash
- Gastrointestinal: Xerostomia, nausea, vomiting, diarrhea, abdominal cramps, weight loss, metallic taste, anorexia
- Hematologic: Mildly myelosuppressive and well tolerated if used without adjunct antineoplastic agents; thrombocytosis has been reported, leukopenia (mainly neutropenia), anemia, thrombocytopenia, decreased hemoglobin, hematocrit, platelets
- Myelosuppressive:
  - WBC: Mild
  - Platelets: Mild
  - Onset (days): 7-10
  - Nadir (days): 14
  - Recovery (days): 21
- Neuromuscular & skeletal: Arthralgia, rigors
- Miscellaneous: Flu-like syndrome, diaphoresis

1% to 10%:

- Central nervous system: Headache, delirium, somnolence, neurotoxicity
- Dermatologic: Alopecia, dry skin
- Gastrointestinal: Stomatitis
- Hepatic: Hepatotoxicity
- Neuromuscular & skeletal: Peripheral neuropathy, leg cramps
- Ocular: Blurred vision
- Miscellaneous: Diaphoresis

<1%:

- Cardiovascular: Tachycardia, arrhythmias, chest pain, hypotension, SVT, edema
- Central nervous system: EEG abnormalities, confusion, sensory neuropathy, fever, confusion, psychiatric effects, depression
- Endocrine & metabolic: Hypothyroidism, increased uric acid level
- Gastrointestinal: Change in taste
- Hepatic: Increased hepatic transaminase, increased ALT and AST
- Local: Sensitivity to injection
- Neuromuscular & skeletal: Myalgia
- Ocular: Visual disturbances
- Renal: Proteinuria, increased BUN/creatinine
- Respiratory: Coughing, dyspnea, cough, nasal congestion
- Miscellaneous: Neutralizing antibodies, usually patient can build up a tolerance to side effects

Overdosage/Toxicology Symptoms of overdose include CNS depression, obtundation, flu-like symptoms, myelosuppression; treatment is supportive

(Continued)

Interferon Alfa-n3 *(Continued)*

Drug Interactions

Increased effect: Cimetidine: May augment the antitumor effects of interferon in melanoma

Increased toxicity:

Vinblastine: Enhances interferon toxicity in several patients; increased incidence of paresthesia has also been noted

Theophylline: Clearance has been reported to be decreased in hepatitis patients receiving interferon

Stability Store solution at 2°C to 8°C (36°F to 46°F); do not freeze or shake solution

Mechanism of Action Interferons interact with cells through high affinity cell surface receptors. Following activation, multiple effects can be detected including induction of gene transcription. Inhibits cellular growth, alters the state of cellular differentiation, interferes with oncogene expression, alters cell surface antigen expression, increases phagocytic activity of macrophages, and augments cytotoxicity of lymphocytes for target cells

Usual Dosage Adults: Inject 250,000 units (0.05 mL) in each wart twice weekly for a maximum of 8 weeks; therapy should not be repeated for at least 3 months after the initial 8-week course of therapy

Administration Inject into base of wart with a small 30-gauge needle

Patient Information Warts are highly contagious until they completely disappear, abstain from sexual activity or use barrier protection; inform nurse or physician if allergy exists to eggs, neomycin, mouse immunoglobulin, or to human interferon alpha; acetaminophen can be used to treat flu-like symptoms

Dosage Forms Injection: 5 million units (1 mL)

Interferon Beta-1a (in ter FEER on BAY ta won aye)

Brand Names Avonex®

Synonyms rIFN-b

Therapeutic Category Interferon

Use Treatment of relapsing forms of multiple sclerosis (MS); to slow the accumulation of physical disability and decrease the frequency of clinical exacerbations

Pregnancy Risk Factor C

Contraindications History of hypersensitivity to natural or recombinant interferon beta, human albumin, or any other component of the formulation

Warnings/Precautions Interferon beta-1a should be used with caution in patients with a history of depression, seizures, or cardiac disease; because its use has not been evaluated during lactation, its use in breast-feeding mothers may not be safe and should be warned against

Adverse Reactions 1% to 10%:

Cardiovascular: CHF (rare), tachycardia, syncope

Central nervous system: Headache, lethargy, depression, emotional lability, anxiety, suicidal ideations, somnolence, agitation, confusion

Dermatologic: Alopecia (rare)

Endocrine & metabolic: Hypocalcemia

Gastrointestinal: Nausea, anorexia, vomiting, diarrhea, chronic weight loss

Hematologic: Leukopenia, thrombocytopenia, anemia (frequent, dose-related, but not usually severe)

Hepatic: Elevated liver enzymes (mild, transient)

Local: Pain/redness at injection site (80%)

Neuromuscular & skeletal: Weakness

Ocular: Retinal toxicity/visual changes

Renal: Elevated BUN and S_{cr}

Miscellaneous: Flu-like syndrome (fever, nausea, malaise, myalgia) occurs in most patients, but is usually controlled by acetaminophen or NSAIDs; dose related abortifacient activity was reported in rhesus monkeys

Overdosage/Toxicology Symptoms of overdose include CNS depression, obtundation, flu-like symptoms, myelosuppression; treatment is supportive

Drug Interactions Decreases clearance of zidovudine thus increasing zidovudine toxicity

Stability The reconstituted product contains no preservative and is for single use only; discard unused portion; store unreconstituted vial or reconstituted vial at 2°C to 8°C (36°F to 46°F); use the reconstituted product within 6 hours

Mechanism of Action Interferon beta differs from naturally occurring human protein by a single amino acid substitution and the lack of carbohydrate side chains; alters the expression and response to surface antigens and can enhance immune cell activities. Properties of interferon beta that modify biologic responses are mediated by cell surface receptor interactions; mechanism in the treatment of MS is unknown.

Pharmacodynamics/Kinetics Limited data due to small doses used

Half-life: 10 hours

Time to peak serum concentration: 3-15 hours

Usual Dosage Adults >18 years: I.M.: 30 mcg once weekly

Administration Reconstitute with 1.1 mL of diluent and swirl gently to dissolve

Monitoring Parameters Hemoglobin, liver function, and blood chemistries

Patient Information Flu-like symptoms are not uncommon following initiation of therapy. Acetaminophen may reduce these symptoms. Do not change the dosage or schedule of administration without medical consultation. Report depression or suicide ideation to physicians. Avoid prolonged exposure to sunlight or sunlamps.

Nursing Implications Patient should be informed of possible side effects, especially depression, suicidal ideations, and the risk of abortion; flu-like symptoms such as chills, fever, malaise, diaphoresis, and myalgia are common

Dosage Forms Powder for injection, lyophilized: 33 mcg [6.6 million units]

Interferon Beta-1b (in ter FEER on BAY ta won bee)

Related Information

Toxicities of Chemotherapeutic Agents *on page 1382*

Brand Names Betaseron®

Synonyms rIFN-b

Therapeutic Category Interferon

Use Reduces the frequency of clinical exacerbations in ambulatory patients with relapsing-remitting multiple sclerosis (MS)

Pregnancy Risk Factor C

Contraindications Hypersensitivity to *E. coli* derived products, natural or recombinant interferon beta, albumin human or any other component of the formulation

Warnings/Precautions The safety and efficacy of interferon beta-1b in chronic progressive MS have not been evaluated; use with caution in women who are breast-feeding; flu-like symptoms complex (ie, myalgia, fever, chills, malaise, sweating) is reported in 53% of patients who receive interferon beta-1b

Adverse Reactions Due to the pivotal position of interferon in the immune system, toxicities can affect nearly every organ system: Injection site reactions, injection site necrosis, flu-like symptoms, menstrual disorders, depression (with suicidal ideations), somnolence, palpitations, peripheral vascular disorders, hypertension, blood dyscrasias, dyspnea, laryngitis, cystitis, gastrointestinal complaints, seizures, headache, and liver enzyme elevations

Overdosage/Toxicology Symptoms of overdose include CNS depression, obtundation, flu-like symptoms, myelosuppression; treatment is supportive

Stability Store solution at 2°C to 8°C (36°F to 46°F); do not freeze or shake solution; use product within 3 hours of reconstitution

Mechanism of Action Interferon beta-1b differs from naturally occurring human protein by a single amino acid substitution and the lack of carbohydrate side chains; alters the expression and response to surface antigens and can enhance immune cell activities. Properties of interferon beta-1b that modify biologic responses are mediated by cell surface receptor interactions; mechanism in the treatment of MS is unknown.

Usual Dosage S.C.:

Children <18 years: Not recommended

Adults >18 years: 0.25 mg (8 million units) every other day

Administration Withdraw 1 mL of reconstituted solution from the vial into a sterile syringe fitted with a 27-gauge needle and inject the solution subcutaneously; sites for self-injection include arms, abdomen, hips, and thighs

Monitoring Parameters Hemoglobin, liver function, and blood chemistries

Patient Information Instruct patients on self-injection technique and procedures. If possible, perform first injection under the supervision of an appropriately qualified healthcare professional. Injection site reactions may occur during therapy. They are usually transient and do not require discontinuation of therapy, but careful assessment of the nature and severity of all reported reactions. Flu-like symptoms are not uncommon following initiation of therapy. Acetaminophen may reduce these symptoms. Do not change the dosage or schedule of administration without medical consultation. Report depression or suicide ideation to physicians. Avoid prolonged exposure to sunlight or sunlamps.

Nursing Implications Patient should be informed of possible side effects, especially depression, suicidal ideations, and the risk of abortion; flu-like symptoms such as chills, fever, malaise, sweating, and myalgia are common

Additional Information May be available only in small supplies; for information on availability and distribution, call the patient information line at 800-580-3837

Dosage Forms Powder for injection, lyophilized: 0.3 mg [9.6 million units]

Interleukin-2 *see* Aldesleukin *on page 40*

Intralipid® *see* Fat Emulsion *on page 505*

Intravenous Fat Emulsion *see* Fat Emulsion *on page 505*

Intron® A *see* Interferon Alfa-2b *on page 665*

Intropin® *see* Dopamine *on page 417*

Inversine® *see* Mecamylamine *on page 766*

Invirase® *see* Saquinavir *on page 1124*

Iobid DM® *see* Guaifenesin and Dextromethorphan *on page 591*

Iodex® [OTC] *see* Povidone-Iodine *on page 1031*

Iodex-p® [OTC] *see* Povidone-Iodine *on page 1031*

Iodinated Glycerol (EYE oh di nay ted GLI ser ole)

Brand Names Iophen®; Organidin®; Par Glycerol®; R-Gen®

Therapeutic Category Expectorant

Use Mucolytic expectorant in adjunctive treatment of bronchitis, bronchial asthma, pulmonary emphysema, cystic fibrosis, or chronic sinusitis

Pregnancy Risk Factor X

Contraindications Hypersensitivity to inorganic iodides, iodinated glycerol, or any component; pregnancy, newborns

Warnings/Precautions Use with caution in patients with thyroid disease or renal impairment

Adverse Reactions

1% to 10%: Gastrointestinal: Diarrhea, nausea, vomiting

<1%:

- Central nervous system: Headache
- Dermatologic: Acne, dermatitis
- Endocrine & metabolic: Acute parotitis, thyroid gland enlargement
- Gastrointestinal: GI irritation
- Ocular: Eyelid edema
- Respiratory: Pulmonary edema
- Miscellaneous: Hypersensitivity

Overdosage/Toxicology Symptoms include metallic taste, swollen eyelids, sneezing, nausea, vomiting, diarrhea

Drug Interactions Increased toxicity: Disulfiram, metronidazole, procarbazine, MAO inhibitors, CNS depressants, lithium

Mechanism of Action Increases respiratory tract secretions by decreasing surface tension and thereby decreases the viscosity of mucus, which aids in removal of the mucus

Pharmacodynamics/Kinetics

Absorption: From GI tract

Distribution: Accumulates in the thyroid gland

Elimination: In urine

Usual Dosage Oral:

Children: Up to 30 mg 4 times/day

Adults: 60 mg 4 times/day

Test Interactions Thyroid function tests may be altered

Patient Information Take with a full glass of water; not for use in coughs lasting longer than 1 week or associated with a fever

Nursing Implications Administer with plenty of fluids; elixir contains 21.75% alcohol; watch for sedation; avoid elixir in children due to high alcohol content

Dosage Forms Organically bound iodine in brackets

Elixir: 60 mg/5 mL [30 mg/5 mL] (120 mL, 480 mL)

Solution: 50 mg/mL [25 mg/mL] (30 mL)

Tablet: 30 mg [15 mg]

Iodochlorhydroxyquin *see* Clioquinol *on page 291*

Iodoquinol (eye oh doe KWIN ole)

Brand Names Yodoxin®

Canadian/Mexican Brand Names Diodoquin® (Canada)

Synonyms Diiodohydroxyquin

Therapeutic Category Amebicide

Use Treatment of acute and chronic intestinal amebiasis; asymptomatic cyst passers; *Blastocystis hominis* infections; ineffective for amebic hepatitis or hepatic abscess

Pregnancy Risk Factor C

Contraindications Known hypersensitivity to iodine or iodoquinol; hepatic damage; pre-existing optic neuropathy

Warnings/Precautions Optic neuritis, optic atrophy, and peripheral neuropathy have occurred following prolonged use; avoid long-term therapy

Adverse Reactions

>10%: Gastrointestinal: Diarrhea, nausea, vomiting, stomach pain

1% to 10%:

- Central nervous system: Fever, chills, agitation, retrograde amnesia, headache
- Dermatologic: Rash, urticaria
- Endocrine & metabolic: Thyroid gland enlargement

Neuromuscular & skeletal: Peripheral neuropathy, weakness
Ocular: Optic neuritis, optic atrophy, visual impairment
Miscellaneous: Itching of rectal area

Overdosage/Toxicology Chronic overdose can result in vomiting, diarrhea, abdominal pain, metallic taste, paresthesias, paraplegia, and loss of vision; can lead to destruction of the long fibers of the spinal cord and optic nerve

Acute overdose: Delirium, stupor, coma, amnesia

Following GI decontamination, treatment is symptomatic

Mechanism of Action Contact amebicide that works in the lumen of the intestine by an unknown mechanism

Pharmacodynamics/Kinetics
Absorption: Oral: Poor and irregular
Metabolism: In the liver
Elimination: High percentage of the dose excreted in feces

Usual Dosage Oral:
Children: 30-40 mg/kg/day (maximum: 650 mg/dose) in 3 divided doses for 20 days; not to exceed 1.95 g/day
Adults: 650 mg 3 times/day after meals for 20 days; not to exceed 2 g/day

Monitoring Parameters Ophthalmologic exam

Test Interactions May increase protein-bound serum iodine concentrations reflecting a decrease in ^{131}I uptake; false-positive ferric chloride test for phenylketonuria

Patient Information May take with food or milk to reduce stomach upset; complete full course of therapy

Nursing Implications Tablets may be crushed and mixed with applesauce or chocolate syrup

Dosage Forms
Powder: 25 g
Tablet: 210 mg, 650 mg

Ionamin® *see* Phentermine *on page 987*
Iophen® *see* Iodinated Glycerol *on previous page*
Iopidine® *see* Apraclonidine *on page 98*
I-Paracaine® *see* Proparacaine *on page 1062*

Ipecac Syrup (IP e kak SIR up)

Therapeutic Category Antidote, Emetic

Use Treatment of acute oral drug overdosage and in certain poisonings

Pregnancy Risk Factor C

Contraindications Do not use in unconscious patients when time elapsed since exposure is >1 hour, patients with no gag reflex; following ingestion of strong bases or acids, volatile oils; when seizures are likely

Warnings/Precautions Do not confuse ipecac syrup with ipecac fluid extract, which is 14 times more potent; use with caution in patients with cardiovascular disease and bulimics; may not be effective in antiemetic overdose

Adverse Reactions
1% to 10%:
Cardiovascular: Cardiotoxicity
Central nervous system: Lethargy
Gastrointestinal: Protracted vomiting, diarrhea
Neuromuscular & skeletal: Myopathy

Overdosage/Toxicology Contains cardiotoxin; symptoms of overdose include tachycardia, CHF, atrial fibrillation, depressed myocardial contractility, myocarditis, diarrhea, persistent vomiting, hypotension

Treatment is activated charcoal, gastric lavage

Drug Interactions
Decreased effect: Activated charcoal, milk, carbonated beverages
Increased toxicity: Phenothiazines (chlorpromazine has been associated with serious dystonic reactions)

Mechanism of Action Irritates the gastric mucosa and stimulates the medullary chemoreceptor trigger zone to induce vomiting

Pharmacodynamics/Kinetics
Onset of action: Within 15-30 minutes
Duration: 20-25 minutes; can last longer, 60 minutes in some cases
Absorption: Significant amounts, mainly when it does not produce emesis
Elimination: Emetine (alkaloid component) may be detected in urine 60 days after excess dose or chronic use

Usual Dosage Oral:
Children:
6-12 months: 5-10 mL followed by 10-20 mL/kg of water; repeat dose one time if vomiting does not occur within 20 minutes

(Continued)

Ipecac Syrup *(Continued)*

1-12 years: 15 mL followed by 10-20 mL/kg of water; repeat dose one time if vomiting does not occur within 20 minutes

If emesis does not occur within 30 minutes after second dose, ipecac must be removed from stomach by gastric lavage

Adults: 15-30 mL followed by 200-300 mL of water; repeat dose one time if vomiting does not occur within 20 minutes

Patient Information Call Poison Center before administering. Patients should be kept active and moving following administration of ipecac; follow dose with 8 oz of water following initial episode; if vomiting, no food or liquids should be ingested for 1 hour

Nursing Implications Do **not** administer to unconscious patients; patients should be kept active and moving following administration of ipecac; if vomiting does not occur after second dose, gastric lavage may be considered to remove ingested substance

Dosage Forms Syrup: 70 mg/mL (15 mL, 30 mL, 473 mL, 4000 mL)

I-Pentolate® *see* Cyclopentolate *on page 323*

I-Phrine® Ophthalmic Solution *see* Phenylephrine *on page 989*

IPOL™ *see* Polio Vaccines *on page 1015*

Ipratropium (i pra TROE pee um)

Brand Names Atrovent®

Synonyms Ipratropium Bromide

Therapeutic Category Anticholinergic Agent; Bronchodilator

Use Anticholinergic bronchodilator in bronchospasm associated with COPD, bronchitis, and emphysema

Pregnancy Risk Factor B

Contraindications Hypersensitivity to atropine or its derivatives

Warnings/Precautions Not indicated for the initial treatment of acute episodes of bronchospasm; use with caution in patients with narrow-angle glaucoma, prostatic hypertrophy, or bladder neck obstruction; ipratropium has not been specifically studied in the elderly, but it is poorly absorbed from the airways and appears to be safe in this population.

Adverse Reactions Note: Ipratropium is poorly absorbed from the lung, so systemic effects are rare

>10%:

Central nervous system: Nervousness, dizziness, fatigue, headache
Gastrointestinal: Nausea, xerostomia, stomach upset
Respiratory: Cough

1% to 10%:

Cardiovascular: Palpitations, hypotension
Central nervous system: Insomnia
Genitourinary: Urinary retention
Neuromuscular & skeletal: Trembling
Ocular: Blurred vision
Respiratory: Nasal congestion

<1%:

Dermatologic: Rash, urticaria
Gastrointestinal: Stomatitis

Overdosage/Toxicology Symptoms of overdose include dry mouth, drying of respiratory secretions, cough, nausea, GI distress, blurred vision or impaired visual accommodation, headache, nervousness

Acute overdosage with ipratropium by inhalation is unlikely since it is so poorly absorbed. However, if poisoning occurs, it can be treated like any other anticholinergic toxicity. An anticholinergic overdose with severe life-threatening symptoms may be treated with physostigmine 1-2 mg (0.5 or 0.02 mg/kg for children) S.C. or I.V., slowly.

Drug Interactions

Increased effect with albuterol

Increased toxicity with anticholinergics or drugs with anticholinergic properties, dronabinol

Mechanism of Action Blocks the action of acetylcholine at parasympathetic sites in bronchial smooth muscle causing bronchodilation

Pharmacodynamics/Kinetics

Onset of bronchodilation: 1-3 minutes after administration
Peak effect: Within 1.5-2 hours
Duration: Up to 4-6 hours
Absorption: Not readily absorbed into the systemic circulation from the surface of the lung or from the GI tract
Distribution: Inhalation: 15% of dose reaches the lower airways

Usual Dosage

Children:

<2 years: Nebulization: 250 mcg 3 times/day

3-14 years: Metered dose inhaler: 1-2 inhalations 3 times/day, up to 6 inhalations/24 hours

Children >12 years and Adults: Nebulization: 500 mcg (1 unit-dose vial) administered 3-4 times/day by oral nebulization, with doses 6-8 hours apart

Children >14 years and Adults: Metered dose inhaler: 2 inhalations 4 times/day every 4-6 hours up to 12 inhalations in 24 hours

Patient Information

Inhaler directions: Effects are enhanced by breath-holding 10 seconds after inhalation; temporary blurred vision may occur if sprayed into eyes; shake canister well before each use of the inhaler; follow instructions for use accompanying the product; close eyes when administering ipratropium; wait at least one full minute between inhalations

Nebulizer directions: Twist open the top of one unit dose vial and squeeze the contents into the nebulizer reservoir. Connect the nebulizer reservoir to the mouthpiece or face mask. Connect the nebulizer to the compressor. Sit in a comfortable, upright position; place the mouthpiece in your mouth or put on the face mask and turn on the compressor. If a face mask is used, care should be taken to avoid leakage around the mask as temporary blurring of vision, precipitation or worsening of narrow-angle glaucoma, or eye pain may occur if the solution comes into direct contact with the eyes. Breathe as calmly, deeply, and evenly as possible until no more mist is formed in the nebulizer chamber (about 5-15 minutes). At this point, the treatment is finished. Clean the nebulizer.

Dosage Forms Solution, as bromide:

Inhalation: 18 mcg/actuation (14 g)

Nasal spray: 0.03% (30 mL)

Nebulizing: 0.02% (2.5 mL)

Ipratropium Bromide *see* Ipratropium *on previous page*

Iproveratril Hydrochloride *see* Verapamil *on page 1297*

Ircon® [OTC] *see* Ferrous Fumarate *on page 513*

Irinotecan (eye rye no TEE kan)

Brand Names Camptosar®

Synonyms Camptothecin-11; CPT-11

Therapeutic Category Antineoplastic Agent, Miscellaneous

Use FDA-approved: Treatment of metastatic carcinoma of the colon or rectum which has recurred or progressed following fluorouracil-based therapy

Unlabeled uses: Clinical trials are assessing efficacy in the treatment of lung cancer (small cell and nonsmall cell), cervical cancer, ovarian cancer, gastric cancer, leukemia, lymphoma

Pregnancy Risk Factor D

Contraindications Hypersensitivity to irinotecan or any component

Warnings/Precautions The U.S. Food and Drug Administration (FDA) currently recommends that procedures for proper handling and disposal of antineoplastic agents be considered

Irinotecan can induce both early and late forms of diarrhea that appear to be mediated by different mechanisms. Early diarrhea (during or within 24 hours of administration) is cholinergic in nature. It can be preceded by complaints of diaphoresis and abdominal cramping and may be ameliorated by the administration of atropine. The elderly (≥65 years of age) are at particular risk for diarrhea. Late diarrhea (occurring >24 hours after administration) can be prolonged and may lead to dehydration and electrolyte imbalance, and can be life-threatening. Late diarrhea should be treated promptly with loperamide. If grade 3 diarrhea (7-9 stools daily, incontinence, or severe cramping) or grade 4 diarrhea (≥10 stools daily, grossly bloody stool, or need for parenteral support), the administration of irinotecan should be delayed until the patient recovers and subsequent doses should be decreased.

Early diarrhea treatment: 0.25-1 mg of intravenous atropine should be considered (unless clinically contraindicated) in patients experiencing diaphoresis, abdominal cramping, or early diarrhea

Late diarrhea treatment: High-dose loperamide: Oral: 4 mg at the first onset of late diarrhea and then 2 mg every 2 hours until the patient is diarrhea-free for at least 12 hours. During the night, the patient may take 4 mg of loperamide every 4 hours. PREMEDICATION WITH LOPERAMIDE IS NOT RECOMMENDED.

Deaths due to sepsis following severe myelosuppression have been reported. Therapy should be discontinued if neutropenic fever occurs or if the absolute neutrophil count is <500/mm³. The dose of irinotecan should be reduced if there

(Continued)

Irinotecan *(Continued)*

is a clinically significant decrease in the total WBC (<200/mm^3), neutrophil count (<1000/mm^3), hemoglobin (<8 g/dL), or platelet count (<100,000/mm^3). Routine administration of a CSF is generally not necessary. Avoid extravasation

Adverse Reactions

>10%:

Cardiovascular: Vasodilation

Central nervous system: Insomnia, dizziness, fever (45.4%)

Dermatologic: Alopecia (60.5%), rash

Gastrointestinal: Irinotecan therapy may induce two different forms of diarrhea. Onset, symptoms, proposed mechanisms and treatment are different. Overall, 56.9% of patients treated experience abdominal pain and/or cramping during therapy. Anorexia, constipation, flatulence, stomatitis, and dyspepsia have also been reported.

Diarrhea: Dose-limiting toxicity with weekly dosing regimen

Early diarrhea (50.7% incidence) usually occurs during or within 24 hours of administration. May be accompanied by symptoms of cramping, vomiting, flushing, and diaphoresis. It is thought to be mediated by cholinergic effects which can be successfully managed with atropine (refer to Warnings/Precautions).

Late diarrhea (87.8% incidence) usually occurs >24 hours after treatment. National Cancer Institute (NCI) grade 3 or 4 diarrhea occurs in 30.6% of patients. Late diarrhea generally occurs with a median of 11 days after therapy and lasts approximately 3 days. Patients experiencing grade 3 or 4 diarrhea were noted to have symptoms a total of 7 days. Correlated with irinotecan or SN-38 levels in plasma and bile. Due to the duration, dehydration and electrolyte imbalances are significant clinical concerns. Loperamide therapy is recommended. The incidence of grade 3 or 4 late diarrhea is significantly higher in patients ≥ 65 years of age: close monitoring and prompt initiation of high-dose loperamide therapy is prudent (refer to Warnings/Precautions).

Emetic potential: Moderately high (86.2% incidence, however, only 12.5% grade 3 or 4 vomiting)

Hematologic: Myelosuppressive: Dose-limiting toxicity with 3 week dosing regimen

Grade 1-4 neutropenia occurred in 53.9% of patients. Patients who had previously received pelvic or abdominal radiation therapy were noted to have a significantly increased incidence of grade 3 or 4 neutropenia. White blood cell count nadir is 15 days after administration and is more frequent than thrombocytopenia. Recovery is usually within 24-28 days and cumulative toxicity has not been observed.

WBC: Mild to severe

Platelets: Mild

Onset (days): 10

Nadir (days): 14-16

Recovery (days): 21-28

Neuromuscular & skeletal: Weakness (75.7%)

Respiratory: Dyspnea (22%), coughing, rhinitis

Miscellaneous: Diaphoresis

1% to 10%: **Irritant chemotherapy**; thrombophlebitis has been reported

Overdosage/Toxicology Symptoms of overdose include bone marrow suppression, leukopenia, thrombocytopenia, nausea, vomiting; treatment is supportive

Drug Interactions

Increased toxicity: Prochlorperazine: Increased incidence of akathisia

Stability

Store intact vials of injection at room temperature and protected from light

Doses should be diluted in D_5W or NS to a final concentration of 0.12-1.1 mg/mL. Due to the relatively acidic pH, irinotecan appears to be more stable in D_5W than NS. D_5W (500 mL) is the preferred diluent for most doses

Standardized dose: Dose/500 mL D_5W

Stability at room temperature (15°C to 30°C/59°F to 86°F): 24 hours

Stability at refrigeration (2°C to 8°C/36°F to 46°F): 48 hours

Standardized dose: Dose/500 mL NS

Stability at room temperature (15°C to 30°C/59°F to 86°F): 24 hours

Stability at refrigeration (2°C to 8°C/36°F to 46°F): NOT RECOMMENDED DUE TO THE OCCURRENCE OF VISIBLE PARTICULATES

Mechanism of Action Irinotecan and its active metabolite (SN-38) bind reversibly to topoisomerase I and stabilize the cleavable complex so that religation of the cleaved DNA strand cannot occur. This results in the accumulation of cleavable complexes and single-strand DNA breaks. This interaction results in double-stranded DNA breaks and cell death consistent with S-phase cell cycle specificity.

Pharmacodynamics/Kinetics

Distribution: Average V_d: 263 L/m²

Protein binding: 30% to 68%; SN-38 is highly protein bound (95%) predominately to albumin

Metabolism: Irinotecan is a water-soluble prodrug of SN-38, which is approximately 1,000 times the potency of the potency of irinotecan. In the liver, irinotecan undergoes metabolic conversion to the active metabolite SN-38; high interpatient variability.

Half-life: Terminal: Irinotecan = 10 hours; SN-38 = 10 hours

Elimination: Irinotecan is eliminated via biliary excretion, urinary excretion, and conversion to SN-38. SN-38 is eliminated via glucuronidation and biliary excretion.

Usual Dosage Refer to individual protocols

Adults: I.V.: Metastatic colon or rectal carcinoma:

Initial: 125 mg/m² I.V. over 90 minutes once weekly for 4 weeks.

After 2 weeks of rest, subsequent courses may be repeated every 6 weeks.

Note: It is recommended that new courses begin only after the granulocyte count recovers to ≥1,500/mm³, the platelet counts recovers to ≥100,000/mm³, and treatment-related diarrhea has fully resolved. Depending on the patient's ability to tolerate therapy, doses should be adjusted in increments of 25-50 mg/m². Irinotecan doses may range 50-150 mg/m². Treatment should be delayed 1-2 weeks to allow for recovery from treatment-related toxicities. If the patient has not recovered after a 2-week delay, consideration should be given to discontinuing irinotecan.

Dosage adjustment for toxicities: See table.

Recommended Irinotecan Dosage Modifications

Toxicity NCI Grade (Value)	During a Course of Therapy*	At the Start of the Next Courses of Therapy* (After Adequate Recovery), Compared to the Starting Dose in the Previous Courses
No toxicity	Maintain dose level	↑ 25 mg/m² up to a maximum dose of 150 mg/m²
Neutropenia		
1 (1500-1900/mm³)	Maintain dose level	Maintain dose level
2 (1000-1400/mm³)	↓ 25 mg/m²	Maintain dose level
3 (500-900/mm³)	Omit dose, then ↓ 25 mg/m² when resolved to ≤ grade 2	↓ 25 mg/m²
4 (<500/mm³)	Omit dose, then ↓ 50 mg/m² when resolved to ≤ grade 2	↓ 50 mg/m²
Neutropenic Fever (grade 4 neutropenia and ≥ grade 2 fever)	Omit dose then ↓ 50 mg/m² when resolved	↓ 50 mg/m²
Other hematologic toxicities	Dose modifications for leukopenia, thrombocytopenia, and anemia during a course of therapy and at the start of subsequent courses of therapy are also based on NCI toxicity criteria and are the same as recommended for neutropenia above.	
Diarrhea		
1 (2-3 stools/day > pretreatment)	Maintain dose level	Maintain dose level
2 (4-6 stools/day > pretreatment)	↓ 25 mg/m²	Maintain, if only grade 2 toxicity
3 (7-9 stools/day > pretreatment)	Omit dose, then ↓ 25 mg/m² when resolved to ≤ grade 2	↓ 25 mg/m², if only grade 3 toxicity
4 (≥10 stools/day > pretreatment)	Omit dose then ↓ 50 mg/m², when resolved to ≤ grade 2	↓ 50 mg/m²
Other nonhematologic toxicities		
1	Maintain dose level	Maintain dose level
2	↓ 25 mg/m²	↓ 25 mg/m²
3	Omit dose, then ↓ 25 mg/m² when resolved to ≤ grade 2	↓ 50 mg/m²
4	Omit dose, then ↓ 50 mg/m² when resolved to ≤ grade 2	↓ 50 mg/m²

*All dose modifications should be based on the worst preceding toxicity

Dosage adjustment in renal impairment: Effects have not been evaluated

(Continued)

Irinotecan *(Continued)*

Dosage adjustment in hepatic impairment:

AUC of irinotecan and SN-38 have been reported to be higher in patients with known hepatic tumor involvement. The manufacturer recommends that no change in dosage or administration be made for patients with liver metastases and normal hepatic function.

Use caution when treating patients with known hepatic dysfunction or hyperbilirubinemia

Administration Administer I.V. infusion over 90 minutes

Monitoring Parameters CBC with differential, platelet count, and hemoglobin with each dose

Patient Information

Patients and patients' caregivers should be informed of the expected toxic effects of irinotecan, particularly of its gastrointestinal manifestations, such as nausea, vomiting, and diarrhea

Each patient should be instructed to have loperamide readily available and to begin treatment for late diarrhea (occurring >24 hours after administration of irinotecan) at the first episode of poorly formed or loose stools or the earliest onset of bowel movements more frequent than normally expected for the patient. Refer to Warnings/Precautions.

The patient should also be instructed to notify the physician if diarrhea occurs. Premedication with loperamide is not recommended. The use of drugs with laxative properties should be avoided because of the potential for exacerbation of diarrhea. Patients should be advised to contact their physician to discuss any laxative use.

Patients should consult their physician if vomiting occurs, fever or evidence of infection develops, or if symptoms of dehydration, such as fainting, lightheadedness, or dizziness, are noted following therapy

Nursing Implications Monitor infusion site for signs of inflammation and avoid extravasation

Extravasation treatment: Flush the site with sterile water and apply ice

Dosage Forms Injection: 20 mg/mL (5 mL)

Iron Dextran Complex (EYE ern DEKS tran KOM pleks)

Related Information

Antacid Drug Interactions *on page 1388*

Brand Names Dexferrum®; InFed™

Therapeutic Category Iron Salt

Use Treatment of microcytic hypochromic anemia resulting from iron deficiency in whom oral administration is infeasible or ineffective

Pregnancy Risk Factor C

Contraindications Hypersensitivity to iron dextran, all anemias that are not involved with iron deficiency, hemochromatosis, hemolytic anemia

Warnings/Precautions Use with caution in patients with history of asthma, hepatic impairment, rheumatoid arthritis; not recommended in children <4 months of age; deaths associated with parenteral administration following anaphylactic-type reactions have been reported; use only in patients where the iron deficient state is not amenable to oral iron therapy. A test dose of 0.5 mL I.V. or I.M. should be given to observe for adverse reactions. Anemia in the elderly is often caused by "anemia of chronic disease" or associated with inflammation rather than blood loss. Iron stores are usually normal or increased, with a serum ferritin >50 ng/mL and a decreased total iron binding capacity. I.V. administration of iron dextran is often preferred over I.M. in the elderly secondary to a decreased muscle mass and the need for daily injections.

Adverse Reactions

Cardiovascular: Cardiovascular collapse, hypotension
Dermatologic: Urticaria
Hematologic: Leukocytosis

>10%:
- Cardiovascular: Flushing
- Central nervous system: Dizziness, fever, headache, pain
- Gastrointestinal: Nausea, vomiting, metallic taste
- Local: Staining of skin at the site of I.M. injection, phlebitis,
- Miscellaneous: Diaphoresis

1% to 10%:
- Gastrointestinal: Diarrhea
- Genitourinary: Discoloration of urine

<1%:
- Central nervous system: Chills
- Local: Phlebitis
- Neuromuscular & skeletal: Arthralgia
- Respiratory: Respiratory difficulty

Miscellaneous: Lymphadenopathy

Note: Diaphoresis, urticaria, arthralgia, fever, chills, dizziness, headache, and nausea may be delayed 24-48 hours after I.V. administration or 3-4 days after I.M. administration

Anaphylactoid reactions: Respiratory difficulties and cardiovascular collapse have been reported and occur most frequently within the first several minutes of administration

Overdosage/Toxicology Symptoms of overdose include erosion of GI mucosa, pulmonary edema, hyperthermia, convulsions, tachycardia, hepatic and renal impairment, coma, hematemesis, lethargy, tachycardia, acidosis, serum Fe level >300 mcg/mL requires treatment of overdose due to severe toxicity

Although rare, if a severe iron overdose (when the serum iron concentration exceeds the total iron-binding capacity) occurs, it may be treated with deferoxamine. Deferoxamine may be administered I.V. (80 mg/kg over 24 hours) or I.M. (40-90 mg/kg every 8 hours).

Drug Interactions Decreased effect with chloramphenicol

Stability Store at room temperature

Stability of parenteral admixture at room temperature (25°C): 3 months
Standard diluent: Dose/250-1000 mL NS
Minimum volume: 250 mL NS

Mechanism of Action The released iron, from the plasma, eventually replenishes the depleted iron stores in the bone marrow where it is incorporated into hemoglobin

Pharmacodynamics/Kinetics

Absorption:
- I.M.: 50% to 90% is promptly absorbed, the balance is slowly absorbed over month
- I.V.: Uptake of iron by the reticuloendothelial system appears to be constant at about 10-20 mg/hour

Elimination: By the reticuloendothelial system and excreted in the urine and feces (via bile)

Usual Dosage I.M. (Z-track method should be used for I.M. injection), I.V.:

A 0.5 mL test dose (0.25 mL in infants) should be given prior to starting iron dextran therapy; total dose should be divided into a daily schedule for I.M., total dose may be given as a single continuous infusion

Iron deficiency anemia: Dose (mL) = 0.0476 x wt (kg) x (normal hemoglobin - observed hemoglobin) + (1 mL/5 kg) to maximum of 14 mL for iron stores

Iron replacement therapy for blood loss: Replacement iron (mg) = blood loss (mL) x hematocrit

Maximum daily dose (can administer total dose at one time I.V.):
- Infants <5 kg: 25 mg iron (0.5 mL)
- Children:
  - 5-10 kg: 50 mg iron (1 mL)
  - 10-50 kg: 100 mg iron (2 mL)
- Adults >50 kg: 100 mg iron (2 mL)

Administration Use Z-track technique for I.M. administration (deep into the upper outer quadrant of buttock); may be administered I.V. bolus at rate ≤50 mg/minute or diluted in 250-1000 mL NS and infused over 1-6 hours; infuse initial 25 mL slowly, observe for allergic reactions; have epinephrine nearby

Monitoring Parameters Hemoglobin, hematocrit, reticulocyte count, serum ferritin

Reference Range

Hemoglobin 14.8 mg % (for weight >15 kg), hemoglobin 12.0 mg % (for weight <15 kg)
Serum iron: 40-160 μg/dL
Total iron binding capacity: 230-430 μg/dL
Transferrin: 204-360 mg/dL
Percent transferrin saturation: 20% to 50%

Test Interactions May cause falsely elevated values of serum bilirubin and falsely decreased values of serum calcium

Dosage Forms Injection: 50 mg/mL (2 mL, 10 mL)

ISD *see* Isosorbide Dinitrate *on page 684*

ISDN *see* Isosorbide Dinitrate *on page 684*

ISG *see* Immune Globulin, Intramuscular *on page 650*

Ismelin® *see* Guanethidine *on page 593*

ISMN *see* Isosorbide Mononitrate *on page 685*

ISMO™ *see* Isosorbide Mononitrate *on page 685*

Ismotic® *see* Isosorbide *on page 683*

Isoamyl Nitrite *see* Amyl Nitrite *on page 90*

Isobamate *see* Carisoprodol *on page 209*
Isocaine® HCl *see* Mepivacaine *on page 783*
Isodine® [OTC] *see* Povidone-Iodine *on page 1031*

Isoetharine (eye soe ETH a reen)

Brand Names Arm-a-Med® Isoetharine; Beta-2®; Bronkometer®; Bronkosol®; Dey-Lute® Isoetharine

Synonyms Isoetharine Hydrochloride; Isoetharine Mesylate

Therapeutic Category Adrenergic Agonist Agent; Bronchodilator; Sympathomimetic

Use Bronchodilator in bronchial asthma and for reversible bronchospasm occurring with bronchitis and emphysema

Pregnancy Risk Factor C

Contraindications Known hypersensitivity to isoetharine

Warnings/Precautions Excessive or prolonged use may result in decreased effectiveness

Adverse Reactions

1% to 10%:
- Cardiovascular: Tachycardia, hypertension, pounding heartbeat
- Central nervous system: Dizziness, lightheadedness, headache, nervousness, insomnia
- Gastrointestinal: Xerostomia, nausea, vomiting
- Neuromuscular & skeletal: Trembling, weakness

<1%: Respiratory: Paradoxical bronchospasm

Overdosage/Toxicology Symptoms of overdose include nausea, vomiting, hypertension, tremors; beta-adrenergic stimulation can cause increased heart rate, decreased blood pressure, and CNS excitation

Heart rate can be treated with beta-blockers, decreased blood pressure can be treated with pure alpha-adrenergic agents, diazepam 0.07 mg/kg can be used for excitation, seizures

Drug Interactions

Decreased effect with beta-blockers
Increased toxicity with other sympathomimetics (eg, epinephrine)

Stability Do not use if solution is discolored or a precipitation is present; **compatible** with sterile water, 0.45% sodium chloride, and 0.9% sodium chloride; protect from light

Mechanism of Action Relaxes bronchial smooth muscle by action on $beta_2$-receptors with very little effect on heart rate

Pharmacodynamics/Kinetics

Peak effect: Inhaler: Within 5-15 minutes
Duration: 1-4 hours
Metabolism: In many tissues including the liver and lungs
Elimination: Renal, primarily (90%) as metabolites

Usual Dosage Treatments are usually not repeated more often than every 4 hours, except in severe cases

Nebulizer: Children: 0.01 mL/kg; minimum dose 0.1 mL; maximum dose: 0.5 mL diluted in 2-3 mL normal saline
Inhalation: Oral: Adults: 1-2 inhalations every 4 hours as needed

Administration Administer around-the-clock to promote less variation in peak and trough serum levels

Monitoring Parameters Heart rate, blood pressure, respiratory rate

Test Interactions ↓ potassium (S)

Patient Information Do not exceed recommended dosage - excessive use may lead to adverse effects or loss of effectiveness. Shake canister well before use. Administer pressurized inhalation during the second half of inspiration, as the airways are open wider and the aerosol distribution is more extensive. If more than one inhalation per dose is necessary, wait at least 1 full minute between inhalations - second inhalation is best delivered after 10 minutes. May cause nervousness, restlessness, insomnia; if these effects continue after dosage reduction, notify physician. Also notify physician if palpitations, tachycardia, chest pain, muscle tremors, dizziness, headache, flushing, or if breathing difficulty persists.

Additional Information

Isoetharine hydrochloride: Arm-a-Med® isoetharine, Beta-2®, Bronkosol®, Dey-Lute® isoetharine
Isoetharine mesylate: Bronkometer®

Dosage Forms

Aerosol, oral, as mesylate: 340 mcg/metered spray
Solution, inhalation, as hydrochloride: 0.062% (4 mL); 0.08% (3.5 mL); 0.1% (2.5 mL, 5 mL); 0.125% (4 mL); 0.167% (3 mL); 0.17% (3 mL); 0.2% (2.5 mL);

0.25% (2 mL, 3.5 mL); 0.5% (0.5 mL); 1% (0.5 mL, 0.25 mL, 10 mL, 14 mL, 30 mL)

Isoetharine Hydrochloride *see* Isoetharine *on previous page*

Isoetharine Mesylate *see* Isoetharine *on previous page*

Isoflurophate (eye soe FLURE oh fate)

Related Information

Glaucoma Drug Therapy Comparison *on page 1410*

Brand Names Floropryl®

Synonyms DFP; Diisopropyl Fluorophosphate; Dyflos; Fluostigmin

Therapeutic Category Cholinergic Agent, Ophthalmic; Ophthalmic Agent, Miotic

Use Treat primary open-angle glaucoma and conditions that obstruct aqueous outflow and to treat accommodative convergent strabismus

Pregnancy Risk Factor X

Contraindications Active uveal inflammation, angle-closure (narrow-angle) glaucoma, known hypersensitivity to isoflurophate, pregnancy

Warnings/Precautions May retard corneal healing; because of the tendency to produce more severe adverse effects, use the lowest dose possible; keep frequency of use to a minimum to avoid cyst formation; some products may contain sulfites

Adverse Reactions

1% to 10%: Ocular: Stinging, burning eyes, myopia, visual blurring

<1%:

Cardiovascular: Bradycardia, hypotension, flushing
Gastrointestinal: Nausea, vomiting, diarrhea
Neuromuscular & skeletal: Muscle weakness
Ocular: Retinal detachment, browache, miosis, twitching eyelids, watering eyes
Respiratory: Dyspnea
Miscellaneous: Diaphoresis

Overdosage/Toxicology Symptoms of overdose include excessive salivation, urinary incontinence, dyspnea, diarrhea, profuse sweating

If systemic effects occur, administer parenteral atropine; for severe muscle weakness; pralidoxime may be used in addition to atropine

Drug Interactions Increased toxicity: Succinylcholine, systemic anticholinesterases, carbamate or organic phosphate insecticides, may decrease cholinesterase levels

Stability Protect from moisture, freezing, excessive heat

Mechanism of Action Cholinesterase inhibitor that causes contraction of the iris and ciliary muscles producing miosis, reduced intraocular pressure, and increased aqueous humor outflow

Pharmacodynamics/Kinetics

Peak IOP reduction: 24 hours
Duration: 1 week
Onset of miosis: Within 5-10 minutes
Duration: Up to 4 weeks

Usual Dosage Adults: Ophthalmic:

Glaucoma: Instill 0.25" strip in eye every 8-72 hours
Strabismus: Instill 0.25" strip to each eye every night for 2 weeks then reduce to 0.25" every other night to once weekly for 2 months

Patient Information Notify physician if abdominal cramps, diarrhea, or salivation occur

Nursing Implications Keep tube tightly closed to prevent absorption of moisture and loss of potency

Dosage Forms Ointment, ophthalmic: 0.025% in polyethylene mineral oil gel (3.5 g)

Isollyl Improved® *see* Butalbital Compound *on page 176*

Isoniazid (eye soe NYE a zid)

Related Information

Antacid Drug Interactions *on page 1388*
Guidelines for the Prevention of Opportunistic Infections in Persons with HIV *on page 1457*
Recommendations for Prophylaxis Against Tuberculosis *on page 1455*
Recommendations of the Advisory Council on the Elimination of Tuberculosis *on page 1483*

Brand Names Laniazid® Oral; Nydrazid® Injection

Canadian/Mexican Brand Names PMS-Isoniazid (Canada)

Synonyms Isonicotinic Acid Hydrazido

Therapeutic Category Antitubercular Agent

(Continued)

Isoniazid *(Continued)*

Use Treatment of susceptible tuberculosis infections and prophylactically to those individuals exposed to tuberculosis

Pregnancy Risk Factor C

Contraindications Acute liver disease; hypersensitivity to isoniazid or any component; previous history of hepatic damage during isoniazid therapy

Warnings/Precautions Use with caution in patients with renal impairment and chronic liver disease. Severe and sometimes fatal hepatitis may occur or develop even after many months of treatment; patients must report any prodromal symptoms of hepatitis, such as fatigue, weakness, malaise, anorexia, nausea, or vomiting. Children with low milk and low meat intake should receive concomitant pyridoxine therapy. Periodic ophthalmic examinations are recommended even when usual symptoms do not occur; pyridoxine is recommended in individuals likely to develop peripheral neuropathies; dose is 10-50 mg/day.

Adverse Reactions

>10%:

- Gastrointestinal: Loss of appetite, nausea, vomiting, stomach pain
- Hepatic: Hepatitis
- Neuromuscular & skeletal: Weakness, peripheral neuritis

1% to 10%:

- Central nervous system: Dizziness, slurred speech, lethargy
- Neuromuscular & skeletal: Hyperreflexia

<1%:

- Central nervous system: Fever, seizures, mental depression, psychosis
- Dermatologic: Rash
- Hematologic: Blood dyscrasias
- Neuromuscular & skeletal: Arthralgia
- Ocular: Blurred vision, loss of vision

Overdosage/Toxicology Symptoms of overdose include nausea, vomiting, slurred speech, dizziness, blurred vision, hallucinations, stupor, coma, intractable seizures, onset of metabolic acidosis is 30 minutes to 3 hours. Because of the severe morbidity and high mortality rates with isoniazid overdose, patients who are asymptomatic after an overdose, should be monitored for 4-6 hours.

Pyridoxine has been shown to be effective in the treatment of intoxication, especially when seizures occur. Pyridoxine I.V. is administered on a milligram to milligram dose. If the amount of isoniazid ingested is unknown, 5 g of pyridoxine should be given over 3-5 minutes and may be followed by an additional 5 g in 30 minutes. Treatment is supportive; may require airway protection, ventilation; diazepam for seizures, sodium bicarbonate for acidosis; forced diuresis and hemodialysis can result in more rapid removal.

Drug Interactions Inhibitor and inducer of cytochrome P-450 2E enzymes

Decreased effect/levels of isoniazid with aluminum salts

Increased toxicity/levels of oral anticoagulants, carbamazepines, cycloserine, hydantoins, hepatically metabolized benzodiazepines; reaction with disulfiram

Stability Protect oral dosage forms from light

Mechanism of Action Unknown, but may include the inhibition of myocolic acid synthesis resulting in disruption of the bacterial cell wall

Pharmacodynamics/Kinetics

Absorption: Oral, I.M.: Rapid and complete; rate can be slowed when orally administered with food

Distribution: Crosses the placenta; appears in breast milk; distributes into all body tissues and fluids including the CSF

Protein binding: 10% to 15%

Metabolism: By the liver with decay rate determined genetically by acetylation phenotype

Half-life:

- Fast acetylators: 30-100 minutes
- Slow acetylators: 2-5 hours; half-life may be prolonged in patients with impaired hepatic function or severe renal impairment

Time to peak serum concentration: Within 1-2 hours

Elimination: In urine (75% to 95%), feces, and saliva

Usual Dosage Oral, I.M. (recommendations often change due to resistant strains and newly developed information; consult *MMWR* for current CDC recommendations):

Children: 10-20 mg/kg/day in 1-2 divided doses (maximum: 300 mg total dose)

- Prophylaxis: 10 mg/kg/day given daily (up to 300 mg total dose) for 6 months

Adults: 5 mg/kg/day given daily (usual dose is 300 mg)

- Disseminated disease: 10 mg/kg/day in 1-2 divided doses
- Treatment should be continued for 9 months with rifampin or for 6 months with rifampin and pyrazinamide
- Prophylaxis: 300 mg/day given daily for 6 months

American Thoracic Society and CDC currently recommend twice weekly therapy as part of a short-course regimen which follows 1-2 months of daily treatment for uncomplicated pulmonary tuberculosis in compliant patients
Children: 20-40 mg/kg/dose (up to 900 mg) twice weekly
Adults: 15 mg/kg/dose (up to 900 mg) twice weekly

Dosing adjustment in hepatic impairment: Dose should be reduced in severe hepatic disease
Hemodialysis: Dialyzable (50% to 100%)

Monitoring Parameters Monitor transaminase levels at baseline 1, 3, 6, and 9 months

Reference Range Therapeutic: 1-7 μg/mL (SI: 7-51 μmol/L); Toxic: 20-710 μg/mL (SI: 146-5176 μmol/L)

Test Interactions False-positive urinary glucose with Clinitest®

Patient Information Report any prodromal symptoms of hepatitis (fatigue, weakness, nausea, vomiting, dark urine, or yellowing of eyes) or any burning, tingling, or numbness in the extremities

Dosage Forms
Injection: 100 mg/mL (10 mL)
Syrup (orange flavor): 50 mg/5 mL (473 mL)
Tablet: 50 mg, 100 mg, 300 mg

Isonicotinic Acid Hydrazide *see* Isoniazid *on page 679*

Isonipecaine Hydrochloride *see* Meperidine *on page 780*

Isoprenaline Hydrochloride *see* Isoproterenol *on this page*

Isoproterenol (eye soe proe TER e nole)

Related Information
Adrenergic Agonists, Cardiovascular Comparison *on page 1385*
Adult ACLS Algorithm, Bradycardia *on page 1514*
Cardiovascular Agents Comparison *on page 1405*

Brand Names Arm-a-Med® Isoproterenol; Dey-Dose® Isoproterenol; Dispos-a-Med® Isoproterenol; Isuprel®; Medihaler-Iso®; Norisodrine®

Synonyms Isoprenaline Hydrochloride; Isoproterenol Hydrochloride; Isoproterenol Sulfate

Therapeutic Category Adrenergic Agonist Agent; Bronchodilator; Sympathomimetic

Use Treatment of reversible airway obstruction as in asthma or COPD; used parenterally in ventricular arrhythmias due to A-V nodal block; hemodynamically compromised bradyarrhythmias or atropine-resistant bradyarrhythmias; temporary use in third degree A-V block until pacemaker insertion; low cardiac output; vasoconstrictive shock states

Pregnancy Risk Factor C

Contraindications Angina, pre-existing cardiac arrhythmias (ventricular); tachycardia or A-V block caused by cardiac glycoside intoxication; allergy to sulfites or isoproterenol or other sympathomimetic amines

Warnings/Precautions Elderly patients, diabetics, renal or cardiovascular disease, hyperthyroidism; excessive or prolonged use may result in decreased effectiveness

Adverse Reactions
>10%:
Central nervous system: Insomnia, restlessness
Gastrointestinal: Dry throat, xerostomia, discoloration of saliva (pinkish-red)
1% to 10%:
Cardiovascular: Flushing of the face or skin, ventricular arrhythmias, tachycardias, profound hypotension, hypertension
Central nervous system: Nervousness, anxiety, dizziness, headache, lightheadedness
Gastrointestinal: Vomiting, nausea
Neuromuscular & skeletal: Trembling, tremor, weakness
Miscellaneous: Diaphoresis
<1%:
Cardiovascular: Arrhythmias, chest pain
Respiratory: Paradoxical bronchospasm

Overdosage/Toxicology Symptoms of overdose include tremors, nausea, vomiting, hypotension; beta-adrenergic stimulation can cause increased heart rate, decreased blood pressure, and CNS excitation

Heart rate can be treated with beta-blockers, decreased blood pressure can be treated with pure alpha-adrenergic agents, diazepam 0.07 mg/kg can be used for excitation, seizures

Drug Interactions Increased toxicity: Sympathomimetic agents may cause headaches and elevate blood pressure; general anesthetics may cause arrhythmias
(Continued)

Isoproterenol *(Continued)*

Stability

Isoproterenol solution should be stored at room temperature; it should not be used if a color or precipitate is present

Exposure to air, light, or increased temperature may cause a pink to brownish pink color to develop

Stability of parenteral admixture at room temperature (25°C) or at refrigeration (4°C): 24 hours

Standard diluent: 2 mg/500 mL D_5W; 4 mg/500 mL D_5W

Minimum volume: 1 mg/100 mL D_5W

Incompatible with alkaline solutions, aminophylline and furosemide

Mechanism of Action Stimulates $beta_1$- and $beta_2$-receptors resulting in relaxation of bronchial, GI, and uterine smooth muscle, increased heart rate and contractility, vasodilation of peripheral vasculature

Pharmacodynamics/Kinetics

Onset of bronchodilation: Oral inhalation: Immediately

Time to peak serum concentration: Oral: Within 1-2 hours

Duration:

- Oral inhalation: 1 hour
- S.C.: Up to 2 hours

Metabolism: By conjugation in many tissues including the liver and lungs

Half-life: 2.5-5 minutes

Elimination: In urine principally as sulfate conjugates

Usual Dosage

Children:

- Bronchodilation: Inhalation: Metered dose inhaler: 1-2 metered doses up to 5 times/day
- Bronchodilation (using 1:200 inhalation solution) 0.01 mL/kg/dose every 4 hours as needed (maximum: 0.05 mL/dose) diluted with NS to 2 mL
- Sublingual: 5-10 mg every 3-4 hours, not to exceed 30 mg/day
- Cardiac arrhythmias: I.V.: Start 0.1 mcg/kg/minute (usual effective dose 0.2-2 mcg/kg/minute)

Adults:

- Bronchodilation: Inhalation: Metered dose inhaler: 1-2 metered doses 4-6 times/day
- Bronchodilation: 1-2 inhalations of a 0.25% solution, no more than 2 inhalations at any one time (1-5 minutes between inhalations); no more than 6 inhalations in any hour during a 24-hour period; maintenance therapy: 1-2 inhalations 4-6 times/day. Alternatively: 0.5% solution via hand bulb nebulizer is 5-15 deep inhalations repeated once in 5-10 minutes if necessary; treatments may be repeated up to 5 times/day.
- Sublingual: 10-20 mg every 3-4 hours; not to exceed 60 mg/day
- Cardiac arrhythmias: I.V.: 5 mcg/minute initially, titrate to patient response (2-20 mcg/minute)
- Shock: I.V.: 0.5-5 mcg/minute; adjust according to response

Administration Administer around-the-clock to promote less variation in peak and trough serum levels; I.V. infusion administration requires the use of an infusion pump

To prepare for infusion:

$$\frac{6 \times \text{weight (kg)} \times \text{desired dose (mcg/kg/min)}}{\text{I.V. infusion rate (mL/h)}} = \text{mg of drug to be added to 100 mL of I.V. fluid}$$

Monitoring Parameters EKG, heart rate, respiratory rate, arterial blood gas, arterial blood pressure, CVP

Patient Information Do not exceed recommended dosage; excessive use may lead to adverse effects or loss of effectiveness. Shake canister well before use. Administer pressurized inhalation during the second half of inspiration, as the airways are open wider and the aerosol distribution is more extensive. If more than one inhalation per dose is necessary, wait at least 1 full minute between inhalations - second inhalation is best delivered after 10 minutes. May cause nervousness, restlessness, insomnia; if these effects continue after dosage reduction, notify physician. Notify physician if palpitations, tachycardia, chest pain, muscle tremors, dizziness, headache, flushing or if breathing difficulty persists. Do not chew or swallow sublingual tablet.

Nursing Implications Elderly may find it useful to utilize a spacer device when using a metered dose inhaler

Additional Information

Isoproterenol hydrochloride: Aerolone®, Dey-Dose® isoproterenol, Dispos-a-Med® isoproterenol, Isopro®, Isuprel®, Norisodrine®, Vapo-Iso®

Isoproterenol sulfate: Medihaler-Iso®

Dosage Forms
Inhalation:
Aerosol: 0.2% (1:500) (15 mL, 22.5 mL); 0.25% (1:400) (15 mL)
Solution for nebulization: 0.031% (4 mL); 0.062% (4 mL); 0.25% (0.5 mL, 30 mL); 0.5% (0.5 mL, 10 mL, 60 mL); 1% (10 mL)
Injection: 0.2 mg/mL (1:5000) (1 mL, 5 mL, 10 mL)
Tablet, sublingual: 10 mg, 15 mg

Isoproterenol Hydrochloride *see* Isoproterenol *on page 681*

Isoproterenol Sulfate *see* Isoproterenol *on page 681*

Isoptin® *see* Verapamil *on page 1297*

Isoptin® SR *see* Verapamil *on page 1297*

Isopto® Atropine *see* Atropine *on page 116*

Isopto® Carbachol Ophthalmic *see* Carbachol *on page 200*

Isopto® Carpine Ophthalmic *see* Pilocarpine *on page 999*

Isopto® Cetamide® Ophthalmic *see* Sulfacetamide Sodium *on page 1171*

Isopto® Cetapred® Ophthalmic *see* Sulfacetamide Sodium and Prednisolone *on page 1172*

Isopto® Eserine *see* Physostigmine *on page 997*

Isopto® Frin Ophthalmic Solution *see* Phenylephrine *on page 989*

Isopto® Homatropine *see* Homatropine *on page 612*

Isopto® Hyoscine *see* Scopolamine *on page 1127*

Isordil® *see* Isosorbide Dinitrate *on next page*

Isosorbide (eye soe SOR bide)

Brand Names Ismotic®

Therapeutic Category Diuretic, Osmotic; Ophthalmic Agent, Osmotic

Use Short-term emergency treatment of acute angle-closure glaucoma and short-term reduction of intraocular pressure prior to and following intraocular surgery; may be used to interrupt an acute glaucoma attack; preferred agent when need to avoid nausea and vomiting

Pregnancy Risk Factor B

Contraindications Severe renal disease, anuria, severe dehydration, acute pulmonary edema, severe cardiac decompensation, known hypersensitivity to isosorbide

Warnings/Precautions Use with caution in patients with impending pulmonary edema and in the elderly due to the elderly's predisposition to dehydration and the fact that they frequently have concomitant diseases which may be aggravated by the use of isosorbide; hypernatremia and dehydration may begin to occur after 72 hours of continuous administration. Maintain fluid/electrolyte balance with multiple doses; monitor urinary output; if urinary output declines, need to review clinical status.

Adverse Reactions
1% to 10%:
Central nervous system: Headache, confusion, disorientation
Gastrointestinal: Vomiting
<1%:
Cardiovascular: Syncope
Central nervous system: Lethargy, vertigo, dizziness, lightheadedness, irritability
Dermatologic: Rash
Endocrine & metabolic: Hypernatremia, hyperosmolarity
Gastrointestinal: Nausea, abdominal/gastric discomfort (infrequently), anorexia
Miscellaneous: Hiccups, thirst

Overdosage/Toxicology Symptoms of overdose include dehydration, hypotension, hyponatremia; general supportive care, fluid administration, electrolyte balance, discontinue agent

Mechanism of Action Elevates osmolarity of glomerular filtrate to hinder the tubular resorption of water and increase excretion of sodium and chloride to result in diuresis; creates an osmotic gradient between plasma and ocular fluids

Pharmacodynamics/Kinetics
Onset of action: Within 10-30 minutes
Peak action: 1-1.5 hours
Duration: 5-6 hours
Distribution: In total body water
Metabolism: Not metabolized
Half-life: 5-9.5 hours
Elimination: By glomerular filtration; see Mechanism of Action

Usual Dosage Adults: Oral: Initial: 1.5 g/kg with a usual range of 1-3 g/kg 2-4 times/day as needed

Monitoring Parameters Monitor for signs of dehydration, blood pressure, renal output, intraocular pressure reduction

(Continued)

Isosorbide *(Continued)*

Nursing Implications Palatability may be improved if poured over ice and sipped

Additional Information Each 220 mL contains isosorbide 100 g, sodium 4.6 mEq, and potassium 0.9 mEq

Dosage Forms Solution: 45% [450 mg/mL] (220 mL)

Isosorbide Dinitrate (eye soe SOR bide dye NYE trate)

Related Information

Heart Failure: Management of Patients With Left-Ventricular Systolic Dysfunction *on page 1533*

Nitrates Comparison *on page 1419*

Brand Names Dilatrate®-SR; Isordil®; Sorbitrate®

Canadian/Mexican Brand Names Apo-ISDN® (Canada); Cedocard-SR® (Canada); Coradur® (Canada); Isoket® (Mexico); Isorbid® (Mexico)

Synonyms ISD; ISDN

Therapeutic Category Antianginal Agent; Nitrate; Vasodilator, Coronary

Use Prevention and treatment of angina pectoris; for congestive heart failure; to relieve pain, dysphagia, and spasm in esophageal spasm with GE reflux

Pregnancy Risk Factor C

Contraindications Severe anemia, closed-angle glaucoma, postural hypotension, cerebral hemorrhage, head trauma, hypersensitivity to isosorbide dinitrate or any component

Warnings/Precautions Use with caution in patients with increased intracranial pressure, hypotension, hypovolemia, glaucoma; sustained release products may be absorbed erratically in patients with GI hypermotility or malabsorption syndrome; do not crush or chew sublingual dosage form; abrupt withdrawal may result in angina; tolerance may develop (adjust dose or change agent)

Adverse Reactions

>10%:

- Cardiovascular: Flushing, postural hypotension
- Central nervous system: Headache, lightheadedness, dizziness
- Neuromuscular & skeletal: Weakness

1% to 10%: Dermatologic: Drug rash, exfoliative dermatitis

<1%:

- Gastrointestinal: Nausea, vomiting
- Hematologic: Methemoglobinemia (overdose)

Overdosage/Toxicology Symptoms of overdose include hypotension, throbbing headache, palpitations, visual disturbances, tachycardia, methemoglobinemia, flushing, diaphoresis, metabolic acidosis, coma. High levels or methemoglobinemia can cause signs and symptoms of hypoxemia.

Treatment consists of placing patient in recumbent position and administering fluids; alpha-adrenergic vasopressors may be required; treat methemoglobinemia with oxygen and methylene blue at a dose of 1-2 mg/kg I.V. slowly.

Mechanism of Action Stimulation of intracellular cyclic-GMP results in vascular smooth muscle relaxation of both arterial and venous vasculature. Increased venous pooling decreases left ventricular pressure (preload) and arterial dilatation decreases arterial resistance (afterload). Therefore, this reduces cardiac oxygen demand by decreasing left ventricular pressure and systemic vascular resistance by dilating arteries. Additionally, coronary artery dilation improves collateral flow to ischemic regions; esophageal smooth muscle is relaxed via the same mechanism.

Pharmacodynamics/Kinetics See table.

Dosage Form	Onset of Action	Duration
Sublingual tablet	2-10 min	1-2 h
Chewable tablet	3 min	0.5-2 h
Oral tablet	45-60 min	4-6 h
Sustained release tablet	30 min	6-12 h

Metabolism: Extensive in the liver to conjugated metabolites, including isosorbide 5-mononitrate (active) and 2-mononitrate (active)

Half-life:

- Parent drug: 1-4 hours
- Metabolite (5-mononitrate): 4 hours

Elimination: In urine and feces

Usual Dosage Adults (elderly should be given lowest recommended daily doses initially and titrate upward):

Angina: Oral: 5-40 mg 4 times/day or 40 mg every 8-12 hours in sustained released dosage form

Congestive heart failure: Oral:
Initial dose: 10 mg 3 times/day
Target dose: 40 mg 3 times/day
Maximum dose: 80 mg 3 times/day
Sublingual: 2.5-10 mg every 4-6 hours
Chew: 5-10 mg every 2-3 hours

Tolerance to nitrate effects develops with chronic exposure

Dose escalation does not overcome this effect. Tolerance can only be overcome by short periods of nitrate absence from the body. Short periods (14 hours) or nitrate withdrawal help minimize tolerance.

Hemodialysis: During hemodialysis, administer dose postdialysis or administer supplemental 10-20 mg dose
Peritoneal dialysis: Supplemental dose is not necessary

See Administration

Administration Do not administer around-the-clock; the first dose of nitrates should be administered in a physician's office to observe for maximal cardiovascular dynamic effects and adverse effects (orthostatic blood pressure drop, headache); when immediate release products are prescribed twice daily - recommend 7 AM and noon; for 3 times/day dosing - recommend 7 AM, noon, and 5 PM; when sustained-release products are indicated, suggest once a day in morning or via twice daily dosing at 8 AM and 2 PM

Monitoring Parameters Monitor for orthostasis

Test Interactions ↓ cholesterol (S)

Patient Information Do not chew or crush sublingual or sustained release dosage form; do not change brands without consulting your pharmacist or physician; keep tablets or capsules in original container and keep container tightly closed; if no relief from sublingual tablets after 15 minutes, report to nearest emergency room or seek emergency help

Nursing Implications 8- to 12-hour nitrate-free interval is needed each day to prevent tolerance

Dosage Forms

Capsule, sustained release: 40 mg
Tablet:
Chewable: 5 mg, 10 mg
Oral: 5 mg, 10 mg, 20 mg, 30 mg
Sublingual: 2.5 mg, 5 mg, 10 mg
Sustained release: 40 mg

Isosorbide Mononitrate (eye soe SOR bide mon oh NYE trate)

Related Information

Nitrates Comparison *on page 1419*

Brand Names IMDUR™; ISMO™; Monoket®

Canadian/Mexican Brand Names Elantan® (Mexico); Mono-Mack® (Mexico)

Synonyms ISMN

Therapeutic Category Antianginal Agent; Nitrate; Vasodilator, Coronary

Use Long-acting metabolite of the vasodilator isosorbide dinitrate used for the prophylactic treatment of angina pectoris

Contraindications Contraindicated due to potential increases in intracranial pressure in patients with head trauma or cerebral hemorrhage; hypersensitivity or idiosyncrasy to nitrates

Warnings/Precautions Postural hypotension, transient episodes of weakness, dizziness, or syncope may occur even with small doses; alcohol accentuates these effects; tolerance and cross-tolerance to nitrate antianginal and hemodynamic effects may occur during prolonged isosorbide mononitrate therapy; (minimized by using the smallest effective dose, by alternating coronary vasodilators or offering drug-free intervals of as little as 12 hours). Excessive doses may result in severe headache, blurred vision, or dry mouth; increased anginal symptoms may be a result of dosage increases.

Adverse Reactions

>10%: Central nervous system: Headache
1% to 10%: Gastrointestinal: Dizziness, nausea, vomiting
<1%:
Cardiovascular: Angina pectoris, arrhythmias, atrial fibrillation, hypotension, palpitations, postural hypotension, premature ventricular contractions, supraventricular tachycardia, syncope, edema
Central nervous system: Malaise, agitation, anxiety, confusion, hypoesthesia, insomnia, nervousness, nightmares
Dermatologic: Pruritus, rash
Gastrointestinal: Abdominal pain, diarrhea, dyspepsia, tenesmus, increased appetite, tooth disorder
Genitourinary: Impotence, polyuria, dysuria
Hematologic: Methemoglobinemia (rarely)

(Continued)

Isosorbide Mononitrate *(Continued)*

Neuromuscular & skeletal: Neck stiffness, rigors, arthralgia, dyscoordination, weakness

Ocular: Blurred vision, diplopia

Respiratory: Bronchitis, pneumonia, upper respiratory tract infection

Miscellaneous: Cold sweat

Overdosage/Toxicology Symptoms of overdose include hypotension, throbbing headache, palpitations, visual disturbances, tachycardia, methemoglobinemia, flushing, diaphoresis, metabolic acidosis, coma. High levels or methemoglobinemia can cause signs and symptoms of hypoxemia.

Treatment consists of placing patient in recumbent position and administering fluids; alpha-adrenergic vasopressors may be required; treat methemoglobinemia with oxygen and methylene blue at a dose of 1-2 mg/kg I.V. slowly.

Stability Tablets should be stored in a tight container at room temperature of 15°C to 30°C (59°F to 86°F)

Mechanism of Action Prevailing mechanism of action for nitroglycerin (and other nitrates) is systemic venodilation, decreasing preload as measured by pulmonary capillary wedge pressure and left ventricular end diastolic volume and pressure; the average reduction in LVEDV is 25% at rest, with a corresponding increase in ejection fractions of 50% to 60%. This effect improves congestive symptoms in heart failure and improves the myocardial perfusion gradient in patients with coronary artery disease.

Pharmacodynamics/Kinetics

Absorption: Oral: Nearly complete and low intersubject variability in its pharmacokinetic parameters and plasma concentrations

Metabolism: Metabolite of isosorbide dinitrate

Half-life: Mononitrate: ~4 hours (8 times that of dinitrate)

Usual Dosage Adults: Oral:

Regular tablet: 20 mg twice daily separated by 7 hours

Extended release tablet (Imdur™): Initial: 30-60 mg once daily; after several days the dosage may be increased to 120 mg/day (given as two 60 mg tablets); daily dose should be taken in the morning upon arising; maximum: 240 mg/day

Asymmetrical dosing regimen of 7 AM and 3 PM or 9 AM and 5 PM to allow for a nitrate-free dosing interval to minimize nitrate tolerance

Dosing adjustment in renal impairment: Not necessary for elderly or patients with altered renal or hepatic function

Dietary Considerations Alcohol: Has been found to exhibit additive effects of this variety

Administration Do not administer around-the-clock; Monoket® and Ismo™ should be scheduled twice daily with doses 7 hours apart (8 AM and 3 PM); Imdur™ may be given once daily

Monitoring Parameters Monitor for orthostasis

Patient Information Dispense drug in easy-to-open container; do not change brands without consulting pharmacist or physician; keep tablets or capsules tightly closed in original container; extended release tablets should not be chewed or crushed and should be swallowed together with a half-glassful of fluid; the antianginal efficacy of tablets can be maintained by carefully following the prescribed schedule of dosing (2 doses taken 7 hours apart); headaches are sometimes a marker of the activity of the drug

Nursing Implications Do not crush; 8- to 12-hour nitrate-free interval is needed each day to prevent tolerance

Dosage Forms

Tablet (Ismo™, Monoket®): 10 mg, 20 mg

Tablet, extended release (Imdur™): 30 mg, 60 mg, 120 mg

Isotretinoin (eye soe TRET i noyn)

Brand Names Accutane®

Canadian/Mexican Brand Names Isotrex® (Canada)

Synonyms 13-*cis*-Retinoic Acid

Therapeutic Category Acne Products; Retinoic Acid Derivative; Vitamin A Derivative; Vitamin, Fat Soluble

Use Treatment of severe recalcitrant cystic and/or conglobate acne unresponsive to conventional therapy

Investigational: Treatment of children with metastatic neuroblastoma or leukemia that does not respond to conventional therapy

Pregnancy Risk Factor X

Contraindications Sensitivity to parabens, vitamin A, or other retinoids; patients who are pregnant or intend to become pregnant during treatment

Warnings/Precautions Use with caution in patients with diabetes mellitus, hypertriglyceridemia; **not to be used in women of childbearing potential** unless woman is capable of complying with effective contraceptive measures;

therapy is normally begun on the second or third day of next normal menstrual period; effective contraception must be used for at least 1 month before beginning therapy, during therapy, and for 1 month after discontinuation of therapy. Because of the high likelihood of teratogenic effects (~20%), do not prescribe isotretinoin for women who are or who are likely to become pregnant while using the drug.

Adverse Reactions

>10%:

Dermatologic: Redness, cheilitis, inflammation of lips, dry skin, pruritus, photosensitivity

Endocrine & metabolic: Increased serum concentration of triglycerides

Gastrointestinal: Xerostomia

Local: Burning

Neuromuscular & skeletal: Bone pain, arthralgia, myalgia

Ocular: Itching eyes

Respiratory: Epistaxis, dry nose

1% to 10%:

Cardiovascular: Facial edema, pallor

Central nervous system: Fatigue, headache, mental depression, hypothermia

Dermatologic: Skin peeling on hands or soles of feet, rash, cellulitis

Endocrine & metabolic: Fluid imbalance, acidosis

Gastrointestinal: Stomach upset

Hepatic: Ascites

Neuromuscular & skeletal: Flank pain

Ocular: Dry eyes, photophobia

Miscellaneous: Lymph disorders

<1%:

Central nervous system: Mood changes, pseudomotor cerebri

Dermatologic: Alopecia, pruritus

Endocrine & metabolic: Hyperuricemia

Gastrointestinal: Xerostomia, anorexia, nausea, vomiting, inflammatory bowel syndrome, bleeding of gums

Hematologic: Increase in erythrocyte sedimentation rate, decrease in hemoglobin and hematocrit

Hepatic: Hepatitis

Ocular: Conjunctivitis, corneal opacities, optic neuritis, cataracts

Overdosage/Toxicology Symptoms of overdose include headache, vomiting, flushing, abdominal pain, ataxia; all signs and symptoms have been transient

Drug Interactions

Decreased effect: Increased clearance of carbamazepine

Increased toxicity: Avoid other vitamin A products; may interfere with medications used to treat hypertriglyceridemia

Stability Store at room temperature and protect from light

Mechanism of Action Reduces sebaceous gland size and reduces sebum production; regulates cell proliferation and differentiation

Pharmacodynamics/Kinetics

Absorption: Oral: Demonstrates biphasic absorption

Distribution: Crosses the placenta; appears in breast milk

Protein binding: 99% to 100%

Metabolism: In the liver; major metabolite: 4-oxo-isotretinoin (active)

Half-life, terminal:

Parent drug: 10-20 hours

Metabolite: 11-50 hours

Time to peak serum concentration: Within 3 hours

Elimination: Equally in urine and feces

Usual Dosage Oral:

Children: Maintenance therapy for neuroblastoma: 100-250 mg/m^2/day in 2 divided doses has been used investigationally

Children and Adults: 0.5-2 mg/kg/day in 2 divided doses (dosages as low as 0.05 mg/kg/day have been reported to be beneficial) for 15-20 weeks or until the total cyst count decreases by 70%, whichever is sooner

Dosing adjustment in hepatic impairment: Dose reductions empirically are recommended in hepatitis disease

Monitoring Parameters CBC with differential and platelet count, baseline sedimentation rate, serum triglycerides, liver enzymes

Patient Information Avoid pregnancy during therapy; effective contraceptive measures must be used since this drug may harm the fetus; there is information from manufacturers about this product that you should receive; discontinue therapy if visual difficulties, abdominal pain, rectal bleeding, diarrhea; exacerbation of acne may occur during first weeks of therapy; avoid use of other vitamin A products; decreased tolerance to contact lenses may occur; do not donate blood

(Continued)

Isotretinoin *(Continued)*

for at least 1 month following stopping of the drug; loss of night vision may occur, avoid prolonged exposure to sunlight; do not double next dose if dose is skipped

Nursing Implications Capsules can be swallowed, or chewed and swallowed. The capsule may be opened with a large needle and the contents placed on applesauce or ice cream for patients unable to swallow the capsule.

Dosage Forms Capsule: 10 mg, 20 mg, 40 mg

Isoxsuprine (eye SOKS syoo preen)

Brand Names Vasodilan®

Canadian/Mexican Brand Names Vadosilan® (Mexico); Vadosilan® 20 (Mexico)

Synonyms Isoxsuprine Hydrochloride

Therapeutic Category Vasodilator

Use Treatment of peripheral vascular diseases, such as arteriosclerosis obliterans and Raynaud's disease

Pregnancy Risk Factor C

Contraindications Presence of arterial bleeding; do not administer immediately postpartum

Adverse Reactions

1% to 10%: Gastrointestinal: Nausea, vomiting

<1%:

Cardiovascular: Chest pain, hypotension

Dermatologic: Rash

Respiratory: Pulmonary edema

Overdosage/Toxicology Symptoms of overdose include hypotension, flushing; vasodilation mediated second to alpha-adrenergic stimulation or direct smooth muscle effects

Treat with I.V. fluids, alpha-adrenergic pressors may be required

Mechanism of Action In studies on normal human subjects, isoxsuprine increases muscle blood flow, but skin blood flow is usually unaffected. Rather than increasing muscle blood flow by beta-receptor stimulation, isoxsuprine probably has a direct action on vascular smooth muscle. The generally accepted mechanism of action of isoxsuprine on the uterus is beta-adrenergic stimulation. Isoxsuprine was shown to inhibit prostaglandin synthetase at high serum concentrations, with low concentrations there was an increase in the P-G synthesis.

Pharmacodynamics/Kinetics

Absorption: Nearly complete

Metabolism: Partially conjugated in the liver

Half-life, serum: 1.25 hours mean

Time to peak serum concentration: Oral, I.M.: Within 1 hour

Elimination: Primarily in urine

Usual Dosage Adults: 10-20 mg 3-4 times/day; start with lower dose in elderly due to potential hypotension

Patient Information May cause skin rash; discontinue use if rash occurs; arise slowly from prolonged sitting or lying position

Dosage Forms Tablet, as hydrochloride: 10 mg, 20 mg

Isoxsuprine Hydrochloride *see* Isoxsuprine *on this page*

Isradipine (iz RA di peen)

Related Information

Calcium Channel Blockers Comparative Actions *on page 1401*

Calcium Channel Blockers Comparative Pharmacokinetics *on page 1402*

Calcium Channel Blockers FDA-Approved Indications *on page 1403*

Brand Names DynaCirc®

Canadian/Mexican Brand Names DynaCirc SRO® (Mexico)

Therapeutic Category Antihypertensive; Calcium Channel Blocker

Use Treatment of hypertension, congestive heart failure, migraine prophylaxis

Pregnancy Risk Factor C

Pregnancy/Breast-Feeding Implications

Clinical effects on the fetus: No data on crossing the placenta

Breast-feeding/lactation: No data on crossing into breast milk. Not recommended due to potential harm to infant.

Contraindications Sinus bradycardia; advanced heart block; ventricular tachycardia; cardiogenic shock, hypotension, congestive heart failure; hypersensitivity to isradipine or any component, hypersensitivity to calcium channel blockers and adenosine; atrial fibrillation or flutter associated with accessory conduction pathways; not to be given within a few hours of I.V. beta-blocking agents

Warnings/Precautions Avoid use in hypotension, congestive heart failure, cardiac conduction defects, PVCs, idiopathic hypertrophic subaortic stenosis; may cause platelet inhibition; do not abruptly withdraw (chest pain); may cause hepatic dysfunction or increased angina; increased intracranial pressure with cranial tumors; elderly may have greater hypotensive effect

Adverse Reactions

>10%: Central nervous system: Headache

1% to 10%:

Cardiovascular: Edema, palpitations, flushing, chest pain, tachycardia, hypotension

Central nervous system: Dizziness, fatigue

Dermatologic: Rash

Gastrointestinal: Nausea, abdominal discomfort, vomiting, diarrhea

Neuromuscular & skeletal: Weakness

Respiratory: Dyspnea

<1%:

Cardiovascular: Heart failure, atrial and ventricular fibrillation, TIAs, A-V block, myocardial infarction, abnormal EKG

Central nervous system: Disturbed sleep

Dermatologic: Pruritus, urticaria, rash

Gastrointestinal: Xerostomia

Genitourinary: Nocturia

Hematologic: Leukopenia

Neuromuscular & skeletal: Foot cramps, paresthesia, numbness

Ocular: Visual disturbance

Respiratory: Cough

Overdosage/Toxicology The primary cardiac symptoms of calcium blocker overdose includes hypotension and bradycardia. The hypotension is caused by peripheral vasodilation, myocardial depression, and bradycardia. Bradycardia results from sinus bradycardia, second- or third-degree atrioventricular block, or sinus arrest with junctional rhythm. Intraventricular conduction is usually not affected so QRS duration is normal (verapamil does prolong the P-R interval and bepridil prolongs the Q-T and may cause ventricular arrhythmias, including torsade de pointes).

The noncardiac symptoms include confusion, stupor, nausea, vomiting, metabolic acidosis and hyperglycemia. Following initial gastric decontamination, if possible, repeated calcium administration may promptly reverse the depressed cardiac contractility (but not sinus node depression or peripheral vasodilation); glucagon, epinephrine, and amrinone may treat refractory hypotension; glucagon and epinephrine also increase the heart rate (outside the U.S., 4-aminopyridine may be available as an antidote); dialysis and hemoperfusion are not effective in enhancing elimination although repeat-dose activated charcoal may serve as an adjunct with sustained-release preparations.

Drug Interactions

Decreased effect:

Isradipine and NSAIDs (diclofenac) may decrease antihypertensive response

Isradipine and lovastatin causes decrease lovastatin effect

Increased toxicity/effect/levels:

Isradipine and beta-blockers may increase cardiovascular adverse effects

Isradipine and cyclosporine may minimally increase cyclosporine levels

Mechanism of Action Inhibits calcium ion from entering the "slow channels" or select voltage-sensitive areas of vascular smooth muscle and myocardium during depolarization, producing a relaxation of coronary vascular smooth muscle and coronary vasodilation; increases myocardial oxygen delivery in patients with vasospastic angina

Pharmacodynamics/Kinetics

Absorption: Oral: 90% to 95%

Protein binding: 95%

Metabolism: In the liver

Bioavailability: Absolute due to first-pass elimination 15% to 24%

Half-life: 8 hours

Time to peak: Serum concentration: 1-1.5 hours

Elimination: Renal excretion by metabolites (cyclic lactone and monoacids)

Usual Dosage Adults: 2.5 mg twice daily; antihypertensive response seen in 2-3 hours; maximal response in 2-4 weeks; increase dose at 2- to 4-week intervals at 2.5-5 mg increments; usual dose range: 5-20 mg/day. **Note**: Most patients show no improvement with doses >10 mg/day except adverse reaction rate increases; therefore, maximal dose in elderly should be 10 mg/day.

Patient Information Do not discontinue abruptly; report any dizziness, shortness of breath, palpitations, or edema

Additional Information Although there is some initial data which may show increased risk of myocardial infarction following treatment of hypertension with calcium antagonists, controlled trials (eg, ALL-HAT) are ongoing to examine the long-term effects of not only calcium antagonists but other antihypertensives in preventing heart disease. Until these studies are completed, patients taking

(Continued)

Isradipine *(Continued)*

calcium antagonists should be encouraged to continue with prescribed antihypertensive regimes, although a switch from high-dose, short-acting agents to sustained release products may be warranted. It is also generally agreed that calcium antagonists should be avoided as the primary treatment for hypertension unless diuretics or beta-blockers are contraindicated and for the primary treatment of angina following acute myocardial infarction.

Dosage Forms Capsule: 2.5 mg, 5 mg

Isuprel® *see* Isoproterenol *on page 681*

Itch-X® [OTC] *see* Pramoxine *on page 1033*

Itraconazole (i tra KOE na zole)

Related Information

Antifungal Agents *on page 1395*

Guidelines for the Prevention of Opportunistic Infections in Persons with HIV *on page 1457*

Brand Names Sporanox®

Canadian/Mexican Brand Names Isox® (Mexico); Itranax® (Mexico)

Therapeutic Category Antifungal Agent, Systemic

Use Treatment of susceptible fungal infections in immunocompromised and immunocompetent patients including blastomycosis and histoplasmosis; also indicated for aspergillosis and onychomycosis of the toenail; approved for treatment of onychomycosis of the fingernail without concomitant toenail infection via a pulse-type dosing regimen; has activity against *Aspergillus, Candida, Coccidioides, Cryptococcus, Sporothrix*, tinea unguium

Oral solution is marketed for oral and esophageal candidiasis

Unlabeled uses: Superficial mycoses including dermatophytoses (eg, tinea capitis), pityriasis versicolor, sebopsoriasis, vaginal and chronic mucocutaneous candidiases; systemic mycoses including candidiasis, meningeal and disseminated cryptococcal infections, paracoccidioidomycosis, coccidioidomycoses; miscellaneous mycoses such as sporotrichosis, chromomycosis, leishmaniasis, fungal keratitis, alternariosis, zygomycosis

Pregnancy Risk Factor C

Contraindications Known hypersensitivity to itraconazole or other azoles; terfenadine

Warnings/Precautions Rare cases of serious cardiovascular adverse event, including death, ventricular tachycardia and torsade de pointes have been observed due to increased terfenadine concentrations induced by itraconazole; patients who develop abnormal liver function tests during fluconazole therapy should be monitored and therapy discontinued if symptoms of liver disease develop

Adverse Reactions

>10%: Gastrointestinal: Nausea

1% to 10%:

- Central nervous system: Headache
- Dermatologic: Rash
- Gastrointestinal: Abdominal pain, vomiting

<1%:

- Cardiovascular: Edema, hypertension
- Central nervous system: Fatigue, fever, malaise, dizziness, somnolence
- Dermatologic: Pruritus
- Endocrine & metabolic: Hypokalemia, decreased libido
- Gastrointestinal: Diarrhea, anorexia
- Genitourinary: Impotence
- Hepatic: Abnormal hepatic function
- Renal: Albuminuria

Overdosage/Toxicology Overdoses are well tolerated; following decontamination, if possible, supportive measures only are required; dialysis is not effective

Drug Interactions Inhibitor of cytochrome P-450 2C and cytochrome P-450 3A enzymes

Decreased effect:

- Decreased serum levels with isoniazid and phenytoin; may cause a decreased effect of oral contraceptives; alternative birth control is recommended
- Decreased/undetectable serum levels with rifampin - **should not be administered concomitantly with rifampin**
- Absorption requires gastric acidity; therefore, antacids, H_2-antagonists (cimetidine and ranitidine), omeprazole, and sucralfate significantly reduce bioavailability resulting in treatment failures and should not be administered concomitantly; amphotericin B or fluconazole should be used instead

Increased toxicity:

- May increase cyclosporine levels (by 50%) when high doses are used

Itraconazole increases lovastatin levels (possibly 20-fold) due to inhibition of CYP3A4

May increase phenytoin serum concentration

May inhibit warfarins metabolism

May increase digoxin serum levels

May increase terfenadine levels - **concomitant administration is not recommended**

Pharmacodynamics/Kinetics

Absorption: Enhanced by food and requires gastric acidity

Distribution: Apparent volume averaged 796±185 L or 10 L/kg; highly lipophilic and tissue concentrations are higher than plasma concentrations. The highest itraconazole concentrations are achieved in adipose, omentum, endometrium, cervical and vaginal mucus, and skin/nails. Aqueous fluids, such as cerebrospinal fluid and urine, contain negligible amounts of itraconazole; steady-state concentrations are achieved in 13 days with multiple administration of itraconazole 100-400 mg/day.

Protein binding: 99.9% bound to plasma proteins; metabolite hydroxy-itraconazole is 99.5% bound to plasma proteins

Metabolism: Extensive by the liver into >30 metabolites including hydroxy-itraconazole which is the major metabolite and appears to have *in vitro* antifungal activity. The main metabolic pathway is oxidation; may undergo saturation metabolism with multiple dosing

Bioavailability: Increased from 40% fasting to 100% postprandial; absolute oral bioavailability: 55%; hypochlorhydria has been reported in HIV-infected patients; therefore, oral absorption in these patients may be decreased

Half-life: After single 200 mg dose: 21±5 hours

Elimination: ~3% to 18% excreted in feces; ~0.03% of parent drug excreted renally and 40% of dose excreted as inactive metabolites in urine

Usual Dosage Oral (absorption is best if taken with food, therefore, it is best to administer itraconazole after meals):

Children: Efficacy and safety have not been established; a small number of patients 3-16 years of age have been treated with 100 mg/day for systemic fungal infections with no serious adverse effects reported

Adults: 200 mg once daily, if obvious improvement or there is evidence of progressive fungal disease, increase the dose in 100 mg increments to a maximum of 400 mg/day; doses >200 mg/day are given in 2 divided doses; length of therapy varies from 1 day to >6 months depending on the condition and mycological response

Onychomycosis: 200 mg twice daily for 1 week each month

Life-threatening infections: Loading dose: 200 mg 3 times/day (600 mg/day) should be given for the first 3 days of therapy

Dosing adjustment in renal impairment: Not necessary

Hemodialysis: Not dialyzable

Dosing adjustment in hepatic impairment: May be necessary, but specific guidelines are not available

Administration Doses >200 mg/day are given in 2 divided doses; do not administer with antacids

Patient Information Take with food; report any signs and symptoms that may suggest liver dysfunction so that the appropriate laboratory testing can be done; signs and symptoms may include unusual fatigue, anorexia, nausea and/or vomiting, jaundice, dark urine, or pale stool

Dosage Forms

Capsule: 100 mg

Solution, oral: 100 mg/10 mL (150 mL)

Extemporaneous Preparations A 40 mg/mL suspension (made by emptying the beads from twenty-four 100 mg capsules, adding 4-5 mL of 95% ethyl alcohol, USP, to the beads and letting it stand for 3-4 minutes to soften beads; grind to a fine powder and allow ethyl alcohol to evaporate; add 15 mL of simple syrup to the powder, triturate well, and transfer contents to an amber bottle; rinse mortar with 15 mL of syrup and transfer contents to the amber bottle; repeat with enough syrup to bring the final volume to 60 mL); measured stability: 35 days when stored in amber bottles under refrigeration. However, bioavailability of this formulation has not been evaluated.

Jacobson PA, Johnson CE, and Walters JR, "Stability of Itraconazole in an Extemporaneously Compounded Oral Liquid," *Am J Health Syst Pharm*, 1995, 52:189-91.

I-Tropine® *see* Atropine *on page 116*

IUDR *see* Idoxuridine *on page 644*

IVIG *see* Immune Globulin, Intravenous *on page 651*

Janimine® *see* Imipramine *on page 648*

Jenamicin® *see* Gentamicin *on page 570*

Jenest-28™ *see* Ethinyl Estradiol and Norethindrone *on page 486*
Junior Strength Motrin® [OTC] *see* Ibuprofen *on page 639*
K+ 10® *see* Potassium Chloride *on page 1024*
Kabikinase® *see* Streptokinase *on page 1159*
Kalcinate® *see* Calcium Gluconate *on page 191*

Kanamycin (kan a MYE sin)

Related Information

Antimicrobial Drugs of Choice *on page 1468*
Recommendations for Prophylaxis Against Tuberculosis *on page 1455*

Brand Names Kantrex®

Canadian/Mexican Brand Names Randikan® (Mexico)

Synonyms Kanamycin Sulfate

Therapeutic Category Antibiotic, Aminoglycoside

Use

Oral: Preoperative bowel preparation in the prophylaxis of infections and adjunctive treatment of hepatic coma (oral kanamycin is not indicated in the treatment of systemic infections); treatment of susceptible bacterial infection including gram-negative aerobes, gram-positive *Bacillus* as well as some mycobacteria

Parenteral: Rarely used in antibiotic irrigations during surgery

Pregnancy Risk Factor D

Contraindications Hypersensitivity to kanamycin or any component or other aminoglycosides

Warnings/Precautions Use with caution in patients with pre-existing renal insufficiency, vestibular or cochlear impairment, myasthenia gravis, conditions which depress neuromuscular transmission

Parenteral aminoglycosides are associated with nephrotoxicity or ototoxicity; the ototoxicity may be proportional to the amount of drug given and the duration of treatment; tinnitus or vertigo are indications of vestibular injury and impending hearing loss; renal damage is usually reversible

Adverse Reactions

>10%: Renal: Nephrotoxicity

1% to 10%:
- Cardiovascular: Edema
- Central nervous system: Neurotoxicity
- Dermatologic: Skin itching, redness, rash
- Otic: Ototoxicity (auditory), ototoxicity (vestibular)

<1%:
- Central nervous system: Drowsiness, headache, pseudomotor cerebri
- Dermatologic: Photosensitivity, erythema
- Gastrointestinal: Anorexia, nausea, vomiting, weight loss, increased salivation, enterocolitis
- Hematologic: Granulocytopenia, agranulocytosis, thrombocytopenia
- Local: Burning, stinging
- Neuromuscular & skeletal: Weakness, tremors, muscle cramps
- Respiratory: Dyspnea

Overdosage/Toxicology Symptoms of overdose include ototoxicity, nephrotoxicity, and neuromuscular toxicity

The treatment of choice following a single acute overdose appears to be the maintenance of good urine output of at least 3 mL/kg/hour. Dialysis is of questionable value in the enhancement of aminoglycoside elimination. If required, hemodialysis is preferred over peritoneal dialysis in patients with normal renal function. Careful hydration may be all that is required to promote diuresis and, therefore, the enhancement of the drug's elimination.

Drug Interactions

Increased toxicity:
- Penicillins, cephalosporins, amphotericin B, diuretics may increase nephrotoxicity
- Neuromuscular blocking agents may increase neuromuscular blockade

Stability Darkening of vials does not indicate loss of potency

Mechanism of Action Interferes with protein synthesis in bacterial cell by binding to ribosomal subunit

Pharmacodynamics/Kinetics

Absorption: Oral: Not absorbed following administration

Relative diffusion of antimicrobial agents from blood into cerebrospinal fluid (CSF): Good only with inflammation (exceeds usual MICs)
- Ratio of CSF to blood level (%):
- Normal meninges: Nil
- Inflamed meninges: 43

Half-life: 2-4 hours, increases in anuria to 80 hours
- End stage renal disease: 40-96 hours

Time to peak serum concentration: I.M.: 1-2 hours

Elimination: Entirely in the kidney, principally by glomerular filtration

Usual Dosage

Children:

Infections: I.M., I.V.: 15-30 mg/kg/day in divided doses every 8 hours

Suppression of bowel flora: Oral: 150-250 mg/kg/day in divided doses administered every 1-6 hours

Adults:

Infections: I.M., I.V.: 5-7.5 mg/kg/dose in divided doses every 8-12 hours

Preoperative intestinal antisepsis: Oral: 1 g every 4-6 hours for 36-72 hours

Hepatic coma: Oral: 8-12 g/day in divided doses

Dosing adjustment/interval in renal impairment:

Cl_{cr} 50-80 mL/minute: Administer 60% to 90% of dose or administer every 8-12 hours

Cl_{cr} 10-50 mL/minute: Administer 30% to 70% of dose or administer every 12 hours

Cl_{cr} <10 mL/minute: Administer 20% to 30% of dose or administer every 24-48 hours

Hemodialysis: Dialyzable (50% to 100%)

Administration Adults: Dilute to 100-200 mL and infuse over 30 minutes; administer around-the-clock to promote less variation in peak and trough serum levels

Monitoring Parameters Serum creatinine and BUN every 2-3 days; peak and trough concentrations; hearing

Reference Range Therapeutic: Peak: 25-35 μg/mL; Trough: 4-8 μg/mL; Toxic: Peak: >35 μg/mL; Trough: >10 μg/mL

Patient Information Report any dizziness or sensations of ringing or fullness in ears

Nursing Implications Aminoglycoside levels in blood taken from Silastic® central catheters can sometime give falsely high readings (sample from alternative lumen or via peripheral stick if possible; otherwise flush very well following administration); hearing should be tested before, during, and after treatment

Dosage Forms

Capsule, as sulfate: 500 mg

Injection, as sulfate:

Pediatric: 75 mg (2 mL)

Adults: 500 mg (2 mL); 1 g (3 mL)

Kanamycin Sulfate *see* Kanamycin *on previous page*

Kantrex® *see* Kanamycin *on previous page*

Kaochlor® *see* Potassium Chloride *on page 1024*

Kaochlor® SF *see* Potassium Chloride *on page 1024*

Kaon® *see* Potassium Gluconate *on page 1026*

Kaon-Cl® *see* Potassium Chloride *on page 1024*

Kaon Cl-10® *see* Potassium Chloride *on page 1024*

Kaopectate® Advanced Formula [OTC] *see* Attapulgite *on page 118*

Kaopectate® II [OTC] *see* Loperamide *on page 739*

Kaopectate® Maximum Strength Caplets *see* Attapulgite *on page 118*

Karidium® *see* Fluoride *on page 536*

Karigel® *see* Fluoride *on page 536*

Karigel®-N *see* Fluoride *on page 536*

Kasof® [OTC] *see* Docusate *on page 415*

Kato® *see* Potassium Chloride *on page 1024*

Kaybovite-1000® *see* Cyanocobalamin *on page 319*

Kay Ciel® *see* Potassium Chloride *on page 1024*

Kayexalate® *see* Sodium Polystyrene Sulfonate *on page 1148*

Kaylixir® *see* Potassium Gluconate *on page 1026*

K+ Care® *see* Potassium Chloride *on page 1024*

KCl *see* Potassium Chloride *on page 1024*

K-Dur® 10 *see* Potassium Chloride *on page 1024*

K-Dur® 20 *see* Potassium Chloride *on page 1024*

Keflex® *see* Cephalexin *on page 239*

Keflin® *see* Cephalothin *on page 241*

Keftab® *see* Cephalexin *on page 239*

Kefurox® *see* Cefuroxime *on page 238*

Kefzol® *see* Cefazolin *on page 220*

Kemadrin® *see* Procyclidine *on page 1054*

Kenacort® *see* Triamcinolone *on page 1255*

Kenaject-40® *see* Triamcinolone *on page 1255*

Kenalog® *see* Triamcinolone *on page 1255*

Kenalog-10® *see* Triamcinolone *on page 1255*

Kenalog-40® *see* Triamcinolone *on page 1255*
Kenalog® H *see* Triamcinolone *on page 1255*
Kenalog® in Orabase® *see* Triamcinolone *on page 1255*
Kenonel® *see* Triamcinolone *on page 1255*
Kerlone® *see* Betaxolol *on page 149*
Kestrone® *see* Estrone *on page 474*
Ketalar® *see* Ketamine *on this page*

Ketamine (KEET a meen)

Related Information
Adult ACLS Algorithm, Electrical Conversion *on page 1515*

Brand Names Ketalar®

Canadian/Mexican Brand Names Ketalin® (Mexico)

Synonyms Ketamine Hydrochloride

Therapeutic Category General Anesthetic

Use Induction of anesthesia; short surgical procedures; dressing changes

Pregnancy Risk Factor D

Contraindications Elevated intracranial pressure; patients with hypertension, aneurysms, thyrotoxicosis, congestive heart failure, angina, psychotic disorders; hypersensitivity to ketamine or any component

Warnings/Precautions Should be used by or under the direct supervision of physicians experienced in administering general anesthetics and in maintenance of an airway, and in the control of respiration. Resuscitative equipment should be available for use.

Postanesthetic emergence reactions which can manifest as vivid dreams, hallucinations and/or frank delirium occur in 12% of patients; these reactions are less common in patients >65 and when given I.M.; emergence reactions, confusion, or irrational behavior may occur up to 24 hours postoperatively and may be reduced by minimization of verbal, tactile, and visual patient stimulation during recovery or by pretreatment with a benzodiazepine. Avoid postsurgery stimulation which may cause agitation and hallucinations in patients.

Adverse Reactions

>10%:
- Cardiovascular: Hypertension, tachycardia, increased cardiac output, paradoxical direct myocardial depression
- Central nervous system: Increased intracranial pressure, vivid dreams, visual hallucinations
- Neuromuscular & skeletal: Tonic-clonic movements, tremors
- Miscellaneous: Emergence reactions, vocalization

1% to 10%:
- Cardiovascular: Bradycardia, hypotension
- Dermatologic: Pain at injection site, skin rash
- Gastrointestinal: Vomiting, anorexia, nausea
- Ocular: Nystagmus, diplopia
- Respiratory: Respiratory depression

<1%:
- Cardiovascular: Cardiac arrhythmias, myocardial depression
- Central nervous system: Increased intracranial pressure, increases in cerebral blood
- Endocrine & metabolic: Increased metabolic rate, increased intraocular pressure
- Gastrointestinal: Hypersalivation
- Neuromuscular & skeletal: Increased skeletal muscle tone, fasciculations
- Ocular: Increased intraocular pressure
- Respiratory: Increased airway resistance, cough reflex may be depressed, decreased bronchospasm, respiratory depression or apnea with large doses or rapid infusions, laryngospasm

Overdosage/Toxicology Symptoms of overdose include respiratory depression with excessive dosing or too rapid administration

Supportive care is the treatment of choice; mechanical support of respiration is preferred

Drug Interactions

Increased effect:
- Barbiturates, narcotics, hydroxyzine increase prolonged recovery
- Nondepolarizing may increase effects

Increased toxicity:
- Muscle relaxants, thyroid hormones may increase blood pressure and heart rate
- Halothane may decrease BP

Stability Do not mix with barbiturates or diazepam → precipitation may occur

Mechanism of Action Produces dissociative anesthesia by direct action on the cortex and limbic system

Pharmacodynamics/Kinetics Duration of action (following a single dose):

Anesthesia:
- I.M.: 12-25 minutes
- I.V.: 5-10 minutes

Analgesia: I.M.: 15-30 minutes

Amnesia: May persist for 1-2 hours

Recovery:
- I.M.: 3-4 hours
- I.V.: 1-2 hours

Usual Dosage Used in combination with anticholinergic agents to decrease hypersalivation

Children:
- Oral: 6-10 mg/kg for 1 dose (mixed in 0.2-0.3 mL/kg of cola or other beverage) given 30 minutes before the procedure
- I.M.: 3-7 mg/kg
- I.V.: Range: 0.5-2 mg/kg, use smaller doses (0.5-1 mg/kg) for sedation for minor procedures; usual induction dosage: 1-2 mg/kg
- Continuous I.V. infusion: Sedation: 5-20 mcg/kg/minute

Adults:
- I.M.: 3-8 mg/kg
- I.V.: Range: 1-4.5 mg/kg; usual induction dosage: 1-2 mg/kg

Children and Adults: Maintenance: Supplemental doses of $^1/_3$ to $^1/_2$ of initial dose

Administration

Oral: Use 100 mg/mL I.V. solution and mix the appropriate dose in 0.2-0.3 mL/kg of cola or other beverage

Parenteral: I.V.: Do not exceed 0.5 mg/kg/minute or administer faster than 60 seconds; do not exceed final concentration of 2 mg/mL

Monitoring Parameters Cardiovascular effects, heart rate, blood pressure, respiratory rate, transcutaneous O_2 saturation

Dosage Forms Injection, as hydrochloride: 10 mg/mL (20 mL, 25 mL, 50 mL); 50 mg/mL (10 mL); 100 mg/mL (5 mL)

Ketamine Hydrochloride *see* Ketamine *on previous page*

Ketoconazole (kee toe KOE na zole)

Related Information

Antacid Drug Interactions *on page 1388*
Antifungal Agents *on page 1395*
Guidelines for the Prevention of Opportunistic Infections in Persons with HIV *on page 1457*

Brand Names Nizoral®

Canadian/Mexican Brand Names Akorazol® (Mexico)

Therapeutic Category Antifungal Agent, Systemic; Antifungal Agent, Topical

Use Treatment of susceptible fungal infections, including candidiasis, oral thrush, blastomycosis, histoplasmosis, paracoccidioidomycosis, chronic mucocutaneous candidiasis, as well as, certain recalcitrant cutaneous dermatophytoses; used topically for treatment of tinea corporis, tinea cruris, tinea versicolor, and cutaneous candidiasis, seborrheic dermatitis

Pregnancy Risk Factor C

Contraindications Hypersensitivity to ketoconazole or any component; CNS fungal infections (due to poor CNS penetration); coadministration with terfenadine or cisapride is contraindicated due to risk of potentially fatal cardiac arrhythmias

Warnings/Precautions Rare cases of serious cardiovascular adverse event, including death, ventricular tachycardia and torsade de pointes have been observed due to increased terfenadine concentrations induced by ketoconazole. Use with caution in patients with impaired hepatic function; has been associated with hepatotoxicity, including some fatalities; perform periodic liver function tests; high doses of ketoconazole may depress adrenocortical function.

Adverse Reactions

Oral:
- 1% to 10%:
  - Dermatologic: Pruritus
  - Gastrointestinal: Nausea, vomiting, abdominal pain
- <1%:
  - Central nervous system: Headache, dizziness, somnolence, fever, chills, bulging fontanelles
  - Endocrine & metabolic: Gynecomastia
  - Gastrointestinal: Diarrhea
  - Genitourinary: Impotence
  - Hematologic: Thrombocytopenia, leukopenia, hemolytic anemia

(Continued)

Ketoconazole *(Continued)*

Ocular: Photophobia

Cream: Severe irritation, pruritus, stinging (~5%)

Shampoo: Increases in normal hair loss, irritation (<1%), abnormal hair texture, scalp pustules, mild dryness of skin, itching, oiliness/dryness of hair

Overdosage/Toxicology Symptoms of overdose include dizziness, headache, nausea, vomiting, diarrhea. Overdoses are well tolerated; treatment includes supportive measures and gastric decontamination

Drug Interactions

Decreased effect:

Decreased ketoconazole serum levels with isoniazid and phenytoin; decreased/undetectable serum levels with rifampin - **should not be administered concomitantly with rifampin**; theophylline serum levels may be decreased

Possible decreased effect of oral contraceptive; suggest alternative method of birth control

Absorption requires gastric acidity; therefore, antacids, H_2-antagonists (cimetidine and ranitidine), omeprazole, and sucralfate significantly reduce bioavailability resulting in treatment failures; should not be administered concomitantly; amphotericin B or fluconazole may be used instead

Increased toxicity:

May increase cyclosporine levels (by 50%) when high doses are used; inhibits warfarin metabolism resulting in increased anticoagulant effect; increases corticosteroid bioavailability and decreases steroid clearance; increases phenytoin, digoxin, terfenadine and cisapride concentrations; **concomitant administration with terfenadine or cisapride is contraindicated**; may significantly increase levels and toxicity of lovastatin and simvastatin due to CYP3A4 inhibition

Mechanism of Action Alters the permeability of the cell wall; inhibits biosynthesis of triglycerides and phospholipids by fungi; inhibits several fungal enzymes that results in a build-up of toxic concentrations of hydrogen peroxide

Pharmacodynamics/Kinetics

Absorption: Oral: Rapid (~75%); no detectable absorption following use of the shampoo

Distribution: Minimal distribution into the CNS

Protein binding: 93% to 96%

Metabolism: Partially in the liver by enzymes to inactive compounds

Bioavailability: Decreases as pH of the gastric contents increases

Half-life, biphasic:

Initial: 2 hours

Terminal: 8 hours

Time to peak serum concentration: 1-2 hours

Elimination: Primarily in feces (57%) with smaller amounts excreted in urine (13%)

Usual Dosage

Oral:

Children >2 years: 5-10 mg/kg/day divided every 12-24 hours for 2-4 weeks

Adults: 200-400 mg/day as a single daily dose

Shampoo: Apply twice weekly for 4 weeks with at least 3 days between each shampoo

Topical: Rub gently into the affected area once daily to twice daily

Dosing adjustment in hepatic impairment: Dose reductions should be considered in patients with severe liver disease

Hemodialysis: Not dialyzable (0% to 5%)

Monitoring Parameters Liver function tests

Patient Information Cream is for topical application to the skin only; avoid contact with the eye; avoid taking antacids at the same time as ketoconazole; may take with food; may cause drowsiness, impair judgment or coordination. Notify physician of unusual fatigue, anorexia, vomiting, dark urine, or pale stools.

Nursing Implications Administer 2 hours prior to antacids to prevent decreased absorption due to the high pH of gastric contents

Dosage Forms

Cream: 2% (15 g, 30 g, 60 g)

Shampoo: 2% (120 mL)

Tablet: 200 mg

Extemporaneous Preparations A 20 mg/mL suspension may be made by pulverizing twelve 200 mg ketoconazole tablets to a fine powder; add 40 mL Ora-Plus® in small portions with thorough mixing; incorporate Ora-Sweet® to make a final volume of 120 mL and mix thoroughly; refrigerate (no stability information is available)

Allen LV, "Ketoconazole Oral Suspension," *US Pharm*, 1993, 18(2):98-9, 101.

Ketoprofen (kee toe PROE fen)

Related Information

Dosing Data for Acetaminophen and NSAIDs *on page 1377*

Nonsteroidal Anti-Inflammatory Agents Comparison *on page 1419*

Brand Names Actron® [OTC]; Orudis®; Orudis® KT [OTC]; Oruvail®

Canadian/Mexican Brand Names Apo-Keto® (Canada); Apo-Keto-E® (Canada); Novo-Keto-EC® (Canada); Nu-Ketoprofen® (Canada); Nu-Ketoprofen-E® (Canada); Orafen (Canada); Rhodis™ (Canada); Rhodis-EC™ (Canada); Rhodis-SR™ (Canada); Rhovail® (Canada); PMS-Ketoprofen (Canada); Keduril® (Mexico); K-Profen® (Mexico); Pro-Fenid® (Mexico); Profenid® 200 (Mexico); Profenid-IM® (Mexico)

Therapeutic Category Analgesic, Nonsteroidal Anti-inflammatory Drug; Anti-inflammatory Agent; Nonsteroidal Anti-inflammatory Agent (NSAID), Oral

Use Acute or long-term treatment of rheumatoid arthritis and osteoarthritis; primary dysmenorrhea; mild to moderate pain

Pregnancy Risk Factor B

Contraindications Known hypersensitivity to ketoprofen or other NSAIDs/aspirin

Warnings/Precautions Use with caution in patients with congestive heart failure, hypertension, decreased renal or hepatic function, history of GI disease (bleeding or ulcers), or those receiving anticoagulants; safety and efficacy in children <6 months of age have not yet been established

Adverse Reactions

>10%:
- Central nervous system: Dizziness
- Dermatologic: Rash
- Gastrointestinal: Abdominal cramps, heartburn, indigestion, nausea

1% to 10%:
- Central nervous system: Headache, nervousness
- Dermatologic: Itching
- Endocrine & metabolic: Fluid retention
- Gastrointestinal: Vomiting
- Otic: Tinnitus

<1%:
- Cardiovascular: Congestive heart failure, hypertension, arrhythmias, tachycardia
- Central nervous system: Confusion, hallucinations, mental depression, drowsiness, insomnia, aseptic meningitis
- Dermatologic: Urticaria, erythema multiforme, toxic epidermal necrolysis, Stevens-Johnson syndrome, angioedema
- Endocrine & metabolic: Polydipsia, hot flashes
- Gastrointestinal: Gastritis, GI ulceration
- Genitourinary: Cystitis, polyuria
- Hematologic: Agranulocytosis, anemia, hemolytic anemia, bone marrow suppression, leukopenia, thrombocytopenia
- Hepatic: Hepatitis
- Neuromuscular & skeletal: Peripheral neuropathy
- Ocular: Toxic amblyopia, blurred vision, conjunctivitis, dry eyes
- Otic: Decreased hearing
- Renal: Acute renal failure
- Respiratory: Allergic rhinitis, shortness of breath, epistaxis

Overdosage/Toxicology Symptoms include apnea, metabolic acidosis, coma, and nystagmus; leukocytosis, renal failure

Management of a nonsteroidal anti-inflammatory drug (NSAID) intoxication is primarily supportive and symptomatic. Fluid therapy is commonly effective in managing the hypotension that may occur following an acute NSAID overdose, except when this is due to an acute blood loss. Seizures tend to be very short-lived and often do not require drug treatment. Although, recurrent seizures should be treated with I.V. diazepam. Since many of the NSAIDs undergo enterohepatic cycling, multiple doses of charcoal may be needed to reduce the potential for delayed toxicities.

Drug Interactions

Decreased effect of diuretics

Increased effect/toxicity with probenecid, lithium

Increased toxicity of methotrexate

Mechanism of Action Inhibits prostaglandin synthesis by decreasing the activity of the enzyme, cyclo-oxygenase, which results in decreased formation of prostaglandin precursors

Pharmacodynamics/Kinetics

Absorption: Almost completely

Metabolism: In the liver

Half-life: 1-4 hours

Time to peak serum concentration: 0.5-2 hours

(Continued)

Ketoprofen *(Continued)*

Elimination: Renal excretion (60% to 75%), primarily as glucuronide conjugates

Usual Dosage Oral:

Children 3 months to 14 years: Fever: 0.5-1 mg/kg every 6-8 hours

Children >12 years and Adults:

Rheumatoid arthritis or osteoarthritis: 50-75 mg 3-4 times/day up to a maximum of 300 mg/day

Mild to moderate pain: 25-50 mg every 6-8 hours up to a maximum of 300 mg/day

Test Interactions ↑ chloride (S), ↑ sodium (S), ↑ bleeding time

Patient Information Take with food; may cause dizziness or drowsiness

Dosage Forms

Capsule (Orudis®): 25 mg, 50 mg, 75 mg

Actron®, Orudis® KT [OTC]: 12.5 mg

Capsule, extended release (Oruvail®): 100 mg, 200 mg

Ketorolac Tromethamine (KEE toe role ak troe METH a meen)

Related Information

Dosing Data for Acetaminophen and NSAIDs *on page 1377*
Nonsteroidal Anti-Inflammatory Agents Comparison *on page 1419*

Brand Names Acular®; Toradol®

Canadian/Mexican Brand Names Dolac® Oral (Mexico); Dolac® Injectable (Mexico)

Therapeutic Category Analgesic, Nonsteroidal Anti-inflammatory Drug; Anti-inflammatory Agent; Nonsteroidal Anti-inflammatory Agent (NSAID), Oral; Nonsteroidal Anti-Inflammatory Agent (NSAID), Parenteral

Use Short-term (<5 days) management of pain; first parenteral NSAID for analgesia; 30 mg provides the analgesia comparable to 12 mg of morphine or 100 mg of meperidine

Pregnancy Risk Factor B (D if used in the 3rd trimester)

Contraindications In patients who have developed nasal polyps, angioedema, or bronchospastic reactions to other NSAIDs, active peptic ulcer disease, recent GI bleeding or perforation, patients with advanced renal disease or risk of renal failure, labor and delivery, nursing mothers, patients with hypersensitivity to ketorolac, aspirin, or other NSAIDs, **prophylaxis before major surgery**, suspected or confirmed cerebrovascular bleeding, hemorrhagic diathesis, concurrent ASA or other NSAIDs, epidural or intrathecal administration, concomitant probenecid

Warnings/Precautions Use extra caution and reduce dosages in the elderly because it is cleared renally somewhat slower, and the elderly are also more sensitive to the renal effects of NSAIDs; use with caution in patients with congestive heart failure, hypertension, decreased renal or hepatic function, history of GI disease (bleeding or ulcers), or those receiving anticoagulants

Adverse Reactions

Genitourinary: Renal impairment

Hematologic: Wound bleeding (with I.M.), postoperative hematomas

1% to 10%:

Cardiovascular: Edema

Central nervous system: Drowsiness, dizziness, headache, pain

Gastrointestinal: Nausea, dyspepsia, diarrhea, gastric ulcers, indigestion

Local: Pain at injection site

Miscellaneous: Diaphoresis (increased)

<1%:

Central nervous system: Mental depression

Dermatologic: Purpura

Gastrointestinal: Aphthous stomatitis, rectal bleeding, peptic ulceration

Ocular: Change in vision

Renal: Oliguria

Respiratory: Dyspnea

Overdosage/Toxicology Symptoms of overdose include diarrhea, pallor, vomiting, labored breathing, apnea, metabolic acidosis, leukocytosis, renal failure

Management of a nonsteroidal anti-inflammatory drug (NSAID) intoxication is primarily supportive and symptomatic. Fluid therapy is commonly effective in managing the hypotension that may occur following an acute NSAID overdose, except when this is due to an acute blood loss. Seizures tend to be very short-lived and often do not require drug treatment; although, recurrent seizures should be treated with I.V. diazepam. Since many of the NSAIDs undergo enterohepatic cycling, multiple doses of charcoal may be needed to reduce the potential for delayed toxicities; NSAIDs are highly bound to plasma proteins; therefore, hemodialysis and peritoneal dialysis are not useful.

Drug Interactions

Decreased effect of diuretics

Increased toxicity: Lithium, methotrexate increased drug level; increased effect/toxicity with salicylates, probenecid

Stability

Ketorolac tromethamine injection should be stored at controlled room temperature and protected from light; injection is clear and has a slight yellow color; precipitation may occur at relatively low pH values

Compatible with NS, D_5W, D_5NS, LR

Incompatible with meperidine, morphine, promethazine, and hydroxyzine

Mechanism of Action Inhibits prostaglandin synthesis by decreasing the activity of the enzyme, cyclo-oxygenase, which results in decreased formation of prostaglandin precursors

Pharmacodynamics/Kinetics

Analgesic effect:
- Onset of action: I.M.: Within 10 minutes
- Peak effect: Within 75-150 minutes
- Duration of action: 6-8 hours

Absorption: Oral: Well absorbed

Time to peak serum concentration: I.M.: 30-60 minutes

Distribution: Crosses placenta; crosses into breast milk; poor penetration into CSF

Protein binding: 99%

Metabolism: In the liver

Half-life: 2-8 hours; increased 30% to 50% in elderly

Elimination: Renal excretion, 61% appearing in the urine as unchanged drug

Usual Dosage

Adults (pain relief usually begins within 10 minutes with parenteral forms):
- Oral: 10 mg every 4-6 hours as needed for a maximum of 40 mg/day; on day of transition from I.M. to oral: maximum oral dose: 40 mg (or 120 mg combined oral and I.M.); maximum 5 days administration
- I.M.: Initial: 30-60 mg, then 15-30 mg every 6 hours as needed for up to 5 days maximum; maximum dose in the first 24 hours: 150 mg with 120 mg/24 hours for up to 5 days total
- I.V.: Initial: 30 mg, then 15-30 mg every 6 hours as needed for up to 5 days **maximum**; maximum daily dose: 120 mg for up to 5 days total
- Ophthalmic: Instill 1 drop in eye(s) 4 times/day

Elderly >65 years: Renal insufficiency or weight <50 kg:
- I.M.: 30 mg, then 15 mg every 6 hours
- I.V.: 15 mg every 6 hours as needed for up to 5 days total; maximum daily dose: 120 mg

Dietary Considerations

Potassium: Hyperkalemia has been reported. The elderly and those with renal insufficiency are at greatest risk. Monitor potassium serum concentration in those at greatest risk. Avoid salt substitutes.

Sodium: Hyponatremia from sodium retention. Suspect secondary to suppression of renal prostaglandin. Monitor serum concentration and fluid status. May need to restrict fluid.

Monitoring Parameters Monitor response (pain, range of motion, grip strength, mobility, ADL function), inflammation; observe for weight gain, edema; monitor renal function (serum creatinine, BUN, urine output); observe for bleeding, bruising; evaluate gastrointestinal effects (abdominal pain, bleeding, dyspepsia); mental confusion, disorientation, CBC, liver function tests

Reference Range Serum concentration: Therapeutic: 0.3-5 µg/mL; Toxic: >5 µg/mL

Test Interactions ↑ chloride (S), ↑ sodium (S), ↑ bleeding time

Patient Information Serious gastrointestinal bleeding can occur as well as ulceration and perforation. Pain may or may not be present. Avoid aspirin and aspirin-containing products while taking this medication. If gastric adverse effects persist, contact physician. May cause drowsiness, dizziness, blurred vision, and confusion. Use caution when performing tasks which require alertness (eg, driving).

Nursing Implications Monitor for signs of pain relief, such as an increased appetite and activity

Dosage Forms

Injection: 15 mg/mL (1 mL); 30 mg/mL (1 mL, 2 mL)

Solution, ophthalmic: 0.5% (5 mL)

Tablet: 10 mg

Key-Pred® *see* Prednisolone *on page 1037*

Key-Pred-SP® *see* Prednisolone *on page 1037*

K-G® Elixir *see* Potassium Gluconate *on page 1026*

KI *see* Potassium Iodide *on page 1027*

K-Ide® *see* Potassium Bicarbonate and Potassium Citrate, Effervescent *on page 1023*

Kinesed® *see* Hyoscyamine, Atropine, Scopolamine, and Phenobarbital *on page 637*

Klaron® Lotion *see* Sulfacetamide Sodium *on page 1171*

K-Lease® *see* Potassium Chloride *on page 1024*

Klonopin™ *see* Clonazepam *on page 297*

K-Lor™ *see* Potassium Chloride *on page 1024*

Klor-Con® *see* Potassium Chloride *on page 1024*

Klor-Con® 8 *see* Potassium Chloride *on page 1024*

Klor-Con® 10 *see* Potassium Chloride *on page 1024*

Klor-Con/25® *see* Potassium Chloride *on page 1024*

Klor-con®/EF *see* Potassium Bicarbonate and Potassium Citrate, Effervescent *on page 1023*

Kloromin® [OTC] *see* Chlorpheniramine *on page 260*

Klorvess® *see* Potassium Chloride *on page 1024*

Klotrix® *see* Potassium Chloride *on page 1024*

K-Lyte® *see* Potassium Bicarbonate and Potassium Citrate, Effervescent *on page 1023*

K-Lyte/Cl® *see* Potassium Chloride *on page 1024*

K-Norm® *see* Potassium Chloride *on page 1024*

Koāte®-HP *see* Antihemophilic Factor (Human) *on page 94*

Koāte®-HS *see* Antihemophilic Factor (Human) *on page 94*

Kolephrin® GG/DM [OTC] *see* Guaifenesin and Dextromethorphan *on page 591*

Konakion® *see* Phytonadione *on page 998*

Kondremul® [OTC] *see* Mineral Oil *on page 841*

Konsyl® [OTC] *see* Psyllium *on page 1075*

Konsyl-D® [OTC] *see* Psyllium *on page 1075*

Konӯne® 80 *see* Factor IX Complex (Human) *on page 502*

K-Phos® Neutral *see* Potassium Phosphate and Sodium Phosphate *on page 1031*

K-Phos® Original *see* Potassium Acid Phosphate *on page 1022*

K-Tab® *see* Potassium Chloride *on page 1024*

Ku-Zyme® HP *see* Pancrelipase *on page 949*

K-Vescent® *see* Potassium Bicarbonate and Potassium Citrate, Effervescent *on page 1023*

Kytril® *see* Granisetron *on page 586*

***L*-3-Hydroxytyrosine** *see* Levodopa *on page 714*

LA-12® *see* Hydroxocobalamin *on page 629*

Labetalol (la BET a lole)

Related Information

Beta-Blockers Comparison *on page 1398*
Therapy of Hypertension *on page 1540*

Brand Names Normodyne®; Trandate®

Canadian/Mexican Brand Names Midotens® (Mexico)

Synonyms Ibidomide Hydrochloride; Labetalol Hydrochloride

Therapeutic Category Antihypertensive; Beta-Adrenergic Blocker

Use Treatment of mild to severe hypertension; I.V. for hypertensive emergencies

Pregnancy Risk Factor C

Pregnancy/Breast-Feeding Implications

Clinical effects on the fetus: Crosses the placenta. Bradycardia, hypotension, hypoglycemia, IUGR. IUGR probably related to maternal hypertension. Available evidence suggests safe use during pregnancy and breast-feeding. Monitor breast-fed infant for symptoms of beta-blockade.

Breast-feeding/lactation: Crosses into breast milk. American Academy of Pediatrics considers COMPATIBLE with breast-feeding.

Contraindications Cardiogenic shock, uncompensated congestive heart failure, bradycardia, pulmonary edema, or heart block

Warnings/Precautions Paradoxical increase in blood pressure has been reported with treatment of pheochromocytoma or clonidine withdrawal syndrome; use with caution in patients with hyper-reactive airway disease, congestive heart failure, diabetes mellitus, hepatic dysfunction; orthostatic hypotension may occur with I.V. administration; patient should remain supine during and for up to 3 hours after I.V. administration; use with caution in impaired hepatic function (discontinue if signs of liver dysfunction occur); may mask the signs and symptoms of hypoglycemia; a lower hemodynamic response rate and higher incidence of toxicity may be observed with administration to elderly patients.

Adverse Reactions

1% to 10%:

Cardiovascular: Congestive heart failure, arrhythmia, reduced peripheral circulation, orthostatic hypotension

Central nervous system: Mental depression, dizziness, drowsiness

Dermatologic: Itching, numbness of skin

Endocrine & metabolic: Decreased sexual ability

Gastrointestinal: Nausea, vomiting, stomach discomfort, abnormal taste

Neuromuscular & skeletal: Weakness

Respiratory: Dyspnea, nasal congestion

<1%:

Cardiovascular: Bradycardia, chest pain

Dermatologic: Rash

Gastrointestinal: Diarrhea

Hepatic: Hepatotoxicity

Neuromuscular & skeletal: Arthralgia

Ocular: Dry eyes

Overdosage/Toxicology Symptoms of intoxication include cardiac disturbances, CNS toxicity, bronchospasm, hypoglycemia and hyperkalemia. The most common cardiac symptoms include hypotension and bradycardia; atrioventricular block, intraventricular conduction disturbances, cardiogenic shock, and systole may occur with severe overdose, especially with membrane-depressant drugs (eg, propranolol); CNS effects include convulsions, coma, and respiratory arrest is commonly seen with propranolol and other membrane-depressant and lipid-soluble drugs.

Treatment includes symptomatic treatment of seizures, hypotension, hyperkalemia and hypoglycemia; bradycardia and hypotension resistant to atropine, isoproterenol or pacing may respond to glucagon; wide QRS defects caused by the membrane-depressant poisoning may respond to hypertonic sodium bicarbonate; repeat-dose charcoal, hemoperfusion, or hemodialysis may be helpful in removal of only those beta-blockers with a small V_d, long half-life or low intrinsic clearance (acebutolol, atenolol, nadolol, sotalol)

Drug Interactions

Decreased effect of beta-blockers with aluminum salts, barbiturates, calcium salts, cholestyramine, colestipol, NSAIDs, penicillins (ampicillin), rifampin, salicylates and sulfinpyrazone due to decreased bioavailability and plasma levels

Beta-blockers may decrease the effect of sulfonylureas

Increased effect/toxicity of beta-blockers with calcium blockers (diltiazem, felodipine, nicardipine), contraceptives, flecainide, haloperidol (propranolol, hypotensive effects), H_2-antagonists (metoprolol, propranolol only by cimetidine, possibly ranitidine), hydralazine (metoprolol, propranolol), loop diuretics (propranolol, not atenolol), MAO inhibitors (metoprolol, nadolol, bradycardia), phenothiazines (propranolol), propafenone (metoprolol, propranolol), quinidine (in extensive metabolizers), ciprofloxacin, thyroid hormones (metoprolol, propranolol, when hypothyroid patient is converted to euthyroid state)

Beta-blockers may increase the effect/toxicity of flecainide, haloperidol (hypotensive effects), hydralazine, phenothiazines, acetaminophen, anticoagulants (propranolol, warfarin), benzodiazepines (not atenolol), clonidine (hypertensive crisis after or during withdrawal of either agent), epinephrine (initial hypertensive episode followed by bradycardia), nifedipine and verapamil lidocaine, ergots (peripheral ischemia), prazosin (postural hypotension)

Beta-blockers may affect the action or levels of ethanol, disopyramide, nondepolarizing muscle relaxants and theophylline although the effects are difficult to predict

Stability

Labetalol should be stored at room temperature or under refrigeration and should be protected from light and freezing; the solution is clear to slightly yellow

Stability of parenteral admixture at room temperature (25°C) and refrigeration temperature (4°C): 3 days

Standard diluent: 500 mg/250 mL D_5W

Minimum volume: 250 mL D_5W

Incompatible with sodium bicarbonate, most stable at pH of 2-4; **incompatible** with alkaline solutions

Mechanism of Action Blocks alpha-, $beta_1$-, and $beta_2$-adrenergic receptor sites; elevated renins are reduced

Pharmacodynamics/Kinetics

Onset of action:

Oral: 20 minutes to 2 hours

I.V.: 2-5 minutes

Peak effect:

Oral: 1-4 hours

I.V.: 5-15 minutes

(Continued)

Labetalol *(Continued)*

Duration:
- Oral: 8-24 hours (dose-dependent)
- I.V.: 2-4 hours

Distribution: Crosses placenta; small amounts in breast milk; moderately lipid soluble, therefore, can enter CNS
- V_d: Adults: 3-16 L/kg; mean: <9.4 L/kg

Protein binding: 50%

Metabolism: Extensive first-pass effect; metabolized in liver primarily via glucuronide conjugation

Bioavailability: Oral: 25%; increased with liver disease, elderly, and concurrent cimetidine

Half-life, normal renal function: 6-8 hours

Elimination: <5% excreted in urine unchanged; possible decreased clearance in neonates/infants

Usual Dosage Due to limited documentation of its use, labetalol should be initiated cautiously in pediatric patients with careful dosage adjustment and blood pressure monitoring

Children:
- Oral: Limited information regarding labetalol use in pediatric patients is currently available in literature. Some centers recommend initial oral doses of 4 mg/kg/day in 2 divided doses. Reported oral doses have started at 3 mg/kg/day and 20 mg/kg/day and have increased up to 40 mg/kg/day.
- I.V., intermittent bolus doses of 0.3-1 mg/kg/dose have been reported
- For treatment of pediatric hypertensive emergencies, initial continuous infusions of 0.4-1 mg/kg/hour with a maximum of 3 mg/kg/hour have been used; administration requires the use of an infusion pump

Adults:
- Oral: Initial: 100 mg twice daily, may increase as needed every 2-3 days by 100 mg until desired response is obtained; usual dose: 200-400 mg twice daily; not to exceed 2.4 g/day
- I.V.: 20 mg or 1-2 mg/kg whichever is lower, IVP over 2 minutes, may administer 40-80 mg at 10-minute intervals, up to 300 mg total dose
- I.V. infusion: Initial: 2 mg/minute; titrate to response up to 300 mg total dose; administration requires the use of an infusion pump
- **I.V. infusion (500 mg/250 mL D_5W)** rates:
  - 1 mg/minute: 30 mL/hour
  - 2 mg/minute: 60 mL/hour
  - 3 mg/minute: 90 mL/hour
  - 4 mg/minute: 120 mL/hour
  - 5 mg/minute: 150 mL/hour
  - 6 mg/minute: 180 mL/hour

Dialysis: Not removed by hemo- or peritoneal dialysis; supplemental dose is not necessary

Dosage adjustment in hepatic impairment: Dosage reduction may be necessary

Monitoring Parameters Blood pressure, standing and sitting/supine, pulse, cardiac monitor and blood pressure monitor required for I.V. administration

Test Interactions False-positive urine catecholamines, VMA if measured by fluorometric or photometric methods; use HPLC or specific catecholamine radioenzymatic technique

Patient Information Do not stop medication without aid of physician; may mask signs and symptoms of diabetes

Dosage Forms
- Injection, as hydrochloride: 5 mg/mL (20 mL, 40 mL, 60 mL)
- Tablet, as hydrochloride: 100 mg, 200 mg, 300 mg

Labetalol Hydrochloride *see* Labetalol *on page 700*

LaBID® *see* Theophylline Salts *on page 1207*

Laboratory Values *see page 1488*

LactiCare-HC® *see* Hydrocortisone *on page 623*

Lactinex® [OTC] *see Lactobacillus acidophilus* and *Lactobacillus bulgaricus on this page*

Lactobacillus acidophilus and *Lactobacillus bulgaricus*

(lak toe ba SIL us as i DOF fil us & lak toe ba SIL us bul GAR i cus)

Brand Names Bacid® [OTC]; Lactinex® [OTC]; More-Dophilus® [OTC]

Canadian/Mexican Brand Names Fermalac® (Canada); Lacteol® Fort (Mexico); Sinuberase® (Mexico)

Therapeutic Category Antidiarrheal

Use Treatment of uncomplicated diarrhea particularly that caused by antibiotic therapy; re-establish normal physiologic and bacterial flora of the intestinal tract

Contraindications Allergy to milk or lactose

Warnings/Precautions Discontinue if high fever present; do not use in children <3 years of age

Adverse Reactions 1% to 10%: Gastrointestinal: Intestinal flatus

Stability Store in the refrigerator

Mechanism of Action Creates an environment unfavorable to potentially pathogenic fungi or bacteria through the production of lactic acid, and favors establishment of an aciduric flora, thereby suppressing the growth of pathogenic microorganisms; helps re-establish normal intestinal flora

Pharmacodynamics/Kinetics

Absorption: Oral: Not absorbed

Distribution: Locally, primarily in the colon

Elimination: In feces

Usual Dosage Children >3 years and Adults: Oral:

Capsules: 2 capsules 2-4 times/day

Granules: 1 packet added to or taken with cereal, food, milk, fruit juice, or water, 3-4 times/day

Powder: 1 teaspoonful daily with liquid

Tablet, chewable: 4 tablets 3-4 times/day; may follow each dose with a small amount of milk, fruit juice, or water

Administration Granules may be added to or given with cereal, food, milk, fruit juice, or water

Patient Information Refrigerate; granules may be added to or taken with cereal, food, milk, fruit juice, or water

Dosage Forms

Capsule: 50s, 100s

Granules: 1 g/packet (12 packets/box)

Powder: 12 oz

Tablet, chewable: 50s

Lactoflavin *see* Riboflavin *on page 1104*

Lactulose (LAK tyoo lose)

Related Information

Laxatives, Classification and Properties *on page 1412*

Brand Names Cephulac®; Cholac®; Chronulac®; Constilac®; Constulose®; Duphalac®; Enulose®; Evalose®; Heptalac®; Lactulose PSE®

Therapeutic Category Ammonium Detoxicant; Laxative, Miscellaneous

Use Adjunct in the prevention and treatment of portal-systemic encephalopathy (PSE); treatment of chronic constipation

Pregnancy Risk Factor B

Contraindications Patients with galactosemia and require a low galactose diet, hypersensitivity to any component

Warnings/Precautions Use with caution in patients with diabetes mellitus; monitor periodically for electrolyte imbalance when lactulose is used >6 months or in patients predisposed to electrolyte abnormalities (eg, elderly); patients receiving lactulose and an oral anti-infective agent should be monitored for possible inadequate response to lactulose

Adverse Reactions

>10%: Gastrointestinal: Flatulence, diarrhea (excessive dose)

1% to 10%: Gastrointestinal: Abdominal discomfort, nausea, vomiting

Overdosage/Toxicology Symptoms of overdose include diarrhea, abdominal pain, hypochloremic alkalosis, dehydration, hypotension, hypokalemia; treatment includes supportive care

Drug Interactions Decreased effect: Oral neomycin, laxatives, antacids

Stability Keep solution at room temperature to reduce viscosity; discard solution if cloudy or very dark

Mechanism of Action The bacterial degradation of lactulose resulting in an acidic pH inhibits the diffusion of NH_3 into the blood by causing the conversion of NH_3 to NH_4+; also enhances the diffusion of NH_3 from the blood into the gut where conversion to NH_4+ occurs; produces an osmotic effect in the colon with resultant distention promoting peristalsis

Pharmacodynamics/Kinetics

Absorption: Oral: Not absorbed appreciably following administration; this is desirable since the intended site of action is within the colon

Metabolism: By colonic flora to lactic acid and acetic acid, requires colonic flora for primary drug activation

Elimination: Primarily in feces and urine (~3%)

Usual Dosage Diarrhea may indicate overdosage and responds to dose reduction

(Continued)

Lactulose *(Continued)*

Prevention of portal systemic encephalopathy (PSE): Oral:

Infants: 2.5-10 mL/day divided 3-4 times/day; adjust dosage to produce 2-3 stools/day

Older Children: Daily dose of 40-90 mL divided 3-4 times/day; if initial dose causes diarrhea, then reduce it immediately; adjust dosage to produce 2-3 stools/day

Constipation:

Children: 5 g/day (7.5 mL) after breakfast

Adults:

Acute PSE:

Oral: 20-30 g (30-45 mL) every 1-2 hours to induce rapid laxation; adjust dosage daily to produce 2-3 soft stools; doses of 30-45 mL may be given hourly to cause rapid laxation, then reduce to recommended dose; usual daily dose: 60-100 g or 20-30 g (30-45 mL), 3-4 times/day

Rectal administration: 200 g (300 mL) diluted with 700 mL of H_2O or NS; administer rectally via rectal balloon catheter and retain 30-60 minutes every 4-6 hours

Constipation: Oral: 15-30 mL/day increased to 60 mL/day if necessary

Monitoring Parameters Blood pressure, standing/supine; serum potassium, bowel movement patterns, fluid status, serum ammonia

Patient Information Lactulose can be taken "as is" or diluted with water, fruit juice or milk, or taken in a food; laxative results may not occur for 24-48 hours

Nursing Implications Dilute lactulose in water, usually 60-120 mL, prior to administering through a gastric or feeding tube

Dosage Forms Syrup: 10 g/15 mL (15 mL, 30 mL, 237 mL, 473 mL, 946 mL, 1890 mL)

Lactulose PSE® *see* Lactulose *on previous page*

Lamictal® *see* Lamotrigine *on next page*

Lamisil® *see* Terbinafine, Topical *on page 1194*

Lamivudine (la MI vyoo deen)

Related Information

Occupational Exposure to HIV *on page 1448*

Brand Names Epivir®

Synonyms 3TC

Therapeutic Category Antiretroviral Agent; Antiviral Agent, Oral; Reverse Transcriptase Inhibitor

Use In combination with zidovudine (or other nucleoside) and often a protease inhibitor for treatment of HIV infection when therapy is warranted based on clinical and/or immunological evidence of disease progression; recommended with zidovudine for prophylaxis of HIV following needle sticks; has also demonstrated positive effects in the treatment of hepatitis B

Pregnancy Risk Factor C

Pregnancy/Breast-Feeding Implications

Use only if the potential benefits outweigh the risks. Combination therapy with zidovudine and lamivudine is currently being investigated to decrease the maternal/fetal transmission of HIV.

HIV-infected mothers are discouraged from breast-feeding to decrease postnatal transmission of HIV

Contraindications Hypersensitivity to any component

Warnings/Precautions A decreased dosage is recommended in patients with renal dysfunction since AUC, C_{max}, and half-life increased with diminishing renal function; use with extreme caution in children with history of pancreatitis or risk factors for development of pancreatitis

Adverse Reactions

>10%:

Central nervous system: Headache, insomnia, malaise, fatigue, pain

Gastrointestinal: Nausea, diarrhea, vomiting

Neuromuscular & skeletal: Peripheral neuropathy, paresthesia

Respiratory: Nasal signs and symptoms, cough

1% to 10%:

Central nervous system: Dizziness, depression, fever, chills

Dermatologic: Rashes

Gastrointestinal: Anorexia, abdominal pain, dyspepsia, elevated amylase

Hematologic: Neutropenia, anemia

Hepatic: Elevated AST, ALT

Neuromuscular & skeletal: Myalgia, arthralgia

<1%:

Gastrointestinal: Pancreatitis

Hematologic: Thrombocytopenia

Hepatic: Hyperbilirubinemia

Overdosage/Toxicology Very limited information is available although there have been no clinical signs or symptoms noted and hematologic tests remained normal in overdose; no antidote is available; unknown dialyzability

Drug Interactions Increased effect: Zidovudine concentrations increase significantly (~39%) with coadministration with lamivudine; trimethoprim/sulfamethoxazole increases lamivudine's AUC and decreases its renal clearance by 44% and 29%, respectively; although the AUC was not significantly affected, absorption of lamivudine was slowed and C_{max} was 40% lower when administered to patients in the fed versus the fasted state

Stability Store solution at 2°C to 25°C tightly closed

Mechanism of Action *In vitro*, lamivudine is phosphorylated to its active 5'-triphosphate metabolite (L-TP), which inhibits HIV reverse transcription via viral DNA chain termination; L-TP also inhibits the RNA- and DNA-dependent DNA polymerase activities of reverse transcriptase

Pharmacodynamics/Kinetics

Absorption: Oral: Rapid in HIV-infected patients

Distribution: V_d: 1.3 L/kg

Protein binding, plasma: <36%

Metabolism: 5.6% metabolized to trans-sulfoxide metabolite

Bioavailability: Absolute; Cp_{max} decreased with food although AUC not significantly affected

- Children: 66%
- Adults: 87%

Half-life:

- Children: 2 hours
- Adults: 5-7 hours

Elimination: Most eliminated unchanged in urine

Usual Dosage Oral:

Children 3 months to 12 years: 4 mg/kg twice daily (maximum: 150 mg twice daily) with zidovudine

Adolescents 12-16 years and Adults: 150 mg twice daily with zidovudine

Prevention of HIV following needle sticks: 150 mg twice daily with zidovudine 200 mg 3 times/day; a protease inhibitor (eg, indinavir) may be added for high risk exposures; begin therapy within 2 hours of exposure if possible

Adults <50 kg: 2 mg/kg twice daily with zidovudine

Dosing interval in renal impairment in patients >16 years:

- Cl_{cr} <50 mL/minute: Administer 150 mg twice daily
- Cl_{cr} 30-49 mL/minute: Administer 150 mg once daily
- Cl_{cr} 15-29 mL/minute: Administer 150 mg first dose, then 100 mg once daily
- Cl_{cr} 5-14 mL/minute: Administer 150 mg first dose, then 50 mg once daily
- Cl_{cr} <5 mL/minute: Administer 50 mg first dose, then 25 mg once daily

Dialysis: No data available

Monitoring Parameters Amylase, bilirubin, liver enzymes, hematologic parameters

Patient Information Patients may still experience illnesses associated with HIV infection; lamivudine is not a cure for HIV infection nor has it been shown to reduce the risk of transmission to others; long-term effects are unknown; take exactly as prescribed; children should be monitored for symptoms of pancreatitis; taken on an empty stomach if possible

Nursing Implications Monitor children for signs and symptoms of pancreatitis; evaluate frequently for opportunistic infection and other complications of HIV; administer on an empty stomach, if possible; adjust dosage in renal failure

Additional Information There are, as yet, no results from clinical trials evaluating the effect of lamivudine, in combination with zidovudine, on progression of HIV infection (eg, incidence of opportunistic infections or survival). Patients may continue to develop infections and other complications of HIV infection and should remain under close physician observation.

Dosage Forms

Solution, oral: 10 mg/mL (240 mL)

Tablets: 150 mg

Lamotrigine (la MOE tri jeen)

Related Information

Anticonvulsants by Seizure Type *on page 1392*

Epilepsy Treatment *on page 1531*

Brand Names Lamictal®

Synonyms BW-430C; LTG

Therapeutic Category Anticonvulsant

Use Partial/secondary generalized seizures in adults; childhood epilepsy **(not approved for use in children <16 years of age)**

Pregnancy Risk Factor C

(Continued)

Lamotrigine *(Continued)*

Contraindications History of hypersensitivity to lamotrigine or any component

Warnings/Precautions Lactation, impaired renal, hepatic, or cardiac function; avoid abrupt cessation, taper over at least 2 weeks if possible. Severe and potentially life-threatening skin rashes have been reported; this appears to occur most frequently in pediatric patients.

Adverse Reactions

1% to 10%:

Central nervous system: Dizziness, sedation, ataxia

Dermatologic: Hypersensitivity rash, Stevens-Johnson syndrome, angioedema

Ocular: Nystagmus, diplopia

Renal: Hematuria

Overdosage/Toxicology

Decontamination: Lavage/activated charcoal with cathartic

Enhancement of elimination: Multiple dosing of activated charcoal may be useful

Drug Interactions

Decreased effect: Acetaminophen (increased renal clearance); carbamazepine, phenobarbital, and phenytoin (increased metabolic clearance)

Increased effect: Valproic acid increases half-life of lamotrigine (decreased metabolic clearance)

Mechanism of Action A triazine derivative which inhibits release of glutamate (an excitatory amino acid) and inhibits voltage-sensitive sodium channels, which stabilizes neuronal membranes

Pharmacodynamics/Kinetics

Distribution: V_d: 1.1 L/kg

Protein binding: 55%

Metabolism: Hepatic and renal

Half-life: 24 hours; increases to 59 hours with concomitant valproic acid therapy; decreases with concomitant phenytoin or carbamazepine therapy to 15 hours

Peak levels: Within 1-4 hours

Elimination: In urine as the glucuronide conjugate

Usual Dosage Oral:

Children: 2-15 mg/kg/day in 2 divided doses

Adults: Initial dose: 50-100 mg/day then titrate to daily maintenance dose of 100-400 mg/day in 1-2 divided daily doses

With concomitant valproic acid therapy: Start initial dose at 25 mg/day then titrate to maintenance dose of 50-200 mg/day in 1-2 divided daily doses

Dietary Considerations Food: Has no effect on absorption, take without regard to meals; drug may cause GI upset

Monitoring Parameters Seizure, frequency and duration, serum levels of concurrent anticonvulsants, hypersensitivity reactions, especially rash

Reference Range Therapeutic range: 2-4 μg/mL

Additional Information Low water solubility

Dosage Forms Tablet: 25 mg, 100 mg, 150 mg, 200 mg

Lamprene® *see* Clofazimine *on page 293*

Lanacane® [OTC] *see* Benzocaine *on page 138*

Lanacort® [OTC] *see* Hydrocortisone *on page 623*

Laniazid® Oral *see* Isoniazid *on page 679*

Lanorinal® *see* Butalbital Compound *on page 176*

Lanoxicaps® *see* Digoxin *on page 385*

Lanoxin® *see* Digoxin *on page 385*

Lansoprazole (lan SOE pra zole)

Brand Names Prevacid®

Therapeutic Category Gastric Acid Secretion Inhibitor

Use Short-term treatment (up to 4 weeks) for healing and symptom relief of active duodenal ulcers (should not be used for maintenance therapy of duodenal ulcers); up to 8 weeks of treatment for all grades of erosive esophagitis (8 additional weeks can be given for incompletely healed esophageal erosions or for recurrence); and long-term treatment of pathological hypersecretory conditions, including Zollinger-Ellison syndrome

Pregnancy Risk Factor B

Contraindications Should not be taken by anyone with a known hypersensitivity to lansoprazole or any of the formulation's components

Warnings/Precautions Liver disease may require dosage reductions

Adverse Reactions

1% to 10%:

Central nervous system: Fatigue, dizziness, headache

Gastrointestinal: Abdominal pain, diarrhea, nausea, increased appetite, hypergastrinoma

<1%:
- Dermatologic: Rash
- Otic: Tinnitus
- Renal: Proteinuria

Overdosage/Toxicology Symptoms of overdose include hypothermia, sedation, convulsions, decreased respiratory rate demonstrated in animals only; treatment is supportive; not dialyzable

Drug Interactions Decreased effect: Ketoconazole, itraconazole, and other drugs dependent upon acid for absorption; theophylline clearance increased slightly; sucralfate delays and reduces lansoprazole absorption by 30%

Stability Lansoprazole is unstable in acidic media (eg, stomach contents) and is, therefore, administered as enteric coated granules in capsule form; the capsule contents (granules) may be given via nasogastric tube when mixed (not crushed) with apple juice

Usual Dosage

Duodenal or gastric ulcer: 30 mg once daily for 4-8 weeks

Erosive esophagitis: 30 mg once daily for 4-8 weeks

Hypersecretory conditions: 30-180 mg once daily, titrated to reduce acid secretion to <10 mEq/hour (5 mEq/hour in patients with prior gastric surgery)

Dosing adjustment in hepatic impairment: May require a dose reduction

Administration For nasogastric tube administration, the capsules can be opened, the granules mixed (not crushed) with 40 mL of apple juice and then injected through the NG tube into the stomach

Monitoring Parameters Patients with Zollinger-Ellison syndrome should be monitored for gastric acid output, which should be maintained at 10 mEq/hour or less during the last hour before the next lansoprazole dose; lab monitoring should include CBC, liver function, renal function, and serum gastrin levels

Patient Information Take before eating; do not crush or chew capsules

Dosage Forms Capsule, delayed release: 15 mg, 30 mg

Lariam® *see* Mefloquine *on page 774*

Larodopa® *see* Levodopa *on page 714*

Lasan™ *see* Anthralin *on page 93*

Lasan HP-1™ *see* Anthralin *on page 93*

Lasix® *see* Furosemide *on page 561*

L-asparaginase *see* Asparaginase *on page 103*

Lassar's Zinc Paste *see* Zinc Oxide *on page 1324*

Latanoprost (la TAN oh prost)

Brand Names Xalatan®

Therapeutic Category Prostaglandin, Ophthalmic

Use Reduction of elevated intraocular pressure in patients with open-angle glaucoma and ocular hypertension who are intolerant of the other IOP lowering medications or insufficiently responsive (failed to achieve target IOP determined after multiple measurements over time) to another IOP lowering medication

Pregnancy Risk Factor C

Contraindications Hypersensitivity to any component of product

Warnings/Precautions Latanoprost may gradually change eye color, increasing the amount of brown pigment in the iris by increasing the number of melanosome in melanocytes. The long-term effects on the melanocytes and the consequences of potential injury to the melanocytes or deposition of pigment granules to other areas of the eye is currently unknown. Patients should be examined regularly, and depending on the clinical situation, treatment may be stopped if increased pigmentation ensues.

There have been reports of bacterial keratitis associated with the use of multiple-dose containers of topical ophthalmic products. Do not administer while wearing contact lenses.

Adverse Reactions

>10%: Ocular: Blurred vision, burning and stinging, conjunctival hyperemia, foreign body sensation, itching, increased pigmentation of the iris, and punctate epithelial keratopathy

1% to 10%:
- Cardiovascular: Chest pain, angina pectoris
- Dermatologic: Rash, allergic skin reaction
- Neuromuscular & skeletal: Myalgia, arthralgia, back pain
- Ocular: Dry eye, excessive tearing, eye pain, lid crusting, lid edema, lid erythema, lid discomfort/pain, photophobia
- Respiratory: Upper respiratory tract infection, cold, flu

<1%: Ocular: Conjunctivitis, diplopia, discharge from the eye, retinal artery embolus, retinal detachment, vitreous hemorrhage from diabetic retinopathy

Overdosage/Toxicology Symptoms include ocular irritation and conjunctival or episcleral hyperemia; treatment should be symptomatic

(Continued)

Latanoprost *(Continued)*

Drug Interactions Decreased effect: *In vitro* studies have shown that precipitation occurs when eye drops containing thimerosal are mixed with latanoprost. If such drugs are used, administer with an interval of at least 5 minutes between applications

Stability Protect from light; store intact bottles under refrigeration (2°C to 8°C/ 36°F to 46°F). Once opened, the container may be stored at room temperature up to 25°C (77°F) for 6 weeks.

Mechanism of Action Latanoprost is a prostaglandin F_2-alpha analog believed to reduce intraocular pressure by increasing the outflow of the aqueous humor

Pharmacodynamics/Kinetics

Onset of effect: 3-4 hours

Maximum effect: 8-12 hours

Absorption: Through the cornea where the isopropyl ester prodrug is hydrolyzed by esterases to the biologically active acid. Peak concentration is reached in 2 hours after topical administration in the aqueous humor.

Distribution: V_d: 0.16 L/kg

Half-life: 17 minutes

Metabolism: Primarily metabolized by the liver via fatty acid beta-oxidation

Elimination: After hepatic metabolism, the metabolites are mainly eliminated via the kidneys

Usual Dosage Adults: Ophthalmic: 1 drop (1.5 mcg) in the affected eye(s) once daily in the evening; do not exceed the once daily dosage because it has been shown that more frequent administration may decrease the IOP lowering effect

Administration If more than one topical ophthalmic drug is being used, administer the drugs at least 5 minutes apart

Patient Information Inform patients about the possibility of iris color change because of an increase of the brown pigment and resultant cosmetically different eye coloration that may occur. Iris pigmentation changes may be more noticeable in patients with green-brown, blue/gray-brown, or yellow-brown irides.

Advise patients to avoid allowing the tip of the dispensing container to contact the eye or surrounding structures because this could cause the tip to become contaminated by common bacteria known to cause ocular infections. Serious damage to the eye and subsequent loss of vision may result from using contaminated solutions.

Advise patients that if they develop any ocular reactions, particularly conjunctivitis and lid reactions, they should immediately seek their physician's advice.

Latanoprost contains benzalkonium chloride, which may be absorbed by contact lenses. Remove contact lenses prior to administration of the solution. Lenses may be reinserted 15 minutes following latanoprost administration.

If more than one topical ophthalmic drug is being used, administer the drugs at least 5 minutes apart.

Dosage Forms Solution, ophthalmic: 0.005% (2.5 mL)

Laxatives, Classification and Properties *see page 1412*

LazerSporin-C® Otic *see* Neomycin, Polymyxin B, and Hydrocortisone *on page 890*

***l*-Bunolol Hydrochloride** *see* Levobunolol *on page 712*

LCR *see* Vincristine *on page 1302*

L-Deprenyl *see* Selegiline *on page 1130*

***L*-Dopa** *see* Levodopa *on page 714*

Ledercillin® VK *see* Penicillin V Potassium *on page 965*

Lente® Iletin® I *see* Insulin Preparations *on page 659*

Lente® Iletin® II *see* Insulin Preparations *on page 659*

Lente® Insulin *see* Insulin Preparations *on page 659*

Lente® L *see* Insulin Preparations *on page 659*

Lescol® *see* Fluvastatin *on page 550*

Leucovorin (loo koe VOR in)

Related Information

Cancer Chemotherapy Regimens *on page 1351*

Guidelines for the Prevention of Opportunistic Infections in Persons with HIV *on page 1457*

Brand Names Wellcovorin®

Synonyms Calcium Leucovorin; Citrovorum Factor; Folinic Acid; 5-Formyl Tetrahydrofolate; Leucovorin Calcium

Therapeutic Category Antidote, Folic Acid Antagonist; Antidote, Methotrexate; Folic Acid Derivative; Vitamin, Water Soluble

Use Antidote for folic acid antagonists (methotrexate [>100 mg/m^2], trimethoprim, pyrimethamine); treatment of megaloblastic anemias when folate is deficient as in infancy, sprue, pregnancy, and nutritional deficiency when oral folate therapy is not possible; in combination with fluorouracil in the treatment of malignancy

Pregnancy Risk Factor C

Contraindications Pernicious anemia or vitamin B_{12} deficient megaloblastic anemias; should **NOT** be administered Intrathecally/Intraventricularly

Warnings/Precautions Use with caution in patients with a history of hypersensitivity

Adverse Reactions

<1%:

Dermatologic: Rash, pruritus, erythema, urticaria

Hematologic: Thrombocytosis

Respiratory: Wheezing

Miscellaneous: Anaphylactoid reactions

Stability

Leucovorin injection should be stored at room temperature and protected from light

Reconstituted solution is stated to be chemically stable for 7 days; reconstitutions with bacteriostatic water for injection, U.S.P., must be used within 7 days. Doses >10 mg/m^2 must be prepared using leucovorin reconstituted with sterile water for injection, U.S.P., and used immediately.

Stability of parenteral admixture at room temperature (25°C): 24 hours

Stability of parenteral admixture at refrigeration temperature (4°C): 4 days

Standard diluent: 50-100 mg/50 mL D_5W

Minimum volume: 50 mL D_5W

Concentrations of >2 mg/mL of leucovorin and >25 mg/mL of fluorouracil are **incompatible** (precipitation occurs)

Mechanism of Action A reduced form of folic acid, but does not require a reduction reaction by an enzyme for activation, allows for purine and thymidine synthesis, a necessity for normal erythropoiesis; leucovorin supplies the necessary cofactor blocked by MTX, enters the cells via the same active transport system as MTX

Pharmacodynamics/Kinetics

Onset of activity:

Oral: Within 30 minutes; rapid, well absorbed but decreases at doses >25 mg

I.V.: Within 5 minutes

Absorption: Oral, I.M.: Rapid

Metabolism: Rapidly converted to (5MTHF) 5-methyl-tetrahydrofolate (active) in the intestinal mucosa and by the liver

Half-life:

Leucovorin: 15 minutes

5MTHF: 33-35 minutes

Elimination: Primarily in urine (80% to 90%) with small losses appearing in feces (5% to 8%)

Usual Dosage Children and Adults:

Treatment of folic acid antagonist overdosage (eg, pyrimethamine or trimethoprim): Oral: 2-15 mg/day for 3 days or until blood counts are normal or 5 mg every 3 days; doses of 6 mg/day are needed for patients with platelet counts <100,000/mm^3

Folate-deficient megaloblastic anemia: I.M.: 1 mg/day

Megaloblastic anemia secondary to congenital deficiency of dihydrofolate reductase: I.M.: 3-6 mg/day

Rescue dose (rescue therapy should start within 24 hours of MTX therapy): I.V.: 10 mg/m^2 to start, then 10 mg/m^2 every 6 hours orally for 72 hours until serum MTX concentration is <10^{-8} molar; if serum creatinine 24 hours after methotrexate is elevated 50% or more above the pre-MTX serum creatinine **or** the serum MTX concentration is >5 x 10^{-6} molar (see graph), increase dose to 100 mg/m^2/dose (preservative-free) every 3 hours until serum methotrexate level is <1 x 10^{-8} molar

Investigational: Post I.T. methotrexate: Oral, I.V.: 12 mg/m^2 as a single dose; post high-dose methotrexate: 100-1000 mg/m^2/dose until the serum methotrexate level is less than 1 x 10^{-7} molar

The drug should be given parenterally instead of orally in patients with GI toxicity, nausea, vomiting, and when individual doses are >25 mg

Administration Leucovorin calcium should be administered I.M. or I.V.; rate of I.V. infusion should not exceed 160 mg/minute

Monitoring Parameters Plasma MTX concentration as a therapeutic guide to high-dose MTX therapy with leucovorin factor rescue

Leucovorin is continued until the plasma MTX level is <1 x 10^{-7} molar

Each dose of leucovorin is increased if the plasma MTX concentration is excessively high (see graph)

(Continued)

Leucovorin *(Continued)*

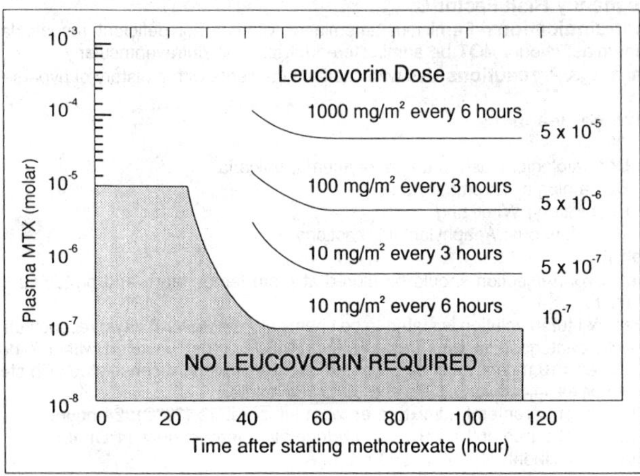

With 4- to 6-hour high-dose MTX infusions, plasma drug values in excess of 5×10^{-5} and 10^{-6} molar at 24 and 48 hours after starting the infusion, respectively, are often predictive of delayed MTX clearance; see graph.

Patient Information Patients should be informed to:

Contact their physician immediately, if they have an allergic reaction after taking leucovorin calcium (trouble breathing, wheezing, fainting, skin rash, or hives)

Let their physician know if they are pregnant or are trying to get pregnant before taking leucovorin calcium

Leucovorin calcium can be taken with or without food

Take exactly as directed; take at evenly spaced times day and night

Dosage Forms

Injection, as calcium: 3 mg/mL (1 mL)

Powder for injection, as calcium: 25 mg, 50 mg, 100 mg, 350 mg

Powder for oral solution, as calcium: 1 mg/mL (60 mL)

Tablet, as calcium: 5 mg, 10 mg, 15 mg, 25 mg

Leucovorin Calcium *see* Leucovorin *on page 708*

Leukeran® *see* Chlorambucil *on page 248*

Leukine™ *see* Sargramostim *on page 1125*

Leuprolide Acetate (loo PROE lide AS e tate)

Related Information

Cancer Chemotherapy Regimens *on page 1351*

Brand Names Lupron®; Lupron Depot®; Lupron Depot-3® Month; Lupron Depot-Ped™

Synonyms Leuprorelin Acetate

Therapeutic Category Gonadotropin Releasing Hormone Analog

Use Palliative treatment of advanced prostate carcinoma (alternative when orchiectomy or estrogen administration are not indicated or are unacceptable to the patient); combination therapy with flutamide for treating metastatic prostatic carcinoma; endometriosis (3.75 mg depot only); central precocious puberty (may be used an agent to treat precocious puberty because of its effect in lowering levels of LH and FSH, testosterone, and estrogen).

Unlabeled uses: Treatment of breast, ovarian, and endometrial cancer; leiomyoma uteri; infertility; prostatic hypertrophy

Pregnancy Risk Factor X

Contraindications Hypersensitivity to leuprolide; spinal cord compression (orchiectomy suggested); undiagnosed abnormal vaginal bleeding; women who are or may be pregnant should not receive Lupron® Depot®

Warnings/Precautions Use with caution in patients hypersensitive to benzyl alcohol; after 6 months use of Depot® leuprolide, vertebral bone density decreased (average 13.5%); long-term safety of leuprolide in children has not been established; urinary tract obstruction may occur upon initiation of therapy. Closely observe patients for weakness, paresthesias, and urinary tract obstruction in first few weeks of therapy. Tumor flare and bone pain may occur at initiation of therapy; transient weakness and paresthesia of lower limbs, hematuria, and urinary tract obstruction in first week of therapy; animal studies have shown dose-related benign pituitary hyperplasia and benign pituitary adenomas after 2 years of use.

Adverse Reactions

>10%:
- Central nervous system: Depression, pain
- Endocrine & metabolic: Hot flashes
- Gastrointestinal: Weight gain, nausea, vomiting

1% to 10%:
- Cardiovascular: Cardiac arrhythmias, edema
- Central nervous system: Dizziness, lethargy, insomnia, headache
- Dermatologic: Rash
- Endocrine: Estrogenic effects (gynecomastia, breast tenderness)
- Gastrointestinal: Nausea, vomiting, diarrhea, GI bleed
- Hematologic: Decreased hemoglobin and hematocrit
- Neuromuscular & skeletal: Paresthesia, myalgia
- Ocular: Blurred vision

<1%:
- Cardiovascular: Myocardial infarction
- Local: Thrombophlebitis
- Respiratory: Pulmonary embolism

Overdosage/Toxicology General supportive care

Stability

Store unopened vials of injection in refrigerator, vial in use can be kept at room temperature (≤30°C/86°F) for several months with minimal loss of potency. Protect from light and store vial in carton until use. Do not freeze.

Depot® may be stored at room temperature. Upon reconstitution, the suspension is stable for 24 hours; does not contain a preservative.

Mechanism of Action Continuous daily administration results in suppression of ovarian and testicular steroidogenesis due to decreased levels of LH and FSH with subsequent decrease in testosterone (male) and estrogen (female) levels

Pharmacodynamics/Kinetics

Onset of action: Serum testosterone levels first increase within 3 days of therapy
Duration: Levels decrease after 2-4 weeks with continued therapy
Metabolism: Destroyed within the GI tract
Bioavailability: Orally not bioavailable; S.C. and I.V. doses are comparable
Half-life: 3-4.25 hours
Elimination: Not well defined

Usual Dosage Requires parenteral administration

Children: Precocious puberty:
- S.C.: 20-45 mcg/kg/day
- I.M. (Depot®) formulation: 0.3 mg/kg/dose given every 28 days
  - ≤25 kg: 7.5 mg
  - >25-37.5 kg: 11.25 mg
  - >37.5 kg: 15 mg

Adults:
- Male: Advanced prostatic carcinoma:
  - S.C.: 1 mg/day **or**
  - I.M., Depot® (suspension): 7.5 mg/dose given monthly (every 28-33 days)
- Female: Endometriosis: I.M., Depot® (suspension): 3.75 mg monthly for up to 6 months

Administration When administering the Depot® form, do not use needles smaller than 22-gauge; reconstitute only with diluent provided

Monitoring Parameters Precocious puberty: GnRH testing (blood LH and FSH levels), testosterone in males and estradiol in females; closely monitor patients with prostatic carcinoma for weakness, paresthesias, and urinary tract obstruction in first few weeks of therapy

Test Interactions Interferes with pituitary gonadotropic and gonadal function tests during and up to 4-8 weeks after therapy

Patient Information Do not discontinue medication without physician's advice

Nursing Implications Patient must be taught aseptic technique and S.C. injection technique. Rotate S.C. injection sites frequently. Disease flare (increased bone pain, urinary retention) can briefly occur with initiation of therapy.

Dosage Forms

Injection: 5 mg/mL (2.8 mL)
Powder for injection (depot):
- Depot®: 3.75 mg, 7.5 mg
- Depot-3® Month: 11.25 mg
- Depot-Ped™: 7.5 mg, 11.25 mg, 15 mg

Leuprorelin Acetate *see* Leuprolide Acetate *on previous page*

Leurocristine *see* Vincristine *on page 1302*

Leustatin™ *see* Cladribine *on page 285*

Levamisole (lee VAM i sole)

Related Information

Cancer Chemotherapy Regimens *on page 1351*

Brand Names Ergamisol®

Synonyms Levamisole Hydrochloride

Therapeutic Category Immune Modulator

Use Adjuvant treatment with fluorouracil in Dukes stage C colon cancer

Pregnancy Risk Factor C

Contraindications Previous hypersensitivity to the drug

Warnings/Precautions Agranulocytosis can occur asymptomatically and flu-like symptoms can occur without hematologic adverse effects; frequent hematologic monitoring is necessary

Adverse Reactions

>10%: Gastrointestinal: Nausea, diarrhea

1% to 10%:

- Cardiovascular: Edema
- Central nervous system: Fatigue, fever, dizziness, headache, somnolence, depression, nervousness, insomnia
- Dermatologic: Dermatitis, alopecia
- Gastrointestinal: Stomatitis, vomiting, anorexia, abdominal pain, constipation, taste perversion
- Hematologic: Leukopenia
- Neuromuscular & skeletal: Rigors, arthralgia, myalgia, paresthesia
- Miscellaneous: Infection

<1%:

- Cardiovascular: Chest pain
- Central nervous system: Anxiety
- Dermatologic: Pruritus, urticaria
- Gastrointestinal: Flatulence, dyspepsia
- Hematologic: Thrombocytopenia, anemia, granulocytopenia
- Ocular: Abnormal tearing, blurred vision, conjunctivitis
- Respiratory: Epistaxis
- Miscellaneous: Altered sense of smell

Overdosage/Toxicology Treatment following decontamination is symptomatic and supportive

Drug Interactions

Increased toxicity/serum levels of phenytoin

Disulfiram-like reaction with alcohol

Mechanism of Action Clinically, combined therapy with levamisole and 5-fluorouracil has been effective in treating colon cancer patients, whereas demonstrable activity has been. Due to the broad range of pharmacologic activities of levamisole, it has been suggested that the drug may act as a biochemical modulator (of fluorouracil, for example, in colon cancer), an effect entirely independent of immune modulation. Further studies are needed to evaluate the mechanisms of action of the drug in cancer patients.

Pharmacodynamics/Kinetics

Absorption: Well absorbed

Metabolism: In the liver, >70%

Half-life, elimination: 2-6 hours

Time to peak serum concentration: 1-2 hours

Elimination: In urine and feces; elimination is virtually complete within 48 hours after an oral dose

Usual Dosage Adults: Oral: Initial: 50 mg every 8 hours for 3 days, then 50 mg every 8 hours for 3 days every 2 weeks (fluorouracil is always given concomitantly)

Dosing adjustment in hepatic impairment: May be necessary in patients with liver disease, but no specific guidelines are available

Monitoring Parameters CBC with platelet count prior to therapy and weekly prior to treatment; LFTs every 3 months

Patient Information Notify physician immediately if flu-like symptoms appear; may cause dizziness, drowsiness, impair judgment or coordination

Dosage Forms Tablet, as base: 50 mg

Levamisole Hydrochloride *see* Levamisole *on this page*

Levaquin® *see* Levofloxacin *on page 717*

Levarterenol Bitartrate *see* Norepinephrine *on page 914*

Levbid® *see* Hyoscyamine *on page 635*

Levlen® *see* Ethinyl Estradiol and Levonorgestrel *on page 484*

Levobunolol (lee voe BYOO noe lole)

Related Information

Glaucoma Drug Therapy Comparison *on page 1410*

Brand Names AKBeta®; Betagan®

Synonyms *l*-Bunolol Hydrochloride; Levobunolol Hydrochloride

Therapeutic Category Beta-Adrenergic Blocker, Ophthalmic

Use To lower intraocular pressure in chronic open-angle glaucoma or ocular hypertension

Pregnancy Risk Factor C

Contraindications Known hypersensitivity to levobunolol; bronchial asthma, severe COPD, sinus bradycardia, second or third degree A-V block, cardiac failure, cardiogenic shock

Warnings/Precautions Use with caution in patients with congestive heart failure, diabetes mellitus, hyperthyroidism; contains metabisulfite. Because systemic absorption does occur with ophthalmic administration, the elderly with other disease states or syndromes that may be affected by a beta-blocker (CHF, COPD, etc) should be monitored closely.

Adverse Reactions

>10%: Ocular: Stinging/burning eyes

1% to 10%:

- Cardiovascular: Bradycardia, arrhythmia, hypotension
- Central nervous system: Dizziness, headache
- Dermatologic: Alopecia, erythema
- Local: Stinging, burning
- Ocular: Blepharoconjunctivitis, conjunctivitis
- Respiratory: Bronchospasm

<1%:

- Dermatologic: Rash, itching
- Ocular: Visual disturbances, keratitis, decreased visual acuity

Overdosage/Toxicology Symptoms of intoxication include cardiac disturbances, CNS toxicity, bronchospasm, hypoglycemia and hyperkalemia. The most common cardiac symptoms include hypotension and bradycardia; atrioventricular block, intraventricular conduction disturbances, cardiogenic shock, and systole may occur with severe overdose, especially with membrane-depressant drugs (eg, propranolol); CNS effects include convulsions, coma, and respiratory arrest is commonly seen with propranolol and other membrane-depressant and lipid-soluble drugs

Treatment includes symptomatic treatment of seizures, hypotension, hyperkalemia and hypoglycemia; bradycardia and hypotension resistant to atropine, isoproterenol or pacing may respond to glucagon; wide QRS defects caused by the membrane-depressant poisoning may respond to hypertonic sodium bicarbonate; repeat-dose charcoal, hemoperfusion, or hemodialysis may be helpful in removal of only those beta-blockers with a small V_d, long half-life or low intrinsic clearance (acebutolol, atenolol, nadolol, sotalol).

Drug Interactions

Increased toxicity:

- Systemic beta-adrenergic blocking agents
- Ophthalmic epinephrine (increased blood pressure/loss of IOP effect)
- Quinidine (sinus bradycardia)
- Verapamil (bradycardia and asystole have been reported)

Mechanism of Action A nonselective beta-adrenergic blocking agent that lowers intraocular pressure by reducing aqueous humor production and possibly increases the outflow of aqueous humor

Pharmacodynamics/Kinetics

Onset of action: Decreases in intraocular pressure (IOP) can be noted within 1 hour

Peak effect: 2-6 hours

Duration: 1-7 days

Elimination: Not well defined

Usual Dosage Adults: Instill 1 drop in the affected eye(s) 1-2 times/day

Monitoring Parameters Intraocular pressure, heart rate, funduscopic exam, visual field testing

Patient Information May sting on instillation, do not touch dropper to eye; visual acuity may be decreased after administration; night vision may be decreased; distance vision may be altered; apply finger pressure between the bridge of the nose and corner of the eye to decrease systemic absorption; assess patient's or caregiver's ability to administer

Nursing Implications Apply finger pressure over nasolacrimal duct to decrease systemic absorption

Dosage Forms Solution, ophthalmic, as hydrochloride: 0.25% (5 mL, 10 mL, 15 mL); 0.5% (2 mL, 5 mL, 10 mL, 15 mL)

Levobunolol Hydrochloride *see* Levobunolol *on previous page*

Levocabastine (LEE voe kab as teen)

Brand Names Livostin®

Canadian/Mexican Brand Names Livostin® Nasal (Mexico); Livostin® Oftalmico (Mexico)

Synonyms Levocabastine Hydrochloride

Therapeutic Category Antiallergic, Ophthalmic; Antihistamine, H_1 Blocker; Antihistamine, H_1 Blocker, Ophthalmic

Use Treatment of allergic conjunctivitis

Pregnancy Risk Factor B

Contraindications Hypersensitivity to any component of product; while soft contact lenses are being worn

Warnings/Precautions Safety and efficacy in children <12 years of age have not been established; not for injection; not for use in patients wearing soft contact lenses during treatment

Adverse Reactions

>10%: Local: Transient burning, stinging, discomfort

1% to 10%:

- Central nervous system: Headache, somnolence, fatigue
- Dermatologic: Rash
- Gastrointestinal: Xerostomia
- Ocular: Blurred vision, eye pain, somnolence, red eyes, eyelid edema
- Respiratory: Dyspnea

Mechanism of Action Potent, selective histamine H_1-receptor antagonist for topical ophthalmic use

Pharmacodynamics/Kinetics Absorption: Topical: Systemically absorbed

Usual Dosage Children >12 years and Adults: Instill 1 drop in affected eye(s) 4 times/day for up to 2 weeks

Dosage Forms Suspension, ophthalmic, as hydrochloride: 0.05% (2.5 mL, 5 mL, 10 mL)

Levocabastine Hydrochloride *see* Levocabastine *on this page*

Levodopa (lee voe DOE pa)

Related Information

Antacid Drug Interactions *on page 1388*

Brand Names Dopar®; Larodopa®

Synonyms *L*-3-Hydroxytyrosine; *L*-Dopa

Therapeutic Category Anti-Parkinson's Agent

Use Treatment of Parkinson's disease; used as a diagnostic agent for growth hormone deficiency

Pregnancy Risk Factor C

Contraindications Hypersensitivity to levodopa or any component; narrow-angle glaucoma, MAO inhibitor therapy, melanomas or any undiagnosed skin lesions

Warnings/Precautions Use with caution in patients with history of myocardial infarction, arrhythmias, asthma, wide-angle glaucoma, peptic ulcer disease; sudden discontinuation of levodopa may cause a worsening of Parkinson's disease; some products may contain tartrazine. Elderly may be more sensitive to CNS effects of levodopa.

Adverse Reactions

>10%:

- Cardiovascular: Orthostatic hypotension, arrhythmias
- Central nervous system: Dizziness, anxiety, confusion, nightmares
- Gastrointestinal: Anorexia, nausea, vomiting, constipation
- Genitourinary: Dysuria
- Neuromuscular & skeletal: Choreiform and involuntary movements
- Ocular: Blepharospasm

1% to 10%:

- Central nervous system: Headache
- Gastrointestinal: Anorexia, diarrhea, xerostomia
- Genitourinary: Discoloration of urine
- Neuromuscular & skeletal: Muscle twitching
- Ocular: Eyelid spasms
- Miscellaneous: Discoloration of sweat

<1%:

- Cardiovascular: Hypertension
- Gastrointestinal: Duodenal ulcer, GI bleeding
- Hematologic: Hemolytic anemia
- Ocular: Blurred vision

Overdosage/Toxicology Symptoms of overdose include palpitations, dysrhythmias, spasms, hypertension

Use fluids judiciously to maintain pressures; may precipitate a variety of arrhythmias

Drug Interactions

Decreased effect:

Hydantoins may decrease effectiveness

Phenothiazines and hypotensive agents may decrease effect of levodopa

Pyridoxine may increase peripheral conversion, may decrease levodopa effectiveness

Increased toxicity with antacids

Monoamine oxidase inhibitors → hypertensive reactions

Mechanism of Action Increases dopamine levels in the brain, then stimulates dopaminergic receptors in the basal ganglia to improve the balance between cholinergic and dopaminergic activity

Pharmacodynamics/Kinetics

Time to peak serum concentration: Oral: 1-2 hours

Metabolism: Majority of drug is peripherally decarboxylated to dopamine; small amounts of levodopa reach the brain where it is also decarboxylated to active dopamine

Half-life: 1.2-2.3 hours

Elimination: Primarily in urine (80%) as dopamine, norepinephrine, and homovanillic acid

Usual Dosage Oral:

Children (administer as a single dose to evaluate growth hormone deficiency):

0.5 g/m^2 **or**

<30 lbs: 125 mg

30-70 lbs: 250 mg

>70 lbs: 500 mg

Adults: 500-1000 mg/day in divided doses every 6-12 hours; increase by 100-750 mg/day every 3-7 days until response or total dose of 8,000 mg is reached

A significant therapeutic response may not be obtained for 6 months

Administration Administer with meals to decrease GI upset

Monitoring Parameters Serum growth hormone concentration

Test Interactions False-positive reaction for urinary glucose with Clinitest®; false-negative reaction using Clinistix®; false-positive urine ketones with Acetest®, Ketostix®, Labstix®

Patient Information Avoid vitamins with B_6 (pyridoxine); can take with food to prevent GI upset; do not stop taking this drug even if you do not think it is working; dizziness, lightheadedness, fainting may occur when you get up from a sitting or lying position.

Nursing Implications Sustained release product should not be crushed

Dosage Forms

Capsule: 100 mg, 250 mg, 500 mg

Tablet: 100 mg, 250 mg, 500 mg

Levodopa and Carbidopa (lee voe DOE pa & kar bi DOE pa)

Related Information

Carbidopa *on page 204*

Brand Names Sinemet®

Canadian/Mexican Brand Names Racovel® (Mexico)

Synonyms Carbidopa and Levodopa

Therapeutic Category Anti-Parkinson's Agent

Use Treatment of parkinsonian syndrome; 50-100 mg/day of carbidopa is needed to block the peripheral conversion of levodopa to dopamine. "On-off" can be managed by giving smaller, more frequent doses of Sinemet® or adding a dopamine agonist or selegiline; when adding a new agent, doses of Sinemet® should usually be decreased.

Pregnancy Risk Factor C

Contraindications Narrow-angle glaucoma, MAO inhibitors, hypersensitivity to levodopa, carbidopa, or any component; do not use in patients with malignant melanoma or undiagnosed skin lesions

Warnings/Precautions Use with caution in patients with history of myocardial infarction, arrhythmias, asthma, wide angle glaucoma, peptic ulcer disease; sudden discontinuation of levodopa may cause a worsening of Parkinson's disease; some tablets may contain tartrazine. The elderly may be more sensitive to the CNS effects of levodopa. Protein in the diet should be distributed throughout the day to avoid fluctuations in levodopa absorption.

Adverse Reactions

>10%:

Cardiovascular: Orthostatic hypotension, palpitations, cardiac arrhythmias

Central nervous system: Confusion, nightmares, dizziness, anxiety

Gastrointestinal: Nausea, vomiting, anorexia, constipation

Neuromuscular & skeletal: Dystonic movements, "on-off", choreiform and involuntary movements

Ocular: Blepharospasm

(Continued)

Levodopa and Carbidopa *(Continued)*

Renal: Dysuria

1% to 10%:

Central nervous system: Headache
Gastrointestinal: Diarrhea, xerostomia
Genitourinary: Discoloration of urine
Neuromuscular & skeletal: Muscle twitching
Ocular: Eyelid spasms
Miscellaneous: Discoloration of sweat

<1%:

Cardiovascular: Hypertension
Central nervous system: Memory loss, nervousness, insomnia, fatigue, hallucinations, ataxia
Gastrointestinal: Duodenal ulcer, GI bleeding
Hematologic: Hemolytic anemia
Ocular: Blurred vision

Overdosage/Toxicology Symptoms of overdose include palpitations, arrhythmias, spasms, hypotension; may cause hypertension or hypotension

Treatment is supportive; initiate gastric lavage, administer I.V. fluids judiciously and monitor EKG; use fluids judiciously to maintain pressures; may precipitate a variety of arrhythmias

Drug Interactions

Decreased effect:

Hydantoins, pyridoxine
Phenothiazines and hypotensive agents may decrease effects of levodopa

Increased toxicity with antacids

Monoamine oxidase inhibitors → hypertensive reactions

Mechanism of Action Parkinson's symptoms are due to a lack of striatal dopamine; levodopa circulates in the plasma to the blood-brain-barrier (BBB), where it crosses, to be converted by striatal enzymes to dopamine; carbidopa inhibits the peripheral plasma breakdown of levodopa by inhibiting its decarboxylation, and thereby increases available levodopa at the BBB

Pharmacodynamics/Kinetics

Carbidopa:

Absorption: Oral: 40% to 70%
Protein binding: 36%
Half-life: 1-2 hours
Elimination: Excreted unchanged

Levodopa:

Absorption: May be decreased if given with a high protein meal
Half-life: 1.2-2.3 hours
Elimination: Primarily in urine (80%) as dopamine, norepinephrine, and homovanillic acid

Usual Dosage Oral:

Adults: Initial: 25/100 2-4 times/day, increase as necessary to a maximum of 200/2000 mg/day

Elderly: Initial: 25/100 twice daily, increase as necessary

Conversion from Sinemet® to Sinemet® CR (50/200): (Sinemet® [total daily dose of levodopa] / Sinemet® CR)

300-400 mg / 1 tablet twice daily
500-600 mg / 1½ tablets twice daily or one 3 times/day
700-800 mg / 4 tablets in 3 or more divided doses
900-1000 mg / 5 tablets in 3 or more divided doses

Intervals between doses of Sinemet® CR should be 4-8 hours while awake

Administration Administer with meals to decrease GI upset

Monitoring Parameters Blood pressure, standing and sitting/supine; symptoms of parkinsonism, dyskinesias, mental status

Test Interactions False-positive reaction for urinary glucose with Clinitest®; false-negative reaction using Clinistix®; false-positive urine ketones with Acetest®, Ketostix®, Labstix®

Patient Information Do not stop taking this drug even if you do not think it is working; take on an empty stomach if possible; if GI distress occurs, take with meals; rise carefully from lying or sitting position as dizziness, lightheadedness, or fainting may occur; do not crush or chew sustained release product

Nursing Implications Space doses evenly over the waking hours; sustained release product should not be crushed

Dosage Forms Tablet:

10/100: Carbidopa 10 mg and levodopa 100 mg
25/100: Carbidopa 25 mg and levodopa 100 mg
25/250: Carbidopa 25 mg and levodopa 250 mg

Sustained release: Carbidopa 25 mg and levodopa 100 mg; carbidopa 50 mg and levodopa 200 mg

Levo-Dromoran® *see* Levorphanol *on page 719*

Levofloxacin (lee voe FLOKS a sin)

Brand Names Levaquin®

Therapeutic Category Antibiotic, Quinolone

Use Acute maxillary sinusitis due to *S. pneumoniae, H. influenzae*, or *M. catarrhalis*; also for acute bacterial exacerbation of chronic bronchitis and community-acquired pneumonia due to *S. aureus, S. pneumoniae, H. influenzae, H. parainfluenza*, or *M. catarrhalis, C. pneumoniae, L. pneumophila*, or *M. pneumoniae*; may be used for uncomplicated skin and skin structure infection (due to *S. aureus* or *S. pyogenes*) and complicated urinary tract infection due to gram-negative enterobacteriae, including acute pyelonephritis (caused by *E. coli*); although clinical efficacy has been similar between levofloxacin and ofloxacin, levofloxacin is more potent and may be given in lower doses

Pregnancy Risk Factor C

Pregnancy/Breast-Feeding Implications Quinolones are known to distribute well into breast milk; consequently, use during lactation should be avoided, if possible; avoid use in pregnant women unless the benefit justifies the potential risk to the fetus

Contraindications Hypersensitivity to sparfloxacin, any component, or other quinolones; pregnancy, lactation

Warnings/Precautions Not recommended in children <18 years of age; other quinolones have caused transient arthropathy in children; CNS stimulation may occur (tremor, restlessness, confusion, and very rarely hallucinations or seizures); use with caution in patients with known or suspected CNS disorders or renal dysfunction; prolonged use may result in superinfection; if an allergic reaction (itching, urticaria, dyspnea, pharyngeal or facial edema, loss of consciousness, tingling, cardiovascular collapse) occurs, discontinue the drug immediately; use caution to avoid possible photosensitivity reactions during and for several days following fluoroquinolone therapy; pseudomembranous colitis may occur and should be considered in patients who present with diarrhea

Adverse Reactions

>1%:

- Central nervous system: Dizziness, headache, insomnia
- Dermatologic: Rash
- Gastrointestinal: Nausea, vomiting, increased transaminases
- Hematologic: Leukopenia, thrombocytopenia
- Neuromuscular & skeletal: Tremor, arthralgia

Overdosage/Toxicology Symptoms of overdose include acute renal failure, seizures

Treatment should include GI decontamination and supportive care; not removed by peritoneal or hemodialysis

Drug Interactions

Decreased effect: Decreased absorption with antacids containing aluminum, magnesium, and/or calcium (by up to 98% if given at the same time); phenytoin serum levels may be reduced by quinolones; antineoplastic agents may also decrease serum levels of fluoroquinolones

Increased toxicity/serum levels: Quinolones cause increased levels of caffeine, warfarin, azlocillin, cyclosporine, and theophylline (one study indicates no effect on theophylline metabolism); azlocillin, cimetidine, and probenecid increases quinolone levels; an increased incidence of seizures may occur with foscarnet

Stability Stable for 72 hours when diluted to 5 mg/mL in a compatible I.V. fluid and stored at room temperature; stable for 14 days when stored at room temperature; stable for 6 months when frozen, do not refreeze; do not thaw in microwave or by bath immersion; **incompatible** with mannitol and sodium bicarbonate

Mechanism of Action As the S (-) enantiomer of the fluoroquinolone, ofloxacin, levofloxacin, inhibits DNA-gyrase in susceptible organisms; inhibits relaxation of supercoiled DNA and promotes breakage of double-stranded DNA

Pharmacodynamics/Kinetics

Absorption: Well absorbed

Distribution: V_d: 1.25 L/kg; CSF concentrations ~15% of serum levels; high concentrations are achieved in prostate and gynecological tissues, sinus, breast milk, and saliva

Protein binding: 50%

Metabolism: Hepatic, minimal

Half-life: 6 hours

Bioavailability: 100%

Time to peak serum concentration: 1 hour

Elimination: Most excreted unchanged in urine

(Continued)

Levofloxacin *(Continued)*

Usual Dosage Adults: Oral, I.V. (infuse I.V. solution over 60 minutes):
- Acute bacterial exacerbation of chronic bronchitis: 500 mg every 24 hours for at least 7 days
- Community acquired pneumonia: 500 mg every 24 hours for 7-14 days
- Acute maxillary sinusitis: 500 mg every 24 hours for 10-14 days
- Uncomplicated skin infections: 500 mg every 24 hours for 7-10 days
- Complicated urinary tract infections include acute pyelonephritis: 250 mg every 24 hours for 10 days

Dosing adjustment in renal impairment:
- Cl_{cr} 20-49 mL/minute: Administer 250 mg every 24 hours (initial: 500 mg)
- Cl_{cr} 10-19 mL/minute: Administer 250 mg every 48 hours (initial: 500 mg for most infections; 250 mg for renal infections)
- Hemodialysis/CAPD: 250 mg every 48 hours (initial: 500 mg)

Monitoring Parameters Evaluation of organ system functions (renal, hepatic, ophthalmologic, and hematopoietic) is recommended periodically during therapy; the possibility of crystalluria should be assessed; WBC and signs of infection

Patient Information May be taken with or without food; drink plenty of fluids; avoid exposure to direct sunlight during therapy and for several days following; do not take antacids within 4 hours before or 2 hours after dosing; contact your physician immediately if signs of allergy occur; do not discontinue therapy until your course has been completed; take a missed dose as soon as possible, unless it is almost time for your next dose.

Nursing Implications Infuse I.V. solutions over 60 minutes

Dosage Forms
- Infusion, in D_5W: 5 mg/mL (50 mL, 100 mL)
- Injection: 25 mg/mL (20 mL)
- Tablet: 250 mg, 500 mg

Levomethadyl Acetate Hydrochloride

(lee voe METH a dil AS e tate hye droe KLOR ide)

Brand Names ORLAAM®

Therapeutic Category Analgesic, Narcotic

Use Management of opiate dependence

Restrictions C-II; must be dispensed in a designated clinic setting only

Warnings/Precautions Not recommended for use outside of the treatment of opiate addiction; shall be dispensed only by treatment programs approved by FDA, DEA, and the designated state authority. Approved treatment programs shall dispense and use levomethadyl in oral form only and according to the treatment requirements stipulated in federal regulations. Failure to abide by these requirements may result in injunction precluding operation of the program, seizure of the drug supply, revocation of the program approval, and possible criminal prosecution.

Adverse Reactions

>10%:
- Cardiovascular: Bradycardia, hypotension
- Central nervous system: Drowsiness
- Gastrointestinal: Nausea, vomiting
- Respiratory: Respiratory depression

1% to 10%:
- Cardiovascular: Peripheral vasodilation, orthostatic hypotension, increased intracranial pressure
- Central nervous system: Dizziness/vertigo, CNS depression, confusion, sedation
- Endocrine & metabolic: Antidiuretic hormone release
- Gastrointestinal: Constipation, biliary tract spasm
- Genitourinary: Urinary tract spasm
- Ocular: Miosis, blurred vision

Drug Interactions Decreased effect/levels with phenobarbital

Usual Dosage Adults: Oral: 20-40 mg 3 times/week, with ranges of 10 mg to as high as 140 mg 3 times/week; always dilute before administration and mix with diluent prior to dispensing

Monitoring Parameters Patient adherence with regimen and avoidance of illicit substances; random drug testing is recommended

Nursing Implications Drug administration and dispensing is to take place in an authorized clinic setting only; can potentially cause Q-T prolongation on EKG (not dose related)

Dosage Forms Solution, oral: 10 mg/mL (474 mL)

Levonorgestrel (LEE voe nor jes trel)

Brand Names Norplant®

Canadian/Mexican Brand Names Microlut® (Mexico)

Therapeutic Category Contraceptive, Implant (Progestin); Contraceptive, Oral (Progestin); Progestin Derivative

Use Prevention of pregnancy. The net cumulative 5-year pregnancy rate for levonorgestrel implant use has been reported to be from 1.5-3.9 pregnancies/100 users. Norplant® is a very efficient, yet reversible, method of contraception. The long duration of action may be particularly advantageous in women who desire an extended period of contraceptive protection without sacrificing the possibility of future fertility.

Pregnancy Risk Factor X

Contraindications Women with undiagnosed abnormal uterine bleeding, hemorrhagic diathesis, known or suspected pregnancy, active hepatic disease, active thrombophlebitis, thromboembolic disorders, or known or suspected carcinoma of the breast

Warnings/Precautions Patients presenting with lower abdominal pain should be evaluated for follicular atresia and ectopic pregnancy

Adverse Reactions

>10%: Hormonal: Prolonged menstrual flow, spotting

1% to 10%:

- Central nervous system: Headache, nervousness, dizziness
- Dermatologic: Dermatitis, acne
- Endocrine & metabolic: Amenorrhea, irregular menstrual cycles, scanty bleeding, breast discharge
- Gastrointestinal: Nausea, change in appetite, weight gain
- Genitourinary: Vaginitis, leukorrhea
- Local: Pain or itching at implant site
- Neuromuscular & skeletal: Myalgia

<1%: Local: Infection at implant site

Overdosage/Toxicology Can result if >6 capsules are *in situ*; symptoms include uterine bleeding irregularities and fluid retention; treatment includes removal of all implanted capsules

Drug Interactions Decreased effect: Carbamazepine/phenytoin

Mechanism of Action First, ovulation is inhibited in about 50% to 60% of implant users from a negative feedback mechanism on the hypothalamus, leading to reduced secretion of follicle stimulating hormone (FSH) and luteinizing hormone (LH). An insufficient luteal phase has also been demonstrated with levonorgestrel administration and may result from defective gonadotropin stimulation of the ovary or from a direct effect of the drug on progesterone synthesis by the corpora lutea.

Pharmacodynamics/Kinetics

Protein binding: Following release from the implant, levonorgestrel enters the blood stream highly bound to sex hormone binding globulin (SHBG), albumin, and alpha$_1$ glycoprotein

Metabolism: In the liver

Half-life, terminal: 11-45 hours

Elimination: In urine primarily as conjugates of sulfate and glucuronide

Usual Dosage Total administration doses (implanted): 216 mg in 6 capsules which should be implanted during the first 7 days of onset of menses subdermally in the upper arm; each Norplant® silastic capsule releases 80 mcg of drug/day for 6-18 months, following which a rate of release of 25-30 mcg/day is maintained for ≤5 years; capsules should be removed by end of 5th year

Patient Information Notify physician if unusual or persistent nausea, vomiting, abdominal pain, dark urine, or pale stools; may cause changes in vision or contact lens tolerability

Dosage Forms Capsule, subdermal implantation: 36 mg (6s)

Levonorgestrel and Ethinyl Estradiol *see* Ethinyl Estradiol and Levonorgestrel *on page 484*

Levophed® *see* Norepinephrine *on page 914*

Levora® *see* Ethinyl Estradiol and Levonorgestrel *on page 484*

Levorphanol (lee VOR fa nole)

Related Information

Narcotic Agonists Comparison *on page 1414*

Dose Equivalents for Opioid Analgesics in Opioid-Naive Adults <50 kg *on page 1376*

Dose Equivalents for Opioid Analgesics in Opioid-Naive Adults ≥50 kg *on page 1375*

Brand Names Levo-Dromoran®

Synonyms Levorphanol Tartrate; Levorphan Tartrate

Therapeutic Category Analgesic, Narcotic

Use Relief of moderate to severe pain; also used parenterally for preoperative sedation and an adjunct to nitrous oxide/oxygen anesthesia; 2 mg levorphanol produces analgesia comparable to that produced by 10 mg of morphine

(Continued)

Levorphanol *(Continued)*

Restrictions C-II

Pregnancy Risk Factor B (D if used for prolonged periods or in high doses at term)

Contraindications Hypersensitivity to levorphanol or any component

Warnings/Precautions Use with caution in patients with hypersensitivity reactions to other phenanthrene derivative opioid agonists (morphine, hydrocodone, hydromorphone, levorphanol, oxycodone, oxymorphone); respiratory diseases including asthma, emphysema, COPD or severe liver or renal insufficiency; some preparations contain sulfites which may cause allergic reactions; may be habit-forming; dextromethorphan has equivalent antitussive activity but has much lower toxicity in accidental overdose. Elderly may be particularly susceptible to the CNS depressant and constipating effects of narcotics.

Adverse Reactions

>10%:

Cardiovascular: Palpitations, hypotension, bradycardia, peripheral vasodilation
Central nervous system: CNS depression, fatigue, drowsiness, dizziness
Dermatologic: Pruritus
Gastrointestinal: Nausea, vomiting
Neuromuscular & skeletal: Weakness

1% to 10%:

Central nervous system: Nervousness, headache, restlessness, anorexia, malaise, confusion
Gastrointestinal: Stomach cramps, xerostomia, constipation
Endocrine & metabolic: Antidiuretic hormone release
Gastrointestinal: Biliary tract spasm
Genitourinary: Decreased urination, urinary tract spasm
Local: Pain at injection site
Ocular: Miosis
Respiratory: Respiratory depression

<1%:

Central nervous system: Paralytic ileus, mental depression, hallucinations, paradoxical CNS stimulation, increased intracranial pressure
Dermatologic: Rash, urticaria
Sensitivity reactions: Histamine release
Miscellaneous: Physical and psychological dependence, histamine release

Overdosage/Toxicology Symptoms of overdose include CNS depression, respiratory depression, miosis, apnea, pulmonary edema, convulsions

Naloxone 2 mg I.V. (0.01 mg/kg for children) with repeat administration as necessary up to a total of 10 mg

Drug Interactions Increased toxicity: CNS depressants increase CNS depression

Stability Store at room temperature, protect from freezing; I.V. is **incompatible** when mixed with aminophylline, barbiturates, heparin, methicillin, phenytoin, sodium bicarbonate

Mechanism of Action Levorphanol tartrate is a synthetic opioid agonist that is classified as a morphinan derivative. Opioids interact with stereospecific opioid receptors in various parts of the central nervous system and other tissues. Analgesic potency parallels the affinity for these binding sites. These drugs do not alter the threshold or responsiveness to pain, but the perception of pain.

Usual Dosage Adults:

Oral: 2 mg every 6-24 hours as needed
S.C.: 2 mg, up to 3 mg if necessary, every 6-8 hours

Dosing adjustment in hepatic disease: Reduction is necessary in patients with liver disease

Dietary Considerations

Alcohol: Additive CNS effects, avoid or limit alcohol; watch for sedation
Food: Glucose may cause hyperglycemia; monitor blood glucose concentrations

Monitoring Parameters Pain relief, respiratory and mental status, blood pressure

Patient Information Avoid alcohol, may cause drowsiness, impaired judgment or coordination; may cause physical and psychological dependence with prolonged use

Nursing Implications Observe patient for excessive sedation, respiratory depression; implement safety measures, assist with ambulation

Dosage Forms

Injection, as tartrate: 2 mg/mL (1 mL, 10 mL)
Tablet, as tartrate: 2 mg

Levorphanol Tartrate *see* Levorphanol *on previous page*

Levorphan Tartrate *see* Levorphanol *on previous page*

Levo-T™ *see* Levothyroxine *on next page*

Levothroid® *see* Levothyroxine *on this page*

Levothyroxine (lee voe thye ROKS een)

Brand Names Eltroxin™; Levo-T™; Levothroid®; Levoxyl™; Synthroid®

Canadian/Mexican Brand Names Eltroxin® (Canada); PMS-Levothyroxine Sodium (Canada); Eutirox® (Mexico); Tiroidine® (Mexico)

Synonyms Levothyroxine Sodium; *L*-Thyroxine Sodium; T_4

Therapeutic Category Thyroid Product

Use Replacement or supplemental therapy in hypothyroidism; some clinicians suggest levothyroxine is the drug of choice for replacement therapy

Pregnancy Risk Factor A

Contraindications Recent myocardial infarction or thyrotoxicosis, uncorrected adrenal insufficiency, hypersensitivity to levothyroxine sodium or any component

Warnings/Precautions Ineffective for weight reduction; high doses may produce serious or even life-threatening toxic effects particularly when used with some anorectic drugs. Use with caution and reduce dosage in patients with angina pectoris or other cardiovascular disease; levothyroxine tablets contain tartrazine dye which may cause allergic reactions in susceptible individuals; use cautiously in elderly since they may be more likely to have compromised cardiovascular functions. Patients with adrenal insufficiency, myxedema, diabetes mellitus and insipidus may have symptoms exaggerated or aggravated; thyroid replacement requires periodic assessment of thyroid status. Chronic hypothyroidism predisposes patients to coronary artery disease.

Adverse Reactions

<1%:

- Cardiovascular: Palpitations, cardiac arrhythmias, tachycardia, chest pain
- Central nervous system: Nervousness, headache, insomnia, fever, ataxia
- Dermatologic: Alopecia
- Endocrine: Changes in menstrual cycle
- Gastrointestinal: Weight loss, increased appetite, diarrhea, abdominal cramps, constipation
- Neuromuscular & skeletal: Myalgia, hand tremors, tremor
- Respiratory: Shortness of breath
- Miscellaneous: Diaphoresis

Overdosage/Toxicology Chronic overdose is treated by withdrawal of the drug; massive overdose may require beta-blockers for increased sympathomimetic activity. Chronic overdose may cause hyperthyroidism, weight loss, nervousness, sweating, tachycardia, insomnia, heat intolerance, menstrual irregularities, palpitations, psychosis, fever; acute overdose may cause fever, hypoglycemia, CHF, unrecognized adrenal insufficiency

Reduce dose or temporarily discontinue therapy; normal hypothalamic-pituitary-thyroid axis will return to normal in 6-8 weeks; serum T_4 levels do not correlate well with toxicity; in massive acute ingestion, reduce GI absorption, administer general supportive care; treat congestive heart failure with digitalis glycosides; excessive adrenergic activity (tachycardia) require propranolol 1-3 mg I.V. over 10 minutes or 80-160 mg orally/day; fever may be treated with acetaminophen.

Drug Interactions

Decreased effect:

- Phenytoin may decrease levothyroxine levels
- Cholestyramine may decrease absorption of levothyroxine
- Increased oral hypoglycemic requirements

Increased effect: Increased effects of oral anticoagulants

Increased toxicity: Tricyclic antidepressants may increase toxic potential of both drugs

Stability Protect tablets from light; do not mix I.V. solution with other I.V. infusion solutions; reconstituted solutions should be used immediately and any unused portions discarded

Mechanism of Action Exact mechanism of action is unknown; however, it is believed the thyroid hormone exerts its many metabolic effects through control of DNA transcription and protein synthesis; involved in normal metabolism, growth, and development; promotes gluconeogenesis, increases utilization and mobilization of glycogen stores, and stimulates protein synthesis, increases basal metabolic rate

Pharmacodynamics/Kinetics

Onset of therapeutic effect:

- Oral: 3-5 days
- I.V. Within 6-8 hours

Peak effect: I.V.: Within 24 hours

Absorption: Oral: Erratic

Metabolism: In the liver to triiodothyronine (active)

Time to peak serum concentration: 2-4 hours

Elimination: In feces and urine

(Continued)

Levothyroxine *(Continued)*

Usual Dosage

Children:

Oral:

0-6 months: 8-10 mcg/kg/day **or** 25-50 mcg/day
6-12 months: 6-8 mcg/kg/day **or** 50-75 mcg/day
1-5 years: 5-6 mcg/kg/day **or** 75-100 mcg/day
6-12 years: 4-5 mcg/kg/day **or** 100-150 mcg/day
>12 years: 2-3 mcg/kg/day **or** ≥150 mcg/day

I.M., I.V.: 50% to 75% of the oral dose

Adults:

Oral: 12.5-50 mcg/day to start, then increase by 25-50 mcg/day at intervals of 2-4 weeks; average adult dose: 100-200 mcg/day

I.M., I.V.: 50% of the oral dose

Myxedema coma or stupor: I.V.: 200-500 mcg one time, then 100-300 mcg the next day if necessary

Thyroid suppression therapy: Oral: 2-6 mcg/kg/day for 7-10 days

Administration

Oral: Administer on an empty stomach

Parenteral: Dilute vial with 5 mL normal saline; use immediately after reconstitution; administer by direct I.V. infusion over 2- to 3-minute period. I.V. form must be prepared immediately prior to administration; should not be admixed with other solutions

Monitoring Parameters Thyroid function test (serum thyroxine, thyrotropin concentrations), resin triiodothyronine uptake (RT_3U), free thyroxine index (FTI), T_4, TSH, heart rate, blood pressure, clinical signs of hypo- and hyperthyroidism; TSH is the most reliable guide for evaluating adequacy of thyroid replacement dosage. TSH may be elevated during the first few months of thyroid replacement despite patients being clinically euthyroid. In cases where T_4 remains low and TSH is within normal limits, an evaluation of "free" (unbound) T_4 is needed to evaluate further increase in dosage

Reference Range Pediatrics: Cord T_4 and values in the first few weeks are much higher, falling over the first months and years. ≥10 years: ~5.8-11 μg/dL (SI: 75-142 nmol/L). Borderline low: ≤4.5-5.7 μg/dL (SI: 58-73 nmol/L); low: ≤4.4 μg/dL (SI: 57 nmol/L); results <2.5 μg/dL (SI: <32 nmol/L) are strong evidence for hypothyroidism.

Approximate adult normal range: 4-12 μg/dL (SI: 51-154 nmol/L). Borderline high: 11.1-13 μg/dL (SI: 143-167 nmol/L); high: ≥13.1 μg/dL (SI: 169 nmol/L). Normal range is increased in women on birth control pills (5.5-12 μg/dL); normal range in pregnancy: ~5.5-16 μg/dL (SI: ~71-206 nmol/L). TSH: 0.4-10 (for those ≥80 years) mIU/L; T_4: 4-12 μg/dL (SI: 51-154 nmol/L); T_3 (RIA) (total T_3): 80-230 ng/dL (SI: 1.2-3.5 nmol/L); T_4 free (free T_4): 0.7-1.8 ng/dL (SI: 9-23 pmol/L).

Test Interactions Many drugs may have effects on thyroid function tests; para-aminosalicylic acid, aminoglutethimide, amiodarone, barbiturates, carbamazepine, chloral hydrate, clofibrate, colestipol, corticosteroids, danazol, diazepam, estrogens, ethionamide, fluorouracil, I.V. heparin, insulin, lithium, methadone, methimazole, mitotane, nitroprusside, oxyphenbutazone, phenylbutazone, PTU, perphenazine, phenytoin, propranolol, salicylates, sulfonylureas, and thiazides

Patient Information Do not change brands without physician's knowledge; report immediately to physician any chest pain, increased pulse, palpitations, heat intolerances, excessive sweating; do not discontinue without notifying your physician

Nursing Implications I.V. form must be prepared immediately prior to administration; should not be admixed with other solutions

Additional Information Levothroid® tablets contain lactose and tartrazine dye

To convert doses: Levothyroxine 0.05-0.06 mg is equivalent to 60 mg thyroid USP; 60 mg thyroglobulin; 4.5 mg thyroid strong; 1 grain (60 mg) liotrix

Dosage Forms

Powder for injection, as sodium, lyophilized: 200 mcg/vial (6 mL, 10 mL); 500 mcg/vial (6 mL, 10 mL)

Tablet, as sodium: 25 mcg, 50 mcg, 75 mcg, 88 mcg, 100 mcg, 112 mcg, 125 mcg, 150 mcg, 175 mcg, 200 mcg, 300 mcg

Levothyroxine Sodium *see* Levothyroxine *on previous page*
Levoxyl™ *see* Levothyroxine *on previous page*
Levsin® *see* Hyoscyamine *on page 635*
Levsinex® *see* Hyoscyamine *on page 635*
Levsin/SL® *see* Hyoscyamine *on page 635*
LH-RH *see* Gonadorelin *on page 583*
l-Hyoscyamine Sulfate *see* Hyoscyamine *on page 635*
Libritabs® *see* Chlordiazepoxide *on page 252*

Librium® *see* Chlordiazepoxide *on page 252*

Lice-Enz® Shampoo [OTC] *see* Pyrethrins *on page 1079*

Lidex® *see* Fluocinonide *on page 534*

Lidex-E® *see* Fluocinonide *on page 534*

Lidocaine (LYE doe kane)

Related Information

Adult ACLS Algorithm, Tachycardia *on page 1512*
Adult ACLS Algorithm, V. Fib and Pulseless V. Tach *on page 1509*
Antiarrhythmic Drugs *on page 1389*
Comparative Pharmacokinetic Properties of Antiarrhythmic Agents *on page 1391*
Pediatric ALS Algorithm, Asystole and Pulseless Arrest *on page 1507*

Brand Names Anestacon®; Dermaflex® Gel; Dilocaine®; Dr Scholl's® Cracked Heel Relief Cream [OTC]; Duo-Trach®; LidoPen® Auto-Injector; Nervocaine®; Octocaine®; Solarcaine® Aloe Extra Burn Relief [OTC]; Xylocaine®; Zilactin-L® [OTC]

Canadian/Mexican Brand Names PMS-Lidocaine Viscous (Canada); Xylocard® (Canada); Pisacina® (Mexico); Xylocaina® (Mexico)

Synonyms Lidocaine Hydrochloride; Lignocaine Hydrochloride

Therapeutic Category Antiarrhythmic Agent, Class I-B; Local Anesthetic, Injectable; Local Anesthetic, Topical

Use Local anesthetic and acute treatment of ventricular arrhythmias from myocardial infarction, cardiac manipulation, digitalis intoxication; topical local anesthetic; drug of choice for ventricular ectopy, ventricular tachycardia, ventricular fibrillation; for pulseless VT or VF preferably administer **after** defibrillation and epinephrine; control of premature ventricular contractions, wide-complex PSVT

Pregnancy Risk Factor C

Contraindications Known hypersensitivity to amide-type local anesthetics; patients with Adams-Stokes syndrome or with severe degree of S-A, A-V, or intraventricular heart block (without a pacemaker)

Warnings/Precautions Avoid use of preparations containing preservatives for spinal or epidural (including caudal) anesthesia. Use extreme caution in patients with hepatic disease, heart failure, marked hypoxia, severe respiratory depression, hypovolemia or shock, incomplete heart block or bradycardia, and atrial fibrillation.

Due to decreases in phase I metabolism and possibly decrease in splanchnic perfusion with age, there may be a decreased clearance or increased half-life in elderly and increased risk for CNS side effects and cardiac effects

Adverse Reactions

1% to 10%:
- Cardiovascular: Hypotension
- Central nervous system: Positional headache
- Miscellaneous: Shivering

<1%:
- Cardiovascular: Heart block, arrhythmias, cardiovascular collapse
- Central nervous system: Lethargy, coma, agitation, slurred speech, seizures, anxiety, euphoria, hallucinations
- Dermatologic: Itching, rash, edema of the skin
- Gastrointestinal: Nausea, vomiting
- Neuromuscular & skeletal: Paresthesias
- Ocular: Blurred vision, diplopia
- Respiratory: Dyspnea, respiratory depression or arrest

Overdosage/Toxicology Has a narrow therapeutic index and severe toxicity may occur slightly above the therapeutic range, especially with other antiarrhythmic drugs; symptoms of overdose include sedation, confusion, coma, seizures, respiratory arrest and cardiac toxicity (sinus arrest, A-V block, asystole, and hypotension); the QRS and Q-T intervals are usually normal, although they may be prolonged after massive overdose; other effects include dizziness, paresthesias, tremor, ataxia, and GI disturbance.

Treatment is supportive, using conventional therapies (fluids, positioning, vasopressors, antiarrhythmics, anticonvulsants); sodium bicarbonate may reverse QRS prolongation, bradyarrhythmias and hypotension; enhanced elimination with dialysis, hemoperfusion or repeat charcoal is not effective.

Drug Interactions

Increased toxicity:
- Concomitant cimetidine or propranolol may result in increased serum concentrations of lidocaine with resultant toxicity
- Effect of succinylcholine may be enhanced

Stability

Lidocaine injection is stable at room temperature

(Continued)

Lidocaine *(Continued)*

Stability of parenteral admixture at room temperature (25°C): Expiration date on premixed bag; out of overwrap stability: 30 days

Standard diluent: 2 g/250 mL D_5W

Mechanism of Action Class IB antiarrhythmic; suppresses automaticity of conduction tissue, by increasing electrical stimulation threshold of ventricle, HIS-Purkinje system, and spontaneous depolarization of the ventricles during diastole by a direct action on the tissues; blocks both the initiation and conduction of nerve impulses by decreasing the neuronal membrane's permeability to sodium ions, which results in inhibition of depolarization with resultant blockade of conduction

Pharmacodynamics/Kinetics

Onset of action (single bolus dose): 45-90 seconds

Duration: 10-20 minutes

Distribution: V_d: Alterable by many patient factors; decreased in CHF and liver disease

Protein binding: 60% to 80%; binds to $alpha_1$ acid glycoprotein

Metabolism: 90% metabolized in liver; active metabolites monoethylglycinexylidide (MEGX) and glycinexylidide (GX) can accumulate and may cause CNS toxicity

Half-life (biphasic): Increased with CHF, liver disease, shock, severe renal disease

Initial: 7-30 minutes

Terminal:

Infants, premature: 3.2 hours

Adults: 1.5-2 hours

Usual Dosage

Topical: Apply to affected area as needed; maximum: 3 mg/kg/dose; do not repeat within 2 hours

Injectable local anesthetic: Varies with procedure, degree of anesthesia needed, vascularity of tissue, duration of anesthesia required, and physical condition of patient; maximum: 4.5 mg/kg/dose; do not repeat within 2 hours

Children: Endotracheal, I.O., I.V.: Loading dose: 1 mg/kg; may repeat in 10-15 minutes x 2 doses; after loading dose, start I.V. continuous infusion 20-50 mcg/kg/minute

Use 20 mcg/kg/minute in patients with shock, hepatic disease, mild congestive heart failure (CHF)

Moderate to severe CHF may require ½ loading dose and lower infusion rates to avoid toxicity

Adults: Antiarrhythmic:

I.V.: 1-1.5 mg/kg bolus over 2-3 minutes; may repeat doses of 0.5-0.75 mg/kg in 5-10 minutes up to a total of 3 mg/kg; continuous infusion: 1-4 mg/minute

I.V. (2 g/250 mL D_5W) infusion rates (infusion pump should be used for I.V. infusion administration):

1 mg/minute: 7 mL/hour

2 mg/minute: 15 mL/hour

3 mg/minute: 21 mL/hour

4 mg/minute: 30 mL/hour

Ventricular fibrillation (after defibrillation and epinephrine): Initial dose: 1.5 mg/kg, may repeat boluses as above; follow with continuous infusion after return of perfusion

Prevention of ventricular fibrillation: I.V.: Initial bolus: 0.5 mg/kg; repeat every 5-10 minutes to a total dose of 2 mg/kg

Refractory ventricular fibrillation: Repeat 1.5 mg/kg bolus may be given 3-5 minutes after initial dose

Endotracheal: 2-2.5 times the I.V. dose

Decrease dose in patients with CHF, shock, or hepatic disease

Dosing adjustment/comments in hepatic disease: Reduce dose in acute hepatitis and decompensated cirrhosis by 50%

Dialysis: Not dialyzable (0% to 5%) by hemo- or peritoneal dialysis; supplemental dose not necessary; supplemental dose is not necessary

Reference Range

Therapeutic: 1.5-5.0 μg/mL (SI: 6-21 μmol/L)

Potentially toxic: >6 μg/mL (SI: >26 μmol/L)

Toxic: >9 μg/mL (SI: >38 μmol/L)

Nursing Implications Local thrombophlebitis may occur in patients receiving prolonged I.V. infusions

Dosage Forms

Cream, as hydrochloride: 2% (56 g)

Injection, as hydrochloride: 0.5% [5 mg/mL] (50 mL); 1% [10 mg/mL] (2 mL, 5 mL, 10 mL, 20 mL, 30 mL, 50 mL); 1.5% [15 mg/mL] (20 mL); 2% [20 mg/mL]

(2 mL, 5 mL, 10 mL, 20 mL, 30 mL, 50 mL); 4% [40 mg/mL] (5 mL); 10% [100 mg/mL] (10 mL); 20% [200 mg/mL] (10 mL, 20 mL)

Injection, as hydrochloride:

I.M. use: 10% [100 mg/mL] (3 mL, 5 mL)

Direct I.V.: 1% [10 mg/mL] (5 mL, 10 mL); 20 mg/mL (5 mL)

I.V. admixture, preservative free: 4% [40 mg/mL] (25 mL, 30 mL); 10% [100 mg/mL] (10 mL); 20% [200 mg/mL] (5 mL, 10 mL)

I.V. infusion, in D_5W: 0.2% [2 mg/mL] (500 mL); 0.4% [4 mg/mL] (250 mL, 500 mL, 1000 mL); 0.8% [8 mg/mL] (250 mL, 500 mL)

Gel, , as hydrochloride, topical: 2% (30 mL); 2.5% (15 mL)

Liquid, as hydrochloride, topical: 2.5% (7.5 mL)

Liquid, as hydrochloride, viscous: 2% (20 mL, 100 mL)

Ointment, as hydrochloride, topical: 2.5% [OTC], 5% (35 g)

Solution, as hydrochloride, topical: 2% (15 mL, 240 mL); 4% (50 mL)

Lidocaine and Epinephrine (LYE doe kane & ep i NEF rin)

Brand Names Octocaine® Injection; Xylocaine® With Epinephrine

Canadian/Mexican Brand Names Pisacaina® (Mexico); Uvega® (Mexico); Xylocaina® (Mexico)

Therapeutic Category Local Anesthetic, Injectable

Use Local infiltration anesthesia; AVS for nerve block

Pregnancy Risk Factor B

Contraindications Hypersensitivity to local anesthetics of the amide type, myasthenia gravis, shock, or cardiac conduction disease

Warnings/Precautions Do not use solutions in distal portions of the body (digits, nose, ears, penis); use with caution in endocrine, heart, hepatic, or thyroid disease

Adverse Reactions Refer to Lidocaine monograph

Overdosage/Toxicology Refer to Lidocaine monograph

Drug Interactions MAO inhibitors, tricyclic antidepressants, vasopressors, ester-type anesthetics

Stability Solutions with epinephrine should be protected from light

Mechanism of Action Lidocaine blocks both the initiation and conduction of nerve impulses via decreased permeability of sodium ions; epinephrine increases the duration of action of lidocaine by causing vasoconstriction (via alpha effects) which slows the vascular absorption of lidocaine

Pharmacodynamics/Kinetics

Peak effect: Within 5 minutes

Duration: ~2 hours, dependent on dose and anesthetic procedure

Usual Dosage

Children: Use lidocaine concentrations of 0.5% to 1% (or even more diluted) to decrease possibility of toxicity; lidocaine dose should not exceed 7 mg/kg/dose; do not repeat within 2 hours

Adults: Dosage varies with the anesthetic procedure, degree of anesthesia needed, vascularity of tissue, duration of anesthesia required, and physical condition of patient

Nursing Implications Before injecting, withdraw syringe plunger to ensure injection is not into vein or artery

Additional Information Contains metabisulfites

Dosage Forms Injection with epinephrine:

1:200,000: Lidocaine hydrochloride 0.5% [5 mg/mL] (50 mL); 1% [10 mg/mL] (30 mL); 1.5% [15 mg/mL] (5 mL, 10 mL, 30 mL); 2% [20 mg/mL] (20 mL)

1:100,000: Lidocaine hydrochloride 1% [10 mg/mL] (20 mL, 50 mL); 2% [20 mg/mL] (1.8 mL, 20 mL, 50 mL)

1:50,000: Lidocaine hydrochloride 2% [20 mg/mL] (1.8 mL)

Lidocaine and Prilocaine (LYE doe kane & PRIL oh kane)

Brand Names EMLA®

Therapeutic Category Analgesic, Topical; Anesthetic, Topical; Local Anesthetic, Topical

Use Topical anesthetic for use on normal intact skin to provide local analgesia for minor procedures such as I.V. cannulation or venipuncture; has also been used for painful procedures such as lumbar puncture and skin graft harvesting

Pregnancy Risk Factor B

Contraindications

Children <1 month of age

Administration on mucous membranes

Administration on broken or inflamed skin

Children with congenital or idiopathic methemoglobinemia, or in children who are receiving medications associated with drug-induced methemoglobinemia [ie,

(Continued)

Lidocaine and Prilocaine *(Continued)*

acetaminophen (overdosage), benzocaine, chloroquine, dapsone, nitrofurantoin, nitroglycerin, nitroprusside, phenazopyridine, phenelzine, phenobarbital, phenytoin, quinine, sulfonamides]

Patients with a documented hypersensitivity to amide type anesthetic agents [ie, lidocaine, prilocaine, dibucaine, mepivacaine, bupivacaine, etidocaine]

Patients with a documented hypersensitivity to any components of EMLA® cream or Tegaderm®

Adverse Reactions

1% to 10%:
- Dermatologic: Angioedema, contact dermatitis
- Local: Burning, stinging

<1%:
- Cardiovascular: Bradycardia, hypotension, shock, edema
- Central nervous system: Nervousness, euphoria, confusion, dizziness, drowsiness, convulsions, CNS excitation
- Dermatologic: Erythema, itching, rash, urticaria
- Hematologic: Methemoglobinemia in infants
- Local: Blanching, alteration in temperature sensation, tenderness
- Neuromuscular & skeletal: Tremors
- Ocular: Blurred vision
- Otic: Tinnitus
- Respiratory: Respiratory depression, bronchospasm

Drug Interactions Increased toxicity:

Class I antiarrhythmic drugs (tocainide, mexiletine): Effects are additive and potentially synergistic

Drugs known to induce methemoglobinemia

Stability Store at room temperature

Mechanism of Action Local anesthetic action occurs by stabilization of neuronal membranes and inhibiting the ionic fluxes required for the initiation and conduction of impulses

Pharmacodynamics/Kinetics

Onset of action: 1 hour for sufficient dermal analgesia

Peak effect: 2-3 hours

Duration: 1-2 hours after removal of the cream

Absorption: Related to the duration of application and to the area over which it is applied
- 3-hour application: 3.6% lidocaine and 6.1% prilocaine were absorbed
- 24-hour application: 16.2% lidocaine and 33.5% prilocaine were absorbed

Distribution: Both cross the blood-brain barrier
- V_d:
  - Lidocaine: 1.1-2.1 L/kg
  - Prilocaine: 0.7-4.4 L/kg

Protein binding:
- Lidocaine: 70%
- Prilocaine: 55%

Metabolism:
- Lidocaine: Metabolized by the liver to inactive and active metabolites
- Prilocaine: Metabolized in both the liver and kidneys

Half-life:
- Lidocaine: 65-150 minutes, prolonged with cardiac or hepatic dysfunction
- Prilocaine: 10-150 minutes, prolonged in hepatic or renal dysfunction

Usual Dosage Children and Adults:

EMLA® cream should not be used in infants under the age of 1 month or in infants, under the age of 12 months, who are receiving treatment with methemogloblin-inducing agents

EMLA® Cream Maximum Recommended Application Area* for Infants and Children Based on Application to Intact Skin

Body Weight (kg)	Maximum Application Area (cm^2)†
<10 kg	100
10-20 kg	600
>20 kg	2000

*These are broad guidelines for avoiding systemic toxicity in applying EMLA® to patients with normal intact skin and with normal renal and hepatic function.

†For more individualized calculation of how much lidocaine and prilocaine may be absorbed, use the following estimates of lidocaine and prilocaine absorption for children and adults:

Estimated mean (±SD) absorption of lidocaine: 0.045 (±0.016) mg/cm²/h.

Estimated mean (±SD) absorption of prilocaine: 0.077 (±0.036) mg/cm²/h.

Choose 2 application sites available for intravenous access

Apply a thick layer (2.5 g/site ~½ of a 5 g tube) of cream to each designated site of intact skin

Cover each site with the occlusive dressing (Tegaderm®)

Mark the time on the dressing

Allow at least 1 hour for optimum therapeutic effect. Remove the dressing and wipe off excess EMLA® cream (gloves should be worn).

Debilitated patients, small children or patients with impaired elimination (ie, hepatic or renal dysfunction): Smaller areas of treatment are recommended

Patient Information Not for ophthalmic use; for external use only. EMLA® may block sensation in the treated skin.

Nursing Implications In small infants and children, an occlusive bandage should be placed over the EMLA® cream to prevent the child from placing the cream in his mouth

Dosage Forms Cream: Lidocaine 2.5% and prilocaine 2.5% [2 Tegaderm® dressings] (5 g, 30 g)

Lidocaine Hydrochloride *see* Lidocaine *on page 723*

LidoPen® Auto-Injector *see* Lidocaine *on page 723*

Lignocaine Hydrochloride *see* Lidocaine *on page 723*

Lincocin® Injection *see* Lincomycin *on this page*

Lincocin® Oral *see* Lincomycin *on this page*

Lincomycin (lin koe MYE sin)

Brand Names Lincocin® Injection; Lincocin® Oral; Lincorex® Injection

Canadian/Mexican Brand Names Princol® (Mexico)

Synonyms Lincomycin Hydrochloride

Therapeutic Category Antibiotic, Macrolide

Use Treatment of susceptible bacterial infections, mainly those caused by streptococci and staphylococci resistant to other agents

Pregnancy Risk Factor B

Contraindications Minor bacterial infections or viral infections, hypersensitivity to lincomycin or any component or clindamycin

Warnings/Precautions Can cause severe and possibly fatal colitis; characterized by severe persistent diarrhea, severe abdominal cramps and, possibly, the passage of blood and mucus; discontinue drug if significant diarrhea occurs; severe hepatic disease

Adverse Reactions

1% to 10%: Gastrointestinal: Nausea, vomiting, diarrhea

<1%:

- Cardiovascular: Hypotension
- Central nervous system: Vertigo
- Dermatologic: Urticaria, rash, Stevens-Johnson syndrome
- Gastrointestinal: Pseudomembranous colitis, glossitis, stomatitis, pruritus ani
- Genitourinary: Vaginitis
- Hematologic: Granulocytopenia, thrombocytopenia, pancytopenia
- Hepatic: Elevation of liver enzymes
- Local: Sterile abscess at I.M. injection site, thrombophlebitis
- Otic: Tinnitus

Overdosage/Toxicology Symptoms of overdose include diarrhea, abdominal cramps; following oral decontamination, treatment is supportive

Drug Interactions

Decreased effect with erythromycin

Increased activity/toxicity of neuromuscular blocking agents

Mechanism of Action Lincosamide antibiotic which was isolated from a strain of *Streptomyces lincolnensis*; lincomycin, like clindamycin, inhibits bacterial protein synthesis by specifically binding on the 50S subunit and affecting the process of peptide chain initiation. Other macrolide antibiotics (erythromycin) also bind to the 50S subunit. Since only one molecule of antibiotic can bind to a single ribosome, the concomitant use of erythromycin and lincomycin is not recommended.

Pharmacodynamics/Kinetics

Absorption: Oral: ~20% to 30%

Distribution: V_d: 23-38 L; CSF levels are higher with inflamed meninges; CSF penetration is poor

Protein binding: 72%

Metabolism: Hepatic

Half-life, elimination: 2-11.5 hours

Time to peak serum concentration:

- Oral: 2-4 hours
- I.M.: 1 hour

Elimination: 5% to 10% excreted unchanged in urine, with 30% to 40% (oral) and 4% to 14% (parenteral) excreted unchanged in feces

(Continued)

Lincomycin *(Continued)*

Usual Dosage

Children >1 month:

Oral: 30-60 mg/kg/day in divided doses every 8 hours

I.M.: 10 mg/kg every 8-12 hours

I.V.: 10-20 mg/kg/day in divided doses every 8-12 hours

Adults:

Oral: 500 mg every 6-8 hours

I.M.: 600 mg every 12-24 hours

I.V.: 600-1 g every 8-12 hours up to 8 g/day

Dosing interval in renal impairment:

Cl_{cr} 10-50 mL/minute: Administer every 6-12 hours

Cl_{cr} <10 mL/minute: Administer every 12 hours

Dosing adjustment in hepatic impairment: Reductions are indicated

Administration Administer oral dosage form with a full glass of water to minimize esophageal ulceration; administer around-the-clock to promote less variation in peak and trough serum levels

Patient Information Report any severe diarrhea immediately and do not take antidiarrheal medication; take each oral dose with a full glass of water; finish all medication; do not skip doses; store capsules in a light-proof container

Dosage Forms

Capsule, as hydrochloride: 250 mg, 500 mg

Injection, as hydrochloride: 300 mg/mL (2 mL, 10 mL)

Lincomycin Hydrochloride *see* Lincomycin *on previous page*

Lincorex® Injection *see* Lincomycin *on previous page*

Lindane (LIN dane)

Brand Names G-well®; Scabene®

Canadian/Mexican Brand Names Hexit® (Canada); Kwellada® (Canada); PMS-Lindane (Canada); Herklin® (Mexico); Scabisan® Shampoo (Mexico)

Synonyms Benzene Hexachloride; Gamma Benzene Hexachloride; Hexachlorocyclohexane

Therapeutic Category Antiparasitic Agent, Topical; Pediculocide; Scabicidal Agent; Shampoos

Use Treatment of scabies (*Sarcoptes scabiei*), *Pediculus capitis* (head lice), and *Pediculus pubis* (crab lice); FDA recommends reserving lindane as a second-line agent or with inadequate response to other therapies

Pregnancy Risk Factor B

Pregnancy/Breast-Feeding Implications There are no well controlled studies in pregnant women; treat no more than twice during a pregnancy

Contraindications Hypersensitivity to lindane or any component; premature neonates; acutely inflamed skin or raw, weeping surfaces

Warnings/Precautions Use with caution in infants and small children, and patients with a history of seizures; avoid contact with face, eyes, mucous membranes, and urethral meatus. Because of the potential for systemic absorption and CNS side effects, lindane should be used with caution; not considered a drug of first choice; consider permethrin or crotamiton agent first.

Adverse Reactions

<1%:

Cardiovascular: Cardiac arrhythmia

Central nervous system: Dizziness, restlessness, seizures, headache, ataxia

Dermatologic: Eczematous eruptions, contact dermatitis, skin and adipose tissue may act as repositories

Gastrointestinal: Nausea, vomiting

Hematologic: Aplastic anemia

Hepatic: Hepatitis

Local: Burning and stinging

Renal: Hematuria

Respiratory: Pulmonary edema

Overdosage/Toxicology Symptoms of overdose include vomiting, restlessness, ataxia, seizures, arrhythmias, pulmonary edema, hematuria, hepatitis. Absorbed through skin and mucous membranes and GI tract, has occasionally caused serious CNS, hepatic and renal toxicity when used excessively for prolonged periods, or when accidental ingestion has occurred

If ingested, perform gastric lavage and general supportive measures; diazepam 0.01 mg/kg can be used to control seizures.

Drug Interactions Increased toxicity: Oil-based hair dressing may increase toxic potential

Mechanism of Action Directly absorbed by parasites and ova through the exoskeleton; stimulates the nervous system resulting in seizures and death of parasitic arthropods

Pharmacodynamics/Kinetics

Absorption: Systemic absorption of up to 13% may occur

Distribution: Stored in body fat and accumulates in brain; skin and adipose tissue may act as repositories

Metabolism: By the liver

Half-life: Children: 17-22 hours

Time to peak serum concentration: Topical: Children: 6 hours

Elimination: In urine and feces

Usual Dosage Children and Adults: Topical:

Scabies: Apply a thin layer of lotion or cream and massage it on skin from the neck to the toes (head to toe in infants). For adults, bathe and remove the drug after 8-12 hours; for children, wash off 6-8 hours after application (for infants, wash off 6 hours after application); repeat treatment in 7 days if lice or nits are still present

Pediculosis, capitis and pubis: 15-30 mL of shampoo is applied and lathered for 4-5 minutes; rinse hair thoroughly and comb with a fine tooth comb to remove nits; repeat treatment in 7 days if lice or nits are still present

Administration Drug should not be administered orally, for topical use only; apply to dry, cool skin

Patient Information Topical use only, do not apply to face, avoid getting in eyes; do **not** apply lotion immediately after a hot, soapy bath. Clothing and bedding should be washed in hot water or by dry cleaning to kill the scabies mite. Combs and brushes may be washed with lindane shampoo then thoroughly rinsed with water. Notify physician if condition worsens; treat sexual contact simultaneously.

Dosage Forms

Cream: 1% (60 g, 454 g)

Lotion: 1% (60 mL, 473 mL, 4000 mL)

Shampoo: 1% (60 mL, 473 mL, 4000 mL)

Lioresal® *see* Baclofen *on page 130*

Liothyronine (lye oh THYE roe neen)

Brand Names Cytomel®; Triostat™

Synonyms Liothyronine Sodium; Sodium *L*-Triiodothyronine; T_3 Sodium

Therapeutic Category Thyroid Product

Use Replacement or supplemental therapy in hypothyroidism, management of nontoxic goiter, chronic lymphocytic thyroiditis, as an adjunct in thyrotoxicosis and as a diagnostic aid; **levothyroxine is recommended for chronic therapy**; although previously thought to benefit cardiac patients with severely reduced fractions, liothyronine injection is no longer considered beneficial

Pregnancy Risk Factor A

Contraindications Recent myocardial infarction or thyrotoxicosis, hypersensitivity to liothyronine sodium or any component, undocumented or uncorrected adrenal insufficiency

Warnings/Precautions Ineffective for weight reduction; high doses may produce serious or even life-threatening toxic effects particularly when used with some anorectic drugs. Use with extreme caution in patients with angina pectoris or other cardiovascular disease (including hypertension) or coronary artery disease; use with caution in elderly patients since they may be more likely to have compromised cardiovascular function. Patients with adrenal insufficiency, myxedema, diabetes mellitus and insipidus may have symptoms exaggerated or aggravated; thyroid replacement requires periodic assessment of thyroid status. Chronic hypothyroidism predisposes patients to coronary artery disease.

Adverse Reactions

<1%:

Cardiovascular: Palpitations, tachycardia, cardiac arrhythmias, chest pain

Central nervous system: Nervousness, insomnia, fever, headache, ataxia

Dermatologic: Alopecia

Endocrine & metabolic: Changes in menstrual cycle

Gastrointestinal: Weight loss, increased appetite, diarrhea, abdominal cramps, constipation

Neuromuscular & skeletal: Myalgia, hand tremors, tremor

Respiratory: Shortness of breath

Miscellaneous: Diaphoresis

Overdosage/Toxicology Chronic overdose may cause hyperthyroidism, weight loss, nervousness, sweating, tachycardia, insomnia, heat intolerance, menstrual irregularities, palpitations, psychosis, fever; acute overdose may cause fever, hypoglycemia, CHF, unrecognized adrenal insufficiency.

(Continued)

Liothyronine *(Continued)*

Reduce dose or temporarily discontinue therapy; normal hypothalamic-pituitary-thyroid axis will return to normal in 6-8 weeks; serum T_4 levels do not correlate well with toxicity

In massive acute ingestion, reduce GI absorption, administer general supportive care; treat congestive heart failure with digitalis glycosides; excessive adrenergic activity (tachycardia) requires propranolol 1-3 mg I.V. over 10 minutes or 80-160 mg orally/day; fever may be treated with acetaminophen.

Drug Interactions

Decreased effect:

Cholestyramine resin may decrease absorption

Antidiabetic drug requirements are increased

Estrogens may increase thyroid requirements

Increased effect: Increased oral anticoagulant effects

Stability Vials must be stored under refrigeration at 2°C to 8°C (36°F to 46°F)

Mechanism of Action Primary active compound is T_3 (triiodothyronine), which may be converted from T_4 (thyroxine) and then circulates throughout the body to influence growth and maturation of various tissues; exact mechanism of action is unknown; however, it is believed the thyroid hormone exerts its many metabolic effects through control of DNA transcription and protein synthesis; involved in normal metabolism, growth, and development; promotes gluconeogenesis, increases utilization and mobilization of glycogen stores, and stimulates protein synthesis, increases basal metabolic rate

Pharmacodynamics/Kinetics

Onset of effect: Within 24-72 hours

Duration: Up to 72 hours

Absorption: Oral: Well absorbed (~85% to 90%)

Metabolism: In the liver to inactive compounds

Half-life: 16-49 hours

Elimination: In urine

Usual Dosage

Congenital hypothyroidism: Children: Oral: 5 mcg/day increase by 5 mcg every 3 days to 20 mcg/day for infants, 50 mcg/day for children 1-3 years of age, and administer adult dose for children >3 years.

Hypothyroidism: Oral:

Adults: 25 mcg/day increase by 12.5-25 mcg/day every 1-2 weeks to a maximum of 100 mcg/day

Elderly: Initial: 5 mcg/day, increase by 5 mcg/day every 1-2 weeks; usual maintenance dose: 25-75 mcg/day

T_3 suppression test: Oral: 75-100 mcg/day for 7 days; use lowest dose for elderly

Myxedema coma: I.V.: 25-50 mcg

Patients with known or suspected cardiovascular disease: 10-20 mcg

Note: Normally, at least 4 hours should be allowed between doses to adequately assess therapeutic response and no more than 12 hours should elapse between doses to avoid fluctuations in hormone levels. Oral therapy should be resumed as soon as the clinical situation has been stabilized and the patient is able to take oral medication. If levothyroxine rather than liothyronine sodium is used in initiating oral therapy, the physician should bear in mind that there is a delay of several days in the onset of levothyroxine activity and that I.V. therapy should be discontinued gradually.

Administration For I.V. use only - **do not administer I.M. or S.C.**

Administer doses at least 4 hours, and no more than 12 hours, apart

Resume oral therapy as soon as the clinical situation has been stabilized and the patient is able to take oral medication

When switching to tablets, discontinue the injectable, initiate oral therapy at a low dosage and increase gradually according to response

If levothyroxine is used for oral therapy, there is a delay of several days in the onset of activity; therefore, discontinue I.V. therapy gradually

Monitoring Parameters T_4, TSH, heart rate, blood pressure, clinical signs of hypo- and hyperthyroidism; TSH is the most reliable guide for evaluating adequacy of thyroid replacement dosage. TSH may be elevated during the first few months of thyroid replacement despite patients being clinically euthyroid. In cases where T_4 remains low and TSH is within normal limits, an evaluation of "free" (unbound) T_4 is needed to evaluate further increase in dosage.

Reference Range Free T_3, serum: 250-390 pg/dL; TSH: 0.4 and up to 10 (≥80 years of age) mIU/L; remains normal in pregnancy

Test Interactions Many drugs may have effects on thyroid function tests; para-aminosalicylic acid, aminoglutethimide, amiodarone, barbiturates, carbamazepine, chloral hydrate, clofibrate, colestipol, corticosteroids, danazol, diazepam, estrogens, ethionamide, fluorouracil, I.V. heparin, insulin, lithium, methadone, methimazole, mitotane, nitroprusside, oxyphenbutazone, phenylbutazone, PTU, perphenazine, phenytoin, propranolol, salicylates, sulfonylureas, and thiazides

Patient Information Do not change brands without physician's knowledge; report immediately to physician any chest pain, increased pulse, palpitations, heat intolerances, excessive sweating; do not discontinue without notifying physician

Additional Information 15-37.5 mcg is equivalent to 0.05-0.06 mg levothyroxine; 60 mg thyroid USP; 45 mg Thyroid Strong®, and 60 mg thyroglobulin

Dosage Forms

Injection, as sodium: 10 mcg/mL (1 mL)

Tablet, as sodium: 5 mcg, 25 mcg, 50 mcg

Liothyronine Sodium *see* Liothyronine *on page 729*

Liotrix (LYE oh triks)

Brand Names Thyrolar®

Synonyms T_3/T_4 Liotrix

Therapeutic Category Thyroid Product

Use Replacement or supplemental therapy in hypothyroidism (uniform mixture of $T_4:T_3$ in 4:1 ratio by weight); little advantage to this product exists and cost is not justified

Pregnancy Risk Factor A

Contraindications Hypersensitivity to liotrix or any component; recent myocardial infarction or thyrotoxicosis, uncomplicated by hypothyroidism; uncorrected adrenal insufficiency, hypersensitivity to active or extraneous constituents

Warnings/Precautions Ineffective for weight reduction; high doses may produce serious or even life-threatening toxic effects particularly when used with some anorectic drugs; use cautiously in patients with pre-existing cardiovascular disease (angina, CHD), elderly since they may be more likely to have compromised cardiovascular function

Adverse Reactions

<1%:

Cardiovascular: Palpitations, tachycardia, cardiac arrhythmias, chest pain

Central nervous system: Nervousness, headache, insomnia, fever, ataxia

Dermatologic: Alopecia

Endocrine & metabolic: Excessive bone loss with overtreatment (excess thyroid replacement), heat intolerance, changes in menstrual cycle

Gastrointestinal: Weight loss, increased appetite, diarrhea, abdominal cramps, vomiting, constipation

Neuromuscular & skeletal: Tremor, myalgia, hand tremors

Respiratory: Shortness of breath

Miscellaneous: Diaphoresis

Overdosage/Toxicology Chronic overdose may cause weight loss, nervousness, sweating, tachycardia, insomnia, heat intolerance, menstrual irregularities, palpitations, psychosis, fever; acute overdose may cause fever, hypoglycemia, CHF, unrecognized adrenal insufficiency

Reduce dose or temporarily discontinue therapy; normal hypothalamic-pituitary-thyroid axis will return to normal in 6-8 weeks; serum T_4 levels do not correlate well with toxicity

In massive acute ingestion, reduce GI absorption, administer general supportive care; treat congestive heart failure with digitalis glycosides; excessive adrenergic activity (tachycardia) require propranolol 1-3 mg I.V. over 10 minutes or 80-160 mg orally/day; fever may be treated with acetaminophen

Drug Interactions

Decreased effect:

Thyroid hormones increase hypoglycemic drug requirements

Phenytoin → clinical lymphothyroidism

Cholestyramine may decrease drug absorption

Increased effect: Increased oral anticoagulant effect

Increased toxicity: Tricyclic antidepressants may increase potential of both drugs

Mechanism of Action The primary active compound is T_3 (triiodothyronine), which may be converted from T_4 (thyroxine) and then circulates throughout the body to influence growth and maturation of various tissues. Liotrix is uniform mixture of synthetic T_4 and T_3 in 4:1 ratio; exact mechanism of action is unknown; however, it is believed the thyroid hormone exerts its many metabolic effects through control of DNA transcription and protein synthesis; involved in normal metabolism, growth, and development; promotes gluconeogenesis, increases utilization and mobilization of glycogen stores and stimulates protein synthesis, increases basal metabolic rate

Pharmacodynamics/Kinetics

Absorption: 50% to 95% from GI tract

Time to peak serum concentration: 12-48 hours

Metabolism: Partially in the liver, kidneys, and intestines

(Continued)

Liotrix *(Continued)*

Half-life: 6-7 days

Elimination: Partially in feces and bile as conjugated metabolites

Usual Dosage Oral:

Congenital hypothyroidism:

Children (dose of T_4 or levothyroxine/day):

0-6 months: 8-10 mcg/kg or 25-50 mcg/day

6-12 months: 6-8 mcg/kg or 50-75 mcg/day

1-5 years: 5-6 mcg/kg or 75-100 mcg/day

6-12 years: 4-5 mcg/kg or 100-150 mcg/day

>12 years: 2-3 mcg/kg or >150 mcg/day

Hypothyroidism (dose of thyroid equivalent):

Adults: 30 mg/day, increasing by 15 mg/day at 2- to 3-week intervals to a maximum of 180 mg/day (usual maintenance dose: 60-120 mg/day)

Elderly: Initial: 15 mg, adjust dose at 2- to 4-week intervals by increments of 15 mg

Monitoring Parameters T_4, TSH, heart rate, blood pressure, clinical signs of hypo- and hyperthyroidism; TSH is the most reliable guide for evaluating adequacy of thyroid replacement dosage. TSH may be elevated during the first few months of thyroid replacement despite patients being clinically euthyroid. In cases where T_4 remains low and TSH is within normal limits, an evaluation of "free" (unbound) T_4 is needed to evaluate further increase in dosage.

Reference Range

TSH: 0.4-10 (for those ≥80 years) mIU/L

T_4: 4-12 μg/dL (SI: 51-154 nmol/L)

T_3 (RIA) (total T_3): 80-230 ng/dL (SI: 1.2-3.5 nmol/L)

T_4 free (Free T_4): 0.7-1.8 ng/dL (SI: 9-23 pmol/L)

Test Interactions Many drugs may have effects on thyroid function tests; para-aminosalicylic acid, aminoglutethimide, amiodarone, barbiturates, carbamazepine, chloral hydrate, clofibrate, colestipol, corticosteroids, danazol, diazepam, estrogens, ethionamide, fluorouracil, I.V. heparin, insulin, lithium, methadone, methimazole, mitotane, nitroprusside, oxyphenbutazone, phenylbutazone, PTU, perphenazine, phenytoin, propranolol, salicylates, sulfonylureas, and thiazides

Patient Information Do not change brands without physician's knowledge; report immediately to physician any chest pain, increased pulse, palpitations, heat intolerances, excessive sweating; do not discontinue without notifying your physician; replacement therapy will be for life; take as a single dose before breakfast

Additional Information Since T_3 is produced by monodeiodination of T_4 in peripheral tissues (80%) and since elderly have decreased T_3 (25% to 40%), little advantage to this product exists and cost is not justified; no advantage over synthetic levothyroxine sodium; 1 grain (60 mg) liotrix is equivalent to 0.05-0.06 mg levothyroxine; 60 mg thyroid USP and thyroglobulin; and 45 mg of Thyroid Strong®

Comparison of Liotrix Products

Liotrix Product	T_4 Content (mcg)	T_3 Content (mcg)	Thyroid Equivalent (mg)
Euthroid® 1/2 grain	30	7.5	30
Euthroid® 1 grain	60	15	60
Euthroid® 2 grain	120	30	120
Euthroid® 3 grain	180	45	180
Thyrolar® 1/4 grain	12.5	3.1	15
Thyrolar® 1/2 grain	25	6.25	30
Thyrolar® 1 grain	50	12.5	60
Thyrolar® 2 grain	100	25	120
Thyrolar® 3 grain	150	37.5	180

Dosage Forms Tablet: 15 mg, 30 mg, 60 mg, 120 mg, 180 mg [thyroid equivalent]

Lipancreatin *see* Pancrelipase *on page 949*

Lipid-Lowering Agents *see page 1413*

Lipitor® *see* Atorvastatin *on page 113*
Liposyn® *see* Fat Emulsion *on page 505*
Liquibid® *see* Guaifenesin *on page 589*
Liqui-Char® [OTC] *see* Charcoal *on page 245*
Liquid Antidote *see* Charcoal *on page 245*
Liquid Paraffin *see* Mineral Oil *on page 841*
Liquid Pred® *see* Prednisone *on page 1039*

Lisinopril (lyse IN oh pril)

Related Information

Angiotensin-Converting Enzyme Inhibitors Comparison *on page 1386*
Heart Failure: Management of Patients With Left-Ventricular Systolic Dysfunction *on page 1533*

Brand Names Prinivil®; Zestril®

Therapeutic Category Angiotensin-Converting Enzyme (ACE) Inhibitors; Antihypertensive

Use Treatment of hypertension, either alone or in combination with other antihypertensive agents; adjunctive therapy in treatment of CHF (afterload reduction); treatment of hemodynamically stable patients within 24 hours of acute myocardial infarction, to improve survival

Pregnancy Risk Factor C (first trimester); D (second and third trimester)

Pregnancy/Breast-Feeding Implications

Clinical effects on the fetus: No data available on crossing the placenta. Cranial defects, hypocalvaria/acalvaria, oligohydramnios, persistent anuria following delivery, hypotension, renal defects, renal dysgenesis/dysplasia, renal failure, pulmonary hypoplasia, limb contractures secondary to oligohydramnios and still-birth reported. ACE inhibitors should be avoided during pregnancy.

Breast-feeding/lactation: Crosses into breast milk. American Academy of Pediatrics considers COMPATIBLE with breast-feeding.

Contraindications Hypersensitivity to lisinopril or any component or other ACE inhibitors

Warnings/Precautions Use with caution and modify dosage in patients with renal impairment (decrease dosage) (especially renal artery stenosis), severe congestive heart failure, or with coadministered diuretic therapy; experience in children is limited. Severe hypotension may occur in patients who are sodium and/or volume depleted, initiate lower doses and monitor closely when starting therapy in these patients.

Adverse Reactions

1% to 10%:

Cardiovascular: Hypotension
Central nervous system: Dizziness, headache, fatigue
Gastrointestinal: Diarrhea
Renal: Increased BUN/serum creatinine
Respiratory: Upper respiratory symptoms, cough

<1%:

Cardiovascular: Chest discomfort, flushing, myocardial infarction, angina pectoris, orthostatic hypotension, rhythm disturbances, tachycardia, peripheral edema, vasculitis, palpitations, syncope
Central nervous system: Fever, malaise, depression, somnolence, insomnia
Dermatologic: Urticaria, pruritus, angioedema
Endocrine & metabolic: Gout
Gastrointestinal: Pancreatitis, abdominal pain, anorexia, constipation, flatulence, xerostomia
Hematologic: Neutropenia, bone marrow suppression
Hepatic: Hepatitis
Neuromuscular & skeletal: Arthralgia, shoulder pain
Ocular: Blurred vision
Respiratory: Bronchitis, sinusitis, pharyngeal pain
Miscellaneous: Diaphoresis

Overdosage/Toxicology Mild hypotension has been the only toxic effect seen with acute overdose. Bradycardia may also occur; hyperkalemia occurs even with therapeutic doses, especially in patients with renal insufficiency and those taking NSAIDs

Following initiation of essential overdose management, toxic symptom treatment and supportive treatment should be initiated. Hypotension usually responds to I.V. fluids or Trendelenburg positioning.

Drug Interactions

Increased toxicity:

Probenecid increases blood levels of captopril
Captopril and diuretics have additive hypotensive effects; see table.

(Continued)

Lisinopril *(Continued)*

Drug-Drug Interactions With ACEIs

Precipitant Drug	Drug (Category) and Effect	Description
Antacids	ACE Inhibitors: decreased	Decreased bioavailability of ACEIs. May be more likely with captopril. Separate administration times by 1-2 hours.
NSAIDs (indomethacin)	ACEIs: decreased	Reduced hypotensive effects of ACEIs. More prominent in low renin or volume dependent hypertensive patients.
Phenothiazines	ACEIs: increased	Pharmacologic effects of ACEIs may be increased.
ACEIs	Allopurinol: increased	Higher risk of hypersensitivity reaction possible when given concurrently. Three case reports of Stevens-Johnson syndrome with captopril.
ACEIs	Digoxin: increased	Increased plasma digoxin levels.
ACEIs	Lithium: increased	Increased serum lithium levels and symptoms of toxicity may occur.
ACEIs	Potassium preps/ potassium sparing diuretics increased	Coadministration may result in elevated potassium levels.

Mechanism of Action Competitive inhibitor of angiotensin-converting enzyme (ACE); prevents conversion of angiotensin I to angiotensin II, a potent vasoconstrictor; results in lower levels of angiotensin II which causes an increase in plasma renin activity and a reduction in aldosterone secretion; a CNS mechanism may also be involved in hypotensive effect as angiotensin II increases adrenergic outflow from CNS; vasoactive kallikreins may be decreased in conversion to active hormones by ACE inhibitors, thus reducing blood pressure

Pharmacodynamics/Kinetics

Peak hypotensive effect: Oral: Within 6 hours

Absorption: Well absorbed; unaffected by food

Distribution: protein binding :25%

Half-life: 11-12 hours

Elimination: Almost entirely excreted in urine as unchanged drug

Usual Dosage

Adults: Initial: 10 mg/day; increase doses 5-10 mg/day at 1- to 2-week intervals; maximum daily dose: 40 mg

Elderly: Initial: 2.5-5 mg/day; increase doses 2.5-5 mg/day at 1- to 2-week intervals; maximum daily dose: 40 mg

Patients taking diuretics should have them discontinued 2-3 days prior to initiating lisinopril if possible; restart diuretic after blood pressure is stable if needed; in patients with hyponatremia (<130 mEq/L), start dose at 2.5 mg/day

Acute myocardial infarction (within 24 hours in hemodynamically stable patients): Oral: 5 mg immediately, then 5 mg at 24 hours, 10 mg at 48 hours, and 10 mg every day thereafter for 6 weeks; patients should continue to receive standard treatments such as thrombolytics, aspirin, and beta-blockers

Dosing adjustment in renal impairment:

Cl_{cr} 10-50 mL/minute: Administer 50% to 75% of normal dose

Cl_{cr} <10 mL/minute: Administer 25% to 50% of normal dose

Hemodialysis: Dialyzable (50%)

Monitoring Parameters Serum calcium levels, BUN, serum creatinine, renal function, WBC, and potassium

Test Interactions May cause false-positive results in urine acetone determinations using sodium nitroprusside reagent; ↑ potassium (S); ↑ serum creatinine/ BUN

Patient Information Notify physician if vomiting, diarrhea, excessive perspiration, or dehydration should occur; also if swelling of face, lips, tongue or difficulty in breathing occurs or if persistent cough develops; do not stop therapy without the advise of the prescriber; do not add a salt substitute (potassium) without physician advice

Nursing Implications May cause depression in some patients; discontinue if angioedema of the face, extremities, lips, tongue, or glottis occurs; watch for hypotensive effects within 1-3 hours of first dose or new higher dose

Dosage Forms Tablet: 2.5 mg, 5 mg, 10 mg, 20 mg, 40 mg

Listermint® with Fluoride [OTC] *see* Fluoride *on page 536*

Lithane® *see* Lithium *on next page*

Lithium (LITH ee um)

Related Information

Antacid Drug Interactions *on page 1388*

Brand Names Eskalith®; Lithane®; Lithobid®; Lithonate®; Lithotabs®

Canadian/Mexican Brand Names Carbolit® (Mexico); Lithellm® 300 (Mexico)

Synonyms Lithium Carbonate; Lithium Citrate

Therapeutic Category Antidepressant; Antimanic Agent

Use Management of acute manic episodes, bipolar disorders, and depression

Pregnancy Risk Factor D

Contraindications Hypersensitivity to lithium or any component; severe cardiovascular or renal disease

Warnings/Precautions Lithium toxicity is closely related to serum levels and can occur at therapeutic doses; serum lithium determinations are required to monitor therapy. Use with caution in patients with cardiovascular or thyroid disease, severe debilitation, dehydration or sodium depletion, or in patients receiving diuretics. Some elderly patients may be extremely sensitive to the effects of lithium; see dosage and therapeutic levels.

Adverse Reactions

>10%:
- Endocrine & metabolic: Polydipsia, stress
- Gastrointestinal: Nausea, diarrhea, abnormal taste
- Neuromuscular & skeletal: Trembling

1% to 10%:
- Central nervous system: Fatigue
- Dermatologic: Rash
- Gastrointestinal: Bloated feeling, weight gain
- Neuromuscular & skeletal: Muscle twitching, weakness

<1%:
- Central nervous system: Lethargy, dizziness, vertigo, pseudotumor cerebri
- Dermatologic: Eruptions
- Endocrine & metabolic: Hypothyroidism, goiter, acneiform, diabetes insipidus
- Gastrointestinal: Anorexia, xerostomia
- Genitourinary: Nonspecific nephron atrophy, renal tubular acidosis
- Hematologic: Leukocytosis
- Neuromuscular & skeletal: Cogwheel rigidity, chronic movements of the limbs, tremor
- Ocular: Vision problems
- Miscellaneous: Discoloration of fingers and toes

Overdosage/Toxicology Symptoms of overdose include sedation, confusion, tremors, joint pain, visual changes, seizures, coma

There is no specific antidote for lithium poisoning. In the acute ingestion following initiation of essential overdose management, correction of fluid and electrolyte imbalances should be commenced. Hemodialysis and whole bowel irrigation is the treatment of choice for severe intoxications; charcoal is ineffective.

Drug Interactions

Decreased effect with xanthines (eg, theophylline, caffeine)

Increased effect/toxicity of CNS depressants, alfentanil, iodide salts increased hypothyroid effect

Increased toxicity with thiazide diuretics (dose may need to be reduced by 30%), NSAIDs, haloperidol, phenothiazines (neurotoxicity), neuromuscular blockers, carbamazepine, fluoxetine, ACE inhibitors

Mechanism of Action Alters cation transport across cell membrane in nerve and muscle cells and influences reuptake of serotonin and/or norepinephrine

Pharmacodynamics/Kinetics

Distribution: V_d: Initial: 0.3-0.4 L/kg, V_{dss}: 0.7-1 L/kg; crosses the placenta; appears in breast milk at 35% to 50% the concentrations in serum

Half-life: 18-24 hours; can increase to more than 36 hours in elderly or patients with renal impairment

Time to peak serum concentration (nonsustained release product): Within 0.5-2 hours following oral absorption

Elimination: 90% to 98% of dose excreted in urine as unchanged drug; other excretory routes include feces (1%) and sweat (4% to 5%)

Usual Dosage Oral: Monitor serum concentrations and clinical response (efficacy and toxicity) to determine proper dose

Children 6-12 years: 15-60 mg/kg/day in 3-4 divided doses; dose not to exceed usual adult dosage

Adults: 300-600 mg 3-4 times/day; usual maximum maintenance dose: 2.4 g/day or 450-900 mg of sustained release twice daily

Elderly: Initial dose: 300 mg twice daily; increase weekly in increments of 300 mg/day, monitoring levels; rarely need to go >900-1200 mg/day

(Continued)

Lithium *(Continued)*

Dosing adjustment in renal impairment:

Cl_{cr} 10-50 mL/minute: Administer 50% to 75% of normal dose

Cl_{cr} <10 mL/minute: Administer 25% to 50% of normal dose

Hemodialysis: Dialyzable (50% to 100%)

Administration Administer with meals to decrease GI upset

Monitoring Parameters Serum lithium every 3-4 days during initial therapy; draw lithium serum concentrations 8-12 hours postdose; renal, hepatic, thyroid, and cardiovascular function; fluid status; serum electrolytes; CBC with differential, urinalysis; monitor for signs of toxicity

Reference Range Levels should be obtained twice weekly until both patient's clinical status and levels are stable then levels may be obtained every 1-2 months

Timing of serum samples: Draw trough just before next dose

Therapeutic levels:

Acute mania: 0.6-1.2 mEq/L (SI: 0.6-1.2 mmol/L)

Protection against future episodes in most patients with bipolar disorder: 0.8-1 mEq/L (SI: 0.8-1.0 mmol/L); a higher rate of relapse is described in subjects who are maintained at <0.4 mEq/L (SI: 0.4 mmol/L)

Elderly patients can usually be maintained at lower end of therapeutic range (0.6-0.8 mEq/L)

Toxic concentration: >2 mEq/L (SI: >2 mmol/L)

Adverse effect levels:

GI complaints/tremor: 1.5-2 mEq/L

Confusion/somnolence: 2-2.5 mEq/L

Seizures/death: >2.5 mEq/L

Test Interactions ↑ calcium (S), glucose, magnesium, potassium (S); ↓ thyroxine (S)

Patient Information Avoid tasks requiring psychomotor coordination until the CNS effects are known, blood level monitoring is required to determine the proper dose; maintain a steady salt and fluid intake especially during the summer months; do not crush or chew slow or extended release dosage form, swallow whole

Nursing Implications Avoid dehydration

Additional Information

Lithium citrate: Cibalith-S®

Lithium carbonate: Eskalith®, Lithane®, Lithobid®, Lithonate®, Lithotabs®

Dosage Forms

Capsule, as carbonate: 150 mg, 300 mg, 600 mg

Syrup, as citrate: 300 mg/5 mL (5 mL, 10 mL, 480 mL)

Tablet, as carbonate: 300 mg

Tablet:

Controlled release, as carbonate: 450 mg

Slow release, as carbonate: 300 mg

Lithium Carbonate *see* Lithium *on previous page*

Lithium Citrate *see* Lithium *on previous page*

Lithobid® *see* Lithium *on previous page*

Lithonate® *see* Lithium *on previous page*

Lithotabs® *see* Lithium *on previous page*

Livostin® *see* Levocabastine *on page 714*

LKV-Drops® [OTC] *see* Vitamins, Multiple *on page 1310*

8-*L*-Lysine Vasopressin *see* Lypressin *on page 750*

LMD® *see* Dextran *on page 363*

Locoid® *see* Hydrocortisone *on page 623*

Lodine® *see* Etodolac *on page 494*

Lodine® XL *see* Etodolac *on page 494*

Lodosyn® *see* Carbidopa *on page 204*

Lodoxamide Tromethamine (loe DOKS a mide troe METH a meen)

Brand Names Alomide®

Therapeutic Category Antiallergic, Ophthalmic

Use Treatment of vernal keratoconjunctivitis, vernal conjunctivitis, and vernal keratitis

Pregnancy Risk Factor B

Contraindications Hypersensitivity to any component of product

Warnings/Precautions Safety and efficacy in children <2 years of age have not been established; not for injection; not for use in patients wearing soft contact lenses during treatment

Adverse Reactions

>10%: Local: Transient burning, stinging, discomfort

1% to 10%:

Central nervous system: Headache

Ocular: Blurred vision, corneal erosion/ulcer, eye pain, corneal abrasion, blepharitis

<1%:

Central nervous system: Dizziness, somnolence

Dermatologic: Rash

Gastrointestinal: Nausea, stomach discomfort

Respiratory: Sneezing, dry nose

Overdosage/Toxicology Symptoms include feeling of warmth of flushing, headache, dizziness, fatigue, sweating, nausea, loose stools, and urinary frequency/urgency; consider emesis in the event of accidental ingestion

Mechanism of Action Mast cell stabilizer that inhibits the *in vivo* type I immediate hypersensitivity reaction to increase cutaneous vascular permeability associated with IgE and antigen-mediated reactions

Pharmacodynamics/Kinetics Absorption: Topical: Very small and undetectable

Usual Dosage Children >2 years and Adults: Instill 1-2 drops in eye(s) 4 times/day for up to 3 months

Dosage Forms Solution, ophthalmic: 0.1% (10 mL)

Loestrin® *see* Ethinyl Estradiol and Norethindrone *on page 486*

Lofene® *see* Diphenoxylate and Atropine *on page 400*

Logen® *see* Diphenoxylate and Atropine *on page 400*

Lomanate® *see* Diphenoxylate and Atropine *on page 400*

Lomefloxacin (loe me FLOKS a sin)

Brand Names Maxaquin®

Synonyms Lomefloxacin Hydrochloride

Therapeutic Category Antibiotic, Quinolone

Use Quinolone antibiotic for skin and skin structure, lower respiratory and urinary tract infections, and sexually transmitted diseases; also indicated for preoperative use to prevent infection in transrectal prostate biopsy

Pregnancy Risk Factor C

Contraindications Hypersensitivity to lomefloxacin or other members of the quinolone group such as nalidixic acid, oxolinic acid, cinoxacin, norfloxacin, and ciprofloxacin; avoid use in children <18 years of age due to association of other quinolones with transient arthropathies

Warnings/Precautions Use with caution in patients with epilepsy or other CNS diseases which could predispose them to seizures

Adverse Reactions

1% to 10%:

Central nervous system: Headache, dizziness

Dermatologic: Photosensitivity

Gastrointestinal: Nausea

<1%:

Cardiovascular: Flushing, chest pain, hypotension, hypertension, edema, syncope, tachycardia, bradycardia, arrhythmia, extrasystoles, cyanosis, cardiac failure, angina pectoris, myocardial infarction, facial edema

Central nervous system: Fatigue, malaise, chills, convulsions, vertigo, coma

Dermatologic: Purpura, rash

Endocrine & metabolic: Gout, hypoglycemia

Gastrointestinal: Abdominal pain, vomiting, flatulence, constipation, xerostomia, discoloration of tongue, abnormal taste

Genitourinary: Urinary disorders, dysuria

Hematologic: Thrombocytopenia, increased fibrinolysis

Neuromuscular & skeletal: Back pain, hyperkinesia, tremor, paresthesias, leg cramps, myalgia, weakness

Otic: Earache

Renal: Hematuria, anuria

Respiratory: Dyspnea, cough, epistaxis

Miscellaneous: Diaphoresis (increased), allergic reaction, flu-like symptoms, decreased heat tolerance, thirst

Overdosage/Toxicology Symptoms of overdose include acute renal failure, seizures

GI decontamination and supportive care; diazepam for seizures; not removed by peritoneal or hemodialysis

Drug Interactions

Decreased effect: Decreased absorption with antacids containing aluminum, magnesium, and/or calcium (by up to 98% if given at the same time)

Increased toxicity/serum levels: Quinolones cause increased levels of caffeine, warfarin, cyclosporine, and theophylline; azlocillin, cimetidine, probenecid increase quinolone levels

(Continued)

Lomefloxacin *(Continued)*

Mechanism of Action Inhibits DNA-gyrase in susceptible organisms thereby inhibits relaxation of supercoiled DNA and promotes breakage of DNA strands. DNA gyrase (topoisomerase II), is an essential bacterial enzyme that maintains the superhelical structure of DNA and is required for DNA replication and transcription, DNA repair, recombination, and transposition.

Pharmacodynamics/Kinetics

Absorption: Well absorbed
Distribution: V_d: 2.4-3.5 L/kg
Protein binding: 20%
Half-life, elimination: 5-7.5 hours
Elimination: Primarily unchanged in urine

Usual Dosage Oral: Adults: 400 mg once daily for 10-14 days

Patient Information Take 1 hour before or 2 hours after meals

Dosage Forms Tablet, as hydrochloride: 400 mg

Lomefloxacin Hydrochloride *see* Lomefloxacin *on previous page*

Lomodix® *see* Diphenoxylate and Atropine *on page 400*

Lomotil® *see* Diphenoxylate and Atropine *on page 400*

Lomustine (loe MUS teen)

Related Information

Antiemetics for Chemotherapy Induced Nausea and Vomiting *on page 1348*
Cancer Chemotherapy Regimens *on page 1351*
Toxicities of Chemotherapeutic Agents *on page 1382*

Brand Names CeeNU®

Synonyms CCNU

Therapeutic Category Antineoplastic Agent, Alkylating Agent (Nitrosourea)

Use Treatment of brain tumors and Hodgkin's disease, non-Hodgkin's lymphoma, melanoma, renal carcinoma, lung cancer, colon cancer

Pregnancy Risk Factor D

Contraindications Hypersensitivity to lomustine or any component

Warnings/Precautions The U.S. Food and Drug Administration (FDA) currently recommends that procedures for proper handling and disposal for antineoplastic agents be considered. Bone marrow suppression, notably thrombocytopenia and leukopenia, may lead to bleeding and overwhelming infections in an already compromised patient; will last for at least 6 weeks after a dose, do not administer courses more frequently than every 6 weeks because the toxicity is cumulative. Use with caution in patients with depressed platelet, leukocyte or erythrocyte counts, liver function abnormalities.

Adverse Reactions

>10%:

Gastrointestinal: Nausea and vomiting occur 3-6 hours after oral administration; this is due to a centrally mediated mechanism, not a direct effect on the GI lining; if vomiting occurs, it is not necessary to replace the dose unless it occurs immediately after drug administration
Emetic potential:
<60 mg: Moderately high (60% to 90%)
≥60 mg: High (>90%)
Time course of nausea/vomiting: Onset: 2-6 hours; Duration: 4-6 hours

Hematologic: Myelosuppression: Anemia; effects occur 4-6 weeks after a dose and may persist for 1-2 weeks
WBC: Moderate
Platelets: Severe
Onset (days): 14
Nadir (weeks): 4-5
Recovery (weeks): 6

1% to 10%:

Central nervous system: Neurotoxicity
Dermatologic: Skin rash
Gastrointestinal: Stomatitis, diarrhea
Hematologic: Anemia

<1%:

Central nervous system: Disorientation, lethargy, ataxia
Dermatologic: Alopecia
Hepatic: Hepatotoxicity
Neuromuscular & skeletal: Dysarthria
Respiratory: Pulmonary fibrosis with cumulative doses >600 mg
Renal: Renal failure

Overdosage/Toxicology Symptoms of overdose include nausea, vomiting, leukopenia; there are no known antidotes; treatment is primarily symptomatic and supportive

Drug Interactions

Decreased effect with phenobarbital, resulting in ↓ efficacy of both drugs

Increased toxicity with cimetidine, reported to cause bone marrow suppression or to potentiate the myelosuppressive effects of lomustine

Stability Refrigerate (<40°C/<104°F)

Mechanism of Action Inhibits DNA and RNA synthesis via carbamylation of DNA polymerase, alkylation of DNA, and alteration of RNA, proteins, and enzymes

Pharmacodynamics/Kinetics

Absorption: Complete from GI tract; appears in plasma within 3 minutes after administration

Distribution: Crosses blood-brain barrier to a greater degree than BNCU and CNS concentrations are equal to that of plasma

Protein binding: 50%

Metabolism: Rapid in the liver by hydroxylation produces at least 2 active metabolites

Half-life: Parent drug: 16-72 hours

Active metabolite: Terminal half-life: 1.3-2 days

Time to peak serum concentration: Active metabolite: Within 3 hours

Elimination: Enterohepatically recycled; excreted in the urine, feces (<5%), and in the expired air (<10%)

Usual Dosage Oral (refer to individual protocols):

Children: 75-150 mg/m^2 as a single dose every 6 weeks; subsequent doses are readjusted after initial treatment according to platelet and leukocyte counts

Adults: 100-130 mg/m^2 as a single dose every 6 weeks; readjust after initial treatment according to platelet and leukocyte counts

With compromised marrow function: Initial dose: 100 mg/m^2 as a single dose every 6 weeks

Repeat courses should only be administered after adequate recovery: WBC >4000 and platelet counts >100,000

Subsequent dosing adjustment based on nadir:

Leukocytes 2000-2900/mm^3, platelets 25,000-74,999/mm^3: Administer 70% of prior dose

Leukocytes <2000/mm^3, platelets <25,000/mm^3: Administer 50% of prior dose

Dosage adjustment in renal impairment:

Cl_{cr} 10-50 mL/minute: Administer 75% of normal dose

Cl_{cr} <10 mL/minute: Administer 50% of normal dose

Hemodialysis: Supplemental dose is not necessary

Peritoneal dialysis: Significant drug removal is unlikely based on physiochemical characteristics

Monitoring Parameters CBC with differential and platelet count, hepatic and renal function tests, pulmonary function tests

Test Interactions Liver function tests

Patient Information Take with fluids on an empty stomach; no food or drink for 2 hours after administration; notify physician if unusual or persistent fever, sore throat, bleeding, bruising, or fatigue occur; contraceptive measures are recommended during therapy

Dosage Forms

Capsule: 10 mg, 40 mg, 100 mg

Dose Pack: 10 mg (2s); 100 mg (2s); 40 mg (2s)

Loniten® *see* Minoxidil *on page 843*

Lonox® *see* Diphenoxylate and Atropine *on page 400*

Lo/Ovral® *see* Ethinyl Estradiol and Norgestrel *on page 489*

Loperamide (loe PER a mide)

Brand Names Diar-aid® [OTC]; Imodium®; Imodium® A-D [OTC]; Kaopectate® II [OTC]; Pepto® Diarrhea Control [OTC]

Canadian/Mexican Brand Names PMS-Loperamine (Canada); Acanol® (Mexico); Pramidal® (Mexico); Raxedin® (Mexico)

Synonyms Loperamide Hydrochloride

Therapeutic Category Antidiarrheal

Use Treatment of acute diarrhea and chronic diarrhea associated with inflammatory bowel disease; chronic functional diarrhea (idiopathic), chronic diarrhea caused by bowel resection or organic lesions; to decrease the volume of ileostomy discharge

Unlabeled use: Treatment of traveler's diarrhea in combination with trimethoprim-sulfamethoxazole (co-trimoxazole) (3 days therapy)

Pregnancy Risk Factor B

(Continued)

Loperamide *(Continued)*

Contraindications Patients who must avoid constipation, diarrhea resulting from some infections, or in patients with pseudomembranous colitis, hypersensitivity to specific drug or component, bloody diarrhea

Warnings/Precautions Large first-pass metabolism, use with caution in hepatic dysfunction; should not be used if diarrhea accompanied by high fever, blood in stool

Adverse Reactions

Central nervous system: Sedation, fatigue, dizziness, drowsiness

Dermatologic: Rash

Gastrointestinal: Nausea, vomiting, constipation, abdominal cramping, xerostomia, abdominal distention

Overdosage/Toxicology Symptoms of overdose include CNS and respiratory depression, gastrointestinal cramping, constipation, GI irritation, nausea, vomiting; overdosage is noted when daily doses approximate 60 mg of loperamide

Treatment of overdose: Gastric lavage followed by 100 g activated charcoal through a nasogastric tube. Monitor for signs of CNS depression; if they occur, administer naloxone 2 mg I.V. (0.01 mg/kg for children) with repeat administration as necessary up to a total of 10 mg.

Drug Interactions Increased toxicity: CNS depressants, phenothiazines, tricyclic antidepressants may potentiate the adverse effects

Mechanism of Action Acts directly on intestinal muscles to inhibit peristalsis and prolongs transit time enhancing fluid and electrolyte movement through intestinal mucosa; reduces fecal volume, increases viscosity, and diminishes fluid and electrolyte loss; demonstrates antisecretory activity; exhibits peripheral action

Pharmacodynamics/Kinetics

Onset of action: Oral: Within 0.5-1 hour

Absorption: Oral: <40%; levels in breast milk expected to be very low

Protein binding: 97%

Metabolism: Hepatic (>50%) to inactive compounds

Half-life: 7-14 hours

Elimination: Fecal and urinary (1%) excretion of metabolites and unchanged drug (30% to 40%)

Usual Dosage Oral:

Children:

- Acute diarrhea: Initial doses (in first 24 hours):
  - 2-6 years: 1 mg 3 times/day
  - 6-8 years: 2 mg twice daily
  - 8-12 years: 2 mg 3 times/day
  - Maintenance: After initial dosing, 0.1 mg/kg doses after each loose stool, but not exceeding initial dosage
- Chronic diarrhea: 0.08-0.24 mg/kg/day divided 2-3 times/day, maximum: 2 mg/dose

Adults: Initial: 4 mg (2 capsules), followed by 2 mg after each loose stool, up to 16 mg/day (8 capsules)

Patient Information Do not take more than 8 capsules or 80 mL in 24 hours; may cause drowsiness; if acute diarrhea lasts longer than 48 hours, consult physician

Nursing Implications Therapy for chronic diarrhea should not exceed 10 days

Dosage Forms

Caplet, as hydrochloride: 2 mg

Capsule, as hydrochloride: 2 mg

Liquid, oral, as hydrochloride: 1 mg/5 mL (60 mL, 90 mL, 120 mL)

Tablet, as hydrochloride: 2 mg

Loperamide Hydrochloride *see* Loperamide *on previous page*

Lopid® *see* Gemfibrozil *on page 569*

Lopressor® *see* Metoprolol *on page 827*

Loprox® *see* Ciclopirox *on page 273*

Lopurin® *see* Allopurinol *on page 47*

Lorabid™ *see* Loracarbef *on this page*

Loracarbef (lor a KAR bef)

Related Information

Cephalosporins by Generation *on page 1447*

Brand Names Lorabid™

Canadian/Mexican Brand Names Carbac® (Mexico)

Therapeutic Category Antibiotic, Carbacephem

Use Infections caused by susceptible organisms involving the respiratory tract, acute otitis media, sinusitis, skin and skin structure, bone and joint, and urinary tract and gynecologic

Pregnancy Risk Factor B

Contraindications Patients with a history of hypersensitivity to loracarbef or cephalosporins

Warnings/Precautions Use with caution in patients with a previous history of hypersensitivity to other beta-lactam antibiotics (eg, penicillins, cephalosporins)

Adverse Reactions

1% to 10%:

Central nervous system: Headache

Dermatologic: Rashes

Gastrointestinal: Diarrhea, nausea, vomiting, abdominal pain, anorexia

Genitourinary: Vaginitis, vaginal moniliasis

<1%:

Cardiovascular: Vasodilation

Central nervous system: Somnolence, nervousness, dizziness

Hematologic: Transient thrombocytopenia, leukopenia, and eosinophilia

Hepatic: Transient elevations of ALT, AST, alkaline phosphatase

Renal: Transient elevations of BUN/creatinine

Overdosage/Toxicology Symptoms of overdose include abdominal discomfort, diarrhea; supportive care only

Drug Interactions Increased serum levels with probenecid

Stability Suspension may be kept at room temperature for 14 days

Mechanism of Action Inhibits bacterial cell wall synthesis by binding to one or more of the penicillin binding proteins (PBPs); inhibits the final transpeptidation step of peptidoglycan synthesis in bacterial cell walls, thus inhibiting cell wall biosynthesis. It is thought that beta-lactam antibiotics inactivate transpeptidase via acylation of the enzyme with cleavage of the CO-N bond of the beta-lactam ring. Upon exposure to beta-lactam antibiotics, bacteria eventually lyse due to ongoing activity of cell wall autolytic enzymes (autolysins and murein hydrolases) while cell wall assembly is arrested.

Pharmacodynamics/Kinetics

Absorption: Oral: Rapid

Half-life, elimination: ~1 hour

Time to peak serum concentration: Oral: Within 1 hour

Elimination: Plasma clearance: ~200-300 mL/minute

Usual Dosage Oral:

Children:

Acute otitis media: 15 mg/kg twice daily for 10 days

Pharyngitis: 7.5-15 mg/kg twice daily for 10 days

Adults: Women:

Uncomplicated urinary tract infections: 200 mg once daily for 7 days

Skin and soft tissue: 200-400 mg every 12-24 hours

Uncomplicated pyelonephritis: 400 mg every 12 hours for 14 days

Dosing comments in renal impairment:

Cl_{cr} ≥50 mL/minute: Administer usual dose

Cl_{cr} 10-49 mL/minute: 50% of usual dose at usual interval or usual dose given half as often

Cl_{cr} <10 mL/minute: Administer usual dose every 3-5 days

Hemodialysis: Doses should be administered after dialysis sessions

Patient Information Take on an empty stomach at least 1 hour before or 2 hours after meals; finish all medication

Dosage Forms

Capsule: 200 mg, 400 mg

Suspension, oral: 100 mg/5 mL (50 mL, 100 mL); 200 mg/5 mL (50 mL, 100 mL)

Loratadine (lor AT a deen)

Brand Names Claritin®

Canadian/Mexican Brand Names Clarityne® (Mexico); Lertamine® (Mexico); Lowadina® (Mexico)

Therapeutic Category Antihistamine, H_1 Blocker; Antihistamine, H_1 Blocker, Nonsedating

Use Relief of nasal and non-nasal symptoms of seasonal allergic rhinitis

Pregnancy Risk Factor B

Contraindications Patients hypersensitive to loratadine or any of its components

Warnings/Precautions Patients with liver impairment should start with a lower dose (10 mg every other day), since their ability to clear the drug will be reduced; use with caution in lactation, safety in children <12 years of age has not been established

Adverse Reactions

>10%:

Central nervous system: Headache, somnolence, fatigue

Gastrointestinal: Xerostomia

1% to 10%:

Cardiovascular: Hypotension, hypertension, palpitations, tachycardia

(Continued)

Loratadine *(Continued)*

Central nervous system: Anxiety, depression
Endocrine & metabolic: Breast pain
Neuromuscular & skeletal: Hyperkinesia, arthralgias
Respiratory: Nasal dryness, pharyngitis, dyspnea
Miscellaneous: Diaphoresis

Overdosage/Toxicology Symptoms of overdose include somnolence, tachycardia, headache

No specific antidote is available, treatment is first decontamination, then symptomatic and supportive; loratadine is not eliminated by dialysis

Drug Interactions

Increased plasma concentrations of loratadine and its active metabolite with ketoconazole; erythromycin increases the AUC of loratadine and its active metabolite; no change in Q-T_c interval was seen

Increased toxicity: Procarbazine, other antihistamines, alcohol

Mechanism of Action Long-acting tricyclic antihistamine with selective peripheral histamine H_1-receptor antagonistic properties

Pharmacodynamics/Kinetics

Onset of action: Within 1-3 hours
Peak effect: 8-12 hours
Duration: >24 hours
Absorption: Rapid
Metabolism: Extensive to an active metabolite
Half-life: 12-15 hours
Elimination: Significant excretion into breast milk

Usual Dosage Children ≥6 years and Adults: Oral: 10 mg/day on an empty stomach

Dosing interval in hepatic impairment: 10 mg every other day to start

Patient Information Drink plenty of water; may cause dry mouth, sedation, drowsiness, and can impair judgment and coordination

Dosage Forms

Solution, oral: 1 mg/mL syrup
Tablet: 10 mg
Rapid-disintegrating tablets: 10 mg (RediTabs®)

Lorazepam (lor A ze pam)

Related Information

Benzodiazepines Comparison *on page 1397*
Convulsive Status Epilepticus *on page 1528*

Brand Names Ativan®

Canadian/Mexican Brand Names Apo-Lorazepam® (Canada); Novo-Lorazepam® (Canada); Nu-Loraz® (Canada); PMS-Lorazepam (Canada); Pro-Lorazepam® (Canada)

Therapeutic Category Antianxiety Agent; Anticonvulsant; Antiemetic; Benzodiazepine; Sedative

Use Management of anxiety, status epilepticus, preoperative sedation, for desired amnesia, and as an antiemetic adjunct

Unapproved uses: Alcohol detoxification, insomnia, psychogenic catatonia, partial complex seizures

Restrictions C-IV

Pregnancy Risk Factor D

Pregnancy/Breast-Feeding Implications

Clinical effects on the fetus: Crosses the placenta. Respiratory depression or hypotonia if administered near time of delivery.

Breast-feeding/lactation: Crosses into breast milk and no data on clinical effects on the infant. American Academy of Pediatrics states MAY BE OF CONCERN.

Contraindications Hypersensitivity to lorazepam or any component; there may be a cross-sensitivity with other benzodiazepines; do not use in a comatose patient, those with pre-existing CNS depression, narrow-angle glaucoma, severe uncontrolled pain, severe hypotension

Warnings/Precautions Use caution in patients with renal or hepatic impairment, organic brain syndrome, myasthenia gravis, or Parkinson's disease. Dilute injection prior to I.V. use with equal volume of compatible diluent (D_5W, 0.9% sodium chloride, sterile water for injection); do **not** inject intra-arterially, arteriospasm and gangrene may occur; injection contains benzyl alcohol 2%, polyethylene glycol and propylene glycol, which may be toxic to newborns in high doses, may reduce effectiveness of ECT; oral doses >0.09 mg/kg produced increased ataxia without increased sedative benefit versus lower doses

Adverse Reactions

Respiratory: Decrease in respiratory rate, apnea, laryngospasm

>10%:
- Cardiovascular: Tachycardia, chest pain
- Central nervous system: Drowsiness, confusion, ataxia, amnesia, slurred speech, paradoxical excitement, rage, headache, depression, anxiety, fatigue, lightheadedness, insomnia
- Dermatologic: Rash
- Endocrine & metabolic: Decreased libido
- Gastrointestinal: Xerostomia, constipation, diarrhea, nausea, vomiting, increased or decreased appetite, decreased salivation
- Local: Phlebitis, pain with injection
- Neuromuscular & skeletal: Dysarthria
- Ocular: Blurred vision, diplopia
- Miscellaneous: Diaphoresis

1% to 10%:
- Cardiovascular: Cardiac arrest, hypotension, bradycardia, cardiovascular collapse, syncope
- Central nervous system: Confusion, nervousness, dizziness, akathisia
- Neuromuscular & skeletal: Rigidity, tremor, muscle cramps
- Dermatologic: Dermatitis
- Gastrointestinal: Weight gain or loss
- Otic: Tinnitus
- Respiratory: Nasal congestion, hyperventilation

<1%:
- Endocrine & metabolic: Menstrual irregularities
- Gastrointestinal: Increased salivation
- Hematologic: Blood dyscrasias
- Neuromuscular & skeletal: Reflex slowing
- Miscellaneous: Physical and psychological dependence with prolonged use

Overdosage/Toxicology Symptoms of overdose include confusion, coma, hypoactive reflexes, dyspnea, labored breathing

Treatment for benzodiazepine overdose is supportive. Rarely is mechanical ventilation required. Flumazenil has been shown to selectively block the binding of benzodiazepines to CNS receptors, resulting in a reversal of benzodiazepine-induced CNS depression but not respiratory depression. Treatment requires support of blood pressure and respiration until drug effects subside.

Drug Interactions
- Decreased effect with oral contraceptives (combination products), cigarette smoking; decreased effect of levodopa
- Increased effect with morphine
- Increased toxicity with alcohol, CNS depressants, MAO inhibitors, loxapine, TCAs

Stability
- Intact vials should be refrigerated, protected from light; do not use discolored or precipitate containing solutions
- May be stored at room temperature for up to 60 days
- Stability of parenteral admixture at room temperature (25°C): 24 hours
- Standard diluent: 1 mg/100 mL D_5W
- I.V. is **incompatible** when administered in the same line with foscarnet, ondansetron, sargramostim

Mechanism of Action Depresses all levels of the CNS, including the limbic and reticular formation, probably through the increased action of gamma-aminobutyric acid (GABA), which is a major inhibitory neurotransmitter in the brain

Pharmacodynamics/Kinetics
- Onset of hypnosis: I.M.: 20-30 minutes
- Duration: 6-8 hours
- Absorption: Oral, I.M.: Prompt following administration
- Distribution: Crosses the placenta; appears in breast milk
  - V_d:
    - Neonates: 0.76 L/kg
    - Adults: 1.3 L/kg
- Protein binding: 85%, free fraction may be significantly higher in elderly
- Metabolism: In the liver to inactive compounds
- Half-life:
  - Neonates: 40.2 hours
  - Older Children: 10.5 hours
  - Adults: 12.9 hours
  - Elderly: 15.9 hours
  - End stage renal disease: 32-70 hours
- Elimination: Urinary excretion and minimal fecal clearance

Usual Dosage
- Antiemetic:
  - Children 2-15 years: I.V.: 0.05 mg/kg (up to 2 mg/dose) prior to chemotherapy
  - Adults: Oral, I.V.: 0.5-2 mg every 4-6 hours as needed

(Continued)

Lorazepam *(Continued)*

Anxiety and sedation:

Infants and Children: Oral, I.V.: Usual: 0.05 mg/kg/dose (range: 0.02-0.09 mg/kg) every 4-8 hours

Adults: Oral: 1-10 mg/day in 2-3 divided doses; usual dose: 2-6 mg/day in divided doses

Insomnia: Adults: Oral: 2-4 mg at bedtime

Preoperative: Adults:

I.M.: 0.05 mg/kg administered 2 hours before surgery; maximum: 4 mg/dose

I.V.: 0.044 mg/kg 15-20 minutes before surgery; usual maximum: 2 mg/dose

Operative amnesia: Adults: I.V.: Up to 0.05 mg/kg; maximum: 4 mg/dose

Status epilepticus: I.V.:

Infants and Children: 0.1 mg/kg slow I.V. over 2-5 minutes, do not exceed 4 mg/single dose; may repeat second dose of 0.05 mg/kg slow I.V. in 10-15 minutes if needed

Adolescents: 0.07 mg/kg slow I.V. over 2-5 minutes; maximum: 4 mg/dose; may repeat in 10-15 minutes

Adults: 4 mg/dose given slowly over 2-5 minutes; may repeat in 10-15 minutes; usual maximum dose: 8 mg

Dietary Considerations Alcohol: Additive CNS depression has been reported with benzodiazepines; avoid or limit alcohol

Administration

Lorazepam may be administered by I.M. or I.V.

I.M.: Should be administered deep into the muscle mass

I.V.: Do not exceed 2 mg/minute or 0.05 mg/kg over 2-5 minutes

Dilute I.V. dose with equal volume of compatible diluent (D_5W, NS, SWI)

Injection must be made slowly with repeated aspiration to make sure the injection is not intra-arterial and that perivascular extravasation has not occurred

Monitoring Parameters Respiratory and cardiovascular status, blood pressure, heart rate, symptoms of anxiety

Reference Range Therapeutic: 50-240 ng/mL (SI: 156-746 nmol/L)

Test Interactions May increase the results of liver function tests

Patient Information Advise patient of potential for physical and psychological dependence with chronic use; advise patient of possible retrograde amnesia after I.V. or I.M. use; will cause drowsiness, impairment of judgment or coordination

Nursing Implications Keep injectable form in the refrigerator; **inadvertent intra-arterial injection may produce arteriospasm resulting in gangrene which may require amputation;** emergency resuscitative equipment should be available when administering by I.V.; prior to I.V. use, lorazepam injection must be diluted with an equal amount of compatible diluent; injection must be made slowly with repeated aspiration to make sure the injection is not intra-arterial and that perivascular extravasation has not occurred; provide safety measures (ie, side rails, night light, and call button); supervise ambulation

Dosage Forms

Injection: 2 mg/mL (1 mL, 10 mL); 4 mg/mL (1 mL, 10 mL)

Solution, oral concentrated, alcohol and dye free: 2 mg/mL (30 mL)

Tablet: 0.5 mg, 1 mg, 2 mg

Lorcet® *see* Hydrocodone and Acetaminophen *on page 620*

Lorcet®-HD *see* Hydrocodone and Acetaminophen *on page 620*

Lorcet® Plus *see* Hydrocodone and Acetaminophen *on page 620*

Loroxide® [OTC] *see* Benzoyl Peroxide *on page 140*

Lortab® *see* Hydrocodone and Acetaminophen *on page 620*

Lortab® ASA *see* Hydrocodone and Aspirin *on page 621*

Losartan (loe SAR tan)

Related Information

Angiotensin-Converting Enzyme Inhibitors Comparison *on page 1386*

Brand Names Cozaar®

Synonyms DuP 753; Losartan Potassium; MK594

Therapeutic Category Angiotensin II Antagonist

Use Treatment of hypertension with or without concurrent use of thiazide diuretics; may prolong survival in heart failure; recommended for patients unable to tolerated ACE inhibitors

Pregnancy Risk Factor C (first trimester); D (second & third trimester)

Pregnancy/Breast-Feeding Implications Avoid use in the nursing mother, if possible, since it is postulated that losartan is excreted in breast milk

Contraindications Hypersensitivity to losartan or any components; pregnancy

Warnings/Precautions Avoid use or use a much smaller dose in patients who are intravascularly volume-depleted; use caution in patients with unilateral or bilateral renal artery stenosis to avoid a decrease in renal function; AUCs of losartan (not the active metabolite) are about 50% greater in patients with Cl_{cr} <30 mL/minute and are doubled in hemodialysis patients

Adverse Reactions

1% to 10%:

- Cardiovascular: Hypotension without reflex tachycardia
- Central nervous system: Dizziness, insomnia
- Endocrine & metabolic: Hyperkalemia
- Gastrointestinal: Diarrhea, dyspepsia
- Hematologic: Slight decreases in hemoglobin and hematocrit
- Neuromuscular & skeletal: Back/leg pain, myalgia
- Renal: Hypouricemia (with large doses)
- Respiratory: Cough (less than ACE inhibitors), nasal congestion, sinus disorders, sinusitis

<1%:

- Cardiovascular: Orthostatic effects, angina, second degree A-V block, CVA, palpitations, sinus bradycardia, tachycardia, flushing, facial edema
- Central nervous system: Anxiety, ataxia, confusion, depression, dream abnormality, migraine headache, sleep disorders, vertigo, fever
- Dermatologic: Alopecia, dermatitis, dry skin, bruising, erythema, photosensitivity, pruritus, rash, urticaria
- Endocrine & metabolic: Gout
- Gastrointestinal: Anorexia, constipation, flatulence, vomiting, abnormal taste, gastritis
- Genitourinary: Impotence, decreased libido, polyuria, nocturia
- Hepatic: Slight elevations of LFTs and bilirubin
- Neuromuscular & skeletal: Paresthesia, tremor; arm, hip, shoulder, and knee pain, joint edema, fibromyalgia, muscle weakness
- Ocular: Blurred vision, burning and stinging eyes, conjunctivitis, decreased visual acuity
- Otic: Tinnitus
- Renal: Urinary tract infection, nocturia, mild increases in BUN/creatinine
- Respiratory: Dyspnea, bronchitis, pharyngeal discomfort, epistaxis, rhinitis, respiratory congestion
- Miscellaneous: Diaphoresis

Overdosage/Toxicology Symptoms may occur with very significant overdosages including hypotension and tachycardia; treatment should be supportive

Drug Interactions

Decreased effect: Phenobarbital, ketoconazole, troleandomycin, sulfaphenazole

Increased effect: Cimetidine, moxonidine

Mechanism of Action As a selective and competitive, nonpeptide angiotensin II receptor antagonist, losartan blocks the vasoconstrictor and aldosterone-secreting effects of angiotensin II; losartan interacts reversibly at the AT1 and AT2 receptors of many tissues and has slow dissociation kinetics; its affinity for the AT1 receptor is 1000 times greater than the AT2 receptor. Angiotensin II receptor antagonists may induce a more complete inhibition of the renin-angiotensin system than ACE inhibitors, they do not affect the response to bradykinin, and are less likely to be associated with nonrenin-angiotensin effects (eg, cough and angioedema). Losartan increases urinary flow rate and in addition to being natriuretic and kaliuretic, increases excretion of chloride, magnesium, uric acid, calcium, and phosphate.

Pharmacodynamics/Kinetics

Onset of effect: 6 hours

Distribution: Does not cross the blood brain barrier, V_d: Losartan: 34 L; E-3174: 12 L

Protein binding: Highly bound to plasma proteins

Metabolism: 14% of an orally administered dose is metabolized by cytochrome P-450 enzymes to an active metabolite E-3174 (40 times more potent than losartan); undergoes substantial first-pass metabolism

Bioavailability: 25% to 33%; AUC of E-3174 is 4 times greater than that of losartan

Half-life:

- Losartan: 1.5-2 hours
- E-3174: 6-9 hours

Time to peak: Peak serum levels of losartan: 1 hour; metabolite, E-3174: 3-4 hours

Elimination: 3% to 8% excreted in urine as unchanged parent or as E-3174, ~35% of a dose is recovered in urine and 60% in feces; total plasma clearance of losartan: 600 mL/minute: its active metabolite: 50 mL/minute

(Continued)

Losartan *(Continued)*

Usual Dosage

Oral: 25-100 mg once or twice daily (adjust dosage at weekly intervals; maximum effect may not be apparent for 3-6 weeks)

Usual initial doses in patients receiving diuretics or those with intravascular volume depletion: 25 mg

Patients not receiving diuretics: 50 mg

Dosing adjustment in renal impairment: None necessary

Dosing adjustment in hepatic impairment or geriatric patients: Reduce the initial dose to 25 mg; divide dosage intervals into two

Hemodialysis: Not removed via hemodialysis

Monitoring Parameters Supine blood pressure, electrolytes, serum creatinine, BUN, urinalysis, symptomatic hypotension and tachycardia, CBC

Patient Information Use caution standing or rising abruptly following a dosage increase; report any symptoms of difficulty breathing, swallowing, swelling of face, lips, extremities, or tongue immediately, as well as symptoms of fever or sore throat; do not use if pregnant

Nursing Implications Observe for symptomatic hypotension and tachycardia especially in patients with CHF; hyponatremia, high-dose diuretics, or severe volume depletion

Additional Information Losartan's effect in African-American patients was notably less than in non-African Americans; and while dosage adjustments are not needed, plasma levels are twice as high in female hypertensives as male hypertensives

Dosage Forms Tablet, film coated, as potassium: 25 mg, 50 mg

Losartan Potassium *see* Losartan *on page 744*

Losec® *see* Omeprazole *on page 925*

Lotensin® *see* Benazepril *on page 136*

Lotrimin® *see* Clotrimazole *on page 302*

Lotrimin® AF Cream [OTC] *see* Clotrimazole *on page 302*

Lotrimin® AF Lotion [OTC] *see* Clotrimazole *on page 302*

Lotrimin® AF Powder [OTC] *see* Miconazole *on page 834*

Lotrimin® AF Solution [OTC] *see* Clotrimazole *on page 302*

Lotrimin® AF Spray Liquid [OTC] *see* Miconazole *on page 834*

Lotrimin® AF Spray Powder [OTC] *see* Miconazole *on page 834*

Lovastatin (LOE va sta tin)

Related Information

Lipid-Lowering Agents *on page 1413*

Brand Names Mevacor®

Synonyms Mevinolin; Monacolin K

Therapeutic Category Antilipemic Agent; HMG-CoA Reductase Inhibitor

Use Adjunct to dietary therapy to decrease elevated serum total and LDL cholesterol concentrations in primary hypercholesterolemia

Pregnancy Risk Factor X

Contraindications Active liver disease, hypersensitivity to lovastatin or any component

Warnings/Precautions May elevate aminotransferases; LFTs should be performed before and every 4- 6 weeks during the first 12-15 months of therapy and periodically thereafter; can also cause myalgia and rhabdomyolysis; use with caution in patients who consume large quantities of alcohol or who have a history of liver disease

Adverse Reactions

Endocrine & metabolic: Gynecomastia

1% to 10%:

Central nervous system: Headache, dizziness

Dermatologic: Rash, pruritus

Endocrine & metabolic: Elevated creatine phosphokinase (CPK)

Gastrointestinal: Flatulence, abdominal pain, cramps, diarrhea, pancreatitis, constipation, nausea, dyspepsia, heartburn

Neuromuscular & skeletal: Myalgia

<1%:

Gastrointestinal: Abnormal taste

Ocular: Blurred vision, myositis, lenticular opacities

Overdosage/Toxicology Very few adverse events; treatment is symptomatic

Drug Interactions

Inhibitor of cytochrome P-450 2C enzymes

Cytochrome P-450 3A enzyme substrate

Increased toxicity: Gemfibrozil (musculoskeletal effects such as myopathy, myalgia, and/or muscle weakness accompanied by markedly elevated CK concentrations, rash, and/or pruritus); clofibrate, niacin (myopathy), erythromycin, cyclosporine, oral anticoagulants (elevated PT)

Increased effect/toxicity of lovastatin (20-fold increase in serum levels) with concurrent itraconazole or ketoconazole; interactions may also occur with simvastatin

Increased effect/toxicity of levothyroxine

Concurrent use of erythromycin and lovastatin may result in elevated lovastatin levels and rhabdomyolysis

Mechanism of Action Lovastatin acts by competitively inhibiting 3-hydroxyl-3-methylglutaryl-coenzyme A (HMG-CoA) reductase, the enzyme that catalyzes the rate-limiting step in cholesterol biosynthesis

Pharmacodynamics/Kinetics

Onset of effect: 3 days of therapy required for LDL cholesterol concentration reductions

Absorption: Oral: 30%

Protein binding: 95%

Half-life: 1.1-1.7 hours

Time to peak serum concentration: Oral: 2-4 hours

Elimination: ~80% to 85% of dose excreted in feces and 10% in urine following liver hydrolysis

Usual Dosage Adults: Oral: Initial: 20 mg with evening meal, then adjust at 4-week intervals; maximum dose: 80 mg/day; before initiation of therapy, patients should be placed on a standard cholesterol-lowering diet for 3-6 months and the diet should be continued during drug therapy

Administration Administer with meals

Monitoring Parameters Plasma triglycerides, cholesterol, and liver function tests

Test Interactions ↑ liver transaminases (S), altered thyroid function tests

Patient Information Promptly report any unexplained muscle pain, tenderness or weakness, especially if accompanied by malaise or fever; do not interrupt, increase, or decrease dose without advice of physician; take with meals

Nursing Implications Urge patient to adhere to cholesterol-lowering diet

Dosage Forms Tablet: 10 mg, 20 mg, 40 mg

Lovenox® *see* Enoxaparin *on page 445*

Low Potassium Diet *see page 1575*

Low-Quel® *see* Diphenoxylate and Atropine *on page 400*

Loxapine (LOKS a peen)

Related Information

Antipsychotic Agents Comparison *on page 1396*

Brand Names Loxitane®

Canadian/Mexican Brand Names Loxapac® (Canada)

Synonyms Loxapine Hydrochloride; Loxapine Succinate; Oxilapine Succinate

Therapeutic Category Antipsychotic Agent

Use Management of psychotic disorders

Pregnancy Risk Factor C

Contraindications Hypersensitivity to chlorpromazine or any component, cross-sensitivity with other phenothiazines may exist; avoid use in patients with narrow-angle glaucoma, bone marrow suppression, severe liver or cardiac disease, severe CNS depression, coma

Warnings/Precautions Watch for hypotension when administering I.M.; safety in children <6 months of age has not been established; use with caution in patients with cardiovascular disease or seizures; benefits of therapy must be weighed against risks of therapy; should not be given I.V.

Adverse Reactions

>10%:

Cardiovascular: Orthostatic hypotension

Central nervous system: Drowsiness, extrapyramidal effects (parkinsonian), confusion, persistent tardive dyskinesia

Gastrointestinal: Xerostomia

Ocular: Blurred vision

1% to 10%:

Dermatologic: Rash

Endocrine & metabolic: Enlargement of breasts

Gastrointestinal: Constipation, nausea, vomiting

<1%:

Cardiovascular: Tachycardia, arrhythmias, abnormal T-waves with prolonged ventricular repolarization

Central nervous system: Neuroleptic malignant syndrome (NMS), sedation, restlessness, anxiety, seizures, altered central temperature regulation

(Continued)

Loxapine *(Continued)*

Dermatologic: Hyperpigmentation, pruritus, photosensitivity
Endocrine & metabolic: Galactorrhea, amenorrhea, gynecomastia
Gastrointestinal: Weight gain, adynamic ileus
Genitourinary: Urinary retention, overflow incontinence, priapism, sexual dysfunction
Hematologic: Agranulocytosis (more often in women between fourth and tenth week of therapy), leukopenia (usually in patients with large doses for prolonged periods)
Hepatic: Cholestatic jaundice
Ocular: Retinal pigmentation

Overdosage/Toxicology Symptoms of overdose include deep sleep, dystonia, agitation, dysrhythmias, extrapyramidal symptoms, hypotension, seizures

Following initiation of essential overdose management, toxic symptom treatment and supportive treatment should be initiated. Hypotension usually responds to I.V. fluids or Trendelenburg positioning. If unresponsive to these measures, the use of a parenteral inotrope may be required (eg, norepinephrine 0.1-0.2 mcg/kg/minute titrated to response). Seizures commonly respond to diazepam (I.V. 5-10 mg bolus in adults every 15 minutes if needed up to a total of 30 mg; I.V. 0.25-0.4 mg/kg/dose up to a total of 10 mg in children) or to phenytoin or phenobarbital. Critical cardiac arrhythmias often respond to I.V. phenytoin (15 mg/kg up to 1 g), while other antiarrhythmics can be used. Neuroleptics often cause extrapyramidal symptoms (eg, dystonic reactions) requiring management with diphenhydramine 1-2 mg/kg (adults) up to a maximum of 50 mg I.M. or I.V. slow push followed by a maintenance dose for 48-72 hours. When these reactions are unresponsive to diphenhydramine, benztropine mesylate I.V. 1-2 mg (adults) may be effective. These agents are generally effective within 2-5 minutes.

Drug Interactions

Decreased effect of guanethidine, phenytoin
Increased toxicity with CNS depressants, metrizamide (increased seizure potential), guanabenz, MAO inhibitors

Mechanism of Action Unclear, thought to be similar to chlorpromazine

Pharmacodynamics/Kinetics

Onset of neuroleptic effect: Oral: Within 20-30 minutes
Peak effect: 1.5-3 hours
Duration: ~12 hours
Metabolism: Hepatic to glucuronide conjugates
Half-life, biphasic:
  Initial: 5 hours
  Terminal: 12-19 hours
Elimination: In urine, and to a smaller degree, feces

Usual Dosage Adults:

Oral: 10 mg twice daily, increase dose until psychotic symptoms are controlled; usual dose range: 60-100 mg/day in divided doses 2-4 times/day; dosages >250 mg/day are not recommended
I.M.: 12.5-50 mg every 4-6 hours or longer as needed and change to oral therapy as soon as possible

Dietary Considerations Alcohol: Additive CNS effect, avoid use

Administration Injectable is for I.M. use only

Test Interactions False-positives for phenylketonuria, amylase, uroporphyrins, urobilinogen, ↑ liver function tests

Patient Information May cause drowsiness; avoid alcoholic beverages; may impair judgment or coordination; may cause photosensitivity; avoid excessive sunlight; do not stop taking without consulting physician

Additional Information

Loxapine hydrochloride: Loxitane® C oral concentrate, Loxitane® IM
Loxapine succinate: Loxitane® capsule

Dosage Forms

Capsule, as succinate: 5 mg, 10 mg, 25 mg, 50 mg
Concentrate, oral, as hydrochloride: 25 mg/mL (120 mL dropper bottle)
Injection, as hydrochloride: 50 mg/mL (1 mL)

Loxapine Hydrochloride *see* Loxapine *on previous page*

Loxapine Succinate *see* Loxapine *on previous page*

Loxitane® *see* Loxapine *on previous page*

Lozol® *see* Indapamide *on page 654*

L-PAM *see* Melphalan *on page 776*

LRH *see* Gonadorelin *on page 583*

L-Sarcolysin *see* Melphalan *on page 776*

LTG *see* Lamotrigine *on page 705*

***L*-Thyroxine Sodium** *see* Levothyroxine *on page 721*

Ludiomil® *see* Maprotiline *on page 759*
Lugol's Solution *see* Potassium Iodide *on page 1027*
Luminal® *see* Phenobarbital *on page 984*
Lupron® *see* Leuprolide Acetate *on page 710*
Lupron Depot® *see* Leuprolide Acetate *on page 710*
Lupron Depot-3® Month *see* Leuprolide Acetate *on page 710*
Lupron Depot-Ped™ *see* Leuprolide Acetate *on page 710*
Luride® *see* Fluoride *on page 536*
Luride® Lozi-Tab® *see* Fluoride *on page 536*
Luride®-SF Lozi-Tab® *see* Fluoride *on page 536*
Luteinizing Hormone Releasing Hormone *see* Gonadorelin *on page 583*
Lutrepulse® *see* Gonadorelin *on page 583*
Luvox® *see* Fluvoxamine *on page 551*
LY170053 *see* Olanzapine *on page 924*

Lymphocyte Immune Globulin (LIM foe site i MYUN GLOB yoo lin)

Brand Names Atgam®

Synonyms Antithymocyte Globulin (Equine); Antithymocyte Immunoglobulin; ATG; Horse Anti-human Thymocyte Gamma Globulin

Therapeutic Category Immunosuppressant Agent

Use Prevention and treatment of acute renal allograft rejection; treatment of moderate to severe aplastic anemia in patients not considered suitable candidates for bone marrow transplantation; prevention of graft-versus-host disease following bone marrow transplantation

Pregnancy Risk Factor C

Contraindications Known hypersensitivity to ATG, thimerosal, or other equine gamma globulins; severe, unremitting leukopenia and/or thrombocytopenia

Warnings/Precautions Must be administered via central line due to chemical phlebitis; should only be used by physicians experienced in immunosuppressive therapy or management of renal transplant patients; adequate laboratory and supportive medical resources must be readily available in the facility for patient management; rash, dyspnea, hypotension, or anaphylaxis precludes further administration of the drug. Dose must be administered over at least 4 hours; patient may need to be pretreated with an antipyretic, antihistamine, and/or corticosteroid.

Adverse Reactions

>10%:
- Central nervous system: Fever, chills
- Dermatologic: Rash
- Hematologic: Leukopenia, thrombocytopenia
- Miscellaneous: Systemic infection

1% to 10%:
- Cardiovascular: Hypotension, hypertension, tachycardia, edema, chest pain
- Central nervous system: Headache, malaise, pain
- Gastrointestinal: Diarrhea, nausea, stomatitis, GI bleeding
- Respiratory: Dyspnea
- Local: Edema or redness at injection site, thrombophlebitis
- Neuromuscular & skeletal: Myalgia, back pain
- Renal: Abnormal renal function tests
- Miscellaneous: Sensitivity reactions: Anaphylaxis may be indicated by hypotension, respiratory distress, serum sickness, viral infection

<1%:
- Central nervous system: Seizures
- Dermatologic: Pruritus, urticaria
- Hematologic: Hemolysis, anemia
- Neuromuscular & skeletal: Arthralgia, weakness
- Renal: Acute renal failure
- Miscellaneous: Lymphadenopathy

Stability

Ampuls must be refrigerated

Dose must be diluted in 0.45% or 0.9% sodium chloride

Diluted solution is stable for 12 hours (including infusion time) at room temperature and 24 hours (including infusion time) at refrigeration

The use of dextrose solutions is not recommended (precipitation may occur)

Standard diluent: Dose/1000 mL NS or 0.45% sodium chloride

Minimum volume: Concentration should not exceed 1 mg/mL for a peripheral line or 4 mg/mL for a central line

Mechanism of Action May involve elimination of antigen-reactive T-lymphocytes (killer cells) in peripheral blood or alteration of T-cell function

(Continued)

Lymphocyte Immune Globulin *(Continued)*

Pharmacodynamics/Kinetics

Distribution: Poorly distributed into lymphoid tissues; binds to circulating lymphocytes, granulocytes, platelets, bone marrow cells

Half-life, plasma: 1.5-12 days

Elimination: ~1% of dose excreted in urine

Usual Dosage An intradermal skin test is recommended prior to administration of the initial dose of ATG; use 0.1 mL of a 1:1000 dilution of ATG in normal saline

First dose: Premedicate with diphenhydramine 50 mg orally 30 minutes prior to and hydrocortisone 100 mg I.V. 15 minutes prior to infusion and acetaminophen 650 mg 2 hours after start of infusion

Children: I.V.:

- Aplastic anemia protocol: 10-20 mg/kg/day for 8-14 days; additional doses may be given every other day for 21 total doses
- Cardiac allograft: 10 mg/kg/day for 7 days
- Renal allograft: 5-25 mg/kg/day

Adults: I.V.:

- Aplastic anemia protocol: 10-20 mg/kg/day for 8-14 days, then administer every other day for 7 more doses **or** 40 mg/kg/day for 4 days
- Rejection prevention: 15 mg/kg/day until therapeutic cyclosporine levels are achieved or 14 days of therapy
- Rejection treatment: 10-15 mg/kg/day for 14 days, then administer every other day for 10-14 days

Administration For I.V. use only; administer via central line; use of high flow veins will minimize the occurrence of phlebitis and thrombosis; administer by slow I.V. infusion through an inline filter with pore size of 0.2-1 micrometer over 4-8 hours at a final concentration not to exceed 4 mg ATG/mL

Monitoring Parameters Lymphocyte profile, CBC with differential and platelet count, vital signs during administration

Nursing Implications For I.V. use only; mild itching and erythema can be treated with antihistamines; infuse dose over at least 4 hours; any severe systemic reaction to the skin test such as generalized rash, tachycardia, dyspnea, hypotension, or anaphylaxis should preclude further therapy; **epinephrine and resuscitative equipment should be nearby.** Patient may need to be pretreated with an antipyretic, antihistamine, and/or corticosteroid.

Dosage Forms Injection: 50 of equine IgG/mL (5 mL)

Lyphocin® *see* Vancomycin *on page 1288*

Lypressin (lye PRES in)

Brand Names Diapid®

Synonyms 8-*L*-Lysine Vasopressin

Therapeutic Category Antidiuretic Hormone Analog; Pituitary Hormone; Vasopressin Analog

Use Controls or prevents signs and complications of neurogenic diabetes insipidus

Pregnancy Risk Factor C

Contraindications Known hypersensitivity to lypressin

Warnings/Precautions Use with caution in patients with coronary artery disease

Adverse Reactions

1% to 10%:

- Cardiovascular: Chest tightness
- Central nervous system: Dizziness, headache
- Endocrine & metabolic: Water intoxication
- Gastrointestinal: Abdominal cramping, increased bowel movements
- Local: Irritation or burning
- Renal: Rhinorrhea, nasal congestion
- Respiratory: Coughing, dyspnea

<1%: Miscellaneous: Inadvertent inhalation

Overdosage/Toxicology Symptoms of overdose include drowsiness, headache, confusion, weight gain, hypertension; systemic toxicity is unlikely to occur from the nasal spray

Drug Interactions Increased effect: Chlorpropamide, clofibrate, carbamazepine → prolongation of antidiuretic effects

Mechanism of Action Increases cyclic adenosine monophosphate (cAMP) which increases water permeability at the renal tubule resulting in decreased urine volume and increased osmolality; causes peristalsis by directly stimulating the smooth muscle in the GI tract

Pharmacodynamics/Kinetics

Onset of antidiuretic effect: Intranasal spray: Within 0.5-2 hours

Duration: 3-8 hours

Metabolism: In the liver and kidneys

Half-life: 15-20 minutes
Elimination: Urinary excretion

Usual Dosage Children and Adults: Instill 1-2 sprays into one or both nostrils whenever frequency of urination increases or significant thirst develops; usual dosage is 1-2 sprays 4 times/day; range: 1 spray/day at bedtime to 10 sprays each nostril every 3-4 hours

Patient Information To control nocturia, an additional dose may be given at bedtime; notify physician if drowsiness, fatigue, headache, shortness of breath, abdominal cramps, or severe nasal irritation occurs

Additional Information Approximately 2 USP posterior pituitary pressor units per spray

Dosage Forms Spray: 0.185 mg/mL (equivalent to 50 USP posterior pituitary units/mL) (8 mL)

Lysodren® *see* Mitotane *on page 848*

Maalox Anti-Gas® [OTC] *see* Simethicone *on page 1136*

Macrobid® *see* Nitrofurantoin *on page 907*

Macrodantin® *see* Nitrofurantoin *on page 907*

Macrodex® *see* Dextran *on page 363*

Mafenide (MA fe nide)

Related Information

Sulfonamide Derivatives *on page 1420*

Brand Names Sulfamylon®

Synonyms Mafenide Acetate

Therapeutic Category Antibacterial, Topical; Antibiotic, Topical

Use Adjunct in the treatment of second and third degree burns to prevent septicemia caused by susceptible organisms such as *Pseudomonas aeruginosa*; prevention of graft loss of meshed autografts on excised burn wounds

Pregnancy Risk Factor C

Contraindications Hypersensitivity to mafenide, sulfites, or any component

Warnings/Precautions Use with caution in patients with renal impairment and in patients with G-6-PD deficiency; prolonged use may result in superinfection

Adverse Reactions

>10%:
- Central nervous system: Pain
- Local: Burning sensation, excoriation

1% to 10%:
- Cardiovascular: Facial edema
- Dermatologic: Rash
- Miscellaneous: Dyspnea

<1%:
- Dermatologic: Erythema
- Endocrine & metabolic: Hyperchloremia, metabolic acidosis
- Hematologic: Bone marrow suppression, hemolytic anemia, bleeding
- Hepatic: Porphyria
- Respiratory: Hyperventilation, tachypnea
- Sensitivity reactions: Hypersensitivity

Mechanism of Action Interferes with bacterial folic acid synthesis through competitive inhibition of para-aminobenzoic acid

Pharmacodynamics/Kinetics

Absorption: Diffuses through devascularized areas and is rapidly absorbed from burned surface
Time to peak serum concentration: Topical: 2-4 hours
Metabolism: To para-carboxybenzene sulfonamide which is a carbonic anhydrase inhibitor
Elimination: In urine as metabolites

Usual Dosage Children and Adults: Topical: Apply once or twice daily with a sterile gloved hand; apply to a thickness of approximately 16 mm; the burned area should be covered with cream at all times

Monitoring Parameters Acid base balance

Patient Information Discontinue and call physician immediately if rash, blisters, or swelling appear while using cream; discontinue if condition persists or worsens while using this product; for external use only

Dosage Forms Cream, topical, as acetate: 85 mg/g (56.7 g, 113.4 g, 411 g)

Mafenide Acetate *see* Mafenide *on this page*

Magnesia Magma *see* Magnesium Hydroxide *on page 753*

Magnesium Citrate (mag NEE zhum SIT rate)

Related Information

Laxatives, Classification and Properties *on page 1413*

Brand Names Evac-Q-Mag® [OTC]

(Continued)

Magnesium Citrate *(Continued)*

Synonyms Citrate of Magnesia

Therapeutic Category Laxative, Saline

Use Evacuation of bowel prior to certain surgical and diagnostic procedures or overdose situations

Pregnancy Risk Factor B

Contraindications Renal failure, appendicitis, abdominal pain, intestinal impaction, obstruction or perforation, diabetes mellitus, complications in gastrointestinal tract, patients with colostomy, ileostomy, ulcerative colitis or diverticulitis

Warnings/Precautions Use with caution in patients with impaired renal function, especially if Cl_{cr} <30 mL/minute (accumulation of magnesium which may lead to magnesium intoxication); use with caution in digitalized patients (may alter cardiac conduction leading to heart block); use with caution in patients with lithium administration; use with caution with neuromuscular blocking agents, CNS depressants

Adverse Reactions

1% to 10%:

Cardiovascular: Hypotension

Endocrine & metabolic: Hypermagnesemia

Gastrointestinal: Abdominal cramps, diarrhea, gas formation

Respiratory: Respiratory depression

Overdosage/Toxicology Serious, potentially life-threatening electrolyte disturbances may occur with long-term use or overdosage due to diarrhea; hypermagnesemia may occur. CNS depression, confusion, hypotension, muscle weakness, blockage of peripheral neuromuscular transmission.

Serum level >4 mEq/L (4.8 mg/dL): Deep tendon reflexes may be depressed

Serum level ≥10 mEq/L (12 mg/dL): Deep tendon reflexes may disappear, respiratory paralysis may occur, heart block may occur

I.V. calcium (5-10 mEq) will reverse respiratory depression or heart block; in extreme cases, peritoneal dialysis or hemodialysis may be required.

Serum level >12 mEq/L may be fatal, serum level ≥10 mEq/L may cause complete heart block

Mechanism of Action Promotes bowel evacuation by causing osmotic retention of fluid which distends the colon with increased peristaltic activity

Pharmacodynamics/Kinetics

Absorption: Oral: 15% to 30%

Elimination: Renal

Usual Dosage Cathartic: Oral:

Children:

<6 years: 0.5 mL/kg up to a maximum of 200 mL repeated every 4-6 hours until stools are clear

6-12 years: 100-150 mL

Adults ≥12 years: ½ to 1 full bottle (120-300 mL)

Reference Range Serum magnesium:

Children: 1.5-1.9 mg/dL ~1.2-1.6 mEq/L

Adults: 2.2-2.8 mg/dL ~1.8-2.3 mEq/L

Test Interactions ↑ magnesium; ↓ protein, ↓ calcium (S), ↓ potassium (S)

Patient Information Take with a glass of water, fruit juice, or citrus flavored carbonated beverage to improve taste, chill before using; report severe abdominal pain to physician

Nursing Implications To increase palatability, manufacturer suggests chilling the solution prior to administration

Additional Information Magnesium content of 5 mL: 3.85-4.71 mEq

Dosage Forms Solution, oral: 300 mL

Magnesium Gluconate (mag NEE zhum GLOO koe nate)

Brand Names Magonate® [OTC]

Therapeutic Category Magnesium Salt

Use Dietary supplement for treatment of magnesium deficiencies

Contraindications Patients with heart block, severe renal disease

Warnings/Precautions Use with caution in patients with impaired renal function; hypermagnesemia and toxicity may occur due to decreased renal clearance of absorbed magnesium

Adverse Reactions

1% to 10%: Gastrointestinal: Diarrhea (excessive dose)

<1%:

Cardiovascular: Hypotension

Endocrine & metabolic: Hypermagnesemia

Gastrointestinal: Abdominal cramps

Neuromuscular & skeletal: Muscle weakness

Respiratory: Respiratory depression

Overdosage/Toxicology Hypermagnesemia rarely occurs after acute or chronic overexposure except in patients with renal insufficiency or massive overdose; moderate toxicity causes nausea, vomiting, weakness, and cutaneous flushing; larger doses cause cardiac conduction abnormalities, hypotension, severe muscle weakness, and lethargy; very high levels cause coma, respiratory arrest, and asystole.

Treatment includes replacing fluid and electrolyte losses caused by excessive catharsis; while there is no specific antidote and treatment is supportive, administration of I.V. calcium may temporarily alleviate respiratory depression; hemodialysis rapidly removes magnesium and is the only route of elimination in anuric patients (hemoperfusion and repeat-dose charcoal are not effective).

Drug Interactions Increased effect of nondepolarizing neuromuscular blockers

Mechanism of Action Magnesium is important as a cofactor in many enzymatic reactions in the body involving protein synthesis and carbohydrate metabolism, (at least 300 enzymatic reactions require magnesium). Actions on lipoprotein lipase have been found to be important in reducing serum cholesterol and on sodium/potassium ATPase in promoting polarization (ie, neuromuscular functioning).

Pharmacodynamics/Kinetics

Absorption: Oral: 15% to 30%

Elimination: Renal

Usual Dosage The recommended dietary allowance (RDA) of magnesium is 4.5 mg/kg which is a total daily allowance of 350-400 mg for adult men and 280-300 mg for adult women. During pregnancy the RDA is 300 mg and during lactation the RDA is 355 mg. Average daily intakes of dietary magnesium have declined in recent years due to processing of food. The latest estimate of the average American dietary intake was 349 mg/day.

Dietary supplement: Oral:

Children: 3-6 mg/kg/day in divided doses 3-4 times/day; maximum: 400 mg/day

Adults: 27-54 mg 2-3 times/day or 100 mg 4 times/day

Dosing in renal impairment: Patients in severe renal failure should not receive magnesium due to toxicity from accumulation. Patients with a Cl_{cr} <25 mL/minute receiving magnesium should be monitored by serum magnesium levels.

Reference Range Serum magnesium:

Children: 1.5-1.9 mg/dL ~1.2-1.6 mEq/L

Adults: 2.2-2.8 mg/dL ~1.8-2.3 mEq/L

Additional Information Magnesium content of 500 mg: 27 mg elemental magnesium

Dosage Forms Tablet: 500 mg [elemental magnesium 27 mg]

Magnesium Hydroxide (mag NEE zhum hye DROKS ide)

Related Information

Laxatives, Classification and Properties *on page 1412*

Brand Names Phillips'® Milk of Magnesia [OTC]

Canadian/Mexican Brand Names Leche De Magnesia Normex (Mexico)

Synonyms Magnesia Magma; Milk of Magnesia; MOM

Therapeutic Category Antacid; Laxative, Saline; Magnesium Salt

Use Short-term treatment of occasional constipation and symptoms of hyperacidity, magnesium replacement therapy

Pregnancy Risk Factor B

Contraindications Patients with colostomy or an ileostomy, intestinal obstruction, fecal impaction, renal failure, appendicitis, hypersensitivity to any component

Warnings/Precautions Use with caution in patients with severe renal impairment, (especially when doses are >50 mEq magnesium/day); hypermagnesemia and toxicity may occur due to decreased renal clearance of absorbed magnesium. Decreased renal function (Cl_{cr} <30 mL/minute) may result in toxicity; monitor for toxicity.

Adverse Reactions

>10%: Gastrointestinal: Diarrhea

1% to 10%:

Cardiovascular: Hypotension

Endocrine & metabolic: Hypermagnesemia

Gastrointestinal: Abdominal cramps

Neuromuscular & skeletal: Muscle weakness

Respiratory: Respiratory depression

Overdosage/Toxicology Magnesium antacids are also laxative and may cause diarrhea and hypokalemia; in patients with renal failure, magnesium may accumulate to toxic levels.

(Continued)

Magnesium Hydroxide *(Continued)*

I.V. calcium (5-10 mEq) will reverse respiratory depression or heart block; in extreme cases, peritoneal dialysis or hemodialysis may be required.

Drug Interactions Decreased effect: Decreased absorption of tetracyclines, digoxin, indomethacin, or iron salts

Mechanism of Action Promotes bowel evacuation by causing osmotic retention of fluid which distends the colon with increased peristaltic activity; reacts with hydrochloric acid in stomach to form magnesium chloride

Pharmacodynamics/Kinetics

Onset of laxative action: 4-8 hours

Elimination: Absorbed magnesium ions (up to 30%) are usually excreted by kidneys, unabsorbed drug is excreted in feces

Usual Dosage Oral:

Laxative:

<2 years: 0.5 mL/kg/dose

2-5 years: 5-15 mL/day or in divided doses

6-12 years: 15-30 mL/day or in divided doses

≥12 years: 30-60 mL/day or in divided doses

Antacid:

Children: 2.5-5 mL as needed up to 4 times/day

Adults: 5-15 mL or 650 mg to 1.3 g tablets up to 4 times/day as needed

Dosing in renal impairment: Patients in severe renal failure should not receive magnesium due to toxicity from accumulation. Patients with a Cl_{cr} <25 mL/minute receiving magnesium should be monitored by serum magnesium levels.

Reference Range Serum magnesium:

Children: 1.5-1.9 mg/dL (1.2-1.6 mEq/L)

Adults: 1.5-2.5 mg/dL (1.2-2.0 mEq/L)

Test Interactions ↑ magnesium; ↓ protein, calcium (S), ↓ potassium (S)

Patient Information Dilute dose in water or juice, shake well

Nursing Implications MOM concentrate is 3 times as potent as regular strength product

Additional Information Magnesium content of 30 mL: 1.05 g (87 mEq)

Dosage Forms

Liquid: 390 mg/5 mL (10 mL, 15 mL, 20 mL, 30 mL, 100 mL, 120 mL, 180 mL, 360 mL, 720 mL)

Liquid, concentrate: 10 mL equivalent to 30 mL milk of magnesia USP

Suspension, oral: 2.5 g/30 mL (10 mL, 15 mL, 30 mL)

Tablet: 300 mg, 600 mg

Magnesium Oxide (mag NEE zhum OKS ide)

Brand Names Maox®

Therapeutic Category Antacid; Electrolyte Supplement, Oral; Laxative, Saline; Magnesium Salt

Use Short-term treatment of occasional constipation and symptoms of hyperacidity

Pregnancy Risk Factor B

Contraindications Patients with colostomy or an ileostomy, appendicitis, ulcerative colitis, diverticulitis, heart block, myocardial damage, serious renal impairment, hepatitis, Addison's disease, hypersensitivity to any component

Warnings/Precautions Hypermagnesemia and toxicity may occur due to decreased renal clearance (Cl_{cr} <30 mL/minute) of absorbed magnesium; monitor serum magnesium level, respiratory rate, deep tendon reflex, renal function when $MgSO_4$ is administered parenterally; use with caution in digitalized patients (may alter cardiac conduction leading heart block); use with caution in patients with lithium administration; elderly, due to disease or drug therapy, may be predisposed to diarrhea; diarrhea may result in electrolyte imbalance; monitor for toxicity

Adverse Reactions

>10%: Gastrointestinal: Diarrhea

1% to 10%:

Cardiovascular: Hypotension, EKG changes

Central nervous system: Mental depression, coma

Gastrointestinal: Nausea, vomiting

Respiratory: Respiratory depression

Overdosage/Toxicology Magnesium antacids are also laxative and may cause diarrhea and hypokalemia. In patients with renal failure, magnesium may accumulate to toxic levels.

I.V. calcium (5-10 mEq) will reverse respiratory depression or heart block; in extreme cases, peritoneal dialysis or hemodialysis may be required.

Drug Interactions Decreased effect: Tetracyclines, digoxin, indomethacin, iron salts, isoniazid, quinolones

Dosing adjustment/comments in renal impairment: Cl_{cr} <25 mL/minute: Do not administer or monitor serum magnesium levels carefully

Administration

Magnesium sulfate may be administered I.M. or I.V.

I.M.: A 25% or 50% concentration may be used for adults and a 20% solution is recommended for children

I.V.: Magnesium may be administered IVP, IVPB or I.V. infusion in an auxiliary medication infusion solution (eg, TPN); when giving I.V. push, must dilute first and should not be given any faster than 150 mg/minute

Maximal rate of infusion: 2 g/hour to avoid hypotension; doses of 4 g/hour have been given in emergencies (eclampsia, seizures); optimally, should add magnesium to I.V. fluids or to IVH, but bolus doses are also effective

For I.V., a concentration <20% should be used and the rate of injection should not exceed 1.5 mL of a 10% solution (or equivalent) per minute

Monitoring Parameters Monitor blood pressure when administering $MgSO_4$ I.V.; serum magnesium levels should be monitored to avoid overdose; monitor for diarrhea; monitor for arrhythmias, hypotension, respiratory and CNS depression during rapid I.V. administration

Reference Range Serum magnesium:

Children: 1.5-1.9 mg/dL (1.2-1.6 mEq/L)

Adults: 1.5-2.5 mg/dL (1.2-2.0 mEq/L)

Note: Serum magnesium is poor reflection of repletional status as the majority of magnesium is intracellular; serum levels may be transiently normal for a few hours after a dose is given, therefore, aim for consistently high normal serum levels in patients with normal renal function for most efficient repletion

Test Interactions ↑ magnesium; ↓ protein, calcium (S), ↓ potassium (S)

Additional Information 10% elemental magnesium; 8.1 mEq magnesium/g; 4 mmol magnesium/g

500 mg $MgSO_4$ = 4.06 mEq magnesium = 49.3 mg elemental magnesium

Dosage Forms

Granules: ~40 mEq magnesium/5 g (240 g)

Injection: 100 mg/mL (20 mL); 125 mg/mL (8 mL); 250 mg/mL (150 mL); 500 mg/mL (2 mL, 5 mL, 10 mL, 30 mL, 50 mL)

Solution, oral: 50% [500 mg/mL] (30 mL)

Magonate® [OTC] *see* Magnesium Gluconate *on page 752*

Maigret-50 *see* Phenylpropanolamine *on page 991*

Malatal® *see* Hyoscyamine, Atropine, Scopolamine, and Phenobarbital *on page 637*

Mallisol® [OTC] *see* Povidone-Iodine *on page 1031*

Malotuss® [OTC] *see* Guaifenesin *on page 589*

Management of Overdosages *see page 1547*

Mandol® *see* Cefamandole *on page 219*

Mandrake *see* Podophyllum Resin *on page 1014*

Manganese (MAN ga nees)

Brand Names Chelated Manganese® [OTC]

Synonyms Manganese Chloride; Manganese Sulfate

Therapeutic Category Trace Elements; Trace Element, Parenteral

Use Trace element added to TPN (total parenteral nutrition) solution to prevent manganese deficiency; orally as a dietary supplement

Pregnancy Risk Factor C

Contraindications High manganese levels; patients with severe liver dysfunction or cholestasis (conjugated bilirubin >2 mg/dL) due to reduced biliary excretion

Overdosage/Toxicology Acute poisoning due to ingestion of manganese or manganese salts is rare owing to poor absorption of manganese. The main symptoms of chronic poisoning, either from injection or usually inhalation of manganese dust or fumes in air, include extrapyramidal symptoms that can lead to progressive deterioration in the central nervous system.

Stability Compatible with electrolytes usually present in amino acid/dextrose solution used for TPN solutions

Mechanism of Action Cofactor in many enzyme systems, stimulates synthesis of cholesterol and fatty acids in liver, and influences mucopolysaccharide synthesis

Pharmacodynamics/Kinetics

Distribution: Concentrated in mitochondria of pituitary gland, pancreas, liver, kidney, and bone

Elimination: Mainly in bile, urinary excretion is negligible

Usual Dosage

Infants: I.V.: 2-10 mcg/kg/day usually administered in TPN solutions

Adults:

Oral: 20-50 mg/day

RDA: 2-5 mg/day

(Continued)

Manganese *(Continued)*

I.V.: 150-800 mcg/day usually administered in TPN solutions

Administration Do not administer I.M. or by direct I.V. injection since the acidic pH of the solution may cause tissue irritations and it is hypotonic

Monitoring Parameters Periodic manganese plasma level

Reference Range 4-14 µg/L

Dosage Forms

Injection, as chloride: 0.1 mg/mL (10 mL)
Injection, as sulfate: 0.1 mg/mL (10 mL, 30 mL)
Tablet: 20 mg, 50 mg

Manganese Chloride *see* Manganese *on previous page*

Manganese Sulfate *see* Manganese *on previous page*

Mannitol (MAN i tole)

Brand Names Osmitrol®; Resectisol®

Synonyms *D*-Mannitol

Therapeutic Category Diuretic, Osmotic

Use Reduction of increased intracranial pressure associated with cerebral edema; promotion of diuresis in the prevention and/or treatment of oliguria or anuria due to acute renal failure; reduction of increased intraocular pressure; promoting urinary excretion of toxic substances; genitourinary irrigant in transurethral prostatic resection or other transurethral surgical procedures

Pregnancy Risk Factor C

Contraindications Severe renal disease (anuria), dehydration, or active intracranial bleeding, severe pulmonary edema or congestion, hypersensitivity to any component

Warnings/Precautions Should not be administered until adequacy of renal function and urine flow is established; cardiovascular status should also be evaluated; do not administer electrolyte-free mannitol solutions with blood

Adverse Reactions

>10%:
- Central nervous system: Headache
- Gastrointestinal: Nausea, vomiting
- Genitourinary: Polyuria

1% to 10%:
- Central nervous system: Dizziness
- Dermatologic: Rash
- Ocular: Blurred vision

<1%:
- Cardiovascular: Circulatory overload, congestive heart failure
- Central nervous system: Convulsions, headache, chills
- Endocrine & metabolic: Fluid and electrolyte imbalance, water intoxication, dehydration and hypovolemia secondary to rapid diuresis
- Gastrointestinal: Xerostomia
- Genitourinary: Dysuria
- Local: Tissue necrosis
- Respiratory: Pulmonary edema
- Miscellaneous: Allergic reactions

Overdosage/Toxicology Symptoms of overdose include polyuria, hypotension, cardiovascular collapse, pulmonary edema, hyponatremia, hypokalemia, oliguria, seizures; increased electrolyte excretion and fluid overload can occur; hemodialysis will clear mannitol and reduce osmolality

Stability Should be stored at room temperature (15°C to 30°C) and protected from freezing; crystallization may occur at low temperatures; do not use solutions that contain crystals, heating in a hot water bath and vigorous shaking may be utilized for resolubilization; cool solutions to body temperature before using

Mechanism of Action Increases the osmotic pressure of glomerular filtrate, which inhibits tubular reabsorption of water and electrolytes and increases urinary output

Pharmacodynamics/Kinetics

Onset of diuresis: Injection: Within 1-3 hours
Onset of reduction in intracerebral pressure: Within 15 minutes
Duration of reduction in intracerebral pressure: 3-6 hours
Distribution: Remains confined to extracellular space (except in extreme concentrations) and does not penetrate the blood-brain barrier
Metabolism: Minimal amounts metabolized in the liver to glycogen
Half-life: 1.1-1.6 hours
Elimination: Primarily excreted unchanged in urine by glomerular filtration

Usual Dosage I.V.:

Children:

Test dose (to assess adequate renal function): 200 mg/kg over 3-5 minutes to produce a urine flow of at least 1 mL/kg for 1-3 hours

Initial: 0.5-1 g/kg

Maintenance: 0.25-0.5 g/kg given every 4-6 hours

Adults:

Test dose (to assess adequate renal function): 12.5 g (200 mg/kg) over 3-5 minutes to produce a urine flow of at least 30-50 mL of urine per hour over the next 2-3 hours

Initial: 0.5-1 g/kg

Maintenance: 0.25-0.5 g/kg every 4-6 hours; usual adult dose: 20-200 g/24 hours

Intracranial pressure: Cerebral edema: 1.5-2 g/kg/dose I.V. as a 15% to 20% solution over ≥30 minutes; maintain serum osmolality 310-320 mOsm/kg

Preoperative for neurosurgery: 1.5-2 g/kg administered 1-1.5 hours prior to surgery

Transurethral irrigation: Use urogenital solution as required for irrigation

Administration In-line 5-micron filter set should always be used for mannitol infusion with concentrations ≥20%; administer test dose (for oliguria) I.V. push over 3-5 minutes; for cerebral edema or elevated ICP, administer over 20-30 minutes

Monitoring Parameters Renal function, daily fluid I & O, serum electrolytes, serum and urine osmolality; for treatment of elevated intracranial pressure, maintain serum osmolality 310-320 mOsm/kg

Nursing Implications Avoid extravasation; crenation and agglutination of red blood cells may occur if administered with whole blood

Additional Information May autoclave or heat to redissolve crystals; mannitol 20% has an approximate osmolarity of 1100 mOsm/L and mannitol 25% has an approximate osmolarity of 1375 mOsm/L

Dosage Forms

Injection: 5% [50 mg/mL] (1000 mL); 10% [100 mg/mL] (500 mL, 1000 mL); 15% [150 mg/mL] (150 mL, 500 mL); 20% [200 mg/mL] (150 mL, 250 mL, 500 mL); 25% [250 mg/mL] (50 mL)

Solution, urogenital: 0.54% [5.4 mg/mL] (2000 mL)

Mantoux *see* Tuberculin Purified Protein Derivative *on page 1276*

Maox® *see* Magnesium Oxide *on page 754*

Maprotiline (ma PROE ti leen)

Related Information

Antidepressant Agents Comparison *on page 1393*

Brand Names Ludiomil®

Synonyms Maprotiline Hydrochloride

Therapeutic Category Antidepressant, Tetracyclic

Use Treatment of depression and anxiety associated with depression

Pregnancy Risk Factor B

Contraindications Narrow-angle glaucoma, hypersensitivity to maprotiline or any component

Warnings/Precautions Use with caution in patients with cardiac conduction disturbances, history of hyperthyroid, renal, or hepatic dysfunction; safe use of tricyclic antidepressants in children <12 years of age has not been established; to avoid cholinergic crisis do not discontinue abruptly in patients receiving high doses chronically

Adverse Reactions

>10%:

Cardiovascular: Orthostatic hypotension

Central nervous system: Drowsiness

Dermatologic: Rash

Gastrointestinal: Xerostomia

Genitourinary: Urinary retention

Neuromuscular & skeletal: Weakness

1% to 10%:

Central nervous system: Insomnia

Gastrointestinal: Constipation, nausea, vomiting, increased appetite and weight gain or loss

Neuromuscular & skeletal: Trembling

<1%:

Central nervous system: Confusion

Endocrine & metabolic: Breast enlargement

Genitourinary: Testicular edema

Hepatic: Cholestatic hepatitis

Ocular: Blurred vision, increased intraocular pressure

(Continued)

Maprotiline *(Continued)*

Otic: Tinnitus

Overdosage/Toxicology Symptoms of overdose include agitation, confusion, hallucinations, urinary retention, hypothermia, hypotension, seizures, ventricular tachycardia

Following initiation of essential overdose management, toxic symptoms should be treated. Ventricular arrhythmias often respond to systemic alkalinization (sodium bicarbonate 0.5-2 mEq/kg I.V.). Arrhythmias unresponsive to this therapy may respond to lidocaine 1 mg/kg I.V. followed by a titrated infusion. Physostigmine (1-2 mg I.V. slowly for adults or 0.5 mg I.V. slowly for children) may be indicated in reversing cardiac arrhythmias that are life-threatening. Seizures usually respond to diazepam I.V. boluses (5-10 mg for adults up to 30 mg or 0.25-0.4 mg/kg/dose for children up to 10 mg/dose). If seizures are unresponsive or recur, phenytoin or phenobarbital may be required.

Drug Interactions

Decreased effect: Barbiturates, phenytoin, carbamazepine

Increased toxicity: CNS depressants, MAO inhibitors (hyperpyretic crisis), anticholinergics, sympathomimetics, thyroid increases cardiotoxicity, phenothiazines (seizures), benzodiazepines

Mechanism of Action Traditionally believed to increase the synaptic concentration of norepinephrine in the central nervous system by inhibition of their reuptake by the presynaptic neuronal membrane. However, additional receptor effects have been found including desensitization of adenyl cyclase, down regulation of beta-adrenergic receptors, and down regulation of serotonin receptors.

Pharmacodynamics/Kinetics

Absorption: Slow

Protein binding: 88%

Metabolism: In the liver to active and inactive compounds

Half-life: 27-58 hours (mean, 43 hours)

Time to peak serum concentration: Within 12 hours

Elimination: In urine (70%) and feces (30%)

Usual Dosage Oral:

Children 6-14 years: 10 mg/day, increase to a maximum daily dose of 75 mg

Adults: 75 mg/day to start, increase by 25 mg every 2 weeks up to 150-225 mg/day; given in 3 divided doses or in a single daily dose

Elderly: Initial: 25 mg at bedtime, increase by 25 mg every 3 days for inpatients and weekly for outpatients if tolerated; usual maintenance dose: 50-75 mg/day, higher doses may be necessary in nonresponders

Dietary Considerations Alcohol: Additive CNS effect, avoid use

Monitoring Parameters Monitor blood pressure and pulse rate prior to and during initial therapy; evaluate mood and somatic complaints; monitor appetite and weight

Reference Range Therapeutic: 200-600 ng/mL (SI: 721-2163 nmol/L); not well established

Patient Information Avoid alcohol ingestion; do not discontinue medication abruptly; may cause drowsiness; full effect may not occur for 3-6 weeks; dry mouth may be helped by sips of water, sugarless gum, or hard candy; rise slowly to avoid dizziness

Nursing Implications May increase appetite and possibly a craving for sweets; often requires 2-3 weeks for therapeutic effects to be seen; severe constipation and urinary retention are possible; urge patient to report symptoms of stomatitis, sialadenitis, and xerostomia; observe seizure precautions

Dosage Forms Tablet, as hydrochloride: 25 mg, 50 mg, 75 mg

Maprotiline Hydrochloride *see* Maprotiline *on previous page*

Marazide® *see* Benzthiazide *on page 141*

Marbaxin® *see* Methocarbamol *on page 805*

Marcaine® *see* Bupivacaine *on page 170*

Marcillin® *see* Ampicillin *on page 85*

Marezine® [OTC] *see* Cyclizine *on page 321*

Margesic® H *see* Hydrocodone and Acetaminophen *on page 620*

Marinol® *see* Dronabinol *on page 432*

Marmine® Injection *see* Dimenhydrinate *on page 395*

Marmine® Oral [OTC] *see* Dimenhydrinate *on page 395*

Marnal® *see* Butalbital Compound *on page 176*

Marthritic® *see* Salsalate *on page 1122*

Masoprocol (ma SOE pro kole)

Brand Names Actinex®

Therapeutic Category Topical Skin Product, Acne

Use Treatment of actinic keratosis

Pregnancy Risk Factor B

Contraindications Hypersensitivity to masoprocol or any component

Warnings/Precautions Occlusive dressings should not be used; for external use only

Adverse Reactions

>10%:

Dermatologic: Erythema, flaking, dryness, itching

Local: Burning

1% to 10%:

Dermatologic: Soreness, rash

Neuromuscular & skeletal: Paresthesia

Ocular: Eye irritation

<1%: Dermatologic: Blistering, excoriation, skin roughness, wrinkling

Mechanism of Action Antiproliferative activity against keratinocytes

Pharmacodynamics/Kinetics Absorption: Topical: <1% to 2%

Usual Dosage Adults: Topical: Wash and dry area; gently massage into affected area every morning and evening for 28 days

Patient Information For external use only; may stain clothing or fabrics; avoid eyes and mucous membranes; do not use occlusive dressings; transient local burning sensation may occur immediately after application; contact physician if oozing or blistering occurs; wash hands immediately after use.

Dosage Forms Cream: 10% (30 g)

Massengill® Medicated Douche w/Cepticin [OTC] *see* Povidone-Iodine *on page 1031*

Matulane® *see* Procarbazine *on page 1049*

Maxair™ *see* Pirbuterol *on page 1009*

Maxaquin® *see* Lomefloxacin *on page 737*

Max-Caro® [OTC] *see* Beta-Carotene *on page 147*

Maxidex® *see* Dexamethasone *on page 356*

Maxiflor® *see* Diflorasone *on page 382*

Maximum Strength Anbesol® [OTC] *see* Benzocaine *on page 138*

Maximum Strength Desenex® Antifungal Cream [OTC] *see* Miconazole *on page 834*

Maximum Strength Nytol® [OTC] *see* Diphenhydramine *on page 399*

Maximum Strength Orajel® [OTC] *see* Benzocaine *on page 138*

Maxipime® *see* Cefepime *on page 221*

Maxitrol® *see* Neomycin, Polymyxin B, and Dexamethasone *on page 889*

Maxivate® *see* Betamethasone *on page 147*

Maxolon® *see* Metoclopramide *on page 824*

Maxzide® *see* Hydrochlorothiazide and Triamterene *on page 618*

May Apple *see* Podophyllum Resin *on page 1014*

Mazicon™ *see* Flumazenil *on page 530*

MCH *see* Microfibrillar Collagen Hemostat *on page 836*

Measles and Rubella Vaccines, Combined

(MEE zels & roo BEL a vak SEENS, kom BINED)

Related Information

Adverse Events and Vaccination *on page 1439*

Immunization Guidelines *on page 1421*

Brand Names M-R-VAX® II

Synonyms Rubella and Measles Vaccines, Combined

Therapeutic Category Vaccine

Use Simultaneous immunization against measles and rubella

Pregnancy Risk Factor X

Contraindications Immune deficiency condition, pregnancy

Warnings/Precautions Pregnancy, immunocompromised persons, history of anaphylactic reaction following receipt of neomycin

Adverse Reactions All serious adverse reactions must be reported to the FDA

>10%:

Central nervous system: Fever <100°F

Dermatologic: Urticaria, rash, local erythema

Local: Burning at injection site, local tenderness

Neuromuscular & skeletal: Arthralgia

1% to 10%:

Central nervous system: Fever between 100°F and 103°F, malaise, headache

Gastrointestinal: Sore throat

Miscellaneous: Allergic reaction (delayed type), lymphadenopathy

<1%:

Central nervous system: Fatigue, convulsions, encephalitis, confusion, severe headache, fever >103°F (prolonged)

(Continued)

Measles and Rubella Vaccines, Combined *(Continued)*

Dermatologic: Itching, reddening of skin (especially around ears and eyes)
Gastrointestinal: Vomiting
Hematologic: Thrombocytopenic purpura
Neuromuscular & skeletal: Stiff neck
Ocular: Diplopia, optic neuritis
Respiratory: Dyspnea
Miscellaneous: Hypersensitivity

The chance of a child having a convulsion after receiving the measles vaccine is small. The risk is up to 5 times greater if the child has ever had a convulsion before or if the child's brother, sister, or parent has ever had a convulsion.

Drug Interactions Whole blood, immune globulin, immunosuppressive drugs should not be given within 1 month of other live virus vaccines except monovalent or trivalent polio vaccine; may temporarily depress tuberculin skin test sensitivity; decreased effect when immune globulin is given within 3 months and with concurrent use of corticosteroids and other immunosuppressant agents

Stability Refrigerate prior to use, use as soon as possible; discard if not used within 8 hours of reconstitution

Usual Dosage Children at 15 months and Adults: S.C.: Inject 0.5 mL into outer aspect of upper arm; no routine booster for rubella

Administration Not for I.V. administration

Patient Information Parents should monitor children closely for fever 5-11 days after vaccination

Females should not become pregnant within 3 months of vaccination

Measles vaccine:

A rash may occur from 1-2 weeks after receiving the measles vaccine; about 5 children out of every 100 will get a rash

A fever ≥103°F after receiving the first shot of measles vaccine, even though the child may not act sick. About 5-15 young children out of every 100 who receive the vaccine get such a fever. This could happen from 1-2 weeks after receiving the vaccine and usually lasts 1-2 days. The fever occurs less often after a second injection.

Rubella vaccine:

Swelling of the lymph glands in the neck or a rash that lasts 1-2 days; this could happen 1-2 weeks after getting the rubella vaccine in about 1/7 children who get the vaccine

Mild pain or stiffness in the joints that may last up to 3 days; this could happen from 1-3 weeks after getting the shot. this problem happens to about 1/100 children and 25/100 adults who are vaccinated. Women have this problem more than men and it may happen in up to 40 women out of every 100. Rarely, pain or stiffness can last for months or longer and can come and go.

Painful swelling of the joints (arthritis) happens to <1/100 children who get the rubella vaccine. About 10/100 adults can also have this problem, which usually lasts a few days to a week. Rarely, this swelling has been reported to last longer, or to come and go. Damage to the joints is very rare.

Pain or numbness, or "pins and needles" feeling in the hands and feet that lasts for a short time; this happens rarely

More serious problems: Children 6 months through 6 years of age who get the vaccines can, in rare cases, have a brief convulsion (fits, seizures, spasms, twitching, jerking, or staring spells). This usually occurs 1-2 weeks later, and usually comes from the fever caused by the measles vaccine. Very rarely, hearing loss has been reported, but it is not known whether hearing loss is caused by these vaccines. Rarely, a person can have inflammation of the brain after receiving the vaccine; this usually clears up completely.

Additional Information Federal law requires that the date of administration, the vaccine manufacturer, lot number of vaccine, and the administering person's name, title and address be entered into the patient's permanent medical record

Adults born before 1957 are generally considered to be immune to measles; all born in or after 1957 without documentation of live vaccine on or after first birthday, physician-diagnosed measles, or laboratory evidence of immunity should be vaccinated with two doses separated by or less than 1 month. For those previously vaccinated with one dose of measles vaccine, revaccination is indicated for students entering institutions of higher learning, for health care workers at time of employment, and for travelers to endemic areas. Guidelines for rubella vaccination are the same with the exception of birth year. All adults should be vaccinated against rubella. A booster dose of rubella vaccine is not necessary. Women who are pregnant when vaccinated or become pregnant within 3 months of vaccination should be consulted on the risks to the fetus; although the risks appear negligible. MMR is the vaccine of choice if recipients are likely to be susceptible to mumps as well as measles and rubella.

Dosage Forms Injection: 1000 $TCID_{50}$ each of live attenuated measles virus vaccine and live rubella virus vaccine

Measles, Mumps, and Rubella Vaccines, Combined

(MEE zels, mumpz & roo BEL a vak SEENS, kom BINED)

Related Information

Adverse Events and Vaccination *on page 1439*

Guidelines for the Prevention of Opportunistic Infections in Persons with HIV *on page 1457*

Immunization Guidelines *on page 1421*

Miscellaneous Vaccination Information *on page 1437*

Recommendations of the Advisory Committee on Immunization Practices (ACIP) *on page 1424*

Recommended Childhood Immunization Schedule - US - January-December, 1997 *on page 1423*

Brand Names M-M-R® II

Synonyms MMR; Mumps, Measles and Rubella Vaccines, Combined; Rubella, Measles and Mumps Vaccines, Combined

Therapeutic Category Vaccine

Use

Measles, mumps, and rubella prophylaxis in children (≥15 months) and adults

For HIV-infected children, MMR should routinely be administered at 15 months of age

Pregnancy Risk Factor X

Contraindications Blood dyscrasias, cancers affecting the bone marrow or lymphatic systems, known hypersensitivity to measles, mumps and rubella vaccine, known hypersensitivity to neomycin, acute infections, and respiratory illness, pregnancy; known hypersensitivity to eggs, chicken or chicken feathers, severely immunocompromised persons

Warnings/Precautions

Females should not become pregnant within 3 months of vaccination

MMR vaccine should not be given within 3 months of immune globulin or whole blood

Have epinephrine available during and after administration

MMR vaccine should not be administered to severely immunocompromised persons

Severely immunocompromised patients and symptomatic HIV-infected patients who are exposed to measles should receive immune globulin, regardless of prior vaccination status

The immunogenicity of measles virus vaccine is decreased if vaccine is administered <6 months after immune globulin

Adverse Reactions All serious adverse reactions must be reported to the FDA

1% to 10%:

Dermatologic: Transient rash, tenderness, erythema, edema

Gastrointestinal: Sore throat

Miscellaneous: Allergic reactions

<1%: Central nervous system: Seizures, malaise, fever

The chance of a child having a convulsion after receiving the measles vaccine is small. The risk is up to 5 times greater if the child has ever had a convulsion before or if the child's brother, sister, or parent has ever had a convulsion.

Drug Interactions Decreased effect when immune globulin is given within 3 months and with concurrent use of corticosteroids and other immunosuppressant agents; decreased effect with concurrent infection, immunoglobulin within 1 month, other live vaccines with the exception of attenuated measles, rubella, or polio

Stability Refrigerate, protect from light prior to reconstitution; use as soon as possible; discard 8 hours after reconstitution

Usual Dosage

Infants <12 months of age: If there is risk of exposure to measles, single-antigen measles vaccine should be administered at 6-11 months of age with a second dose (of MMR) at >12 months of age

Administer S.C. in outer aspect of the upper arm to children ≥15 months of age:

0.5 mL at 15 months of age and then repeated at 4-6 years* of age

In some areas, MMR vaccine may be given at 12 months

*Many experts recommend that this dose of MMR be given at entry to middle school or junior high school

Administration Not for I.V. administration

Test Interactions Temporary suppression of TB skin test reactivity with onset approximately 3 days after administration

Patient Information Females should not become pregnant within 3 months of vaccination

(Continued)

Measles, Mumps, and Rubella Vaccines, Combined *(Continued)*

Measles vaccine:

A rash may occur from 1-2 weeks after receiving the measles vaccine; about 5 children out of every 100 will get a rash

A fever ≥103°F after receiving the first shot of measles vaccine, even though the child may not act sick. About 5-15 young children out of every 100 who receive the vaccine get such a fever. This could happen from 1-2 weeks after receiving the vaccine and usually lasts 1-2 days. The fever occurs less often after a second injection.

Mumps vaccine: A little swelling of the glands in the cheeks and under the jaw that lasts for a few days; this could happen from 1-2 weeks after getting the mumps vaccine; this happens rarely

Rubella vaccine: Swelling of the lymph glands in the neck or a rash that lasts 1-2 days; this could happen 1-2 weeks after getting the rubella vaccine in about 1/7 children who get the vaccine

Mild pain or stiffness in the joints that may last up to 3 days; this could happen from 1-3 weeks after getting the shot. This problem happens to about 1/100 children and 25/100 adults who are vaccinated. Women have this problem more than men and it may happen in up to 40 women out of every 100. Rarely, pain or stiffness can last for months or longer and can come and go.

Painful swelling of the joints (arthritis) happens to <1/100 children who get the rubella vaccine. About 10/100 adults can also have this problem, which usually lasts a few days to a week. Rarely, this swelling has been reported to last longer, or to come and go. Damage to the joints is very rare.

Pain or numbness, or "pins and needles" feeling in the hands and feet that lasts for a short time; this happens rarely

More serious problems: Children 6 months through 6 years of age who get the vaccines can, in rare cases, have a brief convulsion (fits, seizures, spasms, twitching, jerking, or staring spells). This usually occurs 1-2 weeks later, and usually comes from the fever caused by the measles vaccine. Very rarely, hearing loss has been reported, but it is not known whether hearing loss is ever caused by these vaccines. Rarely, a person can have inflammation of the brain after receiving the vaccine. This usually clears up completely. These brain problems have been reported in 1/one million MMR injections.

Additional Information Live, attenuated vaccine. Federal law requires that the date of administration, the vaccine manufacturer, lot number of vaccine, and the administering person's name, title and address be entered into the patient's permanent medical record

Adults born before 1957 are generally considered to be immune to measles and mumps; all born in or after 1957 without documentation of live vaccine on or after first birthday, physician-diagnosed measles or mumps, or laboratory evidence of immunity should be vaccine with two doses separated by no less than 1 month; for those previously vaccinated with one dose of measles vaccine, revaccination is indicated for students entering institutions of higher learning, health care workers at time of employment, and for travelers to endemic areas. Guidelines for rubella vaccination are the same with the exception of birth year; all adults should be vaccinated against rubella. Booster doses of mumps and rubella are not necessary; women who are pregnant when vaccinated or become pregnant within 3 months should be counseled on the risks to the fetus; although the risks appear negligible.

Dosage Forms Injection: 1000 $TCID_{50}$ each of measles virus vaccine and rubella virus vaccine, 5000 $TCID_{50}$ mumps virus vaccine

Measles Virus Vaccine, Live (MEE zels VYE rus vak SEEN, live)

Related Information

Adverse Events and Vaccination *on page 1439*
Immunization Guidelines *on page 1421*
Miscellaneous Vaccination Information *on page 1437*
Prophylaxis for Patients Exposed to Common Communicable Diseases *on page 1452*
Recommendations for Travelers *on page 1442*

Brand Names Attenuvax®

Synonyms More Attenuated Enders Strain; Rubeola Vaccine

Therapeutic Category Vaccine, Live Virus

Use Adults born before 1957 are generally considered to be immune. All those born in or after 1957 without documentation of live vaccine on or after first birthday, physician-diagnosed measles, or laboratory evidence of immunity should be vaccinated, ideally with two doses of vaccine separated by no less than 1 month. For those previously vaccinated with one dose of measles vaccine, revaccination is recommended for students entering colleges and other institutions of higher education, for health care workers at the time of employment, and for international travelers who visit endemic areas.

MMR is the vaccine of choice if recipients are likely to be susceptible to rubella and/or mumps as well as to measles. Persons vaccinated between 1963 and 1967 with a killed measles vaccine, followed by live vaccine within 3 months, or with a vaccine of unknown type should be revaccinated with live measles virus vaccine.

Pregnancy Risk Factor X

Contraindications Pregnant females, known anaphylactoid reaction to eggs, known hypersensitivity to neomycin, acute respiratory infections, activated tuberculosis, immunosuppressed patients

Warnings/Precautions Avoid use in immunocompromised patients; defer administration in presence of acute respiratory or other active infections or inactive, untreated tuberculosis; avoid pregnancy for 3 months following vaccination; history of febrile seizures, hypersensitivity reactions may occur

Adverse Reactions All serious adverse reactions must be reported to the FDA

Central nervous system: Rarely encephalitis, fever, headache

Dermatologic: Rarely urticaria, erythema

>10%:

- Cardiovascular: Edema
- Central nervous system: Fever <100°F
- Local: Burning or stinging, induration

1% to 10%:

- Central nervous system: Fever between 100°F and 103°F
- Miscellaneous: Allergic reaction (delayed type)

<1%:

- Dermatologic: Urticaria, itching, reddening of skin (especially around ears and eyes)
- Central nervous system: Fatigue, convulsions, encephalitis, confusion, severe headache, fever >103°F (prolonged)
- Gastrointestinal: Vomiting, sore throat
- Hematologic: Thrombocytopenic purpura
- Ocular: Diplopia
- Neuromuscular & skeletal: Stiff neck
- Respiratory: Dyspnea
- Miscellaneous: Lymphadenopathy, coryza

Drug Interactions Whole blood, immune globulin, immunosuppressive drugs should not be given within 1 month of other live virus vaccines except monovalent or trivalent polio vaccine; may temporarily depress tuberculin skin test sensitivity

Stability Refrigerate at 2°C to 8°C (36°F to 46°F); discard if left at room temperature for over 8 hours; protect from light

Usual Dosage Children >15 months and Adults: S.C.: 0.5 mL in outer aspect of the upper arm, no routine boosters

Administration Vaccine should not be given I.V.; S.C. injection preferred

Test Interactions May temporarily depress tuberculin skin test sensitivity

Patient Information Parents should monitor children closely for fever for 5-11 days after vaccination; females should not become pregnant within 3 months of vaccination

Measles vaccine:

A rash may occur from 1-2 weeks after receiving the measles vaccine; about 5 children out of every 100 will get a rash

A fever ≥103°F after receiving the first shot of measles vaccine, even though the child may not act sick. About 5-15 young children out of every 100 who receive the vaccine get such a fever. This could happen from 1-2 weeks after receiving the vaccine and usually lasts 1-2 days. The fever occurs less often after a second injection.

Additional Information Federal law requires that the date of administration, the vaccine manufacturer, lot number of vaccine, and the administering person's name, title and address be entered into the patient's permanent medical record

Dosage Forms Injection: 1000 $TCID_{50}$ per dose

Measurin® [OTC] *see* Aspirin *on page 106*

Mebaral® *see* Mephobarbital *on page 781*

Mebendazole (me BEN da zole)

Brand Names Vermox®

Canadian/Mexican Brand Names Helminzole® (Mexico); Mebensole® (Mexico); Revapol® (Mexico); Soltric® (Mexico); Vermicol® (Mexico)

Therapeutic Category Anthelmintic

Use Treatment of pinworms, whipworms, roundworms, and hookworms

(Continued)

Mebendazole *(Continued)*

Pregnancy Risk Factor C

Contraindications Hypersensitivity to mebendazole or any component

Warnings/Precautions Pregnancy and children <2 years of age are relative contraindications since safety has not been established; not effective for hydatid disease

Adverse Reactions

1% to 10%: Gastrointestinal: Abdominal pain, diarrhea, nausea, vomiting

<1%:

Central nervous system: Fever, dizziness, headache
Dermatologic: Rash, itching, alopecia (with high doses)
Hematologic: Neutropenia (sore throat, unusual fatigue)
Neuromuscular & skeletal: Unusual weakness

Overdosage/Toxicology Symptoms of overdose include abdominal pain, altered mental status; GI decontamination and supportive care

Drug Interactions Decreased effect: Anticonvulsants such as carbamazepine and phenytoin may increase metabolism of mebendazole

Mechanism of Action Selectively and irreversibly blocks glucose uptake and other nutrients in susceptible adult intestine-dwelling helminths

Pharmacodynamics/Kinetics

Absorption: Only 2% to 10%
Protein binding: High, 95%
Metabolism: Extensive in the liver
Half-life: 1-11.5 hours
Time to peak serum concentration: Within 2-4 hours
Elimination: Primarily excreted in feces with 5% to 10% eliminated in urine

Usual Dosage Children and Adults: Oral:

Pinworms: 100 mg as a single dose; may need to repeat after 2 weeks; treatment should include family members in close contact with patient

Whipworms, roundworms, hookworms: One tablet twice daily, morning and evening on 3 consecutive days; if patient is not cured within 3-4 weeks, a second course of treatment may be administered

Capillariasis: 200 mg twice daily for 20 days

Dosing adjustment in hepatic impairment: Dosage reduction may be necessary in patients with liver dysfunction

Hemodialysis: Not dialyzable (0% to 5%)

Monitoring Parameters Check for helminth ova in feces within 3-4 weeks following the initial therapy

Test Interactions ↑ LFTs

Patient Information Tablets may be chewed, swallowed whole, or crushed and mixed with food; hygienic precautions should be taken to prevent reinfection such as wearing shoes and washing hands

Dosage Forms Tablet, chewable: 100 mg

Mecamylamine (mek a MIL a meen)

Brand Names Inversine®

Synonyms Mecamylamine Hydrochloride

Therapeutic Category Antihypertensive; Ganglionic Blocking Agent

Use Treatment of moderately severe to severe hypertension and in uncomplicated malignant hypertension

Pregnancy Risk Factor C

Contraindications Coronary insufficiency, pyloric stenosis, glaucoma, uremia, recent myocardial infarction, unreliable, uncooperative patients

Warnings/Precautions Use with caution in patients receiving sulfonamides or antibiotics that cause neuromuscular blockade; use with caution in patients with impaired renal function, previous CNS abnormalities, prostatic hypertrophy, bladder obstruction, or urethral strictive; do not abruptly discontinue

Adverse Reactions

>10%:

Cardiovascular: Postural hypotension
Central nervous system: Drowsiness
Endocrine & metabolic: Decreased sexual ability
Gastrointestinal: Xerostomia
Ocular: Blurred vision, enlarged pupils

1% to 10%:

Gastrointestinal: Loss of appetite, nausea, vomiting
Genitourinary: Dysuria

<1%:

Central nervous system: Convulsions, confusion, mental depression,
Gastrointestinal: Bloating, frequent stools, followed by severe constipation

Neuromuscular & skeletal: Uncontrolled movements of hands, arms, legs, or face, trembling

Respiratory: Shortness of breath

Overdosage/Toxicology Symptoms of overdose include hypotension, nausea, vomiting, urinary retention, constipation. Signs and symptoms are a direct result of ganglionic blockade

Treatment is supportive; pressor amines may be used to correct hypotension; use caution as patients will be unusually sensitive to these agents.

Drug Interactions Increased effect with sulfonamides and antibiotics that cause neuromuscular blockade

Mechanism of Action Mecamylamine is a ganglionic blocker. This agent inhibits acetylcholine at the autonomic ganglia, causing a decrease in blood pressure. Mecamylamine also blocks central nicotinic cholinergic receptors, which inhibits the effects of nicotine and may suppress the desire to smoke.

Usual Dosage Adults: Oral: 2.5 mg twice daily after meals for 2 days; increased by increments of 2.5 mg at intervals ≥2 days until desired blood pressure response is achieved; average daily dose: 25 mg

Dosing adjustment/comments in renal impairment: Use with caution, if at all, although no specific guidelines are available

Patient Information Take after meals at the same time each day; notify physician immediately if frequent loose bowel movements occur; rise slowly from sitting or lying for prolonged periods; do not restrict salt intake

Nursing Implications Check frequently for orthostatic hypotension; aid with ambulation

Dosage Forms Tablet, as hydrochloride: 2.5 mg

Mecamylamine Hydrochloride *see* Mecamylamine *on previous page*

Mechlorethamine (me klor ETH a meen)

Related Information

Antiemetics for Chemotherapy Induced Nausea and Vomiting *on page 1348*
Cancer Chemotherapy Regimens *on page 1351*
Extravasation Management of Chemotherapeutic Agents *on page 1379*
Toxicities of Chemotherapeutic Agents *on page 1382*

Brand Names Mustargen®

Synonyms HN_2; Mechlorethamine Hydrochloride; Mustine; Nitrogen Mustard

Therapeutic Category Antineoplastic Agent, Alkylating Agent; Antineoplastic Agent, Nitrogen Mustard; Vesicant

Use Combination therapy of Hodgkin's disease and malignant lymphomas; non-Hodgkin's lymphoma; palliative treatment of bronchogenic, breast and ovarian carcinoma; may be used by intracavitary injection for treatment of metastatic tumors; pleural and other malignant effusions; topical treatment of mycosis fungoides

Pregnancy Risk Factor D

Contraindications Hypersensitivity to mechlorethamine or any component; pre-existing profound myelosuppression or infection

Warnings/Precautions The U.S. Food and Drug Administration (FDA) currently recommends that procedures for proper handling and disposal of antineoplastic agents be considered. Extravasation of the drug into subcutaneous tissues results in painful inflammation and induration; sloughing may occur. Patients with lymphomas should receive prophylactic allopurinol 2-3 days prior to therapy to prevent complications resulting from tumor lysis.

Adverse Reactions

>10%:

Gastrointestinal: Nausea and vomiting usually occur in nearly 100% of patients and onset is within 30 minutes to 2 hours after administration

Emetic potential: High (>90%)

Time course of nausea/vomiting: Onset: 1-3 hours; duration 2-8 hours

Hematologic: Myelosuppressive: Leukopenia and thrombocytopenia can be severe; caution should be used with patients who are receiving radiotherapy, secondary leukemia

WBC: Severe
Platelets: Severe
Onset (days): 4-7
Nadir (days): 14
Recovery (days): 21

Endocrine & metabolic: Delayed menses, oligomenorrhea, temporary or permanent amenorrhea, impaired spermatogenesis; spermatogenesis may return in patients in remission several years after the discontinuation of chemotherapy, chromosomal abnormalities

Genitourinary: Azoospermia

Otic: Ototoxicity

(Continued)

Mechlorethamine *(Continued)*

Miscellaneous: Precipitation of herpes zoster

1% to 10%:

Central nervous system: Fever, vertigo

Dermatologic: Alopecia

Endocrine & metabolic: Hyperuricemia

Gastrointestinal: Diarrhea, anorexia, metallic taste

Local: Thrombophlebitis/extravasation: May cause local vein discomfort which may be relieved by warm soaks and pain medication. A brown discoloration of veins may occur. Mechlorethamine is a strong vesicant and can cause tissue necrosis and sloughing.

Vesicant chemotherapy

Secondary malignancies: Have been reported after several years in 1% to 6% of patients treated

Neuromuscular & skeletal: Weakness

Otic: Tinnitus

Miscellaneous: Hypersensitivity, anaphylaxis

<1%:

Central nervous system: Vertigo

Dermatologic: Rash

Gastrointestinal: Peptic ulcer

Hematologic: Myelosuppression, hemolytic anemia

Hepatic: Hepatotoxicity

Neuromuscular & skeletal: Peripheral neuropathy

Overdosage/Toxicology Suppression of all formed elements of the blood, uric acid crystals, nausea, vomiting, diarrhea

Sodium thiosulfate is the specific antidote for nitrogen mustard extravasations; treatment of systemic overdose is supportive

Stability Store intact vials at room temperature; dilute powder with 10 mL SWI to a final concentration of 1 mg/mL **Solution is highly unstable**; should be administered within 1 hour of dilution; may be diluted in up to 100 mL NS for intracavitary administration

Standard I.V. dilution:

I.V. push: Dose/syringe (concentration is 1 mg/mL)

Maximum syringe for IVP is 30 mL and syringe should be ≤75% full

MUST BE PREPARED FRESH; solution is stable for only 1 hour after dilution and must be administered within that time period

Mechanism of Action Alkylating agent that inhibits DNA and RNA synthesis via formation of carbonium ions; cross-links strands of DNA, causing miscoding, breakage, and failure of replication; produces interstrand and intrastrand cross-links in DNA resulting in miscoding, breakage, and failure of replication

Pharmacodynamics/Kinetics

Absorption: Incomplete absorption into blood stream following intracavitary administration secondary to rapid deactivation by body fluids

Metabolism: Following I.V. administration, drug undergoes rapid chemical transformation; unchanged drug is undetectable in the blood within a few minutes

Half-life: <1 minute

Elimination: <0.01% of unchanged drug is recovered in urine

Usual Dosage Refer to individual protocols. Dosage should be based on ideal dry weight; the presence of edema or ascites must be considered so that dosage will be based on actual weight unaugmented by these conditions

Children and Adults: MOPP: I.V.: 6 mg/m^2 on days 1 and 8 of a 28-day cycle

Adults:

I.V.: 0.4 mg/kg **OR** 12-16 mg/m^2 for one dose **OR** divided into 0.1 mg/kg/day for 4 days, repeated at 4- to 6-week intervals

Intracavitary: 10-20 mg diluted in 10 mL of SWI or 0.9% sodium chloride

Intrapericardially: 0.2-0.4 mg/kg diluted in up to 100 mL of 0.9% sodium chloride

Hemodialysis: Not removed; supplemental dosing is not required

Peritoneal dialysis: Not removed; supplemental dosing is not required

Topical mechlorethamine has been used in the treatment of cutaneous lesions of mycosis fungoides. A skin test should be performed prior to treatment with the topical preparation to detect sensitivity and possible irritation (use fresh mechlorethamine 0.1 mg/mL and apply over a 3 x 5 cm area of normal skin).

Administration Administer I.V. push through a free flowing I.V. over 1-3 minutes at a concentration not to exceed 1 mg/mL

Monitoring Parameters CBC with differential, hemoglobin, and platelet count

Patient Information Protect skin from contact, will burn and irritate. Any signs of infection, easy bruising or bleeding, shortness of breath, or painful or burning urination should be brought to physician's attention. Nausea, vomiting, or hair loss sometimes occur. The drug may cause permanent sterility and may cause birth defects. The drug may be excreted in breast milk, therefore, an alternative form of feeding your baby should be used.

Nursing Implications Use within 1 hour of preparation; avoid extravasation since mechlorethamine is a potent vesicant

Extravasation treatment: Sodium thiosulfate 1/6 molar solution is the specific antidote for nitrogen mustard extravasations and should be used as follows: Mix 4 mL of 10% sodium thiosulfate with 6 mL of sterile water for injection; inject 5-6 mL of this solution into the existing I.V. line; remove the needle; inject 2-3 mL of the solution S.C. clockwise into the infiltrated area using a 25-gauge needle; change the needle with each new injection; apply ice immediately for 6-12 hours.

Dosage Forms Powder for injection, as hydrochloride: 10 mg

Mechlorethamine Hydrochloride *see* Mechlorethamine *on page 767*

Meclan® *see* Meclocycline *on next page*

Meclizine (MEK li zeen)

Brand Names Antivert®; Antrizine®; Bonine® [OTC]; Dizmiss® [OTC]; Dramamine® II [OTC]; Meni-D®; Ru-Vert-M®; Vergon® [OTC]

Canadian/Mexican Brand Names Bonamine®

Synonyms Meclizine Hydrochloride; Meclozine Hydrochloride

Therapeutic Category Antiemetic; Antihistamine, H_1 Blocker

Use Prevention and treatment of symptoms of motion sickness; management of vertigo with diseases affecting the vestibular system

Pregnancy Risk Factor B

Pregnancy/Breast-Feeding Implications

Clinical effects on the fetus: No data available on crossing the placenta. Probably no effect on the fetus (insufficient data). Available evidence suggests safe use during pregnancy.

Breast-feeding/lactation: No data available

Contraindications Hypersensitivity to meclizine or any component; pregnancy

Warnings/Precautions Use with caution in patients with angle-closure glaucoma, prostatic hypertrophy, pyloric or duodenal obstruction, or bladder neck obstruction; use with caution in hot weather, and during exercise; elderly may be at risk for anticholinergic side effects such as glaucoma, prostatic hypertrophy, constipation, gastrointestinal obstructive disease; if vertigo does not respond in 1-2 weeks, it is advised to discontinue use

Adverse Reactions

>10%:
- Central nervous system: Slight to moderate drowsiness
- Respiratory: Thickening of bronchial secretions

1% to 10%:
- Central nervous system: Headache, fatigue, nervousness, dizziness
- Gastrointestinal: Appetite increase, weight gain, nausea, diarrhea, abdominal pain, xerostomia
- Neuromuscular & skeletal: Arthralgia
- Respiratory: Pharyngitis

<1%:
- Cardiovascular: Palpitations, hypotension
- Central nervous system: Depression, sedation
- Dermatologic: Photosensitivity, rash, angioedema
- Genitourinary: Urinary retention
- Hepatic: Hepatitis
- Neuromuscular & skeletal: Myalgia, tremor, paresthesia
- Ocular: Blurred vision
- Respiratory: Bronchospasm, epistaxis

Overdosage/Toxicology Symptoms of overdose include CNS depression, confusion, nervousness, hallucinations, dizziness, blurred vision, nausea, vomiting, hyperthermia

There is no specific treatment for an antihistamine overdose, however, most of its clinical toxicity is due to anticholinergic effects. For anticholinergic overdose with severe life-threatening symptoms, physostigmine 1-2 mg (0.5 or 0.02 mg/kg for children) I.V., slowly may be given to reverse these effects.

Drug Interactions Increased toxicity: CNS depressants, neuroleptics, anticholinergics

Mechanism of Action Has central anticholinergic action by blocking chemoreceptor trigger zone; decreases excitability of the middle ear labyrinth and blocks conduction in the middle ear vestibular-cerebellar pathways

Pharmacodynamics/Kinetics

Onset of action: Oral: Within 1 hour

Duration: 8-24 hours

Metabolism: Reportedly in the liver

(Continued)

Meclizine *(Continued)*

Half-life: 6 hours
Elimination: As metabolites in urine and as unchanged drug in feces

Usual Dosage Children >12 years and Adults: Oral:
Motion sickness: 12.5-25 mg 1 hour before travel, repeat dose every 12-24 hours if needed; doses up to 50 mg may be needed
Vertigo: 25-100 mg/day in divided doses

Dietary Considerations Alcohol: Additive CNS effect, avoid use

Patient Information Take after meals; do not discontinue drug abruptly; notify physician if adverse GI effects, fever, or heat intolerance occurs; may cause drowsiness; avoid alcohol; adequate fluid intake, sugar free gum or hard candy may help dry mouth; adequate fluid and exercise may help constipation

Dosage Forms
Capsule, as hydrochloride: 15 mg, 25 mg, 30 mg
Tablet, as hydrochloride: 12.5 mg, 25 mg, 50 mg
Tablet, as hydrochloride:
Chewable: 25 mg
Film coated: 25 mg

Meclizine Hydrochloride *see* Meclizine *on previous page*

Meclocycline (me kloe SYE kleen)

Brand Names Meclan®

Synonyms Meclocycline Sulfosalicylate

Therapeutic Category Antibiotic, Topical; Topical Skin Product, Acne

Use Topical treatment of inflammatory acne vulgaris

Pregnancy Risk Factor B

Contraindications Known hypersensitivity to tetracyclines or any component

Warnings/Precautions Use with caution in patients allergic to formaldehyde; for external use only

Adverse Reactions
>10%: Topical: Follicular staining, yellowing of the skin, burning/stinging feeling
1% to 10%: Topical: Pain, redness, skin irritation, dermatitis

Mechanism of Action Inhibits bacterial protein synthesis by binding with the 30S and possibly the 50S ribosomal subunit(s) of susceptible bacteria; may also cause alterations in the cytoplasmic membrane

Pharmacodynamics/Kinetics Absorption: Topical: Very little

Usual Dosage Children >11 years and Adults: Topical: Apply generously to affected areas twice daily

Patient Information Apply generously until skin is wet; avoid contact with eyes, nose, and mouth; stinging may occur with application, but soon stops; if skin is discolored yellow, washing will remove the color

Dosage Forms Cream, topical, as sulfosalicylate: 1% (20 g, 45 g)

Meclocycline Sulfosalicylate *see* Meclocycline *on this page*

Meclofenamate (me kloe fen AM ate)

Related Information
Dosing Data for Acetaminophen and NSAIDs *on page 1377*
Nonsteroidal Anti-Inflammatory Agents Comparison *on page 1419*

Brand Names Meclomen®

Synonyms Meclofenamate Sodium

Therapeutic Category Analgesic, Nonsteroidal Anti-inflammatory Drug; Anti-inflammatory Agent; Nonsteroidal Anti-inflammatory Agent (NSAID), Oral

Use Treatment of inflammatory disorders

Pregnancy Risk Factor B (D if used in the 3rd trimester)

Contraindications Active GI bleeding, ulcer disease, hypersensitivity to aspirin, meclofenamate, or other NSAIDs

Warnings/Precautions May have adverse effects on fetus

Adverse Reactions
>10%:
Central nervous system: Dizziness
Dermatologic: Rash
Gastrointestinal: Abdominal cramps, heartburn, indigestion, nausea
1% to 10%:
Central nervous system: Headache, nervousness
Dermatologic: Itching
Endocrine & metabolic: Fluid retention
Gastrointestinal: Vomiting
Otic: Tinnitus
<1%:
Cardiovascular: Congestive heart failure, hypertension, arrhythmia, tachycardia

Central nervous system: Confusion, hallucinations, aseptic meningitis, mental depression, drowsiness, insomnia
Dermatologic: Urticaria, erythema multiforme, toxic epidermal necrolysis, Stevens-Johnson syndrome, angioedema
Endocrine & metabolic: Polydipsia, hot flashes
Gastrointestinal: Gastritis, GI ulceration
Genitourinary: Cystitis, polyuria
Hematologic: Agranulocytosis, anemia, hemolytic anemia, bone marrow suppression, leukopenia, thrombocytopenia
Hepatic: Hepatitis
Neuromuscular & skeletal: Peripheral neuropathy
Ocular: Toxic amblyopia, blurred vision, conjunctivitis, dry eyes
Otic: Decreased hearing
Renal: Acute renal failure
Respiratory: Allergic rhinitis, shortness of breath, epistaxis

Overdosage/Toxicology Symptoms of overdose include drowsiness, lethargy, nausea, vomiting, seizures, paresthesia, headache, dizziness, GI bleeding, cerebral edema, cardiac arrest, tinnitus

Management of a nonsteroidal anti-inflammatory drug (NSAID) intoxication is primarily supportive and symptomatic. Fluid therapy is commonly effective in managing the hypotension that may occur following an acute NSAID overdose, except when this is due to an acute blood loss. Seizures tend to be very short-lived and often do not require drug treatment. Although, recurrent seizures should be treated with I.V. diazepam. Since many of the NSAID undergo enterohepatic cycling, multiple doses of charcoal may be needed to reduce the potential for delayed toxicities.

Drug Interactions
Decreased effect with aspirin; decreased effect of diuretics, antihypertensives
Increased effect/toxicity of warfarin, methotrexate

Mechanism of Action Inhibits prostaglandin synthesis by decreasing the activity of the enzyme, cyclo-oxygenase, which results in decreased formation of prostaglandin precursors

Pharmacodynamics/Kinetics
Duration of action: 2-4 hours
Distribution: Crosses the placenta
Protein binding: 99%
Half-life: 2-3.3 hours
Time to peak serum concentration: Within 0.5-1.5 hours
Elimination: Principally in urine and in feces as glucuronide conjugates

Usual Dosage Children >14 years and Adults: Oral:
Mild to moderate pain: 50 mg every 4-6 hours, not to exceed 400 mg/day
Rheumatoid arthritis/osteoarthritis: 200-400 mg/day in 3-4 equal doses

Test Interactions ↑ chloride (S), ↑ sodium (S)

Patient Information Take with food, milk, or with antacids

Nursing Implications Should be used for short-term only (<7 days); advise patient to report persistent GI discomfort, sore throat, fever, or malaise

Dosage Forms Capsule, as sodium: 50 mg, 100 mg

Meclofenamate Sodium *see* Meclofenamate *on previous page*

Meclomen® *see* Meclofenamate *on previous page*

Meclozine Hydrochloride *see* Meclizine *on page 769*

Medicinal Carbon *see* Charcoal *on page 245*

Medicinal Charcoal *see* Charcoal *on page 245*

Medigesic® *see* Butalbital Compound *on page 176*

Medihaler-Iso® *see* Isoproterenol *on page 681*

Mediplast® Plaster [OTC] *see* Salicylic Acid *on page 1120*

Medipren® [OTC] *see* Ibuprofen *on page 639*

Medi-Quick® Topical Ointment [OTC] *see* Bacitracin, Neomycin, and Polymyxin B *on page 129*

Medi-Tuss® [OTC] *see* Guaifenesin *on page 589*

Medralone® *see* Methylprednisolone *on page 819*

Medrol® *see* Methylprednisolone *on page 819*

Medroxyprogesterone Acetate

(me DROKS ee proe JES te rone AS e tate)

Brand Names Amen®; Curretab®; Cycrin®; Depo-Provera®; Provera®

Synonyms Acetoxymethylprogesterone; Methylacetoxyprogesterone

Therapeutic Category Contraceptive, Parenteral (Progestin); Progestin Derivative

Use Endometrial carcinoma or renal carcinoma as well as secondary amenorrhea or abnormal uterine bleeding due to hormonal imbalance; prevention of pregnancy

(Continued)

Medroxyprogesterone Acetate *(Continued)*

Pregnancy Risk Factor X

Contraindications Pregnancy, thrombophlebitis; hypersensitivity to medroxyprogesterone or any component; cerebral apoplexy, undiagnosed vaginal bleeding, liver dysfunction

Warnings/Precautions Use with caution in patients with depression, diabetes, epilepsy, asthma, migraines, renal or cardiac dysfunction; pretreatment exams should include PAP smear, physical exam of breasts and pelvic areas. May increase serum cholesterol, LDL, decrease HDL and triglycerides; use of any progestin during the first 4 months of pregnancy is not recommended; monitor patient closely for loss of vision, sudden onset of proptosis, diplopia, migraine, and signs and symptoms of thromboembolic disorders.

Adverse Reactions

>10%:

- Cardiovascular: Edema
- Endocrine & metabolic: Breakthrough bleeding, spotting, changes in menstrual flow, amenorrhea
- Gastrointestinal: Anorexia
- Local: Pain at injection site
- Neuromuscular & skeletal: Weakness

1% to 10%:

- Cardiovascular: Embolism, central thrombosis
- Central nervous system: Mental depression, fever, insomnia
- Dermatologic: Melasma or chloasma, allergic rash with or without pruritus
- Endocrine & metabolic: Changes in cervical erosion and secretions, increased breast tenderness
- Gastrointestinal: Weight gain or loss
- Hepatic: Cholestatic jaundice
- Local: Thrombophlebitis

Overdosage/Toxicology Toxicity is unlikely following single exposures of excessive doses; supportive treatment is adequate in most cases

Drug Interactions Decreased effect: Aminoglutethimide may decrease effects by increasing hepatic metabolism

Mechanism of Action Inhibits secretion of pituitary gonadotropins, which prevents follicular maturation and ovulation, stimulates growth of mammary tissue

Pharmacodynamics/Kinetics

Absorption: I.M.: Slow
Metabolism: Oral: In the liver
Elimination: Oral: In urine and feces

Usual Dosage

Adolescents and Adults: Oral:

- Amenorrhea: 5-10 mg/day for 5-10 days or 2.5 mg/day
- Abnormal uterine bleeding: 5-10 mg for 5-10 days starting on day 16 or 21 of cycle
- Accompanying cyclic estrogen therapy, postmenopausal: 2.5-10 mg the last 10-13 days of estrogen dosing each month

Adults: I.M.:

- Endometrial or renal carcinoma: 400-1000 mg/week
- Contraception: 150 mg every 3 months or 450 mg every 6 months

Dosing adjustment in hepatic impairment: Dose needs to be lowered in patients with alcoholic cirrhosis

Monitoring Parameters Monitor patient closely for loss of vision, sudden onset of proptosis, diplopia, migraine, and signs and symptoms of thromboembolic disorders

Test Interactions Altered thyroid and liver function tests

Patient Information Take this medicine only as directed; do not take more of it and do not take it for a longer period of time; if you suspect you may have become pregnant, stop taking this medicine; notify physician if sudden loss of vision or migraine headache occurs; may cause photosensitivity, wear protective clothing or sunscreen

Nursing Implications Patients should receive a copy of the patient labeling for the drug

Dosage Forms

Injection, suspension: 100 mg/mL (5 mL); 150 mg/mL (1 mL); 400 mg/mL (1 mL, 2.5 mL, 10 mL)
Tablet: 2.5 mg, 5 mg, 10 mg

Medrysone (ME dri sone)

Brand Names HMS Liquifilm®

Therapeutic Category Anti-inflammatory Agent, Ophthalmic; Corticosteroid, Ophthalmic

Use Treatment of allergic conjunctivitis, vernal conjunctivitis, episcleritis, ophthalmic epinephrine sensitivity reaction

Pregnancy Risk Factor C

Contraindications Fungal, viral, or untreated pus-forming bacterial ocular infections; not for use in iritis and uveitis

Warnings/Precautions Prolonged use has been associated with the development of corneal or scleral perforation and posterior subcapsular cataracts; may mask or enhance the establishment of acute purulent untreated infections of the eye; effectiveness and safety have not been established in children. Medrysone is a synthetic corticosteroid; structurally related to progesterone; if no improvement after several days of treatment, discontinue medrysone and institute other therapy; duration of therapy: 3-4 days to several weeks dependent on type and severity of disease; taper dose to avoid disease exacerbation.

Adverse Reactions

1% to 10%: Ocular: Temporary mild blurred vision

<1%: Ocular: Stinging, burning eyes, corneal thinning, increased intraocular pressure, glaucoma, damage to the optic nerve, defects in visual activity, cataracts, secondary ocular infection

Overdosage/Toxicology Systemic toxicity is unlikely from the ophthalmic preparation

Mechanism of Action Decreases inflammation by suppression of migration of polymorphonuclear leukocytes and reversal of increased capillary permeability

Pharmacodynamics/Kinetics

Absorption: Through aqueous humor

Metabolism: Any drug absorbed is metabolized in the liver

Elimination: By the kidneys and feces

Usual Dosage Children and Adults: Ophthalmic: Instill 1 drop in conjunctival sac 2-4 times/day up to every 4 hours; may use every 1-2 hours during first 1-2 days

Monitoring Parameters Intraocular pressure and periodic examination of lens (with prolonged use)

Patient Information Shake well before using, do not touch dropper to the eye

Dosage Forms Solution, ophthalmic: 1% (5 mL, 10 mL)

Mefenamic Acid (me fe NAM ik AS id)

Related Information

Dosing Data for Acetaminophen and NSAIDs *on page 1377*

Nonsteroidal Anti-Inflammatory Agents Comparison *on page 1419*

Brand Names Ponstel®

Canadian/Mexican Brand Names Ponstan® (Canada); Ponstan-500® (Mexico)

Therapeutic Category Analgesic, Nonsteroidal Anti-inflammatory Drug; Anti-inflammatory Agent; Nonsteroidal Anti-inflammatory Agent (NSAID), Oral

Use Short-term relief of mild to moderate pain including primary dysmenorrhea

Pregnancy Risk Factor C

Contraindications Known hypersensitivity to mefenamic acid or other NSAIDs

Warnings/Precautions May have adverse effects on fetus

Adverse Reactions

>10%:

Central nervous system: Dizziness

Dermatologic: Rash

Gastrointestinal: Abdominal cramps, heartburn, indigestion, nausea

1% to 10%:

Central nervous system: Headache, nervousness

Dermatologic: Itching

Endocrine & metabolic: Fluid retention

Gastrointestinal: Vomiting

Otic: Tinnitus

<1%:

Cardiovascular: Congestive heart failure, hypertension, arrhythmias, tachycardia

Central nervous system: Confusion, hallucinations, aseptic meningitis, mental depression, drowsiness, insomnia

Dermatologic: Urticaria, erythema multiforme, toxic epidermal necrolysis, Stevens-Johnson syndrome, angioedema

Endocrine & metabolic: Polydipsia, hot flashes

Gastrointestinal: Gastritis, GI ulceration

Genitourinary: Cystitis, polyuria

Hematologic: Agranulocytosis, anemia, hemolytic anemia, bone marrow suppression, leukopenia, thrombocytopenia

Hepatic: Hepatitis

Neuromuscular & skeletal: Peripheral neuropathy

Ocular: Toxic amblyopia, blurred vision, conjunctivitis, dry eyes

Otic: Decreased hearing

(Continued)

Mefenamic Acid *(Continued)*

Renal: Acute renal failure

Respiratory: Shortness of breath, allergic rhinitis, epistaxis

Overdosage/Toxicology Symptoms of overdose include CNS stimulation, agitation, seizures

Management of a nonsteroidal anti-inflammatory drug (NSAID) intoxication is primarily supportive and symptomatic. Fluid therapy is commonly effective in managing the hypotension that may occur following an acute NSAIDs overdose, except when this is due to an acute blood loss. Seizures tend to be very short-lived and often do not require drug treatment. Although, recurrent seizures should be treated with I.V. diazepam. Since many of the NSAID undergo enterohepatic cycling, multiple doses of charcoal may be needed to reduce the potential for delayed toxicities.

Drug Interactions

Decreased effect of diuretics, antihypertensives; decreased effect with aspirin

Increased effect/toxicity with oral anticoagulants, methotrexate

Mechanism of Action Inhibits prostaglandin synthesis by decreasing the activity of the enzyme, cyclo-oxygenase, which results in decreased formation of prostaglandin precursors

Pharmacodynamics/Kinetics

Peak effect: Oral: Within 2-4 hours

Duration of action: Up to 6 hours

Protein binding: High

Metabolism: Conjugated in the liver

Half-life: 3.5 hours

Elimination: In urine (50%) and feces as unchanged drug and metabolites

Usual Dosage Children >14 years and Adults: Oral: 500 mg to start then 250 mg every 4 hours as needed; maximum therapy: 1 week

Dosing adjustment/comments in renal impairment: Not recommended for use

Test Interactions ↑ chloride (S), ↑ sodium (S), positive Coombs' [direct], false-positive urinary bilirubin

Patient Information Take with food, milk, or with antacids; extended release capsules must be swallowed intact

Dosage Forms Capsule: 250 mg

Mefloquine (ME floe kwin)

Related Information

Prevention of Malaria *on page 1441*

Brand Names Lariam®

Synonyms Mefloquine Hydrochloride

Therapeutic Category Antimalarial Agent

Use Treatment of acute malarial infections and prevention of malaria

Pregnancy Risk Factor C

Contraindications Hypersensitivity to any component

Warnings/Precautions Caution is warranted with lactation; discontinue if unexplained neuropsychiatric disturbances occur, caution in epilepsy patients or in patients with significant cardiac disease. If mefloquine is to be used for a prolonged period, periodic evaluations including liver function tests and ophthalmic examinations should be performed. (Retinal abnormalities have not been observed with mefloquine in humans; however, it has with long-term administration to rats.) In cases of life-threatening, serious, or overwhelming malaria infections due to *Plasmodium falciparum*, patients should be treated with intravenous antimalarial drug. Mefloquine may be given orally to complete the course. Caution should be exercised with regard to driving, piloting airplanes, and operating machines since dizziness, disturbed sense of balance; neuropsychiatric reactions have been reported with mefloquine.

Adverse Reactions

1% to 10%:

Central nervous system: Difficulty concentrating, headache, insomnia, lightheadedness, vertigo

Gastrointestinal: Vomiting, diarrhea, stomach pain, nausea

Ocular: Visual disturbances

Otic: Tinnitus

<1%:

Cardiovascular: Bradycardia, extrasystoles, syncope

Central nervous system: Anxiety, dizziness, confusion, seizures, hallucinations, mental depression, psychosis

Overdosage/Toxicology Symptoms of overdose include vomiting, diarrhea; cardiotoxic; following GI contamination supportive care only

Drug Interactions

Decreased effect of valproic acid

Increased toxicity with beta-blockers; increased toxicity/levels of chloroquine, quinine, quinidine (hold treatment until at least 12 hours after these drugs)

Mechanism of Action Mefloquine is a quinoline-methanol compound structurally similar to quinine; mefloquine's effectiveness in the treatment and prophylaxis of malaria is due to the destruction of the asexual blood forms of the malarial pathogens that affect humans, *Plasmodium falciparum, P. vivax, P. malariae, P. ovale*

Pharmacodynamics/Kinetics

Absorption: Oral: Well absorbed

Distribution: V_d: 19 L/kg; concentrates in erythrocytes; appears in breast milk

Protein binding: 98%

Half-life: 21-22 days

Elimination: ~1.5% to 9% of dose excreted unchanged in urine

Usual Dosage Oral:

Children: Malaria prophylaxis:

- 15-19 kg: 1/4 tablet
- 20-30 kg: 1/2 tablet
- 31-45 kg: 3/4 tablet
- >45 kg: 1 tablet
- Administer weekly starting 1 week before travel, continuing weekly during travel and for 4 weeks after leaving endemic area

Adults:

- Treatment of mild to moderate malaria infection: 5 tablets (1250 mg) as a single dose with at least 8 oz of water
- Malaria prophylaxis: 1 tablet (250 mg) weekly starting 1 week before travel, continuing weekly during travel and for 4 weeks after leaving endemic area

Patient Information Begin therapy before trip and continue after; do not take drug on empty stomach; take with food and at least 8 oz of water; women of childbearing age should use reliable contraception during prophylaxis treatment and for 2 months after the last dose; be aware of signs and symptoms of malaria when traveling to an endemic area. Caution should be exercised with regard to driving, piloting airplanes, and operating machines since dizziness, disturbed sense of balance, or neuropsychiatric reactions have been reported with mefloquine.

Dosage Forms Tablet, as hydrochloride: 250 mg

Mefloquine Hydrochloride *see* Mefloquine *on previous page*

Mefoxin® *see* Cefoxitin *on page 229*

Mega-B® [OTC] *see* Vitamins, Multiple *on page 1310*

Megace® *see* Megestrol Acetate *on this page*

Megestrol Acetate (me JES trole AS e tate)

Brand Names Megace®

Therapeutic Category Antineoplastic Agent, Hormone; Progestin Derivative

Use Palliative treatment of breast and endometrial carcinomas, appetite stimulation, and promotion of weight gain in cachexia

Pregnancy Risk Factor X

Contraindications Hypersensitivity to megestrol or any component

Warnings/Precautions The U.S. Food and Drug Administration (FDA) currently recommends that procedures for proper handling and disposal of antineoplastic agents be considered. Use during the first few months of pregnancy is not recommended. Use with caution in patients with a history of thrombophlebitis. Elderly females may have vaginal bleeding or discharge and need to be forewarned of this side effect and inconvenience.

Adverse Reactions

>10%:

- Cardiovascular: Edema
- Endocrine & metabolic: Breakthrough bleeding and amenorrhea, spotting, changes in menstrual flow
- Neuromuscular & skeletal: Weakness

1% to 10%:

- Central nervous system: Insomnia, depression, fever, headache
- Dermatologic: Allergic rash with or without pruritus, melasma or chloasma, rash, and rarely alopecia
- Endocrine & metabolic: Changes in cervical erosion and secretions, increased breast tenderness, amenorrhea, changes in vaginal bleeding pattern, edema, fluid retention, hyperglycemia
- Gastrointestinal: Weight gain (not attributed to edema or fluid retention), nausea, vomiting, stomach cramps
- Hepatic: Cholestatic jaundice, hepatotoxicity

(Continued)

Megestrol Acetate *(Continued)*

Hematologic: Myelosuppressive:
WBC: None
Platelets: None
Local: Thrombophlebitis
Neuromuscular & skeletal: Carpal tunnel syndrome
Respiratory: Hyperpnea

Overdosage/Toxicology Toxicity is unlikely following simple exposures of excessive doses

Mechanism of Action A synthetic progestin with antiestrogenic properties which disrupt the estrogen receptor cycle. Megace® interferes with the normal estrogen cycle and results in a lower LH titer. May also have a direct effect on the endometrium. Megestrol is an antineoplastic progestin thought to act through an antileutenizing effect mediated via the pituitary.

Pharmacodynamics/Kinetics

Onset of action: At least 2 months of continuous therapy is necessary
Absorption: Oral: Well absorbed
Metabolism: Completely metabolized in the liver to free steroids and glucuronide conjugates
Time to peak serum concentration: Oral: Within 1-3 hours
Half-life, elimination: 15-20 hours
Elimination: In urine as steroid metabolites and inactive compound, some in feces and bile

Usual Dosage Adults: Oral (refer to individual protocols):

Female:
Breast carcinoma: 40 mg 4 times/day
Endometrial: 40-320 mg/day in divided doses; use for 2 months to determine efficacy; maximum doses used have been up to 800 mg/day
Uterine bleeding: 40 mg 2-4 times/day
Male and Female: HIV-related cachexia: Initial dose: 800 mg/day; daily doses of 400 and 800 mg/day were found to be clinically effective

Monitoring Parameters Monitor for tumor response; observe for signs of thromboembolic phenomena; monitor for thromboembolism

Test Interactions Altered thyroid and liver function tests

Patient Information Exposure to megestrol during the first 4 months of pregnancy may pose risks to the fetus; notify physician if sudden loss of vision, double vision, migraine headache occur, or if pain in calves with warmth and tenderness develops; may cause photosensitivity, wear protective clothing or sunscreen

Dosage Forms

Suspension, oral: 40 mg/mL with alcohol 0.06% (236.6 mL)
Tablet: 20 mg, 40 mg

Melanex® *see* Hydroquinone *on page 628*
Mellaril® *see* Thioridazine *on page 1219*
Mellaril-S® *see* Thioridazine *on page 1219*
Melpaque HP® *see* Hydroquinone *on page 628*

Melphalan (MEL fa lan)

Related Information

Antiemetics for Chemotherapy Induced Nausea and Vomiting *on page 1348*
Cancer Chemotherapy Regimens *on page 1351*
Toxicities of Chemotherapeutic Agents *on page 1382*

Brand Names Alkeran®

Synonyms L-PAM; L-Sarcolysin; Phenylalanine Mustard

Therapeutic Category Antineoplastic Agent, Alkylating Agent; Antineoplastic Agent, Nitrogen Mustard

Use Palliative treatment of multiple myeloma and nonresectable epithelial ovarian carcinoma; neuroblastoma, rhabdomyosarcoma, breast cancer

Pregnancy Risk Factor D

Contraindications Hypersensitivity to melphalan or any component; severe bone marrow suppression; patients whose disease was resistant to prior therapy

Warnings/Precautions The U.S. Food and Drug Administration (FDA) currently recommends that procedures for proper handling and disposal for antineoplastic agents be considered. Is potentially mutagenic, carcinogenic, and teratogenic; produces amenorrhea. Reduce dosage or discontinue therapy if leukocyte count $<3000/mm^3$ or platelet count $<100,000/mm^3$; use with caution in patients with bone marrow suppression, impaired renal function, or who have received prior chemotherapy or irradiation; will cause amenorrhea. Toxicity to immunosuppressives is increased in elderly. Start with lowest recommended adult doses. Signs of infection, such as fever and WBC rise, may not occur. Lethargy and confusion may be more prominent signs of infection.

Adverse Reactions

>10%

Hematologic: Myelosuppressive: Leukopenia and thrombocytopenia are the most common effects of melphalan. Irreversible bone marrow failure has been reported.

WBC: Moderate

Platelets: Moderate

Onset (days): 7

Nadir (days): 8-10 and 27-32

Recovery (days): 42-50

Second malignancies: Reported are melphalan more frequently

1% to 10%:

Cardiovascular: Vasculitis

Dermatologic: Vesiculation of skin, alopecia, pruritus, rash

Endocrine & metabolic: SIADH, sterility and amenorrhea

Gastrointestinal: Nausea and vomiting are mild; stomatitis and diarrhea are infrequent

Genitourinary: Bladder irritation, hemorrhagic cystitis

Hematologic: Anemia, agranulocytosis, hemolytic anemia

Respiratory: Pulmonary fibrosis, interstitial pneumonitis

Miscellaneous: Hypersensitivity

Overdosage/Toxicology Symptoms of overdose include hypocalcemia, pulmonary fibrosis, nausea and vomiting, bone marrow suppression

Drug Interactions

Decreased effect: Cimetidine and other H_2-antagonists: The reduction in gastric pH has been reported to ↓ bioavailability of melphalan by 30%

Increased toxicity: Cyclosporine: ↑ incidence of nephrotoxicity

Stability

Tablets/injection: Protect from light, store at room temperature (15°C to 30°C)

The time between reconstitution/dilution and administration of parenteral melphalan must be kept to a minimum (<60 minutes) because reconstituted and diluted solutions are unstable

Injection: Preparation:

Dissolve powder initially with 10 mL of diluent to a concentration of 5 mg/mL. This solution is chemically and physically stable for at least 90 minutes when stored at 25°C (77°F).

Immediately dilute dose in 0.9% sodium chloride to a concentration of 0.1-0.45 mg/mL. This solution is physically and chemically stable for at least 60 minutes at 25°C (77°F). HIGHLY UNSTABLE SOLUTION - administration should occur within one hour of dissolution. Do not refrigeration solution - precipitation occurs.

Standard I.V. dilution:

Dose/250-500 mL NS (concentration of 0.1-0.45 mg/mL)

MUST BE PREPARED FRESH - solution is stable for 1 hour after dilution and must be administered within that time period

Mechanism of Action Alkylating agent which is a derivative of mechlorethamine that inhibits DNA and RNA synthesis via formation of carbonium ions; cross-links strands of DNA

Pharmacodynamics/Kinetics

Absorption: Oral: Variable and incomplete from the GI tract; food interferes with absorption

Distribution: V_d: 0.5-0.6 L/kg throughout total body water

Bioavailability: Unpredictable, decreasing from 85% to 58%

Half-life, terminal: 1.5 hours

Time to peak serum concentration: Reportedly within 2 hours

Elimination: 10% to 30% of a dose excreted unchanged in the urine; 20% to 50% excreted in the stool after oral administration

Usual Dosage

Oral (refer to individual protocols); dose should always be adjusted to patient response and weekly blood counts:

Children: 4-20 mg/m^2/day for 1-21 days

Adults:

Multiple myeloma: 6 mg/day initially adjusted as indicated **or** 0.15 mg/kg/day for 7 days **or** 0.25 mg/kg/day for 4 days; repeat at 4- to 6-week intervals

Ovarian carcinoma: 0.2 mg/kg/day for 5 days, repeat every 4-5 weeks

Intravenous (refer to individual protocols):

Children:

Pediatric rhabdomyosarcoma: 10-35 mg/m^2/dose every 21-28 days

High-dose melphalan with bone marrow transplantation for neuroblastoma: 70-100 mg/m^2/day on day 7 and 6 before BMT, or 140-220 mg/m^2 single dose before BMT **or** 50 mg/m^2/day for 4 days; **or** 70 mg/m^2/day for 3 days

(Continued)

Melphalan *(Continued)*

Adults:

Multiple myeloma: 16 mg/m^2 administered at 2-week intervals for 4 doses, then repeat monthly as per protocol for multiple myeloma

Dosing adjustment in renal impairment:

Cl_{cr} 10-50 mL/minute: Administer at 75% of normal dose

Cl_{cr} <10 mL/minute: Administer at 50% of normal dose

OR

BUN >30 mg/dL: Reduce dose by 50%

Serum creatinine >1.5 mg/dL: Reduce dose by 50%

Hemodialysis: Unknown

CAPD effects: Unknown

CAVH effects: Unknown

Administration

Oral: Administer on an empty stomach

Parenteral: Due to limited stability, complete administration of I.V. dose should occur within 60 minutes of reconstitution

I.V. infusion: I.V. dose is FDA-approved for administration as a single infusion over 15-20 minutes

I.V. bolus: I.V. may be administered via central line and via peripheral vein as a rapid I.V. bolus; there have not been any unexpected or serious adverse events specifically related to rapid I.V. bolus administration; the most common adverse events were transient mild symptoms of hot flush and tingling sensation over the body

Central line: I.V. bolus doses of 17-200 mg/m^2 (reconstituted and not diluted) have been infused over 2-20 minutes

Peripheral line: I.V. bolus doses of 2-23 mg/m^2 (reconstituted and not diluted) have been infused over 1-4 minutes

Monitoring Parameters CBC with differential and platelet count, serum electrolytes, serum uric acid

Test Interactions False-positive Coombs' test [direct]

Patient Information Any signs of infection, easy bruising or bleeding, shortness of breath, or painful or burning urination should be brought to physician's attention. Nausea, vomiting, or hair loss sometimes occur. The drug may cause permanent sterility and may cause birth defects. The drug may be excreted in breast milk, therefore, an alternative form of feeding your baby should be used.

Nursing Implications Avoid skin contact with I.V. formulation

Dosage Forms

Powder for injection: 50 mg

Tablet: 2 mg

Melquin HP® *see* Hydroquinone *on page 628*

Menadol® [OTC] *see* Ibuprofen *on page 639*

Menest® *see* Estrogens, Esterified *on page 473*

Meni-D® *see* Meclizine *on page 769*

Meningococcal Polysaccharide Vaccine, Groups A, C, Y, and W-135

(me NIN joe kok al pol i SAK a ride vak SEEN groops aye, see, why & dubl yoo won thur tee fyve)

Related Information

Immunization Guidelines *on page 1421*

Recommendations for Travelers *on page 1442*

Brand Names Menomune®-A/C/Y/W-135

Therapeutic Category Vaccine, Inactivated Bacteria

Use

Immunization of persons 2 years of age and above in epidemic or endemic areas as might be determined in a population delineated by neighborhood, school, dormitory, or other reasonable boundary. The prevalent serogroup in such a situation should match a serogroup in the vaccine. Individuals at particular high-risk include persons with terminal component complement deficiencies and those with anatomic or functional asplenia.

Travelers visiting areas of a country that are recognized as having hyperendemic or epidemic meningococcal disease

Vaccinations should be considered for household or institutional contacts of persons with meningococcal disease as an adjunct to appropriate antibiotic chemoprophylaxis as well as medical and laboratory personnel at risk of exposure to meningococcal disease

Pregnancy Risk Factor C

Contraindications Children <2 years of age

Warnings/Precautions Patients who undergo splenectomy secondary to trauma or nonlymphoid tumors respond well; however, those asplenic patients with lymphoid tumors who receive either chemotherapy or irradiation respond poorly; pregnancy, unless there is substantial risk of infection.

Adverse Reactions

>10%:

Central nervous system: Pain

Dermatologic: Erythema and induration

Local: Tenderness

1% to 10%: Central nervous system: Headache, malaise, fever, chills

Drug Interactions Decreased effect with administration of immunoglobulin within 1 month

Stability Discard remainder of vaccine within 5 days after reconstitution; store reconstituted vaccine in refrigerator

Mechanism of Action Induces the formation of bactericidal antibodies to meningococcal antigens; the presence of these antibodies is strongly correlated with immunity to meningococcal disease caused by *Neisseria meningitidis* groups A, C, Y and W-135.

Pharmacodynamics/Kinetics

Onset: Antibody levels are achieved within 10-14 days after administration

Duration: Antibodies against group A and C polysaccharides decline markedly (to prevaccination levels) over the first 3 years following a single dose of vaccine, especially in children <4 years of age

Usual Dosage One dose S.C. (0.5 mL); the need for booster is unknown

Nursing Implications Epinephrine 1:1000 should be available to control allergic reaction

Dosage Forms Injection: 10 dose, 50 dose

Menomune®-A/C/Y/W-135 *see* Meningococcal Polysaccharide Vaccine, Groups A, C, Y, and W-135 *on previous page*

Menotropins (men oh TROE pins)

Brand Names Humegon™; Pergonal®

Therapeutic Category Gonadotropin; Ovulation Stimulator

Use Sequentially with hCG to induce ovulation and pregnancy in the infertile woman with functional anovulation; used with hCG in men to stimulate spermatogenesis in those with primary hypogonadotropic hypogonadism

Pregnancy Risk Factor X

Contraindications Primary ovarian failure, overt thyroid and adrenal dysfunction, abnormal bleeding, pregnancy, men with normal urinary gonadotropin concentrations, elevated gonadotropin levels indicating primary testicular failure

Warnings/Precautions Advise patient of frequency and potential hazards of multiple pregnancy; to minimize the hazard of abnormal ovarian enlargement, use the lowest possible dose

Adverse Reactions

Male:

>10%: Endocrine & metabolic: Gynecomastia

1% to 10%: Erythrocytosis (shortness of breath, dizziness, anorexia, syncope, epistaxis)

Female:

>10%:

Endocrine & metabolic: Ovarian enlargement

Gastrointestinal: Abdominal distention

Local: Pain/rash at injection site

1% to 10%: Ovarian hyperstimulation syndrome

<1%:

Cardiovascular: Thromboembolism,

Central nervous system: Pain, febrile reactions

Overdosage/Toxicology Symptoms of overdose include ovarian hyperstimulation

Stability Lyophilized powder may be refrigerated or stored at room temperature; after reconstitution inject immediately, discard any unused portion

Mechanism of Action Actions occur as a result of both follicle stimulating hormone (FSH) effects and luteinizing hormone (LH) effects; menotropins stimulate the development and maturation of the ovarian follicle (FSH), cause ovulation (LH), and stimulate the development of the corpus luteum (LH); in males it stimulates spermatogenesis (LH)

Pharmacodynamics/Kinetics Elimination: ~10% of dose is excreted in the urine unchanged

Usual Dosage Adults: I.M.:

Male: Following pretreatment with hCG, 1 ampul 3 times/week and hCG 2000 units twice weekly until sperm is detected in the ejaculate (4-6 months) then may be increased to 2 ampuls of menotropins (150 units FSH/150 units LH) 3 times/week

(Continued)

Menotropins *(Continued)*

Female: 1 ampul/day (75 units of FSH and LH) for 9-12 days followed by 10,000 units hCG 1 day after the last dose; repeated at least twice at same level before increasing dosage to 2 ampuls (150 units FSH/150 units LH)

Administration I.M. administration only

Patient Information Multiple ovulations resulting in plural gestations have been reported

Dosage Forms Injection:

Follicle stimulating hormone activity 75 units and luteinizing hormone activity 75 units per 2 mL ampul

Follicle stimulating hormone activity 150 units and luteinizing hormone activity 150 units per 2 mL ampul

Mentax® *see* Butenafine *on page 178*

Meperidine (me PER i deen)

Related Information

Adult ACLS Algorithm, Electrical Conversion *on page 1515*

Drugs and Routes of Administration Not Recommended for Treatment of Cancer Pain *on page 1378*

Narcotic Agonists Comparison *on page 1414*

Dose Equivalents for Opioid Analgesics in Opioid-Naive Adults <50 kg *on page 1376*

Dose Equivalents for Opioid Analgesics in Opioid-Naive Adults ≥50 kg *on page 1375*

Brand Names Demerol®

Synonyms Isonipecaine Hydrochloride; Meperidine Hydrochloride; Pethidine Hydrochloride

Therapeutic Category Analgesic, Narcotic

Use Management of moderate to severe pain; adjunct to anesthesia and preoperative sedation

Restrictions C-II

Pregnancy Risk Factor B (D if used for prolonged periods or in high doses at term)

Contraindications Hypersensitivity to meperidine or any component; patients receiving MAO inhibitors presently or in the past 14 days

Warnings/Precautions Use with caution in patients with pulmonary, hepatic, renal disorders, or increased intracranial pressure; use with caution in patients with renal failure or seizure disorders or those receiving high-dose meperidine; normeperidine (an active metabolite and CNS stimulant) may accumulate and precipitate twitches, tremors, or seizures; some preparations contain sulfites which may cause allergic reaction; not recommended as a drug of first choice for the treatment of chronic pain in the elderly due to the accumulation of normeperidine; for acute pain, its use should be limited to 1-2 doses

Adverse Reactions

>10%:

- Cardiovascular: Hypotension
- Central nervous system: Fatigue, drowsiness, dizziness
- Gastrointestinal: Nausea, vomiting, constipation
- Neuromuscular & skeletal: Weakness
- Miscellaneous: Histamine release

1% to 10%:

- Central nervous system: Nervousness, headache, restlessness, malaise, confusion
- Gastrointestinal: Anorexia, stomach cramps, xerostomia, biliary spasm
- Genitourinary: Ureteral spasms, decreased urination
- Local: Pain at injection site
- Respiratory: Dyspnea, shortness of breath

<1%:

- Central nervous system: Mental depression, hallucinations, paradoxical CNS stimulation, increased intracranial pressure
- Dermatologic: Rash, urticaria
- Gastrointestinal: Paralytic ileus
- Miscellaneous: Physical and psychological dependence

Overdosage/Toxicology Symptoms of overdose include CNS depression, respiratory depression, mydriasis, bradycardia, pulmonary edema, chronic tremors, CNS excitability, seizures

Treatment of an overdose includes support of the patient's airway, establishment of an I.V. line, and administration of naloxone 2 mg I.V. (0.01 mg/kg for children) with repeat administration as necessary up to a total of 10 mg.

Drug Interactions

Decreased effect: Phenytoin may decrease the analgesic effects

Increased toxicity: May aggravate the adverse effects of isoniazid; MAO inhibitors, fluoxetine, and other serotonin uptake inhibitors greatly potentiate the effects of meperidine; acute opioid overdosage symptoms can be seen, including severe toxic reactions; CNS depressants, tricyclic antidepressants, phenothiazines may potentiate the effects of meperidine

Stability Meperidine injection should be stored at room temperature and protected from light and freezing; protect oral dosage forms from light

Incompatible with aminophylline, heparin, phenobarbital, phenytoin, and sodium bicarbonate

Mechanism of Action Binds to opiate receptors in the CNS, causing inhibition of ascending pain pathways, altering the perception of and response to pain; produces generalized CNS depression

Pharmacodynamics/Kinetics

Oral, S.C., I.M.:

Onset of analgesic effect: Within 10-15 minutes

Peak effect: Within 1 hour

Duration: 2-4 hours

I.V.: Onset of effects: Within 5 minutes

Distribution: Crosses the placenta; appears in breast milk

Protein binding: 65% to 75%

Metabolism: In the liver

Bioavailability: ~50% to 60%; increased with liver disease

Half-life:

Parent drug: Terminal phase:

Neonates: 23 hours; range: 12-39 hours

Adults: 2.5-4 hours

Adults with liver disease: 7-11 hours

Normeperidine (active metabolite): 15-30 hours; is dependent on renal function and can accumulate with high doses or in patients with decreased renal function

Usual Dosage Doses should be titrated to appropriate analgesic effect; when changing route of administration, note that oral doses are about half as effective as parenteral dose

Children: Oral, I.M., I.V., S.C.: 1-1.5 mg/kg/dose every 3-4 hours as needed; 1-2 mg/kg as a single dose preoperative medication may be used; maximum 100 mg/dose

Adults: Oral, I.M., I.V.: S.C.: 50-150 mg/dose every 3-4 hours as needed

Elderly:

Oral: 50 mg every 4 hours

I.M.: 25 mg every 4 hours

Dosing adjustment in renal impairment:

Cl_{cr} 10-50 mL/minute: Administer at 75% of normal dose

Cl_{cr} <10 mL/minute: Administer at 50% of normal dose

Dosing adjustment/comments in hepatic disease: Increased narcotic effect in cirrhosis; reduction in dose more important for oral than I.V. route

Dietary Considerations

Alcohol: Additive CNS effects, avoid or limit alcohol; watch for sedation

Food: Glucose may cause hyperglycemia; monitor blood glucose concentrations

Administration

Meperidine may be administered I.M. (preferably), S.C., or I.V.

I.V. push should be given slowly, use of a 10 mg/mL concentration has been recommended

Monitoring Parameters Pain relief, respiratory and mental status, blood pressure; observe patient for excessive sedation, CNS depression, seizures, respiratory depression

Reference Range Therapeutic: 70-500 ng/mL (SI: 283-2020 nmol/L); Toxic: >1000 ng/mL (SI: >4043 nmol/L)

Test Interactions ↑ amylase (S), ↑ BSP retention, ↑ CPK (I.M. injections)

Patient Information Avoid alcohol, may cause drowsiness

Dosage Forms

Injection, as hydrochloride:

Multiple dose vials: 50 mg/mL (30 mL); 100 mg/mL (20 mL)

Single dose: 10 mg/mL (5 mL, 10 mL, 30 mL); 25 mg/dose (0.5 mL, 1 mL); 50 mg/dose (1 mL); 75 mg/dose (1 mL, 1.5 mL); 100 mg/dose (1 mL)

Syrup, as hydrochloride: 50 mg/5 mL (500 mL)

Tablet, as hydrochloride: 50 mg, 100 mg

Meperidine Hydrochloride *see* Meperidine *on previous page*

Mephobarbital (me foe BAR bi tal)

Brand Names Mebaral®

Synonyms Methylphenobarbital

Therapeutic Category Anticonvulsant; Barbiturate; Sedative

(Continued)

Mephobarbital *(Continued)*

Use Sedative; treatment of grand mal and petit mal epilepsy

Restrictions C-IV

Pregnancy Risk Factor D

Contraindications Hypersensitivity to mephobarbital, other barbiturates, or any component; pre-existing CNS depression; respiratory depression; severe uncontrolled pain; history of porphyria

Warnings/Precautions Use with caution in patients with renal impairment, pulmonary insufficiency, or hepatic dysfunction; sometimes used in specific patients who have excessive sedation or hyperexcitability from phenobarbital; abrupt withdrawal may precipitate status epilepticus

Adverse Reactions

>10%: Central nervous system: Dizziness, lightheadedness, drowsiness, "hangover" effect

1% to 10%:
- Central nervous system: Confusion, mental depression, unusual excitement, nervousness, faint feeling, headache, insomnia, nightmares
- Gastrointestinal: Constipation, nausea, vomiting

<1%:
- Cardiovascular: Hypotension
- Central nervous system: Hallucinations
- Dermatologic: Rash, exfoliative dermatitis, Stevens-Johnson syndrome, angioedema
- Hematologic: Agranulocytosis, megaloblastic anemia, thrombocytopenia
- Local: Thrombophlebitis
- Respiratory: Respiratory depression
- Miscellaneous: Dependence

Overdosage/Toxicology Symptoms of overdose include CNS depression, respiratory depression, hypothermia, tachycardia, hypotension

Repeated oral doses of activated charcoal significantly reduce the half-life of barbiturates resulting from an enhancement of nonrenal elimination. The usual dose is 30-60 g every 4-6 hours for 3-4 days unless the patient has no bowel movement causing the charcoal to remain in the GI tract. Assure adequate hydration and renal function.

Urinary alkalinization with I.V. sodium bicarbonate also helps to enhance elimination. Hemodialysis or hemoperfusion is of uncertain value. Patients in stage IV coma due to high serum barbiturate levels may require charcoal hemoperfusion.

Drug Interactions

Decreased effect: Phenothiazines, haloperidol, quinidine, cyclosporine, TCAs, corticosteroids, theophylline, ethosuximide, warfarin, oral contraceptives, chloramphenicol, griseofulvin, doxycycline, beta-blockers

Increased effect/toxicity: Propoxyphene, benzodiazepines, CNS depressants, valproic acid, methylphenidate, chloramphenicol

Mechanism of Action Increases seizure threshold in the motor cortex; depresses monosynaptic and polysynaptic transmission in the CNS

Pharmacodynamics/Kinetics

Onset of action: 20-60 minutes
Duration: 6-8 hours
Absorption: Oral: ~50%
Metabolism: By the liver to phenobarbital
Half-life: 34 hours
Elimination: In urine

Usual Dosage Oral:

Epilepsy:
- Children: 6-12 mg/kg/day in 2-4 divided doses
- Adults: 200-600 mg/day in 2-4 divided doses

Sedation:
- Children:
  - <5 years: 16-32 mg 3-4 times/day
  - >5 years: 32-64 mg 3-4 times/day
- Adults: 32-100 mg 3-4 times/day

Dosing adjustment in renal or hepatic impairment: Use with caution and reduce dosages

Reference Range Phenobarbital level should be in the range of 15-40 μg/mL

Test Interactions ↑ alk phos (S), ↑ ammonia (B), ↓ bilirubin (S), ↓ calcium (S)

Patient Information May cause drowsiness, may impair coordination and judgment; do not discontinue abruptly; notify physician of dark urine, pale stools, jaundice, abdominal pain, persistent nausea, and vomiting; do not skip doses

Nursing Implications Observe patient for excessive sedation, respiratory depression; raise bed rails, institute safety precautions, assist with ambulation

Dosage Forms Tablet: 32 mg, 50 mg, 100 mg

Mephyton® *see* Phytonadione *on page 998*

Mepivacaine (me PIV a kane)

Brand Names Carbocaine®; Isocaine® HCl; Polocaine®

Synonyms Mepivacaine Hydrochloride

Therapeutic Category Local Anesthetic, Injectable

Use Local anesthesia by nerve block; infiltration in dental procedures; **not** for use in spinal anesthesia

Pregnancy Risk Factor C

Contraindications Hypersensitivity to mepivacaine or any component or other amide anesthetics, allergy to sodium bisulfate

Warnings/Precautions Use with caution in patients with cardiac disease, renal disease, and hyperthyroidism; convulsions due to systemic toxicity leading to cardiac arrest have been reported presumably due to intravascular injection

Adverse Reactions

<1%:

Cardiovascular: Bradycardia, myocardial depression, hypotension, cardiovascular collapse, edema

Central nervous system: Anxiety, restlessness, disorientation, confusion, seizures, drowsiness, unconsciousness, chills

Dermatologic: Urticaria

Gastrointestinal: Nausea, vomiting

Local: Transient stinging or burning at injection site

Neuromuscular & skeletal: Tremors

Ocular: Blurred vision

Otic: Tinnitus

Respiratory: Respiratory arrest

Miscellaneous: Anaphylactoid reactions, shivering

Overdosage/Toxicology Symptoms of overdose include dizziness, cyanosis, tremors, bronchial spasm

Treatment is primarily symptomatic and supportive. Termination of anesthesia by pneumatic tourniquet inflation should be attempted when the agent is administered by infiltration or regional injection. Seizures commonly respond to diazepam, while hypotension responds to I.V. fluids and Trendelenburg positioning. Bradyarrhythmias (when the heart rate is <60) can be treated with I.V., I.M., or S.C. atropine 15 mcg/kg. With the development of metabolic acidosis, I.V. sodium bicarbonate 0.5-2 mEq/kg and ventilatory assistance should be instituted.

Mechanism of Action Mepivacaine is an amino amide local anesthetic similar to lidocaine; like all local anesthetics, mepivacaine acts by preventing the generation and conduction of nerve impulses

Pharmacodynamics/Kinetics

Onset of action: Epidural: Within 7-15 minutes

Duration: 2-2.5 hours; similar onset and duration is seen following infiltration

Protein binding: 70% to 85%

Metabolism: Chiefly in the liver by N-demethylation, hydroxylation, and glucuronidation

Half-life: 1.9 hours

Elimination: Urinary excretion (95% as metabolites)

Usual Dosage Children and Adults: Injectable local anesthetic: Varies with procedure, degree of anesthesia needed, vascularity of tissue, duration of anesthesia required, and physical condition of patient

Nursing Implications Before injecting, withdraw syringe plunger to ensure injection is not into vein or artery

Dosage Forms Injection, as hydrochloride: 1% [10 mg/mL] (30 mL, 50 mL); 1.5% [15 mg/mL] (30 mL); 2% [20 mg/mL] (20 mL, 50 mL); 3% [30 mg/mL] (1.8 mL)

Mepivacaine Hydrochloride *see* Mepivacaine *on this page*

Meprobamate (me proe BA mate)

Brand Names Equanil®; Miltown®; Neuramate®

Canadian/Mexican Brand Names Apo-Meprobamate® (Canada); Meditran® (Canada); Novo-Mepro® (Canada)

Therapeutic Category Antianxiety Agent

Use Management of anxiety disorders

Unlabeled use: Demonstrated value for muscle contraction, headache, premenstrual tension, external sphincter spasticity, muscle rigidity, opisthotonos-associated with tetanus

Restrictions C-IV

Pregnancy Risk Factor D

(Continued)

Meprobamate *(Continued)*

Contraindications Acute intermittent porphyria; hypersensitivity to meprobamate or any component; do not use in patients with pre-existing CNS depression, narrow-angle glaucoma, or severe uncontrolled pain

Warnings/Precautions Physical and psychological dependence and abuse may occur; not recommended in children <6 years of age; allergic reaction may occur in patients with history of dermatological condition (usually by fourth dose); use with caution in patients with renal or hepatic impairment, or with a history of seizures

Adverse Reactions

>10%: Central nervous system: Drowsiness, ataxia

1% to 10%:

- Central nervous system: Dizziness
- Dermatologic: Rashes
- Gastrointestinal: Diarrhea, vomiting
- Ocular: Blurred vision
- Respiratory: Wheezing

<1%:

- Cardiovascular: Syncope, peripheral edema
- Central nervous system: Paradoxical excitement, confusion, slurred speech, headache, euphoria, chills
- Dermatologic: Purpura, dermatitis, Stevens-Johnson syndrome
- Gastrointestinal: Stomatitis
- Hematologic: Thrombocytopenia, leukopenia
- Renal: Renal failure
- Respiratory: Dyspnea, bronchospasm

Overdosage/Toxicology Symptoms of overdose include drowsiness, lethargy, ataxia, coma, hypotension, shock, death

Treatment is supportive following attempts to enhance drug elimination. Hypotension should be treated with I.V. fluids and/or Trendelenburg positioning. Dialysis and hemoperfusion have not demonstrated significant reductions in blood drug concentrations.

Drug Interactions Increased toxicity: CNS depressants may increase CNS depression

Mechanism of Action Precise mechanism is not yet clear, but many effects have been ascribed to its central depressant actions

Pharmacodynamics/Kinetics

Onset of sedation: Oral: Within 1 hour
Distribution: Crosses the placenta; appears in breast milk
Metabolism: Promptly in the liver
Half-life: 10 hours
Elimination: In urine (8% to 20% as unchanged drug) and feces (10% as metabolites)

Usual Dosage Oral:

Children 6-12 years:
- 100-200 mg 2-3 times/day
- Sustained release: 200 mg twice daily

Adults:
- 400 mg 3-4 times/day, up to 2400 mg/day
- Sustained release: 400-800 mg twice daily

Dosing interval in renal impairment:
- Cl_{cr} 10-50 mL/minute: Administer every 9-12 hours
- Cl_{cr} <10 mL/minute: Administer every 12-18 hours

Hemodialysis: Moderately dialyzable (20% to 50%)

Dosing adjustment in hepatic impairment: Probably necessary in patients with liver disease

Dietary Considerations Alcohol: Additive CNS effect, avoid use

Monitoring Parameters Mental status

Reference Range Therapeutic: 6-12 μg/mL (SI: 28-55 μmol/L); Toxic: >60 μg/mL (SI: >275 μmol/L)

Patient Information May cause drowsiness; avoid alcoholic beverages

Dosage Forms

Capsule, sustained release: 200 mg, 400 mg
Tablet: 200 mg, 400 mg, 600 mg

Mepron™ *see* Atovaquone *on page 114*

Mercaptopurine (mer kap toe PYOOR een)

Related Information

Antiemetics for Chemotherapy Induced Nausea and Vomiting *on page 1348*
Cancer Chemotherapy Regimens *on page 1351*
Toxicities of Chemotherapeutic Agents *on page 1382*

Brand Names Purinethol®

Synonyms 6-Mercaptopurine; 6-MP

Therapeutic Category Antineoplastic Agent, Antimetabolite (Purine)

Use Treatment of acute leukemias (ALL or AML) maintenance therapy

Pregnancy Risk Factor D

Contraindications Hypersensitivity to mercaptopurine or any component; patients whose disease showed prior resistance to mercaptopurine or thioguanine; severe liver disease, severe bone marrow suppression

Warnings/Precautions The U.S. Food and Drug Administration (FDA) currently recommends that procedures for proper handling and disposal of antineoplastic agents be considered. Mercaptopurine may cause birth defects; potentially carcinogenic; adjust dosage in patients with renal impairment or hepatic failure; use with caution in patients with prior bone marrow suppression; patients may be at risk for pancreatitis. Toxicity to immunosuppressives is increased in elderly. Start with lowest recommended adult doses. Signs of infection, such as fever and WBC rise, may not occur. Lethargy and confusion may be more prominent signs of infection.

Adverse Reactions

>10%:

Hepatic: 6-MP can cause an intrahepatic cholestasis and focal centrilobular necrosis manifested as hyperbilirubinemia, increased alkaline phosphatase, and increased AST. This may be dose related, occurring more frequently at doses >2.5 mg/kg/day; jaundice is noted 1-2 months into therapy, but has ranged from 1 week to 8 years.

1% to 10%:

Dermatologic: Hyperpigmentation, rash

Endocrine & metabolic: Hyperuricemia

Gastrointestinal: Nausea, vomiting, diarrhea, stomatitis, anorexia, stomach pain, and mucositis may require parenteral nutrition and dose reduction; 6-TG is less GI toxic than 6-MP

Hematologic: Leukopenia, thrombocytopenia, anemia may occur at high doses

Myelosuppressive:

- WBC: Moderate
- Platelets: Moderate
- Onset (days): 7-10
- Nadir (days): 14
- Recovery (days): 21

Renal: Renal toxicity

<1%:

Central nervous system: Drug fever

Dermatologic: Dry, scaling rash

Gastrointestinal: Glossitis, tarry stools

Hematologic: Eosinophilia

Overdosage/Toxicology Symptoms of overdose include:

Immediate: Nausea, vomiting

Delayed: Bone marrow suppression, hepatic necrosis, gastroenteritis

Drug Interactions

Decreased effect: Warfarin: 6-MP inhibits the anticoagulation effect of warfarin by an unknown mechanism

Increased toxicity:

Allopurinol: Can cause ↑ levels of 6-MP by inhibition of xanthine oxidase; ↓ dose of 6-MP by 75% when both drugs are used concomitantly; seen only with oral 6-MP usage, not with I.V.; may potentiate effect of bone marrow suppression (reduce 6-MP to 25% of dose)

Doxorubicin: Synergistic liver toxicity with 6-MP in >50% of patients, which resolved with discontinuation of the 6-MP

Hepatotoxic drugs: Any agent which could potentially alter the metabolic function of the liver could produce higher drug levels and greater toxicities from either 6-MP or 6-TG

Stability Store at room temperature

Mechanism of Action Purine antagonist which inhibits DNA and RNA synthesis; acts as false metabolite and is incorporated into DNA and RNA, eventually inhibiting their synthesis. 6-MP is substituted for hypoxanthine; must be metabolized to active nucleotides once inside the cell.

Pharmacodynamics/Kinetics

Absorption: Variable and incomplete (16% to 50%)

Distribution: V_d = total body water; CNS penetration is poor

Protein binding: 30%

Metabolism: Undergoes first-pass metabolism in the GI mucosa and liver; metabolized in the liver by xanthine oxidase and methylation to sulfate conjugates, 6-thiouric acid and other inactive compounds

Half-life: Age dependent:

Children: 21 minutes

(Continued)

Mercaptopurine *(Continued)*

Adults: 47 minutes

Time to peak serum concentration: Within 2 hours

Elimination: Prompt excretion in the urine; with high doses of I.V. 6-MP, the renal excretion of unchanged drug is 20% to 40% and can produce hematuria and crystalluria; at conventional doses renal elimination is minor

Usual Dosage Oral (refer to individual protocols):

Children: Maintenance: 75 mg/m²/day given once daily

Adults:

Induction: 2.5-5 mg/kg/day (100-200 mg)

Maintenance: 1.5-2.5 mg/kg/day **OR** 80-100 mg/m²/day given once daily

Elderly: Due to renal decline with age, start with lower recommended doses for adults

Dosing adjustment in renal or hepatic impairment: Dose should be reduced to avoid accumulation, but specific guidelines are not available

Hemodialysis: Removed; supplemental dosing is usually required

Monitoring Parameters CBC with differential and platelet count, liver function tests, uric acid, urinalysis

Patient Information Should not be taken with meals. Nausea and vomiting are rare with usual doses. Any signs of infection, easy bruising or bleeding, shortness of breath, or painful or burning urination should be brought to physician's attention. Nausea, vomiting, or hair loss sometimes occur. The drug may cause permanent sterility and may cause birth defects. The drug may be excreted in breast milk, therefore, an alternative form of feeding your baby should be used. Contraceptive measures are recommended during therapy.

Nursing Implications Adjust dosage in patients with renal insufficiency

Dosage Forms Tablet, scored: 50 mg

Extemporaneous Preparations A 50 mg/mL oral suspension was made by crushing the tablets, mixing with a volume of Cologel® suspending agent equal to ⅓ the final volume, and adding a 2:1 mixture of simple syrup and cherry syrup to make the final volume; stable for 14 days when stored in an amber glass bottle at room temperature

Dressman JB and Poust RI, "Stability of Allopurinol and of Five Antineoplastics in Suspension," *Am J Hosp Pharm*, 1983, 40:616-8.

6-Mercaptopurine *see* Mercaptopurine *on page 784*

Mercapturic Acid *see* Acetylcysteine *on page 28*

Meronem® *see* Meropenem *on this page*

Meropenem (mer oh PEN em)

Brand Names Meronem®; Merrem® I.V.

Therapeutic Category Antibiotic, Carbapenem

Use Intra-abdominal infections (complicated appendicitis and peritonitis) caused by viridans group streptococci, *E. coli, K. pneumoniae, P. aeruginosa, B. fragilis, B. thetaiotamicron,* and *Peptostreptococcus* sp; also indicated for bacterial meningitis in pediatric patients >3 months of age caused by *S. pneumoniae, H. influenzae,* and *N. meningitidis*; meropenem has also been used to treat soft tissue infections, febrile neutropenia, and urinary tract infections

Pregnancy Risk Factor B

Pregnancy/Breast-Feeding Implications Although no teratogenic or infant harm has been found in studies, excretion in breast milk is not known and this drug should be used during pregnancy and lactation only if clearly indicated

Contraindications Patients with known hypersensitivity to meropenem, any component, or other carbapenems (eg, imipenem); patients who have experienced anaphylactic reactions to other beta-lactams

Warnings/Precautions Pseudomembranous colitis and hypersensitivity reactions have occurred and often require immediate drug discontinuation; thrombocytopenia has been reported in patients with significant renal dysfunction; seizures have occurred in patients with underlying neurologic disorders (less frequent than with Primaxin®); safety and efficacy have not been established for children <3 months of age; superinfection possible with long courses of therapy

Adverse Reactions

1% to 10%:

Central nervous system: Headache

Dermatologic: Rash, pruritus

Gastrointestinal: Diarrhea, nausea, vomiting, constipation, oral moniliasis, glossitis

Local: Pain at injection site, phlebitis, thrombophlebitis

Respiratory: Apnea

<1%:

Cardiovascular: Hypotension, heart failure (MI and arrhythmias), tachycardia, hypertension, edema, seizures

Central nervous system: Insomnia, agitation, confusion, hallucinations, depression, seizures, fever
Dermatologic: Urticaria
Gastrointestinal: Anorexia, flatulence, ileus
Genitourinary: Dysuria, RBCs in urine
Hepatic: Cholestatic jaundice, hepatic failure, increase LFTs
Hematologic: Anemia, hypo- and hypercytosis, bleeding events (epistaxis, melena, etc)
Neuromuscular & skeletal: Paresthesia, whole body pain
Renal: Renal failure, elevation of creatinine and BUN

Overdosage/Toxicology No cases of acute overdosage are reported which have resulted in symptoms; supportive therapy recommended; meropenem and metabolite are removable by dialysis

Drug Interactions Increased effect: Probenecid competes with meropenem for active tubular secretion and inhibits the renal excretion of meropenem (half-life increased by 38%)

Stability Store at room temperature; when vials are reconstituted with NaCl/D_5W, they are stable for 2 hours/1 hour at room temperature or for 18 hours/8 hours when refrigerated; when diluted in minibags, they are stable for up to 24 hours refrigerated in NaCl and 6 hours in D_5W

Mechanism of Action Inhibits bacterial cell wall synthesis by binding to several of the penicillin-binding proteins; bactericidal against many gram-positive aerobes and gram-negative aerobes and anaerobes, especially *E. coli, P. aeruginosa*, and *S. aureus*; not bactericidal against *L-monocytogenes*; has significant stability against beta-lactamases with the exception of matallo-beta-lactamases; not effective against MRSA; cross-resistance possible with other strains resistant to carbapenems; may act synergistically with aminoglycosides

Pharmacodynamics/Kinetics
Distribution: V_d: ~0.3 L/kg in adults (0.4-0.5 L/kg in children); penetrates well into most body fluids and tissues; CSF concentrations approximate those of the plasma
Protein binding: 2%
Metabolism: Hepatic; metabolizes to open beta-lactam form (inactive); not metabolized by same enzyme as imipenem which results in toxic metabolite
Half-life:
- Normal renal function: 1-1.5 hours
- Cl_{cr} 30-80 mL/minute: 1.9-3.3 hours
- Cl_{cr} 2-30 mL/minute: 3.82-5.7 hours
- Time to peak tissue concentration: 1 hour following infusion

Elimination: Renal, ~25% as the inactive metabolite

Usual Dosage I.V.:
Children >3 months (<50 kg):
- Intra-abdominal infections: 20 mg/kg every 8 hours (maximum dose: 1 g every 8 hours)
- Meningitis: 40 mg/kg every 8 hours (maximum dose: 2 g every 8 hours)

Children >50 kg:
- Intra-abdominal infections: 1 g every 8 hours
- Meningitis: 2 g every 8 hours

Adults: 1 g every 8 hours

Dosing adjustment in renal impairment: Adults:
- Cl_{cr} 26-50 mL/minute: Administer 1 g every 12 hours
- Cl_{cr} 10-25 mL/minute: Administer 500 mg every 12 hours
- Cl_{cr} <10 mL/minute: Administer 500 mg every 24 hours

Dialysis: Meropenem and its metabolites are readily dialyzable

Additional Information 1 g of meropenem contains 90.2 mg of sodium as sodium carbonate (3.92 mEq)

Dosage Forms
Infusion: 500 mg (100 mL); 1 g (100 mL)
Infusion, ADD-vantage®: 500 mg (15 mL); 1 g (15 mL)
Injection: 25 mg/mL (20 mL); 33.3 mg/mL (30 mL)

Merrem® I.V. *see* Meropenem *on previous page*
Meruvax® II *see* Rubella Virus Vaccine, Live *on page 1119*

Mesalamine (me SAL a meen)

Brand Names Asacol®; Pentasa®; Rowasa®

Synonyms 5-Aminosalicylic Acid; 5-ASA; Fisalamine; Mesalazine

Therapeutic Category 5-Aminosalicylic Acid Derivative; Anti-inflammatory Agent, Rectal

Use
Oral: Remission and treatment of mildly to moderately active ulcerative colitis
Rectal: Treatment of active mild to moderate distal ulcerative colitis, proctosigmoiditis, or proctitis
(Continued)

Mesalamine *(Continued)*

Pregnancy Risk Factor B

Contraindications Known hypersensitivity to mesalamine, sulfasalazine, sulfites, or salicylates

Warnings/Precautions Pericarditis should be considered in patients with chest pain; pancreatitis should be considered in any patient with new abdominal complaints. Elderly may have difficulty administering and retaining rectal suppositories. Given renal function decline with aging, monitor serum creatinine often during therapy.

Adverse Reactions

>10%:

Central nervous system: Headache, malaise

Gastrointestinal: Abdominal pain, cramps, flatulence, gas

1% to 10%: Dermatologic: Alopecia, rash

<1%: Anal irritation, acute intolerance syndrome (bloody diarrhea, severe abdominal cramps, severe headache)

Overdosage/Toxicology Symptoms of overdose include decreased motor activity, diarrhea, vomiting, renal function impairment

Treatment is supportive; emesis, gastric lavage, and follow with activated charcoal slurry

Drug Interactions Decreased effect: Decreased digoxin bioavailability

Stability Unstable in presence of water or light; once foil has been removed, unopened bottles have an expiration of 1 year following the date of manufacture

Mechanism of Action Mesalamine (5-aminosalicylic acid) is the active component of sulfasalazine; the specific mechanism of action of mesalamine is unknown; however, it is thought that it modulates local chemical mediators of the inflammatory response, especially leukotrienes; action appears topical rather than systemic

Pharmacodynamics/Kinetics

Absorption: Rectal: ~15%; variable and dependent upon retention time, underlying GI disease, and colonic pH

Metabolism: In the liver by acetylation to acetyl-5-aminosalicylic acid (active) and to glucuronide conjugates; intestinal metabolism may also occur

Half-life:

5-ASA: 0.5-1.5 hours

Acetyl 5-ASA: 5-10 hours

Time to peak serum concentration: Within 4-7 hours

Elimination: Most metabolites are excreted in urine with <2% appearing in feces

Usual Dosage Adults (usual course of therapy is 3-6 weeks):

Oral:

Capsule: 1 g 4 times/day

Tablet: 800 mg 3 times/day

Retention enema: 60 mL (4 g) at bedtime, retained overnight, approximately 8 hours

Rectal suppository: Insert 1 suppository in rectum twice daily

Some patients may require rectal and oral therapy concurrently

Patient Information Retain enemas for 8 hours or as long as practical; shake bottle well; do not chew or break oral tablets; for suppositories, remove foil wrapper, avoid excessive handling

Nursing Implications Provide patient with copy of mesalamine administration instructions

Dosage Forms

Capsule, controlled release (Pentasa®): 250 mg

Suppository, rectal (Rowasa®): 500 mg

Suspension, rectal (Rowasa®): 4 g/60 mL (7s)

Tablet, enteric coated (Asacol®): 400 mg

Mesalazine *see* Mesalamine *on previous page*

Mesna (MES na)

Related Information

Cancer Chemotherapy Regimens *on page 1351*

Brand Names Mesnex™

Synonyms Sodium 2-Mercaptoethane Sulfonate

Therapeutic Category Antidote, Cyclophosphamide-induced Hemorrhagic Cystitis; Antidote, Ifosfamide-induced Hemorrhagic Cystitis

Use Detoxifying agent used as a protectant against hemorrhagic cystitis induced by ifosfamide and cyclophosphamide

Pregnancy Risk Factor B

Contraindications Hypersensitivity to mesna or other thiol compounds

Warnings/Precautions Examine morning urine specimen for hematuria prior to ifosfamide or cyclophosphamide treatment; if hematuria (>50 RBC/HPF)

develops, reduce the ifosfamide/cyclophosphamide dose or discontinue the drug; will not prevent or alleviate other toxicities associated with ifosfamide or cyclophosphamide and will not prevent hemorrhagic cystitis in all patients. Allergic reactions have been reported in patients with autoimmune disorders. Symptoms ranged from mild hypersensitivity to systemic anaphylactic reactions.

Adverse Reactions

1% to 10%:

Cardiovascular: Hypotension

Central nervous system: Malaise, headache

Gastrointestinal: Diarrhea, nausea, vomiting, bad taste in mouth, soft stools

Neuromuscular & skeletal: Limb pain

<1%: Dermatologic: Skin rash, itching

Drug Interactions

Decreased effect: Warfarin: Questionable alterations in coagulation control

Stability Diluted solutions are chemically and physically stable for 24 hours at room temperature; polypropylene syringes are stable for 9 days at refrigeration or room temperature; injection diluted for oral administration is stable 24 hours at refrigeration

Standard dose: Dose/100-1,000 mL D_5W or NS to a final concentration of 1-20 mg/mL

Incompatible with cisplatin

Compatible with cyclophosphamide, etoposide, lorazepam, potassium chloride, bleomycin, dexamethasone

Mechanism of Action Binds with and detoxifies acrolein and other urotoxic metabolites of ifosfamide and cyclophosphamide; detoxifying agent used to prevent hemorrhagic cystitis induced by ifosfamide and cyclophosphamide. In the kidney, mesna is reduced to a free thiol compound which reacts chemically with the acrolein and 4-hydroxy-ifosfamide resulting in detoxification.

Pharmacodynamics/Kinetics

Absorption: From the GI tract

Peak plasma levels: 2-3 hours after administration

Distribution: No tissue penetration; following glomerular filtration, mesna disulfide is reduced in renal tubules back to mesna

Metabolism: Rapidly oxidized intravascularly to mesna disulfide; mesna disulfide is reduced in renal tubules back to mesna following glomerular filtration.

Half-life:

Parent drug: 24 minutes

Mesna disulfide: 72 minutes

Elimination: Unchanged drug and metabolite are excreted primarily in the urine; time it takes for maximum urinary mesna excretion: 1 hour after I.V. and 2-3 hours after an oral mesna dose

Usual Dosage Children and Adults (refer to individual protocols); oral dose is approximately equivalent to 2 times the I.V. dose

I.V.:

Ifosfamide: 20% W/W of ifosfamide dose 15 minutes before ifosfamide administration and 4 and 8 hours after each dose of ifosfamide; **total daily dose is 60% to 100% of ifosfamide**; for high dose ifosfamide: 20% W/W 15 minutes before ifosfamide administration, and every 3 hours for 3-6 doses, some regimens use up to 160% of the total ifosfamide dose

Cyclophosphamide: 20% W/W of cyclophosphamide dose 15 minutes prior to cyclophosphamide administration and 4 and 8 hours after each dose of cyclophosphamide; **total daily dose = 60% to 200% of cyclophosphamide dose**

Oral: 40% W/W of the ifosfamide or cyclophosphamide agent dose in 3 doses at 4-hour intervals **OR** 20 mg/kg/dose every 4 hours x 3 (oral mesna is not recommended for the first dose before ifosfamide or cyclophosphamide)

Administration For oral administration, injection may be diluted in 1:1, 1:2, 1:10, 1:100 concentrations in carbonated beverages (cola, ginger ale, Pepsi®, Sprite®, Dr Pepper®, etc), juices (apple or orange), or whole milk (chocolate or white), and is stable 24 hours at refrigeration; used in conjunction with ifosfamide; examine morning urine specimen for hematuria prior to ifosfamide or cyclophosphamide treatment

Administer by I.V. infusion over 15-30 minutes or per protocol; mesna can be diluted in D_5W or NS to a final concentration of 1-20 mg/mL

Monitoring Parameters Urinalysis

Test Interactions False-positive urinary ketones with Multistix® or Labstix®

Dosage Forms Injection: 100 mg/mL (2 mL, 4 mL, 10 mL)

Mesnex™ *see* Mesna *on previous page*

Mesoridazine (mez oh RID a zeen)

Related Information

Antipsychotic Agents Comparison *on page 1396*

Brand Names Serentil®

Synonyms Mesoridazine Besylate

Therapeutic Category Antipsychotic Agent; Phenothiazine Derivative

Use Symptomatic management of psychotic disorders, including schizophrenia, behavioral problems, alcoholism as well as reducing anxiety and tension occurring in neurosis

Pregnancy Risk Factor C

Contraindications Hypersensitivity to mesoridazine or any component, cross-sensitivity with other phenothiazines may exist

Warnings/Precautions Safety in children <6 months of age has not been established; use with caution in patients with cardiovascular disease or seizures; benefits of therapy must be weighed against risks of therapy; doses >1 g/day frequently cause pigmentary retinopathy; some products contain sulfites and/or tartrazine; use with caution in patients with narrow-angle glaucoma, bone marrow suppression, severe liver disease

Adverse Reactions

>10%:

- Cardiovascular: Hypotension, orthostatic hypotension
- Central nervous system: Pseudoparkinsonism, akathisia, dystonias, tardive dyskinesia (persistent), dizziness
- Gastrointestinal: Constipation
- Ocular: Pigmentary retinopathy
- Respiratory: Nasal congestion
- Miscellaneous: Diaphoresis (decreased)

1% to 10%:

- Dermatologic: Increased sensitivity to sun, rash
- Endocrine & metabolic: Changes in menstrual cycle, changes in libido, breast pain
- Gastrointestinal: Weight gain, nausea, vomiting, stomach pain
- Genitourinary: Dysuria, ejaculatory disturbances
- Neuromuscular & skeletal: Trembling of fingers

<1%:

- Central nervous system: Neuroleptic malignant syndrome (NMS), impairment of temperature regulation, lowering of seizures threshold
- Dermatologic: Discoloration of skin (blue-gray)
- Endocrine & metabolic: Galactorrhea
- Genitourinary: Priapism
- Hematologic: Agranulocytosis, leukopenia
- Hepatic: Cholestatic jaundice, hepatotoxicity
- Ocular: Cornea and lens changes

Overdosage/Toxicology Symptoms of overdose include deep sleep, coma, extrapyramidal symptoms, abnormal involuntary muscle movements, hypotension

Following initiation of essential overdose management, toxic symptom treatment and supportive treatment should be initiated; hypotension usually responds to I.V. fluids or Trendelenburg positioning. If unresponsive to these measures, the use of a parenteral inotrope may be required. Seizures commonly respond to diazepam (I.V. 5-10 mg bolus in adults every 15 minutes if needed up to a total of 30 mg; I.V. 0.25-0.4 mg/kg/dose up to a total of 10 mg in children) or to phenytoin or phenobarbital. Critical cardiac arrhythmias often respond to I.V. phenytoin (15 mg/kg up to 1 g), while other antiarrhythmics can be used. Extrapyramidal symptoms (eg, dystonic reactions) can be managed with benztropine mesylate I.V. 1-2 mg (adults).

Drug Interactions

- Decreased effect with anticonvulsants, anticholinergics
- Increased toxicity with CNS depressants, metrizamide (increases seizures), propranolol

Mechanism of Action Blockade of postsynaptic CNS dopamine receptors

Pharmacodynamics/Kinetics

- Duration of action: 4-6 hours
- Absorption: Very erratic with oral tablet; oral liquids much more dependable
- Protein binding: 91% to 99%
- Half-life: 24-48 hours
- Time to peak serum concentration: 2-4 hours
- Time to steady-state serum: 4-7 days
- Elimination: In urine

Usual Dosage Concentrate may be diluted just prior to administration with distilled water, acidified tap water, orange or grape juice; do not prepare and store bulk dilutions

Adults:

Oral: 25-50 mg 3 times/day; maximum: 100-400 mg/day

I.M.: Initial: 25 mg, repeat in 30-60 minutes as needed; optimal dosage range: 25-200 mg/day

Hemodialysis: Not dialyzable (0% to 5%)

Dietary Considerations Alcohol: Additive CNS effect, avoid use

Administration Watch for hypotension when administering I.M. or I.V., dilute oral concentration before administering; do not mix oral solutions of mesoridazine and lithium, these oral liquids are incompatible when mixed

Test Interactions ↑ cholesterol (S), ↑ glucose; ↓ uric acid (S)

Patient Information May cause drowsiness or restlessness, avoid alcohol and other CNS depressants; do not alter dosage or discontinue without consulting physician; avoid excessive sunlight, yearly ophthalmic examinations are necessary

Dosage Forms

Injection, as besylate: 25 mg/mL (1 mL)

Liquid, oral, as besylate: 25 mg/mL (118 mL)

Tablet, as besylate: 10 mg, 25 mg, 50 mg, 100 mg

Mesoridazine Besylate *see* Mesoridazine *on previous page*

Mestinon® *see* Pyridostigmine *on page 1079*

Mestranol and Norethindrone (MES tra nole & nor eth IN drone)

Brand Names Genora® 1/50; Nelova™ 1/50M; Norethin™ 1/50M; Norinyl® 1+50; Ortho-Novum™ 1/50

Synonyms Norethindrone and Mestranol

Therapeutic Category Contraceptive, Oral (Low Potency Estrogen, Low Potency Progestin); Contraceptive, Oral (Monophasic); Estrogen Derivative, Oral; Progestin Derivative

Use Prevention of pregnancy; treatment of hypermenorrhea, endometriosis, female hypogonadism [monophasic oral contraceptive]

Pregnancy Risk Factor X

Contraindications Known or suspected breast cancer, undiagnosed abnormal vaginal bleeding, carcinoma of the breast, estrogen-dependent tumor

Warnings/Precautions Use with caution in patients with a history of thromboembolism, stroke, myocardial infarction, liver tumor, hypertension, cardiac, renal or hepatic insufficiency; use of any progestin during the first 4 months of pregnancy is not recommended; risk of cardiovascular side effects increases in those women who smoke cigarettes and in women >35 years of age

Adverse Reactions

>10%:

Cardiovascular: Peripheral edema

Central nervous system: Headache

Endocrine: Enlargement of breasts, breast tenderness, increased libido

Gastrointestinal: Nausea, anorexia, bloating

1% to 10%: Gastrointestinal: Vomiting, diarrhea

<1%:

Cardiovascular: Hypertension, thromboembolism, edema, stroke, myocardial infarction

Central nervous system: Depression, dizziness, anxiety

Dermatologic: Chloasma, melasma, rash

Endocrine: Decreased glucose tolerance, amenorrhea, alterations in frequency and flow of menses, increased triglycerides and LDL

Gastrointestinal: GI distress

Hepatic: Cholestatic jaundice

Ocular: Intolerance to contact lenses

Miscellaneous: Increased susceptibility to *Candida* infection, breast tumors

See tables.

Achieving Proper Hormonal Balance in an Oral Contraceptive

Estrogen		Progestin	
Excess	**Deficiency**	**Excess**	**Deficiency**
Nausea, bloating	Early or midcycle breakthrough bleeding	Increased appetite	Late breakthrough bleeding
Cervical mucorrhea, polyposis	Increased spotting	Weight gain	Amenorrhea
Melasma	Hypomenorrhea	Tiredness, fatigue	Hypermenorrhea
Migraine headache		Hypomenorrhea	
Breast fullness or tenderness		Acne, oily scalp*	
Edema		Hair loss, hirsutism*	
Hypertension		Depression	
		Monilial vaginitis	
		Breast regression	

*Result of androgenic activity of progestins.

(Continued)

Mestranol and Norethindrone *(Continued)*

Pharmacological Effects of Progestins Used in Oral Contraceptives

	Progestin	Estrogen	Antiestrogen	Androgen
Norgestrel/levonorgestrel	+++	0	++	+++
Ethynodiol diacetate	++	+*	+*	+
Norethindrone acetate	+	+	+++	+
Norethindrone	+	+*	+*	+
Norethynodrel	+	+++	0	0

*Has estrogenic effect at low doses; may have antiestrogenic effect at higher doses.
+++ = pronounced effect
++ = moderate effect
+ = slight effect
0 = moderate effect

Overdosage/Toxicology Toxicity is unlikely following single exposures of excessive doses

Any treatment following emesis and charcoal administration should be supportive and symptomatic

Drug Interactions

Decreased effect:

Tetracyclines, penicillins, griseofulvin, rifampin, acetaminophen, barbiturates, hydantoins may increase contraceptive failures

Decreases acetaminophen, estrogen levels, and anticoagulants

Increased toxicity: Increases benzodiazepines, caffeine, metoprolol, theophyllines, and tricyclic antidepressants

Mechanism of Action Combination oral contraceptives inhibit ovulation via a negative feedback mechanism on the hypothalamus, which alters the normal pattern of gonadotropin secretion of a follicle-stimulating hormone (FSH) and luteinizing hormone by the anterior pituitary. The follicular phase FSH and midcycle surge of gonadotropins are inhibited. In addition, oral contraceptives produce alterations in the genital tract, including changes in the cervical mucus, rendering it unfavorable for sperm penetration even if ovulation occurs. Changes in the endometrium may also occur, producing an unfavorable environment for nidation. Oral contraceptive drugs may alter the tubal transport of the ova through the fallopian tubes. Progestational agents may also alter sperm fertility.

Usual Dosage Adults: Female: Oral:

Contraception: 1 tablet daily, beginning on day 5 of menstrual cycle (first day of menstrual flow is day 1). With 20-tablet and 21-tablet packages, new dosing cycle begins 7 days after last tablet taken. With 28-tablet packages, dosage is 1 tablet daily without interruption; extra tablets are placebos or contain iron. If next menstrual period does not begin on schedule, rule out pregnancy before starting new dosing cycle. If menstrual period begins, start new dosing cycle 7 days after last tablet was taken. If all doses have been taken on schedule and one menstrual period is missed, continue dosing cycle. If two consecutive menstrual periods are missed, pregnancy test is required before new dosing cycle is started.

One dose missed: Take as soon as remembered or take 2 tablets next day

Two doses missed: Take 2 tablets as soon as remembered or 2 tablets next 2 days

Three doses missed: Begin new compact of tablets starting on day 1 of next cycle

Patient Information Take exactly as directed; use additional method of birth control during first week of administration of first cycle; photosensitivity may occur

Women should inform their physicians if signs or symptoms of any of the following occur thromboembolic or thrombotic disorders including sudden severe headache or vomiting, disturbance of vision or speech, loss of vision, numbness or weakness in an extremity, sharp or crushing chest pain, calf pain, shortness of breath, severe abdominal pain or mass, mental depression or unusual bleeding

Women should be advised that if they miss one daily dose, they should take the tablet as soon as remembered. If 2 daily doses are missed, 2 tablets should be taken daily for 2 days and the regular schedule resumed. If 3 or more daily doses are missed, therapy should be discontinued. Therapy with a new cycle can be resumed in 7 or 8 days. When any doses are missed, alternative contraceptive methods should be used for the next 2 days or until 2 days into the new cycle.

Women should discontinue taking the medication if they suspect they are pregnant or become pregnant

Nursing Implications Administer at bedtime to minimize occurrence of adverse effects

Additional Information 80 mcg of mestranol is approximately equivalent to 50 mcg of ethinyl estradiol

Dosage Forms Tablet: Mestranol 0.05 mg and norethindrone 1 mg (21s and 28s)

Metacortandralone *see* Prednisolone *on page 1037*

Metahydrin® *see* Trichlormethiazide *on page 1259*

Metamucil® [OTC] *see* Psyllium *on page 1075*

Metamucil® Instant Mix [OTC] *see* Psyllium *on page 1075*

Metandren® *see* Methyltestosterone *on page 821*

Metaprel® *see* Metaproterenol *on this page*

Metaproterenol (met a proe TER e nol)

Brand Names Alupent®; Arm-a-Med® Metaproterenol; Dey-Dose® Metaproterenol; Metaprel®; Prometa®

Synonyms Metaproterenol Sulfate; Orciprenaline Sulfate

Therapeutic Category $Beta_2$-Adrenergic Agonist Agent; Bronchodilator; Sympathomimetic

Use Bronchodilator in reversible airway obstruction due to asthma or COPD; because of its delayed onset of action (1 hour) and prolonged effect (4 or more hours), this may not be the drug of choice for assessing response to a bronchodilator

Pregnancy Risk Factor C

Pregnancy/Breast-Feeding Implications

Clinical effects on the fetus: No data on crossing the placenta. Reported association with polydactyly in 1 study; may be secondary to severe maternal disease or chance.

Breast-feeding/lactation: No data on crossing into breast milk or clinical effects on the infant

Contraindications Hypersensitivity to metaproterenol or any components, pre-existing cardiac arrhythmias associated with tachycardia

Warnings/Precautions Use with caution in patients with hypertension, CHF, hyperthyroidism, CAD, diabetes, or sensitivity to sympathomimetics; excessive prolonged use may result in decreased efficacy or increased toxicity and death; use caution in patients with pre-existing cardiac arrhythmias associated with tachycardia. Metaproterenol has more $beta_1$ activity than other sympathomimetics such as albuterol and, therefore, may no longer be the beta agonist of first choice. All patients should utilize a spacer device when using a metered dose inhaler. Oral use should be avoided due to the increased incidence of adverse effects.

Adverse Reactions

>10%:
- Central nervous system: Nervousness
- Neuromuscular & skeletal: Tremor

1% to 10%:
- Cardiovascular: Tachycardia, palpitations, hypertension
- Central nervous system: Headache, dizziness
- Gastrointestinal: Nausea, vomiting, bad taste
- Neuromuscular & skeletal: Trembling, muscle cramps, weakness
- Respiratory: Coughing
- Miscellaneous: Diaphoresis (increased)

<1%: Paradoxical bronchospasm

Overdosage/Toxicology Symptoms of overdose include angina, arrhythmias, tremor, dry mouth, insomnia; beta-adrenergic stimulation can increase and cause increased heart rate, decreased blood pressure, decreased CNS excitation

In cases of overdose, supportive therapy should be instituted, and prudent use of a cardioselective beta-adrenergic blocker (eg, atenolol or metoprolol) should be considered, keeping in mind the potential for induction of bronchoconstriction in an asthmatic individual. Dialysis has not been shown to be of value in the treatment of an overdose with this agent. Diazepam 0.07 mg/kg can be used for excitation seizures.

Drug Interactions

Decreased effect: Beta-blockers

Increased toxicity: Sympathomimetics, TCAs, MAO inhibitors

Stability Store in tight, light-resistant container; do not use if brown solution or contains a precipitate

Mechanism of Action Relaxes bronchial smooth muscle by action on $beta_2$-receptors with very little effect on heart rate

Pharmacodynamics/Kinetics

Oral:
- Onset of bronchodilation: Within 15 minutes

(Continued)

Metaproterenol *(Continued)*

Peak effect: Within 1 hour
Duration of action: ~1-5 hours
Inhalation:
Onset of effects: Within 60 seconds
Duration of action: Similar (~1-5 hours) regardless of route administered

Usual Dosage

Oral:
Children:
<2 years: 0.4 mg/kg/dose given 3-4 times/day; in infants, the dose can be given every 8-12 hours
2-6 years: 1-2.6 mg/kg/day divided every 6 hours
6-9 years: 10 mg/dose 3-4 times/day
Children >9 years and Adults: 20 mg 3-4 times/day
Elderly: Initial: 10 mg 3-4 times/day, increasing as necessary up to 20 mg 3-4 times/day
Inhalation: Children >12 years and Adults: 2-3 inhalations every 3-4 hours, up to 12 inhalations in 24 hours
Nebulizer:
Infants and Children: 0.01-0.02 mL/kg of 5% solution; minimum dose: 0.1 mL; maximum dose: 0.3 mL diluted in 2-3 mL normal saline every 4-6 hours (may be given more frequently according to need)
Adolescents and Adults: 5-20 breaths of full strength 5% metaproterenol **or** 0.2 to 0.3 mL 5% metaproterenol in 2.5-3 mL normal saline until nebulized every 4-6 hours (can be given more frequently according to need)

Administration Administer around-the-clock to promote less variation in peak and trough serum levels

Monitoring Parameters Assess lung sounds, pulse, and blood pressure before administration and during peak of medication; observe patient for wheezing after administration, if this occurs, call physician; monitor heart rate, respiratory rate, blood pressure, and arterial or capillary blood gases if applicable

Test Interactions ↑ potassium (S)

Patient Information Do not exceed recommended dosage - excessive use may lead to adverse effects or loss of effectiveness. Shake canister well before use. Administer pressurized inhalation during the second half of inspiration, as the airways are open wider and the aerosol distribution is more extensive. If more than one inhalation per dose is necessary, wait at least 1 full minute between inhalations - second inhalation is best delivered after 10 minutes for Alupent®. May cause nervousness, restlessness, insomnia - if these effects continue after dosage reduction, notify physician. Also notify physician if palpitations, tachycardia, chest pain, muscle tremors, dizziness, headache, flushing, or if breathing difficulty persists.

Nursing Implications Do not use solutions for nebulization if they are brown or contain a precipitate; before using, the inhaler must be shaken well

Dosage Forms

Aerosol, oral, as sulfate: 0.65 mg/dose (5 mL, 10 mL)
Solution for inhalation, as sulfate, preservative free: 0.4% [4 mg/mL] (2.5 mL); 0.6% [6 mg/mL] (2.5 mL); 5% [50 mg/mL] (10 mL, 30 mL)
Syrup, as sulfate: 10 mg/5 mL (480 mL)
Tablet, as sulfate: 10 mg, 20 mg

Metaproterenol Sulfate *see* Metaproterenol *on previous page*

Metaraminol (met a RAM i nole)

Related Information

Adrenergic Agonists, Cardiovascular Comparison *on page 1385*

Brand Names Aramine®

Synonyms Metaraminol Bitartrate

Therapeutic Category Adrenergic Agonist Agent; Sympathomimetic

Use Acute hypotensive crisis in the treatment of shock

Pregnancy Risk Factor D

Contraindications Hypersensitivity to metaraminol or any component, cyclopropane or halothane anesthesia, or MAO inhibitors

Warnings/Precautions Can cause cardiac arrhythmias; use with caution in patients with a previous myocardial infarction, hypertension, hyperthyroidism; prolonged use may produce cumulative effects

Adverse Reactions

1% to 10%: Cardiovascular: Tachycardia
<1%:
Cardiovascular: Hypertension, cardiac arrhythmias, flushing
Dermatologic: Blanching of skin, sloughing of tissue
Gastrointestinal: Nausea
Local: Abscess formation

Miscellaneous: Diaphoresis

Overdosage/Toxicology Symptoms of overdose include hypertension, cerebral hemorrhage, cardiac arrest, seizures

Drug Interactions

Decreased effect with TCAs

Increased toxicity with cyclopropane, halothane, MAO inhibitors (hypertensive crisis), digoxin, oxytocin, rauwolfia alkaloids, reserpine

Stability Infusion solutions are stable for 24 hours; I.V. metaraminol is **incompatible** when mixed with amphotericin B, dexamethasone, erythromycin, hydrocortisone, methicillin, penicillin G, prednisolone, thiopental

Mechanism of Action Stimulates alpha-adrenergic receptors to cause vasoconstriction, reflex bradycardia, inhibits GI smooth muscle and vascular smooth muscle supplying skeletal muscle, increases heart rate and force of heart muscle contraction

Pharmacodynamics/Kinetics

Onset of pressor effect:

- I.M.: Within 10 minutes
- I.V.: Within 1-2 minutes
- S.C.: Within 5-20 minutes

Elimination: Has not yet been fully elucidated

Usual Dosage

Children:

- I.M.: 0.01 mg/kg as a single dose
- I.V.: 0.01 mg/kg as a single dose or intravenous infusion of 5 mcg/kg/minute

Adults:

- Prevention of hypotension: I.M., S.C.: 2-10 mg
- Adjunctive treatment of hypotension: I.V.: 15-100 mg in 250-500 mL NS or 5% dextrose in water
- Severe shock: I.V.: 0.5-5 mg direct I.V. injection followed by intravenous infusion of 15-100 mg in 250-500 mL NS or D_5W; may also be administered endotracheally

Administration May be given I.M., I.V., S.C.; however, I.V. is the preferred route because extravasation or local injection can cause necrosis; to prevent necrosis infiltrate area with 10-15 mL of saline containing 5-10 mg of phentolamine

Monitoring Parameters Blood pressure, EKG, PCWP, CVP, pulse, and urine output

Dosage Forms Injection, as bitartrate: 10 mg/mL (10 mL)

Metaraminol Bitartrate *see* Metaraminol *on previous page*

Metastron® *see* Strontium-89 *on page 1165*

Metformin (met FOR min)

Related Information

Hypoglycemic Drugs, Comparison of Oral Agents *on page 1411*

Brand Names Glucophage®

Canadian/Mexican Brand Names Novo-Metformin® (Canada); Glucophage® Forte (Mexico)

Synonyms Metformin Hydrochloride

Therapeutic Category Antidiabetic Agent, Oral; Antihyperglycemic Agent; Hypoglycemic Agent, Oral

Use Management of noninsulin-dependent diabetes mellitus (type II) as monotherapy when hyperglycemia cannot be managed on diet alone. May be used concomitantly with a sulfonylurea when diet and metformin or sulfonylurea alone do not result in adequate glycemic control.

Investigational: Data suggests that some patients with NIDDM with secondary failure to sulfonylurea therapy may obtain significant improvement in metabolic control when metformin in combination with insulin and a sulfonylurea is used in lieu of insulin alone

Pregnancy Risk Factor B

Contraindications Hypersensitivity to metformin or any component; renal disease or renal dysfunction (serum creatinine ≥1.5 mg/dL in males or ≥1.4 mg/dL in females or abnormal clearance) which may also result from conditions such as cardiovascular collapse, acute myocardial infarction, and septicemia; acute or chronic metabolic acidosis with or without coma (including diabetic ketoacidosis); should be temporarily withheld in patients undergoing radiologic studies involving the parenteral administration of iodinated contrast materials (potential for acute alteration in renal function).

Warnings/Precautions Administration of oral antidiabetic drugs has been reported to be associated with increased cardiovascular mortality as compared to treatment with diet alone or diet plus insulin. Metformin is substantially excreted by the kidney - the risk of accumulation and lactic acidosis increases with the degree of impairment of renal function. Patients with renal function below the limit

(Continued)

Metformin *(Continued)*

of normal for their age should not receive metformin. In elderly patients, renal function should be monitored regularly. Use of concomitant medications that may affect renal function (ie, affect tubular secretion) may affect metformin disposition. Therapy should be suspended for any surgical procedures. Avoid use in patients with impaired liver function.

Adverse Reactions

>10%: Gastrointestinal: Anorexia, nausea, vomiting, diarrhea, epigastric fullness, constipation, heartburn

1% to 10%:

Dermatologic: Rash, urticaria, photosensitivity

Miscellaneous: Decreased vitamin B_{12} levels

<1%: Hematologic: Blood dyscrasias, aplastic anemia, hemolytic anemia, bone marrow suppression, thrombocytopenia, agranulocytosis

Overdosage/Toxicology Hypoglycemia has not been observed with ingestions of up to 85 g of metformin, although lactic acidosis has occurred in such circumstances

Metformin is dialyzable with a clearance of up to 170 mL/minute; hemodialysis may be useful for removal of accumulated drug from patients in whom metformin overdosage is suspected

Drug Interactions

Decreased effects: Drugs which tend to produce hyperglycemia (eg, diuretics, corticosteroids, phenothiazines, thyroid products, estrogens, oral contraceptives, phenytoin, nicotinic acid, sympathomimetics, calcium channel blocking drugs, isoniazid) may lead to a loss of glycemic control

Increased effects: Furosemide increased the metformin plasma and blood C_{max} without altering metformin renal clearance in a single dose study

Increased toxicity:

Cationic drugs (eg, amiloride, digoxin, morphine, procainamide, quinidine, quinine, ranitidine, triamterene, trimethoprim, and vancomycin) which are eliminated by renal tubular secretion could have the potential for interaction with metformin by competing for common renal tubular transport systems

Cimetidine increases (by 60%) peak metformin plasma and whole blood concentrations

Mechanism of Action Decreases hepatic glucose production, decreasing intestinal absorption of glucose and improves insulin sensitivity (increases peripheral glucose uptake and utilization)

Pharmacodynamics/Kinetics

Distribution: V_d: 654±358 L

Protein binding: 92% to 99%

Protein binding, plasma: negligible

Bioavailability, absolute: 50% to 60% under fasting conditions; food decreases the extent and slightly delays the absorption; the clinical relevance is unknown

Half-life, plasma elimination: 6.2 hours

Elimination: Renal; tubular secretion is major route

Usual Dosage Oral (allow 1-2 weeks between dose titrations):

Adults:

500 mg tablets: Initial: 500 mg twice daily (given with the morning and evening meals). Dosage increases should be made in increments of one tablet every week, given in divided doses, up to a maximum of 2,500 mg/day. Doses of up to 2000 mg/day may be given twice daily. If a dose of 2,500 mg/day is required, it may be better tolerated 3 times/day (with meals).

850 mg tablets: Initial: 850 mg once daily (given with the morning meal). Dosage increases should be made in increments of one tablet every OTHER week, given in divided doses, up to a maximum of 2550 mg/day. The usual maintenance dose is 850 mg twice daily (with the morning and evening meals). Some patients may be given 850 mg 3 times/day (with meals).

Elderly patients: The initial and maintenance dosing should be conservative, due to the potential for decreased renal function. Generally, elderly patients should not be titrated to the maximum dose of metformin.

Transfer from other antidiabetic agents: No transition period is generally necessary except when transferring from chlorpropamide. When transferring from chlorpropamide, care should be exercised during the first 2 weeks because of the prolonged retention of chlorpropamide in the body, leading to overlapping drug effects and possible hypoglycemia.

Concomitant metformin and oral sulfonylurea therapy: If patients have not responded to 4 weeks of the maximum dose of metformin monotherapy, consideration to a gradual addition of an oral sulfonylurea while continuing metformin at the maximum dose, even if prior primary or secondary failure to a sulfonylurea has occurred.

Dosing adjustment/comments in renal impairment: The plasma and blood half-life of metformin is prolonged and the renal clearance is decreased in proportion to the decrease in creatinine clearance

Dosing adjustment in hepatic impairment: No studies have been conducted

Dietary Considerations

Alcohol: Incidence of lactic acidosis may be increased; avoid or limit use

Food: Food decreases the extent and slightly delays the absorption. Drug may cause GI upset; take with food to decrease GI upset.

Glucose: Decreases blood glucose concentration. Hypoglycemia does not usually occur unless a patient is predisposed. Monitor blood glucose concentration. Exercise caution with administration in patients predisposed to hypoglycemia (eg, cases of reduced caloric intake, strenuous exercise without repletion of calories, alcohol ingestion or when metformin is combined with another oral antidiabetic agent).

Vitamin B_{12}: Decreases absorption of Vitamin B_{12}; monitor for signs and symptoms of vitamin B_{12} deficiency

Folic acid: Decreases absorption of folic acid; monitor for signs and symptoms of folic acid deficiency

Monitoring Parameters Urine for glucose and ketones, fasting blood glucose, hemoglobin A_{1c}, and fructosamine. Initial and periodic monitoring of hematologic parameters (eg, hemoglobin/hematocrit and red blood cell indices) and renal function should be performed, at least annually. While megaloblastic anemia has been rarely seen with metformin, if suspected, vitamin B_{12} deficiency should be excluded.

Reference Range Target range: Adults:

Fasting blood glucose: <120 mg/dL

Glycosylated hemoglobin: <7%

Patient Information Patients must be counseled by someone experienced in diabetes education, signs and symptoms of hyper- and hypoglycemia, exercise and diet, blood glucose monitoring, and other related topics; eat regularly, do not skip meals; carry quick source of sugar; medical alert bracelet. Patients should be counselled against excessive alcohol intake while receiving metformin. Metformin alone does not usually cause hypoglycemia, although it may occur in conjunction with oral sulfonylureas.

Nursing Implications Patients who are NPO may need to have their dose held to avoid hypoglycemia

Dosage Forms Tablet, as hydrochloride: 500 mg, 850 mg

Metformin Hydrochloride *see* Metformin *on page 795*

Methacholine (meth a KOLE leen)

Brand Names Provocholine®

Synonyms Methacholine Chloride

Therapeutic Category Cholinergic Agent; Diagnostic Agent, Bronchial Airway Hyperactivity

Use Diagnosis of bronchial airway hyperactivity in subjects who do not have clinically apparent asthma

Pregnancy Risk Factor C

Contraindications Concomitant use of beta-blockers; hypersensitivity to the drug; because of the potential for severe bronchoconstriction, methacholine challenge should not be performed on any patient with clinically apparent asthma, wheezing, or very low baseline pulmonary function tests (forced expiratory volume in one second less than 70% of predicted value).

Warnings/Precautions Methacholine is a bronchoconstrictor for diagnostic purposes only. Perform inhalation challenge under the supervision of a physician trained in and thoroughly familiar with all aspects of the technique, all contraindications, warnings, and precautions of methacholine challenge and the management of respiratory distress. Have emergency equipment and medication immediately available to treat acute respiratory distress. Administer only by inhalation; severe bronchoconstriction and reduction in respiratory function can result. Patients with severe hyperreactivity of the airways can experience bronchoconstriction at a dosage as low as 0.025 mg/mL (0.125 cumulative units). If severe bronchoconstriction occurs, reverse immediately by administration of a rapid-acting inhaled bronchodilator (beta-agonist).

Adverse Reactions

<1%:

Cardiovascular: Hypotension, complete heart block, substernal pain, tightness of the chest, syncope

Central nervous system: Headache, lightheadedness

Respiratory: Throat irritation, itching, cough, dyspnea, wheezing

Stability Store unreconstituted powder at 59°F to 86°F; store dilutions in refrigerator (36°F to 46°F) for up to 2 weeks

(Continued)

Methacholine *(Continued)*

Mechanism of Action Methacholine chloride is a cholinergic (parasympathomimetic) synthetic analogue of acetylcholine. The drug stimulates muscarinic, postganglionic parasympathetic receptors, which results in smooth muscle contraction of the airways and increased tracheobronchial secretions.

Pharmacodynamics/Kinetics

Onset of action: Rapid

Peak effect: Within 1-4 minutes

Duration: 15-75 minutes or 5 minutes if the methacholine challenge is followed with a beta-agonist agent

Usual Dosage Before inhalation challenge, perform baseline pulmonary function tests; the patient must have an FEV_1 of at least 70% of the predicted value. The following is a suggested schedule for administration of methacholine challenge. Calculate cumulative units by multiplying number of breaths by concentration given. Total cumulative units is the sum of cumulative units for each concentration given. See table.

Vial	Serial Concentration (mg/mL)	No. of Breaths	Cumulative Units per Concentration	Total Cumulative Units
E	0.025	5	0.125	0.125
D	0.25	5	1.25	1.375
C	2.5	5	12.5	13.88
B	10	5	50	63.88
A	25	5	125	188.88

Determine FEV_1 within 5 minutes of challenge, a postive challenge is a 20% reduction in FEV_1

Dosage Forms Powder for reconstitution, inhalation, as chloride: 100 mg/5 mL

Methacholine Chloride *see* Methacholine *on previous page*

Methadone (METH a done)

Related Information

Narcotic Agonists Comparison *on page 1414*

Dose Equivalents for Opioid Analgesics in Opioid-Naive Adults <50 kg *on page 1376*

Dose Equivalents for Opioid Analgesics in Opioid-Naive Adults ≥50 kg *on page 1375*

Brand Names Dolophine®

Canadian/Mexican Brand Names Methadose® (Canada)

Synonyms Methadone Hydrochloride

Therapeutic Category Analgesic, Narcotic

Use Management of severe pain, used in narcotic detoxification maintenance programs

Restrictions C-II

Pregnancy Risk Factor B (D if used for prolonged periods or in high doses at term)

Contraindications Hypersensitivity to methadone or any component

Warnings/Precautions Tablets are to be used only for oral administration and **must not** be used for injection; use with caution in patients with respiratory diseases including asthma, emphysema, or COPD and in patients with severe liver disease; because methadone's effects on respiration last much longer than its analgesic effects, the dose must be titrated slowly; because of its long half-life and risk of accumulation, it is not considered a drug of first choice in the elderly, who may be particularly susceptible to its CNS depressant and constipating effects

Adverse Reactions

Central nervous system: CNS depression

Endocrine & metabolic: Antidiuretic hormone release

Ocular: Miosis

Respiratory: Respiratory depression

>10%:

- Cardiovascular: Palpitations, hypotension, bradycardia, peripheral vasodilation
- Central nervous system: Fatigue, drowsiness, dizziness
- Gastrointestinal: Nausea, vomiting, constipation
- Neuromuscular & skeletal: Weakness
- Miscellaneous: Histamine release

1% to 10%:

- Central nervous system: Nervousness, headache, restlessness, anorexia, malaise, confusion, increased intracranial pressure
- Gastrointestinal: Stomach cramps, xerostomia, biliary tract spasm

Genitourinary: Decreased urination, urinary tract spasm
Local: Pain at injection site
Respiratory: Dyspnea, shortness of breath

<1%:

Central nervous system: Mental depression, hallucinations, paradoxical CNS stimulation
Dermatologic: Pruritus, rash, urticaria
Gastrointestinal: Paralytic ileus
Miscellaneous: Physical and psychological dependence

Overdosage/Toxicology Symptoms of overdose include respiratory depression, CNS depression, miosis, hypothermia, circulatory collapse, convulsions

Naloxone 2 mg I.V. (0.01 mg/kg for children) with repeat administration as necessary up to a total of 10 mg

Drug Interactions

Decreased effect: Phenytoin, pentazocine and rifampin may increase the metabolism of methadone and may precipitate withdrawal

Increased toxicity: CNS depressants, phenothiazines, tricyclic antidepressants, MAO inhibitors may potentiate the adverse effects of methadone

Stability Highly **incompatible** with all other I.V. agents when mixed together

Mechanism of Action Binds to opiate receptors in the CNS, causing inhibition of ascending pain pathways, altering the perception of and response to pain; produces generalized CNS depression

Pharmacodynamics/Kinetics

Oral:

Onset of analgesia: Within 0.5-1 hour
Duration: 6-8 hours, increases to 22-48 hours with repeated doses

Parenteral:

Onset of effect: Within 10-20 minutes
Peak effect: Within 1-2 hours

Distribution: Crosses the placenta; appears in breast milk
Protein binding: 80% to 85%
Metabolism: In the liver (N-demethylation)
Half-life: 15-29 hours, may be prolonged with alkaline pH
Elimination: In urine (<10% as unchanged drug); increased renal excretion with urine pH <6

Usual Dosage Doses should be titrated to appropriate effects

Children: Analgesia:

Oral, I.M., S.C.: 0.7 mg/kg/24 hours divided every 4-6 hours as needed or 0.1-0.2 mg/kg every 4-12 hours as needed; maximum: 10 mg/dose

I.V.: 0.1 mg/kg every 4 hours initially for 2-3 doses, then every 6-12 hours as needed; maximum: 10 mg/dose

Adults:

Analgesia: Oral, I.M., I.V., S.C.: 2.5-10 mg every 3-8 hours as needed, up to 5-20 mg every 6-8 hours

Detoxification: Oral: 15-40 mg/day; should not exceed 21 days and may not be repeated earlier than 4 weeks after completion of preceding course

Maintenance of opiate dependence: Oral: 20-120 mg/day

Dosing adjustment in renal impairment: Cl_{cr} <10 mL/minute: Administer at 50% to 75% of normal dose

Dosing adjustment/comments in hepatic disease: Avoid in severe liver disease

Important note: Methadone accumulates with repeated doses and dosage may need to be adjusted downward after 3-5 days to prevent toxic effects. Some patients may benefit from every 8- to 12-hour dosing interval (pain control).

Dietary Considerations

Alcohol: Additive CNS effects, avoid or limit alcohol; watch for sedation
Food: Glucose may cause hyperglycemia; monitor blood glucose concentrations

Monitoring Parameters Pain relief, respiratory and mental status, blood pressure

Reference Range Therapeutic: 100-400 ng/mL (SI: 0.32-1.29 μmol/L); Toxic: >2 μg/mL (SI: >6.46 μmol/L)

Test Interactions ↑ thyroxine (S), ↑ aminotransferase [ALT (SGPT)/AST (SGOT)] (S)

Patient Information May cause drowsiness, avoid alcohol and other CNS depressants

Nursing Implications Observe patient for excessive sedation, respiratory depression, implement safety measures, assist with ambulation

Dosage Forms

Injection, as hydrochloride: 10 mg/mL (1 mL, 10 mL, 20 mL)

Solution, as hydrochloride:

Oral: 5 mg/5 mL (5 mL, 500 mL); 10 mg/5 mL (500 mL)

(Continued)

Methadone *(Continued)*

Oral, concentrate: 10 mg/mL (30 mL)
Tablet, as hydrochloride: 5 mg, 10 mg
Tablet, dispersible, as hydrochloride: 40 mg

Methadone Hydrochloride *see* Methadone *on page 798*

Methaminodiazepoxide Hydrochloride *see* Chlordiazepoxide *on page 252*

Methamphetamine (meth am FET a meen)

Brand Names Desoxyn®

Synonyms Desoxyephedrine Hydrochloride; Methamphetamine Hydrochloride

Therapeutic Category Amphetamine; Central Nervous System Stimulant, Amphetamine

Use Treatment of narcolepsy, exogenous obesity, abnormal behavioral syndrome in children (minimal brain dysfunction)

Restrictions C-II

Pregnancy Risk Factor C

Contraindications Known hypersensitivity to methamphetamine

Warnings/Precautions Cardiovascular disease, nephritis, angina pectoris, hypertension, glaucoma, patients with a history of drug abuse, known hypersensitivity to amphetamine

Adverse Reactions

>10%:
- Cardiovascular: Arrhythmia
- Central nervous system: False feeling of well being, nervousness, restlessness, insomnia

1% to 10%:
- Cardiovascular: Hypertension
- Central nervous system: Mood or mental changes, dizziness, lightheadedness, headache
- Endocrine & metabolic: Changes in libido
- Gastrointestinal: Diarrhea, nausea, vomiting, stomach cramps, constipation, anorexia, weight loss, xerostomia
- Ocular: Blurred vision
- Miscellaneous: Diaphoresis (increased)

<1%:
- Cardiovascular: Chest pain
- Central nervous system: CNS stimulation (severe), Tourette's syndrome, hyperthermia, seizures, paranoia
- Dermatologic: Rash, urticaria
- Miscellaneous: Tolerance and withdrawal with prolonged use

Overdosage/Toxicology Symptoms of overdose include seizures, hyperactivity, coma, hypertension

There is no specific antidote for amphetamine intoxication and the bulk of the treatment is supportive. Hyperactivity and agitation usually respond to reduced sensory input, however with extreme agitation haloperidol (2-5 mg I.M. for adults) may be required. Hyperthermia is best treated with external cooling measures, or when severe or unresponsive, muscle paralysis with pancuronium may be needed. Hypertension is usually transient and generally does not require treatment unless severe. For diastolic blood pressures >110 mm Hg, a nitroprusside infusion should be initiated. Seizures usually respond to diazepam IVP and/or phenytoin maintenance regimens.

Drug Interactions Increased toxicity with MAO inhibitors (hypertensive crisis)

Usual Dosage

Attention deficit disorder: Children >6 years: 2.5-5 mg 1-2 times/day, may increase by 5 mg increments weekly until optimum response is achieved, usually 20-25 mg/day

Exogenous obesity: Children >12 years and Adults: 5 mg, 30 minutes before each meal; long-acting formulation: 10-15 mg in morning; treatment duration should not exceed a few weeks

Monitoring Parameters Heart rate, respiratory rate, blood pressure, and CNS activity

Patient Information Take during day to avoid insomnia; do not discontinue abruptly, may cause physical and psychological dependence with prolonged use; do not crush or chew extended release tablet

Nursing Implications Dose should not be given in evening or at bedtime; do not crush extended release tablet

Dosage Forms

Tablet, as hydrochloride: 5 mg
Tablet, extended release, as hydrochloride (Gradumet®): 5 mg, 10 mg, 15 mg

Methamphetamine Hydrochloride *see* Methamphetamine *on this page*

Methazolamide (meth a ZOE la mide)

Related Information

Glaucoma Drug Therapy Comparison *on page 1410*
Sulfonamide Derivatives *on page 1420*

Brand Names GlaucTabs®; Neptazane®

Therapeutic Category Carbonic Anhydrase Inhibitor; Diuretic, Carbonic Anhydrase Inhibitor

Use Adjunctive treatment of open-angle or secondary glaucoma; short-term therapy of narrow-angle glaucoma when delay of surgery is desired

Pregnancy Risk Factor C

Contraindications Marked kidney or liver dysfunction, severe pulmonary obstruction, hypersensitivity to methazolamide or any component

Warnings/Precautions Sulfonamide-type reactions, melena, anorexia, nausea, vomiting, constipation, hematuria, glycosuria, urinary frequency, renal colic, renal calculi, crystalluria, polyuria, hepatic insufficiency, various CNS effects, transient myopia, bone marrow suppression, thrombocytopenia/purpura, hemolytic anemia, leukopenia, pancytopenia, agranulocytosis, urticaria, pruritus, rash, Stevens-Johnson syndrome, weight loss, fever, acidosis; use with caution in patients with respiratory acidosis and diabetes mellitus; impairment of mental alertness and/or physical coordination. Malaise and complaints of tiredness and myalgia are signs of excessive dosing and acidosis in the elderly.

Adverse Reactions

>10%:
- Central nervous system: Malaise
- Gastrointestinal: Metallic taste, anorexia
- Genitourinary: Polyuria
- Neuromuscular & skeletal: Weakness

1% to 10%:
- Central nervous system: Mental depression, drowsiness, dizziness
- Genitourinary: Crystalluria

<1%:
- Central nervous system: Fever, headache, seizures, fatigue
- Dermatologic: Rash, sulfonamide rash, Stevens-Johnson syndrome
- Endocrine & metabolic: Hyperchloremic metabolic acidosis, hypokalemia, hyperglycemia
- Gastrointestinal: GI irritation, constipation, xerostomia, black tarry stools
- Hematologic: Bone marrow suppression
- Genitourinary: Dysuria
- Neuromuscular & skeletal: Paresthesia, trembling, unsteadiness
- Ocular: Myopia
- Otic: Tinnitus
- Miscellaneous: Loss of smell, hypersensitivity

Drug Interactions

Increased toxicity:
- May induce hypokalemia which would sensitize a patient to digitalis toxicity
- May increase the potential for salicylate toxicity
- Hypokalemia may be compounded with concurrent diuretic use or steroids
- Primidone absorption may be delayed

Decreased effect: Increased lithium excretion and altered excretion of other drugs by alkalinization of the urine, such as amphetamines, quinidine, procainamide, methenamine, phenobarbital, salicylates

Mechanism of Action Noncompetitive inhibition of the enzyme carbonic anhydrase; thought that carbonic anhydrase is located at the luminal border of cells of the proximal tubule. When the enzyme is inhibited, there is an increase in urine volume and a change to an alkaline pH with a subsequent decrease in the excretion of titratable acid and ammonia.

Pharmacodynamics/Kinetics

- Onset of action: Slow in comparison with acetazolamide (2-4 hours)
- Peak effect: 6-8 hours
- Duration: 10-18 hours
- Absorption: Slowly from GI tract
- Distribution: Distributes well into tissue
- Protein binding: ~55%
- Half-life: ~14 hours
- Elimination: ~25% excreted unchanged in urine

Usual Dosage Adults: Oral: 50-100 mg 2-3 times/day

Patient Information Take with food, report any numbness or tingling in extremities to physician; may cause drowsiness, impaired judgment or coordination

Nursing Implications May cause an alteration in taste, especially when drinking carbonated beverages

Dosage Forms Tablet: 25 mg, 50 mg

Methenamine (meth EN a meen)

Brand Names Hiprex®; Urex®

Canadian/Mexican Brand Names Dehydral® (Canada); Hip-Rex® (Canada); Urasal® (Canada)

Synonyms Hexamethylenetetramine; Methenamine Hippurate; Methenamine Mandelate

Therapeutic Category Antibiotic, Miscellaneous

Use Prophylaxis or suppression of recurrent urinary tract infections; urinary tract discomfort secondary to hypermotility; should not be used to treat infections outside of urinary tract

Pregnancy Risk Factor C

Contraindications Severe dehydration, renal insufficiency, hepatic insufficiency in patients receiving hippurate salt, hypersensitivity to methenamine or any component

Warnings/Precautions Use with caution in patients with hepatic disease, gout, and the elderly; doses of 8 g/day may cause bladder irritation, some products may contain tartrazine; methenamine should not be used to treat infections outside of the lower urinary tract

Adverse Reactions

1% to 10%:

Dermatologic: Rash

Gastrointestinal: Nausea, vomiting, diarrhea, anorexia, abdominal cramping

<1%:

Central nervous system: Headache

Genitourinary: Bladder irritation, crystalluria, dysuria

Hepatic: Elevation in AST and ALT

Renal: Hematuria

Overdosage/Toxicology Well tolerated; treatment includes GI decontamination, if possible, and supportive care

Drug Interactions

Decreased effect: Sodium bicarbonate and acetazolamide will decrease effect secondary to alkalinization of urine

Increased toxicity: Sulfonamides (may precipitate)

Stability Protect from excessive heat

Mechanism of Action Methenamine is hydrolyzed to formaldehyde and ammonia in acidic urine; formaldehyde has nonspecific bactericidal action

Pharmacodynamics/Kinetics

Absorption: Readily absorbed from GI tract

Metabolism: 10% to 30% of the drug will be hydrolyzed by gastric juices unless it is protected by an enteric coating; ~10% to 25% is metabolized in the liver

Half-life: 3-6 hours

Elimination: Occurs via glomerular filtration and tubular secretion with ~70% to 90% of dose excreted unchanged in urine within 24 hours

Usual Dosage Oral:

Children: 6-12 years:

Hippurate: 25-50 mg/kg/day divided every 12 hours

Mandelate: 50-75 mg/kg/day divided every 6 hours

Children >12 years and Adults:

Hippurate: 1 g twice daily

Mandelate: 1 g 4 times/day after meals and at bedtime

Dosing adjustment/comments in renal impairment: Cl_{cr} <50 mL/minute: Avoid use

Administration Administer around-the-clock rather than 4 times/day to promote less variation in peak and trough serum levels

Monitoring Parameters Urinalysis, periodic liver function tests in patients

Test Interactions ↑ catecholamines and VMA (U); ↓ HIAA (U)

Patient Information Take with food to minimize GI upset; take with ascorbic acid to acidify urine; drink sufficient fluids to ensure adequate urine flow. Avoid excessive intake of alkalinizing foods (citrus fruits and milk products) or medication (bicarbonate, acetazolamide); notify physician if skin rash, painful urination or excessive abdominal pain occur.

Nursing Implications Urine should be acidic (pH <5.5) for maximum effect

Dosage Forms

Tablet, as hippurate (Hiprex®, Urex®): 1 g (Hiprex® contains tartrazine dye)

Tablet, as mandelate, enteric coated: 250 mg, 500 mg, 1 g

Methenamine Hippurate *see* Methenamine *on this page*

Methenamine Mandelate *see* Methenamine *on this page*

Methergine® *see* Methylergonovine *on page 817*

Methicillin (meth i SIL in)

Brand Names Staphcillin®

Synonyms Dimethoxyphenyl Penicillin Sodium; Methicillin Sodium; Sodium Methicillin

Therapeutic Category Antibiotic, Penicillin

Use Treatment of susceptible bacterial infections such as osteomyelitis, septicemia, endocarditis, and CNS infections due to penicillinase-producing strains of *Staphylococcus*; other antistaphylococcal penicillins are usually preferred

Pregnancy Risk Factor B

Contraindications Known hypersensitivity to methicillin or any penicillin

Warnings/Precautions Elimination rate will be slow in neonates; modify dosage in patients with renal impairment and in the elderly; use with caution in patients with cephalosporin hypersensitivity

Adverse Reactions

1% to 10%:
- Dermatologic: Rash
- Renal: Acute interstitial nephritis

<1%:
- Central nervous system: Fever
- Dermatologic: Rash
- Genitourinary: Hemorrhagic cystitis
- Hematologic: Eosinophilia, anemia, leukopenia, neutropenia, thrombocytopenia
- Local: Phlebitis
- Miscellaneous: Serum sickness-like reactions

Overdosage/Toxicology Symptoms of penicillin overdose include neuromuscular hypersensitivity (agitation, hallucinations, asterixis, encephalopathy, confusion, and seizures) and electrolyte imbalance with potassium or sodium salts, especially in renal failure

Hemodialysis may be helpful to aid in the removal of the drug from the blood, otherwise most treatment is supportive or symptom directed

Drug Interactions

Decreased effect: Efficacy of oral contraceptives may be reduced

Increased effect: Disulfiram, probenecid may increase penicillin levels, increased effect of anticoagulants

Stability Reconstituted solution is stable for 24 hours at room temperature and 4 days when refrigerated; discard solutions if it has a distinctive hydrogen sulfide odor and/or color turns to a deep orange; **incompatible** with aminoglycosides and tetracyclines

Mechanism of Action Inhibits bacterial cell wall synthesis by binding to one or more of the penicillin binding proteins (PBPs); which in turn inhibits the final transpeptidation step of peptidoglycan synthesis in bacterial cell walls, thus inhibiting cell wall biosynthesis. Bacteria eventually lyse due to ongoing activity of cell wall autolytic enzymes (autolysins and murein hydrolases) while cell wall assembly is arrested.

Pharmacodynamics/Kinetics

Distribution: Crosses the placenta; distributes into milk

Protein binding: 40%

Metabolism: Only partially

Half-life (with normal renal function):
- Neonates:
  - <2 weeks: 2-3.9 hours
  - >2 weeks: 0.9-3.3 hours
- Children 2-16 years: 0.8 hour
- Adults: 0.4-0.5 hour

Time to peak serum concentration:
- I.M.: 0.5-1 hour
- I.V. infusion: Within 5 minutes

Elimination: ~60% to 70% of dose eliminated unchanged in urine within 4 hours by tubular secretion and glomerular filtration

Usual Dosage I.M., I.V.:

Children: 150-200 mg/kg/day divided every 6 hours; 200-400 mg/kg/day divided every 4-6 hours has been used for treatment of severe infections; maximum dose: 12 g/day

Adults: 4-12 g/day in divided doses every 4-6 hours

Dosing interval in renal impairment:
- Cl_{cr} 10-50 mL/minute: Administer every 6-8 hours
- Cl_{cr} <10 mL/minute: Administer every 8-12 hours

Hemodialysis: Not dialyzable (0% to 5%)

(Continued)

Methicillin *(Continued)*

Administration Can be administered IVP at a rate not to exceed 200 mg/minute or intermittent infusion over 20-30 minutes; final concentration for administration should not exceed 20 mg/mL

Test Interactions Interferes with tests for urinary and serum proteins, uric acid, urinary steroids; may cause false-positive Coombs' test; may inactivate aminoglycosides *in vitro*

Dosage Forms Powder for injection, as sodium: 1 g, 4 g, 6 g, 10 g

Methicillin Sodium *see* Methicillin *on previous page*

Methimazole (meth IM a zole)

Brand Names Tapazole®

Synonyms Thiamazole

Therapeutic Category Antithyroid Agent

Use Palliative treatment of hyperthyroidism, return the hyperthyroid patient to a normal metabolic state prior to thyroidectomy, and to control thyrotoxic crisis that may accompany thyroidectomy. The use of antithyroid thioamides is as effective in elderly as they are in younger adults; however, the expense, potential adverse effects, and inconvenience (compliance, monitoring) make them undesirable. The use of radioiodine due to ease of administration and less concern for long-term side effects and reproduction problems (some older males) makes it a more appropriate therapy.

Pregnancy Risk Factor D

Contraindications Hypersensitivity to methimazole or any component, nursing mothers

Warnings/Precautions Use with extreme caution in patients receiving other drugs known to cause myelosuppression particularly agranulocytosis, patients >40 years of age; avoid doses >40 mg/day (↑ myelosuppression); may cause acneiform eruptions or worsen the condition of the thyroid

Adverse Reactions

>10%:
- Central nervous system: Fever
- Dermatologic: Rash
- Hematologic: Leukopenia

1% to 10%:
- Central nervous system: Dizziness
- Gastrointestinal: Nausea, vomiting, stomach pain, abnormal taste
- Hematologic: Agranulocytosis
- Miscellaneous: SLE-like syndrome

<1%:
- Cardiovascular: Edema
- Central nervous system: Drowsiness, vertigo, headache
- Dermatologic: Rash, urticaria, pruritus, alopecia
- Endocrine & metabolic: Goiter
- Gastrointestinal: Constipation, weight gain
- Genitourinary: Nephrotic syndrome
- Hematologic: Thrombocytopenia, aplastic anemia
- Hepatic: Cholestatic jaundice
- Neuromuscular & skeletal: Arthralgia, paresthesia
- Miscellaneous: Swollen salivary glands

Overdosage/Toxicology Symptoms of overdose include nausea, vomiting, epigastric distress, headache, fever, arthralgia, pruritus, edema, pancytopenia, and signs of hypothyroidism; management of overdose is supportive

Drug Interactions Increased toxicity: Iodinated glycerol, lithium, potassium iodide; anticoagulant activity increased

Stability Protect from light

Mechanism of Action Inhibits the synthesis of thyroid hormones by blocking the oxidation of iodine in the thyroid gland, blocking iodine's ability to combine with tyrosine to form thyroxine and triiodothyronine (T_3), does not inactivate circulating T_4 and T_3

Pharmacodynamics/Kinetics

Bioavailability: 80% to 95%

Onset of antithyroid effect: Oral: Within 30-40 minutes

Duration: 2-4 hours

Distribution: Crosses the placenta; appears in breast milk (1:1)

Protein binding: No plasma protein binding

Half-life: 4-13 hours

Elimination: Renally with ~12% excreted in urine within 24 hours

Usual Dosage Oral: Administer in 3 equally divided doses at approximately 8-hour intervals

Children: Initial: 0.4 mg/kg/day in 3 divided doses; maintenance: 0.2 mg/kg/day in 3 divided doses up to 30 mg/24 hours maximum

Adults: Initial: 5 mg every 8 hours; maintenance dose: 5-15 mg/day up to 60 mg/day for severe hyperthyroidism

Adjust dosage as required to achieve and maintain serum T_3, T_4, and TSH levels in the normal range. An elevated T_3 may be the sole indicator of inadequate treatment. An elevated TSH indicates excessive antithyroid treatment.

Monitoring Parameters Monitor for signs of hypothyroidism, hyperthyroidism, T_4, T_3; CBC with differential, liver function (baseline and as needed), serum thyroxine, free thyroxine index

Patient Information Take with meals, take at regular intervals around-the-clock; notify physician if persistent fever, sore throat, fatigue, unusual bleeding or bruising occurs

Dosage Forms Tablet: 5 mg, 10 mg

Methocarbamol (meth oh KAR ba mole)

Brand Names Delaxin®; Marbaxin®; Robaxin®; Robomol®

Therapeutic Category Skeletal Muscle Relaxant

Use Treatment of muscle spasm associated with acute painful musculoskeletal conditions, supportive therapy in tetanus

Pregnancy Risk Factor C

Contraindications Renal impairment, hypersensitivity to methocarbamol or any component

Warnings/Precautions Rate of injection should not exceed 3 mL/minute; solution is hypertonic; avoid extravasation; use with caution in patients with a history of seizures

Adverse Reactions

>10%: Central nervous system: Drowsiness, dizziness, lightheadedness

1% to 10%:

- Cardiovascular: Flushing of face, bradycardia
- Dermatologic: Allergic dermatitis
- Gastrointestinal: Nausea, vomiting
- Ocular: Nystagmus
- Respiratory: Nasal congestion

<1%:

- Cardiovascular: Syncope
- Central nervous system: Convulsions
- Hematologic: Leukopenia
- Local: Pain at injection site, thrombophlebitis
- Ocular: Blurred vision, renal impairment
- Miscellaneous: Allergic manifestations

Overdosage/Toxicology Symptoms of overdose include cardiac arrhythmias, nausea, vomiting, drowsiness, coma

Treatment is supportive following attempts to enhance drug elimination. Hypotension should be treated with I.V. fluids and/or Trendelenburg positioning.

Dialysis and hemoperfusion and osmotic diuresis have all been useful in reducing serum drug concentrations

The patient should be observed for possible relapses due to incomplete gastric emptying

Drug Interactions Increased effect/toxicity with CNS depressants

Mechanism of Action Causes skeletal muscle relaxation by reducing the transmission of impulses from the spinal cord to skeletal muscle

Pharmacodynamics/Kinetics

Onset of muscle relaxation: Oral: Within 30 minutes

Metabolism: In the liver

Half-life: 1-2 hours

Time to peak serum concentration: ~2 hours

Elimination: Metabolites renally excreted

Usual Dosage

Children: Recommended **only** for use in tetanus I.V.: 15 mg/kg/dose or 500 mg/m^2/dose, may repeat every 6 hours if needed; maximum dose: 1.8 g/m^2/day for 3 days only

Adults: Muscle spasm:

Oral: 1.5 g 4 times/day for 2-3 days, then decrease to 4-4.5 g/day in 3-6 divided doses

I.M., I.V.: 1 g every 8 hours if oral not possible

Dosing adjustment/comments in renal impairment: Do not administer parenteral formulation to patients with renal dysfunction

Dietary Considerations Alcohol: Additive CNS effect, avoid use

Administration Maximum rate: 3 mL/minute

(Continued)

Methocarbamol *(Continued)*

Patient Information May cause drowsiness, impair judgment or coordination; avoid alcohol or other CNS depressants; may turn urine brown, black, or green; notify physician of rash, itching, or nasal congestion

Nursing Implications Monitor closely for extravasation of I.V. injection

Dosage Forms

Injection: 100 mg/mL in polyethylene glycol 50% (10 mL)
Tablet: 500 mg, 750 mg

Methohexital (meth oh HEKS i tal)

Related Information

Adult ACLS Algorithm, Electrical Conversion *on page 1515*

Brand Names Brevital® Sodium

Canadian/Mexican Brand Names Brietal® Sodium (Canada)

Synonyms Methohexital Sodium

Therapeutic Category Barbiturate; General Anesthetic

Use Induction and maintenance of general anesthesia for short procedures

Restrictions C-IV

Pregnancy Risk Factor C

Contraindications Porphyria, hypersensitivity to methohexital or any component

Warnings/Precautions Use with extreme caution in patients with liver impairment, asthma, cardiovascular instability

Adverse Reactions

>10%: Local: Pain on I.M. injection

1% to 10%: Gastrointestinal: Cramping, diarrhea, rectal bleeding

<1%:

- Cardiovascular: Hypotension, peripheral vascular collapse
- Central nervous system: Seizures, headache
- Gastrointestinal: Nausea, vomiting
- Hematologic: Hemolytic anemia
- Local: Thrombophlebitis
- Neuromuscular & skeletal: Tremor, twitching, rigidity, involuntary muscle movement, radial nerve palsy
- Respiratory: Apnea, respiratory depression, laryngospasm, coughing
- Miscellaneous: Hiccups

Overdosage/Toxicology Symptoms of overdose include apnea, tachycardia, hypotension; treatment is primarily supportive with mechanical ventilation if needed

Drug Interactions CNS depressants worsen CNS depression

Stability Do not dilute with solutions containing bacteriostatic agents; solutions are alkaline (pH 9.5-11) and **incompatible** with acids (eg, atropine sulfate, succinylcholine, silicone), also **incompatible** with phenol containing solutions and silicone

Mechanism of Action Ultra short-acting I.V. barbiturate anesthetic

Usual Dosage Doses must be titrated to effect

Children 3-12 years:

- I.M.: Preop: 5-10 mg/kg/dose
- I.V.: Induction: 1-2 mg/kg/dose
- Rectal: Preop/induction: 20-35 mg/kg/dose; usual 25 mg/kg/dose; administer as 10% aqueous solution

Adults: I.V.: Induction: 50-120 mg to start; 20-40 mg every 4-7 minutes

Dosing adjustment/comments in hepatic impairment: Lower dosage and monitor closely

Nursing Implications Avoid extravasation or intra-arterial administration

Dosage Forms Injection, as sodium: 500 mg, 2.5 g, 5 g

Methohexital Sodium *see* Methohexital *on this page*

Methotrexate (meth oh TREKS ate)

Related Information

Antiemetics for Chemotherapy Induced Nausea and Vomiting *on page 1348*
Cancer Chemotherapy Regimens *on page 1351*
Toxicities of Chemotherapeutic Agents *on page 1382*

Brand Names Folex® PFS; Rheumatrex®

Canadian/Mexican Brand Names Ledertrexate® (Mexico)

Synonyms Amethopterin; Methotrexate Sodium; MTX

Therapeutic Category Antineoplastic Agent, Antimetabolite; Antineoplastic Agent, Folate Antagonist; Antineoplastic Agent, Irritant; Immunosuppressant Agent

Use Treatment of trophoblastic neoplasms; leukemias; psoriasis; rheumatoid arthritis; breast, head and neck, and lung carcinomas; osteosarcoma; sarcomas; carcinoma of gastric, esophagus, testes; lymphomas

Pregnancy Risk Factor D

Contraindications Hypersensitivity to methotrexate or any component; severe renal or hepatic impairment; pre-existing profound bone marrow suppression in patients with psoriasis or rheumatoid arthritis, alcoholic liver disease, AIDS, pre-existing blood dyscrasias

Warnings/Precautions The U.S. Food and Drug Administration (FDA) currently recommends that procedures for proper handling and disposal of antineoplastic agents be considered. May cause photosensitivity type reaction; reduce dosage in patients with renal or hepatic impairment; drain, ascites and pleural effusions prior to treatment; use with caution in patients with peptic ulcer disease, ulcerative colitis, pre-existing bone marrow suppression; monitor closely for pulmonary disease; use with caution in the elderly

Because of the possibility of severe toxic reactions, fully inform patient of the risks involved; do not use in women of childbearing age unless benefit outweighs risks; may cause hepatotoxicity, fibrosis, and cirrhosis, along with marked bone marrow suppression; death from intestinal perforation may occur

Patients should receive 1-2 L of I.V. fluid prior to initiation of high-dose methotrexate. Patients should receive sodium bicarbonate to alkalinize their urine during and after high-dose methotrexate (urine SG <1.010 and pH >7 should be maintained for at least 24 hours after infusion).

Toxicity to methotrexate or any immunosuppressive is increased in elderly; must monitor carefully. For rheumatoid arthritis and psoriasis, immunosuppressive therapy should only be used when disease is active and less toxic, traditional therapy is ineffective. Recommended doses should be reduced when initiating therapy in elderly due to possible decreased metabolism, reduced renal function, and presence of interacting diseases and drugs.

Methotrexate penetrates slowly into 3rd space fluids, such as pleural effusions or ascites, and exits slowly from these compartments (slower than from plasma)

Adverse Reactions

>10%:

- Cardiovascular: Vasculitis
- Central nervous system (with I.T. administration only):
  - Arachnoiditis: Acute reaction manifested as severe headache, nuchal rigidity, vomiting, and fever; may be alleviated by reducing the dose
  - Subacute toxicity: 10% of patients treated with 12-15 mg/m² of I.T. MTX may develop this in the second or third week of therapy; consists of motor paralysis of extremities, cranial nerve palsy, seizures, or coma. This has also been seen in pediatric cases receiving very high-dose I.V. MTX (when enough MTX can get across into the CSF).
  - Demyelinating encephalopathy: Seen months or years after receiving MTX; usually in association with cranial irradiation or other systemic chemotherapy
- Dermatologic: Reddening of skin
- Endocrine & metabolic: Hyperuricemia, defective oogenesis or spermatogenesis
- Gastrointestinal: Ulcerative stomatitis, glossitis, gingivitis, nausea, vomiting, diarrhea, anorexia, intestinal perforation, mucositis (dose-dependent; appears in 3-7 days after therapy, resolving within 2 weeks)
  - Emetic potential:
  - <100 mg: Moderately low (10% to 30%)
  - ≥100 mg or <250 mg: Moderate (30% to 60%)
  - ≥250 mg: Moderately high (60% to 90%)
- Hematologic: Leukopenia, thrombocytopenia
- Renal: Renal failure, azotemia, nephropathy
- Respiratory: Pharyngitis

1% to 10%:

- Cardiovascular: Vasculitis
- Central nervous system: Dizziness, malaise, encephalopathy, seizures, fever, chills
- Dermatitis: Alopecia, rash, photosensitivity, depigmentation or hyperpigmentation of skin
- Endocrine & metabolic: Diabetes
- Genitourinary: Cystitis
- Hematologic: Hemorrhage
- Myelosuppressive: This is the primary dose-limiting factor (along with mucositis) of MTX; occurs about 5-7 days after MTX therapy, and should resolve within 2 weeks
  - WBC: Mild
  - Platelets: Moderate
  - Onset (days): 7
  - Nadir (days): 10
  - Recovery (days): 21

(Continued)

Methotrexate *(Continued)*

Hepatic: Cirrhosis and portal fibrosis have been associated with chronic MTX therapy; acute elevation of liver enzymes are common after high-dose MTX, and usually resolve within 10 days

Neuromuscular & skeletal: Arthralgia

Ocular: Blurred vision

Renal: Renal dysfunction: Manifested by an abrupt rise in serum creatinine and BUN and a fall in urine output; more common with high-dose MTX, and may be due to precipitation of the drug. The best treatment is prevention: Aggressively hydrate with 3 L/m^2/day starting 12 hours before therapy and continue for 24-36 hours; alkalinize the urine by adding 50 mEq of bicarbonate to each liter of fluid; keep urine flow over 100 mL/hour and urine pH >7.

Respiratory: Pneumonitis: Associated with fever, cough, and interstitial pulmonary infiltrates; treatment is to withhold MTX during the acute reaction

Miscellaneous: Anaphylaxis, decreased resistance to infection

Overdosage/Toxicology Symptoms of overdose include nausea, vomiting, alopecia, melena, renal failure

Antidote: Leucovorin; administer as soon as toxicity is seen; administer 10 mg/m^2 orally or parenterally; follow with 10 mg/m^2 orally every 6 hours for 72 hours. After 24 hours following methotrexate administration, if the serum creatinine is ≥50% pre-methotrexate serum creatinine, increase leucovorin dose to 100 mg/m^2 every 3 hours until serum MTX level is $<5 \times 10^{-8}$M. Hydration and alkalinization may be used to prevent precipitation of MTX or MTX metabolites in the renal tubules. Toxicity in low dose range is negligible, but may present mucositis and mild bone marrow suppression; severe bone marrow toxicity can result from overdose. Neither peritoneal nor hemodialysis have been shown to ↑ elimination. Leucovorin should be administered intravenously, never intrathecally, for over doses of intrathecal methotrexate.

Drug Interactions

Decreased effect:

Corticosteroids: Reported to decrease uptake of MTX into leukemia cells. Administration of these drugs should be separated by 12 hours. Dexamethasone has been reported to not affect methotrexate influx into cells.

Decreases phenytoin, 5-FU

Increased toxicity:

Live virus vaccines → vaccinia infections

Vincristine: Inhibits MTX efflux from the cell, leading to increased and prolonged MTX levels in the cell; the dose of VCR needed to produce this effect is not achieved clinically

Organic acids: Salicylates, sulfonamides, probenecid, and high doses of penicillins compete with MTX for transport and reduce renal tubular secretion. Salicylates and sulfonamides may also displace MTX from plasma proteins, ↑ MTX levels.

Ara-C: Increases formation of the Ara-C nucleotide can occur when MTX precedes Ara-C, thus promoting the action of Ara-C

Cyclosporine: CSA and MTX interfere with each others renal elimination, which may result in increased toxicity

Nonsteroidal anti-inflammatory drugs (NSAIDs): Should not be used during moderate or high-dose methotrexate due to increased and prolonged methotrexate levels may increase toxicity

Stability

Store intact vials at room temperature (15°C to 25°C) and protect from light

Use PRESERVATIVE-FREE preparations for high-dose and intrathecal administration

Dilute powder with D_5W or NS to a concentration of ≤25 mg/mL (20 mg and 50 mg vials) and 50 mg/mL (1 g vial) as follows; solution is stable for 7 days at room temperature

20 mg = 20 mL (1 mg/mL)
50 mg = 5 mL (10 mg/mL)
1 g = 19.4 mL (50 mg/mL)

Further dilution in D_5W or NS is stable for 24 hours at room temperature (21°C to 25°C)

Standard I.V. dilution: Maximum syringe size for IVP is a 30 mL syringe and syringe should be ≤75% full

Doses <149 mg: Administer slow I.V. push
Dose/syringe (concentration ≤25 mg/mL)

Doses of 150-499 mg: Administer IVPB over 20-30 minutes
Dose/50 mL D_5W or NS

Doses of 500-1500 mg: Administer IVPB over ≥60 minutes
Dose/250 mL D_5W or NS

Doses of >1500 mg: Administer IVPB over 1-6 hours
Dose/1000 mL D_5W or NS

Standard I.M. dilution: Dose/syringe (concentration = 25 mg/mL)
I.V. dilutions are stable for 8 days at room temperature (25°C)

Intrathecal solutions in 3-20 mL LR are stable for 7 days at room temperature (30°C); **compatible** with cytarabine and hydrocortisone in LR or NS for 7 days at room temperature (25°C)

Standard intrathecal dilution: Dose/3-5 mL LR +/- methotrexate (12 mg) +/- hydrocortisone (15-25 mg)
Intrathecal dilutions are stable for 7 days at room temperature (25°C) but due to sterility issues, use within 24 hours

Mechanism of Action An antimetabolite that inhibits DNA synthesis and cell reproduction in malignant cells

Folates must be in the reduced form (FH_4) to be active
Folates are activated by dihydrofolate reductase (DHFR)
DHFR is inhibited by MTX (by binding irreversibly), causing an increase in the intracellular dihydrofolate pool (the inactive cofactor) and inhibition of both purine and thymidylate synthesis (TS)
MTX enters the cell through an energy-dependent and temperature-dependent process which is mediated by an intramembrane protein; this carrier mechanism is also used by naturally occurring reduced folates, including folinic acid (leucovorin), making this a competitive process
At high drug concentrations (>20 µM), MTX enters the cell by a second mechanism which is not shared by reduced folates; the process may be passive diffusion or a specific, saturable process, and provides a rationale for high-dose MTX
A small fraction of MTX is converted intracellularly to polyglutamates, which leads to a prolonged inhibition of DHFR

The MOA in the treatment of rheumatoid arthritis is unknown, but may affect immune function

In psoriasis, methotrexate is thought to target rapidly proliferating epithelial cells in the skin

Pharmacodynamics/Kinetics
Absorption:
Oral: Rapid; well absorbed orally at low doses (<30 mg/m^2), incomplete absorption after large doses
I.M. injection: Completely absorbed
Distribution: Drug penetrates slowly into 3rd space fluids, such as pleural effusions or ascites, and exits slowly from these compartments (slower than from plasma); crosses the placenta with small amounts appearing in breast milk; does not achieve therapeutic concentrations in the CSF and must be given intrathecally if given for CNS prophylaxis or treatment; sustained concentrations are retained in the kidney and liver
Protein binding: 50%
Metabolism: <10% metabolized; degraded by intestinal flora to DAMPA by carboxypeptidase; aldehyde oxidase in the liver converts MTX to 7-OH MTX; polyglutamates are produced intracellularly and are just as potent as MTX; their production is dose and duration dependent and are slowly eliminated by the cell once they are formed
Half-life: 8-12 hours with high doses and 3-10 hours with low doses
Time to peak serum concentration:
Oral: 1-2 hours
Parenteral: 30-60 minutes
Elimination: Small amounts excreted in the feces; primarily excreted in the urine (44% to 100%) via glomerular filtration and active transport
Miscellaneous: Cytotoxicity is determined by both drug concentration and duration of cell exposure; extracellular drug concentrations of 1 x 10^{-8}M are required to inhibit thymidylate synthesis; reduced folates are able to rescue cells and reverse MTX toxicity if given within 48 hours of the MTX dose; at concentrations of >10 µM MTX, reduced folates are no longer effective

Usual Dosage Refer to individual protocols. May be administered orally, I.M., intra-arterially, intrathecally, I.V., or S.C.

Leucovorin may be administered concomitantly or within 24 hours of methotrexate - refer to leucovorin monograph for details

Children:
Juvenile rheumatoid arthritis: Oral, I.M.: 5-15 mg/m^2/week as a single dose **or** as 3 divided doses given 12 hours apart
Antineoplastic dosage range:
Oral, I.M.: 7.5-30 mg/m^2/week **or** every 2 weeks
I.V.: 10-12,000 mg/m^2 bolus dosing **or** continuous infusion over 6-42 hours
Pediatric solid tumors (high-dose): I.V.:
<12 years: 12 g/m^2 (dosage range: 12-18 g)
≥12 years: 8 g/m^2 (maximum: 18 g)
(Continued)

Methotrexate *(Continued)*

Methotrexate Dosing Schedules

	Dose	Route	Frequency
Conventional Dose	15-20 mg/m^2	Oral	Twice weekly
	30-50 mg/m^2	Oral, I.V.	Weekly
	15 mg/day for 5 days	Oral, I.M.	Every 2-3 weeks
Intermediate Dose	50-150 mg/m^2	I.V. push	Every 2-3 weeks
	240 mg/m^2*	I.V. infusion	Every 4-7 days
	0.5-1 g/m^2*	I.V. infusion	Every 2-3 weeks
High Dose	1-12 g/m^2*	I.V. infusion	Every 1-3 weeks

*Followed with leucovorin rescue - refer to Leucovorin monograph for details.

Acute lymphocytic leukemia (intermediate-dose): I.V.: Loading: 100 mg/m^2 over 1 hour, followed by a 35-hour infusion of 900 mg/m^2/day

Meningeal leukemia: I.T.: 10-15 mg/m^2 (maximum dose: 15 mg) **or**

≤3 months: 3 mg/dose
4-11 months: 6 mg/dose
1 year: 8 mg/dose
2 years: 10 mg/dose
≥3 years: 12 mg/dose

I.T. doses are prepared with preservative-free MTX only. Hydrocortisone may be added to the I.T. preparation; total volume should range from 3-6 mL. Doses should be repeated at 2- to 5-day intervals until CSF counts return to normal followed by a dose once weekly for 2 weeks then monthly thereafter.

Adults: I.V.: Range is wide from 30-40 mg/m^2/week to 100-7,500 mg/m^2 with leucovorin rescue

Doses NOT requiring leucovorin rescue range from 30-40 mg/m^2 I.V. or I.M. repeated weekly, or oral regimens of 10 mg/m^2 twice weekly

High-dose MTX is considered to be >100 mg/m^2 and can be as high as 1,500-7,500 mg/m^2. These doses REQUIRE leucovorin rescue. Patients receiving doses ≥ 1000 mg/m^2 should have their urine alkalinized with bicarbonate or Bicitra® prior to and following MTX therapy.

Trophoblastic neoplasms: Oral, I.M.: 15-30 mg/day for 5 days; repeat in 7 days for 3-5 courses

Head and neck cancer: Oral, I.M., I.V.: 25-50 mg/m^2 once weekly

Rheumatoid arthritis: Oral: 7.5 mg once weekly **OR** 2.5 mg every 12 hours for 3 doses/week; not to exceed 20 mg/week

Psoriasis: Oral: 2.5-5 mg/dose every 12 hours for 3 dose given weekly **or** Oral, I.M.: 10-25 mg/dose given once weekly

Ectopic pregnancy: I.M./I.V.: 50 mg/m^2 single-dose without leucovorin rescue

Elderly: Rheumatoid arthritis/psoriasis: Oral: Initial: 5 mg once weekly; if nausea occurs, split dose to 2.5 mg every 12 hours for the day of administration; dose may be increased to 7.5 mg/week based on response, not to exceed 20 mg/week

Dosing adjustment in renal impairment:

Cl_{cr} 61-80 mL/minute: Reduce dose to 75% of usual dose
Cl_{cr} 51-60 mL/minute: Reduce dose to 70% of usual dose
Cl_{cr} 10-50 mL/minute: Reduce dose to 30% to 50% of usual dose
Cl_{cr} <10 mL/minute: Avoid use

Hemodialysis: Not dialyzable (0% to 5%); supplemental dose is not necessary
Peritoneal dialysis: Supplemental dose is not necessary

Dosage adjustment in hepatic impairment:

Bilirubin 3.1-5 mg/dL OR AST >180 Units: Administer 75% of usual dose
Bilirubin >5 mg/dL: Do not use

Dietary Considerations Alcohol: Avoid use

Administration

Methotrexate may be administered I.M., I.V., or I.T.; refer to Stability section for I.V. administration recommendations based on dosage

I.V. administration rates:

Doses <149 mg: Administer slow I.V. push
Doses of 150-499 mg: Administer IVPB over 20-30 minutes
Doses of 500-1500 mg: Administer IVPB over ≥60 minutes
Doses of >1500 mg: Administer IVPB over 1-6 hours

Specific dosing schemes vary, but high dose should be followed by leucovorin calcium 24-36 hours after initiation of therapy to prevent toxicity

Renal toxicity can be minimized/prevented by alkalinizing the urine (with sodium bicarbonate) and increasing urine flow (hydration therapy)

Monitoring Parameters For prolonged use (especially rheumatoid arthritis, psoriasis) a baseline liver biopsy, repeated at each 1-1.5 g cumulative dose interval, should be performed; WBC and platelet counts every 4 weeks; CBC and creatinine, LFTs every 3-4 months; chest x-ray

Reference Range Refer to chart in Leucovorin Calcium monograph. Therapeutic levels: Variable; Toxic concentration: Variable; therapeutic range is dependent upon therapeutic approach.

High-dose regimens produce drug levels between 10^{-6}Molar and 10^{-7}Molar 24-72 hours after drug infusion

10^{-6} Molar unit = 1 microMolar unit

Toxic: Low-dose therapy: >9.1 ng/mL; high-dose therapy: >454 ng/mL

Patient Information Any signs of infection, easy bruising or bleeding, shortness of breath, or painful or burning urination should be brought to physician's attention. Nausea, vomiting or hair loss sometimes occur. The drug may cause permanent sterility and may cause birth defects. Pregnancy should be avoided for a minimum of 3 months after completion of therapy in male patients, and at least one ovulatory cycle in female patients. The drug may be excreted in breast milk, therefore, an alternative form of feeding your baby should be used. Food may decrease absorption, therefore, take on an empty stomach; avoid alcohol; avoid prolonged exposure to sun

Additional Information

Sodium content of 100 mg injection: 20 mg (0.86 mEq)
Sodium content of 100 mg (low sodium) injection: 15 mg (0.65 mEq)

Dosage Forms

Injection, as sodium: 2.5 mg/mL (2 mL); 25 mg/mL (2 mL, 4 mL, 8 mL, 10 mL)
Injection, as sodium, preservative free: 25 mg (2 mL, 4 mL, 8 mL, 10 mL)
Powder, for injection: 20 mg, 25 mg, 50 mg, 100 mg, 250 mg, 1 g
Tablet, as sodium: 2.5 mg
Tablet, as sodium, dose pack: 2.5 mg (4 cards with 2, 3, 4, 5, or 6 tablets each)

Methotrexate Sodium *see* Methotrexate *on page 806*

Methoxamine (meth OKS a meen)

Brand Names Vasoxyl®

Synonyms Methoxamine Hydrochloride

Therapeutic Category Adrenergic Agonist Agent; Alpha-Adrenergic Agonist; Sympathomimetic

Use Treatment of hypotension occurring during general anesthesia; to terminate episodes of supraventricular tachycardia; treatment of shock

Pregnancy Risk Factor C

Contraindications Hypersensitivity to methoxamine or any component

Adverse Reactions

1% to 10%:
- Cardiovascular: Hypertension (severe)
- Gastrointestinal: Vomiting

<1%:
- Cardiovascular: Ventricular ectopic beats, fetal bradycardia
- Central nervous system: Headache
- Genitourinary: Urinary urgency
- Miscellaneous: Diaphoresis

Overdosage/Toxicology Symptoms of hypertension and bradycardia

Mechanism of Action Direct-acting sympathomimetic amine with similar actions as phenylephrine; causes vasoconstriction primarily via alpha-adrenergic stimulation

Pharmacodynamics/Kinetics

Adrenergic effect:
- Onset of action: I.M.: Within 15 minutes
- Duration:
  - I.M.: 1.5 hours
  - I.V.: ~1 hour

Pressor activity:
- Onset of action:
  - I.M.: 15-20 minutes
  - I.V.: Within 1-2 minutes
- Duration: ~1-1.5 hours

Elimination: Not well defined

Usual Dosage Adults:

Emergencies: I.V.: 3-5 mg
Supraventricular tachycardia: I.V.: 10 mg
During spinal anesthesia: I.M.: 10-20 mg

Dosage Forms Injection, as hydrochloride: 20 mg/mL (1 mL)

Methoxamine Hydrochloride *see* Methoxamine *on this page*

Methoxsalen (meth OKS a len)

Brand Names 8-MOP®; Oxsoralen®; Oxsoralen-Ultra®

Synonyms Methoxypsoralen; 8-Methoxypsoralen; 8-MOP

Therapeutic Category Psoralen

Use

Oral: Symptomatic control of severe, recalcitrant disabling psoriasis, not responsive to other therapy when to diagnosis has been supported by biopsy. Administer only in conjunction with a schedule of controlled doses of long wave ultraviolet (UV) radiation; also used with long wave ultraviolet (UV) radiation for repigmentation of idiopathic vitiligo.

Topical: Repigmenting agent in vitiligo, used in conjunction with controlled doses of UVA or sunlight

Pregnancy Risk Factor C

Contraindications Diseases associated with photosensitivity, cataract, invasive squamous cell cancer, known hypersensitivity to methoxsalen (psoralens), and children <12 years of age

Warnings/Precautions Family history of sunlight allergy or chronic infections; lotion should only be applied under direct supervision of a physician and should not be dispensed to the patient; for use only if inadequate response to other forms of therapy, serious burns may occur from UVA or sunlight even through glass if dose and or exposure schedule is not maintained; some products may contain tartrazine; use caution in patients with hepatic or cardiac disease

Adverse Reactions

>10%:

Dermatologic: Itching

Gastrointestinal: Nausea

1% to 10%:

Cardiovascular: Severe edema, hypotension

Central nervous system: Nervousness, vertigo, depression

Dermatologic: Painful blistering, burning, and peeling of skin; pruritus, freckling, hypopigmentation, rash, cheilitis, erythema

Neuromuscular & skeletal: Loss of muscle coordination

Overdosage/Toxicology Symptoms of overdose include nausea, severe burns; follow accepted treatment of severe burns; keep room darkened until reaction subsides (8-24 hours or more)

Drug Interactions Increased toxicity: Concomitant therapy with other photosensitizing agents such as anthralin, coal tar, griseofulvin, phenothiazines, nalidixic acid, sulfanilamides, tetracyclines, thiazides

Mechanism of Action Bonds covalently to pyrimidine bases in DNA, inhibits the synthesis of DNA, and suppresses cell division. The augmented sunburn reaction involves excitation of the methoxsalen molecule by radiation in the long-wave ultraviolet light (UVA), resulting in transference of energy to the methoxsalen molecule producing an excited state ("triplet electronic state"). The molecule, in this "triplet state", then reacts with cutaneous DNA.

Pharmacodynamics/Kinetics

Metabolism: In the liver with >90% of dose appearing in urine as metabolites

Bioavailability: May be less with the capsule than with the liquid-encapsulated preparation

Time to peak serum concentration: Oral: 2-4 hours

Usual Dosage

Psoriasis: Adults: Oral: 10-70 mg 1½-2 hours before exposure to ultraviolet light, 2-3 times at least 48 hours apart; dosage is based upon patient's body weight and skin type

Vitiligo: Children >12 years and Adults:

Oral: 20 mg 2-4 hours before exposure to UVA light or sunlight; limit exposure to 15-40 minutes based on skin basic color and exposure

Topical: Apply lotion 1-2 hours before exposure to UVA light, no more than once weekly

Patient Information To reduce nausea, oral drug can be taken with food or milk or in 2 divided doses 30 minutes apart. If burning or blistering or intractable pruritus occurs, discontinue therapy until effects subside. Do not sunbathe for at least 24 hours prior to therapy or 48 hours after PUVA therapy. Avoid direct and indirect sunlight for 8 hours after oral and 12-48 hours after topical therapy. **If sunlight cannot be avoided, protective clothing and/or sunscreens must be worn.** Following oral therapy, wraparound sunglasses with UVA-absorbing properties must be worn for 24 hours. Avoid furocoumarin-containing foods (limes, figs, parsley, celery, cloves, lemon, mustard, carrots); do not exceed prescribed dose or exposure times.

Dosage Forms

Capsule: 10 mg

Lotion: 1% (30 mL)

Methoxypsoralen *see* Methoxsalen *on previous page*

8-Methoxypsoralen *see* Methoxsalen *on previous page*

Methsuximide (meth SUKS i mide)

Related Information

Epilepsy Treatment *on page 1531*

Brand Names Celontin®

Canadian/Mexican Brand Names Celontin® (Canada)

Therapeutic Category Anticonvulsant

Use Control of absence (petit mal) seizures; useful adjunct in refractory, partial complex (psychomotor) seizures

Pregnancy Risk Factor C

Contraindications Known hypersensitivity to methsuximide

Warnings/Precautions Use with caution in patients with hepatic or renal disease; abrupt withdrawal of the drug may precipitate absence status; methsuximide may increase tonic-clonic seizures in patients with mixed seizure disorders; methsuximide must be used in combination with other anticonvulsants in patients with both absence and tonic-clonic seizures

Adverse Reactions

>10%:

- Central nervous system: Ataxia, dizziness, drowsiness, headache
- Dermatologic: Stevens-Johnson syndrome
- Gastrointestinal: Anorexia, nausea, vomiting, weight loss
- Miscellaneous: Hiccups, SLE syndrome

1% to 10%:

- Central nervous system: Aggressiveness, mental depression, nightmares, fatigue
- Neuromuscular & skeletal: Weakness

<1%:

- Central nervous system: Paranoid psychosis
- Dermatologic: Urticaria, exfoliative dermatitis
- Hematologic: Agranulocytosis, leukopenia, aplastic anemia, thrombocytopenia, pancytopenia

Overdosage/Toxicology Acute overdosage can cause CNS depression, ataxia, stupor, coma, hypotension; chronic overdose can cause skin rash, confusion, ataxia, proteinuria, hepatic dysfunction, hematuria

Treatment is supportive; hemoperfusion and hemodialysis may be useful

Stability Protect from high temperature

Mechanism of Action Increases the seizure threshold and suppresses paroxysmal spike-and-wave pattern in absence seizures; depresses nerve transmission in the motor cortex

Pharmacodynamics/Kinetics

Metabolism: Rapidly demethylated in the liver to N-desmethylmethsuximide (active metabolite)

Half-life: 2-4 hours

Time to peak serum concentration: Oral: Within 1-3 hours

Elimination: <1% excreted in urine as unchanged drug

Usual Dosage Oral:

Children: Initial: 10-15 mg/kg/day in 3-4 divided doses; increase weekly up to maximum of 30 mg/kg/day

Adults: 300 mg/day for the first week; may increase by 300 mg/day at weekly intervals up to 1.2 g/day in 2-4 divided doses/day

Monitoring Parameters CBC, hepatic function tests, urinalysis

Reference Range Therapeutic: 10-40 µg/mL (SI: 53-212 µmol/L); Toxic: >40 µg/mL (SI: >212 µmol/L)

Test Interactions ↑ alkaline phosphatase (S); positive Coombs' [direct]; ↓ calcium (S)

Patient Information Take with food; do not discontinue abruptly; may cause drowsiness and impair judgment

Nursing Implications Observe patient for excess sedation

Dosage Forms Capsule: 150 mg, 300 mg

Methyclothiazide (meth i kloe THYE a zide)

Related Information

Sulfonamide Derivatives *on page 1420*

Brand Names Aquatensen®; Enduron®

Therapeutic Category Antihypertensive; Diuretic, Thiazide

Use Management of mild to moderate hypertension; treatment of edema in congestive heart failure and nephrotic syndrome

Pregnancy Risk Factor D

(Continued)

Methyclothiazide *(Continued)*

Contraindications Hypersensitivity to methyclothiazide, other thiazides or sulfonamides, or any component, anuria

Warnings/Precautions Use with caution in renal disease, hepatic disease, gout, lupus erythematosus, diabetes mellitus; some products may contain tartrazine

Adverse Reactions

1% to 10%: Endocrine & metabolic: Hypokalemia

<1%:

- Cardiovascular: Hypotension
- Central nervous system: Drowsiness
- Dermatologic: Photosensitivity, rash
- Endocrine & metabolic: Fluid and electrolyte imbalances (hypocalcemia, hypomagnesemia, hyponatremia), hyperglycemia
- Gastrointestinal: Nausea, vomiting, anorexia
- Genitourinary: Polyuria
- Hematologic: Rarely blood dyscrasias, aplastic anemia, hemolytic anemia, leukopenia, agranulocytosis, thrombocytopenia
- Hepatic: Hepatitis
- Neuromuscular & skeletal: Paresthesia
- Renal: Prerenal azotemia, uremia

Overdosage/Toxicology Symptoms of overdose include hypermotility, diuresis, lethargy; GI decontamination and supportive care; fluids for hypovolemia

Drug Interactions Increased toxicity/levels of lithium

Mechanism of Action Inhibits sodium reabsorption in the distal tubules causing increased excretion of sodium and water, as well as, potassium and hydrogen ions

Pharmacodynamics/Kinetics

Onset of diuresis: Oral: 2 hours
Peak effect: 6 hours
Duration: ~1 day
Distribution: Crosses the placenta; appears in breast milk
Elimination: Unchanged in urine

Usual Dosage Oral:

Children: 0.05-0.2 mg/kg/day
Adults:
- Edema: 2.5-10 mg/day
- Hypertension: 2.5-5 mg/day

Monitoring Parameters Blood pressure, fluids, weight loss, serum potassium

Patient Information May be taken with food or milk; take early in day to avoid nocturia; take the last dose of multiple doses no later than 6 PM unless instructed otherwise. A few people who take this medication become more sensitive to sunlight and may experience skin rash, redness, itching, or severe sunburn, especially if sun block SPF ≥15 is not used on exposed skin areas.

Nursing Implications Assess weight, I & O reports daily to determine fluid loss; take blood pressure with patient lying down and standing

Dosage Forms Tablet: 2.5 mg, 5 mg

Methylacetoxyprogesterone *see* Medroxyprogesterone Acetate *on page 771*

Methyldopa (meth il DOE pa)

Related Information

Therapy of Hypertension *on page 1540*

Brand Names Aldomet®

Canadian/Mexican Brand Names Apo-Methyldopa® (Canada); Dopamet® (Canada); Medimet® (Canada); Novo-Medopa® (Canada); Nu-Medopa® (Canada)

Synonyms Methyldopate Hydrochloride

Therapeutic Category Alpha-Adrenergic Inhibitor; Antihypertensive

Use Management of moderate to severe hypertension

Pregnancy Risk Factor B

Pregnancy/Breast-Feeding Implications

Clinical effects on the fetus: Crosses the placenta. Hypotension reported. A large amount of clinical experience with the use of these drugs for the management of hypertension during pregnancy is available. Available evidence suggests safe use during pregnancy and breast-feeding.

Breast-feeding/lactation: Crosses into breast milk at extremely low levels. American Academy of Pediatrics considers COMPATIBLE with breast-feeding.

Contraindications Hypersensitivity to methyldopa or any component; (oral suspension contains benzoic acid and sodium bisulfite; injection contains sodium bisulfite); liver disease, pheochromocytoma

Warnings/Precautions May rarely produce hemolytic anemia and liver disorders; positive Coombs' test occurs in 10% to 20% of patients (perform periodic

CBCs); sedation usually transient may occur during initial therapy or whenever the dose is increased. Use with caution in patients with previous liver disease or dysfunction, the active metabolites of methyldopa accumulate in uremia. Patients with impaired renal function may respond to smaller doses. Elderly patients may experience syncope (avoid by giving smaller doses). Tolerance may occur usually between the second and third month of therapy. Adding a diuretic or increasing the dosage of methyldopa frequently restores blood pressure control. Because of its CNS effects, methyldopa is not considered a drug of first choice in the elderly.

Adverse Reactions

>10%: Cardiovascular: Peripheral edema

1% to 10%:

- Central nervous system: Drug fever, mental depression, anxiety, nightmares, drowsiness, headache
- Gastrointestinal: Xerostomia

<1%:

- Cardiovascular: Orthostatic hypotension, bradycardia (sinus)
- Central nervous system: Fever, chills, sedation, vertigo, depression, memory lapse
- Dermatologic: Rash
- Endocrine & metabolic: Sodium retention, sexual dysfunction, gynecomastia, hyperprolactinemia
- Gastrointestinal: Colitis, pancreatitis, diarrhea, nausea, vomiting, "black" tongue
- Genitourinary: Decreased libido
- Hematologic: Thrombocytopenia, hemolytic anemia, positive Coombs' test, leukopenia, transient leukopenia or granulocytopenia
- Hepatic: Cholestasis or hepatitis and heptocellular injury, increased liver enzymes, jaundice, cirrhosis
- Neuromuscular & skeletal: Paresthesias, weakness
- Respiratory: Dyspnea
- Miscellaneous: SLE-like syndrome

Overdosage/Toxicology Symptoms of overdose include hypotension, sedation, bradycardia, dizziness, constipation or diarrhea, flatus, nausea, vomiting

Hypotension usually responds to I.V. fluids, Trendelenburg positioning, or vasoconstrictors. Treatment is primarily supportive and symptomatic; can be removed by hemodialysis.

Drug Interactions

Decreased effect: Iron supplements can interact and cause a significant **increase** in blood pressure

Increased toxicity: Lithium may increase lithium toxicity; tolbutamide and levodopa effects/toxicity increased

Stability Injectable dosage form is most stable at acid to neutral pH; stability of parenteral admixture at room temperature (25°C): 24 hours; stability of parenteral admixture at refrigeration temperature (4°C): 4 days; standard diluent: 250-500 mg/100 mL D_5W

Mechanism of Action Stimulation of central alpha-adrenergic receptors by a false transmitter that results in a decreased sympathetic outflow to the heart, kidneys, and peripheral vasculature

Pharmacodynamics/Kinetics

Peak hypotensive effect: Oral, parenteral: Within 3-6 hours

Duration: 12-24 hours

Distribution: Crosses the placenta; appears in breast milk

Protein binding: <15%

Metabolism: Intestinally and in the liver

Half-life: 75-80 minutes

- End stage renal disease: 6-16 hours

Elimination: Most (85%) metabolites appearing in the urine within 24 hours

Usual Dosage

Children:

- Oral: Initial: 10 mg/kg/day in 2-4 divided doses; increase every 2 days as needed to maximum dose of 65 mg/kg/day; do not exceed 3 g/day
- I.V.: 5-10 mg/kg/dose every 6-8 hours up to a total dose of 65 mg/kg/24 hours or 3 g/24 hours

Adults:

- Oral: Initial: 250 mg 2-3 times/day; increase every 2 days as needed; usual dose 1-1.5 g/day in 2-4 divided doses; maximum dose: 3 g/day
- I.V.: 250-1000 mg every 6-8 hours; maximum dose: 1 g every 6 hours

Dosing interval in renal impairment:

- Cl_{cr} >50 mL/minute: Administer every 8 hours
- Cl_{cr} 10-50 mL/minute: Administer every 8-12 hours
- Cl_{cr} <10 mL/minute: Administer every 12-24 hours

(Continued)

Methyldopa *(Continued)*

Hemodialysis: Slightly dialyzable (5% to 20%)

Monitoring Parameters Blood pressure, standing and sitting/lying down, CBC, liver enzymes, Coombs' test (direct); blood pressure monitor required during I.V. administration

Test Interactions Methyldopa interferes with the following laboratory tests: urinary uric acid, serum creatinine (alkaline picrate method), AST (colorimetric method), and urinary catecholamines (falsely high levels)

Patient Information May cause transient drowsiness; may cause urine discoloration; notify physician of unexplained prolonged general tiredness, fever, or jaundice; rise slowly from prolonged sitting or lying position

Nursing Implications Transient sedation or depression may be common for first 72 hours of therapy; usually disappears over time; infuse over 30 minutes; assist with ambulation

Dosage Forms

Injection, as methyldopate hydrochloride: 50 mg/mL (5 mL, 10 mL)
Suspension, oral: 250 mg/5 mL (5 mL, 473 mL)
Tablet: 125 mg, 250 mg, 500 mg

Methyldopate Hydrochloride *see* Methyldopa *on page 814*

Methylene Blue (METH i leen bloo)

Brand Names Urolene Blue®

Therapeutic Category Antidote, Cyanide; Antidote, Drug Induced Methemoglobinemia

Use Antidote for cyanide poisoning and drug-induced methemoglobinemia, indicator dye, chronic urolithiasis.

Unlabeled use: Has been used topically (0.1% solutions) in conjunction with polychromatic light to photoinactivate viruses such as herpes simplex; has been used alone or in combination with vitamin C for the management of chronic urolithiasis

Pregnancy Risk Factor C (D if injected intra-amniotically)

Contraindications Renal insufficiency, hypersensitivity to methylene blue or any component, intraspinal injection

Warnings/Precautions Do not inject S.C. or intrathecally; use with caution in young patients and in patients with G-6-PD deficiency; continued use can cause profound anemia

Adverse Reactions

>10%:
- Gastrointestinal: Fecal discoloration (blue-green)
- Genitourinary: Discoloration of urine (blue-green)

1% to 10%: Hematologic: Anemia

<1%:
- Cardiovascular: Hypertension, precordial pain
- Central nervous system: Dizziness, mental confusion, headache, fever
- Dermatologic: Stains skin
- Gastrointestinal: Nausea, vomiting, abdominal pain
- Genitourinary: Bladder irritation
- Miscellaneous: Diaphoresis

Overdosage/Toxicology Symptoms of overdose include nausea, vomiting, precordial pain, hypertension, methemoglobinemia, cyanosis; overdosage has resulted in methemoglobinemia and cyanosis; treatment is symptomatic and supportive

Mechanism of Action Weak germicide in low concentrations, hastens the conversion of methemoglobin to hemoglobin; has opposite effect at high concentrations by converting ferrous ion of reduced hemoglobin to ferric ion to form methemoglobin; in cyanide toxicity, it combines with cyanide to form cyanmethemoglobin preventing the interference of cyanide with the cytochrome system

Pharmacodynamics/Kinetics

Absorption: Oral: 53% to 97%
Elimination: In bile, feces, and urine

Usual Dosage

Children: NADPH-methemoglobin reductase deficiency: Oral: 1-1.5 mg/kg/day (maximum: 300 mg/day) given with 5-8 mg/kg/day of ascorbic acid

Children and Adults: Methemoglobinemia: I.V.: 1-2 mg/kg or 25-50 mg/m^2 over several minutes; may be repeated in 1 hour if necessary

Adults: Genitourinary antiseptic: Oral: 65-130 mg 3 times/day with a full glass of water (maximum: 390 mg/day)

Administration Administer I.V. undiluted by direct I.V. injection over several minutes

Patient Information May discolor urine and feces blue-green; take oral formulation after meals with a glass of water; skin stains may be removed using a hypochlorite solution

Additional Information Skin stains may be removed using a hypochlorite solution

Dosage Forms

Injection: 10 mg/mL (1 mL, 10 mL)
Tablet: 65 mg

Methylergometrine Maleate *see* Methylergonovine *on this page*

Methylergonovine (meth il er goe NOE veen)

Brand Names Methergine®

Synonyms Methylergometrine Maleate; Methylergonovine Maleate

Therapeutic Category Ergot Alkaloid and Derivative

Use Prevention and treatment of postpartum and postabortion hemorrhage caused by uterine atony or subinvolution

Pregnancy Risk Factor C

Contraindications Induction of labor, threatened spontaneous abortion, hypertension, toxemia, hypersensitivity to methylergonovine or any component, pregnancy

Warnings/Precautions Use caution in patients with sepsis, obliterative vascular disease, hepatic, or renal involvement, hypertension; administer with extreme caution if using I.V.

Adverse Reactions

>10%:
- Cardiovascular: Hypertension
- Central nervous system: Headache, seizures

1% to 10%: Gastrointestinal: Nausea, vomiting

<1%:
- Cardiovascular: Temporary chest pain, palpitations
- Central nervous system: Hallucinations, dizziness
- Endocrine & metabolic: Water intoxication
- Gastrointestinal: Diarrhea
- Local: Thrombophlebitis
- Neuromuscular & skeletal: Leg cramps
- Otic: Tinnitus
- Renal: Hematuria
- Respiratory: Dyspnea, nasal congestion
- Miscellaneous: Diaphoresis, foul taste

Overdosage/Toxicology Symptoms of overdose include prolonged gangrene, numbness in extremities, acute nausea, vomiting, abdominal pain, respiratory depression, hypotension, seizures

Treatment is symptomatic and supportive; hypotension may require pressors; seizures can be treated with benzodiazepines

Mechanism of Action Similar smooth muscle actions as seen with ergotamine; however, it affects primarily uterine smooth muscles producing sustained contractions and thereby shortens the third stage of labor

Pharmacodynamics/Kinetics

Onset of oxytocic effect:
- Oral: 5-10 minutes
- I.M.: 2-5 minutes
- I.V.: Immediately

Duration of action:
- Oral: ~3 hours
- I.M.: ~3 hours
- I.V.: 45 minutes

Absorption: Rapid

Distribution: Rapidly distributed primarily to plasma and extracellular fluid following I.V. administration; distribution to tissues also occurs rapidly

Metabolism: In the liver

Half-life (biphasic):
- Initial: 1-5 minutes
- Terminal: 30 minutes to 2 hours

Time to peak serum concentration: Within 30 minutes to 3 hours

Elimination: In urine and feces

Usual Dosage Adults:

Oral: 0.2 mg 3-4 times/day for 2-7 days

I.M.: 0.2 mg after delivery of anterior shoulder, after delivery of placenta, or during puerperium; may be repeated as required at intervals of 2-4 hours

I.V.: Same dose as I.M., but should not be routinely administered I.V. because of possibility of inducing sudden hypertension and cerebrovascular accident

Administration Administer over no less than 60 seconds

(Continued)

Methylergonovine *(Continued)*

Patient Information May cause nausea, vomiting, dizziness, increased blood pressure, headache, ringing in the ears, chest pain, or shortness of breath

Nursing Implications Ampuls containing discolored solution should not be used

Dosage Forms

Injection, as maleate: 0.2 mg/mL (1 mL)
Tablet, as maleate: 0.2 mg

Methylergonovine Maleate *see* Methylergonovine *on previous page*

Methylmorphine *see* Codeine *on page 306*

Methylone® *see* Methylprednisolone *on next page*

Methylphenidate (meth il FEN i date)

Brand Names Ritalin®; Ritalin-SR®

Canadian/Mexican Brand Names PMS-Methylphenidate (Canada)

Synonyms Methylphenidate Hydrochloride

Therapeutic Category Central Nervous System Stimulant, Nonamphetamine

Use Treatment of attention deficit disorder and symptomatic management of narcolepsy; many unlabeled uses

Restrictions C-II

Pregnancy Risk Factor C

Contraindications Hypersensitivity to methylphenidate or any components; glaucoma, motor tics, Tourette's syndrome, patients with marked agitation, tension, and anxiety

Warnings/Precautions Use with caution in patients with hypertension, dementia (may worsen agitation or confusion) seizures; has high potential for abuse. Treatment should include "drug holidays" or periodic discontinuation in order to assess the patient's requirements and to decrease tolerance and limit suppression of linear growth and weight; it is often useful in treating elderly patients who are discouraged, withdrawn, apathetic, or disinterested in their activities. In particular, it is useful in patients who are starting a rehabilitation program but have resigned themselves to fail; these patients may not have a major depressive disorder; will not improve memory or cognitive function.

Adverse Reactions

>10%:
- Cardiovascular: Tachycardia
- Central nervous system: Nervousness, insomnia
- Gastrointestinal: Anorexia

1% to 10%:
- Central nervous system: Dizziness, drowsiness
- Gastrointestinal: Stomach pain
- Miscellaneous: Hypersensitivity reactions

<1%:
- Cardiovascular: Hypertension, hypotension, palpitations, cardiac arrhythmias
- Central nervous system: Movement disorders, precipitation of Tourette's syndrome, and toxic psychosis (rare), fever, headache, convulsions
- Dermatologic: Rash
- Gastrointestinal: Nausea, weight loss, vomiting
- Endocrine & metabolic: Growth retardation
- Hematologic: Thrombocytopenia, anemia, leukopenia
- Ocular: Blurred vision

Overdosage/Toxicology Symptoms of overdose include vomiting, agitation, tremors, hyperpyrexia, muscle twitching, hallucinations, tachycardia, mydriasis, sweating, palpitations

There is no specific antidote for methylphenidate intoxication and the bulk of the treatment is supportive. Hyperactivity and agitation usually respond to reduced sensory input or benzodiazepines, however, with extreme agitation haloperidol (2-5 mg I.M. for adults) may be required. Hyperthermia is best treated with external cooling measures, or when severe or unresponsive, muscle paralysis with pancuronium may be needed. Hypertension is usually transient and generally does not require treatment unless severe. For diastolic blood pressures >110 mm Hg, a nitroprusside infusion should be initiated. Seizures usually respond to diazepam I.V. and/or phenytoin maintenance regimens.

Drug Interactions

Decreased effect: Effects of guanethidine, bretylium may be antagonized by methylphenidate

Increased toxicity: May increase serum concentrations of tricyclic antidepressants, warfarin, phenytoin, phenobarbital, and primidone; MAO inhibitors may potentiate effects of methylphenidate

Mechanism of Action Blocks the reuptake mechanism of dopaminergic neurons; appears to stimulate the cerebral cortex and subcortical structures similar to amphetamines

Pharmacodynamics/Kinetics

Immediate release tablet:

Peak cerebral stimulation effect: Within 2 hours

Duration: 3-6 hours

Sustained release tablet:

Peak effect: Within 4-7 hours

Duration: 8 hours

Absorption: Slow and incomplete from GI tract

Metabolism: In liver via hydroxylation to ritolinic acid

Half-life: 2-4 hours

Elimination: In urine as metabolites and unchanged drug with 45% to 50% excreted in feces via bile

Usual Dosage Oral: (Discontinue periodically to re-evaluate or if no improvement occurs within 1 month)

Children ≥6 years: Attention deficit disorder: Initial: 0.3 mg/kg/dose or 2.5-5 mg/dose given before breakfast and lunch; increase by 0.1 mg/kg/dose or by 5-10 mg/day at weekly intervals; usual dose: 0.5-1 mg/kg/day; maximum dose: 2 mg/kg/day or 60 mg/day

Adults:

Narcolepsy: 10 mg 2-3 times/day, up to 60 mg/day

Depression: Initial: 2.5 mg every morning before 9 AM; dosage may be increased by 2.5-5 mg every 2-3 days as tolerated to a maximum of 20 mg/day; may be divided (ie, 7 AM and 12 noon), but should not be given after noon; do not use sustained release product

Patient Information Last daily dose should be given several hours before retiring; do not abruptly discontinue; prolonged use may cause dependence

Nursing Implications Do not crush or allow patient to chew sustained release dosage form; to effectively avoid insomnia, dosing should be completed by noon

Dosage Forms

Tablet, as hydrochloride: 5 mg, 10 mg, 20 mg

Tablet, as hydrochloride, sustained release: 20 mg

Methylphenidate Hydrochloride *see* Methylphenidate *on previous page*

Methylphenobarbital *see* Mephobarbital *on page 781*

Methylphenyl Isoxazolyl Penicillin *see* Oxacillin *on page 931*

Methylphytyl Napthoquinone *see* Phytonadione *on page 998*

Methylprednisolone (meth il pred NIS oh lone)

Related Information

Corticosteroids Comparison *on page 1407*

Brand Names Adlone®; A-Methapred®; depMedalone®; Depoject®; Depo-Medrol®; Depopred®; Duralone®; Medralone®; Medrol®; Methylone®; Solu-Medrol®

Canadian/Mexican Brand Names Cryosolona® (Mexico)

Synonyms 6-α-Methylprednisolone; Methylprednisolone Acetate; Methylprednisolone Sodium Succinate

Therapeutic Category Anti-inflammatory Agent; Corticosteroid; Corticosteroid, Systemic; Glucocorticoid

Use Primarily as an anti-inflammatory or immunosuppressant agent in the treatment of a variety of diseases including those of hematologic, allergic, inflammatory, neoplastic, and autoimmune origin

Pregnancy Risk Factor C

Contraindications Serious infections, except septic shock or tuberculous meningitis; known hypersensitivity to methylprednisolone; viral, fungal, or tubercular skin lesions; administration of live virus vaccines

Warnings/Precautions Use with caution in patients with hyperthyroidism, cirrhosis, nonspecific ulcerative colitis, hypertension, osteoporosis, thromboembolic tendencies, CHF, convulsive disorders, myasthenia gravis, thrombophlebitis, peptic ulcer, diabetes; because of the risk of adverse effects, systemic corticosteroids should be used cautiously in the elderly, in the smallest possible dose, and for the shortest possible time

Acute adrenal insufficiency may occur with abrupt withdrawal after long-term therapy or with stress; young pediatric patients may be more susceptible to adrenal axis suppression from topical therapy

Adverse Reactions

>10%:

Central nervous system: Insomnia, nervousness

Gastrointestinal: Increased appetite, indigestion

1% to 10%:

Dermatologic: Hirsutism

Endocrine & metabolic: Diabetes mellitus

Neuromuscular & skeletal: Arthralgia

(Continued)

Methylprednisolone *(Continued)*

Ocular: Cataracts, glaucoma
Respiratory: Epistaxis

<1%:

Cardiovascular: Edema, hypertension
Central nervous system: Vertigo, seizures, psychoses, pseudotumor cerebri, headache, mood swings, delirium, hallucinations, euphoria
Dermatologic: Acne, skin atrophy, bruising, hyperpigmentation
Endocrine & metabolic: Cushing's syndrome, pituitary-adrenal axis suppression, growth suppression, glucose intolerance, hypokalemia, alkalosis, amenorrhea, sodium and water retention, hyperglycemia
Gastrointestinal: Peptic ulcer, nausea, vomiting, abdominal distention, ulcerative esophagitis, pancreatitis
Neuromuscular & skeletal: Muscle weakness, osteoporosis, fractures
Miscellaneous: Hypersensitivity reactions

Overdosage/Toxicology Symptoms of overdose include cushingoid appearance (systemic), muscle weakness (systemic), osteoporosis (systemic) all with long-term use only. When consumed in excessive quantities for prolonged periods, systemic hypercorticism and adrenal suppression may occur; in those cases, discontinuation and withdrawal of the corticosteroid should be done judiciously

Drug Interactions

Inducer of cytochrome P-450 enzymes
Cytochrome P-450 3A enzyme substrate

Decreased effect:
Phenytoin, phenobarbital, rifampin ↑ clearance of methylprednisolone
Potassium depleting diuretics enhance potassium depletion

Increased toxicity:
Skin test antigens, immunizations ↓ response and ↑ potential infections
Methylprednisolone may ↑ circulating glucose levels → may need adjustments of insulin or oral hypoglycemics

Stability

Intact vials of methylprednisolone sodium succinate should be stored at controlled room temperature
Reconstituted solutions of methylprednisolone sodium succinate should be stored at room temperature (15°C to 30°C) and used within 48 hours
Stability of parenteral admixture at room temperature (25°C) and at refrigeration temperature (4°C): 48 hours
Standard diluent (Solu-Medrol®): 40 mg/50 mL D_5W; 125 mg/50 mL D_5W
Minimum volume (Solu-Medrol®): 50 mL D_5W

Mechanism of Action Decreases inflammation by suppression of migration of polymorphonuclear leukocytes and reversal of increased capillary permeability

Pharmacodynamics/Kinetics

Time to obtain peak effect and the duration of these effects is dependent upon the route of administration. See table.

Route	Peak Effect	Duration
Oral	1-2 h	30-36 h
I.M.	4-8 d	1-4 wk
Intra-articular	1 wk	1-5 wk

Distribution: V_d: 0.7 L/kg
Half-life: 3-3.5 hours
Methylprednisolone sodium succinate is highly soluble and has a rapid effect by I.M. and I.V. routes; methylprednisolone acetate has a low solubility and has a sustained I.M. effect

Usual Dosage Only sodium succinate may be given I.V.; methylprednisolone sodium succinate is highly soluble and has a rapid effect by I.M. and I.V. routes. Methylprednisolone acetate has a low solubility and has a sustained I.M. effect.

Children:
Anti-inflammatory or immunosuppressive: Oral, I.M., I.V. (sodium succinate): 0.5-1.7 mg/kg/day **OR** 5-25 mg/m²/day in divided doses every 6-12 hours; "Pulse" therapy: 15-30 mg/kg/dose over ≥30 minutes given once daily for 3 days
Status asthmaticus: I.V. (sodium succinate): Loading dose: 2 mg/kg/dose, then 0.5-1 mg/kg/dose every 6 hours for up to 5 days
Acute spinal cord injury: I.V. (sodium succinate): 30 mg/kg over 15 minutes, followed in 45 minutes by a continuous infusion of 5.4 mg/kg/hour for 23 hours
Lupus nephritis: I.V. (sodium succinate): 30 mg/kg over ≥30 minutes every other day for 6 doses

High-dose therapy for acute spinal cord injury: I.V. bolus: 30 mg/kg over 15 minutes, followed 45 minutes later by an infusion of 5.4 mg/kg/hour for 23 hours

Adults:

Anti-inflammatory or immunosuppressive: Oral: 2-60 mg/day in 1-4 divided doses to start, followed by gradual reduction in dosage to the lowest possible level consistent with maintaining an adequate clinical response

I.M. (sodium succinate): 10-80 mg/day once daily

I.M. (acetate): 10-80 mg every 1-2 weeks

I.V. (sodium succinate): 10-40 mg over a period of several minutes and repeated I.V. or I.M. at intervals depending on clinical response; when high dosages are needed, administer 30 mg/kg over a period of ≥30 minutes and may be repeated every 4-6 hours for 48 hours

Status asthmaticus: I.V. (sodium succinate): Loading dose: 2 mg/kg/dose, then 0.5-1 mg/kg/dose every 6 hours for up to 5 days

High-dose therapy for acute spinal cord injury: I.V. bolus: 30 mg/kg over 15 minutes, followed 45 minutes later by an infusion of 5.4 mg/kg/hour for 23 hours

Lupus nephritis: High-dose "pulse" therapy: I.V. (sodium succinate): 1 g/day for 3 days

Aplastic anemia: I.V. (sodium succinate): 1 mg/kg/day or 40 mg/day (whichever dose is higher), for 4 days. After 4 days, change to oral and continue until day 10 or until symptoms of serum sickness resolve, then rapidly reduce over approximately 2 weeks.

Hemodialysis: Slightly dialyzable (5% to 20%); administer dose posthemodialysis

Intra-articular (acetate): Administer every 1-5 weeks

Large joints: 20-80 mg

Small joints: 4-10 mg

Intralesional (acetate): 20-60 mg every 1-5 weeks

Topical: Apply sparingly 2-4 times/day

Administration

Oral: Administer after meals or with food or milk

Parenteral: Methylprednisolone sodium succinate may be administered I.M. or I.V.; I.V. administration may be IVP over one to several minutes or IVPB or continuous I.V. infusion

I.V.: Succinate:

Low dose: ≤1.8 mg/kg or ≤125 mg/dose: I.V. push over 3-15 minutes

Moderate dose: ≥2 mg/kg or 250 mg/dose: I.V. over 15-30 minutes

High dose: 15 mg/kg or ≥500 mg/dose: I.V. over ≥30 minutes

Doses >15 mg/kg or ≥1 g: Administer over 1 hour

Do **not** administer high-dose I.V. push; hypotension, cardiac arrhythmia, and sudden death have been reported in patients given high-dose methylprednisolone I.V. push over <20 minutes; intermittent infusion over 15-60 minutes; maximum concentration: I.V. push 125 mg/mL

Monitoring Parameters Blood pressure, blood glucose, electrolytes

Test Interactions Interferes with skin tests

Patient Information Do not discontinue or decreasing the drug without contacting your physician; carry an identification card or bracelet advising that you are on steroids; may take with meals to decrease GI upset

Nursing Implications **Acetate salt should not be given I.V.**

Additional Information Sodium content of 1 g sodium succinate injection: 2.01 mEq; 53 mg of sodium succinate salt is equivalent to 40 mg of methylprednisolone base

Methylprednisolone acetate: Depo-Medrol®

Methylprednisolone sodium succinate: Solu-Medrol®

Dosage Forms

Injection, as acetate: 20 mg/mL (5 mL, 10 mL); 40 mg/mL (1 mL, 5 mL, 10 mL); 80 mg/mL (1 mL, 5 mL)

Injection, as sodium succinate: 40 mg (1 mL, 3 mL); 125 mg (2 mL, 5 mL); 500 mg (1 mL, 4 mL, 8 mL, 20 mL); 1000 mg (1 mL, 8 mL, 50 mL); 2000 mg (30.6 mL)

Tablet: 2 mg, 4 mg, 8 mg, 16 mg, 24 mg, 32 mg

Tablet, dose pack: 4 mg (21s)

6-α-Methylprednisolone *see* Methylprednisolone *on page 819*

Methylprednisolone Acetate *see* Methylprednisolone *on page 819*

Methylprednisolone Sodium Succinate *see* Methylprednisolone *on page 819*

Methyltestosterone (meth il tes TOS te rone)

Brand Names Android®; Metandren®; Oreton® Methyl; Testred®; Virilon®

Therapeutic Category Androgen

(Continued)

Methyltestosterone *(Continued)*

Use
Male: Hypogonadism; delayed puberty; impotence and climacteric symptoms
Female: Palliative treatment of metastatic breast cancer; postpartum breast pain and/or engorgement

Restrictions C-III

Pregnancy Risk Factor X

Contraindications Hypersensitivity to methyltestosterone or any component, known or suspected carcinoma of the breast or the prostate

Warnings/Precautions Use with extreme caution in patients with liver or kidney disease or serious heart disease; may accelerate bone maturation without producing compensatory gain in linear growth

Adverse Reactions
>10%:
Cardiovascular: Edema
Males: Virilism, priapism
Females: Virilism, menstrual problems (amenorrhea), breast soreness
Dermatologic: Acne
1% to 10%:
Males: Prostatic hypertrophy, prostatic carcinoma, impotence, testicular
Females: Hirsutism (increase in pubic hair growth) atrophy
Gastrointestinal: GI irritation, nausea, vomiting
Hepatic: Hepatic dysfunction
<1%:
Endocrine & metabolic: Gynecomastia, amenorrhea, hypercalcemia
Hematologic: Leukopenia, polycythemia
Hepatic: Hepatic necrosis, cholestatic hepatitis
Miscellaneous: Hypersensitivity reactions

Overdosage/Toxicology Abnormal liver function tests

Drug Interactions Decreased effect: Oral anticoagulant effect or decrease insulin requirements

Mechanism of Action Stimulates receptors in organs and tissues to promote growth and development of male sex organs and maintains secondary sex characteristics in androgen-deficient males

Pharmacodynamics/Kinetics
Absorption: From GI tract and oral mucosa
Metabolism: Hepatic
Elimination: In urine

Usual Dosage Adults (buccal absorption produces twice the androgenic activity of oral tablets):
Male:
Oral: 10-40 mg/day
Buccal: 5-25 mg/day

Female:
Breast pain/engorgement:
Oral: 80 mg/day for 3-5 days
Buccal: 40 mg/day for 3-5 days
Breast cancer:
Oral: 50-200 mg/day
Buccal: 25-100 mg/day

Patient Information Men should report overly frequent or persistent penile erections; women should report menstrual irregularities; all patients should report persistent GI distress, diarrhea, or jaundice; buccal tablet should not be chewed or swallowed

Nursing Implications In prepubertal children, perform radiographic examination of the hand and wrist every 6 months to determine the rate of bone maturation and to assess the effect of treatment on the epiphyseal centers

Dosage Forms
Capsule: 10 mg
Tablet: 10 mg, 25 mg
Tablet, buccal: 5 mg, 10 mg

Methysergide (meth i SER jide)

Brand Names Sansert®

Synonyms Methysergide Maleate

Therapeutic Category Ergot Alkaloid and Derivative

Use Prophylaxis of vascular headache

Pregnancy Risk Factor X

Contraindications Peripheral vascular disease, severe arteriosclerosis, pulmonary disease, severe hypertension, phlebitis, serious infections, pregnancy

Warnings/Precautions Patients receiving long-term therapy may develop retroperitoneal fibrosis, pleuropulmonary fibrosis and fibrotic thickening of the cardiac valves. Fibrosis occurs rarely when therapy is interrupted for 3-4 weeks every 6 months. Use caution in patients with impairment of renal of hepatic function; some products may contain tartrazine.

Adverse Reactions

>10%:

Cardiovascular: Postural hypotension, peripheral ischemia

Central nervous system: Insomnia

Gastrointestinal: Nausea, vomiting, abdominal pain, diarrhea

1% to 10%:

Cardiovascular: Peripheral edema, tachycardia, bradycardia

Dermatologic: Rash

Gastrointestinal: Heartburn

<1%:

Central nervous system: Overstimulation, drowsiness, mild euphoria, lethargy, mental depression, vertigo, unsteadiness, confusion, hyperesthesia, rebound headache may occur if methysergide is discontinued abruptly

Ocular: Visual disturbances

Respiratory: Fibrosis

Overdosage/Toxicology Symptoms of overdose include hyperactivity, spasms in limbs, impaired mental function, impaired circulation

Mechanism of Action Ergotamine congener, however actions appear to differ; methysergide has minimal ergotamine-like oxytocic or vasoconstrictive properties, and has significantly greater serotonin-like properties

Pharmacodynamics/Kinetics

Metabolism: Undergoes liver metabolism

Half-life, plasma elimination: ~10 hours

Elimination: Not well defined

Usual Dosage Adults: Oral: 4-8 mg/day with meals; if no improvement is noted after 3 weeks, drug is unlikely to be beneficial; must not be given continuously for longer than 6 months, and a drug-free interval of 3-4 weeks must follow each 6-month course

Patient Information Do not take increased doses per day or for longer time than prescribed; take with meals; may cause drowsiness, impair judgment and coordination; arise slowly from prolonged sitting or lying; notify physician if cold, numbness, painful extremities, chest pain, or painful urination occurs

Nursing Implications Advise patient to make position changes slowly

Dosage Forms Tablet, as maleate: 2 mg

Methysergide Maleate *see* Methysergide *on previous page*

Meticorten® *see* Prednisone *on page 1039*

Metimyd® Ophthalmic *see* Sulfacetamide Sodium and Prednisolone *on page 1172*

Metipranolol (met i PRAN oh lol)

Related Information

Glaucoma Drug Therapy Comparison *on page 1410*

Brand Names OptiPranolol®

Synonyms Metipranolol Hydrochloride

Therapeutic Category Beta-Adrenergic Blocker, Ophthalmic

Use Agent for lowering intraocular pressure in patients with chronic open-angle glaucoma

Pregnancy Risk Factor C

Contraindications Bronchial asthma, sinus bradycardia, second and third degree A-V block, cardiac failure, cardiogenic shock, hypersensitivity to betaxolol or any component, pregnancy

Warnings/Precautions Use with caution in patients with cardiac failure or diabetes mellitus, asthma, bradycardia, or A-V block

Adverse Reactions

>10%: Ocular: Mild ocular stinging and discomfort, eye irritation

1% to 10%: Ocular: Blurred vision, browache

<1%:

Cardiovascular: Bradycardia, A-V block, congestive heart failure

Dermatologic: Erythema

Neuromuscular & skeletal: Weakness

Ocular: Conjunctivitis, blepharitis, tearing, itching eyes, keratitis, photophobia, decreased corneal sensitivity

Respiratory: Bronchospasm

Overdosage/Toxicology Symptoms of overdose include bradycardia, hypotension, A-V block

(Continued)

Metipranolol *(Continued)*

Sympathomimetics (eg, epinephrine or dopamine), glucagon or a pacemaker can be used to treat the toxic bradycardia, asystole, and/or hypotension; initially, fluids may be the best treatment for toxic hypotension

Mechanism of Action Beta-adrenoceptor-blocking agent; lacks intrinsic sympathomimetic activity and membrane-stabilizing effects and possesses only slight local anesthetic activity; mechanism of action of metipranolol in reducing intraocular pressure appears to be via reduced production of aqueous humor. This effect may be related to a reduction in blood flow to the iris root-ciliary body. It remains unclear if the reduction in intraocular pressure observed with beta-blockers is actually secondary to beta-adrenoceptor blockade.

Pharmacodynamics/Kinetics

Onset of action: ≤30 minutes

Maximum effects: ~2 hours

Duration of action: Intraocular pressure reduction has persisted for 24 hours following ocular instillation

Metabolism: Rapid and complete to deacetyl metipranolol, an active metabolite

Half-life, elimination: ~3 hours

Usual Dosage Ophthalmic: Adults: Instill 1 drop in the affected eye(s) twice daily

Patient Information Intended for twice daily dosing; keep eye open and do not blink for 30 seconds after instillation; wear sunglasses to avoid photophobic discomfort

Nursing Implications Monitor for systemic effect of beta-blockade

Dosage Forms Solution, ophthalmic, as hydrochloride: 0.3% (5 mL, 10 mL)

Metipranolol Hydrochloride *see* Metipranolol *on previous page*

Metoclopramide (met oh kloe PRA mide)

Brand Names Clopra®; Maxolon®; Octamide®; Reglan®

Canadian/Mexican Brand Names Apo-Metoclop® (Canada); Maxeran® (Canada); Carnotprim Primperan® (Mexico); Carnotprim Primperan® Retard (Mexico); Meclomid® (Mexico); Plasil® (Mexico); Pramotil® (Mexico)

Therapeutic Category Antiemetic

Use Symptomatic treatment of diabetic gastric stasis, gastroesophageal reflux; prevention of nausea associated with chemotherapy or postsurgery and facilitates intubation of the small intestine

Pregnancy Risk Factor B

Pregnancy/Breast-Feeding Implications

Clinical effects on the fetus: Crosses the placenta. Available evidence suggests safe use during pregnancy and breast-feeding.

Breast-feeding/lactation: Crosses into breast milk

Clinical effects on the infant: Increased milk production; 2 reports of mild intestinal discomfort; American Academy of Pediatrics states MAY BE OF CONCERN

Contraindications Hypersensitivity to metoclopramide or any component; GI obstruction, perforation or hemorrhage, pheochromocytoma, history of seizure disorder

Warnings/Precautions Use with caution in patients with Parkinson's disease and in patients with a history of mental illness; dosage and/or frequency of administration should be modified in response to degree of renal impairment; extrapyramidal reactions, depression; may exacerbate seizures in seizure patients; to prevent extrapyramidal reactions, patients may be pretreated with diphenhydramine; elderly are more likely to develop dystonic reactions than younger adults; use lowest recommended doses initially

Adverse Reactions

>10%:

- Central nervous system: Restlessness, drowsiness
- Gastrointestinal: Diarrhea
- Neuromuscular & skeletal: Weakness

1% to 10%:

- Central nervous system: Insomnia, depression
- Dermatologic: Rash
- Endocrine & metabolic: Breast tenderness, prolactin stimulation
- Gastrointestinal: Nausea, xerostomia

<1%:

- Cardiovascular: Tachycardia, hypertension or hypotension
- Central nervous system: Extrapyramidal reactions*, tardive dyskinesia, fatigue, anxiety, agitation
- Gastrointestinal: Constipation
- Hematologic: Methemoglobinemia

***Note:** A recent study suggests the incidence of extrapyramidal reactions due to metoclopramide may be as high as 34% and the incidence appears more often in the elderly

Overdosage/Toxicology Symptoms of overdose include drowsiness, ataxia, extrapyramidal reactions, seizures, methemoglobinemia (in infants); disorientation, muscle hypertonia, irritability, and agitation are common

Metoclopramide often causes extrapyramidal symptoms (eg, dystonic reactions) requiring management with diphenhydramine 1-2 mg/kg (adults) up to a maximum of 50 mg I.M. or I.V. slow push followed by a maintenance dose for 48-72 hours. When these reactions are unresponsive to diphenhydramine, benztropine mesylate I.V. 1-2 mg (adults) may be effective. These agents are generally effective within 2-5 minutes.

Drug Interactions

Decreased effect: Anticholinergic agents antagonize metoclopramide's actions

Increased toxicity: Opiate analgesics may increase CNS depression

Stability Injection is a clear, colorless solution and should be stored at controlled room temperature and protected from freezing; injection is photosensitive and should be protected from light during storage; dilutions do not require light protection if used within 24 hours

Stability of parenteral admixture at room temperature (25°C) and at refrigeration temperature (4°C): 24 hours

Standard diluent: 10-150 mg/50 mL D_5W or NS

Minimum volume: 50 mL D_5W or NS; send 10 mg unmixed to nursing unit

Compatible with diphenhydramine

Mechanism of Action Blocks dopamine receptors in chemoreceptor trigger zone of the CNS; enhances the response to acetylcholine of tissue in upper GI tract causing enhanced motility and accelerated gastric emptying without stimulating gastric, biliary, or pancreatic secretions

Pharmacodynamics/Kinetics

Onset of effect:
- Oral: Within 0.5-1 hour
- I.V.: Within 1-3 minutes

Duration of therapeutic effect: 1-2 hours, regardless of route administered

Distribution: Crosses the placenta; appears in breast milk

Protein binding: 30%

Half-life, normal renal function: 4-7 hours (may be dose-dependent)

Elimination: Primarily as unchanged drug in urine and feces

Usual Dosage

Children:
- Gastroesophageal reflux: Oral: 0.1-0.2 mg/kg/dose up to 4 times/day; efficacy of continuing metoclopramide beyond 12 weeks in reflux has not been determined; total daily dose should not exceed 0.5 mg/kg/day
- Gastrointestinal hypomotility (gastroparesis): Oral, I.M., I.V.: 0.1 mg/kg/dose up to 4 times/day, not to exceed 0.5 mg/kg/day
- Antiemetic (chemotherapy-induced emesis): I.V.: 1-2 mg/kg 30 minutes before chemotherapy and every 2-4 hours
- Facilitate intubation: I.V.:
  - <6 years: 0.1 mg/kg
  - 6-14 years: 2.5-5 mg

Adults:
- Gastroesophageal reflux: Oral: 10-15 mg/dose up to 4 times/day 30 minutes before meals or food and at bedtime; single doses of 20 mg are occasionally needed for provoking situations; efficacy of continuing metoclopramide beyond 12 weeks in reflux has not been determined
- Gastrointestinal hypomotility (gastroparesis):
  - Oral: 10 mg 30 minutes before each meal and at bedtime for 2-8 weeks
  - I.V. (for severe symptoms): 10 mg over 1-2 minutes; 10 days of I.V. therapy may be necessary for best response
- Antiemetic (chemotherapy-induced emesis): I.V.: 1-2 mg/kg 30 minutes before chemotherapy and every 2-4 hours to every 4-6 hours (and usually given with diphenhydramine 25-50 mg I.V./oral)
- Postoperative nausea and vomiting: I.M.: 10 mg near end of surgery; 20 mg doses may be used
- Facilitate intubation: I.V.: 10 mg

Elderly:
- Gastroesophageal reflux: Oral: 5 mg 4 times/day (30 minutes before meals and at bedtime); increase dose to 10 mg 4 times/day if no response at lower dose
- Gastrointestinal hypomotility:
  - Oral: Initial: 5 mg 30 minutes before meals and at bedtime for 2-8 weeks; increase if necessary to 10 mg doses
  - I.V.: Initiate at 5 mg over 1-2 minutes; increase to 10 mg if necessary
- Postoperative nausea and vomiting: I.M.: 5 mg near end of surgery; may repeat dose if necessary

Dosing adjustment in renal impairment:

Cl_{cr} 10-40 mL/minute: Administer at 50% of normal dose

(Continued)

Metoclopramide *(Continued)*

Cl_{cr} <10 mL/minute: Administer at 25% of normal dose

Hemodialysis: Not dialyzable (0% to 5%); supplemental dose is not necessary

Dietary Considerations Alcohol: Additive CNS effect, avoid use

Administration Lower doses of metoclopramide can be given I.V. push undiluted over 1-2 minutes; parenteral doses of up to 10 mg should be given I.V. push; higher doses to be given IVPB; infuse over at least 15 minutes

Monitoring Parameters Periodic renal function test; monitor for dystonic reactions; monitor for signs of hypoglycemia in patients using insulin and those being treated for gastroparesis; monitor for agitation and irritable confusion

Test Interactions ↑ aminotransferase [ALT (SGPT)/AST (SGOT)] (S), ↑ amylase (S)

Patient Information May impair mental alertness or physical coordination; avoid alcohol, barbiturates or other CNS depressants; take 30 minutes before meals; notify physician if involuntary movements occur

Dosage Forms

Injection: 5 mg/mL (2 mL, 10 mL, 30 mL, 50 mL, 100 mL)

Solution, oral, concentrated: 10 mg/mL (10 mL, 30 mL)

Syrup, sugar free: 5 mg/5 mL (10 mL, 480 mL)

Tablet: 5 mg, 10 mg

Metolazone (me TOLE a zone)

Related Information

Heart Failure: Management of Patients With Left-Ventricular Systolic Dysfunction *on page 1533*

Sulfonamide Derivatives *on page 1420*

Brand Names Mykrox®; Zaroxolyn®

Therapeutic Category Antihypertensive; Diuretic, Miscellaneous

Use Management of mild to moderate hypertension; treatment of edema in congestive heart failure and nephrotic syndrome, impaired renal function

Pregnancy Risk Factor D

Contraindications Hypersensitivity to metolazone or any component, other thiazides, and sulfonamide derivatives; patients with hepatic coma, anuria

Warnings/Precautions Use with caution in renal disease, hepatic disease, gout, lupus erythematosus, diabetes mellitus; some products may contain tartrazine. **Mykrox® is not bioequivalent to Zaroxolyn® and should not be interchanged for one another.**

Adverse Reactions

1% to 10%: Endocrine & metabolic: Hypokalemia

<1%:

- Cardiovascular: Hypotension
- Central nervous system: Drowsiness
- Dermatologic: Photosensitivity, rash
- Endocrine & metabolic: Fluid and electrolyte imbalances (hypocalcemia, hypomagnesemia, hyponatremia), hyperglycemia
- Gastrointestinal: Nausea, vomiting, anorexia
- Genitourinary: Polyuria
- Hematologic: Rarely blood dyscrasias, aplastic anemia, hemolytic anemia, leukopenia, agranulocytosis, thrombocytopenia
- Hepatic: Hepatitis
- Neuromuscular & skeletal: Paresthesia
- Renal: Prerenal azotemia, uremia

Overdosage/Toxicology Symptoms of overdose include orthostatic hypotension, dizziness, drowsiness, syncope, hemoconcentration and hemodynamic changes due to plasma volume depletion; treatment is primarily symptomatic and supportive

Drug Interactions

Increased toxicity: Concurrent administration with furosemide may cause excessive volume and electrolyte depletion; increased digitalis glycosides toxicity; increased lithium toxicity

Mechanism of Action Inhibits sodium reabsorption in the distal tubules causing increased excretion of sodium and water, as well as, potassium and hydrogen ions

Pharmacodynamics/Kinetics Same for all routes:

Onset of diuresis: Within 60 minutes

Duration: 12-24 hours

Absorption: Oral: Incomplete

Distribution: Crosses the placenta; appears in breast milk

Protein binding: 95%

Bioavailability: Mykrox® reportedly has highest

Half-life: 6-20 hours, renal function dependent

Elimination: Enterohepatic recycling; 80% to 95% excreted in urine

Usual Dosage Oral:

Children: 0.2-0.4 mg/kg/day divided every 12-24 hours

Adults:

Edema: 5-20 mg/dose every 24 hours

Hypertension: 2.5-5 mg/dose every 24 hours

Hypertension (Mykrox®): 0.5 mg/day; if response is not adequate, increase dose to maximum of 1 mg/day

Dialysis: Not dialyzable (0% to 5%) via hemo- or peritoneal dialysis; supplemental dose is not necessary

Monitoring Parameters Serum electrolytes (potassium, sodium, chloride, bicarbonate), renal function, blood pressure (standing, sitting/supine)

Patient Information May be taken with food or milk; take early in day to avoid nocturia; take the last dose of multiple doses no later than 6 PM unless instructed otherwise. A few people who take this medication become more sensitive to sunlight and may experience skin rash, redness, itching, or severe sunburn, especially if sun block SPF ≥15 is not used on exposed skin areas.

Nursing Implications Assess weight, I & O reports daily to determine fluid loss; take blood pressure with patient lying down and standing

Dosage Forms Tablet:

Zaroxolyn®: 2.5 mg, 5 mg, 10 mg

Mykrox®: 0.5 mg

Extemporaneous Preparations A 1 mg/mL suspension can be made by crushing twenty-four 5 mg tablets. Add a small amount of distilled water. Add 30 mL Cologel and mix well. Add a sufficient amount of 2:1 simple syrup/cherry syrup mixture to make a final volume of 120 mL. Label "shake well". Stability is 2 weeks refrigerated.

Handbook on Extemporaneous Formulations, Bethesda MD: American Society of Hospital Pharmacists, 1987.

Metoprolol (me toe PROE lole)

Related Information

Antiarrhythmic Drugs *on page 1389*

Beta-Blockers Comparison *on page 1398*

Extravasation Treatment of Other Drugs *on page 1381*

Brand Names Lopressor®; Toprol XL®

Canadian/Mexican Brand Names Apo-Metoprolol® (Type L) (Canada); Betaloc® (Canada); Betaloc Durules® (Canada); Novo-Metoprolol® (Canada); Nu-Metop® (Canada); Kenaprol® (Mexico); Lopresor® (Mexico); Proken® M (Mexico); Prolaken® (Mexico); Ritmolol® (Mexico); Seloken® (Mexico); Selopres® (Mexico)

Synonyms Metoprolol Tartrate

Therapeutic Category Antihypertensive; Beta-Adrenergic Blocker

Use Treatment of hypertension and angina pectoris; prevention of myocardial infarction, atrial fibrillation, flutter, symptomatic treatment of hypertrophic subaortic stenosis

Unlabeled use: Treatment of ventricular arrhythmias, atrial ectopy, migraine prophylaxis, essential tremor, aggressive behavior

Pregnancy Risk Factor B

Pregnancy/Breast-Feeding Implications

Clinical effects on the fetus: Crosses the placenta. None; mild IUGR probably secondary to maternal hypertension. Available evidence suggests safe use during pregnancy and breast-feeding. Monitor breast-fed infant for symptoms of beta-blockade.

Breast-Feeding/lactation: Crosses into breast milk. American Academy of Pediatrics considers COMPATIBLE with breast-feeding.

Contraindications Hypersensitivity to beta-blocking agents, uncompensated congestive heart failure; cardiogenic shock; bradycardia (heart rate <45 bpm) or heart block; sinus node dysfunction; A-V conduction abnormalities, systolic blood pressure <100 mm Hg; diabetes mellitus. Although metoprolol primarily blocks $beta_1$-receptors, high doses can result in $beta_2$-receptor blockage; therefore, use with caution in elderly with bronchospastic lung disease.

Warnings/Precautions Use with caution in patients with inadequate myocardial function; those undergoing anesthesia, patients with CHF, myasthenia gravis, impaired hepatic or renal function, severe peripheral vascular disease, bronchospastic disease, diabetes mellitus or hyperthyroidism. Abrupt withdrawal of the drug should be avoided (may result in an exaggerated cardiac beta-adrenergic response, tachycardia, hypertension, ischemia, angina, myocardial infarction, and sudden death), drug should be discontinued over 1-2 weeks; do not use in pregnant or nursing women, may potentiate hypoglycemia in a diabetic patient and mask signs and symptoms; sweating will continue.

(Continued)

Metoprolol *(Continued)*

Adverse Reactions

>10%:

Central nervous system: Mental depression, fatigue, dizziness
Neuromuscular & skeletal: Weakness

1% to 10%:

Cardiovascular: Bradycardia, arrhythmia, reduced peripheral circulation
Gastrointestinal: Heartburn
Respiratory: Wheezing

<1%:

Cardiovascular: Chest pain, heart failure, Raynaud's phenomenon
Central nervous system: Insomnia, nightmares, confusion, headache
Dermatologic: Rash, itching
Endocrine & metabolic: Decreased sexual activity
Gastrointestinal: Constipation, nausea, vomiting, stomach discomfort
Genitourinary: Impotence
Miscellaneous: Cold extremities

Overdosage/Toxicology Symptoms of intoxication include cardiac disturbances, CNS toxicity, bronchospasm, hypoglycemia and hyperkalemia. The most common cardiac symptoms include hypotension and bradycardia; atrioventricular block, intraventricular conduction disturbances, cardiogenic shock, and asystole may occur with severe overdose, especially with membrane-depressant drugs (eg, propranolol); CNS effects include convulsions, coma, and respiratory arrest.

Treatment includes symptomatic treatment of seizures, hypotension, hyperkalemia and hypoglycemia; bradycardia and hypotension resistant to atropine, isoproterenol or pacing, may respond to glucagon; wide QRS defects caused by the membrane-depressant poisoning may respond to hypertonic sodium bicarbonate; repeat-dose charcoal, hemoperfusion, or hemodialysis may be helpful in removal of only those beta-blockers with a small V_d, long half-life or low intrinsic clearance (acebutolol, atenolol, nadolol, sotalol)

Drug Interactions Cytochrome P-450 2D6 enzyme substrate

Decreased effect of beta-blockers with aluminum salts, barbiturates, calcium salts, cholestyramine, colestipol, NSAIDs, penicillins (ampicillin), rifampin, salicylates and sulfinpyrazone due to decreased bioavailability and plasma levels

Beta-blockers may decrease the effect of sulfonylureas

Increased effect/toxicity of beta-blockers with calcium blockers (diltiazem, felodipine, nicardipine), oral contraceptives, flecainide, haloperidol (propranolol, hypotensive effects), H_2-antagonists (metoprolol, propranolol only by cimetidine, possibly ranitidine), hydralazine (metoprolol, propranolol), loop diuretics (propranolol, not atenolol), MAO inhibitors (metoprolol, nadolol, bradycardia), phenothiazines (propranolol), propafenone (metoprolol, propranolol), quinidine (in extensive metabolizers), ciprofloxacin, thyroid hormones (metoprolol, propranolol, when hypothyroid patient is converted to euthyroid state)

Beta-blockers may increase the effect/toxicity of flecainide, haloperidol (hypotensive effects), hydralazine, phenothiazines, acetaminophen, anticoagulants (propranolol, warfarin), benzodiazepines (not atenolol), clonidine (hypertensive crisis after or during withdrawal of either agent), epinephrine (initial hypertensive episode followed by bradycardia), nifedipine and verapamil lidocaine, ergots (peripheral ischemia), prazosin (postural hypotension)

Beta-blockers may affect the action or levels of ethanol, disopyramide, nondepolarizing muscle relaxants and theophylline although the effects are difficult to predict

Mechanism of Action Selective inhibitor of $beta_1$-adrenergic receptors; competitively blocks $beta_1$-receptors, with little or no effect on $beta_2$-receptors at doses <100 mg; does not exhibit any membrane stabilizing or intrinsic sympathomimetic activity

Pharmacodynamics/Kinetics

Peak antihypertensive effect: Oral: Within 1.5-4 hours
Duration: 10-20 hours
Absorption: 95%
Protein binding: 8%
Metabolism: Significant first-pass metabolism; extensively metabolized in the liver
Bioavailability: Oral: 40% to 50%
Half-life: 3-4 hours
End stage renal disease: 2.5-4.5 hours
Elimination: In urine (3% to 10% as unchanged drug)

Usual Dosage

Children: Oral: 1-5 mg/kg/24 hours divided twice daily; allow 3 days between dose adjustments

Adults:

Oral: 100-450 mg/day in 2-3 divided doses, begin with 50 mg twice daily and increase doses at weekly intervals to desired effect

I.V.: 5 mg every 2 minutes for 3 doses in early treatment of myocardial infarction; thereafter administer 50 mg orally every 6 hours 15 minutes after last I.V. dose and continue for 48 hours; then administer a maintenance dose of 100 mg twice daily

Elderly: Oral: Initial: 25 mg/day; usual range: 25-300 mg/day

Hemodialysis: Administer dose posthemodialysis or administer 50 mg supplemental dose; supplemental dose is not necessary following peritoneal dialysis

Dosing adjustment/comments in hepatic disease: Reduced dose probably necessary

Monitoring Parameters Blood pressure, apical and radial pulses, fluid I & O, daily weight, respirations, mental status, and circulation in extremities before and during therapy

Patient Information Do not discontinue medication abruptly, sudden stopping of medication may precipitate or cause angina; consult pharmacist or physician before taking with other adrenergic drugs (eg, cold medications); use with caution while driving or performing tasks requiring alertness; may mask signs of hypoglycemia in diabetics; may be taken without regard to meals

Dosage Forms

Injection, as tartrate: 1 mg/mL (5 mL)

Tablet, as tartrate: 50 mg, 100 mg

Tablet, as tartrate, sustained release: 50 mg, 100 mg, 200 mg

Metoprolol Tartrate *see* Metoprolol *on page 827*

Metreton® *see* Prednisolone *on page 1037*

Metrodin® Injection *see* Urofollitropin *on page 1281*

MetroGel® *see* Metronidazole *on this page*

Metro I.V.® *see* Metronidazole *on this page*

Metronidazole (me troe NI da zole)

Related Information

Antimicrobial Drugs of Choice *on page 1468*

Helicobacter pylori Treatment *on page 1534*

Treatment of Sexually Transmitted Diseases *on page 1485*

Brand Names Flagyl®; MetroGel®; Metro I.V.®; Protostat®

Canadian/Mexican Brand Names Apo-Metronidazole® (Canada); Novo-Nidazol® (Canada); Ameblin® (Mexico); Flagenase® (Mexico); Milezzol® (Mexico); Otrozol® (Mexico); Vatrix-S® (Mexico); Vertisal® (Mexico)

Synonyms Metronidazole Hydrochloride

Therapeutic Category Amebicide; Antibiotic, Anaerobic; Antibiotic, Topical; Antiprotozoal

Use Treatment of susceptible anaerobic bacterial and protozoal infections in the following conditions: amebiasis, symptomatic and asymptomatic trichomoniasis; skin and skin structure infections; CNS infections; intra-abdominal infections; systemic anaerobic infections; topically for the treatment of acne rosacea; treatment of antibiotic-associated pseudomembranous colitis (AAPC); used in combination with other agents (eg, tetracycline, bismuth subsalicylate, and an H_2-antagonist) to treat duodenal ulcer diseased due to *Helicobacter pylori*

Pregnancy Risk Factor B

Contraindications Hypersensitivity to metronidazole or any component, 1st trimester of pregnancy since found to be carcinogenic in rats

Warnings/Precautions Use with caution in patients with liver impairment due to potential accumulation, blood dyscrasias; history of seizures, congestive heart failure, or other sodium retaining states; reduce dosage in patients with severe liver impairment, CNS disease, and severe renal failure (Cl_{cr} <10 mL/minute); if *H. pylori* is not eradicated in patients being treated with metronidazole in a regimen, it should be assumed that metronidazole-resistance has occurred and it should not again be used; seizures and neuropathies have been reported especially with increased doses and chronic treatment; if this occurs, discontinue therapy; candidiasis may worsen during therapy

Adverse Reactions

>10%:

Central nervous system: Dizziness, headache

Gastrointestinal: Nausea, diarrhea, loss of appetite, vomiting

1% to 10%:

Central nervous system: Seizures

Neuromuscular & skeletal: Peripheral neuropathy

<1%:

Central nervous system: Ataxia

Endocrine & metabolic: Disulfiram-type reaction with alcohol

(Continued)

Metronidazole *(Continued)*

Gastrointestinal: Pancreatitis, xerostomia, metallic taste, furry tongue
Genitourinary: Vaginal candidiasis
Hematologic: Leukopenia
Local: Thrombophlebitis
Miscellaneous: Hypersensitivity, change in taste sensation, dark urine

Overdosage/Toxicology Symptoms of overdose include nausea, vomiting, ataxia, seizures, peripheral neuropathy; treatment is symptomatic and supportive

Drug Interactions

Decreased effect: Phenytoin, phenobarbital may decrease metronidazole half-life
Increased toxicity: Alcohol, disulfiram → disulfiram-like reactions; warfarin increases PT prolongation

Stability

Metronidazole injection should be stored at 15°C to 30°C and protected from light
Product may be refrigerated but crystals may form; crystals redissolve on warming to room temperature
Prolonged exposure to light will cause a darkening of the product. However, short-term exposure to normal room light does not adversely affect metronidazole stability. Direct sunlight should be avoided.
Stability of parenteral admixture at room temperature (25°C): Out of overwrap stability: 30 days
Standard diluent: 500 mg/100 mL NS

Mechanism of Action Reduced to a product which interacts with DNA to cause a loss of helical DNA structure and strand breakage resulting in inhibition of protein synthesis and cell death in susceptible organisms

Pharmacodynamics/Kinetics

Absorption:
Oral: Well absorbed
Topical: Concentrations achieved systemically after application of 1 g topically are 10 times less than those obtained after a 250 mg oral dose
Distribution: Excreted in breast milk
Relative diffusion of antimicrobial agents from blood into cerebrospinal fluid (CSF): Adequate with or without inflammation (exceeds usual MICs)
Ratio of CSF to blood level (%):
Normal meninges: 16-43
Inflamed meninges: 100
Protein binding: <20%
Metabolism: 30% to 60% in the liver
Half-life:
Neonates: 25-75 hours
Others: 6-8 hours, increases with hepatic impairment
End stage renal disease: 21 hours
Time to peak serum concentration: Within 1-2 hours
Elimination: Final excretion via the urine (20% to 40% as unchanged drug) and feces (6% to 15%); clearance: 10 mL/minute/1.73 m^2

Usual Dosage

Infants and Children:
Amebiasis: Oral: 35-50 mg/kg/day in divided doses every 8 hours for 10 days
Trichomoniasis: Oral: 15-30 mg/kg/day in divided doses every 8 hours for 7 days
Anaerobic infections:
Oral: 15-35 mg/kg/day in divided doses every 8 hours
I.V.: 30 mg/kg/day in divided doses every 6 hours
Clostridium difficile (antibiotic-associated colitis): Oral: 20 mg/kg/day divided every 6 hours
Maximum dose: 2 g/day
Adults:
Amebiasis: Oral: 500-750 mg every 8 hours for 5-10 days
Trichomoniasis: Oral: 250 mg every 8 hours for 7 days or 2 g as a single dose
Anaerobic infections: Oral, I.V.: 500 mg every 6-8 hours, not to exceed 4 g/day
Antibiotic-associated pseudomembranous colitis: Oral: 250-500 mg 3-4 times/day for 10-14 days
H. pylori: 1 capsule with meals and at bedtime for 14 days in combination with other agents (eg, tetracycline, bismuth subsalicylate, and H_2-antagonist)
Elderly: Use lower end of dosing recommendations for adults, do not administer as a single dose

Topical (acne rosacea therapy): Apply and rub a thin film twice daily, morning and evening, to entire affected areas after washing. Significant therapeutic results should be noticed within 3 weeks. Clinical studies have demonstrated continuing improvement through 9 weeks of therapy.

Dosing adjustment in renal impairment: Cl_{cr} <10 mL/minute: Administer at 50% of dose or every 12 hours

Hemodialysis: Extensively removed by hemodialysis and peritoneal dialysis (50% to 100%); administer dose post hemodialysis; during peritoneal dialysis and continuous arterio-venous or veno-venous hemofiltration (CAVH/CAVHD), dose as for Cl_{cr} <10 mL/minute

Dosing adjustment/comments in hepatic disease: Unchanged in mild liver disease; reduce dosage in severe liver disease

Dietary Considerations

Alcohol: A disulfiram-like reaction characterized by flushing, headache, nausea, vomiting, sweating or tachycardia; patients should be warned to avoid alcohol during and 72 hours after therapy

Food: Peak antibiotic serum concentration lowered and delayed, but total drug absorbed not affected. Take on an empty stomach. Drug may cause GI upset; if GI upset occurs, take with food.

Test Interactions May cause falsely decreased AST and ALT levels

Patient Information Urine may be discolored to a dark or reddish-brown; do not take alcohol for at least 24 hours after the last dose; avoid beverage alcohol or any topical products containing alcohol during therapy; may cause metallic taste; may be taken with food to minimize stomach upset; notify physician if numbness or tingling in extremities; avoid contact of the topical product with the eyes; cleanse areas to be treated well before application

Nursing Implications No Antabuse®-like reactions have been reported after **topical** application, although metronidazole can be detected in the blood; avoid contact between the drug and aluminum in the infusion set

Additional Information Sodium content of 500 mg (I.V.): 322 mg (14 mEq)

Dosage Forms

Capsule: 375 mg
Gel, topical: 0.75% [7.5 mg/mL] (30 g)
Gel, vaginal: 0.75% (5 g applicator delivering 37.5 mg in 70 g tube)
Injection, ready to use: 5 mg/mL (100 mL)
Powder for injection, as hydrochloride: 500 mg
Tablet: 250 mg, 500 mg

Extemporaneous Preparations To prepare metronidazole suspension 50 mg/mL, pulverize ten 250 mg tablets; levigate with a small amount of distilled water; add 10 mL Cologel® and levigate; add sufficient quantity of cherry syrup to total 50 mL and levigate until a uniform mixture is obtained; stable for 30 days if refrigerated

Committee on Extemporaneous Formulations, ASHP Special Interest Group (SIG) on Pediatric Pharmacy Practice, *Handbook on Extemporaneous Formulations*, 1987.

Metronidazole Hydrochloride *see* Metronidazole *on page 829*

Metyrosine (me TYE roe seen)

Brand Names Demser®

Synonyms AMPT; OGMT

Therapeutic Category Tyrosine Hydroxylase Inhibitor

Use Short-term management of pheochromocytoma before surgery, long-term management when surgery is contraindicated or when malignant

Pregnancy Risk Factor C

Contraindications Hypertension of unknown etiology, known hypersensitivity to metyrosine

Warnings/Precautions Maintain fluid volume during and after surgery; use with caution in patients with impaired renal or hepatic function

Adverse Reactions

>10%:
- Central nervous system: Drowsiness, extrapyramidal symptoms
- Gastrointestinal: Diarrhea

1% to 10%:
- Endocrine & metabolic: Galactorrhea, edema of the breasts
- Gastrointestinal: Nausea, vomiting, xerostomia
- Genitourinary: Impotence
- Respiratory: Nasal congestion

<1%:
- Cardiovascular: Lower extremity edema
- Central nervous system: Depression, hallucinations, disorientation, parkinsonism
- Dermatologic: Urticaria
- Genitourinary: Urinary problems
- Hematologic: Anemia, eosinophilia
- Renal: Hematuria
- Miscellaneous: Hyperstimulation after withdrawal

(Continued)

Metyrosine *(Continued)*

Overdosage/Toxicology Signs of overdose include sedation, fatigue, tremor; reducing dose or discontinuation of therapy usually results in resolution of symptoms

Mechanism of Action Blocks the rate-limiting step in the biosynthetic pathway of catecholamines. It is a tyrosine hydroxylase inhibitor, blocking the conversion of tyrosine to dihydroxyphenylalanine. This inhibition results in decreased levels of endogenous catecholamines. Catecholamine biosynthesis is reduced by 35% to 80% in patients treated with metyrosine 1-4 g/day.

Pharmacodynamics/Kinetics

Half-life: 7.2 hours

Elimination: Following oral absorption, excreted primarily unchanged in urine

Usual Dosage Children >12 years and Adults: Oral: Initial: 250 mg 4 times/day, increased by 250-500 mg/day up to 4 g/day; maintenance: 2-3 g/day in 4 divided doses; for preoperative preparation, administer optimum effective dosage for 5-7 days

Dosing adjustment in renal impairment: Adjustment should be considered

Dietary Considerations Alcohol: Additive CNS effect, avoid use

Patient Information Take plenty of fluids each day; may cause drowsiness, impair coordination and judgment; notify physician if drooling, tremors, speech difficulty, or diarrhea occurs; avoid alcohol and central nervous system depressants

Dosage Forms Capsule: 250 mg

Mevacor® *see* Lovastatin *on page 746*

Mevinolin *see* Lovastatin *on page 746*

Mexiletine (MEKS i le teen)

Related Information

Antiarrhythmic Drugs *on page 1389*

Comparative Pharmacokinetic Properties of Antiarrhythmic Agents *on page 1391*

Brand Names Mexitil®

Therapeutic Category Antiarrhythmic Agent, Class I-B

Use Management of serious ventricular arrhythmias; suppression of PVCs

Unlabeled use: Diabetic neuropathy

Pregnancy Risk Factor C

Contraindications Cardiogenic shock, second or third degree heart block, hypersensitivity to mexiletine or any component

Warnings/Precautions Exercise extreme caution in patients with pre-existing sinus node dysfunction; mexiletine can worsen CHF, bradycardias, and other arrhythmias; mexiletine, like other antiarrhythmic agents, is proarrhythmic; CAST study indicates a trend toward increased mortality with antiarrhythmics in the face of cardiac disease (myocardial infarction); elevation of AST/ALT; hepatic necrosis reported; leukopenia, agranulocytopenia, and thrombocytopenia; seizures; alterations in urinary pH may change urinary excretion; electrolyte disturbances (hypokalemia, hyperkalemia, etc) after drug response

Adverse Reactions

>10%:

- Central nervous system: Lightheadedness, dizziness, nervousness
- Neuromuscular & skeletal: Trembling, unsteady gait

1% to 10%:

- Cardiovascular: Chest pain, premature ventricular contractions
- Central nervous system: Confusion, headache, insomnia
- Dermatologic: Rash
- Gastrointestinal: Constipation or diarrhea
- Hepatic: Increased LFTs
- Neuromuscular & skeletal: Weakness, numbness of fingers or toes
- Ocular: Blurred vision
- Otic: Tinnitus
- Respiratory: Shortness of breath

<1%:

- Hematologic: Leukopenia, agranulocytosis, thrombocytopenia, positive antinuclear antibody
- Ocular: Diplopia

Overdosage/Toxicology Has a narrow therapeutic index and severe toxicity may occur slightly above the therapeutic range, especially with other antiarrhythmic drugs; acute ingestion of twice the daily therapeutic dose is potentially life-threatening; symptoms of overdose includes sedation, confusion, coma, seizures, respiratory arrest and cardiac toxicity (sinus arrest, A-V block, asystole, and hypotension); the QRS and Q-T intervals are usually normal, although they may be prolonged after massive overdose; other effects include dizziness, paresthesias, tremor, ataxia, and GI disturbance.

Treatment is supportive, using conventional therapies (fluids, positioning, vasopressors, antiarrhythmics, anticonvulsants); sodium bicarbonate may reverse the QRS prolongation, bradyarrhythmias and hypotension; enhanced elimination with dialysis, hemoperfusion or repeat charcoal is not effective.

Drug Interactions

Decreased plasma levels: Phenobarbital, phenytoin, rifampin, and other hepatic enzyme inducers, cimetidine and drugs which make the urine acidic

Increased effect: Allopurinol

Increased toxicity/levels of caffeine and theophylline

Mechanism of Action Class IB antiarrhythmic, structurally related to lidocaine, which inhibits inward sodium current, decreases rate of rise of phase 0, increases effective refractory period/action potential duration ratio

Pharmacodynamics/Kinetics

Absorption: Elderly have a slightly slower rate of absorption but extent of absorption is the same as young adults

Distribution: V_d: 5-7 L/kg

Protein binding: 50% to 70%

Metabolism: Low first-pass metabolism

Half-life: Adults: 10-14 hours (average: 14.4 hours elderly, 12 hours in younger adults); increase in half-life with hepatic or heart failure

Time to peak: Peak levels attained in 2-3 hours

Elimination: 10% to 15% excreted unchanged in urine; urinary acidification increases excretion, alkalinization decreases excretion

Usual Dosage Adults: Oral: Initial: 200 mg every 8 hours (may load with 400 mg if necessary); adjust dose every 2-3 days; usual dose: 200-300 mg every 8 hours; maximum dose: 1.2 g/day (some patients respond to every 12-hour dosing); patients with hepatic impairment or CHF may require dose reduction; when switching from another antiarrhythmic, initiate a 200 mg dose 6-12 hours after stopping former agents, 3-6 hours after stopping procainamide

Administration Administer around-the-clock rather than 3 times/day to promote less variation in peak and trough serum levels

Reference Range Therapeutic range: 0.5-2 μg/mL; potentially toxic: >2 μg/mL

Test Interactions Abnormal liver function test, positive ANA, thrombocytopenia

Patient Information Take with food or antacid; notify physician of severe or persistent abdominal pain, nausea, vomiting, yellowing of eyes or skin, pale stools, dark urine, or if persistent fever, sore throat, bleeding, or bruising occurs

Dosage Forms Capsule: 150 mg, 200 mg, 250 mg

Mexitil® *see* Mexiletine *on previous page*

Mezlin® *see* Mezlocillin *on this page*

Mezlocillin (mez loe SIL in)

Related Information

Antimicrobial Drugs of Choice *on page 1468*

Brand Names Mezlin®

Synonyms Mezlocillin Sodium

Therapeutic Category Antibiotic, Penicillin

Use Treatment of infections caused by susceptible gram-negative aerobic bacilli (*Klebsiella, Proteus, Escherichia coli, Enterobacter, Pseudomonas aeruginosa, Serratia*) involving the skin and skin structure, bone and joint, respiratory tract, urinary tract, gastrointestinal tract, as well as, septicemia

Pregnancy Risk Factor B

Contraindications Hypersensitivity to mezlocillin, any component, or penicillins

Warnings/Precautions If bleeding occurs during therapy, mezlocillin should be discontinued; dosage modification required in patients with impaired renal function; use with caution in patients with renal impairment or biliary obstruction, or history of allergy to cephalosporins

Adverse Reactions

1% to 10%: Gastrointestinal: Nausea, diarrhea

<1%:

- Central nervous system: Fever, seizures, dizziness, headache
- Dermatologic: Rash, exfoliative dermatitis
- Endocrine & metabolic: Hypokalemia, hypernatremia
- Gastrointestinal: Vomiting
- Hematologic: Eosinophilia, leukopenia, neutropenia, thrombocytopenia, agranulocytosis, hemolytic anemia, prolonged bleeding time, positive Coombs' [direct]
- Hepatic: Hepatotoxicity, elevated liver enzymes
- Renal: Hematuria, elevated BUN/serum creatinine, interstitial nephritis
- Miscellaneous: Serum sickness-like reactions

(Continued)

Mezlocillin *(Continued)*

Overdosage/Toxicology Symptoms of penicillin overdose include neuromuscular hypersensitivity (agitation, hallucinations, asterixis, encephalopathy, confusion, and seizures) and electrolyte imbalance with potassium or sodium salts, especially in renal failure

Hemodialysis may be helpful to aid in the removal of the drug from the blood, otherwise most treatment is supportive or symptom directed

Drug Interactions Aminoglycosides (synergy), probenecid (decreased clearance), vecuronium (increased duration of neuromuscular blockade), heparin (increased risk of bleeding)

Stability Reconstituted solution is stable for 48 hours at room temperature and 7 days when refrigerated; for I.V. infusion in NS or D_5W solution is stable for 48 hours at room temperature, 7 days when refrigerated or 28 days when frozen; after freezing, thawed solution is stable for 48 hours at room temperature or 7 days when refrigerated; if precipitation occurs under refrigeration, warm in water bath (37°C) for 20 minutes and shake well

Mechanism of Action Interferes with bacterial cell wall synthesis during active multiplication causing cell death and resultant bactericidal activity against susceptible bacteria

Pharmacodynamics/Kinetics

Absorption: I.M.: 63%

Distribution: Into bile, heart, peritoneal fluid, sputum, bone; does not cross the blood-brain barrier well unless meninges are inflamed; crosses the placenta; distributes into breast milk at low concentrations

Protein binding: 30%

Metabolism: Minimal

Half-life: Dose dependent:
- Neonates:
  - <7 days: 3.7-4.4 hours
  - >7 days: 2.5 hours
- Children 2-19 years: 0.9 hour
- Adults: 50-70 minutes, increased in renal impairment

Time to peak serum concentration:
- I.M.: 45-90 minutes after administration
- I.V. infusion: Within 5 minutes

Elimination: Principally as unchanged drug in urine, also excreted via bile

Usual Dosage I.M., I.V.:

Children: 200-300 mg/kg/day divided every 4-6 hours; maximum: 24 g/day

Adults:
- Uncomplicated urinary tract infection: 1.5-2 g every 6 hours
- Serious infections: 3-4 g every 4-6 hours

Dosing interval in renal impairment:
- Cl_{cr} 10-30 mL/minute: Administer every 6-8 hours
- Cl_{cr} <10 mL/minute: Administer every 8 hours

Hemodialysis: Moderately dialyzable (20% to 50%)

Dosing adjustment in hepatic impairment: Reduce dose by 50%

Administration Administer around-the-clock rather than 4 times/day, 3 times/day, etc, (ie, 12-6-12-6, not 9-1-5-9) to promote less variation in peak and trough serum levels; administer I.M. injections in large muscle mass, not more than 2 g/injection. I.M. injections given over 12-15 seconds will be less painful

Test Interactions False-positive direct Coombs'; false-positive urinary protein

Nursing Implications Dosage modification is required in patients with impaired renal function

Additional Information Sodium content of 1 g: 42.6 mg (1.85 mEq)

Dosage Forms Powder for injection, as sodium: 1 g, 2 g, 3 g, 4 g, 20 g

Mezlocillin Sodium *see* Mezlocillin *on previous page*

Miacalcin® Injection *see* Calcitonin *on page 181*

Miacalcin® Nasal Spray *see* Calcitonin *on page 181*

Micatin® Topical [OTC] *see* Miconazole *on this page*

Miconazole (mi KON a zole)

Related Information

Antifungal Agents *on page 1395*

Treatment of Sexually Transmitted Diseases *on page 1485*

Brand Names Absorbine® Antifungal Foot Powder [OTC]; Breezee® Mist Antifungal [OTC]; Femizol-M® [OTC]; Fungoid® Creme; Fungoid® Tincture; Lotrimin® AF Powder [OTC]; Lotrimin® AF Spray Liquid [OTC]; Lotrimin® AF Spray Powder [OTC]; Maximum Strength Desenex® Antifungal Cream [OTC]; Micatin® Topical [OTC]; Monistat-Derm™ Topical; Monistat i.v.™ Injection; Monistat™ Vaginal;

Ony-Clear® Spray; Prescription Strength Desenex® [OTC]; Zeasorb-AF® Powder [OTC]

Canadian/Mexican Brand Names Aloid® (Mexico); Daktarin® (Mexico); Dermifun® (Mexico); Fungiquim® (Mexico); Gyno-Daktarin® (Mexico); Gyno-Daktarin® V (Mexico); Neomicol® (Mexico)

Synonyms Miconazole Nitrate

Therapeutic Category Antifungal Agent, Systemic; Antifungal Agent, Topical; Antifungal Agent, Vaginal

Use

I.V.: Treatment of severe systemic fungal infections and fungal meningitis that are refractory to standard treatment

Topical: Treatment of vulvovaginal candidiasis and a variety of skin and mucous membrane fungal infections

Pregnancy Risk Factor C

Contraindications Hypersensitivity to miconazole, fluconazole, ketoconazole, or polyoxyl 35 castor oil or any component

Warnings/Precautions Administer I.V. with caution to patients with hepatic insufficiency; the safety of miconazole in patients <1 year of age has not been established; cardiorespiratory and anaphylaxis have occurred with excessively rapid administration

Adverse Reactions

>10%:

- Central nervous system: Fever, chills
- Dermatologic: Rash, itching
- Gastrointestinal: Anorexia, diarrhea, nausea, vomiting
- Local: Pain at injection site

1% to 10%: Hematologic: Anemia, thrombocytopenia

<1%:

- Cardiovascular: Flushing of face or skin
- Central nervous system: Drowsiness

Overdosage/Toxicology Symptoms of overdose include nausea, vomiting, drowsiness; following GI decontamination, supportive care only

Drug Interactions Warfarin (increased anticoagulant effect), oral sulfonylureas, amphotericin B (decreased antifungal effect of both agents), phenytoin (levels may be increased)

Stability Protect from heat; darkening of solution indicates deterioration; stability of parenteral admixture at room temperature (25°C): 2 days

Mechanism of Action Inhibits biosynthesis of ergosterol, damaging the fungal cell wall membrane, which increases permeability causing leaking of nutrients

Pharmacodynamics/Kinetics

Protein binding: 91% to 93%

Metabolism: In the liver

Half-life, multiphasic:

- Initial: 40 minutes
- Secondary: 126 minutes
- Terminal phase: 24 hours

Elimination: ~50% excreted in feces and <1% in urine as unchanged drug

Usual Dosage

Children:

- I.V.: 20-40 mg/kg/day divided every 8 hours
- Topical: Apply twice daily for up to 1 month

Adults:

- Topical: Apply twice daily for up to 1 month
- I.T.: 20 mg every 1-2 days
- I.V.: Initial: 200 mg, then 1.2-3.6 g/day divided every 8 hours for up to 20 weeks
- Bladder candidal infections: 200 mg diluted solution instilled in the bladder
- Vaginal: Insert contents of 1 applicator of vaginal cream (100 mg) or 100 mg suppository at bedtime for 7 days, or 200 mg suppository at bedtime for 3 days

Hemodialysis: Not dialyzable (0% to 5%)

Administration Administer I.V. dose over 2 hours; administer around-the-clock to promote less variation in peak and trough serum levels

Test Interactions ↑ protein

Patient Information Avoid contact with the eyes; for vaginal product, insert high into vagina and complete full course of therapy; notify physician if itching or burning occur; refrain from intercourse to prevent reinfection

Additional Information

Miconazole: Monistat i.v.™

Miconazole nitrate: Micatin®, Monistat™, Monistat-Derm™

Dosage Forms

Cream:

- Topical, as nitrate: 2% (15 g, 30 g, 56.7 g, 85 g)

(Continued)

Miconazole *(Continued)*

Vaginal, as nitrate: 2% (45 g is equivalent to 7 doses)
Injection: 1% [10 mg/mL] (20 mL)
Lotion, as nitrate: 2% (30 mL, 60 mL)
Powder, topical: 2% (45 g, 90 g, 113 g)
Spray, topical: 2% (105 mL)
Suppository, vaginal, as nitrate: 100 mg (7s); 200 mg (3s)
Tincture: 2% with alcohol (7.39 mL, 29.57 mL)

Miconazole Nitrate *see* Miconazole *on page 834*

MICRhoGAM™ *see* Rh_0(D) Immune Globulin *on page 1101*

Microfibrillar Collagen Hemostat

(mye kro FI bri lar KOL la jen HEE moe stat)

Brand Names Avitene®; Helistat®; Hemotene®

Synonyms Collagen; MCH

Therapeutic Category Hemostatic Agent

Use Adjunct to hemostasis when control of bleeding by ligature is ineffective or impractical

Pregnancy Risk Factor C

Contraindications Closure of skin incisions, contaminated wounds

Warnings/Precautions Fragments of MCH may pass through filters of blood scavenging systems, avoid reintroduction of blood from operative sites treated with MCH; after several minutes remove excess material

Adverse Reactions 1% to 10%: Miscellaneous: Potentiation of infection, allergic reaction, adhesion formation

Mechanism of Action Microfibrillar collagen hemostat is an absorbable topical hemostatic agent prepared from purified bovine corium collagen and shredded into fibrils. Physically, microfibrillar collagen hemostat yields a large surface area. Chemically, it is collagen with hydrochloric acid noncovalently bound to some of the available amino groups in the collagen molecules. When in contact with a bleeding surface, microfibrillar collagen hemostat attracts platelets which adhere to its fibrils and undergo the release phenomenon. This triggers aggregation of the platelets into thrombi in the interstices of the fibrous mass, initiating the formation of a physiologic platelet plug.

Pharmacodynamics/Kinetics Absorption: By animal tissue in 3 months

Usual Dosage Apply dry directly to source of bleeding

Dosage Forms

Fibrous: 1 g, 5 g
Nonwoven web: 70 mm x 70 mm x 1 mm; 70 mm x 35 mm x 1 mm
Sponge: 1" x 2" (10s); 3" x 4" (10s); 9" x 10" (5s)

Micro-K® 10 *see* Potassium Chloride *on page 1024*

Micro-K® Extencaps® *see* Potassium Chloride *on page 1024*

Micro-K® LS® *see* Potassium Chloride *on page 1024*

Micronase® *see* Glyburide *on page 578*

microNefrin® *see* Epinephrine *on page 448*

Microsulfon® *see* Sulfadiazine *on page 1173*

Microzide® *see* Hydrochlorothiazide *on page 617*

Midamor® *see* Amiloride *on page 62*

Midazolam (MID aye zoe lam)

Related Information

Adult ACLS Algorithm, Electrical Conversion *on page 1515*
Benzodiazepines Comparison *on page 1397*

Brand Names Versed®

Canadian/Mexican Brand Names Dormicum® (Mexico)

Synonyms Midazolam Hydrochloride

Therapeutic Category Benzodiazepine; Hypnotic; Sedative

Use Preoperative sedation and provides conscious sedation prior to diagnostic or radiographic procedures

Restrictions C-IV

Pregnancy Risk Factor D

Contraindications Hypersensitivity to midazolam or any component (cross-sensitivity with other benzodiazepines may occur); uncontrolled pain; existing CNS depression; shock; narrow-angle glaucoma

Warnings/Precautions Use with caution in patients with congestive heart failure, renal impairment, pulmonary disease, hepatic dysfunction, the elderly, and those receiving concomitant narcotics; midazolam may cause respiratory depression/arrest; deaths and hypoxic encephalopathy have resulted when these were not promptly recognized and treated appropriately

Adverse Reactions

>10%:

Local: Pain and local reactions at injection site (severity less than diazepam)
Miscellaneous: Hiccups

1% to 10%:

Cardiovascular: Cardiac arrest, hypotension, bradycardia
Central nervous system: Drowsiness, ataxia, amnesia, dizziness, paradoxical excitement, sedation, headache
Gastrointestinal: Nausea, vomiting
Ocular: Blurred vision, diplopia
Respiratory: Respiratory depression, apnea, laryngospasm, bronchospasm
Miscellaneous: Physical and psychological dependence with prolonged use

<1%:

Cardiovascular: Tachycardia
Central nervous system: Delirium
Dermatologic: Rash
Respiratory: Wheezing

Overdosage/Toxicology Symptoms of overdose include respiratory depression, hypotension, coma, stupor, confusion, apnea

Treatment for benzodiazepine overdose is supportive. Rarely is mechanical ventilation required. Flumazenil has been shown to selectively block the binding of benzodiazepines to CNS receptors, resulting in a reversal of benzodiazepine-induced CNS depression; respiratory reaction to hypoxia may not be restored.

Drug Interactions Cytochrome P-450 3A enzyme substrate

Decreased effect: Theophylline may antagonize the sedative effects of midazolam

Increased toxicity: CNS depressants, may increase sedation and respiratory depression; doses of anesthetic agents should be reduced when used in conjunction with midazolam; cimetidine may increase midazolam serum concentrations

If narcotics or other CNS depressants are administered concomitantly, the midazolam dose should be reduced by 30%, if <65 years of age or by at least 50%, if >65 years of age.

Stability Stable for 24 hours at room temperature/refrigeration; admixtures do not require protection from light for short-term storage; **compatible** with NS, D_5W

Standardized dose for continuous infusion: 100 mg/250 mL D_5W or NS; maximum concentration: 0.5 mg/mL

Mechanism of Action Depresses all levels of the CNS, including the limbic and reticular formation, probably through the increased action of gamma-aminobutyric acid (GABA), which is a major inhibitory neurotransmitter in the brain

Pharmacodynamics/Kinetics

I.M.:

Onset of sedation: Within 15 minutes
Peak effect: 0.5-1 hour
Duration: 2 hours mean, up to 6 hours

I.V.: Onset of action: Within 1-5 minutes
Absorption: Oral: Rapid
Distribution: V_d: 0.8-2.5 L/kg; increased with congestive heart failure (CHF) and chronic renal failure
Protein binding: 95%
Metabolism: Extensively in the liver (microsomally)
Bioavailability: 45% mean
Half-life, elimination: 1-4 hours, increased with cirrhosis, CHF, obesity, elderly
Elimination: As glucuronide conjugated metabolites in urine, ~2% to 10% excreted in feces

Usual Dosage The dose of midazolam needs to be individualized based on the patient's age, underlying diseases, and concurrent medications. Decrease dose (by ~30%) if narcotics or other CNS depressants are administered concomitantly. **Personnel and equipment needed for standard respiratory resuscitation should be immediately available during midazolam administration.**

Neonates: Conscious sedation during mechanical ventilation: I.V. continuous infusion: 0.15-1 mcg/kg/minute. Use smallest dose possible; use lower doses (up to 0.5 mcg/kg/minute) for preterm neonates

Infants <2 months and Children: Status epilepticus refractory to standard therapy: I.V.: Loading dose: 0.15 mg/kg followed by a continuous infusion of 1 mcg/kg/minute; titrate dose upward very 5 minutes until clinical seizure activity is controlled; mean infusion rate required in 24 children was 2.3 mcg/kg/minute with a range of 1-18 mcg/kg/minute

Children:

Preoperative sedation:

I.M.: 0.07-0.08 mg/kg 30-60 minutes presurgery

(Continued)

Midazolam *(Continued)*

I.V.: 0.035 mg/kg/dose, repeat over several minutes as required to achieve the desired sedative effect up to a total dose of 0.1-0.2 mg/kg

Conscious sedation during mechanical ventilation: I.V.: Loading dose: 0.05-0.2 mg/kg then follow with initial continuous infusion: 1-2 mcg/kg/minute; titrate to the desired effect; usual range: 0.4-6 mcg/kg/minute

Conscious sedation for procedures:

Oral, Intranasal: 0.2-0.4 mg/kg (maximum: 15 mg) 30-45 minutes before the procedure

I.V.: 0.05 mg/kg 3 minutes before procedure

Adolescents >12 years: I.V.: 0.5 mg every 3-4 minutes until effect achieved

Adults:

Preoperative sedation: I.M.: 0.07-0.08 mg/kg 30-60 minutes presurgery; usual dose: 5 mg

Conscious sedation: I.V.: Initial: 0.5-2 mg slow I.V. over at least 2 minutes; slowly titrate to effect by repeating doses every 2-3 minutes if needed; usual total dose: 2.5-5 mg; use decreased doses in elderly

Healthy Adults <60 years: Some patients respond to doses as low as 1 mg; no more than 2.5 mg should be administered over a period of 2 minutes. Additional doses of midazolam may be administered after a 2-minute waiting period and evaluation of sedation after each dose increment. A total dose >5 mg is generally not needed. If narcotics or other CNS depressants are administered concomitantly, the midazolam dose should be reduced by 30%.

Elderly: I.V.: Conscious sedation: Initial: 0.5 mg slow I.V.; give no more than 1.5 mg in a 2-minute period; if additional titration is needed, give no more than 1 mg over 2 minutes, waiting another 2 or more minutes to evaluate sedative effect; a total dose of >3.5 mg is rarely necessary

Sedation in mechanically intubated patients: I.V. continuous infusion: 100 mg in 250 mL D_5W or NS, (if patient is fluid-restricted, may concentrate up to a maximum of 0.5 mg/mL); initial dose: 1 mg/hour; titrate to reach desired level of sedation

Hemodialysis: Supplemental dose is not necessary

Peritoneal dialysis: Significant drug removal is unlikely based on physiochemical characteristics

Monitoring Parameters Respiratory and cardiovascular status, blood pressure, blood pressure monitor required during I.V. administration

Nursing Implications Midazolam is a short-acting benzodiazepine; recovery occurs within 2 hours in most patients, however, may require up to 6 hours in some cases

Additional Information Sodium content of 1 mL: 0.14 mEq

Dosage Forms Injection, as hydrochloride: 1 mg/mL (2 mL, 5 mL, 10 mL); 5 mg/mL (1 mL, 2 mL, 5 mL, 10 mL)

Extemporaneous Preparations A 2.5 mg/mL oral solution of injectable midazolam in a flavored, dye-free syrup (Syrpalata®) was stable for 56 days at 7°C, 20°C, or 40°C; the oral solution was made by combining the 5 mg/mL injection in a 1:1 ratio with the syrup (Steedman 1992)

Both 2.5 mg/mL and 3 mg/mL oral solutions of injectable midazolam in simple syrup, NF (with peppermint oil for flavoring) were stable for 14 days in amber bottles at room temperature; the 2.5 mg/mL solution was made by adding 15 mL of the 5 mg/mL injection to 14.5 mL of simple syrup, NF and 0.5 mL of peppermint oil; the 3 mg/mL solution was made by adding 18 mL of the 5 mg/mL injection to 11.4 mL of simple syrup, NF and 0.6 mL of peppermint oil (Gregory, 1993)

A liquid gelatin solution of midazolam 1 mg/mL was stable when stored for 14 days at 4°C and for 28 days at -20°C (Bhatt-Mehta, 1993)

Bhatt-Mehta V, Johnson CE, Kostoff L, et al, "Stability of Midazolam Hydrochloride in Extemporaneously Prepared Flavored Gelatin," *Am J Hosp Pharm*, 1993, 50:472-5.

Gregory DF, Koestner JA, and Tobias JD, "Stability of Midazolam Prepared for Oral Administration," *South Med J*, 1993, 86(7):771-6.

Steedman SL, Koonce JR, Wynn JE, et al, "Stability of Midazolam Hydrochloride in a Flavored Dye-Free Oral Solution," *Am J Hosp Pharm*, 1992, 49(3):615-8.

Midazolam Hydrochloride *see* Midazolam *on page 836*

Midodrine (MI doe dreen)

Brand Names ProAmatine™

Synonyms Midodrine Hydrochloride

Therapeutic Category Alpha-Adrenergic Agonist

Use Treatment of symptomatic orthostatic hypotension; investigationally used in managing urinary incontinence

Pregnancy Risk Factor C

Pregnancy/Breast-Feeding Implications No studies are available; use during pregnancy and lactation should be avoided unless the potential benefit outweighs the risk to the fetus

Contraindications Severe organic heart disease, urinary retention, pheochromocytoma, thyrotoxicosis, persistent and significant supine hypertension; hypersensitivity to midodrine or any component; concurrent use of fludrocortisone

Warnings/Precautions Only indicated for patients for whom orthostatic hypotension significantly impairs their daily life. Use is not recommended with supine hypertension and caution should be exercised in patients with diabetes, visual problems, urinary retention (reduce initial dose) or hepatic dysfunction; monitor renal and hepatic function prior to and periodically during therapy; safety and efficacy has not been established in children; discontinue and re-evaluate therapy if signs of bradycardia occur.

Adverse Reactions

>10%:
- Dermatologic: Piloerection, pruritus
- Genitourinary: Urinary urgency, retention, or polyuria
- Neuromuscular & skeletal: Paresthesia

1% to 10%:
- Cardiovascular: Supine hypertension, facial flushing
- Central nervous system: Confusion, anxiety, dizziness, chills
- Dermatologic: Rash, dry skin
- Gastrointestinal: Xerostomia, nausea, abdominal pain
- Genitourinary: Dysuria
- Neuromuscular & skeletal: Pain

<1%:
- Cardiovascular: Flushing
- Central nervous system: Headache, insomnia
- Gastrointestinal: Flatulence
- Neuromuscular & skeletal: Leg cramps
- Ocular: Visual changes

Overdosage/Toxicology Symptoms of overdose include hypertension, piloerection, urinary retention

Treatment is symptomatic following gastric decontamination; alpha-sympatholytics and/or dialysis may be helpful

Drug Interactions Increased effect: Concomitant fludrocortisone results in hypernatremia or an increase in intraocular pressure and glaucoma; bradycardia may be accentuated with concomitant administration of cardiac glycosides, psychotherapeutics, and beta-blockers; alpha-agonists may increase the pressure effects and alpha-antagonists may negate the effects of midodrine

Mechanism of Action Midodrine forms an active metabolite, desglymidodrine, that is an $alpha_1$-agonist. This agent increases arteriolar and venous tone resulting in a rise in standing, sitting, and supine systolic and diastolic blood pressure in patients with orthostatic hypotension.

Pharmacodynamics/Kinetics
- Absorption: Rapid
- Distribution: V_d (desglymidodrine): <1.6 L/kg; poorly distributed across membrane (eg, blood brain barrier)
- Protein binding: Minimal
- Metabolism: Rapid deglycination to desglymidodrine occurs in many tissues and plasma; further metabolism in the liver
- Bioavailability: Absolute, 93%
- Half-life: ~3-4 hours (active drug); 25 minutes (prodrug)
- Time to peak serum concentration: 1-2 hours (active drug); 30 minutes (prodrug)
- Elimination: Renal, minimal (2% to 4%); clearance of desglymidodrine: 385 mL/minute (predominantly by renal secretion)

Usual Dosage Adults: Oral: 10 mg 3 times/day during daytime hours (every 3-4 hours) when patient is upright (maximum: 40 mg/day)

Dosing adjustment in renal impairment: 2.5 mg 3 times/day, gradually increasing as tolerated

Monitoring Parameters Blood pressure, renal and hepatic parameters

Patient Information Use caution with over-the-counter medications which may affect blood pressure (cough and cold, diet, stay-awake medications); avoid taking a particular dose if you are to be supine for any length of time; take your last daily dose 3-4 hours before bedtime to minimize nighttime supine hypertension

Nursing Implications Doses may be given in approximately 3- to 4-hour intervals (eg, shortly before or upon rising in the morning, at midday, in the late

(Continued)

Midodrine *(Continued)*

afternoon not later than 6 PM); avoid dosing after the evening meal or within 4 hours of bedtime; continue therapy only in patients who appear to attain symptomatic improvement during initial treatment; standing systolic blood pressure may be elevated 15-30 mm Hg at 1 hour after a 10 mg dose; some effect may persist for 2-3 hours

Dosage Forms Tablet, as hydrochloride: 2.5 mg, 5 mg

Midodrine Hydrochloride *see* Midodrine *on page 838*
Midol® 200 [OTC] *see* Ibuprofen *on page 639*
Miles Nervine® Caplets [OTC] *see* Diphenhydramine *on page 399*
Milkinol® [OTC] *see* Mineral Oil *on next page*
Milk of Magnesia *see* Magnesium Hydroxide *on page 753*
Milophene® *see* Clomiphene *on page 295*

Milrinone (MIL ri none)

Related Information

Adrenergic Agonists, Cardiovascular Comparison *on page 1385*
Cardiovascular Agents Comparison *on page 1405*

Brand Names Primacor®

Synonyms Milrinone Lactate

Therapeutic Category Phosphodiesterase Enzyme Inhibitor

Use Short-term I.V. therapy of congestive heart failure; used for calcium antagonist intoxication

Pregnancy Risk Factor C

Contraindications Hypersensitivity to drug or amrinone

Warnings/Precautions Severe obstructive aortic or pulmonic valvular disease, history of ventricular arrhythmias; atrial fibrillation, flutter; renal dysfunction

Adverse Reactions

>10%: Cardiovascular: Ventricular arrhythmias

1% to 10%:
- Cardiovascular: Supraventricular arrhythmias, hypotension, angina, chest pain
- Central nervous system: Headache

<1%:
- Cardiovascular: Ventricular fibrillation
- Endocrine & metabolic: Hypokalemia
- Hematologic: Thrombocytopenia
- Neuromuscular & skeletal: Tremor

Overdosage/Toxicology Hypotension should respond to I.V. fluids and Trendelenburg position; use of vasopressors may be required

Stability Colorless to pale yellow solution; store at room temperature and protect from light; stable at 0.2 mg/mL in 0.9% sodium chloride or D_5W for 72 hours at room temperature in normal light

Incompatible with furosemide and procainamide; **compatible** with atropine, calcium chloride, digoxin, epinephrine, lidocaine, morphine, propranolol, and sodium bicarbonate

Standardized dose: 20 mg in 80 mL of 0.9% sodium chloride or D_5W (0.2 mg/mL)

Mechanism of Action Phosphodiesterase inhibitor resulting in vasodilation

Pharmacodynamics/Kinetics

Serum level: I.V.: Following a 125 mcg/kg dose, peak plasma concentrations of ~1000 ng/mL were observed at 2 minutes postinjection, decreasing to <100 ng/mL in 2 hours

Therapeutic effect: Oral: Following doses of 7.5-15 mg, peak hemodynamic effects occurred at 90 minutes

Drug concentration levels:
- Therapeutic:
  - Serum levels of 166 ng/mL, achieved during I.V. infusions of 0.25-1 mcg/kg/minute, were associated with sustained hemodynamic benefit in severe congestive heart failure patients over a 24-hour period
  - Maximum beneficial effects on cardiac output and pulmonary capillary wedge pressure following I.V. infusion have been associated with plasma milrinone concentrations of 150-250 ng/mL
- Toxic: Serum concentrations >250-300 ng/mL have been associated with marked reductions in mean arterial pressure and tachycardia; however, more studies are required to determine the toxic serum levels for milrinone

Distribution: Not known if distributed into breast milk
- V_d at steady-state following I.V. administration as a single bolus: 0.32 L/kg; not significantly bound to tissues
- In patients with severe congestive heart failure (CHF), V_d has been 0.33-0.47 L/kg

Protein binding: ~70% in plasma

Metabolism: 12% hepatic

Half-life, elimination: I.V.: 136 minutes in patients with CHF; patients with severe CHF have a more prolonged half-life, with values ranging from 1.7-2.7 hours. Patients with CHF have a reduction in the systemic clearance of milrinone, resulting in a prolonged elimination half-life. Alternatively, one study reported that 1 month of therapy with milrinone did not change the pharmacokinetic parameters for patients with CHF despite improvement in cardiac function.

Elimination: Following I.V. administration, 85% of dose excreted unchanged in urine within 24 hours; active tubular secretion is a major elimination pathway for milrinone; bolus doses of I.V. milrinone produced systemic clearance values of 25.9±5.7 L/hour (0.37 L/hour/kg); however, in patients with severe congestive heart failure, the clearance is reduced to 0.11-0.13 L/hour/kg. The reduction in clearance may be a result of reduced renal function. Creatinine clearance values were ½ those reported for healthy adults in patients with severe congestive heart failure (52 vs 119 mL/minute).

Usual Dosage Adults: I.V.: Loading dose: 50 mcg/kg administered over 10 minutes followed by a maintenance dose titrated according to the hemodynamic and clinical response, see table.

Maintenance Dosage	Dose Rate (mcg/kg/min)	Total Dose (mg/kg/24 h)
Minimum	0.375	0.59
Standard	0.500	0.77
Maximum	0.750	1.13

Dosing adjustment in renal impairment:

Cl_{cr} 50 mL/minute/1.73 m^2: Administer 0.43 mcg/kg/minute

Cl_{cr} 40 mL/minute/1.73 m^2: Administer 0.38 mcg/kg/minute

Cl_{cr} 30 mL/minute/1.73 m^2: Administer 0.33 mcg/kg/minute

Cl_{cr} 20 mL/minute/1.73 m^2: Administer 0.28 mcg/kg/minute

Cl_{cr} 10 mL/minute/1.73 m^2: Administer 0.23 mcg/kg/minute

Cl_{cr} 5 mL/minute/1.73 m^2: Administer 0.2 mcg/kg/minute

Monitoring Parameters Cardiac monitor and blood pressure monitor required; serum potassium

Therapeutic: Patients should be monitored for improvement in the clinical signs and symptoms of congestive heart failure

Toxic: Patients should be monitored for ventricular arrhythmias and exacerbation of anginal symptoms; during I.V. therapy with milrinone, blood pressure and heart rate should be monitored

Nursing Implications Monitor closely, titrate to blood pressure cardiac index

Dosage Forms Injection, as lactate: 1 mg/mL (5 mL, 10 mL, 20 mL)

Milrinone Lactate *see* Milrinone *on previous page*

Miltown® *see* Meprobamate *on page 783*

Mineral Oil (MIN er al oyl)

Related Information

Laxatives, Classification and Properties *on page 1412*

Brand Names Agoral® Plain [OTC]; Fleet® Mineral Oil Enema [OTC]; Kondremul® [OTC]; Milkinol® [OTC]; Neo-Cultol® [OTC]; Zymenol® [OTC]

Canadian/Mexican Brand Names Lansoyl®, also sugar-free (Canada)

Synonyms Heavy Mineral Oil; Liquid Paraffin; White Mineral Oil

Therapeutic Category Laxative, Lubricant

Use Temporary relief of constipation, to relieve fecal impaction, preparation for bowel studies or surgery

Pregnancy Risk Factor C

Contraindications Patients with colostomy or an ileostomy, appendicitis, ulcerative colitis, diverticulitis

Warnings/Precautions Oral form should be avoided in children <4 years of age; do not administer with food or meals because of the risk of aspiration; prolonged administration of mineral oil may decrease absorption of lipid-soluble vitamins A, D, E, and K.

Adverse Reactions

1% to 10%:

- Gastrointestinal: Nausea, vomiting, diarrhea, abdominal cramps, anal itching
- Respiratory: Lipid pneumonitis with aspiration

Overdosage/Toxicology Aspiration of oils may cause chemical pneumonitis with fever, leukocytosis, x-ray changes

Drug Interactions

Decreased effect of docusate

May impair absorption of fat-soluble vitamins (A,D,K), oral contraceptives, coumarin, sulfonamides

(Continued)

Mineral Oil *(Continued)*

Mechanism of Action Eases passage of stool by decreasing water absorption and lubricating the intestine

Pharmacodynamics/Kinetics

Onset of action: ~6-8 hours

Metabolism: Site of action is the colon

Elimination: In feces

Usual Dosage

Children:

Oral: 5-11 years: 5-20 mL once daily or in divided doses

Rectal: 2-11 years: 30-60 mL as a single dose

Children >12 years and Adults:

Oral: 15-45 mL/day once daily or in divided doses

Rectal: Retention enema, contents of one enema (range 60-150 mL)/day as a single dose

Administration Administer on an empty stomach

Patient Information Do not take with food or meals; do not use if experiencing abdominal pain, nausea, or vomiting; avoid use of stool softeners at the same time

Dosage Forms

Emulsion, oral: 1.4 g/5 mL (480 mL); 2.5 mL/5 mL (420 mL); 2.75 mL/5 mL (480 mL); 4.75 mL/5 mL (240 mL)

Jelly, oral: 2.75 mL/5 mL (180 mL)

Liquid:

Oral: 30 mL, 180 mL, 500 mL, 1000 mL, 4000 mL

Rectal: 133 mL

Minidyne® [OTC] *see* Povidone-Iodine *on page 1031*

Mini-Gamulin® Rh *see* Rh_0(D) Immune Globulin *on page 1101*

Minipress® *see* Prazosin *on page 1036*

Minitran® *see* Nitroglycerin *on page 909*

Minocin® IV Injection *see* Minocycline *on this page*

Minocin® Oral *see* Minocycline *on this page*

Minocycline (mi noe SYE kleen)

Related Information

Antimicrobial Drugs of Choice *on page 1468*

Brand Names Dynacin® Oral; Minocin® IV Injection; Minocin® Oral

Canadian/Mexican Brand Names Apo-Minocycline® (Canada); Syn-Minocycline® (Canada)

Synonyms Minocycline Hydrochloride

Therapeutic Category Antibiotic, Tetracycline Derivative

Use Treatment of susceptible bacterial infections of both gram-negative and gram-positive organisms; acne, meningococcal carrier state

Pregnancy Risk Factor D

Contraindications Hypersensitivity to minocycline, other tetracyclines, or any component; children <8 years of age

Warnings/Precautions Should be avoided in renal insufficiency, children ≤8 years of age, pregnant and nursing women; photosensitivity reactions can occur with minocycline

Adverse Reactions

>10%: Miscellaneous: Discoloration of teeth in children

1% to 10%:

Dermatologic: Photosensitivity

Gastrointestinal: Nausea, diarrhea

<1%:

Cardiovascular: Pericarditis

Central nervous system: Increased intracranial pressure, bulging fontanels in infants

Dermatologic: Dermatologic effects, pruritus, exfoliative dermatitis, rash, pigmentation of nails

Endocrine & metabolic: Diabetes insipidus syndrome

Gastrointestinal: Vomiting, esophagitis, anorexia, abdominal cramps

Neuromuscular & skeletal: Paresthesia

Renal: Acute renal failure, azotemia

Miscellaneous: Superinfections, anaphylaxis

Overdosage/Toxicology Symptoms of overdose include diabetes insipidus, nausea, anorexia, diarrhea; following GI decontamination, supportive care only; fluid support may be required

Drug Interactions

Decreased effect with antacids (aluminum, calcium, zinc, or magnesium), bismuth salts, sodium bicarbonate, barbiturates, carbamazepine, hydantoins; decreased effect of oral contraceptives

Increased effect of warfarin

Mechanism of Action Inhibits bacterial protein synthesis by binding with the 30S and possibly the 50S ribosomal subunit(s) of susceptible bacteria; cell wall synthesis is not affected

Pharmacodynamics/Kinetics

Absorption: Well absorbed

Distribution: Crosses placenta; appears in breast milk; majority of a dose deposits for extended periods in fat

Protein binding: 70% to 75%

Half-life: 15 hours

Elimination: Eventually cleared renally

Usual Dosage

Children >8 years: Oral, I.V.: Initial: 4 mg/kg followed by 2 mg/kg/dose every 12 hours

Adults:

Infection: Oral, I.V.: 200 mg stat, 100 mg every 12 hours not to exceed 400 mg/24 hours

Acne: Oral: 50 mg 1-3 times/day

Hemodialysis: Not dialyzable (0% to 5%)

Administration Infuse I.V. minocycline over 1 hour

Patient Information Avoid unnecessary exposure to sunlight; finish all medication; do not skip doses

Dosage Forms

Capsule, as hydrochloride: 50 mg, 100 mg

Capsule, as hydrochloride (Dynacin®): 50 mg, 100 mg

Capsule, pellet-filled, as hydrochloride (Minocin®): 50 mg, 100 mg

Injection, as hydrochloride (Minocin® IV): 100 mg

Suspension, oral, as hydrochloride (Minocin®)50 mg/5 mL (60 mL)

Minocycline Hydrochloride *see* Minocycline *on previous page*

Minodyl® *see* Minoxidil *on this page*

Minoxidil (mi NOKS i dil)

Related Information

Therapy of Hypertension *on page 1540*

Brand Names Loniten®; Minodyl®; Rogaine® for Men [OTC]; Rogaine® for Women [OTC]

Canadian/Mexican Brand Names Apo-Gain® (Canada); Gen-Minoxidil® (Canada); Regaine® (Mexico)

Therapeutic Category Antihypertensive; Vasodilator

Use Management of severe hypertension (usually in combination with a diuretic and beta-blocker); treatment of male pattern baldness (alopecia androgenetica)

Pregnancy Risk Factor C

Contraindications Pheochromocytoma, hypersensitivity to minoxidil or any component

Warnings/Precautions Use with caution in patients with pulmonary hypertension, significant renal failure, or congestive heart failure; use with caution in patients with coronary artery disease or recent myocardial infarction; renal failure or dialysis patients may require smaller doses; usually used with a beta-blocker (to treat minoxidil-induced tachycardia) and a diuretic (for treatment of water retention/edema); may take 1-6 months for hypertrichosis to totally reverse after minoxidil therapy is discontinued.

Adverse Reactions

>10%:

Cardiovascular: EKG changes, tachycardia, congestive heart failure, edema

Dermatologic: Hypertrichosis (commonly occurs within 1-2 months of therapy)

1% to 10%: Endocrine & metabolic: Fluid and electrolyte imbalance

<1%:

Cardiovascular: Angina, pericardial effusion tamponade

Central nervous system: Dizziness

Endocrine & metabolic: Breast tenderness

Dermatologic: Rashes, headache, coarsening facial features, dermatologic reactions, Stevens-Johnson syndrome, sunburn

Gastrointestinal: Weight gain

Hematologic: Thrombocytopenia, leukopenia

Overdosage/Toxicology Symptoms of overdose include hypotension, tachycardia, headache, nausea, dizziness, weakness syncope, warm flushed skin and palpitations; lethargy and ataxia may occur in children

(Continued)

Minoxidil *(Continued)*

Hypotension usually responds to I.V. fluids, Trendelenburg positioning or vasoconstrictor; treatment is primarily supportive and symptomatic

Drug Interactions Increased toxicity:

Concurrent administration with guanethidine may cause profound orthostatic hypotensive effects

Additive hypotensive effects with other hypotensive agents or diuretics

Mechanism of Action Produces vasodilation by directly relaxing arteriolar smooth muscle, with little effect on veins; effects may be mediated by cyclic AMP; stimulation of hair growth is secondary to vasodilation, increased cutaneous blood flow and stimulation of resting hair follicles

Pharmacodynamics/Kinetics

Onset of hypotensive effect: Oral: Within 30 minutes
Peak effect: Within 2-8 hours
Duration: Up to 2-5 days
Protein binding: None
Metabolism: 88% primarily via glucuronidation
Bioavailability: Oral: 90%
Half-life: Adults: 3.5-4.2 hours
Elimination: 12% excreted unchanged in urine

Usual Dosage

Children <12 years: Hypertension: Oral: Initial: 0.1-0.2 mg/kg once daily; maximum: 5 mg/day; increase gradually every 3 days; usual dosage: 0.25-1 mg/kg/day in 1-2 divided doses; maximum: 50 mg/day

Children >12 years and Adults:

Hypertension: Oral: Initial: 5 mg once daily, increase gradually every 3 days; usual dose: 10-40 mg/day in 1-2 divided doses; maximum: 100 mg/day

Alopecia: Topical: Apply twice daily; 4 months of therapy may be necessary for hair growth

Elderly: Initial: 2.5 mg once daily; increase gradually

Dialysis: Supplemental dose is not necessary via hemo- or peritoneal dialysis

Monitoring Parameters Blood pressure, standing and sitting/supine; fluid and electrolyte balance and body weight should be monitored

Patient Information Topical product must be used every day. Hair growth usually takes 4 months. Notify physician if any of the following occur: Heart rate ≥20 beats per minute over normal; rapid weight gain >5 lb (2 kg); unusual swelling of extremities, face, or abdomen; breathing difficulty, especially when lying down; rise slowly from prolonged lying or sitting; new or aggravated angina symptoms (chest, arm, or shoulder pain); severe indigestion; dizziness, lightheadedness, or fainting; nausea or vomiting may occur. Do not make up for missed doses.

Nursing Implications May cause hirsutism or hypertrichosis; observe for fluid retention and orthostatic hypotension

Dosage Forms

Solution, topical: 2% = 20 mg/metered dose (60 mL)
Tablet: 2.5 mg, 10 mg

Mintezol® *see* Thiabendazole *on page 1213*
Minute-Gel® *see* Fluoride *on page 536*
Miochol® *see* Acetylcholine *on page 27*
Miostat® Intraocular *see* Carbachol *on page 200*

Mirtazapine (mir TAZ a peen)

Brand Names Remeron®

Therapeutic Category Antidepressant, Tetracyclic

Use Treatment of depression

Contraindications Patients with a known hypersensitivity to mirtazapine, use during or within 14 days of monoamine oxidase inhibitor therapy

Warnings/Precautions Hepatic or renal dysfunction, predisposition to conditions that could be exacerbated by hypotension, history of mania or hypomania, seizure disorders, immunocompromized patients, the elderly, or during pregnancy or nursing

Adverse Reactions

>10%:

Central nervous system: Somnolence
Endocrine & metabolic: Increased cholesterol
Gastrointestinal: Constipation, xerostomia, increased appetite, weight gain

1% to 10%:

Cardiovascular: Hypertension, vasodilatation, peripheral edema, edema
Central nervous system: Dizziness, abnormal dreams, abnormal thoughts, confusion, malaise
Endocrine & metabolic: Increased triglycerides

Gastrointestinal: Vomiting, anorexia, eructation, glossitis, cholecystitis
Genitourinary: Polyuria
Neuromuscular & skeletal: Myalgia, back pain, arthralgia, tremor, weakness
Respiratory: Dyspnea
Miscellaneous: Flu-like symptoms, thirst

<1%:
Cardiovascular: Orthostatic hypotension
Central nervous system: Seizures (1 case reported)
Endocrine & metabolic: Dehydration
Gastrointestinal: Weight loss
Hematologic: Agranulocytosis, neutropenia, lymphadenopathy
Hepatic: Liver function test increases

Drug Interactions

Increased toxicity: Impairment of cognitive and motor skills are additive with those produced by alcohol, benzodiazepines, and other CNS depressants; possibly serious or fatal reactions can occur when given with or when given within 14 days of a monoamine oxidase inhibitor.

Mechanism of Action Mirtazapine is a tetracyclic antidepressant that works by its central presynaptic alpha$_2$-adrenergic antagonist effects, which results in increased release of norepinephrine and serotonin. It is also a potent antagonist of 5HT2 and 5HT3 serotonin receptors and H1 histamine receptors and a moderate peripheral alpha$_1$-adrenergic and muscarinic antagonist; it does not inhibit the reuptake of norepinephrine or serotonin.

Pharmacodynamics/Kinetics

Protein binding: 85%
Metabolism: Extensive by cytochrome P-450 enzymes in the liver
Bioavailability: 50%
Half-life: 20-40 hours
Time to peak serum concentration: 2 hours
Elimination: Extensive hepatic metabolism via demethylation and hydroxylation, metabolites eliminated primarily renally (75%) and some via the feces (15%); elimination is hampered with renal dysfunction or hepatic dysfunction.

Usual Dosage Adults: Oral: Initial: 15 mg nightly, titrate up to 15-45 mg/day with dose increases made no more frequently than every 1-2 weeks

Dietary Considerations Alcohol: Additive CNS effect, avoid use

Monitoring Parameters Patients should be monitored for signs of agranulocytosis or severe neutropenia such as sore throat, stomatitis or other signs of infection or a low WBC; monitor for improvement in clinical signs and symptoms of depression, improvement may be observed within 1-4 weeks after initiating therapy

Patient Information Be aware of the risk of developing agranulocytosis; contact physician if any indication of infection occurs (ie, fever, chills, sore throat, mucous membrane ulceration, and especially flu-like symptoms); may impair judgment, thinking, and particularly motor skills; may impair ability to drive, use machinery, or perform tasks that require you remain alert; avoid concurrent alcohol use

Dosage Forms Tablet: 15 mg, 30 mg

Miscellaneous Vaccination Information *see page 1437*

Misoprostol (mye soe PROST ole)

Brand Names Cytotec®

Therapeutic Category Prostaglandin

Use Prevention of NSAID-induced gastric ulcers

Pregnancy Risk Factor X

Contraindications Hypersensitivity to misoprostol or any component

Warnings/Precautions Safety and efficacy have not been established in children <18 years of age; use with caution in patients with renal impairment and the elderly; not to be used in pregnant women or women of childbearing potential unless woman is capable of complying with effective contraceptive measures; therapy is normally begun on the second or third day of next normal menstrual period

Adverse Reactions

>10%: Gastrointestinal: Diarrhea, abdominal pain

1% to 10%:
Central nervous system: Headache
Gastrointestinal: Constipation, flatulence

<1%:
Gastrointestinal: Nausea, vomiting
Genitourinary: Uterine stimulation, vaginal bleeding

Overdosage/Toxicology Symptoms of overdose include sedation, tremor, convulsions, dyspnea, abdominal pain, diarrhea, hypotension, bradycardia
(Continued)

Misoprostol *(Continued)*

Mechanism of Action Misoprostol is a synthetic prostaglandin E_1 analog that replaces the protective prostaglandins consumed with prostaglandin-inhibiting therapies eg, nonsteroidal anti-inflammatory drugs

Pharmacodynamics/Kinetics

Absorption: Oral: Rapid
Metabolism: Rapidly de-esterified to misoprostol acid
Half-life (parent and metabolite combined): 1.5 hours
Time to peak serum concentration (active metabolite): Within 15-30 minutes
Elimination: In urine (64% to 73% in 24 hours) and feces (15% in 24 hours)

Usual Dosage Adults: Oral: 200 mcg 4 times/day with food; if not tolerated, may decrease dose to 100 mcg 4 times/day with food or 200 mcg twice daily with food

Patient Information May cause diarrhea when first being used; take after meals and at bedtime; avoid taking with magnesium-containing antacids

Nursing Implications Incidence of diarrhea may be lessened by having patient take dose right after meals

Dosage Forms Tablet: 100 mcg, 200 mcg

Mithracin® *see* Plicamycin *on page 1011*

Mithramycin *see* Plicamycin *on page 1011*

Mitomycin (mye toe MYE sin)

Related Information

Antiemetics for Chemotherapy Induced Nausea and Vomiting *on page 1348*
Cancer Chemotherapy Regimens *on page 1351*
Extravasation Management of Chemotherapeutic Agents *on page 1379*
Toxicities of Chemotherapeutic Agents *on page 1382*

Brand Names Mutamycin®

Synonyms Mitomycin-C; MTC

Therapeutic Category Antineoplastic Agent, Antibiotic; Antineoplastic Agent, Vesicant; Vesicant

Use Therapy of disseminated adenocarcinoma of stomach or pancreas in combination with other approved chemotherapeutic agents; bladder cancer, colorectal cancer

Pregnancy Risk Factor C

Contraindications Platelet counts <75,000/mm³; leukocyte counts <3,000/mm³ or serum creatinine >1.7 mg/dL; thrombocytopenia, hypersensitivity to mitomycin or any component

Warnings/Precautions The U.S. Food and Drug Administration (FDA) currently recommends that procedures for proper handling and disposal of antineoplastic agents be considered. Use with caution in patients with impaired renal or hepatic function, myelosuppression. Follow hemoglobin, hematocrit, BUN, and creatinine closely after therapy especially after second and subsequent cycles. Bone marrow suppression, notably thrombocytopenia and leukopenia, may contribute to the development of a secondary infection; hemolytic uremic syndrome, a serious and often fatal syndrome, has occurred in patients receiving long-term therapy and is correlated with total dose and total duration of therapy; mitomycin is potentially carcinogenic and teratogenic.

Adverse Reactions

>10%:

Gastrointestinal: **Nausea and vomiting (mild to moderate) seen in almost 100% of patients**; usually begins 1-2 hours after treatment and persists for 3 hours to 4 days; other toxicities include stomatitis, hepatic toxicity, diarrhea, anorexia
Emetic potential: Moderate (30% to 60%)
Time course of nausea/vomiting: Onset: 1-2 hours; Duration: 48-72 hours

Local: Extravasation: May cause severe tissue irritation if infiltrated; can progress to cellulitis, ulceration, and sloughing of tissue. Refer to institutional policy for treatment.
Vesicant chemotherapy

Hematologic: Myelosuppressive: Dose-related toxicity and may be cumulative; related to both total dose (incidence higher at doses >50 mg) and schedule, may occur at anytime within 8 weeks of treatment.
WBC: Moderate
Platelets: Severe
Onset (days): 21
Nadir (days): 36
Recovery (days): 42-56

1% to 10%:

Dermatologic: Discolored fingernails (violet), alopecia
Gastrointestinal: Mouth ulcers
Neuromuscular & skeletal: Extremity paresthesia

Renal: Elevation of creatinine seen in 2% of patients; hemolytic uremic syndrome observed in <10% of patients and is dose-dependent (doses ≥60 mg or >50 mg/m² have higher risk)

Respiratory: Interstitial pneumonitis or pulmonary fibrosis have been noticed in 7% of patients, and it occurs independent of dosing. Manifested as dry cough and progressive dyspnea; usually is responsive to steroid therapy.

<1%:

Cardiovascular: Cardiac failure (in patients treated with doses >30 mg/m²)

Central nervous system: Malaise, fever

Dermatologic: Pruritus, rash

Gastrointestinal: Mouth ulcers

Hematologic: Bone marrow suppression (leukopenia, thrombocytopenia), microangiopathic hemolytic anemia

Local: Thrombophlebitis

Neuromuscular & skeletal: Paresthesia, weakness

Overdosage/Toxicology Symptoms of overdose include bone marrow suppression, nausea, vomiting, alopecia

Drug Interactions

Increased toxicity:

Vinca alkaloids → acute shortness of breath or bronchospasm

Doxorubicin may enhance cardiac toxicity

Stability Store intact vials of lyophilized powder at room temperature

Dilute powder with SWI to a concentration of 0.5 mg/mL as follows: Solution is stable for 7 days at room temperature and 14 days at refrigeration if protected from light

5 mg = 10 mL

20 mg = 40 mL

Further dilution in NS is stable for 24 hours at room temperature

Standard I.V. dilution:

I.V. push: Dose/syringe (concentration = 0.5 mg/mL)

Maximum syringe size for IVP is a 30 mL syringe and syringe should be ≤75% full

Syringe is stable for 7 days at room temperature and 14 days at refrigeration if protected from light

IVPB: Dose/100 mL NS; IVPB solution is stable for 24 hours at room temperature

Mechanism of Action Isolated from *Streptomyces caespitosus*; acts primarily as an alkylating agent and produces DNA cross-linking (primarily with guanine and cytosine pairs); cell-cycle nonspecific; inhibits DNA and RNA synthesis by alkylation and cross-linking the strands of DNA

Pharmacodynamics/Kinetics

Absorption: Fairly well from the GI tract

Distribution: V_d: 22 L/m²; high drug concentrations found in kidney, tongue, muscle, heart, and lung tissue; probably not distributed into the CNS

Metabolism: Hepatic

Half-life: 23-78 minutes

Terminal: 50 minutes

Elimination: Primarily in metabolism, followed by urinary excretion (<10% as unchanged drug) and to a small extent biliary excretion

Usual Dosage Refer to individual protocols

Children and Adults: I.V.:

Single agent therapy: 20 mg/m² every 6-8 weeks

Note: Doses >20 mg/m² have not been shown to be more effective, and are more toxic.

Combination therapy: 10 mg/m² every 6-8 weeks

Bone marrow transplant:

40-50 mg/m²

2-40 mg/m²/day for 3 days

Total cumulative dose should not exceed 50 mg/m²; see table.

Nadir After Prior Dose per mm³		% of Prior Dose to Be Given
Leukocytes	Platelets	
4000	>100,000	100
3000-3999	75,000-99,999	100
2000-2999	25,000-74,999	70
2000	<25,000	50

Dosing adjustment in renal impairment: Cl_{cr} <10 mL/minute: Administer 75% of normal dose

Hemodialysis: Unknown

CAPD effects: Unknown

(Continued)

Mitomycin *(Continued)*

CAVH effects: Unknown

Intravesicular instillations for bladder carcinoma: 20-40 mg/dose (1 mg/mL in sterile aqueous solution) instilled into the bladder for 3 hours repeated up to 3 times/week for up to 20 procedures per course

Administration

Administer slow I.V. push by **central-line only**

Avoid extravasation - severe local tissue necrosis occurs; flush with 5-10 mL of I.V. solution before and after drug administration; IVPB infusions should be closely monitored for adequate vein patency

Monitoring Parameters Platelet count, CBC with differential, hemoglobin, prothrombin time, renal and pulmonary function tests

Patient Information Any signs of infection, easy bruising or bleeding, shortness of breath, or painful or burning urination should be brought to physician's attention. Nausea, vomiting, or hair loss sometimes occur. The drug may cause permanent sterility and may cause birth defects. The drug may be excreted in breast milk, therefore, an alternative form of feeding your baby should be used.

Nursing Implications

Extravasation management:

Care should be taken to avoid extravasation. If extravasation occurs, the site should be observed closely; these injuries frequently cause necrosis; a plastic surgery consult may be required.

Few agents have been effective as antidotes, but there are reports in the literature of some benefit with dimethylsulfoxide (DMSO). Delayed dermal reactions with mitomycin are possible, even in patients who are asymptomatic at time of drug administration.

Dosage Forms Powder for injection: 5 mg, 20 mg, 40 mg

Mitomycin-C *see* Mitomycin *on page 846*

Mitotane (MYE toe tane)

Related Information

Toxicities of Chemotherapeutic Agents *on page 1382*

Brand Names Lysodren®

Synonyms o,p'-DDD

Therapeutic Category Antiadrenal Agent; Antineoplastic Agent, Miscellaneous

Use Treatment of inoperable adrenal cortical carcinoma

Pregnancy Risk Factor C

Contraindications Known hypersensitivity to mitotane

Warnings/Precautions The U.S. Food and Drug Administration (FDA) currently recommends that procedures for proper handling and disposal of antineoplastic agents be considered. Patients should be hospitalized when mitotane therapy is initiated until a stable dose regimen is established. Discontinue temporarily following trauma or shock since the prime action of mitotane is adrenal suppression; exogenous steroids may be indicated since adrenal function may not start immediately. Administer with care to patients with severe hepatic impairment; observe patients for neurotoxicity with prolonged (2 years) use.

Adverse Reactions

>10%:

Central nervous system: Vertigo, mental depression, dizziness; all are reversible with discontinuation of the drug and can occur in 15% to 26% of patients

Dermatologic: Rash (15%) which may subside without discontinuation of therapy, hyperpigmentation

Gastrointestinal: 75% to 80% will experience nausea, vomiting, and anorexia; diarrhea can occur in 20% of patients

Ocular: Diplopia, visual disturbances, blurred vision (reversible with discontinuation)

1% to 10%:

Cardiovascular: Orthostatic hypotension

Central nervous system: Fever

Endocrine & metabolic: Flushing of skin

Genitourinary: Hemorrhagic cystitis

Neuromuscular & skeletal: Myalgia

<1%:

Adrenal insufficiency: May develop and may require steroid replacement

Cardiovascular: Hypertension, flushing

Central nervous system: Lethargy, somnolence, mental depression, irritability, confusion, fatigue, headache, fever, hyperpyrexia

Dermatologic: Rash

Endocrine & metabolic: Hypercholesterolemia

Hematologic: Myelosuppressive: WBC: None; Platelets: None

Neuromuscular & skeletal: Tremor, weakness

Ocular: Lens opacities, toxic retinopathy
Renal: Hypouricemia, hematuria, albuminuria
Respiratory: Shortness of breath, wheezing

Overdosage/Toxicology Symptoms of overdose include diarrhea, vomiting, numbness of limbs, weakness

Drug Interactions

Decreased effect:

Barbiturates, warfarin may be accelerated by induction of the hepatic microsomal enzyme system

Spironolactone has resulted in negation of mitotane's effect

Phenytoin may increase clearance of these drugs by microsomal enzyme stimulation by mitotane

Increased toxicity: CNS depressants may increase CNS depression

Stability Protect from light, store at room temperature

Mechanism of Action Causes adrenal cortical atrophy; drug affects mitochondria in adrenal cortical cells and decreases production of cortisol; also alters the peripheral metabolism of steroids

Pharmacodynamics/Kinetics

Absorption: Oral: ~35% to 40%
Time to peak serum concentration: Within 3-5 hours
Distribution: Stored mainly in fat tissue but is found in all body tissues
Metabolism: Primarily in the liver by hydroxylation and oxidation and other tissues
Half-life: 18-159 days
Elimination: Metabolites excreted in urine and bile

Usual Dosage Oral:

Children: 0.1-0.5 mg/kg or 1-2 g/day in divided doses increasing gradually to a maximum of 5-7 g/day

Adults: Start at 1-6 g/day in divided doses, then increase incrementally to 8-10 g/day in 3-4 divided doses; dose is changed on basis of side effect with aim of giving as high a dose as tolerated; maximum daily dose: 18 g

Dosing adjustment in hepatic impairment: Dose may need to be decreased in patients with liver disease

Dietary Considerations Alcohol: Additive CNS effect, avoid use

Patient Information Patients should be warned that mitotane may impair ability to operate hazardous equipment or drive; avoid alcohol and other CNS depressants; notify physician if rash or darkening of skin, severe nausea, vomiting, depression, flushing, or fever occurs; contraceptive measures are recommended during therapy

Dosage Forms Tablet, scored: 500 mg

Mitoxantrone (mye toe ZAN trone)

Related Information

Antiemetics for Chemotherapy Induced Nausea and Vomiting *on page 1348*
Cancer Chemotherapy Regimens *on page 1351*
Toxicities of Chemotherapeutic Agents *on page 1382*

Brand Names Novantrone®

Synonyms DHAD; Mitoxantrone Hydrochloride

Therapeutic Category Antineoplastic Agent, Anthracycline; Antineoplastic Agent, Antibiotic; Antineoplastic Agent, Irritant; Vesicant

Use FDA approved for the treatment of acute nonlymphocytic leukemia (ANLL) in adults in combination with other agents; mitoxantrone is also found to be very active against various leukemias, lymphoma, and breast cancer, and moderately active against pediatric sarcoma.

Pregnancy Risk Factor D

Contraindications Hypersensitivity to mitoxantrone or any component

Warnings/Precautions The FDA currently recommends that procedures for proper handling and disposal of antineoplastic agents be considered. Dosage should be reduced in patients with impaired hepatobiliary function; use with caution in patients with pre-existing myelosuppression. Predisposing factors for mitoxantrone-induced cardiotoxicity include prior anthracycline therapy, prior cardiovascular disease, and mediastinal irradiation. The risk of developing cardiotoxicity is <3% when the cumulative doses are <100-120 mg/m² in patients with predisposing factors and <160 mg/m² in patients with no predisposing factors.

Adverse Reactions

>10%:

Central nervous system: Headache
Dermatologic: Alopecia
Gastrointestinal: Nausea, vomiting, diarrhea, abdominal pain, mucositis, stomatitis, GI bleeding
Emetic potential: Moderate (31% to 72%)
Genitourinary: Discoloration of urine (blue-green)

(Continued)

Mitoxantrone *(Continued)*

Hepatic: Abnormal LFTs
Respiratory: Coughing, shortness of breath

1% to 10%:

Cardiac toxicity: Much reduced compared to doxorubicin and has been reported primarily in patients who have received prior anthracycline therapy, congestive heart failure, hypotension
Central nervous system: Seizures, fever
Dermatologic: Pruritus, skin desquamation
Hematologic: Myelosuppressive effects of chemotherapy:
WBC: Mild
Platelets: Mild
Onset (days): 7-10
Nadir (days): 14
Recovery (days): 21
Hepatic: Transient elevation of liver enzymes, jaundice
Ocular: Conjunctivitis
Renal: Renal failure

<1%:

Local: Pain or redness at injection site
Irritant chemotherapy with blue skin discoloration

Overdosage/Toxicology Symptoms of overdose include leukopenia, tachycardia, marrow hypoplasia; no known antidote

Stability

Store intact vials at room temperature or refrigeration
Dilute in at least 50 mL of NS or D_5W; solution is stable for 7 days at room temperature or refrigeration
Incompatible with heparin and hydrocortisone

Standard I.V. dilution:
IVPB: Dose/100 mL D_5W or NS
Solution is stable for 7 days at room temperature and refrigeration

Mechanism of Action Analogue of the anthracyclines, but different in mechanism of action, cardiac toxicity, and potential for tissue necrosis; mitoxantrone does intercalate DNA; binds to nucleic acids and inhibits DNA and RNA synthesis by template disordering and steric obstruction; replication is decreased by binding to DNA topoisomerase II (enzyme responsible for DNA helix supercoiling); active throughout entire cell cycle; does not appear to produce free radicals

Pharmacodynamics/Kinetics

Absorption: Oral: Poor
Distribution: V_d: 14 L/kg; distributes into pleural fluid, kidney, thyroid, liver, heart, and red blood cells
Protein binding: 78%
Albumin binding: 76%
Metabolism: In the liver
Half-life: Terminal: 37 hours; may be prolonged with liver impairment
Elimination: Slowly excreted in urine (6% to 11%) and bile as unchanged drug and metabolites

Usual Dosage

Refer to individual protocols. I.V. (may dilute in D_5W or NS):
ANLL leukemias:
Children ≤2 years: 0.4 mg/kg/day once daily for 3-5 days
Children >2 years and Adults: 12 mg/m²/day once daily for 3 days; acute leukemia in relapse: 8-12 mg/m²/day once daily for 4-5 days

Solid tumors:
Children: 18-20 mg/m² every 3-4 weeks **OR** 5-8 mg/m² every week
Adults: 12-14 mg/m² every 3-4 weeks **OR** 2-4 mg/m²/day for 5 days
Maximum total dose: 80-120 mg/m² in patients with predisposing factor and <160 mg in patients with no predisposing factor

Hemodialysis: Supplemental dose is not necessary
Peritoneal dialysis: Supplemental dose is not necessary

Dosing adjustment in hepatic impairment: Official dosage adjustment recommendations have not been established
Moderate dysfunction (bilirubin 1.5-3 mg/dL): Some clinicians recommend a 50% dosage reduction
Severe dysfunction (bilirubin >3.0 mg/dL) have a lower total body clearance and may require a dosage adjustment to 8 mg/m²; some clinicians recommend a dosage reduction to 25% of dose

Dose modifications based on degree of leukopenia or thrombocytopenia; see table.

Granulocyte Count Nadir (cells/mm^2)	Platelet Count Nadir (cells/mm^2)	Total Bilirubin (mg/dL)	Dose Adjustment
>2000	>150,000	<1.5	Increase by 1 mg/m^2
1000-2000	75,000-150,000	<1.5	Maintain same dose
<1000	<75,000	1.5-3	Decrease by 1 mg/m^2

Administration

MUST BE DILUTED prior to administration

Do **not** administer I.V. bolus over <3 minutes; can be administered I.V. intermittent infusion over 15-30 minutes

Avoid extravasation; although has not generally been proven to be a vesicant

Monitoring Parameters CBC, serum uric acid, liver function tests, ECHO

Patient Information May impart a blue-green color to the urine for 24 hours after administration, and patients should be advised to expect this during therapy. Bluish discoloration of the sclera may also occur. Patients should be advised of the signs and symptoms of myelosuppression; report to physician if persistent fever, malaise, sore throat, fatigue, or unusual bleeding or bruising

Nursing Implications Vesicant; avoid extravasation

Dosage Forms Injection, as base: 2 mg/mL (10 mL, 12.5 mL, 15 mL)

Mitoxantrone Hydrochloride *see* Mitoxantrone *on page 849*

Mitran® *see* Chlordiazepoxide *on page 252*

Mitrolan® Chewable Tablet [OTC] *see* Calcium Polycarbophil *on page 195*

Mivacron® *see* Mivacurium *on this page*

Mivacurium (mye va KYOO ree um)

Related Information

Neuromuscular Blocking Agents Comparison *on page 1417*

Brand Names Mivacron®

Synonyms Mivacurium Chloride

Therapeutic Category Neuromuscular Blocker Agent, Nondepolarizing; Skeletal Muscle Relaxant

Use Short-acting nondepolarizing neuromuscular blocking agent; an adjunct to general anesthesia; facilitates endotracheal intubation; provides skeletal muscle relaxation during surgery or mechanical ventilation

Pregnancy Risk Factor C

Contraindications Hypersensitivity to mivacurium chloride or other benzylisoquinolinium agents; pre-existing tachycardia

Adverse Reactions

>10%: Cardiovascular: Flushing of face

1% to 10%: Cardiovascular: Hypotension

<1%:

- Cardiovascular: Bradycardia, tachycardia
- Central nervous system: Dizziness
- Dermatologic: Cutaneous erythema, rash
- Local: Injection site reaction
- Neuromuscular & skeletal: Muscle spasms
- Respiratory: Bronchospasm, wheezing, hypoxemia
- Miscellaneous: Endogenous histamine release

Drug Interactions

Prolonged neuromuscular blockade:

- Inhaled anesthetics
- Local anesthetics
- Calcium channel blockers
- Antiarrhythmics (eg, quinidine or procainamide)
- Antibiotics (eg, aminoglycosides, tetracyclines, vancomycin, clindamycin)
- Immunosuppressants (eg, cyclosporine)

Mechanism of Action Mivacurium is a short-acting, nondepolarizing, neuromuscular-blocking agent. Like other nondepolarizing drugs, mivacurium antagonizes acetylcholine by competitively binding to cholinergic sites on motor endplates in skeletal muscle. This inhibits contractile activity in skeletal muscle leading to muscle paralysis. This effect is reversible with cholinesterase inhibitors such as edrophonium, neostigmine, and physostigmine.

Pharmacodynamics/Kinetics

Onset of neuromuscular blockade effect: I.V.: Within 2-3 minutes

Peak effect: 1.5-8 minutes

Duration of action: Short due to rapid hydrolysis by plasma cholinesterases; recovery from muscular paralysis occurs within 15-30 minutes

Usual Dosage Continuous infusion requires an infusion pump; dose should be based on ideal body weight

(Continued)

Mivacurium *(Continued)*

Children 2-12 years (duration of action is shorter and dosage requirements are higher): 200 mcg/kg I.V. bolus; 5-31 mcg/kg/minute I.V. infusion

Adults: Initial: I.V.: 0.15 mg/kg bolus; for prolonged neuromuscular block, infusions of 1-15 mcg/kg/minute are used

Dosing adjustment in renal impairment: 150 mcg/kg I.V. bolus; duration of action of blockade: 1.5 times longer in ESRD, may decrease infusion rates by as much as 50%, dependent on degree of renal impairment

Dosing adjustment in hepatic impairment: 150 mcg/kg I.V. bolus; duration of blockade: 3 times longer in ESLD, may decrease rate of infusion by as much as 50% in ESLD, dependent on the degree of impairment

Administration Children require higher mivacurium infusion rates than adults; during opioid/nitrous oxide/oxygen anesthesia, the infusion rate required to maintain 89% to 99% neuromuscular block averages 14 mcg/kg/minute (range: 5-31). For adults and children, the amount of infusion solution required per hour depends upon the clinical requirements of the patient, the concentration of mivacurium in the infusion solution, and the patient's weight. The contribution of the infusion solution to the fluid requirements of the patient must be considered. The following tables provide guidelines for delivery in mL/hour (equivalent to microdrops/minute when 60 microdrops = 1 mL) of mivacurium premixed infusion (0.5 mg/mL) and of mivacurium injection (2 mg/mL).

Infusion Rates for Maintenance of Neuromuscular Block During Opioid/ Nitrous Oxide/Oxygen Anesthesia Using Mivacurium Premixed Infusion (0.5 mg/mL)

Patient Weight (kg)	Drug Delivery Rate (mcg/kg/min)									
	4	5	6	7	8	10	14	16	18	20
	Infusion Delivery Rate (mL/h)									
10	5	6	7	8	10	12	17	19	22	24
15	7	9	11	13	14	18	25	29	32	36
20	10	12	15	17	19	24	34	38	43	48
25	12	15	18	21	24	30	42	48	54	60
35	17	21	26	29	34	42	59	67	76	84
50	24	30	36	42	46	60	84	96	108	120
60	29	36	43	50	58	72	101	115	130	144
70	34	42	50	59	67	84	118	134	151	168
80	39	48	58	67	77	96	134	154	173	192
90	44	54	65	76	86	108	151	173	194	216
100	48	60	72	84	96	120	168	192	216	240

Infusion Rates for Maintenance of Neuromuscular Block During Opioid/ Nitrous Oxide/Oxygen Anesthesia Using Mivacurium Injection (2 mg/mL)

Patient Weight (kg)	Drug Delivery Rate (mcg/kg/min)									
	4	5	6	7	8	10	14	16	18	20
	Infusion Delivery Rate (mL/h)									
10	1.2	1.5	1.8	2.1	2.4	3	4.2	4.8	5.4	6
15	1.8	2.3	2.7	3.2	3.6	4.5	6.3	7.2	8.1	9
20	2.4	3	3.6	4.2	4.8	6	8.4	9.5	10.8	12
25	3	3.8	4.5	5.3	6	7.5	10.5	12	13.5	15
35	4.2	5.3	6.3	7.4	8.4	10.5	14.7	16.8	18.9	21
50	6	7.5	9	10.5	12	15	21	24	27	30
60	7.2	9	10.8	12.8	14.4	18	25.2	28.8	32.4	36
70	8.4	10.5	12.6	14.7	16.8	21	29.4	33.6	37.8	42
80	9.6	12	14.4	16.8	19.2	24	33.6	38.4	43.2	48
90	10.8	13.5	16.2	18.9	21.6	27	37.8	43.2	48.6	54
100	12	15	18	21	24	30	42	48	54	60

Nursing Implications Use with caution in patients in whom histamine release would be detrimental (eg, patients with severe cardiovascular disease or asthma)

Dosage Forms

Infusion, as chloride, in D_5W: 0.5 mg/mL (50 mL)

Injection, as chloride: 2 mg/mL (5 mL, 10 mL)

Mivacurium Chloride *see* Mivacurium *on previous page*

MK594 *see* Losartan *on page 744*

MMR *see* Measles, Mumps, and Rubella Vaccines, Combined *on page 763*

M-M-R® II *see* Measles, Mumps, and Rubella Vaccines, Combined *on page 763*

Moban® *see* Molindone *on next page*

Modane® Bulk [OTC] *see* Psyllium *on page 1075*

Modane® Soft [OTC] *see* Docusate *on page 415*

Modicon™ *see* Ethinyl Estradiol and Norethindrone *on page 486*

Modified Dakin's Solution *see* Sodium Hypochlorite Solution *on page 1145*

Modified Shohl's Solution *see* Sodium Citrate and Citric Acid *on page 1144*

Moexipril (mo EKS i pril)

Related Information

Angiotensin-Converting Enzyme Inhibitors Comparison *on page 1386*

Brand Names Univasc®

Synonyms Moexipril Hydrochloride

Therapeutic Category Angiotensin-Converting Enzyme (ACE) Inhibitors

Use Treatment of hypertension, alone or in combination with thiazide diuretics in a once daily dosing regimen

Pregnancy Risk Factor C (1st trimester); D (2nd and 3rd trimesters)

Contraindications Hypersensitivity to moexipril, moexiprilat, or component; hypersensitivity or allergic reactions or angioedema related to an ACE inhibitor

Warnings/Precautions Do not administer in pregnancy; use with caution and modify dosage in patients with renal impairment especially renal artery stenosis, severe congestive heart failure, or with coadministered diuretic therapy; experience in children is limited. Severe hypotension may occur in patients who are sodium and/or volume depleted; initiate lower doses and monitor closely when starting therapy in these patients; ACE inhibitors may be preferred agents in elderly patients with congestive heart failure and diabetes mellitus (diabetic proteinuria is reduced, minimal CNS effects, and enhanced insulin sensitivity), however due to decreased renal function, tolerance must be carefully monitored; if possible, discontinue the diuretic 2-3 days prior to initiating moexipril in patients receiving them to reduce the risk of symptomatic hypotension.

Drug-Drug Interactions With ACEIs

Precipitant Drug	Drug (Category) and Effect	Description
Antacids	ACE Inhibitors: decreased	Decreased bioavailability of ACEIs. May be more likely with captopril. Separate administration times by 1-2 hours.
NSAIDs (indomethacin)	ACEIs: decreased	Reduced hypotensive effects of ACEIs. More prominent in low renin or volume dependent hypertensive patients.
Phenothiazines	ACEIs: increased	Pharmacologic effects of ACEIs may be increased.
ACEIs	Allopurinol: increased	Higher risk of hypersensitivity reaction possible when given concurrently. Three case reports of Stevens-Johnson syndrome with captopril.
ACEIs	Digoxin: increased	Increased plasma digoxin levels.
ACEIs	Lithium: increased	Increased serum lithium levels and symptoms of toxicity may occur.
ACEIs	Potassium preps/ potassium sparing diuretics increased	Coadministration may result in elevated potassium levels.

Adverse Reactions

1% to 10%:

Central nervous system: Headache, dizziness, fatigue

Dermatologic: Rash, pruritus, alopecia, flushing, rash

Endocrine & metabolic: Hyperkalemia

Gastrointestinal: Diarrhea

Genitourinary: Polyuria

Renal: Oliguria, reversible increases in creatinine or BUN

Respiratory: Nonproductive cough (6%), pharyngitis, upper respiratory infections, rhinitis

Miscellaneous: Flu-like symptoms

<1%:

Cardiovascular: Symptomatic hypotension, chest pain, angina, peripheral edema, myocardial infarction, palpitations, arrhythmias

Central nervous system: Sleep disturbances, anxiety, mood changes

Dermatologic: Angioedema, photosensitivity, pemphigus

Endocrine & metabolic: Hypercholesterolemia

Gastrointestinal: Abdominal pain, taste disturbance, constipation, vomiting, xerostomia, changes in appetite, pancreatitis, abnormal taste

(Continued)

Moexipril *(Continued)*

Hematologic: Neutropenia
Hepatic: Elevated LFTs
Neuromuscular & skeletal: Myalgia, arthralgia
Renal: Proteinuria
Respiratory: Bronchospasm, dyspnea

Overdosage/Toxicology Mild hypotension has been the only toxic effect seen with acute overdose; bradycardia may also occur; hyperkalemia occurs even with therapeutic doses, especially in patients with renal insufficiency and those taking NSAIDs

Following initiation of essential overdose management, toxic symptom treatment and supportive treatment should be initiated; hypotension usually responds to I.V. fluids or Trendelenburg positioning.

Drug Interactions See table.
Decreased effect: NSAIDs
Increased levels/toxicity: Lithium

Mechanism of Action Competitive inhibitor of angiotensin-converting enzyme (ACE); prevents conversion of angiotensin I to angiotensin II, a potent vasoconstrictor; results in lower levels of angiotensin II which causes an increase in plasma renin activity and a reduction in aldosterone secretion

Pharmacodynamics/Kinetics
Absorption: Food decreases bioavailability (AUC decreased by ~40%)
Distribution: V_d (moexiprilat): 180 L
Protein binding (plasma):
  Moexipril: 90%
  Moexiprilat: 50% to 70%
Metabolism: Parent drug is metabolized in liver and small intestine to moexiprilat, the 1000 times more potent diacid metabolite; both parent
Bioavailability (moexiprilat): 13%
Half-life:
  Moexipril: 1 hour
  Moexiprilat: 2-10 hours
Time to peak: 1.5 hours
Elimination: 50% appears in the feces

Usual Dosage Adults: Oral: Initial: 7.5 mg once daily (in patients **not** receiving diuretics), one hour prior to a meal **or** 3.75 mg once daily (when combined with thiazide diuretics); maintenance dose: 7.5-30 mg/day in 1 or 2 divided doses one hour before meals

Dosing adjustment in renal impairment: Cl_{cr} ≤40 mL/minute: Patients may be cautiously placed on 3.75 mg once daily, then upwardly titrated to a maximum of 15 mg/day

Monitoring Parameters Blood pressure, heart rate, electrolytes, CBC, symptoms of hypotension

Test Interactions Increases BUN, creatinine, potassium, positive Coombs' [direct]; decreases cholesterol (S); may cause false-positive results in urine acetone determinations using sodium nitroprusside reagent

Patient Information Food may delay and reduce peak serum levels; take on an empty stomach, if possible. Report swelling of the face, mouth, or tongue, rash, or difficulty breathing to your physician immediately; bothersome side effects such as cough, dizziness, diarrhea, tiredness, rash, headache, irregular heartbeat, anxiety, and flu-like symptoms should also be reported; avoid use of this medication if you are pregnant or have had a previous reaction to other ACE inhibitors.

Nursing Implications Observe for symptoms of severe hypotension, especially within the first 2 hours following the initial dose or subsequent increases in dose as well as for signs of hyperkalemia or cough; administer on an empty stomach

Dosage Forms Tablet, as hydrochloride: 7.5 mg, 15 mg

Moexipril Hydrochloride *see* Moexipril *on previous page*

Molindone (moe LIN done)

Related Information
Antipsychotic Agents Comparison *on page 1396*

Brand Names Moban®

Synonyms Molindone Hydrochloride

Therapeutic Category Antipsychotic Agent

Use Management of psychotic disorder

Pregnancy Risk Factor C

Contraindications Narrow-angle glaucoma, hypersensitivity to molindone or any component

Warnings/Precautions Use with caution in patients with cardiovascular disease or seizures, CNS depression, or hepatic impairment

Adverse Reactions

>10%:

Cardiovascular: Orthostatic hypotension

Central nervous system: Akathisia, extrapyramidal effects, persistent tardive dyskinesia

Gastrointestinal: Constipation, xerostomia

Ocular: Blurred vision

Miscellaneous: Diaphoresis (decreased)

1% to 10%:

Central nervous system: Mental depression, altered central temperature regulation

Endocrine & metabolic: Change in menstrual periods, edema of the breasts

<1%:

Cardiovascular: Tachycardia, arrhythmias

Central nervous system: Sedation, drowsiness, restlessness, anxiety, seizures, neuroleptic malignant syndrome (NMS)

Dermatologic: Hyperpigmentation, pruritus, rash, photosensitivity

Endocrine & metabolic: Galactorrhea, gynecomastia

Gastrointestinal: Weight gain

Genitourinary: Urinary retention

Hematologic: Agranulocytosis (more often in women between fourth and tenth weeks of therapy), leukopenia (usually in patients with large doses for prolonged periods)

Ocular: Retinal pigmentation

Overdosage/Toxicology Symptoms of overdose include deep sleep, extrapyramidal symptoms, cardiac arrhythmias, seizures, hypotension

Following initiation of essential overdose management, toxic symptom treatment and supportive treatment should be initiated. Hypotension usually responds to I.V. fluids or Trendelenburg positioning. If unresponsive to these measures, the use of a parenteral inotrope may be required (eg, norepinephrine 0.1-0.2 mcg/kg/minute titrated to response). Seizures commonly respond to diazepam (I.V. 5-10 mg bolus in adults every 15 minutes if needed up to a total of 30 mg; I.V. 0.25-0.4 mg/kg/dose up to a total of 10 mg in children) or to phenytoin or phenobarbital. Critical cardiac arrhythmias often respond to I.V. phenytoin (15 mg/kg up to 1 g), while other antiarrhythmics can be used. Neuroleptics often cause extrapyramidal symptoms (eg, dystonic reactions) requiring management with diphenhydramine 1-2 mg/kg (adults) up to a maximum of 50 mg I.M. or I.V. slow push followed by a maintenance dose for 48-72 hours. When these reactions are unresponsive to diphenhydramine, benztropine mesylate I.V. 1-2 mg (adults) may be effective. These agents are generally effective within 2-5 minutes.

Drug Interactions Increased toxicity: CNS depressants, antihypertensives, anticonvulsants

Mechanism of Action Mechanism of action mimics that of chlorpromazine; however, it produces more extrapyramidal effects and less sedation than chlorpromazine

Pharmacodynamics/Kinetics

Metabolism: In the liver

Half-life: 1.5 hours

Time to peak serum concentration: Oral: Within 1.5 hours

Elimination: Principally in urine and feces (90% within 24 hours)

Usual Dosage Oral:

Children:

3-5 years: 1-2.5 mg/day divided into 4 doses

5-12 years: 0.5-1 mg/kg/day in 4 divided doses

Adults: 50-75 mg/day increase at 3- to 4-day intervals up to 225 mg/day

Dietary Considerations Alcohol: Avoid use

Monitoring Parameters Monitor blood pressure and pulse rate prior to and during initial therapy evaluate mental status; monitor weight

Patient Information Dry mouth may be helped by sips of water, sugarless gum or hard candy; avoid alcohol; very important to maintain established dosage regimen; photosensitivity to sunlight can occur, do not discontinue abruptly; full effect may not occur for 3-4 weeks; full dosage may be taken at bedtime to avoid daytime sedation; report to physician any involuntary movements or feelings of restlessness

Nursing Implications May increase appetite and possibly a craving for sweets; recognize signs of neuroleptic malignant syndrome and tardive dyskinesia

Dosage Forms

Concentrate, oral, as hydrochloride: 20 mg/mL (120 mL)

Tablet, as hydrochloride: 5 mg, 10 mg, 25 mg, 50 mg, 100 mg

Molindone Hydrochloride *see* Molindone *on previous page*

Mol-Iron® [OTC] *see* Ferrous Sulfate *on page 516*

Mollifene® Ear Wax Removing Formula [OTC] *see* Carbamide Peroxide *on page 203*

MOM *see* Magnesium Hydroxide *on page 753*

Mometasone Furoate (moe MET a sone FYOOR oh ate)

Related Information

Corticosteroids Comparison *on page 1407*

Brand Names Elocon®

Canadian/Mexican Brand Names Elocom® (Canada); Elomet® (Mexico)

Therapeutic Category Corticosteroid, Topical (Medium Potency)

Use Relief of the inflammatory and pruritic manifestations of corticosteroid-responsive dermatoses (medium potency topical corticosteroid)

Pregnancy Risk Factor C

Contraindications Hypersensitivity to mometasone or any component; fungal, viral, or tubercular skin lesions, herpes simplex or zoster

Warnings/Precautions Adverse systemic effects may occur when used on large areas of the body, denuded areas, for prolonged periods of time, with an occlusive dressing, and/or in infants or small children

Adverse Reactions

<1%:

Dermatologic: Acne, hypopigmentation, allergic dermatitis, maceration of the skin, skin atrophy, striae, miliaria, itching, folliculitis, hypertrichosis

Endocrine & metabolic: HPA suppression, Cushing's syndrome, growth retardation

Local: Burning, irritation, dryness

Miscellaneous: Secondary infection

Mechanism of Action May depress the formation, release, and activity of endogenous chemical mediators of inflammation (kinins, histamine, liposomal enzymes, prostaglandins). Leukocytes and macrophages may have to be present for the initiation of responses mediated by the above substances. Inhibits the margination and subsequent cell migration to the area of injury, and also reverses the dilatation and increased vessel permeability in the area resulting in decreased access of cells to the sites of injury.

Usual Dosage Adults: Topical: Apply sparingly to area once daily, do not use occlusive dressings

Patient Information Before applying, gently wash area to reduce risk of infection; apply a thin film to cleansed area and rub in gently and thoroughly until medication vanishes; avoid exposure to sunlight, severe sunburn may occur

Nursing Implications For external use only; do not use on open wounds; should not be used in the presence of open or weeping lesions; use sparingly

Dosage Forms

Cream: 0.1% (15 g, 45 g)

Lotion: 0.1% (27.5 mL, 55 mL)

Ointment, topical: 0.1% (15 g, 45 g)

Monacolin K *see* Lovastatin *on page 746*

Monistat-Derm™ Topical *see* Miconazole *on page 834*

Monistat i.v.™ Injection *see* Miconazole *on page 834*

Monistat™ Vaginal *see* Miconazole *on page 834*

Monocid® *see* Cefonicid *on page 224*

Monoclate-P® *see* Antihemophilic Factor (Human) *on page 94*

Monoclonal Antibody *see* Muromonab-CD3 *on page 863*

Monodox® Oral *see* Doxycycline *on page 430*

Mono-Gesic® *see* Salsalate *on page 1122*

Monoket® *see* Isosorbide Mononitrate *on page 685*

Mononine® *see* Factor IX Complex (Human) *on page 502*

Monopril® *see* Fosinopril *on page 557*

Monurol® *see* Fosfomycin *on page 556*

8-MOP *see* Methoxsalen *on page 812*

8-MOP® *see* Methoxsalen *on page 812*

More Attenuated Enders Strain *see* Measles Virus Vaccine, Live *on page 764*

More-Dophilus® [OTC] *see Lactobacillus acidophilus* and *Lactobacillus bulgaricus on page 702*

Moricizine (mor I siz een)

Related Information

Antiarrhythmic Drugs *on page 1389*

Comparative Pharmacokinetic Properties of Antiarrhythmic Agents *on page 1391*

Brand Names Ethmozine®

Synonyms Moricizine Hydrochloride

Therapeutic Category Antiarrhythmic Agent, Class I

Use For treatment of ventricular tachycardia and life-threatening ventricular arrhythmias

Unlabeled use: PVCs, complete and nonsustained ventricular tachycardia

Pregnancy Risk Factor B

Contraindications Pre-existing second or third degree A-V block and in patients with right bundle-branch block when associated with left hemiblock, unless pacemaker is present; cardiogenic shock; known hypersensitivity to the drug

Warnings/Precautions Considering the known proarrhythmic properties and lack of evidence of improved survival for any antiarrhythmic drug in patients without life-threatening arrhythmias, it is prudent to reserve the use for patients with life-threatening ventricular arrhythmias; CAST II trial demonstrated a trend towards decreased survival for patients treated with moricizine; proarrhythmic effects occur as with other antiarrhythmic agents; hypokalemia, hyperkalemia, hypomagnesemia may effect response to class I agents; use with caution in patients with sick-sinus syndrome, hepatic, and renal impairment

Adverse Reactions

>10%: Central nervous system: Dizziness

1% to 10%:

- Cardiovascular: Proarrhythmia, palpitations, cardiac death, EKG abnormalities, congestive heart failure
- Central nervous system: Headache, fatigue, insomnia
- Endocrine & metabolic: Decreased libido
- Gastrointestinal: Nausea, diarrhea, ileus
- Ocular: Blurred vision, periorbital edema
- Respiratory: Dyspnea

<1%:

- Cardiovascular: Ventricular tachycardia, cardiac chest pain, hypotension or hypertension, syncope, supraventricular arrhythmias, myocardial infarction
- Central nervous system: Anxiety, drug fever, confusion, loss of memory, vertigo, anorexia
- Dermatologic: Rash, dry skin
- Gastrointestinal: GI upset, vomiting, dyspepsia, flatulence, bitter taste
- Genitourinary: Urinary retention, urinary incontinence, impotence
- Neuromuscular & skeletal: Tremor
- Otic: Tinnitus
- Respiratory: Apnea
- Miscellaneous: Diaphoresis

Overdosage/Toxicology Has a narrow therapeutic index and severe toxicity may occur slightly above the therapeutic range, especially if combined with other antiarrhythmic drugs. (Acute single ingestion of twice the daily therapeutic dose is life-threatening). Symptoms of overdose include increases in P-R, QRS, Q-T intervals and amplitude of the T wave, A-V block, bradycardia, hypotension, ventricular arrhythmias (monomorphic or polymorphic ventricular tachycardia), and asystole; other symptoms include dizziness, blurred vision, headache, and GI upset.

Treatment is supportive, using conventional treatment (fluids, positioning, anticonvulsants, antiarrhythmics). **Note:** Type Ia antiarrhythmic agents should not be used to treat cardiotoxicity caused by type 1c drugs; sodium bicarbonate may reverse QRS prolongation, bradycardia and hypotension; ventricular pacing may be needed.

Drug Interactions

Decreased levels of theophylline (50%)

Increased levels with cimetidine (50%)

Mechanism of Action Class I antiarrhythmic agent; reduces the fast inward current carried by sodium ions, shortens Phase I and Phase II repolarization, resulting in decreased action potential duration and effective refractory period

Pharmacodynamics/Kinetics

Protein binding, plasma: 95%

Metabolism: Undergoes significant first-pass metabolism absolute

Bioavailability: 38%

Half-life:

- Normal patients: 3-4 hours
- Cardiac disease patients: 6-13 hours

Elimination: Some enterohepatic recycling occurs; 56% is excreted in feces and 39% in urine

Transferred From	Start Ethmozine®
Encainide, propafenone, tocainide, or mexiletine	8-12 hours after last dose
Flecainide	12-24 hours after last dose
Procainamide	3-6 hours after last dose
Quinidine, disopyramide	6-12 hours after last dose

(Continued)

Moricizine *(Continued)*

Usual Dosage Adults: Oral: 200-300 mg every 8 hours, adjust dosage at 150 mg/day at 3-day intervals. See table for dosage recommendations of transferring from other antiarrhythmic agents to Ethmozine®.

Dosing interval in renal or hepatic impairment: Start at 600 mg/day or less

Patient Information Take as directed; do not change dose except from advice of your physician; report any chest pain and irregular heartbeats

Nursing Implications Administering 30 minutes after a meal delays the rate of absorption, resulting in lower peak plasma concentrations

Dosage Forms Tablet, as hydrochloride: 200 mg, 250 mg, 300 mg

Moricizine Hydrochloride *see* Moricizine *on page 856*

Morning After Pill *see* Ethinyl Estradiol and Norgestrel *on page 489*

Morphine Sulfate (MOR feen SUL fate)

Related Information

Adult ACLS Algorithm, Electrical Conversion *on page 1515*

Narcotic Agonists Comparison *on page 1414*

Dose Equivalents for Opioid Analgesics in Opioid-Naive Adults <50 kg *on page 1376*

Dose Equivalents for Opioid Analgesics in Opioid-Naive Adults ≥50 kg *on page 1375*

Brand Names Astramorph™ PF; Duramorph®; MS Contin®; MSIR®; OMS®; Oramorph SR®; RMS®; Roxanol™; Roxanol SR™

Canadian/Mexican Brand Names Epimorph® (Canada); M-Eslon® (Canada); Morphine-HP® (Canada); MST-Continus® (Mexico); MS-IR® (Canada); Statex® (Canada)

Synonyms MS

Therapeutic Category Analgesic, Narcotic

Use Relief of moderate to severe acute and chronic pain; pain of myocardial infarction; relieves dyspnea of acute left ventricular failure and pulmonary edema; preanesthetic medication

Restrictions C-II

Pregnancy Risk Factor B (D if used for prolonged periods or in high doses at term)

Contraindications Known hypersensitivity to morphine sulfate; increased intracranial pressure; severe respiratory depression

Warnings/Precautions Some preparations contain sulfites which may cause allergic reactions; infants <3 months of age are more susceptible to respiratory depression, use with caution and generally in reduced doses in this age group; use with caution in patients with impaired respiratory function or severe hepatic dysfunction and in patients with hypersensitivity reactions to other phenanthrene derivative opioid agonists (codeine, hydrocodone, hydromorphone, levorphanol, oxycodone, oxymorphone). Morphine shares the toxic potential of opiate agonists and usual precautions of opiate agonist therapy should be observed; may cause hypotension in patients with acute myocardial infarction.

Elderly may be particularly susceptible to the CNS depressant and constipating effects of narcotics

Adverse Reactions

Cardiovascular: Flushing

Central nervous system: CNS depression, drowsiness, sedation, increased intracranial pressure

Endocrine & metabolic: Antidiuretic hormone release

Miscellaneous: Physical and psychological dependence, diaphoresis

>10%:

- Cardiovascular: Palpitations, hypotension, bradycardia
- Central nervous system: Dizziness
- Gastrointestinal: Nausea, vomiting, constipation, xerostomia
- Local: Pain at injection site
- Neuromuscular & skeletal: Weakness
- Miscellaneous: Histamine release

1% to 10%:

- Central nervous system: Restlessness, headache, false feeling of well being, confusion
- Gastrointestinal: Anorexia, GI irritation, paralytic ileus
- Genitourinary: Decreased urination
- Neuromuscular & skeletal: Trembling
- Ocular: Vision problems
- Respiratory: Respiratory depression, shortness of breath

<1%:
- Cardiovascular: Peripheral vasodilation
- Central nervous system: Insomnia, mental depression, hallucinations, paradoxical CNS stimulation, increased intracranial pressure
- Dermatologic: Pruritus
- Gastrointestinal: Biliary tract spasm
- Genitourinary: Urinary tract spasm
- Neuromuscular & skeletal: Muscle rigidity
- Ocular: Miosis

Overdosage/Toxicology Symptoms of overdose include respiratory depression, miosis, hypotension, bradycardia, apnea, pulmonary edema

Treatment of an overdose includes support of the patient's airway, establishment of an I.V. line, and administration of naloxone 2 mg I.V. (0.01 mg/kg for children) with repeat administration as necessary up to a total of 10 mg. Primary attention should be directed to ensuring adequate respiratory exchange.

Drug Interactions

Decreased effect: Phenothiazines may antagonize the analgesic effect of morphine and other opiate agonists

Increased toxicity: CNS depressants, tricyclic antidepressants may potentiate the effects of morphine and other opiate agonists; dextroamphetamine may enhance the analgesic effect of morphine and other opiate agonists

Stability Refrigerate suppositories; do not freeze; degradation depends on pH and presence of oxygen; relatively stable in pH ≤4; darkening of solutions indicate degradation; usual concentration for continuous I.V. infusion = 0.1-1 mg/mL in D_5W

Mechanism of Action Binds to opiate receptors in the CNS, causing inhibition of ascending pain pathways, altering the perception of and response to pain; produces generalized CNS depression

Pharmacodynamics/Kinetics

Absorption: Oral: Variable

Metabolism: In the liver via glucuronide conjugation

Half-life:
- Neonates: 4.5-13.3 hours (mean 7.6 hours)
- Adults: 2-4 hours

Elimination: Unchanged in urine; see table.

Dosage Form/Route	Analgesia	
	Peak	Duration
Tablets	1 h	4-5 h
Oral solution	1 h	4-5 h
Extended release tablets	1 h	8-12 h
Suppository	20-60 min	3-7 h
Subcutaneous injection	50-90 min	4-5 h
I.M. injection	30-60 min	4-5 h
I.V. injection	20 min	4-5 h

Usual Dosage Doses should be titrated to appropriate effect; when changing routes of administration in chronically treated patients, please note that oral doses are approximately one-half as effective as parenteral dose

Infants and Children:
- Oral: Tablet and solution (prompt release): 0.2-0.5 mg/kg/dose every 4-6 hours as needed; tablet (controlled release): 0.3-0.6 mg/kg/dose every 12 hours
- I.M., I.V., S.C.: 0.1-0.2 mg/kg/dose every 2-4 hours as needed; usual maximum: 15 mg/dose; may initiate at 0.05 mg/kg/dose
- I.V., S.C. continuous infusion: Sickle cell or cancer pain: 0.025-2 mg/kg/hour; postoperative pain: 0.01-0.04 mg/kg/hour
- Sedation/analgesia for procedures: I.V.: 0.05-0.1 mg/kg 5 minutes before the procedure

Adolescents >12 years: Sedation/analgesia for procedures: I.V.: 3-4 mg and repeat in 5 minutes if necessary

Adults:
- Oral: Prompt release: 10-30 mg every 4 hours as needed; controlled release: 15-30 mg every 8-12 hours
- I.M., I.V., S.C.: 2.5-20 mg/dose every 2-6 hours as needed; usual: 10 mg/dose every 4 hours as needed
- I.V., S.C. continuous infusion: 0.8-10 mg/hour; may increase depending on pain relief/adverse effects; usual range: up to 80 mg/hour
- Epidural: Initial: 5 mg in lumbar region; if inadequate pain relief within 1 hour, administer 1-2 mg, maximum dose: 10 mg/24 hours

(Continued)

Morphine Sulfate *(Continued)*

Intrathecal ($^1/_{10}$ of epidural dose): 0.2-1 mg/dose; repeat doses **not** recommended

Rectal: 10-20 mg every 4 hours

Dosing adjustment in renal impairment:

Cl_{cr} 10-50 mL/minute: Administer at 75% of normal dose

Cl_{cr} <10 mL/minute: Administer at 50% of normal dose

Dosing adjustment/comments in hepatic disease: Unchanged in mild liver disease; substantial extrahepatic metabolism may occur; excessive sedation may occur in cirrhosis

Dietary Considerations

Alcohol: Additive CNS effects, avoid or limit alcohol; watch for sedation

Food:

Glucose may cause hyperglycemia; monitor blood glucose concentrations

Administration of oral morphine solution with food may increase bioavailability (ie, a report of 34% increase in morphine AUC when morphine oral solution followed a high-fat meal). Morphine may cause GI upset. Be consistent when taking morphine with or without meals. Take with food if GI upset.

Administration When giving morphine I.V. push, it is best to first dilute in 4-5 mL of sterile water, and then to administer slowly (eg, 15 mg over 3-5 minutes)

Monitoring Parameters Pain relief, respiratory and mental status, blood pressure

Reference Range Therapeutic: Surgical anesthesia: 65-80 ng/mL (SI: 227-280 nmol/L); Toxic: 200-5000 ng/mL (SI: 700-17,500 nmol/L)

Test Interactions ↑ aminotransferase [ALT (SGPT)/AST (SGOT)] (S)

Patient Information Avoid alcohol, may cause drowsiness, impaired judgment or coordination; may cause physical and psychological dependence with prolonged use

Nursing Implications Do not crush controlled release drug product, observe patient for excessive sedation, respiratory depression; implement safety measures, assist with ambulation; use preservative-free solutions for intrathecal or epidural use

Dosage Forms

Capsule (MSIR®): 15 mg, 30 mg

Capsule, sustained release (Kadian®): 20 mg, 50 mg, 100 mg

Injection: 0.5 mg/mL (10 mL); 1 mg/mL (10 mL, 30 mL, 60 mL); 2 mg/mL (1 mL, 2 mL, 60 mL); 3 mg/mL (50 mL); 4 mg/mL (1 mL, 2 mL); 5 mg/mL (1 mL, 30 mL); 8 mg/mL (1 mL, 2 mL); 10 mg/mL (1 mL, 2 mL, 10 mL); 15 mg/mL (1 mL, 2 mL, 20 mL); 25 mg/mL (4 mL, 10 mL, 20 mL, 40 mL); 50 mg/mL (10 mL, 20 mL, 40 mL)

Injection:

Preservative free (Astramorph™ PF, Duramorph®): 0.5 mg/mL (2 mL, 10 mL); 1 mg/mL (2 mL, 10 mL); 10 mg/mL (20 mL); 25 mg/mL (20 mL)

I.V. via PCA pump: 1 mg/mL (10 mL, 30 mL, 60 mL); 5 mg/mL (30 mL)

I.V. infusion preparation: 25 mg/mL (4 mL, 10 mL, 20 mL)

Solution, oral: 10 mg/5 mL (5 mL, 10 mL, 100 mL, 120 mL, 500 mL); 20 mg/5 mL (5 mL, 100 mL, 120 mL, 500 mL)

MSIR®: 10 mg/5 mL (5 mL, 120 mL, 500 mL); 20 mg/5 mL (5 mL 120 mL, 500 mL); 20 mg/mL (30 mL, 120 mL)

MS/L®: 100 mg/5 mL (120 mL) 20 mg/5 mL

OMS®: 20 mg/mL (30 mL, 120 mL)

Roxanol™: 10 mg/2.5 mL (2.5 mL); 20 mg/mL (1 mL, 1.5 mL, 30 mL, 120 mL, 240 mL)

Suppository, rectal: 5 mg, 10 mg, 20 mg, 30 mg

MS/S®, RMS®, Roxanol™: 5 mg, 10 mg, 20 mg, 30 mg

Tablet: 15 mg, 30 mg

MSIR®: 15 mg, 30 mg

Controlled release:

MS Contin®: 15 mg, 30 mg, 60 mg, 100 mg, 200 mg

Roxanol™ SR: 30 mg

Soluble: 10 mg, 15 mg, 30 mg

Sustained release (Oramorph SR™): 30 mg, 60 mg, 100 mg

Morrhuate Sodium (MOR yoo ate SOW dee um)

Brand Names Scleromate™

Therapeutic Category Sclerosing Agent

Use Treatment of small, uncomplicated varicose veins of the lower extremities

Contraindications Arterial disease, thrombophlebitis, hypersensitivity to morrhuate sodium or any component

Warnings/Precautions Sloughing and necrosis of tissue may occur following extravasation; anaphylactoid and allergic reactions have occurred; this drug should only be administered by a physician familiar with proper injection techniques; a test dose of 0.25-5 mL of a 5% injection should be given 24 hours before full-dose treatment

Adverse Reactions

>10%:

Cardiovascular: Thrombosis, valvular incompetency

Dermatologic: Urticaria

Local: Burning at the site of injection, severe extravasation effects

<1%:

Cardiovascular: Vascular collapse

Central nervous system: Drowsiness, headache, dizziness

Gastrointestinal: Nausea, vomiting

Neuromuscular & skeletal: Weakness

Respiratory: Asthma

Miscellaneous: Anaphylaxis

Stability Refrigerate

Mechanism of Action Both varicose veins and esophageal varices are treated by the thrombotic action of morrhuate sodium. By causing inflammation of the vein's intima, a thrombus is formed. Occlusion secondary to the fibrous tissue and the thrombus results in the obliteration of the vein.

Pharmacodynamics/Kinetics

Onset of action: ~5 minutes

Absorption: Most of the dose stays at the site of injection

Distribution: After treatment of esophageal varices, ~20% of dose distributes to the lungs

Usual Dosage I.V.:

Children 1-18 years: Esophageal hemorrhage: 2, 3, or 4 mL of 5% repeated every 3-4 days until bleeding is controlled, then every 6 weeks until varices obliterated

Adults: 50-250 mg, repeated at 5- to 7-day intervals (50-100 mg for small veins, 150-250 mg for large veins)

Administration For I.V. use only

Nursing Implications Avoid extravasation; use only clear solutions, solution should become clear when warmed

Dosage Forms Injection: 50 mg/mL (5 mL)

Mosco® Liquid [OTC] *see* Salicylic Acid *on page 1120*

Motrin® *see* Ibuprofen *on page 639*

Motrin® IB [OTC] *see* Ibuprofen *on page 639*

6-MP *see* Mercaptopurine *on page 784*

M-R-VAX® II *see* Measles and Rubella Vaccines, Combined *on page 761*

MS *see* Morphine Sulfate *on page 858*

MS Contin® *see* Morphine Sulfate *on page 858*

MSIR® *see* Morphine Sulfate *on page 858*

MTC *see* Mitomycin *on page 846*

MTX *see* Methotrexate *on page 806*

Muco-Fen-LA® *see* Guaifenesin *on page 589*

Mucomyst® *see* Acetylcysteine *on page 28*

Mucosil™ *see* Acetylcysteine *on page 28*

Multiple Vitamins *see* Vitamins, Multiple *on page 1310*

Multitest CMI® *see* Skin Test Antigens, Multiple *on page 1138*

Multivitamins/Fluoride *see* Vitamins, Multiple *on page 1310*

Multi Vit® Drops [OTC] *see* Vitamins, Multiple *on page 1310*

Mumps, Measles and Rubella Vaccines, Combined *see* Measles, Mumps, and Rubella Vaccines, Combined *on page 763*

Mumpsvax® *see* Mumps Virus Vaccine, Live, Attenuated *on this page*

Mumps Virus Vaccine, Live, Attenuated

(mumpz VYE rus vak SEEN, live, a ten YOO ate ed)

Related Information

Immunization Guidelines *on page 1421*

Skin Tests *on page 1501*

Brand Names Mumpsvax®

Therapeutic Category Vaccine, Live Virus

Use Mumps prophylaxis by promoting active immunity

Pregnancy Risk Factor X

Warnings/Precautions Pregnancy, immunocompromised persons, history of anaphylactic reaction following egg ingestion or receipt of neomycin

Adverse Reactions

>10%: Local: Burning or stinging at injection site

(Continued)

Mumps Virus Vaccine, Live, Attenuated *(Continued)*

1% to 10%:
- Central nervous system: Fever ≤100°F
- Dermatologic: Rash
- Endocrine & metabolic: Parotitis

<1%:
- Central nervous system: Convulsions, confusion, severe or continuing headache, fever >103°F
- Genitourinary: Orchitis in postpubescent and adult males
- Hematologic: Thrombocytopenic purpura
- Miscellaneous: Anaphylactic reactions

Drug Interactions Decreased effect with concurrent infection, immunoglobulin with in 1 month, other live vaccines with the exception of attenuated measles, rubella, or polio

Stability Refrigerate, protect from light, discard within 8 hours after reconstitution

Usual Dosage 1 vial (5000 units) S.C. in outer aspect of the upper arm, no booster

Administration Reconstitute only with diluent provided; administer only S.C. on outer aspect of upper arm

Test Interactions Temporary suppression of tuberculosis skin test

Patient Information Pregnancy should be avoided for 3 months following vaccination; a little swelling of the glands in the cheeks and under the jaw may occur that lasts for a few days; this could happen from 1-2 weeks after getting the mumps vaccine; this happens rarely

Additional Information Federal law requires that the date of administration, the vaccine manufacturer, lot number of vaccine, and the administering person's name, title and address be entered into the patient's permanent medical record; all adults without documentation of live vaccine on or after the first birthday or physician-diagnosed mumps, or laboratory evidence or immunity (particularly males and young adults who work in or congregate in hospitals, colleges, and on military bases) should be vaccinated. It is reasonable to consider persons born before 1957 immune, but there is no contraindication to vaccination of older persons. Susceptible travelers should be vaccinated.

Dosage Forms Injection: Single dose

Mupirocin (myoo PEER oh sin)

Brand Names Bactroban®

Canadian/Mexican Brand Names Mupiban® (Mexico)

Synonyms Mupirocin Calcium; Pseudomonic Acid A

Therapeutic Category Antibiotic, Topical

Use Topical treatment of impetigo due to *Staphylococcus aureus*, beta-hemolytic *Streptococcus*, and *S. pyogenes*

Pregnancy Risk Factor B

Contraindications Known hypersensitivity to mupirocin or polyethylene glycol

Warnings/Precautions Potentially toxic amounts of polyethylene glycol contained in the vehicle may be absorbed percutaneously in patients with extensive burns or open wounds; prolonged use may result in over growth of nonsusceptible organisms; for external use only; not for treatment of pressure sores

Adverse Reactions

1% to 10%:
- Dermatologic: Pruritus, rash, erythema, dry skin
- Local: Burning, stinging, tenderness, edema, pain

Stability Do not mix with Aquaphor®, coal tar solution, or salicylic acid

Mechanism of Action Binds to bacterial isoleucyl transfer-RNA synthetase resulting in the inhibition of protein and RNA synthesis

Pharmacodynamics/Kinetics
- Absorption: Topical: Penetrates the outer layers of the skin; systemic absorption minimal through intact skin
- Protein binding: 95%
- Metabolism: Extensively to monic acid, principally in the liver and skin
- Half-life: 17-36 minutes
- Elimination: In urine

Usual Dosage Children and Adults: Topical: Apply small amount to affected area 2-5 times/day for 5-14 days

Patient Information For topical use only; do not apply into the eye; discontinue if rash, itching, or irritation occurs; improvement should be seen in 5 days

Additional Information Not for treatment of pressure sores in elderly; contains polyethylene glycol vehicle

Dosage Forms

Ointment, as calcium:
- Intranasal: 2% (1 g single use tube)

Topical: 2% (15 g)

Mupirocin Calcium *see* Mupirocin *on previous page*

Murine® Ear Drops [OTC] *see* Carbamide Peroxide *on page 203*

Murine® Plus [OTC] *see* Tetrahydrozoline *on page 1205*

Muro 128® Ophthalmic [OTC] *see* Sodium Chloride *on page 1142*

Muromonab-CD3 (myoo roe MOE nab see dee three)

Brand Names Orthoclone OKT®3

Synonyms Monoclonal Antibody; OKT3

Therapeutic Category Immunosuppressant Agent

Use Treatment of acute allograft rejection in renal transplant patients; effective in reversing acute hepatic, cardiac, kidney, pancreas, and bone marrow transplant rejection episodes resistant to conventional treatment

Pregnancy Risk Factor C

Contraindications Patients with known hypersensitivity to OKT3 or any murine product; patients in fluid overload or those with >3% weight gain within 1 week prior to start of OKT3

Warnings/Precautions It is imperative, especially prior to the first few doses, that there be no clinical evidence of volume overload, uncontrolled hypertension, or uncompensated heart failure, including a clear chest X-ray and weight restriction of ≤3% above the patient's minimum weight during the week prior to injection.

May result in an increased susceptibility to infection; dosage of concomitant immunosuppressants should be reduced during OKT_3 therapy; cyclosporine should be ↓ to 50% usual maintenance dose and maintenance therapy resumed about 4 days before stopping OKT_3.

Severe pulmonary edema has occurred in patients with fluid overload.

First dose effect (flu-like symptoms, anaphylactic-type reaction): may occur within 30 minutes to 6 hours up to 24 hours after the first dose and may be minimized by using the recommended regimens. See table.

Suggested Prevention/Treatment of Muromonab-CD_3 First-Dose Effects

Adverse Reaction	Effective Prevention or Palliation	Supportive Treatment
Severe pulmonary edema	Clear chest X-ray within 24 hours pre-injection. Weight restriction to ≤3% gain over 7 days pre-injection.	Prompt intubation and oxygenation 24 hours close observation.
Fever, chills	15 mg/kg methylprednisolone sodium succinate 1 hour pre-injection. Fever reduction to <37.8°C (100°F) 1 hour pre-injection. Acetaminophen (1 g orally) and diphenhydramine (50 mg orally) 1 hour pre-injection.	Cooling blanket Acetaminophen PRN
Respiratory effects	100 mg hydrocortisone sodium succinate 30 minutes post-injection.	Additional 100 mg hydrocortisone sodium succinate PRN wheezing. If respiratory distress give epinephrine 1:1,000 (0.3 mL SC).

Cardiopulmonary resuscitation may be needed. If the patient's temperature is >37.8°C, reduce before administering OKT_3

Adverse Reactions

>10%:
- Cardiovascular: Tachycardia (including ventricular)
- Central nervous system: Dizziness, faintness
- Gastrointestinal: Diarrhea, nausea, vomiting
- Neuromuscular & skeletal: Trembling
- Respiratory: Shortness of breath

1% to 10%:
- Central nervous system: Headache
- Neuromuscular & skeletal: Stiff neck
- Ocular: Photophobia
- Respiratory: Pulmonary edema

<1%:
- Cardiovascular: Hypertension, hypotension, chest pain, tightness
- Central nervous system: Aseptic meningitis, seizures, fatigue, confusion, coma, hallucinations, pyrexia
- Dermatologic: Pruritus, rash
- Neuromuscular & skeletal: Arthralgia, tremor

(Continued)

Muromonab-CD3 *(Continued)*

Renal: Increased BUN and creatinine
Respiratory: Dyspnea, wheezing
Miscellaneous: Sensitivity reactions: Anaphylactic-type reactions, flu-like symptoms (ie, fever, chills), infection

Drug Interactions
Decreased effect: Immunosuppressive drugs; it is recommended ↓ dose of azathioprine to 1 mg/kg and ↓ dose of cyclosporine by 50% until 4 days prior to stopping OKT_3

Stability Refrigerate; do not shake or freeze; stable in Becton Dickinson syringe for 16 hours at room temperature or refrigeration

Mechanism of Action Reverses graft rejection by binding to T-cells and interfering with their function

Pharmacodynamics/Kinetics
Absorption: I.V.: Immediate
Time to steady-state: Trough level: 3-14 days; pretreatment levels are restored within 7 days after treatment is terminated

Usual Dosage I.V. (refer to individual protocols):
Children <30 kg: 2.5 mg/day once daily for 7-14 days
Children >30 kg: 5 mg/day once daily for 7-14 days
OR
Children <12 years: 0.1 mg/kg/day once daily for 10-14 days
Children ≥12 years and Adults: 5 mg/day once daily for 10-14 days
Hemodialysis: Molecular size of OKT_3 is 150,000 daltons; not dialyzed by most standard dialyzers; however, may be dialyzed by high flux dialysis; OKT_3 will be removed by plasmapheresis; administer following dialysis treatments
Peritoneal dialysis: Significant drug removal is unlikely based on physiochemical characteristics

Administration Filter each dose through a low protein-binding 0.22 micron filter (Millex GV) before administration; administer I.V. push over <1 minute at a final concentration of 1 mg/mL

Children and Adults:
Methylprednisolone sodium succinate 15 mg/kg I.V. given prior to first muromonab-CD3 administration and I.V. hydrocortisone sodium succinate 50-100 mg given 30 minutes after administration are strongly recommended to decrease the incidence of reactions to the first dose
Patient temperature should not exceed 37.8°C (100°F) at time of administration

Monitoring Parameters Chest x-ray, weight gain, CBC with differential, temperature, vital signs (blood pressure, temperature, pulse, respiration); immunologic monitoring of T cells, serum levels of OKT3

Reference Range
OKT_3 serum concentrations:
Serum level monitoring should be performed in conjunction with lymphocyte subset determinations; Trough concentration sampling best correlates with clinical outcome. Serial monitoring may provide a better early indicator of inadequate dosing during induction or rejection.
Mean serum trough levels rise during the first 3 days, then average 0.9 mcg/mL on days 3-14
Circulating levels ≥0.8 mcg/mL block the function of cytotoxic T cells *in vitro* and *in vivo*
Several recent analysis have suggested appropriate dosage adjustments of OKT_3 induction course are better determined with OKT_3 serum levels versus lymphocyte subset determination; however, no prospective controlled trials have been performed to validate the equivalency of these tests in predicting clinical outcome.

Lymphocyte subset monitoring: CD3+ cells: Trough sample measurement is preferable and reagent utilized defines reference range.
OKT_3-FITC: <10-50 cells/mm³ or <3% to 5%
CD3(IgG1)-FITC: similar to OKT_3-FITC
Leu-4a: Higher number of CD3+ cells appears acceptable
Dosage adjustments should be made in conjunction with clinical response and based upon trends over several consecutive days

Patient Information Inform patient of expected first dose effects which are markedly reduced with subsequent treatments

Nursing Implications Do not administer I.M., monitor patient closely for 24 hours after the first dose; drugs and equipment for treating pulmonary edema and anaphylaxis should be on hand

Dosage Forms Injection: 5 mg/5 mL

Muroptic-5® [OTC] *see* Sodium Chloride *on page 1142*
Muro's Opcon® *see* Naphazoline *on page 879*

Muse® Pellet *see* Alprostadil *on page 51*

Mus-Lax® *see* Chlorzoxazone *on page 266*

Mustargen® *see* Mechlorethamine *on page 767*

Mustine *see* Mechlorethamine *on page 767*

Mutamycin® *see* Mitomycin *on page 846*

M.V.I.® *see* Vitamins, Multiple *on page 1310*

Myambutol® *see* Ethambutol *on page 478*

Mycelex® *see* Clotrimazole *on page 302*

Mycelex®-7 *see* Clotrimazole *on page 302*

Mycelex®-G *see* Clotrimazole *on page 302*

Mycifradin® Sulfate *see* Neomycin *on page 887*

Mycinettes® [OTC] *see* Benzocaine *on page 138*

Mycitracin® Topical [OTC] *see* Bacitracin, Neomycin, and Polymyxin B *on page 129*

Mycobutin® *see* Rifabutin *on page 1105*

Mycogen II Topical *see* Nystatin and Triamcinolone *on page 920*

Mycolog®-II Topical *see* Nystatin and Triamcinolone *on page 920*

Myconel® Topical *see* Nystatin and Triamcinolone *on page 920*

Mycophenolate (mye koe FEN oh late)

Brand Names CellCept®

Synonyms Mycophenolate Mofetil

Therapeutic Category Immunosuppressant Agent

Use Immunosuppressant used with corticosteroids and cyclosporine to prevent organ rejection in patients receiving allogenic renal transplants. Treatment of rejection in liver transplant patients unable to tolerate tacrolimus or cyclosporine due to neurotoxicity; mild rejection in heart transplant patients. Treatment of moderate-severe psoriasis.

Pregnancy Risk Factor C

Contraindications Hypersensitivity to mycophenolate mofetil, mycophenolic acid or any ingredient

Warnings/Precautions Increased risk for infection and development of lymphoproliferative disorders. Patients should be monitored appropriately and given supportive treatment should these conditions occur. Increased toxicity in patients with renal impairment. Should be used with caution in patients with active peptic ulcer disease.

Adverse Reactions See table.

Drug Interactions

Decreased effect: Antacids decrease C_{max} and AUC, **do not administer together**; cholestyramine decreases AUC, **do not administer together**

Increased toxicity: Acyclovir and ganciclovir levels may elevate due to competition for tubular secretion of these drugs; probenecid may elevate mycophenolate levels due to inhibition of tubular secretion; salicylates: high doses may increase free fraction of mycophenolic acid

Mechanism of Action Inhibition of purine synthesis of human lymphocytes and proliferation of human lymphocytes

Pharmacodynamics/Kinetics

Absorption: Mycophenolate mofetil is hydrolyzed to mycophenolic acid in the liver and gastrointestinal tract; food does not alter the extent of absorption, but the maximum concentration is decreased

Protein binding: 97%

Metabolism: Mycophenolate mofetil is metabolized to the acid form which is pharmacologically active; mycophenolic acid is glucuronidated to an inactive form; enterohepatic cycling of mycophenolic acid may occur.

Elimination: Mycophenolic acid glucuronide is excreted in the urine and bile. 87% of mycophenolic acid dose has been recovered in urine as inactive glucuronide metabolite.

Half-life: 18 hours

Serum concentrations: Correlation of toxicity or efficacy is still being developed, however, one study indicated that 12-hour AUCs of >40 mcg/mL/hour were correlated with efficacy and decreased episodes of rejection

Usual Dosage Oral:

Children: Doses of 15-23 mg/kg given twice daily have been used, further studies are necessary

Adults: 1 g twice daily within 72 hours of transplant (although 3 g/day has been given in some clinical trials, there was decreased tolerability and no efficacy advantage)

Dosage adjustment in renal impairment: Doses >2 g/day are not recommended in these patients because of the possibility for enhanced immunosuppression as well as toxicities

Dosage adjustment for neutropenia: Dose should be decreased or stopped in patients who develop severe neutropenia (ANC <1.3 x $10^3/\mu L$)

Patient Information Take on an empty stomach

Dosage Forms Capsule, as mofetil: 250 mg

Adverse Reactions Reported in >10%

Adverse Reaction	MM 2 g/day	MM 3 g/day
Body as a whole		
Pain	33	31.2
Abdominal pain	12.1-24.7	11.9-27.6
Fever	20.4	23.3
Headache	20.1	16.1
Infection	12.7-18.2	15.6-20.9
Sepsis	17.6-20.8	17.5-19.7
Asthenia	13.7	16.1
Chest pain	13.4	13.3
Back pain	11.6	12.1
Hypertension	17.6-32.4	16.9-28.2
Central nervous system		
Tremor	11	11.8
Insomnia	8.9	11.8
Dizziness	5.7	11.2
Dermatologic		
Acne	10.1	9.7
Rash	7.7	6.4
Gastrointestinal		
Diarrhea	16.4-31	18.8-36.1
Constipation	21.9	18.5
Nausea	19.9	23.6
Dyspepsia	17.6	13.6
Vomiting	12.5	13.6
Nausea & vomiting	10.4	9.7
Oral monoliasis	10.1	12.1
Hemic/Lymphatic		
Anemia	25.6	25.8
Leukopenia	11.5-23.2	16.3-34.5
Thrombocytopenia	10.1	8.2
Hypochromic anemia	7.4	11.5
Leukocytosis	7.1	10.9
Metabolic/Nutritional		
Peripheral edema	28.6	27
Hypercholesterolemia	12.8	8.5
Hypophosphatemia	12.5	15.8
Edema	12.2	11.8
Hypokalemia	10.1	10
Hyperkalemia	8.9	10.3
Hyperglycemia	8.6	12.4
Respiratory		
Infection	15.8-21	13.1-23.9
Dyspnea	15.5	17.3
Cough increase	15.5	13.3
Pharyngitis	9.5	11.2
Bronchitis	8.5	11.9
Pneumonia	3.6	10.6
Urogenital		
UTI	37.2-45.5	37-44.4
Hematuria	14	12.1
Kidney tubular necrosis	6.3	10
Urinary tract disorder	6.7	10.6

Mycophenolate Mofetil *see* Mycophenolate *on page 865*
Mycostatin® *see* Nystatin *on page 919*
Myco-Triacet® II *see* Nystatin and Triamcinolone *on page 920*
Mydfrin® Ophthalmic Solution *see* Phenylephrine *on page 989*
Mydriacyl® *see* Tropicamide *on page 1275*
Mykrox® *see* Metolazone *on page 826*
Mylanta® Gas [OTC] *see* Simethicone *on page 1136*
Myleran® *see* Busulfan *on page 174*
Mylicon® [OTC] *see* Simethicone *on page 1136*
Myochrysine® *see* Gold Sodium Thiomalate *on page 582*
Myotonachol™ *see* Bethanechol *on page 150*
Mysoline® *see* Primidone *on page 1042*
Mytrex® F Topical *see* Nystatin and Triamcinolone *on page 920*
Mytussin® [OTC] *see* Guaifenesin *on page 589*
Mytussin® AC *see* Guaifenesin and Codeine *on page 590*
Mytussin® DM [OTC] *see* Guaifenesin and Dextromethorphan *on page 591*

Nabumetone (na BYOO me tone)

Related Information

Nonsteroidal Anti-Inflammatory Agents Comparison *on page 1419*

Brand Names Relafen®

Therapeutic Category Analgesic, Nonsteroidal Anti-inflammatory Drug; Anti-inflammatory Agent; Nonsteroidal Anti-inflammatory Agent (NSAID), Oral

Use Management of osteoarthritis and rheumatoid arthritis

Unlabeled use: Sunburn, mild to moderate pain

Pregnancy Risk Factor C

Contraindications Hypersensitivity to nabumetone; should not be administered to patients with active peptic ulceration and those with severe hepatic impairment or in patients in whom nabumetone, aspirin, or other NSAIDs have induced asthma, urticaria, or other allergic-type reactions; fatal asthmatic reactions have occurred following NSAID administration

Warnings/Precautions Elderly patients may sometimes require lower doses; patients with impaired renal function may need a dose reduction; use with caution in patients with severe hepatic impairment

Adverse Reactions

>10%:
- Central nervous system: Dizziness
- Dermatologic: Rash
- Gastrointestinal: Abdominal cramps, heartburn, indigestion, nausea

1% to 10%:
- Central nervous system: Headache, nervousness
- Dermatologic: Itching
- Endocrine & metabolic: Fluid retention
- Gastrointestinal: Vomiting
- Otic: Tinnitus

<1%:
- Cardiovascular: Congestive heart failure, hypertension, arrhythmia, tachycardia
- Central nervous system: Confusion, hallucinations, aseptic meningitis, mental depression, drowsiness, insomnia
- Dermatologic: Angioedema, urticaria, erythema multiforme, toxic epidermal necrolysis, Stevens-Johnson syndrome
- Endocrine & metabolic: Polydipsia, hot flashes
- Gastrointestinal: Gastritis, GI ulceration
- Genitourinary: Cystitis, polyuria
- Hematologic: Agranulocytosis, anemia, hemolytic anemia, bone marrow suppression, leukopenia, thrombocytopenia
- Hepatic: Hepatitis
- Neuromuscular & skeletal: Peripheral neuropathy
- Ocular: Toxic amblyopia, blurred vision, conjunctivitis, dry eyes
- Otic: Decreased hearing
- Renal: Acute renal failure
- Respiratory: Allergic rhinitis, shortness of breath, epistaxis

Mechanism of Action Nabumetone is a nonacidic, nonsteroidal anti-inflammatory drug that is rapidly metabolized after absorption to a major active metabolite, 6-methoxy-2-naphthylacetic acid. As found with previous nonsteroidal anti-inflammatory drugs, nabumetone's active metabolite inhibits the cyclo-

(Continued)

Nabumetone *(Continued)*

oxygenase enzyme which is indirectly responsible for the production of inflammation and pain during arthritis by way of enhancing the production of endoperoxides and prostaglandins E_2 and I_2 (prostacyclin). The active metabolite of nabumetone is felt to be the compound primarily responsible for therapeutic effect. Comparatively, the parent drug is a poor inhibitor of prostaglandin synthesis.

Pharmacodynamics/Kinetics

Distribution: Diffusion occurs readily into synovial fluid with peak concentrations in 4-12 hours

Protein binding: >99%

Metabolism: A prodrug being rapidly metabolized to an active metabolite (6-methoxy-2-naphthylacetic acid); extensive first-pass hepatic metabolism

Half-life, elimination: Major metabolite: 24 hours

Time to peak serum concentration: Metabolite: Oral: Within 3-6 hours

Elimination: 80% recovered in urine and 10% in feces, with very little excreted as unchanged compound

Usual Dosage Adults: Oral: 1000 mg/day; an additional 500-1000 mg may be needed in some patients to obtain more symptomatic relief; may be administered once or twice daily

Dosing adjustment in renal impairment: None necessary; however, adverse effects due to accumulation of inactive metabolites of nabumetone that are renally excreted have not been studied and should be considered

Dietary Considerations

Alcohol: May add to irritant action in the stomach, avoid use if possible

Food: Increases the rate but not the extent of oral absorption. Take without regard to meals OR take with food or milk to minimize GI upset.

Patient Information Take this medication at meal times or with food or milk to minimize gastric irritation; inform your physician if you develop stomach disturbances, blurred vision, or other eye symptoms, rash, weight gain, or edema; inform your physician if you pass dark-colored or tarry stools; concomitant use of alcohol should be avoided, if possible, since it may add to the irritant action of nabumetone in the stomach; aspirin should be avoided

Dosage Forms Tablet: 500 mg, 750 mg

NAC *see* Acetylcysteine *on page 28*

***N*-Acetylcysteine** *see* Acetylcysteine *on page 28*

***N*-Acetyl-L-cysteine** *see* Acetylcysteine *on page 28*

N-Acetyl-P-Aminophenol *see* Acetaminophen *on page 19*

NaCl *see* Sodium Chloride *on page 1142*

Nadolol (nay DOE lole)

Related Information

Beta-Blockers Comparison *on page 1398*

Brand Names Corgard®

Canadian/Mexican Brand Names Apo-Nadol® (Canada); Syn-Nadolol® (Canada)

Therapeutic Category Antianginal Agent; Antihypertensive; Beta-Adrenergic Blocker

Use Treatment of hypertension and angina pectoris; prevention of myocardial infarction; prophylaxis of migraine headaches

Pregnancy Risk Factor C

Pregnancy/Breast-Feeding Implications

Clinical effects on the fetus: No data available on crossing the placenta. Bradycardia, hypotension, hypoglycemia, respiratory depression, hypothermia, IUGR reported. IUGR probably related to maternal hypertension. Alternative beta-blockers are preferred for use during pregnancy due to limited data. Monitor breast-fed infant for symptoms of beta-blockade.

Breast-feeding/lactation: Crosses into breast milk. American Academy of Pediatrics considers COMPATIBLE with breast-feeding.

Contraindications Uncompensated congestive heart failure, cardiogenic shock, bradycardia or heart block, hypersensitivity to any component, bronchial asthma, bronchospasms, diabetes mellitus

Warnings/Precautions Increase dosing interval in patients with renal dysfunction; abrupt withdrawal of beta-blockers may result in an exaggerated cardiac beta-adrenergic responsiveness; symptomatology has included reports of tachycardia, hypertension, ischemia, angina, myocardial infarction, and sudden death; it is recommended that patients be tapered gradually off of beta-blockers over a period of 1-2 weeks rather than via abrupt discontinuation; use with caution in patients with bronchial asthma, bronchospasms, CHF, or diabetes mellitus

Adverse Reactions

>10%: Cardiovascular: Bradycardia

1% to 10%:
- Cardiovascular: Reduced peripheral circulation
- Central nervous system: Mental depression, dizziness
- Endocrine & metabolic: Decreased sexual ability
- Gastrointestinal: Constipation
- Neuromuscular & skeletal: Weakness
- Respiratory: Dyspnea, wheezing

<1%:
- Cardiovascular: Congestive heart failure, chest pain, orthostatic hypotension, Raynaud's syndrome, edema
- Central nervous system: Drowsiness, nightmares, vivid dreams, paresthesia of toes and fingers, insomnia, lethargy, fatigue, confusion, headache
- Dermatologic: Itching, rash
- Gastrointestinal: Vomiting, stomach discomfort, diarrhea, nausea
- Genitourinary: Impotence
- Hematologic: Thrombocytopenia
- Ocular: Dry eyes
- Respiratory: Nasal congestion
- Miscellaneous: Cold extremities

Overdosage/Toxicology Symptoms of intoxication include cardiac disturbances, CNS toxicity, bronchospasm, hypoglycemia and hyperkalemia. The most common cardiac symptoms include hypotension and bradycardia; atrioventricular block, intraventricular conduction disturbances, cardiogenic shock, and asystole may occur with severe overdose; CNS effects include convulsions, coma, and respiratory arrest

Treatment includes symptomatic treatment of seizures, hypotension, hyperkalemia and hypoglycemia; bradycardia and hypotension resistant to atropine, isoproterenol or pacing may respond to glucagon; wide QRS defects caused by the membrane-depressant poisoning may respond to hypertonic sodium bicarbonate; repeat-dose charcoal, hemoperfusion, or hemodialysis may be helpful in removal of only those beta-blockers with a small V_d, long half-life or low intrinsic clearance (acebutolol, atenolol, nadolol, sotalol).

Drug Interactions

- Decreased effect of beta-blockers with aluminum salts, barbiturates, calcium salts, cholestyramine, colestipol, NSAIDs, penicillins (ampicillin), rifampin, salicylates and sulfinpyrazone due to decreased bioavailability and plasma levels
- Beta-blockers may decrease the effect of sulfonylureas
- Increased effect/toxicity of beta-blockers with calcium blockers (diltiazem, felodipine, nicardipine), contraceptives, flecainide, haloperidol (propranolol, hypotensive effects), H_2-antagonists (metoprolol, propranolol only by cimetidine, possibly ranitidine), hydralazine (metoprolol, propranolol), loop diuretics (propranolol, not atenolol), MAO inhibitors (metoprolol, nadolol, bradycardia), phenothiazines (propranolol), propafenone (metoprolol, propranolol), quinidine (in extensive metabolizers), ciprofloxacin, thyroid hormones (metoprolol, propranolol, when hypothyroid patient is converted to euthyroid state)
- Beta-blockers may increase the effect/toxicity of flecainide, haloperidol (hypotensive effects), hydralazine, phenothiazines, acetaminophen, anticoagulants (propranolol, warfarin), benzodiazepines (not atenolol), clonidine (hypertensive crisis after or during withdrawal of either agent), epinephrine (initial hypertensive episode followed by bradycardia), nifedipine and verapamil lidocaine, ergots (peripheral ischemia), prazosin (postural hypotension)
- Beta-blockers may affect the action or levels of ethanol, disopyramide, nondepolarizing muscle relaxants and theophylline although the effects are difficult to predict

Mechanism of Action Competitively blocks response to $beta_1$- and $beta_2$-adrenergic stimulation; does not exhibit any membrane stabilizing or intrinsic sympathomimetic activity

Pharmacodynamics/Kinetics

- Duration of effect: 24 hours
- Absorption: Oral: 30% to 40%
- Time to peak serum concentration: Within 2-4 hours persisting for 17-24 hours
- Distribution: Concentration in human breast milk is 4.6 times higher than serum
- Protein binding: 28%
- Half-life: Adults: 10-24 hours; increased half-life with decreased renal function
  - End stage renal disease: 45 hours
- Elimination: Renally unchanged

Usual Dosage Oral:

- Children: No information regarding pediatric dosage is currently available in the literature
- Adults: Initial: 40-80 mg/day, increase dosage gradually by 40-80 mg increments at 3- to 7-day intervals until optimum clinical response is obtained with profound slowing of heart rate; doses up to 160-240 mg/day in angina and 240-

(Continued)

Nadolol *(Continued)*

320 mg/day in hypertension may be necessary; doses as high as 640 mg/day have been used

Elderly: Initial: 20 mg/day; increase doses by 20 mg increments at 3- to 7-day intervals; usual dosage range: 20-240 mg/day

Dosing adjustment in renal impairment:

Cl_{cr} 31-40 mL/minute: Administer every 24-36 hours or administer 50% of normal dose

Cl_{cr} 10-30 mL/minute: Administer every 24-48 hours or administer 50% of normal dose

Cl_{cr} <10 mL/minute: Administer every 40-60 hours or administer 25% of normal dose

Hemodialysis: Moderately dialyzable (20% to 50%); administer dose postdialysis or administer 40 mg supplemental dose

Peritoneal dialysis: Supplemental dose is not necessary

Dosing adjustment/comments in hepatic disease: Reduced dose probably necessary

Patient Information Adhere to dosage regimen; watch for postural hypotension; abrupt withdrawal of the drug should be avoided; take at the same time each day; may mask symptoms of diabetes; sweating will continue

Nursing Implications Patient's therapeutic response may be evaluated by looking at blood pressure, apical and radial pulses

Dosage Forms Tablet: 20 mg, 40 mg, 80 mg, 120 mg, 160 mg

Nafarelin (NAF a re lin)

Brand Names Synarel®

Synonyms Nafarelin Acetate

Therapeutic Category Hormone, Posterior Pituitary; Luteinizing Hormone-Releasing Hormone Analog

Use Treatment of endometriosis, including pain and reduction of lesions; treatment of central precocious puberty (gonadotropin-dependent precocious puberty) in children of both sexes

Pregnancy Risk Factor X

Contraindications Hypersensitivity to GnRH, GnRH-agonist analogs or any components of this product; undiagnosed abnormal vaginal bleeding; pregnancy; lactation

Warnings/Precautions Use with caution in patients with risk factors for decreased bone mineral content, nafarelin therapy may pose an additional risk; hypersensitivity reactions occur in 0.2% of the patients; safety and efficacy in children have not been established

Adverse Reactions

>10%:

Central nervous system: Headache, emotional lability

Dermatologic: Acne

Endocrine & metabolic: Hot flashes, decreased libido, decreased breast size

Genitourinary: Vaginal dryness

Neuromuscular & skeletal: Myalgia

Respiratory: Nasal irritation

1% to 10%:

Cardiovascular: Edema, chest pain

Central nervous system: Insomnia

Dermatologic: Urticaria, rash, pruritus, seborrhea

Respiratory: Shortness of breath

<1%:

Endocrine & metabolic: Increased libido

Gastrointestinal: Weight loss

Stability Store at room temperature; protect from light

Mechanism of Action Potent synthetic decapeptide analogue of gonadotropin-releasing hormone (GnRH; LHRH) which is approximately 200 times more potent than GnRH in terms of pituitary release of luteinizing hormone (LH) and follicle-stimulating hormone (FSH). Effects on the pituitary gland and sex hormones are dependent upon its length of administration. After acute administration, an initial stimulation of the release of LH and FSH from the pituitary is observed; an increase in androgens and estrogens subsequently follows. Continued administration of nafarelin, however, suppresses gonadotrope responsiveness to endogenous GnRH resulting in reduced secretion of LH and FSH and, secondarily, decreased ovarian and testicular steroid production.

Pharmacodynamics/Kinetics

Absorption: Not absorbed from GI tract

Maximum serum concentration: 10-45 minutes

Protein binding: 80% bound to plasma proteins

Usual Dosage

Endometriosis: Adults: Female: 1 spray (200 mcg) in 1 nostril each morning and the other nostril each evening starting on days 2-4 of menstrual cycle for 6 months

Central precocious puberty: Children: Males/Females: 2 sprays (400 mcg) into each nostril in the morning 2 sprays (400 mcg) into each nostril in the evening. If inadequate suppression, may increase dose to 3 sprays (600 mcg) into alternating nostrils 3 times/day.

Patient Information Begin treatment between days 2 and 4 of menstrual cycle; usually menstruation will stop (as well as ovulation), but is not a reliable contraceptive, use of a nonhormonal contraceptive is suggested; full compliance with taking the medicine is very important; do not use nasal decongestant for at least 30 minutes after using nafarelin spray; notify physician if regular menstruation persists

Nursing Implications Do not administer to pregnant or breast-feeding patients; topical nasal decongestant should be used at least 30 minutes after nafarelin use

Additional Information Each spray delivers 200 mcg

Dosage Forms Solution, nasal, as acetate: 2 mg/mL (10 mL)

Nafarelin Acetate *see* Nafarelin *on previous page*

Nafazair® *see* Naphazoline *on page 879*

Nafcil™ *see* Nafcillin *on this page*

Nafcillin (naf SIL in)

Related Information

Antibiotic Treatment of Adults With Infectious Endocarditis *on page 1465*
Bacterial Meningitis Practical Guidelines for Management *on page 1475*
Extravasation Treatment of Other Drugs *on page 1381*

Brand Names Nafcil™; Nallpen®; Unipen®

Synonyms Ethoxynaphthamido Penicillin Sodium; Nafcillin Sodium; Sodium Nafcillin

Therapeutic Category Antibiotic, Penicillin

Use Treatment of susceptible bacterial infections such as osteomyelitis, septicemia, endocarditis, and CNS infections due to penicillinase-producing strains of *Staphylococcus*

Pregnancy Risk Factor B

Contraindications Hypersensitivity to nafcillin or any component or penicillins

Warnings/Precautions Extravasation of I.V. infusions should be avoided; modification of dosage is necessary in patients with both severe renal and hepatic impairment; elimination rate will be slow in neonates; use with caution in patients with cephalosporin hypersensitivity

Adverse Reactions

<1%:

Central nervous system: Fever, pain
Dermatologic: Rash
Gastrointestinal: Nausea, diarrhea
Hematologic: Neutropenia
Local: Thrombophlebitis; oxacillin (less likely to cause phlebitis) is often preferred in pediatric patients
Renal: Acute interstitial nephritis
Miscellaneous: Hypersensitivity reactions

Overdosage/Toxicology Symptoms of penicillin overdose include neuromuscular hypersensitivity (agitation, hallucinations, asterixis, encephalopathy, confusion, and seizures) and electrolyte imbalance with potassium or sodium salts, especially in renal failure

Hemodialysis may be helpful to aid in the removal of the drug from the blood, otherwise most treatment is supportive or symptom directed

Drug Interactions

Decreased effect: Chloramphenicol may decrease nafcillin levels; oral contraceptive may have a decreased effectiveness
Increased effect: Probenecid may increase nafcillin levels
Increased toxicity: Oral anticoagulants, heparin increases risk of bleeding

Stability Refrigerate oral solution after reconstitution; discard after 7 days; reconstituted parenteral solution is stable for 3 days at room temperature and 7 days when refrigerated or 12 weeks when frozen; for I.V. infusion in NS or D_5W, solution is stable for 24 hours at room temperature and 96 hours when refrigerated

Mechanism of Action Interferes with bacterial cell wall synthesis during active multiplication, causing cell wall death and resultant bactericidal activity against susceptible bacteria

Pharmacodynamics/Kinetics

Absorption: Oral: Poor and erratic
(Continued)

Nafcillin *(Continued)*

Distribution: Crosses the placenta
Protein binding: 90%
Half-life:
  Neonates:
    <3 weeks: 2.2-5.5 hours
    4-9 weeks: 1.2-2.3 hours
  Children 1 month to 14 years: 0.75-1.9 hours
  Adults: 0.5-1.5 hours, with normal hepatic function
  End stage renal disease: 1.2 hours
Time to peak serum concentration:
  Oral: Within 2 hours
  I.M.: Within 0.5-1 hour
Elimination: Primarily in bile, and 10% to 30% in urine as unchanged drug; undergoes enterohepatic recycling

Usual Dosage
Children: I.M., I.V.:
  Mild to moderate infections: 50-100 mg/kg/day in divided doses every 6 hours
  Severe infections: 100-200 mg/kg/day in divided doses every 4-6 hours
  Maximum dose: 12 g/day
Adults:
  I.M.: 500 mg every 4-6 hours
  I.V.: 500-2000 mg every 4-6 hours

Dosing adjustment in renal impairment: Not necessary
Dialysis: Not dialyzable (0% to 5%) via hemodialysis; supplemental dosage not necessary with hemo- or peritoneal dialysis or continuous arterio-venous or veno-venous hemofiltration (CAVH/CAVHD)

Administration Administer around-the-clock to promote less variation in peak and trough serum levels

Test Interactions Positive Coombs' test (direct)

Nursing Implications
Extravasation: Use cold packs
  Hyaluronidase (Wydase®): Add 1 mL NS to 150 unit vial to make 150 units/mL of concentration; mix 0.1 mL of above with 0.9 mL NS in 1 mL syringe to make final concentration = 15 units/mL

Additional Information Sodium content of 1 g: 66.7 mg (2.9 mEq)

Dosage Forms
Capsule, as sodium: 250 mg
Powder for injection, as sodium: 500 mg, 1 g, 2 g, 4 g, 10 g
Solution, as sodium: 250 mg/5 mL (100 mL)
Tablet, as sodium: 500 mg

Nafcillin Sodium *see* Nafcillin *on previous page*

Naftifine (NAF ti feen)

Brand Names Naftin®

Synonyms Naftifine Hydrochloride

Therapeutic Category Antifungal Agent, Topical

Use Topical treatment of tinea cruris (jock itch), tinea corporis (ring worm), and tinea pedis (athlete's foot)

Pregnancy Risk Factor B

Contraindications Hypersensitivity to any component

Warnings/Precautions For external use only

Adverse Reactions
>10%: Local: Burning, stinging
1% to 10%:
  Dermatologic: Erythema, itching
  Local: Dryness, irritation

Mechanism of Action Synthetic, broad-spectrum antifungal agent in the allylamine class; appears to have both fungistatic and fungicidal activity. Exhibits antifungal activity by selectively inhibiting the enzyme squalene epoxidase in a dose-dependent manner which results in the primary sterol, ergosterol, within the fungal membrane not being synthesized.

Pharmacodynamics/Kinetics
Absorption: Systemic, 6% for cream, ≤4% for gel
Half-life: 2-3 days
Elimination: Metabolites excreted in urine and feces

Usual Dosage Adults: Topical: Apply cream once daily and gel twice daily (morning and evening) for up to 4 weeks

Patient Information External use only; avoid eyes, mouth, and other mucous membranes; do not use occlusive dressings unless directed to do so; discontinue if irritation or sensitivity develops; wash hands after application

Dosage Forms
Cream, as hydrochloride: 1% (15 g, 30 g, 60 g)
Gel, topical, as hydrochloride: 1% (20 g, 40 g, 60 g)

Naftifine Hydrochloride *see* Naftifine *on previous page*

Naftin® *see* Naftifine *on previous page*

$NaHCO_3$ *see* Sodium Bicarbonate *on page 1140*

Nalbuphine (NAL byoo feen)

Related Information
Drugs and Routes of Administration Not Recommended for Treatment of Cancer Pain *on page 1378*
Narcotic Agonists Comparison *on page 1414*

Brand Names Nubain®

Synonyms Nalbuphine Hydrochloride

Therapeutic Category Analgesic, Narcotic

Use Relief of moderate to severe pain; preoperative analgesia, postoperative and surgical anesthesia, and obstetrical analgesia during labor and delivery

Pregnancy Risk Factor B (D if used for prolonged periods or in high doses at term)

Contraindications Hypersensitivity to nalbuphine or any component, including sulfites

Warnings/Precautions Use with caution in patients with recent myocardial infarction, biliary tract surgery, or sulfite sensitivity; may produce respiratory depression; use with caution in women delivering premature infants; use with caution in patients with a history of drug dependence, head trauma or increased intracranial pressure, decreased hepatic or renal function, or pregnancy

Adverse Reactions
>10%:
Central nervous system: Drowsiness, CNS depression, narcotic withdrawal
Miscellaneous: Histamine release

1% to 10%:
Cardiovascular: Hypotension, flushing
Central nervous system: Dizziness, headache
Dermatologic: Urticaria, rash
Gastrointestinal: Nausea, vomiting, anorexia, xerostomia
Local: Pain at injection site
Neuromuscular & skeletal: Weakness
Respiratory: Pulmonary edema

<1%:
Cardiovascular: Hypertension, tachycardia
Central nervous system: Mental depression, hallucinations, confusion, paradoxical CNS stimulation, nervousness, restlessness, nightmares, insomnia
Gastrointestinal: GI irritation, biliary spasm
Genitourinary: Decreased urination, toxic megacolon, ureteral spasm
Ocular: Blurred vision
Respiratory: Shortness of breath, respiratory depression

Overdosage/Toxicology Symptoms of overdose include CNS depression, respiratory depression, miosis, hypotension, bradycardia

Treatment of an overdose includes support of the patient's airway, establishment of an I.V. line and administration of naloxone 2 mg I.V. (0.01 mg/kg for children) with repeat administration as necessary up to a total of 10 mg.

Drug Interactions Increased toxicity: Barbiturate anesthetics may increase CNS depression

Mechanism of Action Binds to opiate receptors in the CNS, causing inhibition of ascending pain pathways, altering the perception of and response to pain; produces generalized CNS depression

Pharmacodynamics/Kinetics
Peak effect:
I.M.: 30 minutes
I.V.: 1-3 minutes
Metabolism: In the liver
Half-life: 3.5-5 hours
Elimination: Metabolites excreted primarily in feces (via bile) and in urine (~7%)

Usual Dosage I.M., I.V., S.C.:
Children 10 months to 14 years: Premedication: 0.2 mg/kg; maximum: 20 mg/dose
Adults: 10 mg/70 kg every 3-6 hours; maximum single dose: 20 mg; maximum daily dose: 160 mg

Dosing adjustment/comments in hepatic impairment: Use with caution and reduce dose

(Continued)

Nalbuphine *(Continued)*

Dietary Considerations Alcohol: Additive CNS effects, avoid or limit alcohol; watch for sedation

Monitoring Parameters Relief of pain, respiratory and mental status, blood pressure

Patient Information Avoid alcohol, may cause drowsiness, impaired judgment or coordination; may cause physical and psychological dependence with prolonged use; will cause withdrawal in patients currently dependent on narcotics

Nursing Implications Observe patient for excessive sedation, respiratory depression, implement safety measures, assist with ambulation; observe for narcotic withdrawal

Dosage Forms Injection, as hydrochloride: 10 mg/mL (1 mL, 10 mL); 20 mg/mL (1 mL, 10 mL)

Nalbuphine Hydrochloride *see* Nalbuphine *on previous page*

Naldecon® Senior DX [OTC] *see* Guaifenesin and Dextromethorphan *on page 591*

Naldecon® Senior EX [OTC] *see* Guaifenesin *on page 589*

Nalfon® *see* Fenoprofen *on page 509*

Nalidixic Acid (nal i DIKS ik AS id)

Brand Names NegGram®

Synonyms Nalidixinic Acid

Therapeutic Category Antibiotic, Quinolone

Use Treatment of urinary tract infections

Pregnancy Risk Factor B

Contraindications Hypersensitivity to nalidixic acid or any component; infants <3 months of age

Warnings/Precautions Use with caution in patients with impaired hepatic or renal function and prepubertal children; has been shown to cause cartilage degeneration in immature animals; may induce hemolysis in patients with G-6-PD deficiency

Adverse Reactions

>10%: Central nervous system: Dizziness, drowsiness, headache

1% to 10%: Gastrointestinal: Nausea, vomiting

<1%:

- Central nervous system: Increased intracranial pressure, malaise, vertigo, confusion, toxic psychosis, convulsions, fever, chills
- Dermatologic: Rash, urticaria, photosensitivity reactions
- Endocrine & metabolic: Metabolic acidosis
- Hematologic: Leukopenia, thrombocytopenia
- Hepatic: Hepatotoxicity
- Ocular: Visual disturbances

Overdosage/Toxicology Symptoms of overdose include nausea, vomiting, toxic psychosis, convulsions, increased intracranial pressure, metabolic acidosis; severe overdose, intracranial hypertension, increased pressure, and seizures have occurred; after GI decontamination, treatment is symptomatic

Drug Interactions

Decreased effect with antacids

Increased effect of warfarin

Mechanism of Action Inhibits DNA polymerization in late stages of chromosomal replication

Pharmacodynamics/Kinetics

Distribution: Crosses the placenta; appears in breast milk; achieves significant antibacterial concentrations only in the urinary tract

Protein binding: 90%

Metabolism: Partly in the liver

Half-life: 6-7 hours; increases significantly with renal impairment

Time to peak serum concentration: Oral: Within 1-2 hours

Elimination: In urine as unchanged drug and 80% as metabolites; small amounts appear in feces

Usual Dosage Oral:

Children 3 months to 12 years: 55 mg/kg/day divided every 6 hours; suppressive therapy is 33 mg/kg/day divided every 6 hours

Adults: 1 g 4 times/day for 2 weeks; then suppressive therapy of 500 mg 4 times/day

Dosing comments in renal impairment: Cl_{cr} <50 mL/minute: Avoid use

Test Interactions False-positive urine glucose with Clinitest®, false increase in urinary VMA

Patient Information Avoid undue exposure to direct sunlight or use a sunscreen; take 1 hour before meals, but can take with food to decrease GI upset, finish all medication, do not skip doses; if persistent cough occurs, notify physician

Dosage Forms
Suspension, oral (raspberry flavor): 250 mg/5 mL (473 mL)
Tablet: 250 mg, 500 mg, 1 g

Nalidixinic Acid *see* Nalidixic Acid *on previous page*

Nallpen® *see* Nafcillin *on page 871*

***N*-allylnoroxymorphine Hydrochloride** *see* Naloxone *on next page*

Nalmefene (NAL me feen)

Brand Names Revex®

Synonyms Nalmefene Hydrochloride

Therapeutic Category Antidote, Narcotic Agonist

Use Complete or partial reversal of opioid drug effects, including respiratory depression induced by natural or synthetic opioids; reversal of postoperative opioid depression; management of known or suspected opioid overdose (if opioid dependence is suspected, nalmefene should only be used in opioid overdose if the likelihood of overdose is high based on history or the clinical presentation of respiratory depression with concurrent pupillary constriction is present)

Pregnancy Risk Factor B

Pregnancy/Breast-Feeding Implications Limited information available; do not use in pregnant or lactating women if possible

Contraindications Hypersensitivity to nalmefene, naltrexone, or components

Warnings/Precautions May induce symptoms of acute withdrawal in opioid-dependent patients; recurrence of respiratory depression is possible if the opioid involved is long-acting; observe patients until there is no reasonable risk of recurrent respiratory depression; dosage may need to be decreased in renal and hepatic impairment; safety and efficacy have not been established in children; avoid abrupt reversal of opioid effects in patients of high cardiovascular risk or who have received potentially cardiotoxic drugs; animal studies indicate nalmefene may not completely reverse buprenorphine-induced respiratory depression

Adverse Reactions
>10%: Gastrointestinal: Nausea
1% to 10%:
- Cardiovascular: Tachycardia, hypertension
- Central nervous system: Fever, dizziness
- Gastrointestinal: Vomiting
- Miscellaneous: Postoperative pain

<1%:
- Cardiovascular: Hypotension, vasodilation, arrhythmia, bradycardia
- Central nervous system: Headache, chills, nervousness, confusion, somnolence, depression
- Dermatologic: Pruritus
- Gastrointestinal: Diarrhea, xerostomia
- Genitourinary: Urinary retention
- Hepatic: Increased AST
- Neuromuscular & skeletal: Tremor, myoclonus
- Respiratory: Pharyngitis
- Miscellaneous: Withdrawal syndrome

Overdosage/Toxicology No known symptoms in significant overdose; large doses of opioids administered to overcome a full blockade of opioid antagonists, however, has resulted in adverse respiratory and circulatory reactions

Drug Interactions Increased effect: Potential increased risk of seizures exists with use of flumazenil and nalmefene coadministration

Mechanism of Action As a 6-methylene analog of naltrexone, nalmefene acts as a competitive antagonist at opioid receptor sites, preventing or reversing the respiratory depression, sedation, and hypotension induced by opiates; no pharmacologic activity of its own (eg, opioid agonist activity) has been demonstrated

Pharmacodynamics/Kinetics
Onset of action: I.M., S.C.: 5-15 minutes
Distribution: V_d: 8.6 L/kg; rapid
Protein binding: 45%
Metabolism: Hepatic by glucuronide conjugation to metabolites with little or no activity
Bioavailability: I.M., I.V., S.C.: 100%
T_{max}: I.M.: 2.3 hours; I.V.: <2 minutes; S.C.: 1.5 hours
Half-life: 10.8 hours
Time to peak serum concentration: 2.3 hours
Elimination: <5% excreted unchanged in urine, 17% in feces; clearance: 0.8 L/hour/kg

Usual Dosage
Reversal of postoperative opioid depression: Blue labeled product (100 mcg/mL): Titrate to reverse the undesired effects of opioids; initial dose for nonopioid

(Continued)

Nalmefene *(Continued)*

dependent patients: 0.25 mcg/kg followed by 0.25 mcg/kg incremental doses at 2- to 5-minute intervals; after a total dose of >1 mcg/kg, further therapeutic response is unlikely

Management of known/suspected opioid overdose: Green labeled product (1000 mcg/mL): Initial dose: 0.5 mg/70 kg; may repeat with 1 mg/70 kg in 2-5 minutes; further increase beyond a total dose of 1.5 mg/70 kg will not likely result in improved response and may result in cardiovascular stress and precipitated withdrawal syndrome. (If opioid dependency is suspected, administer a challenge dose of 0.1 mg/70 kg; if no withdrawal symptoms are observed in 2 minutes, the recommended doses can be administered.)

Dosing adjustment in renal or hepatic impairment: Not necessary with single uses, however, slow administration (over 60 seconds) of incremental doses is recommended to minimize hypertension and dizziness

Administration Dilute drug (1:1) with diluent and use smaller doses in patients known to be at increased cardiovascular risk; may be administered via I.M. or S.C. routes if I.V. access is not feasible

Nursing Implications Check dosage strength carefully before use to avoid error; monitor patients for signs of withdrawal, especially those physically dependent who are in pain or at high cardiovascular risk

Additional Information Proper steps should be used to prevent use of the incorrect dosage strength; the goal of treatment in the postoperative setting is to achieve reversal of excessive opioid effects without inducing a complete reversal and acute pain

Dosage Forms Injection, as hydrochloride: 100 mcg/mL [blue label] (1 mL); 1000 mcg/mL [green label] (2 mL)

Nalmefene Hydrochloride *see* Nalmefene *on previous page*

Naloxone (nal OKS one)

Related Information

Drugs and Routes of Administration Not Recommended for Treatment of Cancer Pain *on page 1378*

Narcotic Agonists Comparison *on page 1414*

Brand Names Narcan®

Synonyms *N*-allylnoroxymorphine Hydrochloride; Naloxone Hydrochloride

Therapeutic Category Antidote, Narcotic Agonist

Use Reverses CNS and respiratory depression in suspected narcotic overdose; neonatal opiate depression; coma of unknown etiology

Investigational: Shock, PCP and alcohol ingestion

Pregnancy Risk Factor B

Contraindications Hypersensitivity to naloxone or any component

Warnings/Precautions Use with caution in patients with cardiovascular disease; excessive dosages should be avoided after use of opiates in surgery, because naloxone may cause an increase in blood pressure and reversal of anesthesia; may precipitate withdrawal symptoms in patients addicted to opiates, including pain, hypertension, sweating, agitation, irritability, shrill cry, failure to feed

Adverse Reactions

1% to 10%:

- Cardiovascular: Hypertension, hypotension, tachycardia, ventricular arrhythmias
- Central nervous system: Insomnia, irritability, anxiety, narcotic withdrawal
- Dermatologic: Rash
- Gastrointestinal: Nausea, vomiting
- Ocular: Blurred vision
- Miscellaneous: Diaphoresis

Overdosage/Toxicology Naloxone is the drug of choice for respiratory depression that is known or suspected to be caused by an overdose of an opiate or opioid. **Caution:** Naloxone's effects are due to its action on narcotic reversal, not due to any direct effect upon opiate receptors. Therefore, adverse events occur secondarily to reversal (withdrawal) of narcotic analgesia and sedation, which can cause severe reactions.

Drug Interactions Decreased effect of narcotic analgesics

Stability Protect from light; stable in 0.9% sodium chloride and D_5W at 4 mcg/mL for 24 hours; do not mix with alkaline solutions

Mechanism of Action Competes and displaces narcotics at narcotic receptor sites

Pharmacodynamics/Kinetics

Onset of effect:

- Endotracheal, I.M., S.C.: Within 2-5 minutes
- I.V.: Within 2 minutes

Duration: 20-60 minutes; since shorter than that of most opioids, repeated doses are usually needed

Distribution: Crosses the placenta

Metabolism: Primarily by glucuronidation in the liver

Half-life:

Neonates: 1.2-3 hours

Adults: 1-1.5 hours

Elimination: In urine as metabolites

Usual Dosage I.M., I.V. (preferred), intratracheal, S.C.:

Postanesthesia narcotic reversal: Infants and Children: 0.01 mg/kg; may repeat every 2-3 minutes as needed based on response

Opiate intoxication:

Birth (including premature infants) to 5 years or <20 kg: 0.1 mg/kg; repeat every 2-3 minutes if needed; may need to repeat doses every 20-60 minutes

>5 years or ≥20 kg: 2 mg/dose; if no response, repeat every 2-3 minutes; may need to repeat doses every 20-60 minutes

Continuous infusion: I.V.: Children and Adults: If continuous infusion is required, calculate dosage/hour based on effective intermittent dose used and duration of adequate response seen, titrate dose 0.04-0.16 mg/kg/hour for 2-5 days in children, up to 0.8 mg/kg/hour in adults; alternatively, continuous infusion utilizes $^2/_3$ of the initial naloxone bolus on an hourly basis; add 10 times this dose to each liter of D_5W and infuse at a rate of 100 mL/hour; $^1/_2$ of the initial bolus dose should be readministered 15 minutes after initiation of the continuous infusion to prevent a drop in naloxone levels; increase infusion rate as needed to assure adequate ventilation

Narcotic overdose: Adults: I.V.: 0.4-2 mg every 2-3 minutes as needed; may need to repeat doses every 20-60 minutes, if no response is observed after 10 mg, question the diagnosis. **Note:** Use 0.1-0.2 mg increments in patients who are opioid dependent and in postoperative patients to avoid large cardiovascular changes.

Monitoring Parameters Respiratory rate, heart rate, blood pressure

Nursing Implications The use of neonatal naloxone (0.02 mg/mL) is no longer recommended because unacceptable fluid volumes will result, especially to small neonates; the 0.4 mg/mL preparation is available and can be accurately dosed with appropriately sized syringes (1 mL)

Dosage Forms

Injection, as hydrochloride: 0.4 mg/mL (1 mL, 2 mL, 10 mL); 1 mg/mL (2 mL, 10 mL)

Injection, neonatal, as hydrochloride: 0.02 mg/mL (2 mL)

Naloxone Hydrochloride *see* Naloxone *on previous page*

Naltrexone (nal TREKS one)

Related Information

Drugs and Routes of Administration Not Recommended for Treatment of Cancer Pain *on page 1378*

Brand Names ReVia® Oral

Synonyms Naltrexone Hydrochloride

Therapeutic Category Antidote, Narcotic Agonist

Use Adjunct to the maintenance of an opioid-free state in detoxified individual

Pregnancy Risk Factor C

Contraindications Acute hepatitis, liver failure, known hypersensitivity to naltrexone

Warnings/Precautions Dose-related hepatocellular injury is possible; the margin of separation between the apparent safe and hepatotoxic doses appear to be only fivefold or less

Adverse Reactions

>10%:

Central nervous system: Insomnia, nervousness, headache

Gastrointestinal: Abdominal cramping, nausea, vomiting

Neuromuscular & skeletal: Arthralgia

1% to 10%:

Central nervous system: Dizziness

Dermatologic: Rash

Endocrine & metabolic: Polydipsia

Gastrointestinal: Anorexia

Respiratory: Sneezing

<1%:

Central nervous system: Insomnia, irritability, anxiety, narcotic withdrawal

Hematologic: Thrombocytopenia, agranulocytosis, hemolytic anemia

Ocular: Blurred vision

(Continued)

Naltrexone *(Continued)*

Overdosage/Toxicology Symptoms of overdose include clonic-tonic convulsions, respiratory failure; patients receiving up to 800 mg/day for 1 week have shown no toxicity; seizures and respiratory failure have been seen in animals

Mechanism of Action Naltrexone is a cyclopropyl derivative of oxymorphone similar in structure to naloxone and nalorphine (a morphine derivative); it acts as a competitive antagonist at opioid receptor sites

Pharmacodynamics/Kinetics

Duration of action:

50 mg: 24 hours

100 mg: 48 hours

150 mg: 72 hours

Absorption: Oral: Almost completely

Distribution: V_d: 19 L/kg; distributed widely throughout the body but considerable interindividual variation exists

Protein binding: 21%

Metabolism: Undergoes extensive first-pass metabolism to 6-β-naltrexol

Half-life: 4 hours; 6-β-naltrexol: 13 hours

Time to peak serum concentration: Within 60 minutes

Elimination: Principally in urine as metabolites and unchanged drug

Usual Dosage Do not give until patient is opioid-free for 7-10 days as required by urine analysis

Adults: Oral: 25 mg; if no withdrawal signs within 1 hour give another 25 mg; maintenance regimen is flexible, variable and individualized (50 mg/day to 100-150 mg 3 times/week)

Patient Information Will cause narcotic withdrawal; serious overdose can occur after attempts to overcome the blocking effect of naltrexone

Nursing Implications Monitor for narcotic withdrawal

Dosage Forms Tablet, as hydrochloride: 50 mg

Naltrexone Hydrochloride *see* Naltrexone *on previous page*

Nandrolone (NAN droe lone)

Brand Names Androlone®; Androlone®-D; Deca-Durabolin®; Durabolin®; Hybolin™ Decanoate; Hybolin™ Improved; Neo-Durabolic

Synonyms Nandrolone Decanoate; Nandrolone Phenpropionate

Therapeutic Category Androgen

Use Control of metastatic breast cancer; management of anemia of renal insufficiency

Restrictions C-III

Pregnancy Risk Factor X

Contraindications Carcinoma of breast or prostate, nephrosis, pregnancy and infants, hypersensitivity to any component

Warnings/Precautions Monitor diabetic patients carefully; anabolic steroids may cause peliosis hepatis, liver cell tumors, and blood lipid changes with increased risk of arteriosclerosis; use with caution in elderly patients, they may be at greater risk for prostatic hypertrophy; use with caution in patients with cardiac, renal, or hepatic disease or epilepsy

Adverse Reactions

Male:

Postpubertal:

>10%:

Dermatologic: Acne

Endocrine & metabolic: Gynecomastia

Genitourinary: Bladder irritability, priapism

1% to 10%:

Central nervous system: Insomnia, chills

Endocrine & metabolic: Decreased libido, hepatic dysfunction,

Gastrointestinal: Nausea, diarrhea

Genitourinary: Prostatic hypertrophy (elderly)

Hematologic: Iron deficiency anemia, suppression of clotting factors

<1%: Hepatic: Hepatic necrosis, hepatocellular carcinoma

Prepubertal:

>10%:

Dermatologic: Acne

Endocrine & metabolic: Virilism

1% to 10%:

Central nervous system: Chills, insomnia, factors

Dermatologic: Hyperpigmentation

Gastrointestinal: Diarrhea, nausea

Hematologic: Iron deficiency anemia, suppression of clotting

<1%:
Hepatic: Hepatocellular carcinoma
Miscellaneous: Necrosis

Female:
>10%: Endocrine & metabolic: Virilism
1% to 10%:
Central nervous system: Chills, insomnia
Endocrine & metabolic: Hypercalcemia
Gastrointestinal: Nausea, diarrhea
Hematologic: Iron deficiency anemia, suppression of clotting factors
Hepatic: Hepatic dysfunction
<1%: Hepatic: Hepatic necrosis, hepatocellular carcinoma

Drug Interactions Increased toxicity: Oral anticoagulants, insulin, oral hypoglycemic agents, adrenal steroids, ACTH

Mechanism of Action Promotes tissue-building processes, increases production of erythropoietin, causes protein anabolism; increases hemoglobin and red blood cell volume

Pharmacodynamics/Kinetics
Metabolism: In the liver
Elimination: In urine

Usual Dosage Deep I.M. (into gluteal muscle):
Children 2-13 years: (decanoate): 25-50 mg every 3-4 weeks
Adults:
Male:
Breast cancer (phenpropionate): 50-100 mg/week
Anemia of renal insufficiency (decanoate): 100-200 mg/week
Female: 50-100 mg/week
Breast cancer (phenpropionate): 50-100 mg/week
Anemia of renal insufficiency (decanoate): 50-100 mg/week

Administration Inject deeply I.M., preferably into the gluteal muscle

Test Interactions Altered glucose tolerance tests

Patient Information Virilization may occur in female patients; report menstrual irregularities; male patients report persistent penile erections; all patients should report persistent GI distress, diarrhea, dark urine, pale stools, yellow coloring of skin or sclera; diabetic patients should monitor glucose closely

Additional Information Both phenpropionate and decanoate are Injections in oil

Dosage Forms
Injection, as phenpropionate, in oil: 25 mg/mL (5 mL); 50 mg/mL (2 mL)
Injection, as decanoate, in oil: 50 mg/mL (1 mL, 2 mL); 100 mg/mL (1 mL, 2 mL); 200 mg/mL (1 mL)
Injection, repository, as decanoate: 50 mg/mL (2 mL); 100 mg/mL (2 mL); 200 mg/mL (2 mL)

Nandrolone Decanoate *see* Nandrolone *on previous page*

Nandrolone Phenpropionate *see* Nandrolone *on previous page*

Naphazoline (naf AZ oh leen)

Brand Names AK-Con®; Albalon® Liquifilm®; Allerest® Eye Drops [OTC]; Clear Eyes® [OTC]; Comfort® [OTC]; Degest® 2 [OTC]; Estivin® II [OTC]; I-Naphline®; Muro's Opcon®; Nafazair®; Naphcon Forte®; Naphcon® [OTC]; Opcon®; Privine®; VasoClear® [OTC]; Vasocon Regular®

Canadian/Mexican Brand Names Nazil® Ofteno (Mexico)

Synonyms Naphazoline Hydrochloride

Therapeutic Category Adrenergic Agonist Agent, Ophthalmic; Decongestant, Nasal; Nasal Agent, Vasoconstrictor; Ophthalmic Agent, Vasoconstrictor

Use Topical ocular vasoconstrictor; will temporarily relieve congestion, itching, and minor irritation, and to control hyperemia in patients with superficial corneal vascularity

Pregnancy Risk Factor C

Contraindications Hypersensitivity to naphazoline or any component, narrow-angle glaucoma, prior to peripheral iridectomy (in patients susceptible to angle block)

Warnings/Precautions Rebound congestion may occur with extended use; use with caution in the presence of hypertension, diabetes, hyperthyroidism, heart disease, coronary artery disease, cerebral arteriosclerosis, or long-standing bronchial asthma

Adverse Reactions
1% to 10%:
Cardiovascular: Systemic cardiovascular stimulation
Central nervous system: Dizziness, headache, nervousness
Gastrointestinal: Nausea
Local: Transient stinging, nasal mucosa irritation, dryness, rebound congestion
Ocular: Mydriasis, increased intraocular pressure, blurring of vision

(Continued)

Naphazoline *(Continued)*

Respiratory: Sneezing

Overdosage/Toxicology Symptoms of overdose include CNS depression, hypothermia, bradycardia, cardiovascular collapse, apnea, coma

Following initiation of essential overdose management, toxic symptoms should be treated. The patient should be kept warm and monitored for alterations in vital functions. Seizures commonly respond to diazepam (5-10 mg I.V. bolus in adults every 15 minutes if needed up to a total of 30 mg; I.V. 0.25-0.4 mg/kg/dose up to a total of 10 mg for children) or to phenytoin or phenobarbital. Hypotension should be treated with fluids.

Drug Interactions Increased toxicity: Anesthetics (discontinue mydriatic prior to use of anesthetics that sensitize the myocardium to sympathomimetics, ie, cyclopropane, halothane), MAO inhibitors, tricyclic antidepressants → hypertensive reactions

Stability Store in tight, light-resistant containers

Mechanism of Action Stimulates alpha-adrenergic receptors in the arterioles of the conjunctiva and the nasal mucosa to produce vasoconstriction

Pharmacodynamics/Kinetics

Onset of decongestant action: Topical: Within 10 minutes

Duration: 2-6 hours

Elimination: Not well defined

Usual Dosage

Nasal:

- Children:
  - <6 years: Intranasal: Not recommended (especially infants) due to CNS depression
  - 6-12 years: 1 spray of 0.05% into each nostril every 6 hours if necessary; therapy should not exceed 3-5 days
- Children >12 years and Adults: 0.05%, instill 1-2 drops or sprays every 6 hours if needed; therapy should not exceed 3-5 days

Ophthalmic:

- Children <6 years: Not recommended for use due to CNS depression (especially in infants)
- Children >6 years and Adults: Instill 1-2 drops into conjunctival sac of affected eye(s) every 3-4 hours; therapy generally should not exceed 3-4 days

Patient Information Do not use discolored solutions; discontinue eye drops if visual changes or ocular pain occur; notify physician of insomnia, tremor, or irregular heartbeat; stinging, burning, or drying of the nasal mucosa may occur; do not use beyond 72 hours

Nursing Implications Rebound congestion can result with continued use

Dosage Forms Solution, as hydrochloride:

Nasal:

- Drops: 0.05% (20 mL)
- Spray: 0.05% (15 mL)

Ophthalmic: 0.012% (7.5 mL, 30 mL); 0.02% (15 mL); 0.03% (15 mL); 0.1% (15 mL)

Naphazoline Hydrochloride *see* Naphazoline *on previous page*

Naphcon® [OTC] *see* Naphazoline *on previous page*

Naphcon Forte® *see* Naphazoline *on previous page*

Naprelan® *see* Naproxen *on this page*

Naprosyn® *see* Naproxen *on this page*

Naproxen (na PROKS en)

Related Information

Antacid Drug Interactions *on page 1388*

Dosing Data for Acetaminophen and NSAIDs *on page 1377*

Nonsteroidal Anti-Inflammatory Agents Comparison *on page 1419*

Brand Names Aleve® [OTC]; Anaprox®; Naprelan®; Naprosyn®

Canadian/Mexican Brand Names Apo-Naproxen® (Canada); Naxen® (Canada); Novo-Naprox® (Canada); Nu-Naprox® (Canada); Atiquim® (Mexico); Atiflan® (Mexico); Dafloxen® (Mexico); Faraxen® (Mexico); Flanax® (Mexico); Flexen® (Mexico); Flogen® (Mexico); Fuxen® (Mexico); Naprodil® (Mexico); Naxen® (Mexico); Naxil® (Mexico); Pactens® (Mexico): Pronaxil® (Mexico); Supradol® (Mexico); Synflex® (Canada); Synflex® DS (Canada); Velsay® (Mexico)

Synonyms Naproxen Sodium

Therapeutic Category Analgesic, Nonsteroidal Anti-inflammatory Drug; Anti-inflammatory Agent; Antipyretic; Nonsteroidal Anti-inflammatory Agent (NSAID), Oral

Use Management of inflammatory disease and rheumatoid disorders (including juvenile rheumatoid arthritis); acute gout; mild to moderate pain; dysmenorrhea; fever, migraine headache

Pregnancy Risk Factor B (D if used in the 3rd trimester or near delivery)

Contraindications Hypersensitivity to naproxen, aspirin, or other nonsteroidal anti-inflammatory drugs (NSAIDs)

Warnings/Precautions Use with caution in patients with GI disease (bleeding or ulcers), cardiovascular disease (CHF, hypertension), renal or hepatic impairment, and patients receiving anticoagulants; perform ophthalmologic evaluation for those who develop eye complaints during therapy (blurred vision, diminished vision, changes in color vision, retinal changes); NSAIDs may mask signs/symptoms of infections; photosensitivity reported; elderly are at especially high-risk for adverse effects

Adverse Reactions

>10%:

- Central nervous system: Dizziness
- Dermatologic: Pruritus, rash
- Gastrointestinal: Abdominal discomfort, nausea, heartburn, constipation, GI bleeding, ulcers, perforation, indigestion

1% to 10%:

- Central nervous system: Headache, nervousness
- Dermatologic: Itching
- Endocrine & metabolic: Fluid retention
- Gastrointestinal: Vomiting
- Otic: Tinnitus

<1%:

- Cardiovascular: Edema, congestive heart failure, arrhythmias, tachycardia, hypertension
- Central nervous system: Confusion, hallucinations, mental depression, fatigue, drowsiness, insomnia, aseptic meningitis
- Dermatologic: Urticaria, erythema multiforme, toxic epidermal necrolysis, Stevens-Johnson syndrome, angioedema
- Endocrine & metabolic: Polydipsia, hot flashes
- Gastrointestinal: Gastritis, GI ulceration
- Genitourinary: Cystitis, renal dysfunction, polyuria
- Hematologic: Anemia, hemolytic anemia, bone marrow suppression, leukopenia, thrombocytopenia, inhibits platelet aggregation, prolongs bleeding time, agranulocytosis
- Hepatic: Hepatitis
- Neuromuscular & skeletal: Peripheral neuropathy
- Ocular: Toxic amblyopia, blurred vision, conjunctivitis, dry eyes
- Otic: Decreased hearing
- Renal: Acute renal failure
- Respiratory: Shortness of breath, epistaxis, allergic rhinitis

Overdosage/Toxicology Symptoms of overdose include drowsiness, heartburn, vomiting, CNS depression, leukocytosis, renal failure

Management of a nonsteroidal anti-inflammatory drug (NSAID) intoxication is primarily supportive and symptomatic; fluid therapy is commonly effective in managing the hypotension that may occur following an acute NSAID overdose, except when this is due to an acute blood loss. Seizures tend to be very short-lived and often do not require drug treatment; although, recurrent seizures should be treated with I.V. diazepam; since many of the NSAIDs undergo enterohepatic cycling, multiple doses of charcoal may be needed to reduce the potential for delayed toxicities.

Drug Interactions Cytochrome P-450 2C enzyme substrate

Decreased effect of furosemide

Increased toxicity:

- Naproxen could displace other highly protein bound drugs, such as oral anticoagulants, hydantoins, salicylates, sulfonamides, and sulfonylureas
- Naproxen and warfarin may cause a slight increase in free warfarin
- Naproxen and probenecid may cause increased plasma half-life of naproxen
- Naproxen and methotrexate may significantly increase and prolong blood methotrexate concentration, which may be severe or fatal

Mechanism of Action Inhibits prostaglandin synthesis by decreasing the activity of the enzyme, cyclo-oxygenase, which results in decreased formation of prostaglandin precursors

Pharmacodynamics/Kinetics

Analgesia:

- Onset of action: 1 hour
- Duration: Up to 7 hours

Anti-inflammatory:

- Onset of action: Within 2 weeks
- Peak: 2-4 weeks

(Continued)

Naproxen *(Continued)*

Absorption: Oral: Almost 100%

Time to peak serum concentration: Within 1-2 hours and persisting for up to 12 hours

Protein binding: Highly protein bound (>90%); increased free fraction in elderly

Half-life:

Normal renal function: 12-15 hours

End stage renal disease: Unchanged

Usual Dosage Oral:

Children >2 years:

Fever: 2.5-10 mg/kg/dose; maximum: 10 mg/kg/day

Juvenile arthritis: 10 mg/kg/day in 2 divided doses

Adults:

Rheumatoid arthritis, osteoarthritis, and ankylosing spondylitis: 500-1000 mg/day in 2 divided doses; may increase to 1.5 g/day of naproxen base for limited time period

Mild to moderate pain or dysmenorrhea: Initial: 500 mg, then 250 mg every 6-8 hours; maximum: 1250 mg/day naproxen base

Dosing adjustment in hepatic impairment: Reduce dose to 50%

Dietary Considerations

Alcohol: Additive impairment of mental alertness and physical coordination, avoid or limit use

Food: Food may decrease the rate but not the extent of oral absorption. Drug may cause GI upset, bleeding, ulceration, perforation; take with food or milk to minimize GI upset.

Administration Administer with food, milk, or antacids to decrease GI adverse effects

Monitoring Parameters Occult blood loss, periodic liver function test, CBC, BUN, serum creatinine

Test Interactions ↑ chloride (S), ↑ sodium (S), ↑ bleeding time

Patient Information Serious gastrointestinal bleeding can occur as well as ulceration and perforation. Pain may or may not be present. Avoid aspirin and aspirin-containing products while taking this medication. If gastric upset occurs, take with food, milk, or antacid. If gastric adverse effects persist, contact physician. May cause drowsiness, dizziness, blurred vision, and confusion. Use caution when performing tasks which require alertness (eg, driving). Do not take for more than 3 days for fever or 10 days for pain without physician's advice.

Additional Information Naproxen: Naprosyn®; naproxen sodium: Anaprox®; 275 mg of Anaprox® equivalent to 250 mg of Naprosyn®

Dosage Forms

Suspension, oral: 125 mg/5 mL (15 mL, 30 mL, 480 mL)

Tablet, as sodium (Anaprox®): 220 mg (200 mg base); 275 mg (250 mg base); 550 mg (500 mg base)

Tablet:

Aleve®: 200 mg

Naprosyn®: 250 mg, 375 mg, 500 mg

Tablet, controlled release (Naprelan®): 375 mg, 500 mg

Naproxen Sodium *see* Naproxen *on page 880*

Naqua® *see* Trichlormethiazide *on page 1259*

Narcan® *see* Naloxone *on page 876*

Narcotic Agonists Comparison *see page 1414*

Nardil® *see* Phenelzine *on page 982*

Naropin® *see* Ropivacaine *on page 1117*

Nasacort® *see* Triamcinolone *on page 1255*

Nasahist B® *see* Brompheniramine *on page 166*

NāSal™ [OTC] *see* Sodium Chloride *on page 1142*

Nasalcrom® Nasal Solution [OTC] *see* Cromolyn Sodium *on page 317*

Nasalide® Nasal Aerosol *see* Flunisolide *on page 532*

Nasal Moist® [OTC] *see* Sodium Chloride *on page 1142*

Nasarel® Nasal Spray *see* Flunisolide *on page 532*

Natabec® [OTC] *see* Vitamins, Multiple *on page 1310*

Natabec® FA [OTC] *see* Vitamins, Multiple *on page 1310*

Natabec® Rx *see* Vitamins, Multiple *on page 1310*

Natacyn® *see* Natamycin *on next page*

Natalins® [OTC] *see* Vitamins, Multiple *on page 1310*

Natalins® Rx *see* Vitamins, Multiple *on page 1310*

Natamycin (na ta MYE sin)

Brand Names Natacyn®

Synonyms Pimaricin

Therapeutic Category Antifungal Agent, Ophthalmic

Use Treatment of blepharitis, conjunctivitis, and keratitis caused by susceptible fungi (*Aspergillus, Candida*), *Cephalosporium, Curvularia, Fusarium, Penicillium, Microsporum, Epidermophyton, Blastomyces dermatitidis, Coccidioides immitis, Cryptococcus neoformans, Histoplasma capsulatum, Sporothrix schenckii*, and *Trichomonas vaginalis*

Pregnancy Risk Factor C

Contraindications Known hypersensitivity to natamycin or any component

Warnings/Precautions Failure to improve (keratitis) after 7-10 days of administration suggests infection caused by a microorganism not susceptible to natamycin; inadequate as a single agent in fungal endophthalmitis

Adverse Reactions <1%: Ocular: Blurred vision, photophobia, eye pain, eye irritation not present before therapy

Drug Interactions Increased toxicity: Topical corticosteroids (concomitant use contraindicated)

Stability Store at room temperature (8°C to 24°C/46°F to 75°F); protect from excessive heat and light; do not freeze

Mechanism of Action Increases cell membrane permeability in susceptible fungi

Pharmacodynamics/Kinetics

Absorption: Ophthalmic: <2% systemically absorbed

Distribution: Adheres to cornea and is retained in the conjunctival fornices

Usual Dosage Adults: Ophthalmic: Instill 1 drop in conjunctival sac every 1-2 hours, after 3-4 days reduce to one drop 6-8 times/day; usual course of therapy is 2-3 weeks.

Patient Information Shake well before using, do not touch dropper to eye; notify physician if condition worsens or does not improve after 3-4 days

Dosage Forms Suspension, ophthalmic: 5% (15 mL)

Natural Lung Surfactant *see* Beractant *on page 146*

Navane® *see* Thiothixene *on page 1222*

Navelbine® *see* Vinorelbine *on page 1305*

N-B-P® Ointment [OTC] *see* Bacitracin, Neomycin, and Polymyxin B *on page 129*

ND-Stat® *see* Brompheniramine *on page 166*

Nebcin® Injection *see* Tobramycin *on page 1233*

NebuPent™ Inhalation *see* Pentamidine *on page 968*

Nedocromil Sodium (ne doe KROE mil SOW dee um)

Related Information

Asthma, Guidelines for the Diagnosis and Management of *on page 1518*

Estimated Clinical Comparability of Doses for Inhaled Corticosteroids *on page 1522*

Brand Names Tilade® Inhalation Aerosol

Therapeutic Category Antihistamine, Inhalation; Inhalation, Miscellaneous

Use Maintenance therapy in patients with mild to moderate bronchial asthma

Pregnancy Risk Factor B

Contraindications Hypersensitivity to nedocromil or other ingredients in the preparation

Warnings/Precautions Safety and efficacy in children <12 years of age have not been established; if systemic or inhaled steroid therapy is at all reduced, monitor patients carefully; nedocromil is **not** a bronchodilator and, therefore, should not be used for reversal of acute bronchospasm

Adverse Reactions

1% to 10%:

Cardiovascular: Chest pain

Central nervous system: Dizziness, dysphonia, headache, fatigue

Dermatologic: Rash

Gastrointestinal: Nausea, vomiting, dyspepsia, diarrhea, abdominal pain, xerostomia, unpleasant taste

Hepatic: Increased ALT

Neuromuscular & skeletal: Arthritis, tremor

Respiratory: Cough, pharyngitis, rhinitis, bronchitis, upper respiratory infection, bronchospasm, increased sputum production

Stability Store at 2°C to 30°C/36°F to 86°F; do not freeze

Mechanism of Action Inhibits the activation of and mediator release from a variety of inflammatory cell types associated with asthma including eosinophils, neutrophils, macrophages, mast cells, monocytes, and platelets; it inhibits the release of histamine, leukotrienes, and slow-reacting substance of anaphylaxis; it inhibits the development of early and late bronchoconstriction responses to inhaled antigen

(Continued)

Nedocromil Sodium *(Continued)*

Pharmacodynamics/Kinetics

Duration of therapeutic effect: 2 hours
Protein binding, plasma: 89%
Bioavailability: Systemic: 7% to 9% absorption
Half-life: 1.5-2 hours
Elimination: Excreted unchanged in urine

Usual Dosage Children >12 years and Adults: Inhalation: 2 inhalations 4 times/day; may reduce dosage to 2-3 times/day once desired clinical response to initial dose is observed

Additional Information Has no known therapeutic systemic activity when delivered by inhalation

Dosage Forms Aerosol: 1.75 mg/activation (16.2 g)

N.E.E.® 1/35 *see* Ethinyl Estradiol and Norethindrone *on page 486*

Nefazodone (nef AY zoe done)

Related Information

Antidepressant Agents Comparison *on page 1393*

Brand Names Serzone®

Synonyms Nefazodone Hydrochloride

Therapeutic Category Antidepressant

Use Treatment of depression

Pregnancy Risk Factor C

Contraindications Hypersensitivity to nefazodone or any component; concomitant use of any MAO inhibitors, astemizole, or terfenadine

Warnings/Precautions Safety and efficacy in children <18 years of age have not been established; monitor closely and use with extreme caution in patients with cardiac disease, cerebrovascular disease or seizures; very sedating and can be dehydrating; therapeutic effects may take up to 4 weeks to occur; therapy is normally maintained for several months and optimum response is reached to prevent recurrence of depression, discontinue therapy and re-evaluate if priapism occurs

Adverse Reactions

>10%:
- Central nervous system: Headache, drowsiness, insomnia, agitation, dizziness, confusion
- Gastrointestinal: Xerostomia, nausea
- Neuromuscular & skeletal: Tremor

1% to 10%:
- Cardiovascular: Postural hypotension
- Gastrointestinal: Constipation, vomiting
- Neuromuscular & skeletal: Weakness
- Ocular: Blurred vision, amblyopia

<1%:
- Gastrointestinal: Diarrhea
- Genitourinary: Prolonged priapism

Overdosage/Toxicology Symptoms of overdose include drowsiness, vomiting, hypotension, tachycardia, incontinence, coma

Following initiation of essential overdose management, toxic symptoms should be treated. Ventricular arrhythmias often respond to lidocaine 1.5 mg/kg bolus followed by 2 mg/minute infusion with concurrent systemic alkalinization (sodium bicarbonate 0.5-2 mEq/kg I.V.). Seizures usually respond to diazepam I.V. boluses (5-10 mg for adults up to 30 mg or 0.25-0.4 mg/kg/dose for children up to 10 mg/dose). If seizures are unresponsive or recur, phenytoin or phenobarbital may be required. Hypotension is best treated by I.V. fluids and by placing the patient in the Trendelenburg position.

Drug Interactions

Decreased effect: Clonidine, methyldopa, diuretics, oral hypoglycemics, anticoagulants

Increased toxicity: Terfenadine and astemizole (increased concentrations have been associated with serious ventricular arrhythmias and death), fluoxetine, triazolam (reduce triazolam dose by 75%), alprazolam (reduce alprazolam dose by 50%), phenytoin, MAO inhibitors (allow 14 days after MAO inhibitors are stopped or 7 days after nefazodone is stopped); carbamazepine (40% increase); digoxin

Mechanism of Action Inhibits serotonin (5-HT) reuptake and is a potent antagonist at type 2 serotonin (5-HT) receptors; minimal affinity for cholinergic, histaminic, or alpha$_1$-adrenergic receptors

Pharmacodynamics/Kinetics

Onset of effect: Therapeutic effects take at least 2 weeks to appear

Metabolism: In the liver to 3 active metabolites; triazoledione, hydroxynefazodone and m-chlorophenylpiperazine (mCPP)
Half-life: 2-4 hours (parent compound), active metabolites persist longer
Time to peak serum concentration: 30 minutes, prolonged in presence of food
Elimination: Primarily as metabolites in urine and secondarily in feces

Usual Dosage Oral: Adults: 200 mg/day, administered in two divided doses initially, with a range of 300-600 mg/day in two divided doses thereafter

Dietary Considerations Alcohol: Additive CNS effect, avoid use

Reference Range Therapeutic plasma levels have not yet been defined

Patient Information Take shortly after a meal or light snack; can be given at bedtime if drowsiness occurs; optimum effect may take 2-4 weeks to be achieved; avoid alcohol; may cause painful erections (contact physician if this should occur); avoid sudden changes in position

Nursing Implications Dosing after meals may decrease lightheadedness and postural hypotension, but may also decrease absorption and therefore effectiveness; use side rails on bed if administered to the elderly; observe patient's activity and compare with admission level; assist with ambulation; sitting and standing blood pressure and pulse

Dosage Forms Tablet, as hydrochloride: 100 mg, 150 mg, 200 mg, 250 mg

Nefazodone Hydrochloride *see* Nefazodone *on previous page*

NegGram® *see* Nalidixic Acid *on page 874*

Nelfinavir (nel FIN a veer)

Brand Names Viracept®

Therapeutic Category Protease Inhibitor

Use As monotherapy or preferably in combination with nucleoside analogs in the treatment of HIV infection when antiretroviral therapy is warranted

Pregnancy Risk Factor B

Pregnancy/Breast-Feeding Implications Animal studies suggest that nelfinavir may be excreted in human milk; the CDC advises against breast-feeding by HIV-infected mothers to avoid postnatal transmission of the virus to the infant

Contraindications Hypersensitivity to nelfinavir or product components; phenylketonuria; concurrent therapy with terfenadine, astemizole, cisapride, triazolam, or midazolam

Warnings/Precautions Avoid use of powder in phenylketonurics since contains phenylalanine; use extreme caution when administered to patients with hepatic insufficiency since nelfinavir is metabolized in the liver and excreted predominantly in the feces; avoid use, if possible, with terfenadine, astemizole, cisapride, triazolam, or midazolam. Concurrent use with some anticonvulsants may significantly limit nelfinavir's effectiveness.

Adverse Reactions

>10%: Gastrointestinal: Diarrhea

1% to 10%:
- Central nervous system: Decreased concentration
- Dermatologic: Rash
- Gastrointestinal: Nausea, flatulence, abdominal pain
- Neuromuscular & skeletal: Weakness

<1%:
- Central nervous system: Anxiety, depression, dizziness, emotional lability, hyperkinesia, insomnia, migraine, seizures, sleep disorder, somnolence, suicide ideation, fever, headache, malaise
- Dermatologic: Dermatitis, pruritus, urticaria
- Endocrine & metabolic: Increased LFTs, hyperlipemia, hyperuricemia, hypoglycemia
- Gastrointestinal: Anorexia, dyspepsia, epigastric pain, mouth ulceration, GI bleeding, pancreatitis, vomiting
- Genitourinary: Kidney calculus, sexual dysfunction
- Hematologic: Anemia, leukopenia, thrombocytopenia
- Hepatic: Hepatitis
- Neuromuscular & skeletal: Arthralgia, arthritis, cramps, myalgia, myasthenia, myopathy, paresthesia, back pain
- Respiratory: Dyspnea, pharyngitis, rhinitis, sinusitis
- Miscellaneous: Diaphoresis, allergy

Overdosage/Toxicology No data available; however, unabsorbed drug should be removed via gastric lavage and activated charcoal; significant symptoms beyond gastrointestinal disturbances is likely following acute overdose; hemodialysis will not be effective due to high protein binding of nelfinavir

Drug Interactions Unlike other protease inhibitors, nelfinavir may be administered with dapsone, trimethoprim/sulfamethoxazole, clarithromycin, azithromycin, erythromycin, itraconazole, and fluconazole

(Continued)

Nelfinavir *(Continued)*

Increased effect: Nelfinavir inhibits the metabolism of cisapride, terfenadine, and astemizole and should, therefore, not be administered concurrently due to risk of life-threatening cardiac arrhythmias. A 20% increase in rifabutin plasma AUC has been observed when coadministered with nelfinavir (decrease rifabutin's dose by 50%). An increase in midazolam and triazolam serum levels may occur resulting in significant oversedation when administered with nelfinavir. These drugs should not be administered together. Indinavir and ritonavir may increase nelfinavir plasma concentrations resulting in potential increases in side effects (the safety of these combinations have not been established).

Decreased effect: Rifampin decreases nelfinavir's plasma AUC by ~82%; the two drugs should not be administered together. Serum levels of the hormones in oral contraceptives may decrease significantly with administration of nelfinavir. Patients should use alternative methods of contraceptives during nelfinavir therapy. Phenobarbital, phenytoin, and carbamazepine may decrease serum levels and consequently effectiveness of nelfinavir.

Mechanism of Action Inhibits the HIV-1 protease; inhibition of the viral protease prevents cleavage of the gag-pol polyprotein resulting in the production of immature, noninfectious virus; cross-resistance with other protease inhibitors is possible although, as yet, unknown

Pharmacodynamics/Kinetics

Absorption: Food increases plasma concentration-time curve (AUC) by 2- to 3-fold

Distribution: V_d: 2-7 L/kg

Metabolism: Via multiple cytochrome P-450 isoforms (eg, CYP3A); major metabolite has activity comparable to the parent drug

Protein binding: 98%

Half-life: 3.5-5 hours

Time to peak serum concentration: 2-4 hours

Elimination: 98% to 99% excreted in the feces (78% as metabolites and 22% as unchanged nelfinavir); 1% to 2% excreted in the urine

Usual Dosage Oral:

Children 2-13 years: 20-30 mg/kg 3 times/day with a meal or light snack; if tablets are unable to be taken, use oral powder in small amount of water, milk, formula, or dietary supplements; do not use acidic food/juice or store for >6 hours

Adults: 750 mg 3 times/day with meals

Dosing adjustment in renal impairment: No adjustment needed

Dosing adjustment in hepatic impairment: Use caution when administering to patients with hepatic impairment since eliminated predominantly by the liver

Monitoring Parameters Signs and symptoms of infection, LFTs

Patient Information Nelfinavir should be taken with food to increase its absorption; it is not a cure for HIV infection and the long-term effects of the drug are unknown at this time; the drug has not demonstrated a reduction in the risk of transmitting HIV to others. Take the drug as prescribed; if you miss a dose, take it as soon as possible and then return to your usual schedule (never double a dose, however). If tablets are unable to be taken, use oral powder in small amount of water, milk, formula, or dietary supplement; do not use acidic food/juice of store dilution for >6 hours. Use an alternative method of contraception from birth control pills during nelfinavir therapy.

Nursing Implications If diarrhea occurs, it may be treated with loperamide

Dosage Forms

Powder, oral: 50 mg/g (contains 11.2 mg phenylalanine)

Tablet: 250 mg

Nelova™ 0.5/35E *see* Ethinyl Estradiol and Norethindrone *on page 486*

Nelova™ 1/50M *see* Mestranol and Norethindrone *on page 791*

Nelova™ 10/11 *see* Ethinyl Estradiol and Norethindrone *on page 486*

Nembutal® *see* Pentobarbital *on page 970*

Neo-Calglucon® [OTC] *see* Calcium Glubionate *on page 189*

Neo-Cultol® [OTC] *see* Mineral Oil *on page 841*

Neo-Durabolic *see* Nandrolone *on page 878*

Neofed® [OTC] *see* Pseudoephedrine *on page 1074*

Neo-fradin® *see* Neomycin *on next page*

Neoloid® [OTC] *see* Castor Oil *on page 216*

Neomixin® Topical [OTC] *see* Bacitracin, Neomycin, and Polymyxin B *on page 129*

Neomycin (nee oh MYE sin)

Related Information

Antimicrobial Prophylaxis *on page 1445*

Brand Names Mycifradin® Sulfate; Neo-fradin®; Neo-Tabs®

Synonyms Neomycin Sulfate

Therapeutic Category Ammonium Detoxicant; Antibiotic, Aminoglycoside; Antibiotic, Irrigation; Antibiotic, Topical

Use Prepares GI tract for surgery; treat minor skin infections; treat diarrhea caused by *E. coli*; adjunct in the treatment of hepatic encephalopathy, as irrigant during surgery

Pregnancy Risk Factor C

Contraindications Hypersensitivity to neomycin or any component, or other aminoglycosides; patients with intestinal obstruction

Warnings/Precautions Use with caution in patients with renal impairment, pre-existing hearing impairment, neuromuscular disorders; neomycin is more toxic than other aminoglycosides when given parenterally; **do not administer parenterally**; topical neomycin is a contact sensitizer with sensitivity occurring in 5% to 15% of patients treated with the drug; symptoms include itching, reddening, edema, and failure to heal

Adverse Reactions

1% to 10%:
- Dermatologic: Dermatitis, rash, urticaria, erythema
- Local: Burning
- Ocular: Contact conjunctivitis

<1%:
- Gastrointestinal: Nausea, vomiting, diarrhea
- Neuromuscular & skeletal: Neuromuscular blockade
- Otic: Ototoxicity
- Renal: Nephrotoxicity

Overdosage/Toxicology Symptoms of overdose (rare due to poor oral bioavailability) include ototoxicity, nephrotoxicity, and neuromuscular toxicity

The treatment of choice following a single acute overdose appears to be the maintenance of good urine output of at least 3 mL/kg/hour. Dialysis is of questionable value in the enhancement of aminoglycoside elimination. If required, hemodialysis is preferred over peritoneal dialysis in patients with normal renal function. Chelation with penicillin may be of benefit.

Drug Interactions

Decreased effect: May decrease GI absorption of digoxin and methotrexate

Increased effect: Synergistic effects with penicillins

Increased toxicity:
- Oral neomycin may potentiate the effects of oral anticoagulants
- Increased adverse effects with other neurotoxic, ototoxic, or nephrotoxic drugs

Stability Use reconstituted parenteral solutions within 7 days of mixing, when refrigerated

Mechanism of Action Interferes with bacterial protein synthesis by binding to 30S ribosomal subunits

Pharmacodynamics/Kinetics

Absorption: Oral, percutaneous: Poor (3%)

Distribution: V_d: 0.36 L/kg

Metabolism: Slight hepatic

Half-life: 3 hours (age and renal function dependent)

Time to peak serum concentration:
- Oral: 1-4 hours
- I.M.: Within 2 hours

Elimination: In urine (30% to 50% as unchanged drug); 97% of an oral dose eliminated unchanged in feces

Usual Dosage

Children: Oral:
- Preoperative intestinal antisepsis: 90 mg/kg/day divided every 4 hours for 2 days; or 25 mg/kg at 1 PM, 2 PM, and 11 PM on the day preceding surgery as an adjunct to mechanical cleansing of the intestine and in combination with erythromycin base
- Hepatic coma: 50-100 mg/kg/day in divided doses every 6-8 hours or 2.5-7 g/m²/day divided every 4-6 hours for 5-6 days not to exceed 12 g/day

Children and Adults: Topical: Apply ointment 1-4 times/day; topical solutions containing 0.1% to 1% neomycin have been used for irrigation

Adults: Oral:
- Preoperative intestinal antisepsis: 1 g each hour for 4 doses then 1 g every 4 hours for 5 doses; or 1 g at 1 PM, 2 PM, and 11 PM on day preceding surgery as an adjunct to mechanical cleansing of the bowel and oral erythromycin; or 6 g/day divided every 4 hours for 2-3 days

(Continued)

Neomycin *(Continued)*

Hepatic coma: 500-2000 mg every 6-8 hours or 4-12 g/day divided every 4-6 hours for 5-6 days

Chronic hepatic insufficiency: 4 g/day for an indefinite period

Hemodialysis: Dialyzable (50% to 100%)

Monitoring Parameters Renal function tests

Patient Information Notify physician if redness, burning, or itching occurs of if condition does not improve in 3-4 days

Dosage Forms

Cream, as sulfate: 0.5% (15 g)
Injection, as sulfate: 500 mg
Ointment, topical, as sulfate: 0.5% (15 g, 30 g, 120 g)
Solution, oral, as sulfate: 125 mg/5 mL (480 mL)
Tablet, as sulfate: 500 mg [base 300 mg]

Neomycin and Polymyxin B (nee oh MYE sin & pol i MIKS in bee)

Brand Names Neosporin® Cream [OTC]; Neosporin® G.U. Irrigant

Synonyms Polymyxin B and Neomycin

Therapeutic Category Antibiotic, Topical; Antibiotic, Urinary Irrigation

Use Short-term as a continuous irrigant or rinse in the urinary bladder to prevent bacteriuria and gram-negative rod septicemia associated with the use of indwelling catheters; to help prevent infection in minor cuts, scrapes, and burns; treatment of superficial ocular infections involving the conjunctiva or cornea

Pregnancy Risk Factor C (D G.U. irrigant)

Contraindications Known hypersensitivity to neomycin or polymyxin B or any component; ophthalmic use for topical cream

Warnings/Precautions Use with caution in patients with impaired renal function, infants with diaper rash involving large area of abraded skin, dehydrated patients, burn patients, and patients receiving a high-dose for prolonged periods; topical neomycin is a contact sensitizer; contains methylparaben

Adverse Reactions

1% to 10%:

Dermatologic: Contact dermatitis, erythema, rash, urticaria
Genitourinary: Bladder irritation
Local: Burning
Neuromuscular & skeletal: Neuromuscular blockade
Otic: Ototoxicity
Renal: Nephrotoxicity

Overdosage/Toxicology Refer to individual monographs for Neomycin and Polymyxin B

Stability Store irrigation solution in refrigerator; aseptic prepared dilutions (1 mL/1 L) should be stored in the refrigerator and discarded after 48 hours

Mechanism of Action Refer to individual monographs for Neomycin and Polymyxin

Pharmacodynamics/Kinetics Absorption: Topical: Not absorbed following application to intact skin; absorbed through denuded or abraded skin, peritoneum, wounds, or ulcers

Usual Dosage Children and Adults:

Bladder irrigation: **Not for injection**; add 1 mL irrigant to 1 liter isotonic saline solution and connect container to the inflow of lumen of 3-way catheter. Continuous irrigant or rinse in the urinary bladder for up to a maximum of 10 days with administration rate adjusted to patient's urine output; usually no more than 1 L of irrigant is used per day.

Ophthalmic:

Ointment: Instill ½" ribbon into the conjunctival sac every 3-4 hours for acute infections or 2-3 times/day for mild to moderate infections for 7-10 days

Solution: Instill 1-2 drops every 15-30 minutes for acute infections; 1-2 drops every 3-6 hours for mild-moderate infections.

Topical: Apply cream 1-4 times/day to affected area

Monitoring Parameters Urinalysis

Patient Information Notify physician if condition worsens or if rash or irritation develops

Nursing Implications Do not inject irrigant solution; connect irrigation container to the inflow lumen of a 3-way catheter to permit continuous irrigation of the urinary bladder

Dosage Forms

Cream: Neomycin sulfate 3.5 mg and polymyxin B sulfate 10,000 units per g (0.94 g, 15 g)

Solution, irrigant: Neomycin sulfate 40 mg and polymyxin B sulfate 200,000 units per mL (1 mL, 20 mL)

Neomycin, Polymyxin B, and Dexamethasone

(nee oh MYE sin, pol i MIKS in bee, & deks a METH a sone)

Related Information

Toxicities of Chemotherapeutic Agents *on page 1382*

Brand Names AK-Trol®; Dexacidin®; Dexasporin®; Maxitrol®

Therapeutic Category Antibiotic, Ophthalmic; Corticosteroid, Ophthalmic

Use Steroid-responsive inflammatory ocular conditions in which a corticosteroid is indicated and where bacterial infection or a risk of bacterial infection exists

Pregnancy Risk Factor C

Contraindications Hypersensitivity to dexamethasone, polymyxin B, neomycin or any component; herpes simplex, vaccinia, and varicella

Warnings/Precautions Prolonged use may result in glaucoma, defects in visual acuity, posterior subcapsular cataract formation, and secondary ocular infections

Adverse Reactions

1% to 10%:

Dermatologic: Contact dermatitis, delayed wound healing

Ocular: Cutaneous sensitization, eye pain, development of glaucoma, cataract, increased intraocular pressure, optic nerve damage

Overdosage/Toxicology Refer to individual monographs for Neomycin, Polymyxin B, and Dexamethasone

Mechanism of Action Refer to individual monographs for Neomycin Sulfate, Polymyxin B Sulfate, and Dexamethasone

Pharmacodynamics/Kinetics Refer to individual monographs for Neomycin Sulfate, Polymyxin B Sulfate, and Dexamethasone

Usual Dosage Children and Adults: Ophthalmic:

Ointment: Place a small amount (~½") in the affected eye 3-4 times/day or apply at bedtime as an adjunct with drops

Solution: Instill 1-2 drops into affected eye(s) every 3-4 hours; in severe disease, drops may be used hourly and tapered to discontinuation

Monitoring Parameters Intraocular pressure with use >10 days

Patient Information For the eye; shake well before using; tilt head back, place medication in conjunctival sac, and close eyes; do not touch dropper to eye; apply finger pressure on lacrimal sac for 1 minute following instillation; notify physician if condition worsens or does not improve in 3-4 days

Dosage Forms Ophthalmic:

Ointment: Neomycin sulfate 3.5 mg, polymyxin B sulfate 10,000 units and dexamethasone 0.1% per g (3.5 g, 5 g)

Suspension: Neomycin sulfate 3.5 mg, polymyxin B sulfate 10,000 units and dexamethasone 0.1% per mL (5 mL, 10 mL)

Neomycin, Polymyxin B, and Gramicidin

(nee oh MYE sin, pol i MIKS in bee, & gram i SYE din)

Related Information

Antimicrobial Prophylaxis *on page 1445*

Brand Names AK-Spore® Ophthalmic Solution; Neosporin® Ophthalmic Solution; Ocutricin® Ophthalmic Solution

Canadian/Mexican Brand Names Neosporin® Oftalmico (Mexico)

Therapeutic Category Antibiotic, Ophthalmic

Use Treatment of superficial ocular infection, infection prophylaxis in minor skin abrasions

Pregnancy Risk Factor C

Contraindications Hypersensitivity to neomycin, polymyxin B, gramicidin or any component

Warnings/Precautions Symptoms of neomycin sensitization include itching, reddening, edema, failure to heal; prolonged use may result in glaucoma, defects in visual acuity, posterior subcapsular cataract formation, and secondary ocular infections

Adverse Reactions 1% to 10%:

Cardiovascular: Edema

Dermatologic: Itching

Local: Reddening, failure to heal

Ocular: Low grade conjunctivitis

Mechanism of Action Interferes with bacterial protein synthesis by binding to 30S ribosomal subunits; binds to phospholipids, alters permeability, and damages the bacterial cytoplasmic membrane permitting leakage of intracellular constituents

Usual Dosage Children and Adults: Ophthalmic: Instill 1-2 drops 4-6 times/day or more frequently as required for severe infections

Patient Information Tilt head back, place medication in conjunctival sac, and close eyes; apply finger pressure on lacrimal sac for 1 minute following instillation

(Continued)

Neomycin, Polymyxin B, and Gramicidin *(Continued)*

Dosage Forms Solution, ophthalmic: Neomycin sulfate 1.75 mg, polymyxin B sulfate 10,000 units, and gramicidin 0.025 mg per mL (2 mL, 10 mL)

Neomycin, Polymyxin B, and Hydrocortisone

(nee oh MYE sin, pol i MIKS in bee, & hye droe KOR ti sone)

Related Information

Bacitracin, Neomycin, Polymyxin B, and Hydrocortisone *on page 130*

Brand Names AK-Spore H.C.® Ophthalmic Suspension; AK-Spore H.C.® Otic; AntibiOtic® Otic; Bacticort® Otic; Cortatrigen® Otic; Cortisporin® Ophthalmic Suspension; Cortisporin® Otic; Cortisporin® Topical Cream; Drotic® Otic; Ear-Eze® Otic; LazerSporin-C® Otic; Octicair® Otic; Otic-Care® Otic; OtiTricin® Otic; Otocort® Otic; Otomycin-HPN® Otic; Otosporin® Otic; PediOtic® Otic; UAD Otic®

Therapeutic Category Antibiotic, Ophthalmic; Antibiotic, Otic; Antibiotic, Topical; Corticosteroid, Ophthalmic; Corticosteroid, Otic; Corticosteroid, Topical (Low Potency)

Use Steroid-responsive inflammatory condition for which a corticosteroid is indicated and where bacterial infection or a risk of bacterial infection exists

Pregnancy Risk Factor C

Contraindications Known hypersensitivity to hydrocortisone, polymyxin B sulfate or neomycin sulfate; otic use when drum is perforated; herpes simplex, vaccinia, and varicella

Warnings/Precautions Prolonged use can lead to skin thinning, atrophy, sensitization, and development of resistant infections; neomycin may cause cutaneous and conjunctival sensitization; children are more susceptible to topical corticosteroid-induced hypothalamic - pituitary - adrenal axis suppression and Cushing's syndrome. Otic suspension is the preferred otic preparation; otic suspension can be used for the treatment of infections of mastoidectomy and fenestration cavities caused by susceptible organisms; otic solution is used **only** for superficial infections of the external auditory canal (ie, swimmer's ear).

Adverse Reactions

>10%: Hypersensitivity

1% to 10%:

- Dermatologic: Contact dermatitis, erythema, rash, urticaria, itching
- Genitourinary: Bladder irritation
- Local: Burning, pain, edema, stinging
- Neuromuscular & skeletal: Neuromuscular blockade
- Ocular: Elevation of intraocular pressure, glaucoma, cataracts, conjunctival erythema
- Otic: Ototoxicity
- Renal: Nephrotoxicity
- Miscellaneous: Sensitization to neomycin, secondary infections

Overdosage/Toxicology Refer to individual monographs for Neomycin, Polymyxin B, and Hydrocortisone

Mechanism of Action Refer to individual monographs for Neomycin, Polymyxin B, and Hydrocortisone

Usual Dosage Duration of use should be limited to 10 days unless otherwise directed by the physician

Otic solution is used **only** for swimmer's ear (infections of external auditory canal)

Otic:

- Children: Instill 3 drops into affected ear 3-4 times/day
- Adults: Instill 4 drops 3-4 times/day; otic suspension is the preferred otic preparation

Children and Adults:

- Ophthalmic: Drops: Instill 1-2 drops 2-4 times/day, or more frequently as required for severe infections; in acute infections, instill 1-2 drops every 15-30 minutes gradually reducing the frequency of administration as the infection is controlled
- Topical: Apply a thin layer 1-4 times/day

Patient Information

Ophthalmic: May cause sensitivity to bright light; may cause temporary blurring of vision or stinging following administration, but discontinue product and see physician if problems persist or increase; to use, tilt head back and place medication in conjunctival sac and close eyes; apply light pressure on lacrimal sac for 1 minute

Otic: Hold container in hand to warm; if drops are in suspension form, shake well for approximately 10 seconds, lie on your side with affected ear up; for adults hold the ear lobe up and back, for children hold the ear lobe down and back; instill drops in ear without inserting dropper into ear; maintain tilted ear for 2 minutes

Dosage Forms

Cream, topical: Neomycin sulfate 5 mg, polymyxin B sulfate 10,000 units, and hydrocortisone 10 mg per mL (7.5 g)

Solution, otic: Neomycin sulfate 5 mg, polymyxin B sulfate 10,000 units, and hydrocortisone 10 mg per mL (10 mL)

Suspension:

Ophthalmic: Neomycin sulfate 5 mg, polymyxin B sulfate 10,000 units, and hydrocortisone 10 mg per mL (7.5 mL)

Otic: Neomycin sulfate 5 mg, polymyxin B sulfate 10,000 units, and hydrocortisone 10 mg per mL (10 mL)

Neomycin, Polymyxin B, and Prednisolone

(nee oh MYE sin, pol i MIKS in bee, & pred NIS oh lone)

Brand Names Poly-Pred®

Therapeutic Category Antibiotic, Ophthalmic; Corticosteroid, Ophthalmic

Use Steroid-responsive inflammatory ocular condition in which bacterial infection or a risk of bacterial ocular infection exists

Pregnancy Risk Factor C

Contraindications Known hypersensitivity to neomycin, polymyxin B, or prednisolone; dendritic keratitis, viral disease of the cornea and conjunctiva, mycobacterial infection of the eye, fungal disease of the ocular structure, or after uncomplicated removal of a corneal foreign body

Warnings/Precautions Prolonged use may result in overgrowth of nonsusceptible organisms, glaucoma, damage to the optic nerve, defects in visual acuity, and cataract formation; symptoms of neomycin sensitization include itching, reddening, edema, or failure to heal

Adverse Reactions

1% to 10%:

Dermatologic: Cutaneous sensitization, rash, delayed wound healing

Ocular: Increased intraocular pressure, glaucoma, optic nerve damage, cataracts, conjunctival sensitization

Overdosage/Toxicology Refer to individual monographs for Neomycin, Polymyxin B, and Prednisolone

Mechanism of Action Refer to individual monographs for Neomycin, Polymyxin B, and Prednisolone

Pharmacodynamics/Kinetics Refer to individual monographs for Neomycin Sulfate, Polymyxin B Sulfate, and Prednisolone

Usual Dosage Children and Adults: Ophthalmic: Instill 1-2 drops every 3-4 hours; acute infections may require every 30-minute instillation initially with frequency of administration reduced as the infection is brought under control. To treat the lids: Instill 1-2 drops every 3-4 hours, close the eye and rub the excess on the lids and lid margins.

Patient Information Ophthalmic: May cause sensitivity to bright light; may cause temporary blurring of vision or stinging following administration, but discontinue product and see physician if problems persist or increase; to use, tilt head back and place medication in conjunctival sac and close eyes; apply light pressure on lacrimal sac for 1 minute

Nursing Implications Shake suspension before using

Dosage Forms Suspension, ophthalmic: Neomycin sulfate 0.35%, polymyxin B sulfate 10,000 units, and prednisolone acetate 0.5% per mL (5 mL, 10 mL)

Neomycin Sulfate *see* Neomycin *on page 887*

Neopap® [OTC] *see* Acetaminophen *on page 19*

Neoral® *see* Cyclosporine *on page 327*

Neosar® *see* Cyclophosphamide *on page 323*

Neosporin® Cream [OTC] *see* Neomycin and Polymyxin B *on page 888*

Neosporin® G.U. Irrigant *see* Neomycin and Polymyxin B *on page 888*

Neosporin® Ophthalmic Ointment *see* Bacitracin, Neomycin, and Polymyxin B *on page 129*

Neosporin® Ophthalmic Solution *see* Neomycin, Polymyxin B, and Gramicidin *on page 889*

Neosporin® Topical Ointment [OTC] *see* Bacitracin, Neomycin, and Polymyxin B *on page 129*

Neostigmine (nee oh STIG meen)

Brand Names Prostigmin®

Synonyms Neostigmine Bromide; Neostigmine Methylsulfate

Therapeutic Category Antidote, Neuromuscular Blocking Agent; Cholinergic Agent; Diagnostic Agent, Myasthenia Gravis

Use Diagnosis and treatment of myasthenia gravis and prevent and treat postoperative bladder distention and urinary retention; reversal of the effects of nondepolarizing neuromuscular blocking agents after surgery

(Continued)

Neostigmine *(Continued)*

Pregnancy Risk Factor C

Contraindications Hypersensitivity to neostigmine, bromides or any component; GI or GU obstruction

Warnings/Precautions Does **not** antagonize and may prolong the phase I block of depolarizing muscle relaxants (eg, succinylcholine); use with caution in patients with epilepsy, asthma, bradycardia, hyperthyroidism, cardiac arrhythmias, or peptic ulcer; adequate facilities should be available for cardiopulmonary resuscitation when testing and adjusting dose for myasthenia gravis; have atropine and epinephrine ready to treat hypersensitivity reactions; overdosage may result in cholinergic crisis, this must be distinguished from myasthenic crisis; anticholinesterase insensitivity can develop for brief or prolonged periods

Adverse Reactions

Respiratory: Bronchoconstriction

>10%:

- Gastrointestinal: Hyperperistalsis, nausea, vomiting, salivation, diarrhea, stomach cramps
- Miscellaneous: Diaphoresis (increased)

1% to 10%:

- Genitourinary: Urge to urinate
- Ocular: Small pupils, lacrimation
- Respiratory: Increased bronchial secretions

<1%:

- Cardiovascular: A-V block, bradycardia, hypotension, bradyarrhythmias, asystole
- Central nervous system: Dysphoria, restlessness, agitation, seizures, headache, drowsiness
- Local: Thrombophlebitis
- Neuromuscular & skeletal: Muscle spasms, tremor, weakness, fasciculations
- Ocular: Diplopia, miosis
- Respiratory: Laryngospasm, respiratory paralysis
- Miscellaneous: Hypersensitivity, hyper-reactive cholinergic responses

Overdosage/Toxicology Symptoms of overdose include muscle weakness, blurred vision, excessive sweating, tearing and salivation, nausea, vomiting, diarrhea, hypertension, bradycardia, muscle weakness, paralysis

Atropine sulfate injection should be readily available as an antagonist for the effects of neostigmine

Drug Interactions

Decreased effect: Antagonizes effects of nondepolarizing muscle relaxants (eg, pancuronium, tubocurarine); atropine antagonizes the muscarinic effects of neostigmine

Increased effect: Neuromuscular blocking agents effects are increased

Mechanism of Action Inhibits destruction of acetylcholine by acetylcholinesterase which facilitates transmission of impulses across myoneural junction

Pharmacodynamics/Kinetics

Onset of effect:

- I.M.: Within 20-30 minutes
- I.V.: Within 1-20 minutes

Duration:

- I.M.: 2.5-4 hours
- I.V.: 1-2 hours

Absorption: Oral: Poor, <2%

Metabolism: In the liver

Half-life:

- Normal renal function: 0.5-2.1 hours
- End stage renal disease: Prolonged

Elimination: 50% excreted renally as unchanged drug

Usual Dosage

Myasthenia gravis: Diagnosis: I.M.:

- Children: 0.04 mg/kg as a single dose
- Adults: 0.02 mg/kg as a single dose

Myasthenia gravis: Treatment:

- Children:
  - Oral: 2 mg/kg/day divided every 3-4 hours
  - I.M., I.V., S.C.: 0.01-0.04 mg/kg every 2-4 hours
- Adults:
  - Oral: 15 mg/dose every 3-4 hours up to 375 mg/day maximum
  - I.M., I.V., S.C.: 0.5-2.5 mg every 1-3 hours up to 10 mg/24 hours maximum

Reversal of nondepolarizing neuromuscular blockade after surgery in conjunction with atropine: I.V.:

- Infants: 0.025-0.1 mg/kg/dose

Children: 0.025-0.08 mg/kg/dose
Adults: 0.5-2.5 mg; total dose not to exceed 5 mg

Bladder atony: Adults: I.M., S.C.:
Prevention: 0.25 mg every 4-6 hours for 2-3 days
Treatment: 0.5-1 mg every 3 hours for 5 doses after bladder has emptied

Dosing adjustment in renal impairment:
Cl_{cr} 10-50 mL/minute: Administer 50% of normal dose
Cl_{cr} <10 mL/minute: Administer 25% of normal dose

Test Interactions ↑ aminotransferase [ALT (SGPT)/AST (SGOT)] (S), ↑ amylase (S)

Patient Information Side effects are generally due to exaggerated pharmacologic effects; most common are salivation and muscle fasciculations; notify physician if nausea, vomiting, muscle weakness, severe abdominal pain, or difficulty breathing occurs

Nursing Implications In the diagnosis of myasthenia gravis, all anticholinesterase medications should be discontinued for at least 8 hours before administering neostigmine

Additional Information
Neostigmine bromide: Prostigmin® tablet
Neostigmine methylsulfate: Prostigmin® injection

Dosage Forms
Injection, as methylsulfate: 0.25 mg/mL (1 mL); 0.5 mg/mL (1 mL, 10 mL); 1 mg/mL (10 mL)
Tablet, as bromide: 15 mg

Neostigmine Bromide *see* Neostigmine *on page 891*

Neostigmine Methylsulfate *see* Neostigmine *on page 891*

Neo-Synephrine® 12 Hour Nasal Solution [OTC] *see* Oxymetazoline *on page 940*

Neo-Synephrine® Nasal Solution [OTC] *see* Phenylephrine *on page 989*

Neo-Synephrine® Ophthalmic Solution *see* Phenylephrine *on page 989*

Neo-Tabs® *see* Neomycin *on page 887*

Neotricin HC® Ophthalmic Ointment *see* Bacitracin, Neomycin, Polymyxin B, and Hydrocortisone *on page 130*

NeoVadrin® [OTC] *see* Vitamins, Multiple *on page 1310*

Nephrocaps® [OTC] *see* Vitamins, Multiple *on page 1310*

Nephro-Fer™ [OTC] *see* Ferrous Fumarate *on page 513*

Nephrox Suspension [OTC] *see* Aluminum Hydroxide *on page 55*

Neptazane® *see* Methazolamide *on page 801*

Nervocaine® *see* Lidocaine *on page 723*

Nesacaine® *see* Chloroprocaine *on page 254*

Nesacaine®-MPF *see* Chloroprocaine *on page 254*

Nestrex® *see* Pyridoxine *on page 1081*

1-*N*-Ethyl Sisomicin *see* Netilmicin *on this page*

Netilmicin (ne til MYE sin)

Brand Names Netromycin®

Canadian/Mexican Brand Names Netromicina® (Mexico)

Synonyms 1-*N*-Ethyl Sisomicin; Netilmicin Sulfate

Therapeutic Category Antibiotic, Aminoglycoside

Use Short-term treatment of serious or life-threatening infections including septicemia, peritonitis, intra-abdominal abscess, lower respiratory tract infections, urinary tract infections; skin, bone, and joint infections caused by sensitive *Pseudomonas aeruginosa, Escherichia coli, Proteus, Klebsiella, Serratia, Enterobacter, Citrobacter,* and *Staphylococcus*

Pregnancy Risk Factor D

Contraindications Known hypersensitivity to netilmicin (aminoglycosides, bisulfites)

Warnings/Precautions Use with caution in patients with pre-existing renal insufficiency, vestibular or cochlear impairment, myasthenia gravis, hypocalcemia, conditions which depress neuromuscular transmission. Parenteral aminoglycosides are associated with nephrotoxicity or ototoxicity; the ototoxicity may be proportional to the amount of drug given and the duration of treatment; tinnitus or vertigo are indications of vestibular injury and impending hearing loss; renal damage is usually reversible.

Adverse Reactions
>10%:
Central nervous system: Neurotoxicity
Otic: Ototoxicity (auditory), ototoxicity (vestibular)
Renal: Decreased creatinine clearance, nephrotoxicity

(Continued)

Netilmicin *(Continued)*

1% to 10%:

Cardiovascular: Edema

Dermatologic: Skin itching, redness, rash

<1%:

Central nervous system: Drowsiness, headache, pseudomotor cerebri

Dermatologic: Photosensitivity, erythema

Gastrointestinal: Anorexia, nausea, vomiting, weight loss, increased salivation, enterocolitis

Hematologic: Granulocytopenia, agranulocytosis, thrombocytopenia

Local: Burning, stinging

Neuromuscular & skeletal: Weakness, tremors, muscle cramps

Respiratory: Dyspnea

Overdosage/Toxicology Serum level monitoring is recommended. Symptoms of overdose include ototoxicity, nephrotoxicity, and neuromuscular toxicity.

Treatment of choice following a single acute overdose appears to be the maintenance of good urine output of at least 3 mL/kg/hour. Dialysis is of questionable value in the enhancement of aminoglycoside elimination. If required, hemodialysis is preferred over peritoneal dialysis in patients with normal renal function. Careful hydration may be all that is required to promote diuresis and, therefore, the enhancement of the drug's elimination. Chelation with penicillins is experimental.

Drug Interactions Increased toxicity:

Penicillins, cephalosporins, amphotericin B, loop diuretics, vancomycin may increase nephrotoxic potential

Neuromuscular blocking agents may increase neuromuscular blockade

Mechanism of Action Interferes with protein synthesis in bacterial cell by binding to ribosomal subunit

Pharmacodynamics/Kinetics

Absorption: I.M.: Well absorbed

Distribution: V_d: 0.16-0.34 L/kg; distributes into extracellular fluid including serum, abscesses, ascitic, pericardial, pleural, synovial, lymphatic, and peritoneal fluids; high concentrations in urine; crosses placenta

Half-life: 2-3 hours (age and renal function dependent)

Time to peak serum concentration: I.M.: Within 0.5-1 hour

Elimination: By glomerular filtration

Usual Dosage Individualization is critical because of the low therapeutic index. Use of ideal body weight (IBW) for determining the mg/kg/dose appears to be more accurate than dosing on the basis of total body weight (TBW). In morbid obesity, dosage requirement may best be estimated using a dosing weight of IBW + 0.4 (TBW - IBW). Peak and trough plasma drug levels should be determined, particularly in critically ill patients with serious infections or in disease states known to significantly alter aminoglycoside pharmacokinetics (eg, cystic fibrosis, burns, or major surgery).

Once daily dosing: Higher peak serum drug concentration to MIC ratios, demonstrated aminoglycoside postantibiotic effect, decreased renal cortex drug uptake, and improved cost-time efficiency are supportive reasons for the use of once daily dosing regimens for aminoglycosides. Current research indicates these regimens to be as effective for nonlife-threatening infections, with no higher incidence of nephrotoxicity, than those requiring multiple daily doses. Doses are determined by calculating the entire day's dose via usual multiple dose calculation techniques and administering this quantity as a single dose. Doses are then adjusted to maintain mean serum concentrations above the MIC(s) of the causative organism(s). (Example: 4.5-6.5 mg/kg as a single dose; expected Cp_{max}: 10-20 mcg/mL, and Cp_{min}: <1 mcg/mL). Further research is needed for universal recommendation in all patient populations and gram-negative disease; exceptions may include those with known high clearance (eg, children, patients with cystic fibrosis, or burns who may require shorter dosage intervals) and patients with renal function impairment for whom longer than conventional dosage intervals are usually required.

I.M., I.V.:

Children 6 weeks to 12 years: 1-2.5 mg/kg/dose every 8 hours

Children >12 years and Adults: 1.5-2 mg/kg/dose every 8-12 hours

Some clinicians suggest a daily dose of 4-7 mg/kg for all patients with normal renal function. This dose is at least as efficacious with similar, if not less, toxicity than conventional dosing.

Dosing adjustment in renal impairment: Initial dose:

All patients should receive a loading dose of at least 2 mg/kg (subsequent dosing should be base on serum concentrations)

Cl_{cr} ≥60 mL/minute: Administer every 8 hours

Cl_{cr} 40-60 mL/minute: Administer every 12 hours

Cl_{cr} 20-40 mL/minute: Administer every 24 hours

Reference Range

Therapeutic: Peak: 4-10 µg/mL (SI: 8-21 µmol/L); Trough: <2 µg/mL (SI: 4 µmol/L)

Toxic: Peak: >10 µg/mL (SI: >21 µmol/L); Trough: >2 µg/mL (SI: >4.2 µmol/L)

Patient Information Report any dizziness or sensations of ringing or fullness in ears

Nursing Implications When injected into the muscles of paralyzed patients, the results are different than in normal patients, slower absorption and lower peak concentrations probably due to poor circulation in the atrophic muscles, suggest I.V. route; aminoglycoside levels measured in blood taken from Silastic® central catheters can sometime give falsely high readings (draw from alternate lumen or via peripheral stick; otherwise flush well following administration). Monitor serum creatinine and urine output; obtain drug levels after the third dose unless otherwise directed (eg, toxicity suspected, renal dysfunction). Peak levels are drawn 30 minutes after the end of a 30-minute infusion or 1 hour after I.M. injection; trough levels are drawn within 30 minutes before the next dose; give other antibiotic drugs at least 1 hour before or after gentamicin. Hearing should be tested before, during, and after treatment in high-risk patients.

Dosage Forms

Injection, as sulfate: 100 mg/mL (1.5 mL)

Injection, as sulfate:

- Neonatal: 10 mg/mL (2 mL)
- Pediatric: 25 mg/mL (2 mL)

Netilmicin Sulfate *see* Netilmicin *on page 893*

Netromycin® *see* Netilmicin *on page 893*

Neucalm® *see* Hydroxyzine *on page 634*

Neupogen® *see* Filgrastim *on page 518*

Neuramate® *see* Meprobamate *on page 783*

Neuromuscular Blocking Agents Comparison *see page 1417*

Neurontin® *see* Gabapentin *on page 563*

Neut® *see* Sodium Bicarbonate *on page 1140*

Neutra-Phos® *see* Potassium Phosphate and Sodium Phosphate *on page 1031*

Neutra-Phos®-K *see* Potassium Phosphate *on page 1029*

Neutrexin® *see* Trimetrexate Glucuronate *on page 1266*

Neutrogena® Acne Mask [OTC] *see* Benzoyl Peroxide *on page 140*

Nevirapine (ne VYE re peen)

Brand Names Viramune®

Therapeutic Category Antiviral Agent, Oral; Reverse Transcriptase Inhibitor

Use In combination therapy with at least one nucleoside antiretroviral agent for the treatment of HIV-1 in adults

Pregnancy Risk Factor C

Pregnancy/Breast-Feeding Implications Administer nevirapine during pregnancy only if benefits to the mother outweigh the risk to the fetus; avoid use during lactation, if possible

Contraindications Previous hypersensitivity to nevirapine or its components

Warnings/Precautions Severe skin reactions (eg, Stevens-Johnson syndrome) have occurred, usually within 6 weeks. Therapy should be discontinued if any rash which develops does not resolve; although mild to moderate alterations in LFTs are not uncommon, if abnormalities reoccur after temporarily discontinuing therapy, treatment should be permanently halted. Safety and efficacy have not been established in children.

Adverse Reactions

>10%:

- Central nervous system: Headache, fever
- Dermatologic: Rash
- Gastrointestinal: Nausea, diarrhea, abdominal pain
- Hematologic: Thrombocytopenia

1% to 10%:

- Gastrointestinal: Ulcerative stomatitis
- Hematologic: Anemia, thrombocytopenia
- Hepatic: Hepatitis, increased LFTs
- Neuromuscular & skeletal: Peripheral neuropathy, paresthesia, myalgia

Overdosage/Toxicology No toxicities have been reported with acute ingestions of large sums of tablets

Drug Interactions Decreased effect: Rifampin and rifabutin may decrease nevirapine trough concentrations due to induction of CYP3A; since nevirapine may decrease concentrations of protease inhibitors, they should not be administered concomitantly; nevirapine may decrease the effectiveness of oral contraceptives - suggest alternate method of birth control

(Continued)

Nevirapine *(Continued)*

Mechanism of Action As a non-nucleoside reverse transcriptase inhibitor, nevirapine has activity against HIV-1 by binding to reverse transcriptase. It consequently blocks the RNA-dependent and DNA-dependent DNA polymerase activities including HIV-1 replication. It does not require intracellular phosphorylation for antiviral activity. Cross-resistance between nevirapine and HIV protease inhibitors is unlikely although emergence of HIV strains which are cross-resistant between non-nucleoside reverse transcriptase inhibitors have been observed *in vitro.*

Pharmacodynamics/Kinetics

Absorption: Oral: >90%

Distribution: V_d: 1.2-1.4 L/kg; widely distributed; distributes well into breast milk and crosses the placenta; CSF penetration approximates 50% of that found in the plasma

Protein binding, plasma: 50% to 60%

Metabolism: Extensively metabolized via cytochrome P-450 system (hydroxylation to inactive compounds); may undergo enterohepatic recycling

Half-life: Decreases over 2- to 4-week time with chronic dosing due to autoinduction (ie, half-life = 45 hours initially and decreases to 23 hours)

Time to peak serum concentration: 2-4 hours

Elimination: Renal elimination of metabolites; <3% of parent compound excreted in urine

Usual Dosage Adults: Oral:

Initial: 200 mg once daily for 14 days

Maintenance: 200 mg twice daily (in combination with an additional antiretroviral agent)

Monitoring Parameters Liver function tests periodically throughout therapy; observe for CNS side effects

Patient Information Report any right upper quadrant pain, jaundice, or rash to your physician immediately

Nursing Implications May be given with food, antacids, or didanosine; if a therapy is interrupted for >7 days, the dose should be decreased to the initial regimen and increased after 14 days

Dosage Forms Tablet: 200 mg

N.G.T.® Topical *see* Nystatin and Triamcinolone *on page 920*

Niacin (NYE a sin)

Related Information

Lipid-Lowering Agents *on page 1413*

Brand Names Nicobid® [OTC]; Nicolar® [OTC]; Nicotinex [OTC]; Slo-Niacin® [OTC]

Synonyms Nicotinic Acid; Vitamin B_3

Therapeutic Category Antilipemic Agent; Vitamin, Water Soluble

Use Adjunctive treatment of hyperlipidemias; peripheral vascular disease and circulatory disorders; treatment of pellagra; dietary supplement

Pregnancy Risk Factor A (C if used in doses greater than RDA suggested doses)

Contraindications Liver disease, peptic ulcer, severe hypotension, arterial hemorrhaging, hypersensitivity to niacin

Warnings/Precautions Monitor liver function tests, blood glucose; may elevate uric acid levels; use with caution in patients predisposed to gout; large doses should be administered with caution to patients with gallbladder disease, jaundice, liver disease, or diabetes; some products may contain tartrazine

Adverse Reactions

1% to 10%:

- Cardiovascular: Generalized flushing
- Central nervous system: Headache
- Gastrointestinal: Bloating, flatulence, nausea
- Hepatic: Abnormalities of hepatic function tests, jaundice
- Neuromuscular & skeletal: Paresthesia in extremities
- Miscellaneous: Increased sebaceous gland activity, sensation of warmth

<1%:

- Cardiovascular: Tachycardia, syncope, vasovagal attacks
- Central nervous system: Dizziness
- Dermatologic: Rash
- Hepatic: Chronic liver damage
- Ocular: Blurred vision
- Respiratory: Wheezing

Overdosage/Toxicology Symptoms of acute overdose include flushing, GI distress, pruritus; chronic excessive use has been associated with hepatitis; antihistamines may relieve niacin-induced histamine release; otherwise treatment is symptomatic

Drug Interactions

Decreased effect of oral hypoglycemics; may inhibit uricosuric effects of sulfinpyrazone and probenecid

Decreased toxicity (flush) with aspirin

Increased toxicity with lovastatin (myopathy) and possibly with other HMG-CoA reductase inhibitors; adrenergic blocking agents → additive vasodilating effect and postural hypotension

Mechanism of Action Component of two coenzymes which is necessary for tissue respiration, lipid metabolism, and glycogenolysis; inhibits the synthesis of very low density lipoproteins

Pharmacodynamics/Kinetics

Peak serum concentrations: Oral: Within 45 minutes

Metabolism: Depending upon the dose, niacin converts to niacinamide; following this conversion, niacinamide is 30% metabolized in the liver

Half-life: 45 minutes

Elimination: In urine; with larger doses, a greater percentage is excreted unchanged in urine

Usual Dosage Administer I.M., I.V., or S.C. only if oral route is unavailable and use only for vitamin deficiencies (not for hyperlipidemia)

Children: Oral:
- Pellagra: 50-100 mg/dose 3 times/day
- Recommended daily allowances:
  - 0-0.5 years: 5 mg/day
  - 0.5-1 year: 6 mg/day
  - 1-3 years: 9 mg/day
  - 4-6 years: 12 mg/day
  - 7-10 years: 13 mg/day

Children and Adolescents: Oral: Recommended daily allowances:
- Male:
  - 11-14 years: 17 mg/day
  - 15-18 years: 20 mg/day
  - 19-24 years: 19 mg/day
- Female: 11-24 years: 15 mg/day

Adults: Oral:
- Recommended daily allowances:
  - Male: 25-50 years: 19 mg/day; >51 years: 15 mg/day
  - Female: 25-50 years: 15 mg/day; >51 years: 13 mg/day
- Hyperlipidemia: 1.5-6 g/day in 3 divided doses with or after meals
- Pellagra: 50-100 mg 3-4 times/day, maximum: 500 mg/day
- Niacin deficiency: 10-20 mg/day, maximum: 100 mg/day

Administration Administer with food

Monitoring Parameters Blood glucose, liver function tests (with large doses or prolonged therapy), serum cholesterol

Test Interactions False elevations in some fluorometric determinations of urinary catecholamines; false-positive urine glucose (Benedict's reagent)

Patient Information May experience transient cutaneous flushing and sensation of warmth, especially of face and upper body; itching or tingling, and headache may occur, these adverse effects may be decreased by increasing the dose slowly or by taking aspirin or a NSAID 30 minutes to 1 hour prior to taking niacin; may cause GI upset, take with food; if dizziness occurs, avoid sudden changes in posture; report any persistent nausea, vomiting, abdominal pain, dark urine, or pale stools to the physician; do not crush sustained release capsule

Nursing Implications Monitor closely for signs of hepatotoxicity and myositis; avoid sudden changes in posture

Dosage Forms

Capsule, timed release: 125 mg, 250 mg, 300 mg, 400 mg, 500 mg

Elixir: 50 mg/5 mL (473 mL, 4000 mL)

Injection: 100 mg/mL (30 mL)

Tablet: 25 mg, 50 mg, 100 mg, 250 mg, 500 mg

Tablet, timed release: 150 mg, 250 mg, 500 mg, 750 mg

Niacinamide (nye a SIN a mide)

Synonyms Nicotinamide; Vitamin B_3

Therapeutic Category Vitamin, Water Soluble

Use Prophylaxis and treatment of pellagra

Pregnancy Risk Factor A (C if used in doses greater than RDA suggested doses)

Contraindications Liver disease, peptic ulcer, known hypersensitivity to niacin

Warnings/Precautions Large doses should be administered with caution to patients with gallbladder disease or diabetes; monitor blood glucose; may elevate uric acid levels; use with caution in patients predisposed to gout; some products may contain tartrazine

(Continued)

Niacinamide *(Continued)*

Adverse Reactions

1% to 10%:

Gastrointestinal: Bloating, flatulence, nausea
Neuromuscular & skeletal: Paresthesia in extremities
Miscellaneous: Increased sebaceous gland activity

<1%:

Cardiovascular: Tachycardia
Dermatologic: Rash
Ocular: Blurred vision
Respiratory: Wheezing

Overdosage/Toxicology Symptoms of overdose include GI distress

Mechanism of Action Used by the body as a source of niacin; is a component of two coenzymes which is necessary for tissue respiration, lipid metabolism, and glycogenolysis; inhibits the synthesis of very low density lipoproteins

Pharmacodynamics/Kinetics

Absorption: Rapid from GI tract
Metabolism: In the liver
Half-life: 45 minutes
Time to peak serum concentration: 20-70 minutes
Elimination: In urine

Usual Dosage Oral:

Children: Pellagra: 100-300 mg/day in divided doses

Adults: 50 mg 3-10 times/day
Pellagra: 300-500 mg/day
Recommended daily allowance: 13-19 mg/day

Test Interactions False elevations of urinary catecholamines in some fluorometric determinations

Dosage Forms Tablet: 50 mg, 100 mg, 125 mg, 250 mg, 500 mg

Nicardipine (nye KAR de peen)

Related Information

Calcium Channel Blockers Comparative Actions *on page 1401*
Calcium Channel Blockers Comparative Pharmacokinetics *on page 1402*
Calcium Channel Blockers FDA-Approved Indications *on page 1403*
Therapy of Hypertension *on page 1540*

Brand Names Cardene®; Cardene® SR

Canadian/Mexican Brand Names Ridene® (Mexico)

Synonyms Nicardipine Hydrochloride

Therapeutic Category Antianginal Agent; Antihypertensive; Calcium Channel Blocker

Use Chronic stable angina; management of essential hypertension, migraine prophylaxis

Unlabeled use: Congestive heart failure

Pregnancy Risk Factor C

Pregnancy/Breast-Feeding Implications

Clinical effects on the fetus: Crosses the placenta; may exhibit tocolytic effect
Breast-feeding/lactation: No data available

Contraindications Contraindicated in severe hypotension or second and third degree heart block, sinus bradycardia, advanced heart block, ventricular tachycardia, cardiogenic shock, atrial fibrillation or flutter associated with accessory conduction pathways, CHF; hypersensitivity to nicardipine or any component, calcium channel blockers, and adenosine; not to be given within a few hours of I.V. beta-blocking agents

Warnings/Precautions Use with caution in titrating dosages for impaired renal or hepatic function patients; may increase frequency, severity, and duration of angina during initiation of therapy; do not abruptly withdraw (chest pain); elderly may have a greater hypotensive effect

Adverse Reactions

1% to 10%:

Cardiovascular: Flushing, palpitations, tachycardia, pedal edema
Central nervous system: Headache, dizziness, nausea, somnolence
Neuromuscular & skeletal: Weakness

<1%:

Cardiovascular: Edema, tachycardia, syncope, abnormal EKG
Central nervous system: Insomnia, malaise, abnormal dreams
Dermatologic: Rash
Gastrointestinal: Vomiting, constipation, dyspepsia, xerostomia
Genitourinary: Nocturia
Neuromuscular & skeletal: Tremor

Overdosage/Toxicology The primary cardiac symptoms of calcium blocker overdose includes hypotension and bradycardia. The hypotension is caused by peripheral vasodilation, myocardial depression, and bradycardia. Bradycardia results from sinus bradycardia, second- or third-degree atrioventricular block, or sinus arrest with junctional rhythm. Intraventricular conduction is usually not affected so QRS duration is normal (verapamil does prolong the P-R interval and bepridil prolongs the Q-T and may cause ventricular arrhythmias, including torsade de pointes).

The noncardiac symptoms include confusion, stupor, nausea, vomiting, metabolic acidosis and hyperglycemia. Following initial gastric decontamination, if possible, repeated calcium administration may promptly reverse the depressed cardiac contractility (but not sinus node depression or peripheral vasodilation); glucagon, epinephrine, and amrinone may treat refractory hypotension; glucagon and epinephrine also increase the heart rate (outside the U.S., 4-aminopyridine may be available as an antidote); dialysis and hemoperfusion are not effective in enhancing elimination although repeat-dose activated charcoal may serve as an adjunct with sustained-release preparations.

Drug Interactions

Increased toxicity/effect/levels:

Nicardipine and H_2 blockers may increase bioavailability of nicardipine

Nicardipine and propranolol or metoprolol may increase cardiac depressant effects on A-V conduction

Nicardipine and cyclosporine may increase cyclosporine levels

Diltiazem and vecuronium may increase vecuronium levels

Stability Compatible with D_5W, $D_5{}^1\!/_2NS$, D_5NS, and D_5W with 40 mEq potassium chloride; 0.45% and 0.9% NS; **do not** mix with 5% sodium bicarbonate and lactated Ringer's solution; store at room temperature; protect from light; stable for 24 hours at room temperature

Mechanism of Action Inhibits calcium ion from entering the "slow channels" or select voltage-sensitive areas of vascular smooth muscle and myocardium during depolarization, producing a relaxation of coronary vascular smooth muscle and coronary vasodilation; increases myocardial oxygen delivery in patients with vasospastic angina

Pharmacodynamics/Kinetics

Absorption: Oral: Well absorbed, ~100%

Protein binding: 95%

Metabolism: Extensive first-pass metabolism; only metabolized in the liver

Bioavailability: Absolute, 35%

Half-life: 2-4 hours

Time to peak: Peak serum levels occur within 20-120 minutes and an onset of hypotension occurs within 20 minutes

Elimination: As metabolites in urine

Usual Dosage Adults:

Oral: 40 mg 3 times/day (allow 3 days between dose increases)

Oral, sustained release: Initial: 30 mg twice daily, titrate up to 60 mg twice daily

I.V. (dilute to 0.1 mg/mL): Initial: 5 mg/hour increased by 2.5 mg/hour every 15 minutes to a maximum of 15 mg/hour

Dietary Considerations Alcohol: Avoid use

Patient Information Sustained release products should be taken with food (not fatty meal); do not crush; limit caffeine intake; avoid alcohol; notify physician if angina pain is not reduced when taking this drug, irregular heartbeat, shortness of breath, swelling, dizziness, constipation, nausea, or hypotension occur; do not stop therapy without advice of physician

Nursing Implications Monitor closely for orthostasis; ampuls must be diluted before use; do not crush sustained release product

Additional Information Although there is some initial data which may show increased risk of myocardial infarction following treatment of hypertension with calcium antagonists, controlled trials (eg, ALL-HAT) are ongoing to examine the long-term effects of not only calcium antagonists but other antihypertensives in preventing heart disease. Until these studies are completed, patients taking calcium antagonists should be encouraged to continue with prescribed antihypertensive regimens although a switch from high-dose, short-acting agents to sustained release products may be warranted. It is generally agreed that the calcium antagonists should be avoided as primary treatment for hypertension unless diuretics or beta-blockers are contraindicated and for primary treatment of angina following acute myocardial infarction

Dosage Forms

Capsule, as hydrochloride: 20 mg, 30 mg

Capsule, as hydrochloride, sustained release: 30 mg, 45 mg, 60 mg

Injection, as hydrochloride: 2.5 mg/mL (10 mL)

Nicardipine Hydrochloride *see* Nicardipine *on previous page*

N'ice® Vitamin C Drops [OTC] *see* Ascorbic Acid *on page 102*

Nicobid® [OTC] *see* Niacin *on page 896*
Nicoderm® Patch *see* Nicotine *on this page*
Nicolar® [OTC] *see* Niacin *on page 896*
Nicorette® DS Gum *see* Nicotine *on this page*
Nicorette® Gum *see* Nicotine *on this page*
Nicotinamide *see* Niacinamide *on page 897*

Nicotine (nik oh TEEN)

Brand Names Habitrol™ Patch; Nicoderm® Patch; Nicorette® DS Gum; Nicorette® Gum; Nicotrol® NS Nasal Spray; Nicotrol® Patch [OTC]; ProStep® Patch

Canadian/Mexican Brand Names Nicorette™ (Canada); Nicorette™ Plus (Canada); Nicolan® (Mexico); Nicotinell®-TTS (Mexico)

Therapeutic Category Smoking Deterrent

Use Treatment aid to smoking cessation while participating in a behavioral modification program under medical supervision

Pregnancy Risk Factor D (transdermal)/X (chewing gum)

Contraindications Nonsmokers, patients with a history of hypersensitivity or allergy to nicotine or any components used in the transdermal system, pregnant or nursing women, patients who are smoking during the postmyocardial infarction period, patients with life-threatening arrhythmias, or severe or worsening angina pectoris, active temporomandibular joint disease (gum)

Warnings/Precautions Use with caution in oropharyngeal inflammation and in patients with history of esophagitis, peptic ulcer, coronary artery disease, vasospastic disease, angina, hypertension, hyperthyroidism, diabetes, and hepatic dysfunction; nicotine is known to be one of the most toxic of all poisons; while the gum is being used to help the patient overcome a health hazard, it also must be considered a hazardous drug vehicle.

Nicotine nasal spray: Fatal dose: 40 mg

Adverse Reactions

Chewing gum:

>10%:
- Cardiovascular: Tachycardia
- Central nervous system: Headache (mild)
- Gastrointestinal: Nausea, vomiting, indigestion, excessive salivation, belching, increased appetite, mouth or throat soreness
- Neuromuscular & skeletal: Jaw muscle ache
- Miscellaneous: Hiccups

1% to 10%:
- Central nervous system: Insomnia, dizziness, nervousness
- Endocrine & metabolic: Dysmenorrhea
- Gastrointestinal: GI distress, eructation
- Neuromuscular & skeletal: Myalgia
- Respiratory: Hoarseness
- Miscellaneous: Hiccups

<1%:
- Cardiovascular: Atrial fibrillation
- Dermatologic: Erythema, itching
- Miscellaneous: Hypersensitivity reactions

Transdermal systems:

>10%:
- Cardiovascular: Tachycardia
- Central nervous system: Headache (mild)
- Dermatologic: Pruritus, erythema
- Gastrointestinal: Increased appetite

1% to 10%:
- Central nervous system: Insomnia, nervousness
- Endocrine & metabolic: Dysmenorrhea
- Neuromuscular & skeletal: Myalgia

<1%:
- Cardiovascular: Atrial fibrillation
- Dermatologic: Itching
- Miscellaneous: Hypersensitivity reactions

Overdosage/Toxicology Symptoms of overdose include nausea, vomiting, abdominal pain, mental confusion, diarrhea, salivation, tachycardia, respiratory and cardiovascular collapse

Treatment after decontamination is symptomatic and supportive; remove patch, rinse area with water and dry, do not use soap as this may increase absorption.

Mechanism of Action Nicotine is one of two naturally-occurring alkaloids which exhibit their primary effects via autonomic ganglia stimulation. The other alkaloid is lobeline which has many actions similar to those of nicotine but is less potent. Nicotine is a potent ganglionic and central nervous system stimulant, the actions of which are mediated via nicotine-specific receptors. Biphasic actions are observed depending upon the dose administered. The main effect of nicotine in small doses is stimulation of all autonomic ganglia; with larger doses, initial stimulation is followed by blockade of transmission. Biphasic effects are also evident in the adrenal medulla; discharge of catecholamines occurs with small doses, whereas prevention of catecholamines release is seen with higher doses as a response to splanchnic nerve stimulation. Stimulation of the central nervous system (CNS) is characterized by tremors and respiratory excitation. However, convulsions may occur with higher doses, along with respiratory failure secondary to both central paralysis and peripheral blockade to respiratory muscles.

Pharmacodynamics/Kinetics Intranasal nicotine may more closely approximate the time course of plasma nicotine levels observed after cigarette smoking than other dosage forms

Duration of action: Transdermal: 24 hours
Absorption: Transdermal: Slow
Metabolism: In the liver, primarily to cotinine, which is $^{1}/_{5}$ as active.
Half-life, elimination: 4 hours
Time to peak serum concentration: Transdermal: 8-9 hours
Elimination: Via the kidneys; renal clearance is pH-dependent

Usual Dosage

Gum: Chew 1 piece of gum when urge to smoke, up to 30 pieces/day; most patients require 10-12 pieces of gum/day

Transdermal patch (patients should be advised to completely stop smoking upon initiation of therapy): Apply new patch every 24 hours to nonhairy, clean, dry skin on the upper body or upper outer arm; each patch should be applied to a different site

- Initial starting dose: 21 mg/day for 4-8 weeks for most patients
- First weaning dose: 14 mg/day for 2-4 weeks
- Second weaning dose: 7 mg/day for 2-4 weeks
- Initial starting dose for patients <100 pounds, smoke <10 cigarettes/day, have a history of cardiovascular disease: 14 mg/day for 4-8 weeks followed by 7 mg/day for 2-4 weeks
- In patients who are receiving >600 mg/day of cimetidine: Decrease to the next lower patch size
- Benefits of use of nicotine transdermal patches beyond 3 months have not been demonstrated

Spray: 1-2 sprays/hour; do not exceed more than 5 doses (10 sprays) per hour; each dose (2 sprays) contains 1 mg of nicotine. **Warning:** A dose of 40 mg can cause fatalities

Patient Information Instructions for the proper use of the patch should be given to the patient; notify physician if persistent rash, itching, or burning may occur with the patch; do not smoke while wearing patches

Nursing Implications Patients should be instructed to chew slowly to avoid jaw ache and to maximize benefit; patches cannot be cut; use of an aerosol corticosteroid may diminish local irritation under patches

Dosage Forms

Patch, transdermal:
- Habitrol™: 21 mg/day; 14 mg/day; 7 mg/day (30 systems/box)
- Nicoderm®: 21 mg/day; 14 mg/day; 7 mg/day (14 systems/box)
- Nicotrol® [OTC]: 15 mg/day (gradually released over 16 hours)
- ProStep®: 22 mg/day; 11 mg/day (7 systems/box)

Pieces, chewing gum, as polacrilex: 2 mg/square [OTC] (96 pieces/box); 4 mg/square (96 pieces/box)

Spray, nasal: 0.5 mg/actuation [10 mg/mL-200 actuations] (10 mL)

Nicotinex [OTC] *see* Niacin *on page 896*

Nicotinic Acid *see* Niacin *on page 896*

Nicotrol® NS Nasal Spray *see* Nicotine *on previous page*

Nicotrol® Patch [OTC] *see* Nicotine *on previous page*

Nidryl® Oral [OTC] *see* Diphenhydramine *on page 399*

Nifedipine (nye FED i peen)

Related Information

Calcium Channel Blockers Comparative Actions *on page 1401*
Calcium Channel Blockers Comparative Pharmacokinetics *on page 1402*
Calcium Channel Blockers FDA-Approved Indications *on page 1403*

Brand Names Adalat®; Adalat® CC; Procardia®; Procardia XL®

Canadian/Mexican Brand Names Adalat PA® (Canada); Apo-Nifed® (Canada); Gen-Nifedipine® (Canada); Novo-Nifedin® (Canada); Nu-Nifedin® (Canada); Adalat® Oros (Mexico); Adalat® Retard (Mexico); Corogal® (Mexico); Corotrend® (Mexico); Corotrend® Retard (Mexico); Nifedipres® (Mexico); Noviken-N® (Mexico)

Therapeutic Category Antianginal Agent; Antihypertensive; Calcium Channel Blocker

(Continued)

Nifedipine *(Continued)*

Use Angina, including unstable and chronic stable angina (sustained release products only), hypertrophic cardiomyopathy, hypertension (sustained release only), pulmonary hypertension

Pregnancy Risk Factor C

Pregnancy/Breast-Feeding Implications

Use in pregnancy only when clearly needed and when the benefits outweigh the potential hazard to the fetus

Clinical effects on the fetus: No data on crossing the placenta. Hypotension, IUGR reported. IUGR probably related to maternal hypertension. May exhibit tocolytic effects. Available evidence suggests safe use during pregnancy and breast-feeding.

Breast-feeding/lactation: Crosses into breast milk. American Academy of Pediatrics considers COMPATIBLE with breast-feeding.

Contraindications Known hypersensitivity to nifedipine or any other calcium channel blocker and adenosine; sick-sinus syndrome, 2nd or 3rd degree A-V block, hypotension (<90 mm Hg systolic)

Warnings/Precautions Use with caution and titrate dosages for patients with impaired renal or hepatic function; use caution when treating patients with congestive heart failure, sick-sinus syndrome, severe left ventricular dysfunction, hypertrophic cardiomyopathy (especially obstructive), concomitant therapy with beta-blockers or digoxin, edema, or increased intracranial pressure with cranial tumors; do not abruptly withdraw (may cause chest pain); elderly may experience hypotension and constipation more readily. The National Heart, Lung and Blood Institute has advised that elderly patients should not receive short-acting nifedipine, especially at higher doses. Fast-acting agents should not be used in treatment of hypertension, hypertensive crisis, acute myocardial infarction, some forms of unstable angina and chronic stable angina.

Adverse Reactions

>10%:

- Cardiovascular: Flushing
- Central nervous system: Dizziness, lightheadedness, giddiness, headache
- Gastrointestinal: Nausea, heartburn
- Neuromuscular & skeletal: Weakness
- Miscellaneous: Heat sensation

1% to 10%:

- Cardiovascular: Peripheral edema, palpitations, hypotension
- Central nervous system: Nervousness, mood changes
- Gastrointestinal: Sore throat
- Neuromuscular & skeletal: Muscle cramps, tremor
- Respiratory: Dyspnea, cough, nasal congestion

<1%:

- Cardiovascular: Tachycardia, syncope, peripheral edema
- Central nervous system: Fever, chills
- Dermatologic: Dermatitis, urticaria, purpura
- Gastrointestinal: Diarrhea, constipation, gingival hyperplasia
- Hematologic: Thrombocytopenia, leukopenia, anemia
- Neuromuscular & skeletal: Joint stiffness, arthritis with increased ANA
- Ocular: Blurred vision, transient blindness
- Respiratory: Shortness of breath
- Miscellaneous: Diaphoresis

Overdosage/Toxicology The primary cardiac symptoms of calcium blocker overdose include hypotension and bradycardia. The hypotension is caused by peripheral vasodilation, myocardial depression, and bradycardia. Bradycardia results from sinus bradycardia, second- or third-degree atrioventricular block, or sinus arrest with junctional rhythm. Intraventricular conduction is usually not affected so QRS duration is normal.

The noncardiac symptoms include confusion, stupor, nausea, vomiting, metabolic acidosis and hyperglycemia. Following initial gastric decontamination, if possible, repeated calcium administration may promptly reverse the depressed cardiac contractility (but not sinus node depression or peripheral vasodilation); glucagon, epinephrine, and amrinone may treat refractory hypotension; glucagon and epinephrine also increase the heart rate (outside the U.S., 4-aminopyridine may be available as an antidote); dialysis and hemoperfusion are not effective in enhancing elimination although repeat-dose activated charcoal may serve as an adjunct with sustained-release preparations.

Drug Interactions Cytochrome P-450 3A enzyme substrate

Decreased toxicity:

- Nifedipine and phenobarbital may decrease nifedipine levels
- Nifedipine and quinidine may decrease quinidine levels
- Nifedipine and rifampin may decrease nifedipine levels

Increased toxicity:
- Nifedipine and beta-blockers may increase cardiovascular adverse effects
- Nifedipine and H_2-antagonists increase bioavailability and may increase nifedipine serum concentration
- Nifedipine and phenytoin may increase phenytoin levels
- Nifedipine and quinidine may increase nifedipine levels
- Nifedipine and theophylline may increase theophylline levels
- Nifedipine and vincristine may increase vincristine levels

Mechanism of Action Inhibits calcium ion from entering the "slow channels" or select voltage-sensitive areas of vascular smooth muscle and myocardium during depolarization, producing a relaxation of coronary vascular smooth muscle and coronary vasodilation; increases myocardial oxygen delivery in patients with vasospastic angina

Pharmacodynamics/Kinetics

Onset of action:
- Oral: Within 20 minutes
- S.L.: Within 1-5 minutes

Protein binding: 92% to 98% (concentration-dependent)

Metabolism: In the liver to inactive metabolites

Bioavailability:
- Capsules: 45% to 75%
- Sustained release: 65% to 86%

Half-life:
- Adults, normal: 2-5 hours
- Adults with cirrhosis: 7 hours

Elimination: In urine

Usual Dosage Capsule may be punctured and drug solution administered sublingually to reduce blood pressure

Children: Oral, S.L.:
- Hypertensive emergencies: 0.25-0.5 mg/kg/dose
- Hypertrophic cardiomyopathy: 0.6-0.9 mg/kg/24 hours in 3-4 divided doses

Adults:
- Initial: 10 mg 3 times/day as capsules or 30 mg once daily as sustained release
- Usual dose: 10-30 mg 3 times/day as capsules or 30-60 mg once daily as sustained release
- Maximum dose: 120-180 mg/day
- *Increase sustained release at 7- to 14-day intervals*

Dialysis: Not removed by hemo- or peritoneal dialysis; supplemental dose is not necessary

Dosing adjustment in hepatic impairment: Reduce oral dose by 50% to 60% in patients with cirrhosis

Dietary Considerations Alcohol: Avoid use

Monitoring Parameters Heart rate, blood pressure, signs and symptoms of CHF, peripheral edema

Patient Information Sustained release products should not be crushed or chewed; Adalat® CC should be taken on an empty stomach; limit caffeine intake; avoid alcohol; notify physician if angina pain is not reduced when taking this drug, irregular heartbeat, shortness of breath, swelling, dizziness, constipation, nausea, or hypotension occurs; do not stop therapy without advice of physician

Nursing Implications May cause some patients to urinate frequently at night; may cause inflamed gums; capsule may be punctured and drug solution administered sublingually or orally to reduce blood pressure in recumbent patient

Additional Information Although there is some initial data which may show increased risk of myocardial infarction with the treatment of hypertension with calcium antagonists, controlled trial (eg, ALL-HAT) are ongoing to examine the long-term effects of not only these agents but other antihypertensives in preventing heart disease. Until these studies are completed, patients taking calcium antagonists should be encouraged to continue with the prescribed antihypertensive regimens although a switch from high-dose short-acting products to sustained release agents may be warranted. It is also generally agreed that calcium antagonists should be avoided as primary treatment for hypertension unless diuretics or beta-blockers are contraindicated and as primary therapy of angina after acute myocardial infarction.

Dosage Forms
- Capsule, liquid-filled (Adalat®, Procardia®): 10 mg, 20 mg
- Tablet, extended release (Adalat® CC): 30 mg, 60 mg, 90 mg
- Tablet, sustained release (Procardia XL®): 30 mg, 60 mg, 90 mg

Niferex®-PN *see* Vitamins, Multiple *on page 1310*

Nilandron® *see* Nilutamide *on next page*

Nilstat® *see* Nystatin *on page 919*

Nilutamide (ni LU ta mide)

Related Information

Cancer Chemotherapy Regimens *on page 1351*

Brand Names Nilandron®

Canadian/Mexican Brand Names Anandron® (Canada)

Therapeutic Category Antiandrogen; Antineoplastic Agent, Miscellaneous

Use In combination with surgical castration in treatment of metastatic prostatic carcinoma (Stage D_2); for maximum benefit, nilutamide treatment must begin on the same day as or on the day after surgical castration

Pregnancy Risk Factor C

Contraindications Severe hepatic impairment; severe respiratory insufficiency; hypersensitivity to nilutamide or any component of this preparation

Warnings/Precautions The U.S. Food and Drug Administration (FDA) currently recommends that procedures for proper handling and disposal of antineoplastic agents be considered.

Interstitial pneumonitis has been reported in 2% of patients exposed to nilutamide. Patients typically experienced progressive exertional dyspnea, and possibly cough, chest pain and fever. X-rays showed interstitial or alveolo-interstitial changes. The suggestive signs of pneumonitis most often occurred within the first 3 months of nilutamide treatment.

Hepatitis or marked increases in liver enzymes leading to drug discontinuation occurred in 1% of nilutamide patients. There has been a report of elevated hepatic enzymes followed by death in a 65 year old patient treated with nilutamide.

Foreign postmarketing surveillance has revealed isolated cases of aplastic anemia in which a causal relationship with nilutamide could not be ascertained.

13% to 57% of patients receiving nilutamide reported a delay in adaptation to the dark, ranging from seconds to a few minutes. This effect sometimes does not abate as drug treatment is continued. Caution patients who experience this effect about driving at night or through tunnels. This effect can be alleviated by wearing tinted glasses.

Adverse Reactions

>10%:

- Central nervous system: Pain, headache, insomnia
- Gastrointestinal: Nausea, constipation, anorexia
- Genitourinary: Impotence, testicular atrophy, gynecomastia
- Endocrine & metabolic: Loss of libido, hot flashes
- Neuromuscular & skeletal: Weakness
- Ocular: Impaired adaption to dark

1% to 10%:

- Cardiovascular: Hypertension
- Central nervous system: Flu syndrome, fever, dizziness, depression, hypesthesia
- Dermatologic: Alopecia, dry skin, rash
- Gastrointestinal: Dyspepsia, vomiting, abdominal pain
- Genitourinary: Urinary tract infection, hematuria, urinary tract disorder, nocturia
- Respiratory: Dyspnea, upper respiratory infection, pneumonia
- Ocular: Chromatopsia, impaired adaption to light, abnormal vision
- Miscellaneous: Diaphoresis

Overdosage/Toxicology One case of massive overdosage has been published. A 79-year old man attempted suicide by ingesting 13 g of nilutamide. There were no clinical signs or symptoms or changes in parameters such as transaminases or chest x-ray. Maintenance treatment (150 mg/day) was resumed 30 days later.

Management is supportive, dialysis not of benefit; induce vomiting if the patient is alert, general supportive care (including frequent monitoring of the vital signs and close observation of the patient)

Stability Store at room temperature (15°C to 30°C/59°F to 86°F); protect from light

Mechanism of Action Nonsteroidal antiandrogen that inhibits androgen uptake or inhibits binding of androgen in target tissues

Pharmacodynamics/Kinetics

Absorption: Rapid and complete

Distribution: Moderately binds to plasma proteins and low binding to erythrocytes.

Metabolism: Extensive

Half-life: 38-59 hours

Elimination: All metabolites excreted primarily in urine

Usual Dosage Adults: Oral: 6 tablets (50 mg each) once a day for a total daily dose of 300 mg for 30 days followed thereafter by 3 tablets (50 mg each) once a day for a total daily dose of 150 mg

Dietary Considerations Food: Can be taken without regard to food

Monitoring Parameters

Perform routine chest x-rays before treatment, and tell patients to report immediately any dyspnea or aggravation of pre-existing dyspnea. At the onset of dyspnea or worsening of pre-existing dyspnea any time during therapy, interrupt nilutamide until it can be determined if respiratory symptoms are drug-related. Obtain a chest x-ray, and if there are findings suggestive of interstitial pneumonitis, discontinue treatment with nilutamide. The pneumonitis is almost always reversible when treatment is discontinued. If the chest x-ray appears normal, perform pulmonary function tests.

Measure serum hepatic enzyme levels at baseline and at regular intervals (3 months); if transaminases increase over 2-3 times the upper limit of normal, discontinue treatment. Perform appropriate laboratory testing at the first symptom/sign of liver injury (eg, jaundice, dark urine, fatigue, abdominal pain or unexplained GI symptoms) and nilutamide treatment must be discontinued immediately if transaminases exceed 3 times the upper limit of normal.

Dosage Forms Tablet: 50 mg, 100 mg

Nimbex® *see* Cisatracurium *on page 281*

Nimodipine (nye MOE di peen)

Related Information

Calcium Channel Blockers Comparative Actions *on page 1401*

Calcium Channel Blockers Comparative Pharmacokinetics *on page 1402*

Calcium Channel Blockers FDA-Approved Indications *on page 1403*

Brand Names Nimotop®

Therapeutic Category Calcium Channel Blocker

Use Improvement of neurological deficits due to spasm following subarachnoid hemorrhage from ruptured congenital intracranial aneurysms in patients who are in good neurological condition postictus

Pregnancy Risk Factor C

Pregnancy/Breast-Feeding Implications Use in pregnancy only when clearly needed and when the benefits outweigh the potential hazard to the fetus

Clinical effects on the fetus: Teratogenic and embryotoxic effects have been demonstrated in small animals. No well controlled studies have been conducted in pregnant women. Use in pregnancy only when clearly needed and when the benefits outweigh the potential hazard to the fetus.

Breast milk/lactation: Appears in breast milk at levels higher than maternal plasma levels; no recommendations are currently available on breast-feeding

Contraindications Hypersensitivity to nimodipine or any component

Warnings/Precautions Use with caution and titrate dosages for patients with impaired renal or hepatic function; use caution when treating patients with congestive heart failure, sick-sinus syndrome, PVCs, severe left ventricular dysfunction, hypertrophic cardiomyopathy (especially obstructive, IHSS), concomitant therapy with beta-blockers or digoxin, edema, or increased intracranial pressure with cranial tumors; do not abruptly withdraw (may cause chest pain); elderly may experience hypotension and constipation more readily

Adverse Reactions

1% to 10%: Cardiovascular: Reductions in systemic blood pressure

<1%:

- Cardiovascular: Edema, EKG abnormalities, tachycardia, bradycardia
- Central nervous system: Headache, depression
- Dermatologic: Rash, acne
- Gastrointestinal: Diarrhea, nausea
- Hematologic: Hemorrhage
- Hepatic: Hepatitis
- Neuromuscular & skeletal: Muscle cramps
- Respiratory: Dyspnea

Overdosage/Toxicology The primary cardiac symptoms of calcium blocker overdose include hypotension and bradycardia. The hypotension is caused by peripheral vasodilation, myocardial depression, and bradycardia. Bradycardia results from sinus bradycardia, second- or third-degree atrioventricular block, or sinus arrest with junctional rhythm. Intraventricular conduction is usually not affected so QRS duration is normal.

The noncardiac symptoms include confusion, stupor, nausea, vomiting, metabolic acidosis and hyperglycemia. Following initial gastric decontamination, if possible, repeated calcium administration may promptly reverse the depressed cardiac contractility (but not sinus node depression or peripheral vasodilation); glucagon, epinephrine, and amrinone may treat refractory hypotension; glucagon and epinephrine also increase the heart rate (outside the U.S., 4-aminopyridine may be available as an antidote); dialysis and hemoperfusion are not effective in enhancing elimination although repeat-dose activated charcoal may serve as an adjunct with sustained-release preparations.

(Continued)

Nimodipine *(Continued)*

Drug Interactions Cytochrome P-450 3A enzyme substrate

Increased toxicity/effect/levels:

Nimodipine and cimetidine may increase bioavailability of nimodipine

Nimodipine and omeprazole may increase bioavailability of nimodipine

Nimodipine and propranolol may have minimal increase of depressant effects on A-V conduction

Nimodipine and valproic acid may increase nimodipine levels

Mechanism of Action Nimodipine shares the pharmacology of other calcium channel blockers; animal studies indicate that nimodipine has a greater effect on cerebral arterials than other arterials; this increased specificity may be due to the drug's increased lipophilicity and cerebral distribution as compared to nifedipine; inhibits calcium ion from entering the "slow channels" or select voltage sensitive areas of vascular smooth muscle and myocardium during depolarization

Pharmacodynamics/Kinetics

Metabolism: Extensive in the liver

Half-life: 3 hours, increases with reduced renal function

Protein binding: >95%

Bioavailability: 13%

Time to peak serum concentration: Oral: Within 1 hour

Elimination: In feces (32%) and in urine (50% within 4 days)

Usual Dosage Adults: Oral: 60 mg every 4 hours for 21 days, start therapy within 96 hours after subarachnoid hemorrhage

Dialysis: Not removed by hemo- or peritoneal dialysis; supplemental dose is not necessary

Dosing adjustment in hepatic impairment: Reduce dosage to 30 mg every 4 hours in patients with liver failure

Nursing Implications If the capsules cannot be swallowed, the liquid may be removed by making a hole in each end of the capsule with an 18-gauge needle and extracting the contents into a syringe; if given via NG tube, follow with a flush of 30 mL NS

Dosage Forms Capsule, liquid-filled: 30 mg

Nimotop® *see* Nimodipine *on previous page*

Nipent™ *see* Pentostatin *on page 973*

Nisoldipine (NYE sole di peen)

Brand Names Sular®

Therapeutic Category Calcium Channel Blocker

Use Management of hypertension, may be used alone or in combination with other antihypertensive agents

Pregnancy Risk Factor C

Contraindications Hypersensitivity to nisoldipine or any component or other dihydropyridine calcium channel blocker

Warnings/Precautions Increased angina and/or myocardial infarction in patients with coronary artery disease

Adverse Reactions

Cardiovascular: Peripheral edema, tachycardia

Central nervous system: Dizziness, headache

Overdosage/Toxicology The primary cardiac symptoms of calcium blocker overdose includes hypotension and bradycardia. The hypotension is caused by peripheral vasodilation, myocardial depression, and bradycardia. Bradycardia results from sinus bradycardia, second- or third-degree atrioventricular block, or sinus arrest with junctional rhythm. Intraventricular conduction is usually not affected so QRS duration is normal.

The noncardiac symptoms include confusion, stupor, nausea, vomiting, metabolic acidosis and hyperglycemia. Following initial gastric decontamination, if possible, repeated calcium administration may promptly reverse the depressed cardiac contractility (but not sinus node depression or peripheral vasodilation); glucagon, epinephrine, and amrinone may treat refractory hypotension; glucagon and epinephrine also increase the heart rate (outside the U.S., 4-aminopyridine may be available as an antidote); dialysis and hemoperfusion are not effective in enhancing elimination although repeat-dose activated charcoal may serve as an adjunct with sustained release preparations.

Drug Interactions

Increased toxicity:

Nisoldipine and digoxin may increase digoxin effect

Nisoldipine and propranolol may increase cardiovascular adverse effects

Nisoldipine and H_2-antagonists increase bioavailability and may increase nisoldipine serum concentration

Nisoldipine and omeprazole increase bioavailability and may increase nisoldipine serum concentration

Mechanism of Action As a dihydropyridine calcium channel blocker, structurally similar to nifedipine, nisoldipine impedes the movement of calcium ions into vascular smooth muscle and cardiac muscle. Dihydropyridines are potent vasodilators and are not as likely to suppress cardiac contractility and slow cardiac conduction as other calcium antagonists such as verapamil and diltiazem; nisoldipine is 5-10 times as potent a vasodilator as nifedipine.

Pharmacodynamics/Kinetics

Absorption: Well absorbed

Metabolism: Extensive presystemic metabolism in the intestinal wall and the liver; hepatically metabolized to inactive metabolites

Half-life: 7-12 hours

Bioavailability: 5%; T_{max}: 6-12 hours

Elimination: In the urine

Usual Dosage Adults: Oral: Initial: 20 mg once daily, then increase by 10 mg/week (or longer intervals) to attain adequate control of blood pressure; doses >60 mg once daily are not recommended. A starting dose not exceeding 10 mg/day is recommended for the elderly and those with hepatic impairment.

Patient Information Avoid grapefruit products before and after dosing; administration with a high fat meal can lead to excessive peak drug concentrations and should be avoided

Nursing Implications Administer at the same time each day to ensure minimal fluctuation of serum levels

Additional Information Initial data indicate that once daily doses of 10-40 mg are about as effective as hydrochlorothiazide, lisinopril, or amlodipine; doses of 20-60 mg are about as effective as twice daily verapamil in lowering blood pressure in patients with mild to moderate hypertension; although there is some initial data which may show increased risk of myocardial infarction following treatment of hypertension with calcium channel blockers, controlled trials (eg, ALL-HAT) are ongoing to examine the long-term effects of not only the calcium channel blockers, but also other antihypertensives in preventing heart disease. Until done, patients taking these agents should be encouraged to continue with prescribed antihypertension regimens although a switch from high-dose, short-acting agents to sustained release products may be warranted. Most practitioners agree to avoid calcium channel blockers as primary treatment for hypertension unless diuretics or beta-blockers are contraindicated.

Dosage Forms Tablet, extended release: 10 mg, 20 mg, 30 mg, 40 mg

Nitrates Comparison *see page 1419*

Nitro-Bid® *see* Nitroglycerin *on page 909*

Nitrocine® *see* Nitroglycerin *on page 909*

Nitrodisc® *see* Nitroglycerin *on page 909*

Nitro-Dur® *see* Nitroglycerin *on page 909*

Nitrofural *see* Nitrofurazone *on next page*

Nitrofurantoin (nye troe fyoor AN toyn)

Related Information

Antacid Drug Interactions *on page 1388*

Antimicrobial Drugs of Choice *on page 1468*

Brand Names Furadantin®; Furalan®; Furan®; Furanite®; Macrobid®; Macrodantin®

Canadian/Mexican Brand Names Apo-Nitrofurantoin® (Canada); Nephronex® (Canada); Novo-Furan® (Canada); Furadantina® (Mexico); Macrodantina® (Mexico)

Therapeutic Category Antibiotic, Miscellaneous

Use Prevention and treatment of urinary tract infections caused by susceptible gram-negative and some gram-positive organisms; *Pseudomonas, Serratia,* and most species of *Proteus* are generally resistant to nitrofurantoin

Pregnancy Risk Factor B

Contraindications Hypersensitivity to nitrofurantoin or any component; renal impairment; infants <1 month (due to the possibility of hemolytic anemia)

Warnings/Precautions Use with caution in patients with G-6-PD deficiency, patients with anemia, vitamin B deficiency, diabetes mellitus or electrolyte abnormalities; therapeutic concentrations of nitrofurantoin are not attained in urine of patients with Cl_{cr} <40 mL/minute (elderly); use with caution if prolonged therapy is anticipated due to possible pulmonary toxicity

Adverse Reactions

>10%:

Cardiovascular: Chest pains

Central nervous system: Chills, fever

Gastrointestinal: Stomach upset, diarrhea, loss of appetite, vomiting

Respiratory: Cough, dyspnea

(Continued)

Nitrofurantoin *(Continued)*

1% to 10%:
- Central nervous system: Fatigue, drowsiness, headache, dizziness
- Gastrointestinal: Sore throat
- Neuromuscular & skeletal: Weakness, paresthesia, numbness

<1%:
- Dermatologic: Rash, itching
- Hematologic: Hemolytic anemia
- Hepatic: Hepatitis
- Neuromuscular & skeletal: Arthralgia

Overdosage/Toxicology Symptoms of overdose include vomiting; supportive care only

Drug Interactions

Decreased effect: Antacids (decreases absorption of nitrofurantoin)

Increased toxicity: Probenecid (decreases renal excretion of nitrofurantoin)

Mechanism of Action Inhibits several bacterial enzyme systems including acetyl coenzyme A interfering with metabolism and possibly cell wall synthesis

Pharmacodynamics/Kinetics

Absorption: Well absorbed from GI tract; the macrocrystalline form is absorbed more slowly due to slower dissolution, but causes less GI distress

Distribution: V_d: 0.8 L/kg; crosses the placenta; appears in breast milk

Protein binding: ~40%

Metabolism: 60% of drug metabolized by body tissues throughout the body, with exception of plasma, to inactive metabolites

Bioavailability: Increased by presence of food

Half-life: 20-60 minutes; prolonged with renal impairment

Elimination: As metabolites and unchanged drug (40%) in urine and small amounts in bile; renal excretion via glomerular filtration and tubular secretion

Usual Dosage Oral:

Children >1 month: 5-7 mg/kg/day in divided doses every 6 hours; maximum: 400 mg/day

Chronic therapy: 1-2 mg/kg/day in divided doses every 12-24 hours; maximum dose: 100 mg/day

Adults: 50-100 mg/dose every 6 hours

Prophylaxis or chronic therapy: 50-100 mg/dose at bedtime

Dosing adjustment in renal impairment: Cl_{cr} <50 mL/minute: Avoid use

Avoid use in hemo and peritoneal dialysis and continuous arterio-venous or veno-venous hemofiltration (CAVH/CAVHD)

Dietary Considerations Alcohol: Avoid use

Administration Administer around-the-clock rather than 4 times/day to promote less variation in peak and trough serum levels; administer with meals to slow the rate of absorption and decrease adverse effects; suspension may be mixed with water, milk, fruit juice, or infant formula

Monitoring Parameters Signs of pulmonary reaction, signs of numbness or tingling of the extremities, periodic liver function tests

Test Interactions Causes false-positive urine glucose with Clinitest®

Patient Information Take with food or milk; may discolor urine to a dark yellow or brown color; notify physician if fever, chest pain, persistent, nonproductive cough, or difficulty breathing occurs; avoid alcohol

Nursing Implications Higher peak serum levels may cause increased GI upset

Dosage Forms

Capsule: 50 mg, 100 mg

Capsule:
- Extended release: 100 mg
- Macrocrystal: 25 mg, 50 mg, 100 mg
- Macrocrystal/monohydrate: 100 mg

Suspension, oral: 25 mg/5 mL (470 mL)

Nitrofurazone (nye troe FYOOR a zone)

Brand Names Furacin®

Synonyms Nitrofural

Therapeutic Category Antibacterial, Topical

Use Antibacterial agent in second and third degree burns and skin grafting

Pregnancy Risk Factor C

Contraindications Hypersensitivity to nitrofurazone or any component

Warnings/Precautions Use with caution in patients with renal impairment and patients with G-6-PD deficiency

Adverse Reactions Women should inform their physicians if signs or symptoms of any of the following occur thromboembolic or thrombotic disorders including sudden severe headache or vomiting, disturbance of vision or speech, loss of vision, numbness or weakness in an extremity, sharp or crushing chest pain, calf pain, shortness of breath, severe abdominal pain or mass, mental depression or unusual bleeding

Women should discontinue taking the medication if they suspect they are pregnant or become pregnant. Notify physician if area under dermal patch becomes irritated or a rash develops.

Drug Interactions Decreased effect: Sutilains decrease activity of nitrofurazone

Stability Avoid exposure to direct sunlight; excessive heat, strong fluorescent lighting, and alkaline materials

Mechanism of Action A broad antibacterial spectrum; it acts by inhibiting bacterial enzymes involved in carbohydrate metabolism; effective against a wide range of gram-negative and gram-positive organisms; bactericidal against most bacteria commonly causing surface infections including *Staphylococcus aureus, Streptococcus, Escherichia coli, Enterobacter cloacae, Clostridium perfringens, Aerobacter aerogenes*, and *Proteus* sp; not particularly active against most *Pseudomonas aeruginosa* strains and does not inhibit viruses or fungi. Topical preparations of nitrofurazone are readily soluble in blood, pus, and serum and are nonmacerating.

Usual Dosage Children and Adults: Topical: Apply once daily or every few days to lesion or place on gauze

Patient Information Notify physician if condition worsens or if irritation develops

Dosage Forms

Cream: 0.2% (28 g)

Ointment, Soluble dressing, topical: 0.2% (28 g, 56 g, 454 g, 480 g)

Solution, topical: 0.2% (480 mL, 4000 mL)

Nitrogard® *see* Nitroglycerin *on this page*

Nitrogen Mustard *see* Mechlorethamine *on page 767*

Nitroglycerin (nye troe GLI ser in)

Related Information

Adult ACLS Algorithm, Hypotension, Shock *on page 1516*

Cardiovascular Agents Comparison *on page 1405*

Nitrates Comparison *on page 1419*

Therapy of Hypertension *on page 1540*

Brand Names Deponit®; Minitran®; Nitro-Bid®; Nitrocine®; Nitrodisc®; Nitro-Dur®; Nitrogard®; Nitroglyn®; Nitrol®; Nitrolingual®; Nitrong®; Nitrostat®; Transdermal-NTG®; Transderm-Nitro®; Tridil®

Canadian/Mexican Brand Names Cardinit® (Mexico); Nitradisc® (Mexico); Nitroderm-TTS® (Mexico)

Synonyms Glyceryl Trinitrate; Nitroglycerol; NTG

Therapeutic Category Antianginal Agent; Antihypertensive; Nitrate; Vasodilator; Vasodilator, Coronary

Use Treatment and prevention of angina pectoris; I.V. for congestive heart failure (especially when associated with acute myocardial infarction); pulmonary hypertension; hypertensive emergencies occurring perioperatively (especially during cardiovascular surgery)

Pregnancy Risk Factor C

Contraindications Hypersensitivity to nitroglycerin or any component; closed-angle glaucoma; severe anemia, early myocardial infarction, head trauma, cerebral hemorrhage, allergy to adhesive (transdermal), uncorrected hypovolemia (I.V.), inadequate cerebral circulation, increased intracranial pressure, constrictive pericarditis and pericardial tamponade; transdermal NTG is not effective for immediate relief of angina

Warnings/Precautions Do not use extended release preparations in patients with GI hypermotility or malabsorptive syndrome; use with caution in patients with hepatic impairment; available preparations of I.V. nitroglycerin differ in concentration or volume; pay attention to dilution and dosage; I.V. preparations contain alcohol and/or propylene glycol

Adverse Reactions

>10%:

- Cardiovascular: Postural hypotension, flushing
- Central nervous system: Headache, lightheadedness, dizziness
- Neuromuscular & skeletal: Weakness

1% to 10%: Dermatologic: Drug rash, exfoliative dermatitis

<1%:

- Cardiovascular: Reflex tachycardia, bradycardia, coronary vascular insufficiency, arrhythmias
- Dermatologic: Allergic contact dermatitis, exfoliative dermatitis
- Gastrointestinal: Nausea, vomiting
- Hematologic: Methemoglobinemia (overdose)
- Miscellaneous: Diaphoresis, collapse, alcohol intoxication

Overdosage/Toxicology Symptoms of overdose include hypotension, throbbing headache, palpitations, bloody diarrhea, bradycardia, cyanosis, tissue hypoxia,

(Continued)

Nitroglycerin *(Continued)*

metabolic acidosis, clonic convulsions, circulatory collapse, methemoglobinemia with extremely large overdoses

Treatment is supportive and symptomatic; hypotension is treated with fluids and alpha-adrenergic pressors if needed

Drug Interactions

Decreased effect: I.V. nitroglycerin may antagonize the anticoagulant effect of heparin, monitor closely; may need to decrease heparin dosage when nitroglycerin is discontinued

Increased toxicity: Alcohol, beta-blockers, calcium channel blockers may enhance nitroglycerin's hypotensive effect

Stability Doses should be made in glass bottles, Excell® or PAB® containers; adsorption occurs to soft plastic (ie, PVC)

Nitroglycerin diluted in D_5W or NS in glass containers is physically and chemically stable for 48 hours at room temperature and 7 days under refrigeration; in D_5W or NS in Excell®/PAB® containers is physically and chemically stable for 24 hours at room temperature and 14 days under refrigeration

Premixed bottles are stable according to the manufacturer's expiration dating

Standard diluent: 50 mg/250 mL D_5W; 50 mg/500 mL D_5W

Minimum volume: 100 mg/250 mL D_5W; concentration should not exceed 400 mcg/mL

Store sublingual tablets and ointment in tightly closed containers at 15°C to 30°C

Mechanism of Action Reduces cardiac oxygen demand by decreasing left ventricular pressure and systemic vascular resistance; dilates coronary arteries and improves collateral flow to ischemic regions

Pharmacodynamics/Kinetics

Onset and duration of action is dependent upon dosage form administered; see table.

Dosage Form	Onset of Effect	Peak Effect	Duration
Sublingual tablet	1-3 min	4-8 min	30-60 min
Translingual spray	2 min	4-10 min	30-60 min
Buccal tablet	2-5 min	4-10 min	2 h
Sustained release	20-45 min	45-120 min	4-8 h
Topical	15-60 min	30-120 min	2-12 h
Transdermal	40-60 min	60-180 min	18-24 h
I.V. drip	Immediate	Immediate	3-5 min

Protein binding: 60%

Metabolism: Extensive first-pass metabolism

Half-life: 1-4 minutes

Elimination: Excretion of inactive metabolites in urine

Usual Dosage Note: Hemodynamic and antianginal tolerance often develop within 24-48 hours of continuous nitrate administration

Children: Pulmonary hypertension: Continuous infusion: Start 0.25-0.5 mcg/kg/minute and titrate by 1 mcg/kg/minute at 20- to 60-minute intervals to desired effect; usual dose: 1-3 mcg/kg/minute; maximum: 5 mcg/kg/minute

Adults:

Buccal: Initial: 1 mg every 3-5 hours while awake (3 times/day); titrate dosage upward if angina occurs with tablet in place

Oral: 2.5-9 mg 2-4 times/day (up to 26 mg 4 times/day)

I.V.: 5 mcg/minute, increase by 5 mcg/minute every 3-5 minutes to 20 mcg/minute; if no response at 20 mcg/minute increase by 10 mcg/minute every 3-5 minutes, up to 200 mcg/minute

Ointment: 1" to 2" every 8 hours up to 4" to 5" every 4 hours

Patch, transdermal: 0.2-0.4 mg/hour initially and titrate to doses of 0.4-0.8 mg/hour; tolerance is minimized by using a patch-on period of 12-14 hours and patch-off period of 10-12 hours

Sublingual: 0.2-0.6 mg every 5 minutes for maximum of 3 doses in 15 minutes; may also use prophylactically 5-10 minutes prior to activities which may provoke an attack

Translingual: 1-2 sprays into mouth under tongue every 3-5 minutes for maximum of 3 doses in 15 minutes, may also be used 5-10 minutes prior to activities which may provoke an attack prophylactically

May need to use nitrate-free interval (10-12 hours/day) to avoid tolerance development; tolerance may possibly be reversed with acetylcysteine; gradually decrease dose in patients receiving NTG for prolonged period to avoid withdrawal reaction

Monitoring Parameters Blood pressure, heart rate

Patient Information Go to hospital if no relief after 3 sublingual doses; do not swallow or chew sublingual form; do not change brands without notifying your physician or pharmacist; take oral nitrates on an empty stomach; keep tablets and capsules in original container; keep tightly closed; use spray only when lying down; highly flammable; do not inhale spray; do not chew sustained release products; a treatment-free interval of 8-12 hours is recommended each day; take 3 times/day rather than every 8 hours

Nursing Implications I.V. must be prepared in glass bottles and use special sets intended for nitroglycerin; transdermal patches labeled as mg/hour; do not crush sublingual drug product

Dosage Forms

Capsule, sustained release: 2.5 mg, 6.5 mg, 9 mg

Injection: 0.5 mg/mL (10 mL); 0.8 mg/mL (10 mL); 5 mg/mL (1 mL, 5 mL, 10 mL, 20 mL); 10 mg/mL (5 mL, 10 mL)

Ointment, topical (Nitrol®): 2% [20 mg/g] (30 g, 60 g)

Patch, transdermal, topical: Systems designed to deliver 2.5, 5, 7.5, 10, or 15 mg NTG over 24 hours

Spray, translingual: 0.4 mg/metered spray (13.8 g)

Tablet:

- Buccal, controlled release: 1 mg, 2 mg, 3 mg
- Sublingual (Nitrostat®): 0.15 mg, 0.3 mg, 0.4 mg, 0.6 mg
- Sustained release: 2.6 mg, 6.5 mg, 9 mg

Nitroglycerol *see* Nitroglycerin *on page 909*

Nitroglyn® *see* Nitroglycerin *on page 909*

Nitrol® *see* Nitroglycerin *on page 909*

Nitrolingual® *see* Nitroglycerin *on page 909*

Nitrong® *see* Nitroglycerin *on page 909*

Nitropress® *see* Nitroprusside *on this page*

Nitroprusside (nye troe PRUS ide)

Related Information

Adult ACLS Algorithm, Hypotension, Shock *on page 1516*

Cardiovascular Agents Comparison *on page 1405*

Therapy of Hypertension *on page 1540*

Brand Names Nitropress®

Synonyms Nitroprusside Sodium; Sodium Nitroferricyanide; Sodium Nitroprusside

Therapeutic Category Antihypertensive; Vasodilator

Use Management of hypertensive crises; congestive heart failure; used for controlled hypotension to reduce bleeding during surgery

Pregnancy Risk Factor C

Contraindications Hypersensitivity to nitroprusside or components; decreased cerebral perfusion; arteriovenous shunt or coarctation of the aorta (ie, compensatory hypertension)

Warnings/Precautions Use with caution in patients with increased intracranial pressure (head trauma, cerebral hemorrhage); severe renal impairment, hepatic failure, hypothyroidism; use only as an infusion with 5% dextrose in water; continuously monitor patient's blood pressure; excessive amounts of nitroprusside can cause cyanide toxicity (usually in patients with decreased liver function) or thiocyanate toxicity (usually in patients with decreased renal function, or in patients with normal renal function but prolonged nitroprusside use)

Adverse Reactions

1% to 10%:

- Cardiovascular: Excessive hypotensive response, palpitations, substernal distress
- Central nervous system: Disorientation, psychosis, headache, restlessness
- Endocrine & metabolic: Thyroid suppression
- Gastrointestinal: Nausea, vomiting
- Neuromuscular & skeletal: Weakness, muscle spasm
- Otic: Tinnitus
- Respiratory: Hypoxia
- Miscellaneous: Diaphoresis, thiocyanate toxicity

Overdosage/Toxicology Symptoms of overdose include hypotension, vomiting, hyperventilation, tachycardia, muscular twitching, hypothyroidism, cyanide or thiocyanate toxicity. Thiocyanate toxicity includes psychosis, hyperreflexia, confusion, weakness, tinnitus, seizures, and coma; cyanide toxicity includes acidosis (decreased HCO_3, decreased pH, increased lactate), increase in mixed venous blood oxygen tension, tachycardia, altered consciousness, coma, convulsions, and almond smell on breath.

Nitroprusside has been shown to release cyanide *in vivo* with hemoglobin. Cyanide toxicity does not usually occur because of the rapid uptake of cyanide by

(Continued)

Nitroprusside *(Continued)*

erythrocytes and its eventual incorporation into cyanocobalamin. However, prolonged administration of nitroprusside or its reduced elimination can lead to cyanide intoxication. In these situations, airway support with oxygen therapy is germane, followed closely with antidotal therapy of amyl nitrate perles, sodium nitrate 300 mg I.V. (6 mg/kg for children) and sodium thiosulfate 12.5 g I.V. (1.5 mL/kg for children); nitrates should not be administered to neonates and small children. Thiocyanate is dialyzable. May be mixed with sodium thiosulfate in I.V. to prevent cyanide toxicity.

Stability

Nitroprusside sodium should be reconstituted freshly by diluting 50 mg in 250-1000 mL of D_5W

Use only clear solutions; solutions of nitroprusside exhibit a color described as brownish, brown, brownish-pink, light orange, and straw. Solutions are highly sensitive to light. Exposure to light causes decomposition, resulting in a highly colored solution of orange, dark brown or blue. **A blue color indicates almost complete degradation and breakdown to cyanide.**

Solutions should be wrapped with aluminum foil or other opaque material to protect from light (do as soon as possible)

Stability of parenteral admixture at room temperature (25°C) and at refrigeration temperature (4°C): 24 hours

Mechanism of Action Causes peripheral vasodilation by direct action on venous and arteriolar smooth muscle, thus reducing peripheral resistance; will increase cardiac output by decreasing afterload; reduces aortal and left ventricular impedance

Pharmacodynamics/Kinetics

Onset of hypotensive effect: <2 minutes

Duration: Within 1-10 minutes following discontinuation of therapy, effects cease

Metabolism: Nitroprusside is converted to cyanide ions in the bloodstream; decomposes to prussic acid which in the presence of sulfur donor is converted to thiocyanate (liver and kidney rhodanase systems)

Half-life:

Parent drug: <10 minutes

Thiocyanate: 2.7-7 days

Elimination: Thiocyanate renally eliminated

Usual Dosage Administration requires the use of an infusion pump. Average dose: 5 mcg/kg/minute

Children: Pulmonary hypertension: I.V.: Initial: 1 mcg/kg/minute by continuous I.V. infusion; increase in increments of 1 mcg/kg/minute at intervals of 20-60 minutes; titrating to the desired response; usual dose: 3 mcg/kg/minute, rarely need >4 mcg/kg/minute; maximum: 5 mcg/kg/minute.

Adults: I.V. Initial: 0.3-0.5 mcg/kg/minute; increase in increments of 0.5 mcg/kg/minute, titrating to the desired hemodynamic effect or the appearance of headache or nausea; usual dose: 3 mcg/kg/minute; rarely need >4 mcg/kg/minute; maximum: 10 mcg/kg/minute. When >500 mcg/kg is administered by prolonged infusion of faster than 2 mcg/kg/minute, cyanide is generated faster than an unaided patient can handle.

Administration I.V. infusion only, not for direct injection

Monitoring Parameters Blood pressure, heart rate; monitor for cyanide and thiocyanate toxicity; monitor acid-base status as acidosis can be the earliest sign of cyanide toxicity; monitor thiocyanate levels if requiring prolonged infusion (>3 days) or dose ≥4 mcg/kg/minute or patient has renal dysfunction; monitor cyanide blood levels in patients with decreased hepatic function; cardiac monitor and blood pressure monitor required

Reference Range Monitor thiocyanate levels if requiring prolonged infusion (>4 days) or ≥4 µg/kg/minute; not to exceed 100 µg/mL (or 10 mg/dL) plasma thiocyanate

Thiocyanate:

Therapeutic: 6-29 µg/mL

Toxic: 35-100 µg/mL

Fatal: >200 µg/mL

Cyanide: Normal <0.2 µg/mL; normal (smoker): <0.4 µg/mL

Toxic: >2 µg/mL

Potentially lethal: >3 µg/mL

Nursing Implications Brownish solution is usable, discard if bluish in color

Dosage Forms Injection, as sodium: 10 mg/mL (5 mL); 25 mg/mL (2 mL)

Nitroprusside Sodium *see* Nitroprusside *on previous page*

Nitrostat® *see* Nitroglycerin *on page 909*

Nix™ [OTC] *see* Permethrin *on page 978*

Nizatidine (ni ZA ti deen)

Brand Names Axid®; Axid® AR [OTC]

Therapeutic Category Antihistamine, H_2 Blocker; Histamine-2 Antagonist

Use Treatment and maintenance of duodenal ulcer; treatment of gastroesophageal reflux disease (GERD); OTC tablet used for the prevention of meal-induced heartburn, acid indigestion, and sour stomach

Pregnancy Risk Factor C

Contraindications Hypersensitivity to nizatidine or any component of the preparation; hypersensitivity to other H_2-antagonists since a cross-sensitivity has been observed with this class of drugs

Warnings/Precautions Use with caution in children <12 years of age; use with caution in patients with liver and renal impairment; dosage modification required in patients with renal impairment

Adverse Reactions

1% to 10%:

- Central nervous system: Dizziness, headache
- Gastrointestinal: Constipation, diarrhea

<1%:

- Cardiovascular: Bradycardia, tachycardia, palpitations, hypertension
- Central nervous system: Fever, fatigue, seizures, insomnia, drowsiness
- Dermatologic: Acne, pruritus, urticaria, dry skin
- Gastrointestinal: Abdominal discomfort, flatulence, belching, anorexia
- Hematologic: Agranulocytosis, neutropenia, thrombocytopenia
- Hepatic: Increases in AST, ALT
- Neuromuscular & skeletal: Paresthesia, weakness
- Renal: Increases in BUN/creatinine, proteinuria
- Respiratory: Bronchospasm
- Miscellaneous: Allergic reaction

Overdosage/Toxicology Symptoms of overdose include muscular tremors, vomiting, rapid respiration. LD_{50} ~80 mg/kg; treatment is primarily symptomatic and supportive.

Mechanism of Action Nizatidine is an H_2-receptor antagonist. In healthy volunteers, nizatidine has been effective in suppressing gastric acid secretion induced by pentagastrin infusion or food. Nizatidine reduces gastric acid secretion by 29.4% to 78.4%. This compares with a 60.3% reduction by cimetidine. Nizatidine 100 mg is reported to provide equivalent acid suppression as cimetidine 300 mg.

Usual Dosage Adults: Oral:

Active duodenal ulcer:

- Treatment: 300 mg at bedtime or 150 mg twice daily
- Maintenance: 150 mg/day

Meal-induced heartburn, acid indigestion, and sour stomach:

- 75 mg tablet [OTC] twice daily, 30 to 60 minutes prior to consuming food or beverages

Dosing adjustment in renal impairment:

- Cl_{cr} 50-80 mL/minute: Administer 75% of normal dose
- Cl_{cr} 10-50 mL/minute: Administer 50% of normal dose or 150 mg/day for active treatment and 150 mg every other day for maintenance treatment
- Cl_{cr} <10 mL/minute: Administer 25% of normal dose or 150 mg every other day for treatment and 150 mg every 3 days for maintenance treatment

Test Interactions False-positive urine protein using Multistix®, gastric acid secretion test, skin tests allergen extracts, serum creatinine and serum transaminase concentrations, urine protein test

Patient Information May take several days before medication begins to relieve stomach pain; antacids may be taken with nizatidine unless physician has instructed you not to use them; wait 30-60 minutes between taking the antacid and nizatidine; avoid aspirin, cough and cold preparations; avoid use of black pepper, caffeine, alcohol, and harsh spices; may cause drowsiness or impair coordination and judgment

Nursing Implications Giving dose at 6 PM may better suppress nocturnal acid secretion than 10 PM

Dosage Forms

- Capsule: 150 mg, 300 mg
- Tablet [OTC]: 75 mg

Nizoral® *see* Ketoconazole *on page 695*

N-Methylhydrazine *see* Procarbazine *on page 1049*

Nolvadex® *see* Tamoxifen *on page 1189*

Nonsteroidal Anti-Inflammatory Agents Comparison *see page 1419*

No Pain-HP® [OTC] *see* Capsaicin *on page 197*

Noradrenaline *see* Norepinephrine *on next page*

Noradrenaline Acid Tartrate *see* Norepinephrine *on next page*

Norcet® *see* Hydrocodone and Acetaminophen *on page 620*
Norcuron® *see* Vecuronium *on page 1295*
Nordeoxyguanosine *see* Ganciclovir *on page 566*
Nordette® *see* Ethinyl Estradiol and Levonorgestrel *on page 484*
Norditropin® Injection *see* Human Growth Hormone *on page 613*
Nordryl® Injection *see* Diphenhydramine *on page 399*
Nordryl® Oral *see* Diphenhydramine *on page 399*

Norepinephrine (nor ep i NEF rin)

Related Information

Adrenergic Agonists, Cardiovascular Comparison *on page 1385*
Adult ACLS Algorithm, Hypotension, Shock *on page 1516*
Cardiovascular Agents Comparison *on page 1405*
Extravasation Treatment of Other Drugs *on page 1381*

Brand Names Levophed®

Synonyms Levarterenol Bitartrate; Noradrenaline; Noradrenaline Acid Tartrate; Norepinephrine Bitartrate

Therapeutic Category Adrenergic Agonist Agent; Sympathomimetic

Use Treatment of shock which persists after adequate fluid volume replacement

Pregnancy Risk Factor D

Contraindications Hypersensitivity to norepinephrine or sulfites

Warnings/Precautions Blood/volume depletion should be corrected, if possible, before norepinephrine therapy; extravasation may cause severe tissue necrosis, administer into a large vein. The drug should not be given to patients with peripheral or mesenteric vascular thrombosis because ischemia may be increased and the area of infarct extended; use with caution during cyclopropane and halothane anesthesia; use with caution in patients with occlusive vascular disease; some products may contain sulfites

Adverse Reactions

1% to 10%:

- Central nervous system: Dizziness, anxiety, headache, insomnia
- Endocrine & metabolic: Thyroid gland enlargement
- Neuromuscular & skeletal: Trembling

<1%:

- Cardiovascular: Cardiac arrhythmias, palpitations, bradycardia, tachycardia, hypertension, chest pain, pallor, gangrene of extremities
- Gastrointestinal: Vomiting
- Genitourinary: Uterine contractions
- Local: Sloughing at the infusion site
- Ocular: Photophobia
- Respiratory: Respiratory distress
- Miscellaneous: Diaphoresis

Overdosage/Toxicology Symptoms of overdose include hypertension, sweating, cerebral hemorrhage, convulsions

Treatment of extravasation: Infiltrate area of extravasation with phentolamine 5-10 mg in 10-15 mL of saline solution

Drug Interactions

Increased effect with tricyclic antidepressants, MAO inhibitors, antihistamines (diphenhydramine, tripelennamine), guanethidine, ergot alkaloids, and methyldopa

Atropine sulfate may block the reflex bradycardia caused by norepinephrine and enhances the pressor response

Stability Readily oxidized, protect from light, do not use if brown coloration; dilute with D_5W or DS/NS, but not recommended to dilute in normal saline; not stable with alkaline solutions; stability of parenteral admixture at room temperature (25°C): 24 hours

Mechanism of Action Stimulates $beta_1$-adrenergic receptors and alpha-adrenergic receptors causing increased contractility and heart rate as well as vasoconstriction, thereby increasing systemic blood pressure and coronary blood flow; clinically alpha effects (vasoconstriction) are greater than beta effects (inotropic and chronotropic effects)

Pharmacodynamics/Kinetics

Onset of action: I.V.: Very rapid-acting

Duration: Limited

Metabolism: By catechol-o-methyltransferase (COMT) and monoamine oxidase (MAO)

Elimination: In urine (84% to 96% as inactive metabolites)

Usual Dosage Note: Norepinephrine dosage is stated in terms of norepinephrine base and intravenous formulation is norepinephrine bitartrate

Norepinephrine bitartrate 2 mg = norepinephrine base 1 mg

Continuous I.V. infusion:

Children:

Initial: 0.05-0.1 mcg/kg/minute; titrate to desired effect

Maximum dose: 1-2 mcg/kg/minute

Adults: Initiate at 4 mcg/minute and titrate to desired response; 8-12 mcg/minute is usual range

ACLS dosing range: 0.5-30 mcg/minute

Rate of infusion: 4 mg in 500 mL D_5W

2 mcg/minute = 15 mL/hour
4 mcg/minute = 30 mL/hour
6 mcg/minute = 45 mL/hour
8 mcg/minute = 60 mL/hour
10 mcg/minute = 75 mL/hour
12 mcg/minute = 90 mL/hour
14 mcg/minute = 105 mL/hour
16 mcg/minute = 120 mL/hour
18 mcg/minute = 135 mL/hour
20 mcg/minute = 150 mL/hour

Administration Administer into large vein to avoid the potential for extravasation; potent drug, must be diluted prior to use. Rate (mL/hour) = dose (mcg/kg/minute) x weight (kg) x 60 minutes/hour divided by concentration (mcg/mL)

"Rule of 6" method for infusion preparation:

Simplified equation: 0.6 x weight (kg) = amount (mg) of drug to be added to 100 mL of I.V. fluid

When infused at 1 mL/hour, then it will deliver the drug at a rate of 0.1 mcg/kg/minute

Complex equation: 0.6 x desired dose (mcg/kg/minute) x body weight (kg) divided by desired rate (mL/hour) is the mg added to make 100 mL of solution

Nursing Implications Central line administration required; do not administer $NaHCO_3$ through an I.V. line containing norepinephrine; administer into large vein to avoid the potential for extravasation; potent drug, must be diluted prior to use

Extravasation: Use phentolamine as antidote; mix 5 mg with 9 mL of NS; inject a small amount of this dilution into extravasated area; blanching should reverse immediately. Monitor site; if blanching should recur, additional injections of phentolamine may be needed.

Dosage Forms Injection, as bitartrate: 1 mg/mL (4 mL)

Norepinephrine Bitartrate *see* Norepinephrine *on previous page*

Norethin™ 1/35E *see* Ethinyl Estradiol and Norethindrone *on page 486*

Norethin™ 1/50M *see* Mestranol and Norethindrone *on page 791*

Norethindrone Acetate and Ethinyl Estradiol *see* Ethinyl Estradiol and Norethindrone *on page 486*

Norethindrone and Mestranol *see* Mestranol and Norethindrone *on page 791*

Norflex™ *see* Orphenadrine *on page 930*

Norfloxacin (nor FLOKS a sin)

Brand Names Chibroxin™; Noroxin®

Canadian/Mexican Brand Names Floxacin® (Mexico); Oranor® (Mexico)

Therapeutic Category Antibiotic, Ophthalmic; Antibiotic, Quinolone

Use Uncomplicated urinary tract infections and cystitis caused by susceptible gram-negative and gram-positive bacteria; sexually transmitted disease (eg, uncomplicated urethral and cervical gonorrhea) caused by *N. gonorrhoeae*; prostatitis due to *E. coli*; ophthalmic solution for conjunctivitis

Pregnancy Risk Factor C

Contraindications Known hypersensitivity to quinolones

Warnings/Precautions Not recommended in children <18 years of age; other quinolones have caused transient arthropathy in children; CNS stimulation may occur which may lead to tremor, restlessness, confusion, and very rarely to hallucinations or convulsive seizures; use with caution in patients with known or suspected CNS disorders; has rarely caused ruptured tendons (discontinue immediately with signs of inflammation or tendon pain)

Adverse Reactions

1% to 10%:

Central nervous system: Headache, dizziness, fatigue

Gastrointestinal: Nausea

<1%:

Central nervous system: Somnolence, depression, insomnia, fever

Dermatologic: Pruritus, hyperhidrosis, erythema, rash

(Continued)

Norfloxacin *(Continued)*

Gastrointestinal: Abdominal pain, dyspepsia, constipation, flatulence, heartburn, xerostomia, diarrhea, vomiting, loose stools, anorexia, bitter taste, GI bleeding
Hepatic: Increased liver enzymes
Neuromuscular & skeletal: Back pain, ruptured tendons, weakness
Renal: Increased serum creatinine/BUN, acute renal failure

Overdosage/Toxicology Symptoms of overdose include acute renal failure, seizures; following GI decontamination, use supportive measures

Drug Interactions
Decreased effect: Decreased absorption with antacids containing aluminum, magnesium, and/or calcium (by up to 98% if given at the same time)
Increased toxicity/serum levels: Quinolones cause increased levels of caffeine, warfarin, cyclosporine, and theophylline; azlocillin, cimetidine, probenecid increase quinolone levels

Mechanism of Action Norfloxacin is a DNA gyrase inhibitor. DNA gyrase is an essential bacterial enzyme that maintains the superhelical structure of DNA. DNA gyrase is required for DNA replication and transcription, DNA repair, recombination, and transposition; bactericidal

Pharmacodynamics/Kinetics
Absorption: Oral: Rapid, up to 40%
Distribution: Crosses the placenta; small amounts appear in breast milk
Protein binding: 15%
Metabolism: In the liver
Half-life: 4.8 hours (can be higher with reduced glomerular filtration rates)
Time to peak serum concentration: Within 1-2 hours
Elimination: In urine and feces (30%)

Usual Dosage
Ophthalmic: Children >1 year and Adults: Instill 1-2 drops in affected eye(s) 4 times/day for up to 7 days
Oral: Adults:
Urinary tract infections: 400 mg twice daily for 3-21 days depending on severity of infection or organism sensitivity; maximum: 800 mg/day
Uncomplicated gonorrhea: 800 mg as a single dose (CDC recommends as an alternative regimen to ciprofloxacin or ofloxacin)
Prostatitis: 400 mg every 12 hours for 4 weeks

Dosing interval in renal impairment:
Cl_{cr} 10-30 mL/minute: Administer every 24 hours
Cl_{cr} <10 mL/minute: Do not use

Patient Information Tablets should be taken at least 1 hour before or at least 2 hours after a meal with a glass of water; patients receiving norfloxacin should be well hydrated; take all the medication, do not skip doses; do not take with antacids; contact your physician immediately with inflammation or tendon pain

Nursing Implications Hold antacids, sucralfate for 3-4 hours after giving

Dosage Forms
Solution, ophthalmic: 0.3% [3 mg/mL] (5 mL)
Tablet: 400 mg

Norgestrel (nor JES trel)

Brand Names Ovrette®

Therapeutic Category Contraceptive, Oral (Progestin); Progestin Derivative

Use Prevention of pregnancy; **progestin only products have higher risk of failure in contraceptive use**

Pregnancy Risk Factor X

Contraindications Known hypersensitivity to norgestrel; thromboembolic disorders, severe hepatic disease, breast cancer, undiagnosed vaginal bleeding

Warnings/Precautions Discontinue if sudden loss of vision or if diplopia or proptosis occur; use with caution in patients with a history of mental depression; use of any progestin during the first 4 months of pregnancy is not recommended

Adverse Reactions
>10%:
Cardiovascular: Edema
Endocrine & metabolic: Breakthrough bleeding, spotting, changes in menstrual flow, amenorrhea
Gastrointestinal: Anorexia
Neuromuscular & skeletal: Weakness
1% to 10%:
Cardiovascular: Embolism, central thrombosis
Central nervous system: Mental depression, fever, insomnia
Dermatologic: Melasma or chloasma, allergic rash with or without pruritus
Endocrine & metabolic: Changes in cervical erosion and secretions, increased breast tenderness

Gastrointestinal: Weight gain or loss
Hepatic: Cholestatic jaundice
Local: Thrombophlebitis

Overdosage/Toxicology Toxicity is unlikely following single exposures of excessive doses; supportive treatment is adequate in most cases

Drug Interactions Decreased effect: Aminoglutethimide may decrease effects by increasing hepatic metabolism

Mechanism of Action Inhibits secretion of pituitary gonadotropin (LH) which prevents follicular maturation and ovulation

Usual Dosage Administer daily, starting the first day of menstruation, take one tablet at the same time each day, every day of the year. If one dose is missed, take as soon as remembered, then next tablet at regular time; if two doses are missed, take one tablet and discard the other, then take daily at usual time; if three doses are missed, use an additional form of birth control until menses or pregnancy is ruled out

Test Interactions Thyroid function tests, metyrapone test, liver function tests

Patient Information Take this medicine only as directed; do not take more of it and do not take it for a longer period of time; if you suspect you may have become pregnant, stop taking this medicine; report any loss of vision or vision changes immediately; avoid excessive exposure to sunlight

Nursing Implications Patients should receive a copy of the patient labeling

Dosage Forms Tablet: 0.075 mg

Norgestrel and Ethinyl Estradiol *see* Ethinyl Estradiol and Norgestrel *on page 489*

Norinyl® 1+35 *see* Ethinyl Estradiol and Norethindrone *on page 486*

Norinyl® 1+50 *see* Mestranol and Norethindrone *on page 791*

Norisodrine® *see* Isoproterenol *on page 681*

Normal Human Serum Albumin *see* Albumin *on page 37*

Normal Saline *see* Sodium Chloride *on page 1142*

Normal Serum Albumin (Human) *see* Albumin *on page 37*

Normodyne® *see* Labetalol *on page 700*

Noroxin® *see* Norfloxacin *on page 915*

Norpace® *see* Disopyramide *on page 409*

Norplant® *see* Levonorgestrel *on page 718*

Norpramin® *see* Desipramine *on page 352*

Nor-tet® *see* Tetracycline *on page 1203*

Nortriptyline (nor TRIP ti leen)

Related Information

Antidepressant Agents Comparison *on page 1393*

Brand Names Aventyl® Hydrochloride; Pamelor®

Synonyms Nortriptyline Hydrochloride

Therapeutic Category Antidepressant, Tricyclic

Use Treatment of various forms of depression, often in conjunction with psychotherapy. Maximum antidepressant effect may not be seen for 2 or more weeks after initiation of therapy; has also demonstrated effectiveness for chronic pain.

Pregnancy Risk Factor D

Contraindications Narrow-angle glaucoma, avoid use during pregnancy and lactation, hypersensitivity to tricyclic antidepressants

Warnings/Precautions Use with caution in patients with cardiac conduction disturbances, history of hyperthyroid; should not be abruptly discontinued in patients receiving high doses for prolonged periods; use with caution with renal or hepatic impairment

Adverse Reactions

Neuromuscular & skeletal: Tremor

>10%:
- Central nervous system: Dizziness, drowsiness, headache
- Gastrointestinal: Xerostomia, constipation, increased appetite, nausea, unpleasant taste, weight gain
- Neuromuscular & skeletal: Weakness

1% to 10%:
- Cardiovascular: Postural hypotension, arrhythmias, tachycardia, sudden death
- Central nervous system: Confusion, delirium, hallucinations, nervousness, restlessness, parkinsonian syndrome, insomnia
- Endocrine & metabolic: Sexual dysfunction
- Gastrointestinal: Diarrhea, heartburn, constipation
- Genitourinary: Dysuria, urinary retention
- Ocular: Blurred vision, eye pain, increased intraocular pressure
- Neuromuscular & skeletal: Fine muscle tremors
- Miscellaneous: Diaphoresis (excessive)

(Continued)

Nortriptyline *(Continued)*

<1%:

Central nervous system: Anxiety, seizures
Dermatologic: Alopecia, photosensitivity
Endocrine & metabolic: Breast enlargement, galactorrhea, SIADH
Gastrointestinal: Trouble with gums, decreased lower esophageal sphincter tone may cause GE reflux
Genitourinary: Testicular edema
Hematologic: Leukopenia, rarely agranulocytosis, eosinophilia
Hepatic: Increased liver enzymes, cholestatic jaundice
Ocular: Increased intraocular pressure
Otic: Tinnitus
Miscellaneous: Allergic reactions

Overdosage/Toxicology Symptoms of overdose include agitation, confusion, hallucinations, urinary retention, hypothermia, hypotension, seizures, ventricular tachycardia

Following initiation of essential overdose management, toxic symptoms should be treated. Sodium bicarbonate is indicated when QRS interval is >0.10 seconds or QT_c >0.42 seconds. Ventricular arrhythmias and EKG changes (QRS widening) often respond to phenytoin 15-20 mg/kg (adults) with concurrent systemic alkalinization (sodium bicarbonate 0.5-2 mEq/kg I.V.). Arrhythmias unresponsive to this therapy may respond to lidocaine 1 mg/kg I.V. followed by a titrated infusion. Physostigmine (1-2 mg I.V. slowly for adults or 0.5 mg I.V. slowly for children) may be indicated in reversing cardiac arrhythmias that are life-threatening. Seizures usually respond to diazepam I.V. boluses (5-10 mg for adults up to 30 mg or 0.25-0.4 mg/kg/dose for children up to 10 mg/dose). If seizures are unresponsive or recur, phenytoin or phenobarbital may be required.

Drug Interactions Cytochrome P-450 2D6 enzyme substrate

Blocks the uptake of guanethidine and thus prevents the hypotensive effect of guanethidine; may be additive with or may potentiate the action of other CNS depressants such as sedatives or hypnotics; potentiates the pressor and cardiac effects of sympathomimetic agents such as isoproterenol, epinephrine, etc

With MAO inhibitors, hyperpyrexia, hypertension, tachycardia, confusion, seizures, and death have been reported

Additive anticholinergic effect seen with other anticholinergic agents

Cimetidine reduces the metabolism of nortriptyline

May increase prothrombin time in patients stabilized on warfarin

Stability Protect from light

Mechanism of Action Traditionally believed to increase the synaptic concentration of serotonin and/or norepinephrine in the central nervous system by inhibition of their reuptake by the presynaptic neuronal membrane. However, additional receptor effects have been found including desensitization of adenyl cyclase, down regulation of beta-adrenergic receptors, and down regulation of serotonin receptors.

Pharmacodynamics/Kinetics

Onset of action: 1-3 weeks before therapeutic effects are seen
Distribution: V_d: 21 L/kg
Protein binding: 93% to 95%
Metabolism: Undergoes significant first-pass metabolism; primarily detoxified in the liver
Half-life: 28-31 hours
Time to peak serum concentration: Oral: Within 7-8.5 hours
Elimination: As metabolites and small amounts of unchanged drug in urine; small amounts of biliary elimination occur

Usual Dosage Oral:

Nocturnal enuresis:
- Children:
  - 6-7 years (20-25 kg): 10 mg/day
  - 8-11 years (25-35 kg): 10-20 mg/day
  - >11 years (35-54 kg): 25-35 mg/day

Depression:
- Adolescents: 30-50 mg/day in divided doses
- Adults: 25 mg 3-4 times/day up to 150 mg/day
- Elderly:
  - Initial: 10-25 mg at bedtime
  - Dosage can be increased by 25 mg every 3 days for inpatients and weekly for outpatients if tolerated
  - Usual maintenance dose: 75 mg as a single bedtime dose, however, lower or higher doses may be required to stay within the therapeutic window

Dosing adjustment in hepatic impairment: Lower doses and slower titration dependent on individualization of dosage is recommended

Dietary Considerations Alcohol: Additive CNS effect, avoid use

Monitoring Parameters Monitor blood pressure and pulse rate prior to and during initial therapy; evaluate mental status; monitor weight

Reference Range

Plasma levels do not always correlate with clinical effectiveness

Therapeutic: 50-150 ng/mL (SI: 190-570 nmol/L)

Toxic: >500 ng/mL (SI: >1900 nmol/L)

Test Interactions ↑ glucose

Patient Information Avoid alcohol ingestion; do not discontinue medication abruptly; may cause urine to turn blue-green; may cause drowsiness; full effect may not occur for 3-6 weeks; dry mouth may be helped by sips of water, sugarless gum, or hard candy

Nursing Implications May increase appetite and possibly a craving for sweets

Dosage Forms

Capsule, as hydrochloride: 10 mg, 25 mg, 50 mg, 75 mg

Solution, as hydrochloride: 10 mg/5 mL (473 mL)

Nortriptyline Hydrochloride *see* Nortriptyline *on page 917*

Norvasc® *see* Amlodipine *on page 72*

Norvir® *see* Ritonavir *on page 1113*

Norzine® *see* Thiethylperazine *on page 1215*

Nōstrilla® [OTC] *see* Oxymetazoline *on page 940*

Nostril® Nasal Solution [OTC] *see* Phenylephrine *on page 989*

Novafed® *see* Pseudoephedrine *on page 1074*

Novantrone® *see* Mitoxantrone *on page 849*

Novocain® *see* Procaine *on page 1049*

Novolin® 70/30 *see* Insulin Preparations *on page 659*

Novolin® L *see* Insulin Preparations *on page 659*

Novolin® N *see* Insulin Preparations *on page 659*

Novolin® R *see* Insulin Preparations *on page 659*

NP-27® [OTC] *see* Tolnaftate *on page 1243*

NPH Iletin® I *see* Insulin Preparations *on page 659*

NPH Insulin *see* Insulin Preparations *on page 659*

NPH-N *see* Insulin Preparations *on page 659*

NSC 125066 *see* Bleomycin *on page 159*

NTG *see* Nitroglycerin *on page 909*

NTZ® Long Acting Nasal Solution [OTC] *see* Oxymetazoline *on page 940*

Nubain® *see* Nalbuphine *on page 873*

NuLytely® *see* Polyethylene Glycol-Electrolyte Solution *on page 1017*

Numorphan® *see* Oxymorphone *on page 942*

Numzitdent® [OTC] *see* Benzocaine *on page 138*

Numzit Teething® [OTC] *see* Benzocaine *on page 138*

Nupercainal® [OTC] *see* Dibucaine *on page 373*

Nuprin® [OTC] *see* Ibuprofen *on page 639*

Nuquin HP® *see* Hydroquinone *on page 628*

Nuromax® Injection *see* Doxacurium *on page 421*

Nutracort® *see* Hydrocortisone *on page 623*

Nutraplus® [OTC] *see* Urea *on page 1280*

Nutrilipid® *see* Fat Emulsion *on page 505*

Nutropin® AQ Injection *see* Human Growth Hormone *on page 613*

Nutropin® Injection *see* Human Growth Hormone *on page 613*

Nydrazid® Injection *see* Isoniazid *on page 679*

Nystatin (nye STAT in)

Related Information

Antifungal Agents *on page 1395*

Guidelines for the Prevention of Opportunistic Infections in Persons with HIV *on page 1457*

Brand Names Mycostatin®; Nilstat®; Nystat-Rx®; Nystex®; O-V Staticin®

Canadian/Mexican Brand Names Mestatin® (Canada); Nadostine® (Canada); PMS-Nystatin (Canada); Micostatin® (Mexico); Nistaquim® (Mexico)

Therapeutic Category Antifungal Agent, Oral Nonabsorbed; Antifungal Agent, Topical; Antifungal Agent, Vaginal

Use Treatment of susceptible cutaneous, mucocutaneous, and oral cavity fungal infections normally caused by the *Candida* species

Pregnancy Risk Factor B/C (oral)

Contraindications Hypersensitivity to nystatin or any component

Adverse Reactions

1% to 10%: Gastrointestinal: Nausea, vomiting, diarrhea, stomach pain

(Continued)

Nystatin *(Continued)*

<1%: Miscellaneous: Hypersensitivity reactions

Dermatologic: Contact dermatitis, Stevens-Johnson syndrome

Overdosage/Toxicology Symptoms of overdose include nausea, vomiting, diarrhea

Stability Keep vaginal inserts in refrigerator; protect from temperature extremes, moisture, and light

Mechanism of Action Binds to sterols in fungal cell membrane, changing the cell wall permeability allowing for leakage of cellular contents

Pharmacodynamics/Kinetics

Onset of symptomatic relief from candidiasis: Within 24-72 hours

Absorption: Not absorbed through mucous membranes or intact skin; poorly absorbed from the GI tract

Elimination: In feces as unchanged drug

Usual Dosage

Oral candidiasis: Suspension (swish and swallow orally):

Infants: 200,000 units 4 times/day or 100,000 units to each side of mouth 4 times/day

Children and Adults: 400,000-600,000 units 4 times/day; troche: 200,000-400,000 units 4-5 times/day

Adults: 400,000-600,000 units 4 times/day; pastilles: 200,000-400,000 units 4-5 times/day

Mucocutaneous infections: Children and Adults: Topical: Apply 2-3 times/day to affected areas; very moist topical lesions are treated best with powder

Intestinal infections: Adults: Oral tablets: 500,000-1,000,000 units every 8 hours

Vaginal infections: Adults: Vaginal tablets: Insert 1 tablet/day at bedtime for 2 weeks

Patient Information The oral suspension should be swished about the mouth and retained in the mouth for as long as possible (several minutes) before swallowing. For neonates and infants, paint nystatin suspension into recesses of the mouth. Troches must be allowed to dissolve slowly and should not be chewed or swallowed whole. If topical irritation occurs, discontinue; for external use only; do not discontinue therapy even if symptoms are gone

Dosage Forms

Cream: 100,000 units/g (15 g, 30 g)

Ointment, topical: 100,000 units/g (15 g, 30 g)

Powder, for preparation of oral suspension: 50 million units, 1 billion units, 2 billion units, 5 billion units

Powder, topical: 100,000 units/g (15 g)

Suspension, oral: 100,000 units/mL (5 mL, 60 mL, 480 mL)

Tablet:

Oral: 500,000 units

Vaginal: 100,000 units (15 and 30/box with applicator)

Troche: 200,000 units

Nystatin and Triamcinolone (nye STAT in & trye am SIN oh lone)

Brand Names Mycogen II Topical; Mycolog®-II Topical; Myconel® Topical; Myco-Triacet® II; Mytrex® F Topical; N.G.T.® Topical; Tri-Statin® II Topical

Synonyms Triamcinolone and Nystatin

Therapeutic Category Antifungal Agent, Topical; Corticosteroid, Topical (Medium Potency)

Use Treatment of cutaneous candidiasis

Pregnancy Risk Factor C

Contraindications Known hypersensitivity to nystatin or triamcinolone

Warnings/Precautions Avoid use of occlusive dressings; limit therapy to least amount necessary for effective therapy, pediatric patients may be more susceptible to HPA axis suppression due to larger BSA to weight ratio

Adverse Reactions

1% to 10%:

Dermatologic: Dryness, folliculitis, hypertrichosis, acne, hypopigmentation, allergic dermatitis, maceration of the skin, skin atrophy, itching

Local: Burning, irritation

Miscellaneous: Increased incidence of secondary infection

Overdosage/Toxicology Refer to individual monographs for Nystatin and Triamcinolone

Mechanism of Action Refer to individual monographs for Nystatin and Triamcinolone

Pharmacodynamics/Kinetics Refer to individual monographs for Nystatin and Triamcinolone

Usual Dosage Children and Adults: Topical: Apply sparingly 2-4 times/day

Patient Information Before applying, gently wash area to reduce risk of infection; apply a thin film to cleansed area and rub in gently and thoroughly until medication vanishes; avoid exposure to sunlight, severe sunburn may occur

Nursing Implications External use only; do not use on open wounds; apply sparingly to occlusive dressings; should not be used in the presence of open or weeping lesions

Dosage Forms

Cream: Nystatin 100,000 units and triamcinolone acetonide 0.1% (1.5 g, 15 g, 30 g, 60 g, 120 g)

Ointment, topical: Nystatin 100,000 units and triamcinolone acetonide 0.1% (15 g, 30 g, 60 g, 120 g)

Nystat-Rx® *see* Nystatin *on page 919*

Nystex® *see* Nystatin *on page 919*

Nytol® Oral [OTC] *see* Diphenhydramine *on page 399*

Occlusal-HP Liquid *see* Salicylic Acid *on page 1120*

Occupational Exposure to HIV *see page 1448*

Ocean Nasal Mist [OTC] *see* Sodium Chloride *on page 1142*

OCL® *see* Polyethylene Glycol-Electrolyte Solution *on page 1017*

Octamide® *see* Metoclopramide *on page 824*

Octicair® Otic *see* Neomycin, Polymyxin B, and Hydrocortisone *on page 890*

Octocaine® *see* Lidocaine *on page 723*

Octocaine® Injection *see* Lidocaine and Epinephrine *on page 725*

Octreotide Acetate (ok TREE oh tide AS e tate)

Brand Names Sandostatin®

Therapeutic Category Antidiarrheal; Antisecretory Agent; Somatostatin Analog

Use Control of symptoms in patients with metastatic carcinoid and vasoactive intestinal peptide-secreting tumors (VIPomas); pancreatic tumors, gastrinoma, secretory diarrhea

Unlabeled uses: Acromegaly, AIDS-associated secretory diarrhea, control of bleeding of esophageal varices, breast cancer, cryptosporidiosis, Cushing's syndrome, insulinomas, small bowel fistulas, postgastrectomy dumping syndrome, chemotherapy-induced diarrhea, GVHD-induced diarrhea, Zollinger-Ellison syndrome

Pregnancy Risk Factor B

Contraindications Known hypersensitivity to octreotide or any component

Warnings/Precautions Dosage adjustment may be required to maintain symptomatic control; insulin requirements may be reduced as well as sulfonylurea requirements; monitor patients for cholelithiasis, hyper- or hypoglycemia; use with caution in patients with renal impairment

Adverse Reactions

1% to 10%:

Cardiovascular: Flushing, edema

Central nervous system: Fatigue, headache, dizziness, vertigo, anorexia, depression

Endocrine & metabolic: Hypoglycemia or hyperglycemia (1%), hypothyroidism, galactorrhea

Gastrointestinal: Nausea, vomiting, diarrhea, constipation, abdominal pain, cramping, discomfort, fat malabsorption, loose stools, flatulence

Hepatic: Jaundice, hepatitis, increase LFTs, cholelithiasis has occurred, presumably by altering fat absorption and decreasing the motility of the gallbladder

Local: Pain at injection site

Neuromuscular & skeletal: Weakness

<1%:

Cardiovascular: Chest pain, hypertensive reaction

Central nervous system: Anxiety, fever, hyperesthesia

Dermatologic: Alopecia, wheal/erythema, rash

Local: Thrombophlebitis

Neuromuscular & skeletal: Leg cramps, Bell's palsy, muscle cramping

Ocular: Burning eyes

Respiratory: Throat discomfort, rhinorrhea, shortness of breath

Overdosage/Toxicology Symptoms of overdose include hypo- or hyperglycemia, blurred vision, dizziness, drowsiness, loss of motor function; well tolerated bolus doses up to 1000 mcg have failed to produce adverse effects

Drug Interactions Decreased effect: Cyclosporine (case report of a transplant rejection due to reduction of serum cyclosporine levels)

Stability Octreotide is a clear solution and should be stored under refrigeration; ampuls may be stored at room temperature for up to 14 days when protected from light

(Continued)

Octreotide Acetate *(Continued)*

Stability of parenteral admixture in NS at room temperature (25°C) and at refrigeration temperature (4°C): 48 hours

Common diluent: 50-100 mcg/50 mL NS; common diluent for continuous I.V. infusion: 1200 mcg/250 mL NS

Minimum volume: 50 mL NS

Mechanism of Action Mimics natural somatostatin by inhibiting serotonin release, and the secretion of gastrin, VIP, insulin, glucagon, secretin, motilin, and pancreatic polypeptide

Pharmacodynamics/Kinetics

Duration of action: 6-12 hours

Absorption:

Oral: Absorbed but still under study

S.C.: Rapid

Bioavailability: S.C.: 100%

Distribution: V_d: 14 L; 65% bound to lipoproteins

Metabolism: Extensive by the liver

Half-life: 60-110 minutes

Elimination: 32% by the kidney

Usual Dosage Adults: S.C.: Initial: 50 mcg 1-2 times/day and titrate dose based on patient tolerance and response

Carcinoid: 100-600 mcg/day in 2-4 divided doses

VIPomas: 200-300 mcg/day in 2-4 divided doses

Diarrhea: Initial: I.V.: 50-100 mcg every 8 hours; increase by 100 mcg/dose at 48-hour intervals; maximum dose: 500 mcg every 8 hours

Esophageal varices bleeding: I.V. bolus: 25-50 mcg followed by continuous I.V. infusion of 25-50 mcg/hour

Administration

Administer S.C. or I.V.

I.V. administration may be IVP, IVPB, or continuous I.V. infusion

IVP should be administered undiluted over 3 minutes

IVPB should be administered over 15-30 minutes

Continuous I.V. infusion rates have ranged from 25-50 mcg/hour for the treatment of esophageal variceal bleeding

Reference Range Vasoactive intestinal peptide: <75 ng/L; levels vary considerably between laboratories

Nursing Implications Do not use if solution contains particles or is discolored

Dosage Forms Injection: 0.05 mg/mL (1 mL); 0.1 mg/mL (1 mL); 0.2 mg/mL (5 mL); 0.5 mg/mL (1 mL); 1 mg/mL (5 mL)

Ocu-Carpine® Ophthalmic *see* Pilocarpine *on page 999*

OcuClear® Ophthalmic [OTC] *see* Oxymetazoline *on page 940*

Ocu-Dex® *see* Dexamethasone *on page 356*

Ocu-Drop® [OTC] *see* Tetrahydrozoline *on page 1205*

Ocufen® *see* Flurbiprofen *on page 547*

Ocuflox™ *see* Ofloxacin *on this page*

Oculinum® *see* Botulinum Toxin Type A *on page 161*

Ocumycin® *see* Gentamicin *on page 570*

Ocu-Pentolate® *see* Cyclopentolate *on page 323*

Ocupress® *see* Carteolol *on page 212*

Ocusert Pilo-20® Ophthalmic *see* Pilocarpine *on page 999*

Ocusert Pilo-40® Ophthalmic *see* Pilocarpine *on page 999*

Ocusulf-10® Ophthalmic *see* Sulfacetamide Sodium *on page 1171*

Ocutricin® Ophthalmic Solution *see* Neomycin, Polymyxin B, and Gramicidin *on page 889*

Ocutricin® Topical Ointment *see* Bacitracin, Neomycin, and Polymyxin B *on page 129*

Ocu-Tropine® *see* Atropine *on page 116*

Off-Ezy® Wart Remover [OTC] *see* Salicylic Acid *on page 1120*

Ofloxacin (oh FLOKS a sin)

Related Information

Antimicrobial Drugs of Choice *on page 1468*

Treatment of Sexually Transmitted Diseases *on page 1485*

Brand Names Floxin®; Ocuflox™

Canadian/Mexican Brand Names Bactocin® (Mexico); Floxil® (Mexico); Floxstat® (Mexico)

Therapeutic Category Antibiotic, Quinolone

Use Quinolone antibiotic for skin and skin structure, lower respiratory and urinary tract infections, and sexually transmitted diseases (eg, uncomplicated gonorrhea); bacterial conjunctivitis caused by susceptible organisms and corneal ulcers also may be treated. **Note:** Avoid use in treating gonorrhea in travelers from Asia due to growing resistance, consider adding azithromycin or doxycycline.

Pregnancy Risk Factor C

Contraindications Hypersensitivity to ofloxacin or other members of the quinolone group such as nalidixic acid, oxolinic acid, cinoxacin, norfloxacin, and ciprofloxacin

Warnings/Precautions Use with caution in patients with epilepsy or other CNS diseases which could predispose seizures; use with caution in patients with renal impairment; failure to respond to an ophthalmic antibiotic after 2-3 days may indicate the presence of resistant organisms, or another causative agent; use caution with systemic preparation in children <18 years of age due to association of other quinolones with transient arthropathy; has rarely caused ruptured tendons (discontinue immediately with signs of inflammation or tendon pain)

Adverse Reactions

>10%: Gastrointestinal: Nausea

1% to 10%:

- Cardiovascular: Chest pain
- Central nervous system: Headache, insomnia, dizziness, fatigue, somnolence, sleep disorders, nervousness, pyrexia, pain
- Dermatologic: Rash, pruritus
- Gastrointestinal: Diarrhea, vomiting, GI distress, cramps, abdominal cramps, flatulence, abnormal taste, xerostomia, decreased appetite
- Genitourinary: Vaginitis, external genital pruritus in women
- Ocular: Superinfection (ophthalmic), photophobia, lacrimation, dry eyes, stinging, visual disturbances
- Miscellaneous: Trunk pain

<1%:

- Cardiovascular: Syncope, edema, hypertension, palpitations, vasodilation
- Central nervous system: Anxiety, cognitive change, depression, dream abnormality, euphoria, hallucinations, vertigo, chills, malaise, extremity pain
- Gastrointestinal: Weight loss
- Neuromuscular & skeletal: Paresthesia, ruptured tendons, weakness
- Ocular: Photophobia
- Otic: Decreased hearing acuity, tinnitus
- Respiratory: Cough
- Miscellaneous: Thirst

Overdosage/Toxicology Symptoms of overdose include acute renal failure, seizures, nausea, vomiting

Treatment includes GI decontamination, if possible, and supportive care; not removed by peritoneal or hemodialysis

Drug Interactions

Decreased effect: Decreased absorption with antacids containing aluminum, magnesium, and/or calcium (by up to 98% if given at the same time)

Increased toxicity/serum levels: Quinolones cause increased caffeine, warfarin, cyclosporine, procainamide, and theophylline levels; azlocillin, cimetidine, probenecid increase quinolone levels

Mechanism of Action Ofloxacin, a fluorinated quinolone, is a pyridine carboxylic acid derivative which exerts a broad spectrum bactericidal effect. It inhibits DNA gyrase inhibitor, an essential bacterial enzyme that maintains the superhelical structure of DNA. DNA gyrase is required for DNA replication and transcription, DNA repair, recombination, and transposition within the bacteria.

Pharmacodynamics/Kinetics

Absorption: Well absorbed; administration with food causes only minor alterations in absorption

Distribution: V_d: 2.4-3.5 L/kg

Protein binding: 20%

Half-life, elimination 5-7.5 hours

Elimination: Primarily unchanged in urine

Usual Dosage

Children >1 year and Adults: Ophthalmic: Instill 1-2 drops in affected eye(s) every 2-4 hours for the first 2 days, then use 4 times/day for an additional 5 days

Adults: Oral, I.V.: 200-400 mg every 12 hours for 7-10 days for most infections or for 6 weeks for prostatitis

Dosing adjustment/interval in renal impairment:

Cl_{cr} 10-50 mL/minute: Administer 50% of normal dose or administer every 24 hours

Cl_{cr} <10 mL/minute: Administer 25% of normal dose or administer 50% of normal dose every 24 hours

Patient Information Report any skin rash or other allergic reactions; avoid excessive sunlight; do not take with food; do not take within 2 hours of any

(Continued)

Ofloxacin *(Continued)*

products including antacids which contain zinc, magnesium, or aluminum; contact your physician immediately with signs of inflammation or tendon pain

Dosage Forms

Injection: 200 mg (50 mL); 400 mg (10 mL, 20 mL, 100 mL)
Solution, ophthalmic: 0.3% (5 mL)
Tablet: 200 mg, 300 mg, 400 mg

Ogen® *see* Estropipate *on page 475*

OGMT *see* Metyrosine *on page 831*

OKT3 *see* Muromonab-CD3 *on page 863*

Olanzapine (oh LAN za peen)

Brand Names Zyprexa®

Synonyms LY170053

Therapeutic Category Antipsychotic Agent

Use Treatment of the manifestations of psychotic disorders

Warnings/Precautions Use with caution in patients with cardiovascular disease, cerebrovascular disease, hypovolemia, dehydration, seizure disorders, Alzheimers disease, hepatic impairment, prostatic hypertrophy, narrow-angle glaucoma, history of paralytic ileus or a history of breast cancer, the elderly, and in pregnancy or with nursing patients

Adverse Reactions

>10%: Central nervous system: Headache, somnolence, insomnia, agitation, nervousness, hostility, dizziness

1% to 10%:

- Central nervous system: Dystonic reactions, Parkinsonian events, akathisia, anxiety, personality changes, fever
- Gastrointestinal: Xerostomia, constipation, abdominal pain, weight gain
- Neuromuscular & skeletal: Arthralgia
- Ocular: Amblyopia
- Respiratory: Rhinitis, cough, pharyngitis

<1%:

- Cardiovascular: Peripheral edema
- Central nervous system: Tardive dyskinesia, neuroleptic malignant syndrome

Drug Interactions

Decreased effect: Cigarette smoking, levodopa, pergolide, bromocriptine, charcoal, and reduction of effects may be seen with cytochrome P-450 enzyme inducers such as rifampin, omeprazole, carbamazepine

Increased effect: Effects may be potentiated with cytochrome P-450 $1A_2$ inhibitors such as fluvoxamine

Increased toxicity: Increased sedation with alcohol or other CNS depressants, increased risk of hypotension and orthostatic hypotension with antihypertensives

Mechanism of Action Olanzapine is a thienobenzodiazepine neuroleptic; thought to work by antagonizing dopamine and serotonin activities. It is a selective monoaminergic antagonist with high affinity binding to serotonin $5HT2_A$ and $5HT2_C$, dopamine D_{1-4}, muscarinic M_{1-5}, histamine H_1 and alpha$_1$-adrenergic receptor sites.

Usual Dosage Adults >18 years: Oral: Usual starting dose: 5-10 mg once daily; increase to 10 mg once daily within 5-7 days, thereafter adjust by 5 mg/day at 1-week intervals, up to a maximum of 20 mg/day

Dosage Forms Tablet: 5 mg, 7.5 mg, 10 mg

Oleovitamin A *see* Vitamin A *on page 1307*

Oleum Ricini *see* Castor Oil *on page 216*

Olsalazine (ole SAL a zeen)

Brand Names Dipentum®

Synonyms Olsalazine Sodium

Therapeutic Category 5-Aminosalicylic Acid Derivative; Anti-inflammatory Agent

Use Maintenance of remission of ulcerative colitis in patients intolerant to sulfasalazine

Pregnancy Risk Factor C

Contraindications Hypersensitivity to salicylates

Warnings/Precautions Diarrhea is a common adverse effect of olsalazine; use with caution in patients with hypersensitivity to salicylates, sulfasalazine, or mesalamine

Adverse Reactions

>10%: Gastrointestinal: Diarrhea, cramps, abdominal pain

1% to 10%:

- Central nervous system: Headache, fatigue, depression

Dermatologic: Rash, itching
Gastrointestinal: Nausea, dyspepsia, bloating, anorexia
Neuromuscular & skeletal: Arthralgia

<1%:

Central nervous system: Fever
Gastrointestinal: Bloody diarrhea
Hematologic: Blood dyscrasias
Hepatic: Hepatitis

Overdosage/Toxicology Symptoms of overdose include decreased motor activity, diarrhea

Mechanism of Action The mechanism of action appears to be topical rather than systemic

Pharmacodynamics/Kinetics

Absorption: <3%; very little intact olsalazine is systemically absorbed
Protein binding: High
Metabolism: Mostly by colonic bacteria to the active drug, 5-aminosalicylic acid
Half-life, elimination: 56 minutes or 55 hours depending on the analysis used
Elimination: Primarily in feces

Usual Dosage Adults: Oral: 1 g/day in 2 divided doses

Test Interactions ↑ ALT, AST (S)

Patient Information Take with food in evenly divided doses; report any sign of allergic reaction including rash

Dosage Forms Capsule, as sodium: 250 mg

Olsalazine Sodium *see* Olsalazine *on previous page*

Omeprazole (oh ME pray zol)

Related Information

Helicobacter pylori Treatment *on page 1534*

Replaces Losec®

Brand Names Prilosec™

Canadian/Mexican Brand Names Losec® (Canada); Inhibitron® (Mexico); Ozoken® (Mexico); Prazidec® (Mexico); Ulsen® (Mexico)

Therapeutic Category Gastric Acid Secretion Inhibitor

Use Short-term (4-8 weeks) treatment of severe erosive esophagitis (grade 2 or above), diagnosed by endoscopy and short-term treatment of symptomatic gastroesophageal reflux disease (GERD) poorly responsive to customary medical treatment; pathological hypersecretory conditions; peptic ulcer disease; gastric ulcer therapy; approved for combination use in the eradication of *H. pylori* in patients with active duodenal ulcer.

Unlabeled use: Healing NSAID-induced ulcers

Pregnancy Risk Factor C

Pregnancy/Breast-Feeding Implications

Clinical effects on the fetus: Crosses the placenta
Breast-feeding/lactation: No data available. American Academy of Pediatrics makes NO RECOMMENDATION.

Contraindications Known hypersensitivity to omeprazole

Warnings/Precautions In long-term (2-year) studies in rats, omeprazole produced a dose-related increase in gastric carcinoid tumors. While available endoscopic evaluations and histologic examinations of biopsy specimens from human stomachs have not detected a risk from short-term exposure to omeprazole, further human data on the effect of sustained hypochlorhydria and hypergastrinemia are needed to rule out the possibility of an increased risk for the development of tumors in humans receiving long-term therapy. Bioavailability may be increased in the elderly.

Adverse Reactions

1% to 10%:

Cardiovascular: Angina, tachycardia, bradycardia, edema
Central nervous system: Headache (7%), dizziness
Dermatologic: Rash, urticaria, pruritus, dry skin
Gastrointestinal: Diarrhea, nausea, abdominal pain, vomiting, constipation, anorexia, irritable colon, fecal discoloration, esophageal candidiasis, xerostomia, abnormal taste
Genitourinary: Testicular pain, urinary tract infection, polyuria
Neuromuscular & skeletal: Back pain, muscle cramps, myalgia, arthralgia, leg pain, weakness occurred in more frequently than 1% of patients
Renal: Pyuria, proteinuria, hematuria, glycosuria
Respiratory: Cough

<1%:

Cardiovascular: Chest pain
Central nervous system: Fever, fatigue, malaise, apathy, somnolence, nervousness, anxiety, pain
Gastrointestinal: Abdominal swelling

(Continued)

Omeprazole *(Continued)*

Overdosage/Toxicology Symptoms of overdose include hypothermia, sedation, convulsions, decreased respiratory rate demonstrated in animals only; treatment is supportive; not dialyzable

Drug Interactions Cytochrome P-450 1A2 enzyme inducer and cytochrome P-450 IIC enzyme inhibitor

Decreased effect: Decreased ketoconazole; decreased itraconazole

Increased toxicity: Diazepam may increase half-life; increased digoxin, increased phenytoin, increased warfarin

Stability Omeprazole stability is a function of pH; it is rapidly degraded in acidic media, but has acceptable stability under alkaline conditions. Prilosec™ is supplied as capsules for oral administration; each capsule contains 20 mg of omeprazole in the form of enteric coated granules to inhibit omeprazole degradation by gastric acidity; therefore, the manufacturer recommends against extemporaneously preparing it in an oral liquid form for administration via an NG tube.

Mechanism of Action Suppresses gastric acid secretion by inhibiting the parietal cell H+/K+ ATP pump

Pharmacodynamics/Kinetics

Onset of antisecretory action: Oral: Within 1 hour

Peak effect: 2 hours

Duration: 72 hours

Protein binding: 95%

Metabolism: Extensive in the liver

Half-life: 30-90 minutes

Usual Dosage Adults: Oral:

Active duodenal ulcer: 20 mg/day for 4-8 weeks

GERD or severe erosive esophagitis: 20 mg/day for 4-8 weeks

Pathological hypersecretory conditions: 60 mg once daily to start; doses up to 120 mg 3 times/day have been administered; administer daily doses >80 mg in divided doses

Helicobacter pylori: Combination therapy with bismuth subsalicylate, tetracycline, clarithromycin, and H_2-antagonist; or with clarithromycin. Adult dose: Oral: 20 mg twice daily

Gastric ulcers: 40 mg/day for 4-8 weeks

Administration Administration via NG tube should be in an acidic juice; although not recommended by the manufacturer, the extemporaneous oral liquid formulation has been described; it is best to maintain the pH of the solution less than 5.3, this can be accomplished with an acidic beverage such as orange juice or cranberry juice

Patient Information Take before eating; do not chew, crush, or open capsule

Nursing Implications Capsule should be swallowed whole; not chewed, crushed, or opened

Dosage Forms Capsule, delayed release: 10 mg, 20 mg

OmniHIB® *see Haemophilus* b Conjugate Vaccine *on page 595*

Omnipen® *see* Ampicillin *on page 85*

Omnipen®-N *see* Ampicillin *on page 85*

OMS® *see* Morphine Sulfate *on page 858*

Oncaspar® *see* Pegaspargase *on page 956*

Oncovin® *see* Vincristine *on page 1302*

Ondansetron (on DAN se tron)

Brand Names Zofran®

Synonyms Ondansetron Hydrochloride

Therapeutic Category Antiemetic; Serotonin Antagonist

Use May be prescribed for patients who are refractory to or have severe adverse reactions to standard antiemetic therapy. Ondansetron may be prescribed for young patients (ie, <45 years of age who are more likely to develop extrapyramidal reactions to high-dose metoclopramide) who are to receive highly emetogenic chemotherapeutic agents as listed:

Agents with high emetogenic potential (>90%) (dose/m^2):

- Carmustine ≥200 mg
- Cisplatin ≥75 mg
- Cyclophosphamide ≥1000 mg
- Cytarabine ≥1000 mg
- Dacarbazine ≥500 mg
- Ifosfamide ≥1000 mg
- Lomustine ≥60 mg
- Mechlorethamine
- Pentostatin
- Streptozocin

or two agents classified as having high or moderately high emetogenic potential as listed:

Agents with moderately high emetogenic potential (60% to 90%) (dose/m^2):
- Carmustine <200 mg
- Cisplatin <75 mg
- Cyclophosphamide 1000 mg
- Cytarabine 250-1000 mg
- Dacarbazine <500 mg
- Doxorubicin ≥75 mg
- Ifosfamide
- Lomustine <60 mg
- Methotrexate ≥250 mg
- Mitomycin
- Mitoxantrone
- Procarbazine

Ondansetron should not be prescribed for chemotherapeutic agents with a low emetogenic potential (eg, bleomycin, busulfan, cyclophosphamide <1000 mg, etoposide, 5-fluorouracil, vinblastine, vincristine)

Pregnancy Risk Factor B

Pregnancy/Breast-Feeding Implications

Clinical effects on the fetus: No data available on crossing the placenta; no effects on the fetus from 2 case reports

Breast-feeding/lactation: No data available. American Academy of Pediatrics has NO RECOMMENDATION.

Contraindications Hypersensitivity to ondansetron or any component

Warnings/Precautions **Ondansetron should be used on a scheduled basis, not as an "as needed" (PRN) basis,** since data supports the use of this drug in the prevention of nausea and vomiting and not in the rescue of nausea and vomiting. Ondansetron should only be used in the first 24-48 hours of receiving chemotherapy. Data does not support any increased efficacy of ondansetron in delayed nausea and vomiting.

Adverse Reactions

>10%:
- Central nervous system: Headache, fever
- Gastrointestinal: Constipation, diarrhea

1% to 10%:
- Central nervous system: Dizziness
- Gastrointestinal: Abdominal cramps, xerostomia
- Neuromuscular & skeletal: Weakness

<1%:
- Cardiovascular: Tachycardia
- Central nervous system: Lightheadedness, seizures
- Dermatologic: Rash
- Endocrine & metabolic: Hypokalemia
- Hepatic: Transient elevations in serum levels of aminotransferases and bilirubin
- Respiratory: Bronchospasm, shortness of breath, wheezing

Drug Interactions Mild cytochrome P-450 1A2 enzyme substrate, cytochrome P-450 2D6 enzyme substrate, and cytochrome P-450 3A enzyme substrate

Decreased effect: Metabolized by the hepatic cytochrome P-450 enzymes; therefore, the drug's clearance and half-life may be changed with concomitant use of cytochrome P-450 inducers (eg, barbiturates, carbamazepine, rifampin, phenytoin, and phenylbutazone)

Increased toxicity: Inhibitors (eg, cimetidine, allopurinol, and disulfiram)

Stability Injection may be stored between 36°F and 86°F; stable when mixed in 5% dextrose or 0.9% sodium chloride for 48 hours at room temperature; does not need protection from light

Mechanism of Action Selective 5-HT$_3$-receptor antagonist, blocking serotonin, both peripherally on vagal nerve terminals and centrally in the chemoreceptor trigger zone

Pharmacodynamics/Kinetics

Plasma protein binding: 70% to 76%

Metabolism: Extensively by hydroxylation, followed by glucuronide or sulfate conjugation

Half-life:
- Children <15 years: 2-3 hours
- Adults: 4 hours

Elimination: In urine and feces; <10% of parent drug recovered unchanged in urine

(Continued)

Ondansetron *(Continued)*

Usual Dosage

Oral:

Children 4-11 years: 4 mg 30 minutes before chemotherapy; repeat 4 and 8 hours after initial dose

Children >11 years and Adults: 8 mg 30 minutes before chemotherapy; repeat 4 and 8 hours after initial dose or every 8 hours for a maximum of 48 hours

I.V.: Administer either three 0.15 mg/kg doses or a single 32 mg dose; with the 3-dose regimen, the initial dose is given 30 minutes prior to chemotherapy with subsequent doses administered 4 and 8 hours after the first dose. With the single-dose regimen 32 mg is infused over 15 minutes beginning 30 minutes before the start of emetogenic chemotherapy. Dosage should be calculated based on weight:

Children: Pediatric dosing should follow the manufacturer's guidelines for 0.15 mg/kg/dose administered 30 minutes prior to chemotherapy, 4 and 8 hours after the first dose. While not as yet FDA-approved, literature supports the day's total dose administered as a single dose 30 minutes prior to chemotherapy.

Adults:

>80 kg: 12 mg IVPB

45-80 kg: 8 mg IVPB

<45 kg: 0.15 mg/kg/dose IVPB

Dosing in hepatic impairment: Maximum daily dose: 8 mg in cirrhotic patients with severe liver disease

Dietary Considerations

Food: Increases the extent of absorption. The C_{max} and T_{max} does not change much; take without regard to meals

Potassium: Hypokalemia; monitor potassium serum concentration

Nursing Implications First dose should be given 30 minutes prior to beginning chemotherapy

Dosage Forms

Injection, as hydrochloride: 2 mg/mL (20 mL); 32 mg (single-dose vials)

Tablet, as hydrochloride: 4 mg, 8 mg

Extemporaneous Preparations A 0.8 mg/mL syrup may be made by crushing ten 8 mg tablets; flaking of the tablet coating occurs. Mix thoroughly with 50 mL of the suspending vehicle, Ora-Plus (Paddock), in 5 mL increments. Add sufficient volume of any of the following syrups: Cherry syrup USP, Syrpalta® (Humco), Ora-Sweet (Paddock), or Ora-Sweet Sugar-Free (Paddock) to make a final volume of 100 mL. Stability is 42 days refrigerated.

Trissel LA, "Trissel's Stability of Compounded Formulations," American Pharmaceutical Association, 1996.

Ondansetron Hydrochloride *see* Ondansetron *on page 926*

Ony-Clear® Spray *see* Miconazole *on page 834*

Opcon® *see* Naphazoline *on page 879*

o,p'-DDD *see* Mitotane *on page 848*

Operand® [OTC] *see* Povidone-Iodine *on page 1031*

Ophthaine® *see* Proparacaine *on page 1062*

Ophthalgan® *see* Glycerin *on page 580*

Ophthetic® *see* Proparacaine *on page 1062*

Ophthifluor® *see* Fluorescein Sodium *on page 535*

Opium and Belladonna *see* Belladonna and Opium *on page 135*

Opium Tincture (OH pee um TING chur)

Synonyms Deodorized Opium Tincture; DTO

Therapeutic Category Analgesic, Narcotic; Antidiarrheal

Use Treatment of diarrhea or relief of pain

Restrictions C-II

Pregnancy Risk Factor B (D if used for prolonged periods or in high doses at term)

Contraindications Increased intracranial pressure, severe respiratory depression, severe liver or renal insufficiency, known hypersensitivity to morphine sulfate

Warnings/Precautions Opium shares the toxic potential of opiate agonists, and usual precautions of opiate agonist therapy should be observed; some preparations contain sulfites which may cause allergic reactions; infants <3 months of age are more susceptible to respiratory depression, use with caution and generally in reduced doses in this age group; this is **not** paregoric, dose accordingly

Adverse Reactions

>10%:

Cardiovascular: Palpitations, hypotension, bradycardia

Central nervous system: Drowsiness, dizziness
Neuromuscular & skeletal: Weakness

1% to 10%:

Central nervous system: Restlessness, headache, malaise
Genitourinary: Decreased urination
Miscellaneous: Histamine release

<1%:

Cardiovascular: Peripheral vasodilation
Central nervous system: CNS depression, increased intracranial pressure, insomnia, mental depression
Gastrointestinal: Nausea, vomiting, constipation, anorexia, stomach cramps, biliary tract spasm
Genitourinary: Urinary tract spasm
Ocular: Miosis
Respiratory: Respiratory depression
Miscellaneous: Physical and psychological dependence

Overdosage/Toxicology Primary attention should be directed to ensuring adequate respiratory exchange; opiate agonist-induced respiratory depression may be reversed with parenteral naloxone hydrochloride. Naloxone 2 mg I.V. (0.01 mg/kg for children) with repeat administration as necessary up to a total of 10 mg.

Drug Interactions

Decreased effect: Phenothiazines may antagonize the analgesic effect of opiate agonists

Increased toxicity: CNS depressants, MAO inhibitors, tricyclic antidepressants may potentiate the effects of opiate agonists; dextroamphetamine may enhance the analgesic effect of opiate agonists

Mechanism of Action Contains many narcotic alkaloids including morphine; its mechanism for gastric motility inhibition is primarily due to this morphine content; it results in a decrease in digestive secretions, an increase in GI muscle tone, and therefore a reduction in GI propulsion

Pharmacodynamics/Kinetics

Duration of effect: 4-5 hours
Absorption: Variable from GI tract
Metabolism: In the liver
Elimination: Urine

Usual Dosage Oral:

Children:

Diarrhea: 0.005-0.01 mL/kg/dose every 3-4 hours for a maximum of 6 doses/24 hours
Analgesia: 0.01-0.02 mL/kg/dose every 3-4 hours

Adults:

Diarrhea: 0.3-1 mL/dose every 2-6 hours to maximum of 6 mL/24 hours
Analgesia: 0.6-1.5 mL/dose every 3-4 hours

Dietary Considerations Alcohol: Additive CNS effect, avoid use

Monitoring Parameters Observe patient for excessive sedation, respiratory depression, implement safety measures, assist with ambulation

Test Interactions ↑ aminotransferase [ALT (SGPT)/AST (SGOT)] (S)

Patient Information Avoid alcohol, may cause drowsiness, impair judgment, or coordination; may cause physical and psychological dependence with prolonged use

Dosage Forms Liquid: 10% [0.6 mL equivalent to morphine 6 mg]

Opticyl® *see* Tropicamide *on page 1275*

Optigene® [OTC] *see* Tetrahydrozoline *on page 1205*

Optimine® *see* Azatadine *on page 121*

OptiPranolol® *see* Metipranolol *on page 823*

OPV *see* Polio Vaccines *on page 1015*

Orabase®-B [OTC] *see* Benzocaine *on page 138*

Orabase® HCA *see* Hydrocortisone *on page 623*

Orabase®-O [OTC] *see* Benzocaine *on page 138*

Oracit® *see* Sodium Citrate and Citric Acid *on page 1144*

Orajel® Brace-Aid Oral Anesthetic [OTC] *see* Benzocaine *on page 138*

Orajel® Maximum Strength [OTC] *see* Benzocaine *on page 138*

Orajel® Mouth-Aid [OTC] *see* Benzocaine *on page 138*

Orajel® Perioseptic [OTC] *see* Carbamide Peroxide *on page 203*

Oraminic® II *see* Brompheniramine *on page 166*

Oramorph SR® *see* Morphine Sulfate *on page 858*

Orap™ *see* Pimozide *on page 1001*

Orasept® [OTC] *see* Benzocaine *on page 138*

Orasol® [OTC] *see* Benzocaine *on page 138*

Orasone® *see* Prednisone *on page 1039*
Oratect® [OTC] *see* Benzocaine *on page 138*
Orazinc® [OTC] *see* Zinc Supplements *on page 1324*
Orciprenaline Sulfate *see* Metaproterenol *on page 793*
Oretic® *see* Hydrochlorothiazide *on page 617*
Oreton® Methyl *see* Methyltestosterone *on page 821*
ORG 946 *see* Rocuronium *on page 1115*
Organidin® *see* Iodinated Glycerol *on page 670*
Organidin® NR *see* Guaifenesin *on page 589*
Orgaran® *see* Danaparoid *on page 339*
ORG NC 45 *see* Vecuronium *on page 1295*
Orimune® *see* Polio Vaccines *on page 1015*
Orinase® *see* Tolbutamide *on page 1240*
ORLAAM® *see* Levomethadyl Acetate Hydrochloride *on page 718*
Ormazine *see* Chlorpromazine *on page 261*
Ornidyl® *see* Eflornithine *on page 441*

Orphenadrine (or FEN a dreen)

Brand Names Norflex™

Canadian/Mexican Brand Names Disipal™ (Canada); Orfenace (Canada)

Synonyms Orphenadrine Citrate

Therapeutic Category Skeletal Muscle Relaxant

Use Treatment of muscle spasm associated with acute painful musculoskeletal conditions; supportive therapy in tetanus

Pregnancy Risk Factor C

Contraindications Glaucoma, GI obstruction, cardiospasm, myasthenia gravis, hypersensitivity to orphenadrine or any component

Warnings/Precautions Use with caution in patients with CHF or cardiac arrhythmias; some products contain sulfites

Adverse Reactions

>10%:
- Central nervous system: Drowsiness, dizziness
- Ocular: Blurred vision

1% to 10%:
- Cardiovascular: Flushing of face, tachycardia, syncope
- Dermatologic: Rash
- Gastrointestinal: Nausea, vomiting, constipation
- Genitourinary: Decreased urination
- Neuromuscular & skeletal: Weakness
- Ocular: Nystagmus, increased intraocular pressure
- Respiratory: Nasal congestion

<1%:
- Central nervous system: Hallucinations
- Hematologic: Aplastic anemia

Overdosage/Toxicology Symptoms of overdose include blurred vision, tachycardia, confusion, seizures, respiratory arrest, dysrhythmias

There is no specific treatment for an antihistamine overdose, however, most of its clinical toxicity is due to anticholinergic effects. Anticholinesterase inhibitors may be useful by reducing acetylcholinesterase. Anticholinesterase inhibitors include physostigmine, neostigmine, pyridostigmine and edrophonium. For anticholinergic overdose with severe life-threatening symptoms, physostigmine 1-2 mg (0.5 or 0.02 mg/kg for children) I.V., slowly may be given to reverse these effects. Lethal dose is 2-3 g; treatment is symptomatic.

Mechanism of Action Indirect skeletal muscle relaxant thought to work by central atropine-like effects; has some euphorogenic and analgesic properties

Pharmacodynamics/Kinetics
- Peak effect: Oral: Within 2-4 hours
- Duration: 4-6 hours
- Protein binding: 20%
- Metabolism: Extensive
- Half-life: 14-16 hours
- Elimination: Primarily in urine (8% as unchanged drug)

Usual Dosage Adults:
- Oral: 100 mg twice daily
- I.M., I.V.: 60 mg every 12 hours

Dietary Considerations Alcohol: Additive CNS effect, avoid use

Patient Information May cause drowsiness; swallow whole, do not crush or chew sustained release product; avoid alcohol, may impair coordination and judgment

Nursing Implications Do not crush sustained release drug product; raise bed rails, institute safety measures, assist with ambulation

Dosage Forms

Injection, as citrate: 30 mg/mL (2 mL, 10 mL)
Tablet, as citrate: 100 mg
Tablet, as citrate, sustained release: 100 mg

Orphenadrine Citrate *see* Orphenadrine *on previous page*
Orthoclone OKT®3 *see* Muromonab-CD3 *on page 863*
Ortho® Dienestrol *see* Dienestrol *on page 379*
Ortho-Est® *see* Estropipate *on page 475*
Ortho-Novum® 1/35 *see* Ethinyl Estradiol and Norethindrone *on page 486*
Ortho-Novum™ 1/50 *see* Mestranol and Norethindrone *on page 791*
Ortho-Novum® 7/7/7 *see* Ethinyl Estradiol and Norethindrone *on page 486*
Ortho-Novum® 10/11 *see* Ethinyl Estradiol and Norethindrone *on page 486*
Or-Tyl® Injection *see* Dicyclomine *on page 376*
Orudis® *see* Ketoprofen *on page 697*
Orudis® KT [OTC] *see* Ketoprofen *on page 697*
Oruvail® *see* Ketoprofen *on page 697*
Os-Cal® 250 [OTC] *see* Calcium Carbonate *on page 185*
Os-Cal® 500 [OTC] *see* Calcium Carbonate *on page 185*
Osmitrol® *see* Mannitol *on page 758*
Osmoglyn® *see* Glycerin *on page 580*
Osteocalcin® Injection *see* Calcitonin *on page 181*
Otic-Care® Otic *see* Neomycin, Polymyxin B, and Hydrocortisone *on page 890*
OtiTricin® Otic *see* Neomycin, Polymyxin B, and Hydrocortisone *on page 890*
Otocort® Otic *see* Neomycin, Polymyxin B, and Hydrocortisone *on page 890*
Otomycin-HPN® Otic *see* Neomycin, Polymyxin B, and Hydrocortisone *on page 890*
Otosporin® Otic *see* Neomycin, Polymyxin B, and Hydrocortisone *on page 890*
Otrivin® [OTC] *see* Xylometazoline *on page 1315*
Ovcon® 35 *see* Ethinyl Estradiol and Norethindrone *on page 486*
Ovcon® 50 *see* Ethinyl Estradiol and Norethindrone *on page 486*
Ovral® *see* Ethinyl Estradiol and Norgestrel *on page 489*
Ovrette® *see* Norgestrel *on page 916*
O-V Staticin® *see* Nystatin *on page 919*

Oxacillin (oks a SIL in)

Related Information

Antibiotic Treatment of Adults With Infectious Endocarditis *on page 1465*
Bacterial Meningitis Practical Guidelines for Management *on page 1475*

Brand Names Bactocill®; Prostaphlin®

Synonyms Methylphenyl Isoxazolyl Penicillin; Oxacillin Sodium

Therapeutic Category Antibiotic, Penicillin

Use Treatment of susceptible bacterial infections such as osteomyelitis, septicemia, endocarditis, and CNS infections due to penicillinase-producing strains of *Staphylococcus*

Pregnancy Risk Factor B

Contraindications Hypersensitivity to oxacillin or other penicillins or any component

Warnings/Precautions Elimination rate will be slow in neonates; modify dosage in patients with renal impairment and in the elderly; use with caution in patients with cephalosporin hypersensitivity

Adverse Reactions

1% to 10%: Gastrointestinal: Nausea, diarrhea

<1%:

- Central nervous system: Fever
- Dermatologic: Rash
- Gastrointestinal: Vomiting
- Hematologic: Eosinophilia, leukopenia, neutropenia, thrombocytopenia, agranulocytosis, mild leukopenia
- Hepatic: Hepatotoxicity, elevated AST
- Renal: Hematuria, acute interstitial nephritis
- Miscellaneous: Serum sickness-like reactions

Overdosage/Toxicology Symptoms of penicillin overdose include neuromuscular hypersensitivity (agitation, hallucinations, asterixis, encephalopathy, confusion, and seizures) and electrolyte imbalance with potassium or sodium salts, especially in renal failure

Hemodialysis may be helpful to aid in the removal of the drug from the blood, otherwise most treatment is supportive or symptom directed

(Continued)

Oxacillin *(Continued)*

Drug Interactions

Decreased effect: Efficacy of oral contraceptives may be reduced

Increased effect: Disulfiram, probenecid may increase penicillin levels, increased effect of anticoagulants

Stability Reconstituted parenteral solution is stable for 3 days at room temperature and 7 days when refrigerated; for I.V. infusion in NS or D_5W, solution is stable for 6 hours at room temperature

Mechanism of Action Inhibits bacterial cell wall synthesis by binding to one or more of the penicillin binding proteins (PBPs); which in turn inhibits the final transpeptidation step of peptidoglycan synthesis in bacterial cell walls, thus inhibiting cell wall biosynthesis. Bacteria eventually lyse due to ongoing activity of cell wall autolytic enzymes (autolysins and murein hydrolases) while cell wall assembly is arrested.

Pharmacodynamics/Kinetics

Absorption: Oral: 35% to 67%

Distribution: Into bile, synovial and pleural fluids, bronchial secretions; also distributes to peritoneal and pericardial fluids; crosses the placenta and appears in breast milk; penetrates the blood-brain barrier only when meninges are inflamed

Metabolism: In the liver to active metabolites

Half-life:

Children 1 week to 2 years: 0.9-1.8 hours

Adults: 23-60 minutes (prolonged with reduced renal function and in neonates)

Time to peak serum concentration:

Oral: Within 2 hours

I.M.: Within 30-60 minutes

Elimination: By kidneys and to small degree the bile as parent drug and metabolites

Usual Dosage

Infants and Children:

Oral: 50-100 mg/kg/day divided every 6 hours

I.M., I.V.: 150-200 mg/kg/day in divided doses every 6 hours; maximum dose: 12 g/day

Adults:

Oral: 500-1000 mg every 4-6 hours for at least 5 days

I.M., I.V.: 250 mg to 2 g/dose every 4-6 hours

Dosing adjustment in renal impairment: Cl_{cr} <10 mL/minute: Use lower range of the usual dosage

Hemodialysis: Not dialyzable (0% to 5%)

Administration Administer around-the-clock to promote less variation in peak and trough serum levels

Test Interactions May interfere with urinary glucose tests using cupric sulfate (Benedict's solution, Clinitest®); may inactivate aminoglycosides *in vitro*; false-positive urinary and serum proteins

Patient Information Take orally on an empty stomach 1 hour before meals or 2 hours after meals; take all medication, do not skip doses

Additional Information Sodium content of 1 g: 2.8-3.1 mEq

Dosage Forms

Capsule, as sodium: 250 mg, 500 mg

Powder:

For injection, as sodium: 250 mg, 500 mg, 1 g, 2 g, 4 g, 10 g

For oral solution, as sodium: 250 mg/5 mL (100 mL)

Oxacillin Sodium *see* Oxacillin *on previous page*

Oxaprozin (oks a PROE zin)

Brand Names Daypro™

Therapeutic Category Anti-inflammatory Agent; Nonsteroidal Anti-inflammatory Agent (NSAID), Oral

Use Acute and long-term use in the management of signs and symptoms of osteoarthritis and rheumatoid arthritis

Pregnancy Risk Factor C

Contraindications Aspirin allergy, third trimester pregnancy or allergy to oxaprozin, history of GI disease, renal or hepatic dysfunction, bleeding disorders, cardiac failure, elderly, debilitated, nursing mothers

Adverse Reactions

>10%:

Central nervous system: Dizziness

Dermatologic: Rash

Gastrointestinal: Abdominal cramps, heartburn, indigestion, nausea

1% to 10%:
- Cardiovascular: Arrhythmia
- Central nervous system: Nervousness
- Dermatologic: Rash, itching
- Gastrointestinal: GI ulceration, vomiting
- Genitourinary: Vaginal bleeding
- Otic: Tinnitus

<1%:
- Cardiovascular: Chest pain, congestive heart failure, hypertension, tachycardia
- Central nervous system: Convulsions, forgetfulness, mental depression, drowsiness, nervousness, insomnia
- Dermatologic: Urticaria, exfoliative dermatitis, erythema multiforme, Stevens-Johnson syndrome, angioedema
- Gastrointestinal: Stomatitis
- Genitourinary: Cystitis
- Hematologic: Agranulocytosis, anemia, pancytopenia, leukopenia, thrombocytopenia
- Hepatic: Hepatitis
- Neuromuscular & skeletal: Peripheral neuropathy, trembling, weakness
- Ocular: Blurred vision, change in vision
- Otic: Decreased hearing
- Renal: Interstitial nephritis, nephrotic syndrome, renal impairment
- Respiratory: Shortness of breath, wheezing, laryngeal edema, epistaxis
- Miscellaneous: Anaphylaxis, diaphoresis (increased)

Overdosage/Toxicology Symptoms of overdose include acute renal failure, vomiting, drowsiness, leukocytes

Management of a nonsteroidal anti-inflammatory drug (NSAID) intoxication is primarily supportive and symptomatic. Fluid therapy is commonly effective in managing the hypotension that may occur following an acute NSAID overdose, except when this is due to an acute blood loss. Seizures tend to be very short-lived and often do not require drug treatment. Although, recurrent seizures should be treated with I.V. diazepam. Since many of the NSAID undergo enterohepatic cycling, multiple doses of charcoal may be needed to reduce the potential for delayed toxicities.

Drug Interactions Increased toxicity: Aspirin, oral anticoagulants, diuretics

Mechanism of Action Inhibits prostaglandin synthesis by decreasing the activity of the enzyme, cyclo-oxygenase, which results in decreased formation of prostaglandin precursors

Pharmacodynamics/Kinetics
- Absorption: Almost completely
- Protein binding: >99%
- Half-life: 40-50 hours
- Time to peak: 2-4 hours

Usual Dosage Adults: Oral (individualize dosage to lowest effective dose to minimize adverse effects):
- Osteoarthritis: 600-1200 mg once daily
- Rheumatoid arthritis: 1200 mg once daily
- Maximum dose: 1800 mg/day or 26 mg/kg (whichever is lower) in divided doses

Monitoring Parameters Monitor blood, hepatic, renal, and ocular function

Dosage Forms Tablet: 600 mg

Oxazepam (oks A ze pam)

Related Information

Benzodiazepines Comparison *on page 1397*

Brand Names Serax®

Canadian/Mexican Brand Names Apo-Oxazepam® (Canada); Novo-Oxazepam® (Canada); Oxpam® (Canada); PMS-Oxazepam (Canada); Zapex® (Canada)

Therapeutic Category Antianxiety Agent; Anticonvulsant; Benzodiazepine

Use Treatment of anxiety and management of alcohol withdrawal; may also be used as an anticonvulsant in management of simple partial seizures

Restrictions C-IV

Pregnancy Risk Factor D

Contraindications Hypersensitivity to oxazepam or any component, cross-sensitivity with other benzodiazepines may exist

Warnings/Precautions Avoid using in patients with pre-existing CNS depression, severe uncontrolled pain, or narrow-angle glaucoma; use with caution in patients using other CNS depressants and in the elderly

Adverse Reactions

>10%:
- Cardiovascular: Tachycardia, chest pain

(Continued)

Oxazepam *(Continued)*

Central nervous system: Drowsiness, fatigue, ataxia, lightheadedness, memory impairment, insomnia, anxiety, depression, headache
Dermatologic: Rash
Endocrine & metabolic: Decreased libido
Gastrointestinal: Xerostomia, constipation, diarrhea, decreased salivation, nausea, vomiting, increased or decreased appetite
Neuromuscular & skeletal: Dysarthria
Ocular: Blurred vision
Miscellaneous: Diaphoresis

1% to 10%:
Cardiovascular: Syncope, hypotension
Central nervous system: Confusion, nervousness, dizziness, akathisia
Dermatologic: Dermatitis
Gastrointestinal: Increased salivation, weight gain or loss
Neuromuscular & skeletal: Rigidity, tremor, muscle cramps
Ocular: Blurred vision
Otic: Tinnitus
Respiratory: Nasal congestion, hyperventilation

<1%:
Endocrine & metabolic: Menstrual irregularities
Hematologic: Blood dyscrasias
Neuromuscular & skeletal: Reflex slowing
Miscellaneous: Drug dependence

Overdosage/Toxicology Symptoms of overdose include somnolence, confusion, coma, hypoactive reflexes, dyspnea, hypotension, slurred speech, impaired coordination

Treatment for benzodiazepine overdose is supportive. Rarely is mechanical ventilation required. Flumazenil has been shown to selectively block the binding of benzodiazepines to CNS receptors, resulting in a reversal of benzodiazepine-induced CNS depression but not the respiratory depression due to toxicity.

Drug Interactions Increased toxicity with CNS depressants (eg, barbiturates, MAO inhibitors, TCAs, alcohol, narcotics, phenothiazines, and other sedative-hypnotics)

Mechanism of Action Benzodiazepine anxiolytic sedative that produces CNS depression at the subcortical level, except at high doses, whereby it works at the cortical level

Pharmacodynamics/Kinetics
Absorption: Oral: Almost completely
Protein binding: 86% to 99%
Metabolism: In the liver to inactive compounds (primarily as glucuronides)
Half-life: 2.8-5.7 hours
Time to peak serum concentration: Within 2-4 hours
Elimination: Excretion of unchanged drug (50%) and metabolites; excreted without need for liver metabolism

Usual Dosage Oral:
Children: 1 mg/kg/day has been administered
Adults:
Anxiety: 10-30 mg 3-4 times/day
Alcohol withdrawal: 15-30 mg 3-4 times/day
Hypnotic: 15-30 mg
Hemodialysis: Not dialyzable (0% to 5%)

Dietary Considerations Alcohol: Additive CNS effect, avoid use

Monitoring Parameters Respiratory and cardiovascular status

Reference Range Therapeutic: 0.2-1.4 μg/mL (SI: 0.7-4.9 μmol/L)

Patient Information Avoid alcohol and other CNS depressants; avoid activities needing good psychomotor coordination until CNS effects are known; drug may cause physical or psychological dependence; avoid abrupt discontinuation after prolonged use

Nursing Implications Provide safety measures (ie, side rails, night light, and call button); remove smoking materials from area; supervise ambulation

Dosage Forms
Capsule: 10 mg, 15 mg, 30 mg
Tablet: 15 mg

Oxiconazole (oks i KON a zole)

Brand Names Oxistat®

Canadian/Mexican Brand Names Myfungar® (Mexico)

Synonyms Oxiconazole Nitrate

Therapeutic Category Antifungal Agent, Topical

Use Treatment of tinea pedis (athlete's foot), tinea cruris (jock itch), and tinea corporis (ring worm)

Pregnancy Risk Factor B

Contraindications Hypersensitivity to this agent; not for ophthalmic use

Warnings/Precautions May cause irritation during therapy; if a sensitivity to oxiconazole occurs, therapy should be discontinued; avoid contact with eyes or vagina

Adverse Reactions 1% to 10%:

Dermatologic: Itching, erythema

Local: Transient burning, local irritation, stinging, dryness

Mechanism of Action Inhibition of ergosterol synthesis. Effective for treatment of tinea pedis, tinea cruris, and tinea corporis. Active against *Trichophyton rubrum, Trichophyton mentagrophytes, Trichophyton violaceum, Microsporum canis, Microsporum audouini, Microsporum gypseum, Epidermophyton floccosum, Candida albicans*, and *Malassezia furfur.*

Pharmacodynamics/Kinetics

Absorption: In each layer of the dermis; very little is absorbed systemically after one topical dose

Distribution: To each layer of the dermis; excreted in breast milk

Elimination: <0.3% excreted in urine

Usual Dosage Children and Adults: Topical: Apply once to twice daily to affected areas for 2 weeks (tinea corporis/tinea cruris) to 1 month (tinea pedis)

Patient Information External use only; discontinue if sensitivity or chemical irritation occurs, contact physician if condition fails to improve in 3-4 days

Dosage Forms

Cream, as nitrate: 1% (15 g, 30 g, 60 g)

Lotion, as nitrate: 1% (30 mL)

Oxiconazole Nitrate *see* Oxiconazole *on previous page*

Oxilapine Succinate *see* Loxapine *on page 747*

Oxistat® *see* Oxiconazole *on previous page*

Oxpentifylline *see* Pentoxifylline *on page 974*

Oxsoralen® *see* Methoxsalen *on page 812*

Oxsoralen-Ultra® *see* Methoxsalen *on page 812*

Oxtriphylline *see* Theophylline Salts *on page 1207*

Oxy-5® Advanced Formula for Sensitive Skin [OTC] *see* Benzoyl Peroxide *on page 140*

Oxy-5® Tinted [OTC] *see* Benzoyl Peroxide *on page 140*

Oxy-10® Advanced Formula for Sensitive Skin [OTC] *see* Benzoyl Peroxide *on page 140*

Oxy 10® Wash [OTC] *see* Benzoyl Peroxide *on page 140*

Oxybutynin (oks i BYOO ti nin)

Brand Names Ditropan®

Synonyms Oxybutynin Chloride

Therapeutic Category Antispasmodic Agent, Urinary

Use Antispasmodic for neurogenic bladder (urgency, frequency, urge incontinence) and uninhibited bladder

Pregnancy Risk Factor B

Contraindications Glaucoma, myasthenia gravis, partial or complete GI obstruction, GU obstruction, ulcerative colitis, hypersensitivity to drug or specific component, intestinal atony, megacolon, toxic megacolon

Warnings/Precautions Use with caution in patients with urinary tract obstruction, angle-closure glaucoma, hyperthyroidism, reflux esophagitis, heart disease, hepatic or renal disease, prostatic hypertrophy, autonomic neuropathy, ulcerative colitis (may cause ileus and toxic megacolon), hypertension, hiatal hernia. Caution should be used in elderly due to anticholinergic activity (eg, confusion, constipation, blurred vision, and tachycardia).

Adverse Reactions

>10%:

Central nervous system: Drowsiness

Gastrointestinal: Xerostomia, constipation

Miscellaneous: Diaphoresis (decreased)

1% to 10%:

Cardiovascular: Tachycardia, palpitations

Central nervous system: Dizziness, insomnia, fever, headache

Dermatologic: Rash

Endocrine & metabolic: Decreased flow of breast milk, decreased sexual ability, hot flashes

Gastrointestinal: Nausea, vomiting

Genitourinary: Urinary hesitancy or retention

Neuromuscular & skeletal: Weakness

Ocular: Blurred vision, mydriatic effect

(Continued)

Oxybutynin *(Continued)*

<1%:

Ocular: Increased intraocular pressure

Miscellaneous: Allergic reaction

Overdosage/Toxicology Symptoms of overdose include hypotension, circulatory failure, psychotic behavior, flushing, respiratory failure, paralysis, tremor, irritability, seizures, delirium, hallucinations, coma

Symptomatic and supportive treatment; induce emesis or perform gastric lavage followed by charcoal and a cathartic; physostigmine may be required; treat hyperpyrexia with cooling techniques (ice bags, cold applications, alcohol sponges)

Drug Interactions

Increased toxicity:

Additive sedation with CNS depressants and alcohol

Additive anticholinergic effects with antihistamines and anticholinergic agents

Mechanism of Action Direct antispasmodic effect on smooth muscle, also inhibits the action of acetylcholine on smooth muscle (exhibits 1/5 the anticholinergic activity of atropine, but is 4-10 times the antispasmodic activity); does not block effects at skeletal muscle or at autonomic ganglia; increases bladder capacity, decreases uninhibited contractions, and delays desire to void; therefore, decreases urgency and frequency

Pharmacodynamics/Kinetics

Onset of effect: Oral: 30-60 minutes

Peak effect: 3-6 hours

Duration: 6-10 hours

Absorption: Oral: Rapid and well absorbed

Metabolism: In the liver

Half-life: 1-2.3 hours

Time to peak serum concentration: Within 60 minutes

Elimination: In urine

Usual Dosage Oral:

Children:

1-5 years: 0.2 mg/kg/dose 2-4 times/day

>5 years: 5 mg twice daily, up to 5 mg 4 times/day maximum

Adults: 5 mg 2-3 times/day up to 5 mg 4 times/day maximum

Elderly: 2.5-5 mg twice daily; increase by 2.5 mg increments every 1-2 days

Note: Should be discontinued periodically to determine whether the patient can manage without the drug and to minimize resistance to the drug

Monitoring Parameters Incontinence episodes, postvoid residual (PVR)

Test Interactions May suppress the wheal and flare reactions to skin test antigens

Patient Information May impair ability to perform activities requiring mental alertness or physical coordination; alcohol or other sedating drugs may enhance drowsiness

Nursing Implications Raise bed rails, institute safety measures, assist with ambulation

Dosage Forms

Syrup, as chloride: 5 mg/5 mL (473 mL)

Tablet, as chloride: 5 mg

Oxybutynin Chloride *see* Oxybutynin *on previous page*

Oxycodone (oks i KOE done)

Related Information

Dose Equivalents for Opioid Analgesics in Opioid-Naive Adults ≥50 kg *on page 1375*

Brand Names OxyContin®; OxyIR®; Roxicodone™

Canadian/Mexican Brand Names Supeudol® (Canada)

Synonyms Dihydrohydroxycodeinone; Oxycodone Hydrochloride

Therapeutic Category Analgesic, Narcotic

Use Management of moderate to severe pain, normally used in combination with non-narcotic analgesics

Restrictions C-II

Pregnancy Risk Factor B (D if used for prolonged periods or in high doses at term)

Contraindications Hypersensitivity to oxycodone or any component

Warnings/Precautions Use with caution in patients with hypersensitivity reactions to other phenanthrene derivative opioid agonists (morphine, hydrocodone, hydromorphone, levorphanol, oxycodone, oxymorphone); respiratory diseases including asthma, emphysema, COPD, or severe liver or renal insufficiency; some preparations contain sulfites which may cause allergic reactions; may be habit-forming; dextromethorphan has equivalent antitussive activity but has much lower toxicity in accidental overdose

Adverse Reactions

>10%:

Cardiovascular: Hypotension

Central nervous system: Fatigue, drowsiness, dizziness

Gastrointestinal: Nausea, vomiting

Neuromuscular & skeletal: Weakness

1% to 10%:

Central nervous system: Nervousness, headache, restlessness, malaise, confusion

Gastrointestinal: Anorexia, stomach cramps, xerostomia, constipation, biliary spasm

Genitourinary: Ureteral spasms, decreased urination

Local: Pain at injection site

Respiratory: Dyspnea, shortness of breath

<1%:

Central nervous system: Mental depression, hallucinations, paradoxical CNS stimulation, increased intracranial pressure

Dermatologic: Skin rash, urticaria

Gastrointestinal: Paralytic ileus

Miscellaneous: Histamine release, physical and psychological dependence

Overdosage/Toxicology Symptoms of overdose include CNS depression, respiratory depression, miosis

Treatment: Naloxone 2 mg I.V. (0.01 mg/kg for children) with repeat administration as necessary up to a total of 10 mg

Drug Interactions

Decreased effect: Phenothiazines may antagonize the analgesic effect of opiate agonists

Increased toxicity: CNS depressants, monoamine oxidase inhibitors, general anesthetics, and tricyclic antidepressants may potentiate the effects of opiate agonists; dextroamphetamine may enhance the analgesic effect of opiate agonists

Mechanism of Action Binds to opiate receptors in the CNS, causing inhibition of ascending pain pathways, altering the perception of and response to pain; produces generalized CNS depression

Pharmacodynamics/Kinetics

Onset of pain relief: Oral: Within 10-15 minutes

Peak effect: 0.5-1 hour

Duration: 4-5 hours

Metabolism: In the liver

Elimination: In urine

Usual Dosage Oral:

Immediate release:

Children:

6-12 years: 1.25 mg every 6 hours as needed

>12 years: 2.5 mg every 6 hours as needed

Adults: 5 mg every 6 hours as needed

Controlled release: Adults: 10 mg every 12 hours around-the-clock

Dosing adjustment in hepatic impairment: Reduce dosage in patients with severe liver disease

Dietary Considerations Alcohol: Additive CNS effect, avoid use

Monitoring Parameters Pain relief, respiratory and mental status, blood pressure

Reference Range Blood level of 5 mg/L associated with fatality

Patient Information Avoid alcohol; may cause drowsiness, impaired judgment or coordination; may be addicting if used for prolonged periods; do not crush or chew the controlled-release product

Nursing Implications Observe patient for excessive sedation, respiratory depression, implement safety measures, assist with ambulation

Additional Information Prophylactic use of a laxative should be considered

Dosage Forms

Capsule, as hydrochloride, immediate release (OxyIR®): 5 mg

Liquid, oral, as hydrochloride: 5 mg/5 mL (500 mL)

Solution, oral concentrate, as hydrochloride: 20 mg/mL (30 mL)

Tablet, as hydrochloride: 5 mg

Tablet, controlled release, as hydrochloride (OxyContin®): 10 mg, 20 mg, 40 mg, 80 mg

Oxycodone and Acetaminophen

(oks i KOE done & a seet a MIN oh fen)

Related Information

Narcotic Agonists Comparison *on page 1414*

Dose Equivalents for Opioid Analgesics in Opioid-Naive Adults <50 kg *on page 1376*

Dose Equivalents for Opioid Analgesics in Opioid-Naive Adults ≥50 kg *on page 1375*

Brand Names Percocet®; Roxicet® 5/500; Roxilox®; Tylox®

Canadian/Mexican Brand Names Endocet® (Canada); Oxycocet® (Canada); Percocet®-Demi (Canada)

Synonyms Acetaminophen and Oxycodone

Therapeutic Category Analgesic, Narcotic

Use Management of moderate to severe pain

Restrictions C-II

Pregnancy Risk Factor C

Contraindications Hypersensitivity to oxycodone, acetaminophen or any component; severe respiratory depression, severe renal or liver insufficiency

Warnings/Precautions Use with caution in patients with hypersensitivity to other phenanthrene derivative opioid agonists (morphine, codeine, hydrocodone, hydromorphone, oxymorphone, levorphanol), asthma, COPD, severe liver or renal disease; some preparations may contain bisulfites which may cause allergies

Enhanced analgesia has been seen in elderly patients on therapeutic doses of narcotics; duration of action may be increased in the elderly; the elderly may be particularly susceptible to the CNS depressant and constipating effects of narcotics

Adverse Reactions

>10%:

- Cardiovascular: Hypotension
- Central nervous system: Fatigue, drowsiness, dizziness
- Gastrointestinal: Nausea, vomiting
- Neuromuscular & skeletal: Weakness

1% to 10%:

- Central nervous system: Nervousness, headache, restlessness, malaise, confusion
- Gastrointestinal: Anorexia, stomach cramps, xerostomia, constipation, biliary spasm
- Genitourinary: Ureteral spasms, decreased urination
- Local: Pain at injection site
- Respiratory: Dyspnea, shortness of breath

<1%:

- Central nervous system: Mental depression, hallucinations, paradoxical CNS stimulation, increased intracranial pressure
- Dermatologic: Rash, urticaria
- Gastrointestinal: Paralytic ileus
- Hematologic: Blood dyscrasias (neutropenia, pancytopenia, leukopenia)
- Hepatic: Hepatic necrosis with overdosage
- Renal: Renal injury with chronic use
- Miscellaneous: Physical and psychological dependence, hypersensitivity reactions (rare), histamine release

Overdosage/Toxicology Symptoms of overdose include hepatic necrosis, transient azotemia, renal tubular necrosis with acute toxicity, anemia, renal damage, and GI disturbances with chronic toxicity

Consult regional poison control center for additional information. Treatment of an overdose includes support of the patient's airway, establishment of an I.V. line and administration of naloxone 2 mg I.V. with repeat administration as necessary. Mucomyst® (acetylcysteine) 140 mg/kg orally (loading) followed by 70 mg/kg (maintenance) every 4 hours for 17 doses. Therapy should be initiated based upon acetaminophen levels that are suggestive of a high probability of hepatotoxic potential.

Drug Interactions

Decreased effect: Phenothiazines may antagonize the analgesic effect of opiate agonists

Increased toxicity: CNS depressants, tricyclic antidepressants may potentiate the effects of opiate agonists; dextroamphetamine may enhance the analgesic effect of opiate agonists

Mechanism of Action Inhibits the synthesis of prostaglandins in the central nervous system and peripherally blocks pain impulse generation; produces antipyresis from inhibition of hypothalamic heat-regulating center; binds to opiate receptors in the CNS, causing inhibition of ascending pain pathways, altering the perception of and response to pain; produces generalized CNS depression

Usual Dosage Oral (doses should be titrated to appropriate analgesic effects):
- Children: Oxycodone: 0.05-0.15 mg/kg/dose to 5 mg/dose (maximum) every 4-6 hours as needed
- Adults: 1-2 tablets every 4-6 hours as needed for pain
  - Maximum daily dose of acetaminophen: 4 g/day

Dosing adjustment in hepatic impairment: Dose should be reduced in patients with severe liver disease

Dietary Considerations
- Acetaminophen: Refer to acetaminophen monograph
- Oxycodone:
  - Alcohol: Additive CNS effects; avoid or limit alcohol. Watch for sedation.
  - Food: Glucose may cause hyperglycemia; monitor blood glucose concentrations

Administration Administer with food, but high carbohydrate meal may retard absorption rate

Monitoring Parameters Pain relief, respiratory and mental status, blood pressure

Patient Information Do not exceed recommended dosage; do not take for more than 10 days without physician's advice; avoid alcohol, may cause drowsiness, impair judgment or coordination; may cause physical and psychological dependence with prolonged use

Nursing Implications Observe patient for excessive sedation, respiratory depression; implement safety measures, assist with ambulation

Additional Information Oxycodone and acetaminophen: Oxycet®, Percocet®, Roxicet®, Tylox®

Dosage Forms
- Caplet: Oxycodone hydrochloride 5 mg and acetaminophen 500 mg
- Capsule: Oxycodone hydrochloride 5 mg and acetaminophen 500 mg
- Solution, oral: Oxycodone hydrochloride 5 mg and acetaminophen 325 mg per 5 mL (5 mL, 500 mL)
- Tablet: Oxycodone hydrochloride 5 mg and acetaminophen 325 mg

Oxycodone and Aspirin (oks i KOE done & AS pir in)

Related Information

- Narcotic Agonists Comparison *on page 1414*
- Dose Equivalents for Opioid Analgesics in Opioid-Naive Adults <50 kg *on page 1376*
- Dose Equivalents for Opioid Analgesics in Opioid-Naive Adults ≥50 kg *on page 1375*

Brand Names Codoxy®; Percodan®; Percodan®-Demi; Roxiprin®

Canadian/Mexican Brand Names Endodan® (Canada); Oxycodan® (Canada)

Therapeutic Category Analgesic, Narcotic

Use Relief of moderate to moderately severe pain

Restrictions C-II

Pregnancy Risk Factor D

Contraindications Known hypersensitivity to oxycodone or aspirin; severe respiratory depression

Warnings/Precautions Use with caution in patients with hypersensitivity to other phenanthrene derivative opioid agonists (morphine, codeine, hydrocodone, hydromorphone, oxymorphone, levorphanol); children and teenagers should not be given aspirin products if chickenpox or flu symptoms are present; aspirin use has been associated with Reye's syndrome; severe liver or renal insufficiency, pre-existing CNS and depression

Adverse Reactions
- >10%:
  - Cardiovascular: Hypotension
  - Central nervous system: Fatigue, drowsiness, dizziness
  - Gastrointestinal: Nausea, vomiting, heartburn, stomach pains, dyspepsia
  - Neuromuscular & skeletal: Weakness
- 1% to 10%:
  - Central nervous system: Nervousness, headache, restlessness, malaise, confusion
  - Dermatologic: Rash
  - Gastrointestinal: Anorexia, stomach cramps, xerostomia, constipation, biliary spasm, gastrointestinal ulceration
  - Genitourinary: Ureteral spasms, decreased urination
  - Hematologic: Hemolytic anemia
  - Local: Pain at injection site
  - Respiratory: Dyspnea, shortness of breath
  - Miscellaneous: Anaphylactic shock

(Continued)

Oxycodone and Aspirin *(Continued)*

<1%:

Central nervous system: Mental depression, hallucinations, paradoxical CNS stimulation, increased intracranial pressure, insomnia, jitters
Dermatologic: Rash, urticaria
Gastrointestinal: Paralytic ileus
Hematologic: Occult bleeding, prolongation of bleeding time, leukopenia, thrombocytopenia, iron deficiency anemia
Hepatic: Hepatotoxicity
Renal: Impaired renal function
Respiratory: Bronchospasm
Miscellaneous: Physical and psychological dependence, histamine release

Overdosage/Toxicology Symptoms of overdose include CNS and respiratory depression, gastrointestinal cramping, constipation, tinnitus, headache, dizziness, confusion, metabolic acidosis, hyperpyrexia

Consult regional poison control center for additional information. Naloxone 2 mg I.V. (0.01 mg/kg for children) with repeat administration as necessary up to a total of 10 mg; see also Aspirin toxicology.

Drug Interactions

Decreased effect with phenothiazines
Increased effect/toxicity with CNS depressants, TCAs, dextroamphetamine

Mechanism of Action Binds to opiate receptors in the CNS, causing inhibition of ascending pain pathways, altering the perception of and response to pain; produces generalized CNS depression; inhibits prostaglandin synthesis, acts on the hypothalamus heat-regulating center to reduce fever, blocks prostaglandin synthetase action which prevents formation of the platelet-aggregating substance thromboxane A_2

Usual Dosage Oral (based on oxycodone combined salts):

Children: 0.05-0.15 mg/kg/dose every 4-6 hours as needed; maximum: 5 mg/dose (1 tablet Percodan® or 2 tablets Percodan®-Demi/dose)
Adults: Percodan®: 1 tablet every 6 hours as needed for pain or Percodan®-Demi: 1-2 tablets every 6 hours as needed for pain

Dosing adjustment in hepatic impairment: Dose should be reduced in patients with severe liver disease

Dietary Considerations

Oxycodone:
Alcohol: Additive CNS effects; avoid or limit alcohol. Watch for sedation.
Food: Glucose may cause hyperglycemia; monitor blood glucose concentrations

Administration Administer with food, but high carbohydrate meal may retard absorption rate

Monitoring Parameters Pain relief, respiratory and mental status, blood pressure

Patient Information Avoid alcohol, may cause drowsiness, impaired judgment or coordination; may cause physical and psychological dependence with prolonged use; watch for bleeding gums or any signs of GI bleeding; take with food or milk to minimize GI distress, notify physician if ringing in ears or persistent GI pain occurs

Nursing Implications Observe patient for excessive sedation, respiratory depression; implement safety measures, assist with ambulation

Dosage Forms Tablet:

Percodan®: Oxycodone hydrochloride 4.5 mg, oxycodone terephthalate 0.38 mg, and aspirin 325 mg
Percodan®-Demi: Oxycodone hydrochloride 2.25 mg, oxycodone terephthalate 0.19 mg, and aspirin 325 mg

Oxycodone Hydrochloride *see* Oxycodone *on page 936*
OxyContin® *see* Oxycodone *on page 936*
Oxydess® II *see* Dextroamphetamine *on page 365*
OxyIR® *see* Oxycodone *on page 936*

Oxymetazoline (oks i met AZ oh leen)

Brand Names Afrin® Children's Nose Drops [OTC]; Afrin® Nasal Solution [OTC]; Allerest® 12 Hour Nasal Solution [OTC]; Chlorphed®-LA Nasal Solution [OTC]; Dristan® Long Lasting Nasal Solution [OTC]; Duramist Plus® [OTC]; Duration® Nasal Solution [OTC]; Neo-Synephrine® 12 Hour Nasal Solution [OTC]; Nōstrilla® [OTC]; NTZ® Long Acting Nasal Solution [OTC]; OcuClear® Ophthalmic [OTC]; Sinarest® 12 Hour Nasal Solution; Sinex® Long-Acting [OTC]; Twice-A-Day® Nasal [OTC]; Visine® L.R. Ophthalmic [OTC]; 4-Way® Long Acting Nasal Solution [OTC]

Canadian/Mexican Brand Names Drixoral® Nasal (Canada)

Synonyms Oxymetazoline Hydrochloride

Therapeutic Category Adrenergic Agonist Agent; Decongestant, Nasal; Vasoconstrictor, Nasal; Vasoconstrictor, Ophthalmic

Use Symptomatic relief of nasal mucosal congestion and adjunctive therapy of middle ear infections, associated with acute or chronic rhinitis, the common cold, sinusitis, hay fever, or other allergies

Ophthalmic: Relief of redness of eye due to minor eye irritations

Pregnancy Risk Factor C

Contraindications Hypersensitivity to oxymetazoline or any component

Warnings/Precautions Rebound congestion may occur with extended use (>3 days); use with caution in the presence of hypertension, diabetes, hyperthyroidism, heart disease, coronary artery disease, cerebral arteriosclerosis, or long-standing bronchial asthma

Adverse Reactions

>10%:

Local: Transient burning, stinging

Respiratory: Dryness of the nasal mucosa, sneezing

1% to 10%:

Cardiovascular: Rebound congestion with prolonged use, hypertension, palpitations

Central nervous system: Nervousness, dizziness, insomnia, headache

Gastrointestinal: Nausea

Overdosage/Toxicology Symptoms of overdose include CNS depression, hypothermia, bradycardia, cardiovascular collapse, coma, apnea

Following initiation of essential overdose management, toxic symptoms should be treated. Patient should be kept warm and monitored for alterations in vital functions. Seizures commonly respond to diazepam (5-10 mg I.V. bolus in adults every 15 minutes if needed up to a total of 30 mg; I.V. 0.25-0.4 mg/kg/dose up to a total of 10 mg for children) or to phenytoin or phenobarbital. Hypotension should be treated with fluids.

Drug Interactions Increased toxicity: MAO inhibitors

Mechanism of Action Stimulates alpha-adrenergic receptors in the arterioles of the nasal mucosa to produce vasoconstriction

Pharmacodynamics/Kinetics

Onset of effect: Intranasal: Within 5-10 minutes

Duration: 5-6 hours

Metabolism: Metabolic fate is unknown

Usual Dosage Therapy should not exceed 3-5 days

Intranasal:

Children 2-5 years: 0.025% solution: Instill 2-3 drops in each nostril twice daily

Children ≥6 years and Adults: 0.05% solution: Instill 2-3 drops or 2-3 sprays into each nostril twice daily

Ophthalmic: Children ≥6 years and Adults: Instill 1-2 drops into affected eye(s) every 6-12 hours

Patient Information Should not be used for self-medication for longer than 3 days, if symptoms persist, drug should be discontinued and a physician consulted; notify physician of insomnia, tremor, or irregular heartbeat; burning, stinging, or drying of the nasal mucosa may occur

Dosage Forms

Nasal solution, as hydrochloride:

Drops:

Afrin® Children's Nose Drops: 0.025% (20 mL)

Afrin®, NTZ® Long Acting Nasal Solution: 0.05% (15 mL, 20 mL)

Spray: Afrin® Sinus, Allerest® 12 Hours, Chlorphed®-LA, Dristan® Long Lasting, Duration®, 4-Way® Long Acting, Genasal®, Nasal Relief®, Neo-Synephrine® 12 Hour, Nōstrilla®, NTZ® Long Acting Nasal Solution, Sinex® Long-Acting, Twice-A-Day®: 0.05% (15 mL, 30 mL)

Ophthalmic solution, as hydrochloride (OcuClear®, Visine® L.R.): 0.025% (15 mL, 30 mL)

Oxymetazoline Hydrochloride *see* Oxymetazoline *on previous page*

Oxymetholone (oks i METH oh lone)

Brand Names Anadrol®

Canadian/Mexican Brand Names Anapolon® (Canada)

Therapeutic Category Androgen

Use Anemias caused by the administration of myelotoxic drugs

Restrictions C-III

Pregnancy Risk Factor X

Contraindications Carcinoma of breast or prostate, nephrosis, pregnancy, hypersensitivity to any component

Warnings/Precautions Anabolic steroids may cause peliosis hepatis, liver cell tumors, and blood lipid changes with increased risk of arteriosclerosis; monitor diabetic patients carefully; use with caution in elderly patients, they may be at

(Continued)

Oxymetholone *(Continued)*

greater risk for prostatic hypertrophy; use with caution in patients with cardiac, renal, or hepatic disease or epilepsy

Adverse Reactions

Male:

Postpubertal:

>10%:

Dermatologic: Acne

Endocrine & metabolic: Gynecomastia

Genitourinary: Bladder irritability, priapism

1% to 10%:

Central nervous system: Insomnia, chills

Endocrine & metabolic: Decreased libido

Gastrointestinal: Nausea, diarrhea

Genitourinary: Prostatic hypertrophy (elderly)

Hematologic: Iron deficiency anemia, suppression of clotting factors

Hepatic: Hepatic dysfunction

<1%:

Hepatic: Hepatic necrosis, hepatocellular carcinoma

Prepubertal:

>10%:

Dermatologic: Acne

Endocrine & metabolic: Virilism

1% to 10%:

Central nervous system: Chills, insomnia

Dermatologic: Hyperpigmentation

Gastrointestinal: Diarrhea, nausea

Hematologic: Iron deficiency anemia, suppression of clotting factors

<1%: Hepatic: Hepatic necrosis, hepatocellular carcinoma

Female:

>10%: Endocrine & metabolic: Virilism

1% to 10%:

Central nervous system: Chills, insomnia

Endocrine & metabolic: Hypercalcemia

Gastrointestinal: Nausea, diarrhea

Hematologic: Iron deficiency anemia, suppression of clotting factors

Hepatic: Hepatic dysfunction

<1%: Hepatic: Hepatic necrosis, hepatocellular carcinoma

Overdosage/Toxicology Abnormal liver function test

Drug Interactions Increased toxicity: Increased oral anticoagulants, insulin requirements may be decreased

Mechanism of Action Stimulates receptors in organs and tissues to promote growth and development of male sex organs and maintains secondary sex characteristics in androgen-deficient males

Pharmacodynamics/Kinetics

Half-life: 9 hours

Elimination: Primarily in urine

Usual Dosage Adults: Erythropoietic effects: Oral: 1-5 mg/kg/day in 1 daily dose; maximum: 100 mg/day; give for a minimum trial of 3-6 months because response may be delayed

Monitoring Parameters Liver function tests

Test Interactions Altered glucose tolerance tests, altered thyroid function tests, altered metyrapone tests

Dosage Forms Tablet: 50 mg

Oxymorphone (oks i MOR fone)

Related Information

Narcotic Agonists Comparison *on page 1414*

Dose Equivalents for Opioid Analgesics in Opioid-Naive Adults <50 kg *on page 1376*

Dose Equivalents for Opioid Analgesics in Opioid-Naive Adults ≥50 kg *on page 1375*

Brand Names Numorphan®

Synonyms Oxymorphone Hydrochloride

Therapeutic Category Analgesic, Narcotic

Use Management of moderate to severe pain and preoperatively as a sedative and a supplement to anesthesia

Restrictions C-II

Pregnancy Risk Factor B (D if used for prolonged periods or in high doses at term)

Contraindications Hypersensitivity to oxymorphone or any component, increased intracranial pressure; severe respiratory depression

Warnings/Precautions Some preparations contain sulfites which may cause allergic reactions; infants <3 months of age are more susceptible to respiratory depression, use with caution and generally in reduced doses in this age group; use with caution in patients with impaired respiratory function or severe hepatic dysfunction and in patients with hypersensitivity reactions to other phenanthrene derivative opioid agonists (codeine, hydrocodone, hydromorphone, levorphanol, oxycodone, oxymorphone)

Adverse Reactions

>10%:

Cardiovascular: Hypotension

Central nervous system: Fatigue, drowsiness, dizziness

Gastrointestinal: Nausea, vomiting, constipation

Neuromuscular & skeletal: Weakness

Miscellaneous: Histamine release

1% to 10%:

Central nervous system: Nervousness, headache, restlessness, malaise, confusion

Gastrointestinal: Anorexia, stomach cramps, xerostomia, biliary spasm

Genitourinary: Decreased urination, ureteral spasms

Local: Pain at injection site

Respiratory: Dyspnea, shortness of breath

<1%:

Central nervous system: Mental depression, hallucinations, paradoxical CNS stimulation, increased intracranial pressure

Dermatologic: Rash, urticaria

Gastrointestinal: Paralytic ileus

Miscellaneous: Histamine release, physical and psychological dependence

Overdosage/Toxicology Symptoms of overdose include respiratory depression, miosis, hypotension, bradycardia, apnea, pulmonary edema

Treatment of an overdose includes support of the patient's airway, establishment of an I.V. line and administration of naloxone 2 mg I.V. (0.01 mg/kg for children) with repeat administration as necessary up to a total of 10 mg.

Drug Interactions

Decreased effect with phenothiazines

Increased effect/toxicity with CNS depressants, TCAs, dextroamphetamine

Stability Refrigerate suppository

Mechanism of Action Oxymorphone hydrochloride (Numorphan®) is a potent narcotic analgesic with uses similar to those of morphine. The drug is a semisynthetic derivative of morphine (phenanthrene derivative) and is closely related to hydromorphone chemically (Dilaudid®).

Pharmacodynamics/Kinetics

Onset of analgesia:

I.V., I.M., S.C.: Within 5-10 minutes

Rectal: Within 15-30 minutes

Duration of analgesia: Parenteral, rectal: 3-4 hours

Metabolism: Conjugated with glucuronic acid

Elimination: In urine

Usual Dosage Adults:

I.M., S.C.: 0.5 mg initially, 1-1.5 mg every 4-6 hours as needed

I.V.: 0.5 mg initially

Rectal: 5 mg every 4-6 hours

Dietary Considerations Alcohol: Additive CNS effect, avoid use

Monitoring Parameters Respiratory rate, heart rate, blood pressure, CNS activity

Patient Information Avoid alcohol, may cause drowsiness, impaired judgment or coordination; may cause physical and psychological dependence with prolonged use

Nursing Implications Observe patient for excessive sedation, respiratory depression, implement safety measures, assist with ambulation

Dosage Forms

Injection, as hydrochloride: 1 mg (1 mL); 1.5 mg/mL (1 mL, 10 mL)

Suppository, rectal, as hydrochloride: 5 mg

Oxymorphone Hydrochloride *see* Oxymorphone *on previous page*

Oxytetracycline (oks i tet ra SYE kleen)

Brand Names Terramycin® IV; Uri-Tet®

Canadian/Mexican Brand Names Oxitraklin® (Mexico); Terramicina® (Mexico)

Synonyms Oxytetracycline Hydrochloride

Therapeutic Category Antibiotic, Tetracycline Derivative

Use Treatment of susceptible bacterial infections; both gram-positive and gram-negative, as well as, *Rickettsia* and *Mycoplasma* organisms

Pregnancy Risk Factor D

(Continued)

Oxytetracycline *(Continued)*

Contraindications Hypersensitivity to tetracycline or any component

Warnings/Precautions Avoid in children ≤8 years of age, pregnant and nursing women; photosensitivity can occur with oxytetracycline

Adverse Reactions

>10%: Miscellaneous: Discoloration of teeth and enamel hypoplasia (infants)

1% to 10%:
- Dermatologic: Photosensitivity
- Gastrointestinal: Nausea, diarrhea

<1%:
- Cardiovascular: Pericarditis
- Central nervous system: Increased intracranial pressure, bulging fontanels in infants, pseudotumor cerebri
- Dermatologic: Pruritus, exfoliative dermatitis, dermatologic effects
- Endocrine & metabolic: Diabetes insipidus syndrome
- Gastrointestinal: Vomiting, esophagitis, anorexia, abdominal cramps, antibiotic-associated pseudomembranous colitis, staphylococcal enterocolitis
- Hepatic: Hepatotoxicity
- Local: Thrombophlebitis,
- Neuromuscular & skeletal: Paresthesia
- Renal: Renal damage, acute renal failure, azotemia
- Miscellaneous: Superinfections, anaphylaxis, pigmentation of nails, hypersensitivity reactions, candidal superinfection

Overdosage/Toxicology Symptoms of overdose include nausea, anorexia, diarrhea; following GI decontamination, supportive care only

Drug Interactions

Decreased effect with antacids containing aluminum, calcium or magnesium
- Iron and bismuth subsalicylate may decrease doxycycline bioavailability
- Barbiturates, phenytoin, and carbamazepine decrease doxycycline's half-life
- Increased effect of warfarin

Mechanism of Action Inhibits bacterial protein synthesis by binding with the 30S and possibly the 50S ribosomal subunit(s) of susceptible bacteria, cell wall synthesis is not affected

Pharmacodynamics/Kinetics

Absorption:
- Oral: Adequate (~75%)
- I.M.: Poor

Distribution: Crosses the placenta

Metabolism: Small amounts in the liver

Half-life: 8.5-9.6 hours (increases with renal impairment)

Time to peak serum concentration: Within 2-4 hours

Elimination: In urine, while much higher amounts can be found in bile

Usual Dosage

Oral:
- Children: 40-50 mg/kg/day in divided doses every 6 hours (maximum: 2 g/24 hours)
- Adults: 250-500 mg/dose every 6 hours

I.M.:
- Children >8 years: 15-25 mg/kg/day (maximum: 250 mg/dose) in divided doses every 8-12 hours
- Adults: 250-500 mg every 24 hours or 300 mg/day divided every 8-12 hours

Dosing interval in renal impairment: Cl_{cr} <10 mL/minute: Administer every 24 hours or avoid use if possible

Dosing adjustment/comments in hepatic impairment: Avoid use in patients with severe liver disease

Administration Injection for intramuscular use only; do not administer with antacids, iron products, or dairy products; administer 1 hour before or 2 hours after meals

Patient Information Avoid unnecessary exposure to sunlight; do not take with antacids, iron products, or dairy products; finish all medication; do not skip doses; take 1 hour before or 2 hours after meals

Dosage Forms

Capsule, as hydrochloride: 250 mg

Injection, as hydrochloride, with lidocaine 2%: 5% [50 mg/mL] (2 mL, 10 mL); 12.5% [125 mg/mL] (2 mL)

Oxytetracycline Hydrochloride *see* Oxytetracycline *on previous page*

Oxytocin (oks i TOE sin)

Brand Names Pitocin®; Syntocinon®

Canadian/Mexican Brand Names Toesen® (Canada); Oxitopisa® (Mexico); Syntocinon® (Mexico); Xitocin® (Mexico)

Synonyms Pit

Therapeutic Category Oxytocic Agent

Use Induces labor at term; controls postpartum bleeding; nasal preparation used to promote milk letdown in lactating females

Pregnancy Risk Factor X

Contraindications Hypersensitivity to oxytocin or any component; significant cephalopelvic disproportion, unfavorable fetal positions, fetal distress, hypertonic or hyperactive uterus, contraindicated vaginal delivery, prolapse, total placenta previa, and vasa previa

Warnings/Precautions To be used for medical rather than elective induction of labor; may produce antidiuretic effect (ie, water intoxication and excess uterine contractions); high doses or hypersensitivity to oxytocin may cause uterine hypertonicity, spasm, tetanic contraction, or rupture of the uterus; severe water intoxication with convulsions, coma, and death is associated with a slow oxytocin infusion over 24 hours

Adverse Reactions

Fetal: <1%:

- Cardiovascular: Bradycardia, arrhythmias, intracranial hemorrhage
- Central nervous system: Brain damage
- Hepatic: Neonatal jaundice
- Respiratory: Hypoxia
- Miscellaneous: Death

Maternal: <1%:

- Cardiovascular: Cardiac arrhythmias, premature ventricular contractions, hypotension, tachycardia, arrhythmias
- Central nervous system: Seizures, coma
- Endocrine & metabolic: SIADH with hyponatremia
- Gastrointestinal: Nausea, vomiting
- Genitourinary: Pelvic hematoma, postpartum hemorrhage, increased uterine motility
- Hematologic: Fatal afibrinogenemia, increased blood loss
- Miscellaneous: Death, anaphylactic reactions

Overdosage/Toxicology Symptoms of overdose include tetanic uterine contractions, impaired uterine blood flow, amniotic fluid embolism, uterine rupture, SIADH, seizures; treat SIADH via fluid restriction, diuresis, saline administration, and anticonvulsants, if needed

Stability Oxytocin should be stored at room temperature (15°C to 30°C) and protected from freezing; **incompatible** with norepinephrine, prochlorperazine

Mechanism of Action Produces the rhythmic uterine contractions characteristic to delivery and stimulates breast milk flow during nursing

Pharmacodynamics/Kinetics

Onset of uterine contractions: I.V.: Within 1 minute

Duration: <30 minutes

Metabolism: Rapid in the liver and plasma (by oxytocinase) and to a smaller degree the mammary gland

Half-life: 1-5 minutes

Elimination: Renal

Usual Dosage I.V. administration requires the use of an infusion pump

Adults:

- Induction of labor: I.V.: 0.001-0.002 units/minute; increase by 0.001-0.002 units every 15-30 minutes until contraction pattern has been established; maximum dose should not exceed 20 milliunits/minute
- Postpartum bleeding:
  - I.M.: Total dose of 10 units after delivery
  - I.V.: 10-40 units by I.V. infusion in 1000 mL of intravenous fluid at a rate sufficient to control uterine atony
- Promotion of milk letdown: Intranasal: 1 spray or 3 drops in one or both nostrils 2-3 minutes before breast-feeding

Monitoring Parameters Fluid intake and output during administration; fetal monitoring

Additional Information Sodium chloride 0.9% (NS) and dextrose 5% in water (D_5W) have been recommended as diluents; dilute 10-40 units to 1 L in NS, LR, or D_5W

Dosage Forms

Injection: 10 units/mL (1 mL, 10 mL)

Solution, nasal: 40 units/mL (2 mL, 5 mL)

P-071 *see* Cetirizine *on page 244*

Paclitaxel (PAK li taks el)

Related Information

Antiemetics for Chemotherapy Induced Nausea and Vomiting *on page 1348*
Cancer Chemotherapy Regimens *on page 1351*

(Continued)

Paclitaxel *(Continued)*

Toxicities of Chemotherapeutic Agents *on page 1382*

Brand Names Taxol®

Therapeutic Category Antineoplastic Agent, Antimicrotubular; Antineoplastic Agent, Miscellaneous

Use Treatment of metastatic carcinoma of the ovary after failure of first-line or subsequent chemotherapy; treatment of metastatic breast cancer

Pregnancy Risk Factor D

Contraindications History of hypersensitivity to any component

Warnings/Precautions Severe hypersensitivity reactions have been reported with the first or later infusions. Current evidence indicates that prolongation of the infusion (to ≥6 hours) plus premedication may minimize this effect.

Adverse Reactions Irritant chemotherapy

>10%:

- Cardiovascular: Hypotension, abnormal EKG
- Dermatologic: Alopecia
- Gastrointestinal: Nausea, vomiting, diarrhea, mucositis
- Hematologic: Bleeding, neutropenia, leukopenia, thrombocytopenia, anemia, neutropenia is increased with longer infusions
- Hepatic: Abnormal liver function tests
- Neuromuscular & skeletal: Peripheral neuropathy, myalgia
- Miscellaneous: Hypersensitivity reactions, infections

1% to 10%: Cardiovascular: Bradycardia, severe cardiovascular events

Drug Interactions Cytochrome P-450 substrate

Increased toxicity:

- In phase I trials, myelosuppression was more profound when given after cisplatin than with alternative sequence; pharmacokinetic data demonstrates a decrease in clearance of ~33% when administered following cisplatin
- Possibility of an inhibition of metabolism in patients treated with ketoconazole

Stability Store intact vials at room temperature or refrigeration (2°C to 36°C/36°F to 77°F). Further dilution in NS or D_5W to a concentration of 0.3-1.2 mg/mL is stable for up to 27 hours at room temperature (25°C) and ambient light conditions.

PACLITAXEL should be administered in either glass or Excel™/PAB™ containers. Should also use NONPOLYVINYL (nonPVC) tubing (eg, polyethylene) to minimize leaching. Formulated in a vehicle known as Cremophor EL™ (polyoxyethylated castor oil). Cremophor EL™ has been found to leach the plasticizer DEHP from polyvinyl chloride infusion bags or administration sets. Contact of the undiluted concentrate with plasticized polyvinyl chloride (PVC) equipment or devices is not recommended. Administer through I.V. tubing containing an in-line (NOT >0.22 μ) filter; administration through IVEX-2™ filters (which incorporate short inlet and outlet polyvinyl chloride-coated tubing) has not resulted in significant leaching of DEHP.

VISUALLY COMPATIBLE via Y-site: Acyclovir, amikacin, bleomycin, calcium chloride, carboplatin, ceftazidime, ceftriaxone, cimetidine, cisplatin, cyclophosphamide, cytarabine, dexamethasone sodium phosphate, diphenhydramine hydrochloride, doxorubicin, etoposide, famotidine, fluconazole, fluorouracil, ganciclovir, gentamicin, haloperidol lactate, heparin, hydrocortisone sodium succinate, hydrocortisone phosphate hydromorphone, lorazepam, magnesium sulfate, mannitol, meperidine, mesna, methotrexate sodium, metoclopramide hydrochloride, morphine sulfate, ondansetron, potassium chloride, prochlorperazine edisylate, ranitidine hydrochloride, sodium bicarbonate, vancomycin hydrochloride

VISUALLY/CHEMICALLY INCOMPATIBLE via Y-site: Amphotericin B, chlorpromazine, hydroxyzine, methylprednisolone, mitoxantrone

Standard I.V. dilution:

- IVPB: Dose/500-1,000 mL D_5W or NS
- Solutions are stable for 27 hours at room temperature (25°C)

Pharmacodynamics/Kinetics Administered by I.V. infusion and exhibits a biphasic decline in plasma concentrations

Distribution: Initial rapid decline represents distribution to the peripheral compartment and significant elimination of the drug; later phase is due to a relatively slow efflux of paclitaxel from the peripheral compartment; mean steady state: 42-162 L/m^2, indicating extensive extravascular distribution and/or tissue binding

Protein binding: 89% to 98% bound to human serum proteins at concentrations of 0.1-50 mcg/mL

Metabolism: In the liver in animals and evidence suggests hepatic metabolism in humans

Half-life, mean, terminal: 5.3-17.4 hours after 1- and 6-hour infusions at dosing levels of 15-275 mg/m^2

Elimination: Urinary recovery of unchanged drug: 1.3% to 12.6% following 1-, 6-, and 24-hour infusions of 15-275 mg/m²
Mean total body clearance range:
After 1- and 6-hour infusions: 5.8-16.3 L/hour/m²
After 24-hour infusions: 14.2-17.2 L/hour/m²

Usual Dosage Premedication with dexamethasone (20 mg orally or I.V. at 12 and 6 hours **or** 14 and 7 hours before the dose), diphenhydramine (50 mg I.V. 30-60 minutes prior to the dose), and famotidine (I.V. 20 mg 30-60 minutes prior to the dose) is recommended.

Adults: I.V. infusion: Refer to individual protocol
Ovarian carcinoma: 135-175 mg/m² over 1-24 hours administered every 3 weeks
Metastatic breast cancer: Treatment is still undergoing investigation; most protocols have used doses of 175-250 mg/m² over 1-24 hours every 3 weeks

Hemodialysis: Significant drug removal is unlikely based on physiochemical characteristics

Peritoneal dialysis: Significant drug removal is unlikely based on physiochemical characteristics

Dosage adjustment in hepatic impairment:
Total bilirubin ≤1.5 mg/dL and AST >2 X normal limits: Total dose <135 mg/m²
Total bilirubin 1.6-3.0 mg/dL: Total dose ≤75 mg/m²
Total bilirubin ≥3.1 mg/dL: Total dose ≤50 mg/m²

Administration
Anaphylactoid-like reactions have been reported: Corticosteroids (dexamethasone), H_1-antagonists (diphenhydramine), and H_2-antagonists (famotidine), should be administered prior to paclitaxel administration to minimize potential for anaphylaxis
Administer I.V. infusion over 1-24 hours; use of a 0.22 micron in-line filter is recommended during the infusion

Monitoring Parameters Monitor for hypersensitivity reactions

Reference Range Mean maximum serum concentrations: 435-802 ng/mL following 24-hour infusions of 200-275 mg/m² and were approximately 10% to 30% of those following 6-hour infusions of equivalent doses

Patient Information Alopecia occurs in almost all patients

Dosage Forms Injection: 6 mg/mL (5 mL)

Palmitate-A® 5000 [OTC] *see* Vitamin A *on page 1307*

2-PAM *see* Pralidoxime *on page 1032*

Pamelor® *see* Nortriptyline *on page 917*

Pamidronate (pa mi DROE nate)

Brand Names Aredia™

Synonyms Pamidronate Disodium

Therapeutic Category Antidote, Hypercalcemia; Bisphosphonate Derivative

Use FDA-approved: Treatment of hypercalcemia associated with malignancy; treatment of osteolytic bone lesions associated with multiple myeloma or metastatic breast cancer; moderate to severe Paget's disease of bone

Pregnancy Risk Factor C

Contraindications Previous hypersensitivity to pamidronate or other biphosphonates

Warnings/Precautions Use caution in patients with renal impairment as the potential nephrotoxic effects of pamidronate are not known; use caution in patients who are pregnant or in the breast-feeding period; leukopenia has been observed with oral pamidronate and monitoring of white blood cell counts is suggested; vein irritation and thrombophlebitis may occur with infusions. Has not been studied exclusively in the elderly; monitor serum electrolytes periodically since elderly are often receiving diuretics which can result in decreases in serum calcium, potassium, and magnesium.

Adverse Reactions
1% to 10%:
Central nervous system: Malaise, fever, convulsions
Endocrine & metabolic: Hypomagnesemia, hypocalcemia, hypokalemia, fluid overload, hypophosphatemia
Gastrointestinal: GI symptoms, nausea, diarrhea, constipation, anorexia
Hepatic: Abnormal hepatic function
Neuromuscular & skeletal: Bone pain
Respiratory: Dyspnea
<1%:
Central nervous system: Pain
Dermatologic: Angioedema, skin rash
Gastrointestinal: Occult blood in stools, abnormal taste
Hematologic: Leukopenia
(Continued)

Pamidronate *(Continued)*

Neuromuscular & skeletal: Increased risk of fractures
Renal: Nephrotoxicity
Miscellaneous: Hypersensitivity reactions

Overdosage/Toxicology Symptoms of overdose include hypocalcemia, EKG changes, seizures, bleeding, paresthesia, carpopedal spasm, fever

Treat with I.V. calcium gluconate, general supportive care; fever and hypotension can be treated with corticosteroids

Stability

Reconstitute by adding 10 mL of sterile water for injection to each 30 mg vial of lyophilized pamidronate disodium powder, the resulting solution will be 30 mg/10 mL

Pamidronate is **incompatible** with calcium-containing infusion solutions such as Ringer's injection

Pamidronate may be further diluted in 250-1000 mL of 0.45% or 0.9% sodium chloride or 5% dextrose; pamidronate should not be mixed with calcium-containing solutions (eg, Ringer's solution)

Pamidronate [reconstituted solution and infusion solution] is stable at room temperature and under refrigeration (36°F to 46°F or 2°C to 8°C) for 24 hours

Mechanism of Action A biphosphonate which inhibits bone resorption via actions on osteoclasts or on osteoclast precursors. Does not appear to produce any significant effects on renal tubular calcium handling and is poorly absorbed following oral administration (high oral doses have been reported effective); therefore, I.V. therapy is preferred.

Pharmacodynamics/Kinetics

Onset of effect: 24-48 hours
Maximum effect: 5-7 days
Absorption: Poorly from the GI tract; pharmacokinetic studies are lacking
Half-life, unmetabolized: 2.5 hours
Distribution half-life: 1.6 hours
Urinary (elimination) half-life: 2.5 hours
Bone half-life: 300 days
Elimination: Biphasic; ~50% excreted unchanged in urine within 72 hours

Usual Dosage Drug must be diluted properly before administration and infused intravenously slowly (over at least 1 hour). Adults: I.V.:

Hypercalcemia of malignancy:

Moderate cancer-related hypercalcemia (corrected serum calcium: 12-13 mg/dL): 60-90 mg given as a slow infusion over 2-24 hours

Severe cancer-related hypercalcemia (corrected serum calcium: >13.5 mg/dL): 90 mg as a slow infusion over 2-24 hours

A period of 7 days should elapse before the use of second course; repeat infusions every 2-3 weeks have been suggested, however, could be administered every 2-3 months according to the degree and of severity of hypercalcemia and/or the type of malignancy

Osteolytic bone lesions with multiple myeloma: 90 mg in 500 mL D_5W, 0.45% NaCl or 0.9% NaCl administered over 4 hours on a monthly basis

Osteolytic bone lesions with metastatic breast cancer: 90 mg in 250 mL D_5W, 0.45% NaCl or 0.9% NaCl administered over 2 hours repeated every 3-4 weeks

Paget's disease: 30 mg in 500 mL 0.45% NaCl, 0.9% NaCl or D_5W administered over 4 hours for 3 consecutive days

Monitoring Parameters Serum electrolytes, monitor for hypocalcemia for at least 2 weeks after therapy; serum calcium, phosphate, magnesium, potassium, serum creatinine, CBC with differential

Reference Range Calcium (total): Adults: 9.0-11.0 mg/dL (SI: 2.05-2.54 mmol/L), may slightly decrease with aging; Phosphorus: 2.5-4.5 mg/dL (SI: 0.81-1.45 mmol/L)

Patient Information Maintain adequate intake of calcium and vitamin D; report any fever, sore throat, or unusual bleeding to your physician

Dosage Forms Powder for injection, lyophilized, as disodium: 30 mg, 60 mg, 90 mg

Pamidronate Disodium *see* Pamidronate *on previous page*

p-Aminoclonidine *see* Apraclonidine *on page 98*

Pamprin IB® [OTC] *see* Ibuprofen *on page 639*

Panadol® [OTC] *see* Acetaminophen *on page 19*

Panasal® 5/500 *see* Hydrocodone and Aspirin *on page 621*

Pancrease® *see* Pancrelipase *on next page*

Pancrease® MT 4 *see* Pancrelipase *on next page*

Pancrease® MT 10 *see* Pancrelipase *on next page*

Pancrease® MT 16 *see* Pancrelipase *on next page*

Pancrelipase (pan kre LI pase)

Brand Names Cotazym®; Cotazym-S®; Creon 10®; Creon 20®; Ilozyme®; Ku-Zyme® HP; Pancrease®; Pancrease® MT 4; Pancrease® MT 10; Pancrease® MT 16; Protilase®; Ultrase® MT12; Ultrase® MT20; Viokase®; Zymase®

Synonyms Lipancreatin

Therapeutic Category Enzyme, Pancreatic; Pancreatic Enzyme

Use Replacement therapy in symptomatic treatment of malabsorption syndrome caused by pancreatic insufficiency

Pregnancy Risk Factor C

Contraindications Hypersensitivity to pancrelipase or any component, pork protein

Warnings/Precautions Pancrelipase is inactivated by acids; use microencapsulated products whenever possible, since these products permit better dissolution of enzymes in the duodenum and protect the enzyme preparations from acid degradation in the stomach

Adverse Reactions

1% to 10%: High doses:
- Endocrine & metabolic: Hyperuricemia
- Gastrointestinal: Nausea, cramps, constipation, diarrhea
- Genitourinary: Hyperuricosuria
- Ocular: Lacrimation
- Respiratory: Sneezing, bronchospasm

<1%:
- Dermatologic: Rash
- Respiratory: Shortness of breath, bronchospasm
- Miscellaneous: Irritation of the mouth

Overdosage/Toxicology Symptoms of overdose include diarrhea, other transient intestinal upset, hyperuricosuria, hyperuricemia

Drug Interactions

Decreased effect: Calcium carbonate, magnesium hydroxide

Increased effect: H_2-antagonists (eg, ranitidine, cimetidine)

Mechanism of Action Replaces endogenous pancreatic enzymes to assist in digestion of protein, starch and fats

Pharmacodynamics/Kinetics

Absorption: Not absorbed, acts locally in GI tract

Elimination: In feces

Usual Dosage Oral:

Powder: Actual dose depends on the digestive requirements of the patient
- Children <1 year: Start with 1/8 teaspoonful with feedings
- Adults: 0.7 g with meals

Enteric coated microspheres and microtablets: The following dosage recommendations are only an approximation for initial dosages. The actual dosage will depend on the digestive requirements of the individual patient.
- Children:
  - <1 year: 2000 units of lipase with meals
  - 1-6 years: 4000-8000 units of lipase with meals and 4000 units with snacks
  - 7-12 years: 4000-12,000 units of lipase with meals and snacks
- Adults: 4000-16,000 units of lipase with meals and with snacks or 1-3 tablets/capsules before or with meals and snacks; in severe deficiencies, dose may be increased to 8 tablets/capsules

Occluded feeding tubes: One tablet of Viokase® crushed with one 325 mg tablet of sodium bicarbonate (to activate the Viokase®) in 5 mL of water can be instilled into the nasogastric tube and clamped for 5 minutes; then, flushed with 50 mL of tap water

Patient Information Do not chew capsules, microspheres, or microtablets; take before or with meals; avoid inhaling powder dosage form

Dosage Forms

Capsule:
- Cotazym®: Lipase 8000 units, protease 30,000 units, amylase 30,000 units
- Ku-Zyme® HP: Lipase 8000 units, protease 30,000 units, amylase 30,000 units
- Ultrase® MT12: Lipase 12,000 units, protease 39,000 units, amylase 39,000 units
- Ultrase® MT20: Lipase 20,000 units, protease 65,000 units, amylase 65,000 units
- Enteric coated microspheres (Pancrease®): Lipase 4000 units, protease 25,000 units, amylase 20,000 units
- Enteric coated microtablets:
  - Pancrease® MT 4: Lipase 4500 units, protease 12,000 units, amylase 12,000 units
  - Pancrease® MT 10: Lipase 10,000 units, protease 30,000 units, amylase 30,000 units

(Continued)

Pancrelipase *(Continued)*

Pancrease® MT 16: Lipase 16,000 units, protease 48,000 units, amylase 48,000 units
Pancrease® MT 20: Lipase 20,000 units, protease 44,000 units, amylase 56,000 units
Enteric coated spheres:
Cotazym-S®: Lipase 5000 units, protease 20,000 units, amylase 20,000 units
Pancrelipase, Protilase®: Lipase 4000 units, protease 25,000 units, amylase 20,000 units
Zymase®: Lipase 12,000 units, protease 24,000 units, amylase 24,000 units
Delayed release:
Creon 10®: Lipase 10,000 units, protease 37,500 units, amylase 33,200 units
Creon 20®: Lipase 20,000 units, protease 75,000 units, amylase 66,400 units
Powder (Viokase®): Lipase 16,800 units, protease 70,000 units, amylase 70,000 units per 0.7 g
Tablet:
Ilozyme®: Lipase 11,000 units, protease 30,000 units, amylase 30,000 units
Viokase®: Lipase 8000 units, protease 30,000 units, amylase 30,000 units

Pancuronium (pan kyoo ROE nee um)

Related Information
Neuromuscular Blocking Agents Comparison *on page 1417*

Brand Names Pavulon®

Synonyms Pancuronium Bromide

Therapeutic Category Neuromuscular Blocker Agent, Nondepolarizing; Skeletal Muscle Relaxant

Use Drug of choice for neuromuscular blockade except in patients with renal failure, hepatic failure, or cardiovascular instability

Produce skeletal muscle relaxation during surgery after induction of general anesthesia, increase pulmonary compliance during assisted respiration, facilitate endotracheal intubation, preferred muscle relaxant for neonatal cardiac patients, must provide artificial ventilation

Pregnancy Risk Factor C

Contraindications Hypersensitivity to pancuronium, bromide, or any component

Warnings/Precautions Ventilation must be supported during neuromuscular blockade. Electrolyte imbalance alters blockade. Use with caution in patients with myasthenia gravis or other neuromuscular diseases, pre-existing pulmonary, hepatic, renal disease, and in the elderly.

Adverse Reactions
1% to 10%:
Cardiovascular: Elevation in pulse rate, elevation in blood pressure, tachycardia, hypertension
Dermatologic: Rash, itching
Gastrointestinal: Excessive salivation
<1%:
Cardiovascular: Skin flushing, edema
Dermatologic: Erythema
Local: Burning sensation along the vein
Neuromuscular & skeletal: Profound muscle weakness
Respiratory: Wheezing, circulatory collapse, bronchospasm
Miscellaneous: Hypersensitivity reaction

Causes of prolonged neuromuscular blockade:
Excessive drug administration
Cumulative drug effect, decreased metabolism/excretion (hepatic and/or renal impairment)
Accumulation of active metabolites
Electrolyte imbalance (hypokalemia, hypocalcemia, hypermagnesemia, hypernatremia)
Hypothermia
Drug interactions
Increased sensitivity to muscle relaxants (eg, neuromuscular disorders such as myasthenia gravis or polymyositis)

Overdosage/Toxicology Symptoms of overdose include apnea, respiratory depression, cardiovascular collapse; pyridostigmine, neostigmine, or edrophonium in conjunction with atropine will usually antagonize the action of pancuronium

Drug Interactions
Increased toxicity: Magnesium sulfate, furosemide can increase or decrease neuromuscular blockade (dose-dependent)
Prolonged neuromuscular blockade:
Inhaled anesthetics

Local anesthetics
Calcium channel blockers
Antiarrhythmics (eg, quinidine or procainamide)
Antibiotics (eg, aminoglycosides, tetracyclines, vancomycin, clindamycin)
Immunosuppressants (eg, cyclosporine)

Stability Refrigerate; however, is stable for up to 6 months at room temperature; I.V. form is **incompatible** when mixed with diazepam at a Y-site injection

Mechanism of Action Blocks neural transmission at the myoneural junction by binding with cholinergic receptor sites

Pharmacodynamics/Kinetics
Peak effect: I.V.: Within 2-3 minutes
Duration: 40-60 minutes (dose dependent)
Metabolism: 30% to 45% in the liver
Half-life: 110 minutes
Elimination: In urine (55% to 70% as unchanged drug)

Usual Dosage Based on ideal body weight in obese patients. **I.V.:**
Infants >1 month, Children, and Adults: Initial: 0.04-0.1 mg/kg; maintenance dose: 0.02-0.1 mg/kg/dose every 30 minutes to 3 hours as needed

Continuous I.V. infusions are not recommended due to case reports of prolonged paralysis

Dosing adjustment in renal impairment: Elimination half-life is doubled, plasma clearance is reduced and rate of recovery is sometimes much slower
Cl_{cr} 10-50 mL/minute: Administer 50% of normal dose
Cl_{cr} <10 mL/minute: Do not use

Dosing adjustment/comments in hepatic disease: Elimination half-life is doubled, plasma clearance is doubled, recovery time is prolonged, volume of distribution is increased (50%) and results in a slower onset, higher total dosage and prolongation of neuromuscular blockade

Patients with liver disease may develop slow resistance to nondepolarizing muscle relaxant; large doses may be required and problems may arise in antagonism

Monitoring Parameters Heart rate, blood pressure, assisted ventilation status; cardiac monitor, blood pressure monitor, and ventilator required

Dosage Forms Injection, as bromide: 1 mg/mL (10 mL); 2 mg/mL (2 mL, 5 mL)

Pancuronium Bromide *see* Pancuronium *on previous page*
Pandel® *see* Hydrocortisone *on page 623*
Panmycin® *see* Tetracycline *on page 1203*
PanOxyl®-AQ *see* Benzoyl Peroxide *on page 140*
PanOxyl® Bar [OTC] *see* Benzoyl Peroxide *on page 140*
Panscol® [OTC] *see* Salicylic Acid *on page 1120*
Panthoderm® [OTC] *see* Dexpanthenol *on page 361*
Pantothenyl Alcohol *see* Dexpanthenol *on page 361*

Papaverine (pa PAV er een)

Brand Names Genabid®; Pavabid®; Pavatine®

Synonyms Papaverine Hydrochloride

Therapeutic Category Vasodilator

Use
Oral: Relief of peripheral and cerebral ischemia associated with arterial spasm; smooth muscle relaxant
Parenteral: Various vascular spasms associated with muscle spasms as in myocardial infarction, angina, peripheral and pulmonary embolism, peripheral vascular disease, angiospastic states, and visceral spasm (ureteral, biliary, and GI colic); testing for impotence

Pregnancy Risk Factor C

Contraindications Complete atrioventricular block; Parkinson's disease

Warnings/Precautions Use with caution in patients with glaucoma; administer I.V. cautiously since apnea and arrhythmias may result; may, in large doses, depress cardiac conduction (eg, A-V node) leading to arrhythmias; may interfere with levodopa therapy of Parkinson's disease; hepatic hypersensitivity noted with jaundice, eosinophilia, and abnormal LFTs

Adverse Reactions
<1%:
Cardiovascular: Flushing of the face, tachycardias, hypotension, arrhythmias with rapid I.V. use
Central nervous system: Depression, dizziness, vertigo, drowsiness, sedation, lethargy, headache
Dermatologic: Pruritus
Gastrointestinal: Xerostomia, nausea, constipation
Hepatic: Hepatic hypersensitivity
(Continued)

Papaverine *(Continued)*

Local: Thrombosis at the I.V. administration site
Respiratory: Apnea with rapid I.V. use
Miscellaneous: Diaphoresis

Overdosage/Toxicology Symptoms of overdose include nausea, vomiting weakness, gastric distress, ataxia, hepatic dysfunction, drowsiness, nystagmus, hyperventilation, hypotension, hypokalemia; treatment is supportive with conventional therapy (ie, fluids, positioning and vasopressors for hypotension)

Drug Interactions Cytochrome P-450 2D6 enzyme substrate and cytochrome P-450 2C enzyme substrate

Decreased effect: Papaverine decreases the effects of levodopa
Increased toxicity: Additive effects with CNS depressants or morphine

Stability Protect from heat or freezing; refrigerate injection at 2°C to 8°C (35°F to 46°F); solutions should be clear to pale yellow; precipitates with lactated Ringer's

Mechanism of Action Smooth muscle spasmolytic producing a generalized smooth muscle relaxation including: vasodilatation, gastrointestinal sphincter relaxation, bronchiolar muscle relaxation, and potentially a depressed myocardium (with large doses); muscle relaxation may occur due to inhibition or cyclic nucleotide phosphodiesterase, increasing cyclic AMP; muscle relaxation is unrelated to nerve innervation; papaverine increases cerebral blood flow in normal subjects; oxygen uptake is unaltered

Pharmacodynamics/Kinetics

Onset of action: Oral: Rapid
Protein binding: 90%
Metabolism: Rapidly in the liver
Half-life: 0.5-1.5 hours
Elimination: Primarily as metabolites in urine

Usual Dosage

Children: I.M., I.V.: 1.5 mg/kg 4 times/day
Adults:
Oral: 100-300 mg 3-5 times/day
Oral, sustained release: 150-300 mg every 12 hours
I.M., I.V.: 30-120 mg every 3 hours as needed; for cardiac extrasystoles, administer 2 doses 10 minutes apart I.V. or I.M.

Administration Rapid I.V. administration may result in arrhythmias and fatal apnea; administer no faster than over 1-2 minutes

Patient Information May cause dizziness, flushing, headache, constipation, caution when driving or performing tasks needing alertness

Nursing Implications Physically incompatible with Lactated Ringer's injection

Dosage Forms

Capsule, sustained release, as hydrochloride: 150 mg
Tablet, as hydrochloride: 30 mg, 60 mg, 100 mg, 150 mg, 200 mg, 300 mg
Tablet, timed release, as hydrochloride: 200 mg

Papaverine Hydrochloride *see* Papaverine *on previous page*
Para-Aminosalicylate Sodium *see* Aminosalicylate Sodium *on page 66*
Parabromdylamine *see* Brompheniramine *on page 166*
Paracetamol *see* Acetaminophen *on page 19*
Paraflex® *see* Chlorzoxazone *on page 266*
Parafon Forte™ DSC *see* Chlorzoxazone *on page 266*
Paraplatin® *see* Carboplatin *on page 206*

Paregoric (par e GOR ik)

Synonyms Camphorated Tincture of Opium

Therapeutic Category Analgesic, Narcotic; Antidiarrheal

Use Treatment of diarrhea or relief of pain; neonatal opiate withdrawal

Restrictions C-III

Pregnancy Risk Factor B (D when used long-term or in high doses)

Contraindications Hypersensitivity to opium or any component; diarrhea caused by poisoning until the toxic material has been removed

Warnings/Precautions Use with caution in patients with respiratory, hepatic or renal dysfunction, severe prostatic hypertrophy, or history of narcotic abuse; opium shares the toxic potential of opiate agonists, and usual precautions of opiate agonist therapy should be observed; some preparations contain sulfites which may cause allergic reactions; infants <3 months of age are more susceptible to respiratory depression, use with caution and generally in reduced doses in this age group

Adverse Reactions

>10%:
Cardiovascular: Hypotension
Central nervous system: Drowsiness, dizziness
Gastrointestinal: Constipation

Neuromuscular & skeletal: Weakness

1% to 10%:

Central nervous system: Restlessness, headache, malaise

Genitourinary: Ureteral spasms, decreased urination

Miscellaneous: Histamine release

<1%:

Cardiovascular: Peripheral vasodilation

Central nervous system: Insomnia, CNS depression, mental depression, increased intracranial pressure

Gastrointestinal: Anorexia, stomach cramps, nausea, vomiting, biliary tract spasm

Genitourinary: Urinary tract spasm

Ocular: Miosis

Respiratory: Respiratory depression

Miscellaneous: Physical and psychological dependence

Overdosage/Toxicology Symptoms of overdose include hypotension, drowsiness, seizures, respiratory depression

Naloxone 2 mg I.V. (0.01 mg/kg for children) with repeat administration as necessary up to a total of 10 mg

Drug Interactions Increased effect/toxicity with CNS depressants (eg, alcohol, narcotics, benzodiazepines, TCAs, MAO inhibitors, phenothiazine)

Stability Store in light-resistant, tightly closed container

Mechanism of Action Increases smooth muscle tone in GI tract, decreases motility and peristalsis, diminishes digestive secretions

Pharmacodynamics/Kinetics In terms of opium

Metabolism: In the liver

Elimination: In urine, primarily as morphine glucuronide conjugates and as parent compound (morphine, codeine, papaverine, etc)

Usual Dosage Oral:

Neonatal opiate withdrawal: Instill 3-6 drops every 3-6 hours as needed, or initially 0.2 mL every 3 hours; increase dosage by approximately 0.05 mL every 3 hours until withdrawal symptoms are controlled; it is rare to exceed 0.7 mL/dose. Stabilize withdrawal symptoms for 3-5 days, then gradually decrease dosage over a 2- to 4-week period.

Children: 0.25-0.5 mL/kg 1-4 times/day

Adults: 5-10 mL 1-4 times/day

Dietary Considerations Alcohol: Additive CNS effect, avoid use

Test Interactions ↑ aminotransferase [ALT (SGPT)/AST (SGOT)] (S)

Patient Information Avoid alcohol, may cause drowsiness, impaired judgment or coordination; may cause physical and psychological dependence with prolonged use

Nursing Implications Observe patient for excessive sedation, respiratory depression, implement safety measures, assist with ambulation

Additional Information Contains morphine 0.4 mg/mL and alcohol 45%

Dosage Forms Liquid: 2 mg morphine equivalent/5 mL [equivalent to 20 mg opium powder] (5 mL, 60 mL, 473 mL, 4000 mL)

Parenteral Multiple Vitamin *see* Vitamins, Multiple *on page 1310*

Parenteral Nutrition *see page 1494*

Par Glycerol® *see* Iodinated Glycerol *on page 670*

Parlodel® *see* Bromocriptine *on page 165*

Parnate® *see* Tranylcypromine *on page 1249*

Paromomycin (par oh moe MYE sin)

Brand Names Humatin®

Synonyms Paromomycin Sulfate

Therapeutic Category Amebicide

Use Treatment of acute and chronic intestinal amebiasis; preoperatively to suppress intestinal flora; tapeworm infestations; rid bowel of nitrogen-forming bacteria in hepatic coma; treatment of *Cryptosporidium* diarrhea

Pregnancy Risk Factor C

Contraindications Intestinal obstruction, renal failure, known hypersensitivity to paromomycin or components

Warnings/Precautions Use with caution in patients with impaired renal function or possible or proven ulcerative bowel lesions

Adverse Reactions

1% to 10%: Gastrointestinal: Diarrhea, abdominal cramps, nausea, vomiting, heartburn

<1%:

Central nervous system: Headache, vertigo

Dermatologic: Exanthema, rash, pruritus

Gastrointestinal: Steatorrhea, secondary enterocolitis

(Continued)

Paromomycin *(Continued)*

Hematologic: Eosinophilia
Otic: Ototoxicity

Overdosage/Toxicology Symptoms of overdose include nausea, vomiting, diarrhea; following GI decontamination, if possible; care is supportive and symptomatic

Drug Interactions
Decreased effect of digoxin and methotrexate
Increased effect of oral anticoagulants

Mechanism of Action Acts directly on ameba; has antibacterial activity against normal and pathogenic organisms in the GI tract; interferes with bacterial protein synthesis by binding to 30S ribosomal subunits

Pharmacodynamics/Kinetics
Absorption: Not absorbed via oral route
Elimination: 100% unchanged in feces

Usual Dosage Oral:
Intestinal amebiasis: Children and Adults: 25-35 mg/kg/day in 3 divided doses for 5-10 days
Dientamoeba fragilis: Children and Adults: 25-30 mg/kg/day in 3 divided doses for 7 days
Cryptosporidium: Adults with AIDS: 1.5-2.25 g/day in 3-6 divided doses for 10-14 days (occasionally courses of up to 4-8 weeks may be needed)
Tapeworm (fish, dog, bovine, porcine):
Children: 11 mg/kg every 15 minutes for 4 doses
Adults: 1 g every 15 minutes for 4 doses
Hepatic coma: Adults: 4 g/day in 2-4 divided doses for 5-6 days
Dwarf tapeworm: Children and Adults: 45 mg/kg/dose every day for 5-7 days

Patient Information Take full course of therapy; do not skip doses; notify physician if ringing in ears, hearing loss, or dizziness occurs

Dosage Forms Capsule, as sulfate: 250 mg

Paromomycin Sulfate *see* Paromomycin *on previous page*

Paroxetine (pa ROKS e teen)

Related Information
Antidepressant Agents Comparison *on page 1393*

Brand Names Paxil™

Therapeutic Category Antidepressant, Serotonin Reuptake Inhibitor

Use Treatment of depression; treatment of panic disorder and obsessive-compulsive disorder

Pregnancy Risk Factor B

Contraindications Do not use within 14 days of MAO inhibitors

Warnings/Precautions Use cautiously in patients with a history of seizures, mania, renal disease, cardiac disease, suicidal patients, children, or during breast-feeding in lactating women; avoid ECT

Adverse Reactions
>10%:
Central nervous system: Headache, somnolence, dizziness, insomnia
Gastrointestinal: Nausea, xerostomia, constipation, diarrhea
Genitourinary: Ejaculatory disturbances
Neuromuscular & skeletal: Weakness
Miscellaneous: Diaphoresis
1% to 10%:
Cardiovascular: Palpitations, vasodilation, postural hypotension
Central nervous system: Nervousness, anxiety
Endocrine & metabolic: Decreased libido
Gastrointestinal: Anorexia, flatulence, vomiting
Neuromuscular & skeletal: Tremor, paresthesia
<1%:
Cardiovascular: Bradycardia, hypotension
Central nervous system: Migraine, akinesia
Dermatologic: Alopecia
Endocrine & metabolic: Amenorrhea
Gastrointestinal: Gastritis
Hematologic: Anemia, leukopenia
Neuromuscular & skeletal: Arthritis
Ocular: Eye pain
Otic: Ear pain
Respiratory: Asthma
Miscellaneous: Bruxism, thirst

Overdosage/Toxicology Symptoms of overdose include nausea, vomiting, drowsiness, sinus tachycardia, and dilated pupils

There are no specific antidotes, following attempts at decontamination, treatment is supportive and symptomatic; forced diuresis, dialysis, and hemoperfusion are unlikely to be beneficial.

Drug Interactions

Decreased effect: Phenobarbital, phenytoin

Increased toxicity: Alcohol, cimetidine, MAO inhibitors (hyperpyrexic crisis); increased effect/toxicity of TCAs, fluoxetine, sertraline, phenothiazines, class 1C antiarrhythmics, warfarin

Mechanism of Action Paroxetine is a selective serotonin reuptake inhibitor, chemically unrelated to tricyclic, tetracyclic, or other antidepressants; presumably, the inhibition of serotonin reuptake from brain synapse stimulated serotonin activity in the brain

Pharmacodynamics/Kinetics

Metabolism: Extensive following absorption by cytochrome P-450 enzymes

Half-life: 21 hours

Elimination: Metabolites are excreted in bile and urine

Usual Dosage Adults: Oral:

Depression: 20 mg once daily (maximum: 60 mg/day), preferably in the morning; in elderly, debilitated, or patients with hepatic or renal impairment, start with 10 mg/day (maximum: 40 mg/day); adjust doses at 7-day intervals

Panic disorder and obsessive compulsive disorder: Recommended average daily dose: 40 mg, this dosage should be given after an adequate trial on 20 mg/day and then titrating upward

Monitoring Parameters Hepatic and renal function tests, blood pressure, heart rate

Test Interactions ↑ LFTs

Dosage Forms Tablet: 10 mg, 20 mg, 30 mg, 40 mg

PAS *see* Aminosalicylate Sodium *on page 66*

Pathocil® *see* Dicloxacillin *on page 375*

Pavabid® *see* Papaverine *on page 951*

Pavatine® *see* Papaverine *on page 951*

Pavulon® *see* Pancuronium *on page 950*

Paxil™ *see* Paroxetine *on previous page*

PBZ® *see* Tripelennamine *on page 1269*

PBZ-SR® *see* Tripelennamine *on page 1269*

PCA *see* Procainamide *on page 1046*

PCE® *see* Erythromycin *on page 461*

PediaCare® Oral *see* Pseudoephedrine *on page 1074*

Pediaflor® *see* Fluoride *on page 536*

Pediapred® *see* Prednisolone *on page 1037*

PediaProfen™ *see* Ibuprofen *on page 639*

Pediatric ALS Algorithm, Asystole and Pulseless Arrest *see page 1507*

Pediatric ALS Algorithm, Bradycardia *see page 1506*

Pediatric Triban® *see* Trimethobenzamide *on page 1265*

Pediazole® *see* Erythromycin and Sulfisoxazole *on page 463*

PediOtic® Otic *see* Neomycin, Polymyxin B, and Hydrocortisone *on page 890*

PedvaxHIB™ *see Haemophilus* b Conjugate Vaccine *on page 595*

Pegademase Bovine (peg A de mase BOE vine)

Brand Names Adagen™

Therapeutic Category Enzyme, Replacement Therapy

Use Enzyme replacement therapy for adenosine deaminase (ADA) deficiency in patients with severe combined immunodeficiency disease (SCID) who can not benefit from bone marrow transplant; not a cure for SCID, unlike bone marrow transplants, injections must be used the rest of the child's life, therefore is not really an alternative

Pregnancy Risk Factor C

Contraindications Hypersensitivity to pegademase bovine; not to be used as preparatory or support therapy for bone marrow transplantation

Warnings/Precautions Use with caution in patients with thrombocytopenia

Adverse Reactions

<1%:

Central nervous system: Headache

Local: Pain at injection site

Drug Interactions Decreased effect: Vidarabine

Stability Refrigerate at 2°C to 8°C (36°F to 46°F); do not freeze

Mechanism of Action Adenosine deaminase is an enzyme that catalyzes the deamination of both adenosine and deoxyadenosine. Hereditary lack of adenocino deaminase activity results in severe combined immunodeficiency disease, a fatal disorder of infancy characterized by profound defects of both cellular and (Continued)

Pegademase Bovine *(Continued)*

humoral immunity. It is estimated that 25% of patients with the autosomal recessive form of severe combined immunodeficiency lack adenosine deaminase.

Pharmacodynamics/Kinetics

Plasma adenosine deaminase activity generally normalizes after 2-3 weeks of weekly I.M. injections

Absorption: Rapid

Half-life: 48-72 hours

Usual Dosage Children: I.M.: Dose given every 7 days, 10 units/kg the first dose, 15 units/kg the second dose, and 20 units/kg the third dose; maintenance dose: 20 units/kg/week is recommended depending on patient's ADA level; maximum single dose: 30 units/kg

Patient Information Not a cure for SCID; unlike bone marrow transplants, injections must be used the rest of the child's life; frequent blood tests are necessary to monitor effect and adjust the dose as needed

Dosage Forms Injection: 250 units/mL (1.5 mL)

Pegaspargase (peg AS par jase)

Related Information

Cancer Chemotherapy Regimens *on page 1351*

Brand Names Oncaspar®

Synonyms PEG-L-asparaginase

Therapeutic Category Antineoplastic Agent, Miscellaneous; Protein Synthesis Inhibitor

Use Patients with acute lymphoblastic leukemia (ALL) who require L-asparaginase in their treatment regimen, but have developed hypersensitivity to the native forms of L-asparaginase. Use as a single agent should only be undertaken when multi-agent chemotherapy is judged to be inappropriate for the patient.

Pregnancy Risk Factor C

Pregnancy/Breast-Feeding Implications Based on limited reports in humans, the use of asparaginase does not seem to pose a major risk to the fetus when used in the 2nd and 3rd trimesters, or when exposure occurs prior to conception in either females or males. Because of the teratogenicity observed in animals and the lack of human data after 1st trimester exposure, asparaginase should be used cautiously, if at all, during this period.

Contraindications Pancreatitis or a history of pancreatitis; patients who have had significant hemorrhagic events associated with prior L-asparaginase therapy; previous serious allergic reactions, such as generalized urticaria, bronchospasm, laryngeal edema, hypotension, or other unacceptable adverse reactions to pegaspargase.

Warnings/Precautions

The U.S. Food and Drug Administration (FDA) currently recommends that procedures for proper handling and disposal of antineoplastic agents be considered

Hypersensitivity reactions to pegaspargase, including life-threatening anaphylaxis, may occur during therapy, especially in patients with known hypersensitivity to the other forms of L-asparaginase. As a routine precaution, keep patients under observation for 1 hour with resuscitation equipment and other agents necessary to treat anaphylaxis (eg, epinephrine, oxygen, I.V. steroids) available.

Use caution when treating patients with pegaspargase in combination with hepatotoxic agents, especially when liver dysfunction is present

Adverse Reactions

Overall, the adult patients had a somewhat higher incidence of L-asparaginase toxicities, except for hypersensitivity reactions, than the pediatric patients

>10%:

Cardiovascular: Edema

Central nervous system: Pain

Dermatologic: Urticaria, erythema

Gastrointestinal: Pancreatitis, (sometimes fulminant and fatal); increased serum amylase and lipase

Hepatic: Elevations of AST, ALT and bilirubin (direct and indirect); jaundice, ascites and hypoalbuminemia, fatty changes in the liver, liver failure

Local: Induration, tenderness

Neuromuscular & skeletal: Arthralgia

Respiratory: Bronchospasm, dyspnea

Miscellaneous: Hypersensitivity: Acute or delayed, acute anaphylaxis, edema of the lips

>5%:

Cardiovascular: Edema

Central nervous system: Pain, fever, chills, malaise

Dermatologic: Rash

Gastrointestinal: Emetic potential: Mild (>5%)
Hepatic: ALT increase
Respiratory: Dyspnea or bronchospasm

1% to 5%:

Cardiovascular: Hypotension, tachycardia, thrombosis
Central nervous system: Chills
Dermatologic: Lip edema
Endocrine & metabolic: Hyperglycemia requiring insulin (3%)
Gastrointestinal: Abdominal pain, pancreatitis (1%)
Hematologic: Decreased anticoagulant effect, disseminated intravascular coagulation, decreased fibrinogen, hemolytic anemia, leukopenia, pancytopenia, thrombocytopenia, increased thromboplastin
Myelosuppressive effects:
WBC: Mild
Platelets: Mild
Onset (days): 7
Nadir (days): 14
Recovery (days): 21
Local: Injection site hypersensitivity
Respiratory: Dyspnea

Overdosage/Toxicology Symptoms of overdose include nausea, diarrhea

Drug Interactions

Decreased effect: Methotrexate: Asparaginase terminates methotrexate action by inhibition of protein synthesis and prevention of cell entry into the S phase

Increased toxicity:

Aspirin, dipyridamole, heparin, warfarin, NSAIDs: Imbalances in coagulation factors have been noted with the use of pegaspargase - use with caution
Vincristine and prednisone: An increase in toxicity has been noticed when asparaginase is administered with VCR and prednisone
Cyclophosphamide (decreases metabolism)
Mercaptopurine (increases hepatotoxicity)
Vincristine (increases neuropathy)
Prednisone (increases hyperglycemia)

Stability Avoid excessive agitation; do **not** shake; refrigerate at 2°C to 8°C (36°F to 46°F); single-use vial; discard unused portions

Do not use if cloudy or if precipitate is present; do not use if stored at room temperature for >48 hours; do **not** freeze; do not use product if it is known to have been frozen

Standard I.M. dilution: Usually no >2 mL/injection site

Standard I.V. dilution: Dose/100 mL NS or D_5W; stable for 48 hours at room temperature

Mechanism of Action Pegaspargase is a modified version of the enzyme L-asparaginase; the L-asparaginase used in the manufacture of pegaspargase is derived from *Escherichia coli*

Some malignant cells (ie, lymphoblastic leukemia cells and those of lymphocyte derivation) must acquire the amino acid asparagine from surrounding fluid such as blood, whereas normal cells can synthesize their own asparagine. Asparaginase is an enzyme that deaminates asparagine to aspartic acid and ammonia in the plasma and extracellular fluid and therefore deprives tumor cells of the amino acid for protein synthesis.

Pharmacodynamics/Kinetics

Distribution: V_d: 4-5 L/kg; 70% to 80% of plasma volume; does not penetrate the CSF
Metabolism: Systemically degraded, only trace amounts are found in the urine
Half-life: 5.73 days
Elimination: Clearance unaffected by age, renal function, or hepatic function; L-asparaginase was measurable for at least 15 days following initial treatment with pegaspargase

Usual Dosage Refer to individual protocols; dose must be individualized based upon clinical response and tolerance of the patient

I.M. administration is **preferred** over I.V. administration; I.M. administration may decrease the incidence of hepatotoxicity, coagulopathy, and GI and renal disorders

Children: I.M., I.V.:
Body surface area <0.6 m^2: 82.5 IU/kg every 14 days
Body surface area ≥0.6 m^2: 2500 IU/m^2 every 14 days
Adults: I.M., I.V.: 2500 IU/m^2 every 14 days

Hemodialysis: Significant drug removal is unlikely based on physiochemical characteristics

(Continued)

Pegaspargase *(Continued)*

Peritoneal dialysis: Significant drug removal is unlikely based on physiochemical characteristics

Administration

I.M.: Must only be given as a deep intramuscular injection into a large muscle; limit the volume of a single injection site to 2 mL; if the volume to be administered is >2 mL, use multiple injection sites

I.V.: Administer over a period of 1-2 hours in 100 mL of 0.9% sodium chloride or dextrose 5% in water, through an infusion that is already running

Monitoring Parameters Vital signs during administration, CBC, urinalysis, amylase, liver enzymes, prothrombin time, renal function tests, urine dipstick for glucose, blood glucose

Patient Information

Inform patients of the possibility of hypersensitivity reactions, including immediate anaphylaxis

Instruct patients that the simultaneous use of pegaspargase with other drugs that may increase the risk of bleeding should be avoided

Patients should notify their physician of adverse reactions that occur

Nursing Implications Do not filter solution; appropriate agents for maintenance of an adequate airway and treatment of a hypersensitivity reaction (antihistamine, epinephrine, oxygen, I.V. corticosteroids) should be readily available. Be prepared to treat anaphylaxis at each administration; monitor for onset of abdominal pain and mental status changes.

Dosage Forms Injection, preservative free: 750 units/mL

PEG-L-asparaginase *see* Pegaspargase *on page 956*

Pemoline (PEM oh leen)

Brand Names Cylert®

Synonyms Phenylisohydantoin; PIO

Therapeutic Category Central Nervous System Stimulant, Nonamphetamine

Use Treatment of attention deficit disorder with hyperactivity (ADDH); narcolepsy

Restrictions C-IV

Pregnancy Risk Factor B

Contraindications Liver disease; hypersensitivity to pemoline or any component; children <6 years of age; Tourette's syndrome, psychoses

Warnings/Precautions Use with caution in patients with renal dysfunction, hypertension, or a history of abuse

Adverse Reactions

>10%:

Central nervous system: Insomnia

Gastrointestinal: Anorexia, weight loss

1% to 10%:

Central nervous system: Dizziness, drowsiness, mental depression

Dermatologic: Rash

Gastrointestinal: Stomach pain, nausea

<1%:

Central nervous system: Seizures, precipitation of Tourette's syndrome, hallucination, headache, movement disorders

Endocrine & metabolic: Growth reaction

Gastrointestinal: Diarrhea

Hepatic: Increased liver enzymes (usually reversible upon discontinuation), hepatitis, jaundice

Overdosage/Toxicology Symptoms of overdose include tachycardia, hallucinations, agitation

There is no specific antidote for intoxication and the bulk of the treatment is supportive. Hyperactivity and agitation usually respond to reduced sensory input or benzodiazepines, however, with extreme agitation haloperidol (2-5 mg I.M. for adults) may be required. Hyperthermia is best treated with external cooling measures, or when severe or unresponsive, muscle paralysis with pancuronium may be needed.

Drug Interactions

Decreased effect of insulin

Increased effect/toxicity with CNS depressants, CNS stimulants, sympathomimetics

Mechanism of Action Blocks the reuptake mechanism of dopaminergic neurons, appears to act at the cerebral cortex and subcortical structures; CNS and respiratory stimulant with weak sympathomimetic effects; actions may be mediated via increase in CNS dopamine

Pharmacodynamics/Kinetics

Peak effect: 4 hours

Duration: 8 hours

Protein binding: 50%
Metabolism: Partially by the liver
Half-life:
Children: 7-8.6 hours
Adults: 12 hours
Time to peak serum concentration: Oral: Within 2-4 hours
Elimination: In urine; only negligible amounts can be detected in feces

Usual Dosage Children ≥6 years: Oral: Initial: 37.5 mg given once daily in the morning, increase by 18.75 mg/day at weekly intervals; usual effective dose range: 56.25-75 mg/day; maximum: 112.5 mg/day; dosage range: 0.5-3 mg/kg/24 hours; significant benefit may not be evident until third or fourth week of administration

Dosing adjustment/comments in renal impairment: Cl_{cr} <50 mL/minute: Avoid use

Dietary Considerations Alcohol: Additive CNS effect, avoid use

Monitoring Parameters Liver enzymes

Patient Information Avoid caffeine; avoid alcoholic beverages; last daily dose should be given several hours before retiring; do not abruptly discontinue; prolonged use may cause dependence

Nursing Implications Administer medication in the morning

Dosage Forms
Tablet: 18.75 mg, 37.5 mg, 75 mg
Tablet, chewable: 37.5 mg

Penciclovir (pen SYE kloe veer)

Brand Names Denavir®

Therapeutic Category Antiviral Agent, Topical

Use Topical treatment of herpes simplex labialis (cold sores); potentially used for Epstein-Barr virus infections; investigations are ongoing for immunocompromised patients with herpes

Pregnancy Risk Factor B

Contraindications Previous and significant adverse reactions to famciclovir; hypersensitivity to the product or any of its components

Adverse Reactions >1%:
Central nervous system: Headache
Dermatologic: Mild erythema

Mechanism of Action Once phosphorylated in the virus-infected cells to penciclovir triphosphate, this drug competitively inhibits DNA polymerase with respect to the natural substrate deoxyguanosine triphosphate (dGTP) in HSV-1 and HSV-2 strains; this prevents viral replication by inhibition of viral DNA synthesis; some activity has been demonstrated against Epstein-Barr and varicella-zoster virus

Pharmacodynamics/Kinetics
Absorption: Minimally absorbed following topical use
Distribution: V_d: 1.5 L/kg
Protein binding: <20%
Metabolism: Phosphorylated in virus-infected cells by viral thymidine kinase to penciclovir monophosphate, then to penciclovir triphosphate, the active form
Half-life: 2 hours
Elimination: Rapidly excreted unchanged (70%) in urine; clearance: 28 L/hour

Usual Dosage Apply cream at the first sign or symptom of cold sore (eg, tingling, swelling); apply every 2 hours during waking hours for 4 days

Dietary Considerations Food: May decrease rate and extent of absorption although not clinically significant

Monitoring Parameters Reduction in virus shedding, negative cultures for herpes virus; resolution of pain and healing of cold sore lesion

Patient Information Inform your physician if you experience significant burning, itching, stinging, or redness when using this medication

Dosage Forms Cream: 1% [10 mg/g] (2 g)

Penecort® *see* Hydrocortisone *on page 623*
Penetrex™ *see* Enoxacin *on page 445*

Penicillamine (pen i SIL a meen)

Related Information
Antacid Drug Interactions *on page 1388*

Brand Names Cuprimine®; Depen®

Synonyms D-3-Mercaptovaline; β,β-Dimethylcysteine; D-Penicillamine

Therapeutic Category Antidote, Copper Toxicity; Antidote, Lead Toxicity; Chelating Agent, Oral

Use Treatment of Wilson's disease, cystinuria, adjunct in the treatment of rheumatoid arthritis; lead, mercury, copper, and possibly gold poisoning. (**Note:** Oral
(Continued)

Penicillamine *(Continued)*

DMSA is preferable for lead or mercury poisoning); primary biliary cirrhosis; as adjunctive therapy following initial treatment with calcium EDTA or BAL.

Pregnancy Risk Factor D

Contraindications Hypersensitivity to penicillamine or components; renal insufficiency; patients with previous penicillamine-related aplastic anemia or agranulocytosis; concomitant administration with other hematopoietic-depressant drugs (eg, gold, immunosuppressants, antimalarials, phenylbutazone)

Warnings/Precautions Cross-sensitivity with penicillin is possible; therefore, should be used cautiously in patients with a history of penicillin allergy. Patients on penicillamine for Wilson's disease or cystinuria should receive pyridoxine supplementation 25 mg/day; once instituted for Wilson's disease or cystinuria, continue treatment on a daily basis; interruptions of even a few days have been followed by hypersensitivity with reinstitution of therapy. Penicillamine has been associated with fatalities due to agranulocytosis, aplastic anemia, thrombocytopenia, Goodpasture's syndrome, and myasthenia gravis; patients should be warned to report promptly any symptoms suggesting toxicity; approximately 33% of patients will experience an allergic reaction; since toxicity may be dose related, it is recommended not to exceed 750 mg/day in elderly.

Adverse Reactions

>10%:
- Central nervous system: Fever
- Dermatologic: Rash, urticaria, itching
- Gastrointestinal: Hypogeusia
- Neuromuscular & skeletal: Arthralgia

1% to 10%:
- Cardiovascular: Edema of the face, feet, or lower legs
- Central nervous system: Fever, chills
- Gastrointestinal: Weight gain, sore throat
- Genitourinary: Bloody or cloudy urine
- Hematologic: Aplastic or hemolytic anemia, leukopenia, thrombocytopenia
- Miscellaneous: White spots on lips or mouth

<1%:
- Central nervous system: Fatigue
- Dermatologic: Toxic epidermal necrolysis, pemphigus, increased friability of the skin
- Endocrine & metabolic: Iron deficiency
- Gastrointestinal: Nausea, vomiting, anorexia, pancreatitis
- Hepatic: Cholestatic jaundice, hepatitis
- Neuromuscular & skeletal: Myasthenia gravis syndrome, weakness
- Ocular: Optic neuritis
- Otic: Tinnitus
- Renal: Nephrotic syndrome
- Respiratory: Coughing, wheezing
- Miscellaneous: SLE-like syndrome, spitting of blood allergic reactions, lymphadenopathy

Overdosage/Toxicology Symptoms of overdose include nausea and vomiting; following GI decontamination, treatment is supportive

Drug Interactions
- Decreased effect with iron and zinc salts, antacids (magnesium, calcium, aluminum) and food
- Decreased effect/levels of digoxin
- Increased effect of gold, antimalarials, immunosuppressants, phenylbutazone (hematologic, renal toxicity)

Stability Store in tight, well-closed containers

Mechanism of Action Chelates with lead, copper, mercury and other heavy metals to form stable, soluble complexes that are excreted in urine; depresses circulating IgM rheumatoid factor, depresses T-cell but not B-cell activity; combines with cystine to form a compound which is more soluble, thus cystine calculi are prevented

Pharmacodynamics/Kinetics
- Absorption: Oral: 40% to 70%
- Metabolism: Small amounts of hepatic metabolism
- Protein binding: 80% bound to albumin
- Half-life: 1.7-3.2 hours
- Time to peak serum concentration: Within 2 hours
- Elimination: Primarily (30% to 60%) in urine as unchanged drug

Usual Dosage Oral:

Rheumatoid arthritis:
- Children: Initial: 3 mg/kg/day (≤250 mg/day) for 3 months, then 6 mg/kg/day (≤500 mg/day) in divided doses twice daily for 3 months to a maximum of 10 mg/kg/day in 3-4 divided doses

Adults: 125-250 mg/day, may increase dose at 1- to 3-month intervals up to 1-1.5 g/day

Wilson's disease (doses titrated to maintain urinary copper excretion >1 mg/day):
Infants <6 months: 250 mg/dose once daily
Children <12 years: 250 mg/dose 2-3 times/day
Adults: 250 mg 4 times/day

Cystinuria:
Children: 30 mg/kg/day in 4 divided doses
Adults: 1-4 g/day in divided doses every 6 hours

Lead poisoning (continue until blood lead level is <60 μg/dL): Children and Adults: 25-35 mg/kg/d, administered in 3-4 divided doses; initiating treatment at 25% of this dose and gradually increasing to the full dose over 2-3 weeks may minimize adverse reactions

Primary biliary cirrhosis: 250 mg/day to start, increase by 250 mg every 2 weeks up to a maintenance dose of 1 g/day, usually given 250 mg 4 times/day

Arsenic poisoning: Children: 100 mg/kg/day in divided doses every 6 hours for 5 days; maximum: 1 g/day

Dosing adjustment/comments in renal impairment: Cl_{cr} <50 mL/minute: Avoid use

Administration Administer on an empty stomach (1 hour before meals and at bedtime)

Monitoring Parameters Urinalysis, CBC with differential, platelet count, liver function tests; weekly measurements of urinary and blood concentration of the intoxicating metal is indicated (3 months has been tolerated)

CBC: WBC <3500/mm³, neutrophils <2000/mm³ or monocytes >500/mm³ indicate need to stop therapy immediately; quantitative 24-hour urine protein at 1- to 2-week intervals initially (first 2-3 months); urinalysis, LFTs occasionally; platelet counts <100,000/mm³ indicate need to stop therapy until numbers of platelets increase

Test Interactions Positive ANA

Patient Information Take at least 1 hour before a meal on an empty stomach; patients with cystinuria should drink copious amounts of water; notify physician if unusual bleeding or bruising, or persistent fever, sore throat, or fatigue occurs; report any unexplained cough, shortness of breath, or rash; loss of taste may occur; do not skip or miss doses or discontinue without notifying physician

Nursing Implications For patients who cannot swallow, contents of capsules may be administered in 15-30 mL of chilled puréed fruit or fruit juice; patients should be warned to report promptly any symptoms suggesting toxicity

Dosage Forms
Capsule: 125 mg, 250 mg
Tablet: 250 mg

Extemporaneous Preparations A 50 mg/mL suspension may be made by mixing twenty 250 mg capsules with 1 g carboxymethylcellulose, 50 g sucrose, 100 mg citric acid, parabens, and purified water to a total volume of 100 mL; cherry flavor may be added. Stability is 30 days refrigerated.

Nahata MC and Hipple TF, *Pediatric Drug Formulations*, 1st ed, Cincinnati, OH: Harvey Whitney Books Co, 1990.

Penicillin G Benzathine (pen i SIL in jee BENZ a theen)

Related Information
Treatment of Sexually Transmitted Diseases *on page 1485*

Brand Names Bicillin® L-A; Permapen®

Canadian/Mexican Brand Names Megacillin® Susp (Canada); Benzetacil® (Mexico); Benzilfan® (Mexico)

Synonyms Benzathine Benzylpenicillin; Benzathine Penicillin G; Benzylpenicillin Benzathine

Therapeutic Category Antibiotic, Penicillin

Use Active against some gram-positive organisms, few gram-negative organisms such as *Neisseria gonorrhoeae*, and some anaerobes and spirochetes; used only for the treatment of mild to moderately severe infections caused by organisms susceptible to low concentrations of penicillin G or for prophylaxis of infections caused by these organisms; used when patient cannot be kept in a hospital environment and neurosyphilis has been ruled out

The CDC and AAP do not currently recommend the use of penicillin G benzathine to treat congenital syphilis or neurosyphilis due to reported treatment failures and lack of published clinical data on its efficacy

Pregnancy Risk Factor B

Contraindications Known hypersensitivity to penicillin or any component

Warnings/Precautions Use with caution in patients with impaired renal function, seizure disorder, or history of hypersensitivity to other beta-lactams; CDC and
(Continued)

Penicillin G Benzathine *(Continued)*

AAP do not currently recommend the use of penicillin G benzathine to treat congenital syphilis or neurosyphilis due to reported treatment failures and lack of published clinical data on its efficacy

Adverse Reactions

1% to 10%: Local: Local pain

<1%:

Central nervous system: Convulsions, confusion, drowsiness, fever
Dermatologic: Rash
Endocrine & metabolic: Electrolyte imbalance
Hematologic: Hemolytic anemia, positive Coombs' reaction
Local: Thrombophlebitis
Neuromuscular & skeletal: Myoclonus
Renal: Acute interstitial nephritis
Miscellaneous: Jarisch-Herxheimer reaction, hypersensitivity reactions, anaphylaxis

Overdosage/Toxicology Symptoms of penicillin overdose include neuromuscular hypersensitivity (agitation, hallucinations, asterixis, encephalopathy, confusion, and seizures) and electrolyte imbalance with potassium or sodium salts, especially in renal failure

Hemodialysis may be helpful to aid in the removal of the drug from the blood, otherwise most treatment is supportive or symptom directed

Drug Interactions

Decreased effect: Tetracyclines may decrease penicillin effectiveness
Increased effect:

Probenecid may increase penicillin levels
Aminoglycosides → synergistic efficacy

Stability Store in refrigerator

Mechanism of Action Interferes with bacterial cell wall synthesis during active multiplication, causing cell wall death and resultant bactericidal activity against susceptible bacteria

Pharmacodynamics/Kinetics

Absorption: I.M.: Slow
Time to peak serum concentration: Within 12-24 hours; serum levels are usually detectable for 1-4 weeks depending on the dose; larger doses result in more sustained levels rather than higher levels

Usual Dosage I.M.: Administer undiluted injection; higher doses result in more sustained rather than higher levels. Use a penicillin G benzathine-penicillin G procaine combination to achieve early peak levels in acute infections.

Infants and Children:

Group A streptococcal upper respiratory infection: 25,000-50,000 units/kg as a single dose; maximum: 1.2 million units
Prophylaxis of recurrent rheumatic fever: 25,000-50,000 units/kg every 3-4 weeks; maximum: 1.2 million units/dose
Early syphilis: 50,000 units/kg as a single injection; maximum: 2.4 million units
Syphilis of more than 1-year duration: 50,000 units/kg every week for 3 doses; maximum: 2.4 million units/dose

Adults:

Group A streptococcal upper respiratory infection: 1.2 million units as a single dose
Prophylaxis of recurrent rheumatic fever: 1.2 million units every 3-4 weeks or 600,000 units twice monthly
Early syphilis: 2.4 million units as a single dose in 2 injection sites
Syphilis of more than 1-year duration: 2.4 million units in 2 injection sites once weekly for 3 doses
Not indicated as single drug therapy for neurosyphilis, but may be given 1 time/week for 3 weeks following I.V. treatment (refer to Penicillin G monograph for dosing)

Administration Administer by deep I.M. injection in the upper outer quadrant of the buttock do **not** administer I.V., intra-arterially, or S.C.; in children <2 years of age, I.M. injections should be made into the midlateral muscle of the thigh, not the gluteal region; when doses are repeated, rotate the injection site

Test Interactions Positive Coombs' [direct], false-positive urinary and/or serum proteins; false-positive or negative urinary glucose using Clinitest®

Patient Information Report any rash

Dosage Forms Injection: 300,000 units/mL (10 mL); 600,000 units/mL (1 mL, 2 mL, 4 mL)

Penicillin G, Parenteral, Aqueous

(pen i SIL in jee, pa REN ter al, AYE kwee us)

Related Information

Antibiotic Treatment of Adults With Infectious Endocarditis *on page 1465*

Antimicrobial Drugs of Choice *on page 1468*
Antimicrobial Prophylaxis *on page 1445*
Bacterial Meningitis Practical Guidelines for Management *on page 1475*
Desensitization Protocols *on page 1496*
Treatment of Sexually Transmitted Diseases *on page 1485*

Brand Names Pfizerpen®

Canadian/Mexican Brand Names Benzanil® (Mexico); Lentopenil® (Mexico)

Synonyms Benzylpenicillin Potassium; Benzylpenicillin Sodium; Crystalline Penicillin; Penicillin G Potassium; Penicillin G Sodium

Therapeutic Category Antibiotic, Penicillin

Use Active against some gram-positive organisms, generally not *Staphylococcus aureus*; some gram-negative organisms such as *Neisseria gonorrhoeae*, and some anaerobes and spirochetes; although ceftriaxone is now the drug of choice for Lyme disease and gonorrhea

Pregnancy Risk Factor B

Contraindications Known hypersensitivity to penicillin or any component

Warnings/Precautions Avoid intravascular or intra-arterial administration or injection into or near major peripheral nerves or blood vessels since such injections may cause severe and/or permanent neurovascular damage; use with caution in patients with renal impairment (dosage reduction required), pre-existing seizure disorders, or with a history of hypersensitivity to cephalosporins

Adverse Reactions

<1%:

- Central nervous system: Convulsions, confusion, drowsiness, fever
- Dermatologic: Rash
- Endocrine & metabolic: Electrolyte imbalance
- Hematologic: Hemolytic anemia, positive Coombs' reaction
- Local: Thrombophlebitis
- Neuromuscular & skeletal: Myoclonus
- Renal: Acute interstitial nephritis
- Miscellaneous: Jarisch-Herxheimer reaction, hypersensitivity reactions, anaphylaxis

Overdosage/Toxicology Symptoms of penicillin overdose include neuromuscular hypersensitivity (agitation, hallucinations, asterixis, encephalopathy, confusion, and seizures) and electrolyte imbalance with potassium or sodium salts, especially in renal failure

Hemodialysis may be helpful to aid in the removal of the drug from the blood, otherwise most treatment is supportive or symptom directed

Drug Interactions

Decreased effect: Tetracyclines may decrease penicillin effectiveness

Increased effect:

- Probenecid may increase penicillin levels
- Aminoglycosides → synergistic efficacy

Stability

Penicillin G potassium is stable at room temperature

Reconstituted parenteral solution is stable for 7 days when refrigerated (2°C to 15°C)

Penicillin G potassium for I.V. infusion in NS or D_5W, solution is stable for 24 hours at room temperature

Incompatible with aminoglycosides; inactivated in acidic or alkaline solutions

Mechanism of Action Interferes with bacterial cell wall synthesis during active multiplication, causing cell wall death and resultant bactericidal activity against susceptible bacteria

Pharmacodynamics/Kinetics

Time to peak serum concentration:

- I.M.: Within 30 minutes
- I.V. Within 1 hour

Distribution: Crosses the placenta; appears in breast milk; penetration across the blood-brain barrier is poor, despite inflamed meninges

- Relative diffusion of antimicrobial agents from blood into cerebrospinal fluid (CSF): Good only with inflammation (exceeds usual MICs)
- Ratio of CSF to blood level (%):
  - Normal meninges: <1
  - Inflamed meninges: 3-5

Protein binding: 65%

Metabolism: In the liver (30%) to penicilloic acid

Half-life:

- Neonates:
  - <6 days: 3.2-3.4 hours
  - 7-13 days: 1.2-2.2 hours
  - >14 days: 0.9-1.9 hours
- Children and adults with normal renal function: 20-50 minutes

(Continued)

Penicillin G, Parenteral, Aqueous *(Continued)*

End stage renal disease: 3.3-5.1 hours
Elimination: In urine

Usual Dosage I.M., I.V.:

Infants and Children (sodium salt is preferred in children): 100,000-250,000 units/kg/day in divided doses every 4 hours; maximum: 4.8 million units/24 hours

Severe infections: Up to 400,000 units/kg/day in divided doses every 4 hours; maximum dose: 24 million units/day

Adults: 2-24 million units/day in divided doses every 4 hours

Congenital syphilis:

Newborns: 50,000 units/kg/day I.V. every 8-12 hours for 10-14 days
Infants: 50,000 units/kg every 4-6 hours for 10-14 days

Disseminated gonococcal infections or gonococcus ophthalmia (if organism proven sensitive): 100,000 units/kg/day in 2 equal doses (4 equal doses/day for infants >1 week)

Gonococcal meningitis: 150,000 units/kg in 2 equal doses (4 doses/day for infants >1 week)

Dosing interval in renal impairment:

Cl_{cr} 30-50 mL/minute: Administer every 6 hours
Cl_{cr} 10-30 mL/minute: Administer every 8 hours
Cl_{cr} <10 mL/minute: Administer every 12 hours

Hemodialysis: Moderately dialyzable (20% to 50%)

Administration Administer I.M. by deep injection in the upper outer quadrant of the buttock; administer injection around-the-clock to promote less variation in peak and trough levels; while I.M. route is preferred route of administration, large doses should be administered by continuous I.V. infusion; determine volume and rate of fluid administration required in a 24-hour period; add appropriate daily dosage to this fluid

Test Interactions False-positive or negative urinary glucose determination using Clinitest®; positive Coombs' [direct]; false-positive urinary and/or serum proteins

Patient Information Report any rash or shortness of breath

Nursing Implications Dosage modification required in patients with renal insufficiency

Additional Information

Penicillin G potassium: 1.7 mEq of potassium and 0.3 mEq of sodium per 1 million units of penicillin G

Penicillin G sodium: 2 mEq of sodium per 1 million units of penicillin G

Dosage Forms

Injection, as sodium: 5 million units
Injection:

Frozen premixed, as potassium: 1 million units, 2 million units, 3 million units
Powder, as potassium: 1 million units, 5 million units, 10 million units, 20 million units

Penicillin G Potassium *see* Penicillin G, Parenteral, Aqueous *on page 962*

Penicillin G Procaine (pen i SIL in jee PROE kane)

Related Information

Treatment of Sexually Transmitted Diseases *on page 1485*

Brand Names Crysticillin® A.S.; Pfizerpen®-AS; Wycillin®

Canadian/Mexican Brand Names Ayercillin® (Canada); Penicil® (Mexico); Penipot® (Mexico); Penprocilina® (Mexico)

Synonyms APPG; Aqueous Procaine Penicillin G; Procaine Benzylpenicillin; Procaine Penicillin G

Therapeutic Category Antibiotic, Penicillin

Use Moderately severe infections due to *Neisseria gonorrhoeae*, *Treponema pallidum* and other penicillin G-sensitive microorganisms that are susceptible to low but prolonged serum penicillin concentrations

Pregnancy Risk Factor B

Contraindications Known hypersensitivity to penicillin or any component; also contraindicated in patients hypersensitive to procaine

Warnings/Precautions May need to modify dosage in patients with severe renal impairment, seizure disorders, or history of hypersensitivity to cephalosporins; avoid I.V., intravascular, or intra-arterial administration of penicillin G procaine since severe and/or permanent neurovascular damage may occur

Adverse Reactions

>10%: Local: Pain at injection site

<1%:

Cardiovascular: Myocardial depression, vasodilation, conduction disturbances
Central nervous system: CNS stimulation, seizures, confusion, drowsiness
Hematologic: Hemolytic anemia, positive Coombs' reaction

Local: Sterile abscess at injection site
Neuromuscular & skeletal: Myoclonus
Renal: Interstitial nephritis
Miscellaneous: Pseudoanaphylactic reactions, Jarisch-Herxheimer reaction, hypersensitivity reactions

Overdosage/Toxicology Symptoms of penicillin overdose include neuromuscular hypersensitivity (agitation, hallucinations, asterixis, encephalopathy, confusion, and seizures) and electrolyte imbalance with potassium or sodium salts, especially in renal failure

Hemodialysis may be helpful to aid in the removal of the drug from the blood, otherwise most treatment is supportive or symptom directed

Drug Interactions
Decreased effect: Tetracyclines may decrease penicillin effectiveness
Increased effect:
Probenecid may increase penicillin levels
Aminoglycosides → synergistic efficacy

Stability Store in refrigerator

Mechanism of Action Inhibits bacterial cell wall synthesis by binding to one or more of the penicillin binding proteins (PBPs); which in turn inhibits the final transpeptidation step of peptidoglycan synthesis in bacterial cell walls, thus inhibiting cell wall biosynthesis. Bacteria eventually lyse due to ongoing activity of cell wall autolytic enzymes (autolysins and murein hydrolases) while cell wall assembly is arrested.

Pharmacodynamics/Kinetics
Absorption: I.M.: Slowly absorbed
Distribution: Penetration across the blood-brain barrier is poor, despite inflamed meninges; appears in breast milk
Protein binding: 65%
Metabolism: ~30% of a dose is inactivated in the liver
Time to peak serum concentration: Within 1-4 hours; can persist within the therapeutic range for 15-24 hours
Elimination: Renal clearance is delayed in neonates, young infants, and patients with impaired renal function; 60% to 90% of the drug is excreted unchanged via renal tubular excretion

Usual Dosage I.M.:
Children: 25,000-50,000 units/kg/day in divided doses 1-2 times/day; not to exceed 4.8 million units/24 hours
Gonorrhea: 100,000 units/kg (maximum 4.8 million units) one time (in 2 injection sites) along with probenecid 25 mg/kg (maximum: 1 g orally) 30 minutes prior to procaine penicillin
Congenital syphilis: 50,000 units/kg/day for 10-14 days
Adults: 0.6-4.8 million units/day in divided doses every 12-24 hours
Uncomplicated gonorrhea: 1 g probenecid orally, then 4.8 million units procaine penicillin divided into 2 injection sites 30 minutes later
Endocarditis caused by susceptible viridans *Streptococcus* (when used in conjunction with an aminoglycoside): 1.2 million units every 6 hours for 2-4 weeks
Neurosyphilis: I.M.: 2-4 million units/day with 500 mg probenecid by mouth 4 times/day for 10-14 days; **penicillin G aqueous I.V. is the preferred agent**

Hemodialysis: Moderately dialyzable (20% to 50%)

Administration Procaine suspension for deep I.M. injection only; rotate the injection site

Monitoring Parameters Periodic renal and hematologic function tests with prolonged therapy; fever, mental status, WBC count

Test Interactions Positive Coombs' [direct], false-positive urinary and/or serum proteins

Patient Information Notify physician if skin rash, itching, hives, or severe diarrhea occurs

Nursing Implications Renal and hematologic systems should be evaluated periodically during prolonged therapy; do not inject in gluteal muscle in children <2 years of age

Dosage Forms Injection, suspension: 300,000 units/mL (10 mL); 500,000 units/mL (1.2 mL); 600,000 units/mL (1 mL, 2 mL, 4 mL)

Penicillin G Sodium *see* Penicillin G, Parenteral, Aqueous *on page 962*

Penicillin V Potassium (pen i SIL in vee poe TASS ee um)

Related Information
Animal and Human Bites Guidelines *on page 1463*
Antimicrobial Drugs of Choice *on page 1468*
Desensitization Protocols *on page 1496*

Brand Names Beepen-VK®; Betapen® VK; Ledercillin® VK; Pen Vee® K; Robicillin® VK; V-Cillin K®; Veetids®
(Continued)

Penicillin V Potassium *(Continued)*

Canadian/Mexican Brand Names Apo-Pen® VK (Canada); Nadopen-V® (Canada); Novo-Pen-VK® (Canada); Nu-Pen-VK® (Canada); PVF® K (Canada); Anapenil® (Mexico); Pen-Vi-K® (Mexico); Pen-Vee® (Canada)

Synonyms Pen VK; Phenoxymethyl Penicillin

Therapeutic Category Antibiotic, Penicillin

Use Treatment of moderate to severe susceptible bacterial infections; no longer recommended for dental procedure prophylaxis; prophylaxis in rheumatic fever; infections caused by susceptible organisms involving the respiratory tract, otitis media, sinusitis, skin, and urinary tract

Pregnancy Risk Factor B

Contraindications Known hypersensitivity to penicillin or any component

Warnings/Precautions Use with caution in patients with severe renal impairment (modify dosage), history of seizures, or hypersensitivity to cephalosporins

Adverse Reactions

>10%: Gastrointestinal: Mild diarrhea, vomiting, nausea, oral candidiasis

<1%:

Central nervous system: Convulsions, fever
Hematologic: Hemolytic anemia, positive Coombs' reaction
Renal: Acute interstitial nephritis
Miscellaneous: Hypersensitivity reactions, anaphylaxis

Overdosage/Toxicology Symptoms of penicillin overdose include neuromuscular hypersensitivity (agitation, hallucinations, asterixis, encephalopathy, confusion, and seizures) and electrolyte imbalance with potassium or sodium salts, especially in renal failure

Hemodialysis may be helpful to aid in the removal of the drug from the blood, otherwise most treatment is supportive or symptom directed

Drug Interactions

Decreased effect: Tetracyclines may decrease penicillin effectiveness; oral contraceptives

Increased effect:

Probenecid may increase penicillin levels
Aminoglycosides → synergistic efficacy

Stability Refrigerate suspension after reconstitution; discard after 14 days

Mechanism of Action Inhibits bacterial cell wall synthesis by binding to one or more of the penicillin binding proteins (PBPs); which in turn inhibits the final transpeptidation step of peptidoglycan synthesis in bacterial cell walls, thus inhibiting cell wall biosynthesis. Bacteria eventually lyse due to ongoing activity of cell wall autolytic enzymes (autolysins and murein hydrolases) while cell wall assembly is arrested.

Pharmacodynamics/Kinetics

Absorption: Oral: 60% to 73% from GI tract
Distribution: Appears in breast milk
Plasma protein binding: 80%
Half-life: 0.5 hours; prolonged in patients with renal impairment
Time to peak serum concentration: Oral: Within 0.5-1 hour
Elimination: Penicillin V and its metabolites are excreted in urine mainly by tubular secretion

Usual Dosage Oral:

Systemic infections:

Children <12 years: 25-50 mg/kg/day in divided doses every 6-8 hours; maximum dose: 3 g/day
Children ≥12 years and Adults: 125-500 mg every 6-8 hours

Prophylaxis of pneumococcal infections:

Children <5 years: 125 mg twice daily
Children ≥5 years and Adults: 250 mg twice daily

Prophylaxis of recurrent rheumatic fever:

Children <5 years: 125 mg twice daily
Children ≥5 years and Adults: 250 mg twice daily

Dosing interval in renal impairment:

Cl_{cr} 10-50 mL/minute: Administer every 8-12 hours
Cl_{cr} <10 mL/minute: Administer every 12-16 hours

Dietary Considerations Food: Decreases drug absorption rate; decreases drug serum concentration. Take on an empty stomach 1 hour before or 2 hours after meals.

Administration Administer around-the-clock rather than 4 times/day to promote less variation in peak and trough serum levels; administer on an empty stomach to increase oral absorption

Monitoring Parameters Periodic renal and hematologic function tests during prolonged therapy

Test Interactions False-positive or negative urinary glucose determination using Clinitest®; positive Coombs' [direct]; false-positive urinary and/or serum proteins

Patient Information Take on an empty stomach 1 hour before or 2 hours after meals, take until gone, do not skip doses, report any rash or shortness of breath; shake liquid well before use

Additional Information 0.7 mEq of potassium per 250 mg penicillin V; 250 mg equals 400,000 units of penicillin; in Canada a oral suspension is available as a benzathine salt in the strength of 180 mg/5 mL [300,000 units/5 mL] and 300 mg/5 mL [500,000 units/5 mL]; a Canadian tablet is available in 300 mg [500,000 units]

Dosage Forms

Powder for oral solution: 125 mg/5 mL (3 mL, 100 mL, 150 mL, 200 mL); 250 mg/5 mL (100 mL, 150 mL, 200 mL)

Tablet: 125 mg, 250 mg, 500 mg

Penicilloyl-polylysine *see* Benzylpenicilloyl-polylysine *on page 143*

Pentacarinat® Injection *see* Pentamidine *on next page*

Pentaerythritol Tetranitrate (pen ta er ITH ri tole te tra NYE trate)

Brand Names Duotrate®; Peritrate®; Peritrate® SA

Synonyms PETN

Therapeutic Category Antianginal Agent; Nitrate; Vasodilator, Coronary

Use Possibly effective for the prophylactic long-term management of angina pectoris. **Note:** Not indicated to abort acute anginal episodes.

Pregnancy Risk Factor C

Contraindications Known hypersensitivity to pentaerythritol tetranitrate or other nitrates; severe anemia, closed-angle glaucoma, postural hypotension, cerebral hemorrhage, head trauma

Warnings/Precautions Use with caution in patients with hypotension, hypovolemia, or increased intracranial pressure

Adverse Reactions

>10%:

Cardiovascular: Flushing, postural hypotension

Central nervous system: Headache, lightheadedness, dizziness

Neuromuscular & skeletal: Weakness

1% to 10%: Dermatologic: Drug rash, exfoliative dermatitis

<1%:

Gastrointestinal: Nausea, vomiting,

Hematologic: Methemoglobinemia (overdose)

Overdosage/Toxicology Symptoms of overdose include hypotension, throbbing headache, palpitations, bloody diarrhea, bradycardia, cyanosis, tissue hypoxia, metabolic acidosis, clonic convulsions, circulatory collapse. Formation of methemoglobinemia is dose-related and unusual in normal or moderate overdoses.

Treatment is supportive and symptomatic; hypotension is treated with fluids, positioning and alpha-adrenergic pressors if needed; treat methemoglobinemia with oxygen and methylene blue at a dose of 1-2 mg/kg I.V. slowly.

Mechanism of Action Stimulation of intracellular cyclic-GMP results in vascular smooth muscle relaxation of both arterial and venous vasculature. Increased venous pooling decreases left ventricular pressure (preload) and arterial dilatation decreases arterial resistance (afterload). Therefore, this reduces cardiac oxygen demand by decreasing left ventricular pressure and systemic vascular resistance by dilating arteries. Additionally, coronary artery dilation improves collateral flow to ischemic regions; esophageal smooth muscle is relaxed via the same mechanism.

Pharmacodynamics/Kinetics

Onset of hemodynamic effect: Oral: Within 20-60 minutes

Duration: 4-5 hours, or up to 12 hours with the sustained release formulations

Metabolism: In the liver

Half-life: 10 minutes

Elimination: In urine and to a smaller degree in bile

Usual Dosage Adults: Oral: 10-20 mg 4 times/day up to 40 mg 4 times/day before or after meals and at bedtime; sustained release preparation 80 mg twice daily; use lowest recommended doses in elderly initially; titrations up to 240 mg/day are tolerated, however, headache may occur with increasing doses (reduce dose for a few days; if headache returns or is persistent, an analgesic can be used to treat symptoms)

Patient Information Keep tablets in original tightly closed container; do not chew or crush sustained release product; do not change brands without consulting your pharmacist or physician; any angina that persists for more than 20 minutes should be evaluated by a physician immediately

Dosage Forms

Capsule: sustained release: 15 mg, 30 mg

Tablet: 10 mg, 20 mg, 40 mg

(Continued)

Pentaerythritol Tetranitrate *(Continued)*

Tablet, sustained release: 80 mg

Pentam-300® Injection *see* Pentamidine *on this page*

Pentamidine (pen TAM i deen)

Related Information

Guidelines for the Prevention of Opportunistic Infections in Persons with HIV *on page 1457*

Brand Names NebuPent™ Inhalation; Pentacarinat® Injection; Pentam-300® Injection

Canadian/Mexican Brand Names Pentacarinat® (Mexico)

Synonyms Pentamidine Isethionate

Therapeutic Category Antibiotic, Miscellaneous

Use Treatment and prevention of pneumonia caused by *Pneumocystis carinii*; treatment of trypanosomiasis

Pregnancy Risk Factor C

Contraindications Hypersensitivity to pentamidine isethionate or any component (inhalation and injection)

Warnings/Precautions Use with caution in patients with diabetes mellitus, renal or hepatic dysfunction; hypertension or hypotension; leukopenia, thrombocytopenia, asthma, hypo/hypoglycemia

Adverse Reactions

>10%:
- Cardiovascular: Chest pain
- Dermatologic: Rash
- Endocrine & metabolic: Hyperkalemia
- Local: Local reactions at injection site
- Respiratory: Wheezing, dyspnea, coughing, pharyngitis

1% to 10%: Gastrointestinal: Bitter or metallic taste

<1%:
- Cardiovascular: Hypotension, tachycardia
- Central nervous system: Dizziness, fever, fatigue
- Endocrine & metabolic: Hyperglycemia or hypoglycemia, hypocalcemia
- Gastrointestinal: Pancreatitis, vomiting
- Hematologic: Megaloblastic anemia, granulocytopenia, leukopenia, thrombocytopenia
- Renal: Renal insufficiency
- Respiratory: Extrapulmonary pneumocystosis, irritation of the airway
- Miscellaneous: Pneumothorax, Jarisch-Herxheimer-like reaction, mild renal or hepatic injury

Overdosage/Toxicology Symptoms of overdose include hypotension, hypoglycemia, cardiac arrhythmias; treatment is supportive

Stability Do not refrigerate due to the possibility of crystallization; do not use NS as a diluent, NS is **incompatible** with pentamidine; reconstituted solutions (60-100 mg/mL) are stable for 48 hours at room temperature and do not require light protection; diluted solutions (1-2.5 mg/mL) in D_5W are stable for at least 24 hours at room temperature

Mechanism of Action Interferes with RNA/DNA, phospholipids and protein synthesis, through inhibition of oxidative phosphorylation and/or interference with incorporation of nucleotides and nucleic acids into RNA and DNA, in protozoa

Pharmacodynamics/Kinetics

Absorption: I.M.: Well absorbed

Distribution: Systemic accumulation of pentamidine does not appear to occur following inhalation therapy

Half-life, terminal: 6.4-9.4 hours; may be prolonged in patients with severe renal impairment

Elimination: 33% to 66% excreted in urine as unchanged drug

Usual Dosage

Children:
- Treatment: I.M., I.V. (I.V. preferred): 4 mg/kg/day once daily for 10-14 days
- Prevention:
  - I.M., I.V.: 4 mg/kg monthly or every 2 weeks
  - Inhalation (aerosolized pentamidine in children ≥5 years): 300 mg/dose given every 3-4 weeks via Respirgard® II inhaler (8 mg/kg dose has also been used in children <5 years)
- Treatment of trypanosomiasis: I.V.: 4 mg/kg/day once daily for 10 days

Adults:
- Treatment: I.M., I.V. (I.V. preferred): 4 mg/kg/day once daily for 14 days
- Prevention: Inhalation: 300 mg every 4 weeks via Respirgard® II nebulizer

Dialysis: Not removed by hemo or peritoneal dialysis or continuous arterio-venous or veno-venous hemofiltration (CAVH/CAVHD); supplemental dosage is not necessary

Administration Infuse I.V. slowly over a period of at least 60 minutes or administer deep I.M.; patients receiving I.V. or I.M. pentamidine should be lying down and blood pressure should be monitored closely during administration of drug and several times thereafter until it is stable

Monitoring Parameters Liver function tests, renal function tests, blood glucose, serum potassium and calcium, EKG, blood pressure

Patient Information PCP pneumonia may still occur despite pentamidine use; notify physician of fever, shortness of breath, or coughing up blood; maintain adequate fluid intake

Nursing Implications Virtually indetectable amounts are transferred to health-care personnel during aerosol administration; **do not use NS as a diluent**

Dosage Forms

Inhalation, as isethionate: 300 mg

Powder for injection, as isethionate, lyophilized: 300 mg

Pentamidine Isethionate *see* Pentamidine *on previous page*

Pentasa® *see* Mesalamine *on page 787*

Pentazocine (pen TAZ oh seen)

Related Information

Drugs and Routes of Administration Not Recommended for Treatment of Cancer Pain *on page 1378*

Narcotic Agonists Comparison *on page 1414*

Brand Names Talwin®; Talwin® NX

Synonyms Pentazocine Hydrochloride; Pentazocine Lactate

Therapeutic Category Analgesic, Narcotic; Sedative

Use Relief of moderate to severe pain; has also been used as a sedative prior to surgery and as a supplement to surgical anesthesia

Restrictions C-IV

Pregnancy Risk Factor B (D if used for prolonged periods or in high doses at term)

Contraindications Hypersensitivity to pentazocine or any component, increased intracranial pressure (unless the patient is mechanically ventilated)

Warnings/Precautions Use with caution in seizure-prone patients, acute myocardial infarction, patients undergoing biliary tract surgery, patients with renal and hepatic dysfunction, head trauma, increased intracranial pressure, and patients with a history of prior opioid dependence or abuse; pentazocine may precipitate opiate withdrawal symptoms in patients who have been receiving opiates regularly; injection contains sulfites which may cause allergic reaction

Adverse Reactions

>10%:

- Central nervous system: Euphoria, drowsiness
- Gastrointestinal: Nausea, vomiting
- Neuromuscular & skeletal: Weakness

1% to 10%:

- Cardiovascular: Hypotension
- Central nervous system: Malaise, headache, restlessness, nightmares
- Dermatologic: Rash
- Gastrointestinal: Xerostomia
- Genitourinary: Ureteral spasm
- Ocular: Blurred vision
- Respiratory: Dyspnea

<1%:

- Central nervous system: Insomnia, CNS depression, sedation, hallucinations, confusion, disorientation, seizures may occur in seizure-prone patients, increased intracranial pressure
- Cardiovascular: Palpitations, bradycardia, peripheral vasodilation
- Dermatologic: Pruritus
- Endocrine & metabolic: Antidiuretic hormone release
- Gastrointestinal: GI irritation, constipation, biliary tract spasm
- Genitourinary: Urinary tract spasm
- Local: Tissue damage and irritation with I.M./S.C. use
- Ocular: Miosis
- Miscellaneous: Histamine release, physical and psychological dependence

Overdosage/Toxicology Symptoms of overdose include drowsiness, sedation, respiratory depression, coma

Naloxone 2 mg I.V. (0.01 mg/kg for children) with repeat administration as necessary up to a total of 10 mg

(Continued)

Pentazocine *(Continued)*

Drug Interactions May potentiate or reduce analgesic effect of opiate agonist, (eg, morphine) depending on patients tolerance to opiates can precipitate withdrawal in narcotic addicts

Increased effect/toxicity with tripelennamine (can be lethal), CNS depressants (phenothiazines, tranquilizers, anxiolytics, sedatives, hypnotics, or alcohol)

Stability Store at room temperature, protect from heat and from freezing; I.V. form is **incompatible** with aminophylline, amobarbital (and all other I.V. barbiturates), glycopyrrolate (same syringe), heparin (same syringe), nafcillin (Y-site)

Mechanism of Action Binds to opiate receptors in the CNS, causing inhibition of ascending pain pathways, altering the perception of and response to pain; produces generalized CNS depression; partial agonist-antagonist

Pharmacodynamics/Kinetics

Onset of action:

- Oral, I.M., S.C.: Within 15-30 minutes
- I.V.: Within 2-3 minutes

Duration:

- Oral: 4-5 hours
- Parenteral: 2-3 hours

Protein binding: 60%

Metabolism: Large first-pass effect; metabolized in liver via oxidative and glucuronide conjugation pathways

Bioavailability, oral: ~20%; increased to 60% to 70% in patients with cirrhosis

Half-life: 2-3 hours; increased with decreased hepatic function

Elimination: Smaller amounts excreted unchanged in urine

Usual Dosage

Children: I.M., S.C.:

- 5-8 years: 15 mg
- 8-14 years: 30 mg

Children >12 years and Adults: Oral: 50 mg every 3-4 hours; may increase to 100 mg/dose if needed, but should not exceed 600 mg/day

Adults:

- I.M., S.C.: 30-60 mg every 3-4 hours, not to exceed total daily dose of 360 mg
- I.V.: 30 mg every 3-4 hours

Dosing adjustment in renal impairment:

- Cl_{cr} 10-50 mL/minute: Administer 75% of normal dose
- Cl_{cr} <10 mL/minute: Administer 50% of normal dose

Dosing adjustment in hepatic impairment: Reduce dose or avoid use in patients with liver disease

Dietary Considerations Alcohol: Additive CNS effect, avoid use

Administration Rotate injection site for I.M., S.C. use; avoid intra-arterial injection

Monitoring Parameters Relief of pain, respiratory and mental status, blood pressure

Patient Information Avoid alcohol, may cause drowsiness, impaired judgment or coordination; may cause physical and psychological dependence with prolonged use; will cause withdrawal in patients currently dependent on narcotics

Nursing Implications Observe patient for excessive sedation, respiratory depression, implement safety measures, assist with ambulation; observe for narcotic withdrawal

Additional Information Pentazocine hydrochloride: Talwin® NX tablet (with naloxone); naloxone is used to prevent abuse by dissolving tablets in water and using as injection

Dosage Forms

Injection, as lactate: 30 mg/mL (1 mL, 1.5 mL, 2 mL, 10 mL)

Tablet: Pentazocine hydrochloride 50 mg and naloxone hydrochloride 0.5 mg

Pentazocine Hydrochloride *see* Pentazocine *on previous page*

Pentazocine Lactate *see* Pentazocine *on previous page*

Pentobarbital (pen toe BAR bi tal)

Brand Names Nembutal®

Canadian/Mexican Brand Names Nova Rectal®

Synonyms Pentobarbital Sodium

Therapeutic Category Anticonvulsant; Barbiturate; Sedative

Use Short-term treatment of insomnia; preoperative sedation; high-dose barbiturate coma for treatment of increased intracranial pressure or status epilepticus unresponsive to other therapy

Restrictions C-II (capsules, injection); C-III (suppositories)

Pregnancy Risk Factor D

Contraindications Marked liver function impairment or latent porphyria; hypersensitivity to barbiturates or any component

Warnings/Precautions Tolerance to hypnotic effect can occur; do not use for >2 weeks to treat insomnia; taper dose to prevent withdrawal; loading doses of 15-35 mg/kg (given over 1-2 hours) have been utilized in pediatric patients to induce pentobarbital coma, but these higher loading doses often cause hypotension requiring vasopressor therapy. Use of this agent as a hypnotic in the elderly is not recommended due to its long half-life and potential for physical and psychological dependence. Use with caution in patients with hypovolemic shock, congestive heart failure, hepatic impairment, respiratory dysfunction or depression, previous addiction to the sedative/hypnotic group, chronic or acute pain, renal dysfunction; tolerance or psychological and physical dependence may occur with prolonged use.

Adverse Reactions

Renal: Oliguria

>10%:

- Cardiovascular: Cardiac arrhythmias, bradycardia, hypotension, arterial spasm,
- Central nervous system: Drowsiness, lethargy, CNS excitation or depression, impaired judgment, "hangover" effect
- Local: Pain at injection site, thrombophlebitis with I.V. use
- Miscellaneous: Gangrene with inadvertent intra-arterial injection

1% to 10%:

- Central nervous system: Confusion, mental depression, unusual excitement, nervousness, faint feeling, headache, insomnia, nightmares
- Gastrointestinal: Nausea, vomiting, constipation

<1%:

- Cardiovascular: Hypotension
- Central nervous system: Hallucinations, hypothermia
- Dermatologic: Rash, exfoliative dermatitis, Stevens-Johnson syndrome
- Hematologic: Agranulocytosis, thrombocytopenia, megaloblastic anemia
- Local: Thrombophlebitis
- Respiratory: Laryngospasm, respiratory depression, apnea (especially with rapid I.V. use)

Overdosage/Toxicology Symptoms of overdose include unsteady gait, slurred speech, confusion, jaundice, hypothermia, hypotension, respiratory depression, coma

If hypotension occurs, administer I.V. fluids and place the patient in the Trendelenburg position. If unresponsive, an I.V. vasopressor (eg, dopamine, epinephrine) may be required. Forced alkaline diuresis is of no value in the treatment of intoxications with short-acting barbiturates. Charcoal hemoperfusion or hemodialysis may be useful in the harder to treat intoxications, especially in the presence of very high serum barbiturate levels when the patient is in a coma, shock, or renal failure.

Drug Interactions

Decreased effect: Decreased chloramphenicol; decreased doxycycline effects

Increased toxicity: Increased CNS depressants, cimetidine; → ↑ pentobarbital

Stability Protect from light; aqueous solutions are not stable, commercially available vehicle (containing propylene glycol) is more stable; low pH may cause precipitate; use only clear solution

Mechanism of Action Short-acting barbiturate with sedative, hypnotic, and anticonvulsant properties

Pharmacodynamics/Kinetics

Onset of action:

- Oral, rectal: 15-60 minutes
- I.M.: Within 10-15 minutes
- I.V.: Within 1 minute

Duration:

- Oral, rectal: 1-4 hours
- I.V.: 15 minutes

Distribution: V_d:

- Children: 0.8 L/kg
- Adults: 1 L/kg

Protein binding: 35% to 55%

Metabolism: Extensively in liver via hydroxylation and oxidation pathways

Half-life, terminal:

- Children: 25 hours
- Adults, normal: 22 hours; range: 35-50 hours

Elimination: <1% excreted unchanged renally

Usual Dosage

Children:

- Sedative: Oral: 2-6 mg/kg/day divided in 3 doses; maximum: 100 mg/day
- Hypnotic: I.M.: 2-6 mg/kg; maximum: 100 mg/dose

(Continued)

Pentobarbital *(Continued)*

Rectal:
- 2 months to 1 year (10-20 lb): 30 mg
- 1-4 years (20-40 lb): 30-60 mg
- 5-12 years (40-80 lb): 60 mg
- 12-14 years (80-110 lb): 60-120 mg

or
- <4 years: 3-6 mg/kg/dose
- >4 years: 1.5-3 mg/kg/dose

Preoperative/preprocedure sedation: ≥6 months:
- Oral, I.M., rectal: 2-6 mg/kg; maximum: 100 mg/dose
- I.V.: 1-3 mg/kg to a maximum of 100 mg until asleep

Children 5-12 years: Conscious sedation prior to a procedure: I.V.: 2 mg/kg 5-10 minutes before procedures, may repeat one time

Adolescents: Conscious sedation: Oral, I.V.: 100 mg prior to a procedure

Adults:

Hypnotic:
- Oral: 100-200 mg at bedtime or 20 mg 3-4 times/day for daytime sedation
- I.M.: 150-200 mg
- I.V.: Initial: 100 mg, may repeat every 1-3 minutes up to 200-500 mg total dose

Rectal: 120-200 mg at bedtime

Preoperative sedation: I.M.: 150-200 mg

Children and Adults: Barbiturate coma in head injury patients: I.V.: Loading dose: 5-10 mg/kg given slowly over 1-2 hours; monitor blood pressure and respiratory rate; Maintenance infusion: Initial: 1 mg/kg/hour; may increase to 2-3 mg/kg/hour; maintain burst suppression on EEG

Dosing adjustment in hepatic impairment: Reduce dosage in patients with severe liver dysfunction

Dietary Considerations Alcohol: Additive CNS effect, avoid use

Administration Pentobarbital may be administered by deep I.M. or slow I.V. injection. I.M.: No more than 5 mL (250 mg) should be injected at any one site because of possible tissue irritation I.V. push doses can be given undiluted, but should be administered no faster than 50 mg/minute; parenteral solutions are highly alkaline; avoid extravasation; avoid rapid I.V. administration >50 mg/minute; avoid intra-arterial injection

Monitoring Parameters Respiratory status (for conscious sedation, includes pulse oximetry), cardiovascular status, CNS status; cardiac monitor and blood pressure monitor required

Reference Range

Therapeutic:
- Hypnotic: 1-5 μg/mL (SI: 4-22 μmol/L)
- Coma: 10-50 μg/mL (SI: 88-221 μmol/L)

Toxic: >10 μg/mL (SI: >44 μmol/L)

Test Interactions ↑ ammonia (B); ↓ bilirubin (S)

Patient Information Avoid the use of alcohol and other CNS depressants; avoid driving and other hazardous tasks; avoid abrupt discontinuation; may cause physical and psychological dependence; do not alter dose without notifying physician

Nursing Implications Avoid extravasation; institute safety measures to avoid injuries; has many incompatibilities when given I.V.

Additional Information Pentobarbital: Nembutal® elixir pentobarbital sodium: Nembutal® capsule, injection, and suppository

Sodium content of 1 mL injection: 5 mg (0.2 mEq)

Dosage Forms
- Capsule, as sodium (C-II): 50 mg, 100 mg
- Elixir (C-II): 18.2 mg/5 mL (473 mL, 4000 mL)
- Injection, as sodium (C-II): 50 mg/mL (1 mL, 2 mL, 20 mL, 50 mL)
- Suppository, rectal (C-III): 30 mg, 60 mg, 120 mg, 200 mg

Pentobarbital Sodium *see* Pentobarbital *on page 970*

Pentosan Polysulfate Sodium

(PEN toe san pol i SUL fate SOW dee um)

Brand Names Elmiron®

Synonyms PPS

Therapeutic Category Analgesic, Urinary

Use Relief of bladder pain or discomfort due to interstitial cystitis

Pregnancy Risk Factor B

Contraindications Hypersensitivity to pentosan polysulfate sodium or any component

Warnings/Precautions Pentosan polysulfate is a low-molecular weight heparin-like compound with anticoagulant and fibrinolytic effects, therefore, bleeding complications such as ecchymosis, epistaxis and gum bleeding, may occur; patients with the following diseases should be carefully evaluated before initiating therapy: aneurysm, thrombocytopenia, hemophilia, gastrointestinal ulcerations, polyps, diverticula, or hepatic insufficiency; patients undergoing invasive procedures or having signs or symptoms of underlying coagulopathies or other increased risk of bleeding (eg, receiving heparin, warfarin, thrombolytics, or high dose aspirin) should be evaluated for hemorrhage; elevations in transaminases and alopecia can occur

Adverse Reactions

1% to 10%:

- Central nervous system: Headache, dizziness
- Dermatologic: Alopecia, rash
- Gastrointestinal: Diarrhea, nausea, dyspepsia, abdominal pain
- Hepatic: Liver function test abnormalities

<1%:

- Dermatologic: Pruritus, urticaria, photosensitivity, bruising
- Gastrointestinal: Vomiting, mouth ulcer, colitis, esophagitis, gastritis, flatulence, constipation, anorexia, gum bleeding
- Hematologic: Anemia, increased prothrombin time, increased partial thromboplastin time, leukopenia, thrombocytopenia
- Ocular: Conjunctivitis, optic neuritis, amblyopia, retinal hemorrhage
- Otic: Tinnitus
- Respiratory: Pharyngitis, rhinitis, epistaxis, dyspnea
- Miscellaneous: Allergic reactions

Overdosage/Toxicology Overdosage has not been reported; based on the pharmacodynamics, toxicity is likely to include anticoagulation, bleeding, thrombocytopenia, liver function abnormalities and gastric distress. Gastric lavage along with symptomatic and supportive therapy is recommended.

Drug Interactions Although there is no information about potential drug interactions, it is expected that pentosan polysulfate sodium would have at least additive anticoagulant effects when administered with anticoagulant drugs such as warfarin or heparin, and possible similar effects when administered with aspirin or thrombolytics

Mechanism of Action Although pentosan polysulfate sodium is a low-molecular weight heparinoid, it is not known whether these properties play a role in its mechanism of action in treating interstitial cystitis; the drug appears to adhere to the bladder wall mucosa where it may act as a buffer to protect the tissues from irritating substances in the urine.

Pharmacodynamics/Kinetics

Absorption: ~3%

Metabolism: In the liver and spleen

Half-life: 4-8 hours

Elimination: In urine, 3% unchanged drug

Usual Dosage Adults: Oral: 100 mg 3 times/day taken with water 1 hour before or 2 hours after meals

Patients should be evaluated at 3 months and may be continued an additional 3 months if there has been no improvement and if there are no therapy-limiting side effects. **The risks and benefits of continued use beyond 6 months in patients who have not responded is not yet known.**

Patient Information Patients should be advised to take the medication as prescribed and no more frequently; tell patients about the slight anticoagulant effects and the potential for increased bleeding; until more is known about drug interactions, carefully monitor the medication profile of patients receiving pentosan polysulfate sodium for drugs that might increase the anticoagulant effects

Dosage Forms Capsule: 100 mg

Pentostatin (PEN toe stat in)

Related Information

Antiemetics for Chemotherapy Induced Nausea and Vomiting *on page 1348*

Brand Names Nipent™

Synonyms DCF; Deoxycoformycin; 2'-deoxycoformycin

Therapeutic Category Antineoplastic Agent, Antimetabolite (Purine)

Use Treatment of adult patients with alpha-interferon-refractory hairy cell leukemia; non-Hodgkin's lymphoma, cutaneous T-cell lymphoma

Pregnancy Risk Factor D

Contraindications Limited or severely compromised bone marrow reserves (white blood cell count <3000 cells/mm^3)

Warnings/Precautions The FDA currently recommends that procedures for proper handling and disposal of antineoplastic agents be considered. Pregnant (Continued)

Pentostatin *(Continued)*

women or women of childbearing age should be apprised of the potential risk to the fetus; use extreme caution in the presence of renal insufficiency; use with caution in patients with signs or symptoms of impaired hepatic function.

Adverse Reactions

>10%:

Central nervous system: Headache, neurologic disorder, fever, fatigue, chills, pain

Dermatologic: Rash

Gastrointestinal: Vomiting, nausea, anorexia, diarrhea

Hematologic: Leukopenia, anemia, thrombocytopenia

Hepatic: Hepatic disorder, liver function tests (abnormal)

Neuromuscular & skeletal: Myalgia

Respiratory: Coughing

Miscellaneous: Allergic reaction

1% to 10%:

Cardiovascular: Chest pain, arrhythmia, peripheral edema

Central nervous system: Anxiety, confusion, depression, dizziness, insomnia, lethargy, coma, seizures, malaise

Dermatologic: Dry skin, eczema, pruritus

Gastrointestinal: Constipation, flatulence, stomatitis, weight loss

Genitourinary: Dysuria

Hematologic: Myelosuppression

Hepatic: Liver dysfunction

Local: Thrombophlebitis

Neuromuscular & skeletal: Arthralgia, paresthesia, back pain, weakness

Ocular: Abnormal vision, eye pain, keratoconjunctivitis

Otic: Ear pain

Renal: Renal failure, hematuria

Respiratory: Bronchitis, dyspnea, lung edema, pneumonia

Miscellaneous: Death, opportunistic infections, diaphoresis

Overdosage/Toxicology Symptoms of overdose include severe renal, hepatic, pulmonary, and CNS toxicity; supportive therapy

Drug Interactions Increased toxicity: Vidarabine, fludarabine, allopurinol

Stability Vials are stable under refrigeration at 2°C to 8°C; reconstituted vials, or further dilutions, may be stored at room temperature exposed to ambient light; diluted solutions are stable for 24 hours in D_5W or 48 hours in NS or lactated Ringer's at room temperature; infusion with 5% dextrose injection USP or 0.9% sodium chloride injection USP does not interact with PVC-containing administration sets or containers

Mechanism of Action An antimetabolite inhibiting adenosine deaminase (ADA), prevents ADA from controlling intracellular adenosine levels through the irreversible deamination of adenosine and deoxyadenosine. ADA is found to exhibit the highest activity in lymphoid tissue. Patients receiving pentostatin accumulate deoxyadenosine (dAdo) and deoxyadenosine 5′-triphosphate (dATP); accumulation of dATP results in cell death, probably through inhibiting DNA or RNA synthesis. Following a single dose, pentostatin has the ability to inhibit ADA for periods exceeding 1 week.

Pharmacodynamics/Kinetics

Distribution: I.V.: V_d: 36.1 L (20.1 L/m^2); distributes rapidly to body tissues and may obtain plasma concentrations ranging from 12-36 ng following doses of 250 mcg/kg for 4-5 days

Half-life, terminal: 5-15 hours

Elimination: ~50% to 96% is recovered in urine within 24 hours

Usual Dosage Refractory hairy cell leukemia: Adults (refer to individual protocols): 4 mg/m^2 every other week; I.V. bolus over ≥3-5 minutes in D_5W or NS at concentrations ≥2 mg/mL

Dosing interval in renal impairment:

Cl_{cr} <60 mL/minute: Use extreme caution

Cl_{cr} 50-60 mL/minute: 2 mg/m^2/dose

Dosage Forms Powder for injection: 10 mg/vial

Pentothal® Sodium *see* Thiopental *on page 1217*

Pentoxifylline (pen toks I fi leen)

Brand Names Trental®

Canadian/Mexican Brand Names Peridane® (Mexico)

Synonyms Oxpentifylline

Therapeutic Category Blood Viscosity Reducer Agent; Hemorheologic Agent

Use Symptomatic management of peripheral vascular disease, mainly intermittent claudication

Unapproved use: AIDS patients with increased TNF, CVA, cerebrovascular diseases, diabetic atherosclerosis, diabetic neuropathy, gangrene, hemodialysis shunt thrombosis, vascular impotence, cerebral malaria, septic shock, sickle cell syndromes, and vasculitis

Pregnancy Risk Factor C

Contraindications Hypersensitivity to pentoxifylline or any component and other xanthine derivatives

Warnings/Precautions Use with caution in patients with renal impairment or chronic occlusive arterial disease of the limbs

Adverse Reactions

1% to 10%:

- Central nervous system: Dizziness, headache
- Gastrointestinal: Dyspepsia, nausea, vomiting

<1%:

- Cardiovascular: Mild hypotension, angina
- Central nervous system: Agitation
- Ocular: Blurred vision
- Otic: Earache

Overdosage/Toxicology Symptoms of overdose include hypotension, flushing, convulsions, deep sleep, agitation, bradycardia, A-V block

Treatment is supportive; seizures can be treated with diazepam 5-10 mg (0.25-0.4 mg/kg in children); arrhythmias respond to lidocaine

Drug Interactions Increased effect/toxic potential with cimetidine (increased levels) and other H_2-antagonists, warfarin; increased effect of antihypertensives

Mechanism of Action Mechanism of action remains unclear; is thought to reduce blood viscosity and improve blood flow by altering the rheology of red blood cells

Pharmacodynamics/Kinetics

Absorption: Oral: Well absorbed

Metabolism: Undergoes first-pass metabolism in the liver

Half-life:

- Parent drug: 24-48 minutes
- Metabolites: 60-96 minutes

Time to peak serum concentration: Within 2-4 hours

Elimination: Mainly in urine

Usual Dosage Adults: Oral: 400 mg 3 times/day with meals; may reduce to 400 mg twice daily if GI or CNS side effects occur

Test Interactions ↓ calcium (S), ↓ magnesium (S), false-positive theophylline levels

Patient Information Take with food or meals; if GI or CNS side effects continue, contact physician; while effects may be seen in 2-4 weeks, continue treatment for at least 8 weeks

Dosage Forms Tablet, controlled release: 400 mg

Pen.Vee® K *see* Penicillin V Potassium *on page 965*

Pen VK *see* Penicillin V Potassium *on page 965*

Pepcid® *see* Famotidine *on page 504*

Pepcid® AC Acid Controller [OTC] *see* Famotidine *on page 504*

Pepto-Bismol® [OTC] *see* Bismuth *on page 154*

Pepto® Diarrhea Control [OTC] *see* Loperamide *on page 739*

Percocet® *see* Oxycodone and Acetaminophen *on page 938*

Percodan® *see* Oxycodone and Aspirin *on page 939*

Percodan®-Demi *see* Oxycodone and Aspirin *on page 939*

Perdiem® Plain [OTC] *see* Psyllium *on page 1075*

Perfectoderm® Gel [OTC] *see* Benzoyl Peroxide *on page 140*

Pergolide (PER go lide)

Brand Names Permax®

Synonyms Pergolide Mesylate

Therapeutic Category Anti-Parkinson's Agent; Ergot Alkaloid and Derivative

Use Adjunctive treatment to levodopa/carbidopa in the management of Parkinson's Disease

Pregnancy Risk Factor B

Contraindications Known hypersensitivity to pergolide mesylate or other ergot derivatives

Warnings/Precautions Symptomatic hypotension occurs in 10% of patients; use with caution in patients with a history of cardiac arrhythmias, hallucinations, or mental illness

(Continued)

Pergolide *(Continued)*

Adverse Reactions

>10%:

Central nervous system: Dizziness, somnolence, insomnia, confusion, hallucinations, anxiety, dystonia

Gastrointestinal: Nausea, constipation

Neuromuscular & skeletal: Dyskinesia

Respiratory: Rhinitis

1% to 10%:

Cardiovascular: Myocardial infarction, postural hypotension, syncope, arrhythmias, peripheral edema, vasodilation, palpitations, chest pain

Central nervous system: Chills

Gastrointestinal: Diarrhea, abdominal pain, vomiting, xerostomia, anorexia, weight gain

Neuromuscular & skeletal: Weakness

Ocular: Abnormal vision

Respiratory: Dyspnea

Miscellaneous: Flu syndrome

Overdosage/Toxicology Symptoms of overdose include vomiting, hypotension, agitation, hallucinations, ventricular extrasystoles, possible seizures; data on overdose is limited

Treatment is supportive and may require antiarrhythmias and/or neuroleptics for agitation; hypotension, when unresponsive to I.V. fluids or Trendelenburg positioning, often responds to norepinephrine infusions started at 0.1-0.2 mcg/kg/minute followed by a titrated infusion. If signs of CNS stimulation are present, a neuroleptic may be indicated; antiarrhythmics may be indicated, monitor EKG; activated charcoal is useful to prevent further absorption and to hasten elimination.

Drug Interactions

Decreased effect: Dopamine antagonists, metoclopramide

Increased toxicity: Highly plasma protein bound drugs

Mechanism of Action Pergolide is a semisynthetic ergot alkaloid similar to bromocriptine but stated to be more potent and longer-acting; it is a centrally-active dopamine agonist stimulating both D_1 and D_2 receptors

Pharmacodynamics/Kinetics

Absorption: Oral: Well absorbed

Protein binding: Plasma 90%

Metabolism: Extensive in the liver (on first-pass)

Elimination: ~50% excreted in urine and 50% in feces

Usual Dosage When adding pergolide to levodopa/carbidopa, the dose of the latter can usually and should be decreased. Patients no longer responsive to bromocriptine may benefit by being switched to pergolide.

Adults: Oral: Start with 0.05 mg/day for 2 days, then increase dosage by 0.1 or 0.15 mg/day every 3 days over next 12 days, increase dose by 0.25 mg/day every 3 days until optimal therapeutic dose is achieved, up to 5 mg/day maximum; usual dosage range: 2-3 mg/day in 3 divided doses

Monitoring Parameters Blood pressure (both sitting/supine and standing), symptoms of parkinsonism, dyskinesias, mental status

Patient Information Take with food or milk; rise slowly from sitting or lying down; report any confusion or change in mental status

Nursing Implications Monitor closely for orthostasis and other adverse effects; raise bed rails and institute safety measures; aid patient with ambulation, may cause postural hypotension and drowsiness

Dosage Forms Tablet, as mesylate: 0.05 mg, 0.25 mg, 1 mg

Pergolide Mesylate *see* Pergolide *on previous page*

Pergonal® *see* Menotropins *on page 779*

Periactin® *see* Cyproheptadine *on page 330*

Peridex® Oral Rinse *see* Chlorhexidine Gluconate *on page 253*

Perindopril Erbumine (per IN doe pril er BYOO meen)

Brand Names Aceon®

Therapeutic Category Antihypertensive

Use Treatment of stage I or II hypertension and congestive heart failure

Pregnancy Risk Factor D (especially during 2nd and 3rd trimester)

Pregnancy/Breast-Feeding Implications Only small amounts are excreted in breast milk

Contraindications Hypersensitivity to perindopril, perindoprilat, other ACE inhibitors, or any component; pregnancy; history of angioedema with other ACE inhibitors

Warnings/Precautions Use with caution and modify dosage in patients with renal impairment (especially renal artery stenosis), severe congestive heart failure, or with coadministered diuretic therapy, valvular stenosis, hyperkalemia (>5.7 mEq/L); experience in children is limited. Severe hypotension may occur in patients who are sodium and/or volume depleted; initiate lower doses and monitor closely when starting therapy in these patients.

Adverse Reactions

1% to 10%

- Central nervous system: Headache, dizziness, mood and sleep disorders, fatigue
- Dermatologic: Rash, pruritus
- Gastrointestinal: Nausea, epigastric pain, diarrhea, vomiting
- Neuromuscular & skeletal: Muscle cramps
- Respiratory: Cough (incidence is greater in women, 3:1)

<1%:

- Cardiovascular: Hypotension
- Dermatologic: Angioedema, psoriasis
- Endocrine & metabolic: Hyperkalemia
- Gastrointestinal: Taste disturbances
- Genitourinary: Impotence
- Hematologic: Agranulocytosis for all ACE inhibitors (especially in patients with renal impairment or collagen vascular disease), possibly neutropenia
- Ocular: Dry eyes, blurred vision, optic phosphenes
- Renal: Decreases in creatinine clearance in some elderly hypertensive patients or those with chronic renal failure, worsening of renal function in patients with bilateral renal artery stenosis, or furosemide therapy; proteinuria

Overdosage/Toxicology Mild hypotension has been the only toxic effect seen with acute overdose. Bradycardia may also occur; hyperkalemia occurs even with therapeutic doses, especially in patients with renal insufficiency and those taking NSAIDs.

Following initiation of essential overdose management, toxic symptom treatment and supportive treatment should be initiated. Hypotension usually responds to I.V. fluids or Trendelenburg positioning.

Drug Interactions See table.

Drug-Drug Interactions With ACEIs

Precipitant Drug	Drug (Category) and Effect	Description
Antacids	ACE Inhibitors: decreased	Decreased bioavailability of ACEIs. May be more likely with captopril. Separate administration times by 1-2 hours.
NSAIDs (indomethacin)	ACEIs: decreased	Reduced hypotensive effects of ACEIs. More prominent in low renin or volume dependent hypertensive patients.
Phenothiazines	ACEIs: increased	Pharmacologic effects of ACEIs may be increased.
ACEIs	Allopurinol: increased	Higher risk of hypersensitivity reaction possible when given concurrently. Three case reports of Stevens-Johnson syndrome with captopril.
ACEIs	Digoxin: increased	Increased plasma digoxin levels.
ACEIs	Lithium: increased	Increased serum lithium levels and symptoms of toxicity may occur.
ACEIs	Potassium preps/ potassium sparing diuretics increased	Coadministration may result in elevated potassium levels.

Mechanism of Action Competitive inhibitor of angiotensin-converting enzyme (ACE); prevents conversion of angiotensin I to angiotensin II, a potent vasoconstrictor; results in lower levels of angiotensin II which, in turn, causes an increase in plasma renin activity and a reduction in aldosterone secretion

Pharmacodynamics/Kinetics

Distribution: Small amounts of the drug are excreted into breast milk

Protein binding:

- Perindopril: 10% to 20%
- Perindoprilat: 60%

Metabolism: Perindopril is hydrolyzed in liver to active metabolite, perindoprilat (~17% to 20% of a dose) and other inactive metabolites

Bioavailability: Perindopril: 65% to 95%

Half-life:

- Parent drug: 1.5-3 hours
- Metabolite: 25-30 hours

(Continued)

Perindopril Erbumine *(Continued)*

Time to peak: Occurs in 1 and 3-4 hours for perindopril and perindoprilat, respectively after chronic therapy; (maximum perindoprilat serum levels are 2-3 times higher and T_{max} is shorter following chronic therapy); in CHF, the peak of perindoprilat is prolonged to 6 hours

Elimination: 75% of an oral dose is recovered in urine (10% as unchanged drug)

Usual Dosage Adults: Oral:

Congestive heart failure: 4 mg once daily

Hypertension: Initial: 4 mg/day but may be titrated to response; usual range: 4-8 mg/day, maximum: 16 mg/day

Dosing adjustment in renal impairment:

Cl_{cr} >60 mL/minute: 4 mg/day

Cl_{cr} 30-60 mL/minute: 2 mg/day

Cl_{cr} 15-29 mL/minute: 2 mg every other day

Cl_{cr} <15 mL/minute: 2 mg on the day of dialysis

Hemodialysis: Perindopril and its metabolites are dialyzable

Dosing adjustment in hepatic impairment: None needed

Dosing adjustment in geriatric patients: Due to greater bioavailability and lower renal clearance of the drug in elderly subjects, dose reduction of 50% is recommended

Monitoring Parameters Serum creatinine, electrolytes, and WBC with differential initially and repeated at 2-week intervals for at least 90 days

Patient Information Avoid taking with food since the efficacy of the drug may be reduced; immediately report signs of infection (sore throat, fever) perioral swelling, significant orthostatic hypotension, difficulty swallowing/breathing, or signs of anaphylaxis or allergy; inform your physician if you are pregnant or have a history of kidney disease

Nursing Implications A reduction in clinical signs of congestive heart failure (dyspnea, orthopnea, cough) and an improvement in exercise duration are indicative of therapeutic response; a reduction of supine diastolic blood pressure of 10 mm Hg or to 90 mm Hg is indicative of excellent therapeutic response in patients with hypertension; observe for cough, difficulty breathing/swallowing, perioral swelling and signs and symptoms of agranulocytosis; monitor for 6 hours after initial dosing for profound hypotension or first-dose phenomenon

Dosage Forms Tablet: 2 mg, 4 mg, 8 mg

PerioGard® *see* Chlorhexidine Gluconate *on page 253*

Peritrate® *see* Pentaerythritol Tetranitrate *on page 967*

Peritrate® SA *see* Pentaerythritol Tetranitrate *on page 967*

Permapen® *see* Penicillin G Benzathine *on page 961*

Permax® *see* Pergolide *on page 975*

Permethrin (per METH rin)

Brand Names Elimite™; Nix™ [OTC]

Therapeutic Category Antiparasitic Agent, Topical; Scabicidal Agent; Shampoos

Use Single application treatment of infestation with *Pediculus humanus capitis* (head louse) and its nits or *Sarcoptes scabiei* (scabies); indicated for prophylactic use during epidemics of lice

Pregnancy Risk Factor B

Contraindications Known hypersensitivity to pyrethyroid, pyrethrin, or chrysanthemums

Warnings/Precautions Treatment may temporarily exacerbate the symptoms of itching, redness, swelling; for external use only; use during pregnancy only if clearly needed

Adverse Reactions

1% to 10%:

Dermatologic: Pruritus, erythema, rash of the scalp

Local: Burning, stinging, tingling, numbness or scalp discomfort, edema

Mechanism of Action Inhibits sodium ion influx through nerve cell membrane channels in parasites resulting in delayed repolarization and thus paralysis and death of the pest

Pharmacodynamics/Kinetics

Absorption: Topical: Minimal (<2%)

Metabolism: In the liver by ester hydrolysis to inactive metabolites

Elimination: In urine

Usual Dosage Topical: Children >2 months and Adults:

Head lice: After hair has been washed with shampoo, rinsed with water, and towel dried, apply a sufficient volume of topical liquid to saturate the hair and scalp. Leave on hair for 10 minutes before rinsing off with water; remove remaining nits; may repeat in 1 week if lice or nits still present.

Scabies: Apply cream from head to toe; leave on for 8-14 hours before washing off with water; for infants, also apply on the hairline, neck, scalp, temple, and forehead; may reapply in 1 week if live mites appear

Permethrin 5% cream was shown to be safe and effective when applied to an infant <1 month of age with neonatal scabies; time of application was limited to 6 hours before rinsing with soap and water

Patient Information Avoid contact with eyes and mucous membranes during application; shake well before using; notify physician if irritation persists; clothing and bedding should be washed in hot water or dry cleaned to kill the scabies mite

Dosage Forms

Cream: 5% (60 g)

Liquid, topical: 1% (60 mL)

Permitil® *see* Fluphenazine *on page 543*

Peroxin A5® *see* Benzoyl Peroxide *on page 140*

Peroxin A10® *see* Benzoyl Peroxide *on page 140*

Perphenazine (per FEN a zeen)

Related Information

Antipsychotic Agents Comparison *on page 1396*

Brand Names Trilafon®

Canadian/Mexican Brand Names Apo-Perphenazine® (Canada); PMS-Perphenazine (Canada); Leptopsique® (Mexico)

Therapeutic Category Antiemetic; Antipsychotic Agent; Phenothiazine Derivative

Use Management of manifestations of psychotic disorders, depressive neurosis, alcohol withdrawal, nausea and vomiting, nonpsychotic symptoms associated with dementia in elderly, Tourette's syndrome, Huntington's chorea, spasmodic torticollis and Reye's syndrome

Pregnancy Risk Factor C

Contraindications Hypersensitivity to perphenazine or any component, cross-sensitivity with other phenothiazines may exist; avoid use in patients with narrow-angle glaucoma, bone marrow suppression, severe liver or cardiac disease; subcortical brain damage; circulatory collapse; severe hypotension or hypertension

Warnings/Precautions Safety in children <6 months of age has not been established; use with caution in patients with cardiovascular disease or seizures, bone marrow suppression, severe liver or cardiac disease

Adverse Reactions

>10%:

- Cardiovascular: Hypotension, orthostatic hypotension
- Central nervous system: Pseudoparkinsonism, akathisia, dystonias, tardive dyskinesia (persistent), dizziness
- Gastrointestinal: Constipation
- Ocular: Pigmentary retinopathy
- Respiratory: Nasal congestion
- Miscellaneous: Diaphoresis (decreased)

1% to 10%:

- Dermatologic: Increased sensitivity to sun, rash
- Endocrine & metabolic: Changes in menstrual cycle, changes in libido, breast pain
- Gastrointestinal: Weight gain, vomiting, stomach pain, nausea
- Genitourinary: Dysuria, ejaculatory disturbances
- Neuromuscular & skeletal: Trembling of fingers

<1%:

- Central nervous system: Neuroleptic malignant syndrome (NMS), impairment of temperature regulation, lowering of seizures threshold
- Dermatologic: Discoloration of skin (blue gray)
- Endocrine & metabolic: Galactorrhea
- Genitourinary: Priapism
- Hematologic: Agranulocytosis, leukopenia
- Hepatic: Cholestatic jaundice, hepatotoxicity
- Ocular: Cornea and lens changes

Overdosage/Toxicology Symptoms of overdose include deep sleep, dystonia, agitation, coma, abnormal involuntary muscle movements, hypotension, arrhythmias

Following initiation of essential overdose management, toxic symptom treatment and supportive treatment should be initiated. Hypotension usually responds to I.V. fluids or Trendelenburg positioning. If unresponsive to these measures, the use of a parenteral inotrope may be required (eg, norepinephrine 0.1-0.2 mcg/kg/minute titrated to response). Seizures commonly respond to diazepam (I.V. 5-10 mg bolus in adults every 15 minutes if needed up to a total of 30 mg; I.V. 0.25-0.4 mg/kg/dose up to a total of 10 mg in children) or to phenytoin or phenobarbital.

(Continued)

Perphenazine *(Continued)*

Extrapyramidal symptoms (eg, dystonic reactions) may be managed with diphenhydramine. When these reactions are unresponsive to diphenhydramine, benztropine mesylate may be effective.

Drug Interactions Cytochrome P-450 2D6 enzyme substrate

Decreased effect: Anticholinergics, anticonvulsants; decreased effect of guanethidine, epinephrine

Increased toxicity: CNS depressants; increased effect/toxicity of anticonvulsants

Mechanism of Action Blocks postsynaptic mesolimbic dopaminergic receptors in the brain; exhibits a strong alpha-adrenergic blocking effect and depresses the release of hypothalamic and hypophyseal hormones

Pharmacodynamics/Kinetics

Absorption: Oral: Well absorbed

Distribution: Crosses the placenta

Metabolism: In the liver

Half-life: 9 hours

Time to peak serum concentration: Within 4-8 hours

Elimination: In urine and bile

Usual Dosage

Children:

- Psychoses: Oral:
  - 1-6 years: 4-6 mg/day in divided doses
  - 6-12 years: 6 mg/day in divided doses
  - >12 years: 4-16 mg 2-4 times/day
  - I.M.: 5 mg every 6 hours
- Nausea/vomiting: I.M.: 5 mg every 6 hours

Adults:

- Psychoses:
  - Oral: 4-16 mg 2-4 times/day not to exceed 64 mg/day
  - I.M.: 5 mg every 6 hours up to 15 mg/day in ambulatory patients and 30 mg/day in hospitalized patients
- Nausea/vomiting:
  - Oral: 8-16 mg/day in divided doses up to 24 mg/day
  - I.M.: 5-10 mg every 6 hours as necessary up to 15 mg/day in ambulatory patients and 30 mg/day in hospitalized patients
  - I.V. (severe): 1 mg at 1- to 2-minute intervals up to a total of 5 mg

Hemodialysis: Not dialyzable (0% to 5%)

Dosing adjustment in hepatic impairment: Dosage reductions should be considered in patients with liver disease although no specific guidelines are available

Dietary Considerations Alcohol: Additive CNS effect, avoid use

Administration Dilute oral concentration to at least 2 oz with water, juice, or milk; for I.V. use, injection should be diluted to at least 0.5 mg/mL with NS and given at a rate of 1 mg/minute; observe for tremor and abnormal movements or posturing

Reference Range 2-6 nmol/L

Test Interactions ↑ cholesterol (S), ↑ glucose; ↓ uric acid (S)

Patient Information May cause drowsiness, impair judgment and coordination; report any feelings of restlessness or any involuntary movements; avoid alcohol and other CNS depressants; do not alter dose or discontinue without consulting physician

Nursing Implications Monitor for hypotension when administering I.M. or I.V. during the first 3-5 days after initiating therapy or making a dosage adjustment

Dosage Forms

Concentrate, oral: 16 mg/5 mL (118 mL)

Injection: 5 mg/mL (1 mL)

Tablet: 2 mg, 4 mg, 8 mg, 16 mg

Persa-Gel® *see* Benzoyl Peroxide *on page 140*

Persantine® *see* Dipyridamole *on page 406*

Pertofrane® *see* Desipramine *on page 352*

Pertussin® CS [OTC] *see* Dextromethorphan *on page 366*

Pertussin® ES [OTC] *see* Dextromethorphan *on page 366*

Pethidine Hydrochloride *see* Meperidine *on page 780*

PETN *see* Pentaerythritol Tetranitrate *on page 967*

PFA *see* Foscarnet *on page 554*

Pfizerpen® *see* Penicillin G, Parenteral, Aqueous *on page 962*

Pfizerpen®-AS *see* Penicillin G Procaine *on page 964*

PGE$_1$ *see* Alprostadil *on page 51*

PGE$_2$ *see* Dinoprostone *on page 397*

PGI$_2$ *see* Epoprostenol *on page 454*

PGX *see* Epoprostenol *on page 454*

Phanatuss® [OTC] *see* Guaifenesin and Dextromethorphan *on page 591*

Pharmaflur® *see* Fluoride *on page 536*

Phazyme® [OTC] *see* Simethicone *on page 1136*

Phenaphen® With Codeine *see* Acetaminophen and Codeine *on page 21*

Phenazine® *see* Promethazine *on page 1058*

Phenazopyridine (fen az oh PEER i deen)

Brand Names Azo-Standard® [OTC]; Baridium® [OTC]; Prodium® [OTC]; Pyridiate®; Pyridium®; Urodine®; Urogesic®

Canadian/Mexican Brand Names Phenazo® (Canada); Pyronium® (Canada); Vito Reins® (Canada); Azo Wintomylon® (Mexico); Madel® (Mexico); Urovalidin® (Mexico)

Synonyms Phenazopyridine Hydrochloride; Phenylazo Diamino Pyridine Hydrochloride

Therapeutic Category Analgesic, Urinary; Local Anesthetic, Urinary

Use Symptomatic relief of urinary burning, itching, frequency and urgency in association with urinary tract infection or following urologic procedures

Pregnancy Risk Factor B

Contraindications Hypersensitivity to phenazopyridine or any component; kidney or liver disease

Warnings/Precautions Does not treat infection, acts only as an analgesic; drug should be discontinued if skin or sclera develop a yellow color; use with caution in patients with renal impairment. Use of this agent in the elderly is limited since accumulation of phenazopyridine can occur in patients with renal insufficiency. It should not be used in patients with a Cl_{cr} <50 mL/minute.

Adverse Reactions

1% to 10%:
- Central nervous system: Headache, dizziness
- Gastrointestinal: Stomach cramps

<1%:
- Central nervous system: Vertigo
- Dermatologic: Skin pigmentation, rash
- Hematologic: Methemoglobinemia, hemolytic anemia
- Hepatic: Hepatitis
- Renal: Acute renal failure

Overdosage/Toxicology Symptoms of overdose include methemoglobinemia, hemolytic anemia, skin pigmentation, renal and hepatic impairment

Antidote is methylene blue 1-2 mg/kg I.V. for methemoglobinemia

Mechanism of Action An azo dye which exerts local anesthetic or analgesic action on urinary tract mucosa through an unknown mechanism

Pharmacodynamics/Kinetics

Metabolism: In the liver and other tissues

Elimination: In urine (where it exerts its action); renal excretion (as unchanged drug) is rapid and accounts for 65% of the drug's elimination

Usual Dosage Oral:

Children: 12 mg/kg/day in 3 divided doses administered after meals for 2 days

Adults: 100-200 mg 3 times/day after meals for 2 days when used concomitantly with an antibacterial agent

Dosing interval in renal impairment:
- Cl_{cr} 50-80 mL/minute: Administer every 8-16 hours
- Cl_{cr} <50 mL/minute: Avoid use

Test Interactions Phenazopyridine may cause delayed reactions with glucose oxidase reagents (Clinistix®, Tes-Tape®); occasional false-positive tests occur with Tes-Tape®; cupric sulfate tests (Clinitest®) are not affected; interference may also occur with urine ketone tests (Acetest®, Ketostix®) and urinary protein tests; tests for urinary steroids and porphyrins may also occur

Patient Information Take after meals; tablets may color urine orange or red and may stain clothing

Dosage Forms Tablet, as hydrochloride:

Azo-Standard®, Prodium®: 95 mg

Baridium®, Geridium®, Pyridiate®, Pyridium®, Urodine®, Urogesic®: 100 mg

Geridium®, Phenazodine®, Pyridium®, Urodine®: 200 mg

Extemporaneous Preparations A 10 mg/mL suspension may be made by crushing three 200 mg tablets. Mix with a small amount of distilled water or glycerin. Add 20 mL Cologel® and levigate until a uniform mixture is obtained. Add sufficient 2:1 simple syrup/cherry syrup mixture to make a final volume of 60 mL. Store in an amber container. Label "shake well". Stability is 60 days refrigerated.

Handbook on Extemporaneous Formulations, Bethesda MD: American Society of Hospital Pharmacists, 1987.

Phenazopyridine Hydrochloride *see* Phenazopyridine *on previous page*

Phendry® Oral [OTC] *see* Diphenhydramine *on page 399*

Phenelzine (FEN el zeen)

Related Information

Antidepressant Agents Comparison *on page 1393*

Brand Names Nardil®

Synonyms Phenelzine Sulfate

Therapeutic Category Antidepressant, Monoamine Oxidase Inhibitor

Use Symptomatic treatment of atypical, nonendogenous or neurotic depression

The MAO inhibitors are usually reserved for patients who do not tolerate or respond to the traditional "cyclic" or "second generation" antidepressants. The brain activity of monoamine oxidase increases with age and even more so in patients with Alzheimer's disease. Therefore, the MAO inhibitors may have an increased role in patients with Alzheimer's disease who are depressed. Phenelzine is less stimulating than tranylcypromine.

Pregnancy Risk Factor C

Contraindications Pheochromocytoma, hepatic or renal disease, cerebrovascular defect, cardiovascular disease, hypersensitivity to phenelzine or any component, do not use within 5 weeks of fluoxetine or 2 weeks of sertraline or paroxetine discontinuance

Warnings/Precautions Safety in children <16 years of age has not been established; use with caution in patients who are hyperactive, hyperexcitable, or who have glaucoma; avoid use of meperidine within 2 weeks of phenelzine use. Hypertensive crisis may occur with tyramine. See table for foods containing tyramine.

Tyramine-Containing Foods

	Cheese/Dairy Products	
American processed	Cheddar	Roquefort
Blue	Emmenthaler	Sour cream
Boursault	Gruyere	Stilton
Brick, natural	Mozzarella	Yogurt
Brie	Parmesan	
Camembert	Romano	
	Meat/Fish	
Beef or chicken liver, other meats, fish (unrefrigerated, fermented)	Fermented sausages (bologna, pepperoni, salami, summer sausage)	Caviar
Meats prepared with tenderizer	Game meat	Dried fish (salted herring)
		Herring, pickled, spoiled
		Shrimp paste
	Alcoholic Beverages (Undistilled)	
Beer and ale (imports, some nonalcoholic)	Red wine (especially Chianti)	Sherry
	Fruit/Vegetables	
Avocados (especially overripe)	Bananas	Soy sauce
Yeast extracts (Marmite, etc)	Figs, canned (overripe)	Miso soup
	Raisins	Bean curd
	Foods Containing Other Vasopressors	
Fava beans (overripe) — dopamine	Caffeine (eg, coffee, tea, colas) — caffeine	Chocolate — phenylethylamine
		Ginseng

The MAO inhibitors are effective and generally well tolerated by older patients. It is the potential interactions with tyramine or tryptophan-containing foods and other drugs, and their effects on blood pressure that have limited their use.

Adverse Reactions

>10%:

- Cardiovascular: Orthostatic hypotension
- Central nervous system: Drowsiness
- Endocrine & metabolic: Decreased sexual ability
- Neuromuscular & skeletal: Trembling, weakness

Ocular: Blurred vision

1% to 10%:

Cardiovascular: Tachycardia, peripheral edema

Central nervous system: Nervousness, chills

Gastrointestinal: Diarrhea, anorexia, xerostomia, constipation

<1%:

Central nervous system: Parkinsonism syndrome

Hematologic: Leukopenia

Hepatic: Hepatitis

Overdosage/Toxicology Symptoms of overdose include tachycardia, palpitations, muscle twitching, seizures, insomnia, restlessness, transient hypertension, hypotension, drowsiness, hyperpyrexia, coma

Competent supportive care is the most important treatment for an overdose with a monoamine oxidase (MAO) inhibitor. Both hypertension or hypotension can occur with intoxication. Hypotension may respond to I.V. fluids or vasopressors and hypertension usually responds to an alpha-adrenergic blocker. While treating the hypertension, care is warranted to avoid sudden drops in blood pressure, since this may worsen the MAO inhibitor toxicity. Muscle irritability and seizures often respond to diazepam, while hyperthermia is best treated antipyretics and cooling blankets. Cardiac arrhythmias are best treated with phenytoin or procainamide.

Drug Interactions

Increased effect/toxicity of barbiturates, psychotropics, rauwolfia alkaloids, CNS depressants

Increased toxicity with disulfiram (seizures), fluoxetine and other serotonin active agents (increased cardiac effect), tricyclic antidepressants (increased cardiovascular instability), meperidine (increased cardiovascular instability), phenothiazine (hypertensive crisis), sympathomimetics (hypertensive crisis), levodopa (hypertensive crisis), tyramine-containing foods (increased blood pressure), dextroamphetamine

Stability Protect from light

Mechanism of Action Thought to act by increasing endogenous concentrations of epinephrine, norepinephrine, dopamine and serotonin through inhibition of the enzyme (monoamine oxidase) responsible for the breakdown of these neurotransmitters

Pharmacodynamics/Kinetics

Onset of action: Within 2-4 weeks

Absorption: Oral: Well absorbed

Duration: May continue to have a therapeutic effect and interactions 2 weeks after discontinuing therapy

Elimination: In urine primarily as metabolites and unchanged drug

Usual Dosage Oral:

Adults: 15 mg 3 times/day; may increase to 60-90 mg/day during early phase of treatment, then reduce to dose for maintenance therapy slowly after maximum benefit is obtained; takes 2-4 weeks for a significant response to occur

Elderly: Initial: 7.5 mg/day; increase by 7.5-15 mg/day every 3-4 days as tolerated; usual therapeutic dose: 15-60 mg/day in 3-4 divided doses

Dietary Considerations

Alcohol: Additive CNS effect, avoid use

Food: Avoid tyramine-containing foods

Monitoring Parameters Blood pressure, heart rate, diet, weight, mood (if depressive symptoms)

Test Interactions ↓ glucose

Patient Information Avoid tyramine-containing foods: Red wine, cheese (except cottage, ricotta, and cream), smoked or pickled fish, beef or chicken liver, dried sausage, fava or broad bean pods, yeast vitamin supplements; do not begin any prescription or OTC medications without consulting your physician or pharmacist; may take as long as 3 weeks to see effects; report any severe headaches, irregular heartbeats, skin rash, insomnia, sedation, changes in strength; sensations of pain, burning, touch, or vibration; or any other unusual symptoms to your physician; avoid alcohol; get up slowly from chair or bed

Nursing Implications Watch for postural hypotension; monitor blood pressure carefully, especially at therapy onset or if other CNS drugs or cardiovascular drugs are added; check for dietary and drug restriction

Dosage Forms Tablet, as sulfate: 15 mg

Phenelzine Sulfate *see* Phenelzine *on previous page*

Phenerbel-S® *see* Ergotamine *on page 459*

Phenergan® *see* Promethazine *on page 1058*

Phenetron® *see* Chlorpheniramine *on page 260*

Phenobarbital (fee noe BAR bi tal)

Related Information

Anticonvulsants by Seizure Type *on page 1392*
Convulsive Status Epilepticus *on page 1528*
Epilepsy Treatment *on page 1531*
Febrile Seizures *on page 1532*

Brand Names Barbita®; Luminal®; Solfoton®

Canadian/Mexican Brand Names Barbilixir® (Canada); Alepsal® (Mexico)

Synonyms Phenobarbital Sodium; Phenobarbitone; Phenylethylmalonylurea

Therapeutic Category Anticonvulsant; Barbiturate; Hypnotic; Sedative

Use Management of generalized tonic-clonic (grand mal) and partial seizures; neonatal seizures; febrile seizures in children; sedation; may also be used for prevention and treatment of neonatal hyperbilirubinemia and lowering of bilirubin in chronic cholestasis

Restrictions C-IV

Pregnancy Risk Factor D

Pregnancy/Breast-Feeding Implications

Clinical effects on the fetus: Crosses the placenta. Cardiac defect reported; hemorrhagic disease of newborn due to fetal vitamin K depletion may occur; may induce maternal folic acid deficiency; withdrawal symptoms observed in infant following delivery. Epilepsy itself, number of medications, genetic factors, or a combination of these probably influence the teratogenicity of anticonvulsant therapy. Benefit:risk ratio usually favors continued use during pregnancy and breast-feeding.

Breast-feeding/Lactation: Crosses into breast milk

Clinical effects on the infant: Sedation; withdrawal with abrupt weaning reported. American Academy of Pediatrics recommends USE WITH CAUTION.

Contraindications Hypersensitivity to phenobarbital or any component; pre-existing CNS depression, severe uncontrolled pain, porphyria, severe respiratory disease with dyspnea or obstruction

Warnings/Precautions Use with caution in patients with hypovolemic shock, congestive heart failure, hepatic impairment, respiratory dysfunction or depression, previous addiction to the sedative/hypnotic group, chronic or acute pain, renal dysfunction, and the elderly, due to its long half-life and risk of dependence, phenobarbital is not recommended as a sedative in the elderly; tolerance or psychological and physical dependence may occur with prolonged use. **Abrupt withdrawal in patients with epilepsy may precipitate status epilepticus.**

Adverse Reactions

>10%:

- Cardiovascular: Hypotension, cardiac arrhythmias, bradycardia, arterial spasm
- Central nervous system: Dizziness, lightheadedness, "hangover" effect, drowsiness, lethargy, CNS excitation or depression, impaired judgment
- Local: Pain at injection site, thrombophlebitis with I.V. use
- Miscellaneous: Gangrene with inadvertent intra-arterial injection

1% to 10%:

- Central nervous system: Confusion, mental depression, unusual excitement, nervousness, faint feeling, headache, insomnia, nightmares
- Gastrointestinal: Nausea, vomiting, constipation

<1%:

- Cardiovascular: Hypotension
- Central nervous system: Hallucinations, hypothermia
- Dermatologic: Exfoliative dermatitis, Stevens-Johnson syndrome, rash
- Hematologic: Agranulocytosis, megaloblastic anemia, thrombocytopenia
- Respiratory: Laryngospasm, respiratory depression, apnea (especially with rapid I.V. use)

Overdosage/Toxicology Symptoms of overdose include unsteady gait, slurred speech, confusion, jaundice, hypothermia, hypotension, respiratory depression, coma

If hypotension occurs, administer I.V. fluids and place the patient in the Trendelenburg position. If unresponsive, an I.V. vasopressor (eg, dopamine, epinephrine) may be required.

Repeated oral doses of activated charcoal significantly reduce the half-life of phenobarbital resulting from an enhancement of nonrenal elimination. The usual dose is 0.1-1 g/kg every 4-6 hours for 3-4 days unless the patient has no bowel movement causing the charcoal to remain in the GI tract. Assure adequate hydration and renal function. Urinary alkalinization with I.V. sodium bicarbonate also helps to enhance elimination. Hemodialysis or hemoperfusion is of uncertain value. Patients in stage IV coma due to high serum barbiturate levels may require charcoal hemoperfusion.

Drug Interactions Inducer of cytochrome P-450 2B6, cytochrome P-450 2C, cytochrome P-450 2D6, cytochrome P-450 2E, and cytochrome P-450 3A enzymes

Decreased effect: Phenothiazines, haloperidol, quinidine, cyclosporine, tricyclic antidepressants, corticosteroids, theophylline, ethosuximide, warfarin, oral contraceptives, chloramphenicol, griseofulvin, doxycycline, beta-blockers

Increased toxicity: Propoxyphene, benzodiazepines, CNS depressants, valproic acid, methylphenidate, chloramphenicol

Stability Protect elixir from light; not stable in aqueous solutions; use only clear solutions; do not add to acidic solutions, precipitation may occur; I.V. form is **incompatible** with benzquinamide (in syringe), cephalothin, chlorpromazine, hydralazine, hydrocortisone, hydroxyzine, insulin, levorphanol, meperidine, methadone, morphine, norepinephrine, pentazocine, prochlorperazine, promazine, promethazine, ranitidine (in syringe), vancomycin

Mechanism of Action Interferes with transmission of impulses from the thalamus to the cortex of the brain resulting in an imbalance in central inhibitory and facilitatory mechanisms

Pharmacodynamics/Kinetics

Oral:
- Onset of hypnosis: Within 20-60 minutes
- Duration: 6-10 hours

I.V.:
- Onset of action: Within 5 minutes
- Peak effect: Within 30 minutes
- Duration: 4-10 hours

Absorption: Oral: 70% to 90%

Protein binding: 20% to 45%, decreased in neonates

Metabolism: In the liver via hydroxylation and glucuronide conjugation

Half-life:
- Neonates: 45-500 hours
- Infants: 20-133 hours
- Children: 37-73 hours
- Adults: 53-140 hours

Time to peak serum concentration: Oral: Within 1-6 hours

Elimination: 20% to 50% excreted unchanged in urine

Usual Dosage

Children:
- Sedation: Oral: 2 mg/kg 3 times/day
- Hypnotic: I.M., I.V., S.C.: 3-5 mg/kg at bedtime
- Preoperative sedation: Oral, I.M., I.V.: 1-3 mg/kg 1-1.5 hours before procedure

Anticonvulsant: Status epilepticus: **Loading dose:** I.V.:
- Infants and Children: 10-20 mg/kg in a single or divided dose; in select patients may administer additional 5 mg/kg/dose every 15-30 minutes until seizure is controlled or a total dose of 40 mg/kg is reached
- Adults: 300-800 mg initially followed by 120-240 mg/dose at 20-minute intervals until seizures are controlled or a total dose of 1-2 g

Anticonvulsant maintenance dose: Oral, I.V.:
- Infants: 5-8 mg/kg/day in 1-2 divided doses
- Children:
  - 1-5 years: 6-8 mg/kg/day in 1-2 divided doses
  - 5-12 years: 4-6 mg/kg/day in 1-2 divided doses
- Children >12 years and Adults: 1-3 mg/kg/day in divided doses or 50-100 mg 2-3 times/day

Adults:
- Sedation: Oral, I.M.: 30-120 mg/day in 2-3 divided doses
- Hypnotic: Oral, I.M., I.V., S.C.: 100-320 mg at bedtime
- Preoperative sedation: I.M.: 100-200 mg 1-1.5 hours before procedure

Dosing interval in renal impairment: Cl_{cr} <10 mL/minute: Administer every 12-16 hours

Hemodialysis: Moderately dialyzable (20% to 50%)

Dosing adjustment/comments in hepatic disease: Increased side effects may occur in severe liver disease; monitor plasma levels and adjust dose accordingly

Dietary Considerations

Alcohol: Additive CNS effect, avoid use

Food:
- Protein-deficient diets: Increases duration of action of barbiturates. Should not restrict or delete protein from diet unless discussed with physician. Be consistent with protein intake during therapy with barbiturates.
- Fresh fruits containing vitamin C: Displaces drug from binding sites, resulting in increased urinary excretion of barbiturate. Educate patients regarding the

(Continued)

Phenobarbital *(Continued)*

potential for a decreased anticonvulsant effect of barbiturates with consumption of foods high in vitamin C.

Vitamin D: Loss in vitamin D due to malabsorption; increase intake of foods rich in vitamin D. Supplementation of vitamin D may be necessary.

Administration Avoid rapid I.V. administration >50 mg/minute; avoid intra-arterial injection

Monitoring Parameters Phenobarbital serum concentrations, mental status, CBC, LFTs, seizure activity

Reference Range

Therapeutic:

Infants and children: 15-30 μg/mL (SI: 65-129 μmol/L)

Adults: 20-40 μg/mL (SI: 86-172 μmol/L)

Toxic: >40 μg/mL (SI: >172 μmol/L)

Toxic concentration: Slowness, ataxia, nystagmus: 35-80 μg/mL (SI: 150-344 μmol/L)

Coma with reflexes: 65-117 μg/mL (SI: 279-502 μmol/L)

Coma without reflexes: >100 μg/mL (SI: >430 μmol/L)

Test Interactions ↑ ammonia (B); ↓ bilirubin (S), ↑ copper (S), assay interference of LDH, ↑ LFTs

Patient Information Avoid use of alcohol and other CNS depressants; avoid driving and other hazardous tasks; avoid abrupt discontinuation; may cause physical and psychological dependence; do not alter dose without notifying physician

Nursing Implications Parenteral solutions are highly alkaline; avoid extravasation; institute safety measures to avoid injuries; observe patient for excessive sedation and respiratory depression

Additional Information Injectable solutions contain propylene glycol

Sodium content of injection (65 mg, 1 mL): 6 mg (0.3 mEq)

Phenobarbital: Barbita®, Solfoton®

Phenobarbital sodium: Luminal®

Dosage Forms

Capsule: 16 mg

Elixir: 15 mg/5 mL (5 mL, 10 mL, 20 mL); 20 mg/5 mL (3.75 mL, 5 mL, 7.5 mL, 120 mL, 473 mL, 946 mL, 4000 mL)

Injection, as sodium: 30 mg/mL (1 mL); 60 mg/mL (1 mL); 65 mg/mL (1 mL); 130 mg/mL (1 mL)

Powder for injection: 120 mg

Tablet: 8 mg, 15 mg, 16 mg, 30 mg, 32 mg, 60 mg, 65 mg, 100 mg

Phenobarbital Sodium *see* Phenobarbital *on page 984*

Phenobarbitone *see* Phenobarbital *on page 984*

Phenoxybenzamine (fen oks ee BEN za meen)

Brand Names Dibenzyline®

Synonyms Phenoxybenzamine Hydrochloride

Therapeutic Category Alpha-Adrenergic Blocking Agent, Oral; Antihypertensive

Use Symptomatic management of pheochromocytoma; treatment of hypertensive crisis caused by sympathomimetic amines

Unlabeled use: Micturition problems associated with neurogenic bladder, functional outlet obstruction, and partial prostate obstruction

Pregnancy Risk Factor C

Contraindications Conditions in which a fall in blood pressure would be undesirable (eg, shock)

Warnings/Precautions Use with caution in patients with renal impairment, cerebral, or coronary arteriosclerosis, can exacerbate symptoms of respiratory tract infections. Because of the risk of adverse effects, avoid the use of this medication in the elderly if possible.

Adverse Reactions

>10%:

Cardiovascular: Postural hypotension, tachycardia, syncope

Ocular: Miosis

Respiratory: Nasal congestion

1% to 10%:

Cardiovascular: Shock

Central nervous system: Lethargy, headache, confusion, fatigue

Gastrointestinal: Vomiting, nausea, diarrhea, xerostomia

Genitourinary: Inhibition of ejaculation

Neuromuscular & skeletal: Weakness

Overdosage/Toxicology Symptoms of overdose include hypotension, tachycardia, lethargy, dizziness, shock

Hypotension and shock should be treated with fluids and by placing the patient in the Trendelenburg position; only alpha-adrenergic pressors such as norepinephrine should be used; mixed agents such as epinephrine, may cause more hypotension

Drug Interactions

Decreased effect: Alpha agonists

Increased toxicity: Beta-blockers (hypotension, tachycardia)

Mechanism of Action Produces long-lasting noncompetitive alpha-adrenergic blockade of postganglionic synapses in exocrine glands and smooth muscle; relaxes urethra and increases opening of the bladder

Pharmacodynamics/Kinetics

Onset of action: Oral: Within 2 hours

Peak effect: Within 4-6 hours

Duration: Can continue for 4 or more days

Half-life: 24 hours

Elimination: Primarily in urine and feces

Usual Dosage Oral:

Children: Initial: 0.2 mg/kg (maximum: 10 mg) once daily, increase by 0.2 mg/kg increments; usual maintenance dose: 0.4-1.2 mg/kg/day every 6-8 hours, higher doses may be necessary

Adults: Initial: 10 mg twice daily, increase by 10 mg every other day until optimum dose is achieved; usual range: 20-40 mg 2-3 times/day

Dietary Considerations Alcohol: Avoid use

Monitoring Parameters Blood pressure, pulse, urine output, orthostasis

Patient Information Avoid alcoholic beverages; if dizziness occurs, avoid sudden changes in posture; may cause nasal congestion and constricted pupils; may inhibit ejaculation; avoid cough, cold or allergy medications containing sympathomimetics

Nursing Implications Monitor for orthostasis; assist with ambulation

Dosage Forms Capsule, as hydrochloride: 10 mg

Phenoxybenzamine Hydrochloride *see* Phenoxybenzamine *on previous page*

Phenoxymethyl Penicillin *see* Penicillin V Potassium *on page 965*

Phentermine (FEN ter meen)

Brand Names Adipex-P®; Fastin®; Ionamin®; Zantryl®

Canadian/Mexican Brand Names Diminex® (Mexico)

Synonyms Phentermine Hydrochloride

Therapeutic Category Anorexiant

Use Short-term adjunct in exogenous obesity

Restrictions C-IV

Pregnancy Risk Factor C

Contraindications Known hypersensitivity to phentermine

Warnings/Precautions Do not use in children <12 years of age; use with caution in patients with diabetes mellitus, cardiovascular disease, nephritis, angina pectoris, hypertension, glaucoma, patients with a history of drug abuse

Adverse Reactions

>10%:

Cardiovascular: Hypertension

Central nervous system: Euphoria, nervousness, insomnia

1% to 10%:

Central nervous system: Confusion, mental depression, restlessness

Gastrointestinal: Nausea, vomiting, constipation

Endocrine & metabolic: Changes in libido

Hematologic: Blood dyscrasias

Neuromuscular & skeletal: Tremor

Ocular: Blurred vision

<1%:

Cardiovascular: Tachycardia, arrhythmias

Central nervous system: Insomnia, restlessness, nervousness, depression, headache

Dermatologic: Alopecia

Gastrointestinal: Nausea, vomiting, diarrhea, abdominal cramps

Genitourinary: Dysuria, polyuria

Neuromuscular & skeletal: Myalgia, tremor

Respiratory: Dyspnea

Miscellaneous: Diaphoresis (increased)

Overdosage/Toxicology Symptoms of overdose include hyperactivity, agitation, hyperthermia, hypertension, seizures

There is no specific antidote for phentermine intoxication and the bulk of the treatment is supportive. Hyperactivity and agitation usually respond to reduced sensory input, however with extreme agitation haloperidol (2-5 mg I.M. for adults)

(Continued)

Phentermine *(Continued)*

may be required. Hyperthermia is best treated with external cooling measures, or when severe or unresponsive, muscle paralysis with pancuronium may be needed. Hypertension is usually transient and generally does not require treatment unless severe. For diastolic blood pressures >110 mm Hg, a nitroprusside infusion should be initiated. Seizures usually respond to diazepam IVP and/or phenytoin maintenance regimens.

Drug Interactions

Decreased effect of guanethidine; decreased effect with CNS depressants

Increased effect/toxicity with MAO inhibitors (hypertensive crisis), sympathomimetics, CNS stimulants

Mechanism of Action Phentermine is structurally similar to dextroamphetamine and is comparable to dextroamphetamine as an appetite suppressant, but is generally associated with a lower incidence and severity of CNS side effects. Phentermine, like other anorexiants, stimulates the hypothalamus to result in decreased appetite; anorexiant effects are most likely mediated via norepinephrine and dopamine metabolism. However, other CNS effects or metabolic effects may be involved.

Pharmacodynamics/Kinetics

Absorption: Well absorbed; resin absorbed slower and produces more prolonged clinical effects

Half-life: 20 hours

Elimination: Primarily unchanged in urine

Usual Dosage Oral:

Children 3-15 years: 5-15 mg/day for 4 weeks

Adults: 8 mg 3 times/day 30 minutes before meals or food or 15-37.5 mg/day before breakfast or 10-14 hours before retiring

Monitoring Parameters CNS

Patient Information Take during day to avoid insomnia; do not discontinue abruptly, may cause physical and psychological dependence with prolonged use

Nursing Implications Dose should not be given in evening or at bedtime

Dosage Forms

Capsule, as hydrochloride: 15 mg, 18.75 mg, 30 mg, 37.5 mg

Capsule, resin complex, as hydrochloride: 15 mg, 30 mg

Tablet, as hydrochloride: 8 mg, 37.5 mg

Phentermine Hydrochloride *see* Phentermine *on previous page*

Phentolamine (fen TOLE a meen)

Related Information

Extravasation Treatment of Other Drugs *on page 1381*

Therapy of Hypertension *on page 1540*

Brand Names Regitine®

Canadian/Mexican Brand Names Rogitine® (Canada)

Synonyms Phentolamine Mesylate

Therapeutic Category Alpha-Adrenergic Blocking Agent, Parenteral; Antidote, Extravasation; Antihypertensive; Diagnostic Agent, Pheochromocytoma

Use Diagnosis of pheochromocytoma and treatment of hypertension associated with pheochromocytoma or other caused by excess sympathomimetic amines; as treatment of dermal necrosis after extravasation of drugs with alpha-adrenergic effects (norepinephrine, dopamine, epinephrine, dobutamine)

Pregnancy Risk Factor C

Contraindications Hypersensitivity to phentolamine or any component; renal impairment; coronary or cerebral arteriosclerosis

Warnings/Precautions Myocardial infarction, cerebrovascular spasm and cerebrovascular occlusion have occurred following administration; use with caution in patients with gastritis or peptic ulcer, tachycardia, or a history of cardiac arrhythmias

Adverse Reactions

>10%:

Cardiovascular: Hypotension, tachycardia, arrhythmias, reflex tachycardia, anginal pain, orthostatic hypotension

Gastrointestinal: Nausea, vomiting, diarrhea, exacerbation of peptic ulcer, abdominal pain

Respiratory: Nasal congestion

1% to 10%:

Cardiovascular: Flushing of face, syncope

Central nervous system: Dizziness

Neuromuscular & skeletal: Weakness

Respiratory: Nasal congestion

<1%:

Cardiovascular: Myocardial infarction

Central nervous system: Severe headache
Miscellaneous: Exacerbation of peptic ulcer

Overdosage/Toxicology Symptoms of overdose include tachycardia, shock, vomiting, dizziness

Hypotension and shock should be treated with fluids and by placing the patient in the Trendelenburg position; only alpha-adrenergic pressors such as norepinephrine should be used; mixed agents such as epinephrine, may cause more hypotension. Take care not to cause so much swelling of the extremity or digit that a compartment syndrome occurs.

Drug Interactions
Decreased effect: Epinephrine, ephedrine
Increased toxicity: Ethanol (disulfiram reaction)

Stability Reconstituted solution is stable for 48 hours at room temperature and 1 week when refrigerated

Mechanism of Action Competitively blocks alpha-adrenergic receptors to produce brief antagonism of circulating epinephrine and norepinephrine to reduce hypertension caused by alpha effects of these catecholamines; also has a positive inotropic and chronotropic effect on the heart

Pharmacodynamics/Kinetics
Onset of action:
I.M.: Within 15-20 minutes
I.V.: Immediate
Duration:
I.M.: 30-45 minutes
I.V.: 15-30 minutes
Metabolism: In the liver
Half-life: 19 minutes
Elimination: Urine (10% as unchanged drug)

Usual Dosage
Treatment of alpha-adrenergic drug extravasation: S.C.:
Children: 0.1-0.2 mg/kg diluted in 10 mL 0.9% sodium chloride infiltrated into area of extravasation within 12 hours
Adults: Infiltrate area with small amount of solution made by diluting 5-10 mg in 10 mL 0.9% sodium chloride within 12 hours of extravasation
If dose is effective, normal skin color should return to the blanched area within 1 hour

Diagnosis of pheochromocytoma: I.M., I.V.:
Children: 0.05-0.1 mg/kg/dose, maximum single dose: 5 mg
Adults: 5 mg

Surgery for pheochromocytoma: Hypertension: I.M., I.V.:
Children: 0.05-0.1 mg/kg/dose given 1-2 hours before procedure; repeat as needed every 2-4 hours until hypertension is controlled; maximum single dose: 5 mg
Adults: 5 mg given 1-2 hours before procedure and repeated as needed every 2-4 hours

Hypertensive crisis: Adults: 5-20 mg

Administration Infiltrate the area of dopamine extravasation with multiple small injections using only 27- or 30-gauge needles and changing the needle between each skin entry; take care not to cause so much swelling of the extremity or digit that a compartment syndrome occurs

Monitoring Parameters Blood pressure, heart rate

Test Interactions ↑ LFTs rarely

Nursing Implications Monitor patient for orthostasis; assist with ambulation

Dosage Forms Injection, as mesylate: 5 mg/mL (1 mL)

Phentolamine Mesylate *see* Phentolamine *on previous page*

Phenylalanine Mustard *see* Melphalan *on page 776*

Phenylazo Diamino Pyridine Hydrochloride *see* Phenazopyridine *on page 981*

Phenylephrine (fen il EF rin)

Related Information
Adrenergic Agonists, Cardiovascular Comparison *on page 1385*
Extravasation Treatment of Other Drugs *on page 1381*

Brand Names AK-Dilate® Ophthalmic Solution; AK-Nefrin® Ophthalmic Solution; Alconefrin® Nasal Solution [OTC]; Doktors® Nasal Solution [OTC]; I-Phrine® Ophthalmic Solution; Isopto® Frin Ophthalmic Solution; Mydfrin® Ophthalmic Solution; Neo-Synephrine® Nasal Solution [OTC]; Neo-Synephrine® Ophthalmic Solution; Nostril® Nasal Solution [OTC]; Prefrin™ Ophthalmic Solution; Relief® Ophthalmic Solution; Rhinall® Nasal Solution [OTC]; Sinarest® Nasal Solution [OTC]; St. Joseph® Measured Dose Nasal Solution [OTC]; Vicks® Sinex® Nasal Solution [OTC]

(Continued)

Phenylephrine *(Continued)*

Canadian/Mexican Brand Names Dionephrine® (Canada); Novahistine® Decongstant (Canada); Prefrin™ Liquifilm®

Synonyms Phenylephrine Hydrochloride

Therapeutic Category Adrenergic Agonist Agent; Adrenergic Agonist Agent, Ophthalmic; Alpha-Adrenergic Agonist; Nasal Agent, Vasoconstrictor; Ophthalmic Agent, Mydriatic; Sympathomimetic

Use Treatment of hypotension, vascular failure in shock; as a vasoconstrictor in regional analgesia; symptomatic relief of nasal and nasopharyngeal mucosal congestion; as a mydriatic in ophthalmic procedures and treatment of wide-angle glaucoma; supraventricular tachycardia

Pregnancy Risk Factor C

Contraindications Pheochromocytoma, severe hypertension, bradycardia, ventricular tachyarrhythmias; hypersensitivity to phenylephrine or any component; narrow-angle glaucoma (ophthalmic preparation), acute pancreatitis, hepatitis, peripheral or mesenteric vascular thrombosis, myocardial disease, severe coronary disease

Warnings/Precautions Injection may contain sulfites which may cause allergic reaction in some patients; do not use if solution turns brown or contains a precipitate; use with extreme caution in elderly patients, patients with hyperthyroidism, bradycardia, partial heart block, myocardial disease, or severe arteriosclerosis; infuse into large veins to help prevent extravasation which may cause severe necrosis; the 10% ophthalmic solution has caused increased blood pressure in elderly patients and its use should, therefore, be avoided

Adverse Reactions

Nasal:
- >10%: Burning, rebound congestion, sneezing
- 1% to 10%: Stinging, dryness

Ophthalmic:
- >10%: Transient stinging
- 1% to 10%:
  - Central nervous system: Headache, browache
  - Ocular: Blurred vision, photophobia, lacrimation

Systemic:
- >10%: Neuromuscular & skeletal: Tremor
- 1% to 10%:
  - Cardiovascular: Peripheral vasoconstriction hypertension, angina, reflex bradycardia, arrhythmias
  - Central nervous system: Restlessness, excitability

Overdosage/Toxicology Symptoms of overdose include vomiting, hypertension, palpitations, paresthesia, ventricular extrasystoles

Treatment is supportive; in extreme cases, I.V. phentolamine may be used

Drug Interactions

Decreased effect: With alpha- and beta-adrenergic blocking agents

Increased effect: With oxytocic drugs

Increased toxicity: With sympathomimetics, tachycardia or arrhythmias may occur; with MAO inhibitors, actions may be potentiated

Stability Is stable for 48 hours in 5% dextrose in water at pH 3.5-7.5; do not use brown colored solutions

Mechanism of Action Potent, direct-acting alpha-adrenergic stimulator with weak beta-adrenergic activity; causes vasoconstriction of the arterioles of the nasal mucosa and conjunctiva; activates the dilator muscle of the pupil to cause contraction; produces vasoconstriction of arterioles in the body; produces systemic arterial vasoconstriction

Pharmacodynamics/Kinetics

Onset of effect:
- I.M., S.C.: Within 10-15 minutes
- I.V.: Immediate

Duration:
- I.M.: 30 minutes to 2 hours
- I.V.: 15-30 minutes
- S.C.: 1 hour

Metabolism: To phenolic conjugates; metabolized in liver and intestine by monoamine oxidase

Half-life: 2.5 hours

Elimination: Urine (90%)

Usual Dosage

Ophthalmic procedures:
- Infants <1 year: Instill 1 drop of 2.5% 15-30 minutes before procedures
- Children and Adults: Instill 1 drop of 2.5% or 10% solution, may repeat in 10-60 minutes as needed

Nasal decongestant: (therapy should not exceed 5 continuous days)

Children:

2-6 years: Instill 1 drop every 2-4 hours of 0.125% solution as needed

6-12 years: Instill 1-2 sprays or instill 1-2 drops every 4 hours of 0.25% solution as needed

Children >12 years and Adults: Instill 1-2 sprays or instill 1-2 drops every 4 hours of 0.25% to 0.5% solution as needed; 1% solution may be used in adult in cases of extreme nasal congestion; do not use nasal solutions more than 3 days

Hypotension/shock:

Children:

I.M., S.C.: 0.1 mg/kg/dose every 1-2 hours as needed (maximum: 5 mg)

I.V. bolus: 5-20 mcg/kg/dose every 10-15 minutes as needed

I.V. infusion: 0.1-0.5 mcg/kg/minute

Adults:

I.M., S.C.: 2-5 mg/dose every 1-2 hours as needed (initial dose should not exceed 5 mg)

I.V. bolus: 0.1-0.5 mg/dose every 10-15 minutes as needed (initial dose should not exceed 0.5 mg)

I.V. infusion: 10 mg in 250 mL D_5W or NS (1:25,000 dilution) (40 mcg/mL); start at 100-180 mcg/minute (2-5 mL/minute; 50-90 drops/minute) initially; when blood pressure is stabilized, maintenance rate: 40-60 mcg/minute (20-30 drops/minute)

Paroxysmal supraventricular tachycardia: I.V.:

Children: 5-10 mcg/kg/dose over 20-30 seconds

Adults: 0.25-0.5 mg/dose over 20-30 seconds

Administration Concentration and rate of infusion can be calculated using the following formulas: Dilute 0.6 mg x weight (kg) to 100 mL; then the dose in mcg/kg/minute = 0.1 x the infusion rate in mL/hour

Monitoring Parameters Blood pressure, heart rate, arterial blood gases, central venous pressure

Patient Information Nasal decongestant should not be used for >3 days in a row, hereby reducing problems of rebound congestion; notify physician of insomnia, dizziness, tremor, or irregular heartbeat; if symptoms do not improve within 7 days or are accompanied by signs of infection, consult physician

Nursing Implications May cause necrosis or sloughing tissue if extravasation occurs during I.V. administration or S.C. administration

Extravasation: Use phentolamine as antidote; mix 5 mg with 9 mL of NS; inject a small amount of this dilution into extravasated area; blanching should reverse immediately. Monitor site; if blanching should recur, additional injections of phentolamine may be needed.

Dosage Forms

Injection, as hydrochloride (Neo-Synephrine®): 1% [10 mg/mL] (1 mL)

Nasal solution, as hydrochloride:

Drops:

Neo-Synephrine®: 0.125% (15 mL)

Alconefrin® 12: 0.16% (30 mL)

Alconefrin® 25, Neo-Synephrine®, Children's Nostril®, Rhinall®: 0.25% (15 mL, 30 mL, 40 mL)

Alconefrin®, Neo-Synephrine®: 0.5% (15 mL, 30 mL)

Spray:

Alconefrin® 25, Neo-Synephrine®, Rhinall®: 0.25% (15 mL, 30 mL, 40 mL)

Neo-Synephrine®, Nostril®, Sinex®: 0.5% (15 mL, 30 mL)

Neo-Synephrine®: 1% (15 mL)

Ophthalmic solution, as hydrochloride:

AK-Nefrin®, Isopto® Frin, Prefrin™ Liquifilm®, Relief®: 0.12% (0.3 mL, 15 mL, 20 mL)

AK-Dilate®, Mydfrin®, Neo-Synephrine®, Phenoptic®: 2.5% (2 mL, 3 mL, 5 mL, 15 mL)

AK-Dilate®, Neo-Synephrine®, Neo-Synephrine® Viscous: 10% (1 mL, 2 mL, 5 mL, 15 mL)

Phenylephrine Hydrochloride *see* Phenylephrine *on page 989*

Phenylethylmalonylurea *see* Phenobarbital *on page 984*

Phenylisohydantoin *see* Pemoline *on page 958*

Phenylpropanolamine (fen il proe pa NOLE a meen)

Brand Names Acutrim® Precision Release® [OTC]; Control® [OTC]; Dex-A-Diet® [OTC]; Dexatrim® [OTC]; Maigret-50; Prolamine® [OTC]; Propadrine; Propagest® [OTC]; Rhindecon®; Stay Trim® Diet Gum [OTC]; Westrim® LA [OTC]

Synonyms *dl*-Norephedrine Hydrochloride; Phenylpropanolamine Hydrochloride; PPA

Therapeutic Category Adrenergic Agonist Agent; Anorexiant; Decongestant, Sympathomimetic

(Continued)

Phenylpropanolamine *(Continued)*

Use Anorexiant; nasal decongestant

Pregnancy Risk Factor C

Contraindications Known hypersensitivity to drug

Warnings/Precautions Use with caution in patients with high blood pressure, tachyarrhythmias, pheochromocytoma, bradycardia, cardiac disease, arteriosclerosis; do not use for more than 3 weeks for weight loss

Adverse Reactions

>10%: Cardiovascular: Hypertension, palpitations

1% to 10%:

Central nervous system: Insomnia, restlessness, dizziness

Gastrointestinal: Xerostomia, nausea

<1%:

Cardiovascular: Tightness in chest, bradycardia, arrhythmias, angina

Central nervous system: Severe headache, anxiety, nervousness, restlessness

Genitourinary: Dysuria

Overdosage/Toxicology Symptoms of overdose include vomiting, hypertension, palpitations, paresthesia, excitation, seizures

Treatment is supportive; diazepam 5-10 mg I.V. (0.25-0.4 mg/kg for children) may be used for excitation and seizures

Drug Interactions

Decreased effect of antihypertensives

Increased effect/toxicity with MAO inhibitors (hypertensive crisis), beta-blockers (increased pressor effects)

Mechanism of Action Releases tissue stores of epinephrine and thereby produces an alpha- and beta-adrenergic stimulation; this causes vasoconstriction and nasal mucosa blanching; also appears to depress central appetite centers

Pharmacodynamics/Kinetics

Absorption: Oral: Well absorbed

Metabolism: In the liver to norephedrine

Bioavailability: Close to 100%

Half-life: 4.6-6.6 hours

Elimination: In urine primarily as unchanged drug (80% to 90%)

Usual Dosage Oral:

Children: Decongestant:

2-6 years: 6.25 mg every 4 hours

6-12 years: 12.5 mg every 4 hours not to exceed 75 mg/day

Adults:

Decongestant: 25 mg every 4 hours or 50 mg every 8 hours, not to exceed 150 mg/day

Anorexic: 25 mg 3 times/day 30 minutes before meals or 75 mg (timed release) once daily in the morning

Precision release: 75 mg after breakfast

Monitoring Parameters Blood pressure, heart rate

Patient Information Should not be used more than 3 consecutive weeks for weight loss; contact physician for insomnia, tremor, or irregular heartbeat

Nursing Implications Administer dose early in day to prevent insomnia; observe for signs of nervousness, excitability

Dosage Forms

Capsule, as hydrochloride: 37.5 mg

Capsule, as hydrochloride, timed release: 25 mg, 75 mg

Tablet, as hydrochloride: 25 mg

Tablet, as hydrochloride:

Precision release: 75 mg

Timed release: 75 mg

Phenylpropanolamine Hydrochloride *see* Phenylpropanolamine *on previous page*

Phenytoin (FEN i toyn)

Related Information

Antacid Drug Interactions *on page 1388*

Anticonvulsants by Seizure Type *on page 1392*

Convulsive Status Epilepticus *on page 1528*

Epilepsy Treatment *on page 1531*

Extravasation Treatment of Other Drugs *on page 1381*

Brand Names Dilantin®; Diphenylan Sodium®

Canadian/Mexican Brand Names Tremytoine® (Canada)

Synonyms Diphenylhydantoin; DPH; Phenytoin Sodium; Phenytoin Sodium, Extended; Phenytoin Sodium, Prompt

Therapeutic Category Antiarrhythmic Agent, Class I-B; Anticonvulsant

Use Management of generalized tonic-clonic (grand mal), simple partial and complex partial seizures; prevention of seizures following head trauma/neurosurgery; ventricular arrhythmias, including those associated with digitalis intoxication, prolonged Q-T interval and surgical repair of congenital heart diseases in children; also used for epidermolysis bullosa

Pregnancy Risk Factor D

Pregnancy/Breast-Feeding Implications

Clinical effects on the fetus: Crosses the placenta. Cardiac defects and multiple other malformations reported; characteristic pattern of malformations called "fetal hydantoin syndrome"; hemorrhagic disease of newborn due to fetal vitamin K depletion, maternal folic acid deficiency may occur. Epilepsy itself, number of medications, genetic factors, or a combination of these probably influence the teratogenicity of anticonvulsant therapy. Benefit:risk ratio usually favors continued use during pregnancy and breast-feeding.

Breast-feeding/lactation: Crosses into breast milk

Clinical effects on the infant: Methemoglobinemia, drowsiness and decreased sucking reported in 1 case. American Academy of Pediatrics considers COMPATIBLE with breast-feeding.

Contraindications Hypersensitivity to phenytoin, other hydantoins, or any component; heart block, sinus bradycardia

Warnings/Precautions May increase frequency of petit mal seizures; I.V. form may cause hypotension, skin necrosis at I.V. site; avoid I.V. administration in small veins; use with caution in patients with porphyria; discontinue if rash or lymphadenopathy occurs; use with caution in patients with hepatic dysfunction, sinus bradycardia, S-A block, A-V block, or hepatic impairment; elderly may have reduced hepatic clearance and low albumin levels, which will increase the free fraction of phenytoin in the serum and, therefore, the pharmacologic response

Adverse Reactions I.V. effects: Hypotension, bradycardia, cardiac arrhythmias, cardiovascular collapse (especially with rapid I.V. use), venous irritation and pain, thrombophlebitis

Effects not related to plasma phenytoin concentrations: Hypertrichosis, gingival hypertrophy, thickening of facial features, carbohydrate intolerance, folic acid deficiency, peripheral neuropathy, vitamin D deficiency, osteomalacia, systemic lupus erythematosus

Dose-related effects: Nystagmus, blurred vision, diplopia, ataxia, slurred speech, dizziness, drowsiness, lethargy, coma, rash, fever, nausea, vomiting, gum tenderness, confusion, mood changes, folic acid depletion, osteomalacia, hyperglycemia

Related to elevated concentrations:

- >20 mcg/mL: Far lateral nystagmus
- >30 mcg/mL: 45° lateral gaze nystagmus and ataxia
- >40 mcg/mL: Decreased mentation
- >100 mcg/mL: Death

>10%:

- Central nervous system: Psychiatric changes, slurred speech, dizziness, drowsiness
- Gastrointestinal: Constipation, nausea, vomiting, gingival hyperplasia
- Neuromuscular & skeletal: Trembling

1% to 10%:

- Central nervous system: Headache, insomnia
- Dermatologic: Rash
- Gastrointestinal: Anorexia, weight loss
- Hematologic: Leukopenia
- Hepatic: Hepatitis
- Renal: Increase in serum creatinine

<1%:

- Cardiovascular: Hypotension, bradycardia, cardiac arrhythmias, cardiovascular collapse
- Central nervous system: Confusion, fever, ataxia
- Local: Thrombophlebitis
- Neuromuscular & skeletal: Peripheral neuropathy, paresthesia
- Ocular: Diplopia, nystagmus, blurred vision

Rarely seen effects: SLE-like syndrome, lymphadenopathy, hepatitis, Stevens-Johnson syndrome, blood dyscrasias, dyskinesias, pseudolymphoma, lymphoma

Miscellaneous: Venous irritation and pain

Overdosage/Toxicology Symptoms of overdose include unsteady gait, slurred speech, confusion, nausea, hypothermia, fever, hypotension, respiratory depression, coma

Treatment is supportive for hypotension; treat with I.V. fluids and place patient in Trendelenburg position; seizures may be controlled with diazepam 5-10 mg (0.25-0.4 mg/kg in children)

(Continued)

ʼhenytoin *(Continued)*

Drug Interactions

Inducer of cytochrome P-450 2B6 and cytochrome P-450 3A enzymes
Cytochrome P-450 2C enzyme substrate

Decreased effect: Rifampin, cisplatin, vinblastine, bleomycin, folic acid, continuous NG feedings

Absorption is impaired when phenytoin suspension is given concurrently to patients who are receiving continuous nasogastric feedings, discontinuation of enteral feedings results in a marked increase in phenytoin concentrations. A method to resolve this interaction is to divide the daily dose of phenytoin and withhold the administration of nutritional supplements for 1-2 hours before and after each phenytoin dose.

Decreased effect/toxicity of valproic acid, ethosuximide, primidone, warfarin, oral contraceptives, corticosteroids, cyclosporine, theophylline, chloramphenicol, rifampin, doxycycline, quinidine, mexiletine, disopyramide, dopamine, nondepolarizing skeletal muscle relaxants

Increased toxicity: Amiodarone decreases metabolism of phenytoin; disulfiram decreases metabolism of phenytoin; fluconazole, itraconazole increases phenytoin serum concentrations; isoniazid may increase phenytoin serum concentrations

Stability

Phenytoin is stable as long as it remains free of haziness and precipitation

Use only clear solutions; parenteral solution may be used as long as there is no precipitate and it is not hazy, slightly yellowed solution may be used

Refrigeration may cause precipitate, sometimes the precipitate is resolved by allowing the solution to reach room temperature again

Drug may precipitate at a pH <11.5

May dilute with normal saline for I.V. infusion; stability is concentration dependent

Standard diluent: Dose/100 mL NS

Minimum volume: Concentration should be maintained at 1-10 mg/mL secondary to stability problems (stable for 4 hours)

Comments: Maximum rate of infusion: 50 mg/minute

IVPB dose should be administered via an in-line 0.22-5 micron filter because of high potential for precipitation I.V. form is highly **incompatible** with many drugs and solutions such as dextrose in water, some saline solutions, amikacin, bretylium, dobutamine, cephapirin, insulin, levorphanol, lidocaine, meperidine, metaraminol, morphine, norepinephrine, heparin, potassium chloride, vitamin B complex with C

Mechanism of Action Stabilizes neuronal membranes and decreases seizure activity by increasing efflux or decreasing influx of sodium ions across cell membranes in the motor cortex during generation of nerve impulses; prolongs effective refractory period and suppresses ventricular pacemaker automaticity, shortens action potential in the heart

Pharmacodynamics/Kinetics

Absorption: Oral: Slow

Distribution: V_d:

- Neonates:
- Premature: 1-1.2 L/kg
- Full-term: 0.8-0.9 L/kg
- Infants: 0.7-0.8 L/kg
- Children: 0.7 L/kg
- Adults: 0.6-0.7 L/kg

Protein binding:

- Neonates: Up to 20% free
- Infants: Up to 15% free
- Adults: 90% to 95%
- Others: Increased free fraction (decreased protein binding)
- Patients with hyperbilirubinemia, hypoalbuminemia, uremia **(see table)**

Metabolism: Follows dose-dependent capacity-limited (Michaelis-Menten) pharmacokinetics with increased V_{max} in infants >6 months of age and children versus adults

Disease States Resulting in a Decrease in Serum Albumin Concentration	Disease States Resulting in an Apparent Decrease in Affinity of Phenytoin for Serum Albumin
Burns Hepatic cirrhosis Nephrotic syndrome Pregnancy Cystic fibrosis	Renal failure Cl_{cr} <25 mL/min (unbound fraction is increased 2-3 fold in uremia) Jaundice (severe) Other drugs (displacers) Hyperbilirubinemia (total bilirubin >15 mg/dL)

Bioavailability: Dependent upon formulation administered

Time to peak serum concentration (dependent upon formulation administered):

Oral:

Extended-release capsule: Within 4-12 hours

Immediate release preparation: Within 2-3 hours

Elimination: Highly variable clearance dependent upon intrinsic hepatic function and dose administered; increased clearance and decreased serum concentrations with febrile illness; <5% excreted unchanged in urine; major metabolite (via oxidation) HPPA undergoes enterohepatic recycling and elimination in urine as glucuronides

Usual Dosage

Status epilepticus: I.V.:

Infants and Children: Loading dose: 15-20 mg/kg in a single or divided dose; maintenance dose: Initial: 5 mg/kg/day in 2 divided doses, usual doses:

6 months to 3 years: 8-10 mg/kg/day

4-6 years: 7.5-9 mg/kg/day

7-9 years: 7-8 mg/kg/day

10-16 years: 6-7 mg/kg/day, some patients may require every 8 hours dosing

Adults: Loading dose: 15-20 mg/kg in a single or divided dose, followed by 100-150 mg/dose at 30-minute intervals up to a maximum of 1500 mg/24 hours; maintenance dose: 300 mg/day or 5-6 mg/kg/day in 3 divided doses or 1-2 divided doses using extended release

Anticonvulsant: Children and Adults: Oral:

Loading dose: 15-20 mg/kg; based on phenytoin serum concentrations and recent dosing history; administer oral loading dose in 3 divided doses given every 2-4 hours to decrease GI adverse effects and to ensure complete oral absorption; maintenance dose: same as I.V.

Dosing adjustment/comments in renal impairment or hepatic disease: Safe in usual doses in mild liver disease; clearance may be substantially reduced in cirrhosis and plasma level monitoring with dose adjustment advisable. Free phenytoin levels should be monitored closely.

Dietary Considerations

Alcohol: Additive CNS depression has been reported with hydantoins

Alcohol (acute use): Inhibits metabolism of phenytoin; avoid or limit use; watch for sedation

Alcohol (chronic use): Stimulates metabolism of phenytoin; avoid or limit use

Food:

Folic acid: Low erythrocyte and CSF folate concentrations. Phenytoin may decrease mucosal uptake of folic acid; to avoid folic acid deficiency and megaloblastic anemia, some clinicians recommend giving patients on anticonvulsants prophylactic doses of folic acid and cyanocobalamin.

Calcium: Hypocalcemia has been reported in patients taking prolonged high-dose therapy with an anticonvulsant. Phenytoin may decrease calcium absorption. Monitor calcium serum concentration and for bone disorders (eg, rickets, osteomalacia). Some clinicians have given an additional 4,000 Units/week of vitamin D (especially in those receiving poor nutrition and getting no sun exposure) to prevent hypocalcemia.

Fresh fruits containing vitamin C: Displaces drug from binding sites, resulting in increased urinary excretion of hydantoin. Educate patients regarding the potential for a decreased anticonvulsant effect of hydantoins with consumption of foods high in vitamin C.

Vitamin D: Phenytoin interferes with vitamin D metabolism and osteomalacia may result; may need to supplement with vitamin D

Glucose: Hyperglycemia and glycosuria may occur in patients receiving high-dose therapy. Monitor blood glucose concentration, especially in patients with impaired renal function.

Tube feedings: Tube feedings decrease phenytoin bioavailability; to avoid decreased serum levels with continuous NG feeds, hold feedings for 2 hours prior to and 2 hours after phenytoin administration, if possible. There is a variety of opinions on how to administer phenytoin with enteral feedings. BE CONSISTENT throughout therapy.

Administration

Phenytoin may be administered by IVP or IVPB administration

I.M. administration is not recommended due to erratic absorption, pain on injection and precipitation of drug at injection site

S.C. administration is not recommended because of the possibility of local tissue damage

The maximum rate of I.V. administration is 50 mg/minute; highly sensitive patients (eg, elderly, patients with pre-existing cardiovascular conditions) should receive phenytoin more slowly (eg, 20 mg/minute)

An in-line 0.22-5 micron filter is recommended for IVPB solutions due to the high potential for precipitation of the solution; avoid extravasation; following I.V.

(Continued)

Phenytoin *(Continued)*

administration, NS should be injected through the same needle or I.V. catheter to prevent irritation

Monitoring Parameters Blood pressure, vital signs (with I.V. use), plasma phenytoin level, CBC, liver function tests

Reference Range

Therapeutic range:

Total phenytoin: 10-20 μg/mL (children and adults), 8-15 μg/mL (neonates)

Concentrations of 5-10 μg/mL may be therapeutic for some patients but concentrations <5 μg/mL are not likely to be effective

50% of patients show decreased frequency of seizures at concentrations >10 μg/mL

86% of patients show decreased frequency of seizures at concentrations >15 μg/mL

Add another anticonvulsant if satisfactory therapeutic response is not achieved with a phenytoin concentration of 20 μg/mL

Free phenytoin: 1-2.5 μg/mL

Toxic: <30-50 μg/mL (SI: <120-200 μmol/L)

Lethal: >100 μg/mL (SI: >400 μmol/L)

Adjustment of Serum Concentration in Patients With Low Serum Albumin

Measured Total Phenytoin Concentration (mcg/mL)	Patient's Serum Albumin (g/dL)			
	3.5	3	2.5	2
	Adjusted Total Phenytoin Concentration (mcg/mL)*			
5	6	7	8	10
10	13	14	17	20
15	19	21	25	30

*Adjusted concentration = measured total concentration ÷ [(0.2 x albumin) + 0.1].

Adjustment of Serum Concentration in Patients With Renal Failure (Cl_{cr} ≤10 mL/min) (Product Information From Parke-Davis)

Measured Total Phenytoin Concentration (mcg/mL)	Patient's Serum Albumin (g/dL)				
	4	3.5	3	2.5	2
	Adjusted Total Phenytoin Concentration (mcg/mL)*				
5	10	11	13	14	17
10	20	22	25	29	33
15	30	33	38	43	50

*Adjusted concentration = measured total concentration ÷ [(0.1 x albumin) + 0.1].

Test Interactions ↑ glucose, alkaline phosphatase (S); ↓ thyroxine (S), calcium (S)

Patient Information Shake oral suspension well prior to each dose; do not change brand or dosage form without consulting physician; do not skip doses, may cause drowsiness, dizziness, ataxia, loss of coordination or judgment; take with food; maintain good oral hygiene

Additional Information

Phenytoin: Dilantin® chewable tablet and oral suspension

Phenytoin sodium, extended: Dilantin® Kapseal®

Phenytoin sodium, prompt: Diphenylan Sodium® capsule

Sodium content of 1 g injection: 88 mg (3.8 mEq)

Dosage Forms

Capsule, as sodium:

Extended: 30 mg, 100 mg

Prompt: 30 mg, 100 mg

Injection, as sodium: 50 mg/mL (2 mL, 5 mL)

Suspension, oral: 30 mg/5 mL (5 mL, 240 mL); 125 mg/5 mL (5 mL, 240 mL)

Tablet, chewable: 50 mg

Phenytoin Sodium *see* Phenytoin *on page 992*

Phenytoin Sodium, Extended *see* Phenytoin *on page 992*

Phenytoin Sodium, Prompt *see* Phenytoin *on page 992*

Phicon® [OTC] *see* Pramoxine *on page 1033*

Phillips'® Milk of Magnesia [OTC] *see* Magnesium Hydroxide *on page 753*

pHisoHex® *see* Hexachlorophene *on page 610*
Phos-Ex® *see* Calcium Acetate *on page 184*
Phos-Flur® *see* Fluoride *on page 536*
PhosLo® *see* Calcium Acetate *on page 184*
Phosphate, Potassium *see* Potassium Phosphate *on page 1029*
Phospholine Iodide® *see* Echothiophate Iodide *on page 436*
Phosphonoformate *see* Foscarnet *on page 554*
Phosphonoformic Acid *see* Foscarnet *on page 554*
3-Phosphoryloxymethyl Phenytoin Disodium *see* Fosphenytoin *on page 558*
Photofrin® *see* Porfimer *on page 1020*
Phrenilin® *see* Butalbital Compound *on page 176*
Phrenilin® Forte *see* Butalbital Compound *on page 176*
***p*-Hydroxyampicillin** *see* Amoxicillin *on page 77*
Phyllocontin® *see* Theophylline Salts *on page 1207*
Phylloquinone *see* Phytonadione *on next page*

Physostigmine (fye zoe STIG meen)

Related Information
Glaucoma Drug Therapy Comparison *on page 1410*

Brand Names Antilirium®; Isopto® Eserine

Synonyms Eserine Salicylate; Physostigmine Salicylate; Physostigmine Sulfate

Therapeutic Category Antidote, Anticholinergic Agent; Antidote, Belladonna Alkaloids; Cholinergic Agent; Cholinergic Agent, Ophthalmic; Ophthalmic Agent, Miotic

Use Reverse toxic CNS effects caused by anticholinergic drugs; used as miotic in treatment of glaucoma

Pregnancy Risk Factor C

Contraindications Hypersensitivity to physostigmine or any component; GI or GU obstruction; physostigmine therapy of drug intoxications should be used with extreme caution in patients with asthma, gangrene, severe cardiovascular disease, or mechanical obstruction of the GI tract or urogenital tract. In these patients, physostigmine should be used only to treat life-threatening conditions.

Warnings/Precautions Use with caution in patients with epilepsy, asthma, diabetes, gangrene, cardiovascular disease, bradycardia. Discontinue if excessive salivation or emesis, frequent urination or diarrhea occur. Reduce dosage if excessive sweating or nausea occurs. Administer I.V. slowly or at a controlled rate not faster than 1 mg/minute. Due to the possibility of hypersensitivity or overdose/cholinergic crisis, atropine should be readily available; ointment may delay corneal healing, may cause loss of dark adaptation; not intended as a first-line agent for anticholinergic toxicity or Parkinson's disease.

Adverse Reactions

Ophthalmic:
- >10%:
  - Ocular: Lacrimation, marked miosis, blurred vision, eye pain
  - Miscellaneous: Diaphoresis
- 1% to 10%:
  - Central nervous system: Headache, browache
  - Dermatologic: Burning, redness

Systemic:
- >10%:
  - Gastrointestinal: Nausea, salivation, diarrhea, stomach pains
  - Ocular: Lacrimation
  - Miscellaneous: Diaphoresis
- 1% to 10%:
  - Cardiovascular: Palpitations, bradycardia
  - Central nervous system: Restlessness, nervousness, hallucinations, seizures
  - Genitourinary: Frequent urge to urinate
  - Neuromuscular & skeletal: Muscle twitching
  - Ocular: Miosis
  - Respiratory: Dyspnea, bronchospasm, respiratory paralysis, pulmonary edema

Overdosage/Toxicology Symptoms of overdose include muscle weakness, blurred vision, excessive sweating, tearing and salivation, nausea, vomiting, bronchospasm, seizures

If physostigmine is used in excess or in the absence of an anticholinergic overdose, patients may manifest signs of cholinergic toxicity. At this point a cholinergic agent (eg, atropine 0.015-0.05 mg/kg) may be necessary.

Drug Interactions Increased toxicity: Bethanechol, methacholine, succinylcholine may increase neuromuscular blockade with systemic administration

(Continued)

Physostigmine *(Continued)*

Stability Do not use solution if cloudy or dark brown

Mechanism of Action Inhibits destruction of acetylcholine by acetylcholinesterase which facilitates transmission of impulses across myoneural junction and prolongs the central and peripheral effects of acetylcholine

Pharmacodynamics/Kinetics

Onset of action:

Ophthalmic instillation: Within 2 minutes

Parenteral: Within 5 minutes

Absorption: I.M., ophthalmic, S.C.: Readily absorbed

Distribution: Crosses the blood-brain barrier readily and reverses both central and peripheral anticholinergic effects

Duration:

Ophthalmic: 12-48 hours

Parenteral: 0.5-5 hours

Metabolism: In the liver

Half-life: 15-40 minutes

Elimination: Via hydrolysis by cholinesterases

Usual Dosage

Children: Anticholinergic drug overdose: Reserve for life-threatening situations only: I.V.: 0.01-0.03 mg/kg/dose, (maximum: 0.5 mg/minute); may repeat after 5-10 minutes to a maximum total dose of 2 mg or until response occurs or adverse cholinergic effects occur

Adults: Anticholinergic drug overdose:

I.M., I.V., S.C.: 0.5-2 mg to start, repeat every 20 minutes until response occurs or adverse effect occurs

Repeat 1-4 mg every 30-60 minutes as life-threatening signs (arrhythmias, seizures, deep coma) recur; maximum I.V. rate: 1 mg/minute

Ophthalmic:

Ointment: Instill a small quantity to lower fornix up to 3 times/day

Solution: Instill 1-2 drops into eye(s) up to 4 times/day

Test Interactions ↑ aminotransferase [ALT (SGPT)/AST (SGOT)] (S), ↑ amylase (S)

Patient Information Burning or stinging may occur with application; may cause loss of dark adaptation; notify physician if abdominal cramps, sweating, salivation, or cramps occur

Dosage Forms

Injection, as salicylate: 1 mg/mL (2 mL)

Ointment, ophthalmic, as sulfate: 0.25% (3.5 g, 3.7 g)

Physostigmine Salicylate *see* Physostigmine *on previous page*

Physostigmine Sulfate *see* Physostigmine *on previous page*

Phytomenadione *see* Phytonadione *on this page*

Phytonadione (fye toe na DYE one)

Brand Names AquaMEPHYTON®; Konakion®; Mephyton®

Synonyms Methylphytyl Napthoquinone; Phylloquinone; Phytomenadione; Vitamin K_1

Therapeutic Category Vitamin, Fat Soluble

Use Prevention and treatment of hypoprothrombinemia caused by drug-induced or anticoagulant-induced vitamin K deficiency, hemorrhagic disease of the newborn; phytonadione is more effective and is preferred to other vitamin K preparations in the presence of impending hemorrhage; oral absorption depends on the presence of bile salts

Pregnancy Risk Factor C

Contraindications Hypersensitivity to phytonadione or any component

Warnings/Precautions Severe reactions resembling anaphylaxis or hypersensitivity have occurred rarely during or immediately after I.V. administration (even with proper dilution and rate of administration); restrict I.V. administration for emergency use only; ineffective in hereditary hypoprothrombinemia, hypoprothrombinemia caused by severe liver disease; severe hemolytic anemia has been reported rarely in neonates following large doses (10-20 mg) of phytonadione

Adverse Reactions

<1%:

Cardiovascular: Transient flushing reaction, rarely hypotension, cyanosis

Central nervous system: Dizziness (rarely), pain

Gastrointestinal: Abnormal taste, GI upset (oral)

Hematologic: Hemolysis in neonates and in patients with G-6-PD deficiency

Local: Tenderness at injection site

Respiratory: Dyspnea

Miscellaneous: Diaphoresis, anaphylaxis, hypersensitivity reactions

Drug Interactions Decreased effect: Warfarin sodium, dicumarol, anisindione effects antagonized by phytonadione

Stability Protect injection from light at all times; may be autoclaved

Mechanism of Action Promotes liver synthesis of clotting factors (II, VII, IX, X); however, the exact mechanism as to this stimulation is unknown. Menadiol is a water soluble form of vitamin K; phytonadione has a more rapid and prolonged effect than menadione; menadiol sodium diphosphate (K_4) is half as potent as menadione (K_3).

Pharmacodynamics/Kinetics
- Onset of increased coagulation factors:
  - Oral: Within 6-12 hours
  - Parenteral: Within 1-2 hours; patient may become normal after 12-14 hours
- Absorption: Oral: Absorbed from the intestines in the presence of bile
- Metabolism: In the liver rapidly
- Elimination: In bile and urine

Usual Dosage I.V. route should be restricted for emergency use only
- Minimum daily requirement: Not well established
  - Infants: 1-5 mcg/kg/day
  - Adults: 0.03 mcg/kg/day
- Hemorrhagic disease of the newborn:
  - Prophylaxis: I.M., S.C.: 0.5-1 mg within 1 hour of birth
  - Treatment: I.M., S.C.: 1-2 mg/dose/day
- Oral anticoagulant overdose:
  - Infants: I.M., S.C.: 1-2 mg/dose every 4-8 hours
  - Children and Adults: Oral, I.M., I.V., S.C.: 2.5-10 mg/dose; rarely up to 25-50 mg has been used; may repeat in 6-8 hours if given by I.M., I.V., S.C. route; may repeat 12-48 hours after oral route
- Vitamin K deficiency: Due to drugs, malabsorption or decreased synthesis of vitamin K
  - Infants and Children:
    - Oral: 2.5-5 mg/24 hours
    - I.M., I.V.: 1-2 mg/dose as a single dose
  - Adults:
    - Oral: 5-25 mg/24 hours
    - I.M., I.V.: 10 mg

Administration I.V. administration: Dilute in normal saline, D_5W or D_5NS and infuse slowly; rate of infusion should not exceed 1 mg/minute. **This route should be used only if administration by another route is not feasible.** The parenteral preparation has been administered orally to neonates. I.V. administration should not exceed 1 mg/minute; for I.V. infusion, dilute in PF (preservative free) D_5W or normal saline.

Monitoring Parameters PT

Additional Information Injection contains benzyl alcohol 0.9% as preservative

Dosage Forms
- Injection:
  - Aqueous colloidal: 2 mg/mL (0.5 mL); 10 mg/mL (1 mL, 2.5 mL, 5 mL)
  - Aqueous (I.M. only): 2 mg/mL (0.5 mL); 10 mg/mL (1 mL)
- Tablet: 5 mg

Pilagan® Ophthalmic *see* Pilocarpine *on this page*

Pilocar® Ophthalmic *see* Pilocarpine *on this page*

Pilocarpine (pye loe KAR peen)

Related Information

Glaucoma Drug Therapy Comparison *on page 1410*

Brand Names Adsorbocarpine® Ophthalmic; Akarpine® Ophthalmic; Isopto® Carpine Ophthalmic; Ocu-Carpine® Ophthalmic; Ocusert Pilo-20® Ophthalmic; Ocusert Pilo-40® Ophthalmic; Pilagan® Ophthalmic; Pilocar® Ophthalmic; Pilopine HS® Ophthalmic; Piloptic® Ophthalmic; Pilostat® Ophthalmic; Salagen® Oral

Canadian/Mexican Brand Names Minims® Pilocarpine (Canada)

Synonyms Pilocarpine Hydrochloride; Pilocarpine Nitrate

Therapeutic Category Cholinergic Agent; Cholinergic Agent, Ophthalmic; Ophthalmic Agent, Miotic

Use
- Ophthalmic: Management of chronic simple glaucoma, chronic and acute angle-closure glaucoma; counter effects of cycloplegics
- Oral: Symptomatic treatment of xerostomia caused by salivary gland hypofunction resulting from radiotherapy for cancer of the head and neck

Pregnancy Risk Factor C

Contraindications Acute inflammatory disease of anterior chamber, hypersensitivity to pilocarpine or any component

(Continued)

Pilocarpine *(Continued)*

Warnings/Precautions Use with caution in patients with corneal abrasion, CHF, asthma, peptic ulcer, urinary tract obstruction, Parkinson's disease, or narrow-angle glaucoma

Adverse Reactions

>10%: Ocular: Blurred vision, miosis

1% to 10%:

Central nervous system: Headache

Genitourinary: Polyuria

Local: Stinging, burning

Ocular: Ciliary spasm, retinal detachment, browache, photophobia, acute iritis, lacrimation, conjunctival and ciliary congestion early in therapy

Miscellaneous: Hypersensitivity reactions

<1%:

Cardiovascular: Hypertension, tachycardia

Gastrointestinal: Nausea, vomiting, diarrhea, salivation

Miscellaneous: Diaphoresis

Overdosage/Toxicology Symptoms of overdose include bronchospasm, bradycardia, involuntary urination, vomiting, hypotension, tremors

Atropine is the treatment of choice for intoxications manifesting with significant muscarinic symptoms. Atropine I.V. 2-4 mg every 3-60 minutes (or 0.04-0.08 mg I.V. every 5-60 minutes if needed for children) should be repeated to control symptoms and then continued as needed for 1-2 days following the acute ingestion. Epinephrine 0.1-1 mg S.C. may be useful in reversing severe cardiovascular or pulmonary sequel.

Stability Refrigerate gel; store solution at room temperature of 8°C to 30°C (46°F to 86°F) and protect from light

Mechanism of Action Directly stimulates cholinergic receptors in the eye causing miosis (by contraction of the iris sphincter), loss of accommodation (by constriction of ciliary muscle), and lowering of intraocular pressure (with decreased resistance to aqueous humor outflow)

Pharmacodynamics/Kinetics

Ophthalmic instillation:

Miosis:

Onset of effect: Within 10-30 minutes

Duration: 4-8 hours

Intraocular pressure reduction:

Onset of effect: 1 hour required

Duration: 4-12 hours

Ocusert® Pilo application:

Miosis: Onset of effect: 1.5-2 hours

Reduced intraocular pressure:

Onset: Within 1.5-2 hours; miosis within 10-30 minutes

Duration: ~1 week

Usual Dosage Adults:

Ophthalmic:

Nitrate solution: Shake well before using; instill 1-2 drops 2-4 times/day

Hydrochloride solution:

Instill 1-2 drops up to 6 times/day; adjust the concentration and frequency as required to control elevated intraocular pressure

To counteract the mydriatic effects of sympathomimetic agents: Instill 1 drop of a 1% solution in the affected eye

Gel: Instill 0.5" ribbon into lower conjunctival sac once daily at bedtime

Ocular systems: Systems are labeled in terms of mean rate of release of pilocarpine over 7 days; begin with 20 mcg/hour at night and adjust based on response

Oral: 5 mg 3 times/day, titration up to 10 mg 3 times/day may be considered for patients who have not responded adequately

Monitoring Parameters Intraocular pressure, funduscopic exam, visual field testing

Patient Information May sting on instillation; notify physician of sweating, urinary retention; usually causes difficulty in dark adaptation; advise patients to use caution while night driving or performing hazardous tasks in poor illumination; after topical instillation, finger pressure should be applied to lacrimal sac to decrease drainage into the nose and throat and minimize possible systemic absorption

Nursing Implications Usually causes difficulty in dark adaptation; advise patients to use caution while night driving or performing hazardous tasks in poor illumination; finger pressure should be applied to lacrimal sac for 1-2 minutes after instillation to decrease risk of absorption and systemic reactions. Assure the patient or a caregiver can adequately administer ophthalmic medication dosage form.

Additional Information

Ocusert® 20 mcg is approximately equivalent to 0.5% or 1% drops
Ocusert® 40 mcg is approximately equivalent to 2% or 3% drops

Oral: Avoid administering with high fat meal; fat decreases the rate of absorption, maximum concentration and increases the time it takes to reach maximum concentration

Dosage Forms Tablet: 5 mg
See table.

Pilocarpine

Dosage Form	Strength %	1 mL	2 mL	15 mL	30 mL	3.5 g
Gel	4					x
Solution as hydrochloride	0.25			x		
	0.5			x	x	
	1	x	x	x	x	
	2	x	x	x	x	
	3			x	x	
	4	x	x	x	x	
	6			x	x	
	8		x			
	10			x		
Solution as nitrate	1			x		
	2			x		
	4			x		

Ocusert® Pilo-20: Releases 20 mcg/hour for 1 week
Ocusert® Pilo-40: Releases 40 mcg/hour for 1 week

Pilocarpine Hydrochloride *see* Pilocarpine *on page 999*
Pilocarpine Nitrate *see* Pilocarpine *on page 999*
Pilopine HS® Ophthalmic *see* Pilocarpine *on page 999*
Piloptic® Ophthalmic *see* Pilocarpine *on page 999*
Pilostat® Ophthalmic *see* Pilocarpine *on page 999*
Pima® *see* Potassium Iodide *on page 1027*
Pimaricin *see* Natamycin *on page 883*

Pimozide (PI moe zide)

Related Information

Antipsychotic Agents Comparison *on page 1396*

Brand Names Orap™

Therapeutic Category Neuroleptic Agent

Use Suppression of severe motor and phonic tics in patients with Tourette's disorder

Pregnancy Risk Factor C

Contraindications Simple tics other than Tourette's, history of cardiac dysrhythmias, known hypersensitivity to pimozide; use in patients receiving macrolide antibiotics such as clarithromycin, erythromycin, azithromycin, and dirithromycin

Adverse Reactions

>10%:
- Cardiovascular: Tachycardia, orthostatic hypotension
- Central nervous system: Akathisia, akinesia, extrapyramidal effects, drowsiness
- Dermatologic: Rash
- Endocrine & metabolic: Edema of the breasts
- Gastrointestinal: Constipation, xerostomia

1% to 10%:
- Cardiovascular: Facial edema
- Central nervous system: Tardive dyskinesia, mental depression
- Gastrointestinal: Diarrhea, anorexia

<1%:
- Central nervous system: Neuroleptic malignant syndrome (NMS)
- Hematologic: Blood dyscrasias
- Hepatic: Jaundice

Overdosage/Toxicology Symptoms of overdose include hypotension, respiratory depression, EKG abnormalities, extrapyramidal symptoms
(Continued)

Pimozide *(Continued)*

Following attempts at decontamination, treatment is supportive and symptomatic; seizures can be treated with diazepam, phenytoin, or phenobarbital

Drug Interactions Increased effect/toxicity of alfentanil, CNS depressants, guanabenz (increased sedation), MAO inhibitors

Mechanism of Action A potent centrally-acting dopamine-receptor antagonist resulting in its characteristic neuroleptic effects

Pharmacodynamics/Kinetics

Absorption: Oral: 50%
Protein binding: 99%
Metabolism: In the liver with significant first-pass decay
Half-life: 50 hours
Time to peak serum concentration: Within 6-8 hours
Elimination: In urine

Usual Dosage Children >12 years and Adults: Oral: Initial: 1-2 mg/day, then increase dosage as needed every other day; range is usually 7-16 mg/day, maximum dose: 20 mg/day or 0.3 mg/kg/day should not be exceeded

Dosing adjustment in hepatic impairment: Reduction of dose is necessary in patients with liver disease

Test Interactions ↑ prolactin (S)

Patient Information Treatment with pimozide exposes the patient to serious risks; a decision to use pimozide chronically in Tourette's disorder is one that deserves full consideration by the patient (or patient's family) as well as by the treating physician. Because the goal of treatment is symptomatic improvement, the patient's view of the need for treatment and assessment of response are critical in evaluating the impact of therapy and weighing its benefits against the risks. Since the physician is the primary source of information about the use of a drug in any disease, it is recommended that the following information be discussed with patients and/or their families.

Dosage Forms Tablet: 2 mg

Pindolol (PIN doe lole)

Related Information

Beta-Blockers Comparison *on page 1398*

Brand Names Visken®

Canadian/Mexican Brand Names Apo-Pindol® (Canada); Gen-Pindolol® (Canada); Novo-Pindol® (Canada); Nu-Pindol® (Canada); Syn-Pindol® (Canada)

Therapeutic Category Antihypertensive; Beta-Adrenergic Blocker

Use Management of hypertension

Unlabeled use: Ventricular arrhythmias/tachycardia, antipsychotic-induced akathisia, situational anxiety; aggressive behavior associated with dementia

Pregnancy Risk Factor B

Contraindications Uncompensated congestive heart failure, cardiogenic shock, bradycardia or heart block, asthma, COPD; hypersensitivity to any component

Warnings/Precautions Use with caution in patients with inadequate myocardial function, undergoing anesthesia, bronchospastic disease, diabetes mellitus, hyperthyroidism, impaired hepatic function; abrupt withdrawal of the drug should be avoided (may exacerbate symptoms; discontinue over 1-2 weeks); do not use in pregnant or nursing women; may potentiate hypoglycemia in a diabetic patient and mask signs and symptoms

Adverse Reactions

>10%:

- Central nervous system: Anxiety, dizziness, insomnia, fatigue
- Endocrine & metabolic: Decreased sexual ability
- Neuromuscular & skeletal: Arthralgia, weakness, back pain

1% to 10%:

- Cardiovascular: Congestive heart failure, arrhythmia, reduced peripheral circulation
- Central nervous system: Hallucinations, nightmares, vivid dreams
- Dermatologic: Rash, itching
- Gastrointestinal: Diarrhea, nausea, vomiting, stomach discomfort
- Neuromuscular & skeletal: Numbness of extremities
- Respiratory: Dyspnea

<1%:

- Cardiovascular: Bradycardia, chest pain
- Central nervous system: Confusion, mental depression
- Hematologic: Thrombocytopenia
- Ocular: Dry eyes

Overdosage/Toxicology Symptoms of intoxication include cardiac disturbances, CNS toxicity, bronchospasm, hypoglycemia and hyperkalemia. The most common cardiac symptoms include hypotension and bradycardia; atrioventricular block, intraventricular conduction disturbances, cardiogenic shock, and systole may occur with severe overdose, especially with membrane-depressant drugs (eg, propranolol); CNS effects include convulsions, coma, and respiratory arrest is commonly seen with propranolol and other membrane-depressant and lipid-soluble drugs.

Treatment includes symptomatic treatment of seizures, hypotension, hyperkalemia and hypoglycemia; bradycardia and hypotension resistant to atropine, isoproterenol or pacing may respond to glucagon; wide QRS defects caused by the membrane-depressant poisoning may respond to hypertonic sodium bicarbonate; repeat-dose charcoal, hemoperfusion, or hemodialysis may be helpful in removal of only those beta-blockers with a small V_d, long half-life or low intrinsic clearance (acebutolol, atenolol, nadolol, sotalol).

Drug Interactions

Decreased effect of beta-blockers with aluminum salts, barbiturates, calcium salts, cholestyramine, colestipol, NSAIDs, penicillins (ampicillin), rifampin, salicylates and sulfinpyrazone due to decreased bioavailability and plasma levels

Beta-blockers may decrease the effect of sulfonylureas

Increased effect/toxicity of beta-blockers with calcium blockers (diltiazem, felodipine, nicardipine), contraceptives, flecainide, haloperidol (propranolol, hypotensive effects), H_2-antagonists (metoprolol, propranolol only by cimetidine, possibly ranitidine), hydralazine (metoprolol, propranolol), loop diuretics (propranolol, not atenolol), MAO inhibitors (metoprolol, nadolol, bradycardia), phenothiazines (propranolol), propafenone (metoprolol, propranolol), quinidine (in extensive metabolizers), ciprofloxacin, thyroid hormones (metoprolol, propranolol, when hypothyroid patient is converted to euthyroid state)

Beta-blockers may increase the effect/toxicity of flecainide, haloperidol (hypotensive effects), hydralazine, phenothiazines, acetaminophen, anticoagulants (propranolol, warfarin), benzodiazepines (not atenolol), clonidine (hypertensive crisis after or during withdrawal of either agent), epinephrine (initial hypertensive episode followed by bradycardia), nifedipine and verapamil lidocaine, ergots (peripheral ischemia), prazosin (postural hypotension)

Beta-blockers may affect the action or levels of ethanol, disopyramide, nondepolarizing muscle relaxants and theophylline although the effects are difficult to predict

Mechanism of Action Blocks both $beta_1$- and $beta_2$-receptors and has mild intrinsic sympathomimetic activity; pindolol has negative inotropic and chronotropic effects and can significantly slow A-V nodal conduction

Pharmacodynamics/Kinetics

Absorption: Oral: Rapid, 50% to 95%

Protein binding: 50%

Metabolism: In the liver (60% to 65%) to conjugates

Half-life: 2.5-4 hours; increased with renal insufficiency, age, and cirrhosis

Time to peak serum concentration: Within 1-2 hours

Elimination: In urine (35% to 50% unchanged drug)

Usual Dosage

Adults: Initial: 5 mg twice daily, increase as necessary by 10 mg/day every 3-4 weeks; maximum daily dose: 60 mg

Elderly: Initial: 5 mg once daily, increase as necessary by 5 mg/day every 3-4 weeks

Dosing adjustment in renal and hepatic impairment: Reduction is necessary in severely impaired

Monitoring Parameters Blood pressure, standing and sitting/supine, pulse, respiratory function

Patient Information Adhere to dosage regimen; watch for postural hypotension; abrupt withdrawal of the drug should be avoided; take at the same time each day; may mask diabetes symptoms; do not discontinue medication abruptly; consult pharmacist or physician before taking over-the-counter cold preparations

Nursing Implications Evaluate blood pressure, apical and radial pulses; do not discontinue abruptly

Dosage Forms Tablet: 5 mg, 10 mg

Pink Bismuth® [OTC] *see* Bismuth *on page 154*

Pin-Rid® [OTC] *see* Pyrantel Pamoate *on page 1076*

Pin-X® [OTC] *see* Pyrantel Pamoate *on page 1076*

PIO *see* Pemoline *on page 958*

Pipecuronium (pi pe kur OH nee um)

Related Information

Neuromuscular Blocking Agents Comparison *on page 1417*

Brand Names Arduan®

(Continued)

Pipecuronium *(Continued)*

Synonyms Pipecuronium Bromide

Therapeutic Category Neuromuscular Blocker Agent, Nondepolarizing; Skeletal Muscle Relaxant

Use Adjunct to general anesthesia, to provide skeletal muscle relaxation during surgery and to provide skeletal muscle relaxation for endotracheal intubation; recommended only for procedures anticipated to last 90 minutes or longer

Pregnancy Risk Factor C

Contraindications Hypersensitivity to pipecuronium or bromide

Warnings/Precautions Use with caution in patients with renal impairment, obesity, cardiovascular disease, myasthenia gravis, myasthenic syndrome, and in the elderly

Adverse Reactions

1% to 10%: Cardiovascular: Hypotension, bradycardia

<1%:

Cardiovascular: Atrial fibrillation, myocardial ischemia, thrombosis, hypertension, ventricular extrasystole

Central nervous system: CNS depression

Dermatologic: Urticaria

Endocrine & metabolic: Hypoglycemia, hyperkalemia

Neuromuscular & skeletal: Muscle atrophy

Renal: Anuria

Respiratory: Respiratory depression, dyspnea

Overdosage/Toxicology Support ventilation by artificial means; paralysis including cessation of respiration

Drug Interactions Increased effect with enflurane, halothane, isoflurane, ketorolac, quinidine, succinylcholine

Mechanism of Action Pipecuronium bromide is a nondepolarizing neuromuscular blocking agent structurally related to pancuronium and vecuronium. Studies in adult patients have demonstrated that pipecuronium is ~20% to 50% more potent than pancuronium as a neuromuscular blocking agent. The neuromuscular effects and pharmacokinetics of pipecuronium appears to lack vagolytic or autonomic activity and produces minimal cardiovascular effects.

Pharmacodynamics/Kinetics

Onset of action: Effective neuromuscular blockade is generally observed within 2-3 minutes

Metabolism: In the liver primarily to 3-desacetyl-pipecuronium

Half-life, elimination: 2-2.5 hours

Elimination: Renally (40% unchanged drug)

Usual Dosage I.V.:

Children:

3 months to 1 year: Adult dosage

1-14 years: May be less sensitive to effects

Adults: Dose is individualized based on ideal body weight, ranges are 85-100 mcg/kg initially to a maintenance dose of 5-25 mcg/kg

Dosing adjustment in renal impairment:

Cl_{cr} 61-80 mL/minute: 70 mcg/kg

Cl_{cr} 41-60 mL/minute: 55 mcg/kg

Cl_{cr} <40 mL/minute: 50 mcg/kg

Extended duration should be expected

Administration Not recommended for dilution into or administration from large volume I.V. solutions

Dosage Forms Injection, as bromide: 10 mg (10 mL)

Pipecuronium Bromide *see* Pipecuronium *on previous page*

Piperacillin (pi PER a sil in)

Related Information

Antimicrobial Drugs of Choice *on page 1468*

Brand Names Pipracil®

Synonyms Piperacillin Sodium

Therapeutic Category Antibiotic, Penicillin

Use Treatment of susceptible infections such as septicemia, acute and chronic respiratory tract infections, skin and soft tissue infections, and urinary tract infections due to susceptible strains of *Pseudomonas, Proteus,* and *Escherichia coli* and *Enterobacter,* normally used with other antibiotics (ie, aminoglycosides)

Pregnancy Risk Factor B

Contraindications Hypersensitivity to piperacillin or any component or penicillins

Warnings/Precautions Dosage modification required in patients with impaired renal function; history of seizure activity; use with caution in patients with a history of beta-lactam allergy

Adverse Reactions

<1%:

Central nervous system: Convulsions, confusion, drowsiness, fever
Dermatologic: Rash
Endocrine & metabolic: Electrolyte imbalance
Hematologic: Hemolytic anemia, positive Coombs' reaction, abnormal platelet aggregation and prolonged prothrombin time (high doses)
Local: Thrombophlebitis
Neuromuscular: Myoclonus
Renal: Acute interstitial nephritis
Miscellaneous: Hypersensitivity reactions, anaphylaxis, Jarisch-Herxheimer reaction

Overdosage/Toxicology Symptoms of penicillin overdose include neuromuscular hypersensitivity (agitation, hallucinations, asterixis, encephalopathy, confusion, and seizures) and electrolyte imbalance with potassium or sodium salts, especially in renal failure

Hemodialysis may be helpful to aid in the removal of the drug from the blood, otherwise most treatment is supportive or symptom directed

Drug Interactions

Decreased effect: Tetracyclines may decrease penicillin effectiveness; aminoglycosides → physical inactivation of aminoglycosides in the presence of high concentrations of piperacillin and potential toxicity in patients with mild-moderate renal dysfunction

Increased effect:

Probenecid may increase penicillin levels
Neuromuscular blockers may increase duration of blockade
Aminoglycosides → synergistic efficacy

Stability Reconstituted solution is stable (I.V. infusion) in NS or D_5W for 24 hours at room temperature, 7 days when refrigerated or 4 weeks when frozen; after freezing, thawed solution is stable for 24 hours at room temperature or 48 hours when refrigerated; 40 g bulk vial should **not** be frozen after reconstitution; **incompatible** with aminoglycosides

Mechanism of Action Inhibits bacterial cell wall synthesis by binding to one or more of the penicillin binding proteins (PBPs); which in turn inhibits the final transpeptidation step of peptidoglycan synthesis in bacterial cell walls, thus inhibiting cell wall biosynthesis. Bacteria eventually lyse due to ongoing activity of cell wall autolytic enzymes (autolysins and murein hydrolases) while cell wall assembly is arrested.

Pharmacodynamics/Kinetics

Absorption: I.M.: 70% to 80%
Distribution: Crosses the placenta; distributes into milk at low concentrations
Protein binding: 22%
Half-life: Dose-dependent; prolonged with moderately severe renal or hepatic impairment:

Neonates:

1-5 days: 3.6 hours
>6 days: 2.1-2.7 hours

Children:

1-6 months: 0.79 hour
6 months to 12 years: 0.39-0.5 hour

Adults: 36-80 minutes

Time to peak serum concentration: I.M.: Within 30-50 minutes
Elimination: Principally in urine and partially in feces (via bile)

Usual Dosage

Infants and Children: I.M., I.V.: 200-300 mg/kg/day in divided doses every 4-6 hours; maximum dose: 24 g/day

Higher doses have been used in cystic fibrosis: 350-500 mg/kg/day in divided doses every 4 hours

Adults:

I.M.: 2-3 g/dose every 6-12 hours; maximum: 24 g/24 hours
I.V.: 3-4 g/dose every 4-6 hours; maximum: 24 g/24 hours

Dosing interval in renal impairment:

Cl_{cr} 10-50 mL/minute: Administer every 6-8 hours
Cl_{cr} <10 mL/minute: Administer every 8 hours

Hemodialysis: Moderately dialyzable (20% to 50%)

Administration Administer around-the-clock to promote less variation in peak and trough serum levels; administer at least 1 hour apart from aminoglycosides

Test Interactions May interfere with urinary glucose tests using cupric sulfate (Benedict's solution, Clinitest®); may inactivate aminoglycosides *in vitro*; false-positive urinary and serum proteins, positive Coombs' test [diroot]

Additional Information Sodium content of 1 g: 1.85 mEq

(Continued)

Piperacillin *(Continued)*

Dosage Forms Powder for injection, as sodium: 2 g, 3 g, 4 g, 40 g

Piperacillin and Tazobactam Sodium

(pi PER a sil in & ta zoe BAK tam SOW dee um)

Related Information

Antimicrobial Drugs of Choice *on page 1468*

Brand Names Zosyn™

Synonyms Piperacillin Sodium and Tazobactam Sodium

Therapeutic Category Antibiotic, Penicillin

Use Treatment of infections of lower respiratory tract, urinary tract, skin and skin structures, gynecologic, bone and joint infections, and septicemia caused by susceptible organisms. Tazobactam expands activity of piperacillin to include beta-lactamase producing strains of *S. aureus*, *H. influenzae*, Enterobacteriaceae, *Pseudomonas*, *Klebsiella*, *Citrobacter*, *Serratia*, *Bacteroides*, and other gram-negative anaerobes.

Application to nosocomial infections may be limited by restricted activity against gram-negative organisms producing class I beta-lactamases and inactivity against methicillin-resistant *Staphylococcus aureus*

Pregnancy Risk Factor B

Pregnancy/Breast-Feeding Implications Use by the breast-feeding mother may result in diarrhea, candidiasis, or allergic response in the infant

Contraindications Hypersensitivity to penicillins, beta-lactamase inhibitors, or any component

Warnings/Precautions Due to sodium load and to the adverse effects of high serum concentrations of penicillins, dosage modification is required in patients with impaired or underdeveloped renal function; use with caution in patients with seizures or in patients with history of beta-lactam allergy; safety and efficacy have not been established in children <12 years of age

Adverse Reactions

>10%: Gastrointestinal: Diarrhea

1% to 10%:

- Central nervous system: Insomnia, headache
- Dermatologic: Rash, pruritus
- Gastrointestinal: Constipation, nausea, vomiting, dyspepsia
- Hematologic: Leukopenia
- Miscellaneous: Serum sickness-like reaction

<1%:

- Cardiovascular: Hypertension, hypotension, edema
- Central nervous system: Dizziness, agitation, confusion
- Gastrointestinal: Pseudomembranous colitis
- Respiratory: Bronchospasm

Several laboratory abnormalities have rarely been associated with piperacillin/tazobactam including reversible eosinophilia, and neutropenia (associated most often with prolonged therapy), positive direct Coombs' test, prolonged PT and PTT, transient elevations of LFT, increases in creatinine

Overdosage/Toxicology Symptoms of penicillin overdose include neuromuscular hypersensitivity (agitation, hallucinations, asterixis, encephalopathy, confusion, and seizures) and electrolyte imbalance with potassium or sodium salts, especially in renal dysfunction

Hemodialysis may be helpful to aid in the removal of the drug from the blood, otherwise most treatment is supportive or symptom directed

Drug Interactions

Decreased effect: Tetracyclines may decrease penicillin effectiveness; aminoglycosides → physical inactivation of aminoglycosides in the presence of high concentrations of piperacillin and potential toxicity in patients with mild-moderate renal dysfunction

Increased effect:

- Probenecid may increase penicillin levels
- Neuromuscular blockers may increase duration of blockade
- Aminoglycosides → synergistic efficacy

Stability Store at controlled room temperature; after reconstitution, solution is stable in NS or D_5W for 24 hours at room temperature and 7 days when refrigerated; use single dose vials immediately after reconstitution (discard unused portions after 24 hours at room temperature and 48 hours if refrigerated)

Mechanism of Action Piperacillin interferes with bacterial cell wall synthesis during active multiplication, causing cell wall death and resultant bactericidal activity against susceptible bacteria; tazobactam prevents degradation of piperacillin by binding to the active side on beta-lactamase; tazobactam inhibits many beta-lactamases, including staphylococcal penicillinase and Richmond and

Sykes types II, III, IV, and V, including extended spectrum enzymes; it has only limited activity against class I beta-lactamases other than class Ic types

Pharmacodynamics/Kinetics Both AUC and peak concentrations are dose proportional

Distribution: Distributes well into lungs, intestinal mucosa, skin, muscle, uterus, ovary, prostate, gallbladder, and bile; penetration into CSF is low in subject with noninflamed meninges

Metabolism:

Piperacillin: 6% to 9%

Tazobactam: ~26%

Protein binding:

Piperacillin: ~26% to 33%

Tazobactam: 31% to 32%

Half-life:

Piperacillin: 1 hour

Metabolite: 1-1.5 hours

Tazobactam: 0.7-0.9 hour

Elimination: Both piperacillin and tazobactam are directly proportional to renal function

Piperacillin: 50% to 70% eliminated unchanged in urine, 10% to 20% excreted in bile

Tazobactam: Found in urine at 24 hours, with 26% as the inactive metabolite

Hemodialysis removes 30% to 40% of piperacillin and tazobactam; peritoneal dialysis removes 11% to 21% of tazobactam and 6% of piperacillin; hepatic impairment does not affect the kinetics of piperacillin or tazobactam significantly

Usual Dosage

Children <12 years: Not recommended due to lack of data

Children >12 years and Adults:

Severe infections: I.V.: Piperacillin/tazobactam 4/0.5 g every 8 hours or 3/0.375 g every 6 hours

Moderate infections: I.M.: Piperacillin/tazobactam 2/0.25 g every 6-8 hours; treatment should be continued for ≥7-10 days depending on severity of disease

Dosing interval in renal impairment:

Cl_{cr} >40 mL/minute: No change

Cl_{cr} 20-40 mL/minute: Administer 2/0.25 g every 6 hours

Cl_{cr} <20 mL/minute: Administer 2/0.25 g every 8 hours

Hemodialysis: Administer 2/0.25 g every 8 hours with an additional dose of 0.75 g after each dialysis

Administration Administer by I.V. infusion over 30 minutes; reconstitute with 5 mL of diluent per 1 g of piperacillin and then further dilute; compatible diluents include NS, SW, dextran 6%, D_5W, D_5W with potassium chloride 40 mEq, bacteriostatic saline and water; not compatible with lactated Ringer's solution

Monitoring Parameters LFTs, creatinine, BUN, CBC with differential, serum electrolytes, urinalysis, PT, PTT

Test Interactions Positive Coombs' [direct] test 3.8%, ALT, AST, bilirubin, and LDH

Nursing Implications Discontinue primary infusion, if possible, during infusion and administer aminoglycosides separately from Zosyn™

Dosage Forms Injection: Piperacillin sodium 2 g and tazobactam sodium 0.25 g; piperacillin sodium 3 g and tazobactam sodium 0.375 g; piperacillin sodium 4 g and tazobactam sodium 0.5 g (vials at an 8:1 ratio of piperacillin sodium/tazobactam sodium)

Piperacillin Sodium *see* Piperacillin *on page 1004*

Piperacillin Sodium and Tazobactam Sodium *see* Piperacillin and Tazobactam Sodium *on previous page*

Piperazine (PI per a zeen)

Brand Names Vermizine®

Synonyms Piperazine Citrate

Therapeutic Category Anthelmintic

Use Treatment of pinworm and roundworm infections (used as an alternative to first-line agents, mebendazole, or pyrantel pamoate)

Pregnancy Risk Factor B

Contraindications Seizure disorders, liver or kidney impairment, hypersensitivity to piperazine or any component

Warnings/Precautions Use with caution in patients with anemia or malnutrition; avoid prolonged use especially in children

Adverse Reactions

<1%:

Central nervous system: Dizziness, seizures, EEG changes, headache, vertigo

(Continued)

Piperazine *(Continued)*

Gastrointestinal: Nausea, vomiting, diarrhea
Hematologic: Hemolytic anemia
Neuromuscular & skeletal: Weakness
Ocular: Visual impairment
Respiratory: Bronchospasms
Miscellaneous: Hypersensitivity reactions

Drug Interactions Pyrantel pamoate (antagonistic mode of action)

Mechanism of Action Causes muscle paralysis of the roundworm by blocking the effects of acetylcholine at the neuromuscular junction

Pharmacodynamics/Kinetics

Absorption: Well absorbed from GI tract
Time to peak serum concentration: 1 hour
Elimination: In urine as metabolites and unchanged drug

Usual Dosage Oral:

Pinworms: Children and Adults: 65 mg/kg/day (not to exceed 2.5 g/day) as a single daily dose for 7 days; in severe infections, repeat course after a 1-week interval

Roundworms:

Children: 75 mg/kg/day as a single daily dose for 2 days; maximum: 3.5 g/day
Adults: 3.5 g/day for 2 days (in severe infections, repeat course, after a 1-week interval)

Monitoring Parameters Stool exam for worms and ova

Patient Information Take on empty stomach; if severe or persistent headache, loss of balance or coordination, dizziness, vomiting, diarrhea, or rash occurs, contact physician. If used for pinworm infections, all members of the family should be treated.

Nursing Implications Cure rates may be decreased with massive infections or in patients with hypermotility of the GI tract

Dosage Forms

Syrup, as citrate: 500 mg/5 mL (473 mL, 4000 mL)
Tablet, as citrate: 250 mg

Piperazine Citrate *see* Piperazine *on previous page*
Piperazine Estrone Sulfate *see* Estropipate *on page 475*

Pipobroman (pi poe BROE man)

Brand Names Vercyte®

Therapeutic Category Antineoplastic Agent, Alkylating Agent

Use Treat polycythemia vera; chronic myelocytic leukemia (in patients refractory to busulfan)

Pregnancy Risk Factor D

Contraindications Pre-existing bone marrow suppression, hypersensitivity to any component

Warnings/Precautions The U.S. Food and Drug Administration (FDA) currently recommends that procedures for proper handling and disposal of antineoplastic agents be considered; bone marrow suppression may not occur for 4 weeks

Adverse Reactions

1% to 10%:

Dermatologic: Rash
Gastrointestinal: Vomiting, diarrhea, nausea, abdominal cramps
Hematologic: Leukopenia, thrombocytopenia, anemia

Overdosage/Toxicology Symptoms of overdose include severe marrow suppression; supportive therapy is required

Mechanism of Action An alkylating agent considered to be cell-cycle nonspecific and capable of killing tumor cells in any phase of the cell cycle. Alkylating agents form covalent cross-links with DNA thereby resulting in cytotoxic, mutagenic, and carcinogenic effects. The end result of the alkylation process results in the misreading of the DNA code and the inhibition of DNA, RNA, and protein synthesis in rapidly proliferating tumor cells.

Usual Dosage Children >15 years and Adults: Oral:

Polycythemia: 1 mg/kg/day for 30 days; may increase to 1.5-3 mg/kg until hematocrit reduced to 50% to 55%; maintenance: 0.1-0.2 mg/kg/day

Myelocytic leukemia: 1.5-2.5 mg/kg/day until WBC drops to 10,000/mm^3 then start maintenance 7-175 mg/day; stop if WBC falls to <3000/mm^3 or platelets fall to <150,000/mm^3

Monitoring Parameters CBC, liver and renal function tests

Patient Information Notify physician if nausea, vomiting, diarrhea, or rash become severe or if unusual bleeding or bruising, sore throat, or fatigue occur; contraceptives are recommended during therapy

Dosage Forms Tablet: 25 mg

Pipracil® *see* Piperacillin *on page 1004*

Pirbuterol (peer BYOO ter ole)

Brand Names Maxair™

Synonyms Pirbuterol Acetate

Therapeutic Category $Beta_2$-Adrenergic Agonist Agent; Bronchodilator

Use Prevention and treatment of reversible bronchospasm including asthma

Pregnancy Risk Factor C

Contraindications Hypersensitivity to pirbuterol or albuterol

Warnings/Precautions Excessive use may result in tolerance; some adverse reactions may occur more frequently in children 2-5 years of age; use with caution in patients with hyperthyroidism, diabetes mellitus; cardiovascular disorders including coronary insufficiency or hypertension or sensitivity to sympathomimetic amines

Adverse Reactions

>10%:

- Central nervous system: Nervousness, restlessness
- Neuromuscular & skeletal: Trembling

1% to 10%:

- Central nervous system: Headache, dizziness
- Gastrointestinal: Taste changes, vomiting, nausea

<1%:

- Cardiovascular: Hypertension, arrhythmias, chest pain
- Central nervous system: Insomnia
- Dermatologic: Bruising
- Gastrointestinal: Anorexia
- Neuromuscular & skeletal: Numbness in hands, weakness
- Respiratory: Paradoxical bronchospasm

Overdosage/Toxicology Symptoms of overdose include hypertension, tachycardia, angina, hypokalemia

In cases of overdose, supportive therapy should be instituted, and prudent use of a cardioselective beta-adrenergic blocker (eg, atenolol or metoprolol) should be considered, keeping in mind the potential for induction of bronchoconstriction in an asthmatic individual. Dialysis has not been shown to be of value in the treatment of an overdose with this agent.

Drug Interactions

Decreased effect with beta-blockers

Increased toxicity with other beta agonists, MAO inhibitors, TCAs

Mechanism of Action Pirbuterol is a $beta_2$-adrenergic agonist with a similar structure to albuterol, specifically a pyridine ring has been substituted for the benzene ring in albuterol. The increased $beta_2$ selectivity of pirbuterol results from the substitution of a tertiary butyl group on the nitrogen of the side chain, which additionally imparts resistance of pirbuterol to degradation by monoamine oxidase and provides a lengthened duration of action in comparison to the less selective previous beta-agonist agents.

Pharmacodynamics/Kinetics

Peak therapeutic effect:

- Oral: 2-3 hours with peak serum concentration of 6.2-9.8 mcg/L
- Inhalation: 0.5-1 hour

Half-life: 2-3 hours

Metabolism: In the liver

Elimination: 10% kidney excretion as unchanged drug

Usual Dosage Children >12 years and Adults: 2 inhalations every 4-6 hours for prevention; two inhalations at an interval of at least 1-3 minutes, followed by a third inhalation in treatment of bronchospasm, not to exceed 12 inhalations/day

Monitoring Parameters Respiratory rate, heart rate, and blood pressure

Patient Information Patient instructions are available with product. Do not exceed recommended dosage; rinse mouth with water following each inhalation to help with dry throat and mouth.

Nursing Implications Before using, the inhaler must be shaken well; assess lung sounds, pulse, and blood pressure before administration and during peak of medication; observe patient for wheezing after administration, if this occurs, call physician

Dosage Forms Aerosol, oral, as acetate: 0.2 mg per actuation (25.6 g)

Pirbuterol Acetate *see* Pirbuterol *on this page*

Piroxicam (peer OKS i kam)

Related Information

Nonsteroidal Anti-Inflammatory Agents Comparison *on page 1419*

Brand Names Feldene®

Canadian/Mexican Brand Names Apo-Piroxicam® (Canada); Novo-Piroxicam® (Canada); Nu-Pirox® (Canada); Pro-Piroxicam® (Canada); Artyflam® (Mexico);

(Continued)

Piroxicam *(Continued)*

Citoken® (Mexico); Facicam® (Mexico); Flogosan® (Mexico); Oxicanol® (Mexico); Piroxan® (Mexico); Piroxen® (Mexico); Rogal® (Mexico)

Therapeutic Category Analgesic, Nonsteroidal Anti-inflammatory Drug; Anti-inflammatory Agent; Nonsteroidal Anti-inflammatory Agent (NSAID), Oral

Use Management of inflammatory disorders; symptomatic treatment of acute and chronic rheumatoid arthritis, osteoarthritis, and ankylosing spondylitis; also used to treat sunburn

Pregnancy Risk Factor B (D if used in the 3rd trimester)

Contraindications Hypersensitivity to piroxicam, any component, aspirin or other nonsteroidal anti-inflammatory drugs (NSAIDs); active GI bleeding

Warnings/Precautions Use with caution in patients with impaired cardiac function, hypertension, impaired renal function, GI disease (bleeding or ulcers) and patients receiving anticoagulants; elderly have increased risk for adverse reactions to NSAIDs

Adverse Reactions

>10%:
- Central nervous system: Dizziness
- Dermatologic: Rash
- Gastrointestinal: Abdominal cramps, heartburn, indigestion, nausea

1% to 10%:
- Central nervous system: Headache, nervousness
- Dermatologic: Itching
- Endocrine & metabolic: Fluid retention
- Gastrointestinal: Vomiting
- Otic: Tinnitus

<1%:
- Cardiovascular: Congestive heart failure, hypertension, arrhythmias, tachycardia
- Central nervous system: Confusion, hallucinations, aseptic meningitis, mental depression, drowsiness, insomnia
- Dermatologic: Urticaria, erythema multiforme, toxic epidermal necrolysis, Stevens-Johnson syndrome, angioedema
- Endocrine & metabolic: Polydipsia, hot flashes
- Gastrointestinal: Gastritis, GI ulceration
- Genitourinary: Cystitis, polyuria
- Hematologic: Agranulocytosis, anemia, hemolytic anemia, bone marrow suppression, leukopenia, thrombocytopenia
- Hepatic: Hepatitis
- Neuromuscular & skeletal: Peripheral neuropathy
- Ocular: Toxic amblyopia, blurred vision, conjunctivitis, dry eyes
- Otic: Decreased hearing
- Renal: Acute renal failure
- Respiratory: Allergic rhinitis, shortness of breath, epistaxis

Overdosage/Toxicology Symptoms of overdose include nausea, epigastric distress, CNS depression, leukocytosis, renal failure

Management of a nonsteroidal anti-inflammatory drug (NSAID) intoxication is primarily supportive and symptomatic. Fluid therapy is commonly effective in managing the hypotension that may occur following an acute NSAID overdose, except when this is due to an acute blood loss.

Seizures tend to be very short-lived and often do not require drug treatment; although, recurrent seizures should be treated with I.V. diazepam

Since many of the NSAIDs undergo enterohepatic cycling, multiple doses of charcoal may be needed to reduce the potential for delayed toxicities

Drug Interactions

Decreased effect of diuretics, beta-blockers; decreased effect with aspirin, antacids, cholestyramine

Increased effect/toxicity of lithium, warfarin, methotrexate (controversial)

Mechanism of Action Inhibits prostaglandin synthesis, acts on the hypothalamus heat-regulating center to reduce fever, blocks prostaglandin synthetase action which prevents formation of the platelet-aggregating substance thromboxane A_2; decreases pain receptor sensitivity. Other proposed mechanisms of action for salicylate anti-inflammatory action are lysosomal stabilization, kinin and leukotriene production, alteration of chemotactic factors, and inhibition of neutrophil activation. This latter mechanism may be the most significant pharmacologic action to reduce inflammation.

Pharmacodynamics/Kinetics

Onset of analgesia: Oral: Within 1 hour

Peak effect: 3-5 hours

Protein binding: 99%

Metabolism: In the liver

Half-life: 45-50 hours

Elimination: As unchanged drug (5%) and metabolites primarily in urine and to a small degree in feces

Usual Dosage Oral:

Children: 0.2-0.3 mg/kg/day once daily; maximum dose: 15 mg/day

Adults: 10-20 mg/day once daily; although associated with increase in GI adverse effects, doses >20 mg/day have been used (ie, 30-40 mg/day)

Dosing adjustment in hepatic impairment: Reduction of dosage is necessary

Monitoring Parameters Occult blood loss, hemoglobin, hematocrit, and periodic renal and hepatic function tests; periodic ophthalmologic exams with chronic use

Test Interactions ↑ chloride (S), ↑ sodium (S), ↑ bleeding time

Patient Information Take with food, may cause drowsiness or dizziness

Dosage Forms Capsule: 10 mg, 20 mg

p-Isobutylhydratropic Acid *see* Ibuprofen *on page 639*

Pit *see* Oxytocin *on page 944*

Pitocin® *see* Oxytocin *on page 944*

Pitressin® *see* Vasopressin *on page 1293*

Placidyl® *see* Ethchlorvynol *on page 480*

Plague Vaccine (plaig vak SEEN)

Therapeutic Category Vaccine, Inactivated Bacteria

Use Selected travelers to countries reporting cases for whom avoidance of rodents and fleas is impossible; all laboratory and field personnel working with *Yersinia pestis* organisms possibly resistant to antimicrobials; those engaged in *Yersinia pestis* aerosol experiments or in field operations in areas with enzootic plague where regular exposure to potentially infected wild rodents, rabbits, or their fleas cannot be prevented. Prophylactic antibiotics may be indicated following definite exposure, whether or not the exposed persons have been vaccinated.

Pregnancy Risk Factor C

Contraindications Persons with known hypersensitivity to any of the vaccine constituents (see manufacturer's label); patients who have had severe local or systemic reactions to a previous dose; defer immunization in patients with a febrile illness until resolved

Warnings/Precautions Pregnancy, unless there is substantial and unavoidable risk of exposure

Adverse Reactions

1% to 10%:

Central nervous system: Malaise, fever, headache

Dermatologic: Local erythema

<1%:

Cardiovascular: Tachycardia

Gastrointestinal: Nausea, vomiting

Local: Sterile abscess

Drug Interactions Decreased effect with immunoglobulin, other live vaccine used within 1 month

Usual Dosage Three I.M. doses: First dose 1 mL, second dose (0.2 mL) 1 month later, third dose (0.2 mL) 5 months after the second dose; booster doses (0.2 mL) at 1- to 2-year intervals if exposure continues

Administration I.M. into deltoid muscle

Test Interactions Temporary suppression of tuberculosis skin test

Additional Information Federal law requires that the date of administration, the vaccine manufacturer, lot number of vaccine, and the administering person's name, title and address be entered into the patient's permanent medical record

Dosage Forms Injection: 2 mL, 20 mL

Plantago Seed *see* Psyllium *on page 1075*

Plantain Seed *see* Psyllium *on page 1075*

Plaquenil® *see* Hydroxychloroquine *on page 630*

Plasbumin® *see* Albumin *on page 37*

Platinol® *see* Cisplatin *on page 282*

Platinol®-AQ *see* Cisplatin *on page 282*

Plendil® *see* Felodipine *on page 506*

Plicamycin (plye kay MYE sin)

Related Information

Antiemetics for Chemotherapy Induced Nausea and Vomiting *on page 1348*

Cancer Chemotherapy Regimens *on page 1351*

Brand Names Mithracin®

Synonyms Mithramycin

Therapeutic Category Antidote, Hypercalcemia; Antineoplastic Agent, Vesicant; Antineoplastic Agent, Miscellaneous; Vesicant

(Continued)

Plicamycin *(Continued)*

Use Malignant testicular tumors, in the treatment of hypercalcemia and hypercalciuria of malignancy not responsive to conventional treatment; Paget's disease

Pregnancy Risk Factor D

Contraindications Thrombocytopenia, bleeding diatheses, coagulation disorders; bone marrow function impairment; or hypocalcemia

Warnings/Precautions The U.S. Food and Drug Administration (FDA) currently recommends that procedures for proper handling and disposal of antineoplastic agents be considered. Use with caution in patients with hepatic or renal impairment; reduce dosage in patients with renal impairment; discontinue if bleeding or epistaxis occurs. Plicamycin may cause permanent sterility and may cause birth defects.

Adverse Reactions

>10%: Gastrointestinal: Anorexia, stomatitis, nausea, vomiting, diarrhea

Nausea and vomiting occur in almost 100% of patients within the first 6 hours after treatment; incidence increases with rapid injection; stomatitis has also occurred

Time course for nausea/vomiting: Onset 4-6 hours; Duration: 4-24 hours

1% to 10%:

Cardiovascular: Facial flushing

Central nervous system: Fever, headache, depression, drowsiness

Endocrine & metabolic: Hypocalcemia

Hematologic: Myelosuppressive: Mild leukopenia and thrombocytopenia

WBC: Moderate, but uncommon

Platelets: Moderate, rapid onset

Onset (days): 7-10

Nadir (days): 14

Recovery (days): 21

Clotting disorders: May also depress hepatic synthesis of clotting factors, leading to a form of coagulopathy; petechiae, increased prothrombin time, epistaxis, and thrombocytopenia may be seen and may require discontinuation of the drug. Epistasis is frequently the first sign of this bleeding disorder.

Hepatic: Hepatotoxicity

Local: Pain at injection site

Extravasation: Is an irritant; may produce local tissue irritation or cellulitis if infiltrated; if extravasation occurs, follow hospital procedure, discontinue I.V., and apply ice for 24 hours

Irritant chemotherapy

Renal: Azotemia, nephrotoxicity

Miscellaneous: Hemorrhagic diathesis

Overdosage/Toxicology Symptoms of overdose include bone marrow suppression, bleeding syndrome, thrombocytopenia

Supportive therapy; treatment of hemorrhagic episodes should include transfusion of fresh whole blood or packed red blood cells and fresh frozen plasma, vitamin K, and corticosteroids

Drug Interactions

Increased toxicity: Calcitonin, etidronate, glucagon, → additive hypoglycemic effects

Stability Store intact vials under refrigeration (2°C to 8°C); vials are stable at room temperature (<25°C) for up to 3 months. Dilute powder in 4.9 mL SWI to result in a concentration of 500 mcg/mL which is stable for 24 hours at room temperature (25°C) and 48 hours under refrigeration (4°C). Further dilution in 1000 mL D_5W or NS is stable for 24 hours at room temperature.

Standard I.V. dilution: Dose/1000 mL D_5W or NS; solution is stable for 24 hours at room temperature (25°C)

Mechanism of Action Potent osteoclast inhibitor; may inhibit parathyroid hormone effect on osteoclasts; inhibits bone resorption; forms a complex with DNA in the presence of magnesium or other divalent cations inhibiting DNA-directed RNA synthesis

Pharmacodynamics/Kinetics

Decreasing calcium levels:

Onset of action: Within 24 hours

Peak effect: 48-72 hours

Duration: 5-15 days

Distribution: Crosses blood-brain barrier in low concentrations

Protein binding: 0%

Half-life, plasma: 1 hour

Elimination: 90% of dose excreted in urine within the first 24 hours

Usual Dosage Refer to individual protocols. Dose should be diluted in 1 L of D_5W or NS and administered over 4-6 hours

Dosage should be based on the patient's body weight. If a patient has abnormal fluid retention (ie, edema, hydrothorax or ascites), the patient's ideal weight rather than actual body weight should be used to calculate the dose.

Adults: I.V.:
- Testicular cancer: 25-30 mcg/kg/day for 8-10 days
- Blastic chronic granulocytic leukemia: 25 mcg/kg over 2-4 hours every other day for 3 weeks
- Paget's disease: 15 mcg/kg/day once daily for 10 days
- Hypercalcemia:
  - 25 mcg/kg single dose which may be repeated in 48 hours if no response occurs
  - **OR** 25 mcg/kg/day for 3-4 days
  - **OR** 25-50 mcg/kg/dose every other day for 3-8 doses

Dosing adjustment in renal impairment:
- Cl_{cr} 10-50 mL/minute: Decrease dosage to 75% of normal dose
- Cl_{cr} <10 mL/minute: Decrease dosage to 50% of normal dose

Hemodialysis: Unknown
CAPD effects: Unknown
CAVH effects: Unknown

Dosing in hepatic impairment: In the treatment of hypercalcemia in patients with hepatic dysfunction: Reduce dose to 12.5 mcg/kg/day

Administration

Administer I.V. infusion over 4-7 hours via central line

Avoid extravasation; local tissue irritation and cellulitis has been reported

Monitoring Parameters Hepatic and renal function tests, CBC, platelet count, prothrombin time, serum electrolytes

Patient Information Any signs of infection, easy bruising or bleeding, shortness of breath, or painful or burning urination should be brought to physician's attention. Nausea, vomiting, or hair loss sometimes occur. The drug may cause permanent sterility and may cause birth defects. The drug may be excreted in breast milk, therefore, an alternative form of feeding your baby should be used.

Nursing Implications Rapid I.V. infusion has been associated with an increased incidence of nausea and vomiting; an antiemetic given prior to and during plicamycin infusion may be helpful. Avoid extravasation since plicamycin is a strong vesicant.

Dosage Forms Powder for injection: 2.5 mg

Pneumococcal Polysaccharide Vaccine *see* Pneumococcal Vaccine *on this page*

Pneumococcal Vaccine (noo moe KOK al vak SEEN)

Related Information

Guidelines for the Prevention of Opportunistic Infections in Persons with HIV *on page 1457*
Immunization Guidelines *on page 1421*
Miscellaneous Vaccination Information *on page 1437*

Brand Names Pneumovax® 23; Pnu-Imune® 23

Synonyms Pneumococcal Polysaccharide Vaccine

Therapeutic Category Vaccine, Inactivated Bacteria

Use Children >2 years of age and adults who are at increased risk of pneumococcal disease and its complications because of underlying health conditions; older adults, including all those ≥65 years of age

Pregnancy Risk Factor C

Contraindications Active infections, Hodgkin's disease patients, <5 years of age, pregnancy, hypersensitivity to pneumococcal vaccine or any component; (children <5 years of age do not respond satisfactorily to the capsular types of 23 capsular pneumococcal vaccine; the safety of vaccine in pregnant women has not been evaluated; it should not be given during pregnancy unless the risk of infection is high)

Warnings/Precautions Epinephrine injection (1:1000) must be immediately available in the case of anaphylaxis; use caution in individuals who have had episodes of pneumococcal infection within the preceding 3 years (pre-existing pneumococcal antibodies may result in increased reactions to vaccine); may cause relapse in patients with stable idiopathic thrombocytopenia purpura

Adverse Reactions

>10%: Local: Induration and soreness at the injection site (2-3 days)

<1%:
- Central nervous system: Guillain-Barré syndrome, low-grade fever
- Dermatologic: Erythema, rash
- Neuromuscular & skeletal: Paresthesias, myalgia, arthralgia
- Miscellaneous: Anaphylaxis

(Continued)

Pneumococcal Vaccine *(Continued)*

Drug Interactions Decreased effect with immunosuppressive agents, immunoglobulin, other live vaccines within 1 month

Stability Refrigerate

Mechanism of Action Although there are more than 80 known pneumococcal capsular types, pneumococcal disease is mainly caused by only a few types of pneumococci. Pneumococcal vaccine contains capsular polysaccharides of 23 pneumococcal types which represent at least 98% of pneumococcal disease isolates in the United States and Europe. The pneumococcal vaccine with 23 pneumococcal capsular polysaccharide types became available in 1983. The 23 capsular pneumococcal vaccine contains purified capsular polysaccharides of pneumococcal types 1, 2, 3, 4, 5, 8, 9, 12, 14, 17, 19, 20, 22, 23, 26, 34, 43, 51, 56, 57, 67, 70 (American Classification). These are the main pneumococcal types associated with serious infections in the United States.

Usual Dosage Children >2 years and Adults: I.M., S.C.: 0.5 mL

Revaccination should be considered:

1. If ≥6 years since initial vaccination has elapsed, or
2. In patients who received 14-valent pneumococcal vaccine and are at highest risk (asplenic) for fatal infection or
3. At ≥6 years in patients with nephrotic syndrome, renal failure, or transplant recipients, or
4. 3-5 years in children with nephrotic syndrome, asplenia, or sickle cell disease

Administration Do not inject I.V., avoid intradermal, administer S.C. or I.M. (deltoid muscle or lateral midthigh)

Additional Information Federal law requires that the date of administration, the vaccine manufacturer, lot number of vaccine, and the administering person's name, title and address be entered into the patient's permanent medical record; inactivated bacteria vaccine

Dosage Forms Injection: 25 mcg each of 23 polysaccharide isolates/0.5 mL dose (0.5 mL, 1 mL, 5 mL)

Pneumomist® *see* Guaifenesin *on page 589*

Pneumovax® 23 *see* Pneumococcal Vaccine *on previous page*

Pnu-Imune® 23 *see* Pneumococcal Vaccine *on previous page*

Pod-Ben-25® *see* Podophyllum Resin *on this page*

Podocon-25® *see* Podophyllum Resin *on this page*

Podofin® *see* Podophyllum Resin *on this page*

Podophyllum Resin (po DOF fil um REZ in)

Brand Names Pod-Ben-25®; Podocon-25®; Podofin®

Canadian/Mexican Brand Names Podofilm® (Canada)

Synonyms Mandrake; May Apple

Therapeutic Category Keratolytic Agent

Use Topical treatment of benign growths including external genital and perianal warts, papillomas, fibroids; compound benzoin tincture generally is used as the medium for topical application

Pregnancy Risk Factor X

Contraindications Not to be used on birthmarks, moles, or warts with hair growth; cervical, urethral, oral warts; not to be used by diabetic patient or patient with poor circulation; pregnant women

Warnings/Precautions Use of large amounts of drug should be avoided; avoid contact with the eyes as it can cause severe corneal damage; do not apply to moles, birthmarks, or unusual warts; to be applied by a physician only; for external use only; 25% solution should not be applied to or near mucous membranes

Adverse Reactions

Local: Pain and edema at injection site

1% to 10%:

- Dermatologic: Pruritus
- Gastrointestinal: Nausea, vomiting, abdominal pain, diarrhea

<1%:

- Central nervous system: Confusion, lethargy, hallucinations
- Hematologic: Leukopenia, thrombocytopenia
- Hepatic: Hepatotoxicity
- Neuromuscular & skeletal: Peripheral neuropathy
- Renal: Renal failure

Mechanism of Action Directly affects epithelial cell metabolism by arresting mitosis through binding to a protein subunit of spindle microtubules (tubulin)

Usual Dosage Topical:

Children and Adults: 10% to 25% solution in compound benzoin tincture; apply drug to dry surface, use 1 drop at a time allowing drying between drops until area is covered; total volume should be limited to <0.5 mL per treatment session

Condylomata acuminatum: 25% solution is applied daily; use a 10% solution when applied to or near mucous membranes

Verrucae: 25% solution is applied 3-5 times/day directly to the wart

Patient Information Notify physician if undue skin irritation develops; should be applied by a physician

Nursing Implications Shake well before using; solution should be washed off within 1-4 hours for genital and perianal warts and within 1-2 hours for accessible meatal warts; use protective occlusive dressing around warts to prevent contact with unaffected skin

Dosage Forms Liquid, topical: 25% in benzoin (15 mL)

Point-Two® *see* Fluoride *on page 536*

Poladex® *see* Dexchlorpheniramine *on page 359*

Polaramine® *see* Dexchlorpheniramine *on page 359*

Poliomyelitis Vaccine *see* Polio Vaccines *on this page*

Polio Vaccines (POE lee oh vak SEENS)

Related Information

Adverse Events and Vaccination *on page 1439*
Guidelines for the Prevention of Opportunistic Infections in Persons with HIV *on page 1457*
Immunization Guidelines *on page 1421*
Miscellaneous Vaccination Information *on page 1437*
Recommendations of the Advisory Committee on Immunization Practices (ACIP) *on page 1424*
Recommended Childhood Immunization Schedule - US - January-December, 1997 *on page 1423*

Brand Names IPOL™; Orimune®

Synonyms E-IPV; Enhanced-potency Inactivated Poliovirus Vaccine; OPV; Poliomyelitis Vaccine; Poliovirus Vaccine, Live, Trivalent; Sabin; Salk; TOPV

Therapeutic Category Vaccine, Live Virus and Inactivated Virus

Use Oral: Prevention of poliomyelitis for infants (6-12 weeks of age) and all unimmunized children and adolescents through 18 years of age for routine prophylaxis. Persons traveling to areas where wild poliovirus is epidemic or endemic, and certain health personnel.

Although a protective immune response to E-IPV cannot be assured in the immunocompromised individual, E-IPV is recommended because the vaccine is safe and some protection may result from its administration.

Pregnancy Risk Factor C

Contraindications

Oral: Leukemia, lymphoma, or other generalized malignancies; diseases in which cellular immunity is absent or suppressed (hypogammaglobulinemia, agammaglobulinemia); immunosuppressive therapy; diarrhea; parenteral administration

Parenteral: Hypersensitivity to any component including neomycin, streptomycin, or polymyxin B; defer vaccination for persons with acute febrile illness until recovery

Warnings/Precautions Although there is no convincing evidence documenting adverse effects of either OPV or E-IPV on the pregnant woman or developing fetus, it is prudent on theoretical grounds to avoid vaccinating pregnant women. However, if immediate protection against poliomyelitis is needed, OPV is recommended. OPV should not be given to immunocompromised individuals or to persons with known or possibly immunocompromised family members; E-IPV is recommended in such situations.

Adverse Reactions All serious adverse reactions must be reported to the FDA

1% to 10%:

Dermatologic: Rash
Central nervous system: Fever >101.3°F
Local: Tenderness or pain at injection site

<1%:

Central nervous system: Fatigue, fussiness, sleepiness, crying, Guillain-Barré
Dermatologic: Reddening of skin, erythema
Gastrointestinal: Decreased appetite
Neuromuscular & skeletal: Weakness
Respiratory: Dyspnea

Drug Interactions Decreased effect with immunosuppressive agents, immune globulin, other live vaccines within 1 month; may temporarily suppress tuberculin skin test sensitivity (4-6 weeks)

(Continued)

Polio Vaccines *(Continued)*

Usual Dosage

Oral:

Infants:

Primary series: 0.5 mL at 6-12 weeks of age, second dose 6-8 weeks after first dose, and third dose 8-12 months after second dose

Booster: All children who have received primary immunization series, should receive a single follow-up dose and all children who have not should complete primary series

Children (older) and Adults (adolescents through 18 years of age): Two 0.5 mL doses 6-8 weeks apart and a third dose of 0.5 mL 6-12 months after second dose

Subcutaneous: **Enhanced-potency inactivated poliovirus vaccine (E-IPV) is preferred for primary vaccination of adults**, two doses S.C. 4-8 weeks apart, a third dose 6-12 months after the second. For adults with a completed primary series and for whom a booster is indicated, either OPV or E-IPV can be given. If immediate protection is needed, either OPV or E-IPV is recommended.

Administration Do not administer I.V.

Additional Information Federal law requires that the date of administration, the vaccine manufacturer, lot number of vaccine, and the administering person's name, title and address be entered into the patient's permanent medical record

Dosage Forms

Injection (IPOL™, E-IPV, Enhanced-potency Inactivated Poliovirus Vaccine, Poliomyelitis Vaccine, Salk): Suspension of three types of poliovirus (Types 1, 2 and 3) grown in human diploid cell cultures (0.5 mL)

Solution, oral (Orimune®, OPV, Poliovirus Vaccine, Live, Trivalent, Sabin, TOPV): Mixture of type 1, 2, and 3 viruses in monkey kidney tissue (0.5 mL)

Poliovirus Vaccine, Live, Trivalent *see* Polio Vaccines *on previous page*

Polocaine® *see* Mepivacaine *on page 783*

Polycillin® *see* Ampicillin *on page 85*

Polycillin-N® *see* Ampicillin *on page 85*

Polydine® [OTC] *see* Povidone-Iodine *on page 1031*

Polyestradiol (pol i es tra DYE ole)

Synonyms Polyestradiol Phosphate

Therapeutic Category Antineoplastic Agent, Hormone; Estrogen Derivative

Use Palliative treatment of advanced, inoperable carcinoma of the prostate

Pregnancy Risk Factor X

Contraindications Known or suspected estrogen-dependent neoplasm, carcinoma of the breast, active thromboembolic disorders, hypersensitivity to estrogens or any component

Warnings/Precautions Use with caution in patients with migraine, diabetes, cardiac, or renal impairment

Adverse Reactions

>10%:

Cardiovascular: Peripheral edema

Endocrine & metabolic: Enlargement of breasts (female and male), breast tenderness

Gastrointestinal: Nausea, anorexia, bloating

1% to 10%:

Central nervous system: Headache

Endocrine & metabolic: Increased libido (female), decrease libido (male)

Gastrointestinal: Vomiting, diarrhea

<1%:

Cardiovascular: Hypertension, thromboembolism, myocardial infarction, edema

Central nervous system: Depression, dizziness, anxiety, stroke

Dermatologic: Chloasma, melasma, rash

Endocrine: Amenorrhea, alterations in frequency and flow of menses, decreased glucose tolerance, increased triglycerides and LDL

Gastrointestinal: Nausea, GI distress

Hepatic: Cholestatic jaundice

Ocular: Intolerance to contact lenses

Miscellaneous: Increased susceptibility to *Candida* infection, breast tumors

Overdosage/Toxicology Toxicity is unlikely following single exposures of excessive doses; any treatment following emesis and charcoal administration should be supportive and symptomatic

Stability After reconstitution, solution is stable for 10 days at room temperature and protected from direct light

Mechanism of Action Estrogens exert their primary effects on the interphase DNA-protein complex (chromatin) by binding to a receptor (usually located in the cytoplasm of a target cell) and initiating translocation of the hormone-receptor complex to the nucleus

Pharmacodynamics/Kinetics

90% of injected dose leaves blood stream within 24 hours

Passive storage in reticuloendothelial system

Increasing the dose prolongs duration of action

Usual Dosage Adults: Deep I.M.: 40 mg every 2-4 weeks or less frequently; maximum dose: 80 mg

Dosage Forms Powder for injection, as phosphate: 40 mg

Polyestradiol Phosphate *see* Polyestradiol *on previous page*

Polyethylene Glycol-Electrolyte Solution

(pol i ETH i leen GLY kol ee LEK troe lite soe LOO shun)

Related Information

Laxatives, Classification and Properties *on page 1412*

Brand Names Colovage®; CoLyte®; GoLYTELY®; NuLytely®; OCL®

Canadian/Mexican Brand Names Peglyte™ (Canada); Klean-Prep® (Canada)

Synonyms Electrolyte Lavage Solution

Therapeutic Category Cathartic; Laxative, Bowel Evacuant

Use Bowel cleansing prior to GI examination or following toxic ingestion

Pregnancy Risk Factor C

Contraindications Gastrointestinal obstruction, gastric retention, bowel perforation, toxic colitis, megacolon

Warnings/Precautions Safety and efficacy not established in children; do not add flavorings as additional ingredients before use; observe unconscious or semiconscious patients with impaired gag reflex or those who are otherwise prone to regurgitation or aspiration during administration; use with caution in ulcerative colitis, caution against the use of hot loop polypectomy

Adverse Reactions

>10%: Gastrointestinal: Nausea, abdominal fullness, bloating

1% to 10%: Gastrointestinal: Abdominal cramps, vomiting, anal irritation

<1%: Dermatologic: Rash

Drug Interactions Oral medications should not be administered within 1 hour of start of therapy

Stability Use within 48 hours of preparation; refrigerate reconstituted solution; tap water may be used for preparation of the solution; shake container vigorously several times to ensure dissolution of powder

Mechanism of Action Induces catharsis by strong electrolyte and osmotic effects

Pharmacodynamics/Kinetics Onset of effect: Oral: Within 1-2 hours

Usual Dosage The recommended dose for adults is 4 L of solution prior to gastrointestinal examination, as ingestion of this dose produces a satisfactory preparation in >95% of patients. Ideally the patient should fast for approximately 3-4 hours prior to administration, but in no case should solid food be given for at least 2 hours before the solution is given. The solution is usually administered orally, but may be given via nasogastric tube to patients who are unwilling or unable to drink the solution.

Children: Oral: 25-40 mL/kg/hour for 4-10 hours

Adults:

Oral: At a rate of 240 mL (8 oz) every 10 minutes, until 4 liters are consumed or the rectal effluent is clear; rapid drinking of each portion is preferred to drinking small amounts continuously

Nasogastric tube: At a rate of 20-30 mL/minute (1.2-1.8 L/hour); the first bowel movement should occur approximately 1 hour after the start of administration

Monitoring Parameters Electrolytes, serum glucose, BUN, urine osmolality

Patient Information Chilled solution is often more palatable

Nursing Implications Rapid drinking of each portion is preferred over small amounts continuously; first bowel movement should occur in 1 hour; chilled solution often more palatable; do not add flavorings as additional ingredients before use

Dosage Forms Powder, for oral solution: PEG 3350 236 g, sodium sulfate 22.74 g, sodium bicarbonate 6.74 g, sodium chloride 5.86 g and potassium chloride 2.97 g (2000 mL, 4000 mL, 4800 mL, 6000 mL)

Polygam® *see* Immune Globulin, Intravenous *on page 651*

Polygam® S/D *see* Immune Globulin, Intravenous *on page 651*

Polymox® *see* Amoxicillin *on page 77*

Polymyxin B (pol i MIKS in bee)

Brand Names Aerosporin®

Synonyms Polymyxin B Sulfate

Therapeutic Category Antibiotic, Irrigation; Antibiotic, Miscellaneous

Use

Topical: Wound irrigation and bladder irrigation against *Pseudomonas aeruginosa*; used occasionally for gut decontamination

Parenteral use of polymyxin B has mainly been replaced by less toxic antibiotics; it is reserved for life-threatening infections caused by organisms resistant to the preferred drugs.

Pregnancy Risk Factor B

Contraindications Concurrent use of neuromuscular blockers

Warnings/Precautions Use with caution in patients with impaired renal function, (modify dosage) neurotoxic reactions are usually associated with high serum levels, found in patients with impaired renal function. Avoid concurrent or sequential use of other nephrotoxic and neurotoxic drugs, particularly bacitracin and the aminoglycosides. The drug's neurotoxicity can result in respiratory paralysis from neuromuscular blockade, especially when the drug is given soon after anesthesia or muscle relaxants. Polymyxin B sulfate is toxic when given parenterally; avoid parenteral use whenever possible.

Adverse Reactions

<1%:

Cardiovascular: Facial flushing

Central nervous system: Neurotoxicity (irritability, drowsiness, ataxia, perioral paresthesia, numbness of the extremities, and blurring of vision); drug fever

Dermatologic: Urticarial rash

Endocrine & metabolic: Hypocalcemia, hyponatremia, hypokalemia, hypochloremia

Neuromuscular & skeletal: Neuromuscular blockade, weakness

Renal: Nephrotoxicity

Respiratory: Respiratory arrest

Miscellaneous: Anaphylactoid reaction, meningeal irritation with intrathecal administration

Overdosage/Toxicology Symptoms of overdose include respiratory paralysis, ototoxicity, nephrotoxicity; supportive care is indicated as treatment; ventilatory support may be necessary

Drug Interactions Increased/prolonged effect of neuromuscular blocking agents

Stability Parenteral solutions stable for 7 days when refrigerated; discard any unused portion after 72 hours. **Incompatible** with calcium, magnesium, cephalothin, chloramphenicol, heparin, penicillins; aqueous solutions remain stable for 6-12 months under refrigeration

Mechanism of Action Binds to phospholipids, alters permeability, and damages the bacterial cytoplasmic membrane permitting leakage of intracellular constituents

Pharmacodynamics/Kinetics

Absorption: Well absorbed from the peritoneum; minimal absorption from the GI tract (except in neonates) from mucous membranes or intact skin

Distribution: Minimal distribution into the CSF; crosses the placenta

Half-life: 4.5-6 hours, increased with reduced renal function

Time to peak serum concentration: I.M.: Within 2 hours

Elimination: Primarily as unchanged drug (>60%) in urine via glomerular filtration

Usual Dosage

Otic: 1-2 drops, 3-4 times/day; should be used sparingly to avoid accumulation of excess debris

Infants <2 years:

I.M.: 25,000-30,000 units/kg/day divided every 6 hours

I.V.: 30,000-45,000 units/kg/day by continuous I.V. infusion

Intrathecal: 20,000 units/day for 3-4 days, then 25,000 units every other day for at least 2 weeks

Children ≥2 years and Adults:

I.M.: 25,000-30,000 units/kg/day divided every 4-6 hours

I.V.: 15,000-25,000 units/kg/day divided every 12 hours or by continuous infusion

Intrathecal: 50,000 units/day for 3-4 days, then every other day for at least 2 weeks

Total daily dose should not exceed 2,000,000 units/day

Bladder irrigation: Continuous irrigant or rinse in the urinary bladder for up to 10 days using 20 mg (equal to 200,000 units) added to 1 L of normal saline; usually no more than 1 L of irrigant is used per day unless urine flow rate is high; administration rate is adjusted to patient's urine output

Topical irrigation or topical solution: 500,000 units/L of normal saline; topical irrigation should not exceed 2 million units/day in adults

Gut sterilization: Oral: 15,000-25,000 units/kg/day in divided doses every 6 hours

Clostridium difficile enteritis: Oral: 25,000 units every 6 hours for 10 days

Ophthalmic: A concentration of 0.1% to 0.25% is administered as 1-3 drops every hour, then increasing the interval as response indicates to 1-2 drops 4-6 times/day

Dosing adjustment/interval in renal impairment:

Cl_{cr} 20-50 mL/minute: Administer 75% to 100% of normal dose every 12 hours

Cl_{cr} 5-20 mL/minute: Administer 50% of normal dose every 12 hours

Cl_{cr} <5 mL/minute: Administer 15% of normal dose every 12 hours

Reference Range Serum concentrations >5 μg/mL are toxic in adults

Patient Information Report any dizziness or sensations of ringing in the ear, loss of hearing, or any muscle weakness

Nursing Implications Parenteral use is indicated only in life-threatening infections caused by organisms not susceptible to other agents

Additional Information 1 mg = 10,000 units

Dosage Forms

Injection, as sulfate: 500,000 units (20 mL)

Powder for solution, ophthalmic, as sulfate: 500,000 units (20-50 mL diluent)

Polymyxin B and Neomycin *see* Neomycin and Polymyxin B *on page 888*

Polymyxin B Sulfate *see* Polymyxin B *on previous page*

Poly-Pred® *see* Neomycin, Polymyxin B, and Prednisolone *on page 891*

Polysporin® Ophthalmic *see* Bacitracin and Polymyxin B *on page 129*

Polysporin® Topical *see* Bacitracin and Polymyxin B *on page 129*

Polythiazide (pol i THYE a zide)

Related Information

Sulfonamide Derivatives *on page 1420*

Brand Names Renese®

Therapeutic Category Diuretic, Thiazide

Use Adjunctive therapy in treatment of edema and hypertension

Pregnancy Risk Factor D

Contraindications Anuria; hypersensitivity to polythiazide or any other sulfonamide derivatives

Warnings/Precautions Use with caution in renal disease, hepatic disease, gout, lupus erythematosus, diabetes mellitus; some products may contain tartrazine

Adverse Reactions

1% to 10%: Hypokalemia

<1%:

Cardiovascular: Hypotension

Central nervous system: Drowsiness

Dermatologic: Photosensitivity, rash

Endocrine & metabolic: Fluid and electrolyte imbalances (hypocalcemia, hypomagnesemia, hyponatremia), hyperglycemia

Gastrointestinal: Nausea, vomiting, anorexia

Genitourinary: Polyuria

Hematologic: Rarely blood dyscrasias

Hepatic: Hepatitis

Renal: Prerenal azotemia, uremia

Overdosage/Toxicology Symptoms of overdose include hypermotility, diuresis, lethargy; GI decontamination and supportive care

Drug Interactions Increased toxicity/levels of lithium

Mechanism of Action The diuretic mechanism of action of the thiazides is primarily inhibition of sodium, chloride, and water reabsorption in the renal distal tubules, thereby producing diuresis with a resultant reduction in plasma volume. The antihypertensive mechanism of action of the thiazides is unknown. It is known that doses of thiazides produce greater reductions in blood pressure than equivalent diuretic doses of loop diuretics (eg, furosemide). There has been speculation that the thiazides may have some influence on vascular tone mediated through sodium depletion, but this remains to be proven.

Pharmacodynamics/Kinetics

Onset of diuretic effect: Within ~2 hours

Duration: 24-48 hours

Usual Dosage Adults: Oral: 1-4 mg/day

Monitoring Parameters Blood pressure, fluids, weight loss, serum potassium

Test Interactions ↑ ammonia (B), ↑ amylase (S), ↑ calcium (S), ↑ chloride (S), ↑ cholesterol (S), ↑ glucose, ↑ uric acid (S); ↓ chloride (S), ↓ magnesium, ↓ potassium (S), ↓ sodium (S); tyramine and phentolamine tests, histamine tests for pheochromocytoma

Patient Information May be taken with food or milk; take early in day to avoid nocturia; take the last dose of multiple doses no later than 6 PM unless instructed

(Continued)

Polythiazide *(Continued)*

otherwise. A few people who take this medication become more sensitive to sunlight and may experience skin rash, redness, itching, or severe sunburn, especially if sun block SPF ≥15 is not used on exposed skin areas.

Nursing Implications Assess weight, I & O reports daily to determine fluid loss; take blood pressure with patient lying down and standing

Dosage Forms Tablet: 1 mg, 2 mg, 4 mg

Poly-Vi-Flor® *see* Vitamins, Multiple *on page 1310*

Poly-Vi-Sol® [OTC] *see* Vitamins, Multiple *on page 1310*

Pondimin® *see* Fenfluramine *on page 508*

Ponstel® *see* Mefenamic Acid *on page 773*

Pontocaine® *see* Tetracaine *on page 1202*

Porcelana® [OTC] *see* Hydroquinone *on page 628*

Porcelana® Sunscreen [OTC] *see* Hydroquinone *on page 628*

Porfimer (POR fi mer)

Brand Names Photofrin®

Synonyms Porfimer Sodium

Therapeutic Category Antineoplastic Agent, Miscellaneous

Use Esophageal cancer: Photodynamic therapy (PDT) with porfimer for palliation of patients with completely obstructing esophageal cancer, or of patients with partially obstructing esophageal cancer who cannot be satisfactorily treated with Nd:YAG laser therapy

Pregnancy Risk Factor C

Contraindications Porphyria or in patients with known allergies to porphyrins; existing tracheoesophageal or bronchoesophageal fistula; tumors eroding into a major blood vessel

Warnings/Precautions The U.S. Food and Drug Administration (FDA) currently recommends that procedures for proper handling and disposal of antineoplastic agents be considered. If the esophageal tumor is eroding into the trachea or bronchial tree, the likelihood of tracheoesophageal or bronchoesophageal fistula resulting from treatment is sufficiently high that PDT is not recommended. All patients who receive porfimer sodium will be photosensitive and must observe precautions to avoid exposure of skin and eyes to direct sunlight or bright indoor light for 30 days. The photosensitivity is due to residual drug which will be present in all parts of the skin. Exposure of the skin to ambient indoor light is, however, beneficial because the remaining drug will be inactivated gradually and safely through a photobleaching reaction. Patients should not stay in a darkened room during this period and should be encouraged to expose their skin to ambient indoor light. Ocular discomfort has been reported; for 30 days, when outdoors, patients should wear dark sunglasses which have an average white light transmittance of <4%.

Adverse Reactions

>10%:

- Cardiovascular: Atrial fibrillation, chest pain
- Central nervous system: Fever, pain, insomnia
- Dermatologic: Photosensitivity reaction
- Gastrointestinal: abdominal pain, constipation, dysphagia, nausea, vomiting
- Hematologic: Anemia
- Neuromuscular & skeletal: Back pain
- Respiratory: Dyspnea, pharyngitis, pleural effusion, pneumonia, respiratory insufficiency

1% to 10%:

- Cardiovascular: Hypertension, hypotension, edema, cardiac failure, tachycardia, chest pain (substernal)
- Central nervous system: Anxiety, confusion
- Endocrine & metabolic: Dehydration
- Gastrointestinal: Diarrhea, dyspepsia, eructation, esophageal edema, esophageal tumor bleeding, esophageal stricture, esophagitis, hematemesis, melena, weight loss, anorexia
- Genitourinary: Urinary tract infection
- Neuromuscular & skeletal: Weakness
- Respiratory: Coughing, tracheoesophageal fistula
- Miscellaneous: Moniliasis, surgical complication

Overdosage/Toxicology Overdose of laser light following porfimer injection: Increased symptoms and damage to normal tissue might be expected following an overdose of light

Treatment: Effects of overdosage on the duration of photosensitivity are unknown. Laser treatment should not be given if an overdose of porfimer is administered. In the event of an overdose, patients should protect their eyes and skin from direct sunlight or bright indoor lights for 30 days. At this time, patients should test for residual photosensitivity. Porfimer is not dialyzable.

Drug Interactions

Decreased effect: Compounds that quench active oxygen species or scavenge radicals (eg, dimethyl sulfoxide, beta-carotene, ethanol, mannitol) would be expected to decrease PDT activity; allopurinol, calcium channel blockers and some prostaglandin synthesis inhibitors could interfere with porfimer; drugs that decrease clotting, vasoconstriction or platelet aggregation could decrease the efficacy of PDT; glucocorticoid hormones may decrease the efficacy of the treatment

Increased toxicity: Concomitant administration of other photosensitizing agents (eg, tetracyclines, sulfonamides, phenothiazines, sulfonylureas, thiazide diuretics, griseofulvin) could increase the photosensitivity reaction

Stability

Store intact vials at controlled room temperature of 20°C to 25°C/68°F to 77°F

Reconstitute each vial of porfimer with 31.8 mL of either 5% dextrose injection or 0.9% sodium chloride injection resulting in a final concentration of 2.5 mg/mL and a pH of 7-8. Shake well until dissolved. Do not mix porfimer with other drugs in the same solution. Protect the reconstituted product from bright light and use immediately. Reconstituted porfimer is an opaque solution in which detection of particulate matter by visual inspection is extremely difficult.

Mechanism of Action Photosensitizing agent used in the photodynamic therapy (PDT) of tumors: cytotoxic and antitumor actions of porfimer are light and oxygen dependent. Cellular damage caused by porfimer PDT is a consequence of the propagation of radical reactions.

Pharmacodynamics/Kinetics

Distribution: Steady state V_d: 0.49 L/kg

Protein binding, plasma: 90%

Half-life: 250 hours

Time to peak serum concentration: Within 2 hours

Elimination: Total plasma clearance: 0.051 mL/minute/kg

Usual Dosage I.V. (refer to individual protocols):

Children: Safety and efficacy have not been established

Adults: I.V.: 2 mg/kg over 3-5 minutes

Photodynamic therapy is a two-stage process requiring administration of both drug and light. The first stage of PDT is the I.V. injection of porfimer. Illumination with laser light 40-50 hours following the injection with porfimer constitutes the second stage of therapy. A second laser light application may be given 90-120 hours after injection, preceded by gentle debridement of residual tumor.

Patients may receive a second course of PDT a minimum of 30 days after the initial therapy; up to three courses of PDT (each separated by a minimum of 30 days) can be given. Before each course of treatment, evaluate patients for the presence of a tracheoesophageal or bronchoesophageal fistula.

Administration Administer slow I.V. injection over 3-5 minutes; avoid extravasation; if extravasation occurs, take care to protect to protect the area from light. There is no known benefit from injecting the extravasation site with another substance. Wipe up spills with a damp cloth. Avoid skin and eye contact due to the potential for photosensitivity reactions upon exposure to light; use of rubber gloves and eye protection is recommended.

Patient Information Avoid exposure of skin and eyes to direct sunlight or bright indoor light (eg, examination lamps, including dental lamps, operating room lamps, unshaded light bulbs at close proximity) for 30 days after exposure. Exposure of skin to ambient indoor light is beneficial, however, because the remaining drug will be inactivated gradually and safely through a photobleaching reaction. Patients should wear dark sunglasses which have an average white light transmittance of <4% when outdoors.

Dosage Forms Powder for injection, as sodium: 75 mg

Porfimer Sodium *see* Porfimer *on previous page*

Pork NPH Iletin® II *see* Insulin Preparations *on page 659*

Pork Regular Iletin® II *see* Insulin Preparations *on page 659*

Posture® [OTC] *see* Calcium Phosphate, Tribasic *on page 194*

Potasalan® *see* Potassium Chloride *on page 1024*

Potassium Acetate (poe TASS ee um AS e tate)

Therapeutic Category Electrolyte Supplement, Parenteral; Potassium Salt; Vesicant

Use Potassium deficiency; to avoid chloride when high concentration of potassium is needed, source of bicarbonate

Pregnancy Risk Factor C

Contraindications Severe renal impairment, hyperkalemia

(Continued)

Potassium Acetate *(Continued)*

Warnings/Precautions Use with caution in patients with renal disease, hyperkalemia, cardiac disease, metabolic alkalosis; must be administered in patients with adequate urine flow

Adverse Reactions

>10%: Gastrointestinal: Diarrhea, nausea, stomach pain, flatulence, vomiting (oral)

1% to 10%:
- Cardiovascular: Bradycardia
- Endocrine & metabolic: Hyperkalemia
- Neuromuscular & skeletal: Weakness
- Respiratory: Dyspnea
- Local: Local tissue necrosis with extravasation

<1%:
- Cardiovascular: Chest pain
- Central nervous system: Mental confusion
- Endocrine & metabolic: Alkalosis
- Gastrointestinal: Abdominal pain, throat pain
- Local: Phlebitis
- Neuromuscular & skeletal: Paresthesias, paralysis

Overdosage/Toxicology Symptoms of overdose include muscle weakness, paralysis, peaked T waves, flattened P waves, prolongation of chloride. QRS complex, ventricular arrhythmias

Removal of potassium can be accomplished by various means; removal through the GI tract with Kayexalate® administration; by way of the kidney through diuresis, mineralocorticoid administration or increased sodium intake; by hemodialysis or peritoneal dialysis; or by shifting potassium back into the cells by insulin and glucose infusion or administration of sodium bicarbonate; calcium chloride will reverse cardiac effects.

Drug Interactions Increased effect/levels with potassium-sparing diuretics, salt substitutes, ACE inhibitors

Mechanism of Action Potassium is the major cation of intracellular fluid and is essential for the conduction of nerve impulses in heart, brain, and skeletal muscle; contraction of cardiac, skeletal and smooth muscles; maintenance of normal renal function, acid-base balance, carbohydrate metabolism, and gastric secretion

Pharmacodynamics/Kinetics
- Absorption: Absorbed well from upper GI tract
- Distribution: Enters cells via active transport from extracellular fluid
- Elimination: Largely by the kidneys, but also small amount via the skin and feces, with most intestinal potassium being reabsorbed

Usual Dosage I.V. doses should be incorporated into the patient's maintenance I.V. fluids, intermittent I.V. potassium administration should be reserved for severe depletion situations and requires EKG monitoring; doses listed as mEq of potassium

Treatment of hypokalemia: I.V.:
- Children: 2-5 mEq/kg/day
- Adults: 40-100 mEq/day

I.V. intermittent infusion (must be diluted prior to administration):
- Children: 0.5-1 mEq/kg/dose (maximum: 30 mEq) to infuse at 0.3-0.5 mEq/kg/hour (maximum: 1 mEq/kg/hour)
- Adults: 10-20 mEq/dose (maximum: 40 mEq/dose) to infuse over 2-3 hours (maximum: 40 mEq over 1 hour)

Administration Injections must be diluted for I.V. infusions

Nursing Implications Supplements usually not needed with adequate diet; EKG should be monitored continuously during the course of highly concentrate potassium solutions

Additional Information 1 mEq of acetate is equivalent to the alkalinizing effect of 1 mEq of bicarbonate

Dosage Forms Injection: 2 mEq/mL (20 mL, 50 mL, 100 mL); 4 mEq/mL (50 mL)

Potassium Acid Phosphate (poe TASS ee um AS id FOS fate)

Brand Names K-Phos® Original

Therapeutic Category Potassium Salt; Urinary Acidifying Agent

Use Acidifies urine and lowers urinary calcium concentration; reduces odor and rash caused by ammoniacal urine; increases the antibacterial activity of methenamine

Pregnancy Risk Factor C

Contraindications Severe renal impairment, hyperkalemia, hyperphosphatemia, and infected magnesium ammonium phosphate stones

Warnings/Precautions Use with caution in patients receiving other potassium supplementation and in patients with renal insufficiency, or severe tissue breakdown (eg, chemotherapy or hemodialysis)

Adverse Reactions

>10%: Gastrointestinal: Diarrhea, nausea, stomach pain, flatulence, vomiting

1% to 10%:

- Cardiovascular: Bradycardia
- Endocrine & metabolic: Hyperkalemia
- Local: Local tissue necrosis with extravasation
- Neuromuscular & skeletal: Weakness
- Respiratory: Dyspnea

<1%:

- Cardiovascular: Chest pain, arrhythmia, edema
- Central nervous system: Mental confusion, tetany, pain of extremities
- Endocrine & metabolic: Hyperphosphatemia, hypocalcemia, alkalosis
- Gastrointestinal: Abdominal pain, weight gain, throat pain
- Genitourinary: Decreased urine output
- Local: Phlebitis
- Neuromuscular & skeletal: Paresthesias, paralysis, bone pain, arthralgia, weakness of extremities
- Respiratory: Shortness of breath
- Miscellaneous: Thirst

Overdosage/Toxicology Symptoms of overdose include muscle weakness, paralysis, peaked T waves, flattened P waves, prolongation of QRS complex, ventricular arrhythmias

Removal of potassium can be accomplished by various means; removal through the GI tract with Kayexalate® administration; by way of the kidney through diuresis, mineralocorticoid administration or increased sodium intake; by hemodialysis or peritoneal dialysis; or by shifting potassium back into the cells by insulin and glucose infusion or sodium bicarbonate; calcium chloride will reverse cardiac effects.

Drug Interactions

Increased effect/levels with potassium-sparing diuretics, salt substitutes, salicylates, ACE inhibitors

Decreased effect with antacids containing magnesium, calcium or aluminum (bind phosphate and decreased its absorption)

Mechanism of Action The principal intracellular cation; involved in transmission of nerve impulses, muscle contractions, enzyme activity, and glucose utilization

Pharmacodynamics/Kinetics

Absorption: Absorbed well from upper GI tract

Distribution: Enters cells via active transport from extracellular fluid

Elimination: Largely by the kidneys, but also small amount via the skin and feces, with most intestinal potassium being reabsorbed

Usual Dosage Adults: Oral: 1000 mg dissolved in 6-8 oz of water 4 times/day with meals and at bedtime; for best results, soak tablets in water for 2-5 minutes, then stir and swallow

Monitoring Parameters Serum potassium, sodium, phosphate, calcium; serum salicylates (if taking salicylates)

Test Interactions ↓ ammonia (B)

Patient Information Dissolve tablets completely before drinking; avoid taking magnesium, calcium, or aluminum antacids at the same time; patients may pass old kidney stones when starting therapy; notify physician if experiencing nausea, vomiting, or abdominal pain

Dosage Forms Tablet, sodium free: 500 mg [potassium 3.67 mEq]

Potassium Bicarbonate and Potassium Citrate, Effervescent

(poe TASS ee um bye KAR bun ate & poe TASS ee um SIT rate, ef er VES ent)

Brand Names Effer-K™; K-Ide®; Klor-con®/EF; K-Lyte®; K-Vescent®

Synonyms Potassium Citrate and Potassium Bicarbonate, Effervescent

Therapeutic Category Potassium Salt

Use Treatment or prevention of hypokalemia

Pregnancy Risk Factor C

Contraindications Severe renal impairment, hyperkalemia

Warnings/Precautions Use with caution in patients with renal disease, cardiac disease

Adverse Reactions

>10%: Gastrointestinal: Diarrhea, nausea, stomach pain, flatulence, vomiting

1% to 10%:

- Cardiovascular: Bradycardia
- Endocrine & metabolic: Hyperkalemia

(Continued)

Potassium Bicarbonate and Potassium Citrate, Effervescent *(Continued)*

Local: Local tissue necrosis with extravasation
Neuromuscular & skeletal: Weakness
Respiratory: Dyspnea

<1%:

Cardiovascular: Chest pain
Central nervous system: Mental confusion
Endocrine & metabolic: Alkalosis
Gastrointestinal: Abdominal pain, throat pain
Local: Phlebitis
Neuromuscular & skeletal: Paresthesias, paralysis

Overdosage/Toxicology Symptoms of overdose include muscle weakness, paralysis, peaked T waves, flattened P waves, prolongation of QRS complex, ventricular arrhythmias

Removal of potassium can be accomplished by various means; removal through the GI tract with Kayexalate® administration; by way of the kidney through diuresis, mineralocorticoid administration or increased sodium intake; by hemodialysis or peritoneal dialysis; or by shifting potassium back into the cells by insulin and glucose infusion or sodium bicarbonate; calcium chloride will reverse cardiac effects.

Drug Interactions Increased effect/levels with potassium-sparing diuretics, salt substitutes, ACE inhibitors

Mechanism of Action Needed for the conduction of nerve impulses in heart, brain, and skeletal muscle; contraction of cardiac, skeletal and smooth muscles; maintenance of normal renal function

Pharmacodynamics/Kinetics

Absorption: Absorbed well from upper GI tract
Distribution: Enters cells via active transport from extracellular fluid
Elimination: Largely by the kidneys, but also small amount via the skin and feces, with most intestinal potassium being reabsorbed

Usual Dosage Oral:

Children: 1-4 mEq/kg/24 hours in divided doses as required to maintain normal serum potassium

Adults:

Prevention: 16-24 mEq/day in 2-4 divided doses
Treatment: 40-100 mEq/day in 2-4 divided doses

Monitoring Parameters Serum potassium

Test Interactions ↓ ammonia (B)

Patient Information Dissolve completely in 3-8 oz cold water, juice, or other suitable beverage and drink slowly

Dosage Forms

Capsule, extended release: 8 mEq, 10 mEq
Powder for oral solution: 15 mEq/packet; 20 mEq/packet; 25 mEq/packet
Tablet, effervescent: 25 mEq, 50 mEq

Potassium Chloride (poe TASS ee um KLOR ide)

Related Information

Extravasation Treatment of Other Drugs *on page 1381*

Brand Names Cena-K®; Gen-K®; K+ 10®; Kaochlor®; Kaochlor® SF; Kaon-Cl®; Kaon Cl-10®; Kato®; Kay Ciel®; K+ Care®; K-Dur® 10; K-Dur® 20; K-Lease®; K-Lor™; Klor-Con®; Klor-Con® 8; Klor-Con® 10; Klor-Con/25®; Klorvess®; Klotrix®; K-Lyte/Cl®; K-Norm®; K-Tab®; Micro-K® 10; Micro-K® Extencaps®; Micro-K® LS®; Potasalan®; Rum-K®; Slow-K®; Ten-K®

Canadian/Mexican Brand Names Celek® 20 (Mexico); Clor-K-Zaf® (Mexico); Cloruro® De Potasio (Mexico); Kaliolite® (Mexico)

Synonyms KCl

Therapeutic Category Electrolyte Supplement, Oral; Electrolyte Supplement, Parenteral; Potassium Salt; Vesicant

Use Treatment or prevention of hypokalemia

Pregnancy Risk Factor A

Contraindications Severe renal impairment, untreated Addison's disease, heat cramps, hyperkalemia, severe tissue trauma; solid oral dosage forms are contraindicated in patients in whom there is a structural, pathological, and/or pharmacologic cause for delay or arrest in passage through the GI tract; an oral liquid potassium preparation should be used in patients with esophageal compression or delayed gastric emptying time

Warnings/Precautions Use with caution in patients with cardiac disease, severe renal impairment, hyperkalemia

Adverse Reactions

>10%: Gastrointestinal: Diarrhea, nausea, stomach pain, flatulence, vomiting (oral)

1% to 10%:

Cardiovascular: Bradycardia
Endocrine & metabolic: Hyperkalemia
Local: Local tissue necrosis with extravasation, pain at the site of injection
Neuromuscular & skeletal: Weakness
Respiratory: Dyspnea

<1%:

Cardiovascular: Chest pain, arrhythmias, heart block, hypotension
Central nervous system: Mental confusion
Endocrine & metabolic: Alkalosis
Gastrointestinal: Abdominal pain, throat pain
Local: Phlebitis
Neuromuscular & skeletal: Paresthesias, paralysis

Overdosage/Toxicology Symptoms of overdose include muscle weakness, paralysis, peaked T waves, flattened P waves, prolongation of QRS complex, ventricular arrhythmias

Removal of potassium can be accomplished by various means; removal through the GI tract with Kayexalate® administration; by way of the kidney through diuresis, mineralocorticoid administration or increased sodium intake; by hemodialysis or peritoneal dialysis; or by shifting potassium back into the cells by insulin and glucose infusion or sodium bicarbonate; calcium chloride reverses cardiac effects.

Drug Interactions

Increased effect/levels with potassium-sparing diuretics, salt substitutes, ACE inhibitors
Increased effect of digitalis

Stability Store at room temperature, protect from freezing; use only clear solutions; use admixtures within 24 hours

Mechanism of Action Potassium is the major cation of intracellular fluid and is essential for the conduction of nerve impulses in heart, brain, and skeletal muscle; contraction of cardiac, skeletal and smooth muscles; maintenance of normal renal function, acid-base balance, carbohydrate metabolism, and gastric secretion

Pharmacodynamics/Kinetics

Absorption: Absorbed well from upper GI tract
Distribution: Enters cells via active transport from extracellular fluid
Elimination: Largely by the kidneys, but also small amount via the skin and feces, with most intestinal potassium being reabsorbed

Usual Dosage I.V. doses should be incorporated into the patient's maintenance I.V. fluids; intermittent I.V. potassium administration should be reserved for severe depletion situations in patients undergoing EKG monitoring.

Normal daily requirements: Oral, I.V.:

Premature infants: 2-6 mEq/kg/24 hours
Term infants 0-24 hours: 0-2 mEq/kg/24 hours
Infants >24 hours: 1-2 mEq/kg/24 hours
Children: 2-3 mEq/kg/day
Adults: 40-80 mEq/day

Prevention during diuretic therapy: Oral:

Children: 1-2 mEq/kg/day in 1-2 divided doses
Adults: 20-40 mEq/day in 1-2 divided doses

Treatment of hypokalemia: Children:

Oral: 1-2 mEq/kg initially, then as needed based on frequently obtained lab values. If deficits are severe or ongoing losses are great, I.V. route should be considered.

I.V.: 1 mEq/kg over 1-2 hours initially, then repeated as needed based on frequently obtained lab values; severe depletion or ongoing losses may require >200% of normal limit needs

I.V. intermittent infusion: Dose should not exceed 1 mEq/kg/hour, or 40 mEq/hour; if it exceeds 0.5 mEq/kg/hour, physician should be at bedside and patient should have continuous EKG monitoring

Potassium Dosage/Rate of Infusion Guidelines

Serum Potassium⁺	Maximum Infusion Rate	Maximum Concentration	Maximum 24-Hour Dose
>2.5 mEq/L	10 mEq/h	40 mEq/L	200 mEq
<2.5 mEq/L	40 mEq/h	80 mEq/L	400 mEq

(Continued)

Potassium Chloride *(Continued)*

Treatment of hypokalemia: Adults:
- I.V. intermittent infusion: 10-20 mEq/hour, not to exceed 40 mEq/hour and 150 mEq/day. See table.
- Potassium >2.5 mEq/L:
  - Oral: 60-80 mEq/day plus additional amounts if needed
  - I.V.: 10 mEq over 1 hour with additional doses if needed
- Potassium <2.5 mEq/L:
  - Oral: Up to 40-60 mEq initial dose, followed by further doses based on lab values; deficits at a plasma level of 2 mEq/L may be as high as 400-800 mEq of potassium
  - I.V.: Up to 40 mEq over 1 hour, with doses based on frequent lab monitoring; deficits at a plasma level of 2 mEq/L may be as high as 400-800 mEq of potassium

Administration Maximum concentration (peripheral line): 80 mEq/L, usual maximum: 30-40 mEq/L; maximum concentration (central line): 40 mEq/100 mL, most guidelines recommend maximal infusion rates of 5 mEq/hour if patient is **not** on a cardiac monitor and 10 mEq/hour (children: 0.3 mEq/kg/hour) if monitored; may not be given I.V. push or I.V. retrograde; oral liquid potassium supplements should be diluted with water or fruit juice during administration

Monitoring Parameters Serum potassium, glucose, chloride, pH, urine output (if indicated), cardiac monitor (if intermittent infusion or potassium infusion rates >0.25 mEq/kg/hour)

Patient Information Sustained release and wax matrix tablets should be swallowed whole, do not crush or chew; effervescent tablets must be dissolved in water before use; take with food; liquid and granules can be diluted or dissolved in water or juice

Nursing Implications Wax matrix tablets must be swallowed and not allowed to dissolve in mouth

Dosage Forms
- Capsule, controlled release (microcapsulated): 600 mg [8 mEq]; 750 mg [10 mEq]
  - Micro-K® Extencaps®: 600 mg [8 mEq]
  - K-Lease®, K-Norm®, Micro-K® 10: 750 mg [10 mEq]
- Liquid: 10% [20 mEq/15 mL] (480 mL, 4000 mL); 20% [40 mEq/15 mL] (480 mL, 4000 mL)
  - Cena-K®, Kaochlor®, Kaochlor® SF, Kay Ciel®, Klorvess®, Potasalan®: 10% [20 mEq/15 mL] (480 mL, 4000 mL)
  - Rum-K®: 15% [30 mEq/15 mL] (480 mL, 4000 mL)
  - Cena-K®, Kaon-Cl® 20%: 20% [40 mEq/15 mL]
- Crystals for oral suspension, extended release (Micro-K® LS®): 20 mEq per packet
- Powder: 20 mEq per packet (30s, 100s)
  - K+ Care®, K-Lor™: 15 mEq per packet (30s, 100s)
  - Gen-K®, Kato®, Kay Ciel®, K+ Care®, K-Lor™, Klor-Con®: 20 mEq per packet (30s, 100s)
  - K+ Care®, Klor-Con/25®: 25 mEq per packet (30s, 100s)
  - K-Lyte/Cl®: 25 mEq per dose (30s)
- Infusion, concentrate: 0.1 mEq/mL, 0.2 mEq/mL, 0.3 mEq/mL, 0.4 mEq/mL
- Injection, concentrate: 1.5 mEq/mL, 2 mEq/mL, 3 mEq/mL
- Tablet, controlled release (microencapsulated)
  - K-Dur® 10, Ten-K®: 750 mg [10 mEq]
  - K-Dur® 20: 1500 mg [20 mEq]
- Tablet, controlled release (wax matrix): 600 mg [8 mEq]; 750 mg [10 mEq]
  - Kaon-Cl®: 500 mg [6.7 mEq]
  - Klor-Con® 8, Slow-K®: 600 mg [8 mEq]
  - K+ 10®, Kaon Cl-10®, Klor-Con® 10, Klotrix®, K-Tab®: 750 mg [10 mEq]

Potassium Gluconate (poe TASS ee um GLOO coe nate)

Brand Names Kaon®; Kaylixir®; K-G® Elixir

Therapeutic Category Potassium Salt

Use Treatment or prevention of hypokalemia

Pregnancy Risk Factor A

Contraindications Severe renal impairment, untreated Addison's disease, heat cramps, hyperkalemia, severe tissue trauma; solid oral dosage forms are contraindicated in patients in whom there is a structural, pathological, and/or pharmacologic cause for delay or arrest in passage through the GI tract; an oral liquid potassium preparation should be used in patients with esophageal compression or delayed gastric emptying time

Warnings/Precautions Use with caution in patients with cardiac disease, severe renal impairment, hyperkalemia; patients must be on a cardiac monitor during intermittent infusions

Adverse Reactions
>10%: Gastrointestinal: Diarrhea, nausea, stomach pain, flatulence, vomiting (oral)
1% to 10%:
Cardiovascular: Bradycardia
Endocrine & metabolic: Hyperkalemia
Neuromuscular & skeletal: Weakness
Respiratory: Dyspnea
<1%:
Cardiovascular: Chest pain
Central nervous system: Mental confusion
Endocrine & metabolic: Alkalosis
Gastrointestinal: Throat pain
Local: Phlebitis
Neuromuscular & skeletal: Paresthesias, paralysis

Overdosage/Toxicology Symptoms of overdose include muscle weakness, paralysis, peaked T waves, flattened P waves, prolongation of QRS complex, ventricular arrhythmias

Removal of potassium can be accomplished by various means; removal through the GI tract with Kayexalate® administration; by way of the kidney through diuresis, mineralocorticoid administration or increased sodium intake; by hemodialysis or peritoneal dialysis; or by shifting potassium back into the cells by insulin, glucose infusion, or sodium bicarbonate; calcium chloride reverses cardiac effects

Drug Interactions Increased effect/levels with potassium-sparing diuretics, salt substitutes, ACE inhibitors; increased effect of digitalis

Stability Store at room temperature, protect from freezing; use only clear solutions

Mechanism of Action Potassium is the major cation of intracellular fluid and is essential for the conduction of nerve impulses in heart, brain, and skeletal muscle; contraction of cardiac, skeletal and smooth muscles; maintenance of normal renal function, acid-base balance, carbohydrate metabolism, and gastric secretion

Pharmacodynamics/Kinetics
Absorption: Absorbed well from upper GI tract
Distribution: Enters cells via active transport from extracellular fluid
Elimination: Largely by the kidneys, but also small amount via the skin and feces, with most intestinal potassium being reabsorbed

Usual Dosage Oral (doses listed as mEq of potassium):
Normal daily requirement:
Children: 2-3 mEq/kg/day
Adults: 40-80 mEq/day
Prevention of hypokalemia during diuretic therapy:
Children: 1-2 mEq/kg/day in 1-2 divided doses
Adults: 20-40 mEq/day in 1-2 divided doses
Treatment of hypokalemia:
Children: 2-5 mEq/kg/day in 2-4 divided doses
Adults: 40-100 mEq/day in 2-4 divided doses

Monitoring Parameters Serum potassium, chloride, glucose, pH, urine output (if indicated)

Test Interactions ↓ ammonia (B)

Patient Information Take with food, water, or fruit juice; swallow tablets whole; do not crush or chew

Nursing Implications Do not administer liquid full strength, must be diluted in 2-6 parts of water or juice

Additional Information 9.4 g potassium gluconate is approximately equal to 40 mEq potassium (4.3 mEq potassium/g salt)

Dosage Forms
Elixir: 20 mEq/15 mL
K-G®, Kaon®, Kaylixir®: 20 mEq/15 mL
Tablet:
Glu-K®: 2 mEq
Kaon®: 5 mEq

Potassium Iodide (poe TASS ee um EYE oh dide)

Brand Names Pima®; SSKI®; Thyro-Block®

Synonyms KI; Lugol's Solution; Strong Iodine Solution

Therapeutic Category Antithyroid Agent; Cough Preparation; Expectorant

Use Facilitate bronchial drainage and cough; reduce thyroid vascularity prior to thyroidectomy and management of thyrotoxic crisis; block thyroidal uptake of radioactive isotopes of iodine in a radiation emergency

Pregnancy Risk Factor D

(Continued)

Potassium Iodide *(Continued)*

Contraindications Known hypersensitivity to iodine; hyperkalemia, pulmonary tuberculosis, pulmonary edema, bronchitis, impaired renal function

Warnings/Precautions Prolonged use can lead to hypothyroidism; cystic fibrosis patients have an exaggerated response; can cause acne flare-ups, can cause dermatitis, some preparations may contain sodium bisulfite (allergy); use with caution in patients with a history of thyroid disease, patients with renal failure, or GI obstruction

Adverse Reactions

1% to 10%:

Central nervous system: Fever, headache
Dermatologic: Urticaria, acne, angioedema, cutaneous hemorrhage
Endocrine & metabolic: Goiter with hypothyroidism
Gastrointestinal: Metallic taste, GI upset, soreness of teeth and gums
Hematologic: Eosinophilia, hemorrhage (mucosal)
Neuromuscular & skeletal: Arthralgia
Respiratory: Rhinitis
Miscellaneous: Lymph node enlargement

Overdosage/Toxicology Symptoms of overdose include angioedema, laryngeal edema in patients with hypersensitivity; muscle weakness, paralysis, peaked T waves, flattened P waves, prolongation of QRS complex, ventricular arrhythmias

Removal of potassium can be accomplished by various means; removal through the GI tract with Kayexalate® administration; by way of the kidney through diuresis, mineralocorticoid administration or increased sodium intake; by hemodialysis or peritoneal dialysis; or by shifting potassium back into the cells by insulin and glucose infusion.

Drug Interactions Increased toxicity: Lithium → additive hypothyroid effects

Stability Store in tight, light-resistant containers at temperature <40°C; freezing should be avoided

Mechanism of Action Reduces viscosity of mucus by increasing respiratory tract secretions; inhibits secretion of thyroid hormone, fosters colloid accumulation in thyroid follicles

Pharmacodynamics/Kinetics

Onset of action: 24-48 hours
Peak effect: 10-15 days after continuous therapy
Elimination: In euthyroid patient, renal clearance rate is 2 times that of the thyroid

Usual Dosage Oral:

Adults: RDA: 130 mcg

Expectorant:
Children: 60-250 mg every 6-8 hours; maximum single dose: 500 mg
Adults: 300-650 mg 2-3 times/day

Preoperative thyroidectomy: Children and Adults: 50-250 mg (1-5 drops SSKI®) 3 times/day **or** 0.1-0.3 mL (3-5 drops) of strong iodine (Lugol's solution) 3 times/day; administer for 10 days before surgery

Thyrotoxic crisis:
Infants <1 year: 150-250 mg (3-5 drops SSKI®) 3 times/day
Children and Adults: 300-500 mg (6-10 drops SSKI®) 3 times/day or 1 mL strong iodine (Lugol's solution) 3 times/day

Sporotrichosis:
Initial:
Preschool: 50 mg/dose 3 times/day
Children: 250 mg/dose 3 times/day
Adults: 500 mg/dose 3 times/day
Oral increase 50 mg/dose daily
Maximum dose:
Preschool: 500 mg/dose 3 times/day
Children and Adults: 1-2 g/dose 3 times/day
Continue treatment for 4-6 weeks after lesions have completely healed

Monitoring Parameters Thyroid function tests

Patient Information Take after meals with food or milk or dilute with a large quantity of water, fruit juice, milk, or broth; discontinue use if stomach pain, skin rash, metallic taste, or nausea and vomiting occurs

Nursing Implications Must be diluted before administration of 240 mL of water, fruit juice, milk, or broth

Additional Information 10 drops of SSKI® = potassium iodide 500 mg

Dosage Forms

Solution, oral:
SSKI®: 1 g/mL (30 mL, 240 mL)
Lugol's Solution, strong iodine: Potassium iodide 100 mg and iodine 50 mg per mL (120 mL, 473 mL, 4000 mL)

Syrup: 325 mg/5 mL (473 mL, 4000 mL)

Tablet: 130 mg

Potassium Phosphate (poe TASS ee um FOS fate)

Brand Names Neutra-Phos®-K

Synonyms Phosphate, Potassium

Therapeutic Category Electrolyte Supplement, Oral; Electrolyte Supplement, Parenteral; Phosphate Salt; Potassium Salt; Vesicant

Use Treatment and prevention of hypophosphatemia or hypokalemia

Pregnancy Risk Factor C

Contraindications Hyperphosphatemia, hyperkalemia, hypocalcemia, hypomagnesemia, renal failure

Warnings/Precautions Use with caution in patients with renal insufficiency, cardiac disease, metabolic alkalosis; admixture of phosphate and calcium in I.V. fluids can result in calcium phosphate precipitation

Adverse Reactions

>10%: Gastrointestinal: Diarrhea, nausea, stomach pain, flatulence, vomiting

1% to 10%:

- Cardiovascular: Bradycardia
- Endocrine & metabolic: Hyperkalemia
- Neuromuscular & skeletal: Weakness
- Respiratory: Dyspnea

<1%:

- Cardiovascular: Chest pain
- Central nervous system: Mental confusion
- Endocrine & metabolic: Alkalosis
- Gastrointestinal: Abdominal pain, throat pain
- Local: Phlebitis
- Neuromuscular & skeletal: Paresthesias, paralysis
- Renal: Acute renal failure

Overdosage/Toxicology Symptoms of overdose include muscle weakness, paralysis, peaked T waves, flattened P waves, prolongation of QRS complex, ventricular arrhythmias, tetany, calcium-phosphate precipitation

Removal of potassium can be accomplished by various means; removal through the GI tract with Kayexalate® administration; by way of the kidney through diuresis, mineralocorticoid administration or increased sodium intake; by hemodialysis or peritoneal dialysis; or by shifting potassium back into the cells by insulin, glucose infusion, or sodium bicarbonate; calcium chloride reverses cardiac effects.

Drug Interactions

Decreased effect/levels with aluminum and magnesium-containing antacids or sucralfate which can act as phosphate binders

Increased effect/levels with potassium-sparing diuretics, salt substitutes, or ACE-inhibitors; increased effect of digitalis

Stability Store at room temperature, protect from freezing; use only clear solutions; up to 10-15 mEq of calcium may be added per liter before precipitate may occur

Stability of parenteral admixture at room temperature (25°C): 24 hours

Phosphate salts may precipitate when mixed with calcium salts; solubility is improved in amino acid parenteral nutrition solutions; check with a pharmacist to determine compatibility

Usual Dosage I.V. doses should be incorporated into the patient's maintenance I.V. fluids; intermittent I.V. infusion should be reserved for severe depletion situations in patients undergoing continuous EKG monitoring. It is difficult to determine total body phosphorus deficit; the following dosages are empiric guidelines:

Normal requirements elemental phosphorus: Oral:

- 0-6 months: 240 mg
- 6-12 months: 360 mg
- 1-10 years: 800 mg
- >10 years: 1200 mg
- Pregnancy lactation: Additional 400 mg/day

Adults RDA: 800 mg

Treatment: It is difficult to provide concrete guidelines for the treatment of severe hypophosphatemia because the extent of total body deficits and response to therapy are difficult to predict. Aggressive doses of phosphate may result in a transient serum elevation followed by redistribution into intracellular compartments or bone tissue. It is recommended that repletion of severe hypophosphatemia (<1 mg/dL in adults) be done I.V. because large doses of oral phosphate may cause diarrhea and intestinal absorption may be unreliable

(Continued)

Potassium Phosphate *(Continued)*

Pediatric I.V. phosphate repletion:

Children: 0.25-0.5 mmol/kg **administer over 4-6 hours and repeat if symptomatic hypophosphatemia persists**; to assess the need for further phosphate administration, obtain serum inorganic phosphate after administration of the first dose and base further doses on serum levels and clinical status

Adult I.V. phosphate repletion:

Initial dose: 0.08 mmol/kg if recent uncomplicated hypophosphatemia

Initial dose: 0.16 mmol/kg if prolonged hypophosphatemia with presumed total body deficits; increase dose by 25% to 50% if patient symptomatic with severe hypophosphatemia

Do not exceed 0.24 mmol/kg/day; administer over 6 hours by I.V. infusion

With orders for I.V. phosphate, there is considerable confusion associated with the use of millimoles (mmol) versus milliequivalents (mEq) to express the phosphate requirement. Because inorganic phosphate exists as monobasic and dibasic anions, with the mixture of valences dependent on pH, ordering by mEq amounts is unreliable and may lead to large dosing errors. In addition, I.V. phosphate is available in the sodium and potassium salt; therefore, the content of these cations must be considered when ordering phosphate. The most reliable method of ordering I.V. phosphate is by millimoles, then specifying the potassium or sodium salt. For example, an order for 15 mmol of phosphate as potassium phosphate in one liter of normal saline would also provide 22 mEq of potassium.

Phosphate maintenance electrolyte requirement in parenteral nutrition: 2 mmol/kg/24 hours or 35 mmol/kcal/24 hours; maximum: 15-30 mmol/24 hours

Maintenance:

I.V. solutions:

Children: 0.5-1.5 mmol/kg/24 hours I.V. or 2-3 mmol/kg/24 hours orally in divided doses

Adults: 15-30 mmol/24 hours I.V. or 50-150 mmol/24 hours orally in divided doses

Oral:

Children <4 years: 1 capsule (250 mg phosphorus/8 mmol) 4 times/day; dilute as instructed

Children >4 years and Adults: 1-2 capsules (250-500 mg phosphorus/8-16 mmol) 4 times/day; dilute as instructed

Fleet® Phospho®-Soda: Laxative: Oral: Single dose

Children: 5-15 mL

Adults: 20-30 mL mixed with 120 mL cold water

Administration Injection must be diluted in appropriate I.V. solution and volume prior to administration and administered over a minimum of 4 hours

Monitoring Parameters Serum potassium, calcium, phosphate, sodium, cardiac monitor (when intermittent infusion or high-dose I.V. replacement needed)

Test Interactions ↓ ammonia (B)

	Elemental Phosphorous (mg)	Phosphate (mmol)	Na (mEq)	K (mEq)
Oral				
Whole cow's milk per mL		0.29	0.025	0.035
Neutra-Phos®				
capsule				
powder concentrate per 75 mL	250	8	7.1	7.1
Neutra-Phos®-K				
capsule	250	8		14.2
powder				
K-Phos® Neutral tablets	250	8	13	1.1
K-Phos® MF tablets	125.6	4	2.9	1.1
K-Phos® No. 2	250	8	5.8	2.3
K-Phos® Original tablets	114	3.6		3.7
Uro-KP-Neutral® tablets	250	8	10.8	1.3
Intravenous				
K phosphate per mL		3		4.4

Patient Information Do not swallow the capsule; empty contents of capsule into 75 mL (2.5 oz) of water before taking; take with food to reduce the risk of diarrhea

Nursing Implications Capsule must be emptied into 3-4 oz of water before administration

Dosage Forms See table.

Potassium Phosphate and Sodium Phosphate

(poe TASS ee um FOS fate & SOW dee um FOS fate)

Brand Names K-Phos® Neutral; Neutra-Phos®; Uro-KP-Neutral®

Synonyms Sodium Phosphate and Potassium Phosphate

Therapeutic Category Phosphate Salt; Potassium Salt

Use Treatment of conditions associated with excessive renal phosphate loss or inadequate GI absorption of phosphate; to acidify the urine to lower calcium concentrations; to increase the antibacterial activity of methenamine; reduce odor and rash caused by ammonia in urine

Pregnancy Risk Factor C

Contraindications Addison's disease, hyperkalemia, hyperphosphatemia, infected urolithiasis or struvite stone formation, patients with severely impaired renal function

Warnings/Precautions Use with caution in patients with renal disease, hyperkalemia, cardiac disease and metabolic alkalosis

Adverse Reactions

>10%: Gastrointestinal: Diarrhea, nausea, stomach pain, flatulence, vomiting

1% to 10%:

- Cardiovascular: Bradycardia
- Endocrine & metabolic: Hyperkalemia
- Neuromuscular & skeletal: Weakness
- Respiratory: Dyspnea

<1%:

- Cardiovascular: Arrhythmia, chest pain, edema
- Central nervous system: Mental confusion, tetany
- Endocrine & metabolic: Alkalosis
- Gastrointestinal: Weight gain, throat pain
- Genitourinary: Decreased urine output
- Local: Phlebitis
- Neuromuscular & skeletal: Paresthesias, paralysis, pain/weakness of extremities, bone pain, arthralgia
- Renal: Acute renal failure
- Respiratory: Shortness of breath
- Miscellaneous: Thirst

Overdosage/Toxicology Symptoms of overdose include muscle weakness, paralysis, peaked T waves, flattened P waves, prolongation of QRS complex, ventricular arrhythmias, tetany, calcium phosphate precipitation

Removal of potassium can be accomplished by various means; removal through the GI tract with Kayexalate® administration; by way of the kidney through diuresis, mineralocorticoid administration or increased sodium intake; by hemodialysis or peritoneal dialysis; or by shifting potassium back into the cells by insulin and glucose infusion; calcium chloride reverses cardiac effects.

Drug Interactions

Decreased effect/levels with aluminum and magnesium-containing antacids or sucralfate which can act as phosphate binders

Increased effect/levels with potassium-sparing diuretics or ACE-inhibitors; increased effect/levels of digitalis, salicylates

Usual Dosage All dosage forms to be mixed in 6-8 oz of water prior to administration

Children: 2-3 mmol phosphate/kg/24 hours given 4 times/day **or** 1 capsule 4 times/day

Adults: 1-2 capsules (250-500 mg phosphorus/8-16 mmol) 4 times/day after meals and at bedtime

Monitoring Parameters Serum potassium, sodium, calcium, phosphate, EKG

Patient Information Do not swallow, open capsule and dissolve in 6-8 oz of water; powder packets are to be mixed in 6-8 oz of water; tablets should be crushed and mixed in 6-8 oz of water

Nursing Implications Tablets may be crushed and stirred vigorously to speed dissolution

Dosage Forms See table in Potassium Phosphate monograph

Povidone-Iodine (POE vi done EYE oh dyne)

Brand Names ACU-dyne® [OTC]; Aerodine® [OTC]; Betadine® [OTC]; Betagen [OTC]; Biodine [OTC]; Efodine® [OTC]; Iodex® [OTC]; Iodex-p® [OTC]; Isodine® [OTC]; Mallisol® [OTC]; Massengill® Medicated Douche w/Cepticin [OTC];

(Continued)

Povidone-Iodine *(Continued)*

Minidyne® [OTC]; Operand® [OTC]; Polydine® [OTC]; Summer's Eve® Medicated Douche [OTC]; Yeast-Gard® Medicated Douche

Therapeutic Category Antibacterial, Topical; Antifungal Agent, Topical; Antiviral Agent, Topical; Shampoos

Use External antiseptic with broad microbicidal spectrum against bacteria, fungi, viruses, protozoa, and yeasts

Pregnancy Risk Factor D

Contraindications Hypersensitivity to iodine

Warnings/Precautions Highly toxic if ingested; sodium thiosulfate is the most effective chemical antidote; avoid contact with eyes

Adverse Reactions

1% to 10%:
- Dermatologic: Rash, pruritus
- Local: Local edema

<1%: Systemic absorption in extensive burns causing iododerma, metabolic acidosis, and renal impairment

Mechanism of Action Povidone-iodine is known to be a powerful broad spectrum germicidal agent effective against a wide range of bacteria, viruses, fungi, protozoa, and spores.

Pharmacodynamics/Kinetics Absorption: In normal individuals, topical application results in very little systemic absorption; with vaginal administration, however, absorption is rapid and serum concentrations of total iodine and inorganic iodide are increased significantly

Usual Dosage

Shampoo: Apply 2 teaspoons to hair and scalp, lather and rinse; repeat application 2 times/week until improvement is noted, then shampoo weekly

Topical: Apply as needed for treatment and prevention of susceptible microbial infections

Patient Information Do not swallow; avoid contact with eyes

Dosage Forms

Aerosol: 5% (88.7 mL, 90 mL)
Antiseptic gauze pads: 10% (3" x 9")
Cleanser:
- Skin: 7.5% (30 mL, 118 mL)
- Skin, foam: 7.5% (170 g)
- Topical: 60 mL, 240 mL

Concentrate, whirlpool: 3,840 mL
Cream: 5% (14 g)
Douche (10%): 0.5 oz/packet (6 packets/box), 240 mL
Foam, topical (10%): 250 g
Gel:
- Lubricating: 5% (5 g)
- Vaginal (10%): 18 g, 90 g

Liquid: 473 mL
Mouthwash (8%): 177 mL
Ointment, topical: 10% (0.94 g, 3.8 g, 28 g, 30 g, 454 g); 1 g, 1.2 g, 2.7 g packets
Perineal wash concentrate: 1% (240 mL); 10% (236 mL)
Scrub, surgical: 7.5% (15 mL, 473 mL, 946 mL)
Shampoo: 7.5% (118 mL)
Solution:
- Prep: 30 mL, 60 mL, 240 mL, 473 mL, 1000 mL, 4000 mL
- Swab aid: 1%
- Swabsticks: 4"
- Topical: 10% (15 mL, 30 mL, 120 mL, 237 mL, 473 mL, 480 mL, 1000 mL, 4000 mL)

Suppositories, vaginal: 10%

PPA *see* Phenylpropanolamine *on page 991*

PPD *see* Tuberculin Purified Protein Derivative *on page 1276*

PPL *see* Benzylpenicilloyl-polylysine *on page 143*

PPS *see* Pentosan Polysulfate Sodium *on page 972*

Pralidoxime (pra li DOKS eem)

Brand Names Protopam®

Synonyms 2-PAM; Pralidoxime Chloride; 2-Pyridine Aldoxime Methochloride

Therapeutic Category Antidote, Ambenonium; Antidote, Anticholinesterase; Antidote, Neostigmine; Antidote, Organophosphate Poisoning; Antidote, Pyridostigmine

Use Reverse muscle paralysis with toxic exposure to organophosphate anticholinesterase pesticides and chemicals; control of overdose of drugs used to treat myasthenia gravis (ambenonium, neostigmine, pyridostigmine)

Pregnancy Risk Factor C

Contraindications Hypersensitivity to pralidoxime or any component; poisonings due to phosphorus, inorganic phosphates, or organic phosphates without anticholinesterase activity

Warnings/Precautions Use with caution in patients with myasthenia gravis; dosage modification required in patients with impaired renal function may not be effective for treating carbamate intoxication; use with caution in patients receiving theophylline, succinylcholine, phenothiazines, respiratory depressants (eg, narcotics, barbiturates)

Adverse Reactions

>10%: Local: Pain at injection site after I.M. administration

1% to 10%:

- Cardiovascular: Tachycardia, hypertension
- Central nervous system: Dizziness, headache, drowsiness
- Dermatologic: Rash
- Gastrointestinal: Nausea
- Neuromuscular & skeletal: Muscle rigidity, weakness
- Ocular: Blurred vision, diplopia
- Respiratory: Hyperventilation, laryngospasm

Overdosage/Toxicology Symptoms of overdose include blurred vision, nausea, tachycardia, dizziness; supportive therapy, mechanical ventilation may be required

Drug Interactions

Increased effect: Barbiturates (potentiated)

Increased toxicity: Avoid morphine, theophylline, succinylcholine, reserpine and phenothiazines in patients with organophosphate poisoning

Mechanism of Action Reactivates cholinesterase that had been inactivated by phosphorylation due to exposure to organophosphate pesticides by displacing the enzyme from its receptor sites; removes the phosphoryl group from the active site of the inactivated enzyme

Pharmacodynamics/Kinetics

Absorption: Slowly from GI tract

Metabolism: In the liver, not bound to plasma proteins

Half-life: 0.8-2.7 hours

Time to peak serum concentration: I.V.: Within 5-15 minutes

Elimination: 80% to 90% quickly excreted in urine, as metabolites and unchanged drug

Usual Dosage

Poisoning: I.M. (use in conjunction with atropine), I.V.:

- Children: 20-50 mg/kg/dose; repeat in 1-2 hours if muscle weakness has not been relieved, then at 10- to 12-hour intervals if cholinergic signs recur
- Adults: 1-2 g; repeat in 1-2 hours if muscle weakness has not been relieved, then at 10- to 12-hour intervals if cholinergic signs recur

Mild organophosphate poisoning: Oral: Initial: 1-3 g, repeat as needed in 5 hours

Dosing adjustment in renal impairment: Dose should be reduced

Administration Infuse over 15-30 minutes at a rate not to exceed 200 mg/minute; may administer I.M. or S.C. if I.V. is not accessible; reconstitute with 20 mL sterile water (preservative free) resulting in 50 mg/mL solution; dilute in normal saline 20 mg/mL and infuse over 15-30 minutes; if a more rapid onset of effect is desired or in a fluid-restricted situation, the maximum concentration is 50 mg/mL; the maximum rate of infusion is over 5 minutes

Monitoring Parameters Heart rate, respiratory rate, blood pressure, continuous EKG; cardiac monitor and blood pressure monitor required for I.V. administration

Dosage Forms

Injection: 20 mL vial containing 1 g each pralidoxime chloride with one 20 mL ampul diluent, disposable syringe, needle, and alcohol swab

Injection, as chloride: 300 mg/mL (2 mL)

Tablet, as chloride: 500 mg

Pralidoxime Chloride *see* Pralidoxime *on previous page*

PrameGel® [OTC] *see* Pramoxine *on this page*

Pramet® FA *see* Vitamins, Multiple *on page 1310*

Pramilet® FA *see* Vitamins, Multiple *on page 1310*

Pramoxine (pra MOKS een)

Brand Names Anusol® Ointment [OTC]; Fleet® Pain Relief [OTC]; Itch-X® [OTC]; Phicon® [OTC]; PrameGel® [OTC]; Prax® [OTC]; Proctofoam® NS [OTC]; Tronolane® [OTC]; Tronothane® HCl [OTC]

Synonyms Pramoxine Hydrochloride

Therapeutic Category Antipruritic, Topical; Local Anesthetic, Topical

Use Temporary relief of pain and itching associated with anogenital pruritus or irritation; dermatosis, minor burns, or hemorrhoids

(Continued)

Pramoxine *(Continued)*

Pregnancy Risk Factor C

Contraindications Use in eyes or near nose, application over large areas, known hypersensitivity to pramoxine or any component

Warnings/Precautions Use with caution in patients with severe trauma to the local area

Adverse Reactions

1% to 10%:

Dermatologic: Contact dermatitis, angioedema

Local: Burning, stinging

<1%:

Cardiovascular: Edema

Dermatologic: Tenderness, urticaria

Genitourinary: Urethritis

Hematologic: Methemoglobinemia in infants

Mechanism of Action Pramoxine, like other anesthetics, decreases the neuronal membrane's permeability to sodium ions; both initiation and conduction of nerve impulses are blocked, thus depolarization of the neuron is inhibited

Pharmacodynamics/Kinetics

Onset of therapeutic effect: Within 2-5 minutes

Peak effect: 3-5 minutes

Duration: May last for several days

Usual Dosage Adults: Topical: Apply as directed, usually every 3-4 hours to affected area (maximum adult dose: 200 mg)

Patient Information Discontinue if rash appears or if condition worsens or does not improve in 3-4 days

Nursing Implications Apply sparingly, use the minimal effective dose

Dosage Forms

Aerosol foam, as hydrochloride (ProctoFoam® NS): 1% (15 g)

Cream, as hydrochloride:

Prax®: 1% (30 g, 113.4 g, 454 g)

Tronolane®: 1% (30 g, 60 g)

Tronothane® HCl: 1% (28.4 g)

Gel, topical, as hydrochloride:

Itch-X®: 1% (35.4 g)

PrameGel®: 1% (118 g)

Lotion, as hydrochloride (Prax®): 1% (15 mL, 120 mL, 240 mL)

Ointment, as hydrochloride (Anusol®): 1% (30 g)

Pads, as hydrochloride (Fleet® Pain Relief): 1% (100s)

Spray, as hydrochloride (Itch-X®): 1% (60 mL)

Pramoxine Hydrochloride *see* Pramoxine *on previous page*

Pravachol® *see* Pravastatin *on this page*

Pravastatin (PRA va stat in)

Related Information

Lipid-Lowering Agents *on page 1413*

Brand Names Pravachol®

Synonyms Pravastatin Sodium

Therapeutic Category Antilipemic Agent; HMG-CoA Reductase Inhibitor

Use Adjunct to diet for the reduction of elevated total and LDL-cholesterol levels in patients with hypercholesterolemia (Type IIa, IIb, and IIc); used in hypercholesterolemic patients without clinically evident heart disease to reduce the risk of myocardial infarction, to reduce the risk for revascularization, and reduce the risk of death due to cardiovascular causes; now indicated for prevention of first heart attack and reduction of death from cardiovascular disease in patients who are at risk of first heart attack

Pregnancy Risk Factor X

Contraindications Previous hypersensitivity, active liver disease, or persistent, unexplained liver function enzyme elevations; specifically contraindicated in pregnant or lactating females

Warnings/Precautions May elevate aminotransferases; LFTs should be performed before and every 4-6 weeks during the first 12-15 months of therapy and periodically thereafter; can also cause myalgia and rhabdomyolysis; use with caution in patients who consume large quantities of alcohol or who have a history of liver disease

Adverse Reactions

1% to 10%:

Central nervous system: Headache, dizziness

Dermatologic: Rash

Endocrine & metabolic: Elevated creatine phosphokinase (CPK)

Gastrointestinal: Flatulence, abdominal cramps, diarrhea, constipation, nausea, dyspepsia, heartburn
Neuromuscular & skeletal: Myalgia
<1%:
Gastrointestinal: Abnormal taste
Ocular: Lenticular opacities, blurred vision

Overdosage/Toxicology Very little adverse events; treatment is symptomatic

Drug Interactions
Increased effect with cholestyramine
Increased effect/toxicity of oral anticoagulants
Increased toxicity with gemfibrozil, clofibrate
Concurrent use of erythromycin and HMG-CoA reductase inhibitors may result in rhabdomyolysis

Mechanism of Action Pravastatin is a competitive inhibitor of 3-hydroxy-3-methylglutaryl coenzyme A (HMG-CoA) reductase, which is the rate-limiting enzyme involved in *de novo* cholesterol synthesis.

Pharmacodynamics/Kinetics
Absorption: Poor
Metabolism: In the liver to at least two metabolites
Bioavailability: 17%
Half-life, elimination: ~2-3 hours
Time to peak serum concentration: 1-1.5 hours
Elimination: Up to 20% excreted in urine (8% unchanged)

Usual Dosage Adults: Oral: 10-20 mg once daily at bedtime, may increase to 40 mg/day at bedtime

Monitoring Parameters Creatinine phosphokinase due to possibility of myopathy

Patient Information Promptly report any unexplained muscle pain, tenderness or weakness, especially if accompanied by malaise or fever

Nursing Implications Liver enzyme elevations may be observed during therapy with pravastatin; diet, weight reduction, and exercise should be attempted prior to therapy with pravastatin

Dosage Forms Tablet, as sodium: 10 mg, 20 mg, 40 mg

Pravastatin Sodium *see* Pravastatin *on previous page*

Prax® [OTC] *see* Pramoxine *on page 1033*

Praziquantel (pray zi KWON tel)

Brand Names Biltricide®

Therapeutic Category Anthelmintic

Use All stages of schistosomiasis caused by all *Schistosoma* species pathogenic to humans; clonorchiasis, opisthorchiasis, cysticercosis, and many intestinal tapeworms

Pregnancy Risk Factor B

Contraindications Ocular cysticercosis, known hypersensitivity to praziquantel

Warnings/Precautions Use caution in patients with severe hepatic disease; patients with cerebral cysticercosis require hospitalization

Adverse Reactions
1% to 10%:
Central nervous system: Dizziness, drowsiness, headache, malaise
Gastrointestinal: Abdominal pain, loss of appetite, nausea, vomiting
Miscellaneous: Diaphoresis
<1%:
Central nervous system: CSF reaction syndrome in patients being treated for neurocysticercosis, fever
Dermatologic: Rash, urticaria, itching
Gastrointestinal: Diarrhea

Overdosage/Toxicology Symptoms of overdose include dizziness, drowsiness, headache, liver function impairment; treatment is supportive following GI decontamination; administer fast-acting laxative

Mechanism of Action Increases the cell permeability to calcium in schistosomes, causing strong contractions and paralysis of worm musculature leading to detachment of suckers from the blood vessel walls and to dislodgment

Pharmacodynamics/Kinetics
Absorption: Oral: ~80%; CSF concentration is 14% to 20% of plasma concentration
Distribution: CSF concentration is 14% to 20% of plasma concentration; appears in breast milk
Protein binding: ~80%
Metabolism: Extensive first-pass metabolism
Half-life:
Parent drug: 0.8-1.5 hours
Metabolites: 4.5 hours
(Continued)

Praziquantel *(Continued)*

Time to peak serum concentration: Within 1-3 hours
Elimination: Urinary excretion (99% as metabolites)

Usual Dosage Children >4 years and Adults: Oral:
Schistosomiasis: 20 mg/kg/dose 2-3 times/day for 1 day at 4- to 6-hour intervals
Flukes: 25 mg/kg/dose every 8 hours for 1-2 days
Cysticercosis: 50 mg/kg/day divided every 8 hours for 14 days
Tapeworms: 10-20 mg/kg as a single dose (25 mg/kg for *Hymenolepis nana*)

Patient Information Do not chew tablets due to bitter taste; take with food; caution should be used when performing tasks requiring mental alertness, may impair judgment and coordination

Nursing Implications Tablets can be halved or quartered

Dosage Forms Tablet, tri-scored: 600 mg

Prazosin (PRA zoe sin)

Brand Names Minipress®

Canadian/Mexican Brand Names Apo-Prazo® (Canada); Novo-Prazin® (Canada); Nu-Prazo® (Canada)

Synonyms Furazosin; Prazosin Hydrochloride

Therapeutic Category Alpha-Adrenergic Blocking Agent, Oral; Antihypertensive

Use Treatment of hypertension, severe congestive heart failure (in conjunction with diuretics and cardiac glycosides); reduce mortality in stable postmyocardial patients with left ventricular dysfunction (ejection fraction ≤40%)

Unlabeled use: Symptoms of benign prostatic hypertrophy

Pregnancy Risk Factor C

Contraindications Hypersensitivity to prazosin or any component

Warnings/Precautions Marked orthostatic hypotension, syncope, and loss of consciousness may occur with first dose ("first dose phenomenon") occurs more often in patients receiving beta-blockers, diuretics, low sodium diets, or larger first doses (ie, >1 mg/dose in adults); avoid rapid increase in dose; use with caution in patients with renal impairment

Adverse Reactions

>10%:
- Cardiovascular: Orthostatic hypotension
- Central nervous system: Dizziness, lightheadedness, drowsiness, headache, malaise

1% to 10%:
- Cardiovascular: Edema, palpitations
- Central nervous system: Fatigue, nervousness
- Gastrointestinal: Xerostomia
- Genitourinary: Urinary incontinence

<1%:
- Cardiovascular: Angina
- Central nervous system: Nightmares, hypothermia
- Dermatologic: Rash
- Endocrine & metabolic: Sexual dysfunction
- Gastrointestinal: Nausea
- Genitourinary: Priapism, polyuria
- Respiratory: Dyspnea, nasal congestion

Overdosage/Toxicology Symptoms of overdose include hypotension, drowsiness

Hypotension usually responds to I.V. fluids, Trendelenburg positioning or vasoconstrictors; treatment is otherwise supportive and symptomatic

Drug Interactions
Decreased effect (antihypertensive) with NSAIDs
Increased effect (hypotensive) with diuretics and antihypertensive medications (especially beta-blockers)

Mechanism of Action Competitively inhibits postsynaptic alpha-adrenergic receptors which results in vasodilation of veins and arterioles and a decrease in total peripheral resistance and blood pressure

Pharmacodynamics/Kinetics
Onset of hypotensive effect: Within 2 hours
Maximum decrease: 2-4 hours
Duration: 10-24 hours
Distribution: V_d: 0.5 L/kg (hypertensive adults)
Protein binding: 92% to 97%
Metabolism: Extensively in the liver
Bioavailability: Oral: 43% to 82%
Half-life: 2-4 hours; increased with congestive heart failure
Elimination: 6% to 10% excreted renally as unchanged drug

Usual Dosage Oral:

Children: Initial: 5 mcg/kg/dose (to assess hypotensive effects); usual dosing interval: every 6 hours; increase dosage gradually up to maximum of 25 mcg/kg/dose every 6 hours

Adults: Initial: 1 mg/dose 2-3 times/day; usual maintenance dose: 3-15 mg/day in divided doses 2-4 times/day; maximum daily dose: 20 mg

Dietary Considerations Alcohol: Avoid use

Monitoring Parameters Blood pressure, standing and sitting/supine

Test Interactions Increased urinary UMA 17%, norepinephrine metabolite 42%

Patient Information Rise from sitting/lying carefully; may cause dizziness; report if painful, persistent erection occurs; avoid alcohol

Nursing Implications Syncope may occur (usually within 90 minutes of the initial dose)

Dosage Forms Capsule, as hydrochloride: 1 mg, 2 mg, 5 mg

Prazosin Hydrochloride *see* Prazosin *on previous page*

Precose™ *see* Acarbose *on page 16*

Predair® *see* Prednisolone *on this page*

Predaject® *see* Prednisolone *on this page*

Predalone T.B.A.® *see* Prednisolone *on this page*

Predcor® *see* Prednisolone *on this page*

Predcor-TBA® *see* Prednisolone *on this page*

Pred Forte® *see* Prednisolone *on this page*

Pred Mild® *see* Prednisolone *on this page*

Prednicarbate (PRED ni kar bate)

Brand Names Dermatop®

Therapeutic Category Corticosteroid, Topical (Medium Potency)

Use Relief of the inflammatory and pruritic manifestations of corticosteroid-responsive dermatoses (medium potency topical corticosteroid)

Contraindications Hypersensitivity to prednicarbate or any component; fungal, viral, or tubercular skin lesions, herpes simplex or zoster

Warnings/Precautions Systemic absorption of topical corticosteroids has produced reversible HPA axis suppression. This is more likely to occur when the preparation is used on large surface or denuded areas for prolonged periods of time or with an occlusive dressing.

Adverse Reactions

<10%:

Dermatologic: Acne, hypopigmentation, allergic dermatitis, maceration of the skin, skin atrophy, folliculitis, hypertrichosis

Endocrine & metabolic: HPA suppression, Cushing's syndrome, growth retardation

Local: Burning, itching, irritation, dryness

Miscellaneous: Secondary infection

Mechanism of Action Topical corticosteroids have anti-inflammatory, antipruritic, vasoconstrictive, and antiproliferative actions

Usual Dosage Adults: Topical: Apply a thin film to affected area twice daily

Monitoring Parameters Relief of symptoms

Patient Information Use only as prescribed and for no longer than the period prescribed; apply sparingly in a thin film and rub in lightly; avoid contact with eyes; notify physician if condition persists or worsens

Nursing Implications Use sparingly

Additional Information Has been shown that the atrophic activity of prednicarbate is many times less than agents with similar clinical potency, nevertheless, avoid prolonged use on the face

Dosage Forms Cream: 0.1% (15 g, 60 g)

Prednicen-M® *see* Prednisone *on page 1039*

Prednisolone (pred NIS oh lone)

Related Information

Corticosteroids Comparison *on page 1407*

Brand Names AK-Pred®; Articulose-50®; Delta-Cortef®; Econopred®; Econopred® Plus; Hydeltrasol®; Hydeltra-T.B.A.®; Inflamase®; Inflamase® Mild; Key-Pred®; Key-Pred-SP®; Metreton®; Pediapred®; Predair®; Predaject®; Predalone T.B.A.®; Predcor®; Predcor-TBA®; Pred Forte®; Pred Mild®; Prelone®

Canadian/Mexican Brand Names Novo-Prednisolone® (Canada); Fisopred® (Mexico); Sophipren® Ofteno (Mexico)

Synonyms Deltahydrocortisone; Metacortandralone; Prednisolone Acetate; Prednisolone Acetate, Ophthalmic; Prednisolone Sodium Phosphate; Prednisolone Sodium Phosphate, Ophthalmic; Prednisolone Tebutate

(Continued)

Prednisolone *(Continued)*

Therapeutic Category Anti-inflammatory Agent; Anti-inflammatory Agent, Ophthalmic; Corticosteroid; Corticosteroid, Ophthalmic; Corticosteroid, Systemic; Glucocorticoid

Use Treatment of palpebral and bulbar conjunctivitis; corneal injury from chemical, radiation, thermal burns, or foreign body penetration; endocrine disorders, rheumatic disorders, collagen diseases, dermatologic diseases, allergic states, ophthalmic diseases, respiratory diseases, hematologic disorders, neoplastic diseases, edematous states, and gastrointestinal diseases; useful in patients with inability to activate prednisone (liver disease)

Pregnancy Risk Factor C

Contraindications Acute superficial herpes simplex keratitis; systemic fungal infections; varicella; hypersensitivity to prednisolone or any component

Warnings/Precautions Use with caution in patients with hyperthyroidism, cirrhosis, nonspecific ulcerative colitis, hypertension, osteoporosis, thromboembolic tendencies, CHF, convulsive disorders, myasthenia gravis, thrombophlebitis, peptic ulcer, diabetes; acute adrenal insufficiency may occur with abrupt withdrawal after long-term therapy or with stress; young pediatric patients may be more susceptible to adrenal axis suppression from topical therapy. Because of the risk of adverse effects, systemic corticosteroids should be used cautiously in the elderly, in the smallest possible dose, and for the shortest possible time.

Adverse Reactions

>10%:

- Central nervous system: Insomnia, nervousness
- Gastrointestinal: Increased appetite, indigestion

1% to 10%:

- Dermatologic: Hirsutism
- Endocrine & metabolic: Diabetes mellitus
- Neuromuscular & skeletal: Arthralgia
- Ocular: Cataracts, glaucoma
- Respiratory: Epistaxis

<1%:

- Cardiovascular: Edema, hypertension
- Central nervous system: Vertigo, seizures, psychoses, pseudotumor cerebri, headache, mood swings, delirium, hallucinations, euphoria
- Dermatologic: Acne, skin atrophy, bruising, hyperpigmentation
- Endocrine & metabolic: Cushing's syndrome, pituitary-adrenal axis suppression, growth suppression, glucose intolerance, hypokalemia, alkalosis, amenorrhea, sodium and water retention, hyperglycemia
- Gastrointestinal: Peptic ulcer, nausea, vomiting, abdominal distention, ulcerative esophagitis, pancreatitis
- Neuromuscular & skeletal: Muscle weakness, osteoporosis, fractures, muscle wasting
- Miscellaneous: Hypersensitivity reactions

Overdosage/Toxicology When consumed in excessive quantities for prolonged periods, systemic hypercorticism and adrenal suppression may occur, in those cases discontinuation and withdrawal of the corticosteroid should be done judiciously.

Drug Interactions

Inducer of cytochrome P-450 enzymes

Cytochrome P-450 3A enzyme substrate

Decreased effect:

- Barbiturates, phenytoin, rifampin decrease corticosteroid effectiveness
- Decreases salicylates
- Decreases vaccines
- Decreases toxoids effectiveness

Mechanism of Action Decreases inflammation by suppression of migration of polymorphonuclear leukocytes and reversal of increased capillary permeability; suppresses the immune system by reducing activity and volume of the lymphatic system

Pharmacodynamics/Kinetics

Protein binding: 65% to 91% (concentration dependent)

Metabolism: Primarily in the liver, but also metabolized in most tissues, to inactive compounds

Half-life: 3.6 hours

- Biological: 18-36 hours
- End stage renal disease: 3-5 hours

Elimination: In urine principally as glucuronides, sulfates, and unconjugated metabolites

Usual Dosage Dose depends upon condition being treated and response of patient; dosage for infants and children should be based on severity of the disease and response of the patient rather than on strict adherence to dosage indicated by age, weight, or body surface area. Consider alternate day therapy for long-term therapy. Discontinuation of long-term therapy requires gradual withdrawal by tapering the dose.

Children:

Acute asthma:

Oral: 1-2 mg/kg/day in divided doses 1-2 times/day for 3-5 days

I.V. (sodium phosphate salt): 2-4 mg/kg/day divided 3-4 times/day

Anti-inflammatory or immunosuppressive dose: Oral, I.V., I.M. (sodium phosphate salt): 0.1-2 mg/kg/day in divided doses 1-4 times/day

Nephrotic syndrome: Oral:

Initial (first 3 episodes): 2 mg/kg/day **OR** 60 mg/m^2/day (maximum: 80 mg/day) in divided doses 3-4 times/day until urine is protein free for 3 consecutive days (maximum: 28 days); followed by 1-1.5 mg/kg/dose **OR** 40 mg/m^2/dose given every other day for 4 weeks

Maintenance (long-term maintenance dose for frequent relapses): 0.5-1 mg/kg/dose given every other day for 3-6 months

Adults:

Oral, I.V., I.M. (sodium phosphate salt): 5-60 mg/day

Multiple sclerosis (sodium phosphate): Oral: 200 mg/day for 1 week followed by 80 mg every other day for 1 month

Rheumatoid arthritis: Oral: Initial: 5-7.5 mg/day; adjust dose as necessary

Elderly: Use lowest effective dose

Hemodialysis: Slightly dialyzable (5% to 20%); administer dose posthemodialysis

Peritoneal dialysis: Supplemental dose is not necessary

Intra-articular, intralesional, soft-tissue administration:

Tebutate salt: 4-40 mg/dose

Sodium phosphate salt: 2-30 mg/dose

Ophthalmic suspension/solution: Children and Adults: Instill 1-2 drops into conjunctival sac every hour during day, every 2 hours at night until favorable response is obtained, then use 1 drop every 4 hours

Administration Administer oral formulation with food or milk to decrease GI effects

Monitoring Parameters Blood pressure, blood glucose, electrolytes

Test Interactions Response to skin tests

Patient Information Notify surgeon or dentist before surgical repair; may cause GI upset, take orally with food; notify physician if any sign of infection occurs; avoid abrupt withdrawal when on long-term therapy

Nursing Implications Do not administer acetate or tebutate salt I.V.

Additional Information

Sodium phosphate injection: For I.V., I.M., intra-articular, intralesional, or soft tissue administration

Tebutate injection: For intra-articular, intralesional, or soft tissue administration only

Dosage Forms

Injection:

As acetate (for I.M., intralesional, intra-articular, or soft tissue administration only): 25 mg/mL (10 mL, 30 mL); 50 mg/mL (30 mL)

As sodium phosphate (for I.M., I.V., intra-articular, intralesional, or soft tissue administration): 20 mg/mL (2 mL, 5 mL, 10 mL)

As tebutate (for intra-articular, intralesional, soft tissue administration only): 20 mg/mL (1 mL, 5 mL, 10 mL)

Liquid, oral, as sodium phosphate: 5 mg/5 mL (120 mL)

Solution, ophthalmic, as sodium phosphate: 0.125% (5 mL, 10 mL, 15 mL); 1% (5 mL, 10 mL, 15 mL)

Suspension, ophthalmic, as acetate: 0.12% (5 mL, 10 mL); 0.125% (5 mL, 10 mL, 15 mL); 1% (1 mL, 5 mL, 10 mL, 15 mL)

Syrup: 15 mg/5 mL (240 mL)

Tablet: 5 mg

Prednisolone Acetate *see* Prednisolone *on page 1037*

Prednisolone Acetate, Ophthalmic *see* Prednisolone *on page 1037*

Prednisolone Sodium Phosphate *see* Prednisolone *on page 1037*

Prednisolone Sodium Phosphate, Ophthalmic *see* Prednisolone *on page 1037*

Prednisolone Tebutate *see* Prednisolone *on page 1037*

Prednisone (PRED ni sone)

Related Information

Anticonvulsants by Seizure Type *on page 1392*

Cancer Chemotherapy Regimens *on page 1351*

Corticosteroids Comparison *on page 1407*

Brand Names Deltasone®; Liquid Pred®; Meticorten®; Orasone®; Prednicen-M®; Sterapred®

(Continued)

Prednisone *(Continued)*

Canadian/Mexican Brand Names Apo-Prednisone® (Canada); Jaa-Prednisone® (Canada); Novo-Prednisone® (Canada); Wimpred® (Canada)

Synonyms Deltacortisone; Deltadehydrocortisone

Therapeutic Category Anti-inflammatory Agent; Corticosteroid; Corticosteroid, Systemic; Glucocorticoid

Use Treatment of a variety of diseases including adrenocortical insufficiency, hypercalcemia, rheumatic, and collagen disorders; dermatologic, ocular, respiratory, gastrointestinal, and neoplastic diseases; organ transplantation and a variety of diseases including those of hematologic, allergic, inflammatory, and autoimmune in origin; not available in injectable form, prednisolone must be used

Investigational: Prevention of postherpetic neuralgia and relief of acute pain in the early stages

Pregnancy Risk Factor B

Pregnancy/Breast-Feeding Implications

Clinical effects on the fetus: Crosses the placenta. Immunosuppression reported in 1 infant exposed to high dose prednisone plus azathioprine throughout gestation. One report of congenital cataracts. Available evidence suggests safe use during pregnancy.

Breast-feeding/lactation: Crosses into breast milk. No data on clinical effects on the infant. American Academy of Pediatrics considers COMPATIBLE with breast-feeding.

Contraindications Serious infections, except septic shock or tuberculous meningitis; systemic fungal infections; hypersensitivity to prednisone or any component; varicella

Warnings/Precautions Withdraw therapy with gradual tapering of dose, may retard bone growth; use with caution in patients with hypothyroidism, cirrhosis, hypertension, congestive heart failure, ulcerative colitis, thromboembolic disorders, and patients at increased risk for peptic ulcer disease. Because of the risk of adverse effects, systemic corticosteroids should be used cautiously in the elderly, in the smallest possible dose, and for the shortest possible time.

Adverse Reactions

>10%:
- Central nervous system: Insomnia, nervousness
- Gastrointestinal: Increased appetite, indigestion

1% to 10%:
- Dermatologic: Hirsutism
- Endocrine & metabolic: Diabetes mellitus
- Ocular: Cataracts, glaucoma
- Neuromuscular & skeletal: Arthralgia
- Respiratory: Epistaxis

<1%:
- Cardiovascular: Edema, hypertension
- Central nervous system: Vertigo, seizures, psychoses, pseudotumor cerebri, headache, mood swings, delirium, hallucinations, euphoria
- Dermatologic: Acne, skin atrophy, bruising, hyperpigmentation
- Endocrine & metabolic: Cushing's syndrome, pituitary-adrenal axis suppression, growth suppression, glucose intolerance, hypokalemia, alkalosis, amenorrhea, sodium and water retention, hyperglycemia
- Gastrointestinal: Peptic ulcer, nausea, vomiting, abdominal distention, ulcerative esophagitis, pancreatitis
- Neuromuscular & skeletal: Muscle weakness, osteoporosis, fractures, muscle wasting
- Miscellaneous: Hypersensitivity reactions

Overdosage/Toxicology When consumed in excessive quantities for prolonged periods, systemic hypercorticism and adrenal suppression may occur; in those cases, discontinuation and withdrawal of the corticosteroid should be done judiciously.

Drug Interactions

Inducer of cytochrome P-450 enzymes
Cytochrome P-450 3A enzyme substrate

Decreased effect:
- Barbiturates, phenytoin, rifampin decrease corticosteroid effectiveness
- Decreases salicylates
- Decreases vaccines
- Decreases toxoids effectiveness

Mechanism of Action Decreases inflammation by suppression of migration of polymorphonuclear leukocytes and reversal of increased capillary permeability; suppresses the immune system by reducing activity and volume of the lymphatic system; suppresses adrenal function at high doses. Antitumor effects may be related to inhibition of glucose transport, phosphorylation, or induction of cell death in immature lymphocytes. Antiemetic effects are thought to occur due to blockade of cerebral innervation of the emetic center via inhibition of prostaglandin synthesis.

Pharmacodynamics/Kinetics Refer to Prednisolone monograph for complete pharmacokinetic information

Metabolism: Converted rapidly to prednisolone (active)

Prednisone is inactive and must be metabolized to prednisolone which may be impaired in patients with impaired liver function

Half-life: Normal renal function: 2.5-3.5 hours

Usual Dosage Oral:

Dose depends upon condition being treated and response of patient; dosage for infants and children should be based on severity of the disease and response of the patient rather than on strict adherence to dosage indicated by age, weight, or body surface area. Consider alternate day therapy for long-term therapy. Discontinuation of long-term therapy requires gradual withdrawal by tapering the dose.

Children:

- Anti-inflammatory or immunosuppressive dose: 0.05-2 mg/kg/day divided 1-4 times/day
- Acute asthma: 1-2 mg/kg/day in divided doses 1-2 times/day for 3-5 days
  - Alternatively (for 3- to 5-day "burst"):
  - <1 year: 10 mg every 12 hours
  - 1-4 years: 20 mg every 12 hours
  - 5-13 years: 30 mg every 12 hours
  - >13 years: 40 mg every 12 hours
- Asthma long-term therapy (alternative dosing by age):
  - <1 year: 10 mg every other day
  - 1-4 years: 20 mg every other day
  - 5-13 years: 30 mg every other day
  - >13 years: 40 mg every other day
- Nephrotic syndrome: Initial (first 3 episodes): 2 mg/kg/day **OR** 60 mg/m^2/day (maximum: of 80 mg/day) in divided doses 3-4 times/day until urine is protein free for 3 consecutive days (maximum: 28 days); followed by 1-1.5 mg/kg/dose **OR** 40 mg/m^2/dose given every other day for 4 weeks
- Maintenance dose (long-term maintenance dose for frequent relapses): 0.5-1 mg/kg/dose given every other day for 3-6 months

Children and Adults: Physiologic replacement: 4-5 mg/m^2/day

Adults: 5-60 mg/day in divided doses 1-4 times/day

Elderly: Use the lowest effective dose

Hemodialysis: Supplemental dose is not necessary

Peritoneal dialysis: Supplemental dose is not necessary

Administration Administer with meals to decrease gastrointestinal upset

Monitoring Parameters Blood pressure, blood glucose, electrolytes

Test Interactions Response to skin tests

Patient Information Notify surgeon or dentist before surgical repair; may cause GI upset, take with food; notify physician if any sign of infection occurs; avoid abrupt withdrawal when on long-term therapy; do not discontinue or decrease drug without contacting physician, carry an identification card or bracelet advising that you are on steroids

Nursing Implications Withdraw therapy with gradual tapering of dose

Dosage Forms

Solution, oral: Concentrate (30% alcohol): 5 mg/mL (30 mL); Nonconcentrate (5% alcohol): 5 mg/5 mL (5 mL, 500 mL)

Syrup: 5 mg/5 mL (120 mL, 240 mL)

Tablet: 1 mg, 2.5 mg, 5 mg, 10 mg, 20 mg, 50 mg

Prefrin™ Ophthalmic Solution *see* Phenylephrine *on page 989*

Pregnenedione *see* Progesterone *on page 1055*

Pregnyl® *see* Chorionic Gonadotropin *on page 272*

Prelone® *see* Prednisolone *on page 1037*

Premarin® *see* Estrogens, Conjugated *on page 471*

Prenatal Vitamins *see* Vitamins, Multiple *on page 1310*

Prenavite® [OTC] *see* Vitamins, Multiple *on page 1310*

Pre-Par® *see* Ritodrine *on page 1112*

Pre-Pen® *see* Benzylpenicilloyl-polylysine *on page 143*

Prepidil® Vaginal Gel *see* Dinoprostone *on page 397*

Prescription Strength Desenex® [OTC] *see* Miconazole *on page 834*

Pretz® [OTC] *see* Sodium Chloride *on page 1142*

Prevacid® *see* Lansoprazole *on page 706*

Prevention of Bacterial Endocarditis *see page 1449*

Prevention of Hepatitis A Through Active or Passive Immunization *see page 1440*

Prevention of Malaria *see page 1441*

PreviDent® *see* Fluoride *on page 536*

Prilosec™ *see* Omeprazole *on page 925*

Primaclone *see* Primidone *on this page*

Primacor® *see* Milrinone *on page 840*

Primaquine and Chloroquine *see* Chloroquine and Primaquine *on page 255*

Primaquine Phosphate (PRIM a kween FOS fate)

Related Information

Prevention of Malaria *on page 1441*

Synonyms Prymaccone

Therapeutic Category Antimalarial Agent

Use Provides radical cure of *P. vivax* or *P. ovale* malaria after a clinical attack has been confirmed by blood smear or serologic titer and postexposure prophylaxis

Pregnancy Risk Factor C

Contraindications Acutely ill patients who have a tendency to develop granulocytopenia (rheumatoid arthritis, SLE); patients receiving other drugs capable of depressing the bone marrow; patients receiving quinacrine

Warnings/Precautions Use with caution in patients with G-6-PD deficiency, NADH methemoglobin reductase deficiency, acutely ill patients who have a tendency to develop granulocytopenia; patients receiving other drugs capable of depressing the bone marrow; do not exceed recommended dosage

Adverse Reactions

>10%:

Gastrointestinal: Abdominal pain, nausea, vomiting
Hematologic: Hemolytic anemia

1% to 10%: Hematologic: Methemoglobinemia

<1%:

Cardiovascular: Arrhythmias
Central nervous system: Headache
Dermatologic: Pruritus
Hematologic: Leukopenia, agranulocytosis, leukocytosis
Miscellaneous: Interference with visual accommodation

Overdosage/Toxicology Symptoms of acute overdose include abdominal cramps, vomiting, cyanosis, methemoglobinemia (possibly severe), leukopenia, acute hemolytic anemia (often significant), granulocytopenia; with chronic overdose, symptoms include ototoxicity and retinopathy

Following GI decontamination, treatment is supportive (fluids, anticonvulsants, blood transfusions, methylene blue if methemoglobinemia severe - 1-2 mg/kg over several minutes)

Drug Interactions Increased toxicity/levels with quinacrine

Mechanism of Action Eliminates the primary tissue exoerythrocytic forms of *P. falciparum*; disrupts mitochondria and binds to DNA

Pharmacodynamics/Kinetics

Absorption: Oral: Well absorbed
Metabolism: Liver metabolism to carboxyprimaquine, an active metabolite
Half-life: 3.7-9.6 hours
Time to peak serum concentration: Within 1-2 hours
Elimination: Only a small amount of unchanged drug excreted in urine

Usual Dosage Oral:

Children: 0.3 mg base/kg/day once daily for 14 days (not to exceed 15 mg/day) or 0.9 mg base/kg once weekly for 8 weeks not to exceed 45 mg base/week

Adults: 15 mg/day (base) once daily for 14 days or 45 mg base once weekly for 8 weeks

Monitoring Parameters Periodic CBC, visual color check of urine, glucose, electrolytes; if hemolysis suspected - CBC, haptoglobin, peripheral smear, urinalysis dipstick for occult blood

Patient Information Take with meals to decrease adverse GI effects; drug has a bitter taste; notify physician if a darkening of urine occurs or if shortness of breath, weakness or skin discoloration (chocolate cyanosis) occurs; complete full course of therapy

Dosage Forms Tablet: 26.3 mg [15 mg base]

Primatene® Mist [OTC] *see* Epinephrine *on page 448*

Primaxin® *see* Imipenem and Cilastatin *on page 647*

Primidone (PRI mi done)

Related Information

Epilepsy Treatment *on page 1531*

Brand Names Mysoline®

Canadian/Mexican Brand Names Apo-Primidone® (Canada); Sertan® (Canada)

Synonyms Desoxyphenobarbital; Primaclone

Therapeutic Category Anticonvulsant; Barbiturate

Use Management of grand mal, complex partial, and focal seizures

Unlabeled use: Benign familial tremor (essential tremor)

Pregnancy Risk Factor D

Pregnancy/Breast-Feeding Implications

Clinical effects on the fetus: Crosses the placenta. Dysmorphic facial features; hemorrhagic disease of newborn due to fetal vitamin K depletion, maternal folic acid deficiency may occur. Epilepsy itself, number of medications, genetic factors, or a combination of these probably influence the teratogenicity of anticonvulsant therapy. Benefit:risk ratio usually favors continued use during pregnancy and breast-feeding.

Breast-feeding/Lactation: Crosses into breast milk

Clinical effects on the fetus: Sedation; feeding problems reported. American Academy of Pediatrics recommends USE WITH CAUTION.

Contraindications Hypersensitivity to primidone, phenobarbital, or any component; porphyria

Warnings/Precautions Use with caution in patients with renal or hepatic impairment, pulmonary insufficiency; abrupt withdrawal may precipitate status epilepticus

Adverse Reactions

>10%: Central nervous system: Drowsiness, vertigo, ataxia, lethargy, behavior change, sedation, headache

1% to 10%:

Gastrointestinal: Nausea, vomiting, anorexia

Genitourinary: Impotence

<1%:

Central nervous system: Behavior change

Dermatologic: Rash

Hematologic: Leukopenia, malignant lymphoma-like syndrome, megaloblastic anemia

Ocular: Diplopia, nystagmus

Miscellaneous: Systemic lupus-like syndrome

Overdosage/Toxicology Symptoms of overdose include unsteady gait, slurred speech, confusion, jaundice, hypothermia, fever, hypotension, coma, respiratory arrest

Assure adequate hydration and renal function. Urinary alkalinization with I.V. sodium bicarbonate also helps to enhance elimination. Repeated oral doses of activated charcoal significantly reduces the half-life of primidone resulting from an enhancement of nonrenal elimination. The usual dose is 0.1-1 g/kg every 4-6 hours for 3-4 days unless the patient has no bowel movement causing the charcoal to remain in the GI tract. Hemodialysis or hemoperfusion is of uncertain value. Patients in stage IV coma due to high serum drug levels may require charcoal hemoperfusion.

Drug Interactions

Decreased effect: Primidone may decrease serum concentrations of ethosuximide, valproic acid, griseofulvin; phenytoin may decrease primidone serum concentrations

Increased toxicity: Methylphenidate may increase primidone serum concentrations; valproic acid may increase phenobarbital concentrations derived from primidone

Stability Protect from light

Mechanism of Action Decreases neuron excitability, raises seizure threshold similar to phenobarbital; primidone has two active metabolites, phenobarbital and phenylethylmalonamide (PEMA); PEMA may enhance the activity of phenobarbital

Pharmacodynamics/Kinetics

Distribution: V_d: 2-3 L/kg in adults

Protein binding: 99%

Metabolism: In the liver to phenobarbital (active) and phenylethylmalonamide (PEMA)

Bioavailability: 60% to 80%

Half-life (age dependent):

Primidone: 10-12 hours

PEMA: 16 hours

Phenobarbital: 52-118 hours

Time to peak serum concentration: Oral: Within 4 hours

Elimination: Urinary excretion of both active metabolites and unchanged primidone (15% to 25%)

(Continued)

Primidone *(Continued)*

Usual Dosage Oral:

Children <8 years: Initial: 50-125 mg/day given at bedtime; increase by 50-125 mg/day increments every 3-7 days; usual dose: 10-25 mg/kg/day in divided doses 3-4 times/day

Children >8 years and Adults: Initial: 125-250 mg/day at bedtime; increase by 125-250 mg/day every 3-7 days; usual dose: 750-1500 mg/day in divided doses 3-4 times/day with maximum dosage of 2 g/day

Dosing interval in renal impairment:

Cl_{cr} 50-80 mL/minute: Administer every 8 hours

Cl_{cr} 10-50 mL/minute: Administer every 8-12 hours

Cl_{cr} <10 mL/minute: Administer every 12-24 hours

Hemodialysis: Moderately dialyzable (20% to 50%); administer dose postdialysis or administer supplemental 30% dose

Dietary Considerations

Food:

Folic acid: Low erythrocyte and CSF folate concentrations. Megaloblastic anemia has been reported. To avoid folic acid deficiency and megaloblastic anemia, some clinicians recommend giving patients on anticonvulsants prophylactic doses of folic acid and cyanocobalamin.

Protein-deficient diets: Increases duration of action of primidone. Should not restrict or delete protein from diet unless discussed with physician. Be consistent with protein intake during primidone therapy.

Fresh fruits containing vitamin C: Displaces drug from binding sites, resulting in increased urinary excretion of primidone. Educate patients regarding the potential for decreased primidone effect with consumption of foods high in vitamin C.

Monitoring Parameters Serum primidone and phenobarbital concentration, CBC, neurological status. Due to CNS effects, monitor closely when initiating drug in elderly. Monitor CBC at 6-month intervals to compare with baseline obtained at start of therapy. Since elderly metabolize phenobarbital at a slower rate than younger adults, it is suggested to measure both primidone and phenobarbital levels together.

Reference Range Therapeutic: Children <5 years: 7-10 µg/mL (SI: 32-46 µmol/L); Adults: 5-12 µg/mL (SI: 23-55 µmol/L); toxic effects rarely present with levels <10 µg/mL (SI: 46 µmol/L) if phenobarbital concentrations are low. Dosage of primidone is adjusted with reference mostly to the phenobarbital level; Toxic: >15 µg/mL (SI: >69 µmol/L)

Test Interactions ↑ alkaline phosphatase (S); ↓ calcium (S)

Patient Information May cause drowsiness, impair judgment and coordination; do not abruptly discontinue or change dosage without notifying physician; can take with food to avoid GI upset

Nursing Implications Observe patient for excessive sedation; institute safety measures

Dosage Forms

Suspension, oral: 250 mg/5 mL (240 mL)

Tablet: 50 mg, 250 mg

Principen® *see* Ampicillin *on page 85*

Prinivil® *see* Lisinopril *on page 733*

Priscoline® *see* Tolazoline *on page 1239*

Privine® *see* Naphazoline *on page 879*

ProAmatine™ *see* Midodrine *on page 838*

Proaqua® *see* Benzthiazide *on page 141*

Probalan® *see* Probenecid *on this page*

Pro-Banthine® *see* Propantheline *on page 1061*

Probenecid (proe BEN e sid)

Related Information

Treatment of Sexually Transmitted Diseases *on page 1485*

Brand Names Benemid®; Probalan®

Canadian/Mexican Brand Names Benuryl® (Canada); Benecid® Probenecida Valdecasas (Mexico)

Therapeutic Category Uricosuric Agent

Use Prevention of gouty arthritis; hyperuricemia; prolongation of beta-lactam effect (ie, serum levels)

Pregnancy Risk Factor B

Contraindications Hypersensitivity to probenecid or any component; high-dose aspirin therapy; moderate to severe renal impairment; children <2 years of age

Warnings/Precautions Use with caution in patients with peptic ulcer; use extreme caution in the use of probenecid with penicillin in patients with renal insufficiency; probenecid may not be effective in patients with a creatinine clearance <30 to 50 mL/minute; may cause exacerbation of acute gouty attack

Adverse Reactions

>10%:

Central nervous system: Headache
Gastrointestinal: Anorexia, nausea, vomiting
Neuromuscular & skeletal: Gouty arthritis (acute)

1% to 10%:

Cardiovascular: Flushing of face
Central nervous system: Dizziness
Dermatologic: Rash, itching
Gastrointestinal: Sore gums
Genitourinary: Painful urination
Renal: Renal calculi

<1%:

Hematologic: Leukopenia, hemolytic anemia, aplastic anemia
Hepatic: Hepatic necrosis
Renal: Urate nephropathy, nephrotic syndrome
Miscellaneous: Anaphylaxis

Overdosage/Toxicology Symptoms of overdose include nausea, vomiting, tonic-clonic seizures, coma

Activated charcoal is especially effective at binding probenecid, for GI decontamination

Drug Interactions

Decreased effect:

Salicylates (high dose) may decrease uricosuria
Decreased urinary levels of nitrofurantoin may decrease efficacy

Increased toxicity:

Increases methotrexate toxic potential; combination with diflunisal has resulted in 40% decrease in its clearance and as much as a 65% increasing plasma concentrations due to inhibition of diflunisal metabolism; probenecid decreases clearance of beta-lactams such as penicillins and cephalosporins; increases acyclovir, thiopental, benzodiazepines, dapsone, sulfonylureas, zidovudine; avoid concomitant use with ketorolac since its half-life is increased twofold and levels and toxicity are significantly increased

Mechanism of Action Competitively inhibits the reabsorption of uric acid at the proximal convoluted tubule, thereby promoting its excretion and reducing serum uric acid levels; increases plasma levels of weak organic acids (penicillins, cephalosporins, or other beta-lactam antibiotics) by competitively inhibiting their renal tubular secretion

Pharmacodynamics/Kinetics

Onset of action: Effect on penicillin levels reached in about 2 hours
Absorption: Rapid and complete from GI tract
Metabolism: In the liver
Half-life: Normal renal function: 6-12 hours and is dose dependent
Time to peak serum concentration: 2-4 hours
Elimination: In urine

Usual Dosage Oral:

Children:

<2 years: Not recommended
2-14 years: Prolong penicillin serum levels: 25 mg/kg starting dose, then 40 mg/kg/day given 4 times/day
Gonorrhea: <45 kg: 25 mg/kg x 1 (maximum: 1 g/dose) 30 minutes before penicillin, ampicillin or amoxicillin

Adults:

Hyperuricemia with gout: 250 mg twice daily for one week; increase to 250-500 mg/day; may increase by 500 mg/month, if needed, to maximum of 2-3 g/day (dosages may be increased by 500 mg every 6 months if serum urate concentrations are controlled)
Prolong penicillin serum levels: 500 mg 4 times/day
Gonorrhea: 1 g 30 minutes before penicillin, ampicillin or amoxicillin

Dosing adjustment in renal impairment: Cl_{cr} <50 mL/minute: Avoid use

Dietary Considerations Food: Drug may cause GI upset; take with food if GI upset. Drink plenty of fluids.

Monitoring Parameters Uric acid, renal function, CBC

Test Interactions False-positive glucosuria with Clinitest®

Patient Information Take with food or antacids; drink plenty of fluids to reduce the risk of uric acid stones; the frequency of acute gouty attacks may increase during the first 6-12 months of therapy; avoid taking large doses of aspirin or other salicylates

Dosage Forms Tablet: 500 mg

Procainamide (proe kane A mide)

Related Information

Adult ACLS Algorithm, Tachycardia *on page 1512*
Adult ACLS Algorithm, V. Fib and Pulseless V. Tach *on page 1509*
Antiarrhythmic Drugs *on page 1389*
Comparative Pharmacokinetic Properties of Antiarrhythmic Agents *on page 1391*

Brand Names Procanbid®; Procan® SR; Promine®; Pronestyl®; Rhythmin®

Canadian/Mexican Brand Names Apo-Procainamide® (Canada)

Synonyms PCA; Procainamide Hydrochloride; Procaine Amide Hydrochloride

Therapeutic Category Antiarrhythmic Agent, Class I-A

Use Treatment of ventricular tachycardia, premature ventricular contractions, paroxysmal atrial tachycardia, and atrial fibrillation; to prevent recurrence of ventricular tachycardia, paroxysmal supraventricular tachycardia, atrial fibrillation or flutter

Pregnancy Risk Factor C

Contraindications Complete heart block; second or third degree heart block without pacemaker; "torsade de pointes"; hypersensitivity to the drug or procaine, or related drugs; myasthenia gravis; SLE

Warnings/Precautions Use with caution in patients with marked A-V conduction disturbances, bundle-branch block or severe cardiac glycoside intoxication, ventricular arrhythmias with organic heart disease or coronary occlusion, supraventricular tachyarrhythmias unless adequate measures are taken to prevent marked increases in ventricular rates; may accumulate in patients with renal or hepatic dysfunction; some tablets contain tartrazine; injection may contain bisulfite (allergens). Long-term administration leads to the development of a positive antinuclear antibody test in 50% of patients which may result in a lupus erythematosus-like syndrome (in 20% to 30% of patients); discontinue procainamide with SLE symptoms and choose an alternative agent; elderly have reduced clearance and frequent drug interactions.

Adverse Reactions

>10%: Miscellaneous: SLE-like syndrome

1% to 10%:
- Cardiovascular: Tachycardia, arrhythmias, A-V block, Q-T prolongation, widening QRS complex
- Central nervous system: Dizziness, lightheadedness
- Gastrointestinal: Diarrhea

<1%:
- Cardiovascular: Hypotension
- Central nervous system: Confusion, hallucinations, mental depression, disorientation, fever, drug fever
- Dermatologic: Rash
- Gastrointestinal: Nausea, vomiting, GI complaints
- Hematologic: Hemolytic anemia, agranulocytosis, neutropenia, thrombocytopenia, positive Coombs' test
- Neuromuscular & skeletal: Arthralgia, myalgia
- Respiratory: Pleural effusion

Overdosage/Toxicology Has a low toxic:therapeutic ratio and may easily produce fatal intoxication (acute toxic dose: 5 g in adults); symptoms of overdose include sinus bradycardia, sinus node arrest or asystole, P-R, QRS or Q-T interval prolongation, torsade de pointes (polymorphous ventricular tachycardia) and depressed myocardial contractility, which along with alpha-adrenergic or ganglionic blockade, may result in hypotension and pulmonary edema; other effects are seizures, coma, and respiratory arrest.

Treatment is primarily symptomatic and effects usually respond to conventional therapies (fluids, positioning, vasopressors, anticonvulsants, antiarrhythmics). **Note**: Do not use other type 1a or 1c antiarrhythmic agents to treat ventricular tachycardia; sodium bicarbonate may treat wide QRS intervals or hypotension; markedly impaired conduction or high degree A-V block, unresponsive to bicarbonate, indicates consideration of a pacemaker is needed.

Drug Interactions

- Increased plasma/NAPA concentrations with cimetidine, ranitidine, beta-blockers, and amiodarone
- Increased procainamide levels with ofloxacin (21% increase in peak plasma concentrations and 24% increase in AUC) due to inhibition of tubular secretion of procainamide
- Increased effect of skeletal muscle relaxants, quinidine and lidocaine and neuromuscular blockers (succinylcholine)
- Increased NAPA levels/toxicity with trimethoprim

Stability Procainamide may be stored at room temperature up to 27°C; however, refrigeration retards oxidation, which causes color formation. The solution is initially colorless but may turn slightly yellow on standing. Injection of air into the vial causes the solution to darken. Solutions darker than a light amber should be discarded.

Minimum volume: 1 g/250 mL NS/D_5W
Stability of admixture at room temperature in D_5W or NS: 24 hours

Some information indicates that procainamide may be subject to greater decomposition in D_5W unless the admixture is refrigerated or the pH is adjusted. Procainamide is believed to form an association complex with dextrose - the bioavailability of procainamide in this complex is not known and the complex formation is reversible.

Mechanism of Action Decreases myocardial excitability and conduction velocity and may depress myocardial contractility, by increasing the electrical stimulation threshold of ventricle, HIS-Purkinje system and through direct cardiac effects

Pharmacodynamics/Kinetics

Onset of action: I.M. 10-30 minutes
Distribution: V_d:
- Children: 2.2 L/kg
- Adults: 2 L/kg
- Congestive heart failure of shock: Decreased V_d

Protein binding: 15% to 20%
Metabolism: By acetylation in the liver to produce N-acetyl procainamide (NAPA) (active metabolite)
Bioavailability: Oral: 75% to 95%
Half-life:
- Procainamide: (Dependent upon hepatic acetylator, phenotype, cardiac function, and renal function):
  - Children: 1.7 hours
  - Adults: 2.5-4.7 hours
  - Anephric: 11 hours
- NAPA: (Dependent upon renal function):
  - Children: 6 hours
  - Adults: 6-8 hours
  - Anephric: 42 hours

Time to peak serum concentration:
- Capsule: Within 45 minutes to 2.5 hours
- I.M.: 15-60 minutes

Elimination: Urinary excretion (25% as NAPA)

Usual Dosage Must be titrated to patient's response

Children:
- Oral: 15-50 mg/kg/24 hours divided every 3-6 hours; maximum: 4 g/24 hours
- I.M.: 20-30 mg/kg/24 hours divided every 4-6 hours in divided doses; maximum: 4 g/24 hours
- I.V. (infusion requires use of an infusion pump):
- Load: 3-6 mg/kg/dose over 5 minutes not to exceed 100 mg/dose; may repeat every 5-10 minutes to maximum of 15 mg/kg/load
- Maintenance as continuous I.V. infusion: 20-80 mcg/kg/minute; maximum: 2 g/24 hours

Adults:
- Oral: 250-500 mg/dose every 3-6 hours or 500 mg to 1 g every 6 hours sustained release; usual dose: 50 mg/kg/24 hours; maximum: 4 g/24 hours (**Note:** Twice daily dosing approved for Procanbid®)
- I.M.: 0.5-1 g every 4-8 hours until oral therapy is possible
- I.V. (infusion requires use of an infusion pump): Loading dose: 15-18 mg/kg administered as slow infusion over 25-30 minutes or 100-200 mg/dose repeated every 5 minutes as needed to a total dose of 1 g; maintenance dose: 1-6 mg/minute by continuous infusion
- Infusion rate: 2 g/250 mL D_5W/NS (I.V. infusion requires use of an infusion pump):
  - 1 mg/minute: 7 mL/hour
  - 2 mg/minute: 15 mL/hour
  - 3 mg/minute: 21 mL/hour
  - 4 mg/minute: 30 mL/hour
  - 5 mg/minute: 38 mL/hour
  - 6 mg/minute: 45 mL/hour
- Refractory ventricular fibrillation: 30 mg/minute, up to a total of 17 mg/kg; I.V. maintenance infusion: 1-4 mg/minute; monitor levels and do not exceed 3 mg/minute for >24 hours in adults with renal failure
- ACLS guidelines: I.V.: Infuse 20 mg/minute until arrhythmia is controlled, hypotension occurs, QRS complex widens by 50% of its original width, or total of 17 mg/kg is given

Dosing interval in renal impairment:
- Cl_{cr} 10-50 mL/minute: Administer every 6-12 hours
- Cl_{cr} <10 mL/minute: Administer every 8-24 hours

(Continued)

Procainamide *(Continued)*

Dialysis:

Procainamide: Moderately hemodialyzable (20% to 50%): 200 mg supplemental dose posthemodialysis is recommended

N-acetylprocainamide: Not dialyzable (0% to 5%)

Procainamide/N-acetylprocainamide: Not peritoneal dialyzable (0% to 5%)

Procainamide/N-acetylprocainamide: Replace by blood level during continuous arterio-venous or veno-venous hemofiltration (CAVH/CAVHD)

Dosing adjustment in hepatic impairment: Reduce dose 50%

Administration Dilute I.V. with D_5W; maximum rate: 50 mg/minute; administer around-the-clock rather than 4 times/day to promote less variation in peak and trough serum levels

Monitoring Parameters EKG, blood pressure, CBC with differential, platelet count; cardiac monitor and blood pressure monitor required during I.V. administration

Reference Range

Timing of serum samples: Draw trough just before next oral dose; draw 6-12 hours after I.V. infusion has started; half-life is 2.5-5 hours

Therapeutic levels: Procainamide: 4-10 μg/mL; NAPA 15-25 μg/mL; Combined: 10-30 μg/mL

Toxic concentration: Procainamide: >10-12 μg/mL

Patient Information Do not discontinue therapy unless instructed by physician; notify physician or pharmacist if soreness of mouth, throat or gums, unexplained fever, or symptoms of upper respiratory tract infection occur. Do not chew sustained release tablets; some sustained release tablets contain a wax core that slowly releases the drug; when this process is complete, the empty, nonabsorbable wax core is eliminated and may be visible in feces; some sustained release tablets may be broken in half.

Nursing Implications Do not crush sustained release drug product

Dosage Forms

Capsule, as hydrochloride: 250 mg, 375 mg, 500 mg

Injection, as hydrochloride: 100 mg/mL (10 mL); 500 mg/mL (2 mL)

Tablet, as hydrochloride: 250 mg, 375 mg, 500 mg

Tablet, as hydrochloride, sustained release: 250 mg, 500 mg, 750 mg, 1000 mg

Tablet, as hydrochloride, sustained release (Procanbid®): 500 mg, 1000 mg

Extemporaneous Preparations Note: Several formulations have been described, some being more complex; for all formulations, the pH must be 4-6 to prevent degradation; some preparations require adjustment of pH; shake well before use

A suspension of 50 mg/mL can be made with the capsules, distilled water, and a 2:1 simple syrup/cherry syrup mixture; stability 2 weeks under refrigeration; (ASHP, 1987)

Concentrations of 5, 50, and 100 mg/mL oral liquid preparations, (made with the capsules, sterile water for irrigation and cherry syrup) stored at 4°C to 6°C (pH 6) were stable for at least 6 months (Metras, 1992).

A sucrose-based syrup (procainamide 50 mg/mL) made with capsules, distilled water, simple syrup, parabens, and cherry flavoring had a calculated stability of 456 days at 25°C and measured stability of 42 days at 40°C (pH ~5) while a maltitol-based syrup (procainamide 50 mg/mL) made with capsules, distilled water, Lycasin® (a syrup vehicle with 75% w/w maltitol), parabens, sodium bisulfate, saccharin, sodium acetate, pineapple and apricot flavoring, FD & C yellow number 6, (pH adjusted to 5 with glacial acetic acid) had a calculated stability of 97 days at 25°C and a measured stability of 94 days at 40°C. The maltitol-based syrup was more stable than the sucrose-based syrup when temperature was >37°C, but the sucrose-based syrup was more stable at temperatures <37°C (Alexander, 1993).

Alexander KS, Pudipeddi M, and Parker GA, "Stability of Procainamide Hydrochloride Syrups Compounded From Capsules," *Am J Hosp Pharm*, 1993, 50(4):693-8.

Handbook in Extemporaneous Formulations, Bethesda, MD: American Society of Hospital Pharmacists, 1987.

Metras JI, Swenson CF, and MacDermott MP, "Stability of Procainamide Hydrochloride in an Extemporaneously Compounded Oral Liquid," *Am J Hosp Pharm*, 1992, 49(7):1720-4.

Swenson CF, "Importance of Following Instructions When Compounding," *Am J Hosp Pharm*, 1993, 50(2):261.

Procainamide Hydrochloride *see* Procainamide *on page 1046*

Procaine (PROE kane)

Brand Names Novocain®

Synonyms Procaine Hydrochloride

Therapeutic Category Local Anesthetic, Injectable

Use Produces spinal anesthesia and epidural and peripheral nerve block by injection and infiltration methods

Pregnancy Risk Factor C

Contraindications Known hypersensitivity to procaine, PABA, parabens, or other ester local anesthetics

Warnings/Precautions Patients with cardiac diseases, hyperthyroidism, or other endocrine diseases may be more susceptible to toxic effects of local anesthetics; some preparations contain metabisulfite

Adverse Reactions

1% to 10%:

Local: Burning sensation at site of injection, tissue irritation, pain at injection site

<1%:

Central nervous system: Aseptic meningitis resulting in paralysis can occur, CNS stimulation followed by CNS depression, chills

Dermatologic: Discoloration of skin

Gastrointestinal: Nausea, vomiting

Ocular: Miosis

Otic: Tinnitus

Miscellaneous: Anaphylactoid reaction

Overdosage/Toxicology Treatment is primarily symptomatic and supportive. Termination of anesthesia by pneumatic tourniquet inflation should be attempted when the agent is administered by infiltration or regional injection. Seizures commonly respond to diazepam, while hypotension responds to I.V. fluids and Trendelenburg positioning. Bradyarrhythmias (heart rate <60) can be treated with I.V., I.M., or S.C. atropine 15 mcg/kg. With the development of metabolic acidosis, I.V. sodium bicarbonate 0.5-2 mEq/kg and ventilatory assistance should be instituted.

Drug Interactions

Decreased effect of sulfonamides with the PABA metabolite of procaine, chloroprocaine, and tetracaine

Decreased/increased effect of vasopressors, ergot alkaloids, and MAO inhibitors on blood pressure when using anesthetic solutions with a vasoconstrictor

Mechanism of Action Blocks both the initiation and conduction of nerve impulses by decreasing the neuronal membrane's permeability to sodium ions, which results in inhibition of depolarization with resultant blockade of conduction

Pharmacodynamics/Kinetics

Onset of effect: Injection: Within 2-5 minutes

Duration: 0.5-1.5 hours (dependent upon patient, type of block, concentration, and method of anesthesia)

Metabolism: Rapidly hydrolyzed by plasma enzymes to para-aminobenzoic acid and diethylaminoethanol (80% conjugated before elimination)

Half-life: 7.7 minutes

Elimination: In urine as metabolites and some unchanged drug

Usual Dosage Dose varies with procedure, desired depth, and duration of anesthesia, desired muscle relaxation, vascularity of tissues, physical condition, and age of patient

Nursing Implications Prior to instillation of anesthetic agent, withdraw plunger to ensure needle is not in artery or vein; resuscitative equipment should be available when local anesthetics are administered

Dosage Forms Injection, as hydrochloride: 1% [10 mg/mL] (2 mL, 6 mL, 30 mL, 100 mL); 2% [20 mg/mL] (30 mL, 100 mL); 10% (2 mL)

Procaine Amide Hydrochloride *see* Procainamide *on page 1046*

Procaine Benzylpenicillin *see* Penicillin G Procaine *on page 964*

Procaine Hydrochloride *see* Procaine *on this page*

Procaine Penicillin G *see* Penicillin G Procaine *on page 964*

Pro-Cal-Sof® [OTC] *see* Docusate *on page 415*

Procanbid® *see* Procainamide *on page 1046*

Procan® SR *see* Procainamide *on page 1046*

Procarbazine (proe KAR ba zeen)

Related Information

Antiemetics for Chemotherapy Induced Nausea and Vomiting *on page 1348*

Cancer Chemotherapy Regimens *on page 1351*

Toxicities of Chemotherapeutic Agents *on page 1382*

Brand Names Matulane®

Synonyms Benzmethyzin; N-Methylhydrazine; Procarbazine Hydrochloride

(Continued)

Procarbazine *(Continued)*

Therapeutic Category Antineoplastic Agent, Alkylating Agent

Use Treatment of Hodgkin's disease, non-Hodgkin's lymphoma, brain tumor, bronchogenic carcinoma

Pregnancy Risk Factor D

Contraindications Hypersensitivity to procarbazine or any component, or pre-existing bone marrow aplasia, alcohol ingestion

Warnings/Precautions The U.S. Food and Drug Administration (FDA) currently recommends that procedures for proper handling and disposal of antineoplastic agents be considered; Use with caution in patients with pre-existing renal or hepatic impairment; modify dosage in patients with renal or hepatic impairment, or marrow disorders; reduce dosage with serum creatinine >2 mg/dL or total bilirubin >3 mg/dL; procarbazine possesses MAO inhibitor activity. Procarbazine is a carcinogen which may cause acute leukemia; procarbazine may cause infertility.

Adverse Reactions

>10%:

Central nervous system: Mental depression, manic reactions, hallucinations, dizziness, headache, nervousness, insomnia, nightmares, ataxia, disorientation, confusion, seizure, CNS stimulation

Endocrine & metabolic: Amenorrhea

Gastrointestinal: Severe nausea and vomiting occur frequently and may be dose-limiting; anorexia, abdominal pain, stomatitis, dysphagia, diarrhea, and constipation; use a nonphenothiazine antiemetic, when possible

Emetic potential: Moderately high (60% to 90%)

Time course of nausea/vomiting: Onset: 24-27 hours; Duration: variable

Hematologic: Thrombocytopenia, hemolytic anemia

Myelosuppressive: May be dose-limiting toxicity; procarbazine should be discontinued if leukocyte count is <4000 mL or platelet count <100,000 mL

WBC: Moderate

Platelets: Moderate

Onset (days): 14

Nadir (days): 21

Recovery (days): 28

Neuromuscular & skeletal: Weakness, paresthesia, neuropathies, decreased reflexes, foot drop, tremors

Ocular: Nystagmus

Respiratory: Pleural effusion, cough

1% to 10%:

Central nervous system: Headache, anorexia, mental depression

Dermatologic: Alopecia, hyperpigmentation

Gastrointestinal: Diarrhea, stomatitis, constipation

Hepatic: Hepatotoxicity

Neuromuscular & skeletal: Peripheral neuropathy

<1%:

Cardiovascular: Orthostatic hypotension, hypertensive crisis

Central nervous system: Nervousness, irritability, somnolence

Dermatologic: Dermatitis, alopecia, pruritus, hyperpigmentation, hypersensitivity rash

Endocrine & metabolic: Disulfiram-like reaction, cessation of menses

Gastrointestinal: Anorexia

Hepatic: Jaundice

Neuromuscular & skeletal: Arthralgia, myalgia

Ocular: Diplopia, photophobia

Respiratory: Pneumonitis, hoarseness

Miscellaneous: Secondary malignancy, allergic reactions, flu-like syndrome

Overdosage/Toxicology Symptoms of overdose include arthralgia, alopecia, paresthesia, bone marrow suppression, hallucinations, nausea, vomiting, diarrhea, seizures, coma

Treatment is supportive, adverse effects such as marrow toxicity may begin as late as 2 weeks after exposure

Drug Interactions

Increased toxicity:

Procarbazine exhibits weak monoamine oxidase (MAO) inhibitor activity; foods containing high amounts of tyramine should, therefore, be avoided (ie, beer, yogurt, yeast, wine, cheese, pickled herring, chicken liver, and bananas). When a MAO inhibitor is given with food high in tyramine, a hypertensive crisis, intracranial bleeding, and headache have been reported.

Sympathomimetic amines (epinephrine and amphetamines) and antidepressants (tricyclics) should be used cautiously with procarbazine.

Barbiturates, narcotics, phenothiazines, and other CNS depressants can cause somnolence, ataxia, and other symptoms of CNS depression

Alcohol has caused a disulfiram-like reaction with procarbazine; may result in headache, respiratory difficulties, nausea, vomiting, sweating, thirst, hypotension, and flushing

Stability Protect from light

Mechanism of Action Mechanism of action is not clear, methylating of nucleic acids; inhibits DNA, RNA, and protein synthesis; may damage DNA directly and suppresses mitosis; metabolic activation required by host

Pharmacodynamics/Kinetics

Absorption: Oral: Rapid and complete

Distribution: Crosses the blood-brain barrier and distributes into CSF

Metabolism: In the liver and kidney

Half-life: 1 hour

Elimination: In urine and through respiratory tract (<5% as unchanged drug) and 70% as metabolites

Usual Dosage Refer to individual protocols. Dose based on patient's ideal weight if the patient is obese or has abnormal fluid retention. Oral:

Children:

BMT aplastic anemia conditioning regimen: 12.5 mg/kg/dose every other day for 4 doses

Hodgkin's disease: MOPP/IC-MOPP regimens: 100 mg/m²/day for 14 days and repeated every 4 weeks

Neuroblastoma and medulloblastoma: Doses as high as 100-200 mg/m²/day once daily have been used

Adults: Initial: 2-4 mg/kg/day in single or divided doses for 7 days then increase dose to 4-6 mg/kg/day until response is obtained or leukocyte count decreased <4000/mm³ or the platelet count decreased <100,000/mm³; maintenance: 1-2 mg/kg/day

In MOPP, 100 mg/m²/day on days 1-14 of a 28-day cycle

Dosing in renal/hepatic impairment: Use with caution, may result in increased toxicity

Dietary Considerations

Alcohol: Avoid use, including alcohol-containing products

Food: Avoid foods with high tyramine content

Monitoring Parameters CBC with differential, platelet and reticulocyte count, urinalysis, liver function test, renal function test.

Patient Information Avoid food with high tyramine content; obtain a list from your physician or pharmacist; do not take any new prescription or OTC drug without consulting your physician or pharmacist; avoid alcohol and alcohol containing products including topicals; notify physician of persistent fever, sore throat, bleeding, or bruising; may impair judgment and coordination; avoid prolonged exposure to sunlight

Dosage Forms Capsule, as hydrochloride: 50 mg

Procarbazine Hydrochloride *see* Procarbazine *on page 1049*

Procardia® *see* Nifedipine *on page 901*

Procardia XL® *see* Nifedipine *on page 901*

Prochlorperazine (proe klor PER a zeen)

Brand Names Compazine®

Canadian/Mexican Brand Names Nu-Prochlor® (Canada); PMS-Prochlorperazine (Canada); Prorazin® (Canada); Stemetil® (Canada)

Synonyms Prochlorperazine Edisylate; Prochlorperazine Maleate

Therapeutic Category Antiemetic; Antipsychotic Agent; Phenothiazine Derivative

Use Management of nausea and vomiting; acute and chronic psychosis

Pregnancy Risk Factor C

Pregnancy/Breast-Feeding Implications

Clinical effects on the fetus: Crosses the placenta. Isolated reports of congenital anomalies, however some included exposures to other drugs. Available evidence with use of occasional low doses suggests safe use during pregnancy.

Breast-feeding/lactation: No data available. American Academy of Pediatrics considers COMPATIBLE with breast-feeding.

Contraindications Hypersensitivity to prochlorperazine or any component; cross-sensitivity with other phenothiazines may exist; avoid use in patients with narrow-angle glaucoma; bone marrow suppression; severe liver or cardiac disease

Warnings/Precautions Injection contains sulfites which may cause allergic reactions; may impair ability to perform hazardous tasks requiring mental alertness or physical coordination; some products contain tartrazine dye, avoid use in sensitive individuals

(Continued)

Prochlorperazine *(Continued)*

Tardive dyskinesia: Prevalence rate may be 40% in elderly; development of the syndrome and the irreversible nature are proportional to duration and total cumulative dose over time. May be reversible if diagnosed early in therapy.

High incidence of extrapyramidal reactions, especially in children or the elderly, so reserve use in children <5 years of age to those who are unresponsive to other antiemetics; incidence of extrapyramidal reactions is increased with acute illnesses such as chicken pox, measles, CNS infections, gastroenteritis, and dehydration

Drug-induced **Parkinson's syndrome** occurs often. **Akathisia** is the most common extrapyramidal reaction in elderly.

Increased confusion, memory loss, psychotic behavior, and agitation frequently occur as a consequence of anticholinergic effects

Lowers seizure threshold, use cautiously in patients with seizure history

Orthostatic hypotension is due to alpha-receptor blockade, the elderly are at greater risk for orthostatic hypotension

Antipsychotic associated sedation in nonpsychotic patients is extremely unpleasant due to feelings of depersonalization, derealization, and dysphoria

Life-threatening arrhythmias have occurred at therapeutic doses of antipsychotics

Adverse Reactions Incidence of extrapyramidal reactions are higher with prochlorperazine than chlorpromazine

Central nervous system: Sedation, drowsiness, restlessness, anxiety, extrapyramidal reactions, parkinsonian signs and symptoms, seizures, altered central temperature regulation

Dermatologic: Photosensitivity, hyperpigmentation, pruritus, rash

Endocrine & metabolic: Amenorrhea, galactorrhea, gynecomastia

Gastrointestinal: Weight gain, GI upset

Miscellaneous: Anaphylactoid reactions

>10%:

Cardiovascular: Hypotension (especially with I.V. use), orthostatic hypotension, tachycardia, arrhythmias

Central nervous system: Pseudoparkinsonism, akathisia, tardive dyskinesia (persistent), dizziness, dystonias

Gastrointestinal: Xerostomia, constipation

Genitourinary: Urinary retention

Ocular: Pigmentary retinopathy, blurred vision

Respiratory: Nasal congestion

Miscellaneous: Diaphoresis (decreased)

1% to 10%:

Dermatologic: Increased sensitivity to sun, rash

Endocrine & metabolic: Changes in menstrual cycle, breast pain, changes in libido

Gastrointestinal: Nausea, vomiting, stomach pain

Genitourinary: Dysuria, ejaculatory disturbances

Neuromuscular & skeletal: Trembling of fingers

<1%:

Central nervous system: Neuroleptic malignant syndrome (NMS), impairment of temperature regulation, lowering of seizures threshold

Dermatologic: Discoloration of skin (blue-gray)

Endocrine & metabolic: Galactorrhea

Genitourinary: Priapism

Hematologic: Agranulocytosis, leukopenia, thrombocytopenia

Hepatic: Cholestatic jaundice, hepatotoxicity

Ocular: Cornea and lens changes

Overdosage/Toxicology Symptoms of overdose include deep sleep, coma, extrapyramidal symptoms, abnormal involuntary muscle movements, hypotension

Following initiation of essential overdose management, toxic symptom treatment and supportive treatment should be initiated. Hypotension usually responds to I.V. fluids or Trendelenburg positioning. If unresponsive to these measures, the use of a parenteral inotrope may be required (eg, norepinephrine 0.1-0.2 mcg/kg/minute titrated to response). Seizures commonly respond to diazepam (I.V. 5-10 mg bolus in adults every 15 minutes if needed up to a total of 30 mg; I.V. 0.25-0.4 mg/kg/dose up to a total of 10 mg in children) or to phenytoin or phenobarbital. Critical cardiac arrhythmias often respond to I.V. phenytoin (15 mg/kg up to 1 g), while other antiarrhythmics can be used. Extrapyramidal symptoms (eg, dystonic reactions) may require management with diphenhydramine 1-2 mg/kg (adults) up to a maximum of 50 mg I.M. or I.V. slow push followed by a maintenance dose for 48-72 hours. When these reactions are unresponsive to diphenhydramine, benztropine mesylate I.V. 1-2 mg (adults) may be effective. These agents are generally effective within 2-5 minutes.

Drug Interactions Increased toxicity: Additive effects with other CNS depressants; anticonvulsants; epinephrine may cause hypotension

Stability Protect from light; clear or slightly yellow solutions may be used; **incompatible** when mixed with aminophylline, amphotericin B, ampicillin, calcium salts, cephalothin, foscarnet (Y-site), furosemide, hydrocortisone, hydromorphone, methohexital, midazolam, penicillin G, pentobarbital, phenobarbital, thiopental

Mechanism of Action Blocks postsynaptic mesolimbic dopaminergic D_1 and D_2 receptors in the brain, including the medullary chemoreceptor trigger zone; exhibits a strong alpha-adrenergic and anticholinergic blocking effect and depresses the release of hypothalamic and hypophyseal hormones; believed to depress the reticular activating system, thus affecting basal metabolism, body temperature, wakefulness, vasomotor tone and emesis

Pharmacodynamics/Kinetics

Onset of effect:

- Oral: Within 30-40 minutes
- I.M.: Within 10-20 minutes
- Rectal: Within 60 minutes

Duration: Persists longest with I.M. and oral extended-release doses (12 hours); shortest following rectal and immediate release oral administration (3-4 hours)

Distribution: Crosses the placenta; appears in breast milk

Metabolism: Hepatic

Half-life: 23 hours

Elimination: Primarily by hepatic metabolism

Usual Dosage

Antiemetic: Children:

- Oral, rectal:
  - >10 kg: 0.4 mg/kg/24 hours in 3-4 divided doses; **or**
  - 9-14 kg: 2.5 mg every 12-24 hours as needed; maximum: 7.5 mg/day
  - 14-18 kg: 2.5 mg every 8-12 hours as needed; maximum: 10 mg/day
  - 18-39 kg: 2.5 mg every 8 hours or 5 mg every 12 hours as needed; maximum: 15 mg/day
- I.M.: 0.1-0.15 mg/kg/dose; usual: 0.13 mg/kg/dose; change to oral as soon as possible
- I.V.: Not recommended in children <10 kg or <2 years

Antiemetic: Adults:

- Oral: 5-10 mg 3-4 times/day; usual maximum: 40 mg/day
- I.M.: 5-10 mg every 3-4 hours; usual maximum: 40 mg/day
- I.V.: 2.5-10 mg; maximum 10 mg/dose or 40 mg/day; may repeat dose every 3-4 hours as needed
- Rectal: 25 mg twice daily

Antipsychotic:

- Children 2-12 years:
  - Oral, rectal: 2.5 mg 2-3 times/day; increase dosage as needed to maximum daily dose of 20 mg for 2-5 years and 25 mg for 6-12 years
  - I.M.: 0.13 mg/kg/dose; change to oral as soon as possible
- Adults:
  - Oral: 5-10 mg 3-4 times/day; doses up to 150 mg/day may be required in some patients for treatment of severe disturbances
  - I.M.: 10-20 mg every 4-6 hours may be required in some patients for treatment of severe disturbances; change to oral as soon as possible

Dementia behavior (nonpsychotic): Elderly: Initial: 2.5-5 mg 1-2 times/day; increase dose at 4- to 7-day intervals by 2.5-5 mg/day; increase dosing intervals (twice daily, 3 times/day, etc) as necessary to control response or side effects; maximum daily dose should probably not exceed 75 mg in elderly; gradual increases (titration) may prevent some side effects or decrease their severity

Hemodialysis: Not dialyzable (0% to 5%)

Administration Prochlorperazine may be administered I.M. or I.V.

I.M. should be administered into the upper outer quadrant of the buttock

I.V. may be administered IVP or IVPB

IVP should be administered at a concentration of 1 mg/mL at a rate of 1 mg/minute

Test Interactions False-positives for phenylketonuria, urinary amylase, uroporphyrins, urobilinogen

Patient Information May cause drowsiness, impair judgment and coordination; may cause photosensitivity; avoid excessive sunlight; notify physician of involuntary movements or feelings of restlessness

Nursing Implications Avoid skin contact with oral solution or injection, contact dermatitis has occurred; observe for extrapyramidal symptoms

Additional Information

Prochlorperazine: Compazine® suppository

(Continued)

Prochlorperazine *(Continued)*

Prochlorperazine edisylate: Compazine® oral solution and injection
Prochlorperazine maleate: Compazine® capsule and tablet

Dosage Forms

Capsule, sustained action, as maleate: 10 mg, 15 mg, 30 mg
Injection, as edisylate: 5 mg/mL (2 mL, 10 mL)
Suppository, rectal: 2.5 mg, 5 mg, 25 mg (12/box)
Syrup, as edisylate: 5 mg/5 mL (120 mL)
Tablet, as maleate: 5 mg, 10 mg, 25 mg

Prochlorperazine Edisylate *see* Prochlorperazine *on page 1051*

Prochlorperazine Maleate *see* Prochlorperazine *on page 1051*

ProCrit® *see* Epoetin Alfa *on page 451*

Proctocort™ *see* Hydrocortisone *on page 623*

ProctoCream-HC™ *see* Hydrocortisone *on page 623*

Proctofoam® NS [OTC] *see* Pramoxine *on page 1033*

Procyclidine (proe SYE kli deen)

Brand Names Kemadrin®

Canadian/Mexican Brand Names PMS-Procyclidine (Canada); Procyclid® (Canada)

Synonyms Procyclidine Hydrochloride

Therapeutic Category Anticholinergic Agent; Anti-Parkinson's Agent

Use Relieves symptoms of parkinsonian syndrome and drug-induced extrapyramidal symptoms

Pregnancy Risk Factor C

Contraindications Angle-closure glaucoma; safe use in children not established

Warnings/Precautions Use with caution in hot weather or during exercise. Elderly patients frequently develop increased sensitivity and require strict dosage regulation - side effects may be more severe in elderly patients with atherosclerotic changes. Use with caution in patients with tachycardia, cardiac arrhythmias, hypertension, hypotension, prostatic hypertrophy (especially in the elderly) or any tendency toward urinary retention, liver or kidney disorders and obstructive disease of the GI or GU tract. When given in large doses or to susceptible patients, may cause weakness and inability to move particular muscle groups.

Adverse Reactions

>10%:
- Dermatologic: Dry skin
- Gastrointestinal: Constipation, xerostomia, dry throat
- Respiratory: Dry nose
- Miscellaneous: Diaphoresis (decreased)

1% to 10%:
- Dermatologic: Increased sensitivity to light
- Endocrine & metabolic: Decreased flow of breast milk
- Gastrointestinal: Dysphagia

<1%:
- Cardiovascular: Orthostatic hypotension, ventricular fibrillation, tachycardia, palpitations
- Central nervous system: Confusion, drowsiness, headache, loss of memory, fatigue, ataxia
- Dermatologic: Rash
- Gastrointestinal: Bloated feeling, nausea, vomiting
- Genitourinary: Dysuria
- Neuromuscular & skeletal: Weakness
- Ocular: Increased intraocular pain, blurred vision

Overdosage/Toxicology Symptoms of overdose include disorientation, hallucinations, delusions, blurred vision, dysphagia, absent bowel sounds, hyperthermia, hypertension, urinary retention

Anticholinergic toxicity is caused by strong binding of the drug to cholinergic receptors. Anticholinesterase inhibitors reduce acetylcholinesterase, the enzyme that breaks down acetylcholine and thereby allows acetylcholine to accumulate and compete for receptor binding with the offending anticholinergic. For anticholinergic overdose with severe life-threatening symptoms, physostigmine 1-2 mg (0.5 or 0.02 mg/kg for children) S.C. or I.V., slowly may be given to reverse these effects.

Drug Interactions

Decreased effect of psychotropics
Increased toxicity with phenothiazines, meperidine, TCAs

Mechanism of Action Thought to act by blocking excess acetylcholine at cerebral synapses; many of its effects are due to its pharmacologic similarities with atropine

Pharmacodynamics/Kinetics

Onset of effect: Oral: Within 30-40 minutes

Duration: 4-6 hours

Usual Dosage Adults: Oral: 2.5 mg 3 times/day after meals; if tolerated, gradually increase dose, maximum of 20 mg/day if necessary

Dosing adjustment in hepatic impairment: Decrease dose to a twice daily dosing regimen

Dietary Considerations Alcohol: Avoid use

Patient Information Take after meals; do not discontinue drug abruptly; notify physician if adverse GI effects, fever or heat intolerance occurs; may cause drowsiness; avoid alcohol; adequate fluid intake or sugar free gum or hard candy may help dry mouth; adequate fluid and exercise may help constipation

Dosage Forms Tablet, as hydrochloride: 5 mg

Procyclidine Hydrochloride *see* Procyclidine *on previous page*

Prodium® [OTC] *see* Phenazopyridine *on page 981*

Profasi® HP *see* Chorionic Gonadotropin *on page 272*

Profenal® *see* Suprofen *on page 1184*

Profilate® OSD *see* Antihemophilic Factor (Human) *on page 94*

Profilate® SD *see* Antihemophilic Factor (Human) *on page 94*

Profilnine® Heat-Treated *see* Factor IX Complex (Human) *on page 502*

Progestasert® *see* Progesterone *on this page*

Progesterone (proe JES ter one)

Brand Names Progestasert®

Canadian/Mexican Brand Names PMS-Progesterone (Canada); Progesterone Oil (Canada); Utrogestan® (Mexico)

Synonyms Pregnenedione; Progestin

Therapeutic Category Progestin Derivative

Use Intrauterine contraception in women who have had at least 1 child, are in a stable, mutually monogamous relationship, and have no history of pelvic inflammatory disease; amenorrhea; functional uterine bleeding

Pregnancy Risk Factor X

Contraindications Pregnancy, thrombophlebitis, undiagnosed vaginal bleeding, hypersensitivity to progesterone or any component, carcinoma of the breast, cerebral apoplexy

Warnings/Precautions Use with caution in patients with impaired liver function, depression, diabetes, and epilepsy; use of any progestin during the first 4 months of pregnancy is not recommended; monitor closely for loss of vision, proptosis, diplopia, migraine, and signs and symptoms of embolic disorders. Not a progestin of choice in the elderly for hormonal cycling.

Adverse Reactions

Intrauterine device:

>10%:

Cardiovascular: Edema

Endocrine & metabolic: Breakthrough bleeding, spotting, changes in menstrual flow, amenorrhea

Gastrointestinal: Anorexia

Neuromuscular & skeletal: Weakness

1% to 10%:

Cardiovascular: Embolism, central thrombosis

Central nervous system: Mental depression, fever, insomnia

Dermatologic: Melasma or chloasma, allergic rash with or without pruritus

Endocrine: Changes in cervical erosion and secretions, increased breast tenderness

Gastrointestinal: Weight gain or loss

Hepatic: Cholestatic jaundice

Injection (I.M.):

>10% Local: Pain at injection site

1% to 10%: Local: Thrombophlebitis

Overdosage/Toxicology Toxicity is unlikely following single exposures of excessive doses; supportive treatment is adequate in most cases

Drug Interactions Inducer of cytochrome P-450 1A2 enzymes

Decreased effect: Aminoglutethimide may decrease effect by increasing hepatic metabolism

Mechanism of Action Natural steroid hormone that induces secretory changes in the endometrium, promotes mammary gland development, relaxes uterine smooth muscle, blocks follicular maturation and ovulation, and maintains pregnancy

Pharmacodynamics/Kinetics

Duration of action: 24 hours

Half-life: 5 minutes

(Continued)

Progesterone *(Continued)*

Elimination: In urine

Usual Dosage Adults:

Amenorrhea: I.M.: 5-10 mg/day for 6-8 consecutive days

Functional uterine bleeding: I.M.: 5-10 mg/day for 6 doses

Contraception: Female: Intrauterine device: Insert a single system into the uterine cavity; contraceptive effectiveness is retained for 1 year and system must be replaced 1 year after insertion

Monitoring Parameters Before starting therapy, a physical exam including the breasts and pelvis are recommended, also a PAP smear; signs or symptoms of depression, glucose in diabetics

Test Interactions Thyroid function, metyrapone, liver function, coagulation tests, endocrine function tests

Patient Information Notify physician if sudden loss of vision or migraine headache occur or if you suspect you may have become pregnant; may cause photosensitivity, wear protective clothing or sunscreen

Nursing Implications Patients should receive a copy of the patient labeling for the drug; administer deep I.M. only; monitor patient closely for loss of vision, sudden onset of proptosis, diplopia, migraine, and signs and symptoms of embolic disorders

Dosage Forms

Intrauterine system, reservoir: 38 mg in silicone fluid

Injection, in oil: 50 mg/mL (10 mL)

Progestin *see* Progesterone *on previous page*

Proglycem® *see* Diazoxide *on page 371*

Prograf® *see* Tacrolimus *on page 1186*

ProHIBiT® *see Haemophilus* b Conjugate Vaccine *on page 595*

Prokine™ *see* Sargramostim *on page 1125*

Prolamine® [OTC] *see* Phenylpropanolamine *on page 991*

Proleukin® *see* Aldesleukin *on page 40*

Prolixin® *see* Fluphenazine *on page 543*

Prolixin Decanoate® *see* Fluphenazine *on page 543*

Prolixin Enanthate® *see* Fluphenazine *on page 543*

Proloprim® *see* Trimethoprim *on page 1266*

Promazine (PROE ma zeen)

Related Information

Antipsychotic Agents Comparison *on page 1396*

Brand Names Sparine®

Synonyms Promazine Hydrochloride

Therapeutic Category Antiemetic; Antipsychotic Agent; Phenothiazine Derivative

Use Management of manifestations of psychotic disorders; depressive neurosis; alcohol withdrawal; nausea and vomiting; nonpsychotic symptoms associated with dementia in elderly, Tourette's syndrome; Huntington's chorea; spasmodic torticollis and Reye's syndrome

Pregnancy Risk Factor C

Contraindications Hypersensitivity to promazine or any component; severe CNS depression, cross-sensitivity to other phenothiazines may exist; avoid use in patients with narrow-angle glaucoma, blood dyscrasias, severe liver or cardiac disease; subcortical brain damage; circulatory collapse; severe hypotension or hypertension

Warnings/Precautions

Tardive dyskinesia: Prevalence rate may be 40% in elderly; development of the syndrome and the irreversible nature are proportional to duration and total cumulative dose over time. May be reversible if diagnosed early in therapy.

Extrapyramidal reactions are more common in elderly with up to 50% developing these reactions after 60 years of age. These reactions may be more common in dementia patients.

Drug-induced **Parkinson's syndrome** occurs often. **Akathisia** is the most common extrapyramidal reaction in elderly.

Increased confusion, memory loss, psychotic behavior, and agitation frequently occur as a consequence of anticholinergic effects

Orthostatic hypotension is due to alpha-receptor blockade, the elderly are at greater risk for orthostatic hypotension

Antipsychotic associated sedation in nonpsychotic patients is extremely unpleasant due to feelings of depersonalization, derealization, and dysphoria

Life-threatening arrhythmias have occurred at therapeutic doses of antipsychotics; use with caution in patients with narrow-angle glaucoma, severe liver disease or severe cardiac disease

Adverse Reactions

>10%:

- Cardiovascular: Hypotension, orthostatic hypotension
- Central nervous system: Pseudoparkinsonism, akathisia, dystonias, tardive dyskinesia (persistent), dizziness
- Gastrointestinal: Constipation
- Ocular: Pigmentary retinopathy
- Respiratory: Nasal congestion
- Miscellaneous: Diaphoresis (decreased)

1% to 10%:

- Dermatologic: Increased sensitivity to sun, rash
- Endocrine & metabolic: Changes in menstrual cycle, changes in libido, breast pain
- Gastrointestinal: Weight gain, nausea, vomiting, stomach pain
- Genitourinary: Dysuria, ejaculatory disturbances
- Neuromuscular & skeletal: Trembling of fingers

<1%:

- Central nervous system: Neuroleptic malignant syndrome (NMS), impairment of temperature regulation, lowering of seizures threshold
- Dermatologic: Discoloration of skin (blue-gray), pigmentary retinopathy
- Endocrine & metabolic: Galactorrhea
- Genitourinary: Priapism
- Hematologic: Agranulocytosis, leukopenia
- Hepatic: Cholestatic jaundice, hepatotoxicity
- Ocular: Cornea and lens changes

Overdosage/Toxicology Symptoms of overdose include deep sleep, coma, extrapyramidal symptoms, abnormal involuntary muscle movements, hypotension

Following initiation of essential overdose management, toxic symptom treatment and supportive treatment should be initiated. Hypotension usually responds to I.V. fluids or Trendelenburg positioning. If unresponsive to these measures, the use of a parenteral inotrope may be required (eg, norepinephrine 0.1-0.2 mcg/kg/minute titrated to response). Seizures commonly respond to diazepam (I.V. 5-10 mg bolus in adults every 15 minutes if needed up to a total of 30 mg; I.V. 0.25-0.4 mg/kg/dose up to a total of 10 mg in children) or to phenytoin or phenobarbital. Critical cardiac arrhythmias often respond to I.V. phenytoin (15 mg/kg up to 1 g), while other antiarrhythmics can be used. Neuroleptics often cause extrapyramidal symptoms (eg, dystonic reactions) requiring management with diphenhydramine 1-2 mg/kg (adults) up to a maximum of 50 mg I.M. or I.V. slow push followed by a maintenance dose for 48-72 hours. When these reactions are unresponsive to diphenhydramine, benztropine mesylate I.V. 1-2 mg (adults) may be effective. These agents are generally effective within 2-5 minutes.

Stability Protect all dosage forms from light, clear or slightly yellow solutions may be used; should be dispensed in amber or opaque vials/bottles. Solutions may be diluted or mixed with fruit juices or other liquids, but must be administered immediately after mixing

Injection: **Incompatible** when mixed with aminophylline, dimenhydrinate, methohexital, nafcillin, penicillin G, pentobarbital, phenobarbital, sodium bicarbonate, thiopental

Mechanism of Action Blocks postsynaptic mesolimbic dopaminergic D_1 and D_2 receptors in the brain; exhibits a strong alpha-adrenergic blocking and anticholinergic effect, depresses the release of hypothalamic and hypophyseal hormones; believed to depress the reticular activating system thus affecting basal metabolism, body temperature, wakefulness, vasomotor tone, and emesis

Pharmacodynamics/Kinetics The specific pharmacokinetics of promazine are poorly established but probably resemble those of other phenothiazines.

- Absorption: Phenothiazines are only partially absorbed; great variability in plasma levels resulting from a given dose
- Metabolism: Extensively in the liver
- Half-life: Most phenothiazines have long half-lives in the range of 24 hours or more

Usual Dosage Oral, I.M.:

- Children >12 years: Antipsychotic: 10-25 mg every 4-6 hours
- Adults:
  - Psychosis: 10-200 mg every 4-6 hours not to exceed 1000 mg/day
  - Antiemetic: 25-50 mg every 4-6 hours as needed

Hemodialysis: Not dialyzable (0% to 5%)

Administration I.M. injections should be deep injections; if giving I.V., dilute to at least 25 mg/mL and administer slowly

Test Interactions ↑ cholesterol (S), ↑ glucose; ↓ uric acid (S)

(Continued)

Promazine *(Continued)*

Patient Information May cause drowsiness, impair judgment and coordination; may cause photosensitivity; avoid excessive sunlight; notify physician of involuntary movements or feelings of restlessness

Nursing Implications Watch for hypotension

Dosage Forms

Injection, as hydrochloride: 25 mg/mL (10 mL); 50 mg/mL (1 mL, 2 mL, 10 mL)
Tablet, as hydrochloride: 25 mg, 50 mg, 100 mg

Promazine Hydrochloride *see* Promazine *on page 1056*

Prometa® *see* Metaproterenol *on page 793*

Prometh® *see* Promethazine *on this page*

Promethazine (proe METH a zeen)

Related Information

Drugs and Routes of Administration Not Recommended for Treatment of Cancer Pain *on page 1378*

Brand Names Anergan®; Phenazine®; Phenergan®; Prometh®; Prorex®

Synonyms Promethazine Hydrochloride

Therapeutic Category Antiemetic; Antihistamine, H_1 Blocker; Phenothiazine Derivative; Sedative

Use Symptomatic treatment of various allergic conditions, antiemetic, motion sickness, and as a sedative

Pregnancy Risk Factor C

Pregnancy/Breast-Feeding Implications

Clinical effects on the fetus: Crosses the placenta. Possible respiratory depression if drug is administered near time of delivery; behavioral changes, EEG alterations, impaired platelet aggregation reported with use during labor. Available evidence with use of occasional low doses suggests safe use during pregnancy.

Breast-feeding/lactation: No data available. American Academy of Pediatrics makes NO RECOMMENDATION.

Contraindications Hypersensitivity to promethazine or any component; narrow-angle glaucoma

Warnings/Precautions Do not administer S.C. or intra-arterially, necrotic lesions may occur; injection may contain sulfites which may cause allergic reactions in some patients; use with caution in patients with cardiovascular disease, impaired liver function, asthma, sleep apnea, seizures. Rapid I.V. administration may produce a transient fall in blood pressure, rate of administration should not exceed 25 mg/minute; slow I.V. administration may produce a slightly elevated blood pressure. Because promethazine is a phenothiazine (and can, therefore, cause side effects such as extrapyramidal symptoms), it is not considered an antihistamine of choice in the elderly.

Adverse Reactions

Hematologic: Thrombocytopenia
Hepatic: Jaundice

>10%:

- Central nervous system: Slight to moderate drowsiness
- Respiratory: Thickening of bronchial secretions

1% to 10%:

- Central nervous system: Headache, fatigue, nervousness, dizziness
- Gastrointestinal: Xerostomia, abdominal pain, nausea, diarrhea, increased appetite, weight gain
- Neuromuscular & skeletal: Arthralgia
- Respiratory: Pharyngitis

<1%:

- Cardiovascular: Tachycardia, bradycardia, palpitations, hypotension
- Central nervous system: Sedation (pronounced), confusion, excitation, extrapyramidal reactions with high doses, dystonia, faintness with I.V. administration, depression, insomnia
- Dermatologic: Photosensitivity, rash, angioedema
- Genitourinary: Urinary retention
- Hepatic: Hepatitis
- Neuromuscular & skeletal: Tremor, paresthesia, myalgia
- Ocular: Blurred vision
- Respiratory: Irregular respiration, bronchospasm, epistaxis
- Miscellaneous: Allergic reactions

Overdosage/Toxicology Symptoms of overdose include CNS depression, respiratory depression, possible CNS stimulation, dry mouth, fixed and dilated pupils, hypotension

Following initiation of essential overdose management, toxic symptom treatment and supportive treatment should be initiated. Hypotension usually responds to

I.V. fluids or Trendelenburg positioning. If unresponsive to these measures, norepinephrine 0.1-0.2 mcg/kg/minute titrated to response may be tried. Seizures commonly respond to diazepam (I.V. 5-10 mg bolus in adults every 15 minutes if needed up to a total of 30 mg; I.V. 0.25-0.4 mg/kg/dose up to a total of 10 mg in children) or to phenytoin or phenobarbital. Critical cardiac arrhythmias often respond to I.V. phenytoin (15 mg/kg up to 1 g), while other antiarrhythmics can be used. Neuroleptics often cause extrapyramidal symptoms (eg, dystonic reactions) requiring management with diphenhydramine 1-2 mg/kg (adults) up to a maximum of 50 mg I.M. or I.V. slow push followed by a maintenance dose for 48-72 hours. When these reactions are unresponsive to diphenhydramine, benztropine mesylate I.V. 1-2 mg (adults) may be effective. These agents are generally effective within 2-5 minutes.

Drug Interactions Increased toxicity: Epinephrine should not be used together with promethazine since blood pressure may decrease further; additive effects with other CNS depressants

Stability Protect from light and from freezing; **compatible** (when comixed in the same syringe) with atropine, chlorpromazine, diphenhydramine, droperidol, fentanyl, glycopyrrolate, hydromorphone, hydroxyzine hydrochloride, meperidine, midazolam, nalbuphine, pentazocine, prochlorperazine, scopolamine; **incompatible** when mixed with aminophylline, cefoperazone (Y-site), chloramphenicol, dimenhydrinate (same syringe), foscarnet (Y-site), furosemide, heparin, hydrocortisone, methohexital, penicillin G, pentobarbital, phenobarbital, thiopental

Mechanism of Action Blocks postsynaptic mesolimbic dopaminergic receptors in the brain; exhibits a strong alpha-adrenergic blocking effect and depresses the release of hypothalamic and hypophyseal hormones; competes with histamine for the H_1-receptor; reduces stimuli to the brainstem reticular system

Pharmacodynamics/Kinetics

Onset of effect: I.V.: Within 20 minutes (3-5 minutes with I.V. injection)

Duration: 2-6 hours

Metabolism: In the liver

Elimination: Principally as inactive metabolites in urine and in feces

Usual Dosage

Children:

- Antihistamine: Oral, rectal: 0.1 mg/kg/dose every 6 hours during the day and 0.5 mg/kg/dose at bedtime as needed
- Antiemetic: Oral, I.M., I.V., rectal: 0.25-1 mg/kg 4-6 times/day as needed
- Motion sickness: Oral, rectal: 0.5 mg/kg/dose 30 minutes to 1 hour before departure, then every 12 hours as needed
- Sedation: Oral, I.M., I.V., rectal: 0.5-1 mg/kg/dose every 6 hours as needed

Adults:

- Antihistamine (including allergic reactions to blood or plasma):
  - Oral, rectal: 12.5 mg 3 times/day and 25 mg at bedtime
  - I.M., I.V.: 25 mg, may repeat in 2 hours when necessary; switch to oral route as soon as feasible
- Antiemetic: Oral, I.M., I.V., rectal: 12.5-25 mg every 4 hours as needed
- Motion sickness: Oral, rectal: 25 mg 30-60 minutes before departure, then every 12 hours as needed
- Sedation: Oral, I.M., I.V., rectal: 25-50 mg/dose

Hemodialysis: Not dialyzable (0% to 5%)

Administration Avoid I.V. use; if necessary, may dilute to a maximum concentration of 25 mg/mL and infuse at a maximum rate of 25 mg/minute; rapid I.V. administration may produce a transient fall in blood pressure

Test Interactions Alters the flare response in intradermal allergen tests

Patient Information May cause drowsiness, impair judgment and coordination; may cause photosensitivity; avoid excessive sunlight; notify physician of involuntary movements or feelings of restlessness

Dosage Forms

Injection, as hydrochloride: 25 mg/mL (1 mL, 10 mL); 50 mg/mL (1 mL, 10 mL)

Suppository, rectal, as hydrochloride: 12.5 mg, 25 mg, 50 mg

Syrup, as hydrochloride: 6.25 mg/5 mL (5 mL, 120 mL, 240 mL, 480 mL, 4000 mL); 25 mg/5 mL (120 mL, 480 mL, 4000 mL)

Tablet, as hydrochloride: 12.5 mg, 25 mg, 50 mg

Promethazine Hydrochloride *see* Promethazine *on previous page*

Promine® *see* Procainamide *on page 1046*

Promit® *see* Dextran 1 *on page 364*

Pronestyl® *see* Procainamide *on page 1046*

Pronto® Shampoo [OTC] *see* Pyrethrins *on page 1079*

Propacet® *see* Propoxyphene and Acetaminophen *on page 1067*

Propadrine *see* Phenylpropanolamine *on page 991*

Propafenone (proe pa FEEN one)

Related Information

Antiarrhythmic Drugs *on page 1389*

Comparative Pharmacokinetic Properties of Antiarrhythmic Agents *on page 1391*

Brand Names Rythmol®

Canadian/Mexican Brand Names Norfenon® (Mexico)

Synonyms Propafenone Hydrochloride

Therapeutic Category Antiarrhythmic Agent, Class I-C

Use Life-threatening ventricular arrhythmias

Unlabeled use: Supraventricular tachycardias, including those patients with Wolff-Parkinson-White syndrome

Pregnancy Risk Factor C

Contraindications Hypersensitivity to propafenone or any component; uncontrolled congestive heart failure; bronchospastic disorders; cardiogenic shock, conduction disorders (A-V block, sick-sinus syndrome), bradycardia

Warnings/Precautions Until evidence to the contrary, propafenone should be considered acceptable only for the treatment of life-threatening arrhythmias; propafenone may cause new or worsened arrhythmias, worsen CHF, decrease A-V conduction and alter pacemaker thresholds; use with caution in patients with recent myocardial infarction, congestive heart failure, hepatic or renal dysfunction; elderly may be at greater risk for toxicity

Adverse Reactions

>10%:

Central nervous system: Dizziness, drowsiness

Gastrointestinal: Xerostomia

1% to 10%:

Cardiovascular: A-V block (first and second degree), cardiac conduction disturbances, palpitations, congestive heart failure, angina, bradycardia

Central nervous system: Headache, anxiety, loss of balance

Gastrointestinal: Abnormal taste, constipation, nausea, vomiting, abdominal pain, dyspepsia, anorexia, flatulence, diarrhea

Ocular: Blurred vision

Respiratory: Dyspnea

<1%:

Cardiovascular: New or worsened arrhythmias (proarrhythmic effect), bundle-branch block

Central nervous system: Abnormal speech, vision, or dreams

Hematologic: Leukopenia, thrombocytopenia, agranulocytosis

Neuromuscular & skeletal: Paresthesias, numbness

Overdosage/Toxicology Has a narrow therapeutic index and severe toxicity may occur slightly above the therapeutic range, especially if combined with other antiarrhythmic drugs. Acute single ingestion of twice the daily therapeutic dose is life-threatening. Symptoms of overdose include increases in P-R, QRS, Q-T intervals and amplitude of the T wave, A-V block, bradycardia, hypotension, ventricular arrhythmias (monomorphic or polymorphic ventricular tachycardia), and asystole; other symptoms include dizziness, blurred vision, headache, and GI upset.

Treatment is supportive, using conventional treatment (fluids, positioning, anticonvulsants, antiarrhythmics). **Note:** Type Ia antiarrhythmic agents should not be used to treat cardiotoxicity caused by type 1c drugs; sodium bicarbonate may reverse QRS prolongation, bradycardia and hypotension; ventricular pacing may be needed; hemodialysis only of possible benefit for tocainide or flecainide overdose in patients with renal failure.

Drug Interactions

Decreased levels with rifampin

Increased levels with cimetidine, quinidine, and beta-blockers

Increased effect/levels of warfarin, beta-blockers metabolized by the liver, local anesthetics, cyclosporine, and digoxin (**Note:** Reduce dose of digoxin by 25%)

Mechanism of Action Propafenone is a 1C antiarrhythmic agent which possesses local anesthetic properties, blocks the fast inward sodium current, and slows the rate of increase of the action potential. prolongs conduction and refractoriness in all areas of the myocardium, with a slightly more pronounced effect on intraventricular conduction; it prolongs effective refractory period, reduces spontaneous automaticity and exhibits some beta-blockade activity.

Pharmacodynamics/Kinetics

Absorption: Well absorbed

Metabolism: Two genetically determined metabolism groups exist: fast or slow metabolizers; 10% of Caucasians are slow metabolizers

Half-life after a single dose (100-300 mg): 2-8 hours; half-life after chronic dosing ranges from 10-32 hours

Time to peak: Peak levels occur in 2 hours with a 150 mg dose and 3 hours after a 300 mg dose; this agent exhibits nonlinear pharmacokinetics; when dose is increased from 300 mg to 900 mg/day, serum concentrations increase tenfold; this nonlinearity is thought to be due to saturable first-pass hepatic enzyme metabolism

Usual Dosage Adults: Oral: 150 mg every 8 hours, increase at 3- to 4-day intervals up to 300 mg every 8 hours. **Note:** Patients who exhibit significant widening of QRS complex or second or third degree A-V block may need dose reduction.

Dosing adjustment in hepatic impairment: Reduction is necessary

Monitoring Parameters EKG, blood pressure, pulse (particularly at initiation of therapy)

Patient Information Take dose the same way each day, either with or without food; do not double the next dose if present dose is missed; do not discontinue drug or change dose without advice of physician; report any severe or persistent fatigue, sore throat, or any unusual bleeding or bruising; may cause drowsiness and impair coordination and judgment

Nursing Implications Patients should be on a cardiac monitor during initiation of therapy or when dosage is increased; monitor heart sounds and pulses for rate, rhythm and quality

Dosage Forms Tablet, as hydrochloride: 150 mg, 225 mg, 300 mg

Propafenone Hydrochloride *see* Propafenone *on previous page*

Propagest® [OTC] *see* Phenylpropanolamine *on page 991*

Propantheline (proe PAN the leen)

Brand Names Pro-Banthine®

Canadian/Mexican Brand Names Propanthel™

Synonyms Propantheline Bromide

Therapeutic Category Anticholinergic Agent; Antispasmodic Agent, Gastrointestinal; Antispasmodic Agent, Urinary

Use Adjunctive treatment of peptic ulcer, irritable bowel syndrome, pancreatitis, ureteral and urinary bladder spasm; reduce duodenal motility during diagnostic radiologic procedures

Pregnancy Risk Factor C

Contraindications Narrow-angle glaucoma, known hypersensitivity to propantheline; ulcerative colitis; toxic megacolon; obstructive disease of the GI or urinary tract

Warnings/Precautions Use with caution in patients with hyperthyroidism, hepatic, cardiac, or renal disease, hypertension, GI infections, or other endocrine diseases

Adverse Reactions

>10%:
- Dermatologic: Dry skin
- Gastrointestinal: Constipation, xerostomia, dry throat
- Respiratory: Dry nose
- Miscellaneous: Diaphoresis (decreased)

1% to 10%: Gastrointestinal: Dysphagia

<1%:
- Cardiovascular: Tachycardia
- Central nervous system: Confusion, headache, loss of memory, fatigue, drowsiness, nervousness, insomnia
- Dermatologic: Rash
- Gastrointestinal: Bloated feeling, nausea, vomiting
- Genitourinary: Urinary retention
- Neuromuscular & skeletal: Weakness
- Ocular: Increased intraocular pressure, blurred vision

Overdosage/Toxicology Symptoms of overdose include CNS disturbances, flushing, respiratory failure, paralysis, coma, urinary retention, hyperthermia

Anticholinergic toxicity is caused by strong binding of the drug to cholinergic receptors. For anticholinergic overdose with severe life-threatening symptoms, physostigmine 1-2 mg (0.5 or 0.02 mg/kg for children) S.C. or I.V., slowly may be given to reverse these effects.

Drug Interactions

Decreased effect with antacids (decreased absorption); decreased effect of sustained release dosage forms (decreased absorption)

Increased effect/toxicity with anticholinergics, disopyramide, narcotic analgesics, bretylium, type I antiarrhythmics, antihistamines, phenothiazines, TCAs, corticosteroids (increased IOP), CNS depressants (sedation), adenosine, amiodarone, beta-blockers, amoxapine

Mechanism of Action Competitively blocks the action of acetylcholine at postganglionic parasympathetic receptor sites

(Continued)

Propantheline *(Continued)*

Pharmacodynamics/Kinetics

Onset of effect: Oral: Within 30-45 minutes

Duration: 4-6 hours

Metabolism: In the liver and GI tract

Elimination: In urine, bile, and other body fluids

Usual Dosage Oral:

Antisecretory:

Children: 1-2 mg/kg/day in 3-4 divided doses

Adults: 15 mg 3 times/day before meals or food and 30 mg at bedtime

Elderly: 7.5 mg 3 times/day before meals and at bedtime

Antispasmodic:

Children: 2-3 mg/kg/day in divided doses every 4-6 hours and at bedtime

Adults: 15 mg 3 times/day before meals or food and 30 mg at bedtime

Administration Administer before meals so that the drug's peak effect occurs at the proper time (peak inhibition of gastric acid secretion occurs at 1 and 3 hours after dosing in fasting subjects and approximately 2 hours in nonfasting subjects. This correlates well with the time food is no longer in the stomach offering a buffering effect).

Patient Information Take 30 minutes before meals and at bedtime. Maintain good oral hygiene habits, because lack of saliva may increase chance of cavities. Observe caution while driving or performing other tasks requiring alertness, as may cause drowsiness, dizziness, or blurred vision. Notify physician if skin rash, flushing, or eye pain occurs; or if difficulty in urinating, constipation, or sensitivity to light becomes severe or persists.

Dosage Forms Tablet, as bromide: 7.5 mg, 15 mg

Propantheline Bromide *see* Propantheline *on previous page*

Proparacaine (proe PAR a kane)

Brand Names AK-Taine®; Alcaine®; I-Paracaine®; Ophthaine®; Ophthetic®

Canadian/Mexican Brand Names Diocaine

Synonyms Proparacaine Hydrochloride; Proxymetacaine

Therapeutic Category Local Anesthetic, Ophthalmic

Use Anesthesia for tonometry, gonioscopy; suture removal from cornea; removal of corneal foreign body; cataract extraction, glaucoma surgery; short operative procedure involving the cornea and conjunctiva

Pregnancy Risk Factor C

Contraindications Known hypersensitivity to proparacaine

Warnings/Precautions Use with caution in patients with cardiac disease, hyperthyroidism; for typical ophthalmic use only; prolonged use not recommended

Adverse Reactions

1% to 10%: Local: Burning, stinging, redness

<1%:

Cardiovascular: Arrhythmias

Central nervous system: CNS depression

Dermatologic: Allergic contact dermatitis, irritation, sensitization

Ocular: Lacrimation, keratitis, iritis, erosion of the corneal epithelium, conjunctival congestion and hemorrhage, corneal opacification, blurred vision

Miscellaneous: Diaphoresis (increased)

Drug Interactions Increased effect of phenylephrine, tropicamide

Stability Store in tight, light-resistant containers

Mechanism of Action Prevents initiation and transmission of impulse at the nerve cell membrane by decreasing ion permeability through stabilizing

Pharmacodynamics/Kinetics

Onset of action: Within 20 seconds of instillation

Duration: 15-20 minutes

Usual Dosage Children and Adults:

Ophthalmic surgery: Instill 1 drop of 0.5% solution in eye every 5-10 minutes for 5-7 doses

Tonometry, gonioscopy, suture removal: Instill 1-2 drops of 0.5% solution in eye just prior to procedure

Patient Information May slow wound healing; use sparingly, avoid touching or rubbing the eye until anesthesia has worn off

Nursing Implications Do not use if discolored; protect eye from irritating chemicals, foreign bodies, and blink reflex; use eye patch if necessary

Dosage Forms Ophthalmic, solution, as hydrochloride: 0.5% (2 mL, 15 mL)

Proparacaine and Fluorescein (proe PAR a kane & FLURE e seen)

Brand Names Fluoracaine® Ophthalmic

Therapeutic Category Diagnostic Agent, Ophthalmic Dye; Local Anesthetic, Ester Derivative (Ophthalmic); Local Anesthetic, Ophthalmic

Use Anesthesia for tonometry, gonioscopy; suture removal from cornea; removal of corneal foreign body; cataract extraction, glaucoma surgery

Pregnancy Risk Factor C

Contraindications Known hypersensitivity to proparacaine or fluorescein or any component or ester-type local anesthetics

Warnings/Precautions Use with caution in patients with cardiac disease, hyperthyroidism; for topical ophthalmic use only; prolonged use not recommended

Adverse Reactions

1% to 10%: Local: Burning, stinging of eye

<1%:

Dermatologic: Allergic contact dermatitis

Local: Irritation, sensitization, erosion of the corneal epithelium, conjunctival congestion and hemorrhage

Ocular: Keratitis, iritis, corneal opacification

Stability Store in tight, light-resistant containers

Mechanism of Action Prevents initiation and transmission of impulse at the nerve cell membrane by decreasing ion permeability through stabilizing

Pharmacodynamics/Kinetics

Onset of action: Within 20 seconds of instillation

Duration: 15-20 minutes

Usual Dosage

Ophthalmic surgery: Children and Adults: Instill 1 drop in each eye every 5-10 minutes for 5-7 doses

Tonometry, gonioscopy, suture removal: Adults: Instill 1-2 drops in each eye just prior to procedure

Patient Information May slow wound healing; use sparingly, avoid touching or rubbing the eye until anesthesia has worn off

Nursing Implications Do not use if discolored; protect eye from irritating chemicals, foreign bodies, and blink reflex; use eye patch if necessary

Dosage Forms Solution: Proparacaine hydrochloride 0.5% and fluorescein sodium 0.25% (2 mL, 5 mL)

Proparacaine Hydrochloride *see* Proparacaine *on previous page*

Prophylaxis for Patients Exposed to Common Communicable Diseases *see page 1452*

Propine® Ophthalmic *see* Dipivefrin *on page 406*

Proplex® SX-T *see* Factor IX Complex (Human) *on page 502*

Proplex® T *see* Factor IX Complex (Human) *on page 502*

Propofol (PROE po fole)

Brand Names Diprivan®

Therapeutic Category General Anesthetic; Sedative

Use Induction or maintenance of anesthesia for inpatient or outpatient surgery; may be used (for patients >18 years of age who are intubated and mechanically ventilated) as an alternative to benzodiazepines for the treatment of agitation in the intensive care unit; pain should be treated with analgesic agents, propofol must be titrated separately from the analgesic agent; has demonstrated antiemetic properties in the postoperative setting

Pregnancy Risk Factor B

Contraindications

Absolute contraindications:

Patients with a hypersensitivity to propofol

Patients with a hypersensitivity to propofol's emulsion which contains soybean oil, egg phosphatide, and glycerol or any of the components

Patients who are not intubated or mechanically ventilated

Patients who are pregnant or nursing: Propofol is not recommended for obstetrics, including cesarian section deliveries. Propofol crosses the placenta and, therefore, may be associated with neonatal depression.

Relative contraindications:

Pediatric Intensive Care Unit patients: Safety and efficacy of propofol is not established

Patients with severe cardiac disease (ejection fraction <50%) or respiratory disease - propofol may have more profound adverse cardiovascular responses

Patients with a history of epilepsy or seizures

Patients with increased intracranial pressure or impaired cerebral circulation - substantial decreases in mean arterial pressure and subsequent decreases in cerebral perfusion pressure may occur

Patients with hyperlipidemia as evidenced by increased serum triglyceride levels or serum turbidity

Patients who are hypotensive, hypovolemic, or hemodynamically unstable

Warnings/Precautions Use slower rate of induction in the elderly; transient local pain may occur during I.V. injection; perioperative myoclonia has occurred; do

(Continued)

Propofol *(Continued)*

not administer with blood or blood products through the same I.V. catheter; not for obstetrics, including cesarean section deliveries. Safety and effectiveness has not been established in children. Abrupt discontinuation prior to weaning or daily wake up assessments should be avoided. Abrupt discontinuation can result in rapid awakening, anxiety, agitation, and resistance to mechanical ventilation. Use slower rate of induction in the elderly; transient local pain may occur during I.V. injection; perioperative myoclonia has occurred; not for use in neurosurgical anesthesia.

Adverse Reactions

>10%:

Cardiovascular: Hypotension, intravenous propofol produces a dose-related degree of hypotension and decrease in systemic vascular resistance which is not associated with a significant increase in heart rate or decrease in cardiac output

Local: Pain at injection site occurs at an incidence of 28.5% when administered into smaller veins of hand versus 6% when administered into antecubital veins

Respiratory: Apnea (incidence occurs in 50% to 84% of patients and may be dependent on premedication, speed of administration, dose and presence of hyperventilation and hyperoxia)

1% to 10%:

Anaphylaxis: Several cases of anaphylactic reactions have been reported with propofol

Central nervous system: Dizziness, fever, headache; although propofol has demonstrated anticonvulsant activity, several cases of propofol-induced seizures with opisthotonos have occurred

Gastrointestinal: Nausea, vomiting, abdominal cramps

Respiratory: Cough, apnea

Neuromuscular & skeletal: Twitching

Miscellaneous: Hiccups

Overdosage/Toxicology Symptoms of overdose include hypotension, bradycardia, cardiovascular collapse

Treatment is symptomatic and supportive; hypotension usually responds to I.V. fluids and/or Trendelenburg positioning; parenteral inotropes may be needed

Drug Interactions

Increased toxicity:

Neuromuscular blockers:

Atracurium: Anaphylactoid reactions (including bronchospasm) have been reported in patients who have received concomitant atracurium and propofol

Vecuronium: Propofol may potentiate the neuromuscular blockade of vecuronium

Central nervous system depressants: Additive CNS depression and respiratory depression may necessitate dosage reduction when used with: Anesthetics, benzodiazepines, opiates, ethanol, narcotics, phenothiazines

Decreased effect: Theophylline: May antagonize the effect of propofol, requiring dosage increases

Stability

Do not use if there is evidence of separation of phases of emulsion

Store at room temperature 4°C to 22°C (40°F to 72°F), refrigeration is not recommended; protect from light

Propofol may be further diluted in dextrose 5% in water to a concentration ≥2 mg/mL and is stable for 8 hours at room temperature

Y-site **compatible** with D_5LR, D_5NS, D_5W, LR, lidocaine

Soybean fat emulsion is used as a vehicle for propofol. This soybean fat emulsion contains no preservatives. **Strict aseptic technique must be maintained in handling because this vehicle is capable of supporting rapid bacterial growth.**

Mechanism of Action Propofol is a hindered phenolic compound with intravenous general anesthetic properties. The drug is unrelated to any of the currently used barbiturate, opioid, benzodiazepine, arylcyclohexylamine, or imidazole intravenous anesthetic agents.

Pharmacodynamics/Kinetics

Onset of anesthesia: Within 9-51 seconds (average 30 seconds) after bolus infusion (dose dependent)

Duration: 3-10 minutes depending on the dose and the rate of administration

Distribution: V_d: 2-6 mcg/mL during anesthesia; 1-2 mcg/mL upon awakening; large volume of distribution; highly lipophilic

Protein binding: 97% to 99%

Half-life, elimination (biphasic):

Initial: 40 minutes

Terminal: 1-3 days

Metabolism: In the liver to water-soluble sulfate and glucuronide conjugates; total body clearance exceeds liver blood flow

Elimination: ~88% of a propofol dose is recovered in the urine as metabolites (40% as glucuronide metabolite) and <2% of a propofol dose is excreted in the feces

Usual Dosage Dosage must be individualized based on total body weight and titrated to the desired clinical effect; however, as a general guideline:

No pediatric dose has been established; however, induction for children 1-12 years 2-2.8 mg/kg has been used

Induction: I.V.:

Adults ≤55 years, and/or ASA I or II patients: 2-2.5 mg/kg of body weight (approximately 40 mg every 10 seconds until onset of induction)

Elderly, debilitated, hypovolemic, and/or ASA III or IV patients: 1-1.5 mg/kg of body weight (approximately 20 mg every 10 seconds until onset of induction)

Maintenance: I.V. infusion:

Adults ≤55 years, and/or ASA I or II patients: 0.1-0.2 mg/kg of body weight/minute (6-12 mg/kg of body weight/hour)

Elderly, debilitated, hypovolemic, and/or ASA III or IV patients: 0.05-0.1 mg/kg of body weight/minute (3-6 mg/kg of body weight/hour)

I.V. intermittent: 25-50 mg increments, as needed

ICU sedation: Rapid bolus injection should be avoided. Bolus injection can result in hypotension, oxyhemoglobin desaturation, apnea, airway obstruction, and oxygen desaturation. The preferred route of administration is slow infusion. Doses are based on individual need and titrated to response.

Recommended starting dose: 1-3 mg/kg/hour

Adjustments in dose can occur at 3- to 5-minute intervals. An 80% reduction in dose should be considered in elderly, debilitated, and ASA II or IV patients. Once sedation is established, the dose should be decreased for the maintenance infusion period and adjusted to response. The dose required for maintenance is 1.5-4.5 mg/kg/hour or 25-75 mcg/kg/minute. An alternative, but less preferred method of administration is intermittent slow I.V. bolus injection of 10-20 mg, administered over 3-5 minutes.

Monitoring Parameters Cardiac monitor, blood pressure monitor, and ventilator required; serum triglyceride levels should be obtained prior to initiation of therapy (ICU setting) and every 3-7 days, thereafter

Vital signs: Blood pressure, heart rate, cardiac output, pulmonary capillary wedge pressure should be monitored

Test Interactions ↓ cholesterol (S); ↑ porphyrin (U); ↓ cortisol (S), but does not appear to inhibit adrenal responsiveness to ACTH

Nursing Implications **Changes urine color to green**; abrupt discontinuation of infusion may result in rapid awakening of the patient associated with anxiety, agitation, and resistance to mechanical ventilation, making weaning from mechanical ventilation difficult; use a light level of sedation throughout the weaning process until 10-15 minutes before extubation; titrate the infusion rate so the patient awakens slowly. Tubing and any unused portions of propofol vials should be discarded after 12 hours.

Dosage Forms Injection: 10 mg/mL (20 mL, 50 mL, 100 mL)

Propoxyphene (proe POKS i feen)

Related Information

Narcotic Agonists Comparison *on page 1414*

Brand Names Darvon®; Darvon-N®; Dolene®

Canadian/Mexican Brand Names Novo-Propoxyn® (Canada); 624® Tablets (Canada)

Synonyms Dextropropoxyphene; Propoxyphene Hydrochloride; Propoxyphene Napsylate

Therapeutic Category Analgesic, Narcotic

Use Management of mild to moderate pain

Restrictions C-IV

Pregnancy Risk Factor C (D if used for prolonged periods)

Contraindications Hypersensitivity to propoxyphene or any component

Warnings/Precautions Administer with caution in patients dependent on opiates, substitution may result in acute opiate withdrawal symptoms, use with caution in patients with severe renal or hepatic dysfunction; when given in excessive doses, either alone or in combination with other CNS depressants or propoxyphene products, propoxyphene is a major cause of drug-related deaths; **do not exceed recommended dosage**

Adverse Reactions

Hepatic: Increased liver enzymes

(Continued)

Propoxyphene *(Continued)*

>10%:
- Cardiovascular: Hypotension
- Central nervous system: Dizziness, lightheadedness, sedation, paradoxical excitement and insomnia, fatigue, drowsiness
- Gastrointestinal: Nausea, vomiting, constipation
- Neuromuscular & skeletal: Weakness
- Miscellaneous: Histamine release

1% to 10%:
- Central nervous system: Nervousness, headache, restlessness, malaise, confusion
- Gastrointestinal: Anorexia, stomach cramps, xerostomia, biliary spasm
- Genitourinary: Decreased urination, ureteral spasms
- Respiratory: Dyspnea, shortness of breath

<1%:
- Central nervous system: Mental depression hallucinations, paradoxical CNS stimulation, increased intracranial pressure
- Dermatologic: Rash, urticaria
- Gastrointestinal: Paralytic ileus
- Miscellaneous: Psychologic and physical dependence with prolonged use, histamine release

Overdosage/Toxicology Symptoms of overdose include CNS, respiratory depression, hypotension, pulmonary edema, seizures

Treatment of an overdose includes support of the patient's airway; establishment of an I.V. line and administration of naloxone 2 mg I.V. (0.01 mg/kg for children) with repeat administration as necessary up to a total of 10 mg; emesis is not indicated as overdose may cause seizures; charcoal is very effective (>95%) at binding propoxyphene

Drug Interactions

Decreased effect with charcoal, cigarette smoking

Increased toxicity: CNS depressants may potentiate pharmacologic effects; propoxyphene may inhibit the metabolism and increase the serum concentrations of carbamazepine, phenobarbital, MAO inhibitors, tricyclic antidepressants, and warfarin

Mechanism of Action Binds to opiate receptors in the CNS, causing inhibition of ascending pain pathways, altering the perception of and response to pain; produces generalized CNS depression

Pharmacodynamics/Kinetics

Onset of effect: Oral: Within 0.5-1 hour

Duration: 4-6 hours

Metabolism: First-pass effect; metabolized in the liver to an active metabolite (norpropoxyphene) and inactive metabolites

Bioavailability: Oral: 30% to 70%

Half-life: Adults:
- Parent drug: 8-24 hours (mean: ~15 hours)
- Norpropoxyphene: 34 hours

Elimination: 20% to 25% excreted in urine

Usual Dosage Oral:

Children: Doses for children are not well established; doses of the hydrochloride of 2-3 mg/kg/d divided every 6 hours have been used

Adults:
- Hydrochloride: 65 mg every 3-4 hours as needed for pain; maximum: 390 mg/day
- Napsylate: 100 mg every 4 hours as needed for pain; maximum: 600 mg/day

Dosing comments in renal impairment: Cl_{cr} <10 mL/minute: Avoid use

Hemodialysis: Not dialyzable (0% to 5%)

Dosing adjustment in hepatic impairment: Reduced doses should be used

Dietary Considerations

Alcohol: Additive CNS effects, avoid or limit alcohol; watch for sedation

Food: May decrease rate of absorption, but may slightly increase bioavailability
- Glucose may cause hyperglycemia; monitor blood glucose concentrations

Monitoring Parameters Pain relief, respiratory and mental status, blood pressure

Reference Range

Therapeutic: Ranges published vary between laboratories and may not correlate with clinical effect

Therapeutic concentration: 0.1-0.4 µg/mL (SI: 0.3-1.2 µmol/L)

Toxic: >0.5 µg/mL (SI: >1.5 µmol/L)

Test Interactions False-positive methadone test, ↓ glucose (S), ↑ LFTs, ↓ 17-OHCS (U)

Patient Information May cause drowsiness, dizziness, or blurring of vision; avoid alcohol and other sedatives; may take with food; can impair judgment and coordination

Additional Information 100 mg of napsylate = 65 mg of hydrochloride
Propoxyphene hydrochloride: Darvon®
Propoxyphene napsylate: Darvon-N®

Dosage Forms
Capsule, as hydrochloride: 65 mg
Tablet, as napsylate: 100 mg

Propoxyphene and Acetaminophen

(proe POKS i feen & a seet a MIN oh fen)

Brand Names Darvocet-N®; Darvocet-N® 100; Genagesic®; Propacet®; Wygesic®

Synonyms Propoxyphene Hydrochloride and Acetaminophen; Propoxyphene Napsylate and Acetaminophen

Therapeutic Category Analgesic, Narcotic

Use Management of mild to moderate pain

Restrictions C-IV

Usual Dosage Adults: Oral:
Darvocet-N®: 1-2 tablets every 4 hours as needed; maximum: 600 mg propoxyphene napsylate/day
Darvocet-N® 100: 1 tablet every 4 hours as needed; maximum: 600 mg propoxyphene napsylate/day

Monitoring Parameters Monitor pain relief, respiratory and mental status, blood pressure, excessive sedation

Dosage Forms Tablet:
Darvocet-N®: Propoxyphene napsylate 50 mg and acetaminophen 325 mg
Darvocet-N® 100: Propoxyphene napsylate 100 mg and acetaminophen 650 mg
Genagesic®, Wygesic®: Propoxyphene hydrochloride 65 mg and acetaminophen 650 mg

Propoxyphene Hydrochloride *see* Propoxyphene *on page 1065*

Propoxyphene Hydrochloride and Acetaminophen *see* Propoxyphene and Acetaminophen *on this page*

Propoxyphene Napsylate *see* Propoxyphene *on page 1065*

Propoxyphene Napsylate and Acetaminophen *see* Propoxyphene and Acetaminophen *on this page*

Propranolol (proe PRAN oh lole)

Related Information
Antiarrhythmic Drugs *on page 1389*
Beta-Blockers Comparison *on page 1398*
Comparative Pharmacokinetic Properties of Antiarrhythmic Agents *on page 1391*

Brand Names Betachron E-R®; Inderal®; Inderal® LA

Canadian/Mexican Brand Names Apo-Propranolol® (Canada); Detensol® (Canada); Nu-Propranolol® (Canada); PMS-Propranolol (Mexico); Inderalici® (Mexico)

Synonyms Propranolol Hydrochloride

Therapeutic Category Antianginal Agent; Antiarrhythmic Agent, Class II; Antihypertensive; Beta-Adrenergic Blocker

Use Management of hypertension, angina pectoris, pheochromocytoma, essential tremor, tetralogy of Fallot cyanotic spells, and arrhythmias (such as atrial fibrillation and flutter, A-V nodal re-entrant tachycardias, and catecholamine-induced arrhythmias); prevention of myocardial infarction, migraine headache; symptomatic treatment of hypertrophic subaortic stenosis

Unlabeled use: Tremor due to Parkinson's disease, alcohol withdrawal, aggressive behavior, antipsychotic-induced akathisia, esophageal varices bleeding, anxiety, schizophrenia, acute panic, and gastric bleeding in portal hypertension

Pregnancy Risk Factor C

Pregnancy/Breast-Feeding Implications
Clinical effects on the fetus: Crosses the placenta. IUGR, hypoglycemia, bradycardia, respiratory depression, hyper-bilirubinemia, polycythemia, polydactyly reported. IUGR probably related to maternal hypertension. Preterm labor has been reported. Available evidence suggests safe use during pregnancy and breast-feeding. Monitor breast-fed infant for symptoms of beta-blockade.
Breast-feeding/lactation: Crosses into breast milk. American Academy of Pediatrics considers COMPATIBLE with breast-feeding.

Contraindications Uncompensated congestive heart failure, cardiogenic shock, bradycardia or heart block, pulmonary edema, severe hyperactive airway disease or chronic obstructive lung disease, Raynaud's disease, hypersensitivity to beta-blockers

(Continued)

Propranolol *(Continued)*

Warnings/Precautions Safety and efficacy in children have not been established; administer very cautiously to patients with CHF, asthma, diabetes mellitus, hyperthyroidism. Abrupt withdrawal of the drug should be avoided, drug should be discontinued over 1-2 weeks; do not use in pregnant or nursing women; may potentiate hypoglycemia in a diabetic patient and mask signs and symptoms.

Adverse Reactions

>10%:

Cardiovascular: Bradycardia
Central nervous system: Mental depression
Endocrine & metabolic: Decreased sexual ability

1% to 10%:

Cardiovascular: Congestive heart failure, reduced peripheral circulation
Central nervous system: Confusion, hallucinations, dizziness, insomnia, fatigue
Dermatologic: Rash
Gastrointestinal: Diarrhea, nausea, vomiting, stomach discomfort
Neuromuscular & skeletal: Weakness
Respiratory: Wheezing

<1%:

Cardiovascular: Chest pain, hypotension, impaired myocardial contractility, worsening of A-V conduction disturbances
Central nervous system: Nightmares, vivid dreams, lethargy
Dermatologic: Red, scaling, or crusted skin
Endocrine & metabolic: Hypoglycemia, hyperglycemia
Gastrointestinal: GI distress
Hematologic: Leukopenia, thrombocytopenia, agranulocytosis
Respiratory: Bronchospasm
Miscellaneous: Cold extremities

Overdosage/Toxicology Symptoms of intoxication include cardiac disturbances, CNS toxicity, bronchospasm, hypoglycemia and hyperkalemia. The most common cardiac symptoms include hypotension and bradycardia; atrioventricular block, intraventricular conduction disturbances, cardiogenic shock, and systole may occur with severe overdose, especially with membrane-depressant drugs (eg, propranolol); CNS effects include convulsions, coma, and respiratory arrest is commonly seen with propranolol and other membrane-depressant and lipid-soluble drugs.

Treatment includes symptomatic treatment of seizures, hypotension, hyperkalemia and hypoglycemia; bradycardia and hypotension resistant to atropine, isoproterenol or pacing may respond to glucagon; wide QRS defects caused by the membrane-depressant poisoning may respond to hypertonic sodium bicarbonate; repeat-dose charcoal, hemoperfusion, or hemodialysis may be helpful in removal of only those beta-blockers with a small V_d, long half-life or low intrinsic clearance (acebutolol, atenolol, nadolol, sotalol)

Drug Interactions Cytochrome P-450 2D6 enzyme substrate and cytochrome P-450 2C enzyme substrate

Decreased effect:

Aluminum salts, barbiturates, calcium salts, cholestyramine, colestipol, NSAIDs, penicillins (ampicillin), rifampin, salicylates and sulfinpyrazone decrease effect of beta-blockers due to decreased bioavailability and plasma levels

Beta-blockers may decrease the effect of sulfonylureas

Ascorbic acid decreases propranolol Cp_{max} and AUC and increases the T_{max} significantly resulting in a greater decrease in the reduction of heart rate, possibly due to decreased absorption and first pass metabolism (n=5)

Nefazodone decreased peak plasma levels and AUC of propranolol and increases time to reach steady state; monitoring of clinical response is recommended

Increased effect:

Increased effect/toxicity of beta-blockers with calcium blockers (diltiazem, felodipine, nicardipine), contraceptives, flecainide, haloperidol (propranolol, hypotensive effects), H_2-antagonists (metoprolol, propranolol only by cimetidine, possibly ranitidine), hydralazine (metoprolol, propranolol), loop diuretics (propranolol, not atenolol), MAO inhibitors (metoprolol, nadolol, bradycardia), phenothiazines (propranolol), propafenone (metoprolol, propranolol), quinidine (in extensive metabolizers), ciprofloxacin, thyroid hormones (metoprolol, propranolol, when hypothyroid patient is converted to euthyroid state)

Beta-blockers may increase the effect/toxicity of flecainide, haloperidol (hypotensive effects), hydralazine, phenothiazines, acetaminophen, anticoagulants (propranolol, warfarin), benzodiazepines (not atenolol), clonidine (hypertensive crisis after or during withdrawal of either agent), epinephrine (initial hypertensive episode followed by bradycardia), nifedipine and verapamil lidocaine, ergots (peripheral ischemia), prazosin (postural hypotension)

Beta-blockers may affect the action or levels of ethanol, disopyramide, nondepolarizing muscle relaxants and theophylline although the effects are difficult to predict

Stability Compatible in saline, **incompatible** with HCO_3^-; protect injection from light; solutions have maximum stability at pH of 3 and decompose rapidly in alkaline pH; propranolol is stable for 24 hours at room temperature in D_5W or NS

Mechanism of Action Nonselective beta-adrenergic blocker (class II antiarrhythmic); competitively blocks response to $beta_1$- and $beta_2$-adrenergic stimulation which results in decreases in heart rate, myocardial contractility, blood pressure, and myocardial oxygen demand

Pharmacodynamics/Kinetics

Onset of beta-blockade: Oral: Within 1-2 hours

Duration: ~6 hours

Distribution: V_d: 3.9 L/kg in adults; crosses the placenta; small amounts appear in breast milk

Protein binding:

- Newborns: 68%
- Adults: 93%

Metabolism: Extensive first-pass effect; metabolized in the liver to active and inactive compounds

Bioavailability: 30% to 40%; oral bioavailability may be increased in Down syndrome children

Half-life:

- Neonates and Infants: Possible increased half-life
- Children: 3.9-6.4 hours
- Adults: 4-6 hours

Elimination: Primarily in urine (96% to 99%)

Usual Dosage

Tachyarrhythmias:

Oral:

- Children: Initial: 0.5-1 mg/kg/day in divided doses every 6-8 hours; titrate dosage upward every 3-7 days; usual dose: 2-4 mg/kg/day; higher doses may be needed; do not exceed 16 mg/kg/day or 60 mg/day
- Adults: 10-30 mg/dose every 6-8 hours
- Elderly: Initial: 10 mg twice daily; increase dosage every 3-7 days; usual dosage range: 10-320 mg given in 2 divided doses

I.V.:

- Children: 0.01-0.1 mg/kg slow IVP over 10 minutes; maximum dose: 1 mg
- Adults: 1 mg/dose slow IVP; repeat every 5 minutes up to a total of 5 mg

Hypertension: Oral:

- Children: Initial: 0.5-1 mg/kg/day in divided doses every 6-12 hours; increase gradually every 3-7 days; maximum: 2 mg/kg/24 hours
- Adults: Initial: 40 mg twice daily; increase dosage every 3-7 days; usual dose: ≤320 mg divided in 2-3 doses/day; maximum daily dose: 640 mg

Migraine headache prophylaxis: Oral:

- Children: 0.6-1.5 mg/kg/day **or**
  - ≤35 kg: 10-20 mg 3 times/day
  - >35 kg: 20-40 mg 3 times/day
- Adults: Initial: 80 mg/day divided every 6-8 hours; increase by 20-40 mg/dose every 3-4 weeks to a maximum of 160-240 mg/day given in divided doses every 6-8 hours; if satisfactory response not achieved within 6 weeks of starting therapy, drug should be withdrawn gradually over several weeks

Tetralogy spells: Children:

- Oral: 1-2 mg/kg/day every 6 hours as needed, may increase by 1 mg/kg/day to a maximum of 5 mg/kg/day, or if refractory may increase slowly to a maximum of 10-15 mg/kg/day
- I.V.: 0.15-0.25 mg/kg/dose slow IVP; may repeat in 15 minutes

Thyrotoxicosis:

- Adolescents and Adults: Oral: 10-40 mg/dose every 6 hours
- Adults: I.V.: 1-3 mg/dose slow IVP as a single dose

Adults: Oral:

- Angina: 80-320 mg/day in doses divided 2-4 times/day
- Pheochromocytoma: 30-60 mg/day in divided doses
- Myocardial infarction prophylaxis: 180-240 mg/day in 3-4 divided doses
- Hypertrophic subaortic stenosis: 20-40 mg 3-4 times/day
- Essential tremor: 40 mg twice daily initially; maintenance doses: usually 120-320 mg/day

Dosing adjustment in renal impairment:

Cl_{cr} 31-40 mL/minute: Administer every 24-36 hours or administer 50% of normal dose

(Continued)

Propranolol *(Continued)*

Cl_{cr} 10-30 mL/minute: Administer every 24-48 hours or administer 50% of normal dose

Cl_{cr} <10 mL/minute: Administer every 40-60 hours or administer 25% of normal dose

Hemodialysis: Not dialyzable (0% to 5%); supplemental dose is not necessary

Peritoneal dialysis: Supplemental dose is not necessary

Dosing adjustment/comments in hepatic disease: Marked slowing of heart rate may occur in cirrhosis with conventional doses; low initial dose and regular heart rate monitoring

Administration I.V. administration should not exceed 1 mg/minute; I.V. dose much smaller than oral dose

Monitoring Parameters Blood pressure, EKG, heart rate, CNS and cardiac effects

Reference Range Therapeutic: 50-100 ng/mL (SI: 190-390 nmol/L) at end of dose interval

Test Interactions $\uparrow$ thyroxine (S)

Patient Information Do not discontinue abruptly; notify physician if CHF symptoms become worse or side effects develop; take at the same time each day; may mask diabetes symptoms; consult pharmacist or physician before taking with other adrenergic drugs (eg, cold medications); use with caution while driving or performing tasks requiring alertness

Nursing Implications Patient's therapeutic response may be evaluated by looking at blood pressure, apical and radial pulses, fluid I & O, daily weight, respirations, and circulation in extremities before and during therapy

Dosage Forms

Capsule, as hydrochloride, sustained action: 60 mg, 80 mg, 120 mg, 160 mg

Injection, as hydrochloride: 1 mg/mL (1 mL)

Solution, oral, as hydrochloride (strawberry-mint flavor): 4 mg/mL (5 mL, 500 mL); 8 mg/mL (5 mL, 500 mL)

Solution, oral, concentrate, as hydrochloride: 80 mg/mL (30 mL)

Tablet, as hydrochloride: 10 mg, 20 mg, 40 mg, 60 mg, 80 mg, 90 mg

Propranolol Hydrochloride *see* Propranolol *on page 1067*

Propulsid® *see* Cisapride *on page 280*

2-Propylpentanoic Acid *see* Valproic Acid and Derivatives *on page 1285*

Propylthiouracil (proe pil thye oh YOOR a sil)

Canadian/Mexican Brand Names Propyl-Thyracil® (Canada)

Synonyms PTU

Therapeutic Category Antithyroid Agent

Use Palliative treatment of hyperthyroidism as an adjunct to ameliorate hyperthyroidism in preparation for surgical treatment or radioactive iodine therapy and in the management of thyrotoxic crisis. The use of antithyroid thioamides is as effective in elderly as they are in younger adults; however, the expense, potential adverse effects, and inconvenience (compliance, monitoring) make them undesirable. The use of radioiodine, due to ease of administration and less concern for long-term side effects and reproduction problems, makes it a more appropriate therapy.

Pregnancy Risk Factor D

Contraindications Hypersensitivity to propylthiouracil or any component

Warnings/Precautions Use with caution in patients >40 years of age because PTU may cause hypoprothrombinemia and bleeding, use with extreme caution in patients receiving other drugs known to cause agranulocytosis; may cause agranulocytosis, thyroid hyperplasia, thyroid carcinoma (usage >1 year)

Adverse Reactions

>10%:

- Central nervous system: Fever
- Dermatologic: Skin rash
- Hematologic: Leukopenia

1% to 10%:

- Central nervous system: Dizziness
- Gastrointestinal: Nausea, vomiting, loss of taste perception, stomach pain
- Hematologic: Agranulocytosis
- Miscellaneous: SLE-like syndrome

<1%:

- Cardiovascular: Edema, cutaneous vasculitis
- Central nervous system: Drowsiness, vertigo, headache, drug fever
- Dermatologic: Rash, urticaria, pruritus, exfoliative dermatitis, alopecia
- Endocrine & metabolic: Goiter
- Gastrointestinal: Constipation, weight gain, swollen salivary glands
- Hematologic: Agranulocytosis, thrombocytopenia, bleeding, aplastic anemia

Hepatic: Cholestatic jaundice, hepatitis
Neuromuscular & skeletal: Arthralgia, paresthesia, neuritis
Renal: Nephritis

Overdosage/Toxicology Symptoms of overdose include nausea, vomiting, epigastric pain, headache, fever, arthralgia, pruritus, edema, pancytopenia, epigastric distress, headache, fever, CNS stimulation or depression

Treatment is supportive; monitor bone marrow response, forced diuresis, peritoneal and hemodialysis, as well as charcoal hemoperfusion

Drug Interactions Increased effect: Increases anticoagulant activity

Mechanism of Action Inhibits the synthesis of thyroid hormones by blocking the oxidation of iodine in the thyroid gland; blocks synthesis of thyroxine and triiodothyronine

Pharmacodynamics/Kinetics

Onset of action: For significant therapeutic effects 24-36 hours are required
Peak effect: Remissions of hyperthyroidism do not usually occur before 4 months of continued therapy
Protein binding: 75% to 80%
Metabolism: Hepatic
Half-life: 1.5-5 hours
End stage renal disease: 8.5 hours
Time to peak serum concentration: Oral: Within 1 hour; persists for 2-3 hours
Elimination: 35% excreted in urine

Usual Dosage Oral: Administer in 3 equally divided doses at approximately 8-hour intervals. Adjust dosage to maintain T_3, T_4, and TSH levels in normal range; elevated T_3 may be sole indicator of inadequate treatment. Elevated TSH indicates excessive antithyroid treatment.

Children: Initial: 5-7 mg/kg/day in divided doses every 8 hours
or
6-10 years: 50-150 mg/day
>10 years: 150-300 mg/day
Maintenance: $^1/_3$ to $^2/_3$ of the initial dose in divided doses every 8-12 hours. This usually begins after 2 months on an effective initial dose.

Adults: Initial: 300-450 mg/day in divided doses every 8 hours (severe hyperthyroidism may require 600-1200 mg/day); maintenance: 100-150 mg/day in divided doses every 8-12 hours

Elderly: Use lower dose recommendations; initial dose: 150-300 mg/day

Dosing adjustment in renal impairment:
Cl_{cr} 10-50 mL/minute: Administer at 75% of normal dose
Cl_{cr} <10 mL/minute: Administer at 50% of normal dose

Monitoring Parameters CBC with differential, prothrombin time, liver function tests, thyroid function tests (TSH, T_3, T_4); periodic blood counts are recommended chronic therapy

Reference Range See table.

Laboratory Ranges

	Normal Values
Total T_4	5-12 μg/dL
Serum T_3	90-185 ng/dL
Free thyroxine index (FT_4I)	6-10.5
TSH	0.5-4.0 μIU/mL

Patient Information Do not exceed prescribed dosage; take at regular intervals around-the-clock; notify physician or pharmacist if fever, sore throat, unusual bleeding or bruising, headache, or general malaise occurs

Additional Information The use of antithyroid thioamides is as effective in elderly as in younger adults; however, the expense, potential adverse effects, and inconvenience (compliance, monitoring) make them undesirable. The use of radioiodine, due to ease of administration and less concern for long-term side effects and reproduction problems, makes it a more appropriate therapy.

Dosage Forms Tablet: 50 mg

2-Propylvaleric Acid *see* Valproic Acid and Derivatives *on page 1285*
Prorex® *see* Promethazine *on page 1058*
Proscar® *see* Finasteride *on page 520*
ProSom™ *see* Estazolam *on page 467*
Prostacyclin *see* Epoprostenol *on page 454*
Prostaglandin E_1 *see* Alprostadil *on page 51*
Prostaglandin E_2 *see* Dinoprostone *on page 397*
Prostaphlin® *see* Oxacillin *on page 931*

ProStep® Patch *see* Nicotine *on page 900*

Prostigmin® *see* Neostigmine *on page 891*

Prostin/15M® *see* Carboprost Tromethamine *on page 208*

Prostin E_2® Vaginal Suppository *see* Dinoprostone *on page 397*

Prostin VR Pediatric® Injection *see* Alprostadil *on page 51*

Protamine Sulfate (PROE ta meen SUL fate)

Therapeutic Category Antidote, Heparin

Use Treatment of heparin overdosage; neutralize heparin during surgery or dialysis procedures

Pregnancy Risk Factor C

Contraindications Hypersensitivity to protamine or any component

Warnings/Precautions May not be totally effective in some patients following cardiac surgery despite adequate doses; may cause hypersensitivity reaction in patients with a history of allergy to fish (have epinephrine 1:1000 available) and in patients sensitized to protamine (via protamine zinc insulin); too rapid administration can cause severe hypotensive and anaphylactoid-like reactions. Heparin rebound associated with anticoagulation and bleeding has been reported to occur occasionally; symptoms typically occur 8-9 hours after protamine administration, but may occur as long as 18 hours later.

Adverse Reactions

>10%:

Cardiovascular: Sudden fall in blood pressure, bradycardia

Respiratory: Dyspnea

1% to 10%: Hemorrhage

<1%:

Cardiovascular: Hypotension, flushing

Central nervous system: Lassitude

Gastrointestinal: Nausea, vomiting

Respiratory: Pulmonary hypertension

Miscellaneous: Hypersensitivity reactions

Overdosage/Toxicology Symptoms of overdose include hypertension; may cause hemorrhage; doses exceeding 100 mg may cause paradox anticoagulation

Stability Refrigerate, avoid freezing; remains stable for at least 2 weeks at room temperature; **incompatible** with cephalosporins and penicillins

Mechanism of Action Combines with strongly acidic heparin to form a stable complex (salt) neutralizing the anticoagulant activity of both drugs

Pharmacodynamics/Kinetics Onset of effect: I.V. injection: Heparin neutralization occurs within 5 minutes

Usual Dosage Protamine dosage is determined by the dosage of heparin; 1 mg of protamine neutralizes 90 USP units of heparin (lung) and 115 USP units of heparin (intestinal); maximum dose: 50 mg

In the situation of heparin overdosage, since blood heparin concentrations decrease rapidly **after** administration, adjust the protamine dosage depending upon the duration of time since heparin administration as follows:

Time Elapsed	Dose of Protamine (mg) to Neutralize 100 units of Heparin
Immediate	1-1.5
30-60 min	0.5-0.75
>2 h	0.25-0.375

If heparin administered by deep S.C. injection, use 1-1.5 mg protamine per 100 units heparin; this may be done by a portion of the dose (eg, 25-50 mg) given slowly I.V. followed by the remaining portion as a continuous infusion over 8-16 hours (the expected absorption time of the S.C. heparin dose)

Administration For I.V. use only; incompatible with cephalosporins and penicillins; administer slow IVP (50 mg over 10 minutes); rapid I.V. infusion causes hypotension; reconstitute vial with 5 mL sterile water; if using protamine in neonates, reconstitute with preservative-free sterile water for injection; resulting solution equals 10 mg/mL; inject without further dilution over 1-3 minutes; maximum of 50 mg in any 10-minute period

Monitoring Parameters Coagulation test, APTT or ACT, cardiac monitor and blood pressure monitor required during administration

Dosage Forms Injection: 10 mg/mL (5 mL, 10 mL, 25 mL)

Protilase® *see* Pancrelipase *on page 949*

Protopam® *see* Pralidoxime *on page 1032*

Protostat® *see* Metronidazole *on page 829*

Protriptyline (proe TRIP ti leen)

Related Information

Antidepressant Agents Comparison *on page 1393*

Brand Names Vivactil®

Canadian/Mexican Brand Names Triptil® (Canada)

Synonyms Protriptyline Hydrochloride

Therapeutic Category Antidepressant, Tricyclic

Use Treatment of various forms of depression, often in conjunction with psychotherapy

Pregnancy Risk Factor C

Contraindications Narrow-angle glaucoma, hypersensitivity to protriptyline or any component

Warnings/Precautions Use with caution in patients with cardiac conduction disturbances, history of hyperthyroid, seizure disorders, or decreased renal function; safe use of tricyclic antidepressants in children <12 years of age has not been established; protriptyline should not be abruptly discontinued in patients receiving high doses for prolonged periods

Adverse Reactions

>10%:

- Central nervous system: Dizziness, drowsiness, headache
- Gastrointestinal: Xerostomia, constipation, unpleasant taste, weight gain, increased appetite, nausea
- Neuromuscular & skeletal: Weakness

1% to 10%:

- Cardiovascular: Arrhythmias, hypotension
- Central nervous system: Confusion, delirium, hallucinations, nervousness, restlessness, parkinsonian syndrome, insomnia
- Gastrointestinal: Diarrhea, heartburn
- Genitourinary: Dysuria, sexual dysfunction
- Neuromuscular & skeletal: Fine muscle tremors
- Ocular: Blurred vision, eye pain
- Miscellaneous: Diaphoresis (excessive)

<1%:

- Central nervous system: Anxiety, seizures
- Dermatologic: Alopecia, photosensitivity
- Endocrine & metabolic: Breast enlargement, galactorrhea, SIADH
- Gastrointestinal: Trouble with gums, decreased lower esophageal sphincter tone may cause GE reflux
- Genitourinary: Testicular edema
- Hematologic: Agranulocytosis, leukopenia, eosinophilia
- Hepatic: Cholestatic jaundice, increased liver enzymes
- Ocular: Increased intraocular pressure
- Otic: Tinnitus
- Miscellaneous: Allergic reactions

Overdosage/Toxicology Symptoms of overdose include confusion, hallucinations, urinary retention, hypotension, tachycardia, seizures, hyperthermia

Following initiation of essential overdose management, toxic symptoms should be treated. Sodium bicarbonate is indicated when QRS interval is >0.10 seconds or QT_c >0.42 seconds. Ventricular arrhythmias often respond to systemic alkalinization (sodium bicarbonate 0.5-2 mEq/kg I.V.). Arrhythmias unresponsive to this therapy may respond to lidocaine 1 mg/kg I.V. followed by a titrated infusion. Physostigmine (1-2 mg I.V. slowly for adults or 0.5 mg I.V. slowly for children) may be indicated in reversing cardiac arrhythmias that are life-threatening.

Seizures usually respond to diazepam I.V. boluses (5-10 mg for adults up to 30 mg or 0.25-0.4 mg/kg/dose for children up to 10 mg/dose). If seizures are unresponsive or recur, phenytoin or phenobarbital may be required.

Drug Interactions

- Decreased effect of guanethidine; decreased effect with barbiturates, carbamazepine, phenytoin
- Increased toxicity of alcohol, MAO inhibitors, sympathomimetics, CNS depressants, anticholinergics (paralytic ileus and hyperpyrexia); increased toxicity with MAO inhibitors (hyperpyretic crisis, convulsions, and death), cimetidine (increased drug levels)

Mechanism of Action Increases the synaptic concentration of serotonin and/or norepinephrine in the central nervous system by inhibition of their reuptake by the presynaptic neuronal membrane

Pharmacodynamics/Kinetics

- Maximum antidepressant effect: 2 weeks of continuous therapy is commonly required
- Distribution: Crosses the placenta
- Protein binding: 92%

(Continued)

Protriptyline *(Continued)*

Metabolism: Undergoes first-pass metabolism (10% to 25%); extensively metabolized in the liver by N-oxidation, hydroxylation and glucuronidation
Half-life: 54-92 hours, averaging 74 hours
Time to peak serum concentration: Oral: Within 24-30 hours
Elimination: In urine

Usual Dosage Oral:
Adolescents: 15-20 mg/day
Adults: 15-60 mg in 3-4 divided doses
Elderly: 15-20 mg/day

Reference Range Therapeutic: 70-250 ng/mL (SI: 266-950 nmol/L); Toxic: >500 ng/mL (SI: >1900 nmol/L)

Test Interactions ↑ glucose

Patient Information Avoid unnecessary exposure to sunlight; do not discontinue abruptly; take dose in morning to avoid insomnia

Nursing Implications Offer patient sugarless hard candy or gum for dry mouth

Dosage Forms Tablet, as hydrochloride: 5 mg, 10 mg

Protriptyline Hydrochloride *see* Protriptyline *on previous page*

Protropin® Injection *see* Human Growth Hormone *on page 613*

Provatene® [OTC] *see* Beta-Carotene *on page 147*

Proventil® *see* Albuterol *on page 38*

Proventil® HFA *see* Albuterol *on page 38*

Provera® *see* Medroxyprogesterone Acetate *on page 771*

Provocholine® *see* Methacholine *on page 797*

Proxigel® Oral [OTC] *see* Carbamide Peroxide *on page 203*

Proxymetacaine *see* Proparacaine *on page 1062*

Prozac® *see* Fluoxetine *on page 541*

PRP-D *see* *Haemophilus* b Conjugate Vaccine *on page 595*

Prymaccone *see* Primaquine Phosphate *on page 1042*

Pseudoephedrine (soo doe e FED rin)

Brand Names Actifed® Allergy Tablet (Day) [OTC]; Afrin® Tablet [OTC]; Cenafed® [OTC]; Children's Silfedrine® [OTC]; Decofed® Syrup [OTC]; Drixoral® Non-Drowsy [OTC]; Efidac/24® [OTC]; Neofed® [OTC]; Novafed®; PediaCare® Oral; Sudafed® [OTC]; Sudafed® 12 Hour [OTC]; Sufedrin® [OTC]; Triaminic® AM Decongestant Formula [OTC]

Canadian/Mexican Brand Names Balminil® Decongestant (Canada); Eltor® 120 (Canada); PMS-Pseudoephedrine (Canada); Robidrine® (Canada)

Synonyms *d*-Isoephedrine Hydrochloride; Pseudoephedrine Hydrochloride; Pseudoephedrine Sulfate

Therapeutic Category Adrenergic Agonist Agent; Decongestant; Sympathomimetic

Use Temporary symptomatic relief of nasal congestion due to common cold, upper respiratory allergies, and sinusitis; also promotes nasal or sinus drainage

Pregnancy Risk Factor C

Contraindications Hypersensitivity to pseudoephedrine or any component; MAO inhibitor therapy

Warnings/Precautions Use with caution in patients >60 years of age; administer with caution to patients with hypertension, hyperthyroidism, diabetes mellitus, cardiovascular disease, ischemic heart disease, increased intraocular pressure, or prostatic hypertrophy. Elderly patients are more likely to experience adverse reactions to sympathomimetics. Overdosage may cause hallucinations, seizures, CNS depression, and death.

Adverse Reactions

>10%:
- Cardiovascular: Tachycardia, palpitations, arrhythmias
- Central nervous system: Nervousness, transient stimulation, insomnia, excitability, dizziness, drowsiness, headache
- Neuromuscular & skeletal: Tremor

1% to 10%:
- Central nervous system: Headache
- Neuromuscular & skeletal: Weakness
- Miscellaneous: Diaphoresis

<1%:
- Central nervous system: Convulsions, hallucinations
- Gastrointestinal: Nausea, vomiting
- Genitourinary: Dysuria
- Respiratory: Shortness of breath, dyspnea

Overdosage/Toxicology Symptoms of overdose include seizures, nausea, vomiting, cardiac arrhythmias, hypertension, agitation

There is no specific antidote for pseudoephedrine intoxication; the bulk treatment is supportive. Hyperactivity and agitation usually respond to reduced sensory input; however, with extreme agitation, haloperidol (2-5 mg I.M. for adults) may be required. Hyperthermia is best treated with external cooling measures; or when severe or unresponsive, muscle paralysis with pancuronium may be needed. Hypertension is usually transient and generally does not require treatment unless severe. For diastolic blood pressures >110 mm Hg, a nitroprusside infusion should be initiated. Seizures usually respond to diazepam I.V. and/or phenytoin maintenance regimens.

Drug Interactions

Decreased effect of methyldopa, reserpine

Increased toxicity: MAO inhibitors may increase blood pressure effects of pseudoephedrine; propranolol, sympathomimetic agents may increase toxicity

Mechanism of Action Directly stimulates alpha-adrenergic receptors of respiratory mucosa causing vasoconstriction; directly stimulates beta-adrenergic receptors causing bronchial relaxation, increased heart rate and contractility

Pharmacodynamics/Kinetics

Onset of decongestant effect: Oral: 15-30 minutes

Duration: 4-6 hours (up to 12 hours with extended release formulation administration)

Metabolism: Partially in the liver

Half-life: 9-16 hours

Elimination: 70% to 90% of dose excreted in urine as unchanged drug and 1% to 6% as norpseudoephedrine (active); renal elimination is dependent on urine pH and flow rate; alkaline urine decreases renal elimination of pseudoephedrine

Usual Dosage Oral:

Children:

- <2 years: 4 mg/kg/day in divided doses every 6 hours
- 2-5 years: 15 mg every 6 hours; maximum: 60 mg/24 hours
- 6-12 years: 30 mg every 6 hours; maximum: 120 mg/24 hours

Adults: 30-60 mg every 4-6 hours, sustained release: 120 mg every 12 hours; maximum: 240 mg/24 hours

Dosing adjustment in renal impairment: Reduce dose

Test Interactions Interferes with urine detection of amphetamine (false-positive)

Patient Information Do not exceed recommended dosage and do not use for more than 3-5 days; may cause wakefulness or nervousness; take last dose 4-6 hours before bedtime; do not crush sustained release product; consult pharmacist or physician before using

Nursing Implications Do not crush extended release drug product; elderly patients should be counseled about the proper use of over-the-counter cough and cold preparations

Additional Information

Pseudoephedrine hydrochloride: Cenafed® syrup [OTC], Decofed® syrup [OTC], Neofed® [OTC], Novafed®, Sudafed® [OTC], Sudafed® 12 Hour [OTC], Sudafed® tablet [OTC], Sufedrin® [OTC]

Pseudoephedrine sulfate: Afrinol® [OTC]

Dosage Forms

Capsule: 60 mg

Capsule, timed release, as hydrochloride: 120 mg

Drops, oral, as hydrochloride: 7.5 mg/0.8 mL (15 mL)

Liquid, as hydrochloride: 15 mg/5 mL (120 mL); 30 mg/5 mL (120 mL, 240 mL, 473 mL)

Tablet, as hydrochloride: 30 mg, 60 mg

Tablet:

- Timed release, as hydrochloride: 120 mg
- Extended release, as sulfate: 120 mg, 240 mg

Pseudoephedrine and Acrivastine *see* Acrivastine and Pseudoephedrine *on page 29*

Pseudoephedrine and Triprolidine *see* Triprolidine and Pseudoephedrine *on page 1270*

Pseudoephedrine Hydrochloride *see* Pseudoephedrine *on previous page*

Pseudoephedrine Sulfate *see* Pseudoephedrine *on previous page*

Pseudomonic Acid A *see* Mupirocin *on page 862*

Psor-a-set® Soap [OTC] *see* Salicylic Acid *on page 1120*

Psorcon™ *see* Diflorasone *on page 382*

P&S® Shampoo [OTC] *see* Salicylic Acid *on page 1120*

Psyllium (SIL i yum)

Related Information

Laxatives, Classification and Properties *on page 1412*

(Continued)

Psyllium *(Continued)*

Brand Names Effer-Syllium® [OTC]; Fiberall® Powder [OTC]; Fiberall® Wafer [OTC]; Hydrocil® [OTC]; Konsyl-D® [OTC]; Konsyl® [OTC]; Metamucil® [OTC]; Metamucil® Instant Mix [OTC]; Modane® Bulk [OTC]; Perdiem® Plain [OTC]; Reguloid® [OTC]; Serutan® [OTC]; Siblin® [OTC]; Syllact® [OTC]; V-Lax® [OTC]

Canadian/Mexican Brand Names Fibrepur® (Canada); Novo-Mucilax® (Canada); Prodiem® Plain (Canada)

Synonyms Plantago Seed; Plantain Seed; Psyllium Hydrophilic Mucilloid

Therapeutic Category Laxative, Bulk-Producing

Use Treatment of chronic atonic or spastic constipation and in constipation associated with rectal disorders; management of irritable bowel syndrome

Pregnancy Risk Factor C

Contraindications Fecal impaction, GI obstruction, hypersensitivity to psyllium or any component

Warnings/Precautions May contain aspartame which is metabolized in the GI tract to phenylalanine which is contraindicated in individuals with phenylketonuria; use with caution in patients with esophageal strictures, ulcers, stenosis, or intestinal adhesions; elderly may have insufficient fluid intake which may predispose them to fecal impaction and bowel obstruction.

Adverse Reactions

1% to 10%:

Gastrointestinal: Esophageal or bowel obstruction, diarrhea, constipation, abdominal cramps

Respiratory: Bronchospasm

Miscellaneous: Anaphylaxis upon inhalation in susceptible individuals, rhinoconjunctivitis

Overdosage/Toxicology Symptoms of overdose include abdominal pain, diarrhea, constipation

Drug Interactions Decreased effect of warfarin, digitalis, potassium-sparing diuretics, salicylates, tetracyclines, nitrofurantoin

Mechanism of Action Adsorbs water in the intestine to form a viscous liquid which promotes peristalsis and reduces transit time

Pharmacodynamics/Kinetics

Onset of action: 12-24 hour, but full effect may take 2-3 days

Peak effect: May take 2-3 days

Absorption: Oral: Generally not absorbed following administration, small amounts of grain extracts present in the preparation have been reportedly absorbed following colonic hydrolysis

Usual Dosage Oral (administer at least 3 hours before or after drugs):

Children 6-11 years: (Approximately 1/2 adult dosage) 1/2 to 1 rounded teaspoonful in 4 oz glass of liquid 1-3 times/day

Adults: 1-2 rounded teaspoonfuls or 1-2 packets or 1-2 wafers in 8 oz glass of liquid 1-3 times/day

Patient Information Must be mixed in a glass of water or juice; drink a full glass of liquid with each dose; do not use for longer than 1 week without the advice of a physician

Nursing Implications Inhalation of psyllium dust may cause sensitivity to psyllium (runny nose, watery eyes, wheezing)

Additional Information 3.4 g psyllium hydrophilic mucilloid per 7 g powder is equivalent to a rounded teaspoonful or one packet

Sodium content of Metamucil® Instant Mix (orange): 6 mg (0.27 mEq)

Dosage Forms

Granules: 4.03 g per rounded teaspoon (100 g, 250 g); 2.5 g per rounded teaspoon

Powder: Psyllium 50% and dextrose 50% (6.5 g, 325 g, 420 g, 480 g, 500 g)

Powder:

Effervescent: 3 g/dose (270 g, 480 g); 3.4 g/dose (single-dose packets)

Psyllium hydrophilic: 3.4 g per rounded teaspoon (210 g, 300 g, 420 g, 630 g)

Squares, chewable: 1.7 g, 3.4 g

Wafers: 3.4 g

Psyllium Hydrophilic Mucilloid *see* Psyllium *on previous page*

Pteroylglutamic Acid *see* Folic Acid *on page 553*

PTU *see* Propylthiouracil *on page 1070*

Pulmozyme® *see* Dornase Alfa *on page 419*

Purge® [OTC] *see* Castor Oil *on page 216*

Purinethol® *see* Mercaptopurine *on page 784*

Pyrantel Pamoate (pi RAN tel PAM oh ate)

Brand Names Antiminth® [OTC]; Pin-Rid® [OTC]; Pin-X® [OTC]; Reese's® Pinworm Medicine [OTC]

Therapeutic Category Anthelmintic

Use Treatment of roundworm, pinworm, and hookworm infestations, and trichostrongyliasis

Pregnancy Risk Factor C

Contraindications Known hypersensitivity to pyrantel pamoate

Warnings/Precautions Use with caution in patients with liver impairment, anemia, malnutrition, or pregnancy

Adverse Reactions

1% to 10%: Gastrointestinal: Anorexia, nausea, vomiting, abdominal cramps, diarrhea

<1%:

Central nervous system: Dizziness, drowsiness, insomnia, headache
Dermatologic: Rash
Hepatic: Elevated liver enzymes
Gastrointestinal: Tenesmus
Neuromuscular & skeletal: Weakness

Overdosage/Toxicology Symptoms of overdose include anorexia, nausea, vomiting, cramps, diarrhea, ataxia; treatment is supportive following GI decontamination

Drug Interactions Decreased effect with piperazine

Stability Protect from light

Mechanism of Action Causes the release of acetylcholine and inhibits cholinesterase; acts as a depolarizing neuromuscular blocker, paralyzing the helminths

Pharmacodynamics/Kinetics

Absorption: Oral: Poor
Metabolism: Undergoes partial hepatic metabolism
Time to peak serum concentration: Within 1-3 hours
Elimination: In feces (50% as unchanged drug) and urine (7% as unchanged drug)

Usual Dosage Children and Adults (purgation is not required prior to use): Oral:

Roundworm, pinworm, or trichostrongyliasis: 11 mg/kg administered as a single dose; maximum dose: 1 g. (**Note:** For pinworm infection, dosage should be repeated in 2 weeks and all family members should be treated).
Hookworm: 11 mg/kg administered once daily for 3 days

Monitoring Parameters Stool for presence of eggs, worms, and occult blood, serum AST and ALT

Patient Information May mix drug with milk or fruit juice; strict hygiene is essential to prevent reinfection

Nursing Implications Shake well before pouring to assure accurate dosage; protect from light

Dosage Forms

Capsule: 180 mg
Liquid: 50 mg/mL (30 mL); 144 mg/mL (30 mL)
Suspension, oral (caramel-currant flavor): 50 mg/mL (60 mL)

Pyrazinamide (peer a ZIN a mide)

Related Information

Antimicrobial Drugs of Choice *on page 1468*
Recommendations of the Advisory Council on the Elimination of Tuberculosis *on page 1483*

Canadian/Mexican Brand Names PMS-Pyrazinamide (Canada); Tebrazid® (Canada); Braccopril® (Mexico)

Synonyms Pyrazinoic Acid Amide

Therapeutic Category Antitubercular Agent

Use Adjunctive treatment of tuberculosis in combination with other antituberculosis agents

Pregnancy Risk Factor C

Contraindications Severe hepatic damage; hypersensitivity to pyrazinamide or any component; acute gout

Warnings/Precautions Administer with at least one other effective agent for tuberculosis; use with caution in patients with renal failure, chronic gout, diabetes mellitus, or porphyria. Pyrazinamide is used in the 2-month intensive treatment phase of a 6-month treatment plan.

Adverse Reactions

1% to 10%:

Central nervous system: Malaise
Gastrointestinal: Nausea, vomiting, anorexia
Neuromuscular & skeletal: Arthralgia, myalgia

<1%:

Central nervous system: Fever
Dermatologic: Rash, itching, acne, photosensitivity
Endocrine & metabolic: Gout
Genitourinary: Dysuria

(Continued)

Pyrazinamide *(Continued)*

Hematologic: Porphyria, thrombocytopenia
Hepatic: Hepatotoxicity
Renal: Interstitial nephritis

Overdosage/Toxicology Symptoms of overdose include gout, gastric upset, hepatic damage (mild); treatment following GI decontamination is supportive

Mechanism of Action Converted to pyrazinoic acid in susceptible strains of *Mycobacterium* which lowers the pH of the environment

Pharmacodynamics/Kinetics Bacteriostatic or bactericidal depending on the drug's concentration at the site of infection

Absorption: Oral: Well absorbed
Distribution: Widely distributed into body tissues and fluids including the liver, lung, and CSF
Relative diffusion of antimicrobial agents from blood into cerebrospinal fluid (CSF): Adequate with or without inflammation (exceeds usual MICs)
Ratio of CSF to blood level (%):
Inflamed meninges: 100
Protein binding: 50%
Metabolism: In the liver
Half-life: 9-10 hours, increased with reduced renal or hepatic function
End stage renal disease: 9 hours
Time to peak serum concentration: Within 2 hours
Elimination: In urine (4% as unchanged drug)

Usual Dosage Oral (calculate dose on ideal body weight rather than total body weight): **Note:** A four-drug regimen (isoniazid, rifampin, pyrazinamide, and either streptomycin or ethambutol) is preferred for the initial, empiric treatment of TB. When the drug susceptibility results are available, the regimen should be altered as appropriate.

Patients with TB and without HIV infection:

OPTION 1:

Isoniazid resistance rate <4%: Administer daily isoniazid, rifampin, and pyrazinamide for 8 weeks followed by isoniazid and rifampin daily or directly observed therapy (DOT) 2-3 times/week for 16 weeks

If isoniazid resistance rate is not documented, ethambutol or streptomycin should also be administered until susceptibility to isoniazid or rifampin is demonstrated. Continue treatment for at least 6 months or 3 months beyond culture conversion.

OPTION 2: Administer daily isoniazid, rifampin, pyrazinamide, and either streptomycin or ethambutol for 2 weeks followed by DOT 2 times/week administration of the same drugs for 6 weeks, and subsequently, with isoniazid and rifampin DOT 2 times/week administration for 16 weeks

OPTION 3: Administer isoniazid, rifampin, pyrazinamide, and either ethambutol or streptomycin by DOT 3 times/week for 6 months

Patients with TB and with HIV infection:

Administer any of the above OPTIONS 1, 2 or 3, however, treatment should be continued for a total of 9 months and at least 6 months beyond culture conversion

Note: Some experts recommend that the duration of therapy should be extended to 9 months for patients with disseminated disease, miliary disease, disease involving the bones or joints, or tuberculosis lymphadenitis

Children and Adults:
Daily therapy: 15-30 mg/kg/day (maximum: 2 g/day)
Directly observed therapy (DOT): Twice weekly: 50-70 mg/kg (maximum: 4 g)
DOT: 3 times/week: 50-70 mg/kg (maximum: 3 g)
Elderly: Start with a lower daily dose (15 mg/kg) and increase as tolerated

Dosing adjustment in renal impairment: Cl_{cr} <50 mL/minute: Avoid use or reduce dose to 12-20 mg/kg/day

Dialysis: Avoid use in hemo- and peritoneal dialysis as well as continuous arterio-venous or veno-venous hemofiltration (CAVH/CAVHD)

Dosing adjustment in hepatic impairment: Reduce dose

Monitoring Parameters Periodic liver function tests, serum uric acid, sputum culture, chest x-ray 2-3 months into treatment and at completion

Test Interactions Reacts with Acetest® and Ketostix® to produce pinkish-brown color

Patient Information Notify physician if fever, loss of appetite, malaise, nausea, vomiting, darkened urine, pale stools occur; do not stop taking without consulting a physician

Dosage Forms Tablet: 500 mg

Extemporaneous Preparations Pyrazinamide suspension can be compounded with simple syrup or 0.5% methylcellulose with simple syrup at a concentration of 100 mg/mL; the suspension is stable for 2 months at 4°C or 25°C when stored in glass or plastic bottles

To prepare pyrazinamide suspension in 0.5% methylcellulose with simple syrup: Crush 200 pyrazinamide 500 mg tablets and mix with a suspension containing 500 mL of 1% methylcellulose and 500 mL simple syrup. Add to this a suspension containing 140 crushed pyrazinamide tablets in 350 mL of 1% methylcellulose and 350 mL of simple syrup to make 1.7 L of suspension containing pyrazinamide 100 mg/mL in 0.5% methylcellulose with simple syrup.

Nahata MC, Morosco RS, and Peritre SP, "Stability of Pyrazinamide in Two Suspensions," *Am J Health-Syst Pharm*, 1995, 52:1558-60.

Pyrazinoic Acid Amide *see* Pyrazinamide *on page 1077*

Pyrethrins (pye RE thrins)

Brand Names A-200™ Shampoo [OTC]; Barc™ Liquid [OTC]; End Lice® Liquid [OTC]; Lice-Enz® Shampoo [OTC]; Pronto® Shampoo [OTC]; Pyrinex® Pediculicide Shampoo [OTC]; Pyrinyl II® Liquid [OTC]; Pyrinyl Plus® Shampoo [OTC]; R & C® Shampoo [OTC]; RID® Shampoo [OTC]; Tisit® Blue Gel [OTC]; Tisit® Liquid [OTC]; Tisit® Shampoo [OTC]; Triple X® Liquid [OTC]

Canadian/Mexican Brand Names Lice-Enz® (Canada)

Therapeutic Category Antiparasitic Agent, Topical; Pediculocide; Shampoo, Pediculocide

Use Treatment of *Pediculus humanus* infestations (head lice, body lice, pubic lice and their eggs)

Pregnancy Risk Factor C

Contraindications Known hypersensitivity to pyrethrins, ragweed, or chrysanthemums

Warnings/Precautions For external use only; do not use in eyelashes or eyebrows

Adverse Reactions 1% to 10%:

Dermatologic: Pruritus

Local: Burning, stinging, irritation with repeat use

Mechanism of Action Pyrethrins are derived from flowers that belong to the chrysanthemum family. The mechanism of action on the neuronal membranes of lice is similar to that of DDT. Piperonyl butoxide is usually added to pyrethrin to enhance the product's activity by decreasing the metabolism of pyrethrins in arthropods.

Pharmacodynamics/Kinetics

Onset of action: ~30 minutes

Absorption: Topical into the system is minimal

Metabolism: By ester hydrolysis and hydroxylation

Usual Dosage Application of pyrethrins: Topical:

Apply enough solution to completely wet infested area, including hair

Allow to remain on area for 10 minutes

Wash and rinse with large amounts of warm water

Use fine-toothed comb to remove lice and eggs from hair

Shampoo hair to restore body and luster

Treatment may be repeated if necessary once in a 24-hour period

Repeat treatment in 7-10 days to kill newly hatched lice

Patient Information For external use only; avoid touching eyes, mouth, or other mucous membranes; contact physician if irritation occurs or if condition does not improve in 2-3 days

Dosage Forms

Gel, topical: 0.3% (30 g)

Liquid, topical: 0.18% (60 mL); 0.2% (60 mL, 120 mL); 0.3% (60 mL, 118 mL, 120 mL, 177 mL, 237 mL, 240 mL)

Shampoo: 0.3% (59 mL, 60 mL, 118 mL, 120 mL, 240 mL); 0.33% (60 mL, 120 mL)

Pyridiate® *see* Phenazopyridine *on page 981*

2-Pyridine Aldoxime Methochloride *see* Pralidoxime *on page 1032*

Pyridium® *see* Phenazopyridine *on page 981*

Pyridostigmine (peer id oh STIG meen)

Brand Names Mestinon®; Regonol®

Canadian/Mexican Brand Names Mestinon®-SR (Canada)

Synonyms Pyridostigmine Bromide

Therapeutic Category Antidote, Neuromuscular Blocking Agent; Cholinergic Agent

(Continued)

Pyridostigmine *(Continued)*

Use Symptomatic treatment of myasthenia gravis; also used as an antidote for nondepolarizing neuromuscular blockers; not a cure; patient may develop resistance to the drug

Pregnancy Risk Factor C

Contraindications Hypersensitivity to pyridostigmine, bromides, or any component; GI or GU obstruction

Warnings/Precautions Use with caution in patients with epilepsy, asthma, bradycardia, hyperthyroidism, cardiac arrhythmias, or peptic ulcer; adequate facilities should be available for cardiopulmonary resuscitation when testing and adjusting dose for myasthenia gravis; have atropine and epinephrine ready to treat hypersensitivity reactions; overdosage may result in cholinergic crisis, this must be distinguished from myasthenic crisis; anticholinesterase insensitivity can develop for brief or prolonged periods

Adverse Reactions

>10%:
- Gastrointestinal: Diarrhea, nausea, stomach cramps, mouth watering
- Miscellaneous: Diaphoresis (increased)

1% to 10%:
- Genitourinary: Urge to urinate
- Ocular: Small pupils, lacrimation
- Respiratory: Increased bronchial secretions

<1%:
- Cardiovascular: Bradycardia, A-V block
- Central nervous system: Seizures, headache, dysphoria, drowsiness
- Local: Thrombophlebitis
- Neuromuscular & skeletal: Muscle spasms, weakness
- Ocular: Miosis, diplopia
- Respiratory: Laryngospasm, respiratory paralysis
- Miscellaneous: Hypersensitivity, hyper-reactive cholinergic responses

Overdosage/Toxicology Symptoms of overdose include muscle weakness, blurred vision, excessive sweating, tearing and salivation, nausea, vomiting, diarrhea, hypertension, bradycardia, paralysis

Atropine is the treatment of choice for intoxications manifesting with significant muscarinic symptoms. Atropine I.V. 2-4 mg every 3-60 minutes (or 0.04-0.08 mg I.V. every 5-60 minutes if needed for children) should be repeated to control symptoms and then continued as needed for 1-2 days following the acute ingestion.

Drug Interactions

Increased effect of depolarizing neuromuscular blockers (succinylcholine)
Increased toxicity with edrophonium

Stability Protect from light

Mechanism of Action Inhibits destruction of acetylcholine by acetylcholinesterase which facilitates transmission of impulses across myoneural junction

Pharmacodynamics/Kinetics

Onset of action:
- Oral, I.M.: Within 15-30 minutes
- I.V. injection: Within 2-5 minutes

Absorption: Oral: Very poor (10% to 20%) from GI tract
Metabolism: In the liver

Usual Dosage Normally, sustained release dosage form is used at bedtime for patients who complain of morning weakness

Myasthenia gravis:
- Oral:
  - Children: 7 mg/kg/day in 5-6 divided doses
  - Adults: Initial: 60 mg 3 times/day with maintenance dose ranging from 60 mg to 1.5 g/day; sustained release formulation should be dosed at least every 6 hours (usually 12-24 hours)
- I.M., I.V.:
  - Children: 0.05-0.15 mg/kg/dose (maximum single dose: 10 mg)
  - Adults: 2 mg every 2-3 hours or 1/30th of oral dose

Reversal of nondepolarizing neuromuscular blocker: I.M., I.V.:
- Children: 0.1-0.25 mg/kg/dose preceded by atropine
- Adults: 10-20 mg preceded by atropine

Test Interactions ↑ aminotransferase [ALT (SGPT)/AST (SGOT)] (S), ↑ amylase (S)

Patient Information Side effects are generally due to exaggerated pharmacologic effects; most common side effects are salivation and muscle fasciculations; notify physician if nausea, vomiting, muscle weakness, severe abdominal pain, or difficulty breathing occurs

Nursing Implications Do not crush sustained release drug product; observe for cholinergic reactions, particularly when administered I.V.

Dosage Forms

Injection, as bromide: 5 mg/mL (2 mL, 5 mL)
Syrup, as bromide (raspberry flavor): 60 mg/5 mL (480 mL)
Tablet, as bromide: 60 mg
Tablet, as bromide, sustained release: 180 mg

Pyridostigmine Bromide *see* Pyridostigmine *on page 1079*

Pyridoxine (peer i DOKS een)

Related Information

Epilepsy Treatment *on page 1531*
Guidelines for the Prevention of Opportunistic Infections in Persons with HIV *on page 1457*

Brand Names Nestrex®

Canadian/Mexican Brand Names Benadon® (Mexico)

Synonyms Pyridoxine Hydrochloride; Vitamin B_6

Therapeutic Category Antidote, Cycloserine Toxicity; Antidote, Hydralazine Toxicity; Antidote, Isoniazid Toxicity; Vitamin, Water Soluble

Use Prevents and treats vitamin B_6 deficiency, pyridoxine-dependent seizures in infants, adjunct to treatment of acute toxicity from isoniazid, cycloserine, or hydralazine overdose

Pregnancy Risk Factor A (C if dose exceeds RDA recommendation)

Pregnancy/Breast-Feeding Implications

Clinical effects on the fetus: Crosses the placenta; available evidence suggests safe use during pregnancy and breast-feeding
Breast-feeding/lactation: Crosses into breast milk
Clinical effects on the infant: Possible inhibition of lactation at doses >600 mg/day. American Academy of Pediatrics considers COMPATIBLE with breast-feeding.

Contraindications Hypersensitivity to pyridoxine or any component

Warnings/Precautions Dependence and withdrawal may occur with doses >200 mg/day

Adverse Reactions

<1%:
- Central nervous system: Sensory neuropathy, seizures have occurred following I.V. administration of very large doses, headache
- Gastrointestinal: Nausea
- Endocrine & metabolic: Decreased serum folic acid secretions
- Hepatic: Increased AST
- Neuromuscular & skeletal: Paresthesia
- Miscellaneous: Allergic reactions have been reported

Overdosage/Toxicology Ataxia, sensory neuropathy with doses of 50 mg to 2 g daily over prolonged periods

Drug Interactions Decreased serum levels of levodopa, phenobarbital, and phenytoin

Stability Protect from light

Mechanism of Action Precursor to pyridoxal, which functions in the metabolism of proteins, carbohydrates, and fats; pyridoxal also aids in the release of liver and muscle-stored glycogen and in the synthesis of GABA (within the central nervous system) and heme

Pharmacodynamics/Kinetics

Absorption: Enteral, parenteral: Well absorbed from GI tract
Metabolism: Metabolized in 4-pyridoxic acid (active form), and other metabolites
Half-life: 15-20 days

Usual Dosage

Recommended daily allowance (RDA):
- Children:
  - 1-3 years: 0.9 mg
  - 4-6 years: 1.3 mg
  - 7-10 years: 1.6 mg
- Adults:
  - Male: 1.7-2.0 mg
  - Female: 1.4-1.6 mg

Pyridoxine-dependent Infants:
- Oral: 2-100 mg/day
- I.M., I.V., S.C.: 10-100 mg

Dietary deficiency: Oral:
- Children: 5-25 mg/24 hours for 3 weeks, then 1.5-2.5 mg/day in multiple vitamin product
- Adults: 10-20 mg/day for 3 weeks

(Continued)

Pyridoxine *(Continued)*

Drug-induced neuritis (eg, isoniazid, hydralazine, penicillamine, cycloserine):
Oral:
Children:
Treatment: 10-50 mg/24 hours
Prophylaxis: 1-2 mg/kg/24 hours
Adults:
Treatment: 100-200 mg/24 hours
Prophylaxis: 25-100 mg/24 hours

Treatment of seizures and/or coma from acute isoniazid toxicity, a dose of pyridoxine hydrochloride equal to the amount of INH ingested can be given I.M./I.V. in divided doses together with other anticonvulsants; if the amount INH ingested is not known, administer 5 g I.V. pyridoxine

Treatment of acute hydralazine toxicity, a pyridoxine dose of 25 mg/kg in divided doses I.M./I.V. has been used

Reference Range Over 50 ng/mL (SI: 243 nmol/L) (varies considerably with method). A broad range is ~25-80 ng/mL (SI: 122-389 nmol/L). HPLC method for pyridoxal phosphate has normal range of 3.5-18 ng/mL (SI: 17-88 nmol/L).

Test Interactions Urobilinogen

Patient Information Dietary sources of pyridoxine include red meats, bananas, potatoes, yeast, lima beans, whole grain cereals; do not exceed recommended doses

Nursing Implications Burning may occur at the injection site after I.M. or S.C. administration; seizures have occurred following I.V. administration of very large doses

Dosage Forms
Injection, as hydrochloride: 100 mg/mL (10 mL, 30 mL)
Tablet, as hydrochloride: 25 mg, 50 mg, 100 mg
Tablet, as hydrochloride, extended release: 100 mg

Pyridoxine Hydrochloride *see* Pyridoxine *on previous page*

Pyrimethamine (peer i METH a meen)

Related Information
Guidelines for the Prevention of Opportunistic Infections in Persons with HIV *on page 1457*

Brand Names Daraprim®

Canadian/Mexican Brand Names Daraprim® (Mexico)

Therapeutic Category Antimalarial Agent

Use Prophylaxis of malaria due to susceptible strains of plasmodia; used in conjunction with quinine and sulfadiazine for the treatment of uncomplicated attacks of chloroquine-resistant *P. falciparum* malaria; used in conjunction with fast-acting schizonticide to initiate transmission control and suppression cure; synergistic combination with sulfonamide in treatment of toxoplasmosis

Pregnancy Risk Factor C

Contraindications Megaloblastic anemia secondary to folate deficiency; known hypersensitivity to pyrimethamine, chloroguanide; resistant malaria; patients with seizure disorders

Warnings/Precautions When used for more than 3-4 days, it may be advisable to administer leucovorin to prevent hematologic complications; monitor CBC and platelet counts every 2 weeks; use with caution in patients with impaired renal or hepatic function or with possible G-6-PD

Adverse Reactions
1% to 10%:
Gastrointestinal: Anorexia, abdominal cramps, vomiting
Hematologic: Megaloblastic anemia, leukopenia, thrombocytopenia, agranulocytosis

<1%:
Central nervous system: Insomnia, lightheadedness, fever, malaise, seizures, depression
Dermatologic: Rash, dermatitis, abnormal skin pigmentation
Gastrointestinal: Diarrhea, xerostomia, atrophic glossitis
Hematologic: Pulmonary eosinophilia

Overdosage/Toxicology Symptoms of overdose include megaloblastic anemia, leukopenia, thrombocytopenia, anorexia, CNS stimulation, seizures, nausea, vomiting, hematemesis

Following GI decontamination, leucovorin should be administered in a dosage of 5-15 mg/day I.M., I.V., or oral for 5-7 days or as required to reverse symptoms of folic acid deficiency; diazepam 0.1-0.25 mg/kg can be used to treat seizures

Drug Interactions
Decreased effect: Pyrimethamine effectiveness decreased by acid
Increased effect: Sulfonamides (synergy), methotrexate, TMP/SMX

Stability Pyrimethamine tablets may be crushed to prepare oral suspensions of the drug in water, cherry syrup, or sucrose-containing solutions at a concentration of 1 mg/mL; stable at room temperature for 5-7 days

Mechanism of Action Inhibits parasitic dihydrofolate reductase, resulting in inhibition of vital tetrahydrofolic acid synthesis

Pharmacodynamics/Kinetics

Absorption: Oral: Well absorbed

Distribution: V_d: 2.9 L/kg in adults; appears in breast milk

Protein binding: 80%

Half-life: 80-95 hours

Time to peak serum concentration: Within 1.5-8 hours

Usual Dosage

Malaria chemoprophylaxis (for areas where chloroquine-resistant *P. falciparum* exists): Begin prophylaxis 2 weeks before entering endemic area:

Children: 0.5 mg/kg once weekly; not to exceed 25 mg/dose

or

Children:

<4 years: 6.25 mg once weekly

4-10 years: 12.5 mg once weekly

Children >10 years and Adults: 25 mg once weekly

Dosage should be continued for all age groups for at least 6-10 weeks after leaving endemic areas

Chloroquine-resistant *P. falciparum* malaria (when used in conjunction with quinine and sulfadiazine):

Children:

<10 kg: 6.25 mg/day once daily for 3 days

10-20 kg: 12.5 mg/day once daily for 3 days

20-40 kg: 25 mg/day once daily for 3 days

Adults: 25 mg twice daily for 3 days

Toxoplasmosis:

Infants for congenital toxoplasmosis: Oral: 1 mg/kg once daily for 6 months with sulfadiazine then every other month with sulfa, alternating with spiramycin.

Children: Loading dose: 2 mg/kg/day divided into 2 equal daily doses for 1-3 days (maximum: 100 mg/day) followed by 1 mg/kg/day divided into 2 doses for 4 weeks; maximum: 25 mg/day

With sulfadiazine or trisulfapyrimidines: 2 mg/kg/day divided every 12 hours for 3 days followed by 1 mg/kg/day once daily or divided twice daily for 4 weeks given with trisulfapyrimidines or sulfadiazine

Adults: 50-75 mg/day together with 1-4 g of a sulfonamide for 1-3 weeks depending on patient's tolerance and response, then reduce dose by 50% and continue for 4-5 weeks **or** 25-50 mg/day for 3-4 weeks

Monitoring Parameters CBC, including platelet counts twice weekly

Patient Information Take with meals to minimize vomiting; begin malaria prophylaxis at least 1-2 weeks prior to departure; discontinue at first sign of skin rash; notify physician if persistent fever, sore throat, bleeding or bruising occurs; regular blood work may be necessary in patients taking high doses

Dosage Forms Tablet: 25 mg

Extemporaneous Preparations Pyrimethamine tablets may be crushed to prepare oral suspensions of the drug in water, cherry syrup or sucrose-containing solutions at a concentration of 1 mg/mL; stable at room temperature for 5-7 days

McEvoy G, ed. AHFS Drug Information 96. Bethesda, MD: American Society of Health-System Pharmacists; 1996.

Pyrinex® Pediculicide Shampoo [OTC] *see* Pyrethrins *on page 1079*

Pyrinyl II® Liquid [OTC] *see* Pyrethrins *on page 1079*

Pyrinyl Plus® Shampoo [OTC] *see* Pyrethrins *on page 1079*

Quazepam (KWAY ze pam)

Related Information

Benzodiazepines Comparison *on page 1397*

Brand Names Doral®

Therapeutic Category Benzodiazepine; Hypnotic; Sedative

Use Treatment of insomnia; more likely than triazolam to cause daytime sedation and fatigue; is classified as a long-acting benzodiazepine hypnotic (like flurazepam - Dalmane®), this long duration of action may prevent withdrawal symptoms when therapy is discontinued

Restrictions C-IV

Pregnancy Risk Factor X

Contraindications Narrow-angle glaucoma, pregnancy, known hypersensitivity to quazepam

Warnings/Precautions Safety and efficacy in children <18 years of age have not been established; do not use in pregnant women; may cause drug dependency;

(Continued)

Quazepam *(Continued)*

avoid abrupt discontinuance in patients with prolonged therapy or seizure disorders; avoid using in patients with pre-existing CNS depression, severe uncontrolled pain, or narrow-angle glaucoma; use with caution in patients receiving other CNS depressants, in patients with hepatic dysfunction, and the elderly

Adverse Reactions

>10%:

Cardiovascular: Tachycardia, chest pain

Central nervous system: Drowsiness, fatigue, ataxia, lightheadedness, memory impairment, insomnia, anxiety, depression, headache

Dermatologic: Rash

Endocrine & metabolic: Decreased libido

Gastrointestinal: Xerostomia, constipation, diarrhea, decreased salivation, nausea, vomiting, increased or decreased appetite

Neuromuscular & skeletal: Dysarthria

Ocular: Blurred vision

Miscellaneous: Diaphoresis

1% to 10%:

Cardiovascular: Syncope, hypotension

Central nervous system: Confusion, nervousness, dizziness, akathisia

Dermatologic: Dermatitis

Gastrointestinal: Increased salivation, weight gain or loss

Neuromuscular & skeletal: Rigidity, tremor, muscle cramps

Otic: Tinnitus

Respiratory: Nasal congestion, hyperventilation

<1%:

Endocrine & metabolic: Menstrual irregularities

Hematologic: Blood dyscrasias

Neuromuscular & skeletal: Reflex slowing

Miscellaneous: Drug dependence

Overdosage/Toxicology Symptoms of overdose include somnolence, confusion, coma, hypoactive reflexes, dyspnea, hypotension, slurred speech, impaired coordination

Treatment for benzodiazepine overdose is supportive; rarely is mechanical ventilation required; has been shown to selectively block the binding of benzodiazepines to CNS receptors, resulting in a reversal of benzodiazepine-induced CNS depression, but not respiratory depression

Drug Interactions Increased effect/toxicity with CNS depressants (narcotics, alcohol, MAO inhibitors, TCAs, anesthetics, barbiturates, phenothiazines)

Mechanism of Action Depresses all levels of the CNS, including the limbic and reticular formation, probably through the increased action of gamma-aminobutyric acid (GABA), which is a major inhibitory neurotransmitter in the brain

Pharmacodynamics/Kinetics

Absorption: Oral: Rapid

Protein binding: 95%

Metabolism: In the liver to at least one active compound

Half-life:

Parent drug: 25-41 hours

Active metabolite: 40-114 hours

Usual Dosage Adults: Oral: Initial: 15 mg at bedtime, in some patients the dose may be reduced to 7.5 mg after a few nights

Dosing adjustment in hepatic impairment: Dose reduction may be necessary

Dietary Considerations Alcohol: Additive CNS effect, avoid use

Monitoring Parameters Respiratory and cardiovascular status

Patient Information Avoid alcohol and other CNS depressants; avoid activities needing good psychomotor coordination until CNS effects are known; drug may cause physical or psychological dependence; avoid abrupt discontinuation after prolonged use

Nursing Implications Institute safety measures, remove smoking materials from area, supervise ambulation

Dosage Forms Tablet: 7.5 mg, 15 mg

Quelicin® *see* Succinylcholine *on page 1166*

Queltuss® [OTC] *see* Guaifenesin and Dextromethorphan *on page 591*

Questran® *see* Cholestyramine Resin *on page 268*

Questran® Light *see* Cholestyramine Resin *on page 268*

Quibron®-T *see* Theophylline Salts *on page 1207*

Quibron®-T/SR *see* Theophylline Salts *on page 1207*

Quiess® *see* Hydroxyzine *on page 634*

Quinaglute® Dura-Tabs® *see* Quinidine *on page 1087*

Quinalan® *see* Quinidine *on page 1087*

Quinalbarbitone Sodium *see* Secobarbital *on page 1129*

Quinapril (KWIN a pril)

Related Information

Angiotensin-Converting Enzyme Inhibitors Comparison *on page 1386*

Heart Failure: Management of Patients With Left-Ventricular Systolic Dysfunction *on page 1533*

Brand Names Accupril®

Canadian/Mexican Brand Names Acupril® (Mexico)

Synonyms Quinapril Hydrochloride

Therapeutic Category Angiotensin-Converting Enzyme (ACE) Inhibitors; Antihypertensive

Use Management of hypertension and treatment of congestive heart failure; increase circulation in Raynaud's phenomenon; idiopathic edema; believed to improve survival in heart failure

Unlabeled use: Hypertensive crisis, diabetic nephropathy, rheumatoid arthritis, diagnosis of anatomic renal artery stenosis, hypertension secondary to scleroderma renal crisis, diagnosis of aldosteronism, Bartter's syndrome, postmyocardial infarction for prevention of ventricular failure

Pregnancy Risk Factor C (first trimester); D (second and third trimester)

Contraindications Hypersensitivity to quinapril or history of angioedema induced by other ACE inhibitors

Warnings/Precautions Use with caution in patients with renal insufficiency, autoimmune disease, renal artery stenosis; excessive hypotension may be more likely in volume-depleted patients, the elderly, and following the first dose (first dose phenomenon); quinapril should be discontinued if laryngeal stridor or angioedema of the face, tongue, or glottis is observed

Adverse Reactions

1% to 10%:

- Cardiovascular: Hypotension
- Central nervous system: Dizziness, headache, fatigue
- Gastrointestinal: Diarrhea
- Renal: Increased BUN/serum creatinine
- Respiratory: Upper respiratory symptoms, cough

<1%:

- Cardiovascular: Chest discomfort, flushing, myocardial infarction, angina pectoris, orthostatic hypotension, rhythm disturbances, tachycardia, peripheral edema, vasculitis, palpitations, syncope
- Central nervous system: Fever, malaise, depression, somnolence, insomnia
- Dermatologic: Urticaria, pruritus, angioedema
- Endocrine & metabolic: Gout
- Gastrointestinal: Pancreatitis, abdominal pain, anorexia, constipation, flatulence, xerostomia
- Hematologic: Neutropenia, bone marrow suppression
- Hepatic: Hepatitis
- Neuromuscular & skeletal: Arthralgia, shoulder pain
- Ocular: Blurred vision
- Respiratory: Bronchitis, sinusitis, pharyngeal pain
- Miscellaneous: Diaphoresis

Drug-Drug Interactions With ACEIs

Precipitant Drug	Drug (Category) and Effect	Description
Antacids	ACE Inhibitors: decreased	Decreased bioavailability of ACEIs. May be more likely with captopril. Separate administration times by 1-2 hours.
NSAIDs (indomethacin)	ACEIs: decreased	Reduced hypotensive effects of ACEIs. More prominent in low renin or volume dependent hypertensive patients.
Phenothiazines	ACEIs: increased	Pharmacologic effects of ACEIs may be increased.
ACEIs	Allopurinol: increased	Higher risk of hypersensitivity reaction possible when given concurrently. Three case reports of Stevens-Johnson syndrome with captopril.
ACEIs	Digoxin: increased	Increased plasma digoxin levels.
ACEIs	Lithium: increased	Increased serum lithium levels and symptoms of toxicity may occur.
ACEIs	Potassium preps/ potassium sparing diuretics increased	Coadministration may result in elevated potassium levels.

(Continued)

Quinapril *(Continued)*

Overdosage/Toxicology Mild hypotension has been the only toxic effect seen with acute overdose. Bradycardia may also occur; hyperkalemia occurs even with therapeutic doses, especially in patients with renal insufficiency and those taking NSAIDs.

Following initiation of essential overdose management, toxic symptom treatment and supportive treatment should be initiated. Hypotension usually responds to I.V. fluids or Trendelenburg positioning.

Drug Interactions See table.

Stability Store at room temperature; unstable in aqueous solutions; to prepare solution for oral administration, mix prior to administration and use within 10 minutes

Mechanism of Action Competitive inhibitor of angiotensin-converting enzyme (ACE); prevents conversion of angiotensin I to angiotensin II, a potent vasoconstrictor; results in lower levels of angiotensin II which causes an increase in plasma renin activity and a reduction in aldosterone secretion; a CNS mechanism may also be involved in hypotensive effect as angiotensin II increases adrenergic outflow from CNS; vasoactive kallikreins may be decreased in conversion to active hormones by ACE inhibitors, thus reducing blood pressure

Pharmacodynamics/Kinetics

Metabolism: Rapidly hydrolyzed to quinaprilat, the active metabolite

Half-life, elimination:

Quinapril: 0.8 hours

Quinaprilat: 2 hours

Time to peak serum concentration:

Quinapril: 1 hour

Quinaprilat: ~2 hours

Elimination: 50% to 60% of quinapril excreted in urine primarily as quinaprilat

Usual Dosage

Adults: Oral: Initial: 10 mg once daily, adjust according to blood pressure response at peak and trough blood levels; in general, the normal dosage range is 20-80 mg/day

Elderly: Initial: 2.5-5 mg/day; increase dosage at increments of 2.5-5 mg at 1- to 2-week intervals

Dosing adjustment in renal impairment:

Cl_{cr} >60 mL/minute: Administer 10 mg/day

Cl_{cr} 30-60 mL/minute: 5 mg/day

Cl_{cr} 10-30 mL/minute: 2.5 mg/day

Dosing comments in hepatic impairment: In patients with alcoholic cirrhosis, hydrolysis of quinapril to quinaprilat is impaired; however, the subsequent elimination of quinaprilat is unaltered

Patient Information Do not discontinue medication without advice of physician; notify physician if sore throat, swelling, palpitations, cough, chest pains, difficulty swallowing, swelling of face, eyes, tongue, lips; hoarseness, sweating, vomiting, or diarrhea occurs; may cause dizziness, lightheadedness during first few days; may also cause changes in taste perception

Nursing Implications May cause depression in some patients; discontinue if angioedema of the face, extremities, lips, tongue, or glottis occurs; watch for hypotensive effects within 1-3 hours of first dose or new higher dose

Dosage Forms Tablet, as hydrochloride: 5 mg, 10 mg, 20 mg, 40 mg

Quinapril Hydrochloride *see* Quinapril *on previous page*

Quinethazone (kwin ETH a zone)

Related Information

Sulfonamide Derivatives *on page 1420*

Brand Names Hydromox®

Therapeutic Category Antihypertensive; Diuretic, Thiazide

Use Adjunctive therapy in treatment of edema and hypertension

Pregnancy Risk Factor D

Contraindications Anuria; hypersensitivity to sulfonamide-derived drugs

Warnings/Precautions Use with caution in renal disease, hepatic disease, gout, lupus erythematosus, diabetes mellitus; some products may contain tartrazine

Adverse Reactions

1% to 10%: Endocrine & metabolic: Hypokalemia

<1%:

Cardiovascular: Hypotension

Central nervous system: Drowsiness

Dermatologic: Photosensitivity, rash

Endocrine & metabolic: Fluid and electrolyte imbalances (hypocalcemia, hypomagnesemia, hyponatremia), hyperglycemia

Gastrointestinal: Nausea, vomiting, anorexia

Genitourinary: Polyuria

Hematologic: Aplastic anemia, hemolytic anemia, leukopenia, agranulocytosis, thrombocytopenia

Hepatic: Hepatitis

Renal: Prerenal azotemia, uremia

Overdosage/Toxicology Symptoms of overdose include hypermotility, diuresis, lethargy, confusion, muscle weakness; following GI decontamination, therapy is supportive with I.V. fluids, electrolytes, and I.V. pressors if needed

Drug Interactions

Decreased effect of oral hypoglycemics; decreased absorption with cholestyramine and colestipol

Increased effect with furosemide and other loop diuretics

Increased toxicity/levels of lithium

Mechanism of Action Quinethazone is a quinazoline derivative which increases the renal excretion of sodium and chloride and an accompanying volume of water due to inhibition of the tubular mechanism of electrolyte reabsorption.

Pharmacodynamics/Kinetics

Onset of action: 2 hours

Duration: 18-24 hours

Usual Dosage Adults: Oral: 50-100 mg once daily up to a maximum of 200 mg/day

Patient Information May be taken with food or milk; take early in day to avoid nocturia; take the last dose of multiple doses no later than 6 PM unless instructed otherwise. A few people who take this medication become more sensitive to sunlight and may experience skin rash, redness, itching, or severe sunburn, especially if sun block SPF ≥15 is not used on exposed skin areas.

Nursing Implications Assess weight, I & O reports daily to determine fluid loss; take blood pressure with patient lying down and standing

Dosage Forms Tablet: 50 mg

Quinidex® Extentabs® *see* Quinidine *on this page*

Quinidine (KWIN i deen)

Related Information

Adult ACLS Algorithm, Tachycardia *on page 1512*

Antacid Drug Interactions *on page 1388*

Antiarrhythmic Drugs *on page 1389*

Comparative Pharmacokinetic Properties of Antiarrhythmic Agents *on page 1391*

Brand Names Cardioquin®; Quinaglute® Dura-Tabs®; Quinalan®; Quinidex® Extentabs®; Quinora®

Canadian/Mexican Brand Names Quini Durules® (Mexico)

Synonyms Quinidine Gluconate; Quinidine Polygalacturonate; Quinidine Sulfate

Therapeutic Category Antiarrhythmic Agent, Class I-A

Use Prophylaxis after cardioversion of atrial fibrillation and/or flutter to maintain normal sinus rhythm; also used to prevent reoccurrence of paroxysmal supraventricular tachycardia, paroxysmal A-V junctional rhythm, paroxysmal ventricular tachycardia, paroxysmal atrial fibrillation, and atrial or ventricular premature contractions; also has activity against *Plasmodium falciparum* malaria

Pregnancy Risk Factor C

Contraindications Patients with complete A-V block with an A-V junctional or idioventricular pacemaker; patients with intraventricular conduction defects (marked widening of QRS complex); patients with cardiac-glycoside induced A-V conduction disorders; hypersensitivity to the drug or cinchona derivatives

Warnings/Precautions Use with caution in patients with myocardial depression, sick-sinus syndrome, incomplete A-V block, hepatic and/or renal insufficiency, myasthenia gravis; hemolysis may occur in patients with G-6-PD (glucose-6-phosphate dehydrogenase) deficiency; quinidine-induced hepatotoxicity, including granulomatous hepatitis can occur, increased serum AST and alkaline phosphatase concentrations, and jaundice may occur; use with caution in nursing women and elderly

Adverse Reactions

>10%: Gastrointestinal: Bitter taste, diarrhea, anorexia, nausea, vomiting, stomach cramping

1% to 10%:

Cardiovascular: Hypotension, syncope

Central nervous system: Lightheadedness, severe headache

Dermatologic: Rash

Ocular: Blurred vision

Otic: Tinnitus

Respiratory: Wheezing

(Continued)

Quinidine *(Continued)*

<1%:

Cardiovascular: Tachycardia, heart block, ventricular fibrillation, vascular collapse

Central nervous system: Confusion, delirium, fever, vertigo

Dermatologic: Angioedema

Hematologic: Anemia, thrombocytopenic purpura, blood dyscrasias

Otic: Impaired hearing

Respiratory: Respiratory depression

Overdosage/Toxicology Has a low toxic:therapeutic ratio and may easily produce fatal intoxication (acute toxic dose: 1 g in adults); symptoms of overdose include sinus bradycardia, sinus node arrest or asystole, P-R, QRS or Q-T interval prolongation, torsade de pointes (polymorphous ventricular tachycardia) and depressed myocardial contractility, which along with alpha-adrenergic or ganglionic blockade, may result in hypotension and pulmonary edema; other effects are anticholinergic (dry mouth, dilated pupils, and delirium) as well as seizures, coma and respiratory arrest.

Treatment is primarily symptomatic and effects usually respond to conventional therapies (fluids, positioning, vasopressors, anticonvulsants, antiarrhythmics). **Note:** Do not use other type 1a or 1c antiarrhythmic agents to treat ventricular tachycardia; sodium bicarbonate may treat wide QRS intervals or hypotension; markedly impaired conduction or high degree A-V block, unresponsive to bicarbonate, indicates consideration of a pacemaker is needed.

Drug Interactions

Inhibitor of cytochrome P-450 2D6 enzymes

Cytochrome P-450 3A enzyme substrate

Decreased effect: Phenobarbital, phenytoin, and rifampin may decrease quinidine serum concentrations (rifampin may decrease quinidine half-life by 50%, probably by inducing the CYP3A isozyme)

Increased toxicity:

Quinidine potentiates nondepolarizing and depolarizing muscle relaxants; quinidine may increase plasma concentration of digoxin, closely monitor digoxin concentrations, digoxin dosage may need to be reduced (by one-half) when quinidine is initiated, new steady-state digoxin plasma concentrations occur in 5-7 days; quinidine may enhance coumarin anticoagulants

Beta-blockers + quinidine may increase bradycardia

Verapamil, amiodarone, alkalinizing agents, and cimetidine may increase quinidine serum concentrations

Stability Do not use discolored parenteral solution

Mechanism of Action Class 1A antiarrhythmic agent; depresses phase O of the action potential; decreases myocardial excitability and conduction velocity, and myocardial contractility by decreasing sodium influx during depolarization and potassium efflux in repolarization; also reduces calcium transport across cell membrane

Pharmacodynamics/Kinetics

Distribution: V_d: Adults: 2-3.5 L/kg, decreased with congestive heart failure, malaria; increased with cirrhosis; crosses the placenta; appears in breast milk

Protein binding:

Newborns: 60% to 70%; decreased protein binding with cyanotic congenital heart disease, cirrhosis, or acute myocardial infarction

Adults: 80% to 90%

Metabolism: Extensively in the liver (50% to 90%) to inactive compounds

Bioavailability:

Sulfate: 80%

Gluconate: 70%

Plasma half-life:

Children: 2.5-6.7 hours

Adults: 6-8 hours; increased half-life with elderly, cirrhosis, and congestive heart failure

Elimination: In urine (15% to 25% as unchanged drug)

Usual Dosage Dosage expressed in terms of the salt: 267 mg of quinidine gluconate = 200 mg of quinidine sulfate

Children: Test dose for idiosyncratic reaction (sulfate, oral or gluconate, I.M.): 2 mg/kg or 60 mg/m²

Oral (quinidine sulfate): 15-60 mg/kg/day in 4-5 divided doses or 6 mg/kg every 4-6 hours; usual 30 mg/kg/day or 900 mg/m²/day given in 5 daily doses

I.V. **not** recommended (quinidine gluconate): 2-10 mg/kg/dose given at a rate ≤10 mg/minute every 3-6 hours as needed

Adults: Test dose: Oral, I.M.: 200 mg administered several hours before full dosage (to determine possibility of idiosyncratic reaction)

Oral:

Sulfate: 100-600 mg/dose every 4-6 hours; begin at 200 mg/dose and titrate to desired effect (maximum daily dose: 3-4 g)

Gluconate: 324-972 mg every 8-12 hours

I.M.: 400 mg/dose every 4-6 hours

I.V.: 200-400 mg/dose diluted and given at a rate ≤10 mg/minute

Dosing adjustment in renal impairment: Cl_{cr} <10 mL/minute: Administer 75% of normal dose

Hemodialysis: Slightly hemodialyzable (5% to 20%); 200 mg supplemental dose posthemodialysis is recommended

Peritoneal dialysis: Not dialyzable (0% to 5%)

Dosing adjustment/comments in hepatic impairment: Larger loading dose may be indicated, reduce maintenance doses by 50% and monitor serum levels closely

Administration When injecting I.M., aspirate carefully to avoid injection into a vessel; administer around-the-clock to promote less variation in peak and trough serum levels; maximum I.V. infusion rate: 10 mg/minute

Monitoring Parameters Cardiac monitor required during I.V. administration; CBC, liver and renal function tests, should be routinely performed during long-term administration

Reference Range Therapeutic: 2-5 µg/mL (SI: 6.2-15.4 µmol/L). Patient dependent therapeutic response occurs at levels of 3-6 µg/mL (SI: 9.2-18.5 µmol/L). Optimal therapeutic level is method dependent; >6 µg/mL (SI: >18 µmol/L).

Patient Information Do not crush sustained release preparations. Patients should notify their physician if rash, fever, unusual bleeding or bruising, ringing in the ears, visual disturbances, or syncope occurs; seek emergency help if palpitations occur.

Nursing Implications Do not crush sustained release drug product

Additional Information

Quinidine gluconate: Duraquin®, Quinaglute® Dura-Tabs®, Quinalan®, Quinatime®

Quinidine polygalacturonate: Cardioquin®

Quinidine sulfate: Cin-Quin®, Quinidex® Extentabs®, Quinora®

Dosage Forms

Injection, as gluconate: 80 mg/mL (10 mL)

Tablet, as polygalacturonate: 275 mg

Tablet, as sulfate: 200 mg, 300 mg

Tablet:

Sustained action, as sulfate: 300 mg

Sustained release, as gluconate: 324 mg

Extemporaneous Preparations A 10 mg/mL quinidine sulfate solution made with six 200 mg capsules, 15 mL alcohol USP, and citric acid syrup USP qs ad to a total amount of 120 mL is stable for 30 days under refrigeration

Nahata MC and Hipple TF, *Pediatric Drug Formulations*, 2nd ed, Cincinnati, OH: Harvey Whitney Books Co, 1992.

Quinidine Gluconate *see* Quinidine *on page 1087*

Quinidine Polygalacturonate *see* Quinidine *on page 1087*

Quinidine Sulfate *see* Quinidine *on page 1087*

Quinine (KWYE nine)

Brand Names Formula Q®

Synonyms Quinine Sulfate

Therapeutic Category Antimalarial Agent

Use Suppression or treatment of chloroquine-resistant *P. falciparum* malaria; treatment of *Babesia microti* infection; prevention and treatment of nocturnal recumbency leg muscle cramps

Pregnancy Risk Factor D

Contraindications Tinnitus, optic neuritis, G-6-PD deficiency, hypersensitivity to quinine or any component, history of black water fever, and thrombocytopenia with quinine or quinidine

Warnings/Precautions Use with caution in patients with cardiac arrhythmias (quinine has quinidine-like activity) and in patients with myasthenia gravis

Adverse Reactions

>10%:

Central nervous system: Severe headache

Gastrointestinal: Nausea, vomiting, diarrhea

Ocular: Blurred vision

Otic: Tinnitus

<1%:

Cardiovascular: Flushing of the skin, anginal symptoms

Central nervous system: Fever

(Continued)

Quinine *(Continued)*

Dermatologic: Rash, pruritus
Endocrine & metabolic: Hypoglycemia
Gastrointestinal: Epigastric pain
Hematologic: Hemolysis, thrombocytopenia
Hepatic: Hepatitis
Ocular: Nightblindness, diplopia, optic atrophy
Otic: Impaired hearing
Miscellaneous: Hypersensitivity reactions

Overdosage/Toxicology Symptoms of mild toxicity include nausea, vomiting, and cinchonism; severe intoxication may cause ataxia, obtundation, convulsions, coma, and respiratory arrest; with massive intoxication quinidine-like cardiotoxicity (hypotension, QRS and Q-T interval prolongation, A-V block, and ventricular arrhythmias) may be fatal; retinal toxicity occurs 9-10 hours after ingestion (blurred vision, impaired color perception, constriction of visual fields and blindness); other toxic effects include hypokalemia, hypoglycemia, hemolysis and congenital malformations when taken during pregnancy.

Treatment includes symptomatic therapy with conventional agents (anticonvulsants, fluids, positioning, vasoconstrictors, antiarrhythmias). **Note:** Avoid type 1a and 1c antiarrhythmic drugs; treat cardiotoxicity with sodium bicarbonate; dialysis and hemoperfusion procedures are ineffective in enhancing elimination.

Drug Interactions Inhibitor of cytochrome P-450 2D6 enzymes

Decreased effect: Phenobarbital, phenytoin, and rifampin may decrease quinine serum concentrations

Increased toxicity:

Beta-blockers + quinine may increase bradycardia

Quinine may enhance coumarin anticoagulants and potentiate nondepolarizing and depolarizing muscle relaxants;

Quinine may inhibit metabolism of astemizole resulting in toxic levels and potentially life-threatening cardiotoxicity

Quinine may increase plasma concentration of digoxin by as much as 2-fold; closely monitor digoxin concentrations and decrease digoxin dose with initiated of quinine by ½

Verapamil, amiodarone, alkalinizing agents, and cimetidine may increase quinine serum concentrations

Stability Protect from light

Mechanism of Action Depresses oxygen uptake and carbohydrate metabolism; intercalates into DNA, disrupting the parasite's replication and transcription; affects calcium distribution within muscle fibers and decreases the excitability of the motor end-plate region; cardiovascular effects similar to quinidine

Pharmacodynamics/Kinetics

Absorption: Oral: Readily absorbed mainly from the upper small intestine
Protein binding: 70% to 95%
Metabolism: Primarily in the liver
Half-life:
Children: 6-12 hours
Adults: 8-14 hours
Time to peak serum concentration: Within 1-3 hours
Elimination: In bile and saliva with <5% excreted unchanged in urine

Usual Dosage Oral:

Children:

Treatment of chloroquine-resistant malaria: 25 mg/kg/day in divided doses every 8 hours for 3-7 days in conjunction with another agent

Babesiosis: 25 mg/kg/day, (up to a maximum of 650 mg/dose) divided every 8 hours for 7 days

Adults:

Treatment of chloroquine-resistant malaria: 650 mg every 8 hours for 3-7 days in conjunction with another agent

Suppression of malaria: 325 mg twice daily and continued for 6 weeks after exposure

Babesiosis: 650 mg every 6-8 hours for 7 days

Leg cramps: 200-300 mg at bedtime

Dosing interval/adjustment in renal impairment:

Cl_{cr} 10-50 mL/minute: Administer every 8-12 hours or 75% of normal dose

Cl_{cr} <10 mL/minute: Administer every 24 hours or 30% to 50% of normal dose

Dialysis: Not removed by hemo- or peritoneal dialysis or continuous arterio-venous or veno-venous hemofiltration (CAVH/CAVHD); dose for Cl_{cr} <10 mL/minute

Reference Range Toxic: >10 µg/mL

Test Interactions Positive Coombs' [direct]

Patient Information Do not crush sustained release preparations. Avoid use of aluminum-containing antacids because of drug absorption problems; swallow dose whole to avoid bitter taste; may cause night blindness. Patients should notify their physician if rash, fever, unusual bleeding or bruising, ringing in the ears, visual disturbances, or syncope occur; seek emergency help if palpitations occur.

Dosage Forms

Capsule, as sulfate: 64.8 mg, 65 mg, 200 mg, 300 mg, 325 mg
Tablet, as sulfate: 162.5 mg, 260 mg

Quinine Sulfate *see* Quinine *on page 1089*

Quinol *see* Hydroquinone *on page 628*

Quinora® *see* Quinidine *on page 1087*

Quinsana Plus® [OTC] *see* Tolnaftate *on page 1243*

Rabies Immune Globulin (Human)

(RAY beez i MYUN GLOB yoo lin HYU man)

Related Information

Immunization Guidelines *on page 1421*

Brand Names Hyperab®; Imogam®

Synonyms RIG

Therapeutic Category Immune Globulin

Use Part of postexposure prophylaxis of persons with rabies exposure who lack a history or pre-exposure or postexposure prophylaxis with rabies vaccine or a recently documented neutralizing antibody response to previous rabies vaccination; although it is preferable to administer RIG with the first dose of vaccine, it can be given up to 8 days after vaccination

Pregnancy Risk Factor C

Contraindications Inadvertent I.V. administration; allergy to thimerosal or any component

Warnings/Precautions Use with caution in individuals with thrombocytopenia, bleeding disorders, or prior allergic reactions to immune globulins

Adverse Reactions

1% to 10%:
- Central nervous system: Fever (mild)
- Local: Soreness at injection site

<1%:
- Dermatologic: Urticaria, angioedema
- Neuromuscular & skeletal: Stiffness, soreness of muscles
- Miscellaneous: Anaphylactic shock

Drug Interactions

Decreased effect: Live vaccines, corticosteroids, immunosuppressive agents; should not be administered within 3 months

Stability Refrigerate

Mechanism of Action Rabies immune globulin is a solution of globulins dried from the plasma or serum of selected adult human donors who have been immunized with rabies vaccine and have developed high titers of rabies antibody. It generally contains 10% to 18% of protein of which not less than 80% is monomeric immunoglobulin G.

Usual Dosage Children and Adults: I.M.: 20 units/kg in a single dose (RIG should always be administered in conjunction with rabies vaccine (HDCV)); infiltrate ½ of the dose locally around the wound; administer the remainder I.M.

Administration Intramuscular injection only; injection should be made into the deltoid muscle or anterolateral aspect of the thigh

Nursing Implications Severe adverse reactions can occur if patient receives RIG I.V.

Dosage Forms Injection: 150 units/mL (2 mL, 10 mL)

Rabies Virus Vaccine (RAY beez VYE rus vak SEEN)

Related Information

Immunization Guidelines *on page 1421*
Miscellaneous Vaccination Information *on page 1437*
Recommendations for Travelers *on page 1442*

Brand Names Imovax® Rabies I.D. Vaccine; Imovax® Rabies Vaccine

Synonyms HDCV; Human Diploid Cell Cultures Rabies Vaccine; Human Diploid Cell Cultures Rabies Vaccine (Intradermal use)

Therapeutic Category Vaccine, Inactivated Virus

Use Veterinarians, animal handlers, certain laboratory workers, and persons living in or visiting countries for longer than 1 month where rabies is a constant threat.

Complete pre-exposure prophylaxis does not eliminate the need for additional therapy with rabies vaccine after a rabies exposure. The Food and Drug Administration has not approved the I.D. use of rabies vaccine for postexposure prophylaxis. Recommendations for I.D. use of HDCV are currently being discussed. The decision for postexposure rabies vaccination

(Continued)

Rabies Virus Vaccine *(Continued)*

depends on the species of biting animal, the circumstances of biting incident, and the type of exposure (bite, saliva contamination of wound, and so on). The type of and schedule for postexposure prophylaxis depends upon the person's previous rabies vaccination status or the result of a previous or current serologic test for rabies antibody. For postexposure prophylaxis, rabies vaccine should always be administered I.M., **not** I.D.

Pregnancy Risk Factor C

Contraindications Developing febrile illness (during pre-exposure therapy only); allergy to neomycin, gentamicin, or amphotericin B

Warnings/Precautions Rabies vaccine is available only in I.M. form; cannot be given intradermally

Adverse Reactions

>10%:

Cardiovascular: Edema

Central nervous system: Dizziness, malaise, encephalomyelitis, transverse myelitis, fever, pain, headache, neuroparalytic reactions

Dermatologic: Itching, erythema

Gastrointestinal: Nausea, abdominal pain

Local: Local discomfort

Neuromuscular & skeletal: Myalgia

Drug Interactions Decreased effect with immunosuppressive agents, corticosteroids, antimalarial drugs (ie, chloroquine); persons on these drugs should receive RIG (3 doses/1 mL each) by the I.M. route

Stability Refrigerate; reconstituted vaccine should be used immediately

Mechanism of Action Rabies vaccine is an inactivated virus vaccine which promotes immunity by inducing an active immune response. The production of specific antibodies requires about 7-10 days to develop. Rabies immune globulin or antirabies serum, equine (ARS) is given in conjunction with rabies vaccine to provide immune protection until an antibody response can occur.

Pharmacodynamics/Kinetics

Onset of effect: I.M.: Rabies antibody appears in the serum within 7-10 days

Peak effect: Within 30-60 days and persists for at least 1 year

Usual Dosage

Pre-exposure prophylaxis: Two 1 mL doses I.M. 1 week apart, third dose 3 weeks after second. If exposure continues, booster doses can be given every 2 years, or an antibody titer determined and a booster dose given if the titer is inadequate.

Postexposure prophylaxis: All postexposure treatment should begin with immediate cleansing of the wound with soap and water

Persons not previously immunized as above: Rabies immune globulin 20 units/kg body weight, half infiltrated at bite site if possible, remainder I.M.; and 5 doses of rabies vaccine, 1 mL I.M., one each on days 0, 3, 7, 14, 28

Persons who have previously received postexposure prophylaxis with rabies vaccine, received a recommended I.M. pre-exposure series of rabies vaccine or have a previously documented rabies antibody titer considered adequate: Two doses of rabies vaccine, 1 mL I.M., one each on days 0 and 3

Reference Range Antibody titers ≥115 as determined by rapid fluorescent-focus inhibition test are indicative of adequate response; collect titers on day 28 postexposure

Additional Information Federal law requires that the date of administration, the vaccine manufacturer, lot number of vaccine, and the administering person's name, title and address be entered into the patient's permanent medical record

Dosage Forms Injection:

I.M. (HDCV): Rabies antigen 2.5 units/mL (1 mL)

Intradermal: Rabies antigen 0.25 units/mL (1 mL)

Racemic Amphetamine Sulfate *see* Amphetamine *on page 80*

Racemic Epinephrine *see* Epinephrine *on page 448*

Ramipril (ra MI pril)

Related Information

Angiotensin-Converting Enzyme Inhibitors Comparison *on page 1386*

Heart Failure: Management of Patients With Left-Ventricular Systolic Dysfunction *on page 1533*

Brand Names Altace™

Canadian/Mexican Brand Names Ramace® (Mexico); Tritace® (Mexico)

Therapeutic Category Angiotensin-Converting Enzyme (ACE) Inhibitors; Antihypertensive

Use Treatment of hypertension, alone or in combination with thiazide diuretics; treatment of congestive heart failure immediately after myocardial infarction (**Note:** This indication is based on a study involving 2006 patients; a decrease by

26% in all-cause mortality was observed when ramipril was administered 3-10 days after a myocardial infarction)

Pregnancy Risk Factor C (first trimester); D (second and third trimester)

Contraindications Hypersensitivity to ramipril or ramiprilat, or any other angiotensin-converting enzyme inhibitors

Warnings/Precautions Use with caution and modify dosage in patients with renal impairment (decrease dosage) (especially renal artery stenosis), severe congestive heart failure, or with coadministered diuretic; severe hypotension may occur in the elderly and patients who are sodium and/or volume depleted, initiate lower doses and monitor closely when starting therapy in these patients; should be discontinued if laryngeal stridor or angioedema of the face, tongue, or glottis is observed

Adverse Reactions

>10% Respiratory: Cough

1% to 10%:

- Cardiovascular: Tachycardia, chest pain, palpitations
- Central nervous system: Insomnia, headache, dizziness, fatigue, malaise
- Dermatologic: Rash, pruritus, alopecia
- Gastrointestinal: Abnormal taste, abdominal pain, vomiting, nausea, diarrhea, anorexia, constipation
- Neuromuscular & skeletal: Paresthesia
- Renal: Oliguria

<1%:

- Cardiovascular: Hypotension
- Dermatologic: Angioedema
- Endocrine & metabolic: Hyperkalemia
- Hematologic: Neutropenia, agranulocytosis
- Renal: Proteinuria; increased BUN/serum creatinine

Overdosage/Toxicology Mild hypotension has been the only toxic effect seen with acute overdose. Bradycardia may also occur; hyperkalemia occurs even with therapeutic doses, especially in patients with renal insufficiency and those taking NSAIDs.

Following initiation of essential overdose management, toxic symptom treatment and supportive treatment should be initiated. Hypotension usually responds to I.V. fluids or Trendelenburg positioning.

Drug Interactions See table.

Drug-Drug Interactions With ACEIs

Precipitant Drug	Drug (Category) and Effect	Description
Antacids	ACE Inhibitors: decreased	Decreased bioavailability of ACEIs. May be more likely with captopril. Separate administration times by 1-2 hours.
NSAIDs (indomethacin)	ACEIs: decreased	Reduced hypotensive effects of ACEIs. More prominent in low renin or volume dependent hypertensive patients.
Phenothiazines	ACEIs: increased	Pharmacologic effects of ACEIs may be increased.
ACEIs	Allopurinol: increased	Higher risk of hypersensitivity reaction possible when given concurrently. Three case reports of Stevens-Johnson syndrome with captopril.
ACEIs	Digoxin: increased	Increased plasma digoxin levels.
ACEIs	Lithium: increased	Increased serum lithium levels and symptoms of toxicity may occur.
ACEIs	Potassium preps/ potassium sparing diuretics increased	Coadministration may result in elevated potassium levels.

Mechanism of Action Ramipril is an angiotensin-converting enzyme (ACE) inhibitor which prevents the formation of angiotensin II from angiotensin I and exhibits pharmacologic effects that are similar to captopril. Ramipril must undergo enzymatic saponification by esterases in the liver to its biologically active metabolite, ramiprilat. The pharmacodynamic effects of ramipril result from the high-affinity, competitive, reversible binding of ramiprilat to angiotensin-converting enzyme thus preventing the formation of the potent vasoconstrictor angiotensin II. This isomerized enzyme-inhibitor complex has a slow rate of dissociation, which results in high potency and a long duration of action; a CNS mechanism may also be involved in the hypotensive effect as angiotensin II increases adrenergic outflow from CNS; vasoactive kallikreins may be decreased in conversion to active hormones by ACE inhibitors, thus reducing blood pressure

(Continued)

Ramipril *(Continued)*

Pharmacodynamics/Kinetics

Absorption: Well absorbed from GI tract (50% to 60%)

Distribution: Plasma levels decline in a triphasic fashion; rapid decline is a distribution phase to peripheral compartment, plasma protein and tissue ACE (half-life 2-4 hours); 2nd phase is an apparent elimination phase representing the clearance of free ramiprilat (half-life: 9-18 hours); and final phase is the terminal elimination phase representing the equilibrium phase between tissue binding and dissociation (half-life: >50 hours)

Metabolism: Hepatic to the active form, ramiprilat

Half-life: Ramiprilat: >50 hours

Time to peak serum concentration: ~1 hour

Elimination: Ramipril and its metabolites are eliminated primarily through the kidneys (60%) and feces (40%)

Usual Dosage Adults: Oral: 2.5-5 mg once daily, maximum: 20 mg/day

Dosing adjustment in renal impairment:

Cl_{cr} 10-50 mL/minute: Administer 50% to 75% of normal dose

Cl_{cr} <40 mL/minute: Patients should be started on 1.25 mg/day and titrated up to 5 mg/day maximum

Cl_{cr} <10 mL/minute: Administer 25% to 50% of normal dose

Test Interactions Increases BUN, creatinine, potassium, positive Coombs' [direct]; decreases cholesterol (S); may cause false-positive results in urine acetone determinations using sodium nitroprusside reagent

Patient Information Notify physician if vomiting, diarrhea, excessive perspiration, or dehydration should occur; also if swelling of face, lips, tongue, or difficulty in breathing occurs or if persistent cough develops

Nursing Implications May cause depression in some patients; discontinue if angioedema of the face, extremities, lips, tongue, or glottis occurs; watch for hypotensive effects within 1-3 hours of first dose or new higher dose; may be mixed in water, apple juice, or applesauce and will remain stable for 48 hours if refrigerated or 24 hours at room temperature

Dosage Forms Capsule: 1.25 mg, 2.5 mg, 5 mg, 10 mg

Ranitidine Bismuth Citrate (ra NI ti deen BIZ muth SIT rate)

Brand Names Tritec®

Synonyms GR1222311X; RBC

Therapeutic Category Gastrointestinal Agent, Miscellaneous; Histamine-2 Antagonist

Use In combination with clarithromycin for the treatment of active duodenal ulcer associated with *H. pylori* infection; not to be used as monotherapy

Pregnancy Risk Factor C

Contraindications Hypersensitivity to ranitidine or bismuth compounds or components; acute porphyria

Warnings/Precautions Avoid use in patients with Cl_{cr} <25 mL/minute; do not use for maintenance therapy or for >16 weeks/year

Adverse Reactions

>1%:

Central nervous system: Headache (14%), dizziness (1% to 2%)

Gastrointestinal: Diarrhea (9%), nausea/vomiting (3%), constipation, abdominal pain, gastric upset (<10%), darkening of the tongue and/or stool (60% to 70%), taste disturbance (11%)

Miscellaneous: Flu-like symptoms (2%)

<1%:

Dermatologic: Rash, pruritus

Hematologic: Anemia, thrombocytopenia

Hepatic: Elevated LFTs

Drug Interactions See individual monographs

Increased effect: Optimal antimicrobial effects of ranitidine bismuth citrate occur when the drug is taken with food

Mechanism of Action As a complex of ranitidine and bismuth citrate, gastric acid secretion is inhibited by histamine-blocking activity at the parietal cell and the structural integrity of *H. pylori* organisms is disrupted; additionally bismuth reduces the adherence of *H. pylori* to epithelial cells of the stomach and may exert a cytoprotectant effect, inhibiting pepsin, as well. Adequate eradication of *Helicobacter pylori* is achieved with the combination of clarithromycin.

Pharmacodynamics/Kinetics See individual monographs

Absorption:

Bismuth: Minimal systemic absorption (≤1%)

Ranitidine: 50% to 60% (dose-dependent)

Distribution: Ranitidine: 1.7 L/kg

Protein binding:

Bismuth: 90%

Ranitidine: 15%

Metabolism: Ranitidine: Metabolized to N-oxide, S-oxide, and N-desmethyl metabolites

Half-life:

Complex: 5-8 days

Bismuth: 11-28 days

Ranitidine: 3 hours

Time to peak serum concentration:

Bismuth: 1-2 hours

Ranitidine: 0.5-5 hours

Time to peak effect of complex: 1 week

Elimination:

Bismuth: Clearance: 50 mL/minute

Ranitidine: Clearance: 530 mL/minute

~30% of ranitidine and <1% of bismuth is excreted in the urine

Usual Dosage Adults: Oral: 400 mg twice daily for 4 weeks with clarithromycin 500 mg 3 times/day for first 2 weeks

Dosing adjustment in renal impairment: Not recommended with Cl_{cr} <25 mL/minute

Dosing adjustment in hepatic impairment: No dosage change necessary

Monitoring Parameters (13) C-urea breath tests to detect *H. pylori*, endoscopic evidence of ulcer healing, CBCs, LFTs, renal function tests

Patient Information Inform your physician immediately if signs of allergy occur; take medication with food, if possible

Dosage Forms Tablet: 400 mg (ranitidine 162 mg, trivalent bismuth 128 mg, and citrate 110 mg)

Ranitidine Hydrochloride (ra NI ti deen hye droe KLOR ide)

Related Information

Antacid Drug Interactions *on page 1388*

Brand Names Zantac®; Zantac® 75 [OTC]

Canadian/Mexican Brand Names Apo-Ranitidine® (Canada); Novo-Ranidine® (Canada); Nu-Ranit® (Canada); Acloral® (Mexico); Alter-H_2® (Mexico); Anistal® (Mexico); Azantac® (Mexico); Cauteridol® (Mexico); Credaxol® (Mexico); Galidrin® (Mexico); Gastrec® (Mexico); Microtid® (Mexico); Neugal® (Mexico); Ranifur® (Mexico); Ranisen® (Mexico); Zantac-C® (Canada)

Therapeutic Category Antihistamine, H_2 Blocker; Histamine-2 Antagonist

Use Short-term treatment of active duodenal ulcers and benign gastric ulcers; long-term prophylaxis of duodenal ulcer and gastric hypersecretory states, gastroesophageal reflux, recurrent postoperative ulcer, upper GI bleeding, prevention of acid-aspiration pneumonitis during surgery, and prevention of stress-induced ulcers; causes fewer interactions than cimetidine

Pregnancy Risk Factor B

Contraindications Hypersensitivity to ranitidine or any component

Warnings/Precautions Use with caution in children <12 years of age; use with caution in patients with liver and renal impairment; dosage modification required in patients with renal impairment; long-term therapy may cause vitamin B_{12} deficiency

Adverse Reactions

Endocrine & metabolic: Gynecomastia

Hepatic: Hepatitis

Neuromuscular & skeletal: Arthralgia

1% to 10%:

Central nervous system: Dizziness, sedation, malaise, headache, drowsiness

Dermatologic: Rash

Gastrointestinal: Constipation, nausea, vomiting, diarrhea

<1%:

Cardiovascular: Bradycardia, tachycardia

Central nervous system: Fever, confusion

Hematologic: Thrombocytopenia, neutropenia, agranulocytosis

Respiratory: Bronchospasm

Overdosage/Toxicology Symptoms of overdose include muscular tremors, vomiting, rapid respiration, renal failure, CNS depression; treatment is primarily symptomatic and supportive

Drug Interactions

Decreased effect: Variable effects on warfarin; antacids may decrease absorption of ranitidine; ketoconazole and itraconazole absorptions are decreased; may produce altered serum levels of procainamide and ferrous sulfate; decreased effect of nondepolarizing muscle relaxants, cefpodoxime, cyanocobalamin (decreased absorption), diazepam, oxaprozin

Decreased toxicity of atropine

(Continued)

Ranitidine Hydrochloride *(Continued)*

Increased toxicity of cyclosporine (increased serum creatinine), gentamicin (neuromuscular blockade), glipizide, glyburide, midazolam (increased concentrations), metoprolol, pentoxifylline, phenytoin, quinidine

Stability Ranitidine injection should be stored at 4°C to 30°C and protected from light; injection solution is a clear, colorless to yellow solution; slight darkening does not affect potency

Stability at room temperature:

Prepared bags: 2 days

Premixed bags: Manufacturer expiration dating and out of overwrap stability: 15 days

Stability of prepared bags at refrigeration temperature (4°C): 10 days

Solution for I.V. infusion in NS or D_5W is stable for 30 days when frozen; I.V. form is **incompatible** with amphotericin B, clindamycin, diazepam (same syringe), hetastarch (Y-line), hydroxyzine (same syringe), midazolam (same syringe), pentobarbital (same syringe), phenobarbital (same syringe)

Mechanism of Action Competitive inhibition of histamine at H_2-receptors of the gastric parietal cells, which inhibits gastric acid secretion, gastric volume and hydrogen ion concentration reduced

Pharmacodynamics/Kinetics

Absorption: Oral: 50% to 60%

Distribution: Minimally penetrates the blood-brain barrier; appears in breast milk

Protein binding: 15%

Metabolism: In the liver (<10%)

Half-life:

Children 3.5-16 years: 1.8-2 hours

Adults: 2-2.5 hours

End stage renal disease: 6-9 hours

Time to peak serum concentration: Oral: Within 1-3 hours and persisting for 8 hours

Elimination: Primarily in urine (35% as unchanged drug) and in feces

Usual Dosage Giving oral dose at 6 PM may be better than 10 PM bedtime, the highest acid production usually starts at approximately 7 PM, thus giving at 6 PM controls acid secretion better

Children:

Oral: 1.25-2.5 mg/kg/dose every 12 hours; maximum: 300 mg/day

I.M., I.V.: 0.75-1.5 mg/kg/dose every 6-8 hours, maximum daily dose: 400 mg

Continuous infusion: 0.1-0.25 mg/kg/hour (preferred for stress ulcer prophylaxis in patients with concurrent maintenance I.V.s or TPNs)

Adults:

Short-term treatment of ulceration: 150 mg/dose twice daily or 300 mg at bedtime

Prophylaxis of recurrent duodenal ulcer: Oral: 150 mg at bedtime

Gastric hypersecretory conditions:

Oral: 150 mg twice daily, up to 6 g/day

I.M., I.V.: 50 mg/dose every 6-8 hours (dose not to exceed 400 mg/day)

I.V.: 50 mg/dose IVPB every 6-8 hours (dose not to exceed 400 mg/day)

or

Continuous I.V. infusion: Initial: 50 mg IVPB, followed by 6.25 mg/hour titrated to gastric pH >4.0 for prophylaxis or >7.0 for treatment; **continuous I.V. infusion is preferred in patients with active bleeding**

Gastric hypersecretory conditions: Doses up to 2.5 mg/kg/hour (220 mg/hour) have been used

Dosing adjustment in renal impairment:

Cl_{cr} 10-50 mL/minute: Administer at 75% of normal dose or administer every 18-24 hours

Cl_{cr} <10 mL/minute: Administer at 50% of normal dose or administer every 18-24 hours

Hemodialysis: Slightly dialyzable (5% to 20%)

Dosing adjustment/comments in hepatic disease: Unchanged

Administration Ranitidine injection may be administered I.M. or I.V.

I.M.: Injection is given undiluted

I.V. must be diluted and may be administered IVP or IVPB or continuous I.V. infusion

IVP: Ranitidine (usually 50 mg) should be diluted to a total of 20 mL with NS or D_5W and administered over at least 5 minutes

IVPB: administer over 15-20 minutes

Continuous I.V. infusion: Administer at 6.25 mg/hour and titrate dosage based on gastric pH by continuous infusion over 24 hours

Monitoring Parameters AST, ALT, serum creatinine; when used to prevent stress-related GI bleeding, measure the intragastric pH and try to maintain pH

>4; signs and symptoms of peptic ulcer disease, occult blood with GI bleeding, monitor renal function to correct dose; monitor for side effects

Test Interactions False-positive urine protein using Multistix®, gastric acid secretion test, skin test allergen extracts, serum creatinine and serum transaminase concentrations, urine protein test

Patient Information It may take several days before this medicine begins to relieve stomach pain; antacids may be taken with ranitidine unless your physician has told you not to use them; wait 30-60 minutes between taking the antacid and ranitidine; may cause drowsiness, impair judgment, or coordination

Nursing Implications I.M. solution does not need to be diluted before use; monitor creatinine clearance for renal impairment; observe caution in patients with renal function impairment and hepatic function impairment

Dosage Forms

Capsule (GELdose™): 150 mg, 300 mg
Granules, effervescent (EFFERdose™): 150 mg
Infusion, preservative free, in NaCl 0.45%: 1 mg/mL (50 mL)
Injection: 25 mg/mL (2 mL, 10 mL, 40 mL)
Syrup (peppermint flavor): 15 mg/mL (473 mL)
Tablet: 75 mg [OTC]; 150 mg, 300 mg
Tablet, effervescent (EFFERdose™): 150 mg

RBC *see* Ranitidine Bismuth Citrate *on page 1094*

R & C® Shampoo [OTC] *see* Pyrethrins *on page 1079*

Rea-Lo® [OTC] *see* Urea *on page 1280*

Recombinant Human Deoxyribonuclease *see* Dornase Alfa *on page 419*

Recombinant plasminogen activator *see* Reteplase *on page 1100*

Recombivax HB® *see* Hepatitis B Vaccine *on page 607*

Recommendations for Preventing the Spread of Vancomycin Resistance *see page 1480*

Recommendations for Prophylaxis Against Tuberculosis *see page 1455*

Recommendations for Travelers *see page 1442*

Recommendations of the Advisory Committee on Immunization Practices (ACIP) *see page 1424*

Recommendations of the Advisory Council on the Elimination of Tuberculosis *see page 1483*

Recommended Childhood Immunization Schedule - US - January-December, 1997 *see page 1423*

Redisol® *see* Cyanocobalamin *on page 319*

Redux® *see* Dexfenfluramine *on page 360*

Reese's® Pinworm Medicine [OTC] *see* Pyrantel Pamoate *on page 1076*

Regitine® *see* Phentolamine *on page 988*

Reglan® *see* Metoclopramide *on page 824*

Regonol® *see* Pyridostigmine *on page 1079*

Regular (Concentrated) Iletin® II U-500 *see* Insulin Preparations *on page 659*

Regular Iletin® I *see* Insulin Preparations *on page 659*

Regular Insulin *see* Insulin Preparations *on page 659*

Regular Purified Pork Insulin *see* Insulin Preparations *on page 659*

Regulax SS® [OTC] *see* Docusate *on page 415*

Reguloid® [OTC] *see* Psyllium *on page 1075*

Rela® *see* Carisoprodol *on page 209*

Relafen® *see* Nabumetone *on page 867*

Relaxadon® *see* Hyoscyamine, Atropine, Scopolamine, and Phenobarbital *on page 637*

Relief® Ophthalmic Solution *see* Phenylephrine *on page 989*

Remeron® *see* Mirtazapine *on page 844*

Remifentanil (rem i FEN ta nil)

Related Information

Narcotic Agonists Comparison *on page 1414*

Brand Names Ultiva®

Synonyms GI87084B

Therapeutic Category Analgesic, Narcotic

Use Analgesic for use during general anesthesia for continued analgesia

Contraindications Not for intrathecal or epidural administration, due to the presence of glycine in the formulation, it is also contraindicated in patients with a known hypersensitivity to remifentanil, fentanyl or fentanyl analogs; interruption of an infusion will result in offset of effects within 5-10 minutes; the discontinuation of remifentanil infusion should be preceded by the establishment of adequate postoperative analgesia orders, especially for patients in whom postoperative pain is anticipated

(Continued)

Remifentanil *(Continued)*

Warnings/Precautions Remifentanil is not recommended as the sole agent in general anesthesia, because the loss of consciousness cannot be assured and due to the high incidence of apnea, hypotension, tachycardia and muscle rigidity; it should be administered by individuals specifically trained in the use of anesthetic agents and should not be used in diagnostic or therapeutic procedures outside the monitored anesthesia setting; resuscitative and intubation equipment should be readily available

Adverse Reactions

>10%: Gastrointestinal: Nausea, vomiting

1% to 10%:

- Cardiovascular: Hypotension, bradycardia, tachycardia, hypertension
- Central nervous system: Dizziness, headache, agitation, fever
- Dermatologic: Pruritus
- Ocular: Visual disturbances
- Respiratory: Respiratory depression, apnea, hypoxia
- Miscellaneous: Shivering, postoperative pain

Overdosage/Toxicology Symptoms of overdose include apnea, chest wall rigidity, seizures, hypoxemia, hypotension and bradycardia

Support of patient's airway, establish an I.V. line, administer intravenous fluids and administer naloxone 2 mg I.V. (0.01 mg/kg for children) with repeat administration as needed up to a total of 10 mg; glycopyrrolate or atropine may be useful for the treatment of bradycardia or hypotension

Mechanism of Action Binds with stereospecific mu-opioid receptors at many sites within the CNS, increases pain threshold, alters pain reception, inhibits ascending pain pathways

Usual Dosage Adults: I.V. continuous infusion:

During induction: 0.5-1 mcg/kg/minute

During maintenance:

- With nitrous oxide (66%): 0.4 mcg/kg/minute (range: 0.1-2 mcg/kg/min)
- With isoflurane: 0.25 mcg/kg/minute (range: 0.05-2 mcg/kg/min)
- With propofol: 0.25 mcg/kg/minute (range: 0.05-2 mcg/kg/min)

Continuation as an analgesic in immediate postoperative period: 0.1 mcg/kg/minute (range: 0.025-0.2 mcg/kg/min)

Monitoring Parameters Respiratory and cardiovascular status, blood pressure, heart rate

Dosage Forms Powder for injection, lyophilized: 1 mg/3 mL vial, 2 mg/5 mL vial, 5 mg/10 mL vial

Renese® *see* Polythiazide *on page 1019*

ReoPro™ *see* Abciximab *on page 14*

Repan® *see* Butalbital Compound *on page 176*

Reposans-10® *see* Chlordiazepoxide *on page 252*

Resectisol® *see* Mannitol *on page 758*

Reserpine (re SER peen)

Related Information

Therapy of Hypertension *on page 1540*

Canadian/Mexican Brand Names Novo-Reserpine® (Canada)

Therapeutic Category Antihypertensive; Rauwolfia Alkaloid

Use Management of mild to moderate hypertension

Unlabeled use: Management of tardive dyskinesia

Pregnancy Risk Factor C

Contraindications Any ulcerative condition, mental depression, hypersensitivity to reserpine or any component

Warnings/Precautions Discontinue reserpine 7 days before electroshock therapy; use with caution in patients with impaired renal function or peptic ulcer disease, gallstones, and the elderly; at high doses, significant mental depression may occur; some products may contain tartrazine

Adverse Reactions

>10%:

- Central nervous system: Dizziness
- Gastrointestinal: Anorexia, diarrhea, xerostomia, nausea, vomiting
- Respiratory: Nasal congestion

1% to 10%:

- Cardiovascular: Peripheral edema, arrhythmias, bradycardia, chest pain
- Central nervous system: Headache
- Gastrointestinal: Black stools
- Genitourinary: Impotence
- Miscellaneous: Bloody vomit

<1%:

- Cardiovascular: Hypotension

Central nervous system: Drowsiness, fatigue, mental depression, parkinsonism
Dermatologic: Rash
Endocrine & metabolic: Sodium and water retention
Gastrointestinal: Increased gastric acid secretion
Genitourinary: Dysuria
Neuromuscular & skeletal: Trembling of hands/fingers

Overdosage/Toxicology Symptoms of overdose include hypotension, bradycardia, CNS depression, sedation, coma, hypothermia, miosis, tremors, diarrhea, vomiting

Hypotension usually responds to I.V. fluids or Trendelenburg positioning. If unresponsive to these measures, the use of a parenteral inotrope may be required (eg, norepinephrine 0.1-0.2 mcg/kg/minute titrated to response). Anticholinergic agents may be useful in reducing the parkinsonian effects and bradycardia.

Drug Interactions
Decreased effect of indirect-acting sympathomimetics
Increased effect/toxicity of MAO inhibitors, direct-acting sympathomimetics, and tricyclic antidepressants

Stability Protect oral dosage forms from light

Mechanism of Action Reduces blood pressure via depletion of sympathetic biogenic amines (norepinephrine and dopamine); this also commonly results in sedative effects

Pharmacodynamics/Kinetics
Onset of antihypertensive effect: Within 3-6 days
Duration: 2-6 weeks
Absorption: Oral: ~40%
Distribution: Crosses the placenta; appears in breast milk
Protein binding: 96%
Metabolism: Extensively in the liver, >90%
Half-life: 50-100 hours
Elimination: Principal excretion in feces (30% to 60%) and small amounts in urine (10%)

Usual Dosage Oral (full antihypertensive effects may take as long as 3 weeks):
Children: 0.01-0.02 mg/kg/24 hours divided every 12 hours; maximum dose: 0.25 mg/day
Adults: 0.1-0.25 mg/day in 1-2 doses; initial: 0.5 mg/day for 1-2 weeks; maintenance: reduce to 0.1-0.25 mg/day
Elderly: Initial: 0.05 mg once daily, increasing by 0.05 mg every week as necessary

Dosing adjustment in renal impairment: Cl_{cr} <10 mL/minute: Avoid use
Dialysis: Not removed by hemo or peritoneal dialysis; supplemental dose is not necessary

Monitoring Parameters Blood pressure, standing and sitting/supine

Test Interactions ↓ catecholamines (U)

Patient Information Take with food or milk; impotency is reversible; notify physician if a weight gain of more than 5 lb has taken place during therapy; may cause drowsiness, may impair judgment and coordination

Nursing Implications Observe for mental depression and alert family members to report any symptoms

Dosage Forms Tablet: 0.1 mg, 0.25 mg

Respa-DM® *see* Guaifenesin and Dextromethorphan *on page 591*

Respa-GF® *see* Guaifenesin *on page 589*

Respbid® *see* Theophylline Salts *on page 1207*

RespiGam® *see* Respiratory Syncytial Virus Immune Globulin (Intravenous) *on this page*

Respiratory Syncytial Virus Immune Globulin (Intravenous)

(RES peer rah tor ee sin SISH al VYE rus i MYUN GLOB yoo lin in tra VEE nus)

Brand Names RespiGam®

Synonyms RSV-IGIV

Therapeutic Category Immune Globulin

Use Prevention of serious lower respiratory infection caused by respiratory syncytial virus (RSV) in children <24 months of age with bronchopulmonary dysplasia (BPD) or a history of premature birth (≤35 weeks gestation)

Pregnancy Risk Factor C

Contraindications Selective IgA deficiency; history of severe prior reaction to any immunoglobulin preparation

Warnings/Precautions Use caution to avoid fluid overload in patients, particularly infants with BPD, when administering RSV-IGIV; hypersensitivity including anaphylaxis or angioneurotic edema may occur; keep epinephrine 1:1000 readily

(Continued)

Respiratory Syncytial Virus Immune Globulin (Intravenous) *(Continued)*

available during infusion; rare occurrences of aseptic meningitis syndrome have been associated with IGIV treatment, particularly with high doses; observe carefully for signs and symptoms of such and treat promptly

Adverse Reactions

1% to 10%:

- Dermatologic: Rash
- Cardiovascular: Tachycardia, hypertension, hypotension
- Central nervous system: Fever (6%)
- Endocrine & metabolic: Fluid overload
- Gastrointestinal: Vomiting, diarrhea, gastroenteritis
- Local: Injection site inflammation
- Respiratory: Respiratory distress, wheezing, rales, hypoxia, tachypnea

<1%:

- Cardiovascular: Edema, pallor, heart murmur, cyanosis, flushing, palpitations, chest tightness
- Central nervous system: Dizziness, anxiety
- Dermatologic: Eczema, pruritus
- Gastrointestinal: Abdominal cramps
- Neuromuscular & skeletal: Myalgia, arthralgia
- Respiratory: Cough, rhinorrhea, dyspnea

Overdosage/Toxicology Likely symptoms of overdose include those associated with fluid overload; treatment is supportive (eg, diuretics)

Drug Interactions

Decreased toxicity: Antibodies present in IVIG preparations may interfere with the immune response to live virus vaccines (eg, MMR); reimmunization is recommended if such vaccines are administered within 10 months following RSV-IVIG treatment; additionally, it is advised that booster doses of oral polio, DPT, and HIB be considered 3-4 months after the last dose of RSV-IVIG in order to ensure immunity

Stability Store between 2°C and 8°C; do not freeze or shake vial; avoid foaming; discard after single use since it is preservative free

Mechanism of Action RSV-IGIV is a sterile liquid immunoglobulin G containing neutralizing antibody to respiratory syncytial virus. It is effective in reducing the incidence and duration of RSV hospitalization and the severity of RSV illness in high risk infants.

Usual Dosage I.V.: 750 mg/kg/month according to the following infusion schedule:

1.5 mL/kg/hour for 15 minutes, then at 3 mL/kg/hour for the next 15 minutes if the clinical condition does not contraindicate a higher rate, and finally, administer at 6 mL/kg/hour until completion of dose

Monitoring Parameters Monitor for symptoms of allergic reaction; check vital signs, cardiopulmonary status after each rate increase and thereafter at 30-minute intervals until 30 minutes following completion of the infusion

Nursing Implications Observe for signs of intolerance during and after infusion; administer through an I.V. line using a constant infusion pump and through a separate I.V. line, if possible; begin infusion within 6 hours and complete within 12 hours after entering the vial; if needed, RSV-IGIV may be "piggy-backed" into dextrose with or without saline solutions, avoiding dilutions >2:1 with such line configurations

Additional Information Each vial contains 1 to 1.5 mEq sodium

Dosage Forms Injection: 2500 mg RSV immunoglobulin/50 mL vial

Restoril® *see* Temazepam *on page 1190*

Reteplase (RE ta plase)

Brand Names Retevase®

Synonyms Recombinant plasminogen activator; r-PA

Therapeutic Category Thrombolytic Agent

Use Improvement of ventricular function following acute myocardial infarction, for the reduction of the incidence of CHF and the reduction of mortality associated with acute myocardial infarction

Pregnancy Risk Factor C

Contraindications Active internal bleeding, history of cerebrovascular accident, recent intracranial or intraspinal surgery or trauma, intracranial neoplasm, arteriovenous malformations or aneurysm, known bleeding diathesis, severe uncontrolled hypertension, history of severe allergic reactions to reteplase, alteplase, anistreplase or streptokinase

Adverse Reactions

>10%:

- Cardiovascular: Hypotension, arrhythmias, trauma arrhythmias

Hematologic: Bleeding

1% to 10%: Hematologic: Anemia, genitourinary bleeding, gastrointestinal bleeding, injection site bleeding

<1%:

Central nervous system: Intracranial hemorrhage

Miscellaneous: Allergic reactions, anaphylaxis

Overdosage/Toxicology Symptoms of overdose include increased incidence of intracranial bleeding

Drug Interactions

Increased effect: Anticoagulants, aspirin, ticlopidine, dipyridamole, abciximab and heparin are at least additive

Stability Dosage kits should be stored at 2°C to 25°C (36°F to 77°F) and remain sealed until use in order to protect from light

Mechanism of Action Reteplase is a nonglycosylated form of tPA produced by recombinant DNA technology using *E. coli*; it initiates local fibrinolysis by binding to fibrin in a thrombus (clot) and converts entrapped plasminogen to plasmin

Pharmacodynamics/Kinetics

Onset: 30-90 minutes

Half-life: 13-16 minutes

Elimination: Hepatic and renal, cleared from the plasma at a rate of 250-450 mL/minute

Usual Dosage

Children: Not recommended

Adults: 10 units I.V. over 2 minutes, followed by a second dose 30 minutes later of 10 units I.V. over 2 minutes

Withhold second dose if serious bleeding or anaphylaxis occurs

Administration Reteplase should be reconstituted using the diluent, syringe, needle and dispensing pin provided with each kit and the each reconstituted dose should be given I.V. over 2 minutes; no other medication should be added to the injection solution

Monitoring Parameters Monitor for signs of bleeding (hematuria, GI bleeding, gingival bleeding)

Additional Information The dosage of reteplase in clinical trials was expressed in terms of million unit (MU); however, reteplase is being marketed in units (U) with 1 unit equivalent to 1 million units, reteplase units are expressed using a reference standard specific for reteplase and are not comparable with units used for other thrombolytic agents, 10 units is equivalent to 17.4 mg

Dosage Forms

Injection: Powder in vials, each vial contains reteplase 10.8 units; supplied with 2 mL diluent (preservative free)

Retevase® *see* Reteplase *on previous page*

Retin-A™ Micro Topical *see* Tretinoin, Topical *on page 1254*

Retin-A™ Topical *see* Tretinoin, Topical *on page 1254*

Retinoic Acid *see* Tretinoin, Topical *on page 1254*

Retrovir® *see* Zidovudine *on page 1320*

Reversol® *see* Edrophonium *on page 439*

Revex® *see* Nalmefene *on page 875*

Rēv-Eyes™ *see* Dapiprazole *on page 342*

ReVia® Oral *see* Naltrexone *on page 877*

Rezine® *see* Hydroxyzine *on page 634*

Rezulin® *see* Troglitazone *on page 1272*

R-Gel® [OTC] *see* Capsaicin *on page 197*

R-Gen® *see* Iodinated Glycerol *on page 670*

R-Gene® *see* Arginine *on page 100*

rGM-CSF *see* Sargramostim *on page 1125*

Rheaban® [OTC] *see* Attapulgite *on page 118*

Rheomacrodex® *see* Dextran *on page 363*

Rhesonativ® *see* Rh_o(D) Immune Globulin *on this page*

Rheumatrex® *see* Methotrexate *on page 806*

Rhinall® Nasal Solution [OTC] *see* Phenylephrine *on page 989*

Rhindecon® *see* Phenylpropanolamine *on page 991*

Rhinocort™ *see* Budesonide *on page 168*

Rhinosyn-DMX® [OTC] *see* Guaifenesin and Dextromethorphan *on page 591*

Rh_o(D) Immune Globulin (ar aych oh (dee) i MYUN GLOB yoo lin)

Brand Names Gamulin® Rh; HypRho®-D; HypRho®-D Mini-Dose; MICRhoGAM™; Mini-Gamulin® Rh; Rhesonativ®; RhoGAM™

Therapeutic Category Immune Globulin

Use Prevention of isoimmunization in Rh-negative individuals exposed to Rh-positive blood during delivery of an Rh-positive infant, as a result of an abortion,

(Continued)

Rh_o(D) Immune Globulin *(Continued)*

following amniocentesis or abdominal trauma, or following a transfusion accident; prevention of hemolytic disease of the newborn if there is a subsequent pregnancy with an Rh-positive fetus

Pregnancy Risk Factor C

Contraindications Rh_o(D)-positive patient; known hypersensitivity to immune globulins or to thimerosal; transfusion of Rh_o(D)-positive blood in previous 3 months; prior sensitization to Rh_o(D)

Warnings/Precautions Use with caution in patients with thrombocytopenia or bleeding disorders, patients with IgA deficiency; do not inject I.V.; do not administer to neonates

Adverse Reactions

<1%:

- Central nervous system: Lethargy
- Gastrointestinal: Splenomegaly
- Hepatic: Elevated bilirubin
- Local: Pain at the injection site
- Neuromuscular & skeletal: Myalgia
- Miscellaneous: Temperature elevation

Stability Reconstituted solution should be refrigerated and will remain stable for 30 days; solution that have been frozen should be discarded

Mechanism of Action Suppresses the immune response and antibody formation of Rh-negative individuals to Rh-positive red blood cells

Pharmacodynamics/Kinetics

Distribution: Appears in breast milk; however, not absorbed by the nursing infant

Half-life: 23-26 days

Usual Dosage Adults (administered I.M. to mothers **not** to infant) I.M.:

Obstetrical usage: 1 vial (300 mcg) prevents maternal sensitization if fetal packed red blood cell volume that has entered the circulation is <15 mL; if it is more, give additional vials. The number of vials = RBC volume of the calculated fetomaternal hemorrhage divided by 15 mL

Postpartum prophylaxis: 300 mcg within 72 hours of delivery

Antepartum prophylaxis: 300 mcg at approximately 26-28 weeks gestation; followed by 300 mcg within 72 hours of delivery if infant is Rh-positive

Following miscarriage, abortion, or termination of ectopic pregnancy at up to 13 weeks of gestation: 50 mcg ideally within 3 hours, but may be given up to 72 hours after; if pregnancy has been terminated at 13 or more weeks of gestation, administer 300 mcg

Administration Administer I.M. in deltoid muscle; do **not** administer I.V.; the total volume can be given in divided doses at different sites at one time or may be divided and given at intervals, provided the total dosage is given within 72 hours of the fetomaternal hemorrhage or transfusion.

Patient Information Acetaminophen may be taken to ease minor discomfort after vaccination

Dosage Forms

Injection: Each package contains one single dose 300 mcg of Rh_o (D) immune globulin

Injection, microdose: Each package contains one single dose of microdose, 50 mcg of Rh_o (D) immune globulin

Rh_o(D) Immune Globulin (Intravenous-Human)

(ar aych oh (dee) i MYUN GLOB yoo lin in tra VEE nus HYU man)

Brand Names WinRho SD®

Synonyms RhoIGIV

Therapeutic Category Immune Globulin

Use

Prevention of Rh isoimmunization in nonsensitized Rh_o(D) antigen-negative women within 7 hours after spontaneous or induced abortion, amniocentesis, chorionic villus sampling, ruptured tubal pregnancy, abdominal trauma, transplacental hemorrhage, or in the normal course of pregnancy unless the blood type of the fetus or father is known to be Rh_o(D) antigen-negative.

Suppression of Rh isoimmunization in Rh_o(D) antigen-negative female children and female adults in their childbearing years transfused with Rh_o(D) antigen-positive RBCs or blood components containing Rh_o(D) antigen-positive RBCs

Treatment of immune thrombocytopenic purpura (ITP) in nonsplenectomized Rh_o(D) antigen-positive patients

Pregnancy Risk Factor C

Contraindications Hypersensitivity to immune globulin or any component, IgA deficiency

Warnings/Precautions Anaphylactic hypersensitivity reactions can occur; studies indicate that there is no discernible risk of transmitting HIV or hepatitis B; do not administer by S.C. route; use only the I.V. route when treating ITP

Adverse Reactions

1% to 10%:

- Central nervous system: Headache, fever, chills
- Hematologic: Hemolysis (Hg decrease of >2 g/dL in 5% to 10% of ITP patients)
- Local: Slight edema and pain at the injection site

Overdosage/Toxicology No symptoms are likely, however, high doses have been associated with a mild, transient hemolytic anemia; treatment supportive

Drug Interactions

Increased toxicity: Live virus, vaccines (measles, mumps, rubella); do not administer within 3 months after administration of these vaccines

Stability Store at 2°C to 8°C; do not freeze; if not used immediately, store the product at room temperature for 4 hours; do not freeze the reconstituted product; use within 4 hours; discard unused portions

Mechanism of Action The Rh_o(D) antigen is responsible for most cases of Rh sensitization, which occurs when Rh-positive fetal RBCs enter the maternal circulation of an Rh-negative woman. Injection of anti-D globulin results in opsonization of the fetal RBCs, which are then phagocytized in the spleen, preventing immunization of the mother. Injection of anti-D into an Rh-positive patient with ITP coats the patient's own D+ RBCs with antibody and, as they are cleared by the spleen, they saturate the capacity of the spleen to clear antibody-coated cells, sparing antibody-coated platelets. Other proposed mechanisms involve the generation of cytokines following the interaction between antibody-coated RBCs and macrophages.

Pharmacodynamics/Kinetics

Half-life: 24-30 days

Time to peak serum concentration: Peak levels achieved in 2 hours

Usual Dosage

Prevention of Rh isoimmunization: I.V.: 1500 units (300 mcg) at 28 weeks gestation or immediately after amniocentesis if before 34 weeks gestation or after chorionic villus sampling; repeat this dose every 12 weeks during the pregnancy, 600 units (120 mcg) at delivery (within 72 hours) and after invasive intrauterine procedures such as abortion, amniocentesis, or any other manipulation if at >34 weeks gestation. **Note:** If the Rh status of the baby is not known at 72 hours, administer Rh_o(D) immune globulin to the mother at 72 hours after delivery. If >72 hours have elapsed, do not withhold Rh_o(D) immune globulin, but administer as soon as possible, up to 28 days after delivery.

I.M.: Reconstitute vial with 1.25 mL and administer as above

Transfusion: Administer within 72 hours after exposure for treatment of incompatible blood transfusions or massive fetal hemorrhage as follows:

- I.V.: 3000 units (600 mcg) every 8 hours until the total dose is administered (45 units [9 mcg] of Rh+ blood/mL blood; 90 units [18 mcg] Rh+ red cells/mL cells)
- I.M.: 6000 units [1200 mcg] every 12 hours until the total dose is administered (60 units [12 mcg] of Rh+ blood/mL blood; 120 units [24 mcg] Rh+ red cells/mL cells)

Treatment of ITP: I.V.: Initial: 25-50 mcg/kg depending on the patient's Hg concentration; maintenance: 25-60 mcg/kg depending on the clinical response

Administration The product should not be shaken when reconstituting or transporting; reconstitute the product shortly before use with NS, according to the manufacturer's guidelines; do not administer with other products

Nursing Implications Increasing the time of infusion from 1-3 minutes to 15-20 minutes may also help; pretreatment with acetaminophen, diphenhydramine, or prednisone can prevent the fever/chill reaction

Additional Information Rh_o(D) is IgA-depleted and is unlikely to cause an anaphylactic reaction in women with IgA deficiency and anti-IgA antibodies. Although immune globulins for I.M. use, manufactured in the U.S. have never been found to transmit any viral infection, Rh_o(D) is the only Rh_o(D) preparation treated with highly effective solvent detergent method of viral inactivation for hepatitis C, HIV, and hepatitis B; treatment of ITP in Rh+ patients with an intact spleen appears to be about as effective as IVIG

Dosage Forms Injection: 600 units [120 mcg], 1500 units [300 mcg] with 2.5 mL diluent

RhoGAM™ *see* Rh_o(D) Immune Globulin *on page 1101*

RhoIGIV *see* Rh_o(D) Immune Globulin (Intravenous-Human) *on previous page*

rHuEPO-α *see* Epoetin Alfa *on page 451*

Rhulicaine® [OTC] *see* Benzocaine *on page 138*

Rhythmin® *see* Procainamide *on page 1046*

Ribavirin (rye ba VYE rin)

Brand Names Virazole®

Synonyms RTCA; Tribavirin

Therapeutic Category Antiviral Agent, Inhalation Therapy

Use Treatment of patients with respiratory syncytial virus (RSV) infections; may also be used in other viral infections including influenza A and B and adenovirus; specially indicated for treatment of severe lower respiratory tract RSV infections in patients with an underlying compromising condition (prematurity, bronchopulmonary dysplasia and other chronic lung conditions, congenital heart disease, immunodeficiency, immunosuppression), and recent transplant recipients

Pregnancy Risk Factor X

Contraindications Females of childbearing age

Warnings/Precautions Use with caution in patients requiring assisted ventilation because precipitation of the drug in the respiratory equipment may interfere with safe and effective patient ventilation; monitor carefully in patients with COPD and asthma for deterioration of respiratory function. Ribavirin is potentially mutagenic, tumor-promoting, and gonadotoxic.

Adverse Reactions

1% to 10%:

- Central nervous system: Fatigue, headache, insomnia
- Gastrointestinal: Nausea, anorexia
- Hematologic: Anemia

<1%:

- Cardiovascular: Hypotension, cardiac arrest, digitalis toxicity
- Dermatologic: Rash, skin irritation
- Ocular: Conjunctivitis
- Respiratory: Mild bronchospasm, worsening of respiratory function, apnea

Drug Interactions Decreased effect of zidovudine

Stability Do not use any water containing an antimicrobial agent to reconstitute drug; reconstituted solution is stable for 24 hours at room temperature

Mechanism of Action Inhibits replication of RNA and DNA viruses; inhibits influenza virus RNA polymerase activity and inhibits the initiation and elongation of RNA fragments resulting in inhibition of viral protein synthesis

Pharmacodynamics/Kinetics

Absorption: Absorbed systemically from the respiratory tract following nasal and oral inhalation; absorption is dependent upon respiratory factors and method of drug delivery; maximal absorption occurs with the use of the aerosol generator via an endotracheal tube; highest concentrations are found in the respiratory tract and erythrocytes

Metabolism: Occurs intracellularly and may be necessary for drug action

Half-life, plasma:

- Children: 6.5-11 hours
- Adults: 24 hours, much longer in the erythrocyte (16-40 days), which can be used as a marker for intracellular metabolism

Time to peak serum concentration: Inhalation: Within 60-90 minutes

Elimination: Hepatic metabolism is major route of elimination with 40% of the drug cleared renally as unchanged drug and metabolites

Usual Dosage Infants, Children, and Adults:

Aerosol inhalation: Use with Viratek® small particle aerosol generator (SPAG-2) at a concentration of 20 mg/mL (6 g reconstituted with 300 mL of sterile water without preservatives)

Aerosol only: 12-18 hours/day for 3 days, up to 7 days in length

Monitoring Parameters Respiratory function, CBC, reticulocyte count, I & O

Nursing Implications Keep accurate I & O record, discard solutions placed in the SPAG-2 unit at least every 24 hours and before adding additional fluid; healthcare workers who are pregnant or who may become pregnant should be advised of the potential risks of exposure and counseled about risk reduction strategies including alternate job responsibilities; ribavirin may adsorb to contact lenses

Dosage Forms Powder for aerosol: 6 g (100 mL)

Riboflavin (RYE boe flay vin)

Brand Names Riobin®

Synonyms Lactoflavin; Vitamin B_2; Vitamin G

Therapeutic Category Vitamin, Water Soluble

Use Prevent riboflavin deficiency and treat ariboflavinosis

Pregnancy Risk Factor A (C if dose exceeds RDA recommendation)

Warnings/Precautions Riboflavin deficiency often occurs in the presence of other B vitamin deficiencies

Drug Interactions Decreased absorption with probenecid

Mechanism of Action Component of flavoprotein enzymes that work together, which are necessary for normal tissue respiration; also needed for activation of pyridoxine and conversion of tryptophan to niacin

Pharmacodynamics/Kinetics

Absorption: Readily via GI tract, however, food increases extent of GI absorption; GI absorption is decreased in patients with hepatitis, cirrhosis, or biliary obstruction

Metabolism: Metabolic fate unknown

Half-life, biologic: 66-84 minutes

Elimination: 9% excreted unchanged in urine

Usual Dosage Oral:

Riboflavin deficiency:

Children: 2.5-10 mg/day in divided doses

Adults: 5-30 mg/day in divided doses

Recommended daily allowance:

Children: 0.4-1.8 mg

Adults: 1.2-1.7 mg

Test Interactions Large doses may interfere with urinalysis based on spectrometry; may cause false elevations in fluorometric determinations of catecholamines and urobilinogen

Patient Information Take with food; large doses may cause bright yellow or orange urine

Additional Information Dietary sources of riboflavin include liver, kidney, dairy products, green vegetables, eggs, whole grain cereals, yeast, mushroom

Dosage Forms Tablet: 25 mg, 50 mg, 100 mg

Rid-A-Pain® [OTC] *see* Benzocaine *on page 138*

Ridaura® *see* Auranofin *on page 119*

RID® Shampoo [OTC] *see* Pyrethrins *on page 1079*

Rifabutin (rif a BYOO tin)

Related Information

Antimicrobial Drugs of Choice *on page 1468*

Guidelines for the Prevention of Opportunistic Infections in Persons with HIV *on page 1457*

Recommendations for Prophylaxis Against Tuberculosis *on page 1455*

Brand Names Mycobutin®

Synonyms Ansamycin

Therapeutic Category Antibiotic, Miscellaneous; Antitubercular Agent

Use Orphan drug status as adjunctive therapy for the prevention of disseminated *Mycobacterium avium-cellulare* complex (MAC) in patients with advanced HIV infection; studies have shown it to halve the risk of MAC bacteremia in patients with AIDS, to decrease the incidence of fever and fatigue, and prevent deterioration in performance status

Pregnancy Risk Factor B

Contraindications Hypersensitivity to rifabutin or any other rifamycins; rifabutin is contraindicated in patients with a WBC <1000/mm^3 or a platelet count <50,000 mm^3

Warnings/Precautions Rifabutin as a single agent must not be administered to patients with active tuberculosis since its use may lead to the development of tuberculosis that is resistant to both rifabutin and rifampin; rifabutin should be discontinued in patients with AST >500 units/L or if total bilirubin is >3 mg/dL. Use with caution in patients with liver impairment; modification of dosage should be considered in patients with renal impairment.

Adverse Reactions

>10%:

Dermatologic: Rash

Hematologic: Neutropenia, leukopenia

Genitourinary: Discolored urine

1% to 10%:

Central nervous system: Headache

Gastrointestinal: Vomiting, nausea, abdominal pain, diarrhea, anorexia, flatulence, eructation

Hematologic: Anemia, thrombocytopenia

Neuromuscular & skeletal: Myalgia

<1%:

Cardiovascular: Chest pain

Central nervous system: Fever, insomnia

Gastrointestinal: Dyspepsia, flatulence, nausea, vomiting, taste perversion

Overdosage/Toxicology Symptoms of overdose include nausea, vomiting, hepatotoxicity, lethargy, CNS depression; treatment is supportive; hemodialysis will remove rifabutin, its effect on outcome is unknown

(Continued)

Rifabutin *(Continued)*

Drug Interactions Decreased plasma concentration (due to induction of liver enzymes) of verapamil, methadone, digoxin, cyclosporine, corticosteroids, oral anticoagulants, theophylline, barbiturates, chloramphenicol, ketoconazole, oral contraceptives, quinidine, halothane

Mechanism of Action Inhibits DNA-dependent RNA polymerase at the beta subunit which prevents chain initiation

Pharmacodynamics/Kinetics

Absorption: Oral: Readily absorbed 53%

Distribution: V_d: 9.32 L/kg; distributes to body tissues including the lungs, liver, spleen, eyes, and kidneys

Protein binding: 85%

Metabolism: To active and inactive metabolites

Bioavailability: Absolute, 20% in HIV patients

Half life, terminal: 45 hours (range: 16-69 hours)

Peak serum level: Within 2-4 hours

Elimination: Renal and biliary clearance of unchanged drugs is 10%; 30% excreted in feces; 53% in urine as metabolites

Usual Dosage Oral:

Children: Efficacy and safety of rifabutin have not been established in children; a limited number of HIV-positive children with MAC have been given rifabutin for MAC prophylaxis; doses of 5 mg/kg/day have been useful

Adults: 300 mg once daily; for patients who experience gastrointestinal upset, rifabutin can be administered 150 mg twice daily with food

Administration Administer with meals

Monitoring Parameters Periodic liver function tests, CBC with differential, platelet count

Patient Information May discolor urine, tears, sweat, or other body fluids to a red-orange color; take 1 hour before or 2 hours after a meal on an empty stomach; soft contact lenses may be permanently stained; report to physician any severe or persistent flu-like symptoms, nausea, vomiting, dark urine or pale stools, or unusual bleeding or bruising; can be taken with meals or sprinkled on applesauce

Dosage Forms Capsule: 150 mg

Rifadin® *see* Rifampin *on this page*

Rifampicin *see* Rifampin *on this page*

Rifampin (RIF am pin)

Related Information

Antibiotic Treatment of Adults With Infectious Endocarditis *on page 1465*

Antimicrobial Drugs of Choice *on page 1468*

Bacterial Meningitis Practical Guidelines for Management *on page 1475*

Desensitization Protocols *on page 1496*

Guidelines for the Prevention of Opportunistic Infections in Persons with HIV *on page 1457*

Prophylaxis for Patients Exposed to Common Communicable Diseases *on page 1452*

Recommendations for Prophylaxis Against Tuberculosis *on page 1455*

Recommendations of the Advisory Council on the Elimination of Tuberculosis *on page 1483*

Brand Names Rifadin®; Rimactane®

Canadian/Mexican Brand Names Rifadin® (Canada); Rimactane® (Canada); Rofact® (Canada)

Synonyms Rifampicin

Therapeutic Category Antibiotic, Miscellaneous; Antitubercular Agent

Use Management of active tuberculosis; eliminate meningococci from asymptomatic carriers; prophylaxis of *Haemophilus influenzae* type b infection; used in combination with other anti-infectives in the treatment of staphylococcal infections

Pregnancy Risk Factor C

Contraindications Hypersensitivity to rifampin or any component

Warnings/Precautions Use with caution in patients with liver impairment; modification of dosage should be considered in patients with severe liver impairment; use with caution in patients with porphyria; monitor closely if intermittent therapy is used; hypersensitivity reactions and thrombocytopenia occur more frequently in this setting

Adverse Reactions

1% to 10%:

Gastrointestinal: Diarrhea, stomach cramps, fecal discoloration, discoloration of saliva (reddish orange)

Genitourinary: Discoloration of urine

Miscellaneous: Discoloration of sputum, sweat, and tears (reddish orange); fungal overgrowth

<1%:

Central nervous system: Drowsiness, fatigue, ataxia, confusion, fever, headache

Dermatologic: Rash, pruritus

Gastrointestinal: Nausea, vomiting, stomatitis

Hematologic: Eosinophilia, blood dyscrasias (leukopenia, thrombocytopenia)

Hepatic: Hepatitis

Local: Irritation at the I.V. site

Renal: Renal failure

Miscellaneous: Flu-like syndrome

Overdosage/Toxicology Symptoms of overdose include nausea, vomiting, hepatotoxicity, lethargy, CNS depression; treatment is supportive

Drug Interactions Inducer of cytochrome P-450 1A2, cytochrome P-450 2C, cytochrome P-450 2D6, and cytochrome P-450 3A

Decreased effect: Rifampin induces liver enzymes which may decrease the plasma concentration of verapamil, methadone, digoxin, cyclosporine, corticosteroids, oral anticoagulants, haloperidol, theophylline, barbiturates, chloramphenicol, ketoconazole, oral contraceptives, quinidine, halothane

Stability Rifampin powder is reddish brown. Intact vials should be stored at room temperature and protected from excessive heat and light. Reconstituted vials are stable for 24 hours at room temperature

Stability of parenteral admixture at room temperature (25°C) is 4 hours

Comments: Do not use sodium chloride as a diluent, rifampin has a reduced stability in NS

Mechanism of Action Inhibits bacterial RNA synthesis by binding to the beta subunit of DNA-dependent RNA polymerase, blocking RNA transcription

Pharmacodynamics/Kinetics

Absorption: Oral: Well absorbed

Time to peak serum concentration: Oral: 2-4 hours and persisting for up to 24 hours; food may delay or slightly reduce

Distribution: Crosses the blood-brain barrier well

Relative diffusion of antimicrobial agents from blood into cerebrospinal fluid (CSF): Adequate with or without inflammation (exceeds usual MICs)

Ratio of CSF to blood level (%):

Inflamed meninges: 25

Protein binding: 80%

Metabolism: Highly lipophilic; metabolized in the liver, undergoes enterohepatic recycling

Half-life: 3-4 hours, prolonged with hepatic impairment

End stage renal disease: 1.8-11 hours

Elimination: Undergoes enterohepatic recycling; principally excreted unchanged in the feces (60% to 65%) and urine (~30%); excreted unchanged: 15% to 30%; plasma rifampin concentrations are not significantly affected by hemodialysis or peritoneal dialysis

Usual Dosage I.V. infusion dose is the same as for the oral route

Tuberculosis therapy: Oral:

Note: A four-drug regimen (isoniazid, rifampin, pyrazinamide, and either streptomycin or ethambutol) is preferred for the initial, empiric treatment of TB. When the drug susceptibility results are available, the regimen should be altered as appropriate.

Patients with TB and without HIV infection:

OPTION 1:

Isoniazid resistance rate <4%: Administer daily isoniazid, rifampin, and pyrazinamide for 8 weeks followed by isoniazid and rifampin daily or directly observed therapy (DOT) 2-3 times/week for 16 weeks

If isoniazid resistance rate is not documented, ethambutol or streptomycin should also be administered until susceptibility to isoniazid or rifampin is demonstrated. Continue treatment for at least 6 months or 3 months beyond culture conversion.

OPTION 2: Administer daily isoniazid, rifampin, pyrazinamide, and either streptomycin or ethambutol for 2 weeks followed by DOT 2 times/week administration of the same drugs for 6 weeks, and subsequently, with isoniazid and rifampin DOT 2 times/week administration for 16 weeks

OPTION 3: Administer isoniazid, rifampin, pyrazinamide, and either ethambutol or streptomycin by DOT 3 times/week for 6 months

Patients with TB and with HIV infection:

Administer any of the above OPTIONS 1, 2 or 3, however, treatment should be continued for a total of 9 months and at least 6 months beyond culture conversion

(Continued)

Rifampin *(Continued)*

Note: Some experts recommend that the duration of therapy should be extended to 9 months for patients with disseminated disease, miliary disease, disease involving the bones or joints, or tuberculosis lymphadenitis

Infants and Children <12 years of age: Oral:

Daily therapy: 10-20 mg/kg/day in divided doses every 12-24 hours (maximum: 600 mg/day)

Directly observed therapy (DOT): Twice weekly: 10-20 mg/kg (maximum: 600 mg)

DOT: 3 times/week: 10-20 mg/kg (maximum: 600 mg)

Adults: Oral:

Daily therapy: 10 mg/kg/day (maximum: 600 mg/day)

Directly observed therapy (DOT): Twice weekly: 10 mg/kg (maximum: 600 mg)

DOT: 3 times/week: 10 mg/kg (maximum: 600 mg)

H. influenzae prophylaxis: Oral:

Infants and Children: 20 mg/kg/day every 24 hours for 4 days, not to exceed 600 mg/dose

Adults: 600 mg every 24 hours for 4 days

Meningococcal prophylaxis: Oral:

<1 month: 10 mg/kg/day in divided doses every 12 hours for 2 days

Infants and Children: 20 mg/kg/day in divided doses every 12 hours for 2 days

Adults: 600 mg every 12 hours for 2 days

Nasal carriers of *Staphylococcus aureus*: Oral:

Children: 15 mg/kg/day divided every 12 hours for 5-10 days in combination with other antibiotics

Adults: 600 mg/day for 5-10 days in combination with other antibiotics

Synergy for *Staphylococcus aureus* infections: Oral: Adults: 300-600 mg twice daily with other antibiotics

Dosing adjustment in hepatic impairment: Dose reductions are necessary to reduce hepatotoxicity

Administration Administer on an empty stomach (ie, 1 hour prior to, or 2 hours after meals) to increase total absorption

Monitoring Parameters Periodic monitoring of liver function (AST, ALT), CBC; hepatic status and mental status, sputum culture, chest x-ray 2-3 months into treatment

Test Interactions Positive Coombs' reaction [direct], inhibit standard assay's ability to measure serum folate and B_{12}

Patient Information May discolor urine, tears, sweat, or other body fluids to a red-orange color; take 1 hour before or 2 hours after a meal on an empty stomach; soft contact lenses may be permanently stained; report to physician any severe or persistent flu-like symptoms, nausea, vomiting, dark urine or pale stools, or unusual bleeding or bruising

Dosage Forms

Capsule: 150 mg, 300 mg

Injection: 600 mg

Extemporaneous Preparations Rifampin oral suspension can be compounded with simple syrup or wild cherry syrup at a concentration of 10 mg/mL; the suspension is stable for 4 weeks at room temperature or in a refrigerator when stored in a glass amber prescription bottle. However, there are some experts who do not recommend using rifampin syrup formulated from capsules due to conflicting reports indicating that the product is unstable (14.5% to 68% of labeled potency after preparation). It may be preferable to perform trituration, rather than simple mixing in syrup when preparing rifampin oral suspension.

Nahata MC, Morosco RS, and Hipple TF, "Effect of Preparation Method and Storage on Rifampin Concentration in Suspensions," *Ann Pharmacother*, 1994, 28(2):182-5.

rIFN-A *see* Interferon Alfa-2a *on page 663*

rIFN-b *see* Interferon Beta-1a *on page 668*

RIG *see* Rabies Immune Globulin (Human) *on page 1091*

Rilutek® *see* Riluzole *on this page*

Riluzole (RIL yoo zole)

Brand Names Rilutek®

Synonyms 2-Amino-6-Trifluoromethoxy-benzothiazole; RP54274

Therapeutic Category Miscellaneous Product

Use Amyotrophic lateral sclerosis (ALS): Treatment of patients with ALS; riluzole can extend survival or time to tracheostomy

Pregnancy Risk Factor C

Contraindications Severe hypersensitivity reactions to riluzole or any of the tablet components

Warnings/Precautions Among 4000 patients given riluzole for ALS, there were 3 cases of marked neutropenia (ANC <500/mm^3), all seen within the first 2 months of treatment. Use with caution in patients with concomitant renal insufficiency. Use with caution in patients with current evidence or history of abnormal liver function. Monitor liver chemistries.

Adverse Reactions

>10%:

Gastrointestinal: Nausea, abdominal pain, constipation

Hepatic: ALT (SGPT) elevations

Overdosage/Toxicology No specific antidote or treatment information available; treatment should be supportive and directed toward alleviating symptoms

Drug Interactions Cytochrome P-450 1A2 (CYP 1A2) substrate

Decreased effect: Drugs that induce CYP 1A2 (eg, cigarette smoke, charbroiled food, rifampin, omeprazole) could increase the rate of riluzole elimination

Increased toxicity: Inhibitors of CYP 1A2 (eg, caffeine, theophylline, amitriptyline, quinolones) could decrease the rate of riluzole elimination

Stability Protect from bright light

Mechanism of Action Inhibitory effect on glutamate release, inactivation of voltage-dependent sodium channels; and ability to interfere with intracellular events that follow transmitter binding at excitatory amino acid receptors

Pharmacodynamics/Kinetics

Absorption: Well absorbed (90%); a high fat meal decreases absorption of riluzole (decreasing AUC by 20% and peak blood levels by 45%)

Protein binding: 96% bound to plasma proteins, mainly albumin and lipoproteins

Metabolism: Extensively to 6 major and a number of minor metabolites. Metabolism is mostly hepatic and consists of cytochrome P-450 dependent hydroxylation and glucuronidation; principle isozyme is CYP 1A2

Bioavailability: Oral: Absolute (50%)

Usual Dosage Adults: Oral: 50 mg every 12 hours; no increased benefit can be expected from higher daily doses, but adverse events are increased

Dosage adjustment in smoking: Cigarette smoking is known to induce CYP 1A2; patients who smoke cigarettes would be expected to eliminate riluzole faster. There is no information, however, on the effect of, or need for, dosage adjustment in these patients.

Dosage adjustment in special populations: Females and Japanese patients may possess a lower metabolic capacity to eliminate riluzole compared with male and Caucasian subjects, respectively

Dosage adjustment in renal impairment: Use with caution in patients with concomitant renal insufficiency

Dosage adjustment in hepatic impairment: Use with caution in patients with current evidence or history of abnormal liver function indicated by significant abnormalities in serum transaminase, bilirubin or GGT levels. Baseline elevations of several LFTs (especially elevated bilirubin) should preclude use of riluzole.

Monitoring Parameters Monitor serum aminotransferases including ALT levels before and during therapy. Evaluate serum ALT levels every month during the first 3 months of therapy, every 3 months during the remainder of the first year and periodically thereafter. Evaluate ALT levels more frequently in patients who develop elevations. Maximum increases in serum ALT usually occurred within 3 months after the start of therapy and were usually transient when <5 x ULN.

In trials, if ALT levels were <5 x ULN, treatment continued and ALT levels usually returned to below 2 x ULN within 2-6 months. Treatment in studies was discontinued, however, if ALT levels exceed 5 x ULN, so that there is no experience with continued treatment of ALS patients once ALT values exceed 5 x ULN.

If a decision is made to continue treatment in patients when the ALT exceeds 5 x ULN, frequent monitoring (at least weekly) of complete liver function is recommended. Discontinue treatment if ALT exceeds 10 x ULN or if clinical jaundice develops.

Patient Information Take at least 1 hour before or 2 hours after a meal to avoid decreased bioavailability. Report any febrile illness to your physician. Take riluzole at the same time of the day each day. If a dose is missed, take the next tablet as originally planned.

Nursing Implications Warn patients about the potential for dizziness, vertigo or somnolence and advise them not to drive or operate machinery until they have gained sufficient experience on riluzole to gauge whether or not it affects their mental or motor performance adversely. Whether alcohol increases the risk of serious hepatotoxicity with riluzole is unknown; discourage riluzole-treated patients from drinking alcohol in excess.

(Continued)

Riluzole *(Continued)*

Additional Information May be obtained through Rhone-Poulenc Rorer Inc (Collegeville, PA) for compassionate use (through treatment IND process) by calling 800-727-6737 for treatment of amyotrophic lateral sclerosis; may be more effective for amyotrophic lateral sclerosis of bulbar onset; in animal models, riluzole was a potent inhibitor of seizures induced by ouabain

Dosage Forms Tablet: 50 mg

Rimactane® *see* Rifampin *on page 1106*

Rimantadine (ri MAN ta deen)

Related Information

Guidelines for the Prevention of Opportunistic Infections in Persons with HIV *on page 1457*

Brand Names Flumadine®

Synonyms Rimantadine Hydrochloride

Therapeutic Category Antiviral Agent, Oral

Use Prophylaxis (adults and children >1 year) and treatment (adults) of influenza A viral infection

Pregnancy Risk Factor C

Pregnancy/Breast-Feeding Implications Embryotoxic in high dose rat studies; avoid use in nursing mothers due to potential adverse effect in infants; rimantadine is concentrated in milk

Contraindications Hypersensitivity to drugs of the adamantine class, including rimantadine and amantadine

Warnings/Precautions Use with caution in patients with renal and hepatic dysfunction; avoid use, if possible, in patients with recurrent and eczematoid dermatitis, uncontrolled psychosis, or severe psychoneurosis. An increase in seizure incidence may occur in patients with seizure disorders; discontinue drug if seizures occur; consider the development of resistance during rimantadine treatment of the index case as likely if failure of rimantadine prophylaxis among family contact occurs and if index case is a child; viruses exhibit cross-resistance between amantadine and rimantadine.

Adverse Reactions

1% to 10%:

- Cardiovascular: Orthostatic hypotension, edema
- Central nervous system: Dizziness, confusion, headache, insomnia, difficulty in concentrating, anxiety, restlessness, irritability, hallucinations; incidence of CNS side effects may be less than that associated with amantadine
- Gastrointestinal: Nausea, vomiting, xerostomia, abdominal pain, anorexia
- Genitourinary: Urinary retention

Overdosage/Toxicology Agitation, hallucinations, ventricular cardiac arrhythmias (torsade de pointes and PVCs), slurred speech, anticholinergic effects (dry mouth, urinary retention and mydriasis), ataxia, tremor, myoclonus, seizures and death have been reported with amantadine, a related drug

Treatment is symptomatic (do not use physostigmine); tachyarrhythmias may be treated with beta-blockers such as propranolol; dialysis is not recommended except possibly in renal failure

Drug Interactions

- Acetaminophen: Reduction in AUC and peak concentration of rimantadine
- Aspirin: Peak plasma and AUC concentrations of rimantadine are reduced
- Cimetidine: Rimantadine clearance is decreased (~16%)

Mechanism of Action Exerts its inhibitory effect on three antigenic subtypes of influenza A virus (H1N1, H2N2, H3N2) early in the viral replicative cycle, possibly inhibiting the uncoating process; it has no activity against influenza B virus and is 2- to 8-fold more active than amantadine

Pharmacodynamics/Kinetics

- Absorption: Tablet and syrup formulations are equally absorbed; T_{max}: 6 hours
- Metabolism: Extensive in the liver
- Half-life: 25.4 hours (increased in elderly)
- Elimination: <25% of dose excreted in urine as unchanged drug; hemodialysis does not contribute to the clearance of rimantadine; no data exist establishing a correlation between plasma concentration and antiviral effect

Usual Dosage Oral:

Prophylaxis:

- Children <10 years: 5 mg/kg once daily; maximum: 150 mg
- Children >10 years and Adults: 100 mg twice daily; decrease to 100 mg/day in elderly or in patients with severe hepatic or renal impairment (Cl_{cr} ≤10 mL/minute)

Treatment: Adults: 100 mg twice daily; decrease to 100 mg/day in elderly or in patients with severe hepatic or renal impairment (Cl_{cr} ≤10 mL/minute)

Administration Initiation of rimantadine within 48 hours of the onset of influenza A illness halves the duration of illness and significantly reduces the duration of viral shedding and increased peripheral airways resistance; continue therapy for 5-7 days after symptoms begin

Monitoring Parameters Monitor for CNS or GI effects in elderly or patients with renal or hepatic impairment

Dosage Forms

Syrup, as hydrochloride: 50 mg/5 mL (60 mL, 240 mL, 480 mL)

Tablet, as hydrochloride: 100 mg

Rimantadine Hydrochloride *see* Rimantadine *on previous page*

Rimexolone (ri MEKS oh lone)

Brand Names Vexol®

Therapeutic Category Anti-inflammatory Agent, Ophthalmic; Corticosteroid, Ophthalmic

Use Treatment of inflammation after ocular surgery and the treatment of anterior uveitis

Pregnancy Risk Factor C

Contraindications Fungal, viral, or untreated pus-forming bacterial ocular infections; hypersensitivity to any component

Warnings/Precautions Prolonged use has been associated with the development of corneal or scleral perforation and posterior subcapsular cataracts; may mask or enhance the establishment of acute purulent untreated infections of the eye; effectiveness and safety have not been established in children

Adverse Reactions

1% to 10%: Ocular: Temporary mild blurred vision

<1%: Ocular: Stinging, burning eyes, corneal thinning, increased intraocular pressure, glaucoma, damage to the optic nerve, defects in visual activity, cataracts, secondary ocular infection

Overdosage/Toxicology Systemic toxicity is unlikely from the ophthalmic preparation

Mechanism of Action Decreases inflammation by suppression of migration of polymorphonuclear leukocytes and reversal of increased capillary permeability

Pharmacodynamics/Kinetics

Absorption: Through aqueous humor

Metabolism: Any drug absorbed is metabolized in the liver

Elimination: By the kidneys and feces

Usual Dosage Adults: Ophthalmic: Instill 1 drop in conjunctival sac 2-4 times/day up to every 4 hours; may use every 1-2 hours during first 1-2 days

Monitoring Parameters Intraocular pressure and periodic examination of lens (with prolonged use)

Patient Information Shake well before using, do not touch dropper to the eye

Dosage Forms Suspension, ophthalmic: 1% (5 mL, 10 mL)

Riobin® *see* Riboflavin *on page 1104*

Risperdal® *see* Risperidone *on this page*

Risperidone (ris PER i done)

Related Information

Antipsychotic Agents Comparison *on page 1396*

Brand Names Risperdal®

Therapeutic Category Antipsychotic Agent

Use Management of psychotic disorders (eg, schizophrenia); nonpsychotic symptoms associated with dementia in elderly

Contraindications Known hypersensitivity to any component of the product

Adverse Reactions

1% to 10%:

Cardiovascular: Hypotension (especially orthostatic), tachycardia, arrhythmias, abnormal T waves with prolonged ventricular repolarization; EKG changes, syncope

Central nervous system: Sedation (occurs at daily doses ≥20 mg/day), headache, dizziness, restlessness, anxiety, extrapyramidal reactions, dystonic reactions, pseudoparkinson signs and symptoms, tardive dyskinesia, neuroleptic malignant syndrome, altered central temperature regulation

Dermatologic: Photosensitivity (rare)

Endocrine & metabolic: Amenorrhea, galactorrhea, gynecomastia sexual dysfunction (up to 60%)

Gastrointestinal: Constipation, adynamic ileus, GI upset, xerostomia (problem for denture user), nausea and anorexia, weight gain

Genitourinary: Urinary retention, overflow incontinence, priapism

Hematologic: Agranulocytosis, leukopenia (usually in patients with large doses for prolonged periods)

(Continued)

Risperidone *(Continued)*

Hepatic: Cholestatic jaundice

Ocular: Blurred vision, retinal pigmentation, decreased visual acuity (may be irreversible)

<1%: Seizures

Drug Interactions

Increased toxicity: Quinidine, warfarin

May antagonize effects of levodopa; carbamazepine decreases risperidone serum concentrations; clozapine decreases clearance of risperidone

Mechanism of Action Risperidone is a benzisoxazole derivative, mixed serotonin-dopamine antagonist; binds to 5-HT_2-receptors in the CNS and in the periphery with a very high affinity; binds to dopamine-D_2 receptors with less affinity. The binding affinity to the dopamine-D_2 receptor is 20 times lower than the 5-HT_2 affinity. The addition of serotonin antagonism to dopamine antagonism (classic neuroleptic mechanism) is thought to improve negative symptoms of psychoses and reduce the incidence of extrapyramidal side effects.

Pharmacodynamics/Kinetics

Absorption: Oral: Rapid

Metabolism: Extensive by cytochrome P-450

Protein binding: Plasma: 90%

Half-life: 24 hours (risperidone and its active metabolite)

Time to peak: Peak plasma concentrations within 1 hour

Usual Dosage Recommended starting dose: 1 mg twice daily; slowly increase to the optimum range of 4-8 mg/day; daily dosages >10 mg does not appear to confer any additional benefit, and the incidence of extrapyramidal reactions is higher than with lower doses

Dosing adjustment in renal, hepatic impairment, and elderly: Starting dose of 0.5 mg twice daily is advisable

Nursing Implications Monitor and observe for extrapyramidal effects, orthostatic blood pressure changes for 3-5 days after starting or increasing dose

Dosage Forms

Solution, oral: 1 mg/mL

Tablet: 1 mg, 2 mg, 3 mg, 4 mg

Ritalin® *see* Methylphenidate *on page 818*

Ritalin-SR® *see* Methylphenidate *on page 818*

Ritodrine (RI toe dreen)

Brand Names Pre-Par®; Yutopar®

Synonyms Ritodrine Hydrochloride

Therapeutic Category Adrenergic Agonist Agent; Beta$_2$-Adrenergic Agonist Agent; Sympathomimetic; Tocolytic Agent

Use Inhibits uterine contraction in preterm labor

Pregnancy Risk Factor B

Contraindications Do not use before 20th week of pregnancy, cardiac arrhythmias, pheochromocytoma

Warnings/Precautions Monitor hydration status and blood glucose concentrations; fatal maternal pulmonary edema has been reported, sometimes after delivery; fluid overload must be avoided, hydration levels should be monitored closely; if pulmonary edema occurs, the drug should be discontinued; use with caution in patients with moderate pre-eclampsia, diabetes, or migraine; some products may contain sulfites; maternal deaths have been reported in patients treated with ritodrine and concurrent corticosteroids (pulmonary edema)

Adverse Reactions

>10%:

Cardiovascular: Increases in maternal and fetal heart rates and maternal hypertension, palpitations

Endocrine & metabolic: Temporary hyperglycemia

Gastrointestinal: Nausea, vomiting

Neuromuscular & skeletal: Tremor

1% to 10%:

Cardiovascular: Chest pain

Central nervous system: Nervousness, anxiety, restlessness

<1%:

Endocrine & metabolic: Ketoacidosis

Hepatic: Impaired liver function

Miscellaneous: Anaphylactic shock

Overdosage/Toxicology Symptoms of overdose include tachycardia, palpitations, hypotension, nervousness, nausea, vomiting, tremor; use an appropriate beta-blocker as an antidote

Drug Interactions

Decreased effect with beta-blockers

Increased effect/toxicity with meperidine, sympathomimetics, diazoxide, magnesium, betamethasone (pulmonary edema), potassium-depleting diuretics, general anesthetics

Stability Stable for 48 hours at room temperature after dilution in 500 mL of NS, D_5W, or LR I.V. solutions

Mechanism of Action Tocolysis due to its uterine $beta_2$-adrenergic receptor stimulating effects; this agent's $beta_2$ effects can also cause bronchial relaxation and vascular smooth muscle stimulation

Pharmacodynamics/Kinetics

Absorption: Oral: Rapid

Distribution: Crosses the placenta

Protein binding: 32%

Metabolism: In the liver

Half-life: 15 hours

Time to peak serum concentration: Within 0.5-1 hour

Elimination: In urine as unchanged drug and inactive conjugates

Usual Dosage Adults:

I.V.: 50-100 mcg/minute; increase by 50 mcg/minute every 10 minutes; continue for 12 hours after contractions have stopped

Oral: Start 30 minutes before stopping I.V. infusion; 10 mg every 2 hours for 24 hours, then 10-20 mg every 4-6 hours up to 120 mg/day

Hemodialysis: Removed by hemodialysis

Administration Monitor amount of I.V. fluid administered to prevent fluid overload; place patient in left lateral recumbent position to reduce risk of hypotension; use microdrip chamber or I.V. pump to control infusion rate

Monitoring Parameters Hematocrit, serum potassium, glucose, colloidal osmotic pressure, heart rate, and uterine contractions

Patient Information Remain in bed during infusion

Dosage Forms

Injection, as hydrochloride: 10 mg/mL (5 mL); 15 mg/mL (10 mL)

Tablet, as hydrochloride: 10 mg

Ritodrine Hydrochloride *see* Ritodrine *on previous page*

Ritonavir (rye TON a veer)

Brand Names Norvir®

Therapeutic Category Antiretroviral Agent; Antiviral Agent, Oral; Protease Inhibitor

Use Treatment of HIV, especially advanced cases; usually is used as part of triple or double therapy with other nucleoside and protease inhibitors although monotherapy is approved

Pregnancy Risk Factor B

Pregnancy/Breast-Feeding Implications

Administer during pregnancy only if benefits to mother outweigh risks to the fetus

HIV-infected mothers are discouraged from breast-feeding to decrease postnatal transmission of HIV

Contraindications

Increased plasma concentration of amiodarone, astemizole, bepridil, bupropion, cisapride, clozapine, dihydroergotamine, encainide, ergotamine, flecainide, meperidine, pimozide, piroxicam, propafenone, propoxyphene, quinidine, rifabutin, and terfenadine.

Ritonavir co-administration is also expected to produce large increases in these highly metabolized sedatives and hypnotics: Alprazolam, clorazepate, diazepam, estazolam, flurazepam, midazolam, triazolam and zolpidem.

Warnings/Precautions Use caution in patients with hepatic insufficiency; safety and efficacy have not been established in children <16 years of age; use caution with benzodiazepines, antiarrhythmics (flecainide, encainide, bepridil, amiodarone, quinidine) and certain analgesics (meperidine, piroxicam, propoxyphene)

Adverse Reactions

1% to 10%:

Gastrointestinal: Nausea, vomiting, diarrhea, abnormal taste

Neuromuscular & skeletal: Circumoral and peripheral paresthesias, weakness

<1%:

Central nervous system: Headache, confusion

Endocrine & metabolic: Elevated triglycerides, cholesterol

Hepatic: Elevated LFTs

Drug Interactions

Inhibitor of cytochrome P-450 3A, cytochrome P-450 2D6, and cytochrome P-450 2C enzymes

Mild cytochrome P-450 2D6 enzyme substrate and cytochrome P-450 3A enzyme substrate

Stability Refrigerate

(Continued)

Ritonavir *(Continued)*

Contraindicated Medications and Potential Alternatives*

Contraindicated Medications†			Potential Alternatives‡ (these alternatives may not be therapeutically equivalent)		
Drug Class	**Generic Name**	**Brand Name**	**Generic Name**	**Brand Name**	**Exposed Patients**
Analgesic	Meperidine Piroxicam Propoxyphene	Demerol® Feldene® Darvon®	Acetaminophen Aspirin Oxycodone	Tylenol® Percodan®	N=135 N=43 N=23
Cardiovascular (antiarrythmic)	Amiodarone Encainide Flecainide Propafenone Quinidine	Cordarone® Enkaid® Tambocor® Rythmol®	Very limited clinical experience		
Antimycobacterial	Rifabutin	Mycobutin®	Clarithromycin Ethambutol	Biaxin® Myambutol®	N=156§ N=66
Cardiovascular (calcium channel blocker)	Bepridil	Vascor®	Very limited clinical experience		
Cold and allergy (antihistamine)	Astemizole Terfenadine	Hismanal® Seldane®	Loratadine	Clarifin®	N=36
Ergot alkaloid (vasoconstrictor)	Dihydro-ergotamine Ergotamine	D.H.E. 45® various	Very limited clinical experience		
Gastrointestinal	Cisapride	Propulsid®	Very limited clinical experience		
Psychotropic (antidepressant)	Bupropion	Wellbutrin®	Desipramine	Norpramin®	¶
Psychotropic (neuroleptic)	Clozapine Pimozide	Clozaril® Orap™	Very limited clinical experience		
Psychotropic (sedative-hypnotic)	Alprazolam Clorazepate Diazepam Estazolam Flurazepam Midazolam Triazolam Zolpidem	Xanax® Tranxene® Valium® ProSom™ Dalmane® Versed® Halcion® Ambien®	Temazepam Lorazepam	Restoril® Ativan®	N=40 N=33

* During clinical trials, Norvir® was given to patients concomitantly taking a variety of medications. These medications were not evaluated in drug interaction studies. The number of Norvir®-treated patients exposed to each drug is provided in the last column.

† See Contraindications in the drug monograph.

‡ See Warnings/Precautions and Drug Interactions in the drug monograph.

§ Also evaluated in drug interaction study (N=22). See Results of Drug Interaction Studies table.

¶ No clinical experience with combination. Only evaluated in drug interaction study (N=14). See Results of Drug Interaction Studies table.

Results of Drug Interaction Studies

Co-administered Drug	Finding
Clarithromycin	77% increase in clarithromycin AUC; no dosage reduction is necessary in patients with normal renal function; for patients with Cl_{cr} from 30-60 mL/minute, decrease dose by 50%; for patients with Cl_{cr}<30 mL/minute, decrease dose by 75%
Desipramine	145% increase in desipramine AUC; dosage reduction should be considered
Didanosine (ddL)	13% decrease in didanosine AUC; no dosage adjustment is necessary
Ethinyl estradiol	40% decrease in ethinyl estradiol AUC; increase ethinyl estradiol dose or substitute with another contraceptive
Fluconazole	15% increase in ritonavir AUC
Saquinavir	Greater than 20-fold increase in saquinavir AUC
Sulfamethoxazole	20% decrease is sulfamethoxazole AUC; no dosage adjustment is necessary
Theophylline	43% decrease in theophylline AUC; increase in theophylline dose may be required
Zidovudine (AZT)	25% decrease in zidovudine AUC; no dosage adjustment is necessary

Mechanism of Action As a protease inhibitor, ritonavir prevents cleavage of protein precursors essential for HIV infection of new cells and viral replication. Saquinavir- and zidovudine-resistant HIV isolates are generally susceptible to ritonavir. Used in combination therapy, resistance to ritonavir develops slowly; strains resistant to ritonavir are cross-resistant to indinavir and saquinavir.

Pharmacodynamics/Kinetics

Absorption: Well absorbed; T_{max}: 2-4 hours

Distribution: High concentrations are produced in serum and lymph nodes

Protein binding: 98% to 99%

Metabolism: Hepatic; 5 metabolites, low concentration of an active metabolite achieved in plasma (oxidative)

Half-life: 3-5 hours

Elimination: Renal clearance is negligible

Usual Dosage Oral:

Children: Initial: 250 mg/m^2 twice daily; titrate upward to 400 mg/m^2 twice daily

Adults: 600 mg twice daily with meals

Dosing adjustment in renal impairment: None necessary

Dosing adjustment in hepatic impairment: Not determined; caution advised with severe impairment

Monitoring Parameters Signs of infection, LFTs

Patient Information Take with food; liquid formulations usually have an unpleasant taste; consider mixing it with chocolate milk or a liquid nutritional supplement

Dosage Forms

Capsule: 100 mg

Solution: 80 mg/mL (240 mL)

rLFN-α2 *see* Interferon Alfa-2b *on page 665*

rIFN-b *see* Interferon Beta-1b *on page 669*

RMS® *see* Morphine Sulfate *on page 858*

Robafen® AC *see* Guaifenesin and Codeine *on page 590*

Robaxin® *see* Methocarbamol *on page 805*

Robicillin® VK *see* Penicillin V Potassium *on page 965*

Robinul® *see* Glycopyrrolate *on page 581*

Robinul® Forte *see* Glycopyrrolate *on page 581*

Robitet® *see* Tetracycline *on page 1203*

Robitussin® [OTC] *see* Guaifenesin *on page 589*

Robitussin® A-C *see* Guaifenesin and Codeine *on page 590*

Robitussin® Cough Calmers [OTC] *see* Dextromethorphan *on page 366*

Robitussin®-DM [OTC] *see* Guaifenesin and Dextromethorphan *on page 591*

Robitussin® Pediatric [OTC] *see* Dextromethorphan *on page 366*

Robomol® *see* Methocarbamol *on page 805*

Rocaltrol® *see* Calcitriol *on page 183*

Rocephin® *see* Ceftriaxone *on page 236*

Rocuronium (roe kyoor OH nee um)

Related Information

Neuromuscular Blocking Agents Comparison *on page 1417*

Brand Names Zemuron®

Synonyms ORG 946; Rocuronium Bromide

Therapeutic Category Neuromuscular Blocker Agent, Nondepolarizing; Skeletal Muscle Relaxant

Use Inpatient and outpatient use as an adjunct to general anesthesia to facilitate both rapid-sequence and routine tracheal intubation, and to provide skeletal muscle relaxation during surgery or mechanical ventilation

Pregnancy Risk Factor B

Contraindications Known hypersensitivity to rocuronium or vecuronium

Warnings/Precautions Use with caution in patients with cardiovascular or pulmonary disease, hepatic impairment, neuromuscular disease, myasthenia gravis, dehydration (may alter neuromuscular blocking effects); respiratory acidosis, hypomagnesemia, hypokalemia, or hypocalcemia (may enhance actions) and the elderly; ventilation must be supported during neuromuscular blockade

Adverse Reactions

>1%: Cardiovascular: Transient hypotension and hypertension

<1%:

- Cardiovascular: Arrhythmias, abnormal EKG, tachycardia, edema
- Dermatologic: Rash, injection site pruritus
- Gastrointestinal: Nausea, vomiting
- Respiratory: Bronchospasm, wheezing, rhonchi
- Miscellaneous: Hiccups

Overdosage/Toxicology Symptoms of overdose include prolonged skeletal muscle block, muscle weakness and apnea

Treatment is maintenance of a patent airway and controlled ventilation until recovery of normal neuromuscular block is observed, further recovery may be

(Continued)

Rocuronium *(Continued)*

facilitated by administering an anticholinesterase agent (eg, neostigmine, edrophonium, or pyridostigmine) with atropine, to antagonize the skeletal muscle relaxation; support of the cardiovascular system with fluids and pressors may be necessary

Drug Interactions

Decreased effect: Chronic carbamazepine or phenytoin can shorten the duration of neuromuscular blockade; phenylephrine can severely inhibit neuromuscular blockade

Increased effect: Infusion requirements are reduced 35% to 40% during anesthesia with enflurane or isoflurane

Increased toxicity: Aminoglycosides, vancomycin, tetracyclines, bacitracin

Stability Store under refrigeration (2°C to 8°C), do not freeze; when stored at room temperature, it is stable for 30 days; unlike vecuronium, it is stable in 0.9% sodium chloride and 5% dextrose in water, this mixture should be used within 24 hours of preparation

Mechanism of Action Blocks acetylcholine from binding to receptors on motor endplate inhibiting depolarization

Pharmacodynamics/Kinetics

Onset: Good intubation conditions within 1-2 minutes; maximum neuromuscular blockade within 4 minutes

Duration: ~30 minutes (with standard doses, increases with higher doses)

Metabolism: Undergoes minimal hepatic metabolism

Elimination: Primarily through hepatic uptake and biliary excretion

Usual Dosage

Children:

Initial: 0.6 mg/kg under halothane anesthesia produce excellent to good intubating conditions within 1 minute and will provide a median time of 41 minutes of clinical relaxation in children 3 months to 1 year of age, and 27 minutes in children 1-12 years

Maintenance: 0.075-0.125 mg/kg administered upon return of T_1 to 25% of control provides clinical relaxation for 7-10 minutes

Adults:

Tracheal intubation: I.V.:

Initial: 0.6 mg/kg is expected to provide approximately 31 minutes of clinical relaxation under opioid/nitrous oxide/oxygen anesthesia with neuromuscular block sufficient for intubation attained in 1-2 minutes; lower doses (0.45 mg/kg) may be used to provide 22 minutes of clinical relaxation with median time to neuromuscular block of 1-3 minutes; maximum blockade is achieved in <4 minutes

Maximum: 0.9-1.2 mg/kg may be given during surgery under opioid/nitrous oxide/oxygen anesthesia without adverse cardiovascular effects and is expected to provide 58-67 minutes of clinical relaxation; neuromuscular blockade sufficient for intubation is achieved in <2 minutes with maximum blockade in <3 minutes

Maintenance: 0.1, 0.15, and 0.2 mg/kg administered at 25% recovery of control T_1 (defined as 3 twitches of train-of-four) provides a median of 12, 17, and 24 minutes of clinical duration under anesthesia

Rapid sequence intubation: 0.6-1.2 mg/kg in appropriately premedicated and anesthetized patients with excellent or good intubating conditions within 2 minutes

Continuous infusion: Initial: 0.01-0.012 mg/kg/minute only after early evidence of spontaneous recovery of neuromuscular function is evident

Dosing adjustment in hepatic impairment: Reductions are necessary in patients with liver disease

Administration Administer I.V. only

Monitoring Parameters Peripheral nerve stimulator measuring twitch response, heart rate, blood pressure, assisted ventilation status

Nursing Implications Concurrent sedation and analgesia are needed

Additional Information Dose based on actual body weight

Dosage Forms Injection, as bromide: 10 mg/mL

Rocuronium Bromide *see* Rocuronium *on previous page*

Roferon-A® *see* Interferon Alfa-2a *on page 663*

Rogaine® for Men [OTC] *see* Minoxidil *on page 843*

Rogaine® for Women [OTC] *see* Minoxidil *on page 843*

Rolaids® Calcium Rich [OTC] *see* Calcium Carbonate *on page 185*

Romazicon™ *see* Flumazenil *on page 530*

Rondec® Drops *see* Carbinoxamine and Pseudoephedrine *on page 204*

Rondec® Filmtab® *see* Carbinoxamine and Pseudoephedrine *on page 204*

Rondec® Syrup *see* Carbinoxamine and Pseudoephedrine *on page 204*

Rondec-TR® *see* Carbinoxamine and Pseudoephedrine *on page 204*

Ropivacaine (roe PIV a kane)

Brand Names Naropin®

Synonyms Ropivacaine Hydrochloride

Therapeutic Category Local Anesthetic, Injectable

Use Local anesthetic (injectable) for use in surgery, postoperative pain management, and obstetrical procedures when local or regional anesthesia is needed. It can be administered via local infiltration, epidural block and epidural infusion, or intermittent bolus.

Pregnancy Risk Factor B

Contraindications Hypersensitivity to amide-type local anesthetics (eg, bupivacaine, mepivacaine, lidocaine); septicemia, severe hypotension and for spinal anesthesia, in the presence of complete heart block

Warnings/Precautions Use with caution in patients with liver disease, cardiovascular disease, neurological or psychiatric disorders; it is not recommended for use in emergency situations where rapid administration is necessary

Adverse Reactions

>10% (dose and route related):
- Cardiovascular: Hypotension, bradycardia
- Gastrointestinal: Nausea, vomiting
- Neuromuscular & skeletal: Back pain
- Miscellaneous: Shivering

1% to 10% (dose related):
- Cardiovascular: Hypertension, tachycardia, bradycardia
- Central nervous system: Headache, dizziness, anxiety, lightheadedness
- Gastrointestinal: Vomiting
- Neuromuscular & skeletal: Hypoesthesia, paresthesia, circumoral paresthesia
- Otic: Tinnitus
- Respiratory: Apnea

Overdosage/Toxicology Treatment is primarily symptomatic and supportive. Termination of anesthesia by pneumatic tourniquet inflation should be attempted when the agent is administered by infiltration or regional injection.

Seizures commonly respond to diazepam, while hypotension responds to I.V. fluids and Trendelenburg positioning

Bradyarrhythmias (when the heart rate is <60) can be treated with I.V., or S.C. atropine 15 mcg/kg

With the development of metabolic acidosis, I.V. sodium bicarbonate 0.5-2 mEq/kg and ventilatory assistance should be instituted

Methemoglobinemia should be treated with methylene blue 1-2 mg/kg in a 1% sterile aqueous solution I.V. push over 4-6 minutes repeated up to a total dose of 7 mg/kg

Drug Interactions

Increased effect: Other local anesthetics or agents structurally related to the amide-type anesthetics

Increased toxicity (possible but not yet reported): Drugs that decrease cytochrome P-450 1A enzyme function

Mechanism of Action Blocks both the initiation and conduction of nerve impulses by decreasing the neuronal membrane's permeability to sodium ions, which results in inhibition of depolarization with resultant blockade of conduction

Pharmacodynamics/Kinetics

Onset of anesthesia (dependent on route administered): Within 3-15 minutes generally

Duration of action (dependent on dose and route administered): 3-15 hours generally

Metabolism: In the liver

Half-life:
- Epidural: 5-7 hours
- I.V.: 2.4 hours

Elimination: 86% of metabolites are excreted in urine

Usual Dosage Dose varies with procedure, onset and depth of anesthesia desired, vascularity of tissues, duration of anesthesia, and condition of patient

Adults:
- Lumbar epidural for surgery: 15-30 mL of 0.5% to 1%
- Lumbar epidural block for cesarean section: 20-30 mL of 0.5%
- Thoracic epidural block for postoperative pain relief: 5-15 mL of 0.5%
- Major nerve block: 35-50 mL dose of 0.5% (175-250 mg)
- Field block: 1-40 mL dose of 0.5% (5-200 mg)
- Lumbar epidural for labor pain: Initial: 10-20 mL 0.2%; continuous infusion dose: 6-14 mL/hour of 0.2% with incremental injections of 10-15 mL/hour of 0.2% solution

(Continued)

Ropivacaine *(Continued)*

Dosage Forms

Infusion, as hydrochloride: 2 mg/mL (100 mL, 200 mL)

Injection, as hydrochloride (single dose): 2 mg/mL (20 mL); 5 mg/mL (30 mL); 7.5 mg/mL (10 mL, 20 mL); 10 mg/mL (10 mL, 20 mL)

Ropivacaine Hydrochloride *see* Ropivacaine *on previous page*

Rowasa® *see* Mesalamine *on page 787*

Roxanol™ *see* Morphine Sulfate *on page 858*

Roxanol SR™ *see* Morphine Sulfate *on page 858*

Roxicet® 5/500 *see* Oxycodone and Acetaminophen *on page 938*

Roxicodone™ *see* Oxycodone *on page 936*

Roxilox® *see* Oxycodone and Acetaminophen *on page 938*

Roxiprin® *see* Oxycodone and Aspirin *on page 939*

RP54274 *see* Riluzole *on page 1108*

r-PA *see* Reteplase *on page 1100*

RSV-IGIV *see* Respiratory Syncytial Virus Immune Globulin (Intravenous) *on page 1099*

RTCA *see* Ribavirin *on page 1104*

Rubella and Measles Vaccines, Combined *see* Measles and Rubella Vaccines, Combined *on page 761*

Rubella and Mumps Vaccines, Combined

(rue BEL a & mumpz vak SEENS, kom BINED)

Related Information

Adverse Events and Vaccination *on page 1439*

Immunization Guidelines *on page 1421*

Brand Names Biavax®II

Therapeutic Category Vaccine

Use Promote active immunity to rubella and mumps by inducing production of antibodies

Pregnancy Risk Factor X

Contraindications Known hypersensitivity to neomycin, eggs; children <1 year, pregnant women, primary immunodeficient patients, patients receiving immunosuppressant drugs except corticosteroids

Warnings/Precautions Women planning on becoming pregnant in the next 3 months should not be vaccinated

Adverse Reactions

1% to 10%:

Central nervous system: Febrile seizures, fever

Local: Soreness, burning, stinging

Miscellaneous: Allergic reactions

Drug Interactions Immune globulin, whole blood

Stability Refrigerate, discard unused portion within 8 hours, protect from light

Usual Dosage Children >12 months and Adults: 1 vial in outer aspect of the upper arm; children vaccinated before 12 months of age should be revaccinated

Administration Administer S.C. only

Test Interactions Temporary suppression of TB skin test

Patient Information

Mumps vaccine: A little swelling of the glands in the cheeks and under the jaw that lasts for a few days; this could happen from 1-2 weeks after getting the mumps vaccine; this happens rarely

Rubella vaccine: Swelling of the lymph glands in the neck or a rash that lasts 1-2 days; this could happen 1-2 weeks after getting the rubella vaccine in about 1/7 children who get the vaccine

Mild pain or stiffness in the joints that may last up to 3 days; this could happen from 1-3 weeks after getting the shot. this problem happens to about 1/100 children who get the shot and 25/100 adults who get the shot. Women have this problem more than men and it may happen in up to 40 women out of every 100. Rarely, pain or stiffness can last for months or longer and can come and go.

Painful swelling of the joints (arthritis) happens to <1/100 children who get the rubella vaccine. About 10/100 adults can also have this problem, which usually lasts a few days to a week. Rarely, this swelling has been reported to last longer, or to come and go. Damage to the joints is very rare.

Pain or numbness, or "pins and needles" feeling in the hands and feet that lasts for a short time; this happens rarely

Nursing Implications Children immunized before 12 months of age should be reimmunized

Additional Information Federal law requires that the date of administration, the vaccine manufacturer, lot number of vaccine, and the administering person's name, title and address be entered into the patient's permanent medical record

Dosage Forms Injection (mixture of 2 viruses):

1. Wistar RA 27/3 strain of rubella virus
2. Jeryl Lynn (B level) mumps strain grown cell cultures of chick embryo

Rubella, Measles and Mumps Vaccines, Combined *see* Measles, Mumps, and Rubella Vaccines, Combined *on page 763*

Rubella Virus Vaccine, Live (rue BEL a VYE rus vak SEEN, live)

Related Information

Adverse Events and Vaccination *on page 1439*
Immunization Guidelines *on page 1421*

Brand Names Meruvax® II

Synonyms German Measles Vaccine

Therapeutic Category Vaccine, Live Virus

Use All adults, both male and female, lacking documentation of live vaccine on or after first birthday, or laboratory evidence of immunity (particularly women of childbearing age and young adults who work in or congregate in hospitals, colleges, and on military bases) should be vaccinated. Susceptible travelers should be vaccinated.

Pregnancy Risk Factor X

Warnings/Precautions Pregnancy, immunocompromised persons, history of anaphylactic reaction following receipt of neomycin; do not administer with other live vaccines

Adverse Reactions

>10%:
- Dermatologic: Local tenderness and erythema, urticaria, rash
- Neuromuscular & skeletal: Arthralgia

1% to 10%:
- Central nervous system: Malaise, fever, headache
- Gastrointestinal: Sore throat
- Miscellaneous: Lymphadenopathy

<1%:
- Ocular: Optic neuritis
- Miscellaneous: Hypersensitivity, allergic reactions to the vaccine

Drug Interactions Decreased effect when immune globulin is given within 3 months and with concurrent use of corticosteroids and other immunosuppressant agents

Stability Refrigerate, discard reconstituted vaccine after 8 hours; store at 2°C to 8°C (36°F to 46°F); ship vaccine at 10°C; may use dry ice, protect from light

Mechanism of Action Rubella vaccine is a live attenuated vaccine that contains the Wistar Institute RA 27/3 strain, which is adapted to and propagated in human diploid cell culture. It is the only strain of rubella vaccine marketed in the U.S. Antibody titers after immunization last 6 years without significant decline; 90% of those vaccinated have protection for at least 15 years.

Pharmacodynamics/Kinetics

Onset of effect: Antibodies to the vaccine are detectable within 2-4 weeks following immunization

Duration: Protection against both clinical rubella and asymptomatic viremia is probably life-long. Vaccine-induced antibody levels have been shown to persist for at least 10 years without substantial decline. If the present pattern continues, it will provide a basis for the expectation that immunity following vaccination will be permanent. However, continued surveillance will be required to demonstrate this point.

Usual Dosage Children ≥12 months and Adults: S.C.: 0.5 mL in outer aspect of upper arm; children vaccinated before 12 months of age should be revaccinated

Test Interactions May depress tuberculin skin test sensitivity

Patient Information

Swelling of the lymph glands in the neck or a rash that lasts 1-2 days; this could happen 1-2 weeks after getting the rubella vaccine in about 1/7 children who get the vaccine

Mild pain or stiffness in the joints that may last up to 3 days; this could happen from 1-3 weeks after getting the shot. This problem happens to about 1/100 children who get the shot and 25/100 adults who get the shot. Women have this problem more than men and it may happen in up to 40 women out of every 100. Rarely, pain or stiffness can last for months or longer and can come and go.

Painful swelling of the joints (arthritis) happens to <1/100 children who get the rubella vaccine. About 10/100 adults can also have this problem, which usually lasts a few days to a week. Rarely, this swelling has been reported to last longer, or to come and go. Damage to the joints is very rare.

(Continued)

Rubella Virus Vaccine, Live *(Continued)*

Pain or numbness, or "pins and needles" feeling in the hands and feet that lasts for a short time; this happens rarely

Nursing Implications Reconstituted vaccine should be used within 8 hours; S.C. injection only

Additional Information Live virus vaccine: Federal law requires that the date of administration, the vaccine manufacturer, lot number of vaccine, and the administering person's name, title and address be entered into the patient's permanent record

Women who are pregnant when vaccinated or who become pregnant within 3 months of vaccination should be counseled on the theoretical risks to the fetus. The risk of rubella-associated malformations in these women is so small as to be negligible. MMR is the vaccine of choice if recipients are likely to be susceptible to measles or mumps as well as to rubella.

Dosage Forms Injection, single dose: 1000 $TCID_{50}$ (Wistar RA 27/3 Strain)

Rubeola Vaccine *see* Measles Virus Vaccine, Live *on page 764*

Rubex® *see* Doxorubicin *on page 425*

Rubidomycin Hydrochloride *see* Daunorubicin Hydrochloride *on page 345*

Rubramin-PC® *see* Cyanocobalamin *on page 319*

Rufen® *see* Ibuprofen *on page 639*

Rum-K® *see* Potassium Chloride *on page 1024*

Ru-Vert-M® *see* Meclizine *on page 769*

Rythmol® *see* Propafenone *on page 1060*

S5614 *see* Dexfenfluramine *on page 360*

Sabin *see* Polio Vaccines *on page 1015*

Sal-Acid® Plaster [OTC] *see* Salicylic Acid *on this page*

Salactic® Film [OTC] *see* Salicylic Acid *on this page*

Salagen® Oral *see* Pilocarpine *on page 999*

Salbutamol *see* Albuterol *on page 38*

Saleto-200® [OTC] *see* Ibuprofen *on page 639*

Saleto-400® *see* Ibuprofen *on page 639*

Salflex® *see* Salsalate *on page 1122*

Salgesic® *see* Salsalate *on page 1122*

Salicylazosulfapyridine *see* Sulfasalazine *on page 1177*

Salicylic Acid (sal i SIL ik AS id)

Brand Names Clear Away® Disc [OTC]; Compound W® [OTC]; Dr Scholl's® Disk [OTC]; Dr Scholl's® Wart Remover [OTC]; DuoFilm® [OTC]; DuoPlant® Gel [OTC]; Freezone® Solution [OTC]; Gordofilm® Liquid; Mediplast® Plaster [OTC]; Mosco® Liquid [OTC]; Occlusal-HP Liquid; Off-Ezy® Wart Remover [OTC]; Panscol® [OTC]; Psor-a-set® Soap [OTC]; P&S® Shampoo [OTC]; Sal-Acid® Plaster [OTC]; Salactic® Film [OTC]; Sal-Plant® Gel [OTC]; Trans-Ver-Sal® AdultPatch [OTC]; Trans-Ver-Sal® PediaPatch [OTC]; Trans-Ver-Sal® PlantarPatch [OTC]; Wart-Off® [OTC]

Canadian/Mexican Brand Names Acnex® (Canada); Acnomel® (Canada); Trans-Planta® (Canada); Trans-Ver-Sal® (Canada)

Therapeutic Category Keratolytic Agent; Shampoo, Keratolytic

Use Topically for its keratolytic effect in controlling seborrheic dermatitis or psoriasis of body and scalp, dandruff, and other scaling dermatoses; also used to remove warts, corns, and calluses

Pregnancy Risk Factor C

Contraindications Hypersensitivity to salicylic acid or any components; children <2 years of age

Warnings/Precautions Should not be used systemically, severe irritating effect on GI mucosa; use with caution in areas of ischemia; prolonged use over large areas, especially in children, may result in salicylate toxicity; do not apply on irritated, reddened, or infected skin; for external use only; avoid contact with eyes, face, and other mucous membranes

Adverse Reactions

>10%: Local: Burning and irritation at site of exposure on normal tissue

1% to 10%:

Central nervous system: Dizziness, mental confusion, headache

Otic: Tinnitus

Respiratory: Hyperventilation

Overdosage/Toxicology Signs and symptoms of salicylate toxicity include nausea, vomiting, dizziness, tinnitus, loss of hearing, lethargy, diarrhea, psychic disturbances

Mechanism of Action Produces desquamation of hyperkeratotic epithelium via dissolution of the intercellular cement which causes the cornified tissue to swell, soften, macerate, and desquamate. Salicylic acid is keratolytic at concentrations of 3% to 6%; it becomes destructive to tissue at concentrations >6%. Concentrations of 6% to 60% are used to remove corns and warts and in the treatment of psoriasis and other hyperkeratotic disorders.

Pharmacodynamics/Kinetics

Absorption: Absorbed percutaneously, but systemic toxicity is unlikely with normal use

Time to peak serum concentration: Topical: Within 5 hours of application with occlusion

Elimination: Salicyluric acid (52%), salicylate glucuronides (42%), and salicylic acid (6%) are major metabolites identified in urine after percutaneous absorption

Usual Dosage

Lotion, cream, gel: Apply a thin layer to affected area once or twice daily

Plaster: Cut to size that covers the corn or callus, apply and leave in place for 48 hours; do not exceed 5 applications over a 14-day period

Solution: Apply a thin layer directly to wart using brush applicator once daily as directed for 1 week or until wart is removed

Patient Information When applying in concentrations >10%, protect surrounding tissue with petrolatum; do not use on open skin, avoid contact with eyes, mouth, and other mucous membranes

Nursing Implications For warts: Before applying product, soak area in warm water for 5 minutes; dry area thoroughly, then apply medication

Dosage Forms

Cream: 2% (30 g)
Disk: 40%
Gel: 5% (60 g); 6% (30 g); 17% (7.5 g)
Liquid: 13.6% (9.3 mL); 17% (9.3 mL, 13.5 mL, 15 mL); 16.7% (15 mL)
Lotion: 3% (120 mL)
Ointment: 3% (90 g)
Patch, transdermal: 15% (20 mm); 40% (20 mm)
Plaster: 40%
Soap: 2% (97.5 g)
Strip: 40%

Salicylsalicylic Acid *see* Salsalate *on next page*
SalineX® [OTC] *see* Sodium Chloride *on page 1142*
Salk *see* Polio Vaccines *on page 1015*

Salmeterol (sal ME te role)

Brand Names Serevent®

Canadian/Mexican Brand Names Zantirel® (Mexico)

Synonyms Salmeterol Xinafoate

Therapeutic Category Adrenergic Agonist Agent; Beta$_2$-Adrenergic Agonist Agent; Bronchodilator

Use Maintenance treatment of asthma and in prevention of bronchospasm in patients >12 years of age with reversible obstructive airway disease, including patients with symptoms of nocturnal asthma, who require regular treatment with inhaled, short-acting beta$_2$ agonists; prevention of exercise-induced bronchospasm

Pregnancy Risk Factor C

Contraindications Hypersensitivity to salmeterol, adrenergic amines or any ingredients; need for acute bronchodilation

Warnings/Precautions Salmeterol is not meant to relieve acute asthmatic symptoms. Acute episodes should be treated with short-acting beta$_2$ agonist. Do not increase the frequency of salmeterol. Cardiovascular effects are not common with salmeterol when used in recommended doses. All beta agonists may cause elevation in blood pressure, heart rate, and result in excitement (CNS). Use with caution in patients with prostatic hypertrophy, diabetes, cardiovascular disorders, convulsive disorders, thyrotoxicosis, or others who are sensitive to the effects of sympathomimetic amines. Paroxysmal bronchospasm (which can be fatal) has been reported with this and other inhaled agents. If this occurs, discontinue treatment. The elderly may be at greater risk of cardiovascular side effects; safety and efficacy have not been established in children <12 years of age.

Adverse Reactions

>10%:

Central nervous system: Headache

Respiratory: Pharyngitis

1% to 10%:

Cardiovascular: Tachycardia, palpitations, elevation or depression of blood pressure, cardiac arrhythmias

Central nervous system: Nervousness, CNS stimulation, hyperactivity, insomnia, malaise, dizziness

(Continued)

Salmeterol *(Continued)*

Gastrointestinal: GI upset, diarrhea, nausea
Neuromuscular & skeletal: Tremors (may be more common in the elderly), myalgias, back pain, arthralgia
Respiratory: Upper respiratory infection, cough, bronchitis
<1%: Immediate hypersensitivity reactions (rash, urticaria, bronchospasm)

Overdosage/Toxicology
Decontamination: Lavage/activated charcoal
Supportive therapy: Beta-blockers can be used for hyperadrenergic signs (use with caution in patients with bronchospasm)
Prudent use of a cardioselective beta-adrenergic blocker (eg, atenolol or metoprolol); keep in mind the potential for induction of bronchoconstriction in an asthmatic. Dialysis has not been shown to be of value in the treatment of an overdose with this agent.

Drug Interactions
Increased effect: Beta-adrenergic blockers (eg, propranolol)
Decreased toxicity (cardiovascular): MAO inhibitors, tricyclic antidepressants

Stability Store cannister with nozzle down; protect from freezing temperature and direct sunlight The therapeutic effect may decrease when the canister is cold therefore the canister should remain at room temperature. Do not store at temperatures >120°F.

Mechanism of Action Relaxes bronchial smooth muscle by selective action on $beta_2$-receptors with little effect on heart rate; because salmeterol acts locally in the lung, therapeutic effect is not predicted by plasma levels

Pharmacodynamics/Kinetics
Onset of action: 5-20 minutes (average 10 minutes)
Peak effect: 2-4 hours
Duration: 12 hours
Protein binding: 94% to 98%
Metabolism: Hydroxylated in liver
Half-life: 3-4 hours

Usual Dosage
Inhalation: 42 mcg (2 puffs) twice daily (12 hours apart) for maintenance and prevention of symptoms of asthma
Prevention of exercise-induced asthma: 42 mcg (2 puffs) 30-60 minutes prior to exercise; additional doses should not be used for 12 hours

Monitoring Parameters Pulmonary function tests, blood pressure, pulse, CNS stimulation

Patient Information Do not use to treat acute symptoms; do not exceed the prescribed dose of salmeterol; do not stop using inhaled or oral corticosteroids without medical advice even if you "feel better"; shake well before using. Avoid spraying in eyes, remove the canister and rinse the plastic case and cap under warm water and dry daily. Store canister with nozzle end down.

Nursing Implications Not to be used for the relief of acute attacks; monitor lung sounds, pulse, blood pressure. Before using, the inhaler must be shaken well; observe for wheezing after administration; if this occurs, call physician.

Dosage Forms Aerosol, oral, as xinafoate: 21 mcg/spray [60 inhalations] (6.5 g), [120 inhalations] (13 g)

Salmeterol Xinafoate *see* Salmeterol *on previous page*
Salmonine® Injection *see* Calcitonin *on page 181*
Sal-Plant® Gel [OTC] *see* Salicylic Acid *on page 1120*

Salsalate (SAL sa late)

Brand Names Argesic®-SA; Artha-G®; Disalcid®; Marthritic®; Mono-Gesic®; Salflex®; Salgesic®; Salsitab®

Synonyms Disalicylic Acid; Salicylsalicylic Acid

Therapeutic Category Analgesic, Salicylate; Anti-inflammatory Agent; Antipyretic; Nonsteroidal Anti-inflammatory Agent (NSAID), Oral; Salicylate

Use Treatment of minor pain or fever; arthritis

Pregnancy Risk Factor C

Contraindications GI ulcer or bleeding, known hypersensitivity to salsalate

Warnings/Precautions Use with caution in patients with platelet and bleeding disorders, renal dysfunction, erosive gastritis, or peptic ulcer disease, previous nonreaction does not guarantee future safe taking of medication; do not use aspirin in children <16 years of age for chickenpox or flu symptoms due to the association with Reye's syndrome

Adverse Reactions
>10%: Gastrointestinal: Nausea, heartburn, stomach pains, dyspepsia
1% to 10%:
Central nervous system: Fatigue
Dermatologic: Rash

Gastrointestinal: Gastrointestinal ulceration
Hematologic: Hemolytic anemia
Neuromuscular & skeletal: Weakness
Respiratory: Dyspnea
Miscellaneous: Anaphylactic shock

<1%:

Central nervous system: Insomnia, nervousness, jitters
Hematologic: Leukopenia, thrombocytopenia, iron deficiency anemia, does not appear to inhibit platelet aggregation, occult bleeding
Hepatic: Hepatotoxicity
Renal: Impaired renal function
Respiratory: Bronchospasm

Overdosage/Toxicology Symptoms of overdose include respiratory alkalosis, hyperpnea, tachypnea, tinnitus, headache, hyperpyrexia, metabolic acidosis, hypoglycemia, coma. The "Done" nomogram is very helpful for estimating the severity of aspirin poisoning and directing treatment using serum salicylate levels. Treatment can also be based upon symptomatology.

Salicylates

Toxic Symptoms	Treatment
Overdose	Induce emesis with ipecac, and/or lavage with saline, followed with activated charcoal
Dehydration	I.V. fluids with KCl (no D_5W only)
Metabolic acidosis (must be treated)	Sodium bicarbonate
Hyperthermia	Cooling blankets or sponge baths
Coagulopathy/hemorrhage	Vitamin K I.V.
Hypoglycemia (with coma, seizures, or change in mental status)	Dextrose 25 g I.V.
Seizures	Diazepam 5-10 mg I.V.

Drug Interactions

Decreased effect with urinary alkalinizers, antacids, corticosteroids; decreased effect of uricosurics, spironolactone

Increased effect/toxicity of oral anticoagulants, hypoglycemics, methotrexate

Mechanism of Action Inhibits prostaglandin synthesis, acts on the hypothalamus heat-regulating center to reduce fever, blocks prostaglandin synthetase action which prevents formation of the platelet-aggregating substance thromboxane A_2

Pharmacodynamics/Kinetics

Onset of action: Therapeutic effects occur within 3-4 days of continuous dosing
Absorption: Oral: Completely from the small intestine
Metabolism: Hydrolyzed in the liver to 2 moles of salicylic acid (active)
Half-life: 7-8 hours
Elimination: Almost totally excreted renally

Usual Dosage Adults: Oral: 3 g/day in 2-3 divided doses

Dosing comments in renal impairment: In patients with end stage renal disease undergoing hemodialysis: 750 mg twice daily with an additional 500 mg after dialysis

Test Interactions False-negative results for glucose oxidase urinary glucose tests (Clinistix®); false-positives using the cupric sulfate method (Clinitest®); also, interferes with Gerhardt test, VMA determination; 5-HIAA, xylose tolerance test and T_3 and T_4

Patient Information Do not self-medicate with other drug products containing aspirin; use antacids to relieve upset stomach; watch for bleeding gums or any signs of GI bleeding; take with food or milk to minimize GI distress, notify physician if ringing in ears or persistent GI pain occurs

Dosage Forms

Capsule: 500 mg
Tablet: 500 mg, 750 mg

Salsitab® *see* Salsalate *on previous page*

Salt *see* Sodium Chloride *on page 1142*

Salt Poor Albumin *see* Albumin *on page 37*

Saluron® *see* Hydroflumethiazide *on page 626*

Sandimmune® *see* Cyclosporine *on page 327*

Sandoglobulin® *see* Immune Globulin, Intravenous *on page 651*

Sandostatin® *see* Octreotide Acetate *on page 921*

Sani-Supp® [OTC] *see* Glycerin *on page 580*

Sansert® *see* Methysergide *on page 822*

Santyl® *see* Collagenase *on page 311*

Saquinavir (sa KWIN a veer)

Brand Names Invirase®

Synonyms Saquinavir Mesylate

Therapeutic Category Antiretroviral Agent; Antiviral Agent, Oral; Protease Inhibitor

Use Treatment of advanced HIV infection in selected patients; used in combination with other nucleoside analog medications

Pregnancy Risk Factor B

Pregnancy/Breast-Feeding Implications Administer saquinavir during pregnancy only if benefits to the mother outweigh the risk to the fetus. HIV-infected mothers are discouraged from breast-feeding to decrease postnatal transmission of HIV.

Contraindications Hypersensitivity to saquinavir or any components; exposure to direct sunlight without sunscreen or protective clothing

Warnings/Precautions The indication for saquinavir for the treatment of HIV infection is based on changes in surrogate markers. At present, there are no results from controlled clinical trials evaluating its effect on patient survival or the clinical progression of HIV infection (ie, occurrence of opportunistic infections or malignancies); use caution in patients with hepatic insufficiency; safety and efficacy have not been established in children <16 years of age

Adverse Reactions

1% to 10%:

- Dermatologic: Rash
- Endocrine & metabolic: Hyperglycemia, elevated CPK
- Gastrointestinal: Diarrhea, abdominal discomfort, nausea, abdominal pain, buccal mucosa, ulceration
- Neuromuscular & skeletal: Paresthesia, weakness

<1%:

- Central nervous system: Headache, confusion, seizures, ataxia, pain
- Dermatologic: Stevens-Johnson syndrome
- Endocrine & metabolic: Hypoglycemia, hyper- and hypokalemia, low serum amylase
- Gastrointestinal: Upper quadrant abdominal pain
- Hematologic: Acute myeloblastic leukemia, hemolytic anemia, thrombocytopenia
- Hepatic: Jaundice, ascites, exacerbation of chronic liver disease, elevated LFTs, altered AST, ALT, bilirubin, Hg
- Local: Thrombophlebitis

Drug Interactions

Decreased effect: Rifampin may decrease saquinavir's plasma levels and AUC by 40% to 80%; other enzyme inducers may induce saquinavir's metabolism (eg, phenobarbital, phenytoin, dexamethasone, carbamazepine)

Increased effect: Ketoconazole significantly increases plasma levels and AUC of saquinavir; as a known, although not potent inhibitor of the cytochrome P-450 system, saquinavir may decrease the metabolism of terfenadine and astemizole (and result in rare but serious cardiac arrhythmias); other drugs which may have increased adverse effects if coadministered with saquinavir include calcium channel blockers, clindamycin, dapsone, quinidine, and triazolam

Mechanism of Action As an inhibitor of HIV protease, saquinavir prevents the cleavage of viral polyprotein precursors which are needed to generate functional proteins in and maturation of HIV-infected cells

Pharmacodynamics/Kinetics

Absorption: Incomplete; food, especially high fat diets, may increase the absorption and oral bioavailability of saquinavir by five-fold

Distribution: Widely distributed; V_d: 700 L (adults); minimal CSF penetration

Protein binding: 98%

Metabolism: Undergoes extensive first-pass metabolism; 87% undergoes hepatic metabolism via cytochrome P-450 system; no known active metabolites

Bioavailability: 4%

Elimination: 88% in feces, 1% in urine

Usual Dosage Oral: 600 mg 3 times/day within 2 hours after a full meal; use in combination with a nucleoside analog (AZT or ddC)

Monitoring Parameters Signs of infection

Patient Information Saquinavir is not a cure for HIV infection nor has it been found to reduce the transmission of HIV; opportunistic infections and other illnesses associated with AIDS may still occur; take saquinavir within 2 hours after a full meal; avoid direct sunlight when taking saquinavir

Nursing Implications Observe for signs of opportunistic infections and other illnesses associated with HIV; administer on a full stomach, if possible

Additional Information The indication for saquinavir for the treatment of HIV infection is based on changes in surrogate markers. At present, there are no results from controlled clinical trials evaluating the effect of regimens containing saquinavir on patient survival or the clinical progression of HIV infection, such as the occurrence of opportunistic infections or malignancies; in cell culture, saquinavir is additive to synergistic with AZT, ddC, and DDI without enhanced toxicity.

Dosage Forms Capsule, as mesylate: 200 mg

Saquinavir Mesylate *see* Saquinavir *on previous page*

Sargramostim (sar GRAM oh stim)

Related Information

Filgrastim *on page 518*

Brand Names Leukine™; Prokine™

Synonyms GM-CSF; Granulocyte-Macrophage Colony Stimulating Factor; rGM-CSF

Therapeutic Category Colony Stimulating Factor

Use

Myeloid reconstitution after autologous bone marrow transplantation:

Non-Hodgkin's lymphoma (NHL)
Acute lymphoblastic leukemia (ALL)
Hodgkin's lymphoma
Metastatic breast cancer

Myeloid reconstitution after allogeneic bone marrow transplantation

Peripheral stem cell transplantation

Metastatic breast cancer
Non-Hodgkin's lymphoma
Hodgkin's lymphoma
Multiple myeloma

Acute myelogenous leukemia (AML) following induction chemotherapy in older adults to shorten time to neutrophil recovery and to reduce the incidence of severe and life-threatening infections and infections resulting in death

Bone marrow transplant (allogeneic or autologous) failure or engraftment delay

Safety and efficacy of GM-CSF given simultaneously with cytotoxic chemotherapy have not been established. Concurrent treatment may increase myelosuppression.

Pregnancy Risk Factor C

Pregnancy/Breast-Feeding Implications Animal reproduction studies have not been conducted. It is not known whether sargramostim can cause fetal harm when administered to a pregnant woman or can affect reproductive capability. Sargramostim should be given to a pregnant woman only if clearly needed.

Contraindications GM-CSF is contraindicated in the following instances:

Patients with excessive myeloid blasts (>10%) in the bone marrow or peripheral blood

Patients with known hypersensitivity to GM-CSF, yeast-derived products, or any known component of the product

Warnings/Precautions Concomitant use with chemotherapy or radiotherapy, initiate ≥ hours after therapy. One controlled trial reported a higher incidence of grade 3 and 4 infections, grade 3 and 4 thrombocytopenia, and higher mortality in patients who received concurrent GM-CSF. Use with caution in patients with preexisting cardiac problems, hypoxia, fluid retention, pulmonary infiltrates or CHF, renal or hepatic impairment; rapid increase in peripheral blood counts; if ANC >20,000/mm^3, or platelets >500,000/mm^3 decrease dose by 50% or discontinue drug (counts will fall to normal within 3-7 days after discontinuing drug); growth factor potential: caution with myeloid malignancies. Precaution should be exercised in the usage of GM-CSF in any malignancy with myeloid characteristics. GM-CSF can potentially act as a growth factor for any tumor type, particularly myeloid malignancies. Tumors of nonhematopoietic origin may have surface receptors for GM-CSF.

Adverse Reactions

>10%:

"First-dose" effects: Fever, hypotension, tachycardia, rigors, flushing, nausea, vomiting, dyspnea
Central nervous system: Neutropenic fever
Dermatologic: Alopecia
Endocrine & metabolic: Polydipsia
Gastrointestinal: Nausea, vomiting, diarrhea, stomatitis, GI hemorrhage, mucositis
Neuromuscular & skeletal: Bone pain, myalgia

1% to 10%:

Cardiovascular: Chest pain, peripheral edema, capillary leak syndrome
Central nervous system: Headache
Dermatologic: Rash

(Continued)

Sargramostim *(Continued)*

Endocrine & metabolic: Fluid retention
Gastrointestinal: Anorexia, sore throat, stomatitis, constipation
Hematologic: Leukocytosis
Local: Pain at injection site
Neuromuscular & skeletal: Weakness, weakness
Respiratory: Dyspnea, cough

<1%:

Cardiovascular: Hypotension, flushing, pericardial effusion, transient supraventricular arrhythmias, pericarditis
Central nervous system: Malaise, fever, headache
Local: Thrombophlebitis
Neuromuscular & skeletal: Rigors
Miscellaneous: Anaphylactic reaction

Overdosage/Toxicology Symptoms of overdose include dyspnea, malaise, nausea, fever, headache, chills

Discontinue drug, wait for levels to fall, monitor CBC, respiratory symptoms, fluid status. Increase WBC; discontinue drug and wait for levels to fall; monitor for pulmonary edema; toxicity of GM-CSF is dose-dependent. Severe reactions such as capillary leak syndrome are seen at higher doses (>15 mcg/kg/day).

Drug Interactions

Increased toxicity: Lithium, corticosteroids may potentiate myeloproliferative effects

Stability

Sargramostim is available as a sterile, white, preservative-free, lyophilized powder

Sargramostim should be stored at 2°C to 8°C (36°F to 46°F)
Vials should not be frozen or shaken

Sargramostim is stable after dilution in 1 mL of bacteriostatic or nonbacteriostatic sterile water for injection for 30 days at 2°C to 8°C or 25°C

Sargramostim may also be further diluted in 0.9% sodium chloride to a concentration of ≥10 mcg/mL for I.V. infusion administration

This diluted solution is stable for 48 hours at room temperature and refrigeration

If the final concentration of sargramostim is <10 mcg/mL, human albumin should be added to the saline prior to the addition of sargramostim to prevent absorption of the components to the delivery system

It is recommended that 1 mg of human albumin/1 mL of 0.9% sodium chloride (eg, 1 mL of 5% human albumin/50 mL of 0.9% sodium chloride) be added

Standard diluent: Dose ≥250 mcg/25 mL NS

Incompatible with dextrose-containing solutions

Mechanism of Action Stimulates proliferation, differentiation and functional activity of neutrophils, eosinophils, monocytes, and macrophages; see table.

Proliferation/Differentiation	G-CSF (Filgrastim)	GM-CSF (Sargramostim)
Neutrophils	Yes	Yes
Eosinophils	No	Yes
Macrophages	No	Yes
Neutrophil migration	Enhanced	Inhibited

Pharmacodynamics/Kinetics

Onset of action: Increase in WBC in 7-14 days
Duration: WBC will return to baseline within 1 week after discontinuing drug
Half-life: 2 hours
Time to peak serum concentration: S.C.: Within 1-2 hours

Usual Dosage

Children and Adults: I.V. infusion over ≥2 hours or S.C.

Existing clinical data suggest that starting GM-CSF between 24 and 72 hours subsequent to chemotherapy may provide optimal neutrophil recover. Continue therapy until the occurrence of an absolute neutrophil count of 10,000/µL after the neutrophil nadir.

The available data suggest that rounding the dose to the nearest vial size may enhance patient convenience and reduce costs without clinical detriment.

Bone marrow transplantation failure or engraftment delay: I.V.: 250 mcg/m²/day for 14 days. The dose can be repeated after 7 days off therapy if engraftment has not occurred. If engraftment still has not occurred, a third course of 500 mcg/m²/day for 14 days may be tried after another 7 days off therapy. If there is still no engraftment, it is unlikely that further dose escalation be beneficial.

Myeloid reconstitution after peripheral stem cell, allogeneic or autologous bone marrow transplant: I.V.: 250 mcg/m²/day to begin 2-4 hours after the marrow infusion on day 0 of autologous bone marrow transplant or ≥24 hours after chemotherapy or 12 hours after last dose of radiotherapy. If significant adverse effects or "first dose" reaction is seen at this dose, discontinue the drug until toxicity resolves, then restart at a reduced dose of 125 mcg/m²/day.

Length of therapy: Bone marrow transplant patients: GM-CSF should be administered daily for up to 30 days or until the ANC has reached 1,500/mm³ for 3 consecutive days following the expected chemotherapy-induced neutrophil-nadir

Cancer chemotherapy recovery: I.V.: 3-15 mcg/kg/day for 14-21 days; maximum daily dose is 15 mcg/kg/day due to dose-related adverse effects; **discontinue therapy** if the ANC count is >20,000/mm³

Excessive blood counts return to normal or baseline levels within 3-7 days following cessation of therapy

Administration Administer by S.C. (undiluted) or I.V. infusion; I.V. infusion should be over at least 2 hours; **incompatible with dextrose-containing solutions**

Monitoring Parameters Vital signs, weight, CBC with differential, platelets, renal/liver function tests, especially with previous dysfunction, WBC with differential, pulmonary function

Reference Range Excessive leukocytosis: ANC >20,000/mm³ or WBC >50,000 cells/mm³

Patient Information May cause bone pain and first dose reaction

Nursing Implications Can premedicate with analgesics and antipyretics; control bone pain with non-narcotic analgesics; do not shake solution; when administering GM-CSF subcutaneously, rotate injection sites

Additional Information

Reimbursement Hotline (Leukine™): 1-800-321-4669

Professional Services (IMMUNEX): 1-800-334-6273

Dosage Forms Injection: 250 mcg, 500 mcg

Scabene® *see* Lindane *on page 728*

Scalpicin® *see* Hydrocortisone *on page 623*

Sclavo-PPD Solution® *see* Tuberculin Purified Protein Derivative *on page 1276*

Sclavo Test-PPD® *see* Tuberculin Purified Protein Derivative *on page 1276*

Scleromate™ *see* Morrhuate Sodium *on page 860*

Scopolamine (skoe POL a meen)

Related Information

Cycloplegic Mydriatics Comparison *on page 1409*

Brand Names Isopto® Hyoscine; Transderm Scop®

Canadian/Mexican Brand Names Transdermal-V® (Canada)

Synonyms Hyoscine; Scopolamine Hydrobromide

Therapeutic Category Anticholinergic Agent; Anticholinergic Agent, Ophthalmic; Anticholinergic Agent, Transdermal; Ophthalmic Agent, Mydriatic

Use Preoperative medication to produce amnesia and decrease salivation and respiratory secretions to produce cycloplegia and mydriasis; treatment of iridocyclitis, prevention of nausea and vomiting by motion; produces more CNS depression, mydriasis, and cycloplegia but less effective in preventing reflex bradycardia and effecting the intestines than atropine

Pregnancy Risk Factor C

Contraindications Hypersensitivity to scopolamine or any component; narrow-angle glaucoma; acute hemorrhage, gastrointestinal or genitourinary obstruction, thyrotoxicosis, tachycardia secondary to cardiac insufficiency, paralytic ileus

Warnings/Precautions Use with caution with hepatic or renal impairment since adverse CNS effects occur more often in these patients; use with caution in infants and children since they may be more susceptible to adverse effects of scopolamine; use with caution in patients with GI obstruction; anticholinergic agents are not well tolerated in the elderly and their use should be avoided when possible

Adverse Reactions

Ophthalmic:

- >10%: Ocular: Blurred vision, photophobia
- 1% to 10%:
  - Ocular: Local irritation, increased intraocular pressure
  - Respiratory: Congestion
- <1%:
  - Cardiovascular: Vascular congestion, edema
  - Central nervous system: Drowsiness
  - Dermatologic: Eczematoid dermatitis
  - Ocular: Follicular conjunctivitis
  - Miscellaneous: Exudate

(Continued)

Scopolamine *(Continued)*

Systemic:
- >10%:
  - Dermatologic: Dry skin
  - Gastrointestinal: Constipation, xerostomia, dry throat
  - Local: Irritation at injection site
  - Respiratory: Dry nose
  - Miscellaneous: Diaphoresis (decreased)
- 1% to 10%:
  - Dermatologic: Increased sensitivity to light
  - Endocrine & metabolic: Decreased flow of breast milk
  - Gastrointestinal: Dysphagia
- <1%:
  - Cardiovascular: Orthostatic hypotension, ventricular fibrillation, tachycardia, palpitations
  - Central nervous system: Confusion, drowsiness, headache, loss of memory, ataxia, fatigue
  - Dermatologic: Rash
  - Gastrointestinal: Bloated feeling, nausea, vomiting
  - Genitourinary: Dysuria
  - Neuromuscular & skeletal: Weakness
  - Ocular: Increased intraocular pain, blurred vision

Note: Systemic adverse effects have been reported following ophthalmic administration

Overdosage/Toxicology Symptoms of overdose include dilated pupils, flushed skin, tachycardia, hypertension, EKG abnormalities, CNS manifestations resemble acute psychosis; CNS depression, circulatory collapse, respiratory failure, and death can occur

Pure scopolamine intoxication is extremely rare. However, for a scopolamine overdose with severe life-threatening symptoms, physostigmine 1-2 mg (0.5 or 0.02 mg/kg for children) S.C. or I.V. slowly should be given to reverse the toxic effects.

Drug Interactions

Decreased effect of acetaminophen, levodopa, ketoconazole, digoxin, riboflavin, potassium chloride in wax matrix preparations

Increased toxicity: Additive adverse effects with other anticholinergic agents; GI absorption of the following drugs may be affected: acetaminophen, levodopa, ketoconazole, digoxin, riboflavin, potassium chloride wax-matrix preparations

Stability Avoid acid solutions, because hydrolysis occurs at pH <3; **physically compatible** when mixed in the same syringe with atropine, butorphanol, chlorpromazine, dimenhydrinate, diphenhydramine, droperidol, fentanyl, glycopyrrolate, hydromorphone, hydroxyzine, meperidine, metoclopramide, morphine, pentazocine, pentobarbital, perphenazine, prochlorperazine, promazine, promethazine, or thiopental

Mechanism of Action Blocks the action of acetylcholine at parasympathetic sites in smooth muscle, secretory glands and the CNS; increases cardiac output, dries secretions, antagonizes histamine and serotonin

Pharmacodynamics/Kinetics

Onset of effect:
- Oral, I.M.: 0.5-1 hour
- I.V.: 10 minutes

Duration of effect:
- Oral, I.M.: 4-6 hours
- I.V.: 2 hours

Peak effect: 20-60 minutes; it may take 3-7 days for full recovery
Absorption: Well absorbed by all routes of administration
Protein binding: Reversibly bound to plasma proteins
Metabolism: In the liver
Elimination: In urine

Usual Dosage

Preoperatively:
- Children: I.M., S.C.: 6 mcg/kg/dose (maximum: 0.3 mg/dose) or 0.2 mg/m^2 may be repeated every 6-8 hours **or** alternatively:
  - 4-7 months: 0.1 mg
  - 7 months to 3 years: 0.15 mg
  - 3-8 years: 0.2 mg
  - 8-12 years: 0.3 mg
- Adults: I.M., I.V., S.C.: 0.3-0.65 mg; may be repeated every 4-6 hours

Motion sickness: Transdermal: Children >12 years and Adults: Apply 1 disc behind the ear at least 4 hours prior to exposure and every 3 days as needed; effective if applied as soon as 2-3 hours before anticipated need, best if 12 hours before

Ophthalmic:
Refraction:
Children: Instill 1 drop of 0.25% to eye(s) twice daily for 2 days before procedure
Adults: Instill 1-2 drops of 0.25% to eye(s) 1 hour before procedure
Iridocyclitis:
Children: Instill 1 drop of 0.25% to eye(s) up to 3 times/day
Adults: Instill 1-2 drops of 0.25% to eye(s) up to 4 times/day

Administration I.V.: Dilute with an equal volume of sterile water and administer by direct I.V. injection over 2-3 minutes

Patient Information Report any changes of vision; wait 5 minutes after instilling ophthalmic preparation before using any other drops, do not blink excessively, after instilling ophthalmic preparation, apply pressure to the side of the nose near the eye to minimize systemic absorption; put patch on day before traveling; once applied, do not remove the patch for 3 full days; may cause drowsiness, dizziness, and blurred vision; may impair coordination and judgment; report to physician any CNS effects; apply patch behind ear

Nursing Implications Topical disc is programmed to deliver *in vivo* 0.5 mg over 3 days; wash hands before and after applying the disc to avoid drug contact with eyes

Dosage Forms
Disc, transdermal: 1.5 mg/disc (4's)
Injection, as hydrobromide: 0.3 mg/mL (1 mL); 0.4 mg/mL (0.5 mL, 1 mL); 0.86 mg/mL (0.5 mL); 1 mg/mL (1 mL)
Solution, ophthalmic, as hydrobromide: 0.25% (5 mL, 15 mL)

Scopolamine Hydrobromide *see* Scopolamine *on page 1127*
Scot-Tussin® [OTC] *see* Guaifenesin *on page 589*
Scot-Tussin DM® Cough Chasers [OTC] *see* Dextromethorphan *on page 366*
SeaMist® [OTC] *see* Sodium Chloride *on page 1142*
Sebizon® Topical Lotion *see* Sulfacetamide Sodium *on page 1171*

Secobarbital (see koe BAR bi tal)

Brand Names Seconal™

Canadian/Mexican Brand Names Novo-Secobarb® (Canada); Seconal® Sodium (Canada)

Synonyms Quinalbarbitone Sodium; Secobarbital Sodium

Therapeutic Category Barbiturate; Hypnotic; Sedative

Use Short-term treatment of insomnia and as preanesthetic agent

Restrictions C-II

Pregnancy Risk Factor D

Contraindications CNS depression, uncontrolled pain, hypersensitivity to secobarbital or any component

Warnings/Precautions Use with caution in patients with hypovolemic shock, congestive heart failure, hepatic impairment, respiratory dysfunction or depression, previous addiction to the sedative/hypnotic group, chronic or acute pain, renal dysfunction, and the elderly; tolerance or psychological and physical dependence may occur with prolonged use, pregnancy with toxemia or bleeding

Adverse Reactions
>10%:
Central nervous system: Dizziness, lightheadedness, drowsiness, "hangover" effect
Local: Pain at injection site
1% to 10%:
Central nervous system: Confusion, mental depression, unusual excitement, nervousness, faint feeling, headache, insomnia, nightmares
Gastrointestinal: Constipation, nausea, vomiting
<1%:
Cardiovascular: Hypotension
Central nervous system: Hallucinations
Dermatologic: Rash, exfoliative dermatitis, Stevens-Johnson syndrome
Hematologic: Megaloblastic anemia, thrombocytopenia, agranulocytosis
Local: Thrombophlebitis
Respiratory: Respiratory depression

Overdosage/Toxicology Symptoms of overdose include unsteady gait, slurred speech, confusion, jaundice, hypothermia, fever, hypotension, respiratory depression, coma

If hypotension occurs, administer I.V. fluids and place the patient in the Trendelenburg position. If unresponsive, an I.V. vasopressor (eg, dopamine, epinephrine) may be required. Charcoal hemoperfusion or hemodialysis may be useful in the harder to treat intoxications, especially in the presence of very high serum barbiturate levels when the patient is in shock, coma, or renal failure. Forced
(Continued)

Secobarbital *(Continued)*

alkaline diuresis is of no value in the treatment of intoxications with short-acting barbiturates.

Drug Interactions

Decreased effect of betamethasone and other corticosteroids, TCAs, chloramphenicol, estrogens, cyclophosphamide, oral anticoagulants, doxycycline, theophylline

Increased effect/toxicity with CNS depressants, chloramphenicol, chlorpropamide

Stability Do not shake vial during reconstitution, rotate ampul; aqueous solutions are not stable, reconstitute with aqueous polyethylene glycol; aqueous (sterile water) solutions should be used within 30 minutes; do not use bacteriostatic water for injection or lactated Ringer's. I.V. form is **incompatible** when mixed with benzquinamide (in syringe), cimetidine (same syringe), codeine, erythromycin, glycopyrrolate (same syringe), hydrocortisone, insulin, levorphanol, methadone, norepinephrine, pentazocine, phenytoin, sodium bicarbonate, tetracycline, vancomycin

Mechanism of Action Interferes with transmission of impulses from the thalamus to the cortex of the brain resulting in an imbalance in central inhibitory and facilitatory mechanisms

Pharmacodynamics/Kinetics

Onset of hypnosis:

- Oral: Within 1-3 minutes
- I.V. injection: Within 15-30 minutes

Duration: ~15 minutes

Absorption: Oral: Well absorbed (90%)

Distribution: Crosses the placenta; appears in breast milk

Protein binding: 45% to 60%

Metabolism: In the liver

Half-life: 25 hours

Time to peak serum concentration: Within 2-4 hours

Elimination: Renally as inactive metabolites and small amounts as unchanged drug

Usual Dosage Hypnotic:

Children: I.M.: 3-5 mg/kg/dose; maximum: 100 mg/dose

Adults:

- I.M.: 100-200 mg/dose
- I.V.: 50-250 mg/dose

Hemodialysis: Slightly dialyzable (5% to 20%)

Dietary Considerations Alcohol: Additive CNS effect, avoid use

Administration I.V.: Administer undiluted or diluted with sterile water for injection, normal saline, or Ringer's injection; maximum infusion rate: 50 mg/15 seconds; avoid intra-arterial injection

Reference Range Therapeutic: 1-2 μg/mL (SI: 4.2-8.4 μmol/L); Toxic: >5 μg/mL (SI: >21 μmol/L)

Patient Information Avoid the use of alcohol and other CNS depressants; avoid driving and other hazardous tasks; avoid abrupt discontinuation; may cause physical and psychological dependence; do not alter dose without notifying physician

Dosage Forms Injection, as sodium: 50 mg/mL (2 mL)

Secobarbital Sodium *see* Secobarbital *on previous page*

Seconal™ *see* Secobarbital *on previous page*

Secran® *see* Vitamins, Multiple *on page 1310*

Sectral® *see* Acebutolol *on page 17*

Sedapap-10® *see* Butalbital Compound *on page 176*

Seldane® *see* Terfenadine *on page 1196*

Selegiline (seh LEDGE ah leen)

Brand Names Eldepryl®

Canadian/Mexican Brand Names Novo-Selegiline® (Canada)

Synonyms Deprenyl; L-Deprenyl; Selegiline Hydrochloride

Therapeutic Category Anti-Parkinson's Agent

Use Adjunct in the management of parkinsonian patients in which levodopa/carbidopa therapy is deteriorating

Unlabeled use: Early Parkinson's disease

Investigational: Alzheimer's disease

Selegiline is also being studied in Alzheimer's disease. Small studies have shown some improvement in behavioral and cognitive performance in patients, however, further study is needed.

Pregnancy Risk Factor C

Contraindications Known hypersensitivity to selegiline, concomitant use of meperidine

Warnings/Precautions Increased risk of nonselective MAO inhibition occurs with doses >10 mg/day; is a monoamine oxidase inhibitor type "B", there should **not** be a problem with tyramine-containing products as long as the typical doses are employed

Adverse Reactions

>10%:

Central nervous system: Mood changes, dizziness

Gastrointestinal: Nausea, vomiting, xerostomia, abdominal pain

Neuromuscular & skeletal: Dyskinesias

1% to 10%:

Cardiovascular: Orthostatic hypotension, arrhythmias, hypertension

Central nervous system: Hallucinations, confusion, depression, insomnia, agitation, loss of balance

Neuromuscular & skeletal: Increased involuntary movements, bradykinesia, muscle twitches

Miscellaneous: Bruxism

Overdosage/Toxicology Symptoms of overdose include tachycardia, palpitations, muscle twitching, seizures

Competent supportive care is the most important treatment; both hypertension or hypotension can occur with intoxication. Hypotension may respond to I.V. fluids or vasopressors, and hypertension usually responds to an alpha-adrenergic blocker. While treating the hypertension, care is warranted to avoid sudden drops in blood pressure, since this may worsen the MAO inhibitor toxicity. Muscle irritability and seizures often respond to diazepam, while hyperthermia is best treated antipyretics and cooling blankets. Cardiac arrhythmias are best treated with phenytoin or procainamide.

Drug Interactions

Increased toxicity

Meperidine in combination with selegiline has caused agitation, delirium, and death; it may be prudent to avoid other opioids as well

Fluoxetine increases pressor effect

Mechanism of Action Potent monoamine oxidase (MAO) type-B inhibitor; MAO-B plays a major role in the metabolism of dopamine; selegiline may also increase dopaminergic activity by interfering with dopamine reuptake at the synapse

Pharmacodynamics/Kinetics

Onset of therapeutic effects: Within 1 hour

Duration: 24-72 hours

Half-life: 9 minutes

Metabolism: In the liver to amphetamine and methamphetamine

Usual Dosage Oral:

Adults: 5 mg twice daily with breakfast and lunch or 10 mg in the morning

Elderly: Initial: 5 mg in the morning, may increase to a total of 10 mg/day

Monitoring Parameters Blood pressure, symptoms of parkinsonism

Patient Information Do not exceed daily doses of 10 mg; report to physician any involuntary movements or CNS agitation; explain the tyramine reaction to patients and tell them to report severe headaches or other unusual symptoms to physician

Nursing Implications Monoamine oxidase inhibitor type "B"; there should **not** be a problem with tyramine-containing products as long as the typical doses are employed

Dosage Forms Capsule, as hydrochloride: 5 mg

Selegiline Hydrochloride *see* Selegiline *on previous page*

Selenium (se LEE nee um)

Brand Names Sele-Pak®; Selepen®

Canadian/Mexican Brand Names Versel® (Canada)

Therapeutic Category Trace Element, Parenteral

Use Trace metal supplement

Pregnancy Risk Factor C

Contraindications Known hypersensitivity to selenium or any component

Adverse Reactions

1% to 10%:

Central nervous system: Lethargy

Dermatologic: Alopecia or hair discoloration

Gastrointestinal: Vomiting following long-term use on damaged skin; abdominal pain, garlic breath

Local: Irritation

Neuromuscular & skeletal: Tremor

Miscellaneous: Diaphoresis

(Continued)

Selenium *(Continued)*

Overdosage/Toxicology Symptoms of overdose include nausea, vomiting, diarrhea

Mechanism of Action Part of glutathione peroxidase which protects cell components from oxidative damage due to peroxidases produced in cellular metabolism

Pharmacodynamics/Kinetics Elimination: Urine, feces, lungs, skin

Usual Dosage I.V. in TPN solutions:
- Children: 3 mcg/kg/day
- Adults:
  - Metabolically stable: 20-40 mcg/day
  - Deficiency from prolonged TPN support: 100 mcg/day for 24 and 21 days

Dosage Forms Injection: 40 mcg/mL (10 mL, 30 mL)

Selenium Sulfide (se LEE nee um SUL fide)

Brand Names Exsel®; Head & Shoulders® Intensive Treatment [OTC]; Selsun®; Selsun Blue® [OTC]; Selsun Gold® for Women [OTC]

Therapeutic Category Antiseborrheic Agent, Topical; Shampoos

Use Treatment of itching and flaking of the scalp associated with dandruff, to control scalp seborrheic dermatitis; treatment of tinea versicolor

Pregnancy Risk Factor C

Contraindications Known hypersensitivity to selenium or any component

Warnings/Precautions Do not use on damaged skin to avoid any systemic toxicity; avoid topical use in very young children; safety of topical in infants has not been established

Adverse Reactions
- >10%: Dermatologic: Unusual dryness or oiliness of scalp
- 1% to 10%:
  - Central nervous system: Lethargy
  - Dermatologic: Alopecia or hair discoloration
  - Gastrointestinal: Vomiting following long-term use on damaged skin, abdominal pain, garlic breath
  - Local: Irritation
  - Neuromuscular & skeletal: Tremor
  - Miscellaneous: Diaphoresis

Overdosage/Toxicology Symptoms of overdose include nausea, vomiting, diarrhea

Mechanism of Action May block the enzymes involved in growth of epithelial tissue

Pharmacodynamics/Kinetics
- Absorption: Topical: Not absorbed through intact skin, but can be absorbed through damaged skin
- Elimination: Urine, feces, lungs, skin

Usual Dosage Topical:
- Dandruff, seborrhea: Massage 5-10 mL into wet scalp, leave on scalp 2-3 minutes, rinse thoroughly, and repeat application; shampoo twice weekly for 2 weeks initially, then use once every 1-4 weeks as indicated depending upon control
- Tinea versicolor: Apply the 2.5% lotion to affected area and lather with small amounts of water; leave on skin for 10 minutes, then rinse thoroughly; apply every day for 7 days

Patient Information Topical formulations are for external use only; notify physician if condition persists or worsens; avoid contact with eyes; thoroughly rinse after application

Dosage Forms Shampoo: 1% (120 mL, 210 mL, 240 mL, 330 mL); 2.5% (120 mL)

Sele-Pak® *see* Selenium *on previous page*

Selepen® *see* Selenium *on previous page*

Selestoject® *see* Betamethasone *on page 147*

Selsun® *see* Selenium Sulfide *on this page*

Selsun Blue® [OTC] *see* Selenium Sulfide *on this page*

Selsun Gold® for Women [OTC] *see* Selenium Sulfide *on this page*

Semprex-D® *see* Acrivastine and Pseudoephedrine *on page 29*

Sensorcaine® *see* Bupivacaine *on page 170*

Septa® Topical Ointment [OTC] *see* Bacitracin, Neomycin, and Polymyxin B *on page 129*

Septisol® *see* Hexachlorophene *on page 610*

Septra® *see* Co-Trimoxazole *on page 315*

Septra® DS *see* Co-Trimoxazole *on page 315*

Serax® *see* Oxazepam *on page 933*

Serentil® *see* Mesoridazine *on page 790*

Serevent® *see* Salmeterol *on page 1121*
Seromycin® Pulvules® *see* Cycloserine *on page 326*
Serophene® *see* Clomiphene *on page 295*

Sertraline (SER tra leen)

Related Information

Antidepressant Agents Comparison *on page 1393*

Brand Names Zoloft™

Synonyms Sertraline Hydrochloride

Therapeutic Category Antidepressant, Serotonin Reuptake Inhibitor

Use Treatment of major depression; also being studied for use in obesity and obsessive-compulsive disorder

Pregnancy Risk Factor B

Contraindications Hypersensitivity to sertraline or any component

Warnings/Precautions Do not use in combination with monoamine oxidase inhibitor or within 14 days of discontinuing treatment or initiating treatment with a monoamine oxidase inhibitor due to the risk of serotonin syndrome; use with caution in patients with pre-existing seizure disorders, patients in whom weight loss is undesirable, patients with recent myocardial infarction, unstable heart disease, hepatic or renal impairment, patients taking other psychotropic medications, agitated or hyperactive patients as drug may produce or activate mania or hypomania; because the risk of suicide is inherent in depression, patient should be closely monitored until depressive symptoms remit and prescriptions should be written for minimum quantities to reduce the risk of overdose

Adverse Reactions

1% to 10%: In clinical trials, dizziness and nausea were two most frequent side effects that led to discontinuation of therapy

- Cardiovascular: Palpitations
- Central nervous system: Insomnia, agitation, dizziness, headache, somnolence, nervousness, fatigue, pain
- Dermatologic: Dermatological reactions
- Endocrine & metabolic: Sexual dysfunction in men
- Gastrointestinal: Xerostomia, diarrhea or loose stools, nausea, constipation
- Genitourinary: Urinary disorders
- Neuromuscular & skeletal: Tremors
- Ocular: Visual difficulty
- Otic: Tinnitus
- Miscellaneous: Diaphoresis

Overdosage/Toxicology Symptoms of overdose include serious toxicity has not yet been reported, monitor cardiovascular, gastrointestinal, and hepatic functions

Establish and maintain an airway, ensure adequate oxygenation and ventilation. Activated charcoal with 70% sorbitol may be as or more effective than emesis or lavage. Monitoring of cardiac and vital signs is recommended along with general symptomatic and supportive measures. There is no specific antidote for sertraline. Treatment should be aimed at first decontamination, then symptomatic and supportive care; forced diuresis, dialysis, hemoperfusion and exchange transfusion are unlikely to enhance elimination due to sertraline's large volume of distribution.

Drug Interactions

All serotonin reuptake inhibitors are capable of inhibiting cytochrome P-450 IID6 isoenzyme enzyme system. The drugs metabolized by this system include desipramine, dextromethorphan, encainide, haloperidol, imipramine, metoprolol, perphenazine, propafenone, and thioridazine

Increased toxicity:

- MAO inhibitors and possibly with lithium or tricyclic antidepressants → **serotonin syndrome** serotonergic hyperstimulation with the following clinical features: mental status changes, restlessness, myoclonus, hyperreflexia, diaphoresis, diarrhea, shivering, and tremor
- May decrease metabolism/plasma clearance of some drugs (diazepam, tolbutamide) to result in increased duration and pharmacological effects
- May displace highly plasma protein bound drugs from binding sites (eg, warfarin) to result in increased effect

Mechanism of Action Antidepressant with selective inhibitory effects on presynaptic serotonin (5-HT) reuptake

Pharmacodynamics/Kinetics

Absorption: Slow
Protein binding: High
Metabolism: Extensive
Half-life:
- Parent: 24 hours
- Metabolites: 66 hours

Elimination: In both urine and feces

(Continued)

Sertraline *(Continued)*

Usual Dosage Oral:

Adults: Start with 50 mg/day in the morning and increase by 50 mg/day increments every 2-3 days if tolerated to 100 mg/day; additional increases may be necessary; maximum dose: 200 mg/day. If somnolence is noted, administer at bedtime.

Elderly: Start treatment with 25 mg/day in the morning and increase by 25 mg/day increments every 2-3 days if tolerated to 75-100 mg/day; additional increases may be necessary; maximum dose: 200 mg/day

Hemodialysis: Not removed by hemodialysis

Dosage comments in hepatic impairment: Sertraline is extensively metabolized by the liver; caution should be used in patients with hepatic impairment

Test Interactions Minor ↑ triglycerides (S), ↑ LFTs, ↓ uric acid (S)

Patient Information If you are currently on another antidepressant drug, please notify your physician. Although sertraline has not been shown to increase the effects of alcohol, it is recommended that you refrain from drinking while on this medication. If you are pregnant or intend becoming pregnant while on this drug, please alert your physician to this fact. You may experience some weight loss, but it is usually minimal.

Dosage Forms Tablet, as hydrochloride: 25 mg, 50 mg, 100 mg

Sertraline Hydrochloride *see* Sertraline *on previous page*

Serutan® [OTC] *see* Psyllium *on page 1075*

Serzone® *see* Nefazodone *on page 884*

Sevoflurane (see voe FLOO rane)

Brand Names Ultane®

Canadian/Mexican Brand Names Serovane™ (Canada)

Therapeutic Category General Anesthetic

Use General induction and maintenance of anesthesia (inhalation)

Pregnancy Risk Factor B

Contraindications Previous hypersensitivity to sevoflurane or other halogenated anesthetics

Warnings/Precautions Malignant hyperthermia has been reported in susceptible patients, due to its potential for fluoride nephropathy, renal function should be closely monitored, similar to isoflurane, sevoflurane has the potential to increase cerebral blood flow and intracranial pressure and therefore, must be used with caution in patients with pre-existing increases in CSF pressure.

Adverse Reactions

>1%:

Cardiovascular: Bradycardia, hypotension, tachycardia, hypertension

Central nervous system: Agitation, headache, somnolence, dizziness, fever, early emergence movement, hypothermia

Gastrointestinal: Nausea (25%) and vomiting (18%), increased salivation

Respiratory: Laryngospasm, airway obstruction, breath holding, increased cough, apnea

Miscellaneous: Shivering

Drug Interactions

Increased effect: Administration of 50% N_20 reduces the minimum alveolar concentration (MAC) equivalent dose of sevoflurane by 50% in adults and 25% in children; benzodiazepines and opioids also reduce the MAC of sevoflurane

Stability Store at controlled room temperature (15°C to 30°C); use cautiously in low-flow or closed-circuit systems, since sevoflurane is unstable potentially toxic breakdown products have been liberated

Pharmacodynamics/Kinetics Sevoflurane has a low blood/gas partition coefficient and therefore is associated with a rapid onset of anesthesia and recovery

Time to induction: Within 2 minutes

Emergence time: 4 to 14 minutes

Metabolism: In the liver to inorganic fluoride, hexafluoroisopropanol and hexafluoroisopropanol glucuronide

Usual Dosage

Induction: Usually administered in concentrations of 1.8% to 5% in N_2O/O_2. It has also been given via the vital capacity rapid inhalation technique as 4.5% in N_2O/O_2

Maintenance: Surgical levels of anesthesia can usually be obtained with concentrations of 0.75% to 3%

Monitoring Parameters Blood pressure, temperature, heart rate, neuromuscular function, oxygen saturation, endtidal CO_2 and endtidal sevoflurane concentrations should be monitored prior to and throughout anesthesia; the dose of sevoflurane may be adjusted by monitoring blood pressure, since the depth of anesthesia is inversely related to blood pressure in the absence of other complications

Dosage Forms Liquid for inhalation: 250 mL

Siblin® [OTC] *see* Psyllium *on page 1075*

Siladryl® Oral [OTC] *see* Diphenhydramine *on page 399*

Silafed® Syrup [OTC] *see* Triprolidine and Pseudoephedrine *on page 1270*

Silain® [OTC] *see* Simethicone *on next page*

Silphen® Cough [OTC] *see* Diphenhydramine *on page 399*

Siltussin® [OTC] *see* Guaifenesin *on page 589*

Siltussin DM® [OTC] *see* Guaifenesin and Dextromethorphan *on page 591*

Silvadene® *see* Silver Sulfadiazine *on next page*

Silver Nitrate (SIL ver NYE trate)

Synonyms $AgNO_3$

Therapeutic Category Antibiotic, Ophthalmic; Antibiotic, Topical; Cauterizing Agent, Topical; Topical Skin Product, Antibacterial

Use Prevention of gonococcal ophthalmia neonatorum; cauterization of wounds and sluggish ulcers, removal of granulation tissue and warts; aseptic prophylaxis of burns

Pregnancy Risk Factor C

Contraindications Not for use on broken skin or cuts; hypersensitivity to silver nitrate or any component

Warnings/Precautions Do not use applicator sticks on the eyes; repeated applications of the ophthalmic solution into the eye can cause cauterization of the cornea and blindness

Adverse Reactions

>10%:
- Dermatologic: Burning and skin irritation
- Ocular: Chemical conjunctivitis

1% to 10%:
- Dermatologic: Staining of the skin
- Hematologic: Methemoglobinemia
- Ocular: Cauterization of the cornea, blindness

Overdosage/Toxicology Symptoms of overdose include pain and burning of mouth, salivation, vomiting, diarrhea, shock, coma, convulsions, death; blackening of skin and mucous membranes; absorbed nitrate can cause methemoglobinemia

Fatal dose is as low as 2 g

Administer sodium chloride in water (10 g/L) to cause precipitation of silver

Drug Interactions Decreased effect: Sulfacetamide preparations are incompatible

Stability Must be stored in a dry place; exposure to light causes silver to oxidize and turn brown, dipping in water causes oxidized film to readily dissolve

Mechanism of Action Free silver ions precipitate bacterial proteins by combining with chloride in tissue forming silver chloride; coagulates cellular protein to form an eschar; silver ions or salts or colloidal silver preparations can inhibit the growth of both gram-positive and gram-negative bacteria. This germicidal action is attributed to the precipitation of bacterial proteins by liberated silver ions. Silver nitrate coagulates cellular protein to form an eschar, and this mode of action is the postulated mechanism for control of benign hematuria, rhinitis, and recurrent pneumothorax.

Pharmacodynamics/Kinetics

Absorption: Because silver ions readily combine with protein, there is minimal GI and cutaneous absorption of the 0.5% and 1% preparations

Elimination: Although the highest amounts of silver noted on autopsy have been in the kidneys, excretion in urine is minimal

Usual Dosage

Neonates: Ophthalmic: Instill 2 drops immediately after birth (no later than 1 hour after delivery) into conjunctival sac of each eye as a single dose, allow to sit for ≥30 seconds; do not irrigate eyes following instillation of eye drops

Children and Adults:
- Ointment: Apply in an apertured pad on affected area or lesion for approximately 5 days
- Sticks: Apply to mucous membranes and other moist skin surfaces only on area to be treated 2-3 times/week for 2-3 weeks
- Topical solution: Apply a cotton applicator dipped in solution on the affected area 2-3 times/week for 2-3 weeks

Monitoring Parameters With prolonged use, monitor methemoglobin levels

Patient Information Discontinue topical preparation if redness or irritation develop

Nursing Implications Silver nitrate solutions stain skin and utensils

Additional Information Applicators are **not** for ophthalmic use

(Continued)

Silver Nitrate *(Continued)*

Dosage Forms

Applicator sticks: 75% with potassium nitrate 25% (6")
Ointment: 10% (30 g)
Solution:
  Ophthalmic: 1% (wax ampuls)
  Topical: 10% (30 mL); 25% (30 mL); 50% (30 mL)

Silver Sulfadiazine (SIL ver sul fa DYE a zeen)

Related Information

Sulfonamide Derivatives *on page 1420*

Brand Names Silvadene®; SSD™; SSD-AF™; Thermazene™

Canadian/Mexican Brand Names Dermazin® (Canada); Flamazine® (Canada)

Therapeutic Category Antibacterial, Topical

Use Prevention and treatment of infection in second and third degree burns

Pregnancy Risk Factor C

Contraindications Hypersensitivity to silver sulfadiazine or any component; premature infants or neonates <2 months of age because sulfonamides compete with bilirubin for protein binding sites which may displace bilirubin and cause kernicterus

Warnings/Precautions Use with caution in patients with G-6-PD deficiency, renal impairment, or history of allergy to other sulfonamides; sulfadiazine may accumulate in patients with impaired hepatic or renal function; use of analgesic might be needed before application; systemic absorption is significant and adverse reactions may be due to sulfa component

Adverse Reactions

>10%:
  Local: Burning, pain at injection site
1% to 10%:
  Dermatologic: Itching, rash, erythema multiforme, discoloration of skin
  Hematologic: Hemolytic anemia, leukopenia, agranulocytosis, aplastic anemia
  Hepatic: Hepatitis
  Renal: Interstitial nephritis
  Miscellaneous: Allergic reactions may be related to sulfa component
<1%: Dermatologic: Photosensitivity

Drug Interactions Decreased effect: Topical proteolytic enzymes are inactivated

Stability Discard if cream is darkened (reacts with heavy metals resulting in release of silver)

Mechanism of Action Acts upon the bacterial cell wall and cell membrane. Bactericidal for many gram-negative and gram-positive bacteria and is effective against yeast. Active against *Pseudomonas aeruginosa, Pseudomonas maltophilia, Enterobacter* species, *Klebsiella* species, *Serratia* species, *Escherichia coli, Proteus mirabilis, Morganella morganii, Providencia rettgeri, Proteus vulgaris, Providencia* species, *Citrobacter* species, *Acinetobacter calcoaceticus, Staphylococcus aureus, Staphylococcus epidermidis, Enterococcus* species, *Candida albicans, Corynebacterium diphtheriae*, and *Clostridium perfringens*

Pharmacodynamics/Kinetics

Absorption: Significant percutaneous absorption of sulfadiazine can occur especially when applied to extensive burns
Half-life: 10 hours and is prolonged in patients with renal insufficiency
Time to peak serum concentration: Within 3-11 days of continuous therapy
Elimination: ~50% excreted unchanged in urine

Usual Dosage Children and Adults: Topical: Apply once or twice daily with a sterile-gloved hand; apply to a thickness of 1/16"; burned area should be covered with cream at all times

Monitoring Parameters Serum electrolytes, urinalysis, renal function tests, CBC in patients with extensive burns on long-term treatment

Patient Information For external use only; bathe daily to aid in debridement (if not contraindicated); apply liberally to burned areas; for external use only; notify physician if condition persists or worsens

Nursing Implications Evaluate the development of granulation

Additional Information Contains methylparaben and propylene glycol

Dosage Forms Cream, topical: 1% [10 mg/g] (20 g, 25 g, 50 g, 85 g, 400 g, 1000 g)

Simethicone (sye METH i kone)

Brand Names Degas® [OTC]; Flatulex® [OTC]; Gas Relief® [OTC]; Gas-X® [OTC]; Maalox Anti-Gas® [OTC]; Mylanta® Gas [OTC]; Mylicon® [OTC]; Phazyme® [OTC]; Silain® [OTC]

Canadian/Mexican Brand Names Ovol® (Canada)

Synonyms Activated Dimethicone; Activated Methylpolysiloxane

Therapeutic Category Antiflatulent

Use Relieves flatulence and functional gastric bloating, and postoperative gas pains

Pregnancy Risk Factor C

Pregnancy/Breast-Feeding Implications

Clinical effects on the fetus: No data available; available evidence suggests safe use during pregnancy and breast-feeding

Breast-feeding/lactation: No data available

Contraindications Hypersensitivity to drug or components

Warnings/Precautions Not recommended for the treatment of infant colic; do not exceed recommended dosing guidelines

Overdosage/Toxicology Nontoxic orally

Stability Protect from light

Mechanism of Action Decreases the surface tension of gas bubbles thereby disperses and prevents gas pockets in the GI system

Pharmacodynamics/Kinetics Elimination: In feces

Usual Dosage Oral:

Infants: 20 mg 4 times/day

Children <12 years: 40 mg 4 times/day

Children >12 years and Adults: 40-120 mg after meals and at bedtime as needed, not to exceed 500 mg/day

Test Interactions False-negative gastric guaiac

Patient Information Some tablets may be chewed thoroughly before swallowing, follow with a glass of water

Nursing Implications Shake suspension before using; mix with water, infant formula, or other liquids

Dosage Forms

Capsule: 125 mg

Drops, oral: 40 mg/0.6 mL (15 mL, 30 mL)

Tablet: 50 mg, 60 mg, 95 mg

Tablet, chewable: 40 mg, 80 mg, 125 mg

Simron® [OTC] *see* Ferrous Gluconate *on page 515*

Simvastatin (SIM va stat in)

Related Information

Lipid-Lowering Agents *on page 1413*

Brand Names Zocor™

Therapeutic Category Antilipemic Agent; HMG-CoA Reductase Inhibitor

Use Adjunct to dietary therapy to decrease elevated serum total and LDL cholesterol concentrations in primary hypercholesterolemia

Pregnancy Risk Factor X

Contraindications Previous hypersensitivity to simvastatin or lovastatin or other HMG-CoA reductase inhibitors; active liver disease or unexplained elevations of serum transaminases; pregnancy and lactation

Adverse Reactions

1% to 10%:

Central nervous system: Headache, dizziness

Dermatologic: Rash

Endocrine & metabolic: Elevated creatine phosphokinase (CPK)

Gastrointestinal: Flatulence, abdominal cramps, diarrhea, constipation, nausea, dyspepsia, heartburn

Neuromuscular & skeletal: Myalgia

<1%:

Gastrointestinal: Abnormal taste

Ocular: Lenticular opacities, blurred vision

Overdosage/Toxicology Very few adverse events; treatment is symptomatic

Drug Interactions

Increased effect of warfarin, erythromycin, niacin

Increased toxicity of cyclosporin, gemfibrozil

Possibly increased toxicity of simvastatin with itraconazole since itraconazole increases lovastatin levels by as much as 20-fold

Concurrent use of erythromycin and HMG-CoA reductase inhibitors may result in rhabdomyolysis

Stability Tablets should be stored in well closed containers at temperatures between 5°C to 30°C (41°F to 86°F)

Mechanism of Action Simvastatin is a methylated derivative of lovastatin that acts by competitively inhibiting 3-hydroxy-3-methylglutaryl-coenzyme A (HMG-CoA) reductase, the enzyme that catalyzes the rate-limiting step in cholesterol biosynthesis

Pharmacodynamics/Kinetics

Absorption: Oral: Although 85% is absorbed following administration, <5% reaches the general circulation due to an extensive first-pass effect

Time to peak concentrations: 1.3-2.4 hours

(Continued)

Simvastatin *(Continued)*

Protein binding: ~95%

Elimination: 13% excreted in urine and 60% in feces; the elimination half-life is unknown

In patients with severe renal insufficiency, high systemic levels may occur

Usual Dosage Adults: Oral: Start with 5-10 mg/day as a single bedtime dose; if LDL is ≤190 mg/dL start with 5 mg; if LDL >190 mg/dL, start with 10 mg/day; increase every 4 weeks as needed; maximum dose: 40 mg/day

Dosing adjustment/comments in renal impairment: Recommended starting dose: 5 mg; patient should be closely monitored

Monitoring Parameters Creatine phosphokinase levels due to possibility of myopathy; serum cholesterol (total and fractionated)

Patient Information Promptly report any unexplained muscle pain, tenderness or weakness, especially if accompanied by malaise or fever; follow prescribed diet; take with meals

Nursing Implications Liver enzyme elevations may be observed during simvastatin therapy; combination therapy with other hypolipidemic agents may be required to achieve optimal reductions of LDL cholesterol; diet, weight reduction, and exercise should be attempted to control hypercholesterolemia before the institution of simvastatin therapy

Dosage Forms Tablet: 5 mg, 10 mg, 20 mg, 40 mg

Sinarest® 12 Hour Nasal Solution *see* Oxymetazoline *on page 940*

Sinarest® Nasal Solution [OTC] *see* Phenylephrine *on page 989*

Sinemet® *see* Levodopa and Carbidopa *on page 715*

Sinequan® Oral *see* Doxepin *on page 424*

Sinex® Long-Acting [OTC] *see* Oxymetazoline *on page 940*

Sinumist®-SR Capsulets® *see* Guaifenesin *on page 589*

Sinusol-B® *see* Brompheniramine *on page 166*

Sirdalud® *see* Tizanidine *on page 1232*

SK and F 104864 *see* Topotecan *on page 1244*

SKF 104864 *see* Topotecan *on page 1244*

SKF 104864-A *see* Topotecan *on page 1244*

Skin Test Antigens, Multiple (skin test AN tee gens, MUL ti pul)

Brand Names Multitest CMI®

Therapeutic Category Diagnostic Agent, Hypersensitivity Skin Testing

Use Detection of nonresponsiveness to antigens by means of delayed hypersensitivity skin testing

Pregnancy Risk Factor C

Contraindications Infected or inflamed skin, known hypersensitivity to skin test antigens; do not apply at sites involving acneiform, infected or inflamed skin; although severe systemic reactions are rare to diphtheria and tetanus antigens, persons known to have a history of systemic reactions should be tested with this test only after the test heads containing these antigens have been removed

Warnings/Precautions Epinephrine should be available is case of severe reactions. Safety and effectiveness in children <17 years of age have not been established; discard applicator after use, do not reuse.

Adverse Reactions 1% to 10%: Local irritation

Drug Interactions Decreased effect: Drugs or procedures that suppress immunity such as corticosteroids, chemotherapeutic agents, antilymphocyte globulin and irradiation, may possibly cause a loss of reactivity

Stability Keep in refrigerator at 2°C to 8°C (35°F to 46°F)

Usual Dosage Select only test sites that permit sufficient surface area and subcutaneous tissue to allow adequate penetration of all eight points, avoid hairy areas

Press loaded unit into the skin with sufficient pressure to puncture the skin and allow adequate penetration of all points, maintain firm contact for at least 5 seconds, during application the device should not be "rocked" back and forth and side to side without removing any of the test heads from the skin sites

If adequate pressure is applied it will be possible to observe:

1. The puncture marks of the nine tines on each of the eight test heads
2. An imprint of the circular platform surrounding each test head
3. Residual antigen and glycerin at each of the eight sites

If any of the above three criteria are not fully followed, the test results may not be reliable

Reading should be done in good light, read the test sites at both 24 and 48 hours, the largest reaction recorded from the two readings at each test site should be used; if two readings are not possible, a single 48 hour is recommended

A positive reaction from any of the seven delayed hypersensitivity skin test antigens is **induration ≥2 mm** providing there is no induration at the negative control site; the size of the induration reactions with this test may be smaller than those obtained with other intradermal procedures

Nursing Implications Patients should be informed of the types of test site reactions that may be expected. Remove tests from refrigeration approximately 1 hour before use; select only test sites that permit sufficient surface area and subcutaneous tissue to allow adequate penetration of all points on all eight test heads; avoid hairy areas when possible because interpretation of reactions will be more difficult

Additional Information Contains disposable plastic applicator consisting of eight sterile test heads preloaded with the following seven delayed hypersensitivity skin test antigens and glycerin negative control for percutaneous administration

Test Head No. 1 = Tetanus toxoid antigen
Test Head No. 2 = Diphtheria toxoid antigen
Test Head No. 3 = *Streptococcus* antigen
Test Head No. 4 = Tuberculin, old
Test Head No. 5 = Glycerin negative control
Test Head No. 6 = *Candida* antigen
Test Head No. 7 = *Trichophyton* antigen
Test Head No. 8 = *Proteus* antigen

Dosage Forms Individual carton containing one preloaded skin test antigen for cellular hypersensitivity

Skin Tests *see page 1501*
Sleep-eze 3® Oral [OTC] *see* Diphenhydramine *on page 399*
Sleepinal® [OTC] *see* Diphenhydramine *on page 399*
Sleepwell 2-nite® [OTC] *see* Diphenhydramine *on page 399*
Slim-Mint® [OTC] *see* Benzocaine *on page 138*
Slo-bid™ *see* Theophylline Salts *on page 1207*
Slo-Niacin® [OTC] *see* Niacin *on page 896*
Slo-Phyllin® *see* Theophylline Salts *on page 1207*
Slow FE® [OTC] *see* Ferrous Sulfate *on page 516*
Slow-K® *see* Potassium Chloride *on page 1024*

Smallpox Vaccine (SMAL poks vak SEEN)

Therapeutic Category Vaccine, Live Virus

Use There are no indications for the use of smallpox vaccine in the general civilian population. Laboratory workers involved with Orthopoxvirus or in the production and testing of smallpox vaccines should receive regular smallpox vaccinations. For advice on vaccine administration and contraindications, contact the Division of Immunization, CDC, Atlanta, GA 30333 (404-639-3356).

Dosage Forms Injection

SMX-TMP *see* Co-Trimoxazole *on page 315*
SMZ-TMP *see* Co-Trimoxazole *on page 315*
Sodium 2-Mercaptoethane Sulfonate *see* Mesna *on page 788*

Sodium Acetate (SOW dee um AS e tate)

Therapeutic Category Alkalinizing Agent, Parenteral; Electrolyte Supplement, Parenteral; Sodium Salt

Use Sodium source in large volume I.V. fluids to prevent or correct hyponatremia in patients with restricted intake; used to counter acidosis through conversion to bicarbonate

Pregnancy Risk Factor C

Contraindications Alkalosis, hypocalcemia, low sodium diets, edema, cirrhosis

Warnings/Precautions Avoid extravasation, use with caution in patients with hepatic failure

Adverse Reactions

1% to 10%:

Cardiovascular: Thrombosis, hypervolemia
Dermatologic: Chemical cellulitis at injection site (extravasation)
Endocrine & metabolic: Hypernatremia, dilution of serum electrolytes, overhydration, hypokalemia, metabolic alkalosis, hypocalcemia
Gastrointestinal: Gastric distension, flatulence
Local: Phlebitis
Respiratory: Pulmonary edema
Miscellaneous: Congestive conditions

Stability Protect from light, heat, and from freezing; **incompatible** with acids, acidic salts, alkaloid salts, calcium salts, catecholamines, atropine

Usual Dosage Sodium acetate is metabolized to bicarbonate on an equimolar basis outside the liver; administer in large volume I.V. fluids as a sodium source. Refer to Sodium Bicarbonate monograph.

(Continued)

Sodium Acetate *(Continued)*

Maintenance electrolyte requirements of sodium in parenteral nutrition solutions:
Daily requirements: 3-4 mEq/kg/24 hours or 25-40 mEq/1000 kcal/24 hours
Maximum: 100-150 mEq/24 hours

Additional Information Sodium and acetate content of 1 g: 7.3 mEq

Dosage Forms Injection: 2 mEq/mL (20 mL, 50 mL); 4 mEq/mL (50 mL)

Sodium Acid Carbonate *see* Sodium Bicarbonate *on this page*

Sodium Ascorbate (SOW dee um a SKOR bate)

Brand Names Cenolate®

Therapeutic Category Urinary Acidifying Agent; Vitamin, Water Soluble

Use Prevention and treatment of scurvy and to acidify urine

Pregnancy Risk Factor C

Contraindications Large doses during pregnancy

Warnings/Precautions Use with caution in diabetics, patients with renal calculi, and those on sodium-restricted diets

Adverse Reactions

1% to 10%:
Cardiovascular: Hypotension with rapid I.V. administration
Gastrointestinal: Diarrhea
Local: Soreness at injection site
Miscellaneous: Precipitation of cystine, oxalate or urate renal stones

Overdosage/Toxicology Symptoms of overdose include diarrhea, precipitation of cystine, oxalate or urate stones; supportive care only following GI decontamination

Pharmacodynamics/Kinetics

Therapeutic serum levels: 0.4-1.5 mg/dL
Time to peak serum concentration: Oral: Within 2-3 hours
Elimination: Without supplementation, 75 mg of ascorbic acid is excreted in urine daily, increasing to 400 mg within 24 hours with the administration of 1 g/day; hemodialysis and peritoneal dialysis remove significant amounts of the drug and supplementation is suggested following dialysis periods

Usual Dosage Oral, I.V.:

Children:
Scurvy: 100-300 mg/day in divided doses for at least 2 weeks
Urinary acidification: 500 mg every 6-8 hours
Dietary supplement: 35-45 mg/day

Adults:
Scurvy: 100-250 mg 1-2 times/day for at least 2 weeks
Urinary acidification: 4-12 g/day in divided doses
Dietary supplement: 50-60 mg/day
Prevention and treatment of cold: 1-3 g/day

Test Interactions May result in false-positive stool occult blood if given within 72 hours; large doses may cause false-negative urine glucose determination

Patient Information Do not exceed recommended daily allowance

Dosage Forms

Crystals: 1020 mg per 1/4 teaspoonful [ascorbic acid 900 mg]
Injection: 250 mg/mL [ascorbic acid 222 mg/mL] (30 mL); 562.5 mg/mL [ascorbic acid 500 mg/mL] (1 mL, 2 mL)
Tablet: 585 mg [ascorbic acid 500 mg]

Sodium Bicarbonate (SOW dee um bye KAR bun ate)

Related Information

Adult ACLS Algorithm, Asystole *on page 1511*
Adult ACLS Algorithm, Pulseless Electrical Activity *on page 1510*
Adult ACLS Algorithm, V. Fib and Pulseless V. Tach *on page 1509*

Brand Names Neut®

Synonyms Baking Soda; $NaHCO_3$; Sodium Acid Carbonate; Sodium Hydrogen Carbonate

Therapeutic Category Alkalinizing Agent, Oral; Alkalinizing Agent, Parenteral; Antacid; Electrolyte Supplement, Oral; Electrolyte Supplement, Parenteral; Sodium Salt

Use Management of metabolic acidosis; gastric hyperacidity; as an alkalinization agent for the urine; treatment and hyperkalemia

Pregnancy Risk Factor C

Contraindications Alkalosis,hypernatremia, severe pulmonary edema, hypocalcemia, unknown abdominal pain

Warnings/Precautions Rapid administration in neonates and children <2 years of age has led to hypernatremia, decreased CSF pressure and intracranial hemorrhage. **Use of I.V. $NaHCO_3$ should be reserved for documented metabolic acidosis and for hyperkalemia-induced cardiac arrest.** Routine use in cardiac arrest is not recommended. Avoid extravasation, tissue necrosis can occur due to the hypertonicity of $NaHCO_3$. May cause sodium retention especially if renal function is impaired; not to be used in treatment of peptic ulcer; use with caution in patients with CHF, edema, cirrhosis, or renal failure. Not the antacid of choice for the elderly because of sodium content and potential for systemic alkalosis.

Adverse Reactions

>10%: Gastrointestinal: Belching, gastric distension, flatulence

1% to 10%:

- Cardiovascular: Edema, cerebral hemorrhage, aggravation of congestive heart failure
- Central nervous system: Tetany, intracranial acidosis
- Endocrine & metabolic: Metabolic alkalosis, hypernatremia, hypokalemia, hypocalcemia, hyperosmolality
- Respiratory: Pulmonary edema
- Miscellaneous: Increased affinity of hemoglobin for oxygen-reduced pH in myocardial tissue necrosis when extravasated

Overdosage/Toxicology Symptoms of overdose include hypocalcemia, hypokalemia, hypernatremia, seizures

Seizures can be treated with diazepam 0.1-0.25 mg/kg; hypernatremia is resolved through the use of diuretics and free water replacement

Drug Interactions

Decreased effect/levels of lithium, chlorpropamide, salicylates due to urinary alkalinization

Increased toxicity/levels of amphetamines, ephedrine, pseudoephedrine, flecainide, quinidine, quinine due to urinary alkalinization

Stability Store injection at room temperature; protect from heat and from freezing; use only clear solutions; Advise patient of milk-alkali syndrome if use is long-term; observe for extravasation when giving I.V.; **incompatible** with acids, acidic salts, alkaloid salts, calcium salts, catecholamines, atropine

Mechanism of Action Dissociates to provide bicarbonate ion which neutralizes hydrogen ion concentration and raises blood and urinary pH

Pharmacodynamics/Kinetics

Oral:

- Onset of action: Rapid
- Duration: 8-10 minutes

I.V.:

- Onset of action: 15 minutes
- Duration: 1-2 hours

Absorption: Oral: Well absorbed

Elimination: Reabsorbed by kidney and <1% is excreted by urine

Usual Dosage

Cardiac arrest: **Routine use of $NaHCO_3$ is not recommended and should be given only after adequate alveolar ventilation has been established and effective cardiac compressions are provided**

- Infants and Children: I.V.: 0.5-1 mEq/kg/dose repeated every 10 minutes or as indicated by arterial blood gases; rate of infusion should not exceed 10 mEq/minute; neonates and children <2 years of age should receive 4.2% (0.5 mEq/mL) solution
- Adults: I.V.: Initial: 1 mEq/kg/dose one time; maintenance: 0.5 mEq/kg/dose every 10 minutes or as indicated by arterial blood gases

Metabolic acidosis: Dosage should be based on the following formula if blood gases and pH measurements are available:

Infants and Children:

HCO_3^-(mEq) = 0.3 x weight (kg) x base deficit (mEq/L) **or**

HCO_3^-(mEq) = 0.5 x weight (kg) x [24 - serum HCO_3^- (mEq/L)]

Adults:

HCO_3^-(mEq) = 0.2 x weight (kg) x base deficit (mEq/L) **or**

HCO_3^-(mEq) = 0.5 x weight (kg) x [24 - serum HCO_3^- (mEq/L)]

If acid-base status is not available: Dose for older Children and Adults: 2-5 mEq/kg I.V. infusion over 4-8 hours; subsequent doses should be based on patient's acid-base status

Chronic renal failure: Oral: Initiate when plasma HCO_3^- <15 mEq/L

- Children: 1-3 mEq/kg/day
- Adults: Start with 20-36 mEq/day in divided doses, titrate to bicarbonate level of 18-20 mEq/L

Renal tubular acidosis: Oral:

Distal:

- Children: 2-3 mEq/kg/day
- Adults: 0.5-2 mEq/kg/day in 4-5 divided doses

Proximal: Children: Initial: 5-10 mEq/kg/day; maintenance: Increase as required to maintain serum bicarbonate in the normal range

(Continued)

Sodium Bicarbonate *(Continued)*

Urine alkalinization: Oral:

Children: 1-10 mEq (84-840 mg)/kg/day in divided doses every 4-6 hours; dose should be titrated to desired urinary pH

Adults: Initial: 48 mEq (4 g), then 12-24 mEq (1-2 g) every 4 hours; dose should be titrated to desired urinary pH; doses up to 16 g/day (200 mEq) in patients <60 years and 8 g (100 mEq) in patients >60 years

Antacid: Adults: Oral: 325 mg to 2 g 1-4 times/day

Patient Information Avoid chronic use as an antacid (<2 weeks)

Nursing Implications Advise patient of milk-alkali syndrome if use is long-term; observe for extravasation when giving I.V.

Additional Information

Sodium content of injection 50 mL, 8.4% = 1150 mg = 50 mEq; each 6 mg of $NaHCO_3$ contains 12 mEq sodium; 1 mEq $NaHCO_3$ = 84 mg

Each 84 mg of sodium bicarbonate provides 1 mEq of sodium and bicarbonate ions; each gram of sodium bicarbonate provides 12 mEq of sodium and bicarbonate ions

Dosage Forms

Injection: 4% [40 mg/mL = 2.4 mEq/5 mL] (5 mL); 4.2% [42 mg/mL = 5 mEq/10 mL] (10 mL); 7.5% [75 mg/mL = 8.92 mEq/10 mL] (10 mL, 50 mL); 8.4% [84 mg/mL = 10 mEq/10 mL] (10 mL, 50 mL)

Powder: 120 g, 480 g

Tablet: 300 mg [3.6 mEq]; 325 mg [3.8 mEq]; 520 mg [6.3 mEq]; 600 mg [7.3 mEq]; 650 mg [7.6 mEq]

Sodium Chloride (SOW dee um KLOR ide)

Brand Names Adsorbonac® Ophthalmic [OTC]; Afrin® Saline Mist [OTC]; AK-NaCl® [OTC]; Ayr® Saline [OTC]; Breathe Free® [OTC]; Dristan® Saline Spray [OTC]; HuMist® Nasal Mist [OTC]; Muro 128® Ophthalmic [OTC]; Muroptic-5® [OTC]; NāSal™ [OTC]; Nasal Moist® [OTC]; Ocean Nasal Mist [OTC]; Pretz® [OTC]; SalineX® [OTC]; SeaMist® [OTC]

Synonyms NaCl; Normal Saline; Salt

Therapeutic Category Electrolyte Supplement, Oral; Electrolyte Supplement, Parenteral; Lubricant, Ocular; Sodium Salt

Use Prevention of muscle cramps and heat prostration; restoration of sodium ion in hyponatremia; induce abortion; restore moisture to nasal membranes; GU irrigant; reduction of corneal edema; source of electrolytes and water for expansion of the extracellular fluid compartment

Pregnancy Risk Factor C

Contraindications Hypertonic uterus, hypernatremia, fluid retention

Warnings/Precautions Use with caution in patients with congestive heart failure, renal insufficiency, liver cirrhosis, hypertension, edema; sodium toxicity is almost exclusively related to how fast a sodium deficit is corrected; both rate and magnitude are extremely important

Adverse Reactions

1% to 10%:

Cardiovascular: Thrombosis, hypervolemia

Endocrine & metabolic: Hypernatremia, dilution of serum electrolytes, overhydration, hypokalemia

Local: Phlebitis

Respiratory: Pulmonary edema

Miscellaneous: Congestive conditions, extravasation

Overdosage/Toxicology Symptoms of overdose include nausea, vomiting, diarrhea, abdominal cramps, hypocalcemia, hypokalemia, hypernatremia

Hypernatremia is resolved through the use of diuretics and free water replacement

Drug Interactions Decreased levels of lithium

Stability Store injection at room temperature; protect from heat and from freezing; use only clear solutions

Mechanism of Action Principal extracellular cation; functions in fluid and electrolyte balance, osmotic pressure control, and water distribution

Pharmacodynamics/Kinetics

Absorption: Oral, I.V.: Rapid

Distribution: Widely distributed

Elimination: Mainly in urine but also in sweat, tears, and saliva

Usual Dosage

Newborn electrolyte requirement:

Premature: 2-8 mEq/kg/24 hours

Term:

0-48 hours: 0-2 mEq/kg/24 hours

>48 hours: 1-4 mEq/kg/24 hours

Children: I.V.: Hypertonic solutions (>0.9%) should only be used for the initial treatment of acute serious symptomatic hyponatremia; maintenance: 3-4 mEq/kg/day; maximum: 100-150 mEq/day; dosage varies widely depending on clinical condition

Replacement: Determined by laboratory determinations mEq

Sodium deficiency (mEq/kg) = [% dehydration (L/kg)/100 x 70 (mEq/L)] + [0.6 (L/kg) x (140 - serum sodium) (mEq/L)]

Nasal: Use as often as needed

Adults:

GU irrigant: 1-3 L/day by intermittent irrigation

Heat cramps: Oral: 0.5-1 g with full glass of water, up to 4.8 g/day

Replacement I.V.: Determined by laboratory determinations mEq

Sodium deficiency (mEq/kg) = [% dehydration (L/kg)/100 x 70 (mEq/L)] + [0.6 (L/kg) x (140 - serum sodium) (mEq/L)]

To correct acute, serious hyponatremia: mEq sodium = [desired sodium (mEq/L) - actual sodium (mEq/L)] x [0.6 x wt (kg)]; for acute correction use 125 mEq/L as the desired serum sodium; acutely correct serum sodium in 5 mEq/L/dose increments; more gradual correction in increments of 10 mEq/L/day is indicated in the asymptomatic patient

Chloride maintenance electrolyte requirement in parenteral nutrition: 2-4 mEq/kg/24 hours or 25-40 mEq/1000 kcals/24 hours; maximum: 100-150 mEq/24 hours

Sodium maintenance electrolyte requirement in parenteral nutrition: 3-4 mEq/kg/24 hours or 25-40 mEq/1000 kcals/24 hours; maximum: 100-150 mEq/24 hours. See table.

Approximate Deficits of Water and Electrolytes in Moderately Severe Dehydration

Condition	Water (mL/kg)	Sodium (mEq/kg)
Fasting and thirsting	100-120	5-7
Diarrhea		
isonatremic	100-120	8-10
hypernatremic	100-120	2-4
hyponatremic	100-120	10-12
Pyloric stenosis	100-120	8-10
Diabetic acidosis	100-120	9-10

*A **negative** deficit indicates total body **excess** prior to treatment.

Adapted from Behrman RE, Kleigman RM, Nelson WE, et al, eds, *Nelson Textbook of Pediatrics*, 14th ed, WB Saunders Co, 1992.

Ophthalmic:

Ointment: Apply once daily or more often

Solution: Instill 1-2 drops into affected eye(s) every 3-4 hours

Abortifacient: 20% (250 mL) administered by transabdominal intra-amniotic instillation

Monitoring Parameters Serum sodium, potassium, chloride, and bicarbonate levels; I & O, weight

Reference Range Serum/plasma sodium levels:

Neonates:

Full-term: 133-142 mEq/L

Premature: 132-140 mEq/L

Children ≥2 months to Adults: 135-145 mEq/L

Patient Information Blurred vision is common with ophthalmic ointment; may sting eyes when first applied

Nursing Implications Bacteriostatic NS should not be used for diluting or reconstituting drugs for administration in neonates; I.V. infusion of 3% or 5% sodium chloride should not exceed 100 mL/hour and should be administered in a central line only

Dosage Forms

Drops, nasal: 0.9% with dropper

Injection: 0.2% (3 mL); 0.45% (3 mL, 5 mL, 500 mL, 1000 mL); 0.9% (1 mL, 2 mL, 3 mL, 4 mL, 5 mL, 10 mL, 20 mL, 25 mL, 30 mL, 50 mL, 100 mL, 130 mL, 150 mL, 250 mL, 500 mL, 1000 mL); 3% (500 mL); 5% (500 mL); 20% (250 mL); 23.4% (30 mL, 100 mL)

Injection:

Admixtures: 50 mEq (20 mL); 100 mEq (40 mL); 625 mEq (250 mL)

Bacteriostatic: 0.9% (30 mL)

Concentrated: 14.6% (20 mL, 40 mL, 200 mL); 23.4% (10 mL, 20 mL, 30 mL)

Irrigation: 0.45% (500 mL, 1000 mL, 1500 mL); 0.9% (250 mL, 500 mL, 1000 mL, 1500 mL, 2000 mL, 3000 mL, 4000 mL)

(Continued)

Sodium Chloride *(Continued)*

Ointment, ophthalmic: 5% (3.5 g)
Solution:
Irrigation: 0.9% (1000 mL, 2000 mL)
Nasal: 0.4% (15 mL, 50 mL); 0.6% (15 mL); 0.65% (20 mL, 45 mL, 50 mL)
Ophthalmic: 2% (15 mL); 5% (15 mL, 30 mL)
Tablet: 650 mg, 1 g, 2.25 g
Tablet:
Enteric coated: 1 g
Slow release: 600 mg

Sodium Citrate and Citric Acid

(SOW dee um SIT rate & SI trik AS id)

Brand Names Bicitra®; Oracit®

Synonyms Modified Shohl's Solution

Therapeutic Category Alkalinizing Agent, Oral

Use Treatment of metabolic acidosis; alkalinizing agent in conditions where long-term maintenance of an alkaline urine is desirable

Pregnancy Risk Factor C

Contraindications Severe renal insufficiency, sodium-restricted diet

Warnings/Precautions Conversion to bicarbonate may be impaired in patients with hepatic failure, in shock, or who are severely ill

Adverse Reactions

1% to 10%:
Central nervous system: Tetany
Endocrine & metabolic: Metabolic alkalosis, hyperkalemia
Gastrointestinal: Diarrhea, nausea, vomiting

Overdosage/Toxicology Symptoms of overdose include hypokalemia, hypernatremia, tetany, seizures

Hypernatremia is resolved through the use of diuretics and free water replacement

Drug Interactions

Decreased effect/levels of lithium, chlorpropamide, salicylates due to urinary alkalinization

Increased toxicity/levels of amphetamines, ephedrine, pseudoephedrine, flecainide, quinidine, quinine due to urinary alkalinization

Usual Dosage Oral:

Infants and Children: 2-3 mEq/kg/day in divided doses 3-4 times/day **or** 5-15 mL with water after meals and at bedtime

Adults: 15-30 mL with water after meals and at bedtime

Administration Administer after meals

Patient Information Palatability is improved by chilling solution, dilute each dose with 1-3 oz of water and follow with additional water; take after meals to prevent saline laxative effect

Nursing Implications May be ordered as modified Shohl's solution; dilute with 30-90 mL of chilled water to enhance taste

Additional Information 1 mL of Bicitra® contains 1 mEq of sodium and the equivalent of 1 mEq of bicarbonate

Dosage Forms Solution, oral:

Bicitra®: Sodium citrate 500 mg and citric acid 334 mg per 5 mL (15 mL unit dose, 480 mL)
Oracit®: Sodium citrate 490 mg and citric acid 640 mg per 5 mL
Polycitra®: Sodium citrate 500 mg and citric acid 334 mg with potassium citrate 550 mg per 5 mL

Sodium Edetate *see* Edetate Disodium *on page 438*
Sodium Etidronate *see* Etidronate Disodium *on page 493*
Sodium Fluoride *see* Fluoride *on page 536*

Sodium Hyaluronate (SOW dee um hye al yoor ON nate)

Brand Names AMO Vitrax®; Amvisc®; Amvisc® Plus; Healon®; Healon® GV

Synonyms Hyaluronic Acid

Therapeutic Category Ophthalmic Agent, Viscoelastic

Use Surgical aid in cataract extraction, intraocular implantation, corneal transplant, glaucoma filtration, and retinal attachment surgery

Pregnancy Risk Factor C

Contraindications Hypersensitivity to hyaluronate

Warnings/Precautions Do not overfill the anterior chamber; carefully monitor intraocular pressure; risk of hypersensitivity exists

Adverse Reactions 1% to 10%: Ocular: Postoperative inflammatory reactions (iritis, hypopyon), corneal edema, corneal decompensation, transient postoperative increase in IOP

Stability Store in refrigerator (2°C to 8°C); do not freeze

Mechanism of Action Functions as a tissue lubricant and is thought to play an important role in modulating the interactions between adjacent tissues. Sodium hyaluronate is a polysaccharide which is distributed widely in the extracellular matrix of connective tissue in man. (Vitreous and aqueous humor of the eye, synovial fluid, skin, and umbilical cord.) Sodium hyaluronate forms a viscoelastic solution in water (at physiological pH and ionic strength) which makes it suitable for aqueous and vitreous humor in ophthalmic surgery.

Pharmacodynamics/Kinetics

Absorption: Following intravitreous injection, diffusion occurs slowly

Elimination: By way of the Canal of Schlemm

Usual Dosage Depends upon procedure (slowly introduce a sufficient quantity into eye)

Monitoring Parameters Intraocular pressure

Dosage Forms Injection, intraocular:

Healon®: 10 mg/mL (0.4 mL, 0.55 mL, 0.85 mL, 2 mL)

Amvisc®: 12 mg/mL (0.5 mL, 0.8 mL)

Healon® GV: 14 mg/mL (0.55 mL, 0.85 mL)

Amvisc® Plus: 16 mg/mL (0.5 mL, 8 mL)

AMO Vitrax®: 30 mg/mL (0.65 mL)

Sodium Hyaluronate-Chrondroitin Sulfate *see* Chondroitin Sulfate-Sodium Hyaluronate *on page 272*

Sodium Hydrogen Carbonate *see* Sodium Bicarbonate *on page 1140*

Sodium Hypochlorite Solution

(SOW dee um hye poe KLOR ite soe LOO shun)

Synonyms Dakin's Solution; Modified Dakin's Solution

Therapeutic Category Disinfectant, Antibacterial (Topical)

Use Treatment of athlete's foot (0.5%); wound irrigation (0.5%); disinfect utensils and equipment (5%)

Pregnancy Risk Factor C

Contraindications Hypersensitivity

Warnings/Precautions For external use only; avoid eye or mucous membrane contact; do not use on open wounds

Adverse Reactions 1% to 10%: Dissolves blood clots, delays clotting, irritating to skin

Stability Use prepared solution within 7 days

Usual Dosage Topical irrigation

Patient Information External use only

Nursing Implications Dakin's solution may hinder wound healing

Dosage Forms

Solution: 5% (4000 mL)

Solution (modified Dakin's solution):

Full strength: 0.5% (1000 mL)

Half strength: 0.25% (1000 mL)

Quarter strength: 0.125% (1000 mL)

Sodium *L*-Triiodothyronine *see* Liothyronine *on page 729*

Sodium Methicillin *see* Methicillin *on page 803*

Sodium Nafcillin *see* Nafcillin *on page 871*

Sodium Nitroferricyanide *see* Nitroprusside *on page 911*

Sodium Nitroprusside *see* Nitroprusside *on page 911*

Sodium P.A.S. *see* Aminosalicylate Sodium *on page 66*

Sodium Phenylbutyrate (SOW dee um fen il BYOO ti rate)

Brand Names Buphenyl®

Synonyms Ammonapse

Therapeutic Category Miscellaneous Product

Use Adjunctive therapy in the chronic management of patients with urea cycle disorder involving deficiencies of carbamoylphosphate synthetase, ornithine transcarbamylase, or argininosuccinic acid synthetase

Contraindications Previous hypersensitivity to phenylbutyrate, severe hypertension, heart failure or renal dysfunction; phenylbutyrate is not indicated in the treatment of acute hyperammonemia

Warnings/Precautions Since no studies have been conducted in pregnant women, sodium phenylbutyrate should be used cautiously during pregnancy; each 1 gram of drug contains 125 mg of sodium and, therefore, should be used cautiously, if at all, in patients who must maintain a low sodium intake

(Continued)

Sodium Phenylbutyrate *(Continued)*

Adverse Reactions

>10%: Endocrine & metabolic: Amenorrhea, menstrual dysfunction

1% to 10%:

Gastrointestinal: Anorexia, abnormal taste

Miscellaneous: Offensive body odor

Stability Store at room temperature (59°F to 86°F); after opening, containers should be kept tightly closed

Mechanism of Action Sodium phenylbutyrate is a prodrug that, when given orally, is rapidly converted to phenylacetate, which is in turn conjugated with glutamine to form the active compound phenylacetyglutamine; phenylacetyglutamine serves as a substitute for urea and is excreted in the urine whereby it carries with it 2 moles of nitrogen per mole of phenylacetyglutamine and can thereby assist in the clearance of nitrogenous waste in patients with urea cycle disorders

Usual Dosage

Powder: Patients weighing <20 kg: 450-600 mg/kg/day or 9.9-13 g/m^2/day, administered in equally divided amounts with each meal or feeding, four to six times daily; safety and efficacy of doses >20 g/day has not been established

Tablet: Children >20 kg and Adults: 450-600 mg/kg/day or 9.9-13 g/m^2/day, administered in equally divided amounts with each meal; safety and efficacy of doses >20 g/day have not been established

Patient Information It is important that patients understand and follow the dietary restrictions required when treating this disorder, the medication must be taken in strict accordance with the prescribed regimen and the patient should avoid altering the dosage without the prescriber's knowledge; the powder formulation has a very salty taste

Dosage Forms

Powder: 3.2 g [sodium phenylbutyrate 3 g] per teaspoon (500 mL, 950 mL); 9.1 g [sodium phenylbutyrate 8.6 g] per **tablespoon** (500 mL, 950 mL)

Tablet: 500 mg

Sodium Phosphate and Potassium Phosphate *see* Potassium Phosphate and Sodium Phosphate *on page 1031*

Sodium Phosphates (SOW dee um FOS fates)

Related Information

Laxatives, Classification and Properties *on page 1412*

Brand Names Fleet® Enema [OTC]; Fleet® Phospho®-Soda [OTC]

Therapeutic Category Electrolyte Supplement, Parenteral; Laxative, Saline; Phosphate Salt; Sodium Salt

Use Short-term treatment of constipation, evacuation of the colon for rectal and bowel exams; source of sodium and phosphorus; treatment and prevention of hypophosphatemia

Pregnancy Risk Factor C

Contraindications Hyperphosphatemia, hypernatremia, hypocalcemia, renal failure, congestive heart failure, abdominal pain, fecal impaction

Warnings/Precautions Use with caution in patients with renal insufficiency, CHF, sodium restriction, cirrhosis; phosphate salts may precipitate in the presence of calcium; prolonged and/or excessive use of laxative may result in dependence; risks of rapid I.V. infusion include hypocalcemia, hypotension, muscular irritability, calcium deposits, renal function deterioration, and hyperkalemia

Adverse Reactions

1% to 10%:

Cardiovascular: Edema, hypotension

Endocrine & metabolic: Hyperphosphatemia, hypocalcemia, hypernatremia, calcium phosphate precipitation

Gastrointestinal: Nausea, vomiting, diarrhea

Renal: Acute renal failure

Overdosage/Toxicology Symptoms of overdose include tetany, convulsions and neuroexcitability, secondary to the hypocalcemia associated with hyperphosphatemia or hypernatremia; aluminum hydroxide may be administered to adults in doses of 60-200 mL/day; 8-24 capsules (or tablets)/day

The dose should be tailored to the patient (aluminum forms an insoluble compound with the phosphate which is excreted in the stool); hypernatremia is treated with loop diuretics and free water replacement; seizures may require diazepam 0.1-0.25 mg/kg; tetany should be treated with I.V. calcium salts

Drug Interactions Do not administer with magnesium- and aluminum-containing antacids or sucralfate which can bind with phosphate

Stability Phosphate salts may precipitate when mixed with calcium salts; solubility is improved in amino acid parenteral nutrition solutions; check with a pharmacist to determine compatibility

Mechanism of Action As a laxative, exerts osmotic effect in the small intestine by drawing water into the lumen of the gut, producing distention and promoting peristalsis and evacuation of the bowel; phosphorous participates in bone deposition, calcium metabolism, utilization of B complex vitamins, and as a buffer in acid-base equilibrium

Pharmacodynamics/Kinetics

Onset of action:
- Cathartic: 3-6 hours
- Rectal: 2-5 minutes

Absorption: Oral: ~1% to 20%

Elimination:
- Oral phosphate: In feces
- I.V. phosphate: In urine with over 80% of dose reabsorbed by the kidney

Usual Dosage

Normal requirements elemental phosphorus: Oral:
- 0-6 months: 240 mg
- 6-12 months: 360 mg
- 1-10 years: 800 mg
- >10 years: 1200 mg

Pregnancy lactation: Additional 400 mg/day

Adults RDA: 800 mg

I.V. doses should be incorporated into the patient's maintenance I.V. fluids whenever possible; intermittent I.V. infusion should be reserved for severe depletion situations and requires continuous EKG monitoring. It is difficult to determine total body phosphorus deficit due to redistribution into intracellular compartment or bone tissue; (it is recommended that repletion of severe hypophosphatemia (<1 mg/dL in adults) be done via I.V. route since large dose of oral phosphate may cause diarrhea and intestinal absorption may be unreliable). The following dosages are empiric guidelines. **Note:** Doses listed as mmol of phosphate.

Severe hypophosphatemia: I.V.:
- Children:
  - Low dose: 0.08 mmol/kg over 6 hours; use if recent losses and uncomplicated
  - Intermediate dose: 0.16-0.24 mmol/kg over 4-6 hours; use if phosphorus level 0.5-1 mg/dL
  - High dose: 0.36 mmol/kg over 6 hours; use if serum phosphorus <0.5 mg/dL
- Adults: 0.15-0.3 mmol/kg/dose over 12 hours, may repeat as needed to achieve desired serum level
- Maintenance:
  - Children: 0.5-1.5 mmol/kg/24 hours I.V. or 2-3 mmol/kg/24 hours orally in divided doses
  - Adults: 50-70 mmol/24 hours I.V. or 50-150 mmol/24 hours orally in divided doses **or**

Children <4 years: Oral: 1 capsule (250 mg/8 mmol phosphorus) 4 times/day; dilute as instructed

Children >4 years and Adults: Oral: 1-2 capsules (250-500 mg/8-16 mmol phosphorus) 4 times/day; dilute as instructed

Phosphate maintenance electrolyte requirement in parenteral nutrition: 2 mmol/kg/24 hours or 35 mmol/kcal/24 hours; maximum: 15-30 mmol/24 hours

Laxative (Fleet®): Rectal:
- Children 2-12 years: Contents of one 2.25 oz pediatric enema, may repeat
- Children ≥12 years and Adults: Contents of one 4.5 oz enema as a single dose, may repeat

Laxative (Fleet® Phospho®-Soda): Oral:
- Children 5-9 years: 5 mL as a single dose
- Children 10-12 years: 10 mL as a single dose
- Children ≥12 years and Adults: 20-30 mL as a single dose

Administration Rate of I.V. infusion should not exceed 0.05 mmol/kg/hour; risks of rapid I.V. infusion include hypocalcemia, hypotension, muscular irritability, calcium deposits, renal function deterioration, and hyperkalemia

With orders for I.V. phosphate, there is considerable confusion associated with the use of millimoles versus milliequivalents to express the phosphate requirement. Because inorganic phosphate exists as monobasic and dibasic anions, with the mixture of valences dependent on pH, ordering by mEq amounts is unreliable and may lead to large dosing errors. In addition, I.V. phosphate is available in the sodium and potassium salt, therefore, the content of these cations must be considered when ordering phosphate. The most reliable method of ordering I.V. phosphate is by millimoles, then specifying the potassium or sodium salt.

(Continued)

Sodium Phosphates *(Continued)*

Contents of one packet should be diluted in 75 mL water before administration; maintain adequate fluid intake

Monitoring Parameters Serum sodium, phosphorus, calcium, renal function, EKG monitor if severe hypophosphatemia

Reference Range Phosphorous serum levels; it should be noted that serum levels do not accurately reflect intracellular phosphorous levels or extent of total body depletion

Newborns: 4.2-9 mg/dL
Children:
- 1-2 years: 3.8-6.2 mg/dL
- 3-15 years: 3.6-5.6 mg/dL

Adults: 3-4.5 mg/dL

Patient Information May cause diarrhea with the oral preparation; excessive or prolonged use as a laxative may cause dependence

Dosage Forms

Enema: Sodium phosphate 6 g and sodium biphosphate 16 g/100 mL (67.5 mL pediatric enema unit, 135 mL adult enema unit)

Injection: Phosphate 3 mmol and sodium 4 mEq per mL (5 mL, 10 mL, 15 mL, 30 mL, 50 mL)

Solution, oral: Sodium phosphate 18 g and sodium biphosphate 48 g/100 mL (45 mL, 90 mL, 273 mL)

See table.

	Phosphate (mmol)	Sodium (mEq)	Potassium (mEq)
Oral			
Whole cow's milk	0.29/mL	0.025/mL	0.035/mL
Fleet® Phospho®-Soda	4.15/mL	4.8/mL	None
Intravenous			
Sodium phosphate	3/mL	4/mL	None

Sodium Polystyrene Sulfonate

(SOW dee um pol ee STYE reen SUL fon ate)

Related Information

Antacid Drug Interactions *on page 1388*

Brand Names Kayexalate®; SPS®

Therapeutic Category Antidote, Hyperkalemia; Antidote, Potassium

Use Treatment of hyperkalemia

Pregnancy Risk Factor C

Contraindications Hypernatremia, hypersensitivity to any component

Warnings/Precautions Use with caution in patients with severe congestive heart failure, hypertension, edema, or renal failure; avoid using the commercially available liquid product in neonates due to the preservative content; large oral doses may cause fecal impaction (especially in elderly); enema will reduce the serum potassium faster than oral administration, but the oral route will result in a greater reduction over several hours.

Adverse Reactions

>10%: Gastrointestinal: Constipation, loss of appetite, nausea, vomiting

1% to 10%:
- Endocrine & metabolic: Hypokalemia, hypocalcemia, hypomagnesemia, sodium retention
- Gastrointestinal: Fecal impaction

Overdosage/Toxicology Symptoms of overdose include hypokalemia including cardiac dysrhythmias, confusion, irritability, EKG changes, muscle weakness, gastrointestinal effects; treatment is supportive, limited to management of fluid and electrolytes

Mechanism of Action Removes potassium by exchanging sodium ions for potassium ions in the intestine before the resin is passed from the body; exchange capacity is 1 mEq/g *in vivo*, and *in vitro* capacity is 3.1 mEq/g, therefore, a wide range of exchange capacity exists such that close monitoring of serum electrolytes is necessary

Pharmacodynamics/Kinetics

Onset of action: Within 2-24 hours
Absorption: Remains in GI tract
Elimination: Completely in feces (primarily as potassium polystyrene sulfonate)

Usual Dosage

Children:
- Oral: 1 g/kg/dose every 6 hours

Rectal: 1 g/kg/dose every 2-6 hours (In small children and infants, employ lower doses by using the practical exchange ratio of 1 mEq K^+/g of resin as the basis for calculation)

Adults:

Oral: 15 g (60 mL) 1-4 times/day

Rectal: 30-50 g every 6 hours

Monitoring Parameters Serum electrolytes (potassium, sodium, calcium, magnesium), EKG

Reference Range Serum potassium: Adults: 3.5-5.2 mEq/L

Patient Information Mix well in full glass of liquid prior to drinking

Nursing Implications Administer oral (or NG) as ~25% sorbitol solution, never mix in orange juice; enema route is less effective than oral administration; retain enema in colon for at least 30-60 minutes and for several hours, if possible; chilling the oral mixture will increase palatability; enema should be followed by irrigation with normal saline to prevent necrosis

Additional Information 1 g of resin binds approximately 1 mEq of potassium; sodium content of 1 g: 31 mg (1.3 mEq)

Dosage Forms Oral or rectal:

Powder for suspension: 454 g

Suspension: 1.25 g/5 mL with sorbitol 33% and alcohol 0.3% (60 mL, 120 mL, 200 mL, 500 mL)

Sodium Sulamyd® Ophthalmic *see* Sulfacetamide Sodium *on page 1171*

Sodium Sulfacetamide *see* Sulfacetamide Sodium *on page 1171*

Sodium Tetradecyl (SOW dee um tetra DEK il)

Brand Names Sotradecol®

Synonyms Sodium Tetradecyl Sulfate

Therapeutic Category Sclerosing Agent

Use Treatment of small, uncomplicated varicose veins of the lower extremities; endoscopic sclerotherapy in the management of bleeding esophageal varices

Pregnancy Risk Factor C

Contraindications Arterial disease, thrombophlebitis, hypersensitivity to sodium tetradecyl or any component, valvular or deep vein incompetence, phlebitis, migraines, cellulitis, acute infections

Warnings/Precautions Buerger's disease, peripheral arteriosclerosis, avoid extravasation

Adverse Reactions

1% to 10%:

Central nervous system: Headache

Dermatologic: Urticaria, sloughing and tissue necrosis following extravasation

Gastrointestinal: Nausea, vomiting, mucosal lesions

Local: Discoloration at the site of injection, ulceration at the site, pain at injection site

Respiratory: Pulmonary edema

<1%:

Gastrointestinal: Esophageal perforation

Respiratory: Asthma

Stability Store at controlled room temperature in a well-closed container; protect from light

Mechanism of Action Acts by irritation of the vein intimal endothelium

Usual Dosage I.V.: Test dose: 0.5 mL given several hours prior to administration of larger dose; 0.5-2 mL in each vein, maximum: 10 mL per treatment session; 3% solution reserved for large varices

Patient Information Notify physician if chest pain, shortness of breath, or heat, pain, or tenderness in lower extremities

Nursing Implications Observe for signs and symptoms of embolism

Dosage Forms Injection, as sulfate: 1% [10 mg/mL] (2 mL); 3% [30 mg/mL] (2 mL)

Sodium Tetradecyl Sulfate *see* Sodium Tetradecyl *on this page*

Sodium Thiosulfate (SOW dee um thye oh SUL fate)

Brand Names Tinver® Lotion

Therapeutic Category Antidote, Arsenic Toxicity; Antidote, Cyanide; Antifungal Agent, Topical

Use

Parenteral: Used alone or with sodium nitrite or amyl nitrite in cyanide poisoning or arsenic poisoning; reduce the risk of nephrotoxicity associated with cisplatin therapy

Topical: Treatment of tinea versicolor

Pregnancy Risk Factor C

Contraindications Hypersensitivity to any component

(Continued)

Sodium Thiosulfate *(Continued)*

Warnings/Precautions Safety in pregnancy has not been established; discontinue topical use if irritation or sensitivity occurs; rapid I.V. infusion has caused transient hypotension and EKG changes in dogs; can increase risk of thiocyanate intoxication

Adverse Reactions

1% to 10%:

Cardiovascular: Hypotension

Central nervous system: Coma, CNS depression secondary to thiocyanate intoxication, psychosis, confusion

Dermatologic: Contact dermatitis, local irritation

Neuromuscular & skeletal: Weakness

Otic: Tinnitus

Mechanism of Action

Cyanide toxicity: Increases the rate of detoxification of cyanide by the enzyme rhodanese by providing an extra sulfur

Cisplatin toxicity: Complexes with cisplatin to form a compound that is nontoxic to either normal or cancerous cells

Pharmacodynamics/Kinetics

Half-life: 0.65 hour

Elimination: 28.5% excreted unchanged in urine

Usual Dosage

Cyanide and nitroprusside antidote: I.V.:

Children <25 kg: 50 mg/kg after receiving 4.5-10 mg/kg sodium nitrite; a half dose of each may be repeated if necessary

Children >25 kg and Adults: 12.5 g after 300 mg of sodium nitrite; a half dose of each may be repeated if necessary

Cyanide poisoning: I.V.: Dose should be based on determination as with nitrite, at rate of 2.5-5 mL/minute to maximum of 50 mL. See table.

Variation of Sodium Nitrite and Sodium Thiosulfate Dose With Hemoglobin Concentration*

Hemoglobin (g/dL)	Initial Dose Sodium Nitrite (mg/kg)	Initial Dose Sodium Nitrite 3% (mL/kg)	Initial Dose Sodium Thiosulfate 25% (mL/kg)
7	5.8	0.19	0.95
8	6.6	0.22	1.10
9	7.5	0.25	1.25
10	8.3	0.27	1.35
11	9.1	0.30	1.50
12	10.0	0.33	1.65
13	10.8	0.36	1.80
14	11.6	0.39	1.95

*Adapted from Berlin DM Jr, 'The Treatment of Cyanide Poisoning in Children,' *Pediatrics*, 1970, 46:793.

Cisplatin rescue should be given before or during cisplatin administration: I.V. infusion (in sterile water): 12 g/m^2 over 6 hours or 9 g/m^2 I.V. push followed by 1.2 g/m^2 continuous infusion for 6 hours

Arsenic poisoning: I.V.: 1 mL first day, 2 mL second day, 3 mL third day, 4 mL fourth day, 5 mL on alternate days thereafter

Children and Adults: Topical: 20% to 25% solution: Apply a thin layer to affected areas twice daily

Administration I.V.: Inject slowly, over at least 10 minutes; rapid administration may cause hypotension

Monitoring Parameters Monitor for signs of thiocyanate toxicity

Patient Information Avoid topical application near the eyes, mouth, or other mucous membranes; notify physician if condition worsens or burning or irritation occurs; shake well before using

Dosage Forms

Injection: 100 mg/mL (10 mL); 250 mg/mL (50 mL)

Lotion: 25% with salicylic acid 1% and isopropyl alcohol 10% (120 mL, 180 mL)

Sodol® *see* Carisoprodol *on page 209*

Solaquin® [OTC] *see* Hydroquinone *on page 628*

Solaquin Forte® *see* Hydroquinone *on page 628*

Solarcaine® [OTC] *see* Benzocaine *on page 138*

Solarcaine® Aloe Extra Burn Relief [OTC] *see* Lidocaine *on page 723*

Solatene® *see* Beta-Carotene *on page 147*

Solfoton® *see* Phenobarbital *on page 984*
Solganal® *see* Aurothioglucose *on page 120*
Soluble Fluorescein *see* Fluorescein Sodium *on page 535*
Solu-Cortef® *see* Hydrocortisone *on page 623*
Solu-Medrol® *see* Methylprednisolone *on page 819*
Solurex L.A.® *see* Dexamethasone *on page 356*
Soma® *see* Carisoprodol *on page 209*
Soma® Compound *see* Carisoprodol *on page 209*
Somatrem *see* Human Growth Hormone *on page 613*
Somatropin *see* Human Growth Hormone *on page 613*
Sominex® Oral [OTC] *see* Diphenhydramine *on page 399*
Soothe® [OTC] *see* Tetrahydrozoline *on page 1205*
Soprodol® *see* Carisoprodol *on page 209*

Sorbitol (SOR bi tole)

Related Information

Laxatives, Classification and Properties *on page 1412*

Therapeutic Category Genitourinary Irrigant

Use Genitourinary irrigant in transurethral prostatic resection or other transurethral resection or other transurethral surgical procedures; diuretic; humectant; sweetening agent; hyperosmotic laxative; facilitate the passage of sodium polystyrene sulfonate through the intestinal tract

Contraindications Anuria

Warnings/Precautions Use with caution in patients with severe cardiopulmonary or renal impairment and in patients unable to metabolize sorbitol

Adverse Reactions

1% to 10%:

- Cardiovascular: Edema
- Endocrine & metabolic: Fluid and electrolyte losses, lactic acidosis
- Gastrointestinal: Diarrhea, nausea, vomiting, abdominal discomfort, xerostomia

Overdosage/Toxicology Symptoms of overdose include nausea, diarrhea, fluid and electrolyte loss; treatment is supportive to ensure fluid and electrolyte balance

Mechanism of Action A polyalcoholic sugar with osmotic cathartic actions

Pharmacodynamics/Kinetics

Onset of action: About 0.25-1 hour
Absorption: Oral, rectal: Poor
Metabolism: Mainly in the liver to fructose

Usual Dosage Hyperosmotic laxative (as single dose, at infrequent intervals):

Children 2-11 years:
- Oral: 2 mL/kg (as 70% solution)
- Rectal enema: 30-60 mL as 25% to 30% solution

Children >12 years and Adults:
- Oral: 30-150 mL (as 70% solution)
- Rectal enema: 120 mL as 25% to 30% solution
- Adjunct to sodium polystyrene sulfonate: 15 mL as 70% solution orally until diarrhea occurs (10-20 mL/2 hours) or 20-100 mL as an oral vehicle for the sodium polystyrene sulfonate resin

When administered with charcoal:
- Oral:
  - Children: 4.3 mL/kg of 35% sorbitol with 1 g/kg of activated charcoal
  - Adults: 4.3 mL/kg of 70% sorbitol with 1 g/kg of activated charcoal every 4 hours until first stool containing charcoal is passed
- Topical: 3% to 3.3% as transurethral surgical procedure irrigation

Nursing Implications Do not use unless solution is clear

Dosage Forms

Solution: 70%
Solution, genitourinary irrigation: 3% (1500 mL, 3000 mL); 3.3% (2000 mL)

Sorbitrate® *see* Isosorbide Dinitrate *on page 684*
Soridol® *see* Carisoprodol *on page 209*

Sotalol (SOE ta lole)

Related Information

Antiarrhythmic Drugs *on page 1389*
Beta-Blockers Comparison *on page 1398*
Comparative Pharmacokinetic Properties of Antiarrhythmic Agents *on page 1391*

Brand Names Betapace®

Canadian/Mexican Brand Names Sotacor® (Canada)

(Continued)

Sotalol *(Continued)*

Synonyms Sotalol Hydrochloride

Therapeutic Category Antiarrhythmic Agent, Class III; Beta-Adrenergic Blocker

Use Treatment of documented ventricular arrhythmias, such as sustained ventricular tachycardia, that in the judgment of the physician are life-threatening

Unlabeled use: Supraventricular arrhythmias

Pregnancy Risk Factor B

Pregnancy/Breast-Feeding Implications Although there are no adequate and well controlled studies in pregnant women, sotalol has been shown to cross the placenta, and is found in amniotic fluid. There has been a report of subnormal birth weight with sotalol, therefore, sotalol should be used during pregnancy only if the potential benefit outweighs the potential risk.

Contraindications Bronchial asthma, sinus bradycardia, second and third degree A-V block (unless a functioning pacemaker is present), congenital or acquired long Q-T syndromes, cardiogenic shock, uncontrolled congestive heart failure, and previous evidence of hypersensitivity to sotalol

Warnings/Precautions Use with caution in patients with congestive heart failure, peripheral vascular disease, hypokalemia, hypomagnesemia, renal dysfunction, sick-sinus syndrome; abrupt withdrawal may result in return of life-threatening arrhythmias; sotalol can provoke new or worsening ventricular arrhythmias

Adverse Reactions

>10%:

- Cardiovascular: Bradycardia
- Central nervous system: Mental depression
- Endocrine & metabolic: Decreased sexual ability

1% to 10%:

- Cardiovascular: Congestive heart failure, reduced peripheral circulation
- Central nervous system: Mental confusion, hallucinations, anxiety, dizziness, drowsiness, nightmares, insomnia, fatigue
- Dermatologic: Itching
- Gastrointestinal: Constipation, diarrhea, nausea, vomiting, stomach discomfort
- Neuromuscular & skeletal: Weakness
- Respiratory: Dyspnea

<1%:

- Cardiovascular: Chest pain, hypotension (especially with higher doses), Raynaud's phenomenon
- Dermatologic: Rash; red, crusted skin, skin necrosis after extravasation
- Hematologic: Leukopenia
- Local: Phlebitis
- Miscellaneous: Diaphoresis, cold extremities

Overdosage/Toxicology Symptoms of intoxication include cardiac disturbances, CNS toxicity, bronchospasm, hypoglycemia and hyperkalemia. The most common cardiac symptoms include hypotension and bradycardia; atrioventricular block, intraventricular conduction disturbances, cardiogenic shock, and systole may occur with severe overdose, especially with membrane-depressant drugs (eg, propranolol); CNS effects include convulsions, coma, and respiratory arrest is commonly seen with propranolol and other membrane-depressant and lipid-soluble drugs.

Treatment includes symptomatic treatment of seizures, hypotension, hyperkalemia and hypoglycemia; bradycardia and hypotension resistant to atropine, isoproterenol or pacing may respond to glucagon; wide QRS defects caused by the membrane-depressant poisoning may respond to hypertonic sodium bicarbonate; repeat-dose charcoal, hemoperfusion, or hemodialysis may be helpful in removal of only those beta-blockers with a small V_d, long half-life or low intrinsic clearance (acebutolol, atenolol, nadolol, sotalol)

Drug Interactions

Decreased effect of beta-blockers with aluminum salts, barbiturates, calcium salts, cholestyramine, colestipol, NSAIDs, penicillins (ampicillin), rifampin, salicylates and sulfinpyrazone due to decreased bioavailability and plasma levels

Beta-blockers may decrease the effect of sulfonylureas

Increased effect/toxicity of beta-blockers with calcium blockers (diltiazem, felodipine, nicardipine), contraceptives, flecainide, haloperidol (propranolol, hypotensive effects), H_2-antagonists (metoprolol, propranolol only by cimetidine, possibly ranitidine), hydralazine (metoprolol, propranolol), loop diuretics (propranolol, not atenolol), MAO inhibitors (metoprolol, nadolol, bradycardia), phenothiazines (propranolol), propafenone (metoprolol, propranolol), quinidine (in extensive metabolizers), ciprofloxacin, thyroid hormones (metoprolol, propranolol, when hypothyroid patient is converted to euthyroid state)

Beta-blockers may increase the effect/toxicity of flecainide, haloperidol (hypotensive effects), hydralazine, phenothiazines, acetaminophen, anticoagulants (propranolol, warfarin), benzodiazepines (not atenolol), clonidine (hypertensive crisis after or during withdrawal of either agent), epinephrine (initial hypertensive episode followed by bradycardia), nifedipine and verapamil lidocaine, ergots (peripheral ischemia), prazosin (postural hypotension)

Beta-blockers may affect the action or levels of ethanol, disopyramide, nondepolarizing muscle relaxants and theophylline although the effects are difficult to predict

Mechanism of Action

Beta-blocker which contains both beta-adrenoreceptor-blocking (Vaughan Williams Class II) and cardiac action potential duration prolongation (Vaughan Williams Class III) properties

Class II effects: Increased sinus cycle length, slowed heart rate, decreased A-V nodal conduction, and increased A-V nodal refractoriness

Class III effects: Prolongation of the atrial and ventricular monophasic action potentials, and effective refractory prolongation of atrial muscle, ventricular muscle, and atrioventricular accessory pathways in both the antegrade and retrograde directions

Sotalol is a racemic mixture of *d*- and *l*-sotalol; both isomers have similar Class III antiarrhythmic effects while the *l*-isomer is responsible for virtually all of the beta-blocking activity

Sotalol has both $beta_1$- and $beta_2$-receptor blocking activity

The beta-blocking effect of sotalol is a noncardioselective [half maximal at about 80 mg/day and maximal at doses of 320-640 mg/day]. Significant beta-blockade occurs at oral doses as low as 25 mg/day.

The Class III effects are seen only at oral doses ≥160 mg/day

Pharmacodynamics/Kinetics

Onset of action: Rapid, 1-2 hours

Peak effect: 2.5-4 hours

Absorption: Decreased 20% to 30% by meals compared to fasting

Bioavailability: 90% to 100%

Distribution: Low lipid solubility; sotalol is excreted in the milk of laboratory animals and is reported to be present in human milk

Metabolism: Sotalol is **not** metabolized

Protein binding: Not protein bound

Half-life: 12 hours

Elimination: Unchanged through kidney

Serum concentrations have not been systematically evaluated: Concentration-effect curves for the beta-blocking and antiarrhythmic agents of sotalol are different

Serum levels of 340-3,440 ng/mL have shown a 70% to 100% reduction in PVBs

Average serum concentrations associated with significant Q-T prolongation were 2,550 ng/mL

Average serum concentrations associated with maximum heart reduction by 50% was 804 ng/mL

Usual Dosage Sotalol should be initiated and doses increased in a hospital with facilities for cardiac rhythm monitoring and assessment. Proarrhythmic events can occur after initiation of therapy and with each upward dosage adjustment.

Children: Oral: The safety and efficacy of sotalol in children have not been established

Supraventricular arrhythmias: 2-4 mg/kg/24 hours was given in 2 equal doses every 12 hours to 18 infants (≤2 months of age). All infants, except one with chaotic atrial tachycardia, were successfully controlled with sotalol. Ten infants discontinued therapy between the ages of 7-18 months when it was no longer necessary. Median duration of treatment was 12.8 months.

Adults: Oral:

Initial: 80 mg twice daily

Dose may be increased (gradually allowing 2-3 days between dosing increments in order to attain steady-state plasma concentrations and to allow monitoring of Q-T intervals) to 240-320 mg/day

Most patients respond to a total daily dose of 160-320 mg/day in 2-3 divided doses

Some patients, with life-threatening refractory ventricular arrhythmias, may require doses as high as 480-640 mg/day; however, these doses should only be prescribed when the potential benefit outweighs the increased of adverse events

Elderly patients: Age does not significantly alter the pharmacokinetics of sotalol, but impaired renal function in elderly patients can increase the terminal half-life, resulting in increased drug accumulation

Dosing adjustment in renal impairment:

Cl_{cr} >60 mL/minute: Administer every 12 hours

Cl_{cr} 30-60 mL/minute: Administer every 24 hours

Cl_{cr} 10-30 mL/minute: Administer every 36-48 hours

Cl_{cr} <10 mL/minute: Individualize dose

(Continued)

Sotalol *(Continued)*

Dialysis: Hemodialysis would be expected to reduce sotalol plasma concentrations because sotalol is not bound to plasma proteins and does not undergo extensive metabolism; administer dose postdialysis or administer supplemental 80 mg dose; peritoneal dialysis does not remove sotalol; supplemental dose is not necessary

Monitoring Parameters Serum magnesium, potassium, EKG

Patient Information Seek emergency help if palpitations occur; do not discontinue abruptly or change dose without notifying physician; take on an empty stomach

Nursing Implications Initiation of therapy and dose escalation should be done in a hospital with cardiac monitoring; lidocaine and other resuscitative measures should be available

Dosage Forms Tablet, as hydrochloride: 80 mg, 120 mg, 160 mg, 240 mg

Sotalol Hydrochloride *see* Sotalol *on page 1151*

Sotradecol® *see* Sodium Tetradecyl *on page 1149*

Soyacal® *see* Fat Emulsion *on page 505*

SPA *see* Albumin *on page 37*

Spancap® No. 1 *see* Dextroamphetamine *on page 365*

Span-FF® [OTC] *see* Ferrous Fumarate *on page 513*

Sparfloxacin (spar FLOKS a sin)

Brand Names Zagam®

Therapeutic Category Antibiotic, Quinolone

Use Treatment of adults with community-acquired pneumonia caused by *C. pneumoniae, H. influenzae, H. parainfluenza, M. catarrhalis, M. pneumoniae* or *S. pneumoniae*; also for treatment of acute bacterial exacerbations of chronic bronchitis caused by *C. pneumoniae, E. cloacae, H. influenzae, H. parainfluenza, K. pneumoniae, M. catarrhalis, S. aureus* or *S. pneumoniae*; offers a potential advantage over other fluoroquinolones due to enhanced activity (particularly against g (+) cocci and anaerobes) and a long half-life, allowing once daily dosing

Pregnancy Risk Factor C

Pregnancy/Breast-Feeding Implications Quinolones are known to distribute well into breast milk; consequently use during lactation should be avoided if possible; avoid use in pregnant women unless the benefit justifies the potential risk to the fetus

Contraindications Hypersensitivity to sparfloxacin, any component, or other quinolones

Warnings/Precautions Not recommended in children <18 years of age, other quinolones have caused transient arthropathy in children; CNS stimulation may occur (tremor, restlessness, confusion, and very rarely hallucinations or seizures); use with caution in patients with known or suspected CNS disorder or renal dysfunction; prolonged use may result in superinfection; if an allergic reaction (itching, urticaria, dyspnea, pharyngeal or facial edema, loss of consciousness, tingling, cardiovascular collapse) occurs, discontinue the drug immediately; use caution to avoid possible photosensitivity reactions during and for several days following fluoroquinolone therapy; pseudomembranous colitis may occur and should be considered in patients who present with diarrhea

Adverse Reactions

>1%:

- Central nervous system: Insomnia, agitation, sleep disorders, anxiety, delirium
- Gastrointestinal: Diarrhea, abdominal pain, vomiting
- Hematologic: Leukopenia, eosinophilia, anemia
- Hepatic: Increased LFTs

<1%:

- Dermatologic: Photosensitivity, rash
- Neuromuscular & skeletal: Myalgia, arthralgia

Overdosage/Toxicology Symptoms of overdose include acute renal failure, seizures

GI decontamination and supportive care; not removed by peritoneal or hemodialysis

Drug Interactions

Decreased effect: Decreased absorption with antacids containing aluminum, magnesium, and/or calcium (by up to 98% if given at the same time); phenytoin serum levels may be reduced by quinolones; antineoplastic agents may also decrease serum levels of fluoroquinolones

Increased toxicity/serum levels: Quinolones cause increased levels of caffeine, warfarin, azlocillin, cyclosporine, and theophylline (although one study indicates that sparfloxacin may not affect theophylline metabolism), azlocillin, cimetidine, and probenecid increase quinolone levels; an increased incidence of seizures may occur with foscarnet

Mechanism of Action Inhibits DNA-gyrase in susceptible organisms; inhibits relaxation of supercoiled DNA and promotes breakage of double-stranded DNA

Pharmacodynamics/Kinetics

Absorption: Slow and erratic

Distribution: V_d: 4.5 L/kg; distributes into many tissues, including lung, skin, prostate, and gynecological tissue; CSF penetration is limited

Metabolism: Hepatic, major metabolite is inactive glucuronide

Half-life: 16 hours

Time to peak serum concentration: 3-5 hours

Elimination: 7% to 12% excreted in urine as unchanged drug

Usual Dosage Adults: Oral:

Loading dose: 2 tablets (400 mg) on day 1

Maintenance: 1 tablet (200 mg) daily for 10 additional days (total 11 tablets)

Dosing adjustment in renal impairment: Cl_{cr} <50 mL/minute: Administer 400 mg on day 1, then 200 mg every 48 hours for a total of 9 days of therapy (total 6 tablets)

Monitoring Parameters Evaluation of organ system functions (renal, hepatic, ophthalmologic, and hematopoietic) is recommended periodically during therapy; the possibility of crystalluria should be assessed; WBC and signs and symptoms of infection

Patient Information May take with or without food; drink with plenty of fluids; avoid exposure to direct sunlight during therapy and for several days following; do not take antacids within 4 hours before or 2 hours after dosing; contact your physician immediately if signs of allergy occur; do not discontinue therapy until your course has been completed; take a missed dose as soon as possible, unless it is almost time for your next dose

Dosage Forms Tablet: 200 mg

Sparine® *see* Promazine *on page 1056*

Spaslin® *see* Hyoscyamine, Atropine, Scopolamine, and Phenobarbital *on page 637*

Spasmoject® Injection *see* Dicyclomine *on page 376*

Spasmolin® *see* Hyoscyamine, Atropine, Scopolamine, and Phenobarbital *on page 637*

Spasmophen® *see* Hyoscyamine, Atropine, Scopolamine, and Phenobarbital *on page 637*

Spasquid® *see* Hyoscyamine, Atropine, Scopolamine, and Phenobarbital *on page 637*

Spec-T® [OTC] *see* Benzocaine *on page 138*

Spectam® *see* Spectinomycin *on this page*

Spectazole™ *see* Econazole *on page 437*

Spectinomycin (spek ti noe MYE sin)

Related Information

Antimicrobial Drugs of Choice *on page 1468*

Treatment of Sexually Transmitted Diseases *on page 1485*

Brand Names Spectam®; Trobicin®

Synonyms Spectinomycin Hydrochloride

Therapeutic Category Antibiotic, Miscellaneous

Use Treatment of uncomplicated gonorrhea (ineffective against syphilis)

Pregnancy Risk Factor B

Contraindications Hypersensitivity to spectinomycin or any component

Warnings/Precautions Since spectinomycin is ineffective in the treatment of syphilis and may mask symptoms, all patients should be tested for syphilis at the time of diagnosis and 3 months later

Adverse Reactions

<1%:

Central nervous system: Dizziness, headache, chills

Dermatologic: Urticaria, rash, pruritus

Gastrointestinal: Nausea, vomiting

Local: Pain at injection site

Stability Use reconstituted solutions within 24 hours; reconstitute with supplied diluent only

Mechanism of Action A bacteriostatic antibiotic that selectively binds to the 30s subunits of ribosomes, and thereby inhibiting bacterial protein synthesis

Pharmacodynamics/Kinetics

Duration of action: Up to 8 hours

Distribution: V_d: 0.2 L/kg

Half-life: 1.7 hours

Time to peak serum concentration: Within 1 hour

(Continued)

Spectinomycin *(Continued)*

Elimination: Almost entirely as unchanged drug in urine (70% to 100%)

Usual Dosage I.M.:

Children:

<45 kg: 40 mg/kg/dose 1 time

≥45 kg: See adult dose

Children >8 years who are allergic to PCNS/cephalosporins may be treated with oral tetracycline

Adults:

Uncomplicated urethral endocervical or rectal gonorrhea: 2 g deep I.M. or 4 g where antibiotic resistance is prevalent 1 time; 4 g (10 mL) dose should be given as two 5 mL injections, followed by doxycycline 100 mg twice daily for 7 days

Disseminated gonococcal infection: 2 g every 12 hours

Hemodialysis: 50% removed by hemodialysis

Administration For I.M. use only

Dosage Forms Injection, as hydrochloride: 2 g, 4 g

Spectinomycin Hydrochloride *see* Spectinomycin *on previous page*

Spironolactone (speer on oh LAK tone)

Related Information

Heart Failure: Management of Patients With Left-Ventricular Systolic Dysfunction *on page 1533*

Brand Names Aldactone®

Canadian/Mexican Brand Names Novo-Spiroton® (Canada)

Therapeutic Category Antihypertensive; Diuretic, Potassium Sparing

Use Management of edema associated with excessive aldosterone excretion; hypertension; primary hyperaldosteronism; hypokalemia; treatment of hirsutism; cirrhosis of liver accompanied by edema or ascites

Pregnancy Risk Factor D

Pregnancy/Breast-Feeding Implications

Clinical effects on the fetus: No data available on crossing the placenta. 1 report of oral cleft. Generally, use of diuretics during pregnancy is avoided due to risk of decreased placental perfusion.

Breast-feeding/lactation: Crosses into breast milk. American Academy of Pediatrics considers COMPATIBLE with breast-feeding.

Contraindications Hypersensitivity to spironolactone or any component, hyperkalemia, renal failure, anuria, patients receiving other potassium-sparing diuretics or potassium supplements

Warnings/Precautions Use with caution in patients with dehydration, hepatic disease, hyponatremia, renal sufficiency; it is recommended the drug may be discontinued several days prior to adrenal vein catheterization; shown to be tumorigenic in toxicity studies using rats at 25-250 times the usual human dose

Adverse Reactions

1% to 10%:

Cardiovascular: Arrhythmia

Central nervous system: Confusion, nervousness, dizziness, drowsiness, lack of energy, unusual fatigue, headache, fever, chills

Endocrine & metabolic: Hyperkalemia, breast tenderness in females, deepening of voice in females, enlargement of breast in males, inability to achieve or maintain an erection, increased hair growth in females, decreased sexual ability

Gastrointestinal: Diarrhea, nausea, vomiting, stomach cramps, dryness of mouth

Neuromuscular & skeletal: Weakness, numbness or paresthesia in hands, feet, or lips,

Respiratory: Shortness of breath, dyspnea

Miscellaneous: Increased thirst

<1%:

Central nervous system: Ataxia

Dermatologic: Skin rash

Genitourinary: Painful urination, dysuria

Neuromuscular & skeletal: Lower back or side pain

Respiratory: Cough or hoarseness

Miscellaneous: Diaphoresis

Overdosage/Toxicology Symptoms of overdose include drowsiness, confusion, clinical signs of dehydration and electrolyte imbalance, hyperkalemia; ingestion of large amounts of potassium-sparing diuretics, may result in life-threatening hyperkalemia.

This can be treated with I.V. glucose, with concurrent regular insulin; sodium bicarbonate may also be used as a temporary measure. If needed, Kayexalate® oral or rectal solutions in sorbitol may also be used.

Drug Interactions Increased toxicity: Potassium, potassium-sparing diuretics, indomethacin, angiotensin-converting enzymes inhibitors may increase serum potassium levels

Stability Protect from light

Mechanism of Action Competes with aldosterone for receptor sites in the distal renal tubules, increasing sodium chloride and water excretion while conserving potassium and hydrogen ions; may block the effect of aldosterone on arteriolar smooth muscle as well

Pharmacodynamics/Kinetics

Protein binding: 91% to 98%

Metabolism: In the liver to multiple metabolites, including canrenone (active)

Half-life: 78-84 minutes

Time to peak serum concentration: Within 1-3 hours (primarily as the active metabolite)

Elimination: Urinary and biliary excretion

Usual Dosage Administration with food increases absorption. To reduce delay in onset of effect, a loading dose of 2 or 3 times the daily dose may be administered on the first day of therapy. Oral:

Children:

- Diuretic, hypertension: 1.5-3.5 mg/kg/day in divided doses every 6-24 hours
- Diagnosis of primary aldosteronism: 125-375 mg/m^2/day in divided doses
- Vaso-occlusive disease: 7.5 mg/kg/day in divided doses twice daily (not FDA approved)

Adults:

- Edema, hypertension, hypokalemia: 25-200 mg/day in 1-2 divided doses
- Diagnosis of primary aldosteronism: 100-400 mg/day in 1-2 divided doses

Elderly: Initial: 25-50 mg/day in 1-2 divided doses, increasing by 25-50 mg every 5 days as needed

Dosing interval in renal impairment:

Cl_{cr} 10-50 mL/minute: Administer every 12-24 hours

Cl_{cr} <10 mL/minute: Avoid use

Monitoring Parameters Blood pressure, serum electrolytes (potassium, sodium), renal function, I & O ratios and daily weight throughout therapy

Test Interactions May cause false elevation in serum digoxin concentrations measured by RIA

Patient Information Avoid hazardous activity such as driving, until response to drug is known; take with meals or milk; avoid excessive ingestion of foods high in potassium or use of salt substitutes

Nursing Implications Diuretic effect may be delayed 2-3 days and maximum hypertensive may be delayed 2-3 weeks; monitor I & O ratios and daily weight throughout therapy

Dosage Forms Tablet: 25 mg, 50 mg, 100 mg

Extemporaneous Preparations A 5 mg/mL suspension may be made by crushing tablets, levigating with a small amount of distilled water or glycerin; dilute with 1 part Cologel® and 2 parts simple syrup and/or cherry syrup to make the final concentration; stable 60 days when refrigerated

Handbook on Extemporaneous Formulations, Bethesda, MD: American Society of Hospital Pharmacists, 1987.

A 1 mg/mL suspension may be compounded by crushing ten 25 mg tablets, add a small amount of water and soak for 5 minutes; add 50 mL 1.5% carboxymethylcellulose, 100 mL syrup NF, and mix; use a sufficient quantity of purified water to a total volume of 250 mL; stable at room temperature or refrigerated for 3 months

Nahata MC, Morosco RS, and Hipple TF, "Stability of Spironolactone in an Extemporaneously Prepared Suspension at Two Temperatures," *Ann Pharmacother*, 1993, 27:1198-9.

Sporanox® *see* Itraconazole *on page 690*

SPS® *see* Sodium Polystyrene Sulfonate *on page 1148*

S-P-T *see* Thyroid *on page 1223*

SSD™ *see* Silver Sulfadiazine *on page 1136*

SSD-AF™ *see* Silver Sulfadiazine *on page 1136*

SSKI® *see* Potassium Iodide *on page 1027*

Stadol® *see* Butorphanol *on page 179*

Stadol® NS *see* Butorphanol *on page 179*

Stagesic® *see* Hydrocodone and Acetaminophen *on page 620*

Stannous Fluoride *see* Fluoride *on page 536*

Stanozolol (stan OH zoe lole)

Brand Names Winstrol®

Therapeutic Category Anabolic Steroid; Androgen

Use Prophylactic use against hereditary angioedema

Restrictions C-III

Pregnancy Risk Factor X

Contraindications Nephrosis, carcinoma of breast or prostate, pregnancy, hypersensitivity to any component

Warnings/Precautions May stunt bone growth in children; anabolic steroids may cause peliosis hepatis, liver cell tumors, and blood lipid changes with increased risk of arteriosclerosis; monitor diabetic patients carefully; use with caution in elderly patients, they may be at greater risk for prostatic hypertrophy; use with caution in patients with cardiac, renal, or hepatic disease or epilepsy

Adverse Reactions

Male:

Postpubertal:

>10%:

Dermatologic: Acne

Endocrine & metabolic: Gynecomastia

Genitourinary: Bladder irritability, priapism

1% to 10%:

Central nervous system: Insomnia, chills

Endocrine & metabolic: Decreased libido, hepatic dysfunction,

Gastrointestinal: Nausea, diarrhea

Genitourinary: Prostatic hypertrophy (elderly)

Hematologic: Iron deficiency anemia, suppression of clotting factors

<1%: Hepatic: Hepatic necrosis, hepatocellular carcinoma

Prepubertal:

>10%:

Dermatologic: Acne

Endocrine & metabolic: Virilism

1% to 10%:

Central nervous system: Chills, insomnia, factors

Dermatologic: Hyperpigmentation

Gastrointestinal: Diarrhea, nausea

Hematologic: Iron deficiency anemia, suppression of clotting

<1%: Hepatic: Hepatic necrosis, hepatocellular carcinoma

Female:

>10%: Endocrine & metabolic: Virilism

1% to 10%:

Central nervous system: Chills, insomnia

Endocrine & metabolic: Hypercalcemia

Gastrointestinal: Nausea, diarrhea

Hematologic: Iron deficiency anemia, suppression of clotting factors

Hepatic: Hepatic dysfunction

<1%: Hepatic: Hepatic necrosis, hepatocellular carcinoma

Drug Interactions Increased toxicity: ACTH, adrenal steroids may increase risk of edema and acne; stanozolol enhances the hypoprothrombinemic effects of oral anticoagulants; enhances the hypoglycemic effects of insulin and sulfonylureas (oral hypoglycemics)

Mechanism of Action Synthetic testosterone derivative with similar androgenic and anabolic actions

Pharmacodynamics/Kinetics

Metabolism: In an analogous fashion to testosterone

Elimination: In an analogous fashion to testosterone

Usual Dosage

Children: Acute attacks:

<6 years: 1 mg/day

6-12 years: 2 mg/day

Adults: Oral: Initial: 2 mg 3 times/day, may then reduce to a maintenance dose of 2 mg/day or 2 mg every other day after 1-3 months

Dosing adjustment in hepatic impairment: Avoid use in patients with severe liver dysfunction

Patient Information High protein, high caloric diet is suggested, restrict salt intake; glucose tolerance may be altered in diabetics

Dosage Forms Tablet: 2 mg

Staphcillin® *see* Methicillin *on page 803*

Stavudine (STAV yoo deen)

Brand Names Zerit®

Synonyms d4T

Therapeutic Category Antiretroviral Agent; Antiviral Agent, Oral; Reverse Transcriptase Inhibitor

Use Treatment of adults with advanced HIV infection who are intolerant to approved therapies with proven clinical benefit or who have experienced significant clinical or immunologic deterioration while receiving these therapies, or for whom such therapies are contraindicated; often used in combination with zidovudine or other nucleoside (not zalcitabine due to increased toxicity and resistance development) and a protease inhibitor

Pregnancy/Breast-Feeding Implications

Administer during pregnancy only if benefits to mother outweigh risks to the fetus

HIV-infected mothers are discouraged from breast-feeding to decrease potential transmission of HIV

Contraindications Hypersensitivity to stavudine

Warnings/Precautions Use with caution in patients who demonstrate previous hypersensitivity to zidovudine, didanosine, zalcitabine, pre-existing bone marrow suppression, or renal insufficiency, peripheral neuropathy, folic acid or vitamin B^{12} deficiency. Peripheral neuropathy may be the dose limiting side effect.

Adverse Reactions

>10%: Neuromuscular & skeletal: Peripheral neuropathy

1% to 10%:

- Central nervous system: Headache, chills/fever, malaise, insomnia, anxiety, depression, pain
- Gastrointestinal: Nausea, vomiting, diarrhea, pancreatitis, abdominal pain
- Neuromuscular & skeletal: Myalgia, back pain, weakness

Mechanism of Action Inhibits reverse transcriptase of the human immunodeficiency virus (HIV)

Pharmacodynamics/Kinetics

Distribution: V_d: 0.5 L/kg

Peak serum level: 1 hour after administration

Bioavailability: 86.4%

Half-life: 1-1.6 hours

Elimination: Renal (40%)

Usual Dosage Oral:

Children: 2 mg/kg/day

Adults:

- ≥60 kg: 40 mg every 12 hours
- <60 kg: 30 mg every 12 hours
- Dose may be cut in half if symptoms of peripheral neuropathy occur

Dosing adjustment in renal impairment:

- Cl_{cr} >50 mL/minute: ≥60 kg: 40 mg every 12 hours
- Cl_{cr} >50 mL/minute: <60 kg: 30 mg every 12 hours
- Cl_{cr} 26-50 mL/minute: ≥60 kg: 20 mg every 12 hours
- Cl_{cr} 26-50 mL/minute: <60 kg: 15 mg every 12 hours
- Cl_{cr} 10-25 mL/minute: ≥60 kg: 20 mg every 24 hours
- Cl_{cr} 10-25 mL/minute: <60 kg: 15 mg every 24 hours

Monitoring Parameters Monitor liver function tests and signs and symptoms of peripheral neuropathy.

Patient Information Contact physician at first signs or symptoms of peripheral neuropathy

Dosage Forms

Capsule: 15 mg, 20 mg, 30 mg, 40 mg

Solution, oral: Flavored powder provides 200 mL of a 1 mg/mL solution when reconstituted

Stay Trim® Diet Gum [OTC] *see* Phenylpropanolamine *on page 991*

S-T Cort® *see* Hydrocortisone *on page 623*

Stelazine® *see* Trifluoperazine *on page 1261*

Sterapred® *see* Prednisone *on page 1039*

Stilbestrol *see* Diethylstilbestrol *on page 381*

Stilphostrol® *see* Diethylstilbestrol *on page 381*

Stimate™ *see* Desmopressin Acetate *on page 353*

St. Joseph® Cough Suppressant [OTC] *see* Dextromethorphan *on page 366*

St. Joseph® Measured Dose Nasal Solution [OTC] *see* Phenylephrine *on page 989*

Stop® [OTC] *see* Fluoride *on page 536*

Streptase® *see* Streptokinase *on this page*

Streptokinase (strep toe KYE nase)

Brand Names Kabikinase®; Streptase®

Therapeutic Category Thrombolytic Agent

(Continued)

Streptokinase *(Continued)*

Use Thrombolytic agent used in treatment of recent severe or massive deep vein thrombosis, pulmonary emboli, myocardial infarction, and occluded arteriovenous cannulas

Pregnancy Risk Factor C

Contraindications Hypersensitivity to streptokinase or any component; recent streptococcal infection within the last 6 months; any internal bleeding; brain carcinoma; pregnancy; cerebrovascular accident or transient ischemic attack, gastrointestinal bleeding, trauma or surgery, prolonged external cardiac massage, intracranial or intraspinal surgery or trauma within 1 month; arteriovenous malformation or aneurysm; bleeding diathesis; severe hepatic or renal disease; subacute bacterial endocarditis; pericarditis; hemostatic defects; suspected aortic dissection, severe uncontrolled hypertension (BP systolic ≥180 mm Hg, BP diastolic ≥110 mm Hg)

Warnings/Precautions Avoid I.M. injections; use with caution in patients with a history of cardiac arrhythmias, major surgery within last 10 days, GI bleeding, recent trauma, or severe hypertension; antibodies to streptokinase remain for 3-6 months after initial dose, use another thrombolytic enzyme (ie, alteplase) if thrombolytic therapy is indicated in patients with prior streptokinase therapy

Adverse Reactions

>10%:

- Cardiovascular: Hypotension, arrhythmias, trauma arrhythmias
- Dermatologic: Angioneurotic edema
- Hematologic: Surface bleeding, internal bleeding, cerebral hemorrhage
- Ocular: Periorbital swelling
- Respiratory: Bronchospasm
- Miscellaneous: Anaphylaxis

<1%:

- Cardiovascular: Flushing
- Central nervous system: Headache, chills, fever
- Dermatologic: Rash, itching
- Gastrointestinal: Nausea, vomiting
- Hematologic: Anemia
- Neuromuscular & skeletal: Musculoskeletal pain
- Ocular: Eye hemorrhage
- Respiratory: Bronchospasm, epistaxis
- Miscellaneous: Diaphoresis

Overdosage/Toxicology Symptoms of overdose include epistaxis, bleeding gums, hematoma, spontaneous ecchymoses, oozing at catheter site

If uncontrollable bleeding occurs, discontinue infusion; whole blood or blood products may be used to reverse bleeding.

Drug Interactions

Decreased effect: Antifibrinolytic agents (aminocaproic acid) may decrease effectiveness

Increased toxicity: Anticoagulants, antiplatelet agents may increase risk of bleeding

Stability Streptokinase, a white lyophilized powder, may have a slight yellow color in solution due to the presence of albumin; intact vials should be stored at room temperature; reconstituted solutions should be refrigerated and are stable for 24 hours

Stability of parenteral admixture at room temperature (25°C): 8 hours; at refrigeration (4°C): 24 hours

Mechanism of Action Activates the conversion of plasminogen to plasmin by forming a complex, exposing plasminogen-activating site, and cleaving a peptide bond that converts plasminogen to plasmin; plasmin degrades fibrin, fibrinogen and other procoagulant proteins into soluble fragments; effective both outside and within the formed thrombus/embolus

Pharmacodynamics/Kinetics

Onset of action: Activation of plasminogen occurs almost immediately

Duration: Fibrinolytic effects last only a few hours, while anticoagulant effects can persist for 12-24 hours

Half-life: 83 minutes

Elimination: By circulating antibodies and via the reticuloendothelial system

Usual Dosage I.V.:

Children: Safety and efficacy not established; limited studies have used 3500-4000 units/kg over 30 minutes followed by 1000-1500 units/kg/hour

- Clotted catheter: 25,000 units, clamp for 2 hours then aspirate contents and flush with normal saline

Adults: Antibodies to streptokinase remain for at least 3-6 months after initial dose: Administration requires the use of an infusion pump

An intradermal skin test of 100 units has been suggested to predict allergic response to streptokinase. If a positive reaction is not seen after 15-20 minutes, a therapeutic dose may be administered.

Guidelines for acute myocardial infarction (AMI): 1.5 million units over 60 minutes

Administration:

Dilute two 750,000 unit vials of streptokinase with 5 mL dextrose 5% in water (D_5W) each, gently swirl to dissolve

Add this dose of the 1.5 million units to 150 mL D_5W

This should be infused over 60 minutes; an in-line filter ≥0.45 micron should be used

Monitor for the first few hours for signs of anaphylaxis or allergic reaction. **Infusion should be slowed if lowering of 25 mm Hg in blood pressure or terminated if asthmatic symptoms appear.**

Begin heparin 5000-10,000 unit bolus followed by 1000 units/hour approximately 3-4 hours after completion of streptokinase infusion or when PTT is <100 seconds

Guidelines for acute pulmonary embolism (APE): 3 million unit dose over 24 hours

Administration:

Dilute four 750,000 unit vials of streptokinase with 5 mL dextrose 5% in water (D_5W) each, gently swirl to dissolve

Add this dose of 3 million units to 250 mL D_5W, an in-line filter ≥0.45 micron should be used

Administer 250,000 units (23 mL) over 30 minutes followed by 100,000 units/hour (9 mL/hour) for 24 hours

Monitor for the first few hours for signs of anaphylaxis or allergic reaction. **Infusion should be slowed if blood pressure is lowered by 25 mm Hg or if asthmatic symptoms appear.**

Begin heparin 1000 units/hour about 3-4 hours after completion of streptokinase infusion or when PTT is <100 seconds

Monitor PT, PTT, and fibrinogen levels during therapy

Thromboses: 250,000 units to start, then 100,000 units/hour for 24-72 hours depending on location

Cannula occlusion: 250,000 units into cannula, clamp for 2 hours, then aspirate contents and flush with normal saline

Administration Avoid I.M. injections

Monitoring Parameters Blood pressure, PT, APTT, platelet count, hematocrit, fibrinogen concentration, signs of bleeding

Reference Range

Partial thromboplastin time (PTT) activated: 20.4-33.2 seconds

Prothrombin time (PT): 10.9-13.7 seconds (same as control)

Fibrinogen: 200-400 mg/dL

Nursing Implications For I.V. or intracoronary use only; monitor for bleeding every 15 minutes for the first hour of therapy; do not mix with other drugs

Dosage Forms Powder for injection: 250,000 units (5 mL, 6.5 mL); 600,000 units (5 mL); 750,000 units (6 mL, 6.5 mL); 1,500,000 units (6.5 mL, 10 mL, 50 mL)

Streptomycin (strep toe MYE sin)

Related Information

Antimicrobial Drugs of Choice *on page 1468*

Recommendations for Prophylaxis Against Tuberculosis *on page 1455*

Recommendations of the Advisory Council on the Elimination of Tuberculosis *on page 1483*

Synonyms Streptomycin Sulfate

Therapeutic Category Antibiotic, Aminoglycoside; Antitubercular Agent

Use Combination therapy of active tuberculosis; used in combination with other agents for treatment of streptococcal or enterococcal endocarditis, mycobacterial infections, plague, tularemia, and brucellosis. Streptomycin is indicated for persons from endemic areas of drug-resistant *Mycobacterium tuberculosis* or who are HIV infected.

Pregnancy Risk Factor D

Contraindications Hypersensitivity to streptomycin, aminoglycosides, or any component

Warnings/Precautions Use with caution in patients with pre-existing vertigo, tinnitus, hearing loss, neuromuscular disorders, or renal impairment; modify dosage in patients with renal impairment; aminoglycosides are associated with nephrotoxicity or ototoxicity; ototoxicity may be proportional to the amount of drug given and duration of treatment; tinnitus or vertigo are indications of vestibular injury and impending hearing damage; renal damage is usually reversible

(Continued)

Streptomycin *(Continued)*

Adverse Reactions

1% to 10%:

- Neuromuscular & skeletal: Neuromuscular blockade
- Otic: Ototoxicity (auditory), ototoxicity (vestibular)
- Renal: Nephrotoxicity

<1%:

- Cardiovascular: Hypotension
- Central nervous system: Drug fever, headache, drowsiness
- Dermatologic: Rash
- Gastrointestinal: Nausea, vomiting
- Hematologic: Eosinophilia, anemia
- Neuromuscular & skeletal: Paresthesia, tremor, arthralgia, weakness
- Respiratory: Dyspnea

Overdosage/Toxicology Symptoms of overdose include ototoxicity, nephrotoxicity, and neuromuscular toxicity

The treatment of choice following a single acute overdose appears to be the maintenance of good urine output of at least 3 mL/kg/hour. Dialysis is of questionable value in the enhancement of aminoglycoside elimination. If required, hemodialysis is preferred over peritoneal dialysis in patients with normal renal function. Careful hydration may be all that is required to promote diuresis and therefore the enhancement of the drug's elimination. Chelation with penicillins is experimental.

Drug Interactions

Increased/prolonged effect: Depolarizing and nondepolarizing neuromuscular blocking agents

Increased toxicity: Concurrent use of amphotericin, loop diuretics may increase nephrotoxicity

Stability Depending upon manufacturer, reconstituted solution remains stable for 2-4 weeks when refrigerated and 24 hours at room temperature; exposure to light causes darkening of solution without apparent loss of potency

Mechanism of Action Inhibits bacterial protein synthesis by binding directly to the 30S ribosomal subunits causing faulty peptide sequence to form in the protein chain

Pharmacodynamics/Kinetics

Absorption: Oral: Absorbed poorly; usually given parenterally

Time to peak serum concentration: Within 1 hour

Distribution: To extracellular fluid including serum, abscesses, ascitic, pericardial, pleural, synovial, lymphatic, and peritoneal fluids; crosses the placenta and small amounts appear in breast milk

V_d:

- Neonates: <1 week, <1500 g: Up to 0.68 L/kg; ≥1 week, >1500 g: Up to 0.58 L/kg
- Children: 0.2-0.4 L/kg
- Adults: 0.26 L/kg (range, 0.20-0.40 L/kg)

Cystic fibrosis patients: 0.30-0.39 L/kg

Protein binding: 34%

Metabolism: None

Half-life:

- Newborns: 4-10 hours
- Adults: 2-4.7 hours, prolonged with renal impairment

Elimination: Almost completely (90%) excreted as unchanged drug in urine, with small amounts (1%) excreted in the bile, saliva, sweat and tears

Usual Dosage Intramuscular (may also be given intravenous piggyback):

Tuberculosis therapy: **Note:** A four-drug regimen (isoniazid, rifampin, pyrazinamide and either streptomycin or ethambutol) is preferred for the initial, empiric treatment of TB. When the drug susceptibility results are available, the regimen should be altered as appropriate.

Patients with TB and without HIV infection:

OPTION 1:

Isoniazid resistance rate <4%: Administer daily isoniazid, rifampin, and pyrazinamide for 8 weeks followed by isoniazid and rifampin daily or directly observed therapy (DOT) 2-3 times/week for 16 weeks

If isoniazid resistance rate is not documented, ethambutol or streptomycin should also be administered until susceptibility to isoniazid or rifampin is demonstrated. Continue treatment for at least 6 months or 3 months beyond culture conversion.

OPTION 2: Administer daily isoniazid, rifampin, pyrazinamide, and either streptomycin or ethambutol for 2 weeks followed by DOT 2 times/week administration of the same drugs for 6 weeks, and subsequently, with isoniazid and rifampin DOT 2 times/week administration for 16 weeks

OPTION 3: Administer isoniazid, rifampin, pyrazinamide, and either ethambutol or streptomycin by DOT 3 times/week for 6 months

Patients with TB and with HIV infection: Administer any of the above OPTIONS 1, 2 or 3, however, treatment should be continued for a total of 9 months and at least 6 months beyond culture conversion

Note: Some experts recommend that the duration of therapy should be extended to 9 months for patients with disseminated disease, miliary disease, disease involving the bones or joints, or tuberculosis lymphadenitis

Children:
- Daily therapy: 20-30 mg/kg/day (maximum: 1 g/day)
- Directly observed therapy (DOT): Twice weekly: 25-30 mg/kg (maximum: 1.5 g)
- DOT: 3 times/week: 25-30 mg/kg (maximum: 1 g)

Adults:
- Daily therapy: 15 mg/kg/day (maximum: 1 g)
- Directly observed therapy (DOT): Twice weekly: 25-30 mg/kg (maximum: 1.5 g)
- DOT: 3 times/week: 25-30 mg/kg (maximum: 1 g)
- Enterococcal endocarditis: 1 g every 12 hours for 2 weeks, 500 mg every 12 hours for 4 weeks in combination with penicillin
- Streptococcal endocarditis: 1 g every 12 hours for 1 week, 500 mg every 12 hours for 1 week
- Tularemia: 1-2 g/day in divided doses for 7-10 days or until patient is afebrile for 5-7 days
- Plague: 2-4 g/day in divided doses until the patient is afebrile for at least 3 days

Elderly: 10 mg/kg/day, not to exceed 750 mg/day; dosing interval should be adjusted for renal function; some authors suggest not to give more than 5 days/week or give as 20-25 mg/kg/dose twice weekly

Dosing interval in renal impairment:
- Cl_{cr} 10-50 mL/minute: Administer every 24-72 hours
- Cl_{cr} <10 mL/minute: Administer every 72-96 hours

Removed by hemo- and peritoneal dialysis: Administer dose postdialysis

Administration Inject deep I.M. into large muscle mass; I.V. administration is not recommended

Monitoring Parameters Hearing (audiogram), BUN, creatinine; serum concentration of the drug should be monitored; eighth cranial nerve damage is usually preceded by high-pitched tinnitus, roaring noises, sense of fullness in ears, or impaired hearing and may persist for weeks after drug is discontinued

Reference Range
- Therapeutic: Peak: 15-40 μg/mL; Trough: <5 μg/mL
- Toxic: Peak: >50 μg/mL; Trough: >10 μg/mL

Test Interactions False-positive urine glucose with Benedict's solution

Patient Information Report any unusual symptoms of hearing loss, dizziness, roaring noises, or fullness in ears

Dosage Forms Injection, as sulfate: 400 mg/mL (2.5 mL)

Streptomycin Sulfate *see* Streptomycin *on page 1161*

Streptozocin (strep toe ZOE sin)

Related Information

Antiemetics for Chemotherapy Induced Nausea and Vomiting *on page 1348*
Cancer Chemotherapy Regimens *on page 1351*
Toxicities of Chemotherapeutic Agents *on page 1382*

Brand Names Zanosar®

Therapeutic Category Antineoplastic Agent, Alkylating Agent; Vesicant

Use Treat metastatic islet cell carcinoma of the pancreas, carcinoid tumor and syndrome, Hodgkin's disease, palliative treatment of colorectal cancer

Pregnancy Risk Factor C

Warnings/Precautions The U.S. Food and Drug Administration (FDA) currently recommends that procedures for proper handling and disposal of antineoplastic agents be considered. Renal toxicity is dose-related and cumulative and may be severe or fatal; other major toxicities include liver dysfunction, diarrhea, nausea and vomiting. There may be an acute release of insulin during treatment. Keep syringe of $D_{50}W$ at bedside during administration.

Adverse Reactions

>10%:
- Gastrointestinal: Nausea and vomiting in all patients usually 1-4 hours after infusion; diarrhea in 10% of patients; increased LFTs and hypoalbuminemia
  - Emetic potential: High (>90%)
  - Time course of nausea/vomiting: Onset 1-3 hours; Duration: 1-12 hours
- Renal: Renal dysfunction occurs in 65% of patients; proteinuria, decreased Cl_{cr}, increased BUN, hypophosphatemia, and renal tubular acidosis; use caution with patients on other nephrotoxic agents; nephrotoxicity (25% to 75% of patients)

(Continued)

Streptozocin *(Continued)*

1% to 10%:
Gastrointestinal: Diarrhea
Endocrine & metabolic: Hypoglycemia: Seen in 6% of patients; may be prevented with the administration of nicotinamide
Local: Pain at injection site
<1%:
Central nervous system: Confusion, lethargy, depression
Hematologic: Leukopenia, thrombocytopenia
Myelosuppressive:
WBC: Mild
Platelets: Mild
Onset (days): 7
Nadir (days): 14
Recovery (days): 21
Hepatic: Liver dysfunction
Miscellaneous: Secondary malignancy

Overdosage/Toxicology Symptoms of overdose include bone marrow suppression, nausea, vomiting

Treatment of bone marrow suppression is supportive

Drug Interactions
Decreased effect: Phenytoin results in negation of streptozocin cytotoxicity
Increased toxicity: Doxorubicin prolongs half-life and thus prolonged leukopenia and thrombocytopenia

Stability
Store intact vials under refrigeration; vials are stable for one year at room temperature
Dilute powder with 9.5 mL SWI or NS to a concentration of 100 mg/mL which is stable for 48 hours at room temperature and 96 hours under refrigeration
Further dilution in D_5W or NS is stable for 48 hours at room temperature and 96 hours under refrigeration when protected from light

Standard I.V. dilution:
IVPB: Dose/100-250 mL D_5W or NS
Solution is stable for 48 hours at room temperature and 96 hours under refrigeration when protected from light

Mechanism of Action Interferes with the normal function of DNA by alkylation and cross-linking the strands of DNA, and by possible protein modification

Pharmacodynamics/Kinetics
Distribution: Concentrates in the liver, intestine, pancreas, and kidney
Metabolism: Rapidly metabolized and disappears from serum in 4 hours
Half-life: 35-40 minutes
Elimination: Majority (60% to 70%) excreted in the urine as metabolites, and smaller amounts eliminated in bile (1%) and in expired air (5%)

Usual Dosage I.V. (refer to individual protocols):
Children and Adults:
Single agent therapy: 1-1.5 g/m^2 weekly for 6 weeks followed by a 4-week observation period
Combination therapy: 0.5-1 g/m^2 for 5 consecutive days followed by a 4- to 6-week observation period

Dosing adjustment in renal impairment:
Cl_{cr} 10-50 mL/minute: Administer 75% of dose
Cl_{cr} <10 mL/minute: Administer 50% of dose
Hemodialysis: Unknown
CAPD effects: Unknown
CAVH effects: Unknown

Dosing adjustment in hepatic impairment: Dose should be decreased in patients with severe liver disease

Administration
Administer by slow I.V. infusion over 15 minutes to 6 hours
Avoid extravasation

Monitoring Parameters Monitor renal function closely

Patient Information Avoid aspirin; use electric shaver; any signs of infection, easy bruising or bleeding, shortness of breath, or painful or burning urination should be brought to physician's attention. Nausea, vomiting or hair loss sometimes occur. The drug may cause permanent sterility and may cause birth defects. The drug may be excreted in breast milk, therefore, an alternative form of feeding your baby should be used.

Nursing Implications Wear gloves when preparing and administering; avoid extravasation

Dosage Forms Injection: 1 g

Stresstabs® 600 Advanced Formula Tablets [OTC] *see* Vitamins, Multiple *on page 1310*

Strong Iodine Solution *see* Potassium Iodide *on page 1027*

Strontium-89 (STRON shee um atey nine)

Brand Names Metastron®

Synonyms Strontium-89 Chloride

Therapeutic Category Radiopharmaceutical

Use Relief of bone pain in patients with skeletal metastases

Pregnancy Risk Factor D

Contraindications Patients with a history of hypersensitivity to any strontium-containing compounds, or any other component; pregnancy, lactation

Warnings/Precautions Use caution in patients with bone marrow compromise; incontinent patients may require urinary catheterization. Body fluids may remain radioactive up to one week after injection. Not indicated for use in patients with cancer not involving bone and should be used with caution in patients whose platelet counts fall <60,000 or whose white blood cell counts fall <2400. A small number of patients have experienced a transient increase in bone pain at 36-72 hours postdose; this reaction is generally mild and self-limiting. It should be handled cautiously, in a similar manner to other radioactive drugs. Appropriate safety measures to minimize radiation to personnel should be instituted.

Adverse Reactions Most severe reactions of marrow toxicity can be managed by conventional means

Cardiovascular: Flushing (most common after rapid injection)

Central nervous system: Fever and chills (rare)

Hematologic: Thrombocytopenia, leukopenia

Neuromuscular & skeletal: An increase in bone pain may occur (10% to 20% of patients)

Stability Store vial and its contents inside its transportation container at room temperature

Usual Dosage Adults: I.V.: 148 megabecquerel (4 millicurie) administered by slow I.V. injection over 1-2 minutes or 1.5-2.2 megabecquerel (40-60 microcurie)/kg; repeated doses are generally not recommended at intervals <90 days; measure the patient dose by a suitable radioactivity calibration system immediately prior to administration

Monitoring Parameters Routine blood tests

Patient Information Eat and drink normally, there is no need to avoid alcohol or caffeine unless already advised to do so; may be advised to take analgesics until Metastron® begins to become effective; the effect lasts for several months, if pain returns before that, notify medical personnel

Nursing Implications During the first week after injection, strontium-89 will be present in the blood and urine, therefore, the following common sense precautions should be instituted:

1. Where a normal toilet is available, use in preference to a urinal, flush the toilet twice
2. Wipe away any spilled urine with a tissue and flush it away
3. Have patient wash hands after using the toilet
4. Immediately wash any linen or clothes that become stained with blood or urine
5. Wash away any spilled blood if a cut occurs

Dosage Forms Injection, as chloride: 10.9-22.6 mg/mL [148 megabecquerel, 4 millicurie] (10 mL)

Strontium-89 Chloride *see* Strontium-89 *on this page*

Stuartnatal® 1 + 1 *see* Vitamins, Multiple *on page 1310*

Stuart Prenatal® [OTC] *see* Vitamins, Multiple *on page 1310*

Sublimaze® *see* Fentanyl *on page 510*

Succimer (SUKS i mer)

Related Information

Toxicology Information *on page 1553*

Brand Names Chemet®

Therapeutic Category Antidote, Lead Toxicity; Chelating Agent, Oral

Use Treatment of lead poisoning in children with blood levels >45 µg/dL. It is not indicated for prophylaxis of lead poisoning in a lead-containing environment. Following oral administration, succimer is generally well tolerated and produces a linear dose-dependent reduction in serum lead concentrations. This agent appears to offer advantages over existing lead chelating agents.

Pregnancy Risk Factor C

Contraindications Known hypersensitivity to succimer

Warnings/Precautions Caution in patients with renal or hepatic impairment; adequate hydration should be maintained during therapy

(Continued)

Succimer *(Continued)*

Adverse Reactions

>10%:

Central nervous system: Fever

Gastrointestinal: Nausea, vomiting, diarrhea, appetite loss, hemorrhoidal symptoms, metallic taste

Neuromuscular & skeletal: Back pain

1% to 10%:

Central nervous system: Drowsiness, dizziness

Dermatologic: Rash

Endocrine & metabolic: Serum cholesterol

Gastrointestinal: Sore throat

Hepatic: Elevated AST, ALT, alkaline phosphatase

Respiratory: Nasal congestion, cough

Miscellaneous: Flu-like symptoms

<1%: Cardiovascular: Arrhythmias

Overdosage/Toxicology Symptoms of overdose include anorexia, vomiting, nephritis, hepatotoxicity, renal tubular necrosis, GI bleeding

Drug Interactions Not recommended for concomitant administration with edetate calcium disodium or penicillamine

Mechanism of Action Succimer is an analog of dimercaprol. It forms water soluble chelates with heavy metals which are subsequently excreted renally. Initial data have shown encouraging results in the treatment of mercury and arsenic poisoning. Succimer binds heavy metals; however, the chemical form of these chelates is not known.

Pharmacodynamics/Kinetics

Absorption: Rapid but incomplete

Metabolism: Rapidly and extensively to mixed succimer cysteine disulfides

Half-life, elimination: 2 days

Time to peak serum concentration: ~1-2 hours

Elimination: ~25% in urine with peak urinary excretion occurring between 2-4 hours after dosing; of the total amount of succimer eliminated in urine, 90% is eliminated as mixed succimer-cysteine disulfide conjugates; 10% is excreted unchanged; fecal excretion of succimer probably represents unabsorbed drug

Usual Dosage Children and Adults: Oral: 10 mg/kg/dose every 8 hours for an additional 5 days followed by 10 mg/kg/dose every 12 hours for 14 days

Dosing adjustment in renal/hepatic impairment: Administer with caution and monitor closely

Concomitant iron therapy has been reported in a small number of children without the formation of a toxic complex with iron (as seen with dimercaprol); courses of therapy may be repeated if indicated by weekly monitoring of blood lead levels; lead levels should be stabilized <15 µg/dL; 2 weeks between courses is recommended unless more timely treatment is indicated by lead levels

Monitoring Parameters Blood lead levels, serum aminotransferases

Test Interactions False-positive ketones (U) using nitroprusside methods, falsely elevated serum CPK; falsely decreased uric acid measurement

Patient Information Maintain adequate fluid intake; notify physician if rash occurs; capsules may be opened and contents sprinkled on food or put on a spoon

Nursing Implications Adequately hydrate patients; rapid rebound of serum lead levels can occur; monitor closely

Dosage Forms Capsule: 100 mg

Succinylcholine (suks in il KOE leen)

Related Information

Neuromuscular Blocking Agents Comparison *on page 1417*

Brand Names Anectine® Chloride; Anectine® Flo-Pack®; Quelicin®; Sucostrin®

Synonyms Succinylcholine Chloride; Suxamethonium Chloride

Therapeutic Category Cholinergic Agent; Neuromuscular Blocker Agent, Depolarizing; Skeletal Muscle Relaxant

Use Produces skeletal muscle relaxation in procedures of short duration such as endotracheal intubation or endoscopic exams

Pregnancy Risk Factor C

Contraindications Malignant hyperthermia, myopathies associated with elevated serum creatine phosphokinase (CPK) values, narrow-angle glaucoma, hyperkalemia, penetrating eye injuries, disorders of plasma pseudocholinesterase, hypersensitivity to succinylcholine or any component

Warnings/Precautions **Use in pediatrics and adolescents**; use with caution in patients with pre-existing hyperkalemia, paraplegia, extensive or severe burns, extensive denervation of skeletal muscle because of disease or injury to the CNS or with degenerative or dystrophic neuromuscular disease; may increase vagal tone

Adverse Reactions

>10%:

Ocular: Increased intraocular pressure

Miscellaneous: Postoperative stiffness

1% to 10%:

Cardiovascular: Bradycardia, hypotension, cardiac arrhythmias, tachycardia

Gastrointestinal: Intragastric pressure, salivation

<1%:

Cardiovascular: Hypertension

Dermatologic: Rash, itching, erythema

Endocrine & metabolic: Hyperkalemia

Neuromuscular & skeletal: Myalgia

Renal: Myoglobinuria

Respiratory: Apnea, bronchospasm, circulatory collapse

Miscellaneous: Malignant hyperthermia

Causes of prolonged neuromuscular blockade:

Excessive drug administration

Cumulative drug effect, decreased metabolism/excretion (hepatic and/or renal impairment)

Accumulation of active metabolites

Electrolyte imbalance (hypokalemia, hypocalcemia, hypermagnesemia, hypernatremia)

Hypothermia

Drug interactions

Increased sensitivity to muscle relaxants (eg, neuromuscular disorders such as myasthenia gravis or polymyositis)

Overdosage/Toxicology Symptoms of overdose include respiratory paralysis, cardiac arrest

Bradyarrhythmias can often be treated with atropine 0.1 mg (infants); do not treat with anticholinesterase drugs (eg, neostigmine, physostigmine) since this may worsen its toxicity by interfering with its metabolism

Drug Interactions

Increased toxicity: Anticholinesterase drugs (neostigmine, physostigmine, or pyridostigmine) in combination with succinylcholine can cause cardiorespiratory collapse; cyclophosphamide, oral contraceptives, lidocaine, thiotepa, pancuronium, and procaine enhance and prolong the effects of succinylcholine

Prolonged neuromuscular blockade:

Inhaled anesthetics

Local anesthetics

Calcium channel blockers

Antiarrhythmics (eg, quinidine or procainamide)

Antibiotics (eg, aminoglycosides, tetracyclines, vancomycin, clindamycin)

Immunosuppressants (eg, cyclosporine)

Stability

Refrigerate (2°C to 8°C/36°F to 46°F); however, remains stable for 14 days unrefrigerated

Stability of parenteral admixture at refrigeration temperature (4°C): 24 hours in D_5W or NS

I.V. form is **incompatible** when mixed with sodium bicarbonate, pentobarbital, thiopental

Mechanism of Action Acts similar to acetylcholine, produces depolarization of the motor endplate at the myoneural junction which causes sustained flaccid skeletal muscle paralysis produced by state of accommodation that developes in adjacent excitable muscle membranes

Pharmacodynamics/Kinetics

Onset of effect:

I.M.: 2-3 minutes

I.V.: Complete muscular relaxation occurs within 30-60 seconds of injection

Duration:

I.M.: 10-30 minutes

I.V.: 4-6 minutes with single administration

Metabolism: Rapidly hydrolyzed by plasma pseudocholinesterase

Usual Dosage I.M., I.V.:

Small Children: Intermittent: Initial: 2 mg/kg/dose one time; maintenance: 0.3-0.6 mg/kg/dose at intervals of 5-10 minutes as necessary

Older Children and Adolescents: Intermittent: Initial: 1 mg/kg/dose one time; maintenance: 0.3-0.6 mg/kg every 5-10 minutes as needed

Adults: 0.6 mg/kg (range: 0.3-1.1 mg/kg) over 10-30 seconds, up to 150 mg total dose

(Continued)

Succinylcholine *(Continued)*

Maintenance: 0.04-0.07 mg/kg every 5-10 minutes as needed

Continuous infusion: 2.5 mg/minute (or 0.5-10 mg/minute); dilute to concentration of 1-2 mg/mL in D_5W or NS

Note: Pretreatment with atropine may reduce occurrence of bradycardia

Dosing adjustment in hepatic impairment: Dose should be decreased in patients with severe liver disease

Administration I.M. injections should be made deeply, preferably high into deltoid muscle

Monitoring Parameters Cardiac monitor, blood pressure monitor, and ventilator required during administration; temperature, serum potassium and calcium, assisted ventilator status

Test Interactions ↑ potassium (S)

Dosage Forms

Injection, as chloride: 20 mg/mL (10 mL); 50 mg/mL (10 mL); 100 mg/mL (5 mL, 10 mL, 20 mL)

Powder for injection, as chloride: 100 mg, 500 mg, 1 g

Succinylcholine Chloride *see* Succinylcholine *on page 1166*

Sucostrin® *see* Succinylcholine *on page 1166*

Sucralfate (soo KRAL fate)

Brand Names Carafate®

Canadian/Mexican Brand Names Novo-Sucralate® (Canada); Sulcrate® (Canada); Sulcrate® Suspension Plus (Canada); Antepsin® (Mexico)

Synonyms Aluminum Sucrose Sulfate, Basic

Therapeutic Category Gastrointestinal Agent, Miscellaneous

Use Short-term management of duodenal ulcers

Unlabeled uses: Gastric ulcers; maintenance of duodenal ulcers; suspension may be used topically for treatment of stomatitis due to cancer chemotherapy and other causes of esophageal and gastric erosions; GERD, esophagitis, treatment of NSAID mucosal damage, prevention of stress ulcers, postsclerotherapy for esophageal variceal bleeding.

Pregnancy Risk Factor B

Pregnancy/Breast-Feeding Implications

Clinical effects on the fetus: No data available; available evidence suggests safe use during pregnancy and breast-feeding

Breast-feeding/lactation: No data available. American Academy of Pediatrics has NO RECOMMENDATION.

Contraindications Hypersensitivity to sucralfate or any component

Warnings/Precautions Successful therapy with sucralfate should not be expected to alter the posthealing frequency of recurrence or the severity of duodenal ulceration; use with caution in patients with chronic renal failure who have an impaired excretion of absorbed aluminum; may decrease gastric emptying. Because of the potential for sucralfate to alter the absorption of some drugs, separate administration (2 hours before or after) should be considered when alterations in bioavailability are believed to be critical; do not administer antacids within 30 minutes of administration

Adverse Reactions

1% to 10%: Gastrointestinal: Constipation

<1%:

Central nervous system: Dizziness, sleepiness, vertigo

Dermatologic: Rash, pruritus

Gastrointestinal: Diarrhea, nausea, gastric discomfort, indigestion, xerostomia

Neuromuscular & skeletal: Back pain

Overdosage/Toxicology Toxicity is minimal, may cause constipation

Drug Interactions Decreased effect:

Digoxin, phenytoin, theophylline, ciprofloxacin, itraconazole; because of the potential for sucralfate to alter the absorption of some drugs, separate administration (2 hours before or after) should be considered when alterations in bioavailability are believed to be critical

Antacids/cimetidine/ranitidine: Do not administer concomitantly - sucralfate requires gastric acid for its mechanism of action (ie, to form a gel in the stomach as a protective barrier)

Stability Shake well and refrigerate suspension

Mechanism of Action Forms a complex by binding with positively charged proteins in exudates, forming a viscous paste-like, adhesive substance, when combined with gastric acid adheres to the damaged mucosal area. This selectively forms a protective coating that protects the lining against peptic acid, pepsin, and bile salts.

Pharmacodynamics/Kinetics

Onset of action: Paste formation and ulcer adhesion occur within 1-2 hours

Duration: Up to 6 hours

Absorption: Oral: <5%

Distribution: Acts locally at ulcer sites; unbound in the GI tract to aluminum and sucrose octasulfate

Metabolism: Not metabolized

Elimination: Small absorbed amounts are excreted in urine as unchanged compounds

Usual Dosage Oral:

Children: Dose not established, doses of 40-80 mg/kg/day divided every 6 hours have been used

Stomatitis: 2.5-5 mL (1 g/15 mL suspension), swish and spit or swish and swallow 4 times/day

Adults:

Stress ulcer prophylaxis: 1 g 4 times/day

Stress ulcer treatment: 1 g every 4 hours

Duodenal ulcer:

Treatment: 1 g 4 times/day, 1 hour before meals or food and at bedtime for 4-8 weeks, or alternatively 2 g twice daily; treatment is recommended for 4-8 weeks in adults, the elderly will require 12 weeks

Maintenance: Prophylaxis: 1 g twice daily

Stomatitis: 1 g/15 mL suspension, swish and spit or swish and swallow 4 times/day

Dosage comment in renal impairment: Aluminum salt is minimally absorbed (<5%), however, may accumulate in renal failure

Patient Information Take before meals or on an empty stomach; do not take antacids 30 minutes before or after taking sucralfate

Nursing Implications Monitor for constipation; administer 2 hours before or after administration of other oral drugs

Dosage Forms

Suspension, oral: 1 g/10 mL (420 mL)

Tablet: 1 g

Extemporaneous Preparations 100 mL of sucralfate suspension (200 mg/mL) may be prepared by crushing 20 sucralfate (1 g) tablets and mixing with a sufficient quantity of water to bring the volume to 100 mL; sorbitol can replace a portion of the water if desired; the suspension is stable for 14 days when refrigerated

Sucrets® Cough Calmers [OTC] *see* Dextromethorphan *on page 366*

Sudafed® [OTC] *see* Pseudoephedrine *on page 1074*

Sudafed® 12 Hour [OTC] *see* Pseudoephedrine *on page 1074*

Sufedrin® [OTC] *see* Pseudoephedrine *on page 1074*

Sufenta® *see* Sufentanil *on this page*

Sufentanil (soo FEN ta nil)

Related Information

Narcotic Agonists Comparison *on page 1414*

Brand Names Sufenta®

Synonyms Sufentanil Citrate

Therapeutic Category General Anesthetic

Use Analgesic supplement in maintenance of balanced general anesthesia

Restrictions C-II

Pregnancy Risk Factor C

Contraindications Hypersensitivity to sufentanil or any component

Warnings/Precautions Sufentanil can cause severely compromised respiratory depression; use with caution in patients with head injuries, hepatic or renal impairment or with pulmonary disease; sufentanil shares the toxic potential of opiate agonists, precaution of opiate agonist therapy should be observed; rapid I.V. infusion may result in skeletal muscle and chest wall rigidity → impaired ventilation → respiratory distress/arrest; inject slowly over 3-5 minutes; nondepolarizing skeletal muscle relaxant may be required

Adverse Reactions

>10%:

Cardiovascular: Bradycardia, hypotension

Central nervous system: Drowsiness

Gastrointestinal: Nausea, vomiting

Respiratory: Respiratory depression

1% to 10%:

Cardiovascular: Cardiac arrhythmias, orthostatic hypotension

Central nervous system: Confusion, CNS depression

Gastrointestinal: Biliary tract spasm

(Continued)

Sufentanil *(Continued)*

Ocular: Blurred vision

<1%:

Cardiovascular: Circulatory depression

Central nervous system: Convulsions, dysesthesia, paradoxical CNS excitation or delirium; mental depression, dizziness

Dermatologic: Rash, urticaria, itching

Genitourinary: Urinary tract spasm

Respiratory: Laryngospasm, bronchospasm

Miscellaneous: Cold, clammy skin; physical and psychological dependence with prolonged use

Overdosage/Toxicology Naloxone 2 mg I.V. (0.01 mg/kg for children) with repeat administration as necessary up to a total of 10 mg; supportive care includes establishment of respiratory change; naloxone may be used to treat respiratory depression; muscular rigidity may also respond to opiate antagonist therapy or to neuromuscular blocking agents

Drug Interactions Increased effect/toxicity with CNS depressants, beta-blockers

Mechanism of Action Binds with stereospecific receptors at many sites within the CNS, increases pain threshold, alters pain reception, inhibits ascending pain pathways; ultra short-acting narcotic

Pharmacodynamics/Kinetics

Onset of action: 1-3 minutes

Duration: Dose dependent

Metabolism: Primarily by the liver

Usual Dosage

Children <12 years: 10-25 mcg/kg with 100% O_2, maintenance: 25-50 mcg as needed

Adults: Dose should be based on body weight. **Note:** In obese patients (ie, >20% above ideal body weight), use lean body weight to determine dosage.

1-2 mcg/kg with N_2O/O_2 for endotracheal intubation; maintenance: 10-25 mcg as needed

2-8 mcg/kg with N_2O/O_2 more complicated major surgical procedures; maintenance: 10-50 mcg as needed

8-30 mcg/kg with 100% O_2 and muscle relaxant produces sleep; at doses ≥8 mcg/kg maintains a deep level of anesthesia; maintenance: 10-50 mcg as needed

Nursing Implications Patient may develop rebound respiratory depression postoperatively

Dosage Forms Injection, as citrate: 50 mcg/mL (1 mL, 2 mL, 5 mL)

Sufentanil Citrate *see* Sufentanil *on previous page*

Sular® *see* Nisoldipine *on page 906*

Sulbactam and Ampicillin *see* Ampicillin and Sulbactam *on page 87*

Sulconazole (sul KON a zole)

Brand Names Exelderm®

Synonyms Sulconazole Nitrate

Therapeutic Category Antifungal Agent, Imidazole Derivative; Antifungal Agent, Topical

Use Treatment of superficial fungal infections of the skin, including tinea cruris (jock itch), tinea corporis (ringworm), tinea versicolor, and possibly tinea pedis (athlete's foot - cream only)

Pregnancy Risk Factor C

Contraindications Known hypersensitivity to sulconazole

Warnings/Precautions Use with caution in nursing mothers; for external use only

Adverse Reactions 1% to 10%:

Dermatologic: Itching

Local: Burning, stinging, redness

Mechanism of Action Substituted imidazole derivative which inhibits metabolic reactions necessary for the synthesis of ergosterol, an essential membrane component. The end result is usually fungistatic; however, sulconazole may act as a fungicide in *Candida albicans* and parapsilosis during certain growth phases.

Pharmacodynamics/Kinetics

Absorption: Topical: About 8.7% absorbed percutaneously

Elimination: Mostly in urine

Usual Dosage Adults: Topical: Apply a small amount to the affected area and gently massage once or twice daily for 3 weeks (tinea cruris, tinea corporis, tinea versicolor) to 4 weeks (tinea pedis).

Patient Information For external use only; avoid contact with eyes; if burning or irritation develops, notify physician

Dosage Forms

Cream, as nitrate: 1% (15 g, 30 g, 60 g)

Solution, as nitrate, topical: 1% (30 mL)

Sulconazole Nitrate *see* Sulconazole *on previous page*

Sulf-10® Ophthalmic *see* Sulfacetamide Sodium *on this page*

Sulfabenzamide, Sulfacetamide, and Sulfathiazole

(sul fa BENZ a mide, sul fa SEE ta mide & sul fa THYE a zole)

Brand Names Gyne-Sulf®; Sultrin™; Trysul®; Vagilia®; V.V.S.®

Synonyms Triple Sulfa

Therapeutic Category Antibiotic, Vaginal

Use Treatment of *Haemophilus vaginalis* vaginitis

Pregnancy Risk Factor C

Contraindications Hypersensitivity to sulfabenzamide, sulfacetamide, sulfathiazole or any component, renal dysfunction

Warnings/Precautions Associated with Stevens-Johnson syndrome; if local irritation or systemic toxicity develops, discontinue therapy

Adverse Reactions

>10%: Dermatologic: Local irritation, pruritus, urticaria

<1%:

Dermatologic: Stevens-Johnson syndrome

Miscellaneous: Allergic reactions

Mechanism of Action Interferes with microbial folic acid synthesis and growth via inhibition of para-aminobenzoic acid metabolism

Pharmacodynamics/Kinetics

Absorption: Absorption from the vagina is variable and unreliable

Metabolism: Primarily by acetylation

Elimination: By glomerular filtration into urine

Usual Dosage Adults:

Cream: Insert one applicatorful in vagina twice daily for 4-6 days; dosage may then be decreased to ½ to ¼ of an applicatorful twice daily

Tablet: Insert one intravaginally twice daily for 10 days

Patient Information Complete full course of therapy; notify physician if burning, irritation, or signs of a systemic allergic reaction occur

Dosage Forms

Cream, vaginal: Sulfabenzamide 3.7%, sulfacetamide 2.86%, and sulfathiazole 3.42% (78 g with applicator, 90 g, 120 g)

Tablet, vaginal: Sulfabenzamide 184 mg, sulfacetamide 143.75 mg, and sulfathiazole 172.5 mg (20 tablets/box with vaginal applicator)

Sulfacetamide Sodium (sul fa SEE ta mide SOW dee um)

Brand Names AK-Sulf® Ophthalmic; Bleph®-10 Ophthalmic; Cetamide® Ophthalmic; Isopto® Cetamide® Ophthalmic; Klaron® Lotion; Ocusulf-10® Ophthalmic; Sebizon® Topical Lotion; Sodium Sulamyd® Ophthalmic; Sulf-10® Ophthalmic

Synonyms Sodium Sulfacetamide

Therapeutic Category Antibiotic, Ophthalmic; Antibiotic, Sulfonamide Derivative

Use Treatment and prophylaxis of conjunctivitis due to susceptible organisms; corneal ulcers; adjunctive treatment with systemic sulfonamides for therapy of trachoma; topical application in scaling dermatosis (seborrheic); bacterial infections of the skin

Pregnancy Risk Factor C

Contraindications Hypersensitivity to sulfacetamide or any component, sulfonamides; infants <2 months of age

Warnings/Precautions Inactivated by purulent exudates containing PABA; use with caution in severe dry eye; ointment may retard corneal epithelial healing; sulfite in some products may cause hypersensitivity reactions; cross-sensitivity may occur with previous exposure to other sulfonamides given by other routes

Adverse Reactions

1% to 10%: Local: Irritation, stinging, burning

<1%:

Central nervous system: Headache

Dermatologic: Stevens-Johnson syndrome, exfoliative dermatitis, toxic epidermal necrolysis

Ocular: Blurred vision, browache

Sensitivity reactions: Hypersensitivity reactions

Drug Interactions Decreased effect: Silver, gentamicin (antagonism)

Stability Protect from light; discolored solution should not be used; **incompatible** with silver and zinc sulfate; sulfacetamide is inactivated by blood or purulent exudates

(Continued)

Sulfacetamide Sodium *(Continued)*

Mechanism of Action Interferes with bacterial growth by inhibiting bacterial folic acid synthesis through competitive antagonism of PABA

Pharmacodynamics/Kinetics

Half-life: 7-13 hours

Elimination: When absorbed, excreted primarily in urine as unchanged drug

Usual Dosage

Children >2 months and Adults: Ophthalmic:

- Ointment: Apply to lower conjunctival sac 1-4 times/day and at bedtime
- Solution: Instill 1-3 drops several times daily up to every 2-3 hours in lower conjunctival sac during waking hours and less frequently at night

Children >12 years and Adults: Topical:

- Seborrheic dermatitis: Apply at bedtime and allow to remain overnight; in severe cases, may apply twice daily
- Secondary cutaneous bacterial infections: Apply 2-4 times/day until infection clears

Monitoring Parameters Response to therapy

Patient Information Eye drops will burn upon instillation; wait at least 10 minutes before using another eye preparation; may sting eyes when first applied; do not touch container to eye, ointment will cause blurred vision; notify physician if condition does not improve in 3-4 days; may cause sensitivity to sunlight

Nursing Implications Assess whether patient can adequately instill drops or ointment

Dosage Forms

Lotion: 10% (59 mL, 85 mL)

Ointment, ophthalmic: 10% (3.5 g)

Solution, ophthalmic: 10% (1 mL, 2 mL, 2.5 mL, 5 mL, 15 mL); 15% (5 mL, 15 mL); 30% (15 mL)

Sulfacetamide Sodium and Prednisolone

(sul fa SEE ta mide SOW dee um & pred NIS oh lone)

Brand Names AK-Cide® Ophthalmic; Blephamide® Ophthalmic; Cetapred® Ophthalmic; Isopto® Cetapred® Ophthalmic; Metimyd® Ophthalmic; Vasocidin® Ophthalmic

Therapeutic Category Antibiotic, Ophthalmic; Anti-inflammatory Agent, Ophthalmic; Corticosteroid, Ophthalmic

Use Steroid-responsive inflammatory ocular conditions where infection is present or there is a risk of infection; ophthalmic suspension may be used as an otic preparation

Pregnancy Risk Factor C

Contraindications Mycobacteria infections, fungal infections, herpes simplex keratitis, hypersensitivity to sulfacetamide, prednisolone or any component, infants <2 months of age

Warnings/Precautions Inactivated by purulent exudates containing PABA; use with caution in severe dry eyes; ointment may retard corneal epithelial healing; sulfite in some products may cause hypersensitivity reactions

Adverse Reactions

1% to 10%: Local burning, stinging

<1%:

- Central nervous system: Vertigo, seizures, psychoses, pseudotumor cerebri, headache
- Dermatologic: Stevens-Johnson syndrome, skin atrophy
- Endocrine & metabolic: Cushing's syndrome, pituitary-adrenal axis suppression, growth suppression
- Gastrointestinal: Peptic ulcer, nausea, vomiting
- Neuromuscular & skeletal: Muscle weakness, osteoporosis, fractures
- Ocular: Cataracts, glaucoma

Drug Interactions Decreased effect: Silver, gentamicin, vaccines, toxoids

Mechanism of Action Interferes with bacterial growth by inhibiting bacterial folic acid synthesis through competitive antagonism of PABA; decreases inflammation by suppression of migration of polymorphonuclear leukocytes and reversal of increased capillary permeability; suppresses the immune system by reducing activity and volume of the lymphatic system

Pharmacodynamics/Kinetics Refer to Sodium Sulfacetamide and Prednisolone Acetate monographs

Usual Dosage Children >2 months and Adults: Ophthalmic:

Ointment: Apply to lower conjunctival sac 1-4 times/day

Solution: Instill 1-3 drops every 2-3 hours while awake

Patient Information Eye drops will burn upon instillation; wait at least 10 minutes before using another eye preparation; may sting eyes when first applied; do not touch container to eye; ointment will cause blurred vision; notify physician if condition does not improve in 3-4 days; may cause sensitivity to sunlight

Nursing Implications Shake ophthalmic suspension before using; assess whether patient can adequately instill drops or ointment

Dosage Forms

Ointment, ophthalmic:

AK-Cide®, Metimyd®, Vasocidin®: Sulfacetamide sodium 10% and prednisolone acetate 0.5% (3.5 g)

Blephamide®: Sulfacetamide sodium 10% and prednisolone acetate 0.2% (3.5 g)

Cetapred®: Sulfacetamide sodium 10% and prednisolone acetate 0.25% (3.5 g)

Suspension, ophthalmic: Sulfacetamide sodium 10% and prednisolone sodium phosphate 0.25% (5 mL)

Suspension, ophthalmic:

AK-Cide®, Metimyd®: Sulfacetamide sodium 10% and prednisolone acetate 0.5% (5 mL)

Blephamide®: Sulfacetamide sodium 10% and prednisolone acetate 0.2% (2.5 mL, 5 mL, 10 mL)

Isopto® Cetapred®: Sulfacetamide sodium 10% and prednisolone acetate 0.25% (5 mL, 15 mL)

Vasocidin®: Sulfacetamide sodium 10% and prednisolone sodium phosphate: 0.25% (5 mL, 10 mL)

Sulfadiazine (sul fa DYE a zeen)

Related Information

Sulfonamide Derivatives *on page 1420*

Brand Names Microsulfon®

Canadian/Mexican Brand Names Coptin® (Canada)

Therapeutic Category Antibiotic, Sulfonamide Derivative

Use Treatment of urinary tract infections and nocardiosis, rheumatic fever prophylaxis; adjunctive treatment in toxoplasmosis; uncomplicated attack of malaria

Pregnancy Risk Factor B (D at term)

Contraindications Porphyria, hypersensitivity to any sulfa drug or any component, pregnancy at term, children <2 months of age unless indicated for the treatment of congenital toxoplasmosis, sunscreens containing PABA

Warnings/Precautions Use with caution in patients with impaired hepatic function or impaired renal function, G-6-PD deficiency; dosage modification required in patients with renal impairment; fluid intake should be maintained ≥1500 mL/day, or administer sodium bicarbonate to keep urine alkaline; more likely to cause crystalluria because it is less soluble than other sulfonamides

Adverse Reactions

>10%:

Central nervous system: Fever, dizziness, headache

Dermatologic: Itching, rash, photosensitivity

Gastrointestinal: Anorexia, nausea, vomiting, diarrhea

1% to 10%:

Dermatologic: Lyell's syndrome, Stevens-Johnson syndrome

Hematologic: Granulocytopenia, leukopenia, thrombocytopenia, aplastic anemia, hemolytic anemia

Hepatic: Hepatitis

<1%:

Endocrine & metabolic: Thyroid function disturbance

Genitourinary: Crystalluria

Hepatic: Jaundice

Renal: Interstitial nephritis, acute nephropathy, hematuria

Miscellaneous: Serum sickness-like reactions

Overdosage/Toxicology Symptoms of overdose include drowsiness, dizziness, anorexia, abdominal pain, nausea, vomiting, hemolytic anemia, acidosis, jaundice, fever, agranulocytosis; doses of as little as 2-5 g/day may produce toxicity; the aniline radical is responsible for hematologic toxicity; high volume diuresis may aid in elimination and prevention of renal failure

Drug Interactions Decreased effect with PABA or PABA metabolites of drugs (eg, procaine, proparacaine, tetracaine, sunscreens); decreased effect of oral anticoagulants and oral hypoglycemic agents

Stability Tablets may be crushed to prepare oral suspension of the drug in water or with a sucrose-containing solution; aqueous suspension with concentrations of 100 mg/mL should be stored in the refrigerator and used within 7 days

Mechanism of Action Interferes with bacterial growth by inhibiting bacterial folic acid synthesis through competitive antagonism of PABA

Pharmacodynamics/Kinetics

Absorption: Oral: Well absorbed

Distribution: Throughout body tissues and fluids including pleural, peritoneal, synovial, and ocular fluids; distributed throughout total body water; readily diffused into CSF; appears in breast milk

(Continued)

Sulfadiazine *(Continued)*

Metabolism: By N-acetylation

Half-life: 10 hours

Time to peak serum concentration: Within 3-6 hours

Elimination: In urine as metabolites (15% to 40%) and as unchanged drug (43% to 60%)

Usual Dosage Oral:

Congenital toxoplasmosis:

Newborns and Children <2 months: 100 mg/kg/day divided every 6 hours in conjunction with pyrimethamine 1 mg/kg/day once daily and supplemental folinic acid 5 mg every 3 days for 6 months

Children >2 months: 25-50 mg/kg/dose 4 times/day

Toxoplasmosis:

Children: 120-150 mg/kg/day, maximum dose: 6 g/day; divided every 6 hours in conjunction with pyrimethamine 2 mg/kg/day divided every 12 hours for 3 days followed by 1 mg/kg/day once daily (maximum: 25 mg/day) with supplemental folinic acid

Adults: 2-8 g/day divided every 6 hours in conjunction with pyrimethamine 25 mg/day and with supplemental folinic acid

Administration Administer around-the-clock rather than 4 times/day to promote less variation in peak and trough serum levels

Monitoring Parameters Monitor urine output

Patient Information Drink plenty of fluids; take on an empty stomach; avoid prolonged exposure to sunlight or wear protective clothing and sunscreen; notify physician if rash, difficulty breathing, severe or persistent fever, or sore throat occurs

Nursing Implications Maintain adequate hydration

Dosage Forms Tablet: 500 mg

Sulfadoxine and Pyrimethamine

(sul fa DOKS een & peer i METH a meen)

Related Information

Prevention of Malaria *on page 1441*

Brand Names Fansidar®

Therapeutic Category Antimalarial Agent

Use Treatment of *Plasmodium falciparum* malaria in patients in whom chloroquine resistance is suspected; malaria prophylaxis for travelers to areas where chloroquine-resistant malaria is endemic

Pregnancy Risk Factor C

Contraindications Known hypersensitivity to any sulfa drug, pyrimethamine, or any component; porphyria, megaloblastic anemia due to folate deficiency, severe renal insufficiency; children <2 months of age due to competition with bilirubin for protein binding sites, pregnancy at term or during breast-feeding

Warnings/Precautions Use with caution in patients with renal or hepatic impairment, patients with possible folate deficiency, and patients with seizure disorders, increased adverse reactions are seen in patients also receiving chloroquine; fatalities associated with sulfonamides, although rare, have occurred due to severe reactions including Stevens-Johnson syndrome, toxic epidermal necrolysis, hepatic necrosis, agranulocytosis, aplastic anemia and other blood dyscrasias; discontinue use at first sign of rash or any sign of dermatologic reaction; hemolysis occurs in patients with G-6-PD deficiency (reversed by leucovorin)

Adverse Reactions

>10%:

Central nervous system: Ataxia, seizures, headache

Dermatologic: Photosensitivity

Gastrointestinal: Atrophic glossitis, vomiting, gastritis

Hematologic: Megaloblastic anemia, leukopenia, thrombocytopenia, pancytopenia

Neuromuscular & skeletal: Tremors

Miscellaneous: Hypersensitivity

1% to 10%:

Dermatologic: Stevens-Johnson syndrome

Hepatic: Hepatitis

<1%:

Dermatologic: Erythema multiforme, toxic epidermal necrolysis, rash

Endocrine & metabolic: Thyroid function dysfunction

Gastrointestinal: Anorexia, glossitis

Genitourinary: Crystalluria

Hepatic: Hepatic necrosis

Respiratory: Respiratory failure

Overdosage/Toxicology Symptoms of overdose include anorexia, vomiting, CNS stimulation including seizures, megaloblastic anemia, leukopenia, thrombocytopenia, crystalluria; doses of as little as 2-5 g/day may produce toxicity; the aniline radical is responsible for hematologic toxicity

Following GI contamination, leucovorin should be administered (3-9 mg/day for 3 days or as required) to reverse symptoms of folic acid deficiency; high volume diuresis may aid in elimination and prevention of renal failure; diazepam can be used to control seizures

Drug Interactions

Decreased effect with PABA or PABA metabolites of local anesthetics

Increased toxicity with methotrexate, other sulfonamides, co-trimoxazole

Mechanism of Action Sulfadoxine interferes with bacterial folic acid synthesis and growth via competitive inhibition of para-aminiobenzoic acid; pyrimethamine inhibits microbial dihydrofolate reductase, resulting in inhibition of tetrahydrofolic acid synthesis

Pharmacodynamics/Kinetics

Absorption: Oral: Well absorbed

Distribution:

- Pyrimethamine: Widely distributed; mainly concentrated in blood cells, kidneys, lungs, liver, and spleen
- Sulfadoxine: Well distributed like other sulfonamides

Metabolism:

- Pyrimethamine: Hepatic
- Sulfadoxine: None

Half-life:

- Pyrimethamine: 80-95 hours
- Sulfadoxine: 5-8 days

Time to peak serum concentration: Within 2-8 hours

Elimination: In urine as parent compounds and several unidentified metabolites

Usual Dosage Children and Adults: Oral:

Treatment of acute attack of malaria: A single dose of the following number of Fansidar® tablets is used in sequence with quinine or alone:

- 2-11 months: 1/4 tablet
- 1-3 years: 1/2 tablet
- 4-8 years: 1 tablet
- 9-14 years: 2 tablets
- >14 years: 2-3 tablets

Malaria prophylaxis:

The first dose of Fansidar® should be taken 1-2 days before departure to an endemic area (CDC recommends that therapy be initiated 1-2 weeks before such travel), administration should be continued during the stay and for 4-6 weeks after return. Dose = pyrimethamine 0.5 mg/kg/dose and sulfadoxine 10 mg/kg/dose up to a maximum of 25 mg pyrimethamine and 500 mg sulfadoxine/dose weekly.

- 2-11 months: 1/8 tablet weekly **or** 1/4 tablet once every 2 weeks
- 1-3 years: 1/4 tablet once weekly **or** 1/2 tablet once every 2 weeks
- 4-8 years: 1/2 tablet once weekly **or** 1 tablet once every 2 weeks
- 9-14 years: 3/4 tablet once weekly **or** 1 1/2 tablets once every 2 weeks
- >14 years: 1 tablet once weekly **or** 2 tablets once every 2 weeks

Monitoring Parameters CBC and platelet count, and urinalysis should be performed periodically

Patient Information Begin therapy for malaria prophylaxis at least 2 days before departure; drink plenty of fluids; avoid prolonged exposure to the sun; notify physician if rash, sore throat, pallor, shortness of breath, or glossitis occurs

Dosage Forms Tablet: Sulfadoxine 500 mg and pyrimethamine 25 mg

Sulfalax® [OTC] *see* Docusate *on page 415*

Sulfamethoxazole (sul fa meth OKS a zole)

Related Information

Sulfonamide Derivatives *on page 1420*

Brand Names Gantanol®; Urobak®

Canadian/Mexican Brand Names Apo-Sulfamethoxazole® (Canada)

Therapeutic Category Antibiotic, Sulfonamide Derivative

Use Treatment of urinary tract infections, nocardiosis, toxoplasmosis, acute otitis media, and acute exacerbations of chronic bronchitis due to susceptible organisms

Pregnancy Risk Factor B (D at term)

Contraindications Porphyria, hypersensitivity to any sulfa drug or any component, pregnancy during third trimester, children <2 months of age unless indicated for the treatment of congenital toxoplasmosis, sunscreens containing PABA

(Continued)

Sulfamethoxazole *(Continued)*

Warnings/Precautions Maintain adequate fluid intake to prevent crystalluria; use with caution in patients with renal or hepatic impairment, and patients with G-6-PD deficiency; should not be used for group A beta-hemolytic streptococcal infections

Adverse Reactions

>10%:

Central nervous system: Fever, dizziness, headache
Dermatologic: Itching, rash, photosensitivity
Gastrointestinal: Anorexia, nausea, vomiting, diarrhea

1% to 10%:

Dermatologic: Lyell's syndrome, Stevens-Johnson syndrome
Hematologic: Granulocytopenia, leukopenia, thrombocytopenia, aplastic anemia, hemolytic anemia
Hepatic: Hepatitis

<1%:

Cardiovascular: Vasculitis
Endocrine & metabolic: Thyroid function disturbance
Genitourinary: Crystalluria
Hepatic: Jaundice
Renal: Hematuria, acute nephropathy, interstitial nephritis
Miscellaneous: Serum sickness-like reactions

Overdosage/Toxicology Symptoms of overdose include drowsiness, dizziness, anorexia, abdominal pain, nausea, vomiting, hemolytic anemia, acidosis, jaundice, fever, agranulocytosis; the aniline radical is responsible for hematologic toxicity; high volume diuresis may aid in elimination and prevention of renal failure

Drug Interactions

Decreased effect with PABA or PABA metabolites of drugs (ie, procaine, proparacaine, tetracaine)

Increased effect of oral anticoagulants, oral hypoglycemic agents, and methotrexate

Stability Protect from light

Mechanism of Action Interferes with bacterial growth by inhibiting bacterial folic acid synthesis through competitive antagonism of PABA

Pharmacodynamics/Kinetics

Absorption: Oral: 90%
Distribution: Crosses the placenta; readily enters the CSF
Protein binding: 70%
Metabolism: Primarily in the liver, with 10% to 20% as the N-acetylated form in the plasma
Half-life: 9-12 hours, prolonged with renal impairment
Time to peak serum concentration: Within 3-4 hours
Elimination: Unchanged drug (20%) and its metabolites are excreted in urine

Usual Dosage Oral:

Children >2 months: 50-60 mg/kg as single dose followed by 50-60 mg/kg/day divided every 12 hours; maximum: 3 g/24 hours or 75 mg/kg/day
Adults: 2 g stat, 1 g 2-3 times/day; maximum: 3 g/24 hours

Dosing adjustment/interval in renal impairment:

Cl_{cr} 10-50 mL/minute: Administer every 18 hours
Cl_{cr} <10 mL/minute: Administer every 24 hours

Hemodialysis: Moderately dialyzable (20% to 50%)

Administration Administer around-the-clock to promote less variation in peak and trough serum levels

Monitoring Parameters Monitor urine output

Patient Information Drink plenty of fluids; avoid prolonged exposure to sunlight or wear protective clothing; avoid aspirin and vitamin C products, notify physician if rash, unusual bleeding, difficulty breathing, severe or persistent fever, or sore throat occurs

Nursing Implications Maintain adequate hydration

Dosage Forms

Suspension, oral (cherry flavor): 500 mg/5 mL (480 mL)
Tablet: 500 mg

Sulfamethoxazole and Trimethoprim *see* Co-Trimoxazole *on page 315*
Sulfamylon® *see* Mafenide *on page 751*

Sulfanilamide (sul fa NIL a mide)

Brand Names AVC™ Cream; AVC™ Suppository; Vagitrol®

Therapeutic Category Antifungal Agent, Vaginal

Use Treatment of vulvovaginitis caused by *Candida albicans*

Pregnancy Risk Factor B (D at term)

Contraindications Hypersensitivity to sulfanilamide, aminacrine, allantoin or any component

Adverse Reactions

1% to 10%:

Central nervous system: Kernicterus

Dermatologic: Itching, rash, burning, irritation, exfoliative dermatitis, Stevens-Johnson syndrome

Gastrointestinal: Nausea, vomiting

Genitourinary: Crystalluria

Hematologic: Agranulocytosis, hemolytic anemia in patients with severe G-6-PD deficiency

Hepatic: Hepatic toxicity

<1%: Irritation of penis of sexual partner

Mechanism of Action Interferes with microbial folic acid synthesis and growth via inhibition of para-aminiobenzoic acid metabolism

Usual Dosage Adults: Female: Insert one applicatorful intravaginally once or twice daily continued through 1 complete menstrual cycle or insert one suppository intravaginally once or twice daily for 30 days

Patient Information Avoid excessive exposure to sunlight; complete full course of therapy; notify physician if burning or irritation become severe or persist or if allergic symptoms occur

Dosage Forms

Cream, vaginal (AVC™, Vagitrol®): 15% [150 mg/g] (120 g with applicator)

Suppository, vaginal (AVC™): 1.05 g (16s)

Sulfasalazine (sul fa SAL a zeen)

Related Information

Sulfonamide Derivatives *on page 1420*

Brand Names Azulfidine®; Azulfidine® EN-tabs®

Canadian/Mexican Brand Names Apo-Sulfasalazine® (Canada); PMS-Sulfasalazine (Canada); Salazopyrin® (Canada); Salazopyrin EN-Tabs® (Canada); S.A.S® (Canada)

Synonyms Salicylazosulfapyridine

Therapeutic Category 5-Aminosalicylic Acid Derivative; Anti-inflammatory Agent

Use Management of ulcerative colitis; enteric coated tablets are used for for rheumatoid arthritis in patients who inadequately respond to analgesics and NSAIDs

Pregnancy Risk Factor B (D at term)

Contraindications Hypersensitivity to sulfasalazine, sulfa drugs, or any component; porphyria, GI or GU obstruction; hypersensitivity to salicylates; children <2 years of age

Warnings/Precautions Use with caution in patients with renal impairment; impaired hepatic function or urinary obstruction, blood dyscrasias severe allergies or asthma, or G-6-PD deficiency; may cause folate deficiency (consider providing 1 mg/day folate supplement)

Adverse Reactions

>10%:

Central nervous system: Fever, dizziness, headache

Dermatologic: Itching, rash, photosensitivity

Gastrointestinal: Anorexia, nausea, vomiting, diarrhea

Genitourinary: Reversible oligospermia

1% to 10%:

Dermatologic: Lyell's syndrome, Stevens-Johnson syndrome

Hematologic: Granulocytopenia, leukopenia, thrombocytopenia, aplastic anemia, hemolytic anemia

Hepatic: Hepatitis

<1%:

Endocrine & metabolic: Thyroid function disturbance

Genitourinary: Crystalluria

Hepatic: Jaundice

Renal: Interstitial nephritis, acute nephropathy, hematuria

Miscellaneous: Serum sickness-like reactions

Overdosage/Toxicology Symptoms of overdose include drowsiness, dizziness, anorexia, abdominal pain, nausea, vomiting, hemolytic anemia, acidosis, jaundice, fever, agranulocytosis; the aniline radical is responsible for hematologic toxicity; high volume diuresis may aid in elimination and prevention of renal failure

Drug Interactions

Decreased effect with iron, digoxin and PABA or PABA metabolites of drugs (ie, procaine, proparacaine, tetracaine)

Decreased effect of oral anticoagulants, methotrexate, and oral hypoglycemic agents

(Continued)

Sulfasalazine *(Continued)*

Stability Protect from light; shake suspension well

Mechanism of Action Acts locally in the colon to decrease the inflammatory response and systemically interferes with secretion by inhibiting prostaglandin synthesis

Pharmacodynamics/Kinetics

Absorption: 10% to 15% of dose is absorbed as unchanged drug from the small intestine

Distribution: Small amounts appear in feces and breast milk

Metabolism: Following absorption, both components are metabolized in the liver; split into sulfapyridine and 5-aminosalicylic acid (5-ASA) in the colon

Half-life: 5.7-10 hours

Elimination: Primary excretion in urine (as unchanged drug, components, and acetylated metabolites)

Usual Dosage Oral:

Children >2 years: 40-60 mg/kg/day in 3-6 divided doses, not to exceed 6 g/day; maintenance dose: 20-30 mg/kg/day in 4 divided doses; not to exceed 2 g/day

Adults: 1 g 3-4 times/day, 2 g/day maintenance in divided doses (with other analgesics, at least initially); not to exceed 6 g/day

Dosing interval in renal impairment:

Cl_{cr} 10-30 mL/minute: Administer twice daily

Cl_{cr} <10 mL/minute: Administer once daily

Dosing adjustment in hepatic impairment: Avoid use

Administration GI intolerance is common during the first few days of therapy (administer with meals)

Patient Information Maintain adequate fluid intake; take after meals; may cause orange-yellow discoloration of urine and skin; take after meals or with food; do not take with antacids; may permanently stain soft contact lenses yellow; avoid prolonged exposure to sunlight; shake well before using

Nursing Implications Drug commonly imparts an orange-yellow discoloration to urine and skin

Dosage Forms

Suspension, oral: 250 mg/5 mL (473 mL)

Tablet: 500 mg

Tablet, enteric coated: 500 mg

Sulfatrim® *see* Co-Trimoxazole *on page 315*

Sulfinpyrazone (sul fin PEER a zone)

Brand Names Anturane®

Canadian/Mexican Brand Names Antazone® (Canada); Anturan® (Canada); Apo-Sulfinpyrazone® (Canada); Novo-Pyrazone® (Canada); Nu-Sulfinpyrazone® (Canada)

Therapeutic Category Uricosuric Agent

Use Treatment of chronic gouty arthritis and intermittent gouty arthritis

Unlabeled use: To decrease the incidence of sudden death postmyocardial infarction

Pregnancy Risk Factor C

Contraindications Active peptic ulcers, hypersensitivity to sulfinpyrazone, phenylbutazone, or other pyrazoles, GI inflammation, blood dyscrasias

Warnings/Precautions Safety and efficacy not established in children <18 years of age, use with caution in patients with impaired renal function and urolithiasis

Adverse Reactions

>10%: Gastrointestinal: Nausea, vomiting, stomach pain

1% to 10%: Dermatologic: Dermatitis, rash

<1%:

- Cardiovascular: Flushing
- Central nervous system: Dizziness, headache
- Hematologic: Anemia, leukopenia, increased bleeding time (decreased platelet aggregation)
- Hepatic: Hepatic necrosis
- Genitourinary: Polyuria
- Renal: Nephrotic syndrome, uric acid stones

Overdosage/Toxicology Symptoms of overdose include nausea, vomiting, ataxia, respiratory depression, seizures; following GI decontamination, treatment is supportive only

Drug Interactions

Decreased effect/levels of theophylline, verapamil; decreased uricosuric activity with salicylates, niacins

Increased effect of oral hypoglycemics and anticoagulants

Risk of acetaminophen hepatotoxicity is increased, but therapeutic effects may be reduced

Mechanism of Action Acts by increasing the urinary excretion of uric acid, thereby decreasing blood urate levels; this effect is therapeutically useful in treating patients with acute intermittent gout, chronic tophaceous gout, and acts to promote resorption of tophi; also has antithrombic and platelet inhibitory effects

Pharmacodynamics/Kinetics

Absorption: Complete and rapid
Metabolism: Hepatic to two active metabolites
Half-life, elimination: 2.7-6 hours
Time to peak serum concentration: 1.6 hours
Elimination: Renal excretion with 22% to 50% as unchanged drug

Usual Dosage Adults: Oral: 100-200 mg twice daily; maximum daily dose: 800 mg

Dosing adjustment in renal impairment: Cl_{cr} <50 mL/minute: Avoid use

Monitoring Parameters Serum and urinary uric acid, CBC

Test Interactions ↓ uric acid (S)

Patient Information Take with food or antacids; drink plenty of fluids; avoid aspirin and other salicylate products

Dosage Forms

Capsule: 200 mg
Tablet: 100 mg

Sulfisoxazole (sul fi SOKS a zole)

Related Information

Antimicrobial Drugs of Choice *on page 1468*
Sulfonamide Derivatives *on page 1420*
Treatment of Sexually Transmitted Diseases *on page 1485*

Brand Names Gantrisin®

Canadian/Mexican Brand Names Novo-Soxazole® (Canada); Sulfizole® (Canada)

Synonyms Sulfisoxazole Acetyl; Sulphafurazole

Therapeutic Category Antibiotic, Sulfonamide Derivative

Use Treatment of urinary tract infections, otitis media, *Chlamydia*; nocardiosis; treatment of acute pelvic inflammatory disease in prepubertal children; often used in combination with trimethoprim

Pregnancy Risk Factor B (D at term)

Contraindications Hypersensitivity to any sulfa drug or any component, porphyria, pregnancy during third trimester, infants <2 months of age (sulfas compete with bilirubin for protein binding sites), patients with urinary obstruction, sunscreens containing PABA

Warnings/Precautions Use with caution in patients with G-6-PD deficiency (hemolysis may occur), hepatic or renal impairment; dosage modification required in patients with renal impairment; risk of crystalluria should be considered in patients with impaired renal function

Adverse Reactions

>10%:
- Central nervous system: Fever, dizziness, headache
- Dermatologic: Itching, rash, photosensitivity
- Gastrointestinal: Anorexia, nausea, vomiting, diarrhea

1% to 10%:
- Dermatologic: Lyell's syndrome, Stevens-Johnson syndrome
- Hematologic: Granulocytopenia, leukopenia, thrombocytopenia, aplastic anemia, hemolytic anemia
- Hepatic: Hepatitis

<1%:
- Endocrine & metabolic: Thyroid function disturbance
- Genitourinary: Crystalluria
- Hepatic: Jaundice
- Renal: Interstitial nephritis, acute nephropathy, hematuria
- Miscellaneous: Serum sickness-like reactions

Overdosage/Toxicology Symptoms of overdose include drowsiness, dizziness, anorexia, abdominal pain, nausea, vomiting, hemolytic anemia, acidosis, jaundice, fever, agranulocytosis; doses of as little as 2-5 g/day may produce toxicity; the aniline radical is responsible for hematologic toxicity; high volume diuresis may aid in elimination and prevention of renal failure

Drug Interactions

Decreased effect with PABA or PABA metabolites of drugs (ie, procaine, proparacaine, tetracaine), thiopental

Increased effect of oral anticoagulants, methotrexate and oral hypoglycemic agents

Stability Protect from light

(Continued)

Sulfisoxazole *(Continued)*

Mechanism of Action Interferes with bacterial growth by inhibiting bacterial folic acid synthesis through competitive antagonism of PABA

Pharmacodynamics/Kinetics

Absorption: Sulfisoxazole acetyl is hydrolyzed in the GI tract to sulfisoxazole which is readily absorbed

Distribution: Crosses the placenta; excreted into breast milk

Relative diffusion of antimicrobial agents from blood into cerebrospinal fluid (CSF): Adequate with or without inflammation (exceeds usual MICs); routine alkalinization of urine is normally not required; not for use in patients <2 months of age

Ratio of CSF to blood level (%):

Normal meninges: 50-80

Inflamed meninges: 80+

Protein binding: 85% to 88%

Metabolized: In the liver by acetylation and glucuronide conjugation to inactive compounds

Half-life: 4-7 hours, prolonged with renal impairment

Time to peak serum concentration: Within 2-3 hours

Elimination: Primarily in urine (95% within 24 hours), 40% to 60% as unchanged drug

Usual Dosage

Oral (not for use in patients <2 months of age):

Children >2 months: 75 mg/kg stat, followed by 120-150 mg/kg/day in divided doses every 4-6 hours; not to exceed 6 g/day

Pelvic inflammatory disease: 100 mg/kg/day in divided doses every 6 hours; used in combination with ceftriaxone

Chlamydia trachomatis: 100 mg/kg/day in divided doses every 6 hours

Adults: 2-4 g stat, 4-8 g/day in divided doses every 4-6 hours

Pelvic inflammatory disease: 500 mg every 6 hours for 21 days; used in combination with ceftriaxone

Chlamydia trachomatis: 500 mg every 6 hours for 10 days

Elderly: 2 g stat, then 2-8 g/day in divided doses every 6 hours

Ophthalmic: Children and Adults:

Solution: Instill 1-2 drops to affected eye every 2-3 hours

Ointment: Apply small amount to affected eye 1-3 times/day and at bedtime

Dosing interval in renal impairment:

Cl_{cr} 10-50 mL/minutes: Administer every 8-12 hours

Cl_{cr} <10 mL/minute: Administer every 12-24 hours

Hemodialysis: >50% removed by hemodialysis

Administration Administer around-the-clock to promote less variation in peak and trough serum levels

Monitoring Parameters CBC, urinalysis, renal function tests, temperature

Test Interactions False-positive protein in urine; false-positive urine glucose with Clinitest®

Patient Information Take with a glass of water on an empty stomach; avoid prolonged exposure to sunlight; report to physician any sore throat, mouth sores, rash, unusual bleeding, or fever; complete full course of therapy

Nursing Implications Maintain adequate fluid intake; obtain specimen for culture prior to first dose, if possible

Additional Information

Sulfisoxazole: Gantrisin® tablet

Sulfisoxazole acetyl: Gantrisin® pediatric syrup/suspension

Dosage Forms

Suspension, oral, pediatric, as acetyl (raspberry flavor): 500 mg/5 mL (480 mL)

Tablet: 500 mg

Sulfisoxazole Acetyl *see* Sulfisoxazole *on previous page*

Sulfisoxazole and Erythromycin *see* Erythromycin and Sulfisoxazole *on page 463*

Sulfisoxazole and Phenazopyridine

(sul fi SOKS a zole & fen az oh PEER i deen)

Brand Names Azo Gantrisin®

Therapeutic Category Antibiotic, Sulfonamide Derivative; Local Anesthetic, Urinary

Use Treatment of urinary tract infections and nocardiosis

Pregnancy Risk Factor B (D at term)

Contraindications Porphyria, hypersensitivity to any sulfa drug or any component, pregnancy at term, children <2 months of age unless indicated for the treatment of congenital toxoplasmosis, sunscreens containing PABA

Warnings/Precautions Use with caution in patients with G-6-PD deficiency (hemolysis may occur), hepatic or renal impairment; dosage modification required in patients with renal impairment; risk of crystalluria should be considered in patients with impaired renal function; drug should be discontinued if skin or sclera develop a yellow color

Adverse Reactions

>10%:

Central nervous system: Fever, dizziness, headache

Dermatologic: Itching, rash, photosensitivity

Gastrointestinal: Anorexia, nausea, vomiting, diarrhea

1% to 10%:

Dermatologic: Lyell's syndrome, Stevens-Johnson syndrome

Hematologic: Granulocytopenia, leukopenia, thrombocytopenia, aplastic anemia, hemolytic anemia

Hepatic: Hepatitis

<1%:

Endocrine & metabolic: Thyroid function disturbance

Genitourinary: Crystalluria

Hepatic: Jaundice

Renal: Hematuria, acute nephropathy, interstitial nephritis

Miscellaneous: Serum sickness-like reactions

Overdosage/Toxicology Symptoms of overdose include methemoglobinemia, skin pigmentation, renal and hepatic impairment, drowsiness, dizziness, anorexia, abdominal pain, nausea, vomiting, hemolytic anemia, acidosis, jaundice, fever, agranulocytosis; the aniline radical is responsible for hematologic toxicity; high volume diuresis may aid in elimination and prevention of renal failure; methylene blue 1-2 mg/kg I.V. or 100-200 mg ascorbic acid should reduce methemoglobinemia

Drug Interactions

Decreased effect with PABA or PABA metabolites of drugs (ie, procaine, proparacaine, tetracaine), thiopental

Increased effect of oral anticoagulants, methotrexate and oral hypoglycemic agents

Mechanism of Action Interferes with bacterial growth by inhibiting bacterial folic acid synthesis through competitive antagonism of PABA; phenazopyridine exerts local anesthetic or analgesic action on urinary tract mucosa through an unknown mechanism

Pharmacodynamics/Kinetics

Absorption: Sulfisoxazole acetyl is hydrolyzed in the GI tract to sulfisoxazole which is readily absorbed

Distribution: Crosses the placenta; excreted into breast milk

Protein binding: 85% to 88%

Metabolized: In the liver and other tissues by acetylation and glucuronide conjugation to inactive compounds

Half-life: 4-7 hours, prolonged with renal impairment

Time to peak serum concentration: Within 2-3 hours

Elimination: Primarily in urine (95% within 24 hours) where it exerts its action, 40% to 60% as unchanged drug; excretion (as unchanged drug) is rapid and accounts for 65% of the drug's elimination

Usual Dosage Adults: Oral: 4-6 tablets to start, then 2 tablets 4 times/day for 2 days, then continue with sulfisoxazole only

Dosing adjustment/comments in renal impairment: Cl_{cr} <50 mL/minute: Avoid use of phenazopyridine

Administration Administer around-the-clock rather than 4 times/day to promote less variation in peak and trough serum levels

Monitoring Parameters Monitor urine output

Test Interactions Urine tests which depend on spectrometry or color reactions, ↑ creatinine

Patient Information Take with meals, may cause reddish-orange discoloration of urine; staining of contact lenses has also been reported; drink plenty of fluids; take on an empty stomach; avoid prolonged exposure to sunlight or wear protective clothing and sunscreen; notify physician if rash, difficulty breathing, severe or persistent fever, or sore throat occurs

Nursing Implications Maintain adequate hydration

Dosage Forms Tablet: Sulfisoxazole 500 mg and phenazopyridine 50 mg

Sulfonamide Derivatives *see page 1420*

Sulindac (sul IN dak)

Related Information

Nonsteroidal Anti-Inflammatory Agents Comparison *on page 1419*

Brand Names Clinoril®

(Continued)

Sulindac *(Continued)*

Canadian/Mexican Brand Names Apo-Sulin® (Canada); Novo-Sundac® (Canada)

Therapeutic Category Analgesic, Nonsteroidal Anti-inflammatory Drug; Anti-inflammatory Agent; Nonsteroidal Anti-inflammatory Agent (NSAID), Oral

Use Management of inflammatory disease, rheumatoid disorders; acute gouty arthritis; structurally similar to indomethacin but acts like aspirin; safest NSAID for use in mild renal impairment

Pregnancy Risk Factor B (D at term)

Contraindications Hypersensitivity to sulindac, any component, aspirin or other nonsteroidal anti-inflammatory drugs (NSAIDs)

Warnings/Precautions Use with caution in patients with peptic ulcer disease, GI bleeding, bleeding abnormalities, impaired renal or hepatic function, congestive heart failure, hypertension, and patients receiving anticoagulants

Adverse Reactions

>10%:

Central nervous system: Dizziness

Dermatologic: Rash

Gastrointestinal: Abdominal cramps, heartburn, indigestion, nausea

1% to 10%:

Central nervous system: Headache, nervousness

Dermatologic: Itching

Endocrine & metabolic: Fluid retention

Gastrointestinal: Vomiting

Otic: Tinnitus

<1%:

Cardiovascular: Congestive heart failure, hypertension, arrhythmias tachycardia

Central nervous system: Confusion, hallucinations, aseptic meningitis, mental depression, drowsiness, insomnia

Dermatologic: Urticaria, erythema multiforme, toxic epidermal necrolysis, Stevens-Johnson syndrome, angioedema

Endocrine & metabolic: Polydipsia, hot flashes

Gastrointestinal: Gastritis, GI ulceration

Genitourinary: Cystitis, polyuria

Hematologic: Agranulocytosis, anemia, hemolytic anemia, bone marrow suppression, leukopenia, thrombocytopenia

Hepatic: Hepatitis

Neuromuscular & skeletal: Peripheral neuropathy

Ocular: Toxic amblyopia, blurred vision, conjunctivitis, dry eyes

Otic: Decreased hearing

Renal: Acute renal failure

Respiratory: Allergic rhinitis, shortness of breath, epistaxis

Overdosage/Toxicology Symptoms of overdose include dizziness, vomiting, nausea, abdominal pain, hypotension, coma, stupor, metabolic acidosis, leukocytosis, renal failure

Management of a nonsteroidal anti-inflammatory drug (NSAID) intoxication is primarily supportive and symptomatic. Fluid therapy is commonly effective in managing the hypotension that may occur following an acute NSAID overdose, except when this is due to an acute blood loss. Seizures tend to be very short-lived and often do not require drug treatment; although, recurrent seizures should be treated with I.V. diazepam.

Drug Interactions

Decreased effect of diuretics, beta-blockers, hydralazine, captopril

Increased toxicity with probenecid, NSAIDs; increased toxicity of digoxin, methotrexate, lithium, aminoglycosides antibiotics (reported in neonates), cyclosporine (increased nephrotoxicity), potassium-sparing diuretics (hyperkalemia)

Mechanism of Action Inhibits prostaglandin synthesis by decreasing the activity of the enzyme, cyclo-oxygenase, which results in decreased formation of prostaglandin precursors

Pharmacodynamics/Kinetics

Absorption: 90%

Metabolism: Sulindac is a prodrug and, therefore, requires metabolic activation; requires hepatic metabolism to sulfide metabolite (active) for therapeutic effects; also metabolized in the liver to sulfone metabolites (inactive)

Half-life:

Parent drug: 7 hours

Active metabolite: 18 hours

Elimination: Principally in urine (50%) with some biliary excretion (25%)

Usual Dosage Maximum therapeutic response may not be realized for up to 3 weeks. Oral:

Children: Dose not established

Adults: 150-200 mg twice daily or 300-400 mg once daily; not to exceed 400 mg/day

Dosing adjustment in hepatic impairment: Dose reduction is necessary

Dietary Considerations Food: May decrease the rate but not the extent of oral absorption. Drug may cause GI upset, bleeding, ulceration, perforation; take with food or milk to minimize GI upset.

Monitoring Parameters Liver enzymes, BUN, serum creatinine, CBC, blood pressure

Test Interactions ↑ chloride (S), ↑ sodium (S), ↑ bleeding time

Patient Information Take with food or milk; inform dentist or surgeon because of prolonged bleeding time; do not take aspirin; may cause dizziness, drowsiness, impair coordination and judgment

Nursing Implications Observe for edema and fluid retention; monitor blood pressure

Dosage Forms Tablet: 150 mg, 200 mg

Extemporaneous Preparations A suspension of sulindac can be prepared by triturating 1000 mg sulindac (5 x 200 mg tablets) with 50 mg of kelco and 400 mg of Veegum® until a powder mixture is formed; then add 30 mL of sorbitol 35% (prepared from 70% sorbitol) to form a slurry; finally add a sufficient quantity of 35% sorbitol to make a final volume of 100 mL; the final suspension is 10 mg/mL and is stable for 7 days

Sulphafurazole *see* Sulfisoxazole *on page 1179*

Sultrin™ *see* Sulfabenzamide, Sulfacetamide, and Sulfathiazole *on page 1171*

Sumatriptan Succinate (SOO ma trip tan SUKS i nate)

Brand Names Imitrex®

Canadian/Mexican Brand Names Imigran® (Mexico)

Therapeutic Category Antimigraine Agent; Serotonin Agonist

Use Acute treatment of migraine with or without aura

Unlabeled use: Cluster headaches

Pregnancy Risk Factor C

Contraindications

Intravenous administration

Use in patients with ischemic heart disease or Prinzmetal angina, patients with signs or symptoms of ischemic heart disease, uncontrolled HTN.

Use with ergotamine derivatives

Hypersensitivity to any component

Management of hemiplegic or basilar migraine

Warnings/Precautions

Sumatriptan is indicated only in patient populations with a clear diagnosis of migraine

Use with caution in elderly, patients with hepatic or renal impairment; may cause mild, transient elevation of blood pressure; may cause coronary vasospasm

Adverse Reactions

>10%:

- Central nervous system: Dizziness
- Endocrine & metabolic: Hot flashes
- Local: Injection site reaction
- Neuromuscular & skeletal: Paresthesia

1% to 10%:

- Cardiovascular: Tightness in chest
- Central nervous system: Drowsiness, headache
- Dermatologic: Burning sensation
- Gastrointestinal: Abdominal discomfort, mouth discomfort
- Neuromuscular & skeletal: Myalgia, numbness, weakness, neck pain, jaw discomfort
- Miscellaneous: Diaphoresis

<1%:

- Dermatologic: Rashes
- Endocrine & metabolic: Polydipsia, dehydration, dysmenorrhea
- Genitourinary: Dysuria
- Renal: Renal calculus
- Respiratory: Dyspnea
- Miscellaneous: Thirst, hiccups

Drug Interactions Increased toxicity: Ergot-containing drugs

Stability Store at 2°C to 20°C (36°F to 86°F); protect from light

Mechanism of Action Selective agonist for serotonin ($5HT_{-1-D}$ receptor) in cranial arteries to cause vasoconstriction and reduces sterile inflammation associated with antidromic neuronal transmission correlating with relief of migraine

(Continued)

Sumatriptan Succinate *(Continued)*

Pharmacodynamics/Kinetics After S.C. administration:

Distribution: V_d: 50 L
Protein binding: 14% to 21%
Bioavailability: 97%
Half-life:
  Distribution: 15 minutes
  Terminal: 115 minutes
Time to peak serum concentration: 5-20 minutes
Elimination: In urine unchanged (22%), excreted as indole acetic acid metabolite (38%)

Usual Dosage Adults:

Oral: 25 mg (taken with fluids); maximum recommended dose is 100 mg. If a satisfactory response has not been obtained at 2 hours, a second dose of up to 100 mg may be given. Efficacy of this second dose has not been examined. If a headache returns, additional doses may be taken at intervals of at least 2 hours up to a daily maximum of 300 mg. There is no evidence that an initial dose of 100 mg provides substantially greater relief than 25 mg.

S.C.: 6 mg; a second injection may be administered at least 1 hour after the initial dose, but not more than 2 injections in a 24-hour period

Administration

Oral: Should be taken with fluids as soon as symptoms to appear
Do not administer I.V.; may cause coronary vasospasm

Patient Information If pain or tightness in chest or throat occurs, notify physician; females should avoid pregnancy; pain at injection site lasts <1 hour

Nursing Implications If pain or tightness in chest occurs, notify physician; females should avoid pregnancy; pain at injection site lasts <1 hour

Dosage Forms

Injection: 12 mg/mL (0.5 mL, 2 mL)
Tablet: 25 mg, 50 mg

Summer's Eve® Medicated Douche [OTC] *see* Povidone-Iodine *on page 1031*
Sumycin® *see* Tetracycline *on page 1203*
SuperChar® [OTC] *see* Charcoal *on page 245*
Suplical® [OTC] *see* Calcium Carbonate *on page 185*
Supprelin™ *see* Histrelin *on page 611*
Suppress® [OTC] *see* Dextromethorphan *on page 366*
Suprax® *see* Cefixime *on page 222*

Suprofen (soo PROE fen)

Brand Names Profenal®

Therapeutic Category Anti-inflammatory Agent; Nonsteroidal Anti-Inflammatory Agent (NSAID), Ophthalmic

Use Inhibition of intraoperative miosis

Pregnancy Risk Factor C

Contraindications Previous hypersensitivity or intolerance to suprofen; epithelial herpes simplex keratitis; history of hypersensitivity reactions to aspirin or other nonsteroidal anti-inflammatory agents

Warnings/Precautions Use with caution in patients sensitive to acetylsalicylic acid and other NSAIDs; some systemic absorption occurs; use with caution in patients with bleeding tendencies; perform ophthalmic evaluation for those who develop eye complaints during therapy (blurred vision, diminished vision, changes in color vision, retinal changes)

Adverse Reactions

1% to 10%: Topical: Transient burning or stinging, redness, iritis
<1%:
  Systemic: Chemosis, photophobia
  Topical: Discomfort, pain, punctate epithelial staining

Overdosage/Toxicology Not usually a problem; if accidental oral ingestion, dilute with fluids

Drug Interactions Decreased effect: When used concurrently with suprofen, acetylcholine chloride and carbachol may be ineffective

Mechanism of Action Inhibits prostaglandin synthesis, acts on the hypothalamus heat-regulating center to reduce fever, blocks prostaglandin synthetase action which prevents formation of the platelet-aggregating substance thromboxane A_2; decreases pain receptor sensitivity.

Pharmacodynamics/Kinetics

Protein binding: 99%
Metabolism: Occurs in the liver to one major inactive metabolite
Half-life, elimination: 2-4 hours
Time to peak serum concentration: ~1 hour
Elimination: <15% excreted unchanged in urine in 48 hours

Usual Dosage Adults: On day of surgery, instill 2 drops in conjunctival sac at 3, 2, and 1 hour prior to surgery; or 2 drops in sac every 4 hours, while awake, the day preceding surgery

Patient Information Avoid aspirin and aspirin-containing products while taking this medication; get instructions on administration of eye drops

Nursing Implications In elderly, remove contact lenses before administering; assess ability to self-administer

Dosage Forms Solution, ophthalmic: 1% (2.5 mL)

Surfak® [OTC] *see* Docusate *on page 415*

Surmontil® *see* Trimipramine *on page 1267*

Survanta® *see* Beractant *on page 146*

Susano® *see* Hyoscyamine, Atropine, Scopolamine, and Phenobarbital *on page 637*

Sus-Phrine® *see* Epinephrine *on page 448*

Sustaire® *see* Theophylline Salts *on page 1207*

Suxamethonium Chloride *see* Succinylcholine *on page 1166*

Syllact® [OTC] *see* Psyllium *on page 1075*

Symadine® *see* Amantadine *on page 56*

Symmetrel® *see* Amantadine *on page 56*

Synacort® *see* Hydrocortisone *on page 623*

Synacthen *see* Cosyntropin *on page 314*

Synalar® *see* Fluocinolone *on page 533*

Synalar-HP® *see* Fluocinolone *on page 533*

Synalgos® [OTC] *see* Aspirin *on page 106*

Synalgos®-DC *see* Dihydrocodeine Compound *on page 390*

Synarel® *see* Nafarelin *on page 870*

Synemol® *see* Fluocinolone *on page 533*

Synthetic Lung Surfactant *see* Colfosceril Palmitate *on page 310*

Synthroid® *see* Levothyroxine *on page 721*

Syntocinon® *see* Oxytocin *on page 944*

Syprine® *see* Trientine *on page 1260*

Syracol-CF® [OTC] *see* Guaifenesin and Dextromethorphan *on page 591*

Sytobex® *see* Cyanocobalamin *on page 319*

T_3 Sodium *see* Liothyronine *on page 729*

T_3/T_4 Liotrix *see* Liotrix *on page 731*

T_4 *see* Levothyroxine *on page 721*

Tac™-3 *see* Triamcinolone *on page 1255*

Tac™-40 *see* Triamcinolone *on page 1255*

TACE® *see* Chlorotrianisene *on page 259*

Tacrine (TAK reen)

Brand Names Cognex®

Synonyms Tacrine Hydrochloride; Tetrahydroaminoacrine; THA

Therapeutic Category Cholinergic Agent

Use Treatment of mild to moderate dementia of the Alzheimer's type

Pregnancy Risk Factor C

Contraindications Patients previously treated with the drug who developed jaundice and in those who are hypersensitive to tacrine or acridine derivatives

Warnings/Precautions The use of tacrine has been associated with elevations in serum transaminases; serum transaminases (specifically ALT) must be monitored throughout therapy; use extreme caution in patients with current evidence of a history of abnormal liver function tests; use caution in patients with bladder outlet obstruction, asthma, and sick-sinus syndrome (tacrine may cause bradycardia). Also, patients with cardiovascular disease, asthma, or peptic ulcer should use cautiously.

Overdosage/Toxicology General supportive measures; can cause a cholinergic crisis characterized by severe nausea, vomiting, salivation, sweating, bradycardia, hypotension, collapse, and convulsions; increased muscle weakness is a possibility and may result in death if respiratory muscles are involved

Tertiary anticholinergics, such as atropine, may be used as an antidote for overdosage. I.V. atropine sulfate titrated to effect is recommended; initial dose of 1-2 mg I.V. with subsequent doses based upon clinical response. Atypical increases in blood pressure and heart rate have been reported with other cholinomimetics when coadministered with quaternary anticholinergics such as glycopyrrolate.

Drug Interactions Increased effect of theophylline, cimetidine, succinylcholine, cholinesterase inhibitors, or cholinergic agonists

(Continued)

Tacrine *(Continued)*

Usual Dosage Adults: Initial: 10 mg 4 times/day; may increase by 40 mg/day adjusted every 6 weeks; maximum: 160 mg/day; best administered separate from meal times; see table.

Dose Adjustment Based Upon Transaminase Elevations

ALT	Regimen
≤3 x ULN*	Continue titration
>3 to ≤5 x ULN	Decrease dose by 40 mg/day, resume when ALT returns to normal
>5 x ULN	Stop treatment, may rechallenge upon return of ALT to normal

*ULN = upper limit of normal.

Patients with clinical jaundice confirmed by elevated total bilirubin (>3 mg/dL) should not be rechallenged with tacrine

Monitoring Parameters ALT (SGPT) levels and other liver enzymes weekly for at least the first 18 weeks, then monitor once every 3 months

Reference Range In clinical trials, serum concentrations >20 ng/mL were associated with a much higher risk of development of symptomatic adverse effects

Patient Information Effect of tacrine therapy is thought to depend upon its administration at regular intervals, as directed; possibility of adverse effects such as those occurring in close temporal association with the initiation of treatment or an increase in dose (ie, nausea, vomiting, loose stools, diarrhea) and those with a delayed onset (ie, rash, jaundice, changes in the color of stool); inform physician of the emergence of new events or any increase in the severity of existing adverse effects; abrupt discontinuation of the drug or a large reduction in total daily dose (80 mg/day or more) may cause a decline in cognitive function and behavioral disturbances; unsupervised increases in the dose may also have serious consequences; do not change dose without consulting physician

Dosage Forms Capsule, as hydrochloride: 10 mg, 20 mg, 30 mg, 40 mg

Tacrine Hydrochloride *see* Tacrine *on previous page*

Tacrolimus (ta KROE li mus)

Brand Names Prograf®

Synonyms FK506

Therapeutic Category Immunosuppressant Agent

Use Potent immunosuppressive drug used in liver, kidney, heart, lung, or small bowel transplant recipients

Pregnancy Risk Factor C

Pregnancy/Breast-Feeding Implications Because FK-506 does cross into breast milk, breast-feeding is not advised while therapy is ongoing

Contraindications Hypersensitivity to tacrolimus or any component (eg, hydrogenated castor oil, used in the parenteral dosage formulation)

Warnings/Precautions Increased susceptibility to infection and the possible development of lymphoma may occur after administration of tacrolimus; it should not be administered simultaneously with cyclosporine; since the pharmacokinetics show great inter and intrapatient variability over time, monitoring of serum concentrations (trough for oral therapy) is essential to prevent organ rejection and reduce drug-related toxicity; tonic clonic seizures may have been triggered by tacrolimus

Adverse Reactions

>10%:

- Cardiovascular: Hypertension, peripheral edema
- Central nervous system: Headache, insomnia, pain, fever
- Dermatologic: Pruritus
- Endocrine & metabolic: Hypo-/hyperkalemia, hyperglycemia, hypomagnesemia
- Gastrointestinal: Diarrhea, nausea, anorexia, vomiting, abdominal pain
- Hematologic: Anemia, leukocytosis
- Hepatic: LFT abnormalities, ascites
- Neuromuscular & skeletal: Tremors, paresthesias, back pain, weakness
- Renal: Nephrotoxicity, elevated BUN/creatinine
- Respiratory: Pleural effusion, atelectasis, dyspnea

1% to 10%:

- Dermatologic: Rash
- Gastrointestinal: Constipation
- Genitourinary: Urinary tract infection
- Hematologic: Thrombocytopenia
- Renal: Oliguria

Overdosage/Toxicology Symptoms are extensions of pharmacologic activity and listed adverse effects; symptomatic and supportive treatment required, hemodialysis is not effective

Drug Interactions Cytochrome P-450 3A enzyme substrate

Decreased effect: Separate administration of antacids and Carafate® from tacrolimus by at least 2 hours

Increased effect: Cyclosporine is associated with synergistic immunosuppression and ↑ nephrotoxicity

Increased toxicity: Nephrotoxic antibiotics, NSAIDs and amphotericin B potentially ↑ nephrotoxicity

See table.

Dosing Tacrolimus

Condition	Tacrolimus
Switch from I.V. to oral therapy	Threefold increase in dose
T-tube clamping	No change in dose
Pediatric patients	About 2 times higher dose compared to adults
Liver dysfunction	Decrease I.V. dose; decrease oral dose
Renal dysfunction	Does not affect kinetics; decrease dose to decrease levels if renal dysfunction is related to the drug
Dialysis	Not removed
Inhibitors of hepatic metabolism	Decrease dose
Inducers of hepatic metabolism	Monitor drug level; increase dose

Stability Polyvinyl-containing sets (eg, Venoset®, Accuset®) adsorb significant amounts of the drug, and their use may lead to a lower dose being delivered to the patient; tacrolimus capsules should be stored at controlled room temperature (15°C to 30°C). FK506 admixtures prepared in 5% dextrose injection or 0.9% sodium chloride injection should be stored in polyolefin containers or glass bottles. Infusion of FK506 through PVC tubings did not result in decreased concentration of the drug, however, loss by absorption may be more important when lower concentrations of FK506 are used. Stable for 48 hours in D_5W or NS in glass or polyolefin containers.

Mechanism of Action Suppressed humoral immunity (inhibits T-lymphocyte activation); produced by the fungus *Streptomyces tsukubaensis*

Pharmacodynamics/Kinetics

Absorption: Better in small bowel patients with a closed stoma; unlike cyclosporine, clamping of the T-tube in liver transplant patients does not alter trough concentrations or AUC; food within 15 minutes of administration decreases absorption (27%); T_{max}: 0.5-4 hours

Distribution: V_d: 17 L/kg; crosses placenta (placental plasma concentrations are 4 times greater than maternal plasma); breast milk concentrations = plasma concentrations

Protein binding, plasma: 77% (primarily alpha$_1$-glycoprotein); blood:plasma = >4:1

Metabolism: >99% metabolized in liver; 9 less active metabolites

Bioavailability, oral: 5% to 67% (average 30%)

Half-life, elimination: 12 hours (range: 4-40 hours, twice as fast in children)

Elimination: <1% in urine as unchanged drug; elimination from the body is primarily via bile; clearance: 43 mL/kg/minute

Usual Dosage

Children: Patients without pre-existing renal or hepatic dysfunction have required and tolerated higher doses than adults to achieve similar blood concentrations. It is recommended that therapy be initiated at high end of the recommended adult I.V. and oral dosing ranges (0.1 mg/kg/day I.V. and 0.3 mg/kg/day oral). Dosage adjustments may be required.

Adults:

I.V.: Initial (given at least 6 hours after transplantation): 0.05-0.10 mg/kg/day; corticosteroid therapy is advised to enhance immunosuppression. Patients should be switched to oral therapy as soon as possible (within 2-3 days).

Oral (usually 3-4 times the I.V. dose): 0.15-0.30 mg/kg/day in two divided doses administered every 12 hours and given 8-12 hours after discontinuation of the I.V. infusion. Lower tacrolimus doses may be sufficient as maintenance therapy.

Dosing adjustment in renal impairment: Evidence suggests that lower doses should be used; patients should receive doses at the lowest value of the recommended I.V. and oral dosing ranges; further reductions in dose below these ranges may be required

Tacrolimus therapy should usually be delayed up to 48 hours or longer in patients with postoperative oliguria

Hemodialysis: Not removed by hemodialysis; supplemental dose is not necessary

(Continued)

Tacrolimus *(Continued)*

Peritoneal dialysis: Significant drug removal is unlikely based on physiochemical characteristics

Dosing adjustment in hepatic impairment: Use of tacrolimus in liver transplant recipients experiencing post-transplant hepatic impairment may be associated with increased risk of developing renal insufficiency related to high whole blood levels of tacrolimus. The presence of moderate-to-severe hepatic dysfunction (serum bilirubin >2 mg/dL) appears to affect the metabolism of FK506. The half-life of the drug was prolonged and the clearance reduced after I.V. administration. The bioavailability of FK506 was also increased after oral administration. The higher plasma concentrations as determined by ELISA, in patients with severe hepatic dysfunction are probably due to the accumulation of FK506 metabolites of lower activity. These patients should be monitored closely and dosage adjustments should be considered. Some evidence indicates that lower doses could be used in these patients. See table.

Drug Interactions With Tacrolimus

Drugs Which May INCREASE Tacrolimus Blood Levels		
Calcium Channel Blockers	**Antifungal Agents**	**Other Drugs**
Diltiazem Nicardipine Verapamil	Clotrimazole Erythromycin Fluconazole Itraconazole Ketoconazole	Bromocriptine Cimetidine Clarithromycin Cyclosporine Danazol Methylprednisolone Metoclopramide Grapefruit juice
Drugs Which May DECREASE Tacrolimus Blood Levels		
Anticonvulsants	**Antibiotics**	
Carbamazepine Phenobarbital Phenytoin	Rifabutin Rifampin	

Administration Administer by I.V. continuous infusion only (use infusion pump); dilute with 0.9% sodium chloride of D_5W to a concentration of 0.004-0.02 mg/mL prior to administration; use only glass or polyethylene containers for storage; do not mix with acyclovir or ganciclovir due to chemical degradation of tacrolimus (use different ports in multilumen lines); do not alter dose with concurrent T-tube clamping

Monitoring Parameters Renal function, hepatic function, serum electrolytes, glucose and blood pressure, hypersensitivity indicators, neurological responses, and other clinical parameters; since the pharmacokinetics show great inter- and intrapatient variability over time, monitoring of serum concentrations (trough for oral therapy) has proven helpful to prevent organ rejection and reduce drug-related toxicity; measure 3 times/week for first few weeks, then gradually decrease frequency as patient stabilizes

Reference Range Trough levels: 0.5-2 ng/mL (ELISA, plasma, extracted at 37°C) for all transplant procedures (liver, heart, lung, kidney, small bowel) whole blood measurements produce concentration 5-40 times higher than those in serum due to high binding to RBCs (therapeutic range: 5-10 ng/mL, although levels >20 mg/mL may be desirable for short periods to prevent rejection)

Patient Information Separate administration with antacids by at least 2 hours

Nursing Implications For I.V. administration, tacrolimus is dispensed in a 50 mL glass container with no overfill; it is intended to be infused over 12 hours; polyolefin administration sets should be used

Additional Information Each mL of injection contains polyoxyl 60 hydrogenated castor oil (HCO-60), 200 mg and dehydrated alcohol, USP, 80% v/v

Dosage Forms

Capsule: 1 mg, 5 mg

Injection, with alcohol and surfactant: 5 mg/mL (1 mL)

Extemporaneous Preparations Tacrolimus oral suspension can be compounded at a concentration of 0.5 mg/mL; an extemporaneous suspension can be prepared by mixing the contents of six 5-mg tacrolimus capsules with equal amounts of Ora-Plus™ and Simple Syrup, N.F., to make a final volume of 60 mL. The Suspension is stable for 56 days at room temperature in glass or plastic amber prescription bottles.

Esquivel C, So S, McDiarmid S, Andrews W, Colombani P. Suggested guidelines for the use of tacrolimus in pediatric liver transplant patients. *Transplantation* 1996;61(5):847-848.

Foster JA, Jacobson PA, Johnson CE, et al. Stability of tacrolimus in an extemporaneously compounded oral liquid. (Abstract of Meeting Presentation) *American Society of Health-System Pharmacists Annual Meeting* 1996;53:P-52(E)

Tagamet® *see* Cimetidine *on page 275*

Tagamet-HB® [OTC] *see* Cimetidine *on page 275*

Talwin® *see* Pentazocine *on page 969*

Talwin® NX *see* Pentazocine *on page 969*

Tambocor™ *see* Flecainide *on page 522*

Tamoxifen (ta MOKS i fen)

Related Information

Cancer Chemotherapy Regimens *on page 1351*
Toxicities of Chemotherapeutic Agents *on page 1382*

Brand Names Nolvadex®

Canadian/Mexican Brand Names Alpha-Tamoxifen® (Canada); Apo-Tamox® (Canada); Novo-Tamoxifen® (Canada); Tamofen® (Canada); Tamone® (Canada); Bilem® (Mexico); Cryoxifeno® (Mexico); Tamoxan® (Mexico); Taxus® (Mexico)

Synonyms Tamoxifen Citrate

Therapeutic Category Antineoplastic Agents, Hormone Antagonist; Estrogen Receptor Antagonist

Use Palliative or adjunctive treatment of advanced breast cancer

Unlabeled use: Treatment of mastalgia, gynecomastia, male breast cancer, and pancreatic carcinoma. Studies have shown tamoxifen to be effective in the treatment of primary breast cancer in elderly women. Comparative studies with other antineoplastic agents in elderly women with breast cancer had more favorable survival rates with tamoxifen. Initiation of hormone therapy rather than chemotherapy is justified for elderly patients with metastatic breast cancer who are responsive.

Pregnancy Risk Factor D

Contraindications Hypersensitivity to tamoxifen

Warnings/Precautions Use with caution in patients with leukopenia, thrombocytopenia, or hyperlipidemias; ovulation may be induced; "hot flashes" may be countered by Bellergal-S® tablets; decreased visual acuity, retinopathy and corneal changes have been reported with use for more than 1 year at doses above recommended; hypercalcemia in patients with bone metastasis; hepatocellular carcinomas have been reported in animal studies; endometrial hyperplasia and polyps have occurred

Adverse Reactions

>10%:

- Cardiovascular: Flushing
- Dermatologic: Skin rash
- Gastrointestinal: Little to mild nausea (10%), vomiting, weight gain
- Hematologic: Myelosuppressive: Transient thrombocytopenia occurs in ~24% of patients receiving 10-20 mg/day; platelet counts return to normal within several weeks in spite of continued administration; leukopenia has also been reported and does resolve during continued therapy; anemia has also been reported
  - WBC: Rare
  - Platelets: None
- Hepatic: Hepatotoxicity
- Neuromuscular & skeletal: Increased bone and tumor pain and local disease flare shortly after starting therapy; this will subside rapidly, but patients should be aware of this since many may discontinue the drug due to the side effects

1% to 10%:

- Cardiovascular: Thromboembolism: Tamoxifen has been associated with the occurrence of venous thrombosis and pulmonary embolism; arterial thrombosis has also been described in a few case reports
- Central nervous system: Lightheadedness, depression, dizziness, headache, lassitude, mental confusion
- Dermatologic: Rash
- Endocrine & metabolic: Hypercalcemia may occur in patients with bone metastases; galactorrhea and vitamin deficiency, menstrual irregularities
- Genitourinary: Vaginal bleeding or discharge, endometriosis, priapism, possible endometrial cancer
- Neuromuscular & skeletal: Weakness
- Ocular: Ophthalmologic effects (visual acuity changes, cataracts, or retinopathy), corneal opacities

Overdosage/Toxicology Symptoms of overdose include hypercalcemia, edema; general supportive care

Drug Interactions Cytochrome P-450 3A enzyme substrate

(Continued)

Tamoxifen *(Continued)*

Increased toxicity:

Allopurinol results in exacerbation of allopurinol-induced hepatotoxicity

Cyclosporine may result in ↑ cyclosporine serum levels

Warfarin results in significant enhancement of the anticoagulant effects of warfarin; has been speculated that a ↓ in antitumor effect of tamoxifen may also occur due to alterations in the percentage of active tamoxifen metabolites

Mechanism of Action Competitively binds to estrogen receptors on tumors and other tissue targets, producing a nuclear complex that decreases DNA synthesis and inhibits estrogen effects; nonsteroidal agent with potent antiestrogenic properties which compete with estrogen for binding sites in breast and other tissues; cells accumulate in the G_0 and G_1 phases; therefore, tamoxifen is cytostatic rather than cytocidal.

Pharmacodynamics/Kinetics

Absorption: Well absorbed from GI tract

Time to peak serum concentration: Oral: Within 4-7 hours

Distribution: High concentrations found in uterus, endometrial and breast tissue

Metabolism: In the liver

Half-life: 7 days

Elimination: Undergoes enterohepatic recycling; excreted in feces with only small amounts appearing in urine

Usual Dosage Oral (refer to individual protocols):

Adults: 10-20 mg twice daily in the morning and evening

High-dose therapy is under investigation

Monitoring Parameters Monitor WBC and platelet counts, tumor

Test Interactions T_4 elevations (no clinical evidence of hyperthyroidism)

Patient Information This drug will cause an initial "flare" of this disease (increased bone pain and hot flashes) which will subside. Report any vomiting that occurs after taking dose; women should be advised to notify their physician of vaginal bleeding, weakness, mental confusion.

Nursing Implications Increase of bone pain usually indicates a good therapeutic response

Dosage Forms Tablet, as citrate: 10 mg, 20 mg

Tamoxifen Citrate *see* Tamoxifen *on previous page*

Tanac® [OTC] *see* Benzocaine *on page 138*

Tao® *see* Troleandomycin *on page 1274*

Tapazole® *see* Methimazole *on page 804*

TAT *see* Tetanus Antitoxin *on page 1199*

Tavist® *see* Clemastine *on page 289*

Tavist®-1 [OTC] *see* Clemastine *on page 289*

Taxol® *see* Paclitaxel *on page 945*

Taxotere® *see* Docetaxel *on page 413*

Tazicef® *see* Ceftazidime *on page 232*

Tazidime® *see* Ceftazidime *on page 232*

3TC *see* Lamivudine *on page 704*

TCN *see* Tetracycline *on page 1203*

Td *see* Diphtheria and Tetanus Toxoid *on page 402*

Tebamide® *see* Trimethobenzamide *on page 1265*

Tega-Vert® Oral *see* Dimenhydrinate *on page 395*

Tegison® *see* Etretinate *on page 500*

Tegopen® *see* Cloxacillin *on page 303*

Tegretol® *see* Carbamazepine *on page 201*

Tegretol-XR® *see* Carbamazepine *on page 201*

Tegrin®-HC *see* Hydrocortisone *on page 623*

Telachlor® *see* Chlorpheniramine *on page 260*

Teladar® *see* Betamethasone *on page 147*

Teldrin® [OTC] *see* Chlorpheniramine *on page 260*

Teline® *see* Tetracycline *on page 1203*

Temazepam (te MAZ e pam)

Related Information

Benzodiazepines Comparison *on page 1397*

Brand Names Restoril®

Therapeutic Category Benzodiazepine; Hypnotic; Sedative

Use Treatment of anxiety and as an adjunct in the treatment of depression; also may be used in the management of panic attacks; transient insomnia and sleep latency

Restrictions C-IV

Pregnancy Risk Factor X

Contraindications Hypersensitivity to temazepam or any component, severe uncontrolled pain, pre-existing CNS depression, or narrow-angle glaucoma; not to be used in pregnancy or lactation

Warnings/Precautions Safety and efficacy in children <18 years of age have not been established; do not use in pregnant women; may cause drug dependency; avoid abrupt discontinuance in patients with prolonged therapy or seizure disorders; use with caution in patients receiving other CNS depressants, in patients with hepatic dysfunction, and the elderly

Adverse Reactions

>10%:

Cardiovascular: Tachycardia, chest pain

Central nervous system: Drowsiness, fatigue, ataxia, lightheadedness, memory impairment, insomnia, anxiety, depression, headache

Dermatologic: Rash

Endocrine & metabolic: Decreased libido

Gastrointestinal: Xerostomia, constipation, diarrhea, decreased salivation, nausea, vomiting, increased or decreased appetite

Neuromuscular & skeletal: Dysarthria

Ocular: Blurred vision

Miscellaneous: Diaphoresis

1% to 10%:

Cardiovascular: Syncope, hypotension

Central nervous system: Confusion, nervousness, dizziness, akathisia

Dermatologic: Dermatitis

Gastrointestinal: Increased salivation, weight gain or loss

Neuromuscular & skeletal: Rigidity, tremor, muscle cramps

Otic: Tinnitus

Respiratory: Nasal congestion, hyperventilation

<1%:

Endocrine & metabolic: Menstrual irregularities

Hematologic: Blood dyscrasias

Neuromuscular & skeletal: Reflex slowing

Miscellaneous: Drug dependence

Overdosage/Toxicology Symptoms of overdose include somnolence, confusion, coma, hypoactive reflexes, dyspnea, hypotension, slurred speech, impaired coordination

Treatment for benzodiazepine overdose is supportive. Rarely is mechanical ventilation required. Flumazenil has been shown to selectively block the binding of benzodiazepines to CNS receptors, resulting in a reversal of benzodiazepine-induced CNS depression.

Drug Interactions Increased effect of CNS depressants

Mechanism of Action Benzodiazepine anxiolytic sedative that produces CNS depression at the subcortical level, except at high doses, whereby it works at the cortical level; causes minimal change in REM sleep patterns

Pharmacodynamics/Kinetics

Protein binding: 96%

Metabolism: In the liver

Half-life: 9.5-12.4 hours

Time to peak serum concentration: Within 2-3 hours

Elimination: 80% to 90% excreted in urine as inactive metabolites

Usual Dosage Adults: Oral: 15-30 mg at bedtime; 15 mg in elderly or debilitated patients

Dietary Considerations Alcohol: Additive CNS effect, avoid use

Monitoring Parameters Respiratory and cardiovascular status

Reference Range Therapeutic: 26 ng/mL after 24 hours

Patient Information Avoid alcohol and other CNS depressants; avoid activities needing good psychomotor coordination until CNS effects are known; drug may cause physical or psychological dependence; avoid abrupt discontinuation after prolonged use

Nursing Implications Provide safety measures (ie, side rails, night light, and call button); remove smoking materials from area; supervise ambulation

Dosage Forms Capsule: 7.5 mg, 15 mg, 30 mg

Temovate® *see* Clobetasol *on page 292*

Tempra® [OTC] *see* Acetaminophen *on page 19*

Tenex® *see* Guanfacine *on page 594*

Teniposide (ten i POE side)

Related Information

Antiemetics for Chemotherapy Induced Nausea and Vomiting *on page 1348*

Extravasation Management of Chemotherapeutic Agents *on page 1379*

Toxicities of Chemotherapeutic Agents *on page 1382*

(Continued)

Teniposide *(Continued)*

Brand Names Vumon

Synonyms EPT; VM-26

Therapeutic Category Antineoplastic Agent, Podophyllotoxin Derivative; Antineoplastic Agent, Vesicant

Use Treatment of acute lymphocytic leukemia, small cell lung cancer

Pregnancy Risk Factor D

Contraindications Hypersensitivity to teniposide or Cremophor EL (polyoxyethylated castor oil) any component

Warnings/Precautions The U.S. Food and Drug Administration (FDA) currently recommends that procedures for proper handling and disposal of antineoplastic agents be considered. Administer I.V. infusions over a period of at least 30-60 minutes, must be diluted, do not administer IVP. Teniposide contains benzyl alcohol, which has been associated with a fatal "gasping" syndrome in premature infants.

Adverse Reactions

>10%:

- Gastrointestinal: Mucositis, nausea, vomiting, diarrhea
- Hematologic: Myelosuppression, leukopenia, neutropenia, thrombocytopenia
- Miscellaneous: Infection

1% to 10%:

- Cardiovascular: Hypotension
- Central nervous system: Fever
- Dermatologic: Alopecia, rash
- Hematologic: Hemorrhage
- Miscellaneous: Hypersensitivity

<1%:

- Endocrine & metabolic: Metabolic abnormalities
- Hepatic: Hepatic dysfunction
- Neuromuscular & skeletal: Peripheral neurotoxicity
- Renal: Renal dysfunction

Overdosage/Toxicology Symptoms of overdose include bone marrow suppression, leukopenia, thrombocytopenia, nausea, vomiting; treatment is supportive

Drug Interactions Increased toxicity:

Methotrexate: Alteration of MTX transport has been found as a slow efflux of MTX and its polyglutamated form out of the cell, leading to intercellular accumulation of MTX

Sodium salicylate, sulfamethizole, tolbutamide: displace teniposide from protein-binding sites - could cause substantial increases in free drug levels, resulting in potentiation of toxicity

Stability Store ampuls in refrigerator at 2°C to 8°C (36°F to 46°F); reconstituted solutions are stable at room temperature for up to 24 hours after preparation. Teniposide must be diluted with either D_5W or 0.9% sodium chloride solutions to a final concentration of 0.1, 0.2, 0.4 or 1 mg/mL. In order to prevent extraction of the plasticizer DEHP, **solutions should be prepared in non-DEHP-containing containers such as glass or polyolefin containers**. The use of polyvinyl chloride (PVC) containers is not recommended. Administer 1 mg/mL solutions within 4 hours of preparation to reduce the potential for precipitation. Precipitation may occur at any concentration. **Incompatible** with heparin.

Mechanism of Action Inhibits mitotic activity; inhibits cells from entering mitosis

Pharmacodynamics/Kinetics

Distribution: V_d: 0.28 L/kg; distributed mainly into liver, kidneys, small intestine, and adrenals; crosses blood-brain barrier to a limited extent

V_d: 3-11 L (children); 8-44 L (adults)

Protein binding: 99.4%

Metabolism: Extensively in the liver

Half-life: 5 hours

Elimination: In urine (21% as unchanged drug); renal (44%) and fecal (≤10%)

Usual Dosage I.V.:

Children: 130 mg/m²/week, increasing to 150 mg/m² after 3 weeks and up to 180 mg/m² after 6 weeks

Adults: 50-180 mg/m² once or twice weekly for 4-6 weeks or 20-60 mg/m²/day for 5 days

Acute lymphoblastic leukemia (ALL): 165 mg/m² twice weekly for 8-9 doses **or** 250 mg/m² weekly for 4-8 weeks

Small cell lung cancer: 80-90 mg/m²/day for 5 days

Dosage adjustment in renal/hepatic impairment: Data is insufficient, but dose adjustments may be necessary in patient with significant renal or hepatic impairment

Dosage adjustment in Down syndrome patients: Reduce initial dosing; administer the first course at half the usual dose. Patients with both Down syndrome and leukemia may be especially sensitive to myelosuppressive chemotherapy.

Administration Do not use in-line filter during I.V. infusion; slow I.V. infusion over ≥30 minutes

Tenoposide must be diluted with either D_5W or 0.9% sodium chloride solutions to a final concentration of 0.1, 0.2, 0.4, or 1 mg/mL. In order to prevent extraction of the plasticizer DEHP, solutions should be prepared in non-DEHP-containing containers such as glass or polyolefin containers. **The use of polyvinylchloride (PVC) containers is not recommended.**

Patient Information Hair should grow back after treatment

Nursing Implications Monitor blood pressure during infusion; observe for chemical phlebitis at injection site

Additional Information May be available only through investigational protocols

Dosage Forms Injection: 10 mg/mL (5 mL)

Ten-K® *see* Potassium Chloride *on page 1024*

Tenormin® *see* Atenolol *on page 111*

Tensilon® *see* Edrophonium *on page 439*

Tenuate® *see* Diethylpropion *on page 380*

Tenuate® Dospan® *see* Diethylpropion *on page 380*

Tepanil® *see* Diethylpropion *on page 380*

Terazol® *see* Terconazole *on page 1196*

Terazosin (ter AY zoe sin)

Brand Names Hytrin®

Therapeutic Category Alpha-Adrenergic Blocking Agent, Oral; Antihypertensive

Use Management of mild to moderate hypertension; used alone or in combination with other agents such as diuretics or beta-blockers; benign prostate hypertrophy

Pregnancy Risk Factor C

Contraindications Hypersensitivity to terazosin, other alpha-adrenergic antagonists, or any component

Warnings/Precautions Marked orthostatic hypotension, syncope, and loss of consciousness may occur with first dose ("first dose phenomenon"). This reaction is more likely to occur in patients receiving beta-blockers, diuretics, low sodium diets, or first doses >1 mg/dose in adults; avoid rapid increase in dose; use with caution in patients with renal impairment.

Adverse Reactions

>10%:
- Cardiovascular: Orthostatic hypotension
- Central nervous system: Dizziness, lightheadedness, drowsiness, headache, malaise

1% to 10%:
- Cardiovascular: Edema, palpitations
- Central nervous system: Fatigue, nervousness
- Gastrointestinal: Xerostomia
- Genitourinary: Urinary incontinence

<1%:
- Cardiovascular: Angina
- Central nervous system: Nightmares, hypothermia
- Dermatologic: Rash
- Endocrine & metabolic: Sexual dysfunction
- Gastrointestinal: Nausea
- Genitourinary: Priapism, polyuria
- Respiratory: Dyspnea, nasal congestion

Overdosage/Toxicology Symptoms of overdose include hypotension, drowsiness, shock

Hypotension usually responds to I.V. fluids or Trendelenburg positioning; if unresponsive to these measures, the use of a parenteral vasoconstrictor may be required; treatment is primarily supportive and symptomatic

Drug Interactions

Decreased antihypertensive response with NSAIDs

Increased hypotensive effect with diuretics and antihypertensive medications (especially beta-blockers)

Mechanism of Action $Alpha_1$-specific blocking agent with minimal $alpha_2$ effects; this allows peripheral postsynaptic blockade, with the resultant decrease in arterial tone, while preserving the negative feedback loop which is mediated by the peripheral presynaptic $alpha_2$-receptors; terazosin relaxes the smooth muscle of the bladder neck, thus reducing bladder outlet obstruction

Pharmacodynamics/Kinetics

Absorption: Oral: Rapid

Protein binding: 90% to 95%

(Continued)

Terazosin *(Continued)*

Metabolism: Extensively in the liver

Half-life: 9.2-12 hours

Time to peak serum concentration: Within 1 hour

Elimination: Principally in feces (60%) and in urine (40%)

Usual Dosage Adults: Oral:

Hypertension: Initial: 1 mg at bedtime; slowly increase dose to achieve desired blood pressure, up to 20 mg/day; usual dose: 1-5 mg/day

Dosage reduction may be needed when adding a diuretic or other antihypertensive agent; if drug is discontinued for greater than several days, consider beginning with initial dose and retitrate as needed; dosage may be given on a twice daily regimen if response is diminished at 24 hours and hypotensive is observed at 2-4 hours following a dose

Benign prostatic hypertrophy: Initial: 1 mg at bedtime, increasing as needed; most patients require 10 mg day; if no response after 4-6 weeks of 10 mg/day, may increase to 20 mg/day

Monitoring Parameters Standing and sitting/supine blood pressure, especially following the initial dose at 2-4 hours following the dose and thereafter at the trough point to ensure adequate control throughout the dosing interval; urinary symptoms

Patient Information Report any gain of body weight or painful, persistent erection; fainting sometimes occurs after the first dose; rise slowly from prolonged sitting or standing

Dosage Forms

Capsule: 1 mg, 2 mg, 5 mg, 10 mg

Tablet: 1 mg, 2 mg, 5 mg, 10 mg

Terbinafine, Topical (TER bin a feen, TOP i kal)

Brand Names Lamisil®

Therapeutic Category Antifungal Agent, Topical

Use Topical antifungal for the treatment of tinea pedis (athlete's foot), tinea cruris (jock itch), and tinea corporis (ring worm)

Unlabeled use: Cutaneous candidiasis and pityriasis versicolor

Pregnancy Risk Factor B

Contraindications Hypersensitivity to terbinafine or any component

Warnings/Precautions For external use only

Adverse Reactions

1% to 10%:

Dermatologic: Pruritus, contact dermatitis

Local: Irritation, stinging

Stability Store at 5°C to 30°C/41°F to 86°F

Mechanism of Action Synthetic alkylamine derivative which inhibits squalene epoxidases which is a key enzyme in sterol biosynthesis in fungi to result in a deficiency in ergosterol within fungal cell wall and result in fungal cell death

Pharmacodynamics/Kinetics

Absorption: Topical: Limited

Elimination: ~75% of cutaneously absorbed drug excreted in urine; 3.5% of administered dose recovered in urine and feces

Usual Dosage Adults: Topical:

Athlete's foot: Apply to affected area twice daily for at least 1 week, not to exceed 4 weeks

Ringworm and jock itch: Apply to affected area once or twice daily for at least 1 week, not to exceed 4 weeks

Patient Information For external use only; not for oral, ophthalmic, or intravaginal use; if irritation or sensitivity occurs, discontinue use and notify physician

Dosage Forms Cream: 1% (15 g, 30 g)

Terbutaline (ter BYOO ta leen)

Brand Names Brethaire®; Brethine®; Bricanyl®

Synonyms Terbutaline Sulfate

Therapeutic Category Beta$_2$-Adrenergic Agonist Agent; Bronchodilator; Sympathomimetic; Tocolytic Agent

Use Bronchodilator in reversible airway obstruction and bronchial asthma

Pregnancy Risk Factor B

Contraindications Hypersensitivity to terbutaline or any component, cardiac arrhythmias associated with tachycardia, tachycardia caused by digitalis intoxication

Warnings/Precautions Excessive or prolonged use may lead to tolerance; paradoxical bronchoconstriction may occur with excessive use; if it occurs, discontinue terbutaline immediately

Adverse Reactions

>10%:

Central nervous system: Nervousness, restlessness

Neuromuscular & skeletal: Trembling

1% to 10%:

Cardiovascular: Tachycardia, hypertension

Central nervous system: Dizziness, drowsiness, headache, insomnia

Gastrointestinal: Xerostomia, nausea, vomiting, bad taste in mouth

Neuromuscular & skeletal: Muscle cramps, weakness

Miscellaneous: Diaphoresis

<1%:

Cardiovascular: Chest pain, arrhythmias

Respiratory: Paradoxical bronchospasm

Overdosage/Toxicology Symptoms of overdose include seizures, nausea, vomiting, tachycardia, cardiac dysrhythmias, hypokalemia

In cases of overdose, supportive therapy should be instituted; prudent use of a cardioselective beta-adrenergic blocker (eg, atenolol or metoprolol) should be considered, keeping in mind the potential for induction of bronchoconstriction in an asthmatic individual. Dialysis has not been shown to be of value in the treatment of an overdose with this agent.

Drug Interactions

Decreased effect with beta-blockers

Increased toxicity with MAO inhibitors, TCAs

Stability Store injection at room temperature; protect from heat, light, and from freezing; use only clear solutions

Mechanism of Action Relaxes bronchial smooth muscle by action on $beta_2$-receptors with less effect on heart rate

Pharmacodynamics/Kinetics

Onset of action:

Oral: 30-45 minutes

S.C.: Within 6-15 minutes

Protein binding: 25%

Metabolism: In the liver to inactive sulfate conjugates

Bioavailability: S.C. doses are more bioavailable than oral

Half-life: 11-16 hours

Elimination: In urine

Usual Dosage

Children <12 years:

Oral: Initial: 0.05 mg/kg/dose 3 times/day, increased gradually as required; maximum: 0.15 mg/kg/dose 3-4 times/day or a total of 5 mg/24 hours

S.C.: 0.005-0.01 mg/kg/dose to a maximum of 0.3 mg/dose every 15-20 minutes for 3 doses

Nebulization: 0.1-0.3 mg/kg/dose up to a maximum of 10 mg/dose every 4-6 hours

Inhalation: 1-2 inhalations every 4-6 hours

Children >12 years and Adults:

Oral:

12-15 years: 2.5 mg every 6 hours 3 times/day; not to exceed 7.5 mg in 24 hours

>15 years: 5 mg/dose every 6 hours 3 times/day; if side effects occur, reduce dose to 2.5 mg every 6 hours; not to exceed 15 mg in 24 hours

S.C.: 0.25 mg/dose repeated in 15-30 minutes for one time only; a total dose of 0.5 mg should not be exceeded within a 4-hour period

Nebulization: 0.01-0.03 mg/kg/dose every 4-6 hours

Inhalation: 2 inhalations every 4-6 hours; wait 1 minute between inhalations

Dosing adjustment/comments in renal impairment:

Cl_{cr} 10-50 mL/minute: Administer at 50% of normal dose

Cl_{cr} <10 mL/minute: Avoid use

Administration Injection with S.C. use; in oral administration administer around-the-clock to promote less variation in peak and trough serum levels

Monitoring Parameters Serum potassium, heart rate, blood pressure, respiratory rate

Patient Information Precede administration of aerosol adrenocorticoid by 15 minutes; report any decreased effectiveness of drug; do not exceed recommended dose or frequency; may take last dose at 6 PM to avoid insomnia

Dosage Forms

Aerosol, oral, as sulfate: 0.2 mg/actuation (10.5 g)

Injection, as sulfate: 1 mg/mL (1 mL)

Tablet, as sulfate: 2.5 mg, 5 mg

Extemporaneous Preparations A 1 mg/mL suspension made from terbutaline tablets in simple syrup NF is stable 30 days when refrigerated

(Continued)

Terbutaline *(Continued)*

Horner RK and Johnson CE, "Stability of An Extemporaneously Compounded Terbutaline Sulfate Oral Liquid," *Am J Hosp Pharm*, 1991, 48(2):293-5.

Terbutaline Sulfate *see* Terbutaline *on page 1194*

Terconazole (ter KONE a zole)

Related Information

Treatment of Sexually Transmitted Diseases *on page 1485*

Brand Names Terazol®

Canadian/Mexican Brand Names Fungistat® (Mexico); Fungistat® Dual (Mexico)

Synonyms Triaconazole

Therapeutic Category Antifungal Agent, Vaginal

Use Local treatment of vulvovaginal candidiasis

Pregnancy Risk Factor C

Contraindications Known hypersensitivity to terconazole or components of the vaginal cream or suppository

Warnings/Precautions Should be discontinued if sensitization or irritation occurs. Microbiological studies (KOH smear and/or cultures) should be repeated in patients not responding to terconazole in order to confirm the diagnosis and rule out other other pathogens.

Adverse Reactions 1% to 10%: Genitourinary: Vulvar/vaginal burning

Stability Room temperature (13°C to 30°C/59°F to 86°F)

Mechanism of Action Triazole ketal antifungal agent; involves inhibition of fungal cytochrome P-450. Specifically, terconazole inhibits cytochrome P-450-dependent 14-alpha-demethylase which results in accumulation of membrane disturbing 14-alpha-demethylsterols and ergosterol depletion.

Pharmacodynamics/Kinetics Absorption: Extent of systemic absorption after vaginal administration may be dependent on the presence of a uterus; 5% to 8% in women who had a hysterectomy versus 12% to 16% in nonhysterectomy women

Usual Dosage Adults: Female: Insert 1 applicatorful intravaginally at bedtime for 7 consecutive days

Patient Information Insert high into vagina; complete full course of therapy; contact physician if itching or burning occurs

Nursing Implications Watch for local irritation; assist patient in administration, if necessary; assess patient's ability to self-administer, may be difficult in patients with arthritis or limited range of motion

Dosage Forms

Cream, vaginal: 0.4% (45 g); 0.8% (20 g)
Suppository, vaginal: 80 mg (3s)

Terfenadine (ter FEN a deen)

Brand Names Seldane®

Canadian/Mexican Brand Names Apo-Terfenadine® (Canada); Novo-Terfenadine® (Canada); Keneter® (Mexico); Teldane® (Mexico)

Therapeutic Category Antihistamine, H_1 Blocker; Antihistamine, H_1 Blocker, Nonsedating

Use Perennial and seasonal allergic rhinitis and other allergic symptoms including urticaria; has drying effect in patients with asthma

Pregnancy Risk Factor C

Contraindications Hypersensitivity to terfenadine or any component; concomitant use of erythromycin, quinine, ketoconazole, or itraconazole; significant hepatic dysfunction; concomitant use of troleandomycin and clarithromycin

Warnings/Precautions Safety and efficacy in children <12 years of age have not been established; use with caution in patients with a history of cardiac conduction disturbances or cardiac arrhythmias, or those receiving antiarrhythmic medication; do not administer with erythromycin, quinine, ketoconazole, or itraconazole; avoid use in patients with significant hepatic dysfunction; discontinue therapy immediately with signs of cardiotoxicity including syncope

Adverse Reactions

1% to 10%:

- Central nervous system: Headache, fatigue, nervousness, dizziness
- Gastrointestinal: Appetite increase, weight gain, nausea, diarrhea, abdominal pain, xerostomia
- Neuromuscular & skeletal: Arthralgia
- Respiratory: Pharyngitis

<1%:

- Cardiovascular: Edema, palpitations, hypotension, torsade de pointes
- Central nervous system: Depression, slight drowsiness, sedation, paradoxical excitement, insomnia

Dermatologic: Angioedema, photosensitivity, rash
Genitourinary: Urinary retention
Hepatic: Hepatitis
Neuromuscular & skeletal: Myalgia, paresthesia, tremor
Ocular: Blurred vision
Respiratory: Bronchospasm, thickening of bronchial secretions, epistaxis

Overdosage/Toxicology Symptoms of overdose include nausea, confusion, sedation, prolonged Q-T interval, torsade de pointes

Lidocaine has been used successfully to treat cardiac arrhythmias; avoid type I antiarrhythmics, torsade may respond to I.V. magnesium

Drug Interactions Serious cardiac events have occurred with elevated terfenadine levels

Increased effect with pseudoephedrine

Increased toxicity with ketoconazole, itraconazole, fluconazole, metronidazole, miconazole, erythromycin, troleandomycin, quinine, azithromycin, clarithromycin, cimetidine, bepridil, psychotropics, probucol, astemizole, carbamazepine

Stability Keep away from direct sunlight

Mechanism of Action Competes with histamine for H_1-receptor sites on effector cells in the gastrointestinal tract, blood vessels, and respiratory tract; binds to lung receptors significantly greater than it binds to cerebellar receptors, resulting in a reduced sedative potential

Pharmacodynamics/Kinetics

Duration of antihistaminic effect: Up to 12 hours
Metabolism: Extensive first-pass metabolism; metabolized in the liver
Half-life: 16-22 hours
Time to peak serum concentration: Within 1-2 hours
Elimination: Primarily in feces and secondarily in urine

Usual Dosage Oral:

Children:
3-6 years: 15 mg twice daily
6-12 years: 30 mg twice daily
Children >12 years and Adults: 60 mg twice daily

Monitoring Parameters Relief of symptoms

Test Interactions Antigen skin testing procedures

Patient Information Drink plenty of water; may cause dry mouth, sedation, drowsiness, can impair judgment and coordination

Nursing Implications Patient on medications that prolong the Q-T interval should be on a cardiac monitor when starting this drug

Dosage Forms Tablet: 60 mg

Terramycin® IV *see* Oxytetracycline *on page 943*
Tesamone® Injection *see* Testosterone *on next page*
Teslac® *see* Testolactone *on this page*
TESPA *see* Thiotepa *on page 1220*
Tessalon® Perles *see* Benzonatate *on page 140*
Testoderm® Transdermal System *see* Testosterone *on next page*

Testolactone (tes toe LAK tone)

Brand Names Teslac®

Therapeutic Category Antineoplastic Agent, Androgen

Use Palliative treatment of advanced disseminated breast carcinoma

Restrictions C-III

Pregnancy Risk Factor C

Contraindications In men for the treatment of breast cancer; known hypersensitivity to testolactone

Warnings/Precautions The U.S. Food and Drug Administration (FDA) currently recommends that procedures for proper handling and disposal of antineoplastic agents be considered. Use with caution in hepatic, renal, or cardiac disease; prolonged use may cause drug-induced hepatic disease; history or porphyria.

Adverse Reactions

1% to 10%:
Cardiovascular: Edema
Dermatologic: Maculopapular rash
Endocrine & metabolic: Hypercalcemia,
Gastrointestinal: Anorexia, diarrhea, nausea, edema of the tongue
Neuromuscular & skeletal: Paresthesias, peripheral neuropathies

Overdosage/Toxicology Increased toxicity: Increased effects of oral anticoagulants

Mechanism of Action Testolactone is a synthetic testosterone derivative without significant androgen activity. The drug inhibits steroid aromatase activity, thereby blocking the production of estradiol and estrone from androgen precursors such

(Continued)

Testolactone *(Continued)*

as testosterone and androstenedione. Unfortunately, the enzymatic block provided by testolactone is transient and is usually limited to a period of 3 months.

Pharmacodynamics/Kinetics

Absorption: Oral: Absorbed well
Metabolism: In the liver
Elimination: In urine

Usual Dosage Adults: Female: Oral: 250 mg 4 times/day for at least 3 months; desired response may take as long as 3 months

Monitoring Parameters Plasma calcium levels

Test Interactions Plasma estradiol concentrations by RIA

Patient Information Passive exercises should be maintained throughout therapy to keep patient mobile; notify physician if numbness of fingers, toes, or face occurs

Dosage Forms Tablet: 50 mg

Testopel® Pellet *see* Testosterone *on this page*

Testosterone (tes TOS ter one)

Brand Names Androderm® Transdermal System; Andro-L.A.® Injection; Andropository® Injection; Delatest® Injection; Delatestryl® Injection; depAndro® Injection; Depotest® Injection; Depo®-Testosterone Injection; Duratest® Injection; Durathate® Injection; Everone® Injection; Histerone® Injection; Tesamone® Injection; Testoderm® Transdermal System; Testopel® Pellet

Synonyms Aqueous Testosterone; Testosterone Cypionate; Testosterone Enanthate; Testosterone Propionate

Therapeutic Category Androgen

Use Androgen replacement therapy in the treatment of delayed male puberty; postpartum breast pain and engorgement; inoperable breast cancer; male hypogonadism

Restrictions C-III

Pregnancy Risk Factor X

Contraindications Severe renal or cardiac disease, benign prostatic hypertrophy with obstruction, undiagnosed genital bleeding, males with carcinoma of the breast or prostate; hypersensitivity to testosterone or any component

Warnings/Precautions Perform radiographic examination of the hand and wrist every 6 months to determine the rate of bone maturation; may accelerate bone maturation without producing compensating gain in linear growth; has both androgenic and anabolic activity, the anabolic action may enhance hypoglycemia

Adverse Reactions

>10%:
- Dermatologic: Acne
- Endocrine & metabolic: Menstrual problems (amenorrhea), virilism, breast soreness
- Genitourinary: Epididymitis, priapism, bladder irritability

1% to 10%:
- Cardiovascular: Flushing, edema
- Central nervous system: Excitation, aggressive behavior, sleeplessness, anxiety, mental depression, headache
- Dermatologic: Hirsutism (increase in pubic hair growth)
- Gastrointestinal: Nausea, vomiting, GI irritation
- Genitourinary: Prostatic hypertrophy, prostatic carcinoma, impotence, testicular atrophy
- Hepatic: Hepatic dysfunction

<1%:
- Endocrine & metabolic: Gynecomastia, hypercalcemia, hypoglycemia
- Hematologic: Leukopenia, suppression of clotting factors, polycythemia
- Hepatic: Cholestatic hepatitis, hepatic necrosis
- Miscellaneous: Hypersensitivity reactions

Drug Interactions Cytochrome P-450 3A enzyme substrate

Increased toxicity: Effects of oral anticoagulants may be enhanced

Mechanism of Action Principal endogenous androgen responsible for promoting the growth and development of the male sex organs and maintaining secondary sex characteristics in androgen-deficient males

Pharmacodynamics/Kinetics

Duration of effect: Based upon the route of administration and which testosterone ester is used; the cypionate and enanthate esters have the longest duration, up to 2-4 weeks after I.M. administration
Distribution: Crosses the placenta; appears in breast milk
Protein binding: 98% (to transcortin and albumin)
Metabolism: In the liver

Half-life: 10-100 minutes
Elimination: In urine (90%) and feces via bile (6%)

Usual Dosage

Delayed puberty: Males: Children: I.M.: 40-50 mg/m²/dose (cypionate or enanthate) monthly for 6 months
Male hypogonadism: I.M.: 50-400 mg every 2-4 weeks
Initiation of pubertal growth: 40-50 mg/m²/dose (cypionate or enanthate) monthly until the growth rate falls to prepubertal levels (~5 cm/year)
During terminal growth phase: 100 mg/m²/dose (cypionate or enanthate) monthly until growth ceases
Maintenance virilizing dose: 100 mg/m²/dose (cypionate or enanthate) twice monthly or 50-400 mg/dose every 2-4 weeks
Inoperable breast cancer: Adults: I.M.: 200-400 mg every 2-4 weeks
Hypogonadism: Males: Adults:
I.M.:
Testosterone or testosterone propionate: 10-25 mg 2-3 times/week
Testosterone cypionate or enanthate: 50-400 mg every 2-4 weeks
Postpubertal cryptorchism: Testosterone or testosterone propionate: 10-25 mg 2-3 times/week
Topical: Initial: 6 mg/day system applied daily applied on scrotal skin. If scrotal area is inadequate, start with a 4 mg/day system. Transdermal system should be worn for 22-24 hours. Determine total serum testosterone after 3-4 weeks of daily application. If patients have not achieved desired results after 6-8 weeks of therapy, another form of testosterone replacement therapy should be considered.

Dosing adjustment/comments in hepatic disease: Reduce dose

Monitoring Parameters Periodic liver function tests, radiologic examination of wrist and hand every 6 months (when using in prepubertal children)

Reference Range Testosterone, urine: Male: 100-1500 ng/24 hours; Female: 100-500 ng/24 hours

Test Interactions May cause a decrease in creatinine and creatine excretion and an increase in the excretion of 17-ketosteroids, thyroid function tests

Patient Information Virilization may occur in female patients; report menstrual irregularities; male patients report persistent penile erections; all patients should report persistent GI distress, diarrhea, or jaundice

Nursing Implications Warm injection to room temperature and shaking vial will help redissolve crystals that have formed after storage; administer by deep I.M. injection into the upper outer quadrant of the gluteus maximus. Transdermal system should be applied on clean, dry, scrotal skin. Dry-shave scrotal hair for optimal skin contact. Do not use chemical depilatories.

Additional Information

Testosterone (aqueous): Andro®, Histerone®, Tesanone®
Testosterone cypionate: Andro-Cyp®, Andronate®, Depotest®, Depo®-Testosterone, Duratest®
Testosterone enanthate: Andro-L.A.®, Andropository®, Delatestryl®, Durathate®, Everone®, Testrin® P.A.
Testosterone propionate: Testex®

Dosage Forms

Injection:
Aqueous suspension: 25 mg/mL (10 mL, 30 mL); 50 mg/mL (10 mL, 30 mL); 100 mg/mL (10 mL, 30 mL)
In oil, as cypionate: 100 mg/mL (1 mL, 10 mL); 200 mg/mL (1 mL, 10 mL)
In oil, as enanthate: 100 mg/mL (5 mL, 10 mL); 200 mg/mL (5 mL, 10 mL)
In oil, as propionate: 50 mg/mL (10 mL, 30 mL); 100 mg/mL (10 mL, 30 mL)
Pellet: 75 mg (1 pellet per vial)
Transdermal system: 2.5 mg/day; 4 mg/day; 6 mg/day

Testosterone Cypionate *see* Testosterone *on previous page*
Testosterone Enanthate *see* Testosterone *on previous page*
Testosterone Propionate *see* Testosterone *on previous page*
Testred® *see* Methyltestosterone *on page 821*
Tetanus and Diphtheria Toxoid *see* Diphtheria and Tetanus Toxoid *on page 402*

Tetanus Antitoxin (TET a nus an tee TOKS in)

Synonyms TAT

Therapeutic Category Antitoxin

Use Tetanus prophylaxis or treatment of active tetanus only when tetanus immune globulin (TIG) is not available; tetanus immune globulin (Hyper-Tet®) is the preferred tetanus immunoglobulin for the treatment of active tetanus; may be given concomitantly with tetanus toxoid adsorbed when immediate treatment is required, but active immunization is desirable

Pregnancy Risk Factor D

(Continued)

Tetanus Antitoxin *(Continued)*

Contraindications Patients sensitive to equine-derived preparations

Warnings/Precautions Tetanus antitoxin is not the same as tetanus immune globulin; sensitivity testing should be conducted in all individuals regardless of clinical history; have epinephrine 1:1000 available

Adverse Reactions

Dermatologic: Skin eruptions, erythema, urticaria, local pain

Neuromuscular & skeletal: Numbness, arthralgia

Miscellaneous: Serum sickness may develop up to several weeks after injection in 10% of patients, anaphylaxis

Stability Refrigerate, do not freeze

Mechanism of Action Provides passive immunization; solution of concentrated globulins containing antitoxic antibodies obtained from horse serum after immunization against tetanus toxin

Usual Dosage

Prophylaxis: I.M., S.C.:

- Children <30 kg: 1500 units
- Children and Adults ≥30 kg: 3000-5000 units

Treatment: Children and Adults: Inject 10,000-40,000 units into wound; administer 40,000-100,000 units I.V.

Nursing Implications All patients should have sensitivity testing prior to starting therapy with tetanus antitoxin

Dosage Forms Injection, equine: Not less than 400 units/mL (12.5 mL, 50 mL)

Tetanus Immune Globulin (Human)

(TET a nus i MYUN GLOB yoo lin HYU man)

Related Information

Adverse Events and Vaccination *on page 1439*

Immunization Guidelines *on page 1421*

Brand Names Hyper-Tet®

Synonyms TIG

Therapeutic Category Immune Globulin

Use Passive immunization against tetanus; tetanus immune globulin is preferred over tetanus antitoxin for treatment of active tetanus; part of the management of an unclean, wound in a person whose history of previous receipt of tetanus toxoid is unknown or who has received less than three doses of tetanus toxoid; elderly may require TIG more often than younger patients with tetanus infection due to declining antibody titers with age

Pregnancy Risk Factor C

Contraindications Hypersensitivity to tetanus immune globulin, thimerosal, or any immune globulin product or component; patients with IgA deficiency; I.V. administration

Warnings/Precautions Have epinephrine 1:1000 available for anaphylactic reactions; do not administer I.V.

Adverse Reactions

>10%: Local: Pain, tenderness, erythema at injection site

1% to 10%:

- Central nervous system: Fever (mild)
- Dermatologic: Urticaria, angioedema
- Neuromuscular & skeletal: Muscle stiffness
- Miscellaneous: Anaphylaxis reaction

<1%: Sensitization to repeated injections

Drug Interactions Never administer tetanus toxoid and TIG in same syringe (toxoid will be neutralized); toxoid may be given at a separate site; concomitant administration with Td may decrease its immune response, especially in individuals with low prevaccination antibody titers (n=119)

Stability Refrigerate at 2°C to 8°C (36°F to 46°F)

Mechanism of Action Passive immunity toward tetanus

Pharmacodynamics/Kinetics Absorption: Well absorbed

Usual Dosage I.M.:

Prophylaxis of tetanus:

- Children: 4 units/kg; some recommend administering 250 units to small children
- Adults: 250 units

Treatment of tetanus:

- Children: 500-3000 units; some should infiltrate locally around the wound
- Adults: 3000-6000 units

Administration Do not administer I.V.; I.M. use only

Additional Information Tetanus immune globulin (TIG) must not contain <50 units/mL. Protein makes up 10% to 18% of TIG preparations. The great majority of this (≥90%) is IgG. TIG has almost no color or odor and it is a sterile, nonpyrogenic, concentrated preparation of immunoglobulins that has been derived from the plasma of adults hyperimmunized with tetanus toxoid. The pooled material from which the immunoglobulin is derived may be from fewer than 1000 donors. This plasma has been shown to be free of hepatitis B surface antigen.

Dosage Forms Injection: 250 units/mL

Tetanus Toxoid, Adsorbed (TET a nus TOKS oyd, ad SORBED)

Related Information

Adverse Events and Vaccination *on page 1439*
Immunization Guidelines *on page 1421*
Miscellaneous Vaccination Information *on page 1437*
Skin Tests *on page 1501*

Therapeutic Category Toxoid

Use Selective induction of active immunity against tetanus in selected patients. **Note:** Tetanus and diphtheria toxoids for adult use (Td) is the preferred immunizing agent for most adults and for children after their seventh birthday. Young children should receive trivalent DTwP or DTaP (diphtheria/tetanus/pertussis - whole cell or acellular), as part of their childhood immunization program, unless pertussis is contraindicated, then TD is warranted.

Pregnancy Risk Factor C

Contraindications Hypersensitivity to tetanus toxoid or any component (may use the fluid tetanus toxoid to immunize the rare patient who is hypersensitive to aluminum adjuvant); avoid use with chloramphenicol or if neurological signs or symptoms occurred after prior administration; poliomyelitis outbreaks require deferral of immunizations; acute respiratory infections or other active infections may dictate deferral of administration of routine primary immunizing but not emergency doses

Warnings/Precautions Not equivalent to tetanus toxoid fluid; the tetanus toxoid adsorbed is the preferred toxoid for immunization and Td, TD or DTaP/DTwP are the preferred adsorbed forms; avoid injection into a blood vessel; have epinephrine (1:1000) available; not for use in treatment of tetanus infection no for immediate prophylaxis of unimmunized individuals; immunosuppressive therapy or other immunodeficiencies may diminish antibody response, however it is recommended for routine immunization of symptomatic and asymptomatic HIV-infected patients; deferral of immunization until immunosuppressive is discontinued or administration of an additional dose >1 month after treatment is recommended; allergic reactions may occur; epinephrine 1:1000 must be available; use in pediatrics should be deferred until >1 year of age when a history of a CNS disorder is present; elderly may not mount adequate antibody titers following immunization

Adverse Reactions

>10%: Local: Induration/redness at injection site

1% to 10%:
- Central nervous system: Chills, fever
- Local: Sterile abscess at injection site
- Miscellaneous: Allergic reaction

<1%:
- Central nervous system: Fever >103°F, malaise, neurological disturbances
- Local: Blistering at injection site
- Miscellaneous: Arthus-type hypersensitivity reactions

Drug Interactions Decreased response: If primary immunization is started in individuals receiving an immunosuppressive agent or corticosteroids, serologic testing may be needed to ensure adequate antibody response; concurrent use of TIG and tetanus toxoid may delay the development of active immunity by several days

Stability Refrigerate, do not freeze

Mechanism of Action Tetanus toxoid preparations contain the toxin produced by virulent tetanus bacilli (detoxified growth products of *Clostridium tetani*). The toxin has been modified by treatment with formaldehyde so that it has lost toxicity but still retains ability to act as antigen and produce active immunity; the aluminum salt, a mineral adjuvant, delays the rate of absorption and prolongs and enhances its properties; duration ~10 years.

Pharmacodynamics/Kinetics Duration of immunization following primary immunization: ~10 years

Usual Dosage Adults: I.M.:

Primary immunization: 0.5 mL; repeat 0.5 mL at 4-8 weeks after first dose and at 6-12 months after second dose

Routine booster doses are recommended only every 5-10 years

Administration Inject intramuscularly in the area of the vastus lateralis (midthigh laterally) or deltoid

Patient Information A nodule may be palpable at the injection site for a few weeks. DT, Td and T vaccines cause few problems; they may cause mild fever or soreness, swelling, and redness where the shot was given. These problems (Continued)

Tetanus Toxoid, Adsorbed *(Continued)*

usually last 1-2 days, but this does not happen nearly as often as with DTP vaccine. Sometimes, adults who get these vaccines can have a lot of soreness and swelling where the shot was given.

Dosage Forms Injection, adsorbed:

Tetanus 5 Lf units per 0.5 mL dose (0.5 mL, 5 mL)
Tetanus 10 Lf units per 0.5 mL dose (0.5 mL, 5 mL)

Tetanus Toxoid, Fluid (TET a nus TOKS oyd FLOO id)

Related Information

Adverse Events and Vaccination *on page 1439*
Immunization Guidelines *on page 1421*
Skin Tests *on page 1501*

Synonyms Tetanus Toxoid Plain

Therapeutic Category Toxoid

Use Detection of delayed hypersensitivity and assessment of cell-mediated immunity; active immunization against tetanus in the rare adult or child who is allergic to the aluminum adjuvant (a product containing adsorbed tetanus toxoid is preferred)

Pregnancy Risk Factor C

Contraindications Hypersensitivity to tetanus toxoid or any product components

Warnings/Precautions Epinephrine 1:1000 should be readily available; skin test responsiveness may be delayed or reduced in elderly patients

Adverse Reactions Very hypersensitive persons may develop a local reaction at the injection site; urticaria, anaphylactic reactions, shock and death are possible

Drug Interactions

Increased effect: Cimetidine may augment delayed hypersensitivity responses to skin test antigens

Stability Refrigerate

Mechanism of Action Tetanus toxoid preparations contain the toxin produced by virulent tetanus bacilli (detoxified growth products of *Clostridium tetani*). The toxin has been modified by treatment with formaldehyde so that is has lost toxicity but still retains ability to act as antigen and produce active immunity.

Usual Dosage

Anergy testing: Intradermal: 0.1 mL

Primary immunization (**Note:** Td, TD, DTaP/DTwP are recommended): Adults: Inject 3 doses of 0.5 mL I.M. or S.C. at 4- to 8-week intervals; administer fourth dose 6-12 months after third dose

Booster doses: I.M., S.C.: 0.5 mL every 10 years

Administration Must not be used I.V.; for skin testing, use 0.1 mL of 1:100 v/v or 0.02 mL of 1:10 v/v solution

Dosage Forms Injection, fluid:

Tetanus 4 Lf units per 0.5 mL dose (7.5 mL)
Tetanus 5 Lf units per 0.5 mL dose (0.5 mL, 7.5 mL)

Tetanus Toxoid Plain *see* Tetanus Toxoid, Fluid *on this page*

Tetracaine (TET ra kane)

Brand Names Pontocaine®

Synonyms Amethocaine Hydrochloride; Tetracaine Hydrochloride

Therapeutic Category Local Anesthetic, Ester Type; Local Anesthetic, Injectable; Local Anesthetic, Ophthalmic; Local Anesthetic, Oral; Local Anesthetic, Topical

Use Spinal anesthesia; local anesthesia in the eye for various diagnostic and examination purposes; topically applied to nose and throat for various diagnostic procedures; **approximately 10 times more potent than procaine**

Pregnancy Risk Factor C

Contraindications Hypersensitivity to tetracaine or any component; ophthalmic secondary bacterial infection, patients with liver disease, CNS disease, meningitis (if used for epidural or spinal anesthesia), myasthenia gravis

Warnings/Precautions No pediatric dosage recommendations; ophthalmic preparations may delay wound healing; use with caution in patients with cardiac disease and hyperthyroidism

Adverse Reactions

1% to 10%: Dermatologic: Contact dermatitis, burning, stinging, angioedema

<1%:

- Dermatologic: Tenderness, urticaria
- Genitourinary: Urethritis
- Hematologic: Methemoglobinemia in infants

Overdosage/Toxicology Maximum dose is 50 mg

Treatment of overdose is primarily symptomatic and supportive. Termination of anesthesia by pneumatic tourniquet inflation should be attempted when the agent is administered by infiltration or regional injection. Seizures commonly respond to diazepam, while hypotension responds to I.V. fluids and Trendelenburg positioning. Bradyarrhythmias (when the heart rate is less than 60) can be treated with I.V., I.M. or S.C. atropine 15 mcg/kg. With the development of metabolic acidosis, I.V. sodium bicarbonate 0.5-2 mEq/kg and ventilatory assistance should be instituted.

Drug Interactions Decreased effect: Aminosalicylic acid, sulfonamides effects may be antagonized

Stability Store solution in the refrigerator

Mechanism of Action Ester local anesthetic blocks both the initiation and conduction of nerve impulses by decreasing the neuronal membrane's permeability to sodium ions, which results in inhibition of depolarization with resultant blockade of conduction

Pharmacodynamics/Kinetics

Onset of anesthetic effect:

- Ophthalmic instillation: Within 60 seconds
- Topical or spinal injection: Within 3-8 minutes after applied to mucous membranes or when saddle block administered for spinal anesthesia

Duration of action: Topical: 1.5-3 hours

Metabolism: By the liver

Elimination: Renal

Usual Dosage Maximum adult dose: 50 mg

Children: Safety and efficacy have not been established

Adults:

- Ophthalmic (not for prolonged use):
  - Ointment: Apply ½" to 1" to lower conjunctival fornix
  - Solution: Instill 1-2 drops
- Spinal anesthesia:
  - High, medium, low, and saddle blocks: 0.2% to 0.3% solution
  - Prolonged (2-3 hours): 1% solution
  - Subarachnoid injection: 5-20 mg
  - Saddle block: 2-5 mg; a 1% solution should be diluted with equal volume of CSF before administration
- Topical mucous membranes (2% solution): Apply as needed; dose should not exceed 20 mg
- Topical for skin: Ointment/cream: Apply to affected areas as needed

Patient Information Report any rashes; keep refrigerated; may cause transient burning or stinging of eyes upon instillation; do not touch or rub eye until anesthesia (if ophthalmic) has worn off

Nursing Implications Store the solutions in the refrigerator; before injection, withdraw syringe plunger to make sure injection is not into vein or artery

Dosage Forms

Cream, as hydrochloride: 1% (28 g)

Injection, as hydrochloride: 1% [10 mg/mL] (2 mL)

Injection, , as hydrochloride, with dextrose 6%: 0.2% [2 mg/mL] (2 mL); 0.3% [3 mg/mL] (5 mL)

Ointment, as hydrochloride:

- Ophthalmic: 0.5% [5 mg/mL] (3.75 g)
- Topical: 0.5% [5 mg/mL] (28 g)

Powder for injection, as hydrochloride: 20 mg

Solution, as hydrochloride:

- Ophthalmic: 0.5% [5 mg/mL] (1 mL, 2 mL, 15 mL, 59 mL)
- Topical: 2% [20 mg/mL] (30 mL, 118 mL)

Tetracaine Hydrochloride *see* Tetracaine *on previous page*

Tetraclear® [OTC] *see* Tetrahydrozoline *on page 1205*

Tetracosactide *see* Cosyntropin *on page 314*

Tetracycline (tet ra SYE kleen)

Related Information

Antimicrobial Drugs of Choice *on page 1468*

Helicobacter pylori Treatment *on page 1534*

Brand Names Achromycin®; Achromycin® V; Ala-Tet®; Nor-tet®; Panmycin®; Robitet®; Sumycin®; Teline®; Tetracyn®; Tetralan®; Topicycline®

Canadian/Mexican Brand Names Apo-Tetra® (Canada); Novo-Tetra® (Canada); Nu-Tetra® (Canada); Acromicina® (Mexico); Ambotetra® (Mexico); Quimocyclar® (Mexico); Tetra-Atlantis® (Mexico); Zorbenal-G® (Mexico)

Synonyms TCN; Tetracycline Hydrochloride

Therapeutic Category Acne Products; Antibiotic, Ophthalmic; Antibiotic, Tetracycline Derivative; Antibiotic, Topical

Use Treatment of susceptible bacterial infections of both gram-positive and gram-negative organisms; also infections due to *Mycoplasma*, *Chlamydia*, and *Rickettsia*; indicated for acne, exacerbations of chronic bronchitis, and treatment of

(Continued)

Tetracycline *(Continued)*

gonorrhea and syphilis in patients that are allergic to penicillin; used concomitantly with metronidazole, bismuth subsalicylate and an H_2-antagonist for the treatment of duodenal ulcer disease induced by *H. pylori*

Pregnancy Risk Factor D; B (topical)

Pregnancy/Breast-Feeding Implications Excreted in breast milk; avoid use if possible in lactating mothers

Contraindications Hypersensitivity to tetracycline or any component; do not administer to children ≤8 years of age

Warnings/Precautions Use of tetracyclines during tooth development may cause permanent discoloration of the teeth and enamel, hypoplasia and retardation of skeletal development and bone growth with risk being the greatest for children <4 years and those receiving high doses; use with caution in patients with renal or hepatic impairment (eg, elderly) and in pregnancy; dosage modification required in patients with renal impairment since it may increase BUN as an antianabolic agent; pseudotumor cerebri has been reported with tetracycline use (usually resolves with discontinuation); outdated drug can cause nephropathy; superinfection possible; use protective measure to avoid photosensitivity

Adverse Reactions

>10%: Discoloration of teeth and enamel hypoplasia (infants)

1% to 10%:

- Dermatologic: Photosensitivity
- Gastrointestinal: Nausea, diarrhea

<1%:

- Cardiovascular: Pericarditis
- Central nervous system: Increased intracranial pressure, bulging fontanels in infants, pseudotumor cerebri
- Dermatologic: Dermatologic effects, pruritus, pigmentation of nails, exfoliative dermatitis
- Endocrine & metabolic: Diabetes insipidus syndrome
- Gastrointestinal: Vomiting, esophagitis, anorexia, abdominal cramps, antibiotic-associated pseudomembranous colitis, staphylococcal enterocolitis
- Hepatic: Hepatotoxicity
- Local: Thrombophlebitis
- Neuromuscular & skeletal: Paresthesia
- Renal: Acute renal failure, azotemia, renal damage
- Miscellaneous: Superinfections, anaphylaxis, hypersensitivity reactions, candidal superinfection

Overdosage/Toxicology Symptoms of overdose include nausea, anorexia, diarrhea; following GI decontamination, supportive care only

Drug Interactions

Decreased effect: Dairy products, calcium, magnesium or aluminum-containing antacids, oral contraceptives, iron, zinc, sodium bicarbonate, methoxyflurane, penicillins, cimetidine may decrease tetracycline absorption

Although no clinical evidence exists, may bind with bismuth or calcium carbonate, an excipient in bismuth subsalicylate, during treatment for *H. pylori*

Increased toxicity: Methoxyflurane anesthesia when concurrent with tetracycline may cause fatal nephrotoxicity; warfarin with tetracyclines → increased anticoagulation

Stability Outdated tetracyclines have caused a Fanconi-like syndrome; protect oral dosage forms from light

Mechanism of Action Inhibits bacterial protein synthesis by binding with the 30S and possibly the 50S ribosomal subunit(s) of susceptible bacteria; may also cause alterations in the cytoplasmic membrane

Pharmacodynamics/Kinetics

Absorption: Oral: 75%

Distribution: Small amount appears in bile

- Relative diffusion of antimicrobial agents from blood into cerebrospinal fluid (CSF): Good only with inflammation (exceeds usual MICs)
- Ratio of CSF to blood level (%): Inflamed meninges: 25

Protein binding: 20% to 60%

Half-life:

- Normal renal function: 8-11 hours
- End stage renal disease: 57-108 hours

Time to peak serum concentration: Oral: Within 2-4 hours

Elimination: Primary route is the kidney, with 60% of a dose excreted as unchanged drug in the urine; concentrated by liver in bile and feces in biologically active form

Usual Dosage

Children >8 years: Oral: 25-50 mg/kg/day in divided doses every 6 hours; not to exceed 3 g/day

Children >8 years and Adults:
Ophthalmic:
Ointment: Instill every 2-12 hours
Suspension: Instill 1-2 drops 2-4 times/day or more often as needed
Topical: Apply to affected areas 1-4 times/day
Adults: Oral: 250-500 mg/dose every 6 hours

Helicobacter pylori: Clinically effective treatment regimens include triple therapy with amoxicillin or tetracycline, metronidazole, and bismuth subsalicylate; amoxicillin, metronidazole, and H_2-receptor antagonist; or double therapy with amoxicillin and omeprazole. Adult dose: 850 mg 3 times/day to 500 mg 4 times/day

Dosing interval in renal impairment:
Cl_{cr} 50-80 mL/minute: Administer every 8-12 hours
Cl_{cr} 10-50 mL/minute: Administer every 12-24 hours
Cl_{cr} <10 mL/minute: Administer every 24 hours
Dialysis: Slightly dialyzable (5% to 20%) via hemo- and peritoneal dialysis nor via continuous arterio-venous or veno-venous hemofiltration (CAVH/CAVHD); no supplemental dosage necessary

Dosing adjustment in hepatic impairment: Avoid use or maximum dose is 1 g/day

Administration Oral should be given on an empty stomach (ie, 1 hour prior to, or 2 hours after meals) to increase total absorption. Administer at least 1-2 hours prior to, or 4 hours after antacid because aluminum and magnesium cations may chelate with tetracycline and reduce its total absorption. Administer around-the-clock rather than 4 times/day to promote less variation in peak and trough serum levels.

Monitoring Parameters Renal, hepatic, and hematologic function test, temperature, WBC, cultures and sensitivity, appetite, mental status

Test Interactions False-negative urine glucose with Clinistix®

Patient Information Take 1 hour before or 2 hours after meals with adequate amounts of fluid; avoid prolonged exposure to sunlight or sunlamps; avoid taking antacids, iron, or dairy products within 2 hours of taking tetracyclines; report persistent nausea, vomiting, yellow coloring of skin or eyes, dark urine, or pale stools; ophthalmic may cause transient burning or itching; topical is for external use only and may stain skin yellow

Additional Information
Tetracycline: Achromycin® V oral suspension, Sumycin® syrup, Tetralan® syrup
Tetracycline hydrochloride: Achromycin® injection, Achromycin® V capsule, Nortet® capsule, Panmycin® capsule, Robitet® capsule, Sumycin® capsule and tablet, Teline® capsule, Tetracyn® capsule, Tetralan® capsule

Dosage Forms
Capsule, as hydrochloride: 100 mg, 250 mg, 500 mg
Ointment:
Ophthalmic: 1% [10 mg/mL] (3.5 g)
Topical, as hydrochloride: 3% [30 mg/mL] (14.2 g, 30 g)
Solution, topical: 2.2 mg/mL (70 mL)
Suspension:
Ophthalmic: 1% [10 mg/mL] (0.5 mL, 1 mL, 4 mL)
Oral, as hydrochloride: 125 mg/5 mL (60 mL, 480 mL)
Tablet, as hydrochloride: 250 mg, 500 mg

Tetracycline Hydrochloride *see* Tetracycline *on page 1203*

Tetracyn® *see* Tetracycline *on page 1203*

Tetrahydroaminoacrine *see* Tacrine *on page 1185*

Tetrahydrocannabinol *see* Dronabinol *on page 432*

Tetrahydrozoline (tet ra hye DROZ a leen)

Brand Names Collyrium Fresh® [OTC]; Eye-Zine® [OTC]; Murine® Plus [OTC]; Ocu-Drop® [OTC]; Optigene® [OTC]; Soothe® [OTC]; Tetraclear® [OTC]; Tetra-Ide® [OTC]; Tyzine®; Visine® [OTC]; Visine A.C.® [OTC]

Synonyms Tetrahydrozoline Hydrochloride; Tetryzoline

Therapeutic Category Decongestant, Nasal; Decongestant, Ophthalmic; Nasal Agent, Vasoconstrictor; Ophthalmic Agent, Vasoconstrictor; Sympathomimetic

Use Symptomatic relief of nasal congestion and conjunctival congestion

Pregnancy Risk Factor C

Contraindications Narrow-angle glaucoma, patients receiving MAO inhibitors, known hypersensitivity to tetrahydrozoline

Warnings/Precautions Do not use in children <2 years of age; excessive use may cause rebound congestion or chemical rhinitis; use with caution in patients
(Continued)

Tetrahydrozoline *(Continued)*

with hypertension, diabetes, cardiovascular or coronary artery disease; discontinue use prior to the use of anesthetics which sensitize the myocardium to the systemic effects of sympathomimetics

Adverse Reactions

>10%:

Local: Transient stinging

Respiratory: Sneezing

1% to 10%:

Cardiovascular: Tachycardia, palpitations, increased blood pressure, increased heart rate

Central nervous system: Headache

Neuromuscular & skeletal: Tremor

Ocular: Blurred vision

Overdosage/Toxicology Symptoms of overdose include CNS depression, hypothermia, bradycardia, cardiovascular collapse, coma

Following initiation of essential overdose management, toxic symptoms should be treated. The patient should be kept warm and monitored for alterations in vital functions. Seizures commonly respond to diazepam (5-10 mg I.V. bolus in adults every 15 minutes if needed up to a total of 30 mg; I.V. 0.25-0.4 mg/kg/dose up to a total of 10 mg for children) or to phenytoin or phenobarbital; apnea will respond to naloxone.

Drug Interactions

Increased toxicity:

MAO inhibitors can cause an exaggerated adrenergic response if taken concurrently or within 21 days of discontinuing MAO inhibitor

Beta-blockers can cause hypertensive episodes and increased risk of intracranial hemorrhage

Anesthetics

Mechanism of Action Stimulates alpha-adrenergic receptors in the arterioles of the conjunctiva and the nasal mucosa to produce vasoconstriction

Pharmacodynamics/Kinetics

Onset of decongestant effect: Intranasal: Within 4-8 hours

Duration: Ophthalmic vasoconstriction: 2-3 hours

Absorption: Topical: Systemic absorption sometimes occurs

Usual Dosage

Nasal congestion: Intranasal:

Children 2-6 years: Instill 2-3 drops of 0.05% solution every 4-6 hours as needed, no more frequent than every 3 hours

Children >6 years and Adults: Instill 2-4 drops or 3-4 sprays of 0.1% solution every 3-4 hours as needed, no more frequent than every 3 hours

Conjunctival congestion: Ophthalmic: Adults: Instill 1-2 drops in each eye 2-4 times/day

Monitoring Parameters Blood pressure, heart rate, symptom response

Patient Information Remove contact lenses before using in eye, do not use for more than 72 hours unless directed to do so; consult physician if changes in vision or visual acuity occur; do not exceed recommended dosage

Nursing Implications Do not use for >3-4 days without direct physician supervision

Dosage Forms Solution, as hydrochloride:

Nasal: 0.05% (15 mL), 0.1% (30 mL, 473 mL)

Ophthalmic: 0.05% (15 mL)

Tetrahydrozoline Hydrochloride *see* Tetrahydrozoline *on previous page*

Tetra-Ide® [OTC] *see* Tetrahydrozoline *on previous page*

Tetralan® *see* Tetracycline *on page 1203*

Tetramune® *see* Diphtheria, Tetanus Toxoids, Whole-Cell Pertussis, and *Haemophilus Influenzae* Type b Conjugate Vaccines *on page 404*

Tetryzoline *see* Tetrahydrozoline *on previous page*

Texacort™ *see* Hydrocortisone *on page 623*

TG *see* Thioguanine *on page 1216*

6-TG *see* Thioguanine *on page 1216*

T-Gen® *see* Trimethobenzamide *on page 1265*

T-Gesic® *see* Hydrocodone and Acetaminophen *on page 620*

THA *see* Tacrine *on page 1185*

Thalitone® *see* Chlorthalidone *on page 265*

Tham® *see* Tromethamine *on page 1274*

Tham-E® *see* Tromethamine *on page 1274*

THC *see* Dronabinol *on page 432*

Theo-24® *see* Theophylline Salts *on next page*

Theobid® *see* Theophylline Salts *on this page*
Theochron® *see* Theophylline Salts *on this page*
Theoclear® L.A. *see* Theophylline Salts *on this page*
Theo-Dur® *see* Theophylline Salts *on this page*
Theodur-Sprinkle® *see* Theophylline Salts *on this page*
Theolair™ *see* Theophylline Salts *on this page*
Theon® *see* Theophylline Salts *on this page*
Theophylline *see* Theophylline Salts *on this page*

Theophylline Salts (thee OFF i lin salts)

Related Information

Asthma, Guidelines for the Diagnosis and Management of *on page 1518*

Estimated Clinical Comparability of Doses for Inhaled Corticosteroids *on page 1522*

Brand Names Aerolate®; Aerolate III®; Aerolate JR®; Aerolate SR®; Aminophyllin™; Aquaphyllin®; Asmalix®; Bronkodyl®; Choledyl®; Constant-T®; Duraphyl™; Elixophyllin®; Elixophyllin® SR; LaBID®; Phyllocontin®; Quibron®-T; Quibron®-T/SR; Respbid®; Slo-bid™; Slo-Phyllin®; Sustaire®; Theo-24®; Theobid®; Theochron®; Theoclear® L.A.; Theo-Dur®; Theodur-Sprinkle®; Theolair™; Theon®; Theospan®-SR; Theovent®; Truphylline®

Synonyms Aminophylline; Choline Theophyllinate; Ethylenediamine; Oxtriphylline; Theophylline

Therapeutic Category Bronchodilator; Theophylline Derivative

Use Bronchodilator in reversible airway obstruction due to asthma, chronic bronchitis, and emphysema; for neonatal apnea/bradycardia

Pregnancy Risk Factor C

Pregnancy/Breast-Feeding Implications

Clinical effects on the fetus: Crosses the placenta. Transient tachycardia, irritability, vomiting in newborn especially if maternal serum concentrations >20 mcg/mL. Apneic spells attributed to withdrawal in newborn exposed throughout gestation period. Available evidence suggests safe use during pregnancy.

Breast-feeding/lactation: Crosses into breast milk

Clinical effects on the infant: Irritability reported in infants. American Academy of Pediatrics considers COMPATIBLE with breast-feeding.

Contraindications Uncontrolled arrhythmias, hyperthyroidism, peptic ulcers, uncontrolled seizure disorders, hypersensitivity to xanthines or any component

Warnings/Precautions Use with caution in patients with peptic ulcer, hyperthyroidism, hypertension, tachyarrhythmias, and patients with compromised cardiac function; do not inject I.V. solution faster than 25 mg/minute; elderly, acutely ill, and patients with severe respiratory problems, pulmonary edema, or liver dysfunction are at greater risk of toxicity because of reduced drug clearance

Although there is a great intersubject variability for half-lives of methylxanthines (2-10 hours), elderly as a group have slower hepatic clearance. Therefore, use lower initial doses and monitor closely for response and adverse reactions. Additionally, elderly are at greater risk for toxicity due to concomitant disease (eg, CHF, arrhythmias), and drug use (eg, cimetidine, ciprofloxacin, etc).

Adverse Reactions See table.

Theophylline Serum Levels (mcg/mL)*	Adverse Reactions
15-25	GI upset, diarrhea, N/V, abdominal pain, nervousness, headache, insomnia, agitation, dizziness, muscle cramp, tremor
25-35	Tachycardia, occasional PVC
>35	Ventricular tachycardia, frequent PVC, seizure

*Adverse effects do not necessarily occur according to serum levels. Arrhythmia and seizure can occur without seeing the other adverse effects.

Uncommon at serum theophylline concentrations ≤20 mcg/mL

1% to 10%:

- Cardiovascular: Tachycardia
- Central nervous system: Nervousness, restlessness
- Gastrointestinal: Nausea, vomiting

<1%:

- Allergic reactions
- Central nervous system: Insomnia, irritability, seizures
- Dermatologic: Rash
- Gastrointestinal: Gastric irritation
- Neuromuscular & skeletal: Tremor

(Continued)

Theophylline Salts *(Continued)*

Overdosage/Toxicology Symptoms of overdose include tachycardia, extrasystoles, nausea, vomiting, anorexia, tonic-clonic seizures, insomnia, circulatory failure; agitation, irritability, headache

If seizures have not occurred, induce vomiting; ipecac syrup is preferred. Do not induce emesis in the presence of impaired consciousness. Repeated doses of charcoal have been shown to be effective in enhancing the total body clearance of theophylline. Do not repeat charcoal doses if an ileus is present. Charcoal hemoperfusion may be considered if the serum theophylline level exceed 40 mcg/mL, the patient is unable to tolerate repeat oral charcoal administrations, or if severe toxic symptoms are present. Clearance with hemoperfusion is better than clearance from hemodialysis. Administer a cathartic, especially if sustained release agents were used. Phenobarbital administered prophylactically may prevent seizures.

Drug Interactions Cytochrome P-450 1A2 enzyme substrate and cytochrome P-450 2E enzyme substrate (minor)

Decreased effect/increased toxicity: Changes in diet may affect the elimination of theophylline; charcoal-broiled foods may increase elimination, reducing half-life by 50%; see table for factors affecting serum levels.

Factors Reported to Affect Theophylline Serum Levels

Decreased Theophylline Level	Increased Theophylline Level
Smoking (cigarettes, marijuana)	Hepatic cirrhosis
High protein/low carbohydrate diet	Cor pulmonale
Charcoal	CHF
Phenytoin	Fever/viral illness
Phenobarbital	Propranolol
Carbamazepine	Allopurinol (>600 mg/d)
Rifampin	Erythromycin
I.V. isoproterenol	Cimetidine
Aminoglutethimide	Troleandomycin
Barbiturates	Ciprofloxacin
Hydantoins	Oral contraceptives
Ketoconazole	Beta blockers
Sulfinpyrazone	Calcium channel blockers
Isoniazide	Corticosteroids
Loop diuretics	Disulfiram
Sympathomimetics	Ephedrine
	Influenza virus vaccine
	Interferon
	Macrolides
	Mexiletine
	Quinolones
	Thiabendazole
	Thyroid hormones
	Carbamazepine
	Isoniazid
	Loop diuretics

Stability

Theophylline injection should be stored at room temperature and protected from freezing

Stability of parenteral admixture at room temperature (25°C): manufacturer expiration dating; out of overwrap stability: 30 days

Standard diluent: 400 mg theophylline/500 mL D_5W (premixed); 800 mg theophylline/1000 mL D_5W (premixed)

Aminophylline injection [content = 80% theophylline] should be stored at room temperature and protected from freezing and light

Stability of parenteral admixture at room temperature (25°C): 24 hours

Standard diluent: 250 mg aminophylline/100 mL D_5W ; 500 mg aminophylline/100 mL D_5W

Mechanism of Action Causes bronchodilatation, diuresis, CNS and cardiac stimulation, and gastric acid secretion by blocking phosphodiesterase which increases tissue concentrations of cyclic adenine monophosphate (cAMP) which in turn promotes catecholamine stimulation of lipolysis, glycogenolysis, and gluconeogenesis and induces release of epinephrine from adrenal medulla cells

Pharmacodynamics/Kinetics

Absorption: Oral: 100% of a dose is absorbed, depending upon the formulation used

Distribution: V_d: 0.45 L/kg; distributes into breast milk (approximates serum concentration); crosses the placenta

Metabolism: In the liver by demethylation and oxidation

Half-life: Highly variable and dependent upon age, liver function, cardiac function, lung disease, and smoking history

Aminophylline

Patient Group	Approximate Half-Life (h)
Neonates	
Premature	30
Normal newborn	24
Infants	
4-52 weeks	4-30
Children/Adolescents	
1-9 years	2-10 (4 avg)
9-16 years	4-16
Adults	
Nonsmoker	4-16 (8.7 avg)
Smoker	4.4
Cardiac compromised, liver failure	20-30

Dosage Form	Time to Peak	Dosing Interval
Uncoated tablet/syrup	2 h	6 h
Enteric coated tablet	5 h	12 h
Chewable tablet	1-1.5 h	6 h
Extended release	4-7 h	12 h
Intravenous	<30 min	

Elimination: In the urine; adults excrete 10% in urine as unchanged drug; neonates excrete a greater percentage of the dose unchanged in the urine (up to 50%)

Usual Dosage Use ideal body weight for obese patients

Neonates:

Apnea of prematurity: Oral, I.V.: Loading dose: 4 mg/kg (theophylline); 5 mg/kg (aminophylline)

There appears to be a delay in theophylline elimination in infants <1 year of age, especially neonates; both the initial dose and maintenance dosage should be conservative

I.V.: Initial: Maintenance infusion rates:

Neonates:

≤24 days: 0.08 mg/kg/hour theophylline

>24 days: 0.12 mg/kg/hour theophylline

Infants 6-52 weeks: 0.008 (age in weeks) + 0.21 mg/kg/hour theophylline

Approximate I.V. Theophylline Dosage for Treatment of Acute Bronchospasm

Group	Dosage for next 12 h*	Dosage after 12 h*
Infants 6 wk to 6 mo	0.5 mg/kg/h	
Children 6 mo to 1 y	0.6-0.7 mg/kg/h	
Children 1-9 y	0.95 mg/kg/h (1.2 mg/kg/h)	0.79 mg/kg/h (1 mg/kg/h)
Children 9-16 y and young adult smokers	0.79 mg/kg/h (1 mg/kg/h)	0.63 mg/kg/h (0.8 mg/kg/h)
Healthy, nonsmoking adults	0.55 mg/kg/h (0.7 mg/kg/h)	0.39 mg/kg/h (0.5 mg/kg/h)
Older patients and patients with cor pulmonale	0.47 mg/kg/h (0.6 mg/kg/h)	0.24 mg/kg/h (0.3 mg/kg/h)
Patients with congestive heart failure or liver failure	0.39 mg/kg/h (0.5 mg/kg/h)	0.08-0.16 mg/kg/h (0.1-0.2 mg/kg/h)

*Equivalent hydrous aminophylline dosageindicated in parentheses.

(Continued)

Theophylline Salts *(Continued)*

Children:

6 weeks to 6 months: 0.5 mg/kg/hour

6 months to 1 year: 0.6-0.7 mg/kg/hour

Children >1 year and Adults:

Treatment of acute bronchospasm: I.V.: Loading dose (in patients not currently receiving aminophylline or theophylline): 6 mg/kg (based on aminophylline) given I.V. over 20-30 minutes; administration rate should not exceed 25 mg/minute (aminophylline). See table.

Approximate I.V. maintenance dosages are based upon continuous infusions; bolus dosing (often used in children <6 months of age) may be determined by multiplying the hourly infusion rate by 24 hours and dividing by the desired number of doses/day; see table.

Maintenance Dose for Acute Symptoms

Population Group	Oral Theophylline (mg/kg/day)	I.V. Aminophylline
Premature infant or newborn - 6 wk (for apnea/bradycardia)	4	5 mg/kg/day
6 wk - 6 mo	10	12 mg/kg/day or continuous I.V. infusion*
Infants 6 mo-1 y	12-18	15 mg/kg/day or continuous I.V. infusion*
Children 1-9 y	20-24	1 mg/kg/hour
Children 9-12 y, and adolescent daily smokers of cigarettes or marijuana, and otherwise healthy adult smokers <50 y	16	0.9 mg/kg/hour
Adolescents 12-16 y (nonsmokers)	13	0.7 mg/kg/hour
Otherwise healthy nonsmoking adults (including elderly patients)	10 (not to exceed 900 mg/day)	0.5 mg/kg/hour
Cardiac decompensation, cor pulmonale and/or liver dysfunction	5 (not to exceed 400 mg/day)	0.25 mg/kg/hour

*For continuous I.V. infusion divide total daily dose by 24 = mg/kg/hour.

Dosage should be adjusted according to serum level measurements during the first 12- to 24-hour period; see table.

Dosage Adjustment After Serum Theophylline Measurement

Serum Theophylline		Guidelines
Within normal limits	10-20 mcg/mL	Maintain dosage if tolerated. Recheck serum theophylline concentration at 6-12 mo intervals.*
Too high	20-25 mcg/mL	Decrease doses by about 10%. Recheck serum theophylline concentration after 3 d and then at 6-12 mo intervals.*
	25-30 mcg/mL	Skip next dose and decrease subsequent doses by about 25%. Recheck serum theophylline.
	>30 mcg/mL	Skip next 2 doses and decrease subsequent doses by 50%. Recheck serum theophylline.
Too low	7.5-10 mcg/mL	Increase dose by about 25%.† Recheck serum theophylline concentration after 3 d and then at 6-12 mo intervals.*
	5-7.5 mcg/mL	Increase dose by about 25% to the nearest dose increment† and recheck serum theophylline for guidance in further dosage adjustment (another increase will probably be needed, but this provides a safety check).

From Weinberger M and Hendeles L, 'Practical Guide to Using Theophylline,' *J Resp Dis*, 1981, 2:12-27.

*Finer adjustments in dosage may be needed for some patients.

†Dividing the daily dose into 3 doses administered at 8-hour intervals may be indicated if symptoms occur repeatedly at the end of a dosing interval.

Oral theophylline: Initial dosage recommendation: Loading dose (to achieve a serum level of about 10 mcg/mL; loading doses should be given using a rapidly absorbed oral product **not** a sustained release product):

If no theophylline has been administered in the previous 24 hours: 4-6 mg/kg theophylline

If theophylline has been administered in the previous 24 hours: administer 1/2 loading dose or 2-3 mg/kg theophylline can be given in emergencies when serum levels are not available

On the average, for every 1 mg/kg theophylline given, blood levels will rise 2 mcg/mL

Ideally, defer the loading dose if a serum theophylline concentration can be obtained rapidly. However, if this is not possible, exercise clinical judgment. If the patient is not experiencing theophylline toxicity, this is unlikely to result in dangerous adverse effects.

See table.

Oral Theophylline Dosage for Bronchial Asthma*

Age	Initial 3 Days	Second 3 Days	Steady-State Maintenance
<1 y	0.2 x (age in weeks) + 5		0.3 x (age in weeks) + 8
1-9 y	16 up to a maximum of 400 mg/24 h	20	22
9-12 y	16 up to a maximum of 400 mg/24 h	16 up to a maximum of 600 mg/24 h	20 up to a maximum of 800 mg/24 h
12-16 y	16 up to a maximum of 400 mg/24 h	16 up to a maximum of 600 mg/24 h	18 up to a maximum of 900 mg/24 h
Adults	400 mg/24 h	600 mg/24 h	900 mg/24 h

*Dose in mg/kg/24 hours of theophylline.

Increasing dose: The dosage may be increased in approximately 25% increments at 2- to 3-day intervals so long as the drug is tolerated or until the maximum dose is reached

Maintenance dose: In newborns and infants, a fast-release oral product can be used. The total daily dose can be divided every 12 hours in newborns and every 6-8 hours in infants. In children and healthy adults, a slow-release product can be used. The total daily dose can be divided every 8-12 hours.

These recommendations, based on mean clearance rates for age or risk factors, were calculated to achieve a serum level of 10 mcg/mL (5 mcg/mL for newborns with apnea/bradycardia)

Dosage should be adjusted according to serum level

Oral oxtriphylline:

Children 1-9 years: 6.2 mg/kg/dose every 6 hours

Children 9-16 years and Adult smokers: 4.7 mg/kg/dose every 6 hours

Adult nonsmokers: 4.7 mg/kg/dose every 8 hours

Dose should be further adjusted based on serum levels

Dosing adjustment/comments in hepatic disease: Higher incidence of toxic effects including seizures in cirrhosis; plasma levels should be monitored closely during long-term administration in cirrhosis and during acute hepatitis, with dose adjustment as necessary

Hemodialysis: Administer dose posthemodialysis or administer supplemental 50% dose

Peritoneal dialysis: Supplemental dose is not necessary

Continuous arterio-venous or veno-venous hemodiafiltration (CAVH/CAVHD) effects: Supplemental dose is not necessary

Administration Administer oral and I.V. administration around-the-clock to promote less variation in peak and trough serum levels; theophylline injection may be administered by continuous I.V. infusion (requires an infusion pump) or IVPB; maximum rate of I.V. administration of theophylline is 20-25 mg per minute

Monitoring Parameters Heart rate, CNS effects (insomnia, irritability); respiratory rate (COPD patients often have resting controlled respiratory rates in low 20s), serum theophylline level, arterial or capillary blood gases (if applicable)

Reference Range

Sample size: 0.5-1 mL serum (red top tube)

Saliva levels are approximately equal to 60% of plasma levels

Therapeutic levels: 10-20 µg/mL

Neonatal apnea 6-13 µg/mL

Pregnancy: 3-12 µg/mL

Toxic concentration: >20 µg/mL

(Continued)

Theophylline Salts *(Continued)*

Timing of serum samples: If toxicity is suspected, draw a level any time during a continuous I.V. infusion, or 2 hours after an oral dose; if lack of therapeutic is effected, draw a trough immediately before the next oral dose; see table.

Guidelines for Drawing Theophylline Serum Levels

Dosage Form	Time to Draw Level
I.V. bolus	30 min after end of 30 min infusion
I.V. continuous infusion	12-24 h after initiation of infusion
P.O. liquid, fast-release tab	Peak: 1 h postdose after at least 1 day of therapy Trough: Just before a dose after at least one day of therapy
P.O. slow-release product	Peak: 4 h postdose after at least 1 day of therapy Trough: Just before a dose after at least one day of therapy

Test Interactions May elevate uric acid levels

Patient Information Oral preparations should be taken with a full glass of water; capsule forms may be opened and sprinkled on soft foods; do not chew beads; notify physician if nausea, vomiting, severe GI pain, restlessness, or irregular heartbeat occurs; do not drink or eat large quantities of caffeine-containing beverages or food (colas, coffee, chocolate); remain in bed for 15-20 minutes after inserting suppository; do not chew or crush enteric coated or sustained release products; take at regular intervals; notify physician if insomnia, nervousness, irritability, palpitations, seizures occur; do not change brands or doses without consulting physician

Nursing Implications Do not crush sustained release drug products; do not crush enteric coated drug product; encourage patient to drink adequate fluids (2 L/day) to decrease mucous viscosity

Additional Information See table for theophylline content.

Salt	% Theophylline Content
Theophylline anhydrous (eg, most oral solids)	100%
Theophylline monohydrate (eg, oral solutions)	91%
Aminophylline (theophylline) (eg, injection)	80% (79% to 86%)
Oxtriphylline (choline theophylline) (eg, Choledyl®)	64%

Dosage Forms

Aminophylline (79% theophylline):
- Injection: 25 mg/mL (10 mL, 20 mL); 250 mg (equivalent to 187 mg theophylline) per 10 mL; 500 mg (equivalent to 394 mg theophylline) per 20 mL
- Liquid, oral: 105 mg (equivalent to 90 mg theophylline) per 5 mL (240 mL, 500 mL)
- Suppository, rectal: 250 mg (equivalent to 198 mg theophylline); 500 mg (equivalent to 395 mg theophylline)
- Tablet: 100 mg (equivalent to 79 mg theophylline); 200 mg (equivalent to 158 mg theophylline)
- Tablet, controlled release: 225 mg (equivalent to 178 mg theophylline)

Oxtriphylline (64% theophylline):
- Elixir: 100 mg (equivalent to 64 mg theophylline)/5 mL (5 mL, 10 mL, 473 mL)
- Syrup: 50 mg (equivalent to 32 mg theophylline)/5 mL (473 mL)
- Tablet: 100 mg (equivalent to 64 mg theophylline); 200 mg (equivalent to 127 mg theophylline)
- Tablet, sustained release: 400 mg (equivalent to 254 mg theophylline); 600 mg (equivalent to 382 mg theophylline)

Theophylline:
- Capsule:
  - Immediate release: 100 mg, 200 mg
  - Sustained release (8-12 hours): 50 mg, 60 mg, 65 mg, 75 mg, 100 mg, 125 mg, 130 mg, 200 mg, 250 mg, 260 mg, 300 mg
  - Timed release (12 hours): 50 mg, 75 mg, 125 mg, 130 mg, 200 mg, 250 mg, 260 mg
  - Timed release (24 hours): 100 mg, 200 mg, 300 mg
- Injection: Theophylline in 5% dextrose: 200 mg/container (50 mL, 100 mL); 400 mg/container (100 mL, 250 mL, 500 mL, 1000 mL); 800 mg/container (250 mL, 500 mL, 1000 mL)
- Elixir, oral: 80 mg/15 mL (15 mL, 30 mL, 500 mL, 4000 mL)
- Solution, oral: 80 mg/15 mL (15 mL, 18.75 mL, 30 mL, 120 mL, 500 mL, 4000 mL); 150 mg/15 mL (480 mL)

Syrup, oral: 80 mg/15 mL (5 mL, 15 mL, 30 mL, 120 mL, 500 mL, 4000 mL); 150 mg/15 mL (480 mL)

Tablet:

Immediate release: 100 mg, 125 mg, 200 mg, 250 mg, 300 mg

Timed release (8-12 hours): 100 mg, 200 mg, 250 mg, 300 mg, 500 mg

Timed release (8-24 hours): 100 mg, 200 mg, 300 mg, 450 mg

Timed release (12-24 hours): 100 mg, 200 mg, 300 mg

Timed release (24 hours): 400 mg

Theospan®-SR *see* Theophylline Salts *on page 1207*

Theovent® *see* Theophylline Salts *on page 1207*

Therabid® [OTC] *see* Vitamins, Multiple *on page 1310*

TheraCys™ *see* BCG Vaccine *on page 132*

Thera-Flur® *see* Fluoride *on page 536*

Thera-Flur-N® *see* Fluoride *on page 536*

Theragran® [OTC] *see* Vitamins, Multiple *on page 1310*

Theragran® Hematinic® *see* Vitamins, Multiple *on page 1310*

Theragran® Liquid [OTC] *see* Vitamins, Multiple *on page 1310*

Theragran-M® [OTC] *see* Vitamins, Multiple *on page 1310*

Theralax® [OTC] *see* Bisacodyl *on page 153*

Therapeutic Multivitamins *see* Vitamins, Multiple *on page 1310*

Therapy of Hyperlipidemia *see page 1535*

Therapy of Hypertension *see page 1540*

Thermazene™ *see* Silver Sulfadiazine *on page 1136*

Theroxide® Wash [OTC] *see* Benzoyl Peroxide *on page 140*

Thiabendazole (thye a BEN da zole)

Brand Names Mintezol®

Synonyms Tiabendazole

Therapeutic Category Anthelmintic

Use Treatment of strongyloidiasis, cutaneous larva migrans, visceral larva migrans, dracunculiasis, trichinosis, and mixed helminthic infections

Pregnancy Risk Factor C

Contraindications Known hypersensitivity to thiabendazole

Warnings/Precautions Use with caution in patients with renal or hepatic impairment, malnutrition or anemia, or dehydration

Adverse Reactions

>10%:

Central nervous system: Seizures, hallucinations, delirium, dizziness, drowsiness, headache

Gastrointestinal: Anorexia, diarrhea, nausea, vomiting, drying of mucous membranes

Neuromuscular & skeletal: Numbness

Otic: Tinnitus

1% to 10%: Dermatologic: Rash, Stevens-Johnson syndrome

<1%:

Central nervous system: Chills

Genitourinary: Malodor of urine

Hematologic: Leukopenia

Hepatic: Hepatotoxicity

Ocular: Blurred or yellow vision

Renal: Nephrotoxicity

Miscellaneous: Lymphadenopathy, hypersensitivity reactions

Overdosage/Toxicology Symptoms of overdose include altered mental status, visual problems; supportive care only following GI decontamination

Drug Interactions Increased levels of theophylline and other xanthines

Mechanism of Action Inhibits helminth-specific mitochondrial fumarate reductase

Pharmacodynamics/Kinetics

Absorption: Rapid and nearly complete

Metabolism: Rapid

Time to peak serum concentration: Within 1-2 hours

Elimination: In feces (5%) and urine (87%), primarily as conjugated metabolites

Usual Dosage Purgation is not required prior to use; drinking of fruit juice aids in expulsion of worms by removing the mucous to which the intestinal tapeworms attach themselves.

Children and Adults: Oral: 50 mg/kg/day divided every 12 hours; maximum dose: 3 g/day

Strongyloidiasis: For 2 consecutive days

Cutaneous larva migrans: For 2-5 consecutive days

Visceral larva migrans: For 5-7 consecutive days

(Continued)

Thiabendazole *(Continued)*

Trichinosis: For 2-4 consecutive days
Dracunculosis: 50-75 mg/kg/day divided every 12 hours for 3 days

Dosing comments in renal/hepatic impairment: Use with caution

Test Interactions ↑ glucose

Patient Information Take after meals, chew chewable tablet well; may decrease alertness, avoid driving or operating machinery; drinking of fruit juice aids in expulsion of worms by removing the mucous to which the intestinal tapeworms attach themselves

Nursing Implications Purgation is not required prior to use; pinworm infections are easily transmitted, all close family members should be treated

Dosage Forms
Suspension, oral: 500 mg/5 mL (120 mL)
Tablet, chewable (orange flavor): 500 mg

Thiamazole *see* Methimazole *on page 804*

Thiamilate® *see* Thiamine *on this page*

Thiamine (THYE a min)

Brand Names Thiamilate®

Canadian/Mexican Brand Names Betaxin® (Canada); Bewon® (Canada)

Synonyms Aneurine Hydrochloride; Thiamine Hydrochloride; Thiaminium Chloride Hydrochloride; Vitamin B_1

Therapeutic Category Vitamin, Water Soluble

Use Treatment of thiamine deficiency including beriberi, Wernicke's encephalopathy syndrome, and peripheral neuritis associated with pellagra, alcoholic patients with altered sensorium; various genetic metabolic disorders

Pregnancy Risk Factor A (C if dose exceeds RDA recommendation)

Contraindications Hypersensitivity to thiamine or any component

Warnings/Precautions Use with caution with parenteral route (especially I.V.) of administration

Adverse Reactions
<1%:
Cardiovascular: Cardiovascular collapse and death
Central nervous system: Warmth
Dermatologic: Rash, angioedema
Neuromuscular & skeletal: Paresthesia

Stability Protect oral dosage forms from light; **incompatible** with alkaline or neutral solutions and with oxidizing or reducing agents

Mechanism of Action An essential coenzyme in carbohydrate metabolism by combining with adenosine triphosphate to form thiamine pyrophosphate

Pharmacodynamics/Kinetics
Absorption:
Oral: Adequate
I.M.: Rapid and complete
Elimination: Renally as unchanged drug, and as pyrimidine after body storage sites become saturated

Usual Dosage
Recommended daily allowance:
<6 months: 0.3 mg
6 months to 1 year: 0.4 mg
1-3 years: 0.7 mg
4-6 years: 0.9 mg
7-10 years: 1 mg
11-14 years: 1.1-1.3 mg
>14 years: 1-1.5 mg
Thiamine deficiency (beriberi):
Children: 10-25 mg/dose I.M. or I.V. daily (if critically ill), or 10-50 mg/dose orally every day for 2 weeks, then 5-10 mg/dose orally daily for 1 month
Adults: 5-30 mg/dose I.M. or I.V. 3 times/day (if critically ill); then orally 5-30 mg/day in single or divided doses 3 times/day for 1 month
Wernicke's encephalopathy: Adults: Initial: 100 mg I.V., then 50-100 mg/day I.M. or I.V. until consuming a regular, balanced diet
Dietary supplement (depends on caloric or carbohydrate content of the diet):
Infants: 0.3-0.5 mg/day
Children: 0.5-1 mg/day
Adults: 1-2 mg/day
Note: The above doses can be found in multivitamin preparations
Metabolic disorders: Oral: Adults: 10-20 mg/day (dosages up to 4 g/day in divided doses have been used)

Administration Parenteral form may be administered by I.M. or slow I.V. injection

Reference Range Therapeutic: 1.6-4 mg/dL

Test Interactions False-positive for uric acid using the phosphotungstate method and for urobilinogen using the Ehrlich's reagent; large doses may interfere with the spectrophotometric determination of serum theophylline concentration

Patient Information Dietary sources include legumes, pork, beef, whole grains, yeast, fresh vegetables; a deficiency state can occur in as little 3 weeks following total dietary absence

Nursing Implications Single vitamin deficiency is rare; look for other deficiencies

Additional Information Dietary sources include legumes, pork, beef, whole grains, yeast, fresh vegetables; a deficiency state can occur in as little as 3 weeks following total dietary absence

Dosage Forms

Injection, as hydrochloride: 100 mg/mL (1 mL, 2 mL, 10 mL, 30 mL); 200 mg/mL (30 mL)

Tablet, as hydrochloride: 50 mg, 100 mg, 250 mg, 500 mg

Tablet, as hydrochloride, enteric coated: 20 mg

Thiamine Hydrochloride *see* Thiamine *on previous page*

Thiaminium Chloride Hydrochloride *see* Thiamine *on previous page*

Thiethylperazine (thye eth il PER a zeen)

Brand Names Norzine®; Torecan®

Synonyms Thiethylperazine Maleate

Therapeutic Category Antiemetic; Phenothiazine Derivative

Use Relief of nausea and vomiting

Unlabeled use: Treatment of vertigo

Pregnancy Risk Factor X

Contraindications Comatose states, hypersensitivity to thiethylperazine or any component; pregnancy, cross-sensitivity to other phenothiazines may exist

Warnings/Precautions Reduce or discontinue if extrapyramidal effects occur; safety and efficacy in children <12 years of age have not been established; postural hypotension may occur after I.M. injection; the injectable form contains sulfite which may cause allergic reactions in some patients; use caution in patients with narrow-angle glaucoma

Adverse Reactions

>10%:

- Central nervous system: Drowsiness, dizziness
- Gastrointestinal: Xerostomia
- Respiratory: Dry nose

1% to 10%:

- Cardiovascular: Tachycardia, orthostatic hypotension
- Central nervous system: Confusion, convulsions, extrapyramidal effects, tardive dyskinesia, fever, headache
- Hematologic: Agranulocytosis
- Hepatic: Cholestatic jaundice
- Otic: Tinnitus

Overdosage/Toxicology Symptoms of overdose include deep sleep, coma, extrapyramidal symptoms, abnormal involuntary muscle movements, hypotension

Following initiation of essential overdose management, toxic symptom treatment and supportive treatment should be initiated. Hypotension usually responds to I.V. fluids or Trendelenburg positioning. If unresponsive to these measures, use of a parenteral inotrope may be required (eg, norepinephrine 0.1-0.2 mcg/kg/minute titrated to response); avoid epinephrine for thiethylperazine-induced hypotension. Seizures commonly respond to diazepam (I.V. 5-10 mg bolus in adults every 15 minutes if needed up to a total of 30 mg; I.V. 0.25-0.4 mg/kg/dose up to a total of 10 mg in children) or to phenytoin or phenobarbital. Critical cardiac arrhythmias often respond to I.V. phenytoin (15 mg/kg up to 1 g), while other antiarrhythmics can be used. Neuroleptics often cause extrapyramidal symptoms (eg, dystonic reactions) requiring management with diphenhydramine 1-2 mg/kg (adults) up to a maximum of 50 mg I.M. or I.V. slow push followed by a maintenance dose for 48-72 hours. When these reactions are unresponsive to diphenhydramine, benztropine mesylate I.V. 1-2 mg (adults) may be effective. These agents are generally effective within 2-5 minutes.

Drug Interactions Increased effect/toxicity with CNS depressants (eg, anesthetics, opiates, tranquilizers, alcohol), lithium, atropine, epinephrine, MAO inhibitors, TCAs

Mechanism of Action Blocks postsynaptic mesolimbic dopaminergic receptors in the brain; exhibits a strong alpha-adrenergic blocking effect and depresses the release of hypothalamic and hypophyseal hormones; acts directly on chemoreceptor trigger zone and vomiting center

Pharmacodynamics/Kinetics

Onset of antiemetic effect: Within 30 minutes

(Continued)

Thiethylperazine *(Continued)*

Duration of action: ~4 hours

Usual Dosage Children >12 years and Adults:

Oral, I.M., rectal: 10 mg 1-3 times/day as needed

I.V. and S.C. routes of administration are not recommended

Hemodialysis: Not dialyzable (0% to 5%)

Dosing comments in hepatic impairment: Use with caution

Administration Inject I.M. deeply into large muscle mass, patient should be lying down and remain so for at least 1 hour after administration

Patient Information May cause drowsiness, impair judgment and coordination; may cause photosensitivity; avoid excessive sunlight; notify physician of involuntary movements or feelings of restlessness

Nursing Implications Assist with ambulation, observe for extrapyramidal symptoms

Dosage Forms

Injection, as maleate: 5 mg/mL (2 mL)

Suppository, rectal, as maleate: 10 mg

Tablet, as maleate: 10 mg

Thiethylperazine Maleate *see* Thiethylperazine *on previous page*

Thioguanine (thye oh GWAH neen)

Related Information

Antiemetics for Chemotherapy Induced Nausea and Vomiting *on page 1348*

Cancer Chemotherapy Regimens *on page 1351*

Synonyms 2-Amino-6-Mercaptopurine; TG; 6-TG; 6-Thioguanine; Tioguanine

Therapeutic Category Antineoplastic Agent, Antimetabolite (Purine)

Use Remission induction, consolidation, and maintenance therapy of acute myelogenous (nonlymphocytic) leukemia; treatment of chronic myelogenous leukemia and granulocytic leukemia

Pregnancy Risk Factor D

Contraindications History of previous therapy resistance with either thioguanine or mercaptopurine (there is usually complete cross resistance between these two); hypersensitivity to thioguanine or any component

Warnings/Precautions The U.S. Food and Drug Administration (FDA) currently recommends that procedures for proper handling and disposal of antineoplastic agents be considered. Use with caution and reduce dose of thioguanine in patients with renal or hepatic impairment; thioguanine is potentially carcinogenic and teratogenic; myelosuppression may be delayed.

Adverse Reactions

>10%:

- Hematologic: Myelosuppressive:
  - WBC: Moderate
  - Platelets: Moderate
  - Onset (days): 7-10
  - Nadir (days): 14
  - Recovery (days): 21

1% to 10%:

- Dermatologic: Skin rash
- Endocrine & metabolic: Hyperuricemia
- Gastrointestinal: Mild nausea or vomiting, anorexia, stomatitis, diarrhea
  - Emetic potential: Low (<10%)
- Neuromuscular & skeletal: Unsteady gait

<1%:

- Central nervous system: Neurotoxicity
- Dermatologic: Photosensitivity
- Gastrointestinal: Stomatitis
- Hepatic: Hepatitis, jaundice, veno-occlusive hepatic disease

Overdosage/Toxicology Symptoms of overdose include bone marrow suppression, nausea, vomiting, malaise, hypertension, sweating; treatment is supportive; dialysis is not useful

Drug Interactions

Increased toxicity:

- Allopurinol can be used in full doses with 6 TG unlike 6-MP
- Busulfan → hepatotoxicity and esophageal varices

Mechanism of Action Purine analog that is incorporated into DNA and RNA resulting in the blockage of synthesis and metabolism of purine nucleotides

Pharmacodynamics/Kinetics

Absorption: Oral: 30%

Distribution: Crosses placenta

Metabolism: Rapidly and extensively in the liver to 2-amino-6-methylthioguanine (active) and inactive compounds

Half-life, terminal: 11 hours

Time to peak serum concentration: Within 8 hours

Elimination: In urine

Usual Dosage Total daily dose can be given at one time; offers little advantage over mercaptopurine; is sometimes ordered as 6-thioguanine, with 6 being part of the drug name and not some kind of unit or strength

Oral (refer to individual protocols):

Infants and Children <3 years: Combination drug therapy for acute nonlymphocytic leukemia: 3.3 mg/kg/day in divided doses twice daily for 4 days

Children and Adults: 2-3 mg/kg/day calculated to nearest 20 mg or 75-200 mg/m^2/day in 1-2 divided doses for 5-7 days or until remission is attained

Dosing comments in renal or hepatic impairment: Reduce dose

Monitoring Parameters CBC with differential and platelet count, liver function tests, hemoglobin, hematocrit, serum uric acid

Patient Information Avoid exposure to persons with infections. Drink plenty of fluids while taking the drug. May cause diarrhea, fever and weakness. Notify physician if these become pronounced. Notify physician if fever, chills, nausea, vomiting, sore throat, unusual bleeding or bruising, yellow discoloration of the skin or eyes, swelling of the feet or legs, or abdominal, joint, or flank pain occurs. Any signs of infection, easy bruising or bleeding, shortness of breath, or painful or burning urination should be brought to physician's attention. Hair loss sometimes occur. The drug may cause permanent sterility and may cause birth defects. The drug may be excreted in breast milk, therefore, an alternative form of feeding your baby should be used.

Dosage Forms Tablet, scored: 40 mg

Extemporaneous Preparations A 40 mg/mL oral suspension compounded from tablets which were crushed, mixed with a volume of Cologel® suspending agent equal to ¹/₃ the final volume, and brought to the final volume with a 2:1 mixture of simple syrup and cherry syrup was stable for 84 days when stored in an amber bottle at room temperature

Dressman JB and Poust RI, "Stability of Allopurinol and Five Antineoplastics in Suspension," *Am J Hosp Pharm*, 1983, 40:616-8.

6-Thioguanine *see* Thioguanine *on previous page*

Thiopental (thye oh PEN tal)

Brand Names Pentothal® Sodium

Synonyms Thiopental Sodium

Therapeutic Category Anticonvulsant; Barbiturate; General Anesthetic; Sedative

Use Induction of anesthesia; adjunct for intubation in head injury patients; control of convulsive states; treatment of elevated intracranial pressure

Restrictions C-III

Pregnancy Risk Factor C

Contraindications Porphyria (variegate or acute intermittent); known hypersensitivity to thiopental or other barbiturates

Warnings/Precautions Use with caution in patients with asthma, unstable aneurysms, severe cardiovascular disease, hepatic or renal disease, laryngospasm or bronchospasms which can occur; hypotension; extravasation or intra-arterial injection causes necrosis due to pH of 10.6, ensure patient has intravenous access

Adverse Reactions

>10%: Local: Pain on I.M. injection

1% to 10%: Gastrointestinal: Cramping, diarrhea, rectal bleeding

<1%:

Cardiovascular: Hypotension, peripheral vascular collapse, myocardial depression, cardiac arrhythmias, circulatory depression

Central nervous system: Seizures, headache, emergence delirium, prolonged somnolence and recovery, anxiety

Dermatologic: Erythema, pruritus, urticaria

Gastrointestinal: Nausea, vomiting

Hematologic: Hemolytic anemia

Local: Thrombophlebitis

Neuromuscular & skeletal: Tremor, involuntary muscle movement, twitching, rigidity, radial nerve palsy

Respiratory: Respiratory depression, coughing, rhinitis, apnea, laryngospasm, bronchospasm, sneezing, dyspnea

Miscellaneous: Hiccups, anaphylactic reactions

Overdosage/Toxicology Symptoms of overdose include respiratory depression, hypotension, shock

(Continued)

Thiopental *(Continued)*

Hypotension should respond to I.V. fluids and placement of patient in Trendelenburg position; if necessary, pressors such as norepinephrine may be used; patient may require ventilatory support

Drug Interactions Increased toxicity with CNS depressants (especially narcotic analgesics and phenothiazines), salicylates, sulfisoxazole

Stability Reconstituted solutions remain stable for 3 days at room temperature and 7 days when refrigerated; solutions are alkaline and **incompatible** with drugs with acidic pH, such as succinylcholine, atropine sulfate, etc. I.V. form is **incompatible** when mixed with amikacin, codeine, dimenhydrinate, diphenhydramine, hydromorphone, insulin, levorphanol, meperidine, metaraminol, morphine, norepinephrine, penicillin G, prochlorperazine, succinylcholine, tetracycline, benzquinamide, chlorpromazine, glycopyrrolate

Mechanism of Action Interferes with transmission of impulses from the thalamus to the cortex of the brain resulting in an imbalance in central inhibitory and facilitatory mechanisms

Pharmacodynamics/Kinetics

Onset of action: I.V.: Anesthesia occurs in 30-60 seconds

Duration: 5-30 minutes

Distribution: V_d: 1.4 L/kg

Protein binding: 72% to 86%

Metabolism: In the liver primarily to inactive metabolites but pentobarbital is also formed

Half-life: 3-11.5 hours, decreased in children vs adults

Usual Dosage I.V.:

Induction anesthesia:
- Infants: 5-8 mg/kg
- Children 1-12 years: 5-6 mg/kg
- Adults: 3-5 mg/kg

Maintenance anesthesia:
- Children: 1 mg/kg as needed
- Adults: 25-100 mg as needed

Increased intracranial pressure: Children and Adults: 1.5-5 mg/kg/dose; repeat as needed to control intracranial pressure

Seizures:
- Children: 2-3 mg/kg/dose, repeat as needed
- Adults: 75-250 mg/dose, repeat as needed

Rectal administration: (Patient should be NPO for no less than 3 hours prior to administration)

Suggested initial doses of thiopental rectal suspension are:

<3 months: 15 mg/kg/dose

>3 months: 25 mg/kg/dose

Note: The age of a premature infant should be adjusted to reflect the age that the infant would have been if full-term (eg, an infant, now age 4 months, who was 2 months premature should be considered to be a 2-month old infant).

Doses should be rounded downward to the nearest 50 mg increment to allow for accurate measurement of the dose

Inactive or debilitated patients and patients recently medicated with other sedatives, (eg, chloral hydrate, meperidine, chlorpromazine, and promethazine), may require smaller doses than usual

If the patient is not sedated within 15-20 minutes, a single repeat dose of thiopental can be given. The single repeat doses are:

<3 months: <7.5 mg/kg/dose

>3 months: 15 mg/kg/dose

Adults weighing >90 kg should not receive >3 g as a total dose (initial plus repeat doses)

Children weighing >34 kg should not receive >1 g as a total dose (initial plus repeat doses)

Neither adults nor children should receive more than one course of thiopental rectal suspension (initial dose plus repeat dose) per 24-hour period

Dosing adjustment in renal impairment: Cl_{cr} <10 mL/minute: Administer at 75% of normal dose

Note: Accumulation may occur with chronic dosing due to lipid solubility; prolonged recovery may result from redistribution of thiopental from fat stores

Monitoring Parameters Respiratory rate, heart rate, blood pressure

Reference Range Therapeutic: Hypnotic: 1-5 μg/mL (SI: 4.1-20.7 μmol/L); Coma: 30-100 μg/mL (SI: 124-413 μmol/L); Anesthesia: 7-130 μg/mL (SI: 29-536 μmol/L); Toxic: >10 μg/mL (SI: >41 μmol/L)

Test Interactions ↑ potassium (S)

Nursing Implications Monitor vital signs every 3-5 minutes; monitor for respiratory distress; place patient in Sim's position if vomiting, to prevent from aspirating vomitus; avoid extravasation, necrosis may occur

Additional Information Sodium content of 1 g (injection) : 86.8 mg (3.8 mEq)

Dosage Forms

Injection, as sodium: 250 mg, 400 mg, 500 mg, 1 g, 2.5 g, 5 g
Suspension, rectal, as sodium: 400 mg/g (2 g)

Thiopental Sodium *see* Thiopental *on page 1217*

Thiophosphoramide *see* Thiotepa *on next page*

Thioridazine (thye oh RID a zeen)

Related Information

Antipsychotic Agents Comparison *on page 1396*

Brand Names Mellaril®; Mellaril-S®

Canadian/Mexican Brand Names Apo-Thioridazine® (Canada); Novo-Ridazine® (Canada); PMS-Thioridazine (Canada)

Synonyms Thioridazine Hydrochloride

Therapeutic Category Antipsychotic Agent; Phenothiazine Derivative

Use Management of manifestations of psychotic disorders; depressive neurosis; alcohol withdrawal; dementia in elderly; behavioral problems in children

Pregnancy Risk Factor C

Contraindications Severe CNS depression, hypersensitivity to thioridazine or any component; cross-sensitivity to other phenothiazines may exist

Warnings/Precautions Oral formulations may cause stomach upset; may cause thermoregulatory changes; use caution in patients with narrow-angle glaucoma, severe liver or cardiac disease; doses of 1 g/day frequently cause pigmentary retinopathy

Adverse Reactions

>10%:

Central nervous system: Pseudoparkinsonism, akathisia, dystonias, tardive dyskinesia (persistent), dizziness
Cardiovascular: Hypotension, orthostatic hypotension
Gastrointestinal: Constipation
Ocular: Pigmentary retinopathy
Respiratory: Nasal congestion
Miscellaneous: Diaphoresis (decreased)

1% to 10%:

Dermatologic: Increased sensitivity to sun, rash
Endocrine & metabolic: Changes in menstrual cycle, changes in libido, breast pain
Gastrointestinal: Weight gain, nausea, vomiting, stomach pain
Genitourinary: Dysuria, ejaculatory disturbances
Neuromuscular & skeletal: Trembling of fingers

<1%:

Central nervous system: Neuroleptic malignant syndrome (NMS), impairment of temperature regulation, lowering of seizures threshold
Dermatologic: Discoloration of skin (blue-gray)
Endocrine & metabolic: Galactorrhea
Genitourinary: Priapism
Hematologic: Agranulocytosis, leukopenia
Hepatic: Cholestatic jaundice, hepatotoxicity
Ocular: Cornea and lens changes

Overdosage/Toxicology Symptoms of overdose include deep sleep, coma, extrapyramidal symptoms, abnormal involuntary muscle movements, hypotension, arrhythmias

Following initiation of essential overdose management, toxic symptom treatment and supportive treatment should be initiated. Hypotension usually responds to I.V. fluids or Trendelenburg positioning. If unresponsive to these measures, the use of a parenteral inotrope may be required (eg, norepinephrine 0.1-0.2 mcg/kg/minute titrated to response); do not use epinephrine. Seizures commonly respond to diazepam (I.V. 5-10 mg bolus in adults every 15 minutes if needed up to a total of 30 mg; I.V. 0.25-0.4 mg/kg/dose up to a total of 10 mg in children) or to phenytoin or phenobarbital. Neuroleptics often cause extrapyramidal symptoms (eg, dystonic reactions) requiring management with diphenhydramine 1-2 mg/kg (adults) up to a maximum of 50 mg I.M. or I.V. slow push followed by a maintenance dose for 48-72 hours. When these reactions are unresponsive to diphenhydramine, benztropine mesylate I.V. 1-2 mg (adults) may be effective. These agents are generally effective within 2-5 minutes.

Drug Interactions Cytochrome P-450 2D6 enzyme substrate

Decreased effect with anticholinergics
Decreased effect of guanethidine
(Continued)

Thioridazine *(Continued)*

Increased toxicity with CNS depressants, epinephrine (hypotension), lithium (rare), TCA (cardiotoxicity), propranolol, pindolol

Stability Protect all dosage forms from light

Mechanism of Action Blocks postsynaptic mesolimbic dopaminergic receptors in the brain; exhibits a strong alpha-adrenergic blocking effect and depresses the release of hypothalamic and hypophyseal hormones

Pharmacodynamics/Kinetics

Duration of action: 4-5 days

Half-life: 21-25 hours

Time to peak serum concentration: Within 1 hour

Usual Dosage Oral:

Children >2 years: Range: 0.5-3 mg/kg/day in 2-3 divided doses; usual: 1 mg/kg/day; maximum: 3 mg/kg/day

Behavior problems: Initial: 10 mg 2-3 times/day, increase gradually

Severe psychoses: Initial: 25 mg 2-3 times/day, increase gradually

Adults:

Psychoses: Initial: 50-100 mg 3 times/day with gradual increments as needed and tolerated; maximum: 800 mg/day in 2-4 divided doses; if >65 years, initial dose: 10 mg 3 times/day

Depressive disorders, dementia: Initial: 25 mg 3 times/day; maintenance dose: 20-200 mg/day

Hemodialysis: Not dialyzable (0% to 5%)

Dietary Considerations Alcohol: Additive CNS effect, avoid use

Administration Dilute oral concentrate with water or juice before administration

Monitoring Parameters For patients on prolonged therapy: CBC, ophthalmologic exam, blood pressure, liver function tests

Reference Range Therapeutic: 1.0-1.5 μg/mL (SI: 2.7-4.1 μmol/L); Toxic: >10 μg/mL (SI: >27 μmol/L)

Test Interactions False-positives for phenylketonuria, urinary amylase, uroporphyrins, urobilinogen

Patient Information Oral concentrate must be diluted in 2-4 oz of liquid (water, fruit juice, carbonated drinks, milk, or pudding); do not take antacid within 1 hour of taking drug; avoid excess sun exposure; may cause drowsiness, restlessness, avoid alcohol and other CNS depressants; do not alter dosage or discontinue without consulting physician; yearly eye exams are necessary; might discolor urine (pink or reddish brown)

Nursing Implications Avoid skin contact with oral suspension or solution; may cause contact dermatitis

Additional Information

Thioridazine: Mellaril-S® oral suspension

Thioridazine hydrochloride: Mellaril® oral solution and tablet

Dosage Forms

Concentrate, oral: 30 mg/mL (120 mL); 100 mg/mL (3.4 mL, 120 mL)

Suspension, oral: 25 mg/5 mL (480 mL); 100 mg/5 mL (480 mL)

Tablet: 10 mg, 15 mg, 25 mg, 50 mg, 100 mg, 150 mg, 200 mg

Thioridazine Hydrochloride *see* Thioridazine *on previous page*

Thiotepa (thye oh TEP a)

Related Information

Antiemetics for Chemotherapy Induced Nausea and Vomiting *on page 1348*

Cancer Chemotherapy Regimens *on page 1351*

Synonyms TESPA; Thiophosphoramide; Triethylenethiophosphoramide; TSPA

Therapeutic Category Antineoplastic Agent, Alkylating Agent

Use Treatment of superficial tumors of the bladder; palliative treatment of adenocarcinoma of breast or ovary; lymphomas and sarcomas; controlling intracavitary effusions caused by metastatic tumors; I.T. use: CNS leukemia/lymphoma

Pregnancy Risk Factor D

Contraindications Hypersensitivity to thiotepa or any component; severe myelosuppression with leukocyte count <3000/mm^3 or platelet count <150,000/mm^3

Warnings/Precautions The U.S. Food and Drug Administration (FDA) currently recommends that procedures for proper handling and disposal of antineoplastic agents be considered. The drug is potentially mutagenic, carcinogenic, and teratogenic. Reduce dosage in patients with hepatic, renal, or bone marrow damage.

Adverse Reactions

>10%:

Hematopoietic: Dose-limiting toxicity which is dose-related and cumulative; moderate to severe leukopenia and severe thrombocytopenia have occurred.

Anemia and pancytopenia may become fatal, so careful hematologic monitoring is required; intravesical administration may cause bone marrow suppression as well.

Hematologic: Myelosuppressive:

WBC: Moderate

Platelets: Severe

Onset (days): 7-10

Nadir (days): 14

Recovery (days): 28

Local: Pain at injection site

1% to 10%:

Central nervous system: Dizziness, fever, headache

Dermatologic: Alopecia, rash, pruritus, hyperpigmentation with high-dose therapy

Endocrine & metabolic: Hyperuricemia

Gastrointestinal: Anorexia, nausea and vomiting rarely occur

Emetic potential: Low (<10%)

Genitourinary: Hemorrhagic cystitis

Renal: Hematuria

Miscellaneous: Tightness of the throat, allergic reactions

<1%:

Gastrointestinal: Stomatitis

Miscellaneous: Anaphylaxis; Carcinogenesis: Like other alkylating agents, this drug is carcinogenic

Overdosage/Toxicology Symptoms of overdose include nausea, vomiting, precipitation of uric acid in kidney tubules, bone marrow suppression, bleeding

Therapy is supportive only; thiotepa is dialyzable; transfusions of whole blood or platelets have been proven beneficial

Drug Interactions Cytochrome P-450 enzyme substrate

Decreased effect:

Clofibrate, phenobarbital may increase clearance of thiotepa

Increased toxicity:

Other alkylating agents or irradiation concomitantly with thiotepa intensifies toxicity rather than enhancing therapeutic response

Prolonged muscular paralysis and respiratory depression may occur when neuromuscular blocking agents are administered

Succinylcholine and other neuromuscular blocking agents' action can be prolonged due to thiotepa inhibiting plasma pseudocholinesterase

Stability

Store intact vials under refrigeration (2°C to 8°C) and protect from light

Dilute powder 1.5 mL SWI to a concentration of 10.4 mg/mL which is stable for 8 hours at refrigeration

Further dilution in NS should be used immediately

Thiotepa is stable for 24 hours at a concentration of 5 mg/mL in NS at 8°C and 23°C; however, stability decreases significantly at concentrations of ≤ 0.5 mg/mL (<8 hours); concentrations of 1-3 mg/mL are stable 48 hours at 8°C and 24 hours at 23°C

Standard I.V. dilution:

I.V. push: Dose/syringe (concentration = 10 mg/mL)

IVPB: Dose/100-150 mL NS for a final concentration of 1.5-3.5 mg/mL

Further dilution in NS should be used immediately (within 8 hours of preparation)

Standard intravesicular dilution: 60 mg/30-60 mL NS; solution is placed via catheter and retained for two hours for maximum effect

Intrathecal doses of 1-10 mg/m^2 should be diluted to 1-5 mg in NS

Standard intrathecal dilution: 10-15 mg/3-5 mL NS

ALL solutions should be **prepared fresh** and administered within one hour of preparation

Mechanism of Action Alkylating agent that reacts with DNA phosphate groups to produce cross-linking of DNA strands leading to inhibition of DNA, RNA, and protein synthesis; mechanism of action has not been explored as thoroughly as the other alkylating agents, it is presumed that the azridine rings open and react as nitrogen mustard; reactivity is enhanced at a lower pH

Pharmacodynamics/Kinetics

Absorption: Following intracavitary instillation, the drug is unreliably absorbed (10% to 100%) through the bladder mucosa; variable I.M. absorption

Metabolism: Extensively in the liver

Half-life, terminal: 109 minutes with dose-dependent clearance

Elimination: As metabolites and unchanged drug in urine

Usual Dosage Refer to individual protocols. Dosing must be based on the clinical and hematologic response of the patient.

(Continued)

Thiotepa *(Continued)*

Children: Sarcomas: I.V.: 25-65 mg/m^2 as a single dose every 21 days
Adults:
I.M., I.V., S.C.: 30-60 mg/m^2 once per week
I.V. doses of 0.3-0.4 mg/kg by rapid I.V. administration every 1-4 weeks, or 0.2 mg/kg or 6-8 mg/m^2/day for 4-5 days every 2-4 weeks
High-dose therapy for bone marrow transplant: I.V.: 500 mg/m^2; up to 900 mg/m^2
I.M. doses of 15-30 mg in various schedules have been given
Intracavitary: 0.6-0.8 mg/kg
Intrapericardial dose: Usually 15-30 mg

Dosing comments/adjustment in renal impairment: Use with extreme caution, reduced dose may be warranted. Less than 3% of alkylating species are detected in the urine in 24 hours.

Intrathecal: Doses of 1-10 mg/m^2 administered 1-2 times/week in concentrations of 1 mg/mL diluted with preservative-free sterile water for injection

Intravesical: Used for treatment of carcinoma of the bladder; patients should be dehydrated for 8-12 hours prior to treatment; instill 60 mg (in 30-60 mL of NS) into the bladder and retain for a minimum of 2 hours. Patient should be positioned every 15 minutes for maximal area exposure. Instillations usually once a week for 4 weeks. Monitor for bone marrow suppression.

Intratumor: use a 22-gauge needle to inject thiotepa directly into the tumor. Initial dose: 0.6-0.8 mg/kg (diluted to 10 mg/mL) are used every 1-4 weeks; maintenance dose: 0.07-0.8 mg/kg are administered at 1- to 4-week intervals

Ophthalmic: 0.05% solution in LF has been instilled into the eye every 3 hours for 6-8 weeks for the prevention of pterygium recurrence

Administration Administer I.V., intracavitary, and intrathecally; solutions should be filtered through a 0.22 micron filter prior to administration

Monitoring Parameters CBC with differential and platelet count, uric acid, urinalysis

Patient Information Any signs of infection, easy bruising or bleeding, shortness of breath, or painful or burning urination should be brought to physician's attention. Nausea, vomiting, or hair loss sometimes occur. The drug may cause permanent sterility and may cause birth defects. The drug may be excreted in breast milk, therefore, an alternative form of feeding your baby should be used.

Nursing Implications A 1 mg/mL solution is considered isotonic; not a vesicant

Dosage Forms Powder for injection: 15 mg

Thiothixene (thye oh THIKS een)

Related Information

Antipsychotic Agents Comparison *on page 1396*

Brand Names Navane®

Synonyms Tiotixene

Therapeutic Category Antipsychotic Agent; Phenothiazine Derivative

Use Management of psychotic disorders

Pregnancy Risk Factor C

Contraindications Hypersensitivity to thiothixene or any component; cross-sensitivity with other phenothiazines may exist, lactation

Warnings/Precautions Watch for hypotension when administering I.M. or I.V.; safety in children <6 months of age has not been established; use with caution in patients with narrow-angle glaucoma, bone marrow suppression, severe liver or cardiac disease, seizures

Adverse Reactions

>10%:
Cardiovascular: Hypotension, orthostatic hypotension
Central nervous system: Pseudoparkinsonism, akathisia, dystonias, tardive dyskinesia (persistent), dizziness
Gastrointestinal: Constipation
Respiratory: Nasal congestion
Miscellaneous: Diaphoresis (decreased)

1% to 10%:
Dermatologic: Increased sensitivity to sun, rash
Endocrine & metabolic: Changes in menstrual cycle, changes in libido, breast pain
Gastrointestinal: Weight gain, nausea, vomiting, stomach pain
Genitourinary: Dysuria, ejaculatory disturbances
Neuromuscular & skeletal: Trembling of fingers
Ocular: Pigmentary retinopathy

<1%:
Central nervous system: Neuroleptic malignant syndrome (NMS), impairment of temperature regulation, lowering of seizures threshold
Dermatologic: Discoloration of skin (blue-gray)

Endocrine & metabolic: Galactorrhea
Genitourinary: Priapism
Hematologic: Agranulocytosis, leukopenia
Hepatic: Cholestatic jaundice, hepatotoxicity
Ocular: Cornea and lens changes

Overdosage/Toxicology Symptoms of overdose include muscle twitching, drowsiness, dizziness, rigidity, tremor, hypotension, cardiac arrhythmias

Following initiation of essential overdose management, toxic symptom treatment and supportive treatment should be initiated. Hypotension usually responds to I.V. fluids or Trendelenburg positioning. If unresponsive to these measures, the use of a parenteral inotrope may be required (eg, norepinephrine 0.1-0.2 mcg/kg/minute titrated to response). Seizures commonly respond to diazepam (I.V. 5-10 mg bolus in adults every 15 minutes if needed up to a total of 30 mg; I.V. 0.25-0.4 mg/kg/dose up to a total of 10 mg in children) or to phenytoin or phenobarbital. Neuroleptics often cause extrapyramidal symptoms (eg, dystonic reactions) requiring management with diphenhydramine 1-2 mg/kg (adults) up to a maximum of 50 mg I.M. or I.V. slow push followed by a maintenance dose for 48-72 hours. When these reactions are unresponsive to diphenhydramine, benztropine mesylate I.V. 1-2 mg (adults) may be effective. These agents are generally effective within 2-5 minutes.

Drug Interactions
Decreased effect of guanethidine
Increased toxicity with CNS depressants, anticholinergics, alcohol

Stability Refrigerate

Mechanism of Action Elicits antipsychotic activity by postsynaptic blockade of CNS dopamine receptors resulting in inhibition of dopamine-mediated effects; also has alpha-adrenergic blocking activity

Pharmacodynamics/Kinetics
Metabolism: Extensive in the liver
Half-life: >24 hours with chronic use

Usual Dosage
Children <12 years: Oral: 0.25 mg/kg/24 hours in divided doses (dose not well established)

Children >12 years and Adults: Mild to moderate psychosis:
Oral: 2 mg 3 times/day, up to 20-30 mg/day; more severe psychosis: Initial: 5 mg 2 times/day, may increase gradually, if necessary; maximum: 60 mg/day
I.M.: 4 mg 2-4 times/day, increase dose gradually; usual: 16-20 mg/day; maximum: 30 mg/day; change to oral dose as soon as able

Hemodialysis: Not dialyzable (0% to 5%)

Dietary Considerations Alcohol: Additive CNS effect, avoid use

Monitoring Parameters Liver function tests; for patients on prolonged therapy: CBC, ophthalmologic exam

Test Interactions ↑ cholesterol (S), ↑ glucose; ↓ uric acid (S); may cause false-positive pregnancy test

Patient Information May cause drowsiness, restlessness, avoid alcohol and other CNS depressants; do not alter dosage or discontinue without consulting physician

Nursing Implications Observe for extrapyramidal effects; concentrate should be mixed in juice before administration

Dosage Forms
Capsule: 1 mg, 2 mg, 5 mg, 10 mg, 20 mg
Concentrate, oral, as hydrochloride: 5 mg/mL (30 mL, 120 mL)
Injection, as hydrochloride: 2 mg/mL (2 mL)
Powder for injection, as hydrochloride: 5 mg/mL (2 mL)

Thorazine® *see* Chlorpromazine *on page 261*
Thrombate III® *see* Antithrombin III *on page 97*
Thyrar® *see* Thyroid *on this page*
Thyro-Block® *see* Potassium Iodide *on page 1027*

Thyroid (THYE royd)

Brand Names Armour® Thyroid; S-P-T; Thyrar®; Thyroid Strong®

Synonyms Desiccated Thyroid; Thyroid Extract

Therapeutic Category Thyroid Hormone; Thyroid Product

Use Replacement or supplemental therapy in hypothyroidism; pituitary TSH suppressants (thyroid nodules, thyroiditis, multinodular goiter, thyroid cancer), thyrotoxicosis, diagnostic suppression tests

Pregnancy Risk Factor A

Contraindications Recent myocardial infarction or thyrotoxicosis, uncomplicated by hypothyroidism; uncorrected adrenal insufficiency, hypersensitivity to active or extraneous constituents
(Continued)

Thyroid *(Continued)*

Warnings/Precautions Ineffective for weight reduction; high doses may produce serious or even life-threatening toxic effects particularly when used with some anorectic drugs; use cautiously in patients with pre-existing cardiovascular disease (angina, CHD), elderly since they may be more likely to have compromised cardiovascular function. Chronic hypothyroidism predisposes patients to coronary artery disease. Desiccated thyroid contains variable amounts of T_3, T_4, and other triiodothyronine compounds which are more likely to cause cardiac signs and symptoms due to fluctuating levels; should avoid use in elderly for this reason; drug of choice is levothyroxine in the minds of many clinicians.

Adverse Reactions

<1%:

Cardiovascular: Palpitations, tachycardia, cardiac arrhythmias, chest pain

Central nervous system: Nervousness, headache, insomnia, fever, ataxia

Dermatologic: Alopecia

Endocrine & metabolic: Changes in menstrual cycle, shortness of breath

Gastrointestinal: Weight loss, increased appetite, diarrhea, abdominal cramps, vomiting, constipation

Neuromuscular & skeletal: Excessive bone loss with overtreatment (excess thyroid replacement), tremor, hand tremors, myalgia

Miscellaneous: Heat intolerance, diaphoresis

Overdosage/Toxicology Chronic excessive use results in signs and symptoms of hyperthyroidism, weight loss, nervousness, sweating, tachycardia, insomnia, heat intolerance, palpitations, vomiting, psychosis, fever, seizures, angina, arrhythmias, and CHF in those predisposed

Reduce dose or temporarily discontinue therapy; normal hypothalamic-pituitary-thyroid axis will return to normal in 6-8 weeks; serum T_4 levels do not correlate well with toxicity

In massive acute ingestion, reduce GI absorption, administer general supportive care; treat CHF with digitalis glycosides; excessive adrenergic activity (tachycardia) require propranolol 1-3 mg I.V. over 10 minutes or 80-160 mg orally/day; fever may be treated with acetaminophen

Drug Interactions

Decreased effect:

Beta-blocker effect is decreased when patients become euthyroid

Thyroid hormones increase the therapeutic need for oral hypoglycemics or insulin

Estrogens increase TBG, thereby decreasing effect of thyroid replacement

Cholestyramine and colestipol decrease the effect of orally administered thyroid replacement

Serum digitalis concentrations are reduced in hyperthyroidism or when hypothyroid patients are converted to a euthyroid state

Theophylline levels decrease when hypothyroid patients converted to a euthyroid state

Increased toxicity: Thyroid may potentiate the hypoprothrombinemic effect of oral anticoagulants

Mechanism of Action The primary active compound is T_3 (triiodothyronine), which may be converted from T_4 (thyroxine) and then circulates throughout the body to influence growth and maturation of various tissues; exact mechanism of action is unknown; however, it is believed the thyroid hormone exerts its many metabolic effects through control of DNA transcription and protein synthesis; involved in normal metabolism, growth, and development; promotes gluconeogenesis, increases utilization and mobilization of glycogen stores and stimulates protein synthesis, increases basal metabolic rate

Pharmacodynamics/Kinetics

Absorption: T_4 is 48% to 79% absorbed; T_3 is 95% absorbed; desiccated thyroid contains thyroxine, liothyronine, and iodine (primarily bound); following absorption thyroxine is largely converted to liothyronine

Recommended Pediatric Dosage for Congenital Hypothyroidism

Age	Daily Dose (mg)	Daily Dose/kg (mg)
0-6 mo	15-30	4.8-6
6-12 mo	30-45	3.6-4.8
1-5 y	45-60	3-3.6
6-12 y	60-90	2.4-3
>12 y	>90	1.2-1.8

Protein binding: 99% (bound to albumin, thyroxine-binding globulin, and thyroxin-binding prealbumin)

Metabolism: Liothyronine is metabolized in the liver, kidneys, and other tissues to inactive compounds

Half-life:

Liothyronine: 1-2 days

Thyroxine: 6-7 days

Elimination: In urine as conjugated forms

Usual Dosage Oral:

Children: See table.

Adults: Initial: 15-30 mg; increase with 15 mg increments every 2-4 weeks; use 15 mg in patients with cardiovascular disease or myxedema. Maintenance dose: Usually 60-120 mg/day; monitor TSH and clinical symptoms.

Thyroid cancer: Requires larger amounts than replacement therapy

Monitoring Parameters T_4, TSH, heart rate, blood pressure, clinical signs of hypo- and hyperthyroidism; TSH is the most reliable guide for evaluating adequacy of thyroid replacement dosage. TSH may be elevated during the first few months of thyroid replacement despite patients being clinically euthyroid. In cases where T_4 remains low and TSH is within normal limits, an evaluation of "free" (unbound) T_4 is needed to evaluate further increase in dosage.

Reference Range

TSH: 0.4-10 (for those ≥80 years) mIU/L

T_4: 4-12 μg/dL (51-154 nmol/L)

T_3 (RIA) (total T_3): 80-230 ng/dL (1.2-3.5 nmol/L)

T_4 free (free T_4): 0.7-1.8 ng/dL (9-23 pmol/L)

Test Interactions Many drugs may have effects on thyroid function tests; para-aminosalicylic acid, aminoglutethimide, amiodarone, barbiturates, carbamazepine, chloral hydrate, clofibrate, colestipol, corticosteroids, danazol, diazepam, estrogens, ethionamide, fluorouracil, I.V. heparin, insulin, lithium, methadone, methimazole, mitotane, nitroprusside, oxyphenbutazone, phenylbutazone, PTU, perphenazine, phenytoin, propranolol, salicylates, sulfonylureas, and thiazides

Patient Information Do not change brands, dose, or discontinue without physician's knowledge; report immediately to physician any chest pain, increased pulse, palpitations, heat intolerances, excessive sweating; replacement therapy will be for life; take as a single daily dose

Nursing Implications Monitor pulse rate and blood pressure

Additional Information

Equivalent levothyroxine dose: Thyroid USP 60 mg = levothyroxine 0.05-0.06 mg; liothyronine 15-37.5 mcg; liotrix 60 mg

Thyroid Strong® is 50% stronger than thyroid U.S.P.: each grain is equivalent to 1.5 grains of thyroid U.S.P.

Thyrar®: Bovine thyroid

S-P-T®: Pork thyroid suspended in soybean oil

Dosage Forms

Capsule, pork source in soybean oil (S-P-T): 60 mg, 120 mg, 180 mg, 300 mg

Tablet:

Armour® Thyroid: 15 mg, 30 mg, 60 mg, 90 mg, 120 mg, 180 mg, 240 mg, 300 mg

Thyrar® (bovine source): 30 mg, 60 mg, 120 mg

Thyroid Strong® (60 mg is equivalent to 90 mg thyroid USP):

: Regular: 30 mg, 60 mg, 120 mg

: Sugar coated: 30 mg, 60 mg, 120 mg, 180 mg

Thyroid USP: 15 mg, 30 mg, 60 mg, 120 mg, 180 mg, 300 mg

Thyroid Extract *see* Thyroid *on page 1223*

Thyroid Stimulating Hormone *see* Thyrotropin *on this page*

Thyroid Strong® *see* Thyroid *on page 1223*

Thyrolar® *see* Liotrix *on page 731*

Thyrotropic Hormone *see* Thyrotropin *on this page*

Thyrotropin (thye roe TROE pin)

Brand Names Thytropar®

Synonyms Thyroid Stimulating Hormone; Thyrotropic Hormone; TSH

Therapeutic Category Diagnostic Agent, Hypothyroidism; Diagnostic Agent, Thyroid Function

Use Diagnostic aid to differentiate thyroid failure; diagnosis of decreased thyroid reserve, to differentiate between primary and secondary hypothyroidism and between primary hypothyroidism and euthyroidism in patients receiving thyroid replacement

Pregnancy Risk Factor C

Contraindications Coronary thrombosis, untreated Addison's disease, hypersensitivity to thyrotropin or any component

(Continued)

Thyrotropin *(Continued)*

Warnings/Precautions Use with caution in patients with angina pectoris or cardiac failure, patients with hypopituitarism, adrenal cortical suppression as may be seen with corticosteroid therapy; may cause thyroid hyperplasia

Adverse Reactions

<1%:

Cardiovascular: Tachycardia
Central nervous system: Fever, headache
Endocrine & metabolic: Menstrual irregularities
Gastrointestinal: Nausea, vomiting, increased bowel motility
Sensitivity reactions: Anaphylaxis with repeated administration

Overdosage/Toxicology Symptoms of overdose include weight loss, nervousness, sweating, tachycardia, insomnia, heat intolerance, menstrual irregularities, headache, angina pectoris, CHF

Acute massive overdose may require cardiac glycosides for CHF; fever should be controlled with the help of acetaminophen; antiadrenergic agents, particularly propranolol 1-3 mg I.V. every 6 hours or 80-160 mg/day, can be used to treat increased sympathetic activity.

Stability Refrigerate at 2°C to 8°C (36°F to 46°F) after reconstitution; use within 2 weeks

Mechanism of Action Stimulates formation and secretion of thyroid hormone, increases uptake of iodine by thyroid gland

Pharmacodynamics/Kinetics

Half-life: 35 minutes, dependent upon thyroid state
Elimination: Rapidly by the kidney in the urine

Usual Dosage Adults: I.M., S.C.: 10 units/day for 1-3 days; follow by a radioiodine study 24 hours past last injection, no response in thyroid failure, substantial response in pituitary failure

Dosage Forms Injection: 10 units

Thytropar® *see* Thyrotropin *on previous page*

Tiabendazole *see* Thiabendazole *on page 1213*

Tiazac® *see* Diltiazem *on page 393*

Ticar® *see* Ticarcillin *on this page*

Ticarcillin (tye kar SIL in)

Related Information

Antimicrobial Drugs of Choice *on page 1468*

Brand Names Ticar®

Synonyms Ticarcillin Disodium

Therapeutic Category Antibiotic, Penicillin

Use Treatment of susceptible infections such as septicemia, acute and chronic respiratory tract infections, skin and soft tissue infections, and urinary tract infections due to susceptible strains of *Pseudomonas*, *Proteus*, and *Escherichia coli* and *Enterobacter*, normally used with other antibiotics (ie, aminoglycosides)

Pregnancy Risk Factor B

Contraindications Hypersensitivity to ticarcillin or any component or penicillins

Warnings/Precautions Due to sodium load and adverse effects (anemia, neuropsychological changes), use with caution and modify dosage in patients with renal impairment; serious and occasionally severe or fatal hypersensitivity (anaphylactoid) reactions have been reported in patients on penicillin therapy (especially with a history of beta-lactam hypersensitivity and/or a history of sensitivity to multiple allergens); use with caution in patients with seizures

Adverse Reactions

<1%:

Central nervous system: Convulsions, confusion, drowsiness, fever
Dermatologic: Rash
Endocrine & metabolic: Electrolyte imbalance
Hematologic: Hemolytic anemia, positive Coombs' reaction
Local: Thrombophlebitis
Neuromuscular & skeletal: Myoclonus
Renal: Acute interstitial nephritis
Miscellaneous: Hypersensitivity reactions, anaphylaxis, Jarisch-Herxheimer reaction

Overdosage/Toxicology Symptoms of penicillin overdose include neuromuscular hypersensitivity (agitation, hallucinations, asterixis, encephalopathy, confusion, and seizures) and electrolyte imbalance with potassium or sodium salts, especially in renal failure

Hemodialysis may be helpful to aid in the removal of the drug from the blood, otherwise most treatment is supportive or symptom directed

Drug Interactions

Decreased effect: Tetracyclines may decrease penicillin effectiveness; aminoglycosides → physical inactivation of aminoglycosides in the presence of high concentrations of ticarcillin and potential toxicity in patients with mild-moderate renal dysfunction

Increased effect:

Probenecid may increase penicillin levels

Neuromuscular blockers may increase duration of blockade

Aminoglycosides → synergistic efficacy

Stability Reconstituted solution is stable for 72 hours at room temperature and 14 days when refrigerated or 30 days when frozen; for I.V. infusion in NS or D_5W; **incompatible** with aminoglycosides

Mechanism of Action Interferes with bacterial cell wall synthesis during active multiplication, causing cell wall death and resultant bactericidal activity against susceptible bacteria

Pharmacodynamics/Kinetics

Absorption: I.M.: 86%

Distribution: V_d: Neonates: 0.42-0.76 L/kg; distributed into milk at low concentrations; attains high concentrations in bile; minimal concentrations attained in CSF with uninflamed meninges

Protein binding: 45% to 65%

Half-life, adults: 1-1.3 hours, prolonged with renal impairment and/or hepatic impairment

Neonates:

<1 week: 3.5-5.6 hours

1-8 weeks: 1.3-2.2 hours

Children 5-13 years: 0.9 hours

Peak serum levels: I.M.: Within 30-75 minutes

Elimination: Almost entirely in urine as unchanged drug and its metabolites with small amounts excreted in feces (3.5%)

Usual Dosage Ticarcillin is generally given I.M. only for the treatment of uncomplicated urinary tract infections

Infants and Children: I.V.: Serious Infections:200-300 mg/kg/day in divided doses every 4-6 hours; doses as high as 400 mg/kg/day divided every 4 hours have been used in acute pulmonary exacerbations of cystic fibrosis

Maximum dose: 24 g/day

Urinary tract infections: I.M., I.V.: 50-100 mg/kg/day in divided doses every 6-8 hours

Adults: I.V.: 1-4 g every 4-6 hours

Dosing interval in renal impairment:

Cl_{cr} 10-30 mL/minute: Administer every 8 hours

Cl_{cr} <10 mL/minute: Administer every 12 hours

Administration Administer around-the-clock; administer 1 hour apart from aminoglycosides

Monitoring Parameters Serum electrolytes, bleeding time, and periodic tests of renal, hepatic, and hematologic function

Test Interactions False-positive urinary or serum protein, positive Coombs' test

Nursing Implications Draw sample for culture and sensitivity before administering first dose, if possible

Additional Information Sodium content of 1 g: 5.2-6.5 mEq

Dosage Forms Powder for injection, as disodium: 1 g, 3 g, 6 g, 20 g, 30 g

Ticarcillin and Clavulanate Potassium

(tye kar SIL in & klav yoo LAN ate poe TASS ee um)

Related Information

Antimicrobial Drugs of Choice *on page 1468*

Brand Names Timentin®

Synonyms Ticarcillin and Clavulanic Acid

Therapeutic Category Antibiotic, Penicillin

Use Treatment of infections of lower respiratory tract, urinary tract, skin and skin structures, bone and joint, and septicemia caused by susceptible organisms. Clavulanate expands activity of ticarcillin to include beta-lactamase producing strains of *S. aureus*, *H. influenzae*, Enterobacteriaceae, *Klebsiella*, *Citrobacter*, and *Serratia*

Pregnancy Risk Factor B

Contraindications Known hypersensitivity to ticarcillin, clavulanate, or any penicillin

Warnings/Precautions Not approved for use in children <12 years of age; use with caution and modify dosage in patients with renal impairment; serious and occasionally fatal hypersensitivity (anaphylactoid) reactions have been reported in patients on penicillin therapy. These reactions are more likely to occur in individuals with a history of cephalosporin hypersensitivity and/or a history of

(Continued)

Ticarcillin and Clavulanate Potassium *(Continued)*

sensitivity to multiple allergens. There have been reports of individuals with a history of cephalosporin hypersensitivity who have experienced severe reactions when treated with penicillins.

Adverse Reactions

<1%:

Central nervous system: Convulsions, confusion, drowsiness, fever
Dermatologic: Rash
Endocrine & metabolic: Electrolyte imbalance
Hematologic: Hemolytic anemia, positive Coombs' reaction
Local: Thrombophlebitis
Neuromuscular & skeletal: Myoclonus
Renal: Acute interstitial nephritis
Miscellaneous: Hypersensitivity reactions, anaphylaxis, Jarisch-Herxheimer reaction

Overdosage/Toxicology Symptoms of overdose include neuromuscular hypersensitivity and seizures

Hemodialysis may be helpful to aid in the removal of the drug from the blood, otherwise most treatment is supportive or symptom directed

Drug Interactions

Decreased effect: Tetracyclines may decrease penicillin effectiveness; aminoglycosides → physical inactivation of aminoglycosides in the presence of high concentrations of ticarcillin and potential toxicity in patients with mild-moderate renal dysfunction

Increased effect:

Probenecid may increase penicillin levels
Neuromuscular blockers may increase duration of blockade
Aminoglycosides → synergistic efficacy

Stability Reconstituted solution is stable for 6 hours at room temperature and 72 hours when refrigerated; for I.V. infusion in NS is stable for 24 hours at room temperature, 7 days when refrigerated, or 30 days when frozen; darkening of drug indicates loss of potency of clavulanate potassium; **incompatible** with sodium bicarbonate, aminoglycosides

Mechanism of Action Ticarcillin interferes with bacterial cell wall synthesis during active multiplication, causing cell wall death and resultant bactericidal activity against susceptible bacteria; clavulanic acid prevents degradation of ticarcillin by binding to the active site on beta-lactamase

Pharmacodynamics/Kinetics

Distribution: Low concentrations of ticarcillin distribute into the CSF and increase when meninges are inflamed

Protein binding:

Ticarcillin: 45% to 65%
Clavulanic acid: 9% to 30% removed by hemodialysis

Metabolism: Clavulanic acid is metabolized in the liver

Half-life:

Clavulanate: 66-90 minutes
Ticarcillin: 66-72 minutes in patients with normal renal function; clavulanic acid does not affect the clearance of ticarcillin

Elimination: 45% excreted unchanged in urine, whereas 60% to 90% of ticarcillin excreted unchanged in urine

Usual Dosage I.V.:

Children: 200-300 mg of ticarcillin component/kg/day in divided doses every 4-6 hours

Adults: 3.1 g (ticarcillin 3 g plus clavulanic acid 0.1 g) every 4-6 hours; maximum: 18-24 g/day

Urinary tract infections: 3.1 g every 6-8 hours

Dosing interval in renal impairment:

Cl_{cr} 10-30 mL/minute: Administer every 8 hours
Cl_{cr} <10 mL/minute: Administer every 12 hours

Dosing interval in hepatic impairment: Cl_{cr} <10 mL/minute: Administer every 24 hours

Administration Infuse over 30 minutes; administer 1 hour apart from aminoglycosides; administer around-the-clock

Test Interactions Positive Coombs' test, false-positive urinary proteins

Nursing Implications Draw sample for culture and sensitivity prior to first dose if possible

Additional Information Sodium content of 1 g: 4.75 mEq; potassium content of 1 g: 0.15 mEq

Dosage Forms

Infusion, premixed (frozen): Ticarcillin disodium 3 g and clavulanate potassium 0.1 g (100 mL)

Powder for injection: Ticarcillin disodium 3 g and clavulanate potassium 0.1 g (3.1 g, 31 g)

Ticarcillin and Clavulanic Acid *see* Ticarcillin and Clavulanate Potassium *on page 1227*

Ticarcillin Disodium *see* Ticarcillin *on page 1226*

TICE® BCG *see* BCG Vaccine *on page 132*

Ticlid® *see* Ticlopidine *on this page*

Ticlopidine (tye KLOE pi deen)

Brand Names Ticlid®

Synonyms Ticlopidine Hydrochloride

Therapeutic Category Antiplatelet Agent

Use Platelet aggregation inhibitor that reduces the risk of thrombotic stroke in patients who have had a stroke or stroke precursors

Unlabeled use: Protection of aortocoronary bypass grafts, diabetic microangiopathy, ischemic heart disease, prevention of postoperative DVT, reduction of graft loss following renal transplant; reduction of postoperative reocclusion in patients receiving PTCA with stents

Pregnancy Risk Factor B

Contraindications Hypersensitivity to ticlopidine; active bleeding disorders; neutropenia or thrombocytopenia; severe liver impairment

Warnings/Precautions Patients predisposed to bleeding such as those with gastric or duodenal ulcers; patients with underlying hematologic disorders; patients receiving oral anticoagulant therapy or nonsteroidal anti-inflammatory agents (including aspirin); liver disease; patients undergoing lumbar puncture or surgical procedure. Ticlopidine should be discontinued if the absolute neutrophil count falls to $<1200/mm^3$ or if the platelet count falls to $<80,000/mm^3$. If possible, ticlopidine should be discontinued 10-14 days prior to surgery. Use caution when phenytoin or propranolol is used concurrently.

Adverse Reactions

1% to 10%: Dermatologic: Rash

<1%:

- Dermatologic: Bruising
- Gastrointestinal: Diarrhea, nausea, vomiting, GI pain
- Hematologic: Neutropenia, thrombocytopenia
- Hepatic: Increased liver function tests
- Otic: Tinnitus
- Renal: Hematuria
- Respiratory: Epistaxis

Overdosage/Toxicology Symptoms of overdose include ataxia, seizures, vomiting, abdominal pain, hematologic abnormalities; specific treatments are lacking; after decontamination, treatment is symptomatic and supportive

Drug Interactions

Decreased effect with antacids (decreased absorption), corticosteroids; decreased effect of digoxin, cyclosporine

Increased effect/toxicity of aspirin, anticoagulants, antipyrine, theophylline, cimetidine (increased levels), NSAIDs

Mechanism of Action Ticlopidine is an inhibitor of platelet function with a mechanism which is different from other antiplatelet drugs. The drug significantly increases bleeding time. This effect may not be solely related to ticlopidine's effect on platelets. The prolongation of the bleeding time caused by ticlopidine is further increased by the addition of aspirin in *ex vivo* experiments. Although many metabolites of ticlopidine have been found, none have been shown to account for *in vivo* activity.

Pharmacodynamics/Kinetics

Onset of action: Within 6 hours

Peak: Achieved after 3-5 days of oral therapy; serum levels do not correlate with clinical antiplatelet activity

Metabolism: Extensively in the liver and has at least one active metabolite

Half-life, elimination: 24 hours

Usual Dosage Adults: Oral: 1 tablet twice daily with food

Monitoring Parameters Signs of bleeding; CBC with differential every 2 weeks starting the second week through the third month of treatment; more frequent monitoring is recommended for patients whose absolute neutrophil counts have been consistently declining or are 30% less than baseline values. Liver function tests (alkaline phosphatase and transaminases) should be performed in the first 4 months of therapy if liver dysfunction is suspected.

Test Interactions ↑ cholesterol (S), ↑ alkaline phosphatase, ↑ transaminases (S)

Dosage Forms Tablet, as hydrochloride: 250 mg

Ticlopidine Hydrochloride *see* Ticlopidine *on this page*

Ticon® *see* Trimethobenzamide *on page 1265*

TIG *see* Tetanus Immune Globulin (Human) *on page 1200*
Tigan® *see* Trimethobenzamide *on page 1265*
Tilade® Inhalation Aerosol *see* Nedocromil Sodium *on page 883*
Timentin® *see* Ticarcillin and Clavulanate Potassium *on page 1227*

Timolol (TYE moe lole)

Related Information

Antiarrhythmic Drugs *on page 1389*
Beta-Blockers Comparison *on page 1398*
Glaucoma Drug Therapy Comparison *on page 1410*

Brand Names Betimol® Ophthalmic; Blocadren® Oral; Timoptic® Ophthalmic; Timoptic-XE® Ophthalmic

Canadian/Mexican Brand Names Apo-Timol® (Canada); Apo-Timop® (Canada); Gen-Timolol® (Canada); Novo-Timol® (Canada); Nu-Timolol® (Canada); Imot® Ofteno (Mexico); Timoptol® (Mexico); Timoptol® XE (Mexico)

Synonyms Timolol Hemihydrate; Timolol Maleate

Therapeutic Category Antianginal Agent; Antihypertensive; Beta-Adrenergic Blocker; Beta-Adrenergic Blocker, Ophthalmic

Use Ophthalmic dosage form used to treat elevated intraocular pressure such as glaucoma or ocular hypertension; orally for treatment of hypertension and angina and reduce mortality following myocardial infarction and prophylaxis of migraine

Pregnancy Risk Factor C

Contraindications Uncompensated congestive heart failure, cardiogenic shock, bradycardia or heart block, severe chronic obstructive pulmonary disease, asthma, hypersensitivity to beta-blockers

Warnings/Precautions Some products contain sulfites which can cause allergic reactions; tachyphylaxis may develop; use with a miotic in angle-closure glaucoma; use with caution in patients with decreased renal or hepatic function (dosage adjustment required); severe CNS, cardiovascular and respiratory adverse effects have been seen following ophthalmic use; patients with a history of asthma, congestive heart failure, or bradycardia appear to be at a higher risk

Adverse Reactions

Ophthalmic:
- 1% to 10%:
  - Dermatologic: Alopecia
  - Ocular: Burning, stinging of eyes
- <1%:
  - Dermatologic: Rash
  - Ocular: Blepharitis, conjunctivitis, keratitis, vision disturbances

Oral:
- >10%: Endocrine & metabolic: Decreased sexual ability
- 1% to 10%:
  - Cardiovascular: Bradycardia, arrhythmia, reduced peripheral circulation
  - Central nervous system: Dizziness, fatigue
  - Dermatologic: Itching
  - Neuromuscular & skeletal: Weakness
  - Ocular: Burning eyes, stinging of eyes
  - Respiratory: Dyspnea
- <1%:
  - Cardiovascular: Chest pain, congestive heart failure
  - Central nervous system: Hallucinations, mental depression, anxiety, nightmares
  - Dermatologic: Skin rash
  - Gastrointestinal: Diarrhea, nausea, vomiting, stomach discomfort
  - Neuromuscular & skeletal: Numbness in toes and fingers
  - Ocular: Dry sore eyes

Overdosage/Toxicology Symptoms of intoxication include cardiac disturbances, CNS toxicity, bronchospasm, hypoglycemia and hyperkalemia. The most common cardiac symptoms include hypotension and bradycardia; atrioventricular block, intraventricular conduction disturbances, cardiogenic shock, and systole may occur with severe overdose, especially with membrane-depressant drugs (eg, propranolol); CNS effects include convulsions, coma, and respiratory arrest is commonly seen with propranolol and other membrane-depressant and lipid-soluble drugs.

Treatment includes symptomatic treatment of seizures, hypotension, hyperkalemia and hypoglycemia; bradycardia and hypotension resistant to atropine, isoproterenol or pacing may respond to glucagon; wide QRS defects caused by the membrane-depressant poisoning may respond to hypertonic sodium bicarbonate; repeat-dose charcoal, hemoperfusion, or hemodialysis may be helpful in removal of only those beta-blockers with a small V_d, long half-life or low intrinsic clearance (acebutolol, atenolol, nadolol, sotalol).

Drug Interactions Cytochrome P-450 2D6 enzyme substrate

Decreased effect of beta-blockers with aluminum salts, barbiturates, calcium salts, cholestyramine, colestipol, NSAIDs, penicillins (ampicillin), rifampin, salicylates and sulfinpyrazone due to decreased bioavailability and plasma levels

Beta-blockers may decrease the effect of sulfonylureas

Increased effect/toxicity of beta-blockers with calcium blockers (diltiazem, felodipine, nicardipine), contraceptives, flecainide, haloperidol (propranolol, hypotensive effects), H_2-antagonists (metoprolol, propranolol only by cimetidine, possibly ranitidine), hydralazine (metoprolol, propranolol), loop diuretics (propranolol, not atenolol), MAO inhibitors (metoprolol, nadolol, bradycardia), phenothiazines (propranolol), propafenone (metoprolol, propranolol), quinidine (in extensive metabolizers), ciprofloxacin, thyroid hormones (metoprolol, propranolol, when hypothyroid patient is converted to euthyroid state)

Beta-blockers may increase the effect/toxicity of flecainide, haloperidol (hypotensive effects), hydralazine, phenothiazines, acetaminophen, anticoagulants (propranolol, warfarin), benzodiazepines (not atenolol), clonidine (hypertensive crisis after or during withdrawal of either agent), epinephrine (initial hypertensive episode followed by bradycardia), nifedipine and verapamil lidocaine, ergots (peripheral ischemia), prazosin (postural hypotension)

Beta-blockers may affect the action or levels of ethanol, disopyramide, nondepolarizing muscle relaxants and theophylline although the effects are difficult to predict

Mechanism of Action Blocks both $beta_1$- and $beta_2$-adrenergic receptors, reduces intraocular pressure by reducing aqueous humor production or possibly outflow; reduces blood pressure by blocking adrenergic receptors and decreasing sympathetic outflow, produces a negative chronotropic and inotropic activity through an unknown mechanism

Pharmacodynamics/Kinetics

Onset of hypotensive effect: Oral: Within 15-45 minutes

Peak effect: Within 0.5-2.5 hours

Duration of action: ~4 hours; intraocular effects persist for 24 hours after ophthalmic instillation

Protein binding: 60%

Metabolism: Extensive first-pass effect; extensively metabolized in the liver

Half-life: 2-2.7 hours; prolonged with reduced renal function

Elimination: Urinary excretion (15% to 20% as unchanged drug)

Usual Dosage

Children and Adults: Ophthalmic: Initial: 0.25% solution, instill 1 drop twice daily; increase to 0.5% solution if response not adequate; decrease to 1 drop/day if controlled; do not exceed 1 drop twice daily of 0.5% solution

Adults: Oral:

Hypertension: Initial: 10 mg twice daily, increase gradually every 7 days, usual dosage: 20-40 mg/day in 2 divided doses; maximum: 60 mg/day

Prevention of myocardial infarction: 10 mg twice daily initiated within 1-4 weeks after infarction

Migraine headache: Initial: 10 mg twice daily, increase to maximum of 30 mg/day

Patient Information Apply gentle pressure to lacrimal sac during and immediately following instillation (1 minute) to avoid systemic absorption; stop drug if breathing difficulty occurs

Nursing Implications Monitor for systemic effect of beta-blockade even when administering ophthalmic product

Dosage Forms

Gel, as maleate, ophthalmic (Timoptic-XE®): 0.25% (2.5 mL, 5 mL); 0.5% (2.5 mL, 5 mL)

Solution, as hemihydrate, ophthalmic (Betimol®): 0.25% (2.5 mL, 5 mL, 10 mL, 15 mL); 0.5% (2.5 mL, 5 mL, 10 mL, 15 mL)

Solution, as maleate, ophthalmic (Timoptic®): 0.25% (2.5 mL, 5 mL, 10 mL, 15 mL); 0.5% (2.5 mL, 5 mL, 10 mL, 15 mL)

Solution, as maleate, ophthalmic, preservative free, single use (Timoptic® OcuDose®): 0.25%, 0.5%

Tablet, as maleate, (Blocadren®): 5 mg, 10 mg, 20 mg

Timolol Hemihydrate *see* Timolol *on previous page*

Timolol Maleate *see* Timolol *on previous page*

Timoptic® Ophthalmic *see* Timolol *on previous page*

Timoptic-XE® Ophthalmic *see* Timolol *on previous page*

Tinactin® [OTC] *see* Tolnaftate *on page 1243*

Tinactin® for Jock Itch [OTC] *see* Tolnaftate *on page 1243*

Tindal® *see* Acetophenazine *on page 26*

Tine Test *see* Tuberculin Purified Protein Derivative *on page 1276*

Tine Test PPD *see* Tuberculin Purified Protein Derivative *on page 1276*

Ting® [OTC] *see* Tolnaftate *on page 1243*

Tinver® Lotion *see* Sodium Thiosulfate *on page 1149*

Tioconazole (tye oh KONE a zole)

Related Information

Treatment of Sexually Transmitted Diseases *on page 1485*

Brand Names Vagistat® OTC

Therapeutic Category Antifungal Agent, Imidazole Derivative; Antifungal Agent, Vaginal

Use Local treatment of vulvovaginal candidiasis

Pregnancy Risk Factor C

Contraindications Known hypersensitivity to tioconazole

Warnings/Precautions Not effective when applied to the scalp; may interact with condoms and vaginal contraceptive diaphragms; avoid these products for 3 days following treatment

Adverse Reactions

1% to 10%: Genitourinary: Vulvar/vaginal burning

<1%: Genitourinary: Vulvar itching, soreness, edema, or discharge; polyuria

Mechanism of Action A 1-substituted imidazole derivative with a broad antifungal spectrum against a wide variety of dermatophytes and yeasts, usually at a concentration ≤6.25 mg/L; has been demonstrated to be at least as active *in vitro* as other imidazole antifungals. *In vitro*, tioconazole has been demonstrated 2-8 times as potent as miconazole against common dermal pathogens including *Trichophyton mentagrophytes*, *T. rubrum*, *T. erinacei*, *T. tonsurans*, *Microsporum canis*, *Microsporum gypseum*, and *Candida albicans*. Both agents appear to be similarly effective against *Epidermophyton floccosum*.

Pharmacodynamics/Kinetics

Absorption: Intravaginal: Following application small amounts of drug are absorbed systemically (25%) within 2-8 hours; therapeutic levels persist for 3-5 days after single dose

Half-life: 21-24 hours

Elimination: Urine and feces in approximate equal amounts

Usual Dosage Adults: Vaginal: Insert 1 applicatorful in vagina, just prior to bedtime, as a single dose; therapy may extend to 7 days

Patient Information Insert high into vagina; contact physician if itching or burning continues; Vagistat-1 may interact with condoms and vaginal contraceptive diaphragms (ie, weaken latex); do not rely on these products for 3 days following treatment

Dosage Forms Cream, vaginal: 6.5% with applicator (4.6 g)

Tioguanine *see* Thioguanine *on page 1216*

Tiotixene *see* Thiothixene *on page 1222*

Tisit® Blue Gel [OTC] *see* Pyrethrins *on page 1079*

Tisit® Liquid [OTC] *see* Pyrethrins *on page 1079*

Tisit® Shampoo [OTC] *see* Pyrethrins *on page 1079*

Titralac® [OTC] *see* Calcium Carbonate *on page 185*

Tizanidine (tye ZAN i deen)

Brand Names Zanaflex®

Synonyms Sirdalud®

Therapeutic Category Alpha$_2$-Adrenergic Agonist Agent

Use Skeletal muscle relaxant used for treatment of muscle spasticity; although not approved for these indications it has been shown to be effective for tension headaches, low back pain and trigeminal neuralgia in a limited number of trials

Pregnancy Risk Factor C

Contraindications Previous hypersensitivity to tizanidine

Warnings/Precautions Reduce dose in patients with liver or renal disease; use with caution in patients with hypotension or cardiac disease

Adverse Reactions

>10%:

- Cardiovascular: Hypotension
- Central nervous system: Sedation, daytime drowsiness, somnolence
- Gastrointestinal: Xerostomia

1% to 10%:

- Cardiovascular: Bradycardia, syncope
- Central nervous system: Fatigue, dizziness, anxiety, nervousness, insomnia
- Dermatologic: Pruritus, skin rash
- Gastrointestinal: Nausea, vomiting, dyspepsia, constipation, diarrhea
- Hepatic: Elevation of liver enzymes
- Neuromuscular & skeletal: Muscle weakness, tremor

<1%:

- Cardiovascular: Palpitations, ventricular extrasystoles

Central nervous system: Psychotic-like symptoms, visual hallucinations, delusions

Hepatic: Hepatic failure

Overdosage/Toxicology Symptoms of overdose include dry mouth, bradycardia, hypotension

Treatment: Lavage (within 2 hours of ingestion) with activated charcoal; benzodiazepines for seizure control; atropine can be given for treatment of bradycardia; flumazenil has been used to reverse coma successfully; forced diuresis is not helpful; multiple dosing of activated charcoal may be helpful. Following attempts to enhance drug elimination, hypotension should be treated with I.V. fluids and/or Trendelenburg positioning.

Drug Interactions

Increased effect: Oral contraceptives

Increased toxicity: Additive hypotensive effects may be seen with diuretics, other alpha adrenergic agonists, or antihypertensives; CNS depression with alcohol, baclofen or other CNS depressants

Mechanism of Action An $alpha_2$-adrenergic agonist agent which decreases excitatory input to alpha motor neurons; an imidazole derivative chemically-related to clonidine, which acts as a centrally acting muscle relaxant with $alpha_2$-adrenergic agonist properties; acts on the level of the spinal cord

Pharmacodynamics/Kinetics

Duration: 3-6 hours

Metabolism: Some liver metabolism

Bioavailability: 98%

Half-life: 4-8 hours

Time to peak serum concentration: 1-5 hours

Usual Dosage

Adults: 2-4 mg 3 times/day

Usual initial dose: 4 mg, may increase by 2-4 mg as needed for satisfactory reduction of muscle tone every 6-8 hours to a maximum of three doses in any 24 hour period

Maximum dose: 36 mg/day

Dosing adjustment in renal/hepatic impairment: Reduce dosage

Monitoring Parameters Monitor liver function (aminotransferases) at baseline, 1, 3, 6 months and then periodically thereafter

Dosage Forms Tablet: 4 mg

TMP *see* Trimethoprim *on page 1266*

TMP-SMX *see* Co-Trimoxazole *on page 315*

TMP-SMZ *see* Co-Trimoxazole *on page 315*

TobraDex® *see* Tobramycin and Dexamethasone *on page 1236*

Tobramycin (toe bra MYE sin)

Related Information

Antimicrobial Drugs of Choice *on page 1468*

Antimicrobial Prophylaxis *on page 1445*

Bacterial Meningitis Practical Guidelines for Management *on page 1475*

Brand Names AKTob® Ophthalmic; Nebcin® Injection; Tobrex® Ophthalmic

Canadian/Mexican Brand Names Tobra® (Mexico); Trazil® Often y Trazil® Ungena (Mexico)

Synonyms Tobramycin Sulfate

Therapeutic Category Antibiotic, Aminoglycoside; Antibiotic, Ophthalmic

Use Treatment of documented or suspected *Pseudomonas aeruginosa* infection; infection with a nonpseudomonal enteric bacillus which is more sensitive to tobramycin than gentamicin based on susceptibility tests; empiric therapy in cystic fibrosis and immunocompromised patients; topically used to treat superficial ophthalmic infections caused by susceptible bacteria

Pregnancy Risk Factor C

Contraindications Hypersensitivity to tobramycin or other aminoglycosides or components

Warnings/Precautions Use with caution in patients with renal impairment (dosage modification required), pre-existing auditory or vestibular impairment, and in patients with neuromuscular disorders; aminoglycosides are associated with nephrotoxicity or ototoxicity; the ototoxicity may be proportional to the amount of drug given and the duration of treatment; tinnitus or vertigo are indications of vestibular injury and impending hearing loss; renal damage is usually reversible

Adverse Reactions

1% to 10%:

Renal: Nephrotoxicity

Neuromuscular & skeletal: Neurotoxicity (neuromuscular blockade)

Otic: Ototoxicity (auditory), ototoxicity (vestibular)

(Continued)

Tobramycin *(Continued)*

<1%:

Cardiovascular: Hypotension
Central nervous system: Drug fever, headache, drowsiness
Dermatologic: Rash
Gastrointestinal: Nausea, vomiting
Hematologic: Eosinophilia, anemia
Neuromuscular & skeletal: Paresthesia, tremor, arthralgia, weakness
Ocular: Lacrimation, itching eyes, edema of the eyelid, keratitis
Respiratory: Dyspnea

Overdosage/Toxicology Symptoms of overdose include ototoxicity, nephrotoxicity, and neuromuscular toxicity

The treatment of choice following a single acute overdose appears to be the maintenance of good urine output of at least 3 mL/kg/hour. Dialysis is of questionable value in the enhancement of aminoglycoside elimination. If required, hemodialysis is preferred over peritoneal dialysis in patients with normal renal function. Careful hydration may be all that is required to promote diuresis and therefore the enhancement of the drug's elimination. Chelation with penicillins is investigational.

Drug Interactions

Increased effect: Extended spectrum penicillins (synergistic)
Increased toxicity:
- Neuromuscular blockers increase neuromuscular blockade
- Amphotericin B, cephalosporins, loop diuretics may increase risk of nephrotoxicity

Stability

Tobramycin is stable at room temperature both as the clear, colorless solution and as the dry powder; reconstituted solutions remain stable for 24 hours at room temperature and 96 hours when refrigerated

Stability of parenteral admixture at room temperature (25°C) and at refrigeration temperature (4°C): 48 hours

Standard diluent: Dose/100 mL NS

Minimum volume: 50 mL NS

Incompatible with penicillins

Mechanism of Action Interferes with bacterial protein synthesis by binding to 30S and 50S ribosomal subunits resulting in a defective bacterial cell membrane

Pharmacodynamics/Kinetics

Absorption: I.M.: Rapid and complete
Time to peak serum concentration:
- I.M.: Within 30-60 minutes
- I.V.: Within 30 minutes

Distribution: Crosses the placenta
- V_d: 0.2-0.3 L/kg; Pediatric patients: 0.2-0.7 L/kg; see table.

Aminoglycoside Penetration Into Various Tissues

Site	Extent of Distribution
Eye	Poor
CNS	Poor (<25%)
Pleural	Excellent
Bronchial secretions	Poor
Sputum	Fair (10%-50%)
Pulmonary tissue	Excellent
Ascitic fluid	Variable (43%-132%)
Peritoneal fluid	Poor
Bile	Variable (25%-90%)
Bile with obstruction	Poor
Synovial fluid	Excellent
Bone	Poor
Prostate	Poor
Urine	Excellent
Renal tissue	Excellent

Relative diffusion of antimicrobial agents from blood into cerebrospinal fluid (CSF): Minimal even with inflammation

Ratio of CSF to blood level (%):
- Normal meninges: Nil
- Inflamed meninges: 14-23

Protein binding: <30%

Half-life:

Neonates:

≤1200 g: 11 hours

>1200 g: 2-9 hours

Adults: 2-3 hours, directly dependent upon glomerular filtration rate

Adults with impaired renal function: 5-70 hours

Elimination: With normal renal function, about 90% to 95% of a dose is excreted in the urine within 24 hours

Usual Dosage Individualization is critical because of the low therapeutic index

Use of ideal body weight (IBW) for determining the mg/kg/dose appears to be more accurate than dosing on the basis of total body weight (TBW)

In morbid obesity, dosage requirement may best be estimated using a dosing weight of IBW + 0.4 (TBW - IBW)

Initial and periodic peak and trough plasma drug levels should be determined, particularly in critically ill patients with serious infections or in disease states known to significantly alter aminoglycoside pharmacokinetics (eg, cystic fibrosis, burns, or major surgery); 2-3 serum level measurements should be obtained after the initial dose to measure the half-life in order to determine the frequency of subsequent doses

Once daily dosing: Higher peak serum drug concentration to MIC ratios, demonstrated aminoglycoside postantibiotic effect, decreased renal cortex drug uptake, and improved cost-time efficiency are supportive reasons for the use of once daily dosing regimens for aminoglycosides. Current research indicates these regimens to be as effective for nonlife-threatening infections, with no higher incidence of nephrotoxicity, than those requiring multiple daily doses. Doses are determined by calculating the entire day's dose via usual multiple dose calculation techniques and administering this quantity as a single dose. Doses are then adjusted to maintain mean serum concentrations above the MIC(s) of the causative organism(s). (Example: 2.5-5 mg/kg as a single dose; expected Cp_{max}: 10-20 mcg/mL and Cp_{min}: <1 mcg/mL). Further research is needed for universal recommendation in all patient populations and gram-negative disease; exceptions may include those with known high clearance (eg, children, patients with cystic fibrosis, or burns who may require shorter dosage intervals) and patients with renal function impairment for whom longer than conventional dosage intervals are usually required.

Infants and Children <5 years: I.M., I.V.: 2.5 mg/kg/dose every 8 hours

Children >5 years: 1.5-2.5 mg/kg/dose every 8 hours

Note: Some patients may require larger or more frequent doses if serum levels document the need (ie, cystic fibrosis or febrile granulocytopenic patients).

Adults: I.M., I.V.:

Severe life-threatening infections: 2-2.5 mg/kg/dose

Urinary tract infection: 1.5 mg/kg/dose

Synergy (for gram-positive infections): 1 mg/kg/dose

Children and Adults: Ophthalmic: Instill 1-2 drops of solution every 4 hours; apply ointment 2-3 times/day; for severe infections apply ointment every 3-4 hours, or solution 2 drops every 30-60 minutes initially, then reduce to less frequent intervals

Dosing interval in renal impairment:

Cl_{cr} ≥60 mL/minute: Administer every 8 hours

Cl_{cr} 40-60 mL/minute: Administer every 12 hours

Cl_{cr} 20-40 mL/minute: Administer every 24 hours

Cl_{cr} 10-20 mL/minute: Administer every 48 hours

Cl_{cr} <10 mL/minute: Administer every 72 hours

Hemodialysis: Dialyzable; 30% removal of aminoglycosides occurs during 4 hours of HD - administer dose after dialysis and follow levels

Continuous arterio-venous or veno-venous hemofiltration (CAVH/CAVHD): Dose as for Cl_{cr} of 10-15 mL/minute and follow levels

Administration in CAPD fluid:

Gram-negative infection: 4-8 mg/L (4-8 mcg/mL) of CAPD fluid

Gram-positive infection (ie, synergy): 3-4 mg/L (3-4 mcg/mL) of CAPD fluid

Administration IVPB/I.M.: Dose as for Cl_{cr} <10 mL/minute and follow levels

Dosing adjustment/comments in hepatic disease: Monitor plasma concentrations

Dietary Considerations Calcium, magnesium, potassium: Renal wasting may cause hypocalcemia, hypomagnesemia, and/or hypokalemia

Monitoring Parameters Urinalysis, urine output, BUN, serum creatinine, peak and trough plasma tobramycin levels; be alert to ototoxicity; hearing should be tested before and during treatment

(Continued)

Tobramycin *(Continued)*

Reference Range

Timing of serum samples: Draw peak 30 minutes after 30-minute infusion has been completed or 1 hour following I.M. injection or beginning of infusion; draw trough immediately before next dose

Therapeutic levels:

Peak:

Serious infections: 6-8 μg/mL (SI: 12-17 mg/L)

Life-threatening infections: 8-10 μg/mL (SI: 17-21 mg/L)

Urinary tract infections: 4-6 μg/mL (SI: 7-12 mg/L)

Synergy against gram-positive organisms: 3-5 μg/mL

Trough:

Serious infections: 0.5-1 μg/mL

Life-threatening infections: 1-2 μg/mL

Monitor serum creatinine and urine output; obtain drug levels after the third dose unless otherwise directed

Test Interactions ↑ protein, ↓ magnesium, ↑ BUN, AST (SGOT), ALT (SGPT), alkaline phosphatase, creatinine, ↓ potassium, sodium, calcium (S)

Patient Information Report symptoms of superinfection; for eye drops - no other eye drops 5-10 minutes before or after tobramycin; report any dizziness or sensations of ringing or fullness in ears

Nursing Implications Eye solutions: Allow 5 minutes between application of "multiple-drop" therapy; obtain drug levels after the third dose; peak levels are drawn 30 minutes after the end of a 30-minute infusion or 1 hour after initiation of infusion or I.M. injection; the trough is drawn just before the next dose; administer penicillins or cephalosporins at least 1 hour apart from tobramycin

Dosage Forms

Injection, as sulfate (Nebcin®): 10 mg/mL (2 mL); 40 mg/mL (1.5 mL, 2 mL)

Ointment, ophthalmic (Tobrex®): 0.3% (3.5 g)

Powder for injection (Nebcin®): 40 mg/mL (1.2 g vials)

Solution, ophthalmic: 0.3% (5 mL)

AKTob®, Tobrex®: 0.3% (5 mL)

Tobramycin and Dexamethasone

(toe bra MYE sin & deks a METH a sone)

Brand Names TobraDex®

Synonyms Dexamethasone and Tobramycin

Therapeutic Category Antibiotic, Ophthalmic; Corticosteroid, Ophthalmic

Use Treatment of external ocular infection caused by susceptible gram-negative bacteria and steroid responsive inflammatory conditions of the palpebral and bulbar conjunctiva, lid, cornea, and anterior segment of the globe

Pregnancy Risk Factor B

Contraindications Known hypersensitivity to tobramycin or dexamethasone, most viral diseases of the cornea, fungal diseases, use after uncomplicated removal of a corneal foreign body

Adverse Reactions 1% to 10%:

Dermatologic: Allergic contact dermatitis

Ocular: Delayed wound healing, lacrimation, itching eyes, edema of eyelid, keratitis, increased intraocular pressure, glaucoma, cataract formation

Overdosage/Toxicology Symptoms of overdose include punctate keratitis, erythema, increased lacrimation, edema, lid itching

Flush eye with copious amounts of fluid at low pressure for 15 minutes

Drug Interactions Refer to individual monographs for Dexamethasone and Tobramycin

Mechanism of Action Refer to individual monographs for Dexamethasone and Tobramycin

Pharmacodynamics/Kinetics

Absorption: Into the aqueous humor

Time to peak serum concentration: 1-2 hours after instillation in the cornea and aqueous humor

Usual Dosage Children and Adults: Ophthalmic: Instill 1-2 drops of solution every 4 hours; apply ointment 2-3 times/day; for severe infections apply ointment every 3-4 hours, or solution 2 drops every 30-60 minutes initially, then reduce to less frequent intervals

Patient Information Shake well before using; tilt head back, place medication in conjunctival sac and close eyes, apply light finger pressure on lacrimal sac for 1 minute following instillation, notify physician if condition fails to improve or worsens

Dosage Forms

Ointment, ophthalmic: Tobramycin 0.3% and dexamethasone 0.1% (3.5 g)

Suspension, ophthalmic: Tobramycin 0.3% and dexamethasone 0.1% (2.5 mL, 5 mL)

Tobramycin Sulfate *see* Tobramycin *on page 1233*

Tobrex® Ophthalmic *see* Tobramycin *on page 1233*

Tocainide (toe KAY nide)

Related Information

Antiarrhythmic Drugs *on page 1389*

Comparative Pharmacokinetic Properties of Antiarrhythmic Agents *on page 1391*

Brand Names Tonocard®

Synonyms Tocainide Hydrochloride

Therapeutic Category Antiarrhythmic Agent, Class I-B

Use Suppress and prevent symptomatic life-threatening ventricular arrhythmias

Unlabeled use: Trigeminal neuralgia

Pregnancy Risk Factor C

Contraindications Second or third degree A-V block without a pacemaker, hypersensitivity to tocainide, amide-type anesthetics, or any component

Warnings/Precautions May exacerbate some arrhythmias (ie, atrial fibrillation/flutter); use with caution in CHF patients; administer with caution in patients with pre-existing bone marrow failure, cytopenia, severe renal or hepatic disease

Adverse Reactions

>10%:

Central nervous system: Nervousness, confusion, ataxia, dizziness
Gastrointestinal: Nausea, anorexia
Neuromuscular & skeletal: Tremor

1% to 10%:

Cardiovascular: Hypotension, tachycardia
Dermatologic: Rash
Gastrointestinal: Vomiting, diarrhea
Neuromuscular & skeletal: Arthralgia, myalgia, paresthesia
Ocular: Blurred vision

<1%:

Cardiovascular: Bradycardia, palpitations
Hematologic: Agranulocytosis, anemia, leukopenia, neutropenia
Respiratory: Respiratory arrest
Miscellaneous: Diaphoresis

Overdosage/Toxicology Has a narrow therapeutic index and severe toxicity may occur slightly above the therapeutic range, especially with other antiarrhythmic drugs; and acute ingestion of twice the daily therapeutic dose is potentially life-threatening; symptoms of overdose include sedation, confusion, coma, seizures, respiratory arrest and cardiac toxicity (sinus arrest, A-V block, asystole, and hypotension); the QRS and Q-T intervals are usually normal, although they may be prolonged after massive overdose; other effects include dizziness, paresthesias, tremor, ataxia, and GI disturbance.

Treatment is supportive, using conventional therapies (fluids, positioning, vasopressors, antiarrhythmics, anticonvulsants); sodium bicarbonate may reverse the QRS prolongation (if present), bradyarrhythmias, and hypotension; enhanced elimination with dialysis, hemoperfusion or repeat charcoal is not effective.

Drug Interactions

Decreased plasma levels: Phenobarbital, phenytoin, rifampin, and other hepatic enzyme inducers, cimetidine and drugs which make the urine acidic
Increased effect of tocainide, allopurinol
Increased toxicity/levels of caffeine and theophylline

Mechanism of Action Class 1B antiarrhythmic agent; suppresses automaticity of conduction tissue, by increasing electrical stimulation threshold of ventricle, HIS-Purkinje system, and spontaneous depolarization of the ventricles during diastole by a direct action on the tissues; blocks both the initiation and conduction of nerve impulses by decreasing the neuronal membrane's permeability to sodium ions, which results in inhibition of depolarization with resultant blockade of conduction

Pharmacodynamics/Kinetics

Absorption: Oral: Extensive, 99% to 100%
Distribution: V_d: 1.62-3.2 L/kg
Protein binding: 10% to 20%
Metabolism: In the liver to inactive metabolites; first-pass effect is negligible
Half-life: 11-14 hours, prolonged with renal and hepatic impairment with half-life increased to 23-27 hours
Time to peak: Peak serum levels occur within 30-160 minutes
Elimination: In urine (40% to 50% as unchanged drug)

Usual Dosage Adults: Oral: 1200-1800 mg/day in 3 divided doses, up to 2400 mg/day

(Continued)

Tocainide *(Continued)*

Dosing adjustment in renal impairment: Cl_{cr} <30 mL/minute: Administer 50% of normal dose or 600 mg once daily

Hemodialysis: Moderately dialyzable (20% to 50%)

Dosing adjustment in hepatic impairment: Maximum daily dose: 1200 mg

Reference Range Therapeutic: 5-12 μg/mL (SI: 22-52 μmol/L)

Patient Information Report any unusual bleeding, fever, sore throat, or any breathing difficulties; do not discontinue or alter dose without notifying physician; may cause drowsiness, dizziness, impair judgment, and coordination

Nursing Implications Monitor for tremor; titration of dosing and initiation of therapy require cardiac monitoring

Dosage Forms Tablet, as hydrochloride: 400 mg, 600 mg

Tocainide Hydrochloride *see* Tocainide *on previous page*

Tofranil® *see* Imipramine *on page 648*

Tofranil-PM® *see* Imipramine *on page 648*

Tolazamide (tole AZ a mide)

Related Information

Hypoglycemic Drugs, Comparison of Oral Agents *on page 1411*

Sulfonamide Derivatives *on page 1420*

Brand Names Tolinase®

Therapeutic Category Antidiabetic Agent, Oral; Antihyperglycemic Agent; Hypoglycemic Agent, Oral; Sulfonylurea Agent

Use Adjunct to diet for the management of mild to moderately severe, stable, noninsulin-dependent (type II) diabetes mellitus

Pregnancy Risk Factor D

Contraindications Type I diabetes therapy (IDDM), hypersensitivity to sulfonylureas, diabetes complicated by ketoacidosis

Warnings/Precautions False-positive response has been reported in patients with liver disease, idiopathic hypoglycemia of infancy, severe malnutrition, acute pancreatitis, renal dysfunction. Transferring a patient from one sulfonylurea to another does not require a priming dose; doses >1000 mg/day normally do not improve diabetic control. Has not been studied in older patients; however, except for drug interactions, it appears to have a safe profile and decline in renal function does not affect its pharmacokinetics. How "tightly" an elderly patient's blood glucose should be controlled is controversial; however, a fasting blood sugar <150 mg/dL is now an acceptable end point. Such a decision should be based on the patient's functional and cognitive status, how well they recognize hypoglycemic or hyperglycemic symptoms, and how to respond to them and their other disease states.

Adverse Reactions

>10%:

- Central nervous system: Headache, dizziness
- Gastrointestinal: Anorexia, nausea, vomiting, diarrhea, constipation, heartburn, epigastric fullness

1% to 10%: Dermatologic: Rash, urticaria, photosensitivity

<1%:

- Endocrine & metabolic: Hypoglycemia
- Hematologic: Aplastic anemia, hemolytic anemia, bone marrow suppression, thrombocytopenia, agranulocytosis
- Hepatic: Cholestatic jaundice
- Renal: Diuretic effect

Overdosage/Toxicology Symptoms of overdose include low blood sugar, tingling of lips and tongue, nausea, yawning, confusion, agitation, tachycardia, sweating, convulsions, stupor, and coma; intoxications with sulfonylureas can cause hypoglycemia and are best managed with glucose administration (oral for milder hypoglycemia or by injection in more severe forms)

Drug Interactions

Increased toxicity: Monitor patient closely; large number of drugs interact with sulfonylureas including salicylates, anticoagulants, H_2-antagonists, TCAs, MAO inhibitors, beta-blockers, thiazides

Mechanism of Action Stimulates insulin release from the pancreatic beta cells; reduces glucose output from the liver; insulin sensitivity is increased at peripheral target sites

Pharmacodynamics/Kinetics

Onset of action: Oral: Within 4-6 hours

Duration: 10-24 hours

Protein binding: >98% ionic/nonionic

Metabolism: Extensively in the liver to one active and three inactive metabolites

Half-life: 7 hours

Elimination: Renal

Usual Dosage Oral (doses >1000 mg/day normally do not improve diabetic control):

Adults: Initial: 100 mg/day, increase at 2- to 4-week intervals; maximum dose: 1000 mg; administer as a single or twice daily dose
Conversion from insulin → tolazamide
10 units day = 100 mg/day
20-40 units/day = 250 mg/day
>40 units/day = 250 mg/day and 50% of insulin dose
Doses >500 mg/day should be given in 2 divided doses

Dosing comments in hepatic impairment: Initial and maintenance doses should be conservative

Dietary Considerations Alcohol: Avoid use

Monitoring Parameters Signs and symptoms of hypoglycemia, (fatigue, sweating, numbness of extremities); urine for glucose and ketones; fasting blood glucose; hemoglobin A_{1c} or fructosamine

Reference Range Target range:
Fasting blood glucose:
Adults: 80-140 mg/dL
Geriatrics: 100-150 mg/dL
Glycosylated hemoglobin: <7%

Patient Information Tablets may be crushed; take drug at the same time each day; avoid alcohol; recognize signs and symptoms of hyper- and hypoglycemia; report any persistent or severe sore throat, fever, malaise, unusual bleeding, or bruising; can take with food; do not skip meals; carry a quick sugar source; medical alert bracelet

Nursing Implications Patients who are anorexic or NPO may need to have their dose held to avoid hypoglycemia

Dosage Forms Tablet: 100 mg, 250 mg, 500 mg

Tolazoline (tole AZ oh leen)

Brand Names Priscoline®

Synonyms Benzazoline Hydrochloride; Tolazoline Hydrochloride

Therapeutic Category Alpha-Adrenergic Blocking Agent, Parenteral

Use Treatment of persistent pulmonary vasoconstriction and hypertension of the newborn (persistent fetal circulation), peripheral vasospastic disorders

Pregnancy Risk Factor C

Contraindications Hypersensitivity to tolazoline; known or suspected coronary artery disease

Warnings/Precautions Stimulates gastric secretion and may activate stress ulcers; therefore, use with caution in patients with gastritis, peptic ulcer; use with caution in patients with mitral stenosis

Adverse Reactions
>10%:
Cardiovascular: Hypotension,
Endocrine & metabolic: Hypochloremic alkalosis
Gastrointestinal: GI bleeding, abdominal pain
Hematologic: Thrombocytopenia
Local: Burning at injection site
Renal: Acute renal failure, oliguria
1% to 10%:
Cardiovascular: Peripheral vasodilation, tachycardia
Gastrointestinal: Nausea, diarrhea
Neuromuscular & skeletal: Increased pilomotor activity
<1%:
Cardiovascular: Hypertension, tachycardia, arrhythmias
Hematologic: Increased agranulocytosis, pancytopenia
Ocular: Mydriasis
Respiratory: Pulmonary hemorrhage
Miscellaneous: Increased secretions

Overdosage/Toxicology Symptoms of overdose include hypotension, shock, flushing; I.V. fluids and Trendelenburg position for hypotension; if pressors are required, use direct-acting alpha agonists (norepinephrine)

Drug Interactions
Decreased effect (vasopressor) of epinephrine followed by a rebound increase in blood pressure
Increased toxicity: Disulfiram reaction may possibly be seen with concomitant ethanol use

Stability Compatible in D_5W, $D_{10}W$, and saline solutions

Mechanism of Action Competitively blocks alpha-adrenergic receptors to produce brief antagonism of circulating epinephrine and norepinephrine; reduces hypertension caused by catecholamines and causes vascular smooth muscle
(Continued)

Tolazoline *(Continued)*

relaxation (direct action); results in peripheral vasodilation and decreased peripheral resistance

Pharmacodynamics/Kinetics

Half-life: Neonates: 3-10 hours, increased half-life with decreased renal function, oliguria

Time to peak serum concentration: Within 30 minutes

Elimination: Excreted rapidly in urine primarily as unchanged drug

Usual Dosage

Neonates: Initial: I.V.: 1-2 mg/kg over 10-15 minutes via scalp vein or upper extremity; maintenance: 1-2 mg/kg/hour; use lower maintenance doses in patients with decreased renal function. Also used in neonates for acute vasospasm "cath toes" at 0.25 mg/kg/hour (no load); maximum dose: 6-8 mg/kg/hour

Dosing interval in renal impairment in newborns: Urine output <0.9 mL/kg/hour: Decrease dose to 0.08 mg/kg/hour for every 1 mg/kg of loading dose

Adults: Peripheral vasospastic disorder: I.M., I.V., S.C.: 10-50 mg 4 times/day

Dietary Considerations Alcohol: Avoid use

Monitoring Parameters Vital signs, blood gases, cardiac monitor

Patient Information Side effects decrease with continued therapy; avoid alcohol

Nursing Implications Dilute in D_5W; monitor blood pressure for hypotension; observe limbs for change in color; do not mix with any other drug in syringe or bag

Dosage Forms Injection, as hydrochloride: 25 mg/mL (4 mL)

Tolazoline Hydrochloride *see* Tolazoline *on previous page*

Tolbutamide (tole BYOO ta mide)

Related Information

Hypoglycemic Drugs, Comparison of Oral Agents *on page 1411*

Sulfonamide Derivatives *on page 1420*

Brand Names Orinase®

Canadian/Mexican Brand Names Apo-Tolbutamide® (Canada); Mobenol® (Canada); Novo-Butamide® (Canada); Artosin® (Mexico); Diaval® (Mexico); Rastinon® (Mexico)

Synonyms Tolbutamide Sodium

Therapeutic Category Antidiabetic Agent, Oral; Antihyperglycemic Agent; Diagnostic Agent, Hypoglycemia; Diagnostic Agent, Insulinoma; Hypoglycemic Agent, Oral; Sulfonylurea Agent

Use Adjunct to diet for the management of mild to moderately severe, stable, noninsulin-dependent (type II) diabetes mellitus

Pregnancy Risk Factor D

Contraindications Diabetes complicated by ketoacidosis, therapy of IDDM, hypersensitivity to sulfonylureas

Warnings/Precautions False-positive response has been reported in patients with liver disease, idiopathic hypoglycemia of infancy, severe malnutrition, acute pancreatitis. Because of its low potency and short duration, it is a useful agent in the elderly if drug interactions can be avoided. How "tightly" an elderly patient's blood glucose should be controlled is controversial; however, a fasting blood sugar <150 mg/dL is now an acceptable end point. Such a decision should be based on the patient's functional and cognitive status, how well they recognize hypoglycemic or hyperglycemic symptoms, and how to respond to them and their other disease states.

Adverse Reactions

>10%:

Central nervous system: Headache, dizziness

Gastrointestinal: Constipation, diarrhea, heartburn, anorexia, epigastric fullness

1% to 10%: Dermatologic: Rash, urticaria, photosensitivity

<1%:

Cardiovascular: Venospasm

Endocrine & metabolic: SIADH, disulfiram-type reactions

Hematologic: Thrombocytopenia, agranulocytosis, hypoglycemia, leukopenia, aplastic anemia, hemolytic anemia, bone marrow suppression

Hepatic: Cholestatic jaundice

Local: Thrombophlebitis

Otic: Tinnitus

Miscellaneous: Hypersensitivity reaction

Overdosage/Toxicology Symptoms of overdose include low blood sugar, tingling of lips and tongue, nausea, yawning, confusion, agitation, tachycardia, sweating, convulsions, stupor, and coma

Treatment: I.V. glucose (12.5-25 g), epinephrine for anaphylaxis

Drug Interactions

Increased effects with salicylates, probenecid, MAO inhibitors, chloramphenicol, insulin, phenylbutazone, antidepressants, metformin, H_2-antagonists, and others

Decreased effects:

Hypoglycemic effects may be decreased by beta-blockers, cholestyramine, hydantoins, thiazides, rifampin, and others

Ethanol may decrease the half-life of tolbutamide

Stability Use parenteral formulation within 1 hour following reconstitution

Mechanism of Action Stimulates insulin release from the pancreatic beta cells; reduces glucose output from the liver; insulin sensitivity is increased at peripheral target sites, suppression of glucagon may also contribute

Pharmacodynamics/Kinetics

Peak hypoglycemic action:

Oral: 1-3 hours

I.V.: 30 minutes

Duration:

Oral: 6-24 hours

I.V.: 3 hours

Time to peak serum concentration: 3-5 hours

Absorption: Oral: Rapid

Distribution: V_d: 6-10 L

Protein binding: 95% to 97% (principally to albumin) ionic/nonionic

Metabolism/Elimination: Hepatic metabolism to hydroxymethyltolbutamide (mildly active) and carboxytolbutamide (inactive) both rapidly excreted renally, less 2% excreted in the urine unchanged; metabolism does not appear to be affected by age

Increased plasma concentrations and volume of distribution secondary to decreased albumin concentrations and less protein binding have been reported.

Half-life:

Plasma: 4-25 hours

Elimination: 4-9 hours

Usual Dosage Divided doses may increase gastrointestinal side effects

Adults:

Oral: Initial: 500-1000 mg 1-3 times/day; usual dose should not be more than 2 g/day

I.V. bolus: 1 g over 2-3 minutes

Elderly: Oral: Initial: 250 mg 1-3 times/day; usual: 500-2000 mg; maximum: 3 g/day

Dosing adjustment in hepatic impairment: Dose reduction is necessary

Hemodialysis: Not dialyzable (0% to 5%)

Dietary Considerations Alcohol: Avoid use

Monitoring Parameters Fasting blood glucose, hemoglobin A_{1c} or fructosamine

Reference Range Target range:

Fasting blood glucose: <120 mg/dL

Adults: 80-140 mg/dL

Geriatrics: 100-150 mg/dL

Glycosylated hemoglobin: <7%

Patient Information Tablets may be crushed; take drug at the same time each day; avoid alcohol; recognize signs and symptoms of hyper- and hypoglycemia; report any persistent or severe sore throat, fever, malaise, unusual bleeding, or bruising; can take with food

Nursing Implications Patients who are anorexic or NPO may need to have their dose held to avoid hypoglycemia

Additional Information Sodium content of 1 g vial: 3.5 mEq

Dosage Forms

Injection, diagnostic, as sodium: 1 g (20 mL)

Tablet: 250 mg, 500 mg

Tolbutamide Sodium *see* Tolbutamide *on previous page*

Tolectin® 200 *see* Tolmetin *on this page*

Tolectin® 400 *see* Tolmetin *on this page*

Tolectin® DS *see* Tolmetin *on this page*

Tolinase® *see* Tolazamide *on page 1238*

Tolmetin (TOLE met in)

Related Information

Antacid Drug Interactions *on page 1388*

Nonsteroidal Anti-Inflammatory Agents Comparison *on page 1419*

Brand Names Tolectin® 200; Tolectin® 400; Tolectin® DS

(Continued)

Tolmetin *(Continued)*

Canadian/Mexican Brand Names Novo-Tolmetin® (Canada)

Synonyms Tolmetin Sodium

Therapeutic Category Analgesic, Nonsteroidal Anti-inflammatory Drug; Anti-inflammatory Agent; Nonsteroidal Anti-inflammatory Agent (NSAID), Oral

Use Treatment of rheumatoid arthritis and osteoarthritis, juvenile rheumatoid arthritis

Pregnancy Risk Factor C (D at term)

Contraindications Known hypersensitivity to tolmetin or any component, aspirin, or other nonsteroidal anti-inflammatory drugs (NSAIDs)

Warnings/Precautions Use with caution in patients with upper GI disease, impaired renal function, congestive heart failure, hypertension, and patients receiving anticoagulants; if GI upset occurs with tolmetin, take with antacids other than sodium bicarbonate

Adverse Reactions

>10%:
- Central nervous system: Dizziness
- Dermatologic: Rash
- Gastrointestinal: Abdominal cramps, heartburn, indigestion, nausea

1% to 10%:
- Central nervous system: Headache, nervousness
- Dermatologic: Itching
- Endocrine & metabolic: Fluid retention
- Gastrointestinal: Vomiting
- Otic: Tinnitus

<1%:
- Cardiovascular: Congestive heart failure, hypertension, arrhythmias, tachycardia
- Central nervous system: Confusion, hallucinations, aseptic meningitis, mental depression, drowsiness, insomnia
- Dermatologic: Urticaria, erythema multiforme, toxic epidermal necrolysis, Stevens-Johnson syndrome, angioedema
- Endocrine & metabolism: Polydipsia, hot flashes
- Gastrointestinal: Gastritis, GI ulceration
- Genitourinary: Cystitis, polyuria
- Hematologic: Agranulocytosis, anemia, hemolytic anemia, bone marrow suppression, leukopenia, thrombocytopenia
- Hepatic: Hepatitis
- Neuromuscular & skeletal: Peripheral neuropathy
- Ocular: Toxic amblyopia, blurred vision, conjunctivitis, dry eyes
- Otic: Decreased hearing
- Renal: Acute renal failure
- Respiratory: Allergic rhinitis, shortness of breath, epistaxis

Overdosage/Toxicology Symptoms of overdose include lethargy, mental confusion, dizziness, leukocytosis, renal failure

Management of a nonsteroidal anti-inflammatory drug (NSAID) intoxication is primarily supportive and symptomatic. Fluid therapy is commonly effective in managing the hypotension that may occur following an acute NSAID overdose, except when this is due to an acute blood loss. Seizures tend to be very short-lived and often do not require drug treatment; although, recurrent seizures should be treated with I.V. diazepam. Since many of the NSAID undergo enterohepatic cycling, multiple doses of charcoal may be needed to reduce the potential for delayed toxicities.

Drug Interactions

Decreased effect with aspirin; decreased effect of thiazides, furosemide

Increased toxicity of digoxin, methotrexate, cyclosporine, lithium, insulin, sulfonylureas, potassium-sparing diuretics, aspirin

Mechanism of Action Inhibits prostaglandin synthesis by decreasing the activity of the enzyme, cyclo-oxygenase, which results in decreased formation of prostaglandin precursors

Pharmacodynamics/Kinetics

- Absorption: Oral: Well absorbed
- Bioavailability: Food/milk decreases total bioavailability by 16%
- Time to peak serum concentration: Within 30-60 minutes

Usual Dosage Oral:

Children ≥2 years:
- Anti-inflammatory: Initial: 20 mg/kg/day in 3 divided doses, then 15-30 mg/kg/day in 3 divided doses
- Analgesic: 5-7 mg/kg/dose every 6-8 hours

Adults: 400 mg 3 times/day; usual dose: 600 mg to 1.8 g/day; maximum: 2 g/day

Monitoring Parameters Occult blood loss, CBC, liver enzymes, BUN, serum creatinine, periodic liver function test

Test Interactions ↑ protein, ↑ bleeding time

Patient Information Take with food, milk, or water; may cause drowsiness, impair judgment or coordination

Additional Information Sodium content of 200 mg: 0.8 mEq

Dosage Forms

Capsule, as sodium (Tolectin® DS): 400 mg

Tablet, as sodium (Tolectin®): 200 mg, 600 mg

Tolmetin Sodium *see* Tolmetin *on page 1241*

Tolnaftate (tole NAF tate)

Brand Names Absorbine® Antifungal [OTC]; Absorbine® Jock Itch [OTC]; Absorbine Jr.® Antifungal [OTC]; Aftate® for Athlete's Foot [OTC]; Aftate® for Jock Itch [OTC]; Blis-To-Sol® [OTC]; Breezee® Mist Antifungal [OTC]; Dr Scholl's Athlete's Foot [OTC]; Dr Scholl's Maximum Strength Tritin [OTC]; Genaspor® [OTC]; NP-27® [OTC]; Quinsana Plus® [OTC]; Tinactin® [OTC]; Tinactin® for Jock Itch [OTC]; Ting® [OTC]; Zeasorb-AF® Powder [OTC]

Canadian/Mexican Brand Names Pitrex® (Canada); Tinaderm® (Mexico)

Therapeutic Category Antifungal Agent, Topical

Use Treatment of tinea pedis, tinea cruris, tinea corporis, tinea manuum, tinea versicolor infections

Pregnancy Risk Factor C

Contraindications Known hypersensitivity to tolnaftate; nail and scalp infections

Warnings/Precautions Cream is not recommended for nail or scalp infections; keep from eyes; if no improvement within 4 weeks, treatment should be discontinued. Usually not effective alone for the treatment of infections involving hair follicles or nails.

Adverse Reactions

1% to 10%:

Dermatologic: Pruritus, contact dermatitis

Local: Irritation, stinging

Mechanism of Action Distorts the hyphae and stunts mycelial growth in susceptible fungi

Pharmacodynamics/Kinetics Onset of action: Response may be seen 24-72 hours after initiation of therapy

Usual Dosage Children and Adults: Topical: Wash and dry affected area; apply 1-3 drops of solution or a small amount of cream or powder and rub into the affected areas 2-3 times/day for 2-4 weeks

Monitoring Parameters Resolution of skin infection

Patient Information Avoid contact with the eyes; apply to clean dry area; consult the physician if a skin irritation develops or if the skin infection worsens or does not improve after 10 days of therapy; does not stain skin or clothing

Nursing Implications Itching, burning, and soreness are usually relieved within 24-72 hours

Dosage Forms

Aerosol, topical:

Liquid: 1% (59.2 mL, 90 mL, 120 mL)

Powder: 1% (56.7 g, 100 g, 105 g, 150 g)

Cream: 1% (15 g, 30 g)

Gel, topical: 1% (15 g)

Powder, topical: 1% (45 g, 90 g)

Solution, topical: 1% (10 mL)

Tolu-Sed® DM [OTC] *see* Guaifenesin and Dextromethorphan *on page 591*

Tonocard® *see* Tocainide *on page 1237*

Topamax® *see* Topiramate *on this page*

Topicort® *see* Desoximetasone *on page 355*

Topicort®-LP *see* Desoximetasone *on page 355*

Topicycline® *see* Tetracycline *on page 1203*

Topiramate (toe PYE ra mate)

Related Information

Anticonvulsants by Seizure Type *on page 1392*

Brand Names Topamax®

Therapeutic Category Anticonvulsant, Miscellaneous

Use Adjunctive therapy for partial onset seizures in adults; topiramate has also been granted orphan drug status for the treatment of Lennox-Gastaut syndrome

Pregnancy Risk Factor C

Pregnancy/Breast-Feeding Implications In studies of rats topiramate has been shown to be secreted in milk; however, it has not been studied in humans

Contraindications Patients with a known hypersensitivity to any components of this drug

(Continued)

Topiramate *(Continued)*

Warnings/Precautions Avoid abrupt withdrawal of topiramate therapy, it should be withdrawn slowly to minimize the potential of increased seizure frequency; the risk of kidney stones is about 2-4 times that of the untreated population, the risk of this event may be reduced by increasing fluid intake; use cautiously in patients with hepatic or renal impairment, during pregnancy or in nursing mothers.

Adverse Reactions

>10%:

Central nervous system: Fatigue, dizziness, ataxia, somnolence, psychomotor slowing, nervousness, memory difficulties, speech problems

Gastrointestinal: Nausea

Neuromuscular & skeletal: Paresthesia, tremor

Ocular: Nystagmus

Respiratory: Upper respiratory infections

1% to 10%:

Cardiovascular: Chest pain, edema

Central nervous system: Language problems, abnormal coordination, confusion, depression, difficulty concentrating, hypoesthesia

Endocrine & metabolic: Hot flashes

Gastrointestinal: Dyspepsia, abdominal pain, anorexia, constipation, xerostomia, gingivitis, weight loss

Neuromuscular & skeletal: Myalgia, weakness, back pain, leg pain, rigors

Otic: Decreased hearing

Renal: Nephrolithiasis

Respiratory: Pharyngitis, sinusitis, epistaxis

Miscellaneous: Flu-like symptoms

Overdosage/Toxicology Activated charcoal has not been shown to adsorb topiramate and is therefore not recommended; hemodialysis can remove drug, however, most cases do not require removal and instead is best treated with supportive measures

Drug Interactions

Decreased effect: Phenytoin can decrease topiramate levels by as much as 48%, carbamazepine reduces it by 40% and valproic acid reduces topiramate by 14%; digoxin levels and norethindrone blood levels are decreased when coadministered with topiramate

Increased toxicity: Concomitant administration with other CNS depressants will increase its sedative effects; coadministration with other carbonic anhydrase inhibitors may increase the chance of nephrolithiasis

Mechanism of Action Mechanism is not fully understood, it is thought to decrease seizure frequency by blocking sodium channels in neurons, enhancing GABA activity and by blocking glutamate activity

Pharmacodynamics/Kinetics

Absorption: Good; unaffected by food

Protein binding: 13% to 17%

Metabolism: Minimal, less than 5% of metabolites are active

Bioavailability: 80%

Half-life: Mean: 21 hours in adults

Time to peak serum concentration: ~2-4 hours

Elimination: Primarily eliminated unchanged in the urine

Dialyzable: ~30%

Usual Dosage

Adults: Initial: 50 mg/day; titrate by 50 mg/day at 1-week intervals to target dose of 200 mg twice daily; usual maximum dose: 1600 mg/day

Dosing adjustment in renal impairment: Cl_{cr} <70 mL/minute: Administer 50% dose and titrate more slowly

Dosing adjustment in hepatic impairment: Clearance may be minimally reduced

Dosage Forms Tablet: 25 mg, 100 mg, 200 mg

TOPO *see* Topotecan *on this page*

Toposar® Injection *see* Etoposide *on page 496*

Topotecan (toe poe TEE kan)

Brand Names Hycamtin®

Synonyms Hycamptamine; SK and F 104864; SKF 104864; SKF 104864-A; TOPO; Topotecan Hydrochloride; TPT

Therapeutic Category Antineoplastic Agent, Antibiotic

Use Treatment of metastatic carcinoma of the ovary after failure of initial or subsequent chemotherapy

Unlabeled use: Under investigation for the treatment of nonsmall cell lung cancer, small cell lung cancer, sarcoma (pediatrics)

Pregnancy Risk Factor D

Contraindications Hypersensitivity to any component, pregnancy, breast-feeding

Warnings/Precautions The U.S. Food and Drug Administration (FDA) currently recommends that procedures for proper handling and disposal of antineoplastic agents be considered; monitor bone marrow function

Adverse Reactions

>10%:

Central nervous system: Headache

Dermatologic: Alopecia (reversible)

Gastrointestinal: Nausea, vomiting, diarrhea

Emetic potential: Moderately low (10% to 30%)

Hematologic: Myelosuppressive: Principle dose-limiting toxicity; white blood cell count nadir is 8-11 days after administration and is more frequent than thrombocytopenia (at lower doses); recover is usually within 21 days and cumulative toxicity has not been noted

WBC: Mild to severe

Platelets: Mild (at low doses)

Nadir (days): 8-11

Recovery (days): 14-21

1% to 10%:

Neuromuscular & skeletal: Paresthesia

Respiratory: Dyspnea

<1%: Local: Mild erythema and bruising

Drug Interactions

Increased toxicity: Filgrastim (G-CSF): Prolonged/severe neutropenia and thrombocytopenia; concomitant administration with other antineoplastics has been associated with increased morbidity/mortality - not recommended (eg, cisplatin)

Stability

Store intact vials of lyophilized powder for injection at room temperature and protected from light. Topotecan should be initially reconstituted with 4 mL SWI. This solution is stable for 24 hours at room temperature. Topotecan should be further diluted in 100 mL D_5W. This solution is stable for 24 hours at room temperature.

Standard I.V. dilution: Dose/100 mL D_5W; stability is pH dependent; although topotecan may be further diluted in 0.9% NaCl, stability is longer in D_5W

Mechanism of Action Inhibits topoisomerase I (an enzyme which relaxes torsionally strained-coiled duplex DNA) to prevent DNA replication and translocation; topotecan acts in S phase

Pharmacodynamics/Kinetics

Absorption: Oral: ~30%

Distribution: V_{dss} of the lactone is high (mean: 87.3 L/mm^2; range: 25.6-186 L/mm^2), suggesting wide distribution and/or tissue sequestering

Metabolism: Topotecan (TPT) undergoes a rapid, pH-dependent opening of the lactone ring to yield a relatively inactive hydroxy acid in plasma.

Half-life: 3 hours

Protein binding: 35%

Elimination: Primarily renal, with 30% of dose eliminated within 24 hours

Usual Dosage Refer to individual protocols

Adults:

Metastatic ovarian cancer: IVPB: 1.5 mg/m^2/day for 5 days; repeated every 21 days (neutrophil count should be >1500/mm^3 and platelet count should be >100,000/mm^3)

Dosage adjustment for hematological effects: If neutrophil count <1500/mm^3, reduce dose by 0.25 mg/m^2/day for 5 days for next cycle

Dosing adjustment in renal impairment:

Cl_{cr} 20-39 mL/minute: Administer 50% of normal dose

Cl_{cr} <20 mL/minute: Do not use, insufficient data available

Hemodialysis: Supplemental dose is not necessary

CAPD effects: Unknown

CAVH effects: Unknown

Dosing adjustment in hepatic impairment: Bilirubin 1.5-10 mg/dL: Dosage adjustment is not necessary

Administration Administer lower doses IVPB over 30 minutes

Monitoring Parameters CBC with differential and platelet count and renal function tests

Test Interactions None known

Patient Information Any signs of infection, easy bruising or bleeding, shortness of breath, painful or burning urination should be brought to the physician's attention. Nausea, vomiting, or hair loss sometimes occur. The drug may cause permanent sterility and may cause birth defects. The drug may be excreted in breast milk, therefore, an alternative form of feeding your baby should be used.

(Continued)

Topotecan *(Continued)*

Additional Information Constituted vial: When constituted with 2 mL of sterile water for injection, USP, each mL contains topotecan 2.5 mg and mannitol 50 mg with a pH of approximately 3.5. Final infusion preparation: Topotecan constituted solution should be further diluted in 5% dextrose injection. Topotecan should NOT be diluted in buffered solutions.

Dosage Forms Powder for injection, as hydrochloride, lyophilized: 4 mg (base)

Topotecan Hydrochloride *see* Topotecan *on page 1244*
Toprol XL® *see* Metoprolol *on page 827*
TOPV *see* Polio Vaccines *on page 1015*
Toradol® *see* Ketorolac Tromethamine *on page 698*
Torecan® *see* Thiethylperazine *on page 1215*
Tornalate® *see* Bitolterol *on page 158*

Torsemide (TOR se mide)

Related Information

Sulfonamide Derivatives *on page 1420*

Brand Names Demadex®

Therapeutic Category Antihypertensive; Diuretic, Loop

Use Management of edema associated with congestive heart failure and hepatic or renal disease; used alone or in combination with antihypertensives in treatment of hypertension; I.V. form is indicated when rapid onset is desired

Pregnancy Risk Factor B

Pregnancy/Breast-Feeding Implications A decrease in fetal weight, an increase in fetal resorption, and delayed fetal ossification has occurred in animal studies

Contraindications Anuria; hypersensitivity to torsemide or any component, or other sulfonylureas; safety in children <18 years has not been established

Warnings/Precautions Excessive diuresis may result in dehydration, acute hypotensive or thromboembolic episodes and cardiovascular collapse; rapid injection, renal impairment, or excessively large doses may result in ototoxicity; SLE may be exacerbated; sudden alterations in electrolyte balance may precipitate hepatic encephalopathy and coma in patients with hepatic cirrhosis and ascites; monitor carefully for signs of fluid or electrolyte imbalances, especially hypokalemia in patients at risk for such (eg, digitalis therapy, history of ventricular arrhythmias, elderly, etc), hyperuricemia, hypomagnesemia, or hypocalcemia; use caution with exposure to ultraviolet light.

Adverse Reactions

>10%: Cardiovascular: Orthostatic hypotension

1% to 10%:

- Central nervous system: Headache, dizziness, vertigo, pain
- Dermatologic: Photosensitivity, urticaria
- Endocrine & metabolic: Electrolyte imbalance, dehydration, hyperuricemia
- Gastrointestinal: Diarrhea, loss of appetite, stomach cramps, pancreatitis
- Ocular: Blurred vision

<1%:

- Dermatologic: Rash
- Endocrine & metabolic: Gout
- Gastrointestinal: Pancreatitis, nausea
- Hepatic: Hepatic dysfunction
- Hematologic: Agranulocytosis, leukopenia, anemia, thrombocytopenia
- Local: Redness at injection site
- Otic: Ototoxicity
- Renal: Nephrocalcinosis, prerenal azotemia, interstitial nephritis

Overdosage/Toxicology Symptoms include electrolyte depletion, volume depletion, hypotension, dehydration, circulatory collapse; electrolyte depletion may be manifested by weakness, dizziness, mental confusion, anorexia, lethargy, vomiting, and cramps

Following GI decontamination, treatment is supportive; hypotension responds to fluids and Trendelenburg position

Drug Interactions

- Aminoglycosides: Ototoxicity may be increased; anticoagulant activity is enhanced
- Beta-blockers: Plasma concentrations of beta-blockers may be increased
- Cisplatin: Ototoxicity may be increased
- Digitalis: Arrhythmias may occur with diuretic-induced electrolyte disturbances
- Lithium: Plasma concentrations of lithium may be increased
- NSAIDs: Torsemide efficacy may be decreased
- Probenecid: Torsemide action may be reduced
- Salicylates: Diuretic action may be impaired in patients with cirrhosis and ascites

Sulfonylureas: Glucose tolerance may be decreased
Thiazides: Synergistic effects may result

Mechanism of Action Inhibits reabsorption of sodium and chloride in the ascending loop of Henle and distal renal tubule, interfering with the chloride-binding cotransport system, thus causing increased excretion of water, sodium, chloride, magnesium, and calcium; does not alter GFR, renal plasma flow, or acid-base balance

Pharmacodynamics/Kinetics

Onset of diuresis: 30-60 minutes
Peak effect: 1-4 hours
Duration: ~6 hours
Absorption: Oral: Rapid
Protein binding: Plasma: ~97% to 99%
Metabolism: Hepatic by cytochrome P-450, 80%
Bioavailability: 80% to 90%
Half-life: 2-4; 7-8 hours in cirrhosis (dose modification appears unnecessary)
Elimination: 20% eliminated unchanged in urine; hemodialysis does not accelerate removal

Usual Dosage Adults: Oral, I.V.:

Congestive heart failure: 10-20 mg once daily; may increase gradually for chronic treatment by doubling dose until the diuretic response is apparent (for acute treatment, I.V. dose may be repeated every 2 hours with double the dose as needed)
Chronic renal failure: 20 mg once daily; increase as described above
Hepatic cirrhosis: 5-10 mg once daily with an aldosterone antagonist or a potassium-sparing diuretic; increase as described above
Hypertension: 5 mg once daily; increase to 10 mg after 4-6 weeks if an adequate hypotensive response is not apparent; if still not effective, an additional antihypertensive agent may be added

Administration I.V. injections should be given over ≥2 minutes; the oral form may be given regardless of meal times; patients may be switched from the I.V. form to the oral and vice-versa with no change in dose; no dosage adjustment is needed in the elderly or patients with hepatic impairment

Monitoring Parameters Renal function, electrolytes, and fluid status (weight and I & O), blood pressure

Patient Information May be taken with food or milk; rise slowly from a lying or sitting position to minimize dizziness, lightheadedness or fainting; also use extra care when exercising, standing for long periods of time, and during hot weather; take dose in the morning or early in the evening to prevent nocturia; use caution with exposure to ultraviolet light

Additional Information 10-20 mg torsemide is approximately equivalent to furosemide 40 mg or bumetanide 1 mg

Dosage Forms

Injection: 10 mg/mL (2 mL, 5 mL)
Tablet: 5 mg, 10 mg, 20 mg, 100 mg

Totacillin® *see* Ampicillin *on page 85*
Totacillin®-N *see* Ampicillin *on page 85*
Touro Ex® *see* Guaifenesin *on page 589*
Toxicities of Chemotherapeutic Agents *see page 1382*
Toxicology Information *see page 1553*
Toxidromes *see page 1561*
t-PA *see* Alteplase *on page 53*
TPT *see* Topotecan *on page 1244*
Tracrium® *see* Atracurium *on page 115*

Tramadol (TRA ma dole)

Brand Names Ultram®

Canadian/Mexican Brand Names Tradol® (Mexico)

Synonyms Tramadol Hydrochloride

Therapeutic Category Analgesic, Miscellaneous

Use Relief of moderate to moderately severe pain

Pregnancy Risk Factor C

Contraindications Previous hypersensitivity to tramadol or any components; do not give to opioid-dependent patients; concurrent use of monoamine oxidase inhibitors; acute alcohol intoxication; concurrent use of centrally acting analgesics, opioids, or psychotropic drugs

Warnings/Precautions Elderly patients and patients with chronic respiratory disorders may be at greater risk of adverse events; liver disease; patients with myxedema, hypothyroidism, or hypoadrenalism should use tramadol with caution and at reduced dosages; not recommended during pregnancy or in nursing

(Continued)

Tramadol *(Continued)*

mothers; increased incidence of seizures may occur in patients receiving concurrent tricyclic antidepressants

Adverse Reactions

>1%:

Central nervous system: Dizziness, headache, somnolence, stimulation, restlessness

Gastrointestinal: Nausea, diarrhea, constipation, vomiting, dyspepsia

Neuromuscular & skeletal: Weakness

Miscellaneous: Diaphoresis

<1%:

Cardiovascular: Palpitations

Respiratory: Respiratory depression

Overdosage/Toxicology Symptoms of overdose include CNS and respiratory depression, gastrointestinal cramping, constipation

Naloxone 2 mg I.V. (0.01 mg/kg children) with repeat administration as needed up to 18 mg

Drug Interactions

Decreased effects: Carbamazepine (decreases half-life by 33% to 50%)

Increased toxicity: Monoamine oxidase inhibitors and tricyclic antidepressants (seizures); quinidine (inhibits cytochrome P-450IID6, thereby increases tramadol serum concentrations); cimetidine (tramadol half-life increased 20% to 25%)

Mechanism of Action Binds to μ-opiate receptors in the CNS causing inhibition of ascending pain pathways, altering the perception of and response to pain; also inhibits the reuptake of norepinephrine and serotonin, which also modifies the ascending pain pathway

Usual Dosage Adults: Oral: 50-100 mg every 4-6 hours, not to exceed 400 mg/day

Monitoring Parameters Monitor patient for pain, respiratory rate, and look for signs of tolerance and, therefore, abuse potential; monitor blood pressure and pulse rate, especially in patients on higher doses

Reference Range 100-300 ng/mL; however, serum level monitoring is not required

Patient Information Avoid driving or operating machinery until the effect of drug wears off; tramadol has not been fully evaluated for its abuse potential, report cravings to your physician immediately

Dosage Forms Tablet, as hydrochloride: 50 mg

Tramadol Hydrochloride *see* Tramadol *on previous page*

Trandate® *see* Labetalol *on page 700*

Tranexamic Acid (tran eks AM ik AS id)

Brand Names Cyklokapron®

Therapeutic Category Antihemophilic Agent

Use Short-term use (2-8 days) in hemophilia patients during and following tooth extraction to reduce or prevent hemorrhage, has also been used as an alternative to aminocaproic acid for subarachnoid hemorrhage

Pregnancy Risk Factor B

Contraindications Acquired defective color vision, active intravascular clotting

Warnings/Precautions Dosage modification required in patients with renal impairment; ophthalmic exam before and during therapy required if patient is treated beyond several days; caution in patients with cardiovascular, renal, or cerebrovascular disease; when used for subarachnoid hemorrhage, ischemic complications may occur

Adverse Reactions

>10%: Gastrointestinal: Nausea, diarrhea, vomiting

1% to 10%:

Cardiovascular: Hypotension, thrombosis

Ocular: Blurred vision

<1%: Endocrine & metabolic: Unusual menstrual discomfort

Stability Incompatible with solutions containing penicillin

Mechanism of Action Forms a reversible complex that displaces plasminogen from fibrin resulting in inhibition of fibrinolysis; it also inhibits the proteolytic activity of plasmin

Pharmacodynamics/Kinetics

Half-life: 2-10 hours

Elimination: Primarily as unchanged drug (>90%) in urine

Usual Dosage Children and Adults: I.V.: 10 mg/kg immediately before surgery, then 25 mg/kg/dose orally 3-4 times/day for 2-8 days

Alternatively:

Oral: 25 mg/kg 3-4 times/day beginning 1 day prior to surgery

I.V.: 10 mg/kg 3-4 times/day in patients who are unable to take oral

Dosing adjustment/interval in renal impairment:

Cl_{cr} 50-80 mL/minute: Administer 50% of normal dose or 10 mg/kg twice daily I.V. or 15 mg/kg twice daily orally

Cl_{cr} 10-50 mL/minute: Administer 25% of normal dose or 10 mg/kg/day I.V. or 15 mg/kg/day orally

Cl_{cr} <10 mL/minute: Administer 10% of normal dose or 10 mg/kg/dose every 48 hours I.V. or 15 mg/kg/dose every 48 hours orally

Administration Use plastic syringe only for I.V. push

Reference Range 5-10 μg/mL is required to decrease fibrinolysis

Patient Information Report any signs of bleeding or myopathy, changes in vision; GI upset usually disappears when dose is reduced

Nursing Implications Dosage modification required in patients with renal impairment

Dosage Forms

Injection: 100 mg/mL (10 mL)

Tablet: 500 mg

Transamine Sulphate *see* Tranylcypromine *on this page*

Transdermal-NTG® *see* Nitroglycerin *on page 909*

Transderm-Nitro® *see* Nitroglycerin *on page 909*

Transderm Scop® *see* Scopolamine *on page 1127*

***trans*-Retinoic Acid** *see* Tretinoin, Topical *on page 1254*

Trans-Ver-Sal® AdultPatch [OTC] *see* Salicylic Acid *on page 1120*

Trans-Ver-Sal® PediaPatch [OTC] *see* Salicylic Acid *on page 1120*

Trans-Ver-Sal® PlantarPatch [OTC] *see* Salicylic Acid *on page 1120*

Tranxene® *see* Clorazepate *on page 301*

Tranylcypromine (tran il SIP roe meen)

Related Information

Antidepressant Agents Comparison *on page 1393*

Brand Names Parnate®

Synonyms Transamine Sulphate; Tranylcypromine Sulfate

Therapeutic Category Antidepressant, Monoamine Oxidase Inhibitor

Use Symptomatic treatment of depressed patients refractory to or intolerant to tricyclic antidepressants or electroconvulsive therapy; has a more rapid onset of therapeutic effect than other MAO inhibitors, but causes more severe hypertensive reactions

Pregnancy Risk Factor C

Contraindications Uncontrolled hypertension, known hypersensitivity to tranylcypromine, pheochromocytoma, cardiovascular disease, severe renal or hepatic impairment, pheochromocytoma

Warnings/Precautions Safety in children <16 years of age has not been established; use with caution in patients who are hyperactive, hyperexcitable, or who have glaucoma, suicidal tendencies, diabetes, elderly

Adverse Reactions

1% to 10%: Cardiovascular: Orthostatic hypotension

<1%:

Cardiovascular: Edema, hypertensive crises

Central nervous system: Drowsiness, hyperexcitability, headache

Dermatologic: Rash, photosensitivity

Gastrointestinal: Xerostomia, constipation

Genitourinary: Urinary retention

Hepatic: Hepatitis

Ocular: Blurred vision

Overdosage/Toxicology Symptoms of overdose include tachycardia, palpitations, muscle twitching, seizures, insomnia, transient hypotension, hypertension, hyperpyrexia, coma

Competent supportive care is the most important treatment for an overdose with a monoamine oxidase (MAO) inhibitor. Both hypertension or hypotension can occur with intoxication. Hypotension may respond to I.V. fluids or vasopressors, and hypertension usually responds to an alpha-adrenergic blocker. While treating the hypertension, care is warranted to avoid sudden drops in blood pressure, since this may worsen the MAO inhibitor toxicity. Muscle irritability and seizures often respond to diazepam, while hyperthermia is best treated antipyretics and cooling blankets. Cardiac arrhythmias are best treated with phenytoin or procainamide.

Drug Interactions

Decreased effect of antihypertensives

(Continued)

Tranylcypromine *(Continued)*

Increased toxicity with disulfiram (seizures), fluoxetine and other serotonin-active agents (eg, paroxetine, sertraline), TCAs (cardiovascular instability), meperidine (cardiovascular instability), phenothiazine (hypertensive crisis), sympathomimetics (hypertensive crisis), sumatriptan (hypothetical), CNS depressants, levodopa (hypertensive crisis), tyramine-containing foods (eg, aged foods), dextroamphetamine (psychosis)

Mechanism of Action Inhibits the enzymes monoamine oxidase A and B which are responsible for the intraneuronal metabolism of norepinephrine and serotonin and increasing their availability to postsynaptic neurons; decreased firing rate of the locus ceruleus, reducing norepinephrine concentration in the brain; agonist effects of serotonin

Pharmacodynamics/Kinetics

Onset of action: 2-3 weeks are required of continued dosing to obtain full therapeutic effect

Half-life: 90-190 minutes

Time to peak serum concentration: Within 2 hours

Elimination: In urine

Usual Dosage Adults: Oral: 10 mg twice daily, increase by 10 mg increments at 1- to 3-week intervals; maximum: 60 mg/day

Dosing comments in hepatic impairment: Use with care and monitor plasma levels and patient response closely

Dietary Considerations

Alcohol: Avoid use

Food: Avoid tyramine-containing foods

Monitoring Parameters Blood pressure, blood glucose

Test Interactions ↓ glucose

Patient Information Tablets may be crushed; avoid alcohol; do not discontinue abruptly; avoid foods high in tyramine (eg, aged cheeses, Chianti wine, raisins, liver, bananas, chocolate, yogurt, sour cream); discuss list of drugs and foods to avoid with pharmacist or physician; arise slowly from prolonged sitting or lying

Nursing Implications Assist with ambulation during initiation of therapy; monitor blood pressure closely, patients should be cautioned against eating foods high in tyramine or tryptophan (cheese, wine, beer, pickled herring, dry sausage)

Dosage Forms Tablet, as sulfate: 10 mg

Tranylcypromine Sulfate *see* Tranylcypromine *on previous page*

Trasylol® *see* Aprotinin *on page 99*

Trazodone (TRAZ oh done)

Related Information

Antidepressant Agents Comparison *on page 1393*

Brand Names Desyrel®

Synonyms Trazodone Hydrochloride

Therapeutic Category Antidepressant

Use Treatment of depression

Pregnancy Risk Factor C

Contraindications Hypersensitivity to trazodone or any component

Warnings/Precautions Safety and efficacy in children <18 years of age have not been established; monitor closely and use with extreme caution in patients with cardiac disease or arrhythmias. Very sedating, but little anticholinergic effects; therapeutic effects may take up to 4 weeks to occur; therapy is normally maintained for several months after optimum response is reached to prevent recurrence of depression.

Adverse Reactions

>10%:
- Central nervous system: Dizziness, headache, confusion
- Gastrointestinal: Nausea, bad taste in mouth, xerostomia
- Neuromuscular & skeletal: Muscle tremors

1% to 10%:
- Gastrointestinal: Diarrhea, constipation
- Neuromuscular & skeletal: Weakness
- Ocular: Blurred vision

<1%:
- Cardiovascular: Hypotension, tachycardia, bradycardia
- Central nervous system: Agitation, seizures, extrapyramidal reactions
- Dermatologic: Rash
- Genitourinary: Prolonged priapism, urinary retention
- Hepatic: Hepatitis

Overdosage/Toxicology Symptoms of overdose include drowsiness, vomiting, hypotension, tachycardia, incontinence, coma, priapism

Following initiation of essential overdose management, toxic symptoms should be treated. Ventricular arrhythmias often respond to lidocaine 1.5 mg/kg bolus followed by 2 mg/minute infusion with concurrent systemic alkalinization (sodium bicarbonate 0.5-2 mEq/kg I.V.). Seizures usually respond to diazepam I.V. boluses (5-10 mg for adults up to 30 mg or 0.25-0.4 mg/kg/dose for children up to 10 mg/dose). If seizures are unresponsive or recur, phenytoin or phenobarbital may be required. Hypotension is best treated by I.V. fluids and by placing the patient in the Trendelenburg position.

Drug Interactions

Decreased effect: Clonidine, methyldopa, anticoagulants

Increased toxicity: Fluoxetine; increased effect/toxicity of phenytoin, CNS depressants, MAO inhibitors; digoxin serum levels increase

Mechanism of Action Inhibits reuptake of serotonin and norepinephrine by the presynaptic neuronal membrane and desensitization of adenyl cyclase, down regulation of beta-adrenergic receptors, and down regulation of serotonin receptors

Pharmacodynamics/Kinetics

Onset of effect: Therapeutic effects take 1-3 weeks to appear

Protein binding: 85% to 95%

Metabolism: In the liver

Half-life: 4-7.5 hours, 2 compartment kinetics

Time to peak serum concentration: Within 30-100 minutes, prolonged in the presence of food (up to 2.5 hours)

Elimination: Primarily in urine and secondarily in feces

Usual Dosage Oral: Therapeutic effects may take up to 4 weeks to occur; therapy is normally maintained for several months after optimum response is reached to prevent recurrence of depression

Children 6-18 years: Initial: 1.5-2 mg/kg/day in divided doses; increase gradually every 3-4 days as needed; maximum: 6 mg/kg/day in 3 divided doses

Adolescents: Initial: 25-50 mg/day; increase to 100-150 mg/day in divided doses

Adults: Initial: 150 mg/day in 3 divided doses (may increase by 50 mg/day every 3-7 days); maximum: 600 mg/day

Elderly: 25-50 mg at bedtime with 25-50 mg/day dose increase every 3 days for inpatients and weekly for outpatients, if tolerated; usual dose: 75-150 mg/day

Dietary Considerations Alcohol: Avoid use

Reference Range

Plasma levels do not always correlate with clinical effectiveness

Therapeutic: 0.5-2.5 μg/mL

Potentially toxic: >2.5 μg/mL

Toxic: >4 μg/mL

Patient Information Take shortly after a meal or light snack, can be given as bedtime dose if drowsiness occurs; avoid alcohol; be aware of possible photosensitivity reaction; report any prolonged or painful erection

Nursing Implications Dosing after meals may decrease lightheadedness and postural hypotension; use side rails on bed if administered to the elderly; observe patient's activity and compare with admission level; assist with ambulation; sitting and standing blood pressure and pulse

Dosage Forms Tablet, as hydrochloride: 50 mg, 100 mg, 150 mg, 300 mg

Trazodone Hydrochloride *see* Trazodone *on previous page*

Treatment of Sexually Transmitted Diseases *see page 1485*

Trecator®-SC *see* Ethionamide *on page 491*

Trendar® [OTC] *see* Ibuprofen *on page 639*

Trental® *see* Pentoxifylline *on page 974*

Tretinoin, Oral (TRET i noyn, oral)

Brand Names Vesanoid®

Synonyms All-*trans*-Retinoic Acid

Therapeutic Category Antineoplastic Agent, Miscellaneous; Retinoic Acid Derivative; Vitamin A Derivative; Vitamin, Fat Soluble

Use Acute promyelocytic leukemia (APL): Induction of remission in patients with APL, French American British (FAB) classification M3 (including the M3 variant), characterized by the presence of the t(15;17) translocation or the presence of the PML/RARα gene who are refractory to or who have relapsed from anthracycline chemotherapy, or for whom anthracycline-based chemotherapy is contraindicated. Tretinoin is for the induction of remission only. All patients should receive an accepted form of remission consolidation or maintenance therapy for APL after completion of induction therapy with tretinoin.

Pregnancy Risk Factor D

Contraindications Sensitivity to parabens, vitamin A, or other retinoids

Warnings/Precautions Patients with acute promyelocytic leukemia (APL) are at high risk and can have severe adverse reactions to tretinoin. Administer under

(Continued)

Tretinoin, Oral *(Continued)*

the supervision of a physician who is experienced in the management of patients with acute leukemia and in a facility with laboratory and supportive services sufficient to monitor drug tolerance and to protect and maintain a patient compromised by drug toxicity, including respiratory compromise.

About 25% of patients with APL treated with tretinoin have experienced a syndrome called the retinoic acid-APL (RA-APL) syndrome characterized by fever, dyspnea, weight gain, radiographic pulmonary infiltrates and pleural or pericardial effusions. This syndrome has occasionally been accompanied by impaired myocardial contractility and episodic hypotension. It has been observed with or without concomitant leukocytosis. Endotracheal intubation and mechanical ventilation have been required in some cases due to progressive hypoxemia, and several patients have expired with multiorgan failure. The syndrome usually occurs during the first month of treatment, with some cases reported following the first dose.

Management of the syndrome has not been defined, but high-dose steroids given at the first suspicion of RA-APL syndrome appear to reduce morbidity and mortality. At the first signs suggestive of the syndrome, immediately initiate high-dose steroids (dexamethasone 10 mg I.V.) every 12 hours for 3 days or until resolution of symptoms, regardless of the leukocyte count. The majority of patients do not require termination of tretinoin therapy during treatment of the RA-APL syndrome.

During treatment, ~40% of patients will develop rapidly evolving leukocytosis. Rapidly evolving leukocytosis is associated with a higher risk of life-threatening complications.

If signs and symptoms of the RA-APL syndrome are present together with leukocytosis, initiate treatment with high-dose steroids immediately. Consider adding full-dose chemotherapy (including an anthracycline, if not contraindicated) to the tretinoin therapy on day 1 or 2 for patients presenting with a WBC count of $>5 \times 10^9/L$ or immediately, for patients presenting with a WBC count of $<5 \times 10^9/L$, if the WBC count reaches $\geq 6 \times 10^9/L$ by day 5, or $\geq 10 \times 10^9/L$ by day 10 or $\geq 15 \times 10^9/L$ by day 28.

Not to be used in women of childbearing potential unless woman is capable of complying with effective contraceptive measures; therapy is normally begun on the second or third day of next normal menstrual period; two reliable methods of effective contraception must be used during therapy and for 1 month after discontinuation of therapy, unless abstinence is the chosen method. Within one week prior to the institution of tretinoin therapy, the patient should have blood or urine collected for a serum or urine pregnancy test with a sensitivity of at least 50 mIU/L. When possible, delay tretinoin therapy until a negative result from this test is obtained. When a delay is not possible, place the patient on two reliable forms of contraception. Repeat pregnancy testing and contraception counseling monthly throughout the period of treatment.

Initiation of therapy with tretinoin may be based on the morphological diagnosis of APL. Confirm the diagnosis of APL by detection of the t(15;17) genetic marker by cytogenetic studies. If these are negative, PML/RARα fusion should be sought using molecular diagnostic techniques. The response rate of other AML subtypes to tretinoin has not been demonstrated.

Retinoids have been associated with pseudotumor cerebri (benign intracranial hypertension), especially in children. Early signs and symptoms include papilledema, headache, nausea, vomiting and visual disturbances.

Up to 60% of patients experienced hypercholesterolemia or hypertriglyceridemia, which were reversible upon completion of treatment.

Elevated liver function test results occur in 50% to 60% of patients during treatment. Carefully monitor liver function test results during treatment and give consideration to a temporary withdrawal of tretinoin if test results reach >5 times the upper limit of normal.

Adverse Reactions Virtually all patients experience some drug-related toxicity, especially headache, fever, weakness and fatigue. These adverse effects are seldom permanent or irreversible nor do they usually require therapy interruption

>10%:

- Cardiovascular: Arrhythmias, flushing, hypotension, hypertension, peripheral edema, chest discomfort, edema
- Central nervous system: Dizziness, anxiety, insomnia, depression, confusion, malaise, pain
- Dermatologic: Burning, redness, cheilitis, inflammation of lips, dry skin, pruritus, photosensitivity
- Endocrine & metabolic: Increased serum concentration of triglycerides

Gastrointestinal: GI hemorrhage, abdominal pain, other GI disorders, diarrhea, constipation, dyspepsia, abdominal distention, weight gain or loss, anorexia, xerostomia
Hematologic: Hemorrhage, disseminated intravascular coagulation
Local: Phlebitis, injection site reactions
Neuromuscular & skeletal: Bone pain, arthralgia, myalgia, paresthesia
Ocular: Itching of eye
Renal: Renal insufficiency
Respiratory: Upper respiratory tract disorders, dyspnea, respiratory insufficiency, pleural effusion, pneumonia, rales, expiratory wheezing, dry nose
Miscellaneous: Infections, shivering

1% to 10%:
Cardiovascular: Cardiac failure, cardiac arrest, myocardial infarction, enlarged heart, heart murmur, ischemia, stroke, myocarditis, pericarditis, pulmonary hypertension, secondary cardiomyopathy, cerebral hemorrhage, pallor
Central nervous system: Intracranial hypertension, agitation, hallucination, agnosia, aphasia, cerebellar edema, cerebellar disorders, convulsions, coma, CNS depression, encephalopathy, hypotaxia, no light reflex, neurologic reaction, spinal cord disorder, unconsciousness, dementia, forgetfulness, somnolence, slow speech, hypothermia
Dermatologic: Skin peeling on hands or soles of feet, rash, cellulitis
Endocrine & metabolic: Fluid imbalance, acidosis
Gastrointestinal: Hepatosplenomegaly, ulcer, unspecified liver disorder
Genitourinary: Dysuria, polyuria, enlarged prostate
Hepatic: Ascites, hepatitis
Neuromuscular & skeletal: Tremor, leg weakness, hyporeflexia, dysarthria, facial paralysis, hemiplegia, flank pain, asterixis, abnormal gait
Ocular: Dry eyes, photophobia
Renal: Acute renal failure, renal tubular necrosis
Respiratory: Lower respiratory tract disorders, pulmonary infiltration, bronchial asthma, pulmonary/larynx edema, unspecified pulmonary disease
Miscellaneous: Face edema, lymph disorders

<1%:
Central nervous system: Mood changes, pseudomotor cerebri
Dermatologic: Alopecia, pruritus
Endocrine & metabolic: Hyperuricemia
Gastrointestinal: Xerostomia, anorexia, nausea, vomiting, inflammatory bowel syndrome, bleeding of gums
Hematologic: Increase in erythrocyte sedimentation rate, decrease in hemoglobin and hematocrit
Hepatic: Hepatitis
Ocular: Conjunctivitis, corneal opacities, optic neuritis, cataracts

Overdosage/Toxicology Symptoms of overdose include transient headache, facial flushing, cheilosis, abdominal pain, dizziness and ataxia; all signs and symptoms have been transient and have resolved without apparent residual effects

Drug Interactions Metabolized by the hepatic cytochrome P-450 system: All drugs that induce or inhibit this system would be expected to interact with tretinoin cytochrome P-450 2C9 substrate

Increased toxicity: Ketoconazole increases the mean plasma AUC of tretinoin

Mechanism of Action Retinoid that induces maturation of acute promyelocytic leukemia (APL) cells in cultures; induces cytodifferentiation and decreased proliferation of APL cells

Pharmacodynamics/Kinetics
Protein binding: >95%
Metabolism: In the liver via cytochrome P-450 enzymes
Half-life, terminal:
Parent drug: 0.5-2 hours
Time to peak serum concentration: Within 1-2 hours
Elimination: Equally in urine and feces

Usual Dosage Oral:
Children: There are limited clinical data on the pediatric use of tretinoin. Of 15 pediatric patients (age range: 1-16 years) treated with tretinoin, the incidence of complete remission was 67%. Safety and efficacy in pediatric patients <1 year of age have not been established. Some pediatric patients experience severe headache and pseudotumor cerebri, requiring analgesic treatment and lumbar puncture for relief. Increased caution is recommended. Consider dose reduction in children experiencing serious or intolerable toxicity; however, the efficacy and safety of tretinoin at doses <45 mg/m^2/day have not been evaluated.

Adults: 45 mg/m^2/day administered as two evenly divided doses until complete remission is documented. Discontinue therapy 30 days after achievement of

(Continued)

Tretinoin, Oral *(Continued)*

complete remission or after 90 days of treatment, whichever occurs first. If after initiation of treatment the presence of the t(15;17) translocation is not confirmed by cytogenetics or by polymerase chain reaction studies and the patient has not responded to tretinoin, consider alternative therapy.

Note: Tretinoin is for the induction of remission only. Optimal consolidation or maintenance regimens have not been determined. All patients should therefore receive a standard consolidation or maintenance chemotherapy regimen for APL after induction therapy with tretinoin unless otherwise contraindicated.

Monitoring Parameters Monitor the patient's hematologic profile, coagulation profile, liver function test results and triglyceride and cholesterol levels frequently

Patient Information Avoid pregnancy during therapy; effective contraceptive measures must be used since this drug may harm the fetus; there is information from manufacturers about this product that you should receive; discontinue therapy if visual difficulties, abdominal pain, rectal bleeding, diarrhea; avoid use of other vitamin A products; decreased tolerance to contact lenses may occur; loss of night vision may occur, avoid prolonged exposure to sunlight

Dosage Forms Capsule: 10 mg

Tretinoin, Topical (TRET i noyn, TOP i kal)

Brand Names Retin-A™ Micro Topical; Retin-A™ Topical

Canadian/Mexican Brand Names Retisol-A® (Canada); Stieva-A® (Canada); Stieva-A Forte® (Canada); Stieva-A® (Mexico); Stieva-A® 0.025% (Mexico)

Synonyms Retinoic Acid; *trans*-Retinoic Acid; Vitamin A Acid

Therapeutic Category Acne Products; Retinoic Acid Derivative; Vitamin A Derivative; Vitamin, Topical

Use Treatment of acne vulgaris, photodamaged skin, and some skin cancers

Pregnancy Risk Factor C

Pregnancy/Breast-Feeding Implications Oral tretinoin is teratogenic and fetotoxic in rats at doses 1000 and 500 times the topical human dose, respectively; however, tretinoin does not appear to be teratogenic when used topically since it is rapidly metabolized by the skin

Contraindications Hypersensitivity to tretinoin or any component; sunburn

Warnings/Precautions Use with caution in patients with eczema; avoid excessive exposure to sunlight and sunlamps; avoid contact with abraded skin, mucous membranes, eyes, mouth, angles of the nose

Adverse Reactions

1% to 10%:

- Cardiovascular: Edema
- Dermatologic: Excessive dryness, erythema, scaling of the skin, hyperpigmentation or hypopigmentation, photosensitivity, initial acne flare-up
- Local: Stinging, blistering

Overdosage/Toxicology Toxic signs of an overdose commonly respond to drug discontinuation, and generally return to normal spontaneously within a few days to weeks.

When confronted with signs of increased intracranial pressure, treatment with mannitol (0.25 g/kg I.V. up to 1 g/kg/dose repeated every 5 minutes as needed), dexamethasone (1.5 mg/kg I.V. load followed with 0.375 mg/kg every 6 hours for 5 days), and/or hyperventilation should be employed.

Drug Interactions Increased toxicity: Sulfur, benzoyl peroxide, salicylic acid, resorcinol (potentiates adverse reactions seen with tretinoin)

Mechanism of Action Keratinocytes in the sebaceous follicle become less adherent which allows for easy removal; inhibits microcomedone formation and eliminates lesions already present

Pharmacodynamics/Kinetics

Absorption: Topical: Minimum absorption occurs

Metabolism: Of the small amount absorbed, metabolism occurs in the liver

Elimination: In bile and urine

Usual Dosage Children >12 years and Adults: Topical: Begin therapy with a weaker formulation of tretinoin (0.025% cream or 0.01% gel) and increase the concentration as tolerated; apply once daily before retiring or on alternate days; if stinging or irritation develop, decrease frequency of application

Patient Information Thoroughly wash hands after applying; avoid hydration of skin immediately before application; minimize exposure to sunlight; avoid washing face more frequently than 2-3 times/day; if severe irritation occurs, discontinue medication temporarily and adjust dose when irritation subsides; avoid using topical preparations with high alcoholic content during treatment period; do not exceed prescribed dose

Nursing Implications Observe for signs of hypersensitivity, blistering, excessive dryness; do not apply to mucous membranes

Dosage Forms

Cream (Retin-A™): 0.025% (20 g, 45 g); 0.05% (20 g, 45 g); 0.1% (20 g, 45 g)
Gel, topical (Retin-A™): 0.01% (15 g, 45 g); 0.025% (15 g, 45 g)
Gel, topical (Retin-A™ Micro): 0.1% (20 g, 45 g)
Liquid, topical (Retin-A™): 0.05% (28 mL)

Triacet® *see* Triamcinolone *on this page*

Triacetyloleandomycin *see* Troleandomycin *on page 1274*

Triaconazole *see* Terconazole *on page 1196*

Triam-A® *see* Triamcinolone *on this page*

Triamcinolone (trye am SIN oh lone)

Related Information

Asthma, Guidelines for the Diagnosis and Management of *on page 1518*
Corticosteroids Comparison *on page 1407*
Estimated Clinical Comparability of Doses for Inhaled Corticosteroids *on page 1522*

Brand Names Amcort®; Aristocort®; Aristocort® A; Aristocort® Forte; Aristocort® Intralesional; Aristospan® Intra-Articular; Aristospan® Intralesional; Atolone®; Azmacort™; Delta-Tritex®; Flutex®; Kenacort®; Kenaject-40®; Kenalog®; Kenalog-10®; Kenalog-40®; Kenalog® H; Kenalog® in Orabase®; Kenonel®; Nasacort®; Tac™-3; Tac™-40; Triacet®; Triam-A®; Triam Forte®; Triderm®; Tri-Kort®; Trilog®; Trilone®; Trisoject®

Synonyms Triamcinolone Acetonide, Aerosol; Triamcinolone Acetonide, Parenteral; Triamcinolone Diacetate, Oral; Triamcinolone Diacetate, Parenteral; Triamcinolone Hexacetonide; Triamcinolone, Oral

Therapeutic Category Anti-inflammatory Agent; Anti-inflammatory Agent, Inhalant; Corticosteroid, Inhalant; Corticosteroid, Intranasal; Corticosteroid, Systemic; Corticosteroid, Topical (Medium Potency); Corticosteroid, Topical (High Potency); Glucocorticoid

Use

Inhalation: Control of bronchial asthma and related bronchospastic conditions.
Systemic: Adrenocortical insufficiency, rheumatic disorders, allergic states, respiratory diseases, systemic lupus erythematosus, and other diseases requiring anti-inflammatory or immunosuppressive effects
Topical: Inflammatory dermatoses responsive to steroids

Pregnancy Risk Factor C

Pregnancy/Breast-Feeding Implications

Clinical effects on the fetus: No data on crossing the placenta or effect on fetus
Breast-feeding/lactation: No data on crossing into breast milk or clinical effects on the infant

Contraindications Known hypersensitivity to triamcinolone; systemic fungal infections; serious infections (except septic shock or tuberculous meningitis); primary treatment of status asthmaticus

Warnings/Precautions Fatalities have occurred due to adrenal insufficiency in asthmatic patients during and after transfer from systemic corticosteroids to aerosol steroids; several months may be required for recovery from this syndrome; during this period, aerosol steroids do **not** provide the increased systemic steroid requirement needed to treat patients having trauma, surgery or infections; avoid using higher than recommended dose

Use with caution in patients with hypothyroidism, cirrhosis, nonspecific ulcerative colitis and patients at increased risk for peptic ulcer disease; do not use occlusive dressings on weeping or exudative lesions and general caution with occlusive dressings should be observed; discontinue if skin irritation or contact dermatitis should occur; do not use in patients with decreased skin circulation; avoid the use of high potency steroids on the face

Because of the risk of adverse effects, systemic corticosteroids should be used cautiously in the elderly, in the smallest possible dose, and for the shortest possible time. Azmacort™ (metered dose inhaler) comes with its own spacer device attached and may be easier to use in older patients.

Adverse Reactions

>10%:
- Central nervous system: Insomnia, nervousness
- Gastrointestinal: Increased appetite, indigestion

1% to 10%:
- Ocular: Cataracts
- Endocrine & metabolic: Diabetes mellitus hirsutism
- Neuromuscular & skeletal: Arthralgia
- Respiratory: Epistaxis

<1%:
- Central nervous system: Fatigue, seizures, mood swings, headache, delirium, hallucinations, euphoria

(Continued)

Triamcinolone *(Continued)*

Dermatologic: Itching, hypertrichosis, skin atrophy, hyperpigmentation, hypopigmentation, acne, bruising

Endocrine & metabolic: Amenorrhea, sodium and water retention, Cushing's syndrome, hyperglycemia, bone growth suppression

Gastrointestinal: Oral candidiasis, dry throat, xerostomia, peptic ulcer, abdominal distention, ulcerative esophagitis, pancreatitis

Local: Burning

Neuromuscular & skeletal: Osteoporosis, muscle wasting

Respiratory: Hoarseness, wheezing, cough

Miscellaneous: Hypersensitivity reactions

Overdosage/Toxicology When consumed in excessive quantities, systemic hypercorticism and adrenal suppression may occur, in those cases discontinuation and withdrawal of the corticosteroid should be done judiciously

Drug Interactions

Decreased effect: Barbiturates, phenytoin, rifampin ↑ metabolism of triamcinolone; vaccine and toxoid effects may be reduced

Increased toxicity: Salicylates may increase risk of GI ulceration

Mechanism of Action Decreases inflammation by suppression of migration of polymorphonuclear leukocytes and reversal of increased capillary permeability; suppresses the immune system by reducing activity and volume of the lymphatic system; suppresses adrenal function at high doses

Pharmacodynamics/Kinetics

Duration of action: Oral: 8-12 hours

Absorption: Topical: Systemic absorption may occur

Time to peak: I.M.: Within 8-10 hours

Half-life, biologic: 18-36 hours

Usual Dosage In general, single I.M. dose of 4-7 times oral dose will control patient from 4-7 days up to 3-4 weeks

Children 6-12 years:

Oral inhalation: 1-2 inhalations 3-4 times/day, not to exceed 12 inhalations/day

I.M. (acetonide or hexacetonide): 0.03-0.2 mg/kg at 1- to 7-day intervals

Intra-articular, intrabursal, or tendon-sheath injection: 2.5-15 mg, repeated as needed

Children >12 years and Adults:

Intranasal: 2 sprays in each nostril once daily; may increase after 4-7 days up to 4 sprays once daily or 1 spray 4 times/day in each nostril

Topical: Apply a thin film 2-3 times/day

Oral: 4-48 mg/day

I.M. (acetonide or hexacetonide): 60 mg (of 40 mg/mL), additional 20-100 mg doses (usual: 40-80 mg) may be given when signs and symptoms recur, best at 6-week intervals to minimize HPA suppression

Intra-articular (hexacetonide): 2-20 mg every 3-4 weeks

Intralesional (diacetate or acetonide - use 10 mg/mL): 1 mg/injection site, may be repeated one or more times/week depending upon patient's response; maximum: 30 mg at any one time; may use multiple injections if they are more than 1 cm apart

Intra-articular, intrasynovial, and soft-tissue (diacetate or acetonide - use 10 mg/mL or 40 mg/mL) 2.5-40 mg depending upon location, size of joints, and degree of inflammation; repeat when signs and symptoms recur

Sublesionally (as acetonide): Up to 1 mg per injection site and may be repeated one or more times weekly; multiple sites may be injected if they are 1 cm or more apart, not to exceed 30 mg

See table.

Triamcinolone Dosing

	Acetonide	Diacetate	Hexacetonide
Intrasynovial	2.5-40 mg	5-40 mg	
Intralesional	2.5-40 mg	5-48 mg	Up to 0.5 mg/sq inch affected area
Sublesional	1-30 mg		
Systemic I.M.	2.5-60 mg/d	~40 mg/wk	20-100 mg
Intra-articular		5-40 mg	2-20 mg average
large joints	5-15 mg		10-20 mg
small joints	2.5-5 mg		2-6 mg
Tendon sheaths	10-40 mg		
Intradermal	1 mg/site		

Oral inhalation: 2 inhalations 3-4 times/day, not to exceed 16 inhalations/day

Patient Information
Inhaler: Rinse mouth and throat after use to prevent candidiasis
Topical: Apply sparingly to affected area, rub in until drug disappears, do not use on open skin
Report any change in body weight; do not discontinue or decrease the drug without contacting your physician; carry an identification card or bracelet advising that you are on steroids; may take with meals to decrease GI upset

Nursing Implications Once daily doses should be given in the morning; evaluate clinical response and mental status; may mask signs and symptoms of infection; inject I.M. dose deep in large muscle mass, avoid deltoid; avoid S.C. dose; a thin film is effective topically and avoid topical application on the face; do not occlude area unless directed

Additional Information 16 mg triamcinolone is equivalent to 100 mg cortisone (no mineralocorticoid activity)

Dosage Forms
Aerosol:
Oral inhalation: 100 mcg/metered spray (20 g)
Topical, as acetonide: 0.2 mg/2 second spray (23 g, 63 g)
Cream, as acetonide: 0.025% (15 g, 30 g, 60 g, 80 g, 120 g, 240 g); 0.1% (15 g, 20 g, 30 g, 60 g, 80 g, 90 g, 120 g, 240 g); 0.5% (15 g, 20 g, 30 g, 120 g, 240 g)
Injection, as acetonide: 3 mg/mL (5 mL); 10 mg/mL (5 mL); 40 mg/mL (1 mL, 5 mL, 10 mL)
Injection, as diacetate: 25 mg/mL (5 mL); 40 mg/mL (1 mL, 5 mL)
Injection, as hexacetonide: 5 mg/mL (5 mL); 20 mg/mL (1 mL, 5 mL)
Lotion, as acetonide: 0.025% (60 mL); 0.1% (15 mL, 60 mL)
Ointment, topical, as acetonide: 0.025% (15 g, 28 g, 30 g, 57 g, 80 g, 113 g, 240 g); 0.1% (15 g, 28 g, 57 g, 60 g, 80 g, 113 g, 240 g, 454 g); 0.5% (15 g, 28 g, 57 g, 113 g, 240 g)
Spray, intranasal acetonide: 55 mcg per actuation (100 sprays/canister) (15 mg canister)
Syrup: 4 mg/5 mL (120 mL)
Tablet: 1 mg, 2 mg, 4 mg, 8 mg

Triamcinolone Acetonide, Aerosol *see* Triamcinolone *on page 1255*

Triamcinolone Acetonide, Parenteral *see* Triamcinolone *on page 1255*

Triamcinolone and Nystatin *see* Nystatin and Triamcinolone *on page 920*

Triamcinolone Diacetate, Oral *see* Triamcinolone *on page 1255*

Triamcinolone Diacetate, Parenteral *see* Triamcinolone *on page 1255*

Triamcinolone Hexacetonide *see* Triamcinolone *on page 1255*

Triamcinolone, Oral *see* Triamcinolone *on page 1255*

Triam Forte® *see* Triamcinolone *on page 1255*

Triaminic® AM Decongestant Formula [OTC] *see* Pseudoephedrine *on page 1074*

Triamterene (trye AM ter een)

Related Information
Heart Failure: Management of Patients With Left-Ventricular Systolic Dysfunction *on page 1533*

Brand Names Dyrenium®

Therapeutic Category Antihypertensive; Diuretic, Potassium Sparing

Use Alone or in combination with other diuretics to treat edema and hypertension; decreases potassium excretion caused by kaliuretic diuretics

Pregnancy Risk Factor D

Pregnancy/Breast-Feeding Implications
Clinical effects on the fetus: No data available. Generally, use of diuretics during pregnancy is avoided due to risk of decreased placental perfusion.
Breast-feeding/lactation: No data available

Contraindications Hyperkalemia, renal impairment, hypersensitivity to triamterene or any component; do not administer to patients receiving spironolactone or amiloride

Warnings/Precautions Use with caution in patients with severe hepatic encephalopathy, patients with diabetes, renal dysfunction, a history of renal stones, or those receiving potassium supplements or ACE inhibitors

Adverse Reactions
1% to 10%:
Cardiovascular: Hypotension, edema, congestive heart failure, bradycardia
Central nervous system: Dizziness, headache, fatigue
Dermatologic: Rash
Gastrointestinal: Constipation, nausea
Respiratory: Dyspnea
<1%:
Cardiovascular: Flushing
(Continued)

Triamterene *(Continued)*

Endocrine & metabolic: Hyperkalemia, dehydration, hyponatremia, gynecomastia, hyperchloremic metabolic acidosis, postmenopausal bleeding

Genitourinary: Inability to achieve or maintain an erection

Overdosage/Toxicology Symptoms of overdose include drowsiness, confusion, clinical signs of dehydration, electrolyte imbalance, and hypotension; ingestion of large amounts of potassium-sparing diuretics, may result in life-threatening hyperkalemia.

This can be treated with I.V. glucose, with concurrent regular insulin, I.V. sodium bicarbonate. If needed, Kayexalate® oral or rectal solutions in sorbitol may also be used.

Drug Interactions

Increased risk of hyperkalemia if given together with amiloride, spironolactone, angiotensin-converting enzyme (ACE) inhibitors

Increased toxicity of amantadine (possibly by decreasing its renal excretion)

Mechanism of Action Competes with aldosterone for receptor sites in the distal renal tubules, increasing sodium, chloride, and water excretion while conserving potassium and hydrogen ions; may block the effect of aldosterone on arteriolar smooth muscle as well

Pharmacodynamics/Kinetics

Onset of action: Diuresis occurs within 2-4 hours

Duration: 7-9 hours

Absorption: Oral: Unreliable

Usual Dosage Oral:

Children: 2-4 mg/kg/day in 1-2 divided doses; maximum: 300 mg/day

Adults: 100-300 mg/day in 1-2 divided doses; maximum dose: 300 mg/day

Dosing comments in renal impairment: Cl_{cr} <10 mL/minute: Avoid use

Dosing adjustment in hepatic impairment: Dose reduction is recommended in patients with cirrhosis

Monitoring Parameters Blood pressure, serum electrolytes, renal function, weight, I & O

Test Interactions Interferes with fluorometric assay of quinidine

Patient Information Take in the morning; take the last dose of multiple doses no later than 6 PM unless instructed otherwise; take after meals; notify physician if weakness, headache or nausea occurs; avoid excessive ingestion of food high in potassium or use of salt substitute; may increase blood glucose; may impart a blue fluorescence color to urine

Nursing Implications Observe for hyperkalemia; assess weight and I & O daily to determine weight loss; if ordered once daily, dose should be given in the morning

Dosage Forms Capsule: 50 mg, 100 mg

Triapin® *see* Butalbital Compound *on page 176*

Triazolam (trye AY zoe lam)

Related Information

Benzodiazepines Comparison *on page 1397*

Brand Names Halcion®

Canadian/Mexican Brand Names Apo-Triazo® (Canada); Gen-Triazolam® (Canada); Novo-Triolam® (Canada); Nu-Triazo® (Canada)

Therapeutic Category Benzodiazepine; Hypnotic; Sedative

Use Short-term treatment of insomnia

Restrictions C-IV

Pregnancy Risk Factor X

Contraindications Hypersensitivity to triazolam, or any component, cross-sensitivity with other benzodiazepines may occur; severe uncontrolled pain; pre-existing CNS depression; narrow-angle glaucoma; not to be used in pregnancy or lactation

Warnings/Precautions May cause drug dependency; avoid abrupt discontinuance in patients with prolonged therapy or seizure disorders; not considered a drug of choice in the elderly

Adverse Reactions

>10%:

Cardiovascular: Tachycardia, chest pain

Central nervous system: Drowsiness, fatigue, ataxia, lightheadedness, memory impairment, insomnia, anxiety, depression, headache

Dermatologic: Rash

Endocrine & metabolic: Decreased libido

Gastrointestinal: Xerostomia, decreased salivation, constipation, nausea, vomiting, diarrhea, increased or decreased appetite

Neuromuscular & skeletal: Dysarthria

Ocular: Blurred vision
Miscellaneous: Diaphoresis

1% to 10%:
Cardiovascular: Syncope, hypotension
Central nervous system: Confusion, nervousness, dizziness, akathisia
Dermatologic: Dermatitis
Gastrointestinal: Weight gain or loss, increased salivation, muscle cramps
Neuromuscular & skeletal: Rigidity, tremor
Otic: Tinnitus
Respiratory: Nasal congestion, hyperventilation

<1%:
Endocrine & metabolic: Menstrual irregularities
Hematologic: Blood dyscrasias
Neuromuscular & skeletal: Reflex slowing
Miscellaneous: Drug dependence

Overdosage/Toxicology Symptoms of overdose include somnolence, confusion, coma, diminished reflexes, dyspnea, and hypotension

Treatment for benzodiazepine overdose is supportive. Rarely is mechanical ventilation required. Flumazenil has been shown to selectively block the binding of benzodiazepines to CNS receptors, resulting in a reversal of benzodiazepine-induced CNS depression but not always respiratory depression.

Drug Interactions
Decreased effect with phenytoin, phenobarbital
Increased effect/toxicity with CNS depressants, cimetidine, erythromycin

Mechanism of Action Depresses all levels of the CNS, including the limbic and reticular formation, probably through the increased action of gamma-aminobutyric acid (GABA), which is a major inhibitory neurotransmitter in the brain

Pharmacodynamics/Kinetics
Onset of hypnotic effect: Within 15-30 minutes
Duration: 6-7 hours
Distribution: V_d: 0.8-1.8 L/kg
Protein binding: 89%
Metabolism: Extensively in the liver
Half-life: 1.7-5 hours
Elimination: In urine as unchanged drug and metabolites

Usual Dosage Onset of action is rapid, patient should be in bed when taking medication. Oral:
Children <18 years: Dosage not established
Adults: 0.125-0.25 mg at bedtime

Dosing adjustment/comments in hepatic impairment: Reduce dose or avoid use in cirrhosis

Dietary Considerations Alcohol: Additive CNS effect, avoid use

Monitoring Parameters Respiratory and cardiovascular status

Patient Information Avoid alcohol and other CNS depressants; avoid activities needing good psychomotor coordination until CNS effects are known; drug may cause physical or psychological dependence; avoid abrupt discontinuation after prolonged use

Nursing Implications Patients may require assistance with ambulation; lower doses in the elderly are usually effective; institute safety measures

Dosage Forms Tablet: 0.125 mg, 0.25 mg

Triban® *see* Trimethobenzamide *on page 1265*

Tribavirin *see* Ribavirin *on page 1104*

Tricalcium Phosphate *see* Calcium Phosphate, Tribasic *on page 194*

Trichlormethiazide (trye klor meth EYE a zide)

Related Information
Sulfonamide Derivatives *on page 1420*

Brand Names Metahydrin®; Naqua®

Therapeutic Category Antihypertensive; Diuretic, Thiazide

Use Management of mild to moderate hypertension; treatment of edema in congestive heart failure and nephrotic syndrome

Pregnancy Risk Factor D

Contraindications Hypersensitivity to trichlormethiazide, other thiazides and sulfonamides, or any component

Warnings/Precautions Use with caution in renal disease, hepatic disease, gout, lupus erythematosus, diabetes mellitus; some products may contain tartrazine

Adverse Reactions
1% to 10%: Hypokalemia

<1%:
Cardiovascular: Hypotension
Dermatologic: Photosensitivity

(Continued)

Trichlormethiazide *(Continued)*

Endocrine & metabolic: Fluid and electrolyte imbalances (hypocalcemia, hypomagnesemia, hyponatremia); hyperglycemia
Hematologic: Rarely blood dyscrasias
Renal: Prerenal azotemia

Overdosage/Toxicology Symptoms of overdose include hypermotility, diuresis, lethargy, confusion, muscle weakness

Following GI decontamination, therapy is supportive with I.V. fluids, electrolytes, and I.V. pressors if needed

Drug Interactions

Decreased effect of oral hypoglycemics; decreased absorption with cholestyramine and colestipol
Increased effect with furosemide and other loop diuretics
Increased toxicity/levels of lithium

Mechanism of Action The diuretic mechanism of action of the thiazides is primarily inhibition of sodium, chloride, and water reabsorption in the renal distal tubules, thereby producing diuresis with a resultant reduction in plasma volume. The antihypertensive mechanism of action of the thiazides is unknown. It is known that doses of thiazides produce greater reduction in blood pressure than equivalent diuretic doses of loop diuretics. There has been speculation that the thiazides may have some influence on vascular tone mediated through sodium depletion, but this remains to be proven.

Pharmacodynamics/Kinetics

Onset of of diuretic effect: Within 2 hours
Peak: 4 hours
Duration: 12-24 hours

Usual Dosage Oral:

Children >6 months: 0.07 mg/kg/24 hours or 2 mg/m²/24 hours
Adults: 1-4 mg/day

Dosing adjustment in renal impairment: Reduced dosage is necessary

Test Interactions ↑ ammonia (B), ↑ amylase (S), ↑ calcium (S), ↑ chloride (S), ↑ cholesterol (S), ↑ glucose, ↑ uric acid (S); ↓ chloride (S), ↓ magnesium, ↓ potassium (S), ↓ sodium (S)

Patient Information May be taken with food or milk; take early in day to avoid nocturia; take the last dose of multiple doses no later than 6 PM unless instructed otherwise. A few people who take this medication become more sensitive to sunlight and may experience skin rash, redness, itching, or severe sunburn, especially if sun block SPF ≥15 is not used on exposed skin areas.

Nursing Implications Assess weight, I & O reports daily to determine fluid loss; take blood pressure with patient lying down and standing

Dosage Forms Tablet: 2 mg, 4 mg

Trichloroacetaldehyde Monohydrate *see* Chloral Hydrate *on page 247*
Tricosal® *see* Choline Magnesium Trisalicylate *on page 269*
Triderm® *see* Triamcinolone *on page 1255*
Tridesilon® *see* Desonide *on page 354*
Tridil® *see* Nitroglycerin *on page 909*

Trientine (TRYE en teen)

Replaces Cuprid®
Brand Names Syprine®
Synonyms Trientine Hydrochloride
Therapeutic Category Antidote, Copper Toxicity; Chelating Agent, Oral
Use Treatment of Wilson's disease in patients intolerant to penicillamine
Pregnancy Risk Factor C
Contraindications Rheumatoid arthritis, biliary cirrhosis, cystinuria, known hypersensitivity to trientine
Warnings/Precautions May cause iron deficiency anemia; monitor closely; use with caution in patients with reactive airway disease
Adverse Reactions

1% to 10%:
Endocrine & metabolic: Iron deficiency
Hematologic: Anemia

<1%:
Central nervous system: Malaise
Gastrointestinal: Heartburn, epigastric pain
Local: Tenderness, thickening and fissuring of skin
Neuromuscular & skeletal: Muscle cramps
Miscellaneous: SLE

Overdosage/Toxicology Overdosage is unknown; a single 30 g ingestion resulted in no toxicity; following GI decontamination, treatment is supportive

Drug Interactions Decreased effect with iron and possibly other mineral supplements

Mechanism of Action Trientine hydrochloride is an oral chelating agent structurally dissimilar from penicillamine and other available chelating agents; an effective oral chelator of copper used to induce adequate cupriuresis

Usual Dosage Oral (administer on an empty stomach):

Children <12 years: 500-750 mg/day in divided doses 2-4 times/day; maximum: 1.5 g/day

Adults: 750-1250 mg/day in divided doses 2-4 times/day; maximum dose: 2 g/day

Patient Information Take 1 hour before or 2 hours after meals and at least 1 hour apart from any drug, food, or milk; do not chew capsule, swallow whole followed by a full glass of water; notify physician of any fever or skin changes; any skin exposed to the contents of a capsule should be promptly washed with water

Dosage Forms Capsule, as hydrochloride: 250 mg

Trientine Hydrochloride *see* Trientine *on previous page*

Triethanolamine Polypeptide Oleate-Condensate

(trye eth a NOLE a meen pol i PEP tide OH lee ate-KON den sate)

Brand Names Cerumenex®

Therapeutic Category Otic Agent, Cerumenolytic

Use Removal of ear wax (cerumen)

Pregnancy Risk Factor C

Contraindications Perforated tympanic membrane or otitis media, hypersensitivity to product or any component

Warnings/Precautions Avoid undue exposure to peridural skin during administration and the flushing out of ear canal; discontinue if sensitization or irritation occurs

Adverse Reactions

<1%:

Dermatologic: Mild erythema and pruritus, severe eczematoid reactions

Local: Localized dermatitis

Mechanism of Action Emulsifies and disperses accumulated cerumen

Pharmacodynamics/Kinetics Onset of effect: Produces slight disintegration of very hard ear wax by 24 hours

Usual Dosage Children and Adults: Otic: Fill ear canal, insert cotton plug; allow to remain 15-30 minutes; flush ear with lukewarm water as a single treatment; if a second application is needed for unusually hard impactions, repeat the procedure

Monitoring Parameters Evaluate hearing before and after instillation of medication

Patient Information For external use in the ear only; warm to body temperature before using to improve effect; avoid touching dropper to any surface; hold ear lobe up and back; lie on your side or tilt the affected ear up for ease of administration; fill ear canal, let stand for 15-30 minutes, then flush

Nursing Implications Warm solution to body temperature before using; avoid undue exposure of the drug to the periauricular skin

Dosage Forms Solution, otic: 6 mL, 12 mL

Triethylenethiophosphoramide *see* Thiotepa *on page 1220*

Trifluoperazine (trye floo oh PER a zeen)

Related Information

Antipsychotic Agents Comparison *on page 1396*

Brand Names Stelazine®

Canadian/Mexican Brand Names Flupazine® (Mexico)

Synonyms Trifluoperazine Hydrochloride

Therapeutic Category Antianxiety Agent; Antipsychotic Agent; Phenothiazine Derivative

Use Treatment of psychoses and management of nonpsychotic anxiety

Pregnancy Risk Factor C

Contraindications Hypersensitivity to trifluoperazine or any component, cross-sensitivity with other phenothiazines may exist, coma, circulatory collapse, history of blood dyscrasias

Warnings/Precautions Safety in children <6 months of age has not been established; use with caution in patients with cardiovascular disease, seizures, hepatic dysfunction, narrow-angle glaucoma, or bone marrow suppression; watch for hypotension when administering I.M. or I.V.; use with caution in patients with myasthenia gravis or Parkinson's disease

(Continued)

Trifluoperazine *(Continued)*

Adverse Reactions

>10%:

Cardiovascular: Hypotension, orthostatic hypotension

Central nervous system: Pseudoparkinsonism, akathisia, dystonias, tardive dyskinesia (persistent), dizziness

Gastrointestinal: Constipation

Ocular: Pigmentary retinopathy

Respiratory: Nasal congestion

Miscellaneous: Diaphoresis (decreased)

1% to 10%:

Genitourinary: Dysuria, ejaculatory disturbances

Dermatologic: Increased sensitivity to sun, rash

Endocrine & metabolic: Changes in menstrual cycle, changes in libido, breast pain

Gastrointestinal: Weight gain, nausea, vomiting, stomach pain

Neuromuscular & skeletal: Trembling of fingers

<1%:

Central nervous system: Neuroleptic malignant syndrome (NMS), impairment of temperature regulation, lowering of seizures threshold

Dermatologic: Discoloration of skin (blue-gray)

Endocrine & metabolic: Galactorrhea

Genitourinary: Priapism

Hematologic: Agranulocytosis, leukopenia

Hepatic: Cholestatic jaundice, hepatotoxicity

Ocular: Cornea and lens changes

Overdosage/Toxicology Symptoms of overdose include deep sleep, coma, extrapyramidal symptoms, abnormal involuntary muscle movements, hypo- or hypertension, cardiac arrhythmias

Following initiation of essential overdose management, toxic symptom treatment and supportive treatment should be initiated. Hypotension usually responds to I.V. fluids or Trendelenburg positioning. If unresponsive to these measures, the use of a parenteral inotrope may be required (eg, norepinephrine 0.1-0.2 mcg/kg/minute titrated to response). Seizures commonly respond to diazepam (I.V. 5-10 mg bolus in adults every 15 minutes if needed up to a total of 30 mg; I.V. 0.25-0.4 mg/kg/dose up to a total of 10 mg in children) or to phenytoin or phenobarbital. Neuroleptics often cause extrapyramidal symptoms (eg, dystonic reactions) requiring management with diphenhydramine 1-2 mg/kg (adults) up to a maximum of 50 mg I.M. or I.V. slow push followed by a maintenance dose for 48-72 hours. When these reactions are unresponsive to diphenhydramine, benztropine mesylate I.V. 1-2 mg (adults) may be effective. These agents are generally effective within 2-5 minutes. Cardiac arrhythmias are treated with lidocaine 1-2 mg/kg bolus followed by a maintenance infusion.

Drug Interactions

Decreased effect of anticonvulsants (increases requirements), guanethidine, anticoagulants; decreased effect with anticholinergics

Increased effect/toxicity with CNS depressants, metrizamide (increases seizures), propranolol, lithium (rare encephalopathy)

Stability Store injection at room temperature; protect from heat and from freezing; use only clear or slightly yellow solutions

Mechanism of Action Blocks postsynaptic mesolimbic dopaminergic receptors in the brain; exhibits a strong alpha-adrenergic blocking effect and depresses the release of hypothalamic and hypophyseal hormones

Pharmacodynamics/Kinetics

Metabolism: Extensive in the liver

Half-life: >24 hours with chronic use

Usual Dosage

Children 6-12 years: Psychoses:

Oral: Hospitalized or well supervised patients: Initial: 1 mg 1-2 times/day, gradually increase until symptoms are controlled or adverse effects become troublesome; maximum: 15 mg/day

I.M.: 1 mg twice daily

Adults:

Psychoses:

Outpatients: Oral: 1-2 mg twice daily

Hospitalized or well supervised patients: Initial: 2-5 mg twice daily with optimum response in the 15-20 mg/day range; do not exceed 40 mg/day

I.M.: 1-2 mg every 4-6 hours as needed up to 10 mg/24 hours maximum

Nonpsychotic anxiety: Oral: 1-2 mg twice daily; maximum: 6 mg/day; therapy for anxiety should not exceed 12 weeks; do not exceed 6 mg/day for longer than 12 weeks when treating anxiety; agitation, jitteriness, or insomnia may be confused with original neurotic or psychotic symptoms

Hemodialysis: Not dialyzable (0% to 5%)

Administration Administer I.M. injection deep in upper outer quadrant of buttock

Reference Range Therapeutic response and blood levels have not been established

Test Interactions ↑ cholesterol (S), ↑ glucose; ↓ uric acid (S)

Patient Information This drug usually requires several weeks for a full therapeutic response to be seen. Avoid excessive exposure to sunlight tanning lamps; concentrate must be diluted in 2-4 oz of liquid (water, carbonated drinks, fruit juices, tomato juice, milk, or pudding); wash hands if undiluted concentrate is spilled on skin to prevent contact dermatosis

Nursing Implications Watch for hypotension when administering I.M. or I.V.; observe for extrapyramidal effects

Dosage Forms

Concentrate, oral, as hydrochloride: 10 mg/mL (60 mL)
Injection, as hydrochloride: 2 mg/mL (10 mL)
Tablet, as hydrochloride: 1 mg, 2 mg, 5 mg, 10 mg

Trifluoperazine Hydrochloride *see* Trifluoperazine *on page 1261*

Trifluorothymidine *see* Trifluridine *on this page*

Trifluridine (trye FLURE i deen)

Brand Names Viroptic®

Synonyms F_3T; Trifluorothymidine

Therapeutic Category Antiviral Agent, Ophthalmic

Use Treatment of primary keratoconjunctivitis and recurrent epithelial keratitis caused by herpes simplex virus types I and II

Pregnancy Risk Factor C

Contraindications Known hypersensitivity to trifluridine or any component

Warnings/Precautions Mild local irritation of conjunctival and cornea may occur when instilled but usually transient effects

Adverse Reactions

1% to 10%: Local: Burning, stinging

<1%:

- Cardiovascular: Hyperemia
- Ocular: Palpebral edema, epithelial keratopathy, keratitis, stromal edema, increased intraocular pressure
- Miscellaneous: Hypersensitivity reactions

Stability Refrigerate at 2°C to 8°C (36°F to 46°F); storage at room temperature may result in a solution altered pH which could result in ocular discomfort upon administration and/or decreased potency

Mechanism of Action Interferes with viral replication by incorporating into viral DNA in place of thymidine, inhibiting thymidylate synthetase resulting in the formation of defective proteins

Pharmacodynamics/Kinetics Absorption: Ophthalmic instillation: Systemic absorption is negligible, while corneal penetration is adequate

Usual Dosage Adults: Instill 1 drop into affected eye every 2 hours while awake, to a maximum of 9 drops/day, until re-epithelialization of corneal ulcer occurs; then use 1 drop every 4 hours for another 7 days; do **not** exceed 21 days of treatment; if improvement has not taken place in 7-14 days, consider another form of therapy

Patient Information Notify physician if improvement is not seen after 7 days, condition worsens, or if irritation occurs; do not discontinue without notifying the physician, do not exceed recommended dosage

Dosage Forms Solution, ophthalmic: 1% (7.5 mL)

Trihexy® *see* Trihexyphenidyl *on this page*

Trihexyphenidyl (trye heks ee FEN i dil)

Brand Names Artañe®; Trihexy®

Canadian/Mexican Brand Names Apo-Trihex® (Canada); Novo-Hexidyl® (Canada); PMS-Trihexyphenidyl (Canada); Trihexyphen® (Canada); Hipokinon® (Mexico)

Synonyms Benzhexol Hydrochloride; Trihexyphenidyl Hydrochloride

Therapeutic Category Anticholinergic Agent; Anti-Parkinson's Agent

Use Adjunctive treatment of Parkinson's disease; also used in treatment of drug-induced extrapyramidal effects and acute dystonic reactions

Pregnancy Risk Factor C

Contraindications Hypersensitivity to trihexyphenidyl or any component, patients with narrow-angle glaucoma; pyloric or duodenal obstruction, stenosing peptic ulcers; bladder neck obstructions; achalasia; myasthenia gravis

Warnings/Precautions Use with caution in hot weather or during exercise. Elderly patients require strict dosage regulation. Use with caution in patients with

(Continued)

Trihexyphenidyl *(Continued)*

tachycardia, cardiac arrhythmias, hypertension, hypotension, prostatic hypertrophy or any tendency toward urinary retention, liver or kidney disorders, and obstructive disease of the GI or GU tract. May exacerbate mental symptoms when used to treat extrapyramidal reactions When given in large doses or to susceptible patients, may cause weakness.

Adverse Reactions

>10%:
- Dermatologic: Dry skin
- Gastrointestinal: Constipation, xerostomia, dry throat
- Respiratory: Dry nose
- Miscellaneous: Diaphoresis (decreased)

1% to 10%:
- Dermatologic: Increased sensitivity to light
- Endocrine & metabolic: Decreased flow of breast milk
- Gastrointestinal: Dysphagia

<1%:
- Cardiovascular: Orthostatic hypotension, ventricular fibrillation, tachycardia, palpitations
- Central nervous system: Confusion, drowsiness, headache, loss of memory, fatigue, ataxia
- Dermatologic: Rash
- Gastrointestinal: Bloated feeling, nausea, vomiting
- Genitourinary: Dysuria
- Neuromuscular & skeletal: Weakness
- Ocular: Increased intraocular pain, blurred vision

Overdosage/Toxicology Symptoms of overdose include blurred vision, urinary retention, tachycardia

Anticholinergic toxicity is caused by strong binding of the drug to cholinergic receptors. Anticholinesterase inhibitors reduce acetylcholinesterase; for anticholinergic overdose with severe life-threatening symptoms, physostigmine 1-2 mg (0.5 or 0.02 mg/kg for children) S.C. or I.V., slowly may be given to reverse these effects

Drug Interactions

Decreased effect of levodopa

Increased toxicity with narcotic analgesics, phenothiazines, TCAs, quinidine, levodopa; anticholinergics

Mechanism of Action Thought to act by blocking excess acetylcholine at cerebral synapses; many of its effects are due to its pharmacologic similarities with atropine

Pharmacodynamics/Kinetics

Peak effect: Within 1 hour

Half-life: 3.3-4.1 hours

Time to peak serum concentration: Within 1-1.5 hours

Elimination: Primarily in urine

Usual Dosage Adults: Oral: Initial: 1-2 mg/day, increase by 2 mg increments at intervals of 3-5 days; usual dose: 5-15 mg/day in 3-4 divided doses

Dietary Considerations Alcohol: Additive CNS effect, avoid use

Monitoring Parameters IOP monitoring and gonioscopic evaluations should be performed periodically

Patient Information Take after meals or with food if GI upset occurs; do not discontinue drug abruptly; notify physician if adverse GI effects, rapid or pounding heartbeat, confusion, eye pain, rash, fever or heat intolerance occurs. Observe caution when performing hazardous tasks or those that require alertness such as driving, as may cause drowsiness. Avoid alcohol and other CNS depressants. May cause dry mouth - adequate fluid intake or hard sugar free candy may relieve. Difficult urination or constipation may occur - notify physician if effects persist; may increase susceptibility to heat stroke.

Nursing Implications Tolerated best if given in 3 daily doses and with food; high doses may be divided into 4 doses, at meal times and at bedtime; patients may be switched to sustained-action capsules when stabilized on conventional dosage forms

Dosage Forms

Capsule, as hydrochloride, sustained release: 5 mg

Elixir, as hydrochloride: 2 mg/5 mL (480 mL)

Tablet, as hydrochloride: 2 mg, 5 mg

Trihexyphenidyl Hydrochloride *see* Trihexyphenidyl *on previous page*

Tri-Kort® *see* Triamcinolone *on page 1255*

Trilafon® *see* Perphenazine *on page 979*

Tri-Levlen® *see* Ethinyl Estradiol and Levonorgestrel *on page 484*

Trilisate® *see* Choline Magnesium Trisalicylate *on page 269*

Trilog® *see* Triamcinolone *on page 1255*

Trilone® *see* Triamcinolone *on page 1255*

Trimazide® *see* Trimethobenzamide *on this page*

Trimethobenzamide (trye meth oh BEN za mide)

Brand Names Arrestin®; Pediatric Triban®; Tebamide®; T-Gen®; Ticon®; Tigan®; Triban®; Trimazide®

Synonyms Trimethobenzamide Hydrochloride

Therapeutic Category Antiemetic

Use Control of nausea and vomiting (especially for long-term antiemetic therapy); less effective than phenothiazines but may be associated with fewer side effects

Pregnancy Risk Factor C

Contraindications Hypersensitivity to trimethobenzamide, benzocaine, or any component; injection contraindicated in children and suppositories are contraindicated in premature infants or neonates

Warnings/Precautions May mask emesis due to Reye's syndrome or mimic CNS effects of Reye's syndrome in patients with emesis of other etiologies; use in patients with acute vomiting should be avoided

Adverse Reactions

>10%: Central nervous system: Drowsiness

1% to 10%:

- Cardiovascular: Hypotension
- Central nervous system: Dizziness, headache
- Gastrointestinal: Diarrhea
- Neuromuscular & skeletal: Muscle cramps

<1%:

- Central nervous system: Mental depression, convulsions, opisthotonus
- Dermatologic: Hypersensitivity skin reactions
- Hematologic: Blood dyscrasias
- Hepatic: Hepatic impairment

Overdosage/Toxicology Symptoms of overdose include hypotension, seizures, CNS depression, cardiac arrhythmias, disorientation, confusion

Following initiation of essential overdose management, toxic symptom treatment and supportive treatment should be initiated. Hypotension usually responds to I.V. fluids or Trendelenburg positioning. If unresponsive to these measures, the use of a parenteral inotrope may be required (eg, norepinephrine 0.1-0.2 mcg/kg/minute titrated to response). Seizures commonly respond to diazepam (I.V. 5-10 mg bolus in adults every 15 minutes, if needed, up to a total of 30 mg; I.V. 0.25-0.4 mg/kg/dose up to a total of 10 mg in children) or to phenytoin or phenobarbital. Critical cardiac arrhythmias often respond to lidocaine 1-2 mg/kg bolus followed by a maintenance infusion. Extrapyramidal symptoms (eg, dystonic reactions) may be managed with diphenhydramine 1-2 mg/kg (adults) up to a maximum of 50 mg I.M. or I.V. slow push followed by a maintenance dose for 48-72 hours. When these reactions are unresponsive to diphenhydramine, benztropine mesylate I.V. 1-2 mg (adults) may be effective. These agents are generally effective within 2-5 minutes.

Drug Interactions Antagonism of oral anticoagulants may occur

Stability Store injection at room temperature; protect from heat and from freezing; use only clear solutions

Mechanism of Action Acts centrally to inhibit the medullary chemoreceptor trigger zone

Pharmacodynamics/Kinetics

Onset of antiemetic effect:

- Oral: Within 10-40 minutes
- I.M.: Within 15-35 minutes

Duration: 3-4 hours

Absorption: Rectal: ~60%

Usual Dosage Rectal use is contraindicated in neonates and premature infants

Children:

- Rectal: <14 kg: 100 mg 3-4 times/day
- Oral, rectal: 14-40 kg: 100-200 mg 3-4 times/day

Adults:

- Oral: 250 mg 3-4 times/day
- I.M., rectal: 200 mg 3-4 times/day

Patient Information May cause drowsiness, impair judgment and coordination; report any restlessness or involuntary movements to physician

Nursing Implications Use only clear solution; observe for extrapyramidal and anticholinergic effects

Dosage Forms

- Capsule, as hydrochloride: 100 mg, 250 mg
- Injection, as hydrochloride: 100 mg/mL (2 mL, 20 mL)
- Suppository, rectal, as hydrochloride: 100 mg, 200 mg

Trimethobenzamide Hydrochloride *see* Trimethobenzamide *on previous page*

Trimethoprim (trye METH oh prim)

Brand Names Proloprim®; Trimpex®

Synonyms TMP

Therapeutic Category Antibiotic, Miscellaneous

Use Treatment of urinary tract infections; acute otitis media in children; acute exacerbations of chronic bronchitis in adults; in combination with other agents for treatment of toxoplasmosis, *Pneumocystis carinii*

Pregnancy Risk Factor C

Contraindications Hypersensitivity to trimethoprim or any component, megaloblastic anemia due to folate deficiency

Warnings/Precautions Use with caution in patients with impaired renal or hepatic function or with possible folate deficiency

Adverse Reactions

>10%: Dermatologic: Rash, pruritus

1% to 10%: Hematologic: Megaloblastic anemia

<1%:

- Central nervous system: Fever
- Dermatologic: Exfoliative dermatitis
- Gastrointestinal: Nausea, vomiting, epigastric distress
- Hematologic: Thrombocytopenia, neutropenia, leukopenia
- Hepatic: Cholestatic jaundice, increased LFTs
- Renal: Elevation of BUN/serum creatinine

Overdosage/Toxicology Symptoms of acute toxicity includes: nausea, vomiting, confusion, dizziness; chronic overdose results in bone marrow suppression

Treatment of acute overdose is supportive following GI decontamination; treatment of chronic overdose is use of oral leucovorin 5-15 mg/day

Drug Interactions Increased effect/toxicity/levels of phenytoin

Mechanism of Action Inhibits folic acid reduction to tetrahydrofolate, and thereby inhibits microbial growth

Pharmacodynamics/Kinetics

Absorption: Oral: Readily and extensive

Protein binding: 42% to 46%

Metabolism: Partially in the liver

Half-life: 8-14 hours, prolonged with renal impairment

Time to peak serum concentration: Within 1-4 hours

Elimination: Significantly in urine (60% to 80% as unchanged drug)

Usual Dosage Oral:

Children: 4 mg/kg/day in divided doses every 12 hours

Adults: 100 mg every 12 hours or 200 mg every 24 hours

Dosing interval in renal impairment:

- Cl_{cr} 15-30 mL/minute: Administer 100 mg every 18 hours or 50 mg every 12 hours
- Cl_{cr} <15 mL/minute: Administer 100 mg every 24 hours or avoid use

Hemodialysis: Moderately dialyzable (20% to 50%)

Reference Range Therapeutic: Peak: 5-15 mg/L; Trough: 2-8 mg/L

Patient Information Take with milk or food; report any skin rash, persistent or severe fatigue, fever, sore throat, or unusual bleeding or bruising; complete full course of therapy

Dosage Forms Tablet: 100 mg, 200 mg

Trimethoprim and Sulfamethoxazole *see* Co-Trimoxazole *on page 315*

Trimethylpsoralen *see* Trioxsalen *on page 1269*

Trimetrexate Glucuronate (tri me TREKS ate gloo KYOOR oh nate)

Related Information

Toxicities of Chemotherapeutic Agents *on page 1382*

Brand Names Neutrexin®

Therapeutic Category Antineoplastic Agent, Folate Antagonist

Use Alternative therapy for the treatment of moderate-to-severe *Pneumocystis carinii* pneumonia (PCP) in immunocompromised patients, including patients with acquired immunodeficiency syndrome (AIDS), who are intolerant of, or are refractory to, co-trimoxazole therapy or for whom co-trimoxazole and pentamidine are contraindicated (concurrent folinic acid [leucovorin] must always be administered); not as effective as co-trimoxazole, however, much fewer treatment-limiting adverse effects

Contraindications Previous hypersensitivity to trimetrexate or methotrexate, severe existing myelosuppression

Warnings/Precautions Must be administered with concurrent leucovorin to avoid potentially serious or life-threatening toxicities; leucovorin therapy must extend for 72 hours past the last dose of trimetrexate; use with caution in patients with mild myelosuppression, severe hepatic or renal dysfunction, hypoproteinemia, hypoalbuminemia, or previous extensive myelosuppressive therapies

Adverse Reactions

1% to 10%:

Central nervous system: Seizures, fever
Dermatologic: Rash
Gastrointestinal: Stomatitis, nausea, vomiting
Hematologic: Neutropenia, thrombocytopenia, anemia
Hepatic: Elevated liver function tests
Neuromuscular & skeletal: Peripheral neuropathy
Renal: Increased serum creatinine
Miscellaneous: Flu-like illness, hypersensitivity reactions

Drug Interactions

Decreased effect of pneumococcal vaccine
Increased toxicity (infection rates) of yellow fever vaccine

Stability Reconstituted I.V. solution is stable for 24 hours at room temperature or 7 days when refrigerated; intact vials should be refrigerated at 2°C to 8°C

Mechanism of Action Exerts an antimicrobial effect through potent inhibition of the enzyme dihydrofolate reductase (DHFR)

Pharmacodynamics/Kinetics

Distribution: V_d: 0.62 L/kg
Metabolism: Extensive in the liver
Half-life: 15-17 hours

Usual Dosage Adults: I.V.: 45 mg/m^2 once daily over 60 minutes for 21 days; it is necessary to reduce the dose in patients with liver dysfunction, although no specific recommendations exist

Administration Reconstituted solution should be filtered (0.22 μM) prior to further dilution; final solution should be clear, hue will range from colorless to pale yellow; trimetrexate forms a precipitate instantly upon contact with chloride ion or leucovorin, therefore it should not be added to solutions containing sodium chloride or other anions; trimetrexate and leucovorin solutions **must** be administered separately; intravenous lines should be flushed with at least 10 mL of D_5W between trimetrexate and leucovorin

Monitoring Parameters Check and record patient's temperature daily; absolute neutrophil counts (ANC), platelet count, renal function tests (serum creatinine, BUN), hepatic function tests (ALT, AST, alkaline phosphatase)

Patient Information Report promptly any fever, rash, flu-like symptoms, numbness or tingling in the extremities, nausea, vomiting, abdominal pain, mouth sores, increased bruising or bleeding, black tarry stools

Nursing Implications Notify primary physician if there is:

Fever ≥103°F
Generalized rash
Seizures
Bleeding from any site
Uncontrolled nausea/vomiting
Laboratory abnormalities which warrant dose modification
Any other clinical adverse event or laboratory abnormality occurring in therapy which is judged as serious for that patient or which causes unexplained effects or concern
Initiate "Bleeding Precautions" for platelet counts ≤50,000/mm^3
Initiate "Infection Control Measures" for absolute neutrophil counts (ANC) ≤1000/mm^3

Additional Information Not a vesicant; methotrexate derivative

Dosage Forms Powder for injection: 25 mg

Trimipramine (trye MI pra meen)

Related Information

Antidepressant Agents Comparison *on page 1393*

Brand Names Surmontil®

Canadian/Mexican Brand Names Apo-Trimip® (Canada); Novo-Tripramine® (Canada); Nu-Trimipramine® (Canada); Rhotrimine® (Canada)

Synonyms Trimipramine Maleate

Therapeutic Category Antidepressant, Tricyclic

Use Treatment of various forms of depression, often in conjunction with psychotherapy

Pregnancy Risk Factor C

Contraindications Narrow-angle glaucoma; avoid use during pregnancy and lactation

Warnings/Precautions Use with caution in patients with cardiovascular disease, conduction disturbances, seizure disorders, urinary retention, hyperthyroidism or those receiving thyroid replacement; avoid use during lactation; use with caution

(Continued)

Trimipramine *(Continued)*

in pregnancy; do not discontinue abruptly in patients receiving chronic high-dose therapy

Adverse Reactions

>10%:

- Central nervous system: Dizziness, drowsiness, headache
- Gastrointestinal: Xerostomia, constipation, increased appetite, nausea, unpleasant taste, weight gain
- Neuromuscular & skeletal: Weakness

1% to 10%:

- Cardiovascular: Arrhythmias, hypotension
- Central nervous system: Confusion, delirium, hallucinations, nervousness, restlessness, parkinsonian syndrome, insomnia
- Endocrine & metabolic: Sexual dysfunction
- Gastrointestinal: Diarrhea, heartburn
- Genitourinary: Dysuria
- Neuromuscular & skeletal: Fine muscle tremors
- Ocular: Blurred vision, eye pain
- Miscellaneous: Diaphoresis (excessive)

<1%:

- Central nervous system: Anxiety, seizures
- Dermatologic: Alopecia, photosensitivity
- Endocrine & metabolic: Breast enlargement, galactorrhea, SIADH
- Gastrointestinal: Trouble with gums, decreased lower esophageal sphincter tone may cause GE reflux
- Genitourinary: Testicular edema
- Hematologic: Agranulocytosis, leukopenia, eosinophilia
- Hepatic: Cholestatic jaundice, increased liver enzymes
- Ocular: Increased intraocular pressure
- Otic: Tinnitus
- Miscellaneous: Allergic reactions

Overdosage/Toxicology Symptoms of overdose include agitation, confusion, hallucinations, urinary retention, hypothermia, hypotension, tachycardia, cardiac arrhythmias

Following initiation of essential overdose management, toxic symptoms should be treated. Sodium bicarbonate is indicated when QRS interval is >0.10 seconds or QT_c >0.42 seconds. Ventricular arrhythmias and EKG changes (QRS widening) often respond to systemic alkalinization (sodium bicarbonate 0.5-2 mEq/kg I.V.). Arrhythmias unresponsive to this therapy may respond to lidocaine 1 mg/kg I.V. followed by a titrated infusion. Physostigmine (1-2 mg I.V. slowly for adults or 0.5 mg I.V. slowly for children) may be indicated in reversing cardiac arrhythmias that are life-threatening. Seizures usually respond to diazepam I.V. boluses (5-10 mg for adults up to 30 mg or 0.25-0.4 mg/kg/dose for children up to 10 mg/dose). If seizures are unresponsive or recur, phenytoin or phenobarbital may be required.

Drug Interactions

Decreased effect of guanethidine, clonidine; decreased effect with barbiturates, carbamazepine, phenytoin

Increased effect/toxicity with MAO inhibitors (hyperpyretic crises), CNS depressants, alcohol (CNS depression), methylphenidate (increased levels), cimetidine (decreased clearance), anticholinergics

Mechanism of Action Increases the synaptic concentration of serotonin and/or norepinephrine in the central nervous system by inhibition of their reuptake by the presynaptic neuronal membrane

Pharmacodynamics/Kinetics

- Therapeutic plasma levels: Oral: Occurs within 6 hours
- Protein binding: 95%
- Metabolism: Undergoes significant first-pass metabolism; metabolized in the liver
- Half-life: 20-26 hours
- Elimination: In urine

Usual Dosage Adults: Oral: 50-150 mg/day as a single bedtime dose up to a maximum of 200 mg/day outpatient and 300 mg/day inpatient

Dietary Considerations Alcohol: Avoid use

Monitoring Parameters Blood pressure and pulse rate prior to and during initial therapy; evaluate mental status; monitor weight

Test Interactions ↑ glucose

Patient Information Avoid unnecessary exposure to sunlight; avoid alcohol ingestion; do not discontinue medication abruptly; may cause urine to turn blue-green; may cause drowsiness; can use sugarless gum or hard candy for dry mouth; full effect may not occur for 4-6 weeks

Nursing Implications May increase appetite; may cause drowsiness, raise bed rails, institute safety precautions

Dosage Forms Capsule, as maleate: 25 mg, 50 mg, 100 mg

Trimipramine Maleate *see* Trimipramine *on page 1267*

Trimox® *see* Amoxicillin *on page 77*

Trimpex® *see* Trimethoprim *on page 1266*

Tri-Norinyl® *see* Ethinyl Estradiol and Norethindrone *on page 486*

Triofed® Syrup [OTC] *see* Triprolidine and Pseudoephedrine *on next page*

Triostat™ *see* Liothyronine *on page 729*

Trioxsalen (trye OKS a len)

Brand Names Trisoralen®

Synonyms Trimethylpsoralen

Therapeutic Category Psoralen

Use In conjunction with controlled exposure to ultraviolet light or sunlight for repigmentation of idiopathic vitiligo; increasing tolerance to sunlight with albinism; enhance pigmentation

Pregnancy Risk Factor C

Contraindications Hypersensitivity to psoralens, melanoma, a history of melanoma, or other diseases associated with photosensitivity; porphyria, acute lupus erythematosus; patients <12 years of age

Warnings/Precautions Serious burns from UVA or sunlight can occur if dosage or exposure schedules are exceeded; patients must wear protective eye wear to prevent cataracts; use with caution in patients with severe hepatic or cardiovascular disease

Adverse Reactions

>10%:

Dermatologic: Itching

Gastrointestinal: Nausea

1% to 10%:

Central nervous system: Dizziness, headache, mental depression, insomnia, nervousness

Dermatologic: Severe burns from excessive sunlight or ultraviolet exposure

Gastrointestinal: Gastric discomfort

Mechanism of Action Psoralens are thought to form covalent bonds with pyrimidine bases in DNA which inhibit the synthesis of DNA. This reaction involves excitation of the trioxsalen molecule by radiation in the long-wave ultraviolet light (UVA) resulting in transference of energy to the trioxsalen molecule producing an excited state. Binding of trioxsalen to DNA occurs only in the presence of ultraviolet light. The increase in skin pigmentation produced by trioxsalen and UVA radiation involves multiple changes in melanocytes and interaction between melanocytes and keratinocytes. In general, melanogenesis is stimulated but the size and distribution of melanocytes is unchanged.

Pharmacodynamics/Kinetics

Peak photosensitivity: 2 hours

Duration: Skin sensitivity to light remains for 8-12 hours

Absorption: Rapid

Half-life, elimination: ~2 hours

Usual Dosage Children >12 years and Adults: Oral: 10 mg/day as a single dose, 2-4 hours before controlled exposure to UVA (for 15-35 minutes) or sunlight; do not continue for longer than 14 days

Patient Information To minimize gastric discomfort, tablets may be taken with milk or after a meal; wear sunglasses during exposure and a light-screening lipstick; do not exceed dose or exposure duration

Dosage Forms Tablet: 5 mg

Tripedia® *see* Diphtheria, Tetanus Toxoids, and Acellular Pertussis Vaccine *on page 403*

Tripedia/ActHIB *see* Diphtheria, Tetanus Toxoids, Whole-Cell Pertussis, and *Haemophilus Influenzae* Type b Conjugate Vaccines *on page 404*

Tripelennamine (tri pel EN a meen)

Brand Names PBZ®; PBZ-SR®

Canadian/Mexican Brand Names Pyribenzamine® (Canada)

Synonyms Tripelennamine Citrate; Tripelennamine Hydrochloride

Therapeutic Category Antihistamine, H_1 Blocker

Use Perennial and seasonal allergic rhinitis and other allergic symptoms including urticaria

Pregnancy Risk Factor B

Contraindications Hypersensitivity to tripelennamine or any component

Warnings/Precautions Use with caution in patients with narrow-angle glaucoma, bladder neck obstruction, symptomatic prostatic hypertrophy, asthmatic attacks, and stenosing peptic ulcer

(Continued)

Tripelennamine *(Continued)*

Adverse Reactions

>10%:

Central nervous system: Slight to moderate drowsiness

Respiratory: Thickening of bronchial secretions

1% to 10%:

Central nervous system: Headache, fatigue, nervousness, dizziness

Gastrointestinal: Appetite increase, weight gain, nausea, diarrhea, abdominal pain, xerostomia

Neuromuscular & skeletal: Arthralgia

Respiratory: Pharyngitis

<1%:

Cardiovascular: Edema, palpitations, hypotension

Central nervous system: Depression, sedation, paradoxical excitement, insomnia

Dermatologic: Angioedema, photosensitivity, rash

Genitourinary: Urinary retention

Hepatic: Hepatitis

Neuromuscular & skeletal: Myalgia, paresthesia, tremor

Ocular: Blurred vision

Respiratory: Bronchospasm, epistaxis

Overdosage/Toxicology Symptoms of overdose include CNS stimulation or depression; flushed skin, mydriasis, ataxia, athetosis, dry mouth

There is no specific treatment for an antihistamine overdose, however, most of its clinical toxicity is due to anticholinergic effects. For anticholinergic overdose with severe life-threatening symptoms, physostigmine 1-2 mg (0.5 or 0.02 mg/kg for children) I.V., slowly may be given to reverse these effects.

Drug Interactions Increased effect/toxicity with alcohol, CNS depressants, MAO inhibitors

Mechanism of Action Competes with histamine for H_1-receptor sites on effector cells in the gastrointestinal tract, blood vessels, and respiratory tract

Pharmacodynamics/Kinetics

Onset of antihistaminic effect: Within 15-30 minutes

Duration: 4-6 hours (up to 8 hours with PBZ-SR®)

Metabolism: Almost completely in the liver

Elimination: In urine

Usual Dosage Oral:

Infants and Children: 5 mg/kg/day in 4-6 divided doses, up to 300 mg/day maximum

Adults: 25-50 mg every 4-6 hours, extended release tablets 100 mg morning and evening up to 100 mg every 8 hours

Dietary Considerations Alcohol: Additive CNS effect, avoid use

Patient Information Do not crush extended release tablets; urinary hesitancy can be reduced if patient voids just prior to taking drug; may cause drowsiness; swallow whole, do not crush or chew sustained release product; avoid alcohol, may impair coordination and judgment

Nursing Implications Raise bed rails, institute safety measures, assist with ambulation

Dosage Forms

Elixir, as citrate: 37.5 mg/5 mL [equivalent to 25 mg hydrochloride] (473 mL)

Tablet, as hydrochloride: 25 mg, 50 mg

Tablet, extended release, as hydrochloride: 100 mg

Tripelennamine Citrate *see* Tripelennamine *on previous page*

Tripelennamine Hydrochloride *see* Tripelennamine *on previous page*

Triphasil® *see* Ethinyl Estradiol and Levonorgestrel *on page 484*

Triple Antibiotic® Topical *see* Bacitracin, Neomycin, and Polymyxin B *on page 129*

Triple Sulfa *see* Sulfabenzamide, Sulfacetamide, and Sulfathiazole *on page 1171*

Triple X® Liquid [OTC] *see* Pyrethrins *on page 1079*

Triposed® Syrup [OTC] *see* Triprolidine and Pseudoephedrine *on this page*

Triposed® Tablet [OTC] *see* Triprolidine and Pseudoephedrine *on this page*

Triprolidine and Pseudoephedrine

(trye PROE li deen & soo doe e FED rin)

Related Information

Pseudoephedrine *on page 1074*

Brand Names Actagen® Syrup [OTC]; Actagen® Tablet [OTC]; Allercon® Tablet [OTC]; Allerfrin® Syrup [OTC]; Allerfrin® Tablet [OTC]; Allerphed Syrup [OTC]; Aprodine® Syrup [OTC]; Aprodine® Tablet [OTC]; Cenafed® Plus Tablet [OTC]; Genac® Tablet [OTC]; Silafed® Syrup [OTC]; Triofed® Syrup [OTC]; Triposed® Syrup [OTC]; Triposed® Tablet [OTC]

Synonyms Pseudoephedrine and Triprolidine

Therapeutic Category Antihistamine, H_1 Blocker; Sympathomimetic

Use Temporary relief of nasal congestion, decongest sinus openings, running nose, sneezing, itching of nose or throat and itchy, watery eyes due to common cold, hay fever, or other upper respiratory allergies

Pregnancy Risk Factor C

Contraindications MAO therapy, hypertension, coronary artery disease, hypersensitivity to pseudoephedrine or any component

Warnings/Precautions Use with caution in patients >60 years of age; use with caution in patients with high blood pressure, heart disease, diabetes, asthma, or thyroid disease

Adverse Reactions

>10%:

- Cardiovascular: Tachycardia
- Central nervous system: Slight to moderate drowsiness, nervousness, insomnia, transient stimulation
- Respiratory: Thickening of bronchial secretions

1% to 10%:

- Central nervous system: Headache, fatigue, dizziness
- Gastrointestinal: Appetite increase, weight gain, nausea, diarrhea, abdominal pain, xerostomia
- Genitourinary: Dysuria
- Neuromuscular & skeletal: Arthralgia, weakness
- Respiratory: Pharyngitis
- Miscellaneous: Diaphoresis

<1%:

- Central nervous system: Depression, hallucinations, convulsions, paradoxical excitement, sedation
- Cardiovascular: Edema, palpitations, hypotension
- Dermatologic: Angioedema, rash, photosensitivity
- Genitourinary: Urinary retention
- Hepatic: Hepatitis
- Neuromuscular & skeletal: Myalgia, paresthesia, tremor
- Ocular: Blurred vision
- Respiratory: Bronchospasm, shortness of breath, dyspnea, epistaxis

Overdosage/Toxicology Symptoms of overdose include hallucinations, CNS depression, seizures, death

There is no specific antidote for pseudoephedrine intoxication and the bulk of the treatment is supportive. Hyperactivity and agitation usually respond to reduced sensory input, however with extreme agitation haloperidol (2-5 mg I.M. for adults) may be required. Hyperthermia is best treated with external cooling measures, or when severe or unresponsive, muscle paralysis with pancuronium may be needed. Hypertension is usually transient and generally does not require treatment unless severe. For diastolic blood pressures >110 mm Hg, a nitroprusside infusion should be initiated. Seizures usually respond to diazepam I.V. and/or phenytoin maintenance regimens.

Drug Interactions

- Decreased effect of guanethidine, reserpine, methyldopa
- Increased toxicity with MAO inhibitors (hypertensive crisis), sympathomimetics, CNS depressants, alcohol (sedation)

Mechanism of Action (Refer to Pseudoephedrine monograph.) Triprolidine is a member of the propylamine (alkylamine) chemical class of H_1-antagonist antihistamines. As such, it is considered to be relatively less sedating than traditional antihistamines of the ethanolamine, phenothiazine, and ethylenediamine classes of antihistamines. Triprolidine has a shorter half-life and duration of action than most of the other alkylamine antihistamines. Like all H_1-antagonist antihistamines, the mechanism of action of triprolidine is believed to involve competitive blockade of H_1-receptor sites resulting in the inability of histamine to combine with its receptor sites and exert its usual effects on target cells. Antihistamines do not interrupt any effects of histamine which have already occurred. Therefore, these agents are used more successfully in the prevention rather than the treatment of histamine-induced reactions.

Usual Dosage Oral:

Children:

- Syrup:
  - 4 months to 2 years: 1.25 mL 3-4 times/day
  - 2-4 years: 2.5 mL 3-4 times/day
  - 4-6 years: 3.75 mL 3-4 times/day
  - 6-12 years: 5 mL every 4-6 hours; do not exceed 4 doses in 24 hours
- Tablet: ½ every 4-6 hours; do not exceed 4 doses in 24 hours

Children >12 years and Adults:

- Syrup: 10 mL every 4-6 hours; do not exceed 4 doses in 24 hours
- Tablet: 1 every 4-6 hours; do not exceed 4 doses in 24 hours

(Continued)

Triprolidine and Pseudoephedrine *(Continued)*

Test Interactions ↑ amylase, lipase

Dosage Forms

Capsule: Triprolidine hydrochloride 2.5 mg and pseudoephedrine hydrochloride 60 mg

Capsule, extended release: Triprolidine hydrochloride 5 mg and pseudoephedrine hydrochloride 120 mg

Syrup: Triprolidine hydrochloride 1.25 mg and pseudoephedrine hydrochloride 30 mg per 5 mL

Tablet: Triprolidine hydrochloride 2.5 mg and pseudoephedrine hydrochloride 60 mg

TripTone® Caplets® [OTC] *see* Dimenhydrinate *on page 395*

Tris Buffer *see* Tromethamine *on page 1274*

Troglitazone (TROE gli to zone)

Related Information

Hypoglycemic Drugs, Comparison of Oral Agents *on page 1411*

Brand Names Rezulin®

Therapeutic Category Antidiabetic Agent; Antihyperglycemic Agent; Hypoglycemic Agent, Oral

Use Type II diabetes: For use in patients with type II diabetes currently on insulin therapy whose hyperglycemia is inadequately controlled (HbA_{1C} >8.5%) despite insulin therapy of over 30 Units/day given as multiple injections.

Management of type II diabetes should include diet control. Caloric restriction, weight loss and exercise are essential for the proper treatment of the diabetic patient. This is important not only the primary treatment of type II diabetes but in maintaining the efficacy of drug therapy. Prior to initiation of troglitazone therapy, investigate secondary causes of poor glycemic control (eg, infection or poor injection technique).

Either monotherapy or combination therapy with sulfonylureas, for patients with type II diabetes

Investigational: A study showed troglitazone may be beneficial in the productive and metabolic consequences of polycystic ovary syndrome (PCOS) (400 mg/day) and less essential hypertension with NIDDM, but more studies are needed.

Pregnancy Risk Factor B

Contraindications Hypersensitivity to troglitazone or any component

Warnings/Precautions Patients with New York Heart Association (NYHA) Class III and IV cardiac status were not studied during clinical trials. Heart enlargement without microscopic changes has been observed in rodents at exposures exceeding 14 times the AUC of the 400 mg human dose. Caution is advised during the administration of troglitazone to patients with NYHA Class III or IV cardiac status.

During all clinical studies, a total of 20 troglitazone-treated patients were withdrawn from treatment because of liver function test abnormalities. Two of the 20 patients developed reversible jaundice. Both had liver biopsies that were consistent with an idiosyncratic drug reaction.

Patients on troglitazone who develop jaundice or whose laboratory results indicate liver injury should stop taking the drug. Approximately 2% of patients can expect to stop taking the drug because of elevated liver enzymes.

Because of its mechanism of action, troglitazone is active only in the presence of insulin. Therefore, do not use in type I diabetes or for the treatment of diabetic ketoacidosis.

Patients receiving troglitazone in combination with insulin may be at risk for hypoglycemia, and a reduction in the dose of insulin may be necessary. Hypoglycemia has not been observed during the administration of troglitazone as monotherapy and would not be expected based on the mechanism of action.

Across all clinical studies, hemoglobin declined by 3% to 4% in troglitazone-treated patients compared with 1% to 2% with placebo. White blood cell counts also declined slightly in troglitazone-treated patients compared with those treated with placebo. These changes occurred within the first 4-8 weeks of therapy. Levels stabilized and remained unchanged for ≤ 2 years of continuing therapy. These changes may be due to the dilutional effects of increased plasma volume and have not been associated with any significant hematologic clinical effects.

Adverse Reactions

>10%:

Central nervous system: Headache, pain

Miscellaneous: Infection

1% to 10%:

Cardiovascular: Peripheral edema

Central nervous system: Dizziness

Gastrointestinal: Nausea, diarrhea, pharyngitis
Genitourinary: Urinary tract infection
Neuromuscular & skeletal: Neck pain, weakness
Respiratory: Rhinitis

Drug Interactions Cytochrome P-450 3A4 Enzyme Inducer

Decreased effects:

Cholestyramine: Concomitant administration of cholestyramine with troglitazone reduces the absorption of troglitazone by 70%; CO-ADMINISTRATION OF CHOLESTYRAMINE AND TROGLITAZONE IS NOT RECOMMENDED.

Oral contraceptives: Administration of troglitazone with an oral contraceptive containing ethinyl estradiol and norethindrone reduced the plasma concentrations of both by 30%. These changes could result in loss of contraception.

Terfenadine: Coadministration of troglitazone with terfenadine decreases plasma concentrations of terfenadine and its active metabolite by 50% to 70% and may reduce the effectiveness of terfenadine

Increased toxicity:

Sulfonylureas (glyburide): Co-administration of troglitazone with glyburide may further decrease plasma glucose levels

Mechanism of Action Thiazolidinedione antidiabetic agent that lowers blood glucose by improving target cell response to insulin, without increasing pancreatic insulin secretion. It has a unique mechanism of action that is dependent on the presence of insulin for activity. Troglitazone decreases hepatic glucose output and increases insulin-dependent glucose disposal in skeletal muscle and possible liver and adipose tissue.

Pharmacodynamics/Kinetics

Absorption: Food increases absorption by 30% to 85%
Distribution: V_d:10.5-26.5 L/kg
Protein binding: >99%, to serum albumin
Metabolism: Extensive; inhibitor of cytochrome P-450 1A1, 1A2, 2A6, 2B6, 2D6, 2E1, and 3A4 isoenzymes
Bioavailability: Absolute
Half-life, plasma elimination: 16-34 hours
Time to peak plasma concentrations: 2-3 hours
Elimination: 85% in feces and 3% in urine

Usual Dosage Oral (take with meals):

Adults:

Continue the current insulin dose upon initiation of troglitazone therapy.

Initiate therapy at 200 mg once daily in patients on insulin therapy. For patients not responding adequately, increase the dose after 2-4 weeks. The usual dose is 400 mg/day; maximum recommended dose: 600 mg/day.

It is recommended that the insulin dose be decreased by 10% to 25% when fasting plasma glucose concentrations decrease to <120 mg/dL in patients receiving concomitant insulin and troglitazone. Individualize further adjustments based on glucose-lowering response.

Elderly: Steady-state pharmacokinetics of troglitazone and metabolites in healthy elderly subjects were comparable to those seen in young adults

Dosing adjustment/comments in renal impairment: Dose adjustment is not necessary

Dosing adjustment in hepatic impairment: Use with caution in patients with hepatic disease

Monitoring Parameters Urine for glucose and ketones, fasting blood glucose, hemoglobin A_{1c}, and fructosamine. Serum transaminase levels should be checked routinely within the first 1-2 months of therapy, then every 3 months during the first year of treatment, and periodically thereafter. Additionally, liver function tests should be performed on any patient on troglitazone who develops symptoms of liver dysfunction, such as nausea, vomiting, abdominal pain, fatigue, loss of appetite, or dark urine.

Reference Range Target range: Adults:

Fasting blood glucose: <120 mg/dL
Glycosylated hemoglobin: <7%

Patient Information

Notify physician if symptoms of liver dysfunction such as nausea, vomiting, abdominal pain, fatigue, loss of appetite, or dark urine occur

Take troglitazone with meals. If the dose is missed at the usual meal, take it at the next meal. If the dose is missed on one day, do not double the dose the following day.

It is important to adhere to dietary instructions and to have blood glucose and glycosylated hemoglobin tested regularly. During periods of stress such as fever, trauma, infection or surgery, insulin requirements may change and patients should seek the advice of their physician.

(Continued)

Troglitazone *(Continued)*

When using combination therapy with insulin, explain the risks of hypoglycemia, its symptoms, treatment and predisposing conditions to patients and their family members.

Nursing Implications Patients who are NPO may need to have their dose held to avoid hypoglycemia

Dosage Forms Tablet: 200 mg, 400 mg

Troleandomycin (troe lee an doe MYE sin)

Brand Names Tao®

Synonyms Triacetyloleandomycin

Therapeutic Category Antibiotic, Macrolide

Use Adjunct in the treatment of corticosteroid-dependent asthma due to its steroid-sparing properties; antibiotic with spectrum of activity similar to erythromycin

Pregnancy Risk Factor C

Contraindications Hypersensitivity to troleandomycin, other macrolides, or any component

Warnings/Precautions Use with caution in patients with impaired hepatic function; chronic hepatitis may occur in patients with long or repetitive courses

Adverse Reactions

>10%: Gastrointestinal: Abdominal cramping and discomfort

1% to 10%:

- Dermatologic: Urticaria, rashes
- Gastrointestinal: Nausea, vomiting, diarrhea

<1%:

- Gastrointestinal: Rectal burning
- Hepatic: Cholestatic jaundice

Overdosage/Toxicology Symptoms of overdose include nausea, vomiting, diarrhea, hearing loss; following GI decontamination, treatment is supportive

Drug Interactions Increased effect/toxicity/levels of carbamazepine, ergot alkaloids, methylprednisolone, oral contraceptives, theophylline, and triazolam; contraindicated with terfenadine due to decreased metabolism of this agent and resultant risk of cardiac arrhythmias and death

Mechanism of Action Decreases methylprednisolone clearance from a linear first order decline to a nonlinear decline in plasma concentration. TAO® also has an undefined action independent of its effects on steroid elimination. Inhibits RNA-dependent protein synthesis at the chain elongation step; binds to the 50S ribosomal subunit resulting in blockage of transpeptidation.

Pharmacodynamics/Kinetics

Time to peak serum concentration: Within 2 hours

Elimination: 10% to 25% of dose excreted in urine as active drug; also excreted in feces via bile

Usual Dosage Oral:

Children 7-13 years: 25-40 mg/kg/day divided every 6 hours (125-250 mg every 6 hours)

- Adjunct in corticosteroid-dependent asthma: 14 mg/kg/day in divided doses every 6-12 hours not to exceed 250 mg every 6 hours; dose is tapered to once daily then alternate day dosing

Children >13 years and adults: 250-500 mg 4 times/day

Administration Administer around-the-clock instead of 4 times/day

Monitoring Parameters Hepatic function tests

Patient Information Complete full course of therapy; notify physician if persistent or severe abdominal pain, nausea, vomiting, jaundice, darkened urine, or fever occurs

Dosage Forms Capsule: 250 mg

Tromethamine (troe METH a meen)

Brand Names Tham®; Tham-E®

Synonyms Tris Buffer; Tris(hydroxymethyl)aminomethane

Therapeutic Category Alkalinizing Agent, Parenteral

Use Correction of metabolic acidosis associated with cardiac bypass surgery or cardiac arrest; to correct excess acidity of stored blood that is preserved with acid citrate dextrose; to prime the pump-oxygenator during cardiac bypass surgery; indicated in infants needing alkalinization after receiving maximum sodium bicarbonate (8-10 mEq/kg/24 hours); (advantage of Tham® is that it alkalinizes without increasing pCO_2 and sodium)

Pregnancy Risk Factor C

Contraindications Uremia or anuria; chronic respiratory acidosis

Warnings/Precautions Reduce dose and monitor pH carefully in renal impairment; drug should not be given for a period of longer than 24 hours unless for a life-threatening situation

Adverse Reactions

1% to 10%:

Cardiovascular: Venospasm

Local: Tissue irritation, necrosis with extravasation

<1%:

Endocrine & metabolic: Hyperosmolality of serum, hyperkalemia, hypoglycemia

Hematologic: Increased blood coagulation time

Hepatic: Liver cell destruction from direct contact with Tham®

Respiratory: Apnea, respiratory depression

Overdosage/Toxicology Symptoms of overdose include alkalosis, hypokalemia, respiratory depression, hypoglycemia; supportive therapy is required to correct electrolyte, osmolality, and abnormalities

Mechanism of Action Acts as a proton acceptor, which combines with hydrogen ions to form bicarbonate buffer, to correct acidosis

Pharmacodynamics/Kinetics

Absorption: 30% of dose is not ionized

Elimination: Rapidly eliminated by kidneys (>75% in 3 hours)

Usual Dosage Dose depends on buffer base deficit; when deficit is known: tromethamine (mL of 0.3 M solution) = body weight (kg) x base deficit (mEq/L); when base deficit is not known: 3-6 mL/kg/dose I.V. (1-2 mEq/kg/dose)

Metabolic acidosis with cardiac arrest:

I.V.: 3.5-6 mL/kg (1-2 mEq/kg/dose) into large peripheral vein; 500-1000 mL if needed in adults

I.V. continuous drip: Infuse slowly by syringe pump over 3-6 hours

Excess acidity of acid citrate dextrose priming blood: 14-70 mL of 0.3 molar solution added to each 500 mL of blood

Dosing comments in renal impairment: Use with caution and monitor for hyperkalemia and EKG

Administration May administer undiluted; infuse into as large a vein as possible; not effective if given orally

Monitoring Parameters Serum electrolytes, arterial blood gases, serum pH, blood sugar, EKG monitoring, renal function tests

Reference Range Blood pH: 7.35-7.45

Nursing Implications If extravasation occurs, aspirate as much fluid as possible, then infiltrate area with procaine 1% to which hyaluronidase has been added

Additional Information 1 mM = 120 mg = 3.3 mL = 1 mEq of Tham®

Dosage Forms

Injection: 36 mg/mL (500 mL)

Powder for injection: 240 mg/mL (150 mL)

Tronolane® [OTC] *see* Pramoxine *on page 1033*

Tronothane® HCl [OTC] *see* Pramoxine *on page 1033*

Tropicacyl® *see* Tropicamide *on this page*

Tropicamide (troe PIK a mide)

Related Information

Cycloplegic Mydriatics Comparison *on page 1409*

Brand Names Mydriacyl®; Opticyl®; Tropicacyl®

Synonyms Bistropamide

Therapeutic Category Ophthalmic Agent, Mydriatic

Use Short-acting mydriatic used in diagnostic procedures; as well as preoperatively and postoperatively; treatment of some cases of acute iritis, iridocyclitis, and keratitis

Pregnancy Risk Factor C

Contraindications Glaucoma, hypersensitivity to tropicamide or any component

Warnings/Precautions Use with caution in infants and children since tropicamide may cause potentially dangerous CNS disturbances; tropicamide may cause an increase in intraocular pressure

Adverse Reactions

1% to 10%:

Cardiovascular: Tachycardia, vascular congestion, edema

Central nervous system: Parasympathetic stimulations, drowsiness, headache

Dermatologic: Eczematoid dermatitis

Gastrointestinal: Xerostomia

Local: Transient stinging

Ocular: Blurred vision, photophobia with or without corneal staining, increased intraocular pressure, follicular conjunctivitis

Overdosage/Toxicology Symptoms of overdose include blurred vision, urinary retention, tachycardia, cardiorespiratory collapse

(Continued)

Tropicamide *(Continued)*

Antidote is physostigmine, pilocarpine; anticholinergic toxicity is caused by strong binding of the drug to cholinergic receptors. For anticholinergic overdose with severe life-threatening symptoms, physostigmine 1-2 mg (0.5 or 0.02 mg/kg for children) S.C. or I.V., slowly may be given to reverse systemic effects.

Stability Store in tightly closed containers

Mechanism of Action Prevents the sphincter muscle of the iris and the muscle of the ciliary body from responding to cholinergic stimulation

Pharmacodynamics/Kinetics

Onset of mydriasis: ~20-40 minutes

Duration: ~6-7 hours

Onset of cycloplegia: Within 30 minutes

Duration: <6 hours

Usual Dosage Children and Adults (individuals with heavily pigmented eyes may require larger doses):

Cycloplegia: Instill 1-2 drops (1%); may repeat in 5 minutes

Exam must be performed within 30 minutes after the repeat dose; if the patient is not examined within 20-30 minutes, instill an additional drop

Mydriasis: Instill 1-2 drops (0.5%) 15-20 minutes before exam; may repeat every 30 minutes as needed

Monitoring Parameters Ophthalmic exam

Patient Information If irritation persists or increases, discontinue use, may cause blurred vision and increased light sensitivity

Nursing Implications Finger pressure should be applied on the lacrimal sac for 1-2 minutes following topical instillation of the solution

Dosage Forms Solution, ophthalmic: 0.5% (2 mL, 15 mL); 1% (2 mL, 3 mL, 15 mL)

Truphylline® *see* Theophylline Salts *on page 1207*

Trusopt® *see* Dorzolamide *on page 419*

Trysul® *see* Sulfabenzamide, Sulfacetamide, and Sulfathiazole *on page 1171*

TSH *see* Thyrotropin *on page 1225*

TSPA *see* Thiotepa *on page 1220*

TST *see* Tuberculin Purified Protein Derivative *on this page*

Tuberculin Purified Protein Derivative

(too BER kyoo lin PURE eh fide PRO teen dah RIV ah tiv)

Related Information

Prophylaxis for Patients Exposed to Common Communicable Diseases *on page 1452*

Skin Tests *on page 1501*

Brand Names Aplisol®; Aplitest®; Sclavo-PPD Solution®; Sclavo Test-PPD®; Tine Test PPD; Tubersol®

Synonyms Mantoux; PPD; Tine Test; TST; Tuberculin Skin Test

Therapeutic Category Diagnostic Agent, Skin Test

Use Skin test in diagnosis of tuberculosis, cell-mediated immunodeficiencies

Pregnancy Risk Factor C

Contraindications 250 TU strength should not be used for initial testing

Warnings/Precautions Do not administer I.V. or S.C.; epinephrine (1:1000) should be available to treat possible allergic reactions

Adverse Reactions

1% to 10%:

Central nervous system:

Dermatologic: Ulceration, necrosis, vesiculation

Local: Pain at injection site

Miscellaneous: Necrosis

Drug Interactions

Decreased effect: Reaction may be suppressed in patients receiving systemic corticosteroids, aminocaproic acid, or within 4-6 weeks following immunization with live or inactivated viral vaccines

Stability Refrigerate; Tubersol™ opened vials are stable for up to 24 hours at <75°F

Mechanism of Action Tuberculosis results in individuals becoming sensitized to certain antigenic components of the *M. tuberculosis* organism. Culture extracts called tuberculins are contained in tuberculin skin test preparations. Upon intracutaneous injection of these culture extracts, a classic delayed (cellular) hypersensitivity reaction occurs. This reaction is characteristic of a delayed course (peak occurs >24 hours after injection, induration of the skin secondary to cell infiltration, and occasional vesiculation and necrosis). Delayed hypersensitivity reactions to tuberculin may indicate infection with a variety of nontuberculosis mycobacteria, or vaccination with the live attenuated mycobacterial strain of *M. bovis* vaccine, BCG, in addition to previous natural infection with *M. tuberculosis*.

Pharmacodynamics/Kinetics

Onset of action: Delayed hypersensitivity reactions to tuberculin usually occur within 5-6 hours following injection

Peak effect: Become maximal at 48-72 hours

Duration: Reactions subside over a few days

Usual Dosage Children and Adults: Intradermal: 0.1 mL about 4" below elbow; use 1/4" to 1/2" or 26- or 27-gauge needle; significant reactions are ≥5 mm in diameter

Interpretation of induration of tuberculin skin test injections: Positive: ≥10 mm; inconclusive: 5-9 mm; negative: <5 mm

Interpretation of induration of Tine test injections: Positive: >2 mm and vesiculation present; inconclusive: <2 mm (give patient Mantoux test of 5 TU/0.1 mL - base decisions on results of Mantoux test); negative: <2 mm or erythema of any size (no need for retesting unless person is a contact of a patient with tuberculosis or there is clinical evidence suggestive of the disease)

Patient Information Return to physician for reaction interpretation at 48-72 hours

Nursing Implications Test dose: 0.1 mL intracutaneously; store in refrigerator; examine site at 48-72 hours after administration; whenever tuberculin is administered, a record should be made of the administration technique (Mantoux method, disposable multiple-puncture device), tuberculin used (OT or PPD), manufacturer and lot number of tuberculin used, date of administration, date of test reading, and the size of the reaction in millimeters (mm).

Dosage Forms Injection:

First test strength: 1 TU/0.1 mL (1 mL)

Intermediate test strength: 5 TU/0.1 mL (1 mL, 5 mL, 10 mL)

Second test strength: 250 TU/0.1 mL (1 mL)

Tine: 5 TU each test

Tuberculin Skin Test *see* Tuberculin Purified Protein Derivative *on previous page*

Tubersol® *see* Tuberculin Purified Protein Derivative *on previous page*

Tubocurarine (too boe kyoor AR een)

Related Information

Neuromuscular Blocking Agents Comparison *on page 1417*

Synonyms *d*-Tubocurarine Chloride; Tubocurarine Chloride

Therapeutic Category Neuromuscular Blocker Agent, Nondepolarizing; Skeletal Muscle Relaxant

Use Adjunct to anesthesia to induce skeletal muscle relaxation

Pregnancy Risk Factor C

Contraindications Hypersensitivity to tubocurarine or any component; patients in whom histamine release is a definite hazard

Warnings/Precautions Use with caution in patients with renal impairment, respiratory depression, impaired hepatic or endocrine function, myasthenia gravis, and the elderly; ventilation must be supported during neuromuscular blockade; rapid administration may cause histamine release resulting in respiratory depression and bronchospasm

Adverse Reactions

1% to 10%: Cardiovascular: Hypotension

<1%:

Cardiovascular: Edema, circulatory collapse, cardiac arrhythmias, increased heart rate or bradycardia, skin flushing

Dermatologic: Rash, itching, erythema

Gastrointestinal: Increased salivation, decreased GI motility

Respiratory: Bronchospasm

Miscellaneous: Hypersensitivity reactions, allergic reactions

Overdosage/Toxicology Symptoms of overdose include prolonged skeletal muscle weakness and apnea, cardiovascular collapse

Use neostigmine, edrophonium or pyridostigmine with atropine to antagonize skeletal muscle relaxation; support of ventilation and the cardiovascular system through mechanical means, fluids, and pressors may be necessary.

Drug Interactions Increased effect/toxicity with aminoglycosides, ketamine, magnesium sulfate, verapamil, quinidine, clindamycin, furosemide

Stability Refrigerate; **incompatible** with barbiturates

Mechanism of Action Blocks acetylcholine from binding to receptors on motor endplate inhibiting depolarization

Pharmacodynamics/Kinetics Elimination: ~33% to 75% of parenteral dose is excreted unchanged in urine in 24 hours; ~10% excreted in bile

Usual Dosage I.V.:

Children and Adults: 0.2-0.4 mg/kg as a single dose; maintenance: 0.04-0.2 mg/kg/dose as needed to maintain paralysis

Alternative adult dose: 6-9 mg once daily, then 3-4.5 mg as needed to maintain paralysis

(Continued)

Tubocurarine *(Continued)*

Dosing adjustment/comments in renal impairment: May accumulate with multiple doses and reductions in subsequent doses is recommended

Cl_{cr} 50-80 mL/minute: Administer 75% of normal dose

Cl_{cr} 10-50 mL/minute: Administer 50% of normal dose

Cl_{cr} <10 mL/minute: Avoid use

Dosing comments in hepatic impairment: Larger doses may be necessary

Administration May also administer I.M.; administer I.V. undiluted over 60-90 seconds and flush I.V. cannula with NS or D_5W

Monitoring Parameters Mean arterial pressure, heart rate, respiratory status, serum potassium

Dosage Forms Injection, as chloride: 3 mg/mL [3 units/mL] (5 mL, 10 mL, 20 mL)

Tubocurarine Chloride *see* Tubocurarine *on previous page*
Tums® [OTC] *see* Calcium Carbonate *on page 185*
Tusibron® [OTC] *see* Guaifenesin *on page 589*
Tusibron-DM® [OTC] *see* Guaifenesin and Dextromethorphan *on page 591*
Tuss-DM® [OTC] *see* Guaifenesin and Dextromethorphan *on page 591*
Tussigon® *see* Hydrocodone and Homatropine *on page 622*
Tussi-Organidin® DM NR *see* Guaifenesin and Dextromethorphan *on page 591*
Tussi-Organidin® NR *see* Guaifenesin and Codeine *on page 590*
Tusstat® Syrup *see* Diphenhydramine *on page 399*
Twice-A-Day® Nasal [OTC] *see* Oxymetazoline *on page 940*
Twilite® Oral [OTC] *see* Diphenhydramine *on page 399*
Two-Dyne® *see* Butalbital Compound *on page 176*
Tylenol® [OTC] *see* Acetaminophen *on page 19*
Tylenol® With Codeine *see* Acetaminophen and Codeine *on page 21*
Tylox® *see* Oxycodone and Acetaminophen *on page 938*

Typhoid Vaccine (TYE foid vak SEEN)

Related Information

Immunization Guidelines *on page 1421*

Recommendations for Travelers *on page 1442*

Brand Names Vivotif Berna™

Synonyms Typhoid Vaccine Live Oral Ty21a

Therapeutic Category Vaccine, Inactivated Bacteria

Use

Parenteral: Promotes active immunity to typhoid fever for patients intimately exposed to a typhoid carrier or foreign travel to a typhoid fever endemic area

Oral: For immunization of children >6 years and adults who expect intimate exposure of or household contact with typhoid fever, travelers to areas of world with risk of exposure to typhoid fever, and workers in microbiology laboratories with expected frequent contact with *S. typhi*

Typhoid vaccine: Live, attenuated TY21a typhoid vaccine should not be administered to immunocompromised persons, including those known to be infected with HIV. Parenteral inactivated vaccine is a theoretically safer alternative for this group.

Pregnancy Risk Factor C

Contraindications Acute respiratory or other active infections, previous sensitivity to typhoid vaccine, congenital or acquired immunodeficient state, acute febrile illness, acute GI illness, other active infection, persistent diarrhea or vomiting

Warnings/Precautions Postpone use in presence of acute infection; use during pregnancy only when clearly needed, immune deficiency conditions; not all recipients of typhoid vaccine will be fully protected against typhoid fever. Travelers should take all necessary precautions to avoid contact or ingestion of potentially contaminated food or water sources. Unless a complete immunization schedule is followed, an optimum immune response may not be achieved.

Adverse Reactions

Oral:

1% to 10%:

Dermatologic: Rash

Gastrointestinal: Abdominal discomfort, stomach cramps, diarrhea, nausea, vomiting

<1%: Anaphylactic reaction

Injection: >10%:

Dermatologic: Local tenderness, erythema, induration

Neuromuscular & skeletal: Myalgia

Drug Interactions Simultaneous administration with other vaccines which cause local or systemic adverse effects should be avoided

Decreased effect with concurrent use of sulfonamides or other antibiotics

Stability Refrigerate, do not freeze; potency is not harmed if mistakenly placed in freezer; however, remove from freezer as soon as possible and place in refrigerator; can still be used if exposed to temperature ≤80°F

Mechanism of Action Virulent strains of *Salmonella typhi* cause disease by penetrating the intestinal mucosa and entering the systemic circulation via the lymphatic vasculature. One possible mechanism of conferring immunity may be the provocation of a local immune response in the intestinal tract induced by oral ingesting of a live strain with subsequent aborted infection. The ability of *Salmonella typhi* to produce clinical disease (and to elicit an immune response) is dependent on the bacteria having a complete lipopolysaccharide. The live attenuate Ty21a strain lacks the enzyme UDP-4-galactose epimerase so that lipopolysaccharide is only synthesized under conditions that induce bacterial autolysis. Thus, the strain remains avirulent despite the production of sufficient lipopolysaccharide to evoke a protective immune response. Despite low levels of lipopolysaccharide synthesis, cells lyse before gaining a virulent phenotype due to the intracellular accumulation of metabolic intermediates.

Pharmacodynamics/Kinetics

Oral:

- Onset of immunity to *Salmonella typhi*: Within about 1 week
- Duration: ~5 years

Parenteral: Duration of immunity: ~3 years

Usual Dosage

S.C.:

- Children 6 months to 10 years: 0.25 mL; repeat in ≥4 weeks (total immunization is 2 doses)
- Children >10 years and Adults: 0.5 mL; repeat dose in ≥4 weeks (total immunization is 2 doses)
- Booster: 0.25 mL every 3 years for children 6 months to 10 years and 0.5 mL every 3 years for children >10 years and adults

Oral: Adults:

- Primary immunization: 1 capsule on alternate days (day 1, 3, 5, and 7)
- Booster immunization: Repeat full course of primary immunization every 5 years

Patient Information Oral capsule should be taken 1 hour before a meal with cold or lukewarm drink, do not chew, swallow whole; systemic adverse effects may persist for 1-2 days. Take all 4 doses exactly as directed on alternate days to obtain a maximal response.

Nursing Implications The doses of vaccine are different between S.C. and intradermal; S.C. injection only should be used

Additional Information Inactivated bacteria vaccine; federal law requires that the date of administration, the vaccine manufacturer, lot number of vaccine, and the administering person's name, title and address be entered into the patient's permanent medical record

Dosage Forms

Capsule, enteric coated: Viable *S. typhi* Ty21a Colony-forming units 2-6 x 10^9 and nonviable *S. typhi* Ty21a Colony-forming units 50 x 10^9 with sucrose, ascorbic acid, amino acid mixture, lactose and magnesium stearate

Injection: 1.5 mL

Typhoid Vaccine Live Oral Ty21a *see* Typhoid Vaccine *on previous page*

Tyramine Content of Foods *see page 1577*

Tyzine® *see* Tetrahydrozoline *on page 1205*

UAD Otic® *see* Neomycin, Polymyxin B, and Hydrocortisone *on page 890*

UCB-P071 *see* Cetirizine *on page 244*

U-Cort™ Cortifoam® *see* Hydrocortisone *on page 623*

Ultane® *see* Sevoflurane *on page 1134*

Ultiva® *see* Remifentanil *on page 1097*

Ultracef® *see* Cefadroxil *on page 218*

Ultram® *see* Tramadol *on page 1247*

Ultra Mide® *see* Urea *on next page*

Ultrase® MT12 *see* Pancrelipase *on page 949*

Ultrase® MT20 *see* Pancrelipase *on page 949*

Ultravate™ *see* Halobetasol *on page 598*

Unasyn® *see* Ampicillin and Sulbactam *on page 87*

Unguentine® [OTC] *see* Benzocaine *on page 138*

Uni-Bent® Cough Syrup *see* Diphenhydramine *on page 399*

Unicap® [OTC] *see* Vitamins, Multiple *on page 1310*

Unipen® *see* Nafcillin *on page 871*

Uni-Pro® [OTC] *see* Ibuprofen *on page 639*

Uni-tussin® [OTC] *see* Guaifenesin *on page 589*

Uni-tussin® DM [OTC] *see* Guaifenesin and Dextromethorphan *on page 591*

Univasc® *see* Moexipril *on page 853*
Unna's Boot *see* Zinc Gelatin *on page 1323*
Unna's Paste *see* Zinc Gelatin *on page 1323*
Urabeth® *see* Bethanechol *on page 150*

Uracil Mustard (YOOR a sil MUS tard)

Therapeutic Category Antineoplastic Agent, Alkylating Agent; Antineoplastic Agent, Nitrogen Mustard

Use Palliative treatment in symptomatic chronic lymphocytic leukemia; non-Hodgkin's lymphomas, chronic myelocytic leukemia, mycosis fungoides, thrombocytosis, polycythemia vera, ovarian carcinoma

Pregnancy Risk Factor X

Contraindications Severe leukopenia, thrombocytopenia, aplastic anemia; in patients whose bone marrow is infiltrated with malignant cells; hypersensitivity to any component

Warnings/Precautions The U.S. Food and Drug Administration (FDA) currently recommends that procedures for proper handling and disposal of antineoplastic agents be considered. Impaired kidney or liver function. The drug should be discontinued if intractable vomiting or diarrhea, precipitous falls in leukocyte or platelet count, or myocardial ischemia occurs. Use with caution in patients who have had high-dose pelvic radiation or previous use of alkylating agents. Patient should be hospitalized during initial course of therapy; may impair fertility in men and women; use with caution in patients with pre-existing marrow suppression.

Adverse Reactions

>10%:
- Gastrointestinal: Nausea, vomiting, diarrhea
- Hematologic: Myelosuppressive; leukopenia and thrombocytopenia nadir: 2-4 weeks, anemia

1% to 10%:
- Central nervous system: Mental depression, nervousness
- Dermatologic: Hyperpigmentation, alopecia
- Endocrine & metabolic: Hyperuricemia

<1%:
- Dermatologic: Pruritus
- Gastrointestinal: Stomatitis, hepatotoxicity

Overdosage/Toxicology Symptoms of overdose include diarrhea, vomiting, severe marrow suppression; no specific antidote to marrow toxicity is available

Mechanism of Action Polyfunctional alkylating agent. The basic reaction of uracil mustard, like that of any alkylating agent, is the replacement of the hydrogen in a reacting chemical with an alkyl group; cell cycle-phase nonspecific antineoplastic agent; exact site of drug action within the cell is not known, but the nucleoproteins of the cell nucleus are believed to be involved.

Pharmacodynamics/Kinetics
- Absorption: Oral
- Elimination: <1% detected in urine

Usual Dosage Oral (do not administer until 2-3 weeks after maximum effect of any previous x-ray or cytotoxic drug therapy of the bone marrow is obtained):

- Children: 0.3 mg/kg in a single weekly dose for 4 weeks
- Adults: 0.15 mg/kg in a single weekly dose for 4 weeks
  - Thrombocytosis: 1-2 mg/day for 14 days

Patient Information Notify physician of persistent or severe nausea, diarrhea, fever, sore throat, chills, bleeding, or bruising

Dosage Forms Capsule: 1 mg

Urea (yoor EE a)

Brand Names Amino-Cerv™ Vaginal Cream; Aquacare® [OTC]; Carmol® [OTC]; Nutraplus® [OTC]; Rea-Lo® [OTC]; Ultra Mide®; Ureacin®-20 [OTC]; Ureacin®-40; Ureaphil®

Canadian/Mexican Brand Names Onyvul® (Canada); Uremol® (Canada); Urisec® (Canada); Velvelan® (Canada)

Synonyms Carbamide

Therapeutic Category Diuretic, Osmotic; Keratolytic Agent; Topical Skin Product

Use Reduces intracranial pressure and intraocular pressure; topically promotes hydration and removal of excess keratin in hyperkeratotic conditions and dry skin; mild cervicitis

Pregnancy Risk Factor C

Contraindications Severely impaired renal function, hepatic failure; active intracranial bleeding, sickle cell anemia, topical use in viral skin disease

Warnings/Precautions Urea should not be used near the eyes; use with caution if applied to face, broken, or inflamed skin; use with caution in patients with mild hepatic or renal impairment

Adverse Reactions

>10%: Gastrointestinal: Nausea, vomiting

1% to 10%:

Central nervous system: Headache

Local: Transient stinging, local irritation, tissue necrosis from extravasation of I.V. preparation

<1%: Endocrine & metabolic: Electrolyte imbalance

Overdosage/Toxicology Increased BUN, decreased renal function; treatment is supportive

Drug Interactions Decreased effect/toxicity/levels of lithium

Mechanism of Action Elevates plasma osmolality by inhibiting tubular reabsorption of water, thus enhancing the flow of water into extracellular fluid

Pharmacodynamics/Kinetics

Onset of therapeutic effect: I.V.: Maximum effects within 1-2 hours

Duration: 3-6 hours (diuresis can continue for up to 10 hours)

Distribution: Crosses the placenta; appears in breast milk

Half-life: 1 hour

Elimination: Excreted unchanged in urine

Usual Dosage

Children: I.V. slow infusion:

<2 years: 0.1-0.5 g/kg

>2 years: 0.5-1.5 g/kg

Adults:

I.V. infusion: 1-1.5 g/kg by slow infusion (1-2½ hours); maximum: 120 g/24 hours

Topical: Apply 1-3 times/day

Vaginal: Insert 1 applicatorful in vagina at bedtime for 2-4 weeks

Patient Information Moisturizing effect is enhanced by applying to the skin while it is still moist after washing or bathing; for external use only

Nursing Implications Do not infuse into leg veins; injection dosage form may be used orally, mix with carbonated beverages, jelly or jam, to mask unpleasant flavor

Dosage Forms

Cream:

Topical: 2% [20 mg/mL] (75 g); 10% [100 mg/mL] (75 g, 90 g, 454 g); 20% [200 mg/mL] (45 g, 75 g, 90 g, 454 g); 30% [300 mg/mL] (60 g, 454 g); 40% (30 g)

Vaginal: 8.34% [83.4 mg/g] (82.5 g)

Injection: 40 g/150 mL

Lotion: 2% (240 mL); 10% (180 mL, 240 mL, 480 mL); 15% (120 mL, 480 mL); 25% (180 mL)

Ureacin®-20 [OTC] *see* Urea *on previous page*

Ureacin®-40 *see* Urea *on previous page*

Urea Peroxide *see* Carbamide Peroxide *on page 203*

Ureaphil® *see* Urea *on previous page*

Urecholine® *see* Bethanechol *on page 150*

Urex® *see* Methenamine *on page 802*

Urispas® *see* Flavoxate *on page 521*

Uri-Tet® *see* Oxytetracycline *on page 943*

Urobak® *see* Sulfamethoxazole *on page 1175*

Urodine® *see* Phenazopyridine *on page 981*

Urofollitropin (yoor oh fol li TROE pin)

Brand Names Fertinex® Injection; Metrodin® Injection

Canadian/Mexican Brand Names Fertinorm® H.P. (Mexico)

Therapeutic Category Gonadotropin; Ovulation Stimulator

Use Induction of ovulation in patients with polycystic ovarian disease and to stimulate the development of multiple oocytes

Pregnancy Risk Factor X

Contraindications Prior hypersensitivity to the drug; high levels of both LH and FSH indicating primary ovarian failure; uncontrolled thyroid or adrenal dysfunction; organic intracranial lesion such as a pituitary tumor; presence of any cause of infertility other than anovulation, unless the patient is a candidate for *in vitro* fertilization; abnormal bleeding of undetermined nature; ovarian cysts or enlargement not due to polycystic ovarian disease; pregnancy; may cause fetal harm when administered to pregnant women

Warnings/Precautions Use lowest dose possible to avoid abnormal ovarian enlargement; if hyperstimulation occurs, discontinue use and hospitalize patient; use with caution in patients with a history of thromboembolism

Adverse Reactions

>10%:

Endocrine & metabolic: Ovarian enlargement

(Continued)

Urofollitropin *(Continued)*

Local: Edema at injection site, pain at injection site

1% to 10%:

Cardiovascular: Arterial thromboembolism
Central nervous system: Fever, chills
Dermatologic: Rash
Gastrointestinal: Nausea, vomiting, abdominal pain, diarrhea
Miscellaneous: Hyperstimulation syndrome

Overdosage/Toxicology Symptoms of overdose include possible hyperstimulation and multiple gestations; supportive care to maintain fluid and electrolyte imbalance may be needed

Stability Protect from light; refrigerate at 3°C to 25°C (37°F to 77°F)

Mechanism of Action Preparation of follicle-stimulating hormone 75 units with <1 unit of luteinizing hormone (LH) which is isolated from the urine of postmenopausal women. Follicle-stimulating hormone plays a role in the development of follicles. Elevated FSH levels early in the normal menstrual cycle are thought to play a significant role in recruiting a cohort of follicles for maturation. A single follicle is enriched with FSH receptors and becomes dominant over the rest of the recruited follicles. The increased number of FSH receptors allows it to grow despite declining FSH levels. This dominant follicle secretes low levels of estrogen and inhibin which further reduces pituitary FSH output. The ovarian stroma, under the influence of luteinizing hormone, produces androgens which the dominant follicle uses as precursors for estrogens.

Pharmacodynamics/Kinetics

Half-life, elimination: 3.9 hours and 70.4 hours (FSH has two half-lives)

Elimination:

Renal clearance: 0.75 mL/minute
Metabolic: 17.2 mL/minute

Usual Dosage Adults: Female: I.M.: 75 units/day for 7-12 days, used with hCG may repeat course of treatment 2 more times

Dosage Forms Injection: 0.83 mg [75 units FSH activity] (2 mL); 1.66 mg [150 units FSH activity]

Urogesic® *see* Phenazopyridine *on page 981*

Urokinase (yoor oh KIN ase)

Brand Names Abbokinase®

Canadian/Mexican Brand Names Ukidan® (Mexico)

Therapeutic Category Thrombolytic Agent

Use Thrombolytic agent used in treatment of recent severe or massive deep vein thrombosis, pulmonary emboli, myocardial infarction, and occluded arteriovenous cannulas; more expensive than streptokinase; not useful on thrombi over 1 week old

Pregnancy Risk Factor B

Contraindications Hypersensitivity to urokinase or any component; active internal bleeding; CVA (within 2 months); brain carcinoma, bacterial endocarditis, anticoagulant therapy, intracranial or intraspinal surgery, surgery or trauma within past 10 days

Warnings/Precautions Use with caution in patients with severe hypertension, recent L.P., patients receiving I.M. administration of medications, patients with trauma or surgery in the last 10 days

Adverse Reactions

>10%:

Cardiovascular: Hypotension, arrhythmias
Dermatologic: Angioneurotic edema
Hematologic: Bleeding at sites of percutaneous trauma
Ocular: Periorbital swelling
Respiratory: Bronchospasm
Miscellaneous: Anaphylaxis

<1%:

Central nervous system: Headache, chills
Dermatologic: Rash
Gastrointestinal: Nausea, vomiting
Hematologic: Anemia
Ocular: Eye hemorrhage
Respiratory: Bronchospasm, epistaxis
Miscellaneous: Diaphoresis

Overdosage/Toxicology Symptoms of overdose include epistaxis, bleeding gums, hematoma, spontaneous ecchymoses, oozing at catheter site. In case of overdose, stop infusion, reverse bleeding with blood products that contain clotting factors.

Drug Interactions Increased toxicity (increased bleeding) with anticoagulants, antiplatelet drugs, aspirin, indomethacin, dextran

Stability Store in refrigerator; reconstitute by gently rolling and tilting; do not shake; contains no preservatives, should not be reconstituted until immediately before using, discard unused portion; stable at room temperature for 24 hours after reconstitution

Mechanism of Action Promotes thrombolysis by directly activating plasminogen to plasmin, which degrades fibrin, fibrinogen, and other procoagulant plasma proteins

Pharmacodynamics/Kinetics

Onset of action: I.V.: Fibrinolysis occurs rapidly

Duration: 4 or more hours

Half-life: 10-20 minutes

Elimination: Cleared by the liver with a small amount excreted in urine and bile

Usual Dosage

Children and Adults: Deep vein thrombosis: I.V.: Loading: 4400 units/kg over 10 minutes, then 4400 units/kg/hour for 12 hours

Adults:

Myocardial infarction: Intracoronary: 750,000 units over 2 hours (6000 units/minute over up to 2 hours)

Occluded I.V. catheters:

5000 units (use only Abbokinase® Open Cath) in each lumen over 1-2 minutes, leave in lumen for 1-4 hours, then aspirate; may repeat with 10,000 units in each lumen if 5000 units fails to clear the catheter; **do not infuse into the patient**; volume to instill into catheter is equal to the volume of the catheter

I.V. infusion: 200 units/kg/hour in each lumen for 12-48 hours at a rate of at least 20 mL/hour

Dialysis patients: 5000 units is administered in each lumen over 1-2 minutes; leave urokinase in lumen for 1-2 days, then aspirate

Clot lysis (large vessel thrombi): Loading: I.V.: 4400 units/kg over 10 minutes, increase to 6000 units/kg/hour; maintenance: 4400-6000 units/kg/hour adjusted to achieve clot lysis or patency of affected vessel; doses up to 50,000 units/kg/hour have been used. **Note:** Therapy should be initiated as soon as possible after diagnosis of thrombi and continued until clot is dissolved (usually 24-72 hours).

Acute pulmonary embolism: Three treatment alternatives: 3 million unit dosage

Alternative 1: 12-hour infusion: 4400 units/kg (2000 units/lb) bolus over 10 minutes followed by 4400 units/kg/hour (2000 units/lb); begin heparin 1000 units/hour approximately 3-4 hours after completion of urokinase infusion or when PTT is <100 seconds

Alternative 2: 2-hour infusion: 1 million unit bolus over 10 minutes followed by 2 million units over 110 minutes; begin heparin 1000 units/hour approximately 3-4 hours after completion of urokinase infusion or when PTT is <100 seconds

Alternative 3: Bolus dose only: 15,000 units/kg over 10 minutes; begin heparin 1000 units/hour approximately 3-4 hours after completion of urokinase infusion or when PTT is <100 seconds

Administration Use 0.22 or 0.45 micron filter during I.V. therapy

Monitoring Parameters CBC, reticulocyte count, platelet count, DIC panel (fibrinogen, plasminogen, FDP, D-dimer, PT, PTT), thrombosis panel (AT-III, protein C), urinalysis, ACT

Dosage Forms

Powder for injection: 250,000 units (5 mL)

Powder for injection, catheter clear: 5000 units (1 mL)

Uro-KP-Neutral® *see* Potassium Phosphate and Sodium Phosphate *on page 1031*

Urolene Blue® *see* Methylene Blue *on page 816*

Ursodeoxycholic Acid *see* Ursodiol *on this page*

Ursodiol (ER soe dye ole)

Brand Names Actigall™

Synonyms Ursodeoxycholic Acid

Therapeutic Category Gallstone Dissolution Agent

Use Gallbladder stone dissolution

Pregnancy Risk Factor B

Contraindications Not to be used with cholesterol, radiopaque, bile pigment stones, or stones >20 mm in diameter; allergy to bile acids

Warnings/Precautions Gallbladder stone dissolution may take several months of therapy; complete dissolution may not occur and recurrence of stones within 5 years has been observed in 50% of patients; use with caution in patients with a nonvisualizing gallbladder and those with chronic liver disease; not recommended for children

(Continued)

Ursodiol *(Continued)*

Adverse Reactions

1% to 10%: Gastrointestinal: Diarrhea

<1%:

Central nervous system: Fatigue, headache

Dermatologic: Pruritus, rash

Gastrointestinal: Nausea, vomiting, dyspepsia, metallic taste, abdominal pain, biliary pain, constipation

Overdosage/Toxicology Symptoms of overdose include diarrhea; no specific therapy for diarrhea and for overdose

Drug Interactions Decreased effect with aluminum-containing antacids, cholestyramine, colestipol, clofibrate, oral contraceptives (estrogens)

Mechanism of Action Decreases the cholesterol content of bile and bile stones by reducing the secretion of cholesterol from the liver and the fractional reabsorption of cholesterol by the intestines

Pharmacodynamics/Kinetics

Metabolism: Undergoes extensive enterohepatic recycling; following hepatic conjugation and biliary secretion, the drug is hydrolyzed to active ursodiol, where it is recycled or transformed to lithocholic acid by colonic microbial flora

Half-life: 100 hours

Elimination: In feces via bile

Usual Dosage Adults: Oral: 8-10 mg/kg/day in 2-3 divided doses; use beyond 24 months is not established; obtain ultrasound images at 6-month intervals for the first year of therapy; 30% of patients have stone recurrence after dissolution

Monitoring Parameters ALT, AST, sonogram

Patient Information Frequent blood work necessary to follow drug effects; report any persistent nausea, vomiting, abdominal pain

Dosage Forms Capsule: 300 mg

Extemporaneous Preparations A 60 mg/mL ursodiol suspension may be made by opening twelve 300 mg capsules and wetting with sufficient glycerin and triturating to make a fine paste; gradually add 45 mL of simple syrup in three steps:

1. Add 15 mL to paste, triturate well and transfer to 2 oz amber bottle
2. Rinse mortar with 10 mL simple syrup and add to amber bottle
3. Repeat step 2 with sufficient syrup to make 60 mL final volume; label "Shake Well and Store in Refrigerator"; 35-day stability

Urticort® *see* Betamethasone *on page 147*

Vagilia® *see* Sulfabenzamide, Sulfacetamide, and Sulfathiazole *on page 1171*

Vagistat® OTC *see* Tioconazole *on page 1232*

Vagitrol® *see* Sulfanilamide *on page 1176*

Valacyclovir (val ay SYE kloe veer)

Brand Names Valtrex®

Therapeutic Category Antiviral Agent, Oral

Use Treatment of herpes zoster (shingles) in immunocompetent patients; episodic treatment of recurrent genital herpes in immunocompetent patients; for first episode genital herpes

Pregnancy Risk Factor B

Pregnancy/Breast-Feeding Implications Teratogenicity registry, thus far, has shown no increased rate of birth defects than that of the general population; however, the registry is small and use during pregnancy is only warranted if the potential benefit to the mother justifies the risk of the fetus; avoid use in breast-feeding, if possible, since the drug distributes in high concentrations in breast milk

Contraindications Hypersensitivity to the drug or any component

Warnings/Precautions Thrombotic thrombocytopenic purpura/hemolytic uremic syndrome has occurred in immunocompromised patients; use caution and adjust the dose in elderly patients or those with renal insufficiency; safety and efficacy in children have not been established

Adverse Reactions

>10%: Gastrointestinal: Nausea

1% to 10%:

Central nervous system: Headache, dizziness

Gastrointestinal: Diarrhea, constipation, abdominal pain, anorexia

Neuromuscular & skeletal: Weakness

Overdosage/Toxicology Precipitation in the renal tubules may occur; treatment includes hemodialysis, especially if compromised renal function develops

Drug Interactions Decreased toxicity: Cimetidine and/or probenecid has decreased the rate but not the extent of valacyclovir conversion to acyclovir

Mechanism of Action Valacyclovir, the L-valyl ester of acyclovir, is rapidly converted to acyclovir before it exerts its antiviral activity against HSV-1, HSV-2, or VZV. It is most active against HSV-1 and least against VZV due to its varied affinity for thymidine kinase. Thymidine kinase converts it into acyclovir monophosphate; this is then converted into the diphosphate and triphosphate forms. Acyclovir triphosphate inhibits replication of herpes viral DNA via competitive inhibition of herpes viral DNA polymerase, incorporation and termination of the growing viral DNA chain, and inactivation of the viral DNA polymerase.

Pharmacodynamics/Kinetics

Absorption: Rapid and converted to acyclovir and L-valine by first-pass/hepatic metabolism

Protein binding: 17.9%; nonlinear relationship between dose and plasma concentrations

Metabolism: Converted to acyclovir and L-valine by first-pass metabolism and hepatic metabolism (not microsomal); inactive metabolites formed

Bioavailability: 54.5%

Half-life:

Normal renal function: 2.5-3.3 hours

End stage renal disease: 14 hours removed partially by hemodialysis, half-life during dialysis: 4 hours; liver disease may decrease rate bot not extent of conversion to acyclovir (half-life not affected)

Elimination: Acyclovir excreted predominantly in urine (88.6%)

Usual Dosage Oral: Adults:

Shingles: 1 g 3 times/day for 7 days

Genital herpes: 500 mg twice daily

Dosing interval in renal impairment:

Cl_{cr}: 30-49 mL/minute: 1 g every 12 hours

Cl_{cr} 10-29 mL/minute: 1 g every 24 hours

Cl_{cr} <10 mL/minute: 500 mg every 24 hours

Hemodialysis: 33% removed during 4-hour session

Peritoneal dialysis: Limited information available; supplemental doses not required

Patient Information Begin use as soon as possible following development of signs of herpes zoster; take with plenty of fluids; may take without regard to meals

Nursing Implications Observe for CNS changes; avoid dehydration; begin therapy at the earliest sign of zoster infection (within 48 hours of the rash)

Dosage Forms Caplets: 500 mg

Valadol® [OTC] *see* Acetaminophen *on page 19*

Valergen® Injection *see* Estradiol *on page 468*

Valisone® *see* Betamethasone *on page 147*

Valium® *see* Diazepam *on page 369*

Valpin® 50 *see* Anisotropine *on page 91*

Valproate Semisodium *see* Valproic Acid and Derivatives *on this page*

Valproate Sodium *see* Valproic Acid and Derivatives *on this page*

Valproic Acid *see* Valproic Acid and Derivatives *on this page*

Valproic Acid and Derivatives

(val PROE ik AS id & dah RIV ah tives)

Related Information

Anticonvulsants by Seizure Type *on page 1392*

Epilepsy Treatment *on page 1531*

Brand Names Depakene®; Depakote®

Canadian/Mexican Brand Names Atemperator-S® (Mexico); Cryoval® (Mexico); Epival® (Mexico and Canada); Leptilan® (Mexico); Valprosid® (Mexico)

Synonyms Dipropylacetic Acid; Divalproex Sodium; DPA; 2-Propylpentanoic Acid; 2-Propylvaleric Acid; Valproate Semisodium; Valproate Sodium; Valproic Acid

Therapeutic Category Anticonvulsant

Use Management of simple and complex absence seizures; mixed seizure types; myoclonic and generalized tonic-clonic (grand mal) seizures; may be effective in partial seizures, infantile spasms, bipolar disorder; prevention of migraine headaches

Pregnancy Risk Factor D

Pregnancy/Breast-Feeding Implications

Clinical effects on the fetus: Crosses the placenta. Neural tube, cardiac, facial (characteristic pattern of dysmorphic facial features), skeletal, multiple other defects reported. Epilepsy itself, number of medications, genetic factors, or a combination of these probably influence the teratogenicity of anticonvulsant therapy. Risk of neural tube defects with use during first 30 days of pregnancy warrants discontinuation prior to pregnancy and through this period of possible.

(Continued)

Valproic Acid and Derivatives *(Continued)*

Breast-feeding/lactation: Crosses into breast milk. American Academy of Pediatrics considers COMPATIBLE with breast-feeding.

Contraindications Hypersensitivity to valproic acid or derivatives or any component; hepatic dysfunction

Warnings/Precautions Hepatic failure resulting in fatalities has occurred in patients; children <2 years of age are at considerable risk; monitor patients closely for appearance of malaise, weakness, facial edema, anorexia, jaundice, and vomiting; may cause severe thrombocytopenia, bleeding; hepatotoxicity has been reported after 3 days to 6 months of therapy; tremors may indicate overdosage; use with caution in patients receiving other anticonvulsants

Adverse Reactions

1% to 10%:

- Endocrine & metabolic: Change in menstrual cycle
- Gastrointestinal: Abdominal cramps, anorexia, diarrhea, nausea, vomiting, weight gain

<1%:

- Central nervous system: Drowsiness, ataxia, irritability, confusion, restlessness, hyperactivity, headache, malaise
- Dermatologic: Alopecia, erythema multiforme
- Endocrine & metabolic: Hyperammonemia
- Gastrointestinal: Pancreatitis
- Hematologic: Thrombocytopenia, prolongation of bleeding time
- Hepatic: Transient increased liver enzymes, liver failure
- Neuromuscular & skeletal: Tremor
- Ocular: Nystagmus, spots before eyes

Overdosage/Toxicology Symptoms of overdose include coma, deep sleep, motor restlessness, visual hallucinations

Supportive treatment is necessary; naloxone has been used to reverse CNS depressant effects, but may block action of other anticonvulsants

Drug Interactions

Decreased effect of phenytoin, clonazepam, diazepam; decreased effect with phenobarbital, primidone, phenytoin, carbamazepine

Increased effect/toxicity with CNS depressants, alcohol, aspirin (bleeding), warfarin (bleeding)

Mechanism of Action Causes increased availability of gamma-aminobutyric acid (GABA), an inhibitory neurotransmitter, to brain neurons or may enhance the action of GABA or mimic its action at postsynaptic receptor sites

Pharmacodynamics/Kinetics

Protein binding: 80% to 90% (dose dependent)

Metabolism: Extensively in the liver

Half-life (increased in neonates and patients with liver disease):

- Children: 4-14 hours
- Adults: 8-17 hours

Time to peak serum concentration: Within 1-4 hours; 3-5 hours after divalproex (enteric coated)

Elimination: 2% to 3% excreted unchanged in urine

Usual Dosage

Epilepsy: Children and Adults:

- Oral: Initial: 10-15 mg/kg/day in 1-3 divided doses; increase by 5-10 mg/kg/day at weekly intervals until therapeutic levels are achieved; maintenance: 30-60 mg/kg/day in 2-3 divided doses
  - Children receiving more than 1 anticonvulsant (ie, polytherapy) may require doses up to 100 mg/kg/day in 3-4 divided doses
- Rectal: Dilute syrup 1:1 with water for use as a retention enema; loading dose: 17-20 mg/kg one time; maintenance: 10-15 mg/kg/dose every 8 hours

Mania: Adults: 750 mg/day in 1-3 divided doses

Hemodialysis: Not dialyzable (0% to 5%)

Dosing adjustment/comments in hepatic impairment: Reduce dose

Dietary Considerations

Alcohol: Additive CNS depression, avoid or limit alcohol

Food:

- Valproic acid may cause GI upset; take with large amount of water or food to decrease GI upset. May need to split doses to avoid GI upset.
- Food may delay but does not affect the extent of absorption
  - Coated particles of divalproex sodium may be mixed with semisolid food (eg, applesauce or pudding) in patients having difficulty swallowing; particles should be swallowed and not chewed
  - Valproate sodium oral solution will generate valproic acid in carbonated beverages and may cause mouth and throat irritation; do not mix valproate sodium oral solution with carbonated beverages
- Milk: No effect on absorption; may take with milk

Sodium: SIADH and water intoxication; monitor fluid status. May need to restrict fluid.

Monitoring Parameters Liver enzymes, CBC with platelets

Reference Range Therapeutic: 50-100 µg/mL (SI: 350-690 µmol/L); Toxic: >200 µg/mL (SI: >1390 µmol/L). Seizure control may improve at levels >100 µg/mL (SI: 690 µmol/L), but toxicity may occur at levels of 100-150 µg/mL (SI: 690-1040 µmol/L).

Test Interactions False-positive result for urine ketones

Patient Information Take with food or milk; do not chew, break, or crush the tablet or capsule; do not administer with carbonated drinks; report any sore throat, fever or fatigue, bleeding or bruising that is severe or that persists; may cause drowsiness, impair judgment or coordination

Nursing Implications Do not crush enteric coated drug product or capsules

Additional Information Sodium content of valproate sodium syrup (5 mL): 23 mg (1 mEq)

Divalproex sodium: Depakote®
Valproate sodium: Depakene® syrup
Valproic acid: Depakene® capsule

Dosage Forms

Capsule, sprinkle, as divalproex sodium (Depakote® Sprinkle®): 125 mg
Capsule, as valproic acid (Depakene®): 250 mg
Syrup, as sodium valproate (Depakene®): 250 mg/5 mL (5 mL, 50 mL, 480 mL)
Tablet, delayed release, as divalproex sodium (Depakote®): 125 mg, 250 mg, 500 mg

Valsartan (val SAR tan)

Brand Names Diovan®

Therapeutic Category Angiotensin II Antagonist

Use Alone or in combination with other antihypertensive agents in treating essential hypertension; may have an advantage over losartan due to minimal metabolism requirements and consequent use in mild to moderate hepatic impairment

Pregnancy Risk Factor X

Pregnancy/Breast-Feeding Implications Although no human data exist, valsartan is known to be excreted in animal breast milk and should be avoided in lactating mothers if possible

Contraindications Hypersensitivity to valsartan or any components, pregnancy, severe hepatic insufficiency, biliary cirrhosis or biliary obstruction, primary hyperaldosteronism, bilateral renal artery stenosis

Warnings/Precautions Use extreme caution with concurrent administration of potassium-sparing diuretics or potassium supplements, in patients with mild-moderate hepatic dysfunction (adjust dose), in those who may be sodium/water depleted (eg, on high-dose diuretics), and in the elderly; avoid use in patients with congestive heart failure, unilateral renal artery stenosis, aortic/mitral valve stenosis, coronary artery disease, or hypertrophic cardiomyopathy, if possible

Adverse Reactions Similar incidence to placebo; independent of race, age, and gender

>1%:

Central nervous system: Headache, dizziness, drowsiness, ataxia
Endocrine & metabolic: Decreased libido
Gastrointestinal: Diarrhea, abdominal pain, nausea, abnormal taste
Genitourinary: Polyuria
Hematologic: Neutropenia
Hepatic: Increased LFTs
Neuromuscular & skeletal: Arthralgia
Respiratory: Cough, upper respiratory infection, rhinitis, sinusitis, pharyngitis

<1%:

Hematologic: Anemia
Renal: Increased Cr

Overdosage/Toxicology Only mild toxicity (hypotension, bradycardia, hyperkalemia) has been reported with large overdoses (up to 5 g of captopril and 300 mg of enalapril); no fatalities have been reported. Treatment is symptomatic (eg, fluids).

Drug Interactions

Decreased effect: Phenobarbital, ketoconazole, troleandomycin, sulfaphenazole
Increased effect: Cimetidine, moxonidine

Mechanism of Action As a prodrug, valsartan produces direct antagonism of the angiotensin II (AT2) receptors, unlike the angiotensin-converting enzyme inhibitors. It displaces angiotensin II from the AT1 receptor and produces its blood pressure lowering effects by antagonizing AT1-induced vasoconstriction, aldosterone release, catecholamine release, arginine vasopressin release, water intake, and hypertrophic responses. This action results in more efficient blockado

(Continued)

Valsartan *(Continued)*

of the cardiovascular effects of angiotensin II and fewer side effects than the ACE inhibitors.

Pharmacodynamics/Kinetics

Distribution: V_d: 17 L (adults)
Protein binding: 94% to 97%
Metabolism: Metabolized to an inactive metabolite
Bioavailability: 23%
Half-life: 9 hours
Time to peak serum concentration: 2 hours (maximal effect: 4-6 hours)
Elimination: 13% and 83% excreted as unchanged drug in urine and feces, respectively

Usual Dosage Adults: 80 mg/day; may be increased to 160 mg if needed (maximal effects observed in 4-6 weeks)

Dosing adjustment in renal impairment: No dosage adjustment necessary if Cl_{cr} >10 mL/minute

Dosing adjustment in hepatic impairment (mild - moderate): ≤80 mg/day
Dialysis: Not significantly removed

Monitoring Parameters Baseline and periodic electrolyte panels, renal and liver function tests, urinalysis; symptoms of hypotension or hypersensitivity

Patient Information Do not stop taking this medication unless instructed by a physician, do not take this medication during pregnancy or lactation; take a missed dose as soon as possible unless it is almost time for your next dose; call your physician immediately if you have symptoms of allergy or develop side effects including headache and dizziness

Dosage Forms Capsule: 80 mg, 160 mg

Valtrex® *see* Valacyclovir *on page 1284*
Vamate® *see* Hydroxyzine *on page 634*
Vancenase® *see* Beclomethasone *on page 133*
Vancenase® AQ *see* Beclomethasone *on page 133*
Vanceril® *see* Beclomethasone *on page 133*
Vancocin® *see* Vancomycin *on this page*
Vancoled® *see* Vancomycin *on this page*

Vancomycin (van koe MYE sin)

Related Information

Antibiotic Treatment of Adults With Infectious Endocarditis *on page 1465*
Antimicrobial Drugs of Choice *on page 1468*
Antimicrobial Prophylaxis *on page 1445*
Bacterial Meningitis Practical Guidelines for Management *on page 1475*
Prevention of Bacterial Endocarditis *on page 1449*
Recommendations for Preventing the Spread of Vancomycin Resistance *on page 1480*

Brand Names Lyphocin®; Vancocin®; Vancoled®

Canadian/Mexican Brand Names Vancocin® CP (Canada); Balcoran® (Mexico); Vanmicina® (Mexico)

Synonyms Vancomycin Hydrochloride

Therapeutic Category Antibiotic, Miscellaneous

Use Treatment of patients with the following infections or conditions:

Infections due to documented or suspected methicillin-resistant *S. aureus* or beta-lactam resistant coagulase negative *Staphylococcus*

Serious or life-threatening infections (ie, endocarditis, meningitis) due to documented or suspected staphylococcal or streptococcal infections in patients who are allergic to penicillins and/or cephalosporins

Empiric therapy of infections associated with gram-positive organisms; used orally for staphylococcal enterocolitis or for antibiotic-associated pseudomembranous colitis produced by *C. difficile*

Pregnancy Risk Factor C

Contraindications Hypersensitivity to vancomycin or any component; avoid in patients with previous severe hearing loss

Warnings/Precautions Use with caution in patients with renal impairment or those receiving other nephrotoxic or ototoxic drugs; dosage modification required in patients with impaired renal function (especially elderly)

Adverse Reactions

Oral:

>10%: Gastrointestinal: Bitter taste, nausea, vomiting

1% to 10%:

Central nervous system: Chills, drug fever
Hematologic: Eosinophilia

<1%:

Cardiovascular: Vasculitis

Hematologic: Thrombocytopenia

Otic: Ototoxicity

Renal: Renal failure, interstitial nephritis

Parenteral:

>10%:

Cardiovascular: Hypotension accompanied by flushing

Dermatologic: Erythematous rash on face and upper body (red neck or red man syndrome)

1% to 10%:

Central nervous system: Chills, drug fever

Hematologic: Eosinophilia

<1%:

Cardiovascular: Vasculitis

Otic: Ototoxicity

Hematologic: Thrombocytopenia

Renal: Renal failure

Overdosage/Toxicology Symptoms of overdose include ototoxicity, nephrotoxicity

There is no specific therapy for an overdosage with vancomycin. Care is symptomatic and supportive in nature. Peritoneal filtration and hemofiltration (not dialysis) have been shown to reduce the serum concentration of vancomycin; high flux dialysis may remove up to 25%.

Drug Interactions Increased toxicity: Anesthetic agents

Stability

Vancomycin reconstituted intravenous solutions are stable for 14 days at room temperature or refrigeration

Stability of parenteral admixture at room temperature (25°C) or refrigeration temperature (4°C): 7 days

Standard diluent: 500 mg/150 mL D_5W; 750 mg/250 mL D_5W; 1 g/250 mL D_5W

Minimum volume: Maximum concentration is 5 mg/mL to minimize thrombophlebitis

Incompatible with heparin, phenobarbital

After the oral solution is reconstituted, it should be refrigerated and used within 2 weeks

Mechanism of Action Inhibits bacterial cell wall synthesis by blocking glycopeptide polymerization through binding tightly to D-alanyl-D-alanine portion of cell wall precursor

Pharmacodynamics/Kinetics

Absorption:

Oral: Poor

I.M.: Erratic

Intraperitoneal: Can result in 38% absorption systemically

Distribution: Widely distributed in body tissues and fluids except for CSF

Relative diffusion of antimicrobial agents from blood into cerebrospinal fluid (CSF): Good only with inflammation (exceeds usual MICs)

Ratio of CSF to blood level (%):

Normal meninges: Nil

Inflamed meninges: 20-30

Protein binding: 10%-50%

Half-life (biphasic): Terminal:

Newborns: 6-10 hours

Infants and Children 3 months to 4 years: 4 hours

Children >3 years: 2.2-3 hours

Adults: 5-11 hours, prolonged significantly with reduced renal function

End stage renal disease: 200-250 hours

Time to peak serum concentration: I.V.: Within 45-65 minutes

Elimination: As unchanged drug in the urine via glomerular filtration (80% to 90%); oral doses are excreted primarily in the feces

Usual Dosage Initial dosage recommendation: I.V.:

Infants >1 month and Children: 10 mg/kg/dose every 6 hours

Infants >1 month and Children with staphylococcal central nervous system infection: 10 mg/kg/dose every 6 hours

Adults (select dosage based on weight):

<60 kg: 750 mg

60-100 kg: 1 g

100-120 kg: 1.25 g

>120 kg: 1.5 g

Dosing interval in renal impairment:

Cl_{cr} >90 mL/minute: Administer every 12 hours

Cl_{cr} 40-90 mL/minute: Administer every 24 hours

(Continued)

Vancomycin *(Continued)*

Cl_{cr} 30-40 mL/minute: Administer every 48 hours
Cl_{cr} 20-30 mL/minute: Administer every 72 hours
Cl_{cr} 10-20 mL/minute: Administer every 96 hours
Cl_{cr} <10 mL/minute: Administer every 5-7 days

Hemodialysis: Not dialyzable (0% to 5%); generally not removed; exception minimal-moderate removal by some of the newer high-flux filters

Continuous ambulatory peritoneal dialysis (CAPD): Not significantly removed; administration via CAPD fluid: 15-30 mg/L (15-30 mcg/mL) of CAPD fluid

Continuous arteriovenous hemofiltration: Dose similar to Cl_{cr} of approximately 10-15 mL/minute

Dosing adjustments/comments in hepatic impairment: Reduce dose by 60%

Antibiotic lock technique (for catheter infections): 2 mg/mL in SWI/NS or D_5W; instill 3-5 mL into catheter port as a flush solution instead of heparin lock (**Note:** Do not mix with any other solutions)

Intrathecal: Vancomycin is available as a powder for injection and may be diluted to 1-5 mg/mL concentration in preservative-free 0.9% sodium chloride for administration into the CSF

Children: 5-20 mg/day
Adults: 20 mg/day

Oral: Pseudomembranous colitis produced by *C. difficile*:

Children: 40 mg/kg/day in divided doses every 6-8 hours, added to fluids
Adults: 125 mg 4 times/day

Monitoring Parameters Periodic renal function tests, urinalysis, serum vancomycin concentrations, WBC, audiogram

Reference Range

Timing of serum samples: Draw peak 1 hour after 1-hour infusion has completed; draw trough just before next dose

Therapeutic levels: Peak: 25-40 µg/mL; Trough: 5-12 µg/mL

Toxic: >80 µg/mL (SI: >54 µmol/L)

Patient Information Report pain at infusion site, dizziness, fullness or ringing in ears with I.V. use; nausea or vomiting with oral use; complete full course of therapy

Nursing Implications Obtain drug levels after the third dose unless otherwise directed; peaks are drawn 1 hour after the completion of a 1- to 2-hour infusion; troughs are obtained just before the next dose; slow I.V. infusion rate if maculopapular rash appears on face, neck, trunk, and upper extremities (Red man reaction)

Dosage Forms

Capsule, as hydrochloride: 125 mg, 250 mg
Powder for oral solution, as hydrochloride: 1 g, 10 g
Powder for injection, as hydrochloride: 500 mg, 1 g, 2 g, 5 g, 10 g

Vancomycin Hydrochloride *see* Vancomycin *on page 1288*
Vanoxide® [OTC] *see* Benzoyl Peroxide *on page 140*
Vantin® *see* Cefpodoxime *on page 230*
Vaponefrin® *see* Epinephrine *on page 448*
VAQTA® *see* Hepatitis A Vaccine *on page 606*

Varicella Virus Vaccine (var i SEL a VYE rus vak SEEN)

Related Information

Immunization Guidelines *on page 1421*
Miscellaneous Vaccination Information *on page 1437*
Recommended Childhood Immunization Schedule - US - January-December, 1997 *on page 1423*

Brand Names Varivax®

Synonyms Chicken Pox Vaccine; Varicella-Zoster Virus (VZV) Vaccine

Therapeutic Category Vaccine, Live Virus

Use The American Association of Pediatrics recommends that the chickenpox vaccine should be given to all healthy children between 12 months and 18 years; children between 12 months and 13 years who have not been immunized or who have not had chickenpox should receive 1 vaccination while children 13-18 years of age require 2 vaccinations 4-8 weeks apart; the vaccine has been added to the childhood immunization schedule for infants 12-28 months of age and children 11-12 years of age who have not been vaccinated previously or who have not had the disease; it is recommended to be given with the measles, mumps, and rubella (MMR) vaccine

Pregnancy Risk Factor C

Pregnancy/Breast-Feeding Implications Varivax® should not be administered to pregnant females and pregnancy should be avoided for 3 months following vaccination; use during breast-feeding should be avoided

Contraindications Hypersensitivity to any component of the vaccine, including gelatin; a history of anaphylactoid reaction to neomycin; individuals with blood dyscrasias, leukemia, lymphomas, or other malignant neoplasms affecting the bone marrow or lymphatic systems; those receiving immunosuppressive therapy; primary and acquired immunodeficiency states; a family history of congenital or hereditary immunodeficiency; active untreated tuberculosis; febrile illness; pregnancy; I.V. injection

Warnings/Precautions

Children and adolescents with acute lymphoblastic leukemia in remission can receive the vaccine under an investigational protocol (215-283-0897); no clinical data are available or efficacy in children <12 months of age

Immediate treatment for anaphylactoid reaction should be available during vaccine use; defer vaccination for at least 5 months following blood or plasma transfusions, immune globulin (IgG), or VZIG (avoid IgG or IVIG use for 2 months following vaccination); salicylates should be avoided for 5 weeks after vaccination; vaccinated individuals should not have close association with susceptible high risk individuals (newborns, pregnant women, immunocompromised persons) following vaccination

Adverse Reactions

1% to 10%:

Central nervous system: Pain, fever, irritability/nervousness, fatigue, disturbed sleep, headache, malaise, chills

Dermatologic: Redness, rash, pruritus, generalized varicella-like rash,

Gastrointestinal: Diarrhea, loss of appetite, vomiting, abdominal pain, nausea

Hematologic: Hematoma

Local: Induration and stiffness at the injection site

Neuromuscular & skeletal: Myalgia, arthralgia

Otic: Otitis

Respiratory: Upper respiratory illness, cough

Miscellaneous: Lymphadenopathy, allergic reactions

<1%:

Central nervous system: Febrile seizures (causality not established)

Respiratory: Pneumonitis

Drug Interactions Clinical studies show that Varivax® can be administered concomitantly with MMR and limited data indicate that DTP and Pedvax® HIB may also be administered together (using separate sites and syringes)

Decreased effect: The effect of the vaccine may be decreased and the risk of varicella disease in individuals who are receiving immunosuppressant drugs may be increased

Increased effect: Salicylates may increase the risk of Reye's following varicella vaccination

Stability Store in freezer (-15°C), store diluent separately at room temperature or in refrigerator; discard if reconstituted vaccine is not used within 30 minutes

Mechanism of Action As a live, attenuated vaccine, varicella virus vaccine offers active immunity to disease caused by the varicella-zoster virus

Pharmacodynamics/Kinetics

Onset of action: Approximately 4-6 weeks postvaccination

Duration: Lowest breakthrough rates (0.2% to 2.9%) exist in the first 2 years following postvaccination, with slightly higher rates in the third through the fifth year

Usual Dosage S.C.:

Children 12 months to 12 years: 0.5 mL

Children 12 years to Adults: 2 doses of 0.5 mL separated by 4-8 weeks

Administration Inject S.C. into the outer aspect of the upper arm, if possible

Monitoring Parameters Rash, fever

Patient Information Report any adverse reactions to the health care provider or Vaccine Adverse Event Reporting System (1-800-822-7967); avoid pregnancy for 3 months following vaccination; avoid salicylates for 5 weeks after vaccination; avoid close association with susceptible high risk individuals following vaccination

Nursing Implications Obtain the previous immunization history (including allergic reactions) to previous vaccines; do not inject into a blood vessel; use the supplied diluent only for reconstitution; inject immediately after reconstitution

Additional Information Minimum potency level: 1350 plaque forming units (PFU)/0.5 mL

Dosage Forms Powder for injection, lyophilized powder, preservative free: 1350 plaque forming units (PFU)/0.5 mL (0.5 mL single-dose vials)

Varicella-Zoster Immune Globulin (Human)

(var i SEL a- ZOS ter i MYUN GLOB yoo lin HYU man)

Related Information

Guidelines for the Prevention of Opportunistic Infections in Persons with HIV *on page 1457*

(Continued)

Varicella-Zoster Immune Globulin (Human) *(Continued)*

Immunization Guidelines *on page 1421*
Miscellaneous Vaccination Information *on page 1437*
Prophylaxis for Patients Exposed to Common Communicable Diseases *on page 1452*

Synonyms VZIG

Therapeutic Category Immune Globulin

Use Passive immunization of susceptible immunodeficient patients after exposure to varicella; most effective if begun within 72 hours of exposure; there is no evidence VZIG modifies established varicella-zoster infections.

Restrict administration to those patients meeting the following criteria:

- Neoplastic disease (eg, leukemia or lymphoma)
- Congenital or acquired immunodeficiency
- Immunosuppressive therapy with steroids, antimetabolites or other immunosuppressive treatment regimens
- Newborn of mother who had onset of chickenpox within 5 days before delivery or within 48 hours after delivery
- Premature (≥28 weeks gestation) whose mother has no history of chickenpox
- Premature (<28 weeks gestation or ≤1000 g VZIG) regardless of maternal history

One of the following types of exposure to chickenpox or zoster patient(s) may warrant administration:

- Continuous household contact
- Playmate contact (>1 hour play indoors)
- Hospital contact (in same 2-4 bedroom or adjacent beds in a large ward or prolonged face-to-face contact with an infectious staff member or patient)
- Susceptible to varicella-zoster
- Age <15 years; administer to immunocompromised adolescents and adults and to other older patients on an individual basis

An acceptable alternative to VZIG prophylaxis is to treat varicella, if it occurs, with high-dose I.V. acyclovir

Age is the most important risk factor for reactivation of varicella zoster; persons <50 years of age have incidence of 2.5 cases per 1000, whereas those 60-79 have 6.5 cases per 1000 and those >80 years have 10 cases per 1000

Pregnancy Risk Factor C

Contraindications **Not** for prophylactic use in immunodeficient patients with history of varicella, unless patient's immunosuppression is associated with bone marrow transplantation; **not** recommended for nonimmunodeficient patients, including pregnant women, because the severity of chickenpox is much less than in immunosuppressed patients; allergic response to gamma globulin or anti-immunoglobulin; sensitivity to thimerosal; persons with IgA deficiency; do not administer to patients with thrombocytopenia or coagulopathies

Warnings/Precautions VZIG is not indicated for prophylaxis or therapy of normal adults who are exposed to or who develop varicella; it is not indicated for treatment of herpes zoster. Do not inject I.V.

Adverse Reactions

1% to 10%: Local: Discomfort at the site of injection (pain, redness, edema)

<1%:

- Central nervous system: Malaise, headache
- Dermatologic: Rash, angioedema
- Gastrointestinal: GI symptoms
- Respiratory: Respiratory symptom
- Miscellaneous: Anaphylactic shock

Drug Interactions Decreased effect: Live virus vaccines (do not administer within 3 months of immune globulin administration)

Stability Refrigerate at 2°C to 8°C (36°F to 46°F)

Mechanism of Action The exact mechanism has not been clarified but the antibodies in varicella-zoster immune globulin most likely neutralize the varicella-zoster virus and prevent its pathological actions

VZIG Dose Based on Weight

Weight of Patient		Dose	
kg	lb	Units	No. of Vials
0-10	0-22	125	1
10.1-20	22.1-44	250	2
20.1-30	44.1-66	375	3
30.1-40	66.1-88	500	4
>40	>88	625	5

Usual Dosage High risk susceptible patients who are exposed again more than 3 weeks after a prior dose of VZIG should receive another full dose; there is no evidence VZIG modifies established varicella-zoster infections.

I.M.: Administer by deep injection in the gluteal muscle or in another large muscle mass. Inject 125 units/10 kg (22 lb); maximum dose: 625 units (5 vials); minimum dose: 125 units; do not administer fractional doses. Do not inject I.V. See table.

Administration Do not inject I.V.; administer deep I.M. into the gluteal muscle or other large muscle mass. For patients ≤10 kg, administer 1.25 mL at a single site; for patients >10 kg, administer no more than 2.5 mL at a single site. Administer entire contents of each vial

Dosage Forms Injection: 125 units of antibody in single dose vials

Varicella-Zoster Virus (VZV) Vaccine *see* Varicella Virus Vaccine *on page 1290*

Varivax® *see* Varicella Virus Vaccine *on page 1290*

Vascor® *see* Bepridil *on page 144*

Vasocidin® Ophthalmic *see* Sulfacetamide Sodium and Prednisolone *on page 1172*

VasoClear® [OTC] *see* Naphazoline *on page 879*

Vasocon Regular® *see* Naphazoline *on page 879*

Vasodilan® *see* Isoxsuprine *on page 688*

Vasopressin (vay soe PRES in)

Brand Names Pitressin®

Canadian/Mexican Brand Names Pressyn® (Canada)

Synonyms ADH; Antidiuretic Hormone; 8-Arginine Vasopressin; Vasopressin Tannate

Therapeutic Category Antidiuretic Hormone Analog; Hormone, Posterior Pituitary; Vesicant

Use Treatment of diabetes insipidus; prevention and treatment of postoperative abdominal distention; differential diagnosis of diabetes insipidus

Unlabeled use: Adjunct in the treatment of GI hemorrhage and esophageal varices

Pregnancy Risk Factor B

Contraindications Hypersensitivity to vasopressin or any component

Warnings/Precautions Use with caution in patients with seizure disorders, migraine, asthma, vascular disease, renal disease, cardiac disease; chronic nephritis with nitrogen retention. Goiter with cardiac complications, arteriosclerosis; I.V. infiltration may lead to severe vasoconstriction and localized tissue necrosis; also, gangrene of extremities, tongue, and ischemic colitis. Elderly patients should be cautioned not to increase their fluid intake beyond that sufficient to satisfy their thirst in order to avoid water intoxication and hyponatremia; under experimental conditions, the elderly have shown to have a decreased responsiveness to vasopressin with respect to its effects on water homeostasis

Adverse Reactions

1% to 10%:

Cardiovascular: Increased blood pressure, bradycardia, arrhythmias, venous thrombosis, vasoconstriction with higher doses, angina

Central nervous system: Pounding in the head, fever, vertigo

Dermatologic: Urticaria, circumoral pallor

Gastrointestinal: Flatulence, abdominal cramps, nausea, vomiting

Neuromuscular & skeletal: Tremor

Miscellaneous: Diaphoresis

<1%:

Cardiovascular: Myocardial infarction

Endocrine & metabolic: Water intoxication

Miscellaneous: Allergic reaction

Overdosage/Toxicology Symptoms of overdose include drowsiness, weight gain, confusion, listlessness, water intoxication

Water intoxication requires withdrawal of the drug; severe intoxication may require osmotic diuresis and loop diuretics

Drug Interactions

Decreased effect: Lithium, epinephrine, demeclocycline, heparin, and alcohol block antidiuretic activity to varying degrees

Increased effect: Chlorpropamide, phenformin, urea and fludrocortisone potentiate antidiuretic response

Stability Store injection at room temperature; protect from heat and from freezing; use only clear solutions

Mechanism of Action Increases cyclic adenosine monophosphate (cAMP) which increases water permeability at the renal tubule resulting in decreased

(Continued)

Vasopressin *(Continued)*

urine volume and increased osmolality; causes peristalsis by directly stimulating the smooth muscle in the GI tract

Pharmacodynamics/Kinetics

Nasal:
- Onset of action: 1 hour
- Duration: 3-8 hours

Parenteral: Duration of action: I.M., S.C.: 2-8 hours

Absorption: Destroyed by trypsin in GI tract, must be administered parenterally or intranasally

Nasal:
- Metabolism: In the liver, kidneys
- Half-life: 15 minutes
- Elimination: In urine

Parenteral:
- Metabolism: Most of dose metabolized by liver and kidneys
- Half-life: 10-20 minutes
- Elimination: 5% of S.C. dose (aqueous) excreted unchanged in urine after 4 hours

Usual Dosage

Diabetes insipidus (highly variable dosage; titrated based on serum and urine sodium and osmolality in addition to fluid balance and urine output):

I.M., S.C.:
- Children: 2.5-10 units 2-4 times/day as needed
- Adults: 5-10 units 2-4 times/day as needed (dosage range 5-60 units/day)

Continuous I.V. infusion: Children and Adults: 0.5 milliunit/kg/hour (0.0005 unit/kg/hour); double dosage as needed every 30 minutes to a maximum of 0.01 unit/kg/hour

Intranasal: Administer on cotton pledget or nasal spray

Abdominal distention (aqueous): Adults: I.M.: 5 mg stat, 10 mg every 3-4 hours

GI hemorrhage: I.V. infusion: Dilute aqueous in NS or D_5W to 0.1-1 unit/mL
- Children: Initial: 0.002-0.005 units/kg/minute; titrate dose as needed; maximum: 0.01 unit/kg/minute; continue at same dosage (if bleeding stops) for 12 hours, then taper off over 24-48 hours
- Adults: Initial: 0.2-0.4 unit/minute, then titrate dose as needed, if bleeding stops; continue at same dose for 12 hours, taper off over 24-48 hours

Dosing adjustment in hepatic impairment: Some patients respond to much lower doses with cirrhosis

Administration

I.V. infusion administration requires the use of an infusion pump and should be administered in a peripheral line to minimize adverse reactions on coronary arteries

Infusion rates: 100 units (aqueous) in 500 mL D_5W rate

0.1 unit/minute: 30 mL/hour
0.2 unit/minute: 60 mL/hour
0.3 unit/minute: 90 mL/hour
0.4 unit/minute: 120 mL/hour
0.5 unit/minute: 150 mL/hour
0.6 unit/minute: 180 mL/hour

Monitoring Parameters Serum and urine sodium, urine output, fluid input and output, urine specific gravity, urine and serum osmolality

Reference Range Plasma: 0-2 pg/mL (SI: 0-2 ng/L) if osmolality <285 mOsm/L; 2-12 pg/mL (SI: 2-12 ng/L) if osmolality >290 mOsm/L

Patient Information Side effects such as abdominal cramps and nausea may be reduced by drinking a glass of water with each dose

Nursing Implications Watch for signs of I.V. infiltration and gangrene; elderly patients should be cautioned not to increase their fluid intake beyond that sufficient to satisfy their thirst in order to avoid water intoxication and hyponatremia; under experimental conditions, the elderly have shown to have a decreased responsiveness to vasopressin with respect to its effects on water homeostasis

Dosage Forms Injection, aqueous: 20 pressor units/mL (0.5 mL, 1 mL)

Vasopressin Tannate *see* Vasopressin *on previous page*

Vasotec® *see* Enalapril *on page 442*

Vasotec® I.V. *see* Enalapril *on page 442*

Vasoxyl® *see* Methoxamine *on page 811*

V-Cillin K® *see* Penicillin V Potassium *on page 965*

VCR *see* Vincristine *on page 1302*

Vecuronium (ve KYOO roe nee um)

Related Information

Neuromuscular Blocking Agents Comparison *on page 1417*

Brand Names Norcuron®

Synonyms ORG NC 45

Therapeutic Category Neuromuscular Blocker Agent, Nondepolarizing; Skeletal Muscle Relaxant

Use Adjunct to anesthesia, to facilitate intubation, and provide skeletal muscle relaxation during surgery or mechanical ventilation

Pregnancy Risk Factor C

Contraindications Known hypersensitivity to vecuronium

Warnings/Precautions Use with caution in patients with hepatic impairment, neuromuscular disease, myasthenia gravis, and the elderly; ventilation must be supported during neuromuscular blockade

Adverse Reactions

<1%:

Cardiovascular: Tachycardia, flushing, edema, hypotension, circulatory collapse, bradycardia

Dermatologic: Rash, itching

Miscellaneous: Hypersensitivity reaction

Overdosage/Toxicology Symptoms of overdose include prolonged skeletal muscle weakness and apnea cardiovascular collapse

Use neostigmine, edrophonium, or pyridostigmine with atropine to antagonize skeletal muscle relaxation; support of ventilation and the cardiovascular system through mechanical means, fluids, and pressors may be necessary

Drug Interactions Increased toxicity/effect with aminoglycosides, ketamine, magnesium sulfate, verapamil, quinidine, clindamycin, furosemide

Stability Stable for 5 days at room temperature when reconstituted with bacteriostatic water; stable for 24 hours at room temperature when reconstituted with preservative-free sterile water (avoid preservatives in neonates); do not mix with alkaline drugs

Mechanism of Action Blocks acetylcholine from binding to receptors on motor endplate inhibiting depolarization

Pharmacodynamics/Kinetics

Good intubation conditions within 2.5-3 minutes; maximum neuromuscular blockade within 3-5 minutes

Elimination: Vecuronium bromide and its metabolite(s) appear to be excreted principally in feces via biliary eliminations; the drug and its metabolite(s) are also excreted in urine

Usual Dosage I.V. (do not administer I.M.):

Infants >7 weeks to 1 year: Initial: 0.08-0.1 mg/kg/dose; maintenance: 0.05-0.1 mg/kg/every hour as needed

Children >1 year and Adults: Initial: 0.08-0.1 mg/kg/dose; maintenance: 0.05-0.1 mg/kg/every hour as needed; may be administered with caution as a continuous infusion at 0.075 mg/kg/hour (concern has been raised of drug-induced myopathies in ICU setting)

Note: Children (1-10 years) may require slightly higher initial doses and slightly more frequent supplementation

Dosing adjustment in hepatic impairment: Dose reductions are necessary in patients with liver disease

Administration Administer undiluted I.V. injection as a single bolus

Monitoring Parameters Blood pressure, heart rate

Dosage Forms Powder for injection: 10 mg (5 mL, 10 mL)

Veetids® *see* Penicillin V Potassium *on page 965*

Velban® *see* Vinblastine *on page 1300*

Velosef® *see* Cephradine *on page 243*

Velosulin® Human *see* Insulin Preparations *on page 659*

Veltane® *see* Brompheniramine *on page 166*

Venlafaxine (VEN la faks een)

Related Information

Antidepressant Agents Comparison *on page 1393*

Brand Names Effexor®

Therapeutic Category Antidepressant, Serotonin Reuptake Inhibitor

Use Treatment of depression in adults

Unapproved use: Obsessive-compulsive disorder

Pregnancy Risk Factor C

Contraindications Do not use concomitantly with MAO inhibitors, contraindicated in patients with hypersensitivity to venlafaxine or other components

(Continued)

Venlafaxine *(Continued)*

Warnings/Precautions Venlafaxine is associated with sustained increases in blood pressure (10-15 mm Hg SDBP); venlafaxine may actuate mania or hypomania and seizures. Concurrent therapy with a monoamine oxidase inhibitor may result in serious or fatal reactions; at least 14 days should elapse between treatment with an MAO inhibitor and venlafaxine. Patients with cardiovascular disorders or a recent myocardial infarction probably should only receive venlafaxine if the benefits of therapy outweigh the risks.

Adverse Reactions

≥10%:

Central nervous system: Headache, somnolence, dizziness, insomnia, nervousness

Gastrointestinal: Nausea, xerostomia, constipation

Genitourinary: Abnormal ejaculation

Neuromuscular & skeletal: Weakness, neck pain

Miscellaneous: Diaphoresis

1% to 10%:

Cardiovascular: Palpitations, hypertension, sinus tachycardia

Central nervous system: Anxiety

Gastrointestinal: Weight loss, anorexia, vomiting, diarrhea, dysphagia

Genitourinary: Impotence

Neuromuscular & skeletal: Tremor

Ocular: Blurred vision

<1%:

Central nervous system: Seizures

Otic: Ear pain

Overdosage/Toxicology Symptoms of overdose include somnolence and occasionally tachycardia

Most overdoses resolve with only supportive treatment. Use of activated charcoal, inductions of emesis, or gastric lavage should be considered for acute ingestion; forced diuresis, dialysis, and hemoperfusion not effective due to large volume of distribution

Drug Interactions Increased toxicity: Cimetidine MAO inhibitors (hyperpyrexic crisis); TCAs, fluoxetine, sertraline, phenothiazine, class 1C antiarrhythmics, warfarin; venlafaxine is a weak inhibitor of cytochrome P-450-IID6, which is responsible for metabolizing antipsychotics, antiarrhythmics, TCAs, and beta-blockers. Therefore, interactions with these agents are possible, however, less likely than with more potent enzyme inhibitors.

Mechanism of Action Venlafaxine and its active metabolite o-desmethylvenlafaxine (ODV) are potent inhibitors of neuronal serotonin and norepinephrine reuptake and weak inhibitors of dopamine reuptake; causes beta-receptor down regulation and reduces adenylcyclase coupled beta-adrenergic systems in the brain

Pharmacodynamics/Kinetics

Absorption: Oral: 92% to 100%

Protein binding: Bound to human plasma 27% to 30%; steady-state achieved within 3 days of multiple dose therapy

Metabolism: In the liver by cytochrome P-450 enzyme system to active metabolite, O-desmyethyl-venlafaxine (ODV)

Half-life: 3-7 hours (venlafaxine) and 11-13 hours (ODV)

Time to peak: 1-2 hours

Elimination: Primarily by renal route

Usual Dosage Adults: Oral: 75 mg/day, administered in 2 or 3 divided doses, taken with food; dose may be increased in 75 mg/day increments at intervals of at least 4 days, up to 225-375 mg/day

Dosing adjustment in renal impairment: Cl_{cr} 10-70 mL/minute: Decrease dose by 25%; decrease total daily dose by 50% if dialysis patients; dialysis patients should receive dosing after completion of dialysis

Dosing adjustment in moderate hepatic impairment: Reduce total dosage by 25%

Dietary Considerations

Alcohol: Additive CNS effect, avoid use

Food: May be taken without regard to food

Monitoring Parameters Blood pressure should be regularly monitored, especially in patients with a high baseline blood pressure

Reference Range Peak serum level of 163 ng/mL (325 ng/mL of ODV metabolite) obtained after a 150 mg oral dose

Test Interactions ↑ thyroid, ↑ uric acid, ↑ glucose, ↑ potassium, ↑ AST, ↑ cholesterol (S)

Patient Information Avoid use of alcohol; use caution when operating hazardous machinery; if a rash or shortness of breath occurs while using venlafaxine, contact physician immediately

Nursing Implications Causes mean increase in heart rate of 4 beats/minute; tapering to minimize symptoms of discontinuation is recommended when the drug is discontinued; tapering should be over a 2-week period if the patient has received it longer than 6 weeks

Dosage Forms Tablet: 25 mg, 37.5 mg, 50 mg, 75 mg, 100 mg

Venoglobulin®-I *see* Immune Globulin, Intravenous *on page 651*

Venoglobulin®-S *see* Immune Globulin, Intravenous *on page 651*

Ventolin® *see* Albuterol *on page 38*

Ventolin® Rotocaps® *see* Albuterol *on page 38*

VePesid® Injection *see* Etoposide *on page 496*

VePesid® Oral *see* Etoposide *on page 496*

Verapamil (ver AP a mil)

Related Information

Adult ACLS Algorithm, Tachycardia *on page 1512*
Antiarrhythmic Drugs *on page 1389*
Calcium Channel Blockers Comparative Actions *on page 1401*
Calcium Channel Blockers Comparative Pharmacokinetics *on page 1402*
Calcium Channel Blockers FDA-Approved Indications *on page 1403*
Comparative Pharmacokinetic Properties of Antiarrhythmic Agents *on page 1391*
Therapy of Hypertension *on page 1540*

Brand Names Calan®; Calan® SR; Covera-HS®; Isoptin®; Isoptin® SR; Verelan®

Canadian/Mexican Brand Names Apo-Verap® (Canada); Novo-Veramil® (Canada); Nu-Verap® (Canada); Dilacoran® (Mexico); Dilacoran-HTA® (Mexico); Dilacoran-Retard® (Mexico); Veraken® (Mexico); Verdilac® (Mexico)

Synonyms Iproveratril Hydrochloride; Verapamil Hydrochloride

Therapeutic Category Antianginal Agent; Antiarrhythmic Agent, Class IV; Antihypertensive; Calcium Channel Blocker

Use Orally used for treatment of angina pectoris (vasospastic, chronic stable, unstable) and hypertension; I.V. for supraventricular tachyarrhythmias (PSVT, atrial fibrillation, atrial flutter); only Covera-HS® is approved for both hypertension and angina as a sustained release product

Pregnancy Risk Factor C

Pregnancy/Breast-Feeding Implications Use in pregnancy only when clearly needed and when the benefits outweigh the potential hazard to the fetus

Clinical effects on the fetus: Crosses the placenta. 1 report of suspected heart block when used to control fetal supraventricular tachycardia. May exhibit tocolytic effects.

Breast-feeding/lactation: Crosses into breast milk. American Academy of Pediatrics considers COMPATIBLE with breast-feeding.

Contraindications Sinus bradycardia; advanced heart block; ventricular tachycardia; cardiogenic shock; hypersensitivity to verapamil or any component; atrial fibrillation or flutter associated with accessory conduction pathways

Warnings/Precautions Use with caution in sick-sinus syndrome, severe left ventricular dysfunction, hepatic or renal impairment, hypertrophic cardiomyopathy (especially obstructive), abrupt withdrawal may cause increased duration and frequency of chest pain; avoid I.V. use in neonates and young infants due to severe apnea, bradycardia, or hypotensive reactions; elderly may experience more constipation and hypotension. Monitor EKG and blood pressure closely in patients receiving I.V. therapy particularly in patients with supraventricular tachycardia.

Adverse Reactions

1% to 10%:

- Cardiovascular: Bradycardia; first, second, or third degree A-V block; congestive heart failure, hypotension, peripheral edema
- Central nervous system: Dizziness, lightheadedness, nausea, fatigue
- Dermatologic: Rash
- Gastrointestinal: Constipation
- Neuromuscular & skeletal: Weakness

<1%:

- Cardiovascular: Chest pain, hypotension (excessive), tachycardia, flushing
- Endocrine & metabolic: Galactorrhea
- Gastrointestinal: Gingival hyperplasia

Overdosage/Toxicology The primary cardiac symptoms of calcium blocker overdose includes hypotension and bradycardia. The hypotension is caused by peripheral vasodilation, myocardial depression, and bradycardia. Bradycardia results from sinus bradycardia, second- or third-degree atrioventricular block, or

(Continued)

Verapamil *(Continued)*

sinus arrest with junctional rhythm. Intraventricular conduction is usually not affected so QRS duration is normal (verapamil does prolong the P-R interval and bepridil prolongs the Q-T and may cause ventricular arrhythmias, including torsade de pointes).

The noncardiac symptoms include confusion, stupor, nausea, vomiting, metabolic acidosis and hyperglycemia. Following initial gastric decontamination, if possible, repeated calcium administration may promptly reverse the depressed cardiac contractility (but not sinus node depression or peripheral vasodilation); glucagon, epinephrine, and amrinone may treat refractory hypotension; glucagon and epinephrine also increase the heart rate (outside the U.S., 4-aminopyridine may be available as an antidote); dialysis and hemoperfusion are not effective in enhancing elimination although repeat-dose activated charcoal may serve as an adjunct with sustained-release preparations.

Drug Interactions

Cytochrome P-450 2D6 enzyme substrate
Cytochrome P-450 3A4 enzyme substrate
Hepatic enzyme inhibitor

Decreased effect: Phenobarbital and rifampin may decrease verapamil serum concentrations by increased hepatic metabolism

Increased toxicity:
- Verapamil and amiodarone may increase cardiotoxicity
- Verapamil and aspirin may cause bruising
- Verapamil and cimetidine may cause increased bioavailability of verapamil
- Verapamil and beta-blockers may cause increased cardiac depressant effects on A-V conduction
- Verapamil and carbamazepine may cause increased carbamazepine levels
- Verapamil and cyclosporine may cause increased cyclosporine levels
- Verapamil and digoxin may cause increased digoxin levels
- Verapamil and doxorubicin may cause increased doxorubicin levels
- Verapamil and theophylline may cause increased pharmacologic actions of theophylline secondary to decreased clearance of theophylline
- Verapamil and vecuronium may cause increased vecuronium levels

Disopyramide: Avoid combination with disopyramide, discontinue disopyramide 48 hours before starting therapy, do not restart until 24 hours after verapamil has been discontinued

Stability Store injection at room temperature; protect from heat and from freezing; use only clear solutions; **compatible** in solutions of pH of 3-6, but may precipitate in solutions having a pH ≥6

Mechanism of Action Inhibits calcium ion from entering the "slow channels" or select voltage-sensitive areas of vascular smooth muscle and myocardium during depolarization; produces a relaxation of coronary vascular smooth muscle and coronary vasodilation; increases myocardial oxygen delivery in patients with vasospastic angina; slows automaticity and conduction of A-V node.

Pharmacodynamics/Kinetics

Oral (nonsustained tablets):
- Peak effect: 2 hours
- Duration: 6-8 hours

I.V.:
- Peak effect: 1-5 minutes
- Duration: 10-20 minutes

Protein binding: 90%
Metabolism: In the liver; extensive first-pass effect
Bioavailability: Oral: 20% to 30%
Half-life:
- Infants: 4.4-6.9 hours
- Adults: Single dose: 2-8 hours, increased up to 12 hours with multiple dosing; increased half-life with hepatic cirrhosis

Elimination: 70% of dose excreted in urine (3% to 4% as unchanged drug) and 16% in feces

Usual Dosage

Children: SVT:
- I.V.:
  - <1 year: 0.1-0.2 mg/kg over 2 minutes; repeat every 30 minutes as needed
  - 1-16 years: 0.1-0.3 mg/kg over 2 minutes; maximum: 5 mg/dose, may repeat dose in 15 minutes if adequate response not achieved; maximum for second dose: 10 mg/dose
- Oral (dose not well established):
  - 1-5 years: 4-8 mg/kg/day in 3 divided doses **or** 40-80 mg every 8 hours
  - >5 years: 80 mg every 6-8 hours

Adults:

SVT: I.V.: 5-10 mg (approximately 0.075-0.15 mg/kg), second dose of 10 mg (~0.15 mg/kg) may be given 15-30 minutes after the initial dose if patient tolerates, but does not respond to initial dose

Angina: Oral: Initial dose: 80-120 mg twice daily (elderly or small stature: 40 mg twice daily); range: 240-480 mg/day in 3-4 divided doses

Hypertension: 80 mg 3 times/day or 240 mg/day (sustained release); range: 240-480 mg/day (no evidence of additional benefit in doses >360 mg/day)

Note: One time per day dosing is recommended at bedtime with Covera-HS®

Dosing adjustment in renal impairment: Cl_{cr} <10 mL/minute: Administer at 50% to 75% of normal dose

Dialysis: Not dialyzable (0% to 5 %) via hemo or peritoneal dialysis; supplemental dose is not necessary

Dosing adjustment/comments in hepatic disease: Reduce dose in cirrhosis, reduce dose to 20% to 50% of normal and monitor EKG

Administration Administer around-the-clock to promote less variation in peak and trough serum levels; I.V. rate of infusion: Over 2 minutes

Monitoring Parameters Monitor blood pressure closely

Reference Range Therapeutic: 50-200 ng/mL (SI: 100-410 nmol/L) for parent; under normal conditions norverapamil concentration is the same as parent drug. Toxic: >90 µg/mL

Patient Information Sustained release products should be taken with food and not crushed; limit caffeine intake; notify physician if angina pain is not reduced when taking this drug, or if irregular heartbeat or shortness of breath occurs

Nursing Implications Do not crush sustained release drug product

Additional Information Although there is some initial data which may show increased risk of myocardial infarction with the treatment of hypertension with calcium antagonists, controlled trial (eg, ALL-HAT) are ongoing to examine the long-term effects of not only these agents but other antihypertensives in preventing heart disease. Until these studies are completed, patients taking calcium antagonists should be encouraged to continue with the prescribed antihypertensive regimens although a switch from high-dose short-acting products to sustained release agents may be warranted. It is also generally agreed that calcium antagonists should be avoided as primary treatment for hypertension unless diuretics or beta-blockers are contraindicated and as primary therapy of angina after acute myocardial infarction.

Dosage Forms

Capsule, , as hydrochloride, sustained release (Verelan®): 120 mg, 180 mg, 240 mg, 360 mg

Injection, as hydrochloride: 2.5 mg/mL (2 mL, 4 mL)

Isoptin®: 2.5 mg/mL (2 mL, 4 mL)

Tablet, as hydrochloride: 40 mg, 80 mg, 120 mg

Calan®, Isoptin®: 40 mg, 80 mg, 120 mg

Tablet, as hydrochloride, sustained release: 180 mg, 240 mg

Calan® SR, Isoptin® SR: 120 mg, 180 mg, 240 mg

Covera-HS®: 180 mg, 240 mg

Extemporaneous Preparations A 50 mg/mL oral suspension may be made using twenty 80 mg verapamil tablets, 3 mL of purified water USP, 8 mL of methylcellulose 1% and simple syrup qs ad to 32 mL; the expected stability is 30 days under refrigeration; shake well before use

Nahata MC and Hipple TF, *Pediatric Drug Formulations*, 2nd ed, Cincinnati, OH: Harvey Whitney Books Co, 1992.

Verapamil Hydrochloride *see* Verapamil *on page 1297*

Verazinc® [OTC] *see* Zinc Supplements *on page 1324*

Vercyte® *see* Pipobroman *on page 1008*

Verelan® *see* Verapamil *on page 1297*

Vergon® [OTC] *see* Meclizine *on page 769*

Vermizine® *see* Piperazine *on page 1007*

Vermox® *see* Mebendazole *on page 765*

Versed® *see* Midazolam *on page 836*

Vesanoid® *see* Tretinoin, Oral *on page 1251*

Vexol® *see* Rimexolone *on page 1111*

Vibazine® *see* Buclizine *on page 167*

Vibramycin® Injection *see* Doxycycline *on page 430*

Vibramycin® Oral *see* Doxycycline *on page 430*

Vibra-Tabs® *see* Doxycycline *on page 430*

Vicks Children's Chloraseptic® [OTC] *see* Benzocaine *on page 138*

Vicks Chloraseptic® Sore Throat [OTC] *see* Benzocaine *on page 138*

Vicks Formula 44® [OTC] *see* Dextromethorphan *on page 366*

Vicks Formula 44® Pediatric Formula [OTC] *see* Dextromethorphan *on page 366*

Vicks® Pediatric Formula 44E [OTC] *see* Guaifenesin and Dextromethorphan *on page 591*

Vicks® Sinex® Nasal Solution [OTC] *see* Phenylephrine *on page 989*

Vicks Vatronol® *see* Ephedrine *on page 446*

Vicodin® *see* Hydrocodone and Acetaminophen *on page 620*

Vicodin® ES *see* Hydrocodone and Acetaminophen *on page 620*

Vicon Forte® *see* Vitamins, Multiple *on page 1310*

Vicon® Plus [OTC] *see* Vitamins, Multiple *on page 1310*

Vidarabine (vye DARE a been)

Brand Names Vira-A®

Canadian/Mexican Brand Names Adena® a Ungena (Mexico)

Synonyms Adenine Arabinoside; Ara-A; Arabinofuranosyladenine; Vidarabine Monohydrate

Therapeutic Category Antiviral Agent, Ophthalmic

Use Treatment of acute keratoconjunctivitis and epithelial keratitis due to herpes simplex virus; herpes simplex conjunctivitis

Pregnancy Risk Factor C

Contraindications Hypersensitivity to vidarabine or any component

Adverse Reactions Ocular: Burning eyes, lacrimation, keratitis, photophobia, foreign body sensation, uveitis

Mechanism of Action Inhibits viral DNA synthesis by blocking DNA polymerase

Usual Dosage Children and Adults: Ophthalmic: Keratoconjunctivitis: Instill ½" of ointment in lower conjunctival sac 5 times/day every 3 hours while awake until complete re-epithelialization has occurred, then twice daily for an additional 7 days

Patient Information Do not use eye make-up when on this medication for ophthalmic infection; use sunglasses if photophobic reaction occurs; may cause blurred vision; notify physician if improvement not seen after 7 days or if condition worsens

Dosage Forms Ointment, ophthalmic, as monohydrate: 3% [30 mg/mL = 28 mg/mL base] (3.5 g)

Vidarabine Monohydrate *see* Vidarabine *on this page*

Vi-Daylin® [OTC] *see* Vitamins, Multiple *on page 1310*

Vi-Daylin/F® *see* Vitamins, Multiple *on page 1310*

Videx® *see* Didanosine *on page 377*

Vinblastine (vin BLAS teen)

Related Information

Antiemetics for Chemotherapy Induced Nausea and Vomiting *on page 1348*
Cancer Chemotherapy Regimens *on page 1351*
Extravasation Management of Chemotherapeutic Agents *on page 1379*
Toxicities of Chemotherapeutic Agents *on page 1382*

Brand Names Alkaban-AQ®; Velban®

Synonyms Vinblastine Sulfate; Vincaleukoblastine; VLB

Therapeutic Category Antineoplastic Agent, Vesicant; Antineoplastic Agent, Vinca Alkaloid; Vesicant

Use Treatment of Hodgkin's and non-Hodgkin's lymphoma, testicular, lung, head and neck, breast, and renal carcinomas, Mycosis fungoides, Kaposi's sarcoma, histiocytosis, choriocarcinoma, and idiopathic thrombocytopenic purpura

Pregnancy Risk Factor D

Contraindications For I.V. use only; **I.T. use may result in death**; severe bone marrow suppression or presence of bacterial infection not under control prior to initiation of therapy

Warnings/Precautions The U.S. Food and Drug Administration (FDA) currently recommends that procedures for proper handling and disposal of antineoplastic agents be considered. Avoid extravasation; dosage modification required in patients with impaired liver function and neurotoxicity. Using small amounts of drug daily for long periods may increase neurotoxicity and is therefore not advised. For I.V. use only. **Intrathecal administration may result in death**. Use with caution in patients with cachexia or ulcerated skin; monitor closely for shortness of breath or bronchospasm in patients receiving mitomycin C.

Adverse Reactions

>10%:

Dermatologic: Alopecia

Gastrointestinal: Nausea and vomiting are most common and are easily controlled with standard antiemetics; constipation, diarrhea (less common), stomatitis, abdominal cramps, anorexia, metallic taste
Emetic potential: Moderate (30% to 60%)

Hematologic: May cause severe bone marrow suppression and is the dose-limiting toxicity of VLB (unlike vincristine); severe granulocytopenia and thrombocytopenia may occur following the administration of VLB and nadir 7-10 days after treatment

Myelosuppressive:

WBC: Moderate - severe
Platelets: Moderate - severe
Onset (days): 4-7
Nadir (days): 4-10
Recovery (days): 17

1% to 10%:

Cardiovascular: Hypertension, Raynaud's phenomenon
Central nervous system: Depression, malaise, headache, seizures
Dermatologic: Rash, photosensitivity, alopecia, dermatitis
Endocrine & metabolic: Hyperuricemia
Extravasation: VLB is a vesicant and can cause tissue irritation and necrosis if infiltrated; if extravasation occurs, follow institutional policy, which may include hyaluronidase and hot compresses
Gastrointestinal: Paralytic ileus, stomatitis
Genitourinary: Urinary retention
Local: **Vesicant chemotherapy**
Neuromuscular & skeletal: Jaw pain, myalgia, paresthesia
Respiratory: Bronchospasm

<1%:

Central nervous system: Neurologic: VLB rarely produces neurotoxicity at clinical doses; however, neurotoxicity may be seen, especially at high doses; if it occurs, symptoms are similar to VCR toxicity (ie, peripheral neuropathy, loss of deep tendon reflexes, headache, weakness, urinary retention, and GI symptoms, tachycardia, orthostatic hypotension, convulsions)
Gastrointestinal: Hemorrhagic colitis

Overdosage/Toxicology Symptoms of overdose include bone marrow suppression, mental depression, paresthesia, loss of deep reflexes, neurotoxicity

There is no information regarding the effectiveness of dialysis. There are no antidotes for vinblastine; treatment is supportive and symptomatic, including fluid restriction or hypertonic saline (3% sodium chloride) for drug-induced secretion of inappropriate antidiuretic hormone (SIADH), diazepam or phenytoin for seizures, laxatives for constipation, and antiemetics for toxic emesis

Drug Interactions Cytochrome P-450 3A enzyme substrate

Decreased effect:

Phenytoin plasma levels may be reduced with concomitant combination chemotherapy with vinblastine
Alpha-interferon enhances interferon toxicity; phenytoin may ↓ plasma levels

Increased toxicity:

Previous or simultaneous use with mitomycin-C has resulted in acute shortness of breath and severe bronchospasm within minutes or several hours after *Vinca* alkaloid injection and may occur up to 2 weeks after the dose of mitomycin
Mitomycin-C in combination with administration of VLB may cause acute shortness of breath and severe bronchospasm, onset may be within minutes or several hours after VLB injection

Stability

Store intact vials under refrigeration (2°C to 8°C) and protect from light; further dilution in D_5W or NS is stable for 21 days at room temperature (25°C) and refrigeration (4°C)

Standard I.V. dilution:

I.V. push: Dose/syringe (concentration = 1 mg/mL)

Maximum syringe size for IVP is a 30 mL syringe and syringe should be ≤75% full

CIV: Dose/250-1000 mL D_5W or NS

Solutions are stable for 21 days at room temperature (25°C) and refrigeration (4°C)

PROTECT FROM LIGHT

Mechanism of Action VLB binds to tubulin and inhibits microtubule formation, therefore, arresting the cell at metaphase by disrupting the formation of the mitotic spindle; it is specific for the M and S phases; binds to microtubular protein of the mitotic spindle causing metaphase arrest

Pharmacodynamics/Kinetics

Absorption: Not reliably absorbed from the GI tract and must be given I.V.
Distribution: V_d: 27.3 L/kg; binds extensively to tissues; does not penetrate CNS or other fatty tissues; distributes to the liver
Protein binding: 99% rapidly
Metabolism: Hepatic metabolism to an active metabolite
(Continued)

Vinblastine *(Continued)*

Half-life (biphasic):
Initial 0.164 hours
Terminal: 25 hours
Elimination: Biliary excretion (95%); <1% eliminated unchanged in urine

Usual Dosage Refer to individual protocols. Varies depending upon clinical and hematological response. Administer at intervals of at least 7 days and only after leukocyte count has returned to at least 4,000/mm^3; maintenance therapy should be titrated according to leukocyte count. Dosage should be reduced in patients with recent exposure to radiation therapy or chemotherapy; single doses in these patients should not exceed 5.5 mg/m^2.

Children and Adults: I.V.: 4-20 mg/m^2 (0.1-0.5 mg/kg) every 7-10 days **or** 5-day continuous infusion of 1.4-1.8 mg/m^2/day **or** 0.1-0.5 mg/kg/week

Dosing adjustment in hepatic impairment:
Serum bilirubin 1.5-3.0 mg/dL or AST 60-180 units: Administer 50% of normal dose
Serum bilirubin 3.0-5.0 mg/dL: Administer 25% of dose
Serum bilirubin >5.0 mg/dL or AST >180 units: Omit dose

Administration
FATAL IF GIVEN INTRATHECALLY
IVP over at least one minute is desired route of administration because of potential for extravasation. However, has also been administered CIV - **CENTRAL LINE ONLY** for CIV administration.
Avoid extravasation
Protect from light

Monitoring Parameters CBC with differential and platelet count, serum uric acid, hepatic function tests

Patient Information Hair may be lost during treatment but will regrow to its pretreatment extent even with continued treatment; report any bleeding; examine mouth daily and report soreness to a physician; jaw pain or pain in the organs containing tumor tissue; avoid constipation. Any signs of infection, easy bruising or bleeding, shortness of breath, or painful or burning urination should be brought to physician's attention. Nausea, vomiting or hair loss sometimes occur. The drug may cause permanent sterility and may cause birth defects. The drug may be excreted in breast milk, therefore, an alternative form of feeding your baby should be used.

Nursing Implications May be administered by I.V. push or into a free flowing I.V.; monitor for life-threatening bronchospasm (most likely to occur if patient is also taking mitomycin). Maintain adequate hydration; allopurinol may be given to prevent uric acid nephropathy; may cause sloughing upon extravasation.

Extravasation treatment:
Mix 250 units hyaluronidase was 6 mL of NS
Inject the hyaluronidase solution subcutaneously through 6 clockwise injections into the infiltrated area using a 25-gauge needle; change the needle with each new injection
Apply heat immediately for 1 hour; repeat 4 times/day for 3-5 days
Application of cold or hydrocortisone is contraindicated

Dosage Forms
Injection, as sulfate: 1 mg/mL (10 mL)
Powder for injection, as sulfate: 10 mg

Vinblastine Sulfate *see* Vinblastine *on page 1300*
Vincaleukoblastine *see* Vinblastine *on page 1300*
Vincasar® PFS *see* Vincristine *on this page*

Vincristine (vin KRIS teen)

Related Information
Antiemetics for Chemotherapy Induced Nausea and Vomiting *on page 1348*
Cancer Chemotherapy Regimens *on page 1351*
Extravasation Management of Chemotherapeutic Agents *on page 1379*
Toxicities of Chemotherapeutic Agents *on page 1382*

Brand Names Oncovin®; Vincasar® PFS

Synonyms LCR; Leurocristine; VCR; Vincristine Sulfate

Therapeutic Category Antineoplastic Agent, Vesicant; Antineoplastic Agent, Vinca Alkaloid; Vesicant

Use Treatment of leukemias, Hodgkin's disease, non-Hodgkin's lymphomas, Wilms' tumor, neuroblastoma, rhabdomyosarcoma

Pregnancy Risk Factor D

Contraindications Hypersensitivity to vincristine or any component; **for I.V. use only, fatal if given intrathecally**; patients with demyelinating form of Charcot-Marie-Tooth syndrome

Warnings/Precautions The U.S. Food and Drug Administration (FDA) currently recommends that procedures for proper handling and disposal of antineoplastic agents be considered. Dosage modification required in patients with impaired hepatic function or who have pre-existing neuromuscular disease; avoid extravasation; use with caution in the elderly; avoid eye contamination; observe closely for shortness of breath, bronchospasm, especially in patients treated with mitomycin C. For I.V. use only; **intrathecal administration results in death**; administer allopurinol to prevent uric acid nephropathy; not to be used with radiation.

Adverse Reactions

>10%:

Dermatologic: Alopecia occurs in 20% to 70% of patients

Extravasation: VCR is a vesicant and can cause tissue irritation and necrosis if infiltrated; if extravasation occurs, follow institutional policy, which may include hyaluronidase and hot compresses

Vesicant chemotherapy

1% to 10%:

Cardiovascular: Orthostatic hypotension or hypertension, hypertension, hypotension

Central nervous system: Motor difficulties, seizures, headache, CNS depression, cranial nerve paralysis, fever

Dermatologic: Rash

Endocrine & metabolic: Hyperuricemia

SIADH: Rarely occurs, but may be related to the neurologic toxicity; may cause symptomatic hyponatremia with seizures; the increase in serum ADH concentration usually subsides within 2-3 days after onset

Gastrointestinal: Constipation and possible paralytic ileus secondary to neurologic toxicity; oral ulceration, abdominal cramps, anorexia, metallic taste, bloating, nausea, vomiting, weight loss, diarrhea

Emetic potential: Low (<10%)

Local: Phlebitis

Neurologic: Alterations in mental status such as depression, confusion, or insomnia; constipation, paralytic ileus, and urinary tract disturbances may occur. All patients should be on a prophylactic bowel management regimen. Cranial nerve palsies, headaches, jaw pain, optic atrophy with blindness have been reported. Intrathecal administration of VCR has uniformly caused death; VCR should **never** be administered by this route. Neurologic effects of VCR may be additive with those of other neurotoxic agents and spinal cord irradiation.

Neuromuscular & skeletal: Jaw pain, leg pain, myalgia, cramping, numbness, weakness

Peripheral neuropathy: Frequently the dose-limiting toxicity of VCR. Most frequent in patients >40 years of age; occurs usually after an average of 3 weekly doses, but may occur after just one dose. Manifested as loss of the deep tendon reflexes in the lower extremities, numbness, tingling, pain, paresthesias of the fingers and toes (stocking glove sensation), and "foot drop" or "wrist drop"

Ocular: Photophobia

<1%:

Gastrointestinal: Stomatitis

Hematologic: Myelosuppressive: Occasionally mild leukopenia and thrombocytopenia may occur

WBC: Rare

Platelets: Rare

Onset (days): 7

Nadir (days): 10

Recovery (days): 21

Overdosage/Toxicology Symptoms of overdose include bone marrow suppression, mental depression, paresthesia, loss of deep reflexes, alopecia, nausea, severe symptoms may occur with 3-4 mg/m^2

There are no antidotes for vincristine; treatment is supportive and symptomatic, including fluid restriction or hypertonic saline (3% sodium chloride) for drug-induced secretion of inappropriate antidiuretic hormone (SIADH), diazepam or phenytoin for seizures, laxatives for constipation, and antiemetics for toxic emesis; case reports suggest that folinic acid may be helpful in treating vincristine overdose; it is suggested that 100 mg folinic acid be given I.V. every 3 hours for 24 hours, then every 6 hours for 48 hours; this is in addition to supportive care; the use of pyridoxine, leucovorin factor, cyanocobalamin or thiamine have been used with little success for drug-induced peripheral neuropathy

Drug Interactions Cytochrome P-450 3A enzyme substrate

Decreased effect: Phenytoin levels may decrease with combination chemotherapy

(Continued)

Vincristine *(Continued)*

Increased toxicity:

Digoxin plasma levels and renal excretion may decrease with combination chemotherapy including vincristine

Vincristine should be given 12-24 hours before asparaginase to minimize toxicity (may decrease the hepatic clearance of vincristine)

Acute pulmonary reactions may occur with mitomycin-C. Previous or simultaneous use with mitomycin-C has resulted in acute shortness of breath and severe bronchospasm within minutes or several hours after *Vinca* alkaloid injection and may occur up to 2 weeks after the dose of mitomycin.

Stability Store intact vials at refrigeration (2°C to 8°C). Further dilution in NS or D_5W is stable for 21 days at room temperature (25°C) and refrigeration (4°C)

Compatible with doxorubicin, bleomycin, cytarabine, fluorouracil, methotrexate, metoclopramide

Standard I.V. dilution:

I.V. push: Dose/syringe (concentration: 1 mg/mL)

Maximum syringe size for IVP is 30 mL syringe and syringe should be ≤75% full

IVPB: Dose/50 mL D_5W

Mechanism of Action Binds to microtubular protein of the mitotic spindle causing metaphase arrest; cell-cycle phase specific in the M and S phases

Pharmacodynamics/Kinetics

Absorption: Oral: Poor

Distribution: Poor penetration into the CSF; rapidly removed from the blood stream and tightly bound to tissues; penetrates blood-brain barrier poorly

Protein binding: 75%

Metabolism: Extensively in the liver

Half-life: Terminal: 24 hours

Elimination: Primarily in the bile (~80%); <1% excreted unchanged in urine

Usual Dosage Refer to individual protocols as dosages vary with protocol used. Adjustments are made depending upon clinical and hematological response and upon adverse reactions

Children: I.V. (maximum single dose: 2 mg):

≤10 kg or BSA <1 m^2: 0.05 mg/kg once weekly

2 mg/m^2; may repeat every week

Adults: I.V.: 0.4-1.4 mg/m^2 (up to 2 mg maximum); may repeat every week

Dosing adjustment in hepatic impairment:

Serum bilirubin 1.5-3.0 mg/dL or AST 60-180 units: Administer 50% of normal dose

Serum bilirubin 3.0-5.0 mg/dL: Administer 25% of dose

Serum bilirubin >5.0 mg/dL or AST >180 units: Omit dose

The average total dose per course of treatment should be around 2-2.5 mg; some recommend capping the dose at 2 mg maximum to reduce toxicity; however, it is felt that this measure can reduce the efficacy of the drug

Administration

FATAL IF GIVEN INTRATHECALLY

IVP over at least one minute is desired route of administration because of potential for extravasation. However, has also been administered IVPB over 15 minutes - **CENTRAL LINE ONLY** for IVPB administration.

Avoid extravasation

Protect from light

Monitoring Parameters Serum electrolytes (sodium), hepatic function tests, neurologic examination, CBC, serum uric acid

Patient Information Maintain adequate fluid intake; rinse mouth with water 3-4 times/day, brush teeth with soft brush and floss with waxed floss; loss of hair occurs in approximately 70% of patients; report any nerve effects to physician; stool softener should be used for constipation prophylaxis; report to physician any persistent or severe fever, sore throat, bleeding, or bruising; shortness of breath

Nursing Implications Observe for life-threatening bronchospasm after administration; use of rectal thermometer or rectal tubing should be avoided to prevent injury to rectal mucosa

Extravasation treatment:

Mix 250 Units hyaluronidase was 6 mL of NS

Inject the hyaluronidase solution subcutaneously through 6 clockwise injections into the infiltrated area using a 25-gauge needle; change the needle with each new injection

Apply heat immediately for 1 hour; repeat 4 times/day for 3-5 days

Application of cold or hydrocortisone is contraindicated

Dosage Forms Injection, as sulfate: 1 mg/mL (1 mL, 2 mL, 5 mL)

Vincristine Sulfate *see* Vincristine *on page 1302*

Vinorelbine (vi NOR el been)

Related Information

Antiemetics for Chemotherapy Induced Nausea and Vomiting *on page 1348*
Cancer Chemotherapy Regimens *on page 1351*
Toxicities of Chemotherapeutic Agents *on page 1382*

Brand Names Navelbine®

Synonyms Vinorelbine Tartrate

Therapeutic Category Antineoplastic Agent, Vesicant; Antineoplastic Agent, Vinca Alkaloid; Vesicant

Use Treatment of nonsmall cell lung cancer (as a single agent or in combination with cisplatin)

Unlabeled use: Breast cancer, ovarian carcinoma (cisplatin-resistant), Hodgkin's disease

Pregnancy Risk Factor D

Contraindications For I.V. use only; **I.T. use may result in death**; severe bone marrow suppression (granulocyte counts <1000 cells/mm^3) or presence of bacterial infection not under control prior to initiation of therapy

Warnings/Precautions The U.S. Food and Drug Administration (FDA) currently recommends that procedures for proper handling and disposal of antineoplastic agents be considered. Avoid extravasation; dosage modification required in patients with impaired liver function and neurotoxicity. Frequently monitor patients for myelosuppression both during and after therapy. Granulocytopenia is dose-limiting. **Intrathecal administration may result in death**. Use with caution in patients with cachexia or ulcerated skin.

Adverse Reactions

>10%:

- Dermatologic: Alopecia (12%)
- Gastrointestinal: Nausea and vomiting are most common and are easily controlled with standard antiemetics; constipation, diarrhea, stomatitis, abdominal cramps, anorexia, metallic taste
  - Emetic potential: Moderate (30% to 60%)
- Hematologic: May cause severe bone marrow suppression and is the dose-limiting toxicity of vinorelbine; severe granulocytopenia may occur following the administration of vinorelbine
- Myelosuppressive:
  - WBC: Moderate - severe
  - Onset (days): 4-7
  - Nadir (days): 7-10
  - Recovery (days): 14-21
- Neuromuscular and skeletal: Peripheral neuropathy (20% to 25%)

1% to 10%:

- Central nervous system: Fatigue
- Extravasation: Vesicant and can cause tissue irritation and necrosis if infiltrated; if extravasation occurs, follow institutional policy, which may include hyaluronidase and hot compresses
  - **Vesicant chemotherapy**
- Neuromuscular & skeletal: Mild-moderate peripheral neuropathy manifested by paresthesia and hyperesthesia, loss of deep tendon reflexes; myalgia, arthralgia, jaw pain

<1%:

- Gastrointestinal: Hemorrhagic colitis
- Neuromuscular & skeletal: Severe peripheral neuropathy (generally reversible)

Overdosage/Toxicology Symptoms of overdose include bone marrow suppression, mental depression, paresthesia, loss of deep reflexes, neurotoxicity

There are no antidotes for vinorelbine. Treatment is supportive and symptomatic, including fluid restriction or hypertonic saline (3% sodium chloride) for drug-induced secretion of inappropriate antidiuretic hormone (SIADH), diazepam or phenytoin for seizures, laxatives for constipation, and antiemetics for toxic emesis.

Drug Interactions

Increased toxicity:

- Previous or simultaneous use with mitomycin-C has resulted in acute shortness of breath and severe bronchospasm within minutes or several hours after *Vinca* alkaloid injection and may occur up to 2 weeks after the dose of mitomycin
- Cisplatin: Incidence of granulocytopenia is significantly higher than with single-agent vinorelbine

Stability Store intact vials under refrigeration (2°C to 8°C) and protect from light; vials are stable at room temperature for up to 72 hours. Further dilution in D_5W or NS is stable for 24 hours at room temperature.

(Continued)

Vinorelbine *(Continued)*

Standard I.V. dilution:

I.V. push: Dose/syringe (concentration = 1.5-3 mg/mL)

Maximum syringe size for IVP is a 30 mL syringe and syringe should be ≤75% full

IVPB: Dose/50-250 mL D_5W or NS (concentration = 0.5-2 mg/mL)

Solutions are stable for 24 hours at room temperature

Mechanism of Action Semisynthetic vinca alkaloid which binds to tubulin and inhibits microtubule formation, therefore, arresting the cell at metaphase by disrupting the formation of the mitotic spindle; it is specific for the M and S phases; binds to microtubular protein of the mitotic spindle causing metaphase arrest

Pharmacodynamics/Kinetics

Absorption: Not reliably absorbed from the GI tract and must be given I.V.

Distribution: V_d: 25.4-40.1 L/kg; binds extensively to human platelets and lymphocytes (79.6% to 91.2%)

Metabolism: Extensive hepatic metabolism to an active metabolite (deacetylvinorelbine)

Half-life (triphasic):

Terminal: 27.7-43.6 hours

Mean plasma clearance: 0.97-1.26 L/hour/kg

Elimination: Feces (46%) and urine (18%)

Usual Dosage Refer to individual protocols; varies depending upon clinical and hematological response

Adults: I.V.: 30 mg/m^2 every 7 days

Dosage adjustment in hematological toxicity: Granulocyte counts should be ≥1000 cells/mm^3 prior to the administration of vinorelbine. Adjustments in the dosage of vinorelbine should be based on granulocyte counts obtained on the day of treatment as follows:

Granulocytes ≥1500 cells/mm^3 on day of treatment: Administer 30 mg/m^2

Granulocytes 1000-1499 cells/mm^3 on day of treatment: Administer 15 mg/m^2

Granulocytes <1000 cells/mm^3 on day of treatment: Do not administer. Repeat granulocyte count in one week; if 3 consecutive doses are held because granulocyte count is <1000 cells/mm^3, discontinue vinorelbine

For patients who, during treatment, have experienced fever and/or sepsis while granulocytopenic or had 2 consecutive weekly doses held due to granulocytopenia, subsequent doses of vinorelbine should be:

22.5 mg/m^2 for granulocytes ≥1500 cells/mm^3

11.25 mg/m^2 for granulocytes 1000-1499 cells/mm^3

Dosage adjustment in renal impairment: No dose adjustments are required for renal insufficiency. If moderate or severe neurotoxicity develops, discontinue vinorelbine.

Dosing adjustment in hepatic impairment: Vinorelbine should be administered with caution in patients with hepatic insufficiency. In patients who develop hyperbilirubinemia during treatment with vinorelbine, the dose should be adjusted for total bilirubin as follows:

Serum bilirubin ≤2 mg/dL: Administer 30 mg/m^2

Serum bilirubin 2.1-3 mg/dL: Administer 15 mg/m^2

Serum bilirubin >3 mg/dL: Administer 7.5 mg/m^2

Dosing adjustment in patients with concurrent hematologic toxicity and hepatic impairment: Administer the lower doses determined from the above recommendations

Administration

FATAL IF GIVEN INTRATHECALLY

Administer IVPB over 20-30 minutes or I.V. push over 6-10 minutes

CENTRAL LINE ONLY for IVPB administration

Avoid extravasation

Monitoring Parameters CBC with differential and platelet count, serum uric acid, hepatic function tests

Patient Information Hair may be lost during treatment but will regrow to its pretreatment extent even with continued treatment; report any bleeding; examine mouth daily and report soreness to a physician; jaw pain or pain in the organs containing tumor tissue; avoid constipation. Any signs of infection, easy bruising or bleeding, shortness of breath, or painful or burning urination should be brought to physician's attention. Nausea, vomiting or hair loss sometimes occur. The drug may cause permanent sterility and may cause birth defects. The drug may be excreted in breast milk, therefore, an alternative form of feeding your baby should be used.

Nursing Implications

Extravasation treatment:

Mix 250 units hyaluronidase was 6 mL of NS

Inject the hyaluronidase solution subcutaneously through 6 clockwise injections into the infiltrated area using a 25-gauge needle; change the needle with each new injection

Apply heat immediately for one hour; repeat 4 times/day for 3-5 days

Application of cold or hydrocortisone is contraindicated.

Monitor for life-threatening bronchospasm (most likely to occur if patient is also taking mitomycin). Maintain adequate hydration; allopurinol may be given to prevent uric acid nephropathy; may cause sloughing upon extravasation

Dosage Forms Injection, as tartrate: 10 mg/mL (1 mL, 5 mL)

Vinorelbine Tartrate *see* Vinorelbine *on page 1305*

Vioform® [OTC] *see* Clioquinol *on page 291*

Viokase® *see* Pancrelipase *on page 949*

Viosterol *see* Ergocalciferol *on page 456*

Vira-A® *see* Vidarabine *on page 1300*

Viracept® *see* Nelfinavir *on page 885*

Viramune® *see* Nevirapine *on page 895*

Virazole® *see* Ribavirin *on page 1104*

Virilon® *see* Methyltestosterone *on page 821*

Viroptic® *see* Trifluridine *on page 1263*

Viscoat® *see* Chondroitin Sulfate-Sodium Hyaluronate *on page 272*

Visine® [OTC] *see* Tetrahydrozoline *on page 1205*

Visine A.C.® [OTC] *see* Tetrahydrozoline *on page 1205*

Visine® L.R. Ophthalmic [OTC] *see* Oxymetazoline *on page 940*

Visken® *see* Pindolol *on page 1002*

Vistacon-50® *see* Hydroxyzine *on page 634*

Vistaquel® *see* Hydroxyzine *on page 634*

Vistaril® *see* Hydroxyzine *on page 634*

Vistazine® *see* Hydroxyzine *on page 634*

Vistide® *see* Cidofovir *on page 274*

Vita-C® [OTC] *see* Ascorbic Acid *on page 102*

Vitamin A (VYE ta min aye)

Brand Names Aquasol A®; Del-Vi-A®; Palmitate-A® 5000 [OTC]

Canadian/Mexican Brand Names Arovit® (Mexico); A-Vicon® (Mexico); A-Vitex® (Mexico)

Synonyms Oleovitamin A

Therapeutic Category Vitamin, Fat Soluble

Use Treatment and prevention of vitamin A deficiency

Pregnancy Risk Factor A (X if dose exceeds RDA recommendation)

Contraindications Hypervitaminosis A, hypersensitivity to vitamin A or any component

Warnings/Precautions Evaluate other sources of vitamin A while receiving this product; patients receiving >25,000 units/day should be closely monitored for toxicity

Adverse Reactions

1% to 10%:

Central nervous system: Irritability, vertigo, lethargy, malaise, fever, headache

Dermatologic: Drying or cracking of skin

Endocrine & metabolic: Hypercalcemia

Gastrointestinal: Weight loss

Ocular: Visual changes

Miscellaneous: Hypervitaminosis A

Overdosage/Toxicology Symptoms of chronic overdose (adults: 25,000 units/day for 2-3 weeks) include increased intracranial pressure (headache, altered mental status, blurred vision), bulging fontanelles in infants, jaundice, ascites, cutaneous desquamation; symptoms of acute overdose (12,000 units/kg) include nausea, vomiting, and diarrhea; toxic signs of an overdose commonly respond to drug discontinuation and generally return to normal spontaneously within a few days to weeks.

When confronted with signs of increased intracranial pressure, treatment with dexamethasone (1.5 mg/kg I.V. load followed with 0.375 mg/kg every 6 hours for 5 days), and/or hyperventilation may be employed; forced diuresis, dialysis, and hemoperfusion are of no clinical benefit.

Drug Interactions

Decreased effect: Cholestyramine decreases absorption of vitamin A; neomycin and mineral oil may also interfere with vitamin A absorption

(Continued)

Vitamin A *(Continued)*

Increased toxicity: Retinoids may have additive adverse effects

Stability Protect from light

Mechanism of Action Needed for bone development, growth, visual adaptation to darkness, testicular and ovarian function, and as a cofactor in many biochemical processes

Pharmacodynamics/Kinetics

Absorption: Vitamin A in dosages **not** exceeding physiologic replacement is well absorbed after oral administration; water miscible preparations are absorbed more rapidly than oil preparations; large oral doses, conditions of fat malabsorption, low protein intake, or hepatic or pancreatic disease reduces oral absorption

Distribution: Following oral absorption, large amounts concentrate for storage in the liver; appears in breast milk

Metabolism: Conjugated with glucuronide, undergoes enterohepatic circulation

Elimination: In feces via biliary elimination

Usual Dosage

RDA:

<1 year: 375 mcg
1-3 years: 400 mcg
4-6 years: 500 mcg*
7-10 years: 700 mcg*
>10 years: 800-1000 mcg*
Male: 1000 mcg
Female: 800 mcg
* mcg retinol equivalent (0.3 mcg retinol = 1 unit vitamin A)

Vitamin A supplementation in measles (recommendation of the World Health Organization): Children: Oral: Administer as a single dose; repeat the next day and at 4 weeks for children with ophthalmologic evidence of vitamin A deficiency:

6 months to 1 year: 100,000 units
>1 year: 200,000 units

Note: Use of vitamin A in measles is recommended only for patients 6 months to 2 years of age hospitalized with measles and its complications **or** patients >6 months of age who have any of the following risk factors and who are not already receiving vitamin A: immunodeficiency, ophthalmologic evidence of vitamin A deficiency including night blindness, Bitot's spots or evidence of xerophthalmia, impaired intestinal absorption, moderate to severe malnutrition including that associated with eating disorders, or recent immigration from areas where high mortality rates from measles have been observed

Note: Monitor patients closely; dosages >25,000 units/kg have been associated with toxicity

Severe deficiency with xerophthalmia: Oral:

Children 1-8 years: 5000-10,000 units/kg/day for 5 days or until recovery occurs

Children >8 years and Adults: 500,000 units/day for 3 days, then 50,000 units/day for 14 days, then 10,000-20,000 units/day for 2 months

Deficiency (without corneal changes): Oral:

Infants <1 year: 100,000 units every 4-6 months

Children 1-8 years: 200,000 units every 4-6 months

Children >8 years and Adults: 100,000 units/day for 3 days then 50,000 units/day for 14 days

Malabsorption syndrome (prophylaxis): Children >8 years and Adults: Oral: 10,000-50,000 units/day of water miscible product

Dietary supplement: Oral:

Infants up to 6 months: 1500 units/day

Children:

6 months to 3 years: 1500-2000 units/day
4-6 years: 2500 units/day
7-10 years: 3300-3500 units/day

Children >10 years and Adults: 4000-5000 units/day

Reference Range 1 RE = 1 retinol equivalent; 1 RE = 1 μg retinol or 6 mg beta-carotene; Normal levels of Vitamin A in serum = 80-300 units/mL

Patient Information Avoid use of mineral oil when taking drug; take with food; notify physician if nausea, vomiting, anorexia, malaise, drying or cracking of skin or lips, irritability, headache, or loss of hair occurs

Nursing Implications Do not administer by I.V. push; patients receiving >25,000 units/day should be closely monitored for toxicity

Additional Information 1 mg equals 3333 units

Dosage Forms

Capsule: 10,000 units [OTC], 25,000 units, 50,000 units

Drops, oral (water miscible) [OTC]: 5000 units/0.1 mL (30 mL)

Injection: 50,000 units/mL (2 mL)
Tablet [OTC]: 5000 units

Vitamin A Acid *see* Tretinoin, Topical *on page 1254*

Vitamin B_1 *see* Thiamine *on page 1214*

Vitamin B_2 *see* Riboflavin *on page 1104*

Vitamin B_3 *see* Niacin *on page 896*

Vitamin B_3 *see* Niacinamide *on page 897*

Vitamin B_6 *see* Pyridoxine *on page 1081*

Vitamin B_{12} *see* Cyanocobalamin *on page 319*

Vitamin B_{12} *see* Hydroxocobalamin *on page 629*

Vitamin C *see* Ascorbic Acid *on page 102*

Vitamin D_2 *see* Ergocalciferol *on page 456*

Vitamin E (VYE ta min ee)

Brand Names Amino-Opti-E® [OTC]; Aquasol E® [OTC]; E-Complex-600® [OTC]; E-Vitamin® [OTC]; Vita-Plus® E Softgels® [OTC]; Vitec® [OTC]; Vite E® Creme [OTC]

Synonyms *d*-Alpha Tocopherol; *dl*-Alpha Tocopherol

Therapeutic Category Vitamin, Fat Soluble; Vitamin, Topical

Use Prevention and treatment hemolytic anemia secondary to vitamin E deficiency, dietary supplement

Pregnancy Risk Factor A (C if dose exceeds RDA recommendation)

Contraindications Hypersensitivity to drug or any components

Warnings/Precautions May induce vitamin K deficiency; necrotizing enterocolitis has been associated with oral administration of large dosages (eg, >200 units/day) of a hyperosmolar vitamin E preparation in low birth weight infants

Adverse Reactions

<1%:

Central nervous system: Headache
Dermatologic: Contact dermatitis with topical preparation
Gastrointestinal: Nausea, diarrhea, intestinal cramps
Neuromuscular & skeletal: Weakness
Ocular: Blurred vision
Miscellaneous: Gonadal dysfunction

Drug Interactions

Decreased absorption with mineral oil
Delayed absorption of iron
Increased effect of oral anticoagulants

Stability Protect from light

Mechanism of Action Prevents oxidation of vitamin A and C; protects polyunsaturated fatty acids in membranes from attack by free radicals and protects red blood cells against hemolysis

Pharmacodynamics/Kinetics

Absorption: Oral: Depends upon the presence of bile; absorption is reduced in conditions of malabsorption, in low birth weight premature infants, and as dosage increases; water miscible preparations are better absorbed than oil preparations

Distribution: Distributes to all body tissues, especially adipose tissue, where it is stored

Metabolism: In the liver to glucuronides

Elimination: In feces and bile

Usual Dosage One unit of vitamin E = 1 mg *dl*-alpha-tocopherol acetate. Oral:

Vitamin E deficiency:

Children (with malabsorption syndrome): 1 unit/kg/day of water miscible vitamin E (to raise plasma tocopherol concentrations to the normal range within 2 months and to maintain normal plasma concentrations)

Adults: 60-75 units/day

Prevention of vitamin E deficiency: Adults: 30 units/day

Prevention of retinopathy of prematurity or BPD secondary to O_2 therapy: (American Academy of Pediatrics considers this use investigational and routine use is not recommended):

Retinopathy prophylaxis: 15-30 units/kg/day to maintain plasma levels between 1.5-2 µg/mL (may need as high as 100 units/kg/day)

Cystic fibrosis, beta-thalassemia, sickle cell anemia may require higher daily maintenance doses:

Cystic fibrosis: 100-400 units/day
Beta-thalassemia: 750 units/day

Sickle cell: 450 units/day

Recommended daily allowance:

Premature infants ≤3 months: 17 mg (25 units)

(Continued)

Vitamin E *(Continued)*

Infants:
≤6 months: 3 mg (4.5 units)
6-12 months: 4 mg (6 units)
Children:
1-3 years: 6 mg (9 units)
4-10 years: 7 mg (10.5 units)
Children >11 years and Adults:
Male: 10 mg (15 units)
Female: 8 mg (12 units)
Topical: Apply a thin layer over affected area

Reference Range Therapeutic: 0.8-1.5 mg/dL (SI: 19-35 μmol/L), some method variation

Patient Information Drops can be placed directly in the mouth or mixed with cereal, fruit juice, or other food; take only the prescribed dose. Vitamin E toxicity appears as blurred vision, diarrhea, dizziness, flu-like symptoms, nausea, headache; swallow capsules whole, do not crush or chew

Dosage Forms
Capsule: 100 units, 200 units, 330 mg, 400 units, 500 units, 600 units, 1000 units
Capsule, water miscible: 73.5 mg, 147 mg, 165 mg, 330 mg, 400 units
Cream: 50 mg/g (15 g, 30 g, 60 g, 75 g, 120 g, 454 g)
Drops, oral: 50 mg/mL (12 mL, 30 mL)
Liquid, topical: 10 mL, 15 mL, 30 mL, 60 mL
Lotion: 120 mL
Oil: 15 mL, 30 mL, 60 mL
Ointment, topical: 30 mg/g (45 g, 60 g)
Tablet: 200 units, 400 units

Vitamin G *see* Riboflavin *on page 1104*

Vitamin K_1 *see* Phytonadione *on page 998*

Vitamin K Content in Selected Foods *see page 1578*

Vitamin, Multiple, Prenatal *see* Vitamins, Multiple *on this page*

Vitamin, Multiple, Therapeutic *see* Vitamins, Multiple *on this page*

Vitamin, Multiple With Iron *see* Vitamins, Multiple *on this page*

Vitamins, Multiple (VYE ta mins, MUL ti pul)

Brand Names Adeflor®; Allbee® With C; Becotin® Pulvules®; Berocca®; Cefol® Filmtab®; Chromagen® OB [OTC]; Eldercaps® [OTC]; Filibon® [OTC]; Florvite®; Iberet-Folic-500®; LKV-Drops® [OTC]; Mega-B® [OTC]; Multi Vit® Drops [OTC]; M.V.I.®; M.V.I.®-12; M.V.I.® Concentrate; M.V.I.® Pediatric; Natabec® [OTC]; Natabec® FA [OTC]; Natabec® Rx; Natalins® [OTC]; Natalins® Rx; NeoVadrin® [OTC]; Nephrocaps® [OTC]; Niferex®-PN; Poly-Vi-Flor®; Poly-Vi-Sol® [OTC]; Pramet® FA; Pramilet® FA; Prenavite® [OTC]; Secran®; Stresstabs® 600 Advanced Formula Tablets [OTC]; Stuartnatal® 1 + 1; Stuart Prenatal® [OTC]; Therabid® [OTC]; Theragran® [OTC]; Theragran® Hematinic®; Theragran® Liquid [OTC]; Theragran-M® [OTC]; Tri-Vi-Flor®; Unicap® [OTC]; Vicon Forte®; Vicon® Plus [OTC]; Vi-Daylin® [OTC]; Vi-Daylin/F®

Synonyms B Complex; B Complex With C; Children's Vitamins; Hexavitamin; Multiple Vitamins; Multivitamins/Fluoride; Parenteral Multiple Vitamin; Prenatal Vitamins; Therapeutic Multivitamins; Vitamin, Multiple, Prenatal; Vitamin, Multiple, Therapeutic; Vitamin, Multiple With Iron

Therapeutic Category Vitamin

Use Dietary supplement

Pregnancy Risk Factor A (C if used in doses above RDA recommendation)

Contraindications Hypersensitivity to product components

Warnings/Precautions RDA values are not requirements, but are recommended daily intakes of certain essential nutrients; periodic dental exams should be performed to check for dental fluorosis; use with caution in patients with severe renal or liver failure

Adverse Reactions 1% to 10%: Hypervitaminosis; refer to individual vitamin entries for individual reactions

Usual Dosage
Infants 1.5-3 kg: I.V.: 3.25 mL/24 hours (M.V.I.® Pediatric)
Children:
Oral:
≤2 years: Drops: 1 mL/day (premature infants may get 0.5-1 mL/day)
>2 years: Chew 1 tablet/day
≥4 years: 5 mL/day liquid
I.V.: >3 kg and <11 years: 5 mL/24 hours (M.V.I.® Pediatric)
Adults:
Oral: 1 tablet/day or 5 mL/day liquid
I.V.: >11 years: 5 mL of vials 1 and 2 (M.V.I.®-12)/one TPN bag/day

Multivitamin Products Available

Product	Content Given Per	A IU	D IU	E IU	C mg	FA mg	B_1 mg	B_2 mg	B_3 mg	B_6 mg	B_{12} mcg	Other
Theragran®	5 mL liquid	10,000	400		200		10	10	100	4.1	5	B_5 21.4 mg
Vi-Daylin®	1 mL drops	1500	400	4.1	35		0.5	0.6	8	0.4	1.5	Alcohol <0.5%
Vi-Daylin® Iron	1 mL	1500	400	4.1	35		0.5	0.6	8	0.4		Fe 10 mg
Albee® with C	tablet				300		15	10.2		5		Niacinamide 50 mg, pantothenic acid 10 mg
Vitamin B Complex	tablet					400 mcg	1.5	1.7		2	6	Niacinamide 20 mg
Hexavitamin	cap/tab	5000	400		75		2	3	20			
Iberet®-Folic - 500	tablet				500	0.8	6	6	30	5	25	B_5 10 mg, Fe 105 mg
Stuartnatal 1+1	tablet	4000	400	11	120	1	1.5	3	20	10	12	Cu, Zn 25 mg, Fe 65 mg, Ca 200 mg
Theragran® M	tablet	5000	400	30	90	0.4	3	3.4	30	3	9	Cl, Cr, I, K, B_5 10 mg, Mg, Mn, Mo, P, Se, Zn 15 mg, Fe 27 mg, biotin 30 mcg, beta-carotene 1250 IU
Vi-Daylin®	tablet	2500	400	15	60	0.3	1.05	1.2	13.5	1.05	4.5	
M.V.I.-12 injection	5 mL	3300	200	10	100	0.4	3	3.6	40	4	5	B_5 15 mg, biotin 60 mcg
M.V.I.-12 unit vial	20 mL											
M.V.I. pediatric powder	5 mL	2300	400	7	80	0.14	1.2	1.4	17	1	1	B_5 5 mg, biotin 20 mcg, vitamin K 200 mcg

(Continued)

I.V. solutions: 10 mL/24 hours (M.V.I.®-12)

Reference Range Recommended daily allowances are published by Food and Nutrition Board, National Research Council - National Academy of Sciences and are revised periodically. RDA quantities apply only to healthy persons and are not intended to cover therapeutic nutrition requirements in disease or other abnormal states (ie, metabolic disorders, weight reduction, chronic disease, drug therapy).

Patient Information Take only amount prescribed

Nursing Implications Doses may be higher for burn or cystic fibrosis patients

Dosage Forms See table.

Vita-Plus® E Softgels® [OTC] *see* Vitamin E *on page 1309*

Vitec® [OTC] *see* Vitamin E *on page 1309*

Vite E® Creme [OTC] *see* Vitamin E *on page 1309*

Vitrasert® *see* Ganciclovir *on page 566*

Vivactil® *see* Protriptyline *on page 1073*

Vivelle™ Transdermal *see* Estradiol *on page 468*

Vivotif Berna™ *see* Typhoid Vaccine *on page 1278*

V-Lax® [OTC] *see* Psyllium *on page 1075*

VLB *see* Vinblastine *on page 1300*

VM-26 *see* Teniposide *on page 1191*

Volmax® *see* Albuterol *on page 38*

Voltaren® *see* Diclofenac *on page 373*

Voltaren-XR® *see* Diclofenac *on page 373*

VōSol® *see* Acetic Acid *on page 24*

VP-16 *see* Etoposide *on page 496*

VP-16-213 *see* Etoposide *on page 496*

Vumon *see* Teniposide *on page 1191*

V.V.S.® *see* Sulfabenzamide, Sulfacetamide, and Sulfathiazole *on page 1171*

VZIG *see* Varicella-Zoster Immune Globulin (Human) *on page 1291*

Warfarin (WAR far in)

Brand Names Coumadin®

Canadian/Mexican Brand Names Warfilone® (Canada)

Synonyms Warfarin Sodium

Therapeutic Category Anticoagulant

Use Prophylaxis and treatment of venous thrombosis, pulmonary embolism and thromboembolic disorders; atrial fibrillation with risk of embolism and as an adjunct in the prophylaxis of systemic embolism after myocardial infarction

Unlabeled use: Prevention of recurrent transient ischemic attacks and to reduce risk of recurrent myocardial infarction

Pregnancy Risk Factor D

Pregnancy/Breast-Feeding Implications

Effects on the infant: Oral anticoagulants cross the placenta and produce fetal abnormalities. Warfarin should not be used during pregnancy because of significant risks. Adjusted-dose heparin can be given safely throughout pregnancy in patients with venous thromboembolism.

Breast-feeding/lactation: Warfarin does not pass into breast milk and can be given to nursing mothers

Contraindications Hypersensitivity to warfarin or any component; severe liver or kidney disease; open wounds; uncontrolled bleeding; GI ulcers; neurosurgical procedures; malignant hypertension, pregnancy

Warnings/Precautions

Do not switch brands once desired therapeutic response has been achieved

Use with caution in patients with active tuberculosis or diabetes

Concomitant use with vitamin K may decrease anticoagulant effect; monitor carefully

Concomitant use with NSAIDs or aspirin may cause severe GI irritation and also increase the risk of bleeding due to impaired platelet function

Salicylates may further increase warfarin's effect by displacing it from plasma protein binding sites

Patients with protein C or S deficiency are at increased risk of skin necrosis syndrome

Before committing an elderly patient to long-term anticoagulation therapy, their risk for bleeding complications secondary to falls, drug interactions, living situation, and cognitive status should be considered. The risk for bleeding complications decreases with the duration of therapy and may increase with advancing age.

If a patient is to undergo an invasive surgical procedure (dental to actual minor/major surgery), warfarin should be stopped 3 days before the scheduled surgery date and the INR/PT should be checked prior to the procedure

Adverse Reactions

1% to 10%:

Dermatologic: Skin lesions, alopecia, skin necrosis

Gastrointestinal: Anorexia, nausea, vomiting, stomach cramps, diarrhea

Hematologic: Hemorrhage, leukopenia, unrecognized bleeding sites (eg, colon cancer) may be uncovered by anticoagulation

Respiratory: Hemoptysis

<1%:

Central nervous system: Fever

Dermatologic: Rash

Gastrointestinal: Anorexia

Hematologic: Agranulocytosis

Hepatic: Hepatotoxicity

Renal: Renal damage

Miscellaneous: Mouth ulcers, discolored toes (blue or purple)

Overdosage/Toxicology See table.

INR	Patient Situation	Action
>3 and ≤6	No bleeding or need for rapid reversal (ie, no need for surgery)	Omit next few warfarin doses and restart at lower dose when INR ≤3.0
>6 and <10.0	No bleeding but in need of rapid reversal for surgery	Stop warfarin and give phytonadione 0.5-1 mg I.V.; repeat 0.5 mg phytonadione I.V. if INR >3 after 24 hours; restart warfarin at a lower dose
>10.0 and <20.0	No bleeding	Stop warfarin, give phytonadione 3-5 mg I.V.; check INR every 6-12 hours; repeat phytonadione if needed; reassess need and dose of warfarin
>20.0	Serious bleeding or warfarin overdose	Stop warfarin, give phytonadione 10 mg I.V.; check INR every 6 hours, if needed, repeat phytonadione every 12 hours and give plasma transfusion or factor concentrate; consider giving heparin if warfarin still indicated

Symptoms of overdose include internal or external hemorrhage, hematuria. Avoid emesis and lavage to avoid the possible trauma and incidental bleeding. When overdose occurs, the drug should be immediately discontinued and vitamin K_1 (phytonadione) may be administered 1-5 mg I.V. for children or up to 25 mg I.V. for adults. When hemorrhaging occurs, fresh frozen plasma transfusions can help control bleeding by replacing clotting factors. In urgent bleeding, prothrombin complex concentrates may be needed.

Drug Interactions Cytochrome P-450 2C enzyme substrate

Stability Protect from light; injection is stable for 4 hours at room temperature after reconstitution with 2.7 mL of sterile water

Mechanism of Action Interferes with hepatic synthesis of vitamin K-dependent coagulation factors (II, VII, IX, X)

Pharmacodynamics/Kinetics

Onset of anticoagulation effect: Oral: Within 36-72 hours

Peak effect: Within 5-7 days

Absorption: Oral: Rapid

Metabolism: In the liver

Half-life: 42 hours, highly variable among individuals
(Continued)

Warfarin *(Continued)*

Decreased Anticoagulant Effects

Induction of Enzymes		Increased Procoagulant Factors	Decreased Drug Absorption	Other
Barbiturates Carbamazepine Glutethimide Griseofulvin	Nafcillin Phenytoin Rifampin	Estrogens Oral contraceptives Vitamin K (including nutritional supplements)	Aluminum hydroxide Cholestyramine* Colestipol*	Ethchlorvynol Griseofulvin Spironolactone† Sucralfate

Decreased anticoagulant effect may occur when these drugs are administered with oral anticoagulants.

*Cholestyramine and colestipol may increase the anticoagulant effect by binding vitamin K in the gut; yet, the decreased drug absorption appears to be of more concern.

†Diuretic-induced hemoconcentration with subsequent concentration of clotting factors has been reported to decrease the effects of oral anticoagulants.

Enhanced Anticoagulant Effects

Decrease Vitamin K	Displace Anticoagulant	Inhibit Metabolism	Other
Oral antibiotics Can ↑ or ↓ an INR Check an INR 3 days after patient begins antibiotics to see the INR value and adjust the warfarin dose accordingly	Chloral hydrate Clofibrate Diazoxide Ethacrynic acid Miconazole Nalidixic acid Phenylbutazone Salicylates Sulfonamides Sulfonylureas Triclofos	Alcohol (acute ingestion)* Allopurinol Amiodarone Chloramphenicol Chlorpropamide Cimetidine Co-trimoxazole Disulfiram Metronidazole Phenylbutazone Phenytoin Propoxyphene Sulfinpyrazone Sulfonamides Tolbutamide	Acetaminophen Anabolic steroids Clofibrate Danazol Erythromycin Gemfibrozil Glucagon Influenza vaccine Ketoconazole Propranolol Ranitidine Sulindac Thyroid drugs

* The hypoprothrombinemic effect of oral anticoagulants has been reported to be both increased and decreased during chronic and excessive alcohol ingestion. Data are insufficient to predict the direction of this interaction in alcoholic patients.

Increased Bleeding Tendency

Inhibit Platelet Aggregation	Inhibit Procoagulant Factors	Ulcerogenic Drugs
Cephalosporins Dipyridamole Indomethacin Oxyphenbutazone Penicillin, parenteral Phenylbutazone Salicylates Sulfinpyrazone	Antimetabolites Quinidine Quinine Salicylates	Adrenal corticosteroids Indomethacin Oxyphenbutazone Phenylbutazone Potassium products Salicylates

Use of these agents with oral anticoagulants may increase the chances of hemorrhage.

Usual Dosage

Oral:

Infants and Children: 0.05-0.34 mg/kg/day; infants <12 months of age may require doses at or near the high end of this range; consistent anticoagulation may be difficult to maintain in children <5 years of age

Adults: 5-15 mg/day for 2-5 days, then adjust dose according to results of prothrombin time; usual maintenance dose ranges from 2-10 mg/day

I.V. (administer as a slow bolus injection): 2-5 mg/day

Dosing adjustment/comments in hepatic disease: Monitor effect at usual doses; the response to oral anticoagulants may be markedly enhanced in obstructive jaundice (due to reduced vitamin K absorption) and also in hepatitis and cirrhosis (due to decreased production of vitamin K-dependent clotting factors); prothrombin index should be closely monitored

Dietary Considerations

Alcohol: Chronic use of alcohol inhibits warfarin metabolism; avoid or limit use

Food:

Vitamin K: Foods high in vitamin K (eg, beef liver, pork liver, green tea and leafy green vegetables) inhibit anti-coagulant effect. Do not change dietary habits once stabilized on warfarin therapy; a balanced diet with a consistent intake of vitamin K is essential; avoid large amounts of alfalfa, asparagus, broccoli, Brussels sprouts, cabbage, cauliflower, green teas, kale, lettuce, spinach, turnip greens, watercress. It is recommended that the diet contain a CONSISTENT vitamin K content of 70-140 mcg/day. Check with physician before changing diet.

Vitamin E: May increase warfarin effect; do not change dietary habits or vitamin supplements once stabilized on warfarin therapy

Administration Administer as a slow bolus injection over 1-2 minutes; avoid all I.M. injections

Monitoring Parameters Prothrombin time, hematocrit, INR

Reference Range

Therapeutic: 2-5 µg/mL (SI: 6.5-16.2 µmol/L)

Prothrombin time should be $1\frac{1}{2}$ to 2 times the control or INR should be ↑ 2 to 3 times based upon indication

Normal prothrombin time: 10-13 seconds

Test Interactions Warfarin ↑ PTT

Patient Information Do not take with food; report any signs of bleeding; avoid hazardous activities; use soft toothbrush; urine may turn red/orange; carry Medi-Alert® ID identifying drug usage; be sure of other drugs and foods to avoid; report any bleeding to physician at once; notify physician if urine turns dark brown or if red or tar black stools occur

Dosage Forms

Powder for injection, as sodium, lyophilized: 2 mg, 5 mg

Tablet, as sodium: 1 mg, 2 mg, 2.5 mg, 4 mg, 5 mg, 7.5 mg, 10 mg

Warfarin Sodium *see* Warfarin *on page 1312*

Wart-Off® [OTC] *see* Salicylic Acid *on page 1120*

4-Way® Long Acting Nasal Solution [OTC] *see* Oxymetazoline *on page 940*

Wellbutrin® *see* Bupropion *on page 172*

Wellbutrin® SR *see* Bupropion *on page 172*

Wellcovorin® *see* Leucovorin *on page 708*

Westcort® *see* Hydrocortisone *on page 623*

Westrim® LA [OTC] *see* Phenylpropanolamine *on page 991*

White Mineral Oil *see* Mineral Oil *on page 841*

Wigraine® *see* Ergotamine *on page 459*

40 Winks® [OTC] *see* Diphenhydramine *on page 399*

WinRho SD® *see* Rh_o(D) Immune Globulin (Intravenous-Human) *on page 1102*

Winstrol® *see* Stanozolol *on page 1158*

Wycillin® *see* Penicillin G Procaine *on page 964*

Wydase® *see* Hyaluronidase *on page 614*

Wygesic® *see* Propoxyphene and Acetaminophen *on page 1067*

Wymox® *see* Amoxicillin *on page 77*

Wytensin® *see* Guanabenz *on page 592*

Xalatan® *see* Latanoprost *on page 707*

Xanax® *see* Alprazolam *on page 49*

Xylocaine® *see* Lidocaine *on page 723*

Xylocaine® With Epinephrine *see* Lidocaine and Epinephrine *on page 725*

Xylometazoline (zye loe met AZ oh leen)

Brand Names Otrivin® [OTC]

Synonyms Xylometazoline Hydrochloride

Therapeutic Category Adrenergic Agonist Agent; Decongestant, Nasal; Nasal Agent, Vasoconstrictor; Sympathomimetic

Use Symptomatic relief of nasal and nasopharyngeal mucosal congestion

Pregnancy Risk Factor C

Contraindications Known hypersensitivity to xylometazoline hydrochloride, narrow-angle glaucoma, patients receiving MAO inhibitors

Warnings/Precautions Do not use in children <2 years of age; excessive use may cause rebound congestion or chemical rhinitis; use with caution in patients with hypertension, diabetes, cardiovascular or coronary artery disease

Adverse Reactions

1% to 10%:

Cardiovascular: Palpitations

Central nervous system: Drowsiness, dizziness, seizures, headache

Ocular: Blurred vision, ocular irritation, photophobia

Miscellaneous: Diaphoresis

Overdosage/Toxicology Symptoms of overdose include CNS depression, hypothermia, bradycardia, cardiovascular collapse, coma, respiratory depression, apnea; following initiation of essential overdose management, toxic symptoms should be treated

(Continued)

Xylometazoline *(Continued)*

The patient should be kept warm and monitored for alterations in vital functions. Seizures commonly respond to diazepam (5-10 mg I.V. bolus in adults every 15 minutes if needed up to a total of 30 mg; I.V. 0.25-0.4 mg/kg/dose up to a total of 1 mg for children) or to phenytoin or phenobarbital. Apnea may respond to naloxone.

Mechanism of Action Stimulates alpha-adrenergic receptors in the arterioles of the conjunctiva and the nasal mucosa to produce vasoconstriction

Pharmacodynamics/Kinetics

Onset of action: Intranasal: Local vasoconstriction occurs within 5-10 minutes

Duration: 5-6 hours

Usual Dosage

Children 2-12 years: Instill 2-3 drops (0.05%) in each nostril every 8-10 hours

Children >12 years and Adults: Instill 2-3 drops or sprays (0.1%) in each nostril every 8-10 hours

Patient Information Do not exceed recommended dosage; do not use for more than 4 consecutive days

Dosage Forms Solution, nasal, as hydrochloride: 0.05% [0.5 mg/mL] (20 mL); 0.1% [1 mg/mL] (15 mL, 20 mL)

Xylometazoline Hydrochloride *see* Xylometazoline *on previous page*

Yeast-Gard® Medicated Douche *see* Povidone-Iodine *on page 1031*

Yellow Fever Vaccine (YEL oh FEE ver vak SEEN)

Related Information

Immunization Guidelines *on page 1421*

Recommendations for Travelers *on page 1442*

Brand Names YF-VAX®

Therapeutic Category Vaccine, Live Virus

Use Selected persons traveling or living in areas where yellow fever infection exists. Some countries require a valid international Certification of Vaccination showing receipt of vaccine; if a pregnant woman is to be vaccinated only to satisfy an international requirement, efforts should be made to obtain a waiver letter.

Pregnancy Risk Factor D

Contraindications Sensitivity to egg or chick embryo protein; pregnant women, children <6 months of age unless in high risk area

Adverse Reactions

>10%: Central nervous system: Fever, malaise

1% to 10%:

- Central nervous system: Headache
- Neuromuscular & skeletal: Myalgia

<1%:

- Central nervous system: Encephalitis in very young infants (rare)
- Miscellaneous: Anaphylaxis

Drug Interactions Administer yellow fever vaccine at least 1 month apart from other live virus vaccines; defer vaccination for 3 weeks following blood, plasma, or immune globulin

Stability Yellow fever vaccine is shipped with dry ice; do not use vaccine unless shipping case contains some dry ice on arrival; maintain vaccine continuously at a temperature between 0°C to 5°C (32°F to 41°F)

Usual Dosage One dose S.C. 10 days to 10 years before travel, booster every 10 years

Patient Information Immunity develops by the tenth day and **WHO** requires revaccination every 10 years to maintain travelers' vaccination certificates

Nursing Implications Sterilize and discard all unused rehydrated vaccine and containers after 1 hour; avoid vigorous shaking

Additional Information Federal law requires that the date of administration, the vaccine manufacturer, lot number of vaccine, and the administering person's name, title and address be entered into the patient's permanent medical record

Dosage Forms Injection: Not less than 5.04 Log_{10} Plaque Forming Units (PFU) per 0.5 mL

YF-VAX® *see* Yellow Fever Vaccine *on this page*

Yodoxin® *see* Iodoquinol *on page 670*

Yutopar® *see* Ritodrine *on page 1112*

Zafirlukast (za FIR loo kast)

Related Information

Asthma, Guidelines for the Diagnosis and Management of *on page 1518*

Brand Names Accolate®

Therapeutic Category Leukotriene Receptor Antagonist

Use Prophylaxis and chronic treatment of asthma in adults and children ≥12 years of age

Pregnancy Risk Factor B

Pregnancy/Breast-Feeding Implications At 2,000 mg/kg/day in rats, maternal toxicity and deaths were seen with increased incidence of early fetal resorption. Spontaneous abortions occurred in cynomolgus monkeys at a maternally toxic dose of 2,000 mg/kg/day orally. there are no adequate and well controlled trials in pregnant women. Zafirlukast is excreted in breast milk; do not administer to nursing women

Contraindications Hypersensitivity to zafirlukast or any of its inactive ingredients

Warnings/Precautions The clearance of zafirlukast is reduced in patients with stable alcoholic cirrhosis such that the Cmax and AUC are approximately 50% to 60% greater than those of normal adults.

Zafirlukast is not indicated for use in the reversal of bronchospasm in acute asthma attacks, including status asthmaticus. Therapy with zafirlukast can be continued during acute exacerbations of asthma.

An increased proportion of zafirlukast patients >55 years old reported infections as compared to placebo-treated patients. these infections were mostly mild or moderate in intensity and predominantly affected the respiratory tract. Infections occurred equally in both sexes, were dose-proportional to total milligrams of zafirlukast exposure and were associated with coadministration of inhaled corticosteroids.

Although the frequency of hepatic transaminase elevations was comparable between zafirlukast and placebo-treated patients, a single case of symptomatic hepatitis and hyperbilirubinemia, without other attributable cause, occurred in patient who had received 40 mg/day of zafirlukast for 100 days. In this patient, the liver enzymes returned to normal within 3 months of stopping zafirlukast.

Adverse Reactions

>10%: Central nervous system: Headache (12.9%)

1% to 10%:

- Central nervous system: Dizziness, pain, fever
- Gastrointestinal: Nausea, diarrhea, abdominal pain, vomiting, dyspepsia
- Neuromuscular & skeletal: Myalgia, weakness

Overdosage/Toxicology Symptoms of overdose: There is no experience to date with zafirlukast overdose in humans; use supportive treatment measures

Drug Interactions Cytochrome P-450 2C9 and 3A4 isoenzyme inhibitor

Decreased effect:

- Erythromycin: Coadministration of a single dose of zafirlukast with erythromycin to steady state results in decreased mean plasma levels of zafirlukast by 40% due to a decrease in zafirlukast bioavailability.
- Terfenadine: Coadministration of zafirlukast with terfenadine to steady state results in a decrease in the mean Cmax (66%) and AUC (54%) of zafirlukast. No effect of zafirlukast on terfenadine plasma concentrations or ECG parameters was seen.
- Theophylline: Coadministration of zafirlukast at steady state with a single dose of liquid theophylline preparations results in decreased mean plasma levels of zafirlukast by 30%, but no effects on plasma theophylline levels were observed.

Increased effect: Aspirin: Coadministration of zafirlukast with aspirin results in mean increased plasma levels of zafirlukast by 45%

Increased toxicity: Warfarin: Coadministration of zafirlukast with warfarin results in a clinically significant increase in prothrombin time (PT). Closely monitor prothrombin times of patients on oral warfarin anticoagulant therapy and zafirlukast, and adjust anticoagulant dose accordingly.

Stability Store tablets at controlled room temperature (20°C to 25°C; 68°F to 77°F); protect from light and moisture; dispense in original airtight container

Mechanism of Action Zafirlukast is a selectively and competitive leukotriene-receptor antagonist (LTRA) of leukotriene D4 and E4 (LTD4 and LTE4), components of slow-reacting substance of anaphylaxis (SRSA). Cysteinyl leukotriene production and receptor occupation have been correlated with the pathophysiology of asthma, including airway edema, smooth muscle constriction and altered cellular activity associated with the inflammatory process, which contribute to the signs and symptoms of asthma.

Pharmacodynamics/Kinetics

Absorption: Food reduces bioavailability by 40%

Protein binding: >99%, predominantly albumin

Metabolism: extensively metabolized by liver via cytochrome P-450 2C9 enzyme pathway.

Half-life: 10 hours

Time to peak serum concentration: 3 hours

Elimination: Urinary excretion (10%) and feces

(Continued)

Zafirlukast *(Continued)*

Usual Dosage Oral:

Children <12 years: Safety and effectiveness has not been established

Adults: 20 mg twice daily

Elderly: The mean dose (mg/kg) normalized AUC and Cmax increase and plasma clearance decreases with increasing age. In patients >65 years of age, there is an 2-3 fold greater Cmax and AUC compared to younger adults.

Dosing adjustment in renal impairment: There are no apparent differences in the pharmacokinetics between renally impaired patients and normal subjects.

Dosing adjustment in hepatic impairment: In patients with hepatic impairment (ie, biopsy-proven cirrhosis), there is a 50% to 60% greater Cmax and AUC compared to normal subjects.

Administration Take at least 1 hour before or 2 hours after a meal

Patient Information Take regularly as prescribed, even during symptom-free periods. Do not use to treat acute episodes of asthma. Do not decrease the dose or stop taking any other antiasthma medications unless instructed by a physician. Nursing women should not take zafirlukast.

Dosage Forms Tablet: 20 mg

Zagam® *see* Sparfloxacin *on page 1154*

Zalcitabine (zal SITE a been)

Brand Names Hivid®

Synonyms ddC; Dideoxycytidine

Therapeutic Category Antiretroviral Agent; Antiviral Agent, Oral; Reverse Transcriptase Inhibitor

Use Treatment as monotherapy in HIV-infected adults with advanced disease who cannot tolerate zidovudine or whose disease has progressed despite it; for the treatment of selected patients with advanced AIDS in combination with zidovudine; due to possible toxicity or resistance combination with didanosine or stavudine should be avoided

Pregnancy Risk Factor C

Pregnancy/Breast-Feeding Implications

Administer during pregnancy only if benefits to mother outweigh risks to the fetus

HIV-infected mothers are discouraged from breast-feeding to decrease potential transmission of HIV

Contraindications Hypersensitivity to the drug or any component of the product

Warnings/Precautions Approved for monotherapy or use in combination with zidovudine; careful monitoring of pancreatic enzymes and liver function tests in patients with a history of pancreatitis, increased amylase, those on parenteral nutrition or with a history of ethanol abuse; discontinue use immediately if pancreatitis is suspected; lactic acidosis and severe hepatomegaly and failure have rarely occurred with zalcitabine resulting in fatality; use with caution in patients on digitalis, congestive heart failure, renal failure, hyperphosphatemia; zalcitabine can cause severe peripheral neuropathy; avoid use, if possible, in patients with pre-existing neuropathy

Adverse Reactions

>10%: Gastrointestinal: Oral ulcers

1% to 10%:

- Cardiovascular: Chest pain
- Central nervous system: Headache, dizziness, myalgia, foot pain, fatigue
- Hematologic: Anemia (occurs as early as 2-4 weeks), granulocytopenia (usually after 6-8 weeks)
- Dermatologic: Rash, pruritus
- Gastrointestinal: Nausea, dysphagia, anorexia, abdominal pain, vomiting, diarrhea, weight loss
- Respiratory: Pharyngitis

<1%:

- Cardiovascular: Edema, hypertension, palpitations, syncope, atrial fibrillation, tachycardia, heart racing
- Central nervous system: Night sweats, fever, pain, malaise
- Endocrine & metabolic: Hyperglycemia, hypocalcemia
- Gastrointestinal: Constipation, pancreatitis (see Warnings)
- Hepatic: Jaundice, hepatitis, hepatomegaly, hepatic failure (see Warnings)
- Neuromuscular & skeletal: Myositis, peripheral neuropathy (see Warnings), weakness
- Respiratory: Epistaxis

Overdosage/Toxicology Symptoms of overdose include delayed peripheral neurotoxicity; following oral decontamination, treatment is supportive

Drug Interactions Increased toxicity:

Amphotericin, foscarnet, and aminoglycosides may potentiate the risk of developing peripheral neuropathy or other toxicities associated with zalcitabine by interfering with the renal elimination of zalcitabine

Other drugs associated with peripheral neuropathy include chloramphenicol, cisplatin, dapsone, disulfiram, ethionamide, glutethimide, gold, hydralazine, iodoquinol, isoniazid, metronidazole, nitrofurantoin, phenytoin, ribavirin, and vincristine

Concomitant use of zalcitabine with didanosine is not recommended

Stability Tablets should be stored in tightly closed bottles at 59°F to 86°F

Mechanism of Action Purine nucleoside analogue, zalcitabine or 2′,3′-dideoxycitidine (ddC) has been found to have *in vitro* activity and is reported to be successful against HIV in short-term clinical trials. Intracellularly, ddc is converted to active metabolite ddCTP; lack the presence of the 3′-hydroxyl group necessary for phosphodiester linkages during DNA replication. As a result viral replication is prematurely terminated. ddCTP acts as a competitor for binding sites on the HIV-RNA dependent DNA polymerase (reverse transcriptase) to further contribute to inhibition of viral replication.

Pharmacodynamics/Kinetics

Absorption: Food decreases absorption by 39%

Distribution: CSF levels are 20% of serum levels

Protein binding: Minimal, 1% to 2%

Metabolism: Intracellularly to active triphosphorylated agent; no significant hepatic metabolism

Bioavailability: >80%

Half-life: 2.9 hours

Elimination: Renal, >70% unchanged

Usual Dosage Safety and efficacy in children <13 years of age have not been established

Adults: Monotherapy:

≥60 kg: 0.75 mg every 8 hours (2.25 mg total daily dose)

<60 kg: 0.375 mg every 8 hours

Combination therapy: 0.75 mg every 8 hours, given together with 200 mg of zidovudine (ie, total daily dose: 2.25 mg of zalcitabine and 600 mg of zidovudine); if zalcitabine is permanently discontinued or interrupted due to toxicities, decrease zidovudine dose to 100 mg every 4 hours

Dosing adjustment in renal impairment: Since renal excretion appears to be the major route of elimination, zalcitabine's elimination may be prolonged in patients with poor renal function

Cl_{cr} 10-40 mL/minute: Daily dose may be adjusted to 0.75 mg every 12 hours

Cl_{cr} <10 mL/minute: Further reduce dose to 0.75 mg every 24 hours

Hemodialysis: Hemodialysis reduces plasma levels by 50%

Dosing in hepatic impairment: Zalcitabine could possibly exacerbate existing liver dysfunction in patients with a previous history of liver disease or alcohol abuse. An increase in liver function tests was observed in patients on zalcitabine therapy; caution should be exercised in patients with hepatic impairment.

Dosing adjustment in peripheral neuropathy: Zalcitabine should be discontinued in patients developing peripheral neuropathy; the drug may be reinitiated at 50% of the dose every 8 hours only if all findings related to the neuropathy improve to the point of classification as mild symptomatology; therapy must be permanently discontinued if severe symptoms occur; Note: zalcitabine-associated peripheral neuropathy may continue to worsen despite interruption of therapy

If other moderate to severe adverse effects occur such as increased LFTs, therapy with zalcitabine or both zalcitabine and zidovudine, if in combination therapy, should be discontinued until the reaction resolves; treatment may be reinitiated at lower doses; if the reaction recurs, discontinue therapy completely.

Dosing adjustment in hematologic toxicities: Zalcitabine may need to be discontinued in patients with poor bone marrow reserve if significant anemia (Hg = 7.5/dL or a reduction >25% from baseline) or granulocytopenia (granulocyte count <750/mm^3 or a reduction >50% from baseline) occur; therapy should not be reinitiated until evidence of marrow recovery is obvious. For less severe blood dyscrasias, a reduction in the zidovudine dose may be adequate; dose modification in patients who develop significant anemia, may not eliminate the need for transfusion; if recovery of the marrow does occur, however, gradual increases in dose may be tolerated

Monitoring Parameters Renal function, CD4 counts, CBC, serum amylase, triglyceride, calcium (see Zidovudine monograph)

Patient Information Zalcitabine is not a cure; if numbness or tingling occurs, or if persistent, severe abdominal pain, nausea, or vomiting occur, notify physician. Women of childbearing age should use effective contraception while on zalcitabine; take on an empty stomach, if possible.

Dosage Forms Tablet: 0.375 mg, 0.75 mg

Zanaflex® *see* Tizanidine *on page 1232*
Zanosar® *see* Streptozocin *on page 1163*
Zantac® *see* Ranitidine Hydrochloride *on page 1095*
Zantac® 75 [OTC] *see* Ranitidine Hydrochloride *on page 1095*
Zantryl® *see* Phentermine *on page 987*
Zarontin® *see* Ethosuximide *on page 491*
Zaroxolyn® *see* Metolazone *on page 826*
Zeasorb-AF® Powder [OTC] *see* Miconazole *on page 834*
Zeasorb-AF® Powder [OTC] *see* Tolnaftate *on page 1243*
Zebeta® *see* Bisoprolol *on page 156*
Zefazone® *see* Cefmetazole *on page 223*
Zemuron® *see* Rocuronium *on page 1115*
Zerit® *see* Stavudine *on page 1158*
Zestril® *see* Lisinopril *on page 733*

Zidovudine (zye DOE vyoo deen)

Related Information
Occupational Exposure to HIV *on page 1448*

Brand Names Retrovir®

Canadian/Mexican Brand Names Apo-Zidovudine® (Canada); Novo-AZT® (Canada); Dipedyne® (Mexico); Kenamil® (Mexico); Retrovir-AZT® (Mexico)

Synonyms Azidothymidine; AZT; Compound S

Therapeutic Category Antiretroviral Agent; Antiviral Agent, Oral; Antiviral Agent, Parenteral; Reverse Transcriptase Inhibitor

Use Management of patients with HIV infections who have had at least one episode of *Pneumocystis carinii* pneumonia or who have CD4 cell counts ≤500/mm^3; patients who have HIV-related symptoms or who are asymptomatic with abnormal laboratory values indicating HIV-related immunosuppression; for prevention of maternal/fetal HIV transmission in a subpopulation of HIV-infected women and their offspring (recommended for HIV-infected women with CD4+ cell counts >200/mm^3), no prior history of extensive zidovudine administration, no clinical indication for antiretroviral therapy and whose pregnancy is between 14 and 34 weeks' gestation when therapy is initiated; often used in combination therapy with other nucleosides such as zalcitabine didanosine or lamivudine (a protease inhibitor can also be added for "triple therapy"); indicated for prevention of HIV infection after needle sticks

Pregnancy Risk Factor C

Pregnancy/Breast-Feeding Implications Administer during pregnancy only if benefits to mother outweigh risks to the fetus. HIV-infected mothers are discouraged from breast-feeding to decrease potential transmission of HIV.

Contraindications Life-threatening hypersensitivity to zidovudine or any component

Warnings/Precautions Use with caution in patients with impaired renal or hepatic function; reduce dosage or interrupt therapy in patients with anemia and/or granulocytopenia and myopathy; often associated with hematologic toxicity including granulocytopenia, thrombocytopenia, and severe anemia requiring transfusions; zidovudine has been shown to be carcinogenic in rats and mice

Adverse Reactions

>10%:
- Central nervous system: Severe headache, insomnia
- Gastrointestinal: Nausea
- Hematologic: Anemia, leukopenia, neutropenia

1% to 10%:
- Dermatologic: Rash, hyperpigmentation of nails (bluish-brown)
- Hematologic: Changes in platelet count

<1%:
- Central nervous system: Neurotoxicity, confusion, mania, seizures
- Gastrointestinal: Anorexia
- Hematologic: Bone marrow suppression, granulocytopenia, thrombocytopenia, pancytopenia
- Hepatic: Hepatotoxicity, cholestatic jaundice
- Local: Tenderness
- Neuromuscular & skeletal: Myopathy, weakness

Overdosage/Toxicology Symptoms of overdose include nausea, vomiting, ataxia, granulocytopenia

Erythropoietin, thymidine, and cyanocobalamin have been used experimentally to treat zidovudine-induced hematopoietic toxicity, yet none are presently specified as the agent of choice. Treatment is supportive.

Drug Interactions

Increased toxicity: Coadministration with drugs that are nephrotoxic (amphotericin B), cytotoxic (flucytosine, vincristine, vinblastine, doxorubicin, interferon), inhibit glucuronidation or excretion (acetaminophen, cimetidine, indomethacin, lorazepam, probenecid, aspirin), or interfere with RBC/WBC number or function (acyclovir, ganciclovir, pentamidine, dapsone); although the AUC was unaffected, the rate of absorption and peak plasma concentrations were increased significantly when zidovudine was administered with clarithromycin (n=18); valproic acid increased AZT's AUC by 80% and decreased clearance by 38% (believed due to inhibition first pass metabolism)

Decreased toxicity: Administration with a fatty meal decreased zidovudine's AUC and peak plasma concentration

Stability After dilution to ≤4 mg/mL, the solution is physically and chemically stable for 24 hours at room temperature and 48 hours if refrigerated; attempt to administer diluted solution within 8 hours, if stored at room temperature or 24 hours if refrigerated to minimize potential for microbially contaminated solutions; store undiluted vials at room temperature and protect from light

Mechanism of Action Zidovudine is a thymidine analog which interferes with the HIV viral RNA dependent DNA polymerase resulting in inhibition of viral replication

Pharmacodynamics/Kinetics

Absorption: Oral: Well absorbed (66% to 70%)

Distribution: Significant penetration into the CSF; crosses the placenta

Relative diffusion of antimicrobial agents from blood into cerebrospinal fluid (CSF): Adequate with or without inflammation (exceeds usual MICs)

Ratio of CSF to blood level (%): Normal meninges: ~60

Protein binding: 25% to 38%

Metabolism: Extensive first-pass metabolism; metabolized in the liver via glucuronidation to inactive metabolites

Half-life: Terminal: 60 minutes

Time to peak serum concentration: Within 30-90 minutes

Elimination: Urinary excretion (63% to 95%); following oral administration, 72% to 74% of the drug is excreted in the urine as metabolites and 14% to 18% as unchanged drug

Usual Dosage

Prevention of maternal-fetal HIV transmission:

Neonatal: Oral: 2 mg/kg/dose every 6 hours for 6 weeks beginning 8-12 hours after birth; infants unable to receive oral dosing may receive 1.5 mg/kg I.V. infused over 30 minutes every 6 hours

Maternal (>14 weeks gestation): Oral: 100 mg 5 times/day until the start of labor; during labor and delivery, administer zidovudine I.V. at 2 mg/kg over 1 hour followed by a continuous I.V. infusion of 1 mg/kg/hour until the umbilical cord is clamped

Asymptomatic/symptomatic HIV infection:

Children 3 months to 12 years:

Oral: 90-180 mg/m^2/dose every 6 hours; maximum: 200 mg every 6 hours

I.V.: 1-2 mg/kg/dose (infused over 1 hour) administered every 4 hours around-the-clock (6 doses/day)

Adults:

Asymptomatic HIV infection: Oral: 100 mg every 4 hours while awake (500 mg/day)

Symptomatic HIV infection:

Oral: Initial: 200 mg every 4 hours (1200 mg/day), then after 1 month, 100 mg every 4 hours (600 mg/day)

I.V.: 1-2 mg/kg/dose (infused over 1 hour) administered every 4 hours around-the-clock (6 doses/day)

Prevention of HIV following needle sticks: 200 mg 3 times/day plus lamivudine 150 mg twice daily; a protease inhibitor (eg, indinavir) may be added for high risk exposures; begin therapy within 2 hours of exposure if possible

Patients should receive I.V. therapy only until oral therapy can be administered

Combination therapy with zalcitabine: Oral: 200 mg with zalcitabine 0.75 mg every 8 hours

Dosing interval in renal impairment: Cl_{cr} <10 mL/minute: Administer 100 mg every 4 hours

Hemodialysis: At least partially removed by hemo- and peritoneal dialysis; administer dose after hemodialysis or administer 100 mg supplemental dose; during CAPD, dose as for Cl_{cr} <10 mL/minute; during continuous arterio-venous or veno-venous hemofiltration (CAVH/CAVHD), administer 100 mg every 4 hours

Dosing adjustment in hepatic impairment: Reduce dose by 50% or double dosing interval in patients with cirrhosis

Dosage adjustment in anemia/granulocytopenia:

Significant anemia (hemoglobin <7.5 g/dL or reduction >25% of baseline) or significant granulocytopenia (granulocyte count <750/mm^3 or reduction >50%

(Continued)

Zidovudine *(Continued)*

from baseline) may require a dose interruption until evidence of marrow recovery is observed

For less severe anemia or granulocytopenia, dose reduction may be adequate

See also Zalcitabine monograph regarding dosage adjustment in combination therapy

Administration Administer around-the-clock to promote less variation in peak and trough serum levels

Monitoring Parameters Monitor CBC and platelet count at least every 2 weeks, MCV, serum creatinine kinase, CD4 cell count; observe for appearance of opportunistic infections

Patient Information Take 30 minutes before or 1 hour after a meal with a glass of water; take zidovudine exactly as prescribed; take around-the-clock; limit acetaminophen-containing analgesics; report all side effects to you physician; zidovudine therapy has not been shown to reduce the risk of transmission of HIV to others nor will is cure HIV infections; opportunistic infections and other illnesses may still occur; maternal/fetal transmission may appear in some cases despite therapy; transfusion, dose modifications and even drug discontinuation may be needed if blood disorders such as anemia occur.

Dosage Forms

Capsule: 100 mg
Injection: 10 mg/mL (20 mL)
Syrup (strawberry flavor): 50 mg/5 mL (240 mL)
Tablet: 300 mg

Zilactin-L® [OTC] *see* Lidocaine *on page 723*

ZilaDent® [OTC] *see* Benzocaine *on page 138*

Zileuton (zye LOO ton)

Related Information

Asthma, Guidelines for the Diagnosis and Management of *on page 1518*

Brand Names Zyflo®

Therapeutic Category Leukotriene Receptor Antagonist

Use Prophylaxis and chronic treatment of asthma in adults and children ≥ 12 years of age

Pregnancy Risk Factor C

Pregnancy/Breast-Feeding Implications Developmental studies indicated adverse effects (reduced body weight and increased skeletal variations) in rats at an oral dose of 300 mg/kg/day. There are no adequate and well controlled studies in pregnant women. Zileuton and its metabolites are excreted in rat milk; it is not known if zileuton is excreted in breast milk.

Contraindications Active liver disease or transaminase elevations greater than or equal to three times the upper limit of normal (≥3 x ULN), hypersensitivity to zileuton or any of its active ingredients

Warnings/Precautions Elevations of one or more liver function tests may occur during therapy. These laboratory abnormalities may progress, remain unchanged or resolve with continued therapy. Use with caution in patients who consume substantial quantities of alcohol or have a past history of liver disease. Zileuton is not indicated for use in the reversal of bronchospasm in acute asthma attacks, including status asthmaticus. Zileuton can be continued during acute exacerbations of asthma.

Adverse Reactions

>10%:

Central nervous system: Headache (24.6%)
Hepatic: ALT elevation (12%)

1% to 10%:

Cardiovascular: Chest pain
Central nervous system: Pain, dizziness, fever, insomnia, malaise, nervousness, somnolence
Gastrointestinal: Dyspepsia, nausea, abdominal pain, constipation, flatulence
Hematologic: Low white blood cell count
Neuromuscular & skeletal: Myalgia, arthralgia, weakness
Ocular: Conjunctivitis

Overdosage/Toxicology Symptoms of overdose: Human experience is limited. Oral minimum lethal doses in mice and rats were 500-1000 and 300-1000 mg/kg, respectively (providing >3 and 9 times the systemic exposure achieved at the maximum recommended human daily oral dose, respectively). No deaths occurred, but nephritis was reported in dogs at an oral dose of 1,000 mg/kg.

Treat symptomatically; institute supportive measures as required. If indicated, achieve elimination of unabsorbed drug by emesis or gastric lavage; observe usual precautions to maintain the airway. Zileuton is NOT removed by dialysis.

Drug Interactions Cytochrome P-450 1A2, 2C9 and 3A4 enzyme substrate

Increased toxicity:

Propranolol: Doubling of propranolol AUC and consequent increased beta-blocker activity

Terfenadine: Decrease in clearance of terfenadine leading to increase in AUC

Theophylline: Doubling of serum theophylline concentrations - reduce theophylline dose and monitor serum theophylline concentrations closely.

Warfarin: Clinically significant increases in prothrombin time (PT) - monitor PT closely

Mechanism of Action Specific inhibitor of 5-lipoxygenase and thus inhibits leukotriene (LTB1, LTC1, LTD1 and LTE1) formation. Leukotrienes are substances that induce numerous biological effects including augmentation of neutrophil and eosinophil migration, neutrophil and monocyte aggregation, leukocyte adhesion, increased capillary permeability and smooth muscle contraction.

Pharmacodynamics/Kinetics

Absorption: Oral: Rapidly absorbed

Distribution: 1.2 L/kg

Protein binding: 93%

Metabolism: Several metabolites in plasma and urine; metabolized by the cytochrome P-450 isoenzymes 1A2, 2C9 and 3A4

Bioavailability: Absolute bioavailability is unknown

Half-life: 2.5 hours

Time to peak serum concentration: 1.7 hours

Elimination: Predominantly via metabolism

Dialyzable: Not removed (>0.5%)

Usual Dosage Oral:

Adults: 600 mg 4 times/day with meals and at bedtime

Elderly: Zileuton pharmacokinetics were similar in healthy elderly subjects (>65 years) compared with healthy younger adults (18-40 years)

Dosing adjustment in renal impairment: Dosing adjustment is not necessary in renal impairment or renal failure (even during dialysis)

Dosing adjustment in hepatic impairment: Contraindicated in patients with active liver disease

Administration Can be administered without regard to meals (ie, with or without food)

Monitoring Parameters Evaluate hepatic transaminases at initiation of and during therapy with zileuton. Monitor serum ALT before treatment begins, one-a-month for the first 3 months, every 2-3 months for the remainder of the first year and periodically thereafter for patients receiving long-term zileuton therapy. If symptoms of liver dysfunction (right upper quadrant pain, nausea, fatigue, lethargy, pruritus, jaundice or "flu-like" symptoms) develop or transaminase elevations >5 times the ULN occur, discontinue therapy and follow transaminase levels until normal.

Patient Information Inform patients that zileuton is indicated for the chronic treatment of asthma and to take regularly as prescribed even during symptom-free periods. Zileuton is not a bronchodilator; do not use to treat acute episodes of asthma. When taking zileuton, do not decrease the dose or stop taking any other antiasthma medications unless instructed by a physician.

While using zileuton, seek medical attention if short-acting bronchodilators are needed more often than usual or if more than the maximum number of inhalations of short-acting bronchodilator treatment prescribed for a 24-period are needed.

The most serious side effect of zileuton is elevation of liver enzyme tests. While taking zileuton, patients must have liver enzyme tests monitored on a regular basis. If patients experience signs or symptoms of liver dysfunction (right upper quadrant pain, nausea, fatigue, lethargy, pruritus, jaundice, or "flu-like" symptoms), contact a physician immediately.

Zileuton can interact with other drugs. While taking zileuton, consult a physician before starting or stopping any prescription or nonprescription medicines.

Dosage Forms Tablet: 600 mg

Zinacef® *see* Cefuroxime *on page 238*

Zinca-Pak® *see* Zinc Supplements *on next page*

Zincate® *see* Zinc Supplements *on next page*

Zinc Chloride *see* Zinc Supplements *on next page*

Zinc Gelatin (zingk JEL ah tin)

Brand Names Gelucast®

Synonyms Dome Paste Bandage; Unna's Boot; Unna's Paste; Zinc Gelatin Boot

Therapeutic Category Topical Skin Product

Use As a protectant and to support varicosities and similar lesions of the lower limbs

(Continued)

Zinc Gelatin *(Continued)*

Contraindications Hypersensitivity to any component

Adverse Reactions 1% to 10%: Local: Irritation

Usual Dosage Apply externally as an occlusive boot

Nursing Implications After a period of about 2 weeks, the dressing is removed by soaking in warm water

Dosage Forms Bandage: 3" x 10 yards, 4" x 10 yards

Zinc Gelatin Boot *see* Zinc Gelatin *on previous page*

Zinc Gluconate *see* Zinc Supplements *on this page*

Zinc Oxide (zingk OKS ide)

Synonyms Base Ointment; Lassar's Zinc Paste

Therapeutic Category Topical Skin Product

Use Protective coating for mild skin irritations and abrasions, soothing and protective ointment to promote healing of chapped skin, diaper rash

Contraindications Hypersensitivity to any component

Warnings/Precautions Do not use in eyes; for external use only

Adverse Reactions 1% to 10%: Local: Skin sensitivity, irritation

Stability Avoid prolonged storage at temperatures >30°C

Mechanism of Action Mild astringent with weak antiseptic properties

Usual Dosage Infants, Children, and Adults: Topical: Apply as required for affected areas several times daily

Patient Information If irritation develops, discontinue use and consult a physician; paste is easily removed with mineral oil; for external use only; do not use in the eyes

Dosage Forms

Ointment, topical: 20% in white ointment (480 g)
Paste, topical: 25% in white petrolatum (480 g)

Zinc Oxide, Cod Liver Oil, and Talc

(zingk OKS ide, kod LIV er oyl, & talk)

Brand Names Desitin® [OTC]

Therapeutic Category Topical Skin Product

Use Relief of diaper rash, superficial wounds and burns, and other minor skin irritations

Contraindications Hypersensitivity to any component

Adverse Reactions 1% to 10%: Local: Skin sensitivity, irritation

Usual Dosage Topical: Apply thin layer as needed

Patient Information If condition persists, or if rash, irritation or sensitivity develops, discontinue and contact physician; for external use only

Dosage Forms Ointment, topical: Zinc oxide, cod liver oil and talc in a petrolatum and lanolin base (30 g, 60 g, 120 g, 240 g, 270 g)

Zinc Sulfate *see* Zinc Supplements *on this page*

Zinc Supplements (zink SUP la ments)

Brand Names Eye-Sed® [OTC]; Orazinc® [OTC]; Verazinc® [OTC]; Zinca-Pak®; Zincate®

Synonyms Zinc Chloride; Zinc Gluconate; Zinc Sulfate

Therapeutic Category Mineral, Oral; Mineral, Parenteral; Trace Elements

Use Cofactor for replacement therapy to different enzymes helps maintain normal growth rates, normal skin hydration and senses of taste and smell; zinc supplement (oral and parenteral); may improve wound healing in those who are deficient. May be useful to promote wound healing in patients with pressure sores.

Pregnancy Risk Factor C

Contraindications Hypersensitivity to any component

Warnings/Precautions Do not take undiluted by direct injection into a peripheral vein because of potential for phlebitis, tissue irritation, and potential to increase renal loss of minerals from a bolus injection; administration of zinc in absence of copper may decrease plasma levels; excessive dose may increase HDL and impair immune system function

Adverse Reactions

<1%:

Cardiovascular: Hypotension
Gastrointestinal: Indigestion, nausea, vomiting
Hematologic: Neutropenia, leukopenia
Hepatic: Jaundice
Respiratory: Pulmonary edema

Overdosage/Toxicology Symptoms of overdose include hypotension, pulmonary edema, diarrhea, vomiting, oliguria, nausea, gastric ulcers, restlessness, dizziness, profuse sweating, decreased consciousness, blurred vision, tachycardia, hypothermia, hyperamylasemia, jaundice.

This agent is corrosive and emesis or gastric lavage should be avoided, instead dilute rapidly with milk or water. Calcium disodium edetate or dimercaprol can be very effective at binding zinc. Supportive care should always be instituted.

Drug Interactions

Decreased effect: Decreased penicillamine, decreased tetracycline effect reduced, iron decreased uptake of zinc, bran products, dairy products reduce absorption of zinc

Mechanism of Action Provides for normal growth and tissue repair, is a cofactor for more than 70 enzymes; ophthalmic astringent and weak antiseptic due to precipitation of protein and clearing mucus from outer surface of the eye

Pharmacodynamics/Kinetics

Absorption: Poor from gastrointestinal tract (20% to 30%)
Elimination: In feces with only traces appearing in urine

Usual Dosage Clinical response may not occur for up to 6-8 weeks

Zinc sulfate:
- RDA: Oral:
  - Birth to 6 months: 3 mg elemental zinc/day
  - 6-12 months: 5 mg elemental zinc/day
  - 1-10 years: 10 mg elemental zinc/day (44 mg zinc sulfate)
  - ≥11 years: 15 mg elemental zinc/day (65 mg zinc sulfate)
- Zinc deficiency: Oral:
  - Infants and Children: 0.5-1 mg elemental zinc/kg/day divided 1-3 times/day; somewhat larger quantities may be needed if there is impaired intestinal absorption or an excessive loss of zinc
  - Adults: 110-220 mg zinc sulfate (25-50 mg elemental zinc)/dose 3 times/day
- Parenteral: TPN: I.V. infusion (chloride or sulfate):

Supplemental to I.V. solutions (clinical response may not occur for up to 6-8 weeks):
- Premature Infants <1500 g, up to 3 kg: 300 mcg/kg/day
- Full-term Infants and Children ≤5 years: 100 mcg/kg/day

or
- Premature Infants: 400 mcg/kg/day
- Term <3 months: 250 mcg/kg/day
- Term >3 months: 100 mcg/kg/day
- Children: 50 mcg/kg/day
- Adults:
  - Stable with fluid loss from small bowel: 12.2 mg zinc/liter TPN or 17.1 mg zinc/kg (added to 1000 mL I.V. fluids) of stool or ileostomy output
  - Metabolically stable: 2.5-4 mg/day, add 2 mg/day for acute catabolic states

Dietary Considerations Food: Avoid foods high in calcium or phosphorus

Administration Administer oral formulation with food if GI upset occurs

Monitoring Parameters Patients on TPN therapy should have periodic serum copper and serum zinc levels, skin integrity

Reference Range

Serum: 50-150 μg/dL (<20 μg/dL as solid test with dermatitis followed by alopecia)
Therapeutic: 66-110 μg/dL (SI: 10-16.8 μmol/L)

Patient Information Take with food if GI upset occurs, but avoid foods high in calcium, phosphorous, or phytate; do not exceed recommended dose; if irritation persists or continues with ophthalmic use, notify physician

Nursing Implications Do not administer undiluted by direct injection into a peripheral vein because of potential for phlebitis, tissue irritation, and potential to increase renal loss of minerals from a bolus injection

Dosage Forms

Zinc carbonate, complex: Liquid: 15 mg/mL (30 mL)
Zinc chloride: Injection: 1 mg/mL (10 mL)
Zinc gluconate (14.3% zinc): Tablet: 10 mg (elemental zinc 1.4 mg), 15 mg (elemental zinc 2 mg), 50 mg (elemental zinc 7 mg), 78 mg (elemental zinc 11 mg)
Zinc sulfate (23% zinc):
- Capsule: 110 mg (elemental zinc 25 mg), 220 mg (elemental zinc 50 mg)
- Injection: 1 mg/mL (10 mL, 30 mL); 4 mg/mL (10 mL); 5 mg/mL (5 mL, 10 mL)
- Tablet: 66 mg (elemental zinc 15 mg), 110 mg (elemental zinc 25 mg), 200 mg (elemental zinc 45 mg)

Zinecard® *see* Dexrazoxane *on page 362*
Zithromax™ *see* Azithromycin *on page 124*
Zocor™ *see* Simvastatin *on page 1137*

Zofran® *see* Ondansetron *on page 926*

Zoladex® *see* Goserelin *on page 584*

Zolicef® *see* Cefazolin *on page 220*

Zoloft™ *see* Sertraline *on page 1133*

Zolpidem (zole PI dem)

Brand Names Ambien™

Synonyms Zolpidem Tartrate

Therapeutic Category Hypnotic; Sedative

Use Short-term treatment of insomnia

Restrictions C-IV

Pregnancy Risk Factor B

Contraindications Lactation

Warnings/Precautions Closely monitor elderly or debilitated patients for impaired cognitive or motor performance; not recommended for use in children <18 years of age

Adverse Reactions

1% to 10%:

- Central nervous system: Headache, drowsiness, dizziness
- Gastrointestinal: Nausea, diarrhea
- Neuromuscular & skeletal: Myalgia

<1%:

- Central nervous system: Amnesia, confusion
- Gastrointestinal: Vomiting
- Neuromuscular & skeletal: Falls, tremor

Overdosage/Toxicology Symptoms of overdose include coma and hypotension. Treatment for overdose is supportive. Rarely is mechanical ventilation required. Flumazenil has been shown to selectively block binding to CNS receptors, resulting in a reversal of CNS depression but not always respiratory depression.

Drug Interactions Increased effect/toxicity with alcohol, CNS depressants

Mechanism of Action Structurally dissimilar to benzodiazepine, however, has much or all of its actions explained by its effects on benzodiazepine (BZD) receptors, especially the omega-1 receptor; retains hypnotic and much of the anxiolytic properties of the BZD, but has reduced effects on skeletal muscle and seizure threshold.

Pharmacodynamics/Kinetics

- Onset of action: 30 minutes
- Duration: 6-8 hours
- Absorption: Rapid
- Distribution: Very low amounts secreted into breast milk
- Protein binding: 92%
- Metabolism: Hepatic to inactive metabolites
- Half-life: 2-2.6 hours, in cirrhosis increased to 9.9 hours

Usual Dosage Duration of therapy should be limited to 7-10 days

- Adults: Oral: 10 mg immediately before bedtime; maximum dose: 10 mg
- Elderly: 5 mg immediately before bedtime
- Hemodialysis: Not dialyzable
- **Dosing adjustment in hepatic impairment:** Decrease dose to 5 mg

Dietary Considerations Alcohol: Additive CNS effect, avoid use

Monitoring Parameters Respiratory, cardiac and mental status

Reference Range 80-150 ng/mL

Patient Information Avoid alcohol and other CNS depressants while taking this medication; for fastest onset, take on an empty stomach; may cause drowsiness

Nursing Implications Patients may require assistance with ambulation; lower doses in the elderly are usually effective; institute safety measures

Dosage Forms Tablet, as tartrate: 5 mg, 10 mg

Zonalon® Topical Cream *see* Doxepin *on page 424*

ZORprin® *see* Aspirin *on page 106*

Zostrix® [OTC] *see* Capsaicin *on page 197*

Zosyn™ *see* Piperacillin and Tazobactam Sodium *on page 1006*

Zovia® *see* Ethinyl Estradiol and Ethynodiol Diacetate *on page 482*

Zovirax® *see* Acyclovir *on page 30*

Zurinol® *see* Allopurinol *on page 47*

Zyban® *see* Bupropion *on page 172*

Zydone® *see* Hydrocodone and Acetaminophen *on page 620*

Zyflo® *see* Zileuton *on page 1322*

Zyloprim® *see* Allopurinol *on page 47*

Zymase® *see* Pancrelipase *on page 949*

Zymenol® [OTC] *see* Mineral Oil *on page 841*

Zyprexa® *see* Olanzapine *on page 924*

Zyrtec™ *see* Cetirizine *on page 244*

APPENDIX TABLE OF CONTENTS

TOXICOLOGY

MISCELLANEOUS

ABBREVIATIONS COMMONLY USED IN MEDICAL ORDERS

Abbreviation	From	Meaning
āā, aa	ana	of each
ac	ante cibum	before meals or food
ad	ad	to, up to
a.d.	aurio dextra	right ear
ad lib	ad libitum	at pleasure
a.l.	aurio laeva	left ear
AM	ante meridiem	morning
amp		ampul
amt		amount
aq	aqua	water
aq. dest.	aqua destillata	distilled water
a.s.	aurio sinister	left ear
ASAP		as soon as possible
a.u.	aures utrae	each ear
bid	bis in die	twice daily
bm		bowel movement
bp		blood pressure
BSA		body surface area
c	cong	a gallon
c̄	cum	with
cal		calorie
cap	capsula	capsule
cc		cubic centimeter
cm		centimeter
comp	compositus	compound
cont		continue
d	dies	day
d/c		discontinue
dil	dilue	dilute
disp	dispensa	dispense
div	divide	divide
dtd	dentur tales doses	give of such a dose
elix, el	elixir	elixir
emp		as directed
et	et	and
ex aq		in water
f, ft	fac, fiat, fiant	make, let be made
FDA		Food and Drug Administration
g	gramma	gram
gr	granum	grain
gtt	gutta	a drop
h	hora	hour
hs	hora somni	at bedtime
I.M.		intramuscular
I.V.		intravenous
kcal		kilocalorie
kg		kilogram
L		liter
liq	liquor	a liquor, solution
mcg		microgram
mEq		milliequivalent
mg		milligram
mixt	mixtura	a mixture
mL		milliliter
mm		millimeter
M	misce	mix
m. dict	more dictor	as directed
NF		National Formulary
no.	numerus	number
noc	nocturnal	in the night

(continued)

Abbreviation	From	Meaning
non rep	non repetatur	do not repeat, no refills
NPO		nothing by mouth
O, Oct	octarius	a pint
o.d.	oculus dexter	right eye
o.l.	oculus laevus	left eye
o.s.	oculus sinister	left eye
o.u.	oculo uterque	each eye
pc, post cib	post cibos	after meals
per		through or by
PM	post meridiem	afternoon or evening
P.O.	per os	by mouth
P.R.	per rectum	rectally
prn	pro re nata	as needed
pulv	pulvis	a powder
q		every
qad	quoque alternis die	every other day
qd		every day
qh	quiaque hora	every hour
qid	quater in die	four times a day
qod		every other day
qs	quantum sufficiat	a sufficient quantity
qs ad		a sufficient quantity to make
qty		quantity
qv	quam volueris	as much as you wish
Rx	recipe	take, a recipe
rep	repetatur	let it be repeated
$\bar{s}$	sine	without
sa	secundum artem	according to art
sat	sataratus	saturated
S.C.		subcutaneous
sig	signa	label, or let it be printed
sol	solutio	solution
solv		dissolve
$\overline{ss}$	semis	one-half
sos	si opus sit	if there is need
stat	statim	at once, immediately
supp	suppositorium	suppository
syr	syrupus	syrup
tab	tabella	tablet
tal		such
tid	ter in die	three times a day
tr, tinct	tincture	tincture
trit		triturate
tsp		teaspoonful
ung	unguentum	ointment
USAN		United States Adopted Names
USP		United States Pharmacopeia
u.d., ut dict	ut dictum	as directed
v.o.		verbal order
w.a.		while awake
x3		3 times
x4		4 times

APOTHECARY/METRIC EQUIVALENTS

Liquid Measures

Basic equivalent: 1 fluid ounce = 30 mL

Examples:

1 gallon	3800 mL	15 minims	1 mL
1 quart	960 mL	10 minims	0.6 mL
1 pint	480 mL	1 gallon	128 fluid ounces
8 fluid ounces	240 mL	1 quart	32 fluid ounces
4 fluid ounces	120 mL	1 pint	16 fluid ounces

Approximate Household Equivalents

1 teaspoonful	5 mL
1 tablespoonful	15 mL

Weights

Basic equivalents:

1 ounce = 30 g   15 grains = 1 g

Examples:

4 ounces	120 g	1/100 grain	600 mcg
2 ounces	60 g	1/150 grain	400 mcg
10 grains	600 mg	1/200 grain	300 mcg
7 1/2 grains	500 mg	16 ounces	1 pound
1 grain	60 mg		

Metric Conversions

Basic equivalents:

1 g	1000 mg	1 mg	1000 mcg

Examples:

5 g	5000 mg	5 mg	5000 mcg
0.5 g	500 mg	0.5 mg	500 mcg
0.05 g	50 mg	0.05 mg	50 mcg

Exact Equivalents

1 gram (g)	15.43 grains	0.1 mg	1/600 gr
1 milliliter (mL)	16.23 minims	0.12 mg	1/500 gr
1 minim	0.06 milliliter	0.15 mg	1/400 gr
1 grain (gr)	64.8 milligrams	0.2 mg	1/300 gr
1 ounce (oz)	31.1 grams	0.5 mg	1/120 gr
1 ounce (oz)	28.35	0.8 mg	1/80 gr
1 pound (lb)	453.6 grams	1 mg	1/65 gr
1 kilogram (kg)	2.2 pounds		

Solids*

1/4 grain	15 mg	5 grains	300 mg
1/2 grain	30 mg	10 grains	600 mg
1 1/2 grain	100 mg		

*Use exact equivalents for compounding and calculations requiring a high degree of accuracy.

AVERAGE WEIGHTS AND SURFACE AREAS

Average Weight and Surface Area of Preterm Infants, Term Infants, and Children

Age	Average Weight (kg)*	Approximate Surface Area (m^2)
Weeks Gestation		
26	0.9-1	0.1
30	1.3-1.5	0.12
32	1.6-2	0.15
38	2.9-3	0.2
40 (term infant at birth)	3.1-4	0.25
Months		
3	5	0.29
6	7	0.38
9	8	0.42
Year		
1	10	0.49
2	12	0.55
3	15	0.64
4	17	0.74
5	18	0.76
6	20	0.82
7	23	0.90
8	25	0.95
9	28	1.06
10	33	1.18
11	35	1.23
12	40	1.34
Adults	70	1.73

*Weights from age 3 months and older are rounded off to the nearest kilogram.

BODY SURFACE AREA OF ADULTS AND CHILDREN

Calculating Body Surface Area in Children

In a child of average size, find weight and corresponding surface area on the boxed scale to the left; or, use the nomogram to the right. Lay a straightedge on the correct height and weight points for the child, then read the intersecting point on the surface area scale.

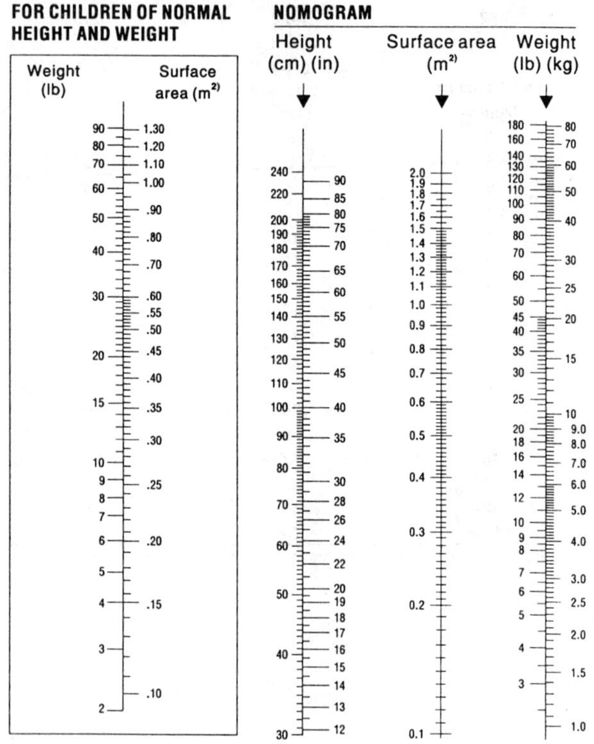

BODY SURFACE AREA FORMULA
(Adult and Pediatric)

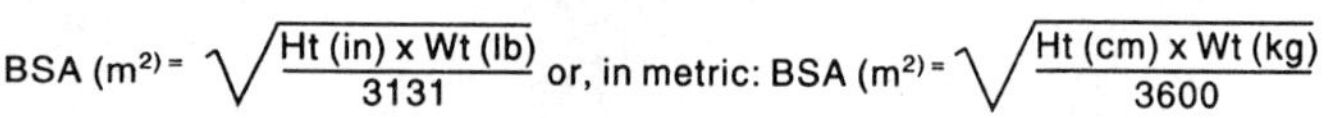

$$BSA\ (m^2) = \sqrt{\frac{Ht\ (in) \times Wt\ (lb)}{3131}}$$ or, in metric: $$BSA\ (m^2) = \sqrt{\frac{Ht\ (cm) \times Wt\ (kg)}{3600}}$$

References
Lam TK, Leung DT, *N Engl J Med*, 1988, 318:1130, (Letter).
Mosteller RD, "Simplified Calculation of Body Surface Area", *N Engl J Med*, 1987, 317:1098.

IDEAL BODY WEIGHT CALCULATION

Adults (18 years and older)

IBW (male) = 50 + (2.3 x height in inches over 5 feet)
IBW (female) = 45.5 + (2.3 x height in inches over 5 feet)

*IBW is in kg.

Children

a. 1-18 years
$$\text{IBW} = \frac{(\text{height}^2 \times 1.65)}{1000}$$
*IBW is in kg.
Height is in cm

b. 5 feet and taller
IBW (male) = 39 + (2.27 x height in inches over 5 feet)
IBW (female) = 42.2 + (2.27 x height in inches over 5 feet)

*IBW is in kg.

MILLIEQUIVALENT AND MILLIMOLE CALCULATIONS

Definitions

mole	=	gram molecular weight of a substance (aka molar weight)
millimole (mM)	=	milligram molecular weight of a substance (a millimole is 1/1000 of a mole)
equivalent weight	=	gram weight of a substance which will combine with or replace one gram (one mole) of hydrogen; an equivalent weight can be determined by dividing the molar weight of a substance by its ionic valence
milliequivalent (mEq)	=	milligram weight of a substance which will combine with or replace one milligram (one millimole) of hydrogen (a milliequivalent is 1/1000 of an equivalent)

Calculations

$$\text{moles} = \frac{\text{weight of a substance (grams)}}{\text{molecular weight of that substance (grams)}}$$

$$\text{millimoles} = \frac{\text{weight of a substance (milligrams)}}{\text{molecular weight of that substance (milligrams)}}$$

$$\text{equivalents} = \text{moles x valence of ion}$$

$$\text{milliequivalents} = \text{millimoles x valence of ion}$$

$$\text{moles} = \frac{\text{equivalents}}{\text{valence of ion}}$$

$$\text{millimoles} = \frac{\text{milliequivalents}}{\text{valence of ion}}$$

$$\text{millimoles} = \text{moles x 1000}$$

$$\text{milliequivalents} = \text{equivalents x 1000}$$

Note: Use of equivalents and milliequivalents is valid only for those substances which have fixed ionic valences (eg, sodium, potassium, calcium, chlorine, magnesium bromine, etc). For substances with variable ionic valences (eg, phosphorous), a reliable equivalent value cannot be determined. In these instances, one should calculate millimoles (which are fixed and reliable) rather than milliequivalents.

MILLIEQUIVALENT CONVERSIONS

To convert mg/100 mL to mEq/L the following formula may be used:

$$\frac{\text{(mg/100 mL) x 10 x valence}}{\text{atomic weight}} = \text{mEq/L}$$

To convert mEq/L to mg/100 mL the following formula may be used:

$$\frac{\text{(mEq/L) x atomic weight}}{\text{10 x valence}} = \text{mg/100 mL}$$

To convert mEq/L to volume of percent of a gas the following formula may be used:

$$\frac{\text{(mEq/L) x 22.4}}{10} = \text{volume percent}$$

Valences and Atomic Weights of Selected Ions

Substance	Electrolyte	Valence	Molecular Wt
Calcium	Ca^{++}	2	40
Chloride	Cl^{-}	1	35.5
Magnesium	Mg^{++}	2	24
Phosphate	HPO_4^{-}(80%)	1.8	96*
pH = 7.4	$H_2PO_4^{-}$(20%)	1.8	96*
Potassium	K^{+}	1	39
Sodium	Na^{+}	1	23
Sulfate	SO_4^{-}	2	96*

*The molecular weight of phosphorus only is 31, and sulfur only is 32.

Approximate Milliequivalents — Weights of Selected Ions

Salt	mEq/g Salt	Mg Salt/mEq
Calcium carbonate ($CaCO_3$)	20	50
Calcium chloride ($CaCl_2$ – $2H_2O$)	14	73
Calcium gluconate (Ca gluconate$_2$ – $1H_2O$)	4	224
Calcium lactate (Ca lactate$_2$ – $5H_2O$)	6	154
Magnesium sulfate ($MgSO_4$)	16	60
Magnesium sulfate ($MgSO_4$ – $7H_2O$)	8	123
Potassium acetate (K acetate)	10	98
Potassium chloride (KCl)	13	75
Potassium citrate (K_3 citrate – $1H_2O$)	9	108
Potassium iodide (KI)	6	166
Sodium bicarbonate ($NaHCO_3$)	12	84
Sodium chloride (NaCl)	17	58
Sodium citrate (Na_3 citrate – $2H_2O$)	10	98
Sodium iodine (NaI)	7	150
Sodium lactate (Na lactate)	9	112

CORRECTED SODIUM

Corrected Na^+ = measured Na^++ [1.5 x (glucose - 150 divided by 100)]

Note: Do not correct for glucose <150.

WATER DEFICIT

Water deficit = 0.6 x body weight [1 - (140 divided by Na^+)]

Note: Body weight is estimated weight in kg when fully hydrated; **Na^+** is serum or plasma sodium. Use corrected Na^+ if necessary. Consult medical references for recommendations for replacement of deficit.

TOTAL SERUM CALCIUM CORRECTED FOR ALBUMIN LEVEL

[(Normal albumin - patient's albumin) x 0.8] + patient's measured total calcium

ACID-BASE ASSESSMENT

Henderson-Hasselbalch Equation

$$pH = 6.1 + \log (HCO_3^- / (0.03)(pCO_2))$$

Alveolar Gas Equation

P_iO_2 = f_iO_2 x (total atmospheric pressure – vapor pressure of H_2O at 37°C)

= f_iO_2 x (760 mm Hg – 47 mm Hg)

P_AO_2 = $P_iO_2 - P_ACO_2 / R$

Alveolar/arterial oxygen gradient = $P_AO_2 - P_aO_2$

Normal ranges:

Children	15-20 mm Hg
Adults	20-25 mm Hg

where:

P_iO_2	=	Oxygen partial pressure of inspired gas (mm Hg) (150 mm Hg in room air at sea level)
f_iO_2	=	Fractional pressure of oxygen in inspired gas (0.21 in room air)
P_AO_2	=	Alveolar oxygen partial pressure
P_ACO_2	=	Alveolar carbon dioxide partial pressure
P_aO_2	=	Arterial oxygen partial pressure
R	=	Respiratory exchange quotient (typically 0.8, increases with high carbohydrate diet, decreases with high fat diet)

Acid-Base Disorders

Acute metabolic acidosis (<12 h duration):

$$PaCO_2 \text{ expected} = 1.5 (HCO_3^-) + 8 \pm 2$$

or

$$\text{expected change in pCO} = (1\text{-}1.5) \times \text{change in } HCO_3^-$$

Acute metabolic alkalosis (<12 h duration):

$$\text{expected change in } pCO_2 = (0.5\text{-}1) \times \text{change in } HCO_3^-$$

Acute respiratory acidosis (<6 h duration):

$$\text{expected change in } HCO_3^- = 0.1 \times pCO_2$$

Acute respiratory acidosis (>6 h duration):

$$\text{expected change in } HCO_3^- = 0.4 \times \text{change in } pCO_2$$

Acute respiratory alkalosis (<6 h duration):

$$\text{expected change in } HCO_3^- = 0.2 \times \text{change in } pCO_2$$

Acute respiratory alkalosis (>6 h duration):

$$\text{expected change in } HCO_3^- = 0.5 \times \text{change in } pCO_2$$

ACID-BASE EQUATION

H^+ (in mEq/L) = (24 x P_aCO_2) divided by HCO_3-

Aa GRADIENT

Aa Gradient [(713)(F_iO_2- (P_aCO_2 divided by 0.8))] - P_aO_2

Aa gradient	=	alveolar-arterial oxygen gradient
F_iO_2	=	inspired oxygen (expressed as a fraction)
P_aCO_2	=	arterial partial pressure carbon dioxide (mm Hg)
P_aO_2	=	arterial partial pressure oxygen (mm Hg)

OSMOLALITY

Definition: The summed concentrations of all osmotically active solute particles.

Preducted serum osmolality =

$2\ Na^+$ + glucose (mg/dL) / 18 + BUN (mg/dL) / 2.8

The normal range of serum osmolality is 285-295 mOsm/L.

Differential diagnosis of increased serum osmolal gap (>10 mOsm/L)

Medications and toxins

- Alcohols (ethanol, methanol, isopropanol, glycerol, ethylene glycol)
- Mannitol
- Paraldehyde

Calculated Osm

Osmolal gap = measured Osm - calculated Osm

0 to +10: Normal

>10: Abnormal

<0: Probable lab or calculation error

For Drugs Causing Increased Osmolar Gap, see "Toxicology Information" section in this Appendix.

BICARBONATE DEFICIT

HCO_3^- deficit = (0.4 x wt in kg) x (HCO_3^- desired – HCO_3^- measured)

Note: In clinical practice, the calculated quantity may differ markedly from the actual amount of bicarbonate needed or that which may be safely administered.

ANION GAP

Definition: The difference in concentration between unmeasured cation and anion equivalents in serum.

Anion gap = $Na^+ - Cl^- - HCO_3^-$

(The normal anion gap is 10-14 mEq/L)

Differential Diagnosis of Increased Anion Gap Acidosis

Organic anions

- Lactate (sepsis, hypovolemia, seizures, large tumor burden)
- Pyruvate
- Uremia
- Ketoacidosis (β-hydroxybutyrate and acetoacetate)
- Amino acids and their metabolites
- Other organic acids

Inorganic anions

- Hyperphosphatemia
- Sulfates
- Nitrates

For Medications and Toxins Affecting the Anion Gap, see "Toxicology Information" section in this Appendix.

Differential Diagnosis of Decreased Anion Gap

- Organic cations
  - Hypergammaglobulinemia
- Inorganic cations
  - Hyperkalemia
  - Hypercalcemia
  - Hypermagnesemia
- Medications and toxins
  - Lithium
- Hypoalbuminemia

RETICULOCYTE INDEX

(% retic divided by 2) x (patients Hct divided by normal Hct) or (% retic divided by 2) x (patient's Hgb divided by normal Hgb)

Normal index: 1.0
Good marrow response: 2.0-6.0

PEDIATRIC DOSAGE ESTIMATIONS

Dosage Estimations Based on Weight:

Augsberger's rule:

(1.5 x weight in kg + 10) % of adult dose = child's approximate dose

Clark's rule:

$$\frac{\text{weight (in pounds)}}{150} \times \text{adult dose} = \text{child's approximate dose}$$

Dosage Estimations Based on Age:

Augsberger's rule:

(4 x age in years + 20) % of adult dose = child's approximate dose

Bastedo's rule:

$$\frac{\text{age in years} + 3}{30} \times \text{adult dose} = \text{child's approximate dose}$$

Cowling's rule:

$$\frac{\text{age at next birthday (in years)}}{24} \times \text{adult dose} = \text{child's approximate dose}$$

Dilling's rule:

$$\frac{\text{age (in years)}}{20} \times \text{adult dose} = \text{child's approximate dose}$$

Fried's rule for infants (younger than 1 year):

$$\frac{\text{age (in months)}}{150} \times \text{adult dose} = \text{infant's approximate dose}$$

Young's rule:

$$\frac{\text{age (in years)}}{\text{age} + 12} \times \text{adult dose} = \text{child's approximate dose}$$

POUNDS/KILOGRAMS CONVERSION

1 pound = 0.45359 kilograms
1 kilogram = 2.2 pounds

lb	= kg	lb	= kg	lb	= kg
1	0.45	70	31.75	140	63.50
5	2.27	75	34.02	145	65.77
10	4.54	80	36.29	150	68.04
15	6.80	85	38.56	155	70.31
20	9.07	90	40.82	160	72.58
25	11.34	95	43.09	165	74.84
30	13.61	100	45.36	170	77.11
35	15.88	105	47.63	175	79.38
40	18.14	110	49.90	180	81.65
45	20.41	115	52.16	185	83.92
50	22.68	120	54.43	190	86.18
55	24.95	125	56.70	195	88.45
60	27.22	130	58.91	200	90.72
65	29.48	135	61.24		

TEMPERATURE CONVERSION

Celsius to Fahrenheit = (°C x 9/5) + 32 = °F
Fahrenheit to Celsius = (°F -32) x 5/9 = °C

°C	= °F	°C	= °F	°C	= °F
100.0	212.0	39.0	102.2	36.8	98.2
50.0	122.0	38.8	101.8	36.6	97.9
41.0	105.8	38.6	101.5	36.4	97.5
40.8	105.4	38.4	101.1	36.2	97.2
40.6	105.1	38.2	100.8	36.0	96.8
40.4	104.7	38.0	100.4	35.8	96.4
40.2	104.4	37.8	100.1	35.6	96.1
40.0	104.0	37.6	99.7	35.4	95.7
39.8	103.6	37.4	99.3	35.2	95.4
39.6	103.3	37.2	99.0	35.0	95.0
39.4	102.9	37.0	98.6	0	32.0
39.2	102.6				

LIVER DISEASE, PUGH'S MODIFICATION OF CHILD'S CLASSIFICATION FOR SEVERITY

Parameter	Points for Increasing Abnormality 1	2	3
Encephalopathy	None	1 or 2	3 or 4
Ascites	Absent	Slight	Moderate
Bilirubin (mg/dL)	<2.9	2.9-5.8	>5.8
Albumin (g/dL)	>3.5	2.8-3.5	<2.8
Prothrombin time (seconds over control)	1-4	4-6	>6

Scores:

Mild hepatic impairment = <6 points.
Moderate hepatic impairment = 6-10 points.
Severe hepatic impairment = >10 points.

LIVER DISEASE, CONSIDERATIONS FOR DRUG DOSE ADJUSTMENT

Extent of Change in Drug Dose	Conditions or Requirements to Be Satisfied
No or minor change	Mild liver disease
	Extensive elimination of drug by kidneys and no renal dysfunction
	Elimination by pathways of metabolism spared by liver disease
	Drug is enzyme-limited and given acutely
	Drug is flow/enzyme-sensitive and only given acutely by I.V. route
	No alteration in drug sensitivity
Decrease in dose up to 25%	Elimination by the liver does not exceed 40% of the dose; no renal dysfunction
	Drug is flow-limited and given by I.V. route, with no large change in protein binding
	Drug is flow/enzyme-limited and given acutely by oral route
	Drug has a large therapeutic ratio
>25% decrease in dose	Drug metabolism is affected by liver disease; drug administered chronically
	Drug has a narrow therapeutic range; protein binding altered significantly
	Drug is flow-limited and given orally
	Drug is eliminated by kidneys and renal function severely affected
	Altered sensitivity to drug due to liver disease

Reference

Arns PA, Wedlund PJ, and Branch RA, "Adjustment of Medications in Liver Failure," *The Pharmacologic Approach to the Critically Ill Patient*, 2nd ed, Chernow B, ed, Baltimore, MD: Williams & Wilkins, 1988, 85-111.

CREATININE CLEARANCE ESTIMATING METHODS IN PATIENTS WITH STABLE RENAL FUNCTION

These formulas provide an acceptable estimate of the patient's creatinine clearance **except** in the following instances.

- Patient's serum creatinine is changing rapidly (either up or down).
- Patients are markedly emaciated.

In above situations, certain assumptions have to be made.

- In patients with rapidly rising serum creatinines (ie, >0.5-0.7 mg/dL/day), it is best to assume that the patient's creatinine clearance is probably <10 mL/minute.
- In emaciated patients, although their actual creatinine clearance is less than their calculated creatinine clearance (because of decreased creatinine production), it is not possible to easily predict how much less.

Infants

Estimation of creatinine clearance using serum creatinine and body length (to be used when an adequate timed specimen cannot be obtained). **Note:** This formula may not provide an accurate estimation of creatinine clearance for infants younger than 6 months of age and for patients with severe starvation or muscle wasting.

$Cl_{cr} = K \times L/S_{cr}$

where:

Cl_{cr} = creatinine clearance in mL/minute/1.73 m^2
K = constant of proportionality that is age specific

Age	K
Low birth weight ≤1 y	0.33
Full-term ≤1 y	0.45
2-12 y	0.55
13-21 y female	0.55
13-21 y male	0.70

L = length in cm
S_{cr} = serum creatinine concentration in mg/dL

Reference

Schwartz GJ, Brion LP, and Spitzer A, "The Use of Plasma Creatinine Concentration for Estimating Glomerular Filtration Rate in Infants, Children and Adolescents," *Ped Clin N Amer*, 1987, 34:571-90.

Children (1-18 years)

Method 1: (Traub SL and Johnson CE, *Am J Hosp Pharm*, 1980, 37:195-201)

$$Cl_{cr} = \frac{0.48 \times (\text{height}) \times BSA}{S_{cr} \times 1.73}$$

where

BSA = body surface area in m^2
Cl_{cr} = creatinine clearance in mL/min
S_{cr} = serum creatinine in mg/dL
Height = in cm

Method 2: Nomogram (Traub SL and Johnson CE, *Am J Hosp Pharm*, 1980, 37:195-201)

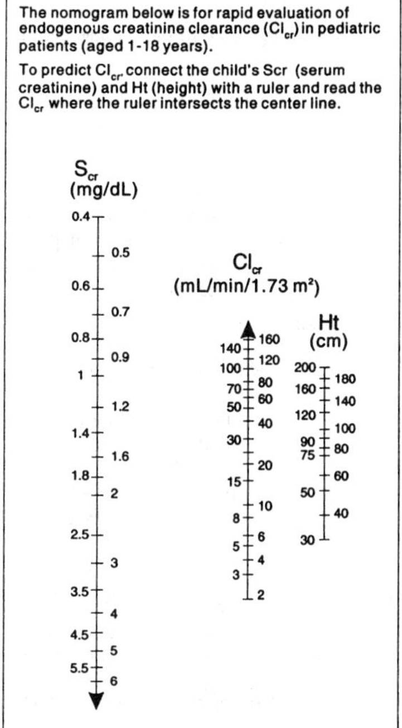

The nomogram below is for rapid evaluation of endogenous creatinine clearance (Cl_{cr}) in pediatric patients (aged 1-18 years).
To predict Cl_{cr}, connect the child's Scr (serum creatinine) and Ht (height) with a ruler and read the Cl_{cr} where the ruler intersects the center line.
S_{cr} (mg/dL)
Cl_{cr} (mL/min/1.73 m^2)
Ht (cm)

Adults (18 years and older)

(Cockroft DW and Gault MH, *Nephron*, 1976, 16:31-41)

Estimated creatinine clearance (Cl_{cr}):
(mL/min)

$$\text{Male} = \frac{(140 - \text{age})\ \text{IBW (kg)}}{72 \times \text{serum creatinine}}$$

$$\text{Female} = \text{estimated } Cl_{cr} \text{ male} \times 0.85$$

Note: The use of the patient's ideal body weight (IBW) is recommended for the above formula except when the patient's actual body weight is less than ideal. Use of the IBW is especially important in obese patients.

RENAL FUNCTION TESTS

Endogenous creatinine clearance vs age (timed collection)

Creatinine clearance (mL/min/1.73 m²) = (Cr_uV/Cr_sT) (1.73/A)

where:

Cr_u	=	urine creatinine concentration (mg/dL)
V	=	total urine collected during sampling period (mL)
Cr_s	=	serum creatinine concentration (mg/dL)
T	=	duration of sampling period (min) (24 h = 1440 min)
A	=	body surface area (m²)

Age-specific normal values

5-7 d	50.6±5.8 mL/min/1.73 m²
1-2 mo	64.6±5.8 mL/min/1.73 m²
5-8 mo	87.7±11.9 mL/min/1.73 m²
9-12 mo	86.9±8.4 mL/min/1.73 m²
≥18 mo	
male	124±26 mL/min/1.73 m²
female	109±13.5 mL/min/1.73 m²
Adults	
male	105±14 mL/min/1.73 m²
female	95±18 mL/min/1.73 m²

Note: In patients with renal failure (creatinine clearance <25 mL/min), creatinine clearance may be elevated over GFR because of tubular secretion of creatinine.

Calculation of Creatinine Clearance From a 24-Hour Urine Collection

Equation 1:

$$Cl_{cr} = \frac{(U) \times (V)}{P}$$

Cl_{cr}	=	creatinine clearance
U	=	urine concentration of creatinine
V	=	total urine volume in the collection
P	=	plasma creatinine concentration

Equation 2:

$$Cl_{cr} = \frac{(\text{total urine volume}) \times (\text{urine Cr concentration}) \times 100}{(\text{serum creatinine}) \times (\text{time of urine collection in minutes})}$$

Occasionally, a patient will have a 12- or 24-hour urine collection done for direct calculation of creatinine clearance. Although a urine collection for 24 hours is best, it is difficult to do since many urine collections occur for a much shorter period. A 24-hour urine collection is the desired duration of urine collection because the urine excretion of creatinine is diurnal and thus the measured creatinine clearance will vary throughout the day as the creatinine in the urine varies. When the urine collection is less than 24 hours, the total excreted creatinine will be affected by the time of the day during which the collection is performed. A 24-hour urine collection is sufficient to be able to accurately average the diurnal creatinine excretion variations. If a patient has 24 hours of urine collected for creatinine clearance, equation 1 can be used for calculating the creatinine clearance. To use equation 1 to calculate the creatinine clearance, it will be necessary to know the duration of urine collection, the urine collection volume, the urine creatinine concentration, and the serum creatinine value that reflects the urine collection period. In most cases, a serum creatinine concentration is drawn anytime during the day, but it is best to have the value drawn halfway through the collection period.

Amylase/Creatinine Clearance Ratio*

$$\frac{Amylase_u \times creatinine_p}{Amylase_p \times creatinine_u} \times 100$$

u = urine; p = plasma

Serum BUN/Serum Creatinine Ratio

Serum BUN (mg/dL:serum creatinine (mg/dL))

Normal BUN:creatinine ratio is 10-15

BUN:creatinine ratio >20 suggests prerenal azotemia (also seen with high urea-generation states such as GI bleeding)

BUN:creatinine ratio <5 may be seen with disorders affecting urea biosynthesis such as urea cycle enzyme deficiencies and with hepatitis.

Fractional Sodium Excretion

Fractional sodium secretion (FENa) = $Na_uCr_s/Na_sCr_u \times 100\%$

where:

Na_u	=	urine sodium (mEq/L)
Na_s	=	serum sodium (mEq/L)
Cr_u	=	urine creatinine (mg/dL)
Cr_s	=	serum creatinine (mg/dL)

FENa <1% suggests prerenal failure

FENa >2% suggest intrinsic renal failure

(for newborns, normal FENa is approximately 2.5%)

Note: Disease states associated with a falsely elevated FENa include severe volume depletion (>10%), early acute tubular necrosis and volume depletion in chronic renal disease. Disorders associated with a lowered FENa include acute glomerulonephritis, hemoglobinuric or myoglobinuric renal failure, nonoliguric acute tubular necrosis and acute urinary tract obstruction. In addition, FENa may be <1% in patients with acute renal failure **and** a second condition predisposing to sodium retention (eg, burns, congestive heart failure, nephrotic syndrome).

Urine Calcium/Urine Creatinine Ratio (spot sample)

Urine calcium (mg/dL): urine creatinine (mg/dL)

Normal values <0.21 (mean values 0.08 males, 0.06 females)

Premature infants show wide variability of calcium:creatinine ratio, and tend to have lower thresholds for calcium loss than older children. Prematures without nephrolithiasis had mean Ca:Cr ratio of 0.75±0.76. Infants with nephrolithiasis had mean Ca:Cr ratio of 1.32±1.03 (Jacinto, et al, *Pediatrics*, vol 81, p 31.)

Urine Protein/Urine Creatinine Ratio (spot sample)

P_u/Cr_u	Total Protein Excretion ($mg/m^2/d$)
0.1	80
1	800
10	8000

where:

P_u = urine protein concentration (mg/dL)
Cr_u = urine creatinine concentration (mg/dL)

ANTIEMETICS FOR CHEMOTHERAPY INDUCED NAUSEA AND VOMITING

Basic Principles of Antiemetic Therapy

1. Rule out other causes of nausea and vomiting before prescribing antiemetics.
2. Evaluate the relative emetic potential of antineoplastic drugs and choose antiemetics accordingly.
3. Treat delayed nausea and vomiting with **scheduled antiemetics** for a period of several days.
4. **Combination antiemetic regimens** provide greater protection against chemotherapy induced emesis than do single agents.
5. Head off trouble before it starts by initiating an aggressive antiemetic regimen before giving highly emetogenic chemotherapy.

Time Course of Nausea and Vomiting

Drug	Onset (h)	Duration (h)
Azacitidine	1-3	3-4
Carboplatin	2-6	1-48
Carmustine	2-6	4-6
Cisplatin	1-4	12-96
Cyclophosphamide	6-8	8-24
Cytarabine	1-3	3-8
Dacarbazine	1-2	2-4
Dactinomycin	2-5	4-24
Daunorubicin	1-3	4-24
Doxorubicin	1-3	4-24
Ifosfamide	2-3	12-72
Lomustine	2-6	4-6
Mechlorethamine	1-3	2-8
Mitomycin	1-2	3-4
Plicamycin	4-6	4-24
Streptozocin	1-3	1-12

Emetogenic Potential of Single Chemotherapeutic Agents

Class I
Low (<10%)

Asparaginase
Bleomycin
Busulfan
Busulfan (oral)
Chlorambucil
Cladribine
Cyclophosphamide (oral)
Cytarabine
Docetaxel
Etoposide
Floxuridine
Fludarabine
Melphalan <100 mg/m^2
Mercaptopurine
Paclitaxel
Thioguanine (oral)
Thiotepa <60 mg
Vincristine

Class II
Moderately Low (10% to 30%)

Bleomycin
Busulfan 1 mg/kg (oral)
Cytarabine ≤20 mg
Doxorubicin ≤20 mg
Etoposide
Fluorouracil <1000 mg
Methotrexate <100 mg
Thiotepa >200 mg
Topotecan

Class III
Moderate (30% to 60%)

Azacitidine
Carboplatin
Cisplatin ≤25 mg/m^2/day
Cyclophosphamide <1 g
Daunorubicin
Doxorubicin <75 mg or >20 mg
Fluorouracil ≥1000 mg
Gemcitabine
Idarubicin
Methotrexate <250 mg or ≥100 mg
Mitoxantrone
Paclitaxel
Teniposide
Vinblastine
Vinorelbine

Class IV
Moderately High (60% to 90%)

Carmustine <200 mg
Cisplatin <75 mg
Cyclophosphamide 1 g
Cytarabine 250 mg to 1 g
Dacarbazine <500 mg
Doxorubicin ≥75 mg
Hexamethyl melamine
Ifosfamide
Irinotecan (dose-limiting_
Lomustine <60 mg
Methotrexate ≥250 mg
Mitomycin
Procarbazine

Class V
High (>90%)

Carmustine ≥200 mg
Cisplatin ≥75 mg
Cyclophosphamide >1 g
Cytarabine >1 g
Dacarbazine ≥500 mg
Dactinomycin
Lomustine ≥60 mg
Mechlorethamine
Melphalan ≥100 mg/m^2
Pentostatin
Streptozocin
Thiotepa ≥100 mg/m^2

Types of Antiemetic Drugs

Anticholinergic drugs

- Scopolamine (Transderm-Scop®)

Antihistamines

- Diphenhydramine (Benadryl®)

Benzodiazepines

- Alprazolam (Xanax®)
- Lorazepam (Ativan®)

Butyrophenones

- Domperidone (Motilium®) (investigational)
- Droperidol (Inapsine®)
- Haloperidol (Haldol®)

Cannabinoids

- Dronabinol (Marinol®)
- Nabilone (Cesamet®)

Corticosteroids

- Dexamethasone (Decadron®)
- Methylprednisolone (Medrol®)

Phenothiazines

- Chlorpromazine (Thorazine®)
- Perphenazine (Trilafon®)
- Prochlorperazine (Compazine®)
- Promethazine (Phenergan®)
- Thiethylperazine (Torecan®)

Serotonin antagonists

- Dolasetron (Anzemet®) (investigational)
- Granisetron (Kytril®)
- Ondansetron (Zofran®)
- Tropisetron (Navoban®) (investigational)

Substituted benzamides

- Alizapride (Plitican®) (investigational)
- Cisapride (Propulsid®)
- Metoclopramide (Reglan®)
- Trimethobenzamide (Tigan®)

Potency of Antiemetic Drugs

Potency	Type of Antiemetic Drug
Active against highly emetogenic chemotherapy	Serotonin antagonist Substituted benzamide (high dose)
Active against mildly or moderately emetogenic chemotherapy	Butyrophenone Cannabinoid Corticosteroid Phenothiazine
Minimally active	Anticholinergic agent Antihistamine Benzodiazepine

Initial Doses in Selected Antiemetic Regimens*

Antiemetic Regimen	Adult Dose	Pediatric Dose
For moderately emetogenic chemotherapy		
Dexamethasone	I.V.: 10-20 mg	I.V.: 10 mg/m²/dose for the first dose, then 5 mg/m²/dose q6h as needed
Dronabinol	P.O.: 10 mg	P.O.: 5 mg/m² starting 6-8 hours before chemotherapy and q4-6 hours after; to be continued for 12 hours after therapy discontinuation
Ondansetron	P.O.: 8 mg or I.V.: 10 mg	P.O.: 4-12 y: 4 mg 30 minutes before treatment; repeat 4 and 8 hours after initial dose >12 y: See adult dose I.V.: 10 mg/m²/dose for the first dose, then 5 mg/m²/dose q6h as needed
Prochlorperazine	P.O.: 5-10 mg; I.V.: 5-10 mg, or 25 mg by rectal suppository	P.O./P.R.: 0.4 mg/kg/24 hours in 3-4 divided doses I.M.: 0.1-0.15 mg/kg/dose
For highly emetogenic chemotherapy†		
Dexamethasone	I.V.: 20 mg	I.V.: 20 mg/m²/dose for the first dose, then 5-10 mg/m²/dose q6h as needed
Diphenhydramine	I.V.: 25-50 mg q2h x 2	I.V.: ≤50 mg/m² q2h x 2
Lorazepam	I.V.: 1-2 mg	I.V.: 2-15 y: 0.05 mg/kg (≤2 mg/dose) prior to chemotherapy
Metoclopramide	I.V.: 3 mg/kg of body weight q2h x 2	I.V.: 1-2 mg/kg 30 minutes before chemotherapy q2-4h
Ondansetron	I.V.: 32 mg (in divided doses)	I.V.: 0.45 mg/kg as single dose 30 minutes prior to chemotherapy or 0.15 mg/kg 30 minutes before and 0.15 mg/kg at 4 and 8 hours after treatment

Adapted with revisions from *N Engl J Med*, 1993, 329:1790-6.

*Antiemetic regimens for moderately emetogenic chemotherapy consist of single drugs; regimens for highly emetogenic chemotherapy consist of drugs given in combination (denoted by brackets).

†Use combination therapy.

Combinations of Antiemetic Drugs Resulting in Decreased Toxicity of the Primary Drug

Primary Antiemetic Drug	Effective Secondary Drug
Phenothiazine	Antihistamine
Butyrophenone	Antihistamine
Substituted benzamide	Antihistamine Corticosteroid Benzodiazepine
Cannabinoid	Phenothiazine

Combinations of Antiemetic Drugs Resulting in Improved Efficacy of the Primary Antiemetic Drug

Primary Antiemetic Drug	Effective Secondary Drug
Serotonin antagonist	Corticosteroid Phenothiazine Butyrophenone
Substituted benzamide	Corticosteroid Corticosteroid with anticholinergic drug
Phenothiazine	Corticosteroid
Butyrophenone	Corticosteroid
Cannabinoid	Corticosteroid
Corticosteroid	Benzodiazepine

CANCER CHEMOTHERAPY REGIMENS

ADULT REGIMENS

Breast Cancer

AC

Doxorubicin (Adriamycin®), I.V., 45 mg/m^2, day 1
Cyclophosphamide, I.V., 500 mg/m^2, day 1

Repeat cycle every 21 days

ACe

Doxorubicin (Adriamycin®), I.V., 40 mg/m^2, day 1
Cyclophosphamide, P.O., 200 mg/m^2/day, days 1-3 or 3-6

Repeat cycle every 21-28 days

CAF

Cyclophosphamide, P.O., 100 mg/m^2, days 1-14
Doxorubicin (Adriamycin®), I.V., 30 mg/m^2, days 1 & 8
Fluorouracil, I.V., 400-500 mg/m^2, days 1 & 8

Repeat cycle every 28 days

or

Cyclophosphamide, I.V., 500 mg/m^2, day 1
Doxorubicin (Adriamycin®), I.V., 50 mg/m^2, day 1
Fluorouracil, I.V., 500 mg/m^2, day 1

Repeat cycle every 21 days

or Dose Intensification of CAF*

Cyclophosphamide, I.V., 600 mg/m^2, day 1
Doxorubicin (Adriamycin®), I.V., 60 mg/m^2, day 1
Fluorouracil, I.V., 600 mg/m^2, day 1
G-CSF, I.V./S.C., 5 mcg/kg/dose

Repeat cycle every 21 days

*Preliminary data presented at ASCO (March, 1992) suggests better response with dose intensification.

CFM

Cyclophosphamide, I.V., 500 mg/m^2, day 1
Fluorouracil, I.V., 500 mg/m^2, day 1
Mitoxantrone, I.V., 10 mg/m^2, day 1

Repeat cycle every 21 days

CFPT

Cyclophosphamide, I.V., 150 mg/m^2, days 1-5
Fluorouracil, I.V., 300 mg/m^2, days 1-5
Prednisone, P.O., 10 mg tid, days 1-7
Tamoxifen, P.O., 10 mg bid, days 1-42

Repeat cycle every 42 days

CMF

Cyclophosphamide, P.O., 100 mg/m^2, days 1-14
Methotrexate, I.V., 40-60 mg/m^2, days 1 & 8
Fluorouracil, I.V., 400-600 mg/m^2, days 1 & 8

Repeat cycle every 28 days

or

Cyclophosphamide, I.V., 600 mg/m^2, days 1 & 8
Methotrexate, I.V., 40-60 mg/m^2, days 1 & 8
Fluorouracil, I.V., 400-600 mg/m^2, days 1 & 8

Repeat cycle every 28 days

CMFP

Cyclophosphamide, P.O., 100 mg/m^2, days 1-14
Methotrexate, I.V., 40-60 mg/m^2, days 1 & 8
Fluorouracil, I.V., 600-700 mg/m^2, days 1 & 8
Prednisone, P.O., 40 mg (first 3 cycles only), days 1-14

Repeat cycle every 28 days

CMFVP (Cooper's)

Cyclophosphamide, P.O., 2-2.5 mg/kg/day for 9 months
Methotrexate, I.V., 0.7 mg/kg/wk for 8 weeks then every other week for 7 months
Fluorouracil, I.V., 12 mg/kg/wk for 8 weeks then every other week for 7 months
Vincristine, I.V., 0.035 mg/kg (max: 2 mg/wk) for 5 weeks then once monthly

Prednisone, P.O., 0.75 mg/kg/day, taper over next 40 days, discontinue, days 1-10

or

Cyclophosphamide, I.V., 400 mg/m², day 1
Methotrexate, I.V., 30 mg/m², days 1 & 8
Fluorouracil, I.V., 400 mg/m², days 1 & 8
Vincristine, I.V., 1 mg, days 1 & 8
Prednisone, P.O., 20 mg qid, days 1-7

Repeat cycle every 28 days

FAC

Fluorouracil, I.V., 500 mg/m², days 1 & 8
Doxorubicin (Adriamycin®), I.V., 50 mg/m², day 1
Cyclophosphamide, I.V., 500 mg/m², day 1

Repeat cycle every 21 days

IMF

Ifosfamide, I.V., 1.5 g/m², days 1 & 8
Mesna, I.V., 20% of ifosfamide dose, give immediately before and 4 and 8 hours after ifosfamide infusion, days 1 & 8
Methotrexate, I.V., 40 mg/m², days 1 & 8
Fluorouracil, I.V., 600 mg/m², days 1 & 8

Repeat cycle every 28 days

NFL

Mitoxantrone (Novantrone®), I.V., 12 mg/m², day 1
Fluorouracil, I.V., 350 mg/m², days 1-3, given after leucovorin calcium
Leucovorin calcium, I.V., 300 mg/m², days 1-3

or

Mitoxantrone (Novantrone®), I.V., 10 mg/m², day 1
Fluorouracil, I.V., 1000 mg/m² continuous infusion, given after leucovorin calcium, days 1-3
Leucovorin calcium, I.V., 100 mg/m², days 1-3

Repeat cycle every 21 days

VATH

Vinblastine, I.V., 4.5 mg/m², day 1
Doxorubicin (Adriamycin®), I.V., 45 mg/m², day 1
Thiotepa, I.V., 12 mg/m², day 1
Fluoxymesterone (Halotestin®), P.O., 30 mg qd, days 1-21

Repeat cycle every 21 days

Single-Agent Regimens

Doxorubicin, I.V., 60 mg/m², every 3 weeks

or

Doxorubicin, I.V., 20 mg/m², every week

or

Doxorubicin, I.V., 20 mg/m² continuous infusion, days 1-3, every 3 weeks

Mitomycin C, I.V., 8-10 mg/m², every 6-8 weeks

Paclitaxel, I.V., 175 mg/m² over 3-24 h, every 21 d
Patient must be premedicated with:
Dexamethasone 20 mg P.O., 12 and 6 h prior
Diphenhydramine 50 mg I.V., 30 min prior
Cimetidine 300 mg I.V., or ranitidine 50 mg I.V., 30 min prior

Vinblastine, I.V., 12 mg/m², every 3-4 weeks

Colon Cancer

F-CL

Fluorouracil, I.V., 375 mg/m², days 1-5
Leucovorin calcium, I.V., 200 mg/m², days 1-5

Repeat cycle every 28 days

or

Fluorouracil, I.V., 500 mg/m² weekly 1 h after initiating the calcium leucovorin infusion for 6 weeks
Leucovorin calcium, I.V., 500 mg/m², over 2 h, weekly for 6 weeks

Two-week break, then repeat cycle

FLe

Fluorouracil, I.V., 450 mg/m² for 5 days, then, after a pause of 4 weeks, 450 mg/m², weekly for 48 weeks
Levamisole, P.O., 50 mg tid for 3 days, repeated every 2 weeks for 1 year

FMV

Fluorouracil, I.V., 10 mg/kg/day, days 1-5
Methyl-CCNU, P.O., 175 mg/m^2, day 1
Vincristine, I.V., 1 mg/m^2 (max: 2 mg), day 1
Repeat cycle every 35 days

FU/LV

Fluorouracil, I.V., 370-400 mg/m^2/day, days 1-5
Leucovorin calcium, I.V., 200 mg/m^2/day, commence infusion 15 min prior to fluorouracil infusion, days 1-5
Repeat cycle every 21 days

or

Fluorouracil, I.V., 1000 mg/m^2/day by continuous infusion, days 1-4
Leucovorin calcium, I.V., 200 mg/m^2/day, days 1-4
Repeat cycle every 28 days

Weekly 5FU/LV

Fluorouracil, I.V., 600 mg/m^2 over 1 h given after leucovorin, repeat weekly x 6 then 2-week rest period = 1 cycle, days 1, 8, 15, 22, 29, 36
Leucovorin calcium, I.V., 500 mg/m^2 over 2 h, days 1, 8, 15, 22, 29, 36
Repeat cycle every 56 days

5FU/LDLF

Fluorouracil, I.V., 370 mg/m^2/day, days 1-5
Leucovorin calcium, I.V., 20-25 mg/m^2/day, days 1-5
Repeat cycle every 28 days

Gastric Cancer

EAP

Etoposide, I.V., 120 mg/m^2, days 4, 5, 6
Doxorubicin (Adriamycin®), I.V., 20 mg/m^2, days 1, 7
Cisplatin (Platinol®), I.V., 40 mg/m^2, days 2, 8
Repeat cycle every 21 days

ELF

Etoposide, I.V., 120 mg/m^2, days 1-3
Leucovorin calcium, I.V., 300 mg/m^2, days 1-3
Fluorouracil, I.V., 500 mg/m^2, days 1-3
Repeat cycle every 21-28 days

FAM

Fluorouracil, I.V., 600 mg/m^2, days 1, 8, 29, & 36
Doxorubicin (Adriamycin®), I.V., 30 mg/m^2, days 1 & 29
Mitomycin C, I.V., 10 mg/m^2, day 1
Repeat cycle every 56 days

FAME

Fluorouracil, I.V., 350 mg/m^2, days 1-5, 36-40
Doxorubicin (Adriamycin®), I.V., 40 mg/m^2, days 1 & 36
Methyl-CCNU, P.O., 150 mg/m^2, day 1
Repeat cycle every 70 days

FAMTX

Methotrexate, IVPB, 1500 mg/m^2, day 1
Fluorouracil, IVPB, 1500 mg/m^2 1 h after methotrexate, day 1
Leucovorin calcium, P.O., 15 mg/m^2 q6h x 48 h 24 h after methotrexate, day 2
Doxorubicin (Adriamycin®), IVPB, 30 mg/m^2, day 15
Repeat cycle every 28 days

FCE

Fluorouracil, I.V., 900 mg/m^2/day continuous infusion, days 1-5
Cisplatin, I.V., 20 mg/m^2, days 1-5
Etoposide, I.V., 90 mg/m^2, days 1, 3, & 5
Repeat cycle every 21 days

PFL

Cisplatin (Platinol®), I.V., 25 mg/m^2 continuous infusion, days 1-5
Fluorouracil, I.V., 800 mg/m^2 continuous infusion, days 2-5
Leucovorin calcium, I.V., 500 mg/m^2 continuous infusion, days 1-5
Repeat cycle every 28 days

Genitourinary Cancer

Bladder

CAP

Cyclophosphamide, I.V., 400 mg/m^2, day 1
Doxorubicin (Adriamycin®), I.V., 40 mg/m^2, day 1
Cisplatin (Platinol®), I.V., 60 mg/m^2, day 1

Repeat cycle every 21 days

CISCA

Cisplatin, I.V., 70-100 mg/m^2, day 2
Cyclophosphamide, I.V., 650 mg/m^2, day 1
Doxorubicin (Adriamycin®), I.V., 50 mg/m^2, day 1

Repeat cycle every 21-28 days

CMV

Cisplatin, I.V., 100 mg/m^2 over 4 h start 12 h after MTX, day 2
Methotrexate, I.V., 30 mg/m^2, days 1 & 8
Vinblastine, I.V., 4 mg/m^2, days 1 & 8

Repeat cycle every 21 days

m-PFL

Methotrexate, I.V., 60 mg/m^2, day 1
Cisplatin (Platinol®), I.V., 25 mg/m^2 continuous infusion, days 2-6
Fluorouracil, I.V., 800 mg/m^2 continuous infusion, days 2-6
Leucovorin calcium, I.V., 500 mg/m^2 continuous infusion, days 2-6

Repeat cycle every 28 days for 4 cycles

MVAC

Methotrexate, I.V., 30 mg/m^2, days 1, 15, 22
Vinblastine, I.V., 3 mg/m^2, days 2, 15, 22
Doxorubicin (Adriamycin®), I.V., 30 mg/m^2, day 2
Cisplatin, I.V., 70 mg/m^2, day 2

Repeat cycle every 28 days

Prostate

FL

Flutamide, P.O., 250 mg tid, days 1-28
Leuprolide acetate, S.C., 1 mg qd, days 1-28

Repeat cycle every 28 days

or

Flutamide, P.O., 250 mg tid, days 1-28
Leuprolide acetate depot, I.M., 7.5 mg, day 1

Repeat cycle every 28 days

FZ

Flutamide, P.O., 250 mg tid
Goserelin acetate (Zoladex®), S.C., 3.6 mg implant, every 28 days

L-VAM

Leuprolide acetate, S.C., 1 mg qd, days 1-28
Vinblastine, I.V., 1.5 mg/m^2/day continuous infusion, days 2-7
Doxorubicin (Adriamycin®), I.V., 50 mg/m^2 continuous infusion, day 1
Mitomycin C, I.V., 10 mg/m^2, day 2

Repeat cycle every 28 days

Testicular, Induction, Good Risk

BEP

Bleomycin, I.V., 30 units, days 2, 9, 16
Etoposide, I.V., 100 mg/m^2, days 1-5
Cisplatin (Platinol®), I.V., 20 mg/m^2, days 1-5

Repeat cycle every 21 days

PE

Cisplatin (Platinol®), I.V., 20 mg/m^2, days 1-5
Etoposide, I.V., 100 mg/m^2, days 1-5

Repeat cycle every 21 days

PVB

Cisplatin (Platinol®), I.V., 20 mg/m^2, days 1-5
Vinblastine, I.V., 6 mg/m^2, days 1, 2
Bleomycin, I.V., 30 units, weekly

Repeat cycle every 21-28 days

Testicular, Induction, Poor Risk

VIP

Etoposide (VePesid®), I.V., 75 mg/m^2, days 1-5
Ifosfamide, I.V., 1.2 g/m^2, days 1-5
Cisplatin (Platinol®), I.V., 20 mg/m^2, days 1-5
Mesna, I.V., 120 mg/m^2 then 1200 mg/m^2/day continuous infusion, days 1-5

Repeat cycle every 21 days

VIP (Einhorn)

Vinblastine, I.V., 0.11 mg/kg, days 1-2
Ifosfamide, I.V., 1200 mg/m^2, days 1-5
Cisplatin (Platinol®), I.V., 20 mg/m^2, days 1-5
Mesna, I.V., 120 mg/m^2, then 1200 mg/m^2/day continuous infusion, days 1-5

Repeat cycle every 21 days

Testicular, Induction, Salvage

VAB VI

Vinblastine, I.V., 4 mg/m^2, day 1
Dactinomycin (Actinomycin D), I.V., 1 mg/m^2, day 1
Bleomycin, I.V., 30 units push day 1, then 20 units/m^2/day continuous infusion, days 1-3
Cisplatin, I.V., 120 mg/m^2, day 4
Cyclophosphamide, I.V., 600 mg/m^2, day 1

Repeat cycle every 21 days

VBP (PVB)

Vinblastine, I.V., 6 mg/m^2, days 1 & 2
Bleomycin, I.V., 30 units, days 1, 8, 15, (22)
Cisplatin (Platinol®), I.V., 20 mg/m^2, days 1-5

Repeat cycle every 21-28 days

Gestational Trophoblastic Cancer

DMC

Dactinomycin, I.V., 0.37 mg/m^2, days 1-5
Methotrexate, I.V., 11 mg/m^2, days 1-5
Cyclophosphamide, I.V., 110 mg/m^2, days 1-5

Repeat cycle every 21 days

Head and Neck Cancer

CAP

Cyclophosphamide, I.V., 500 mg/m^2, day 1
Doxorubicin (Adriamycin®), I.V., 50 mg/m^2, day 1
Cisplatin (Platinol®), I.V., 50 mg/m^2, day 1

Repeat cycle every 28 days

CF

Cisplatin, I.V., 100 mg/m^2, day 1
Fluorouracil, I.V., 1000 mg/m^2/day continuous infusion, days 1-5

Repeat cycle every 21-28 days

CF

Carboplatin, I.V., 400 mg/m^2, day 1
Fluorouracil, I.V., 1000 mg/m^2/day continuous infusion, days 1-5

Repeat cycle every 21-28 days

COB

Cisplatin, I.V., 100 mg/m^2, day 1
Vincristine (Oncovin®), I.V., 1 mg/m^2, days 2 & 5
Bleomycin, I.V., 30 units/day continuous infusion, days 2-5

Repeat cycle every 21 days

5-FU HURT

Hydroxyurea, P.O., 1000 mg q12h x 11 doses; start PM of admission, give 2 hours prior to radiation therapy, days 0-5
Fluorouracil, I.V., 800 mg/m^2/day continuous infusion, start AM after admission, days 1-5
Paclitaxel, I.V., 5-25 mg/m^2/day continuous infusion, start AM after admission; dose escalation study — refer to protocol, days 1-5
G-CSF, S.C., 5 mcg/kg/day, days 6-12, start ≥12 hours after completion of 5-FU infusion

5-7 cycles may be administered

MAP

Mitomycin C, I.V., 8 mg/m^2, day 1
Doxorubicin (Adriamycin®), I.V., 40 mg/m^2, day 1
Cisplatin (Platinol®), I.V., 60 mg/m^2, day 1

Repeat cycle every 28 days

MBC (MBD)

Methotrexate, I.M./I.V., 40 mg/m^2, days 1 & 15
Bleomycin, I.M./I.V., 10 units, days 1, 8, 15
Cisplatin, I.V., 50 mg/m^2, day 4

Repeat cycle every 21 days

MF

Methotrexate, I.V., 125-250 mg/m^2, day 1
Fluorouracil, I.V., 600 mg/m^2 beginning 1 h after methotrexate, day 1
Leucovorin calcium, I.V./P.O., 10 mg/m^2 q6h x 5 doses beginning 24 h after methotrexate

Repeat cycle every 7 days

PFL

Cisplatin (Platinol®), I.V., 100 mg/m^2, day 1
Fluorouracil, I.V., 600-800 mg/m^2/day continuous infusion, days 1-5
Leucovorin calcium, I.V., 200-300 mg/m^2/day, days 1-5

Repeat cycle every 21 days

PFL+IFN

Cisplatin (Platinol®), I.V., 100 mg/m^2, day 1
Fluorouracil, I.V., 640 mg/m^2/day continuous infusion, days 1-5
Leucovorin calcium, P.O., 100 mg q4h, days 1-5
Interferon alfa-2b, S.C., 2 x 10^6 units/m^2, days 1-6

Wayne State

Cisplatin (Platinol®), I.V., 100 mg/m^2 over 30 minutes, day 1
Fluorouracil, I.V., 1000 mg/m^2 continuous infusion, days 1-4 (or 5)

Repeat cycle every 21 days

Single-Agent Regimens

Carboplatin, I.V., 300-400 mg/m^2, over 2 hours every 21-28 days
Methotrexate, I.V., 40 mg/m^2, every week, escalating day 14 by 5 mg/m^2/wk as tolerated
Cisplatin I.V., 100 mg/m^2, every 28 days divided into 1, 2, or 4 equal doses per month

Leukemias

Acute Lymphoblastic, Induction

DVP

Daunorubicin, I.V., 45 mg/m^2, days 1, 2, 3, 14
Vincristine, I.V., 2 mg/m^2 (max: 2 mg), days 1, 8, 15, 22
Prednisone, P.O., 45 mg/m^2, days 1-28 (35)

DVPA

Daunorubicin, I.V., 50 mg/m^2, days 1-3
Vincristine, I.V., 2 mg, days 1, 8, 15, 22
Prednisone, P.O., 60 mg/m^2, days 1-28
Asparaginase, I.M., 6000 units/m^2, days 17-28

VAD

Vincristine, I.V., 0.4 mg continuous infusion, days 1-4
Doxorubicin (Adriamycin®), I.V., 12 mg/m^2 continuous infusion, days 1-4
Dexamethasone, P.O., 40 mg, days 1-4, 9-12, 17-20

VP

Vincristine, I.V., 2 mg/m^2/wk for 4-6 weeks (max: 2 mg)
Prednisone, P.O., 60 mg/m^2/day in divided doses for 4 weeks, taper weeks 5-7

VP-L-Asparaginase

Vincristine, I.V., 2 mg/m^2/wk for 4-6 wk (max: 2 mg)
Prednisone, P.O., 60 mg/m^2/day for 4-6 wk, then taper
L-asparaginase, I.V., 10,000 units/m^2/day

no known acronym

Cyclophosphamide, I.V., 1200 mg/m^2, day 1
Daunorubicin, I.V., 45 mg/m^2, days 1-3
Prednisone, P.O., 60 mg/m^2, days 1-21
Vincristine, I.V., 2 mg/m^2, weekly

L-asparaginase, I.V., 6000 units/m^2, 3 times/wk

or

Pegaspargase, I.M./I.V., 2500 units/m^2, every 14 days if patient develops hypersensitivity to native L-asparaginase

Acute Lymphoblastic, Maintenance

MM

Mercaptopurine, P.O., 50-75 mg/m^2, days 1-7
Methotrexate, P.O./I.V., 20 mg/m^2, day 1

Repeat cycle every 7 days

MMC (MTX + MP + CTX)*

Methotrexate, I.V., 20 mg/m^2/wk
Mercaptopurine, P.O., 50 mg/m^2/day
Cyclophosphamide, I.V., 200 mg/m^2/wk

*Continue all 3 drugs until relapse of disease or after 3 years of remission.

Acute Lymphoblastic, Relapse

AVDP

Asparaginase, I.V., 15,000 units/m^2, days 1-5, 8-12, 15-19, 22-26
Vincristine, I.V., 2 mg/m^2 (max: 2 mg), days 8, 15, 22
Daunorubicin, I.V., 30-60 mg/m^2, days 8, 15, 22
Prednisone, P.O., 40 mg/m^2, days 8-12, 15-19, 22-26

Acute Myeloid Leukemia

5+2

Induction
Cytarabine (Ara-C), I.V., 100-200 mg/m^2 continuous infusion, days 1-5
Daunorubicin, I.V., 45 mg/m^2, days 1-2

7+3

Induction
Cytarabine, I.V., 100-200 mg/m^2/day continuous infusion, days 1-7
Daunorubicin, I.V., 45 mg/m^2/day, days 1-3

Modified 7+3 (considerations in elderly patients)
Cytarabine, I.V., 100 mg/m^2/day continuous infusion, days 1-7
Daunorubicin, I.V., 30 mg/m^2/day, days 1-3

D-3+7

Induction
Daunorubicin, I.V., 45 mg/m^2, days 1-3
Cytarabine (Ara-C), I.V., 100-200 mg/m^2 continuous infusion, days 1-7

DAT/DCT

Induction
Daunorubicin, I.V., 60 mg/m^2/day, days 1-3
Cytarabine (Ara-C), I.V., 200 mg/m^2/day continuous infusion, days 1-5
Thioguanine, P.O., 100 mg/m^2 q12h, days 1-5

Modified DAT (considerations in elderly patients)
Daunorubicin, I.V., 50 mg/m^2, day 1
Cytarabine (Ara-C), S.C., 100 mg/m^2/day q12h, days 1-5
Thioguanine, P.O., 100 mg/m^2 q12h, days 1-5

HDAC

Induction
Cytarabine, I.V., 3 g/m^2 I.V. over 2-3 h q12h x 12 doses, days 1-6

Modified (considerations in elderly patients)
Cytarabine, I.V., 2 g/m^2 I.V. over 2-3 h q12h x 12 doses, days 1-6

HiDAC

Consolidation
Cytarabine (Ara-C), I.V., 3000 mg/m^2 q12h, days 1-6

or

Cytarabine (Ara-C), I.V., 3000 mg/m^2 q12h, days 1, 3, 5

I-3+7

Induction
Idarubicin, I.V., 12 mg/m^2, days 1-3
Cytarabine (Ara-C), I.V., 100 mg/m^2 continuous infusion, days 1-7

IC

Induction
Idarubicin (Idamycin®), I.V., 12 mg/m²/day, days 1-3
Cytarabine, I.V., 100-200 mg/m²/day continuous infusion, days 1-7

LDAC

Considerations in Elderly Patients
Cytarabine, S.C., 10 mg/m² bid, days 10-21

MC

Induction
Mitoxantrone, I.V., 12 mg/m²/day, days 1-3
Cytarabine, I.V., 100-200 mg/m²/day continuous infusion, days 1-7

Consolidation
Mitoxantrone, I.V., 12 mg/m², days 1-2
Cytarabine (Ara-C), I.V., 100 mg/m² continuous infusion, days 1-5

Repeat cycle every 28 days

MV

Induction
Mitoxantrone, I.V., 10 mg/m²/day, days 1-5
Etoposide (VePesid®), I.V., 100 mg/m²/day, days 1-3

Acute Nonlymphoblastic, Consolidation

CD

Cytarabine, I.V., 3000 mg/m² q12h, days 1-6
Daunorubicin, I.V., 30 mg/m²/day, days 7-9

Chronic Lymphocytic Leukemia

CHL + PRED

Chlorambucil, P.O., 0.4 mg/kg/day for 1 day every other week
Prednisone, P.O., 100 mg/day for 2 days every other week; adjust dosage according to blood counts every 2 weeks prior to therapy; increase initial dose of 0.4 mg/kg by 0.1 mg/kg every 2 weeks until toxicity or disease control is achieved

CVP

Cyclophosphamide, P.O., 400 mg/m²/day, days 1-5
Vincristine (Oncovin®), I.V., 1.4 mg/m² (max: 2 mg), day 1
Prednisone, P.O., 100 mg/m², days 1-5

Repeat cycle every 21 days

Fludarabine, I.V., 25-30 mg/m² over 30 min, days 1-5

Repeat cycle every 28 days

Cladribine (2-CdA) for fludarabine resistant, I.V., 0.1 mg/kg/day continuous infusion, days 1-7

Repeat cycle every 28 days

Lung Cancer

Small Cell

ACE/CAE

Doxorubicin (Adriamycin®), I.V., 45 mg/m², day 1
Cyclophosphamide, I.V., 1000 mg/m², day 1
Etoposide, I.V., 50 mg/m²/day, days 1-5

Repeat cycle every 21 days

CAV

Cyclophosphamide, I.V., 1000 mg/m², day 1
Doxorubicin (Adriamycin®), I.V., 50 mg/m², day 1
Vincristine, I.V., 1.4 mg/m² (max: 2 mg), day 1

Repeat cycle every 3 weeks

CAVE

Cyclophosphamide, I.V., 750 mg/m², day 1
Doxorubicin (Adriamycin®), I.V., 50 mg/m², day 1
Vincristine, I.V., 1.4 mg/m² (max: 2 mg), day 1
Etoposide, I.V., 60-100 mg/m², days 1-3

Repeat cycle every 3 weeks

CHOR*

Cyclophosphamide, I.V., 750 mg/m²/day, days 1 & 22
Doxorubicin (Adriamycin®), I.V., 50 mg/m²/day, days 1 & 22

Vincristine, I.V., 1 mg, days 1, 8, 15, 22
Radiation, total dose 3000 rad, 10 daily fractions over 2 weeks beginning with day 36, days 1, 8, 15, 22

CMC-High Dose*

Cyclophosphamide, I.V., 1000 mg/m²/day, days 1 & 29
Methotrexate, I.V., 15 mg/m²/day twice weekly for 6 weeks, days 1 & 29
Lomustine (CCNU), P.O., 100 mg/m², day 1

*If disease responds, proceed to maintenance therapy.

CODE

Cisplatin, I.V., 25 mg/m², every week for 9 weeks
Vincristine (Oncovin®), I.V., 1 mg/m², weeks 1, 2, 4, 6, 8
Doxorubicin, I.V., 25 mg/m², weeks 1, 3, 5, 7, 9
Etoposide, I.V., 80 mg/m², weeks 1, 3, 5, 7, 9

COPE

Cyclophosphamide, I.V., 750 mg/m², day 1
Vincristine (Oncovin®), I.V., 1.4 mg/m² (max: 2 mg), day 3
Cisplatin (Platinol®), I.V., 20 mg/m², days 1-3
Etoposide, I.V., 100 mg/m², days 1-3

Repeat cycle every 21 days

EC

Etoposide, I.V., 60-100 mg/m², days 1-3
Carboplatin, I.V., 400 mg/m², day 1

Repeat cycle every 28 days

EP

Etoposide, I.V., 75-100 mg/m², days 1-3
Cisplatin (Platinol®), I.V., 75-100 mg/m², day 1

Repeat cycle every 21-28 days

MICE (ICE)

Mesna uroprotection, I.V. at 20% of ifosfamide doses given immediately before and at 4 and 8 hours after ifosfamide infusion
Ifosfamide, I.V., 2000 mg/m², days 1-3
Carboplatin, I.V., 300-350 mg/m², day 1
Etoposide, I.V., 60-100 mg/m², days 1-3

PE

Cisplatin (Platinol®), I.V., 50 mg/m², day 1
Etoposide, I.V., 60 mg/m², days 1-5

Repeat cycle every 21-28 days

or

Cisplatin (Platinol®), I.V., 75 mg/m², day 2
Etoposide, I.V., 125 mg/m², days 1, 3, & 5

Repeat cycle every 28 days

or

Cisplatin (Platinol®), I.V., 100 mg/m², day 1
Etoposide, I.V., 100 mg/m², days 1-3

Repeat cycle every 28 days

POCC

Procarbazine, P.O., 100 mg/m²/day, days 1-14
Vincristine (Oncovin®), I.V., 2 mg/day (max: 2 mg), days 1 & 8
Cyclophosphamide, I.V., 600 mg/m²/day, days 1 & 8
Lomustine (CCNU), P.O., 60 mg/m², day 1

Repeat cycle every 28 days

VAC (CAV) (Induction)

Vincristine, I.V., 2 mg/m², day 1
Doxorubicin (Adriamycin®), I.V., 50 mg/m², day 1
Cyclophosphamide, I.V., 750 mg/m², day 1

Repeat cycle every 21 days x 4 cycles

VC

Etoposide (VePesid®), I.V., 100-200 mg/m², days 1-3
Carboplatin, I.V., 50-125 mg/m², days 1-3

Repeat cycle every 28 days

Single-Agent Regimen

Etoposide, P.O., 160 mg/m², days 1-5

Repeat cycle every 28 days

Nonsmall Cell

CAMP

Cyclophosphamide, I.V., 300 mg/m^2, days 1 & 8
Doxorubicin (Adriamycin®), I.V., 20 mg/m^2, days 1 & 8
Methotrexate, I.V., 15 mg/m^2, days 1 & 8
Procarbazine, P.O., 100 mg/m^2, days 1-10

Repeat cycle every 28 days

CAP

Cyclophosphamide, I.V., 400 mg/m^2, day 1
Doxorubicin (Adriamycin®), I.V., 40 mg/m^2, day 1
Cisplatin (Platinol®), I.V., 60 mg/m^2, day 1

Repeat cycle every 28 days

CV

Cisplatin, I.V., 60-80 mg/m^2, day 1
Etoposide (VePesid®), I.V., 120 mg/m^2, days 4, 6, & 8

Repeat cycle every 21-28 days

CVI

Carboplatin, I.V., 300 mg/m^2, day 1
Etoposide (VePesid®), I.V., 60-100 mg/m^2, day 1
Ifosfamide, I.V., 1.5 g/m^2, days 1, 3 & 5
Mesna, I.V., 20% of ifosfamide dose, given immediately before and 4 and 8 hours after ifosfamide infusion, days 1, 3 & 5

Repeat cycle every 28 days

EP

Etoposide, I.V., 75-100 mg/m^2, days 1-3
Cisplatin (Platinol®), I.V., 75-100 mg/m^2, day 1

Repeat cycle every 21-28 days

FAM

Fluorouracil, I.V., 600 mg/m^2, days 1, 8, 28, & 36
Doxorubicin (Adriamycin®), I.V., 30 mg/m^2, days 1 & 28
Mitomycin C, I.V., 10 mg/m^2, day 1

Repeat cycle every 56 days

FOMi*

Fluorouracil, I.V., 300 mg/m^2/day, days 1-4
Vincristine (Oncovin®), I.V., 2 mg, day 1
Mitomycin C, I.V., 10 mg/m^2, day 1

*Repeat at 3-week intervals for 3 courses; thereafter, every 6 weeks.

FOMi/CAP

Fluorouracil, I.V., 300 mg/m^2, days 1-4
Vincristine, I.V., 2 mg, day 1
Mitomycin C, I.V., 10 mg/m^2, day 1
Cyclophosphamide, I.V., 400 mg/m^2, day 28
Doxorubicin (Adriamycin®), I.V., 40 mg/m^2, day 28
Cisplatin, I.V., 40 mg/m^2, day 28

Repeat cycle every 56 days

MACC

Methotrexate, I.V., 40 mg/m^2, day 1
Doxorubicin (Adriamycin®), I.V., 40 mg/m^2, day 1
Cyclophosphamide, I.V., 400 mg/m^2, day 1
Lomustine, P.O., 30 mg/m^2, day 1

Repeat cycle every 21 days

MICE (ICE)

Mesna uroprotection, I.V. at 20% of ifosfamide doses given immediately before and at 4 and 8 hours after ifosfamide infusion
Ifosfamide, I.V., 2000 mg/m^2, days 1-3
Carboplatin, I.V., 300-350 mg/m^2, day 1
Etoposide, I.V., 60-100 mg/m^2, day 1

MVP

Mitomycin, I.V., 8 mg/m^2, days 1, 29, 71
Vinblastine, I.V., 4.5 mg/m^2, days 15, 22, 29, then every 2 weeks
Cisplatin (Platinol®), I.V., 120 mg/m^2, days 1, 29, then every 6 weeks

PFL

Cisplatin (Platinol®), I.V., 25 mg/m^2, days 1-5
Fluorouracil, I.V., 800 mg/m^2 continuous infusion, days 2-5
Leucovorin calcium, I.V., 500 mg/m^2 continuous infusion, days 1-5

Repeat cycle every 28 days

Single-Agent Regimen

Vinorelbine (Navelbine®), I.V., 30 mg/m^2, every week

Lymphoma

Hodgkin's

ABVD

Doxorubicin (Adriamycin®), I.V., 25 mg/m^2, days 1 & 15
Bleomycin, I.V., 10 units/m^2, days 1 & 15
Vinblastine, I.V., 6 mg/m^2, days 1 & 15
Dacarbazine, I.V., 150 mg/m^2, days 1-5

Repeat cycle every 28 days

or

Dacarbazine, I.V., 375 mg/m^2, days 1 & 15

ChIVPP

Chlorambucil, P.O., 6 mg/m^2, days 1-14 (max: 10 mg/day)
Vinblastine, I.V., 6 mg/m^2, days 1-8 (max: 10 mg dose)
Procarbazine, P.O., 50 mg/m^2, days 1-14 (max: 150 mg/day)
Prednisone, P.O., 40 mg/m^2, days 1-14 (25 mg/m^2 for children)

CVPP

Lomustine (CCNU), P.O., 75 mg/m^2, day 1
Vinblastine, I.V., 4 mg/m^2, days 1, 8
Procarbazine, P.O., 100 mg/m^2, days 1-14
Prednisone, P.O., 30 mg/m^2, days 1-14 (cycles 1 & 4 only)

Repeat cycle every 28 days

DHAP

Dexamethasone, P.O./I.V., 40 mg, days 1-4
Cytarabine (Ara-C), I.V., 2 g/m^2, q12h for 2 doses, day 2
Cisplatin (Platinol®), I.V., 100 mg/m^2 continuous infusion, day 1

Repeat cycle every 3-4 weeks

EVA

Etoposide, I.V., 100 mg/m^2, days 1-3
Vinblastine, I.V., 6 mg/m^2, day 1
Doxorubicin (Adriamycin®), I.V., 50 mg/m^2, day 1

Repeat cycle every 28 days

MOPP

Mechlorethamine, I.V., 6 mg/m^2, days 1 & 8
Vincristine (Oncovin®), I.V., 1.4 mg/m^2 (max: 2.5 mg), days 1 & 8
Procarbazine, P.O., 100 mg/m^2, days 1-14
Prednisone, P.O., 40 mg/m^2 (cycles 1 & 4 only), days 1-14

Repeat cycle every 28 days

MOPP/ABV Hybrid

Mechlorethamine, I.V., 6 mg/m^2, day 1
Vincristine (Oncovin®), I.V., 1.4 mg/m^2 (max: 2 mg), day 1
Procarbazine, P.O., 100 mg/m^2, days 1-7
Prednisone, P.O., 40 mg/m^2, days 1-14
Doxorubicin (Adriamycin®), I.V., 35 mg/m^2, day 8
Bleomycin, I.V., 10 units/m^2, day 8
Vinblastine, I.V., 6 mg/m^2, day 8

Repeat cycle every 28 days

MVPP

Mechlorethamine, I.V., 6 mg/m^2, days 1 & 8
Vinblastine, I.V., 6 mg/m^2, days 1 & 8
Procarbazine, P.O., 100 mg/m^2, days 1-14
Prednisone, P.O., 40 mg/m^2, days 1-14

Repeat cycle every 42 days

NOVP

Mitoxantrone (Novantrone®), I.V., 10 mg/m^2, day 1
Vincristine (Oncovin®), I.V., 2 mg, day 8
Vinblastine, I.V., 6 mg/m^2, day 1
Prednisone, P.O., 100 mg/m^2, days 1-5

Repeat cycle every 21 days

Stanford V

Mechlorethamine, I.V., 6 mg/m^2, weeks 1, 5, 9
Doxorubicin, I.V., 25 mg/m^2, weeks 1, 3, 5, 7, 9, 11
Vinblastine, I.V., 6 mg/m^2, weeks 1, 3, 5, 7, 9, 11
Vincristine, I.V., 1.4 mg/m^2, weeks 2, 4, 6, 8, 10, 12
Bleomycin, I.V., 5 units/m^2, weeks 2, 4, 6, 8, 10, 12

Etoposide, I.V., 60 mg/m^2 x 2, weeks 3, 7, 11
Prednisone, P.O., 40 mg/m^2, daily, dose tapered over the last 15 days

Non-Hodgkin's

BACOP

Bleomycin, I.V., 5 units/m^2, days 15 & 22
Doxorubicin (Adriamycin®), I.V., 25 mg/m^2, days 1 & 8
Cyclophosphamide, I.V., 650 mg/m^2, days 1 & 8
Vincristine (Oncovin®), I.V., 1.4 mg/m^2 (max: 2 mg), days 1 & 8
Prednisone, P.O., 60 mg/m^2, days 15-28

Repeat cycle every 28 days

CHOP

Cyclophosphamide, I.V., 750 mg/m^2, day 1
Doxorubicin (Hydroxydaunomycin), I.V., 50 mg/m^2, day 1
Vincristine (Oncovin®), I.V., 1.4 mg/m^2 (max: 2 mg), day 1
Prednisone, P.O., 100 mg/m^2, days 1-5

Repeat cycle every 21 days

CHOP-Bleo

Cyclophosphamide, I.V., 750 mg/m^2, day 1
Doxorubicin (Hydroxydaunomycin), I.V., 50 mg/m^2, day 1
Vincristine (Oncovin®), I.V., 2 mg, days 1 & 5
Prednisone, P.O., 100 mg, days 1-5
Bleomycin, I.V., 15 units, days 1 & 5

Repeat cycle every 21-28 days

COMLA

Cyclophosphamide, I.V., 1500 mg/m^2, day 1
Vincristine (Oncovin®), I.V., 1.4 mg/m^2 (max: 2.5 mg), days 1, 8, 15
Methotrexate, I.V., 120 mg/m^2, days 22, 29, 36, 43, 50, 57, 64, 71
Leucovorin calcium rescue, P.O., 25 mg/m^2, q6h for 4 doses, beginning 24 hours after each methotrexate dose
Cytarabine (Ara-C), I.V., 300 mg/m^2, days 22, 29, 36, 43, 50, 57, 64, 71

Repeat cycle every 21 days

COP

Cyclophosphamide, I.V., 800-1000 mg/m^2, day 1
Vincristine (Oncovin®), I.V., 1.4 mg/m^2 (max: 2 mg), day 1
Prednisone, P.O., 60 mg/m^2, days 1-5

Repeat cycle every 21 days

COP-BLAM

Cyclophosphamide, I.V., 400 mg/m^2, day 1
Vincristine (Oncovin®), I.V., 1 mg/m^2, day 1
Prednisone, P.O., 40 mg/m^2, days 1-10
Bleomycin, I.V., 15 mg, day 14
Doxorubicin (Adriamycin®), I.V., 40 mg/m^2, day 1
Procarbazine (Matulane®), P.O., 100 mg/m^2, days 1-10

COPP (or "C" MOPP)

Cyclophosphamide, I.V., 400-650 mg/m^2, days 1 & 8
Vincristine (Oncovin®), I.V., 1.4-1.5 mg/m^2 (max: 2 mg), days 1 & 8
Procarbazine, P.O., 100 mg/m^2, days 1-14
Prednisone, P.O., 40 mg/m^2, days 1-14

Repeat cycle every 28 days

CVP

Cyclophosphamide, P.O., 400 mg/m^2, days 1-5
Vincristine, I.V., 1.4 mg/m^2 (max: 2 mg), day 1
Prednisone, P.O., 100 mg/m^2, days 1-5

Repeat cycle every 21 days

DHAP

Dexamethasone (Decadron®), I.V., 10 mg q6h, days 1-4
Cytarabine (Ara-C), I.V., 2 g/m^2 q12h x 2 doses, day 2
Cisplatin (Platinol®), I.V., 100 mg/m^2 continuous infusion, day 1

Repeat cycle every 21-28 days

ESHAP

Etoposide, I.V., 60 mg/m^2, days 1-4
Cisplatin, I.V., 25 mg/m^2 continuous infusion, days 1-4
Cytarabine (Ara-C), I.V., 2 g/m^2, immediately following completion of etoposide and cisplatin therapy
Methylprednisolone, I.V., 500 mg/day, days 1-4

Repeat cycle every 21-28 days

IMVP-16

Ifosfamide, I.V., 4 g/m^2 continuous infusion over 24 h, day 1
Mesna, I.V., 800 mg/m^2 bolus prior to ifosfamide, then 4 g/m^2 continuous infusion over 12 hours concurrent w/ifosfamide; then 2.4 g/m^2 continuous infusion over 12 hours after ifosfamide infusion, day 1
Methotrexate, I.V., 30 mg/m^2, days 3 & 10
Etoposide (VePesid®), I.V., 100 mg/m^2, days 1-3

Repeat cycle every 21-28 days

MACOP-B

Methotrexate, I.V., 100 mg/m^2 weeks 2, 6, 10
Doxorubicin (Adriamycin®), I.V., 50 mg/m^2 weeks 1, 3, 5, 7, 9, 11
Cyclophosphamide, I.V., 350 mg/m^2 weeks 1, 3, 5, 7, 9, 11
Vincristine (Oncovin®), I.V., 1.4 mg/m^2 (max: 2 mg) weeks 2, 4, 8, 10, 12
Bleomycin, I.V., 10 units/m^2, weeks 4, 8, 12
Prednisone, P.O., 75 mg/day tapered over 15 d, days 1-15
Leucovorin calcium, P.O., 15 mg q6h x 6 doses 24 h after methotrexate, weeks 2, 6, 10

m-BACOD

Methotrexate, I.V., 200 mg/m^2, days 8 & 15
Leucovorin calcium, P.O., 10 mg/m^2 q6h x 8 doses beginning 24 h after each methotrexate dose, days 8 & 15
Bleomycin, I.V., 4 units/m^2, day 1
Doxorubicin (Adriamycin®), I.V., 45 mg/m^2, day 1
Cyclophosphamide, I.V., 600 mg/m^2, day 1
Vincristine (Oncovin®), I.V., 1 mg/m^2, day 1
Dexamethasone, P.O., 6 mg/m^2, days 1-5

Repeat cycle every 21 days

m-BACOS

Methotrexate, I.V., 1 g/m^2, day 2
Bleomycin, I.V., 10 units/m^2, day 1
Doxorubicin (Adriamycin®), I.V., 50 mg/m^2 continuous infusion, day 1
Cyclophosphamide, I.V., 750 mg/m^2, day 1
Vincristine (Oncovin®), I.V., 1.4 mg/m^2 (max: 2 mg), day 1
Leucovorin calcium rescue, P.O., 15 mg q6h for 8 doses, starting 24 hours after methotrexate
Methylprednisolone, I.V., 500 mg, days 1-3

Repeat cycle every 21-25 days

MINE

Mesna, I.V., 1.33 g/m^2/day concurrent with ifosfamide dose, then 500 mg P.O. 4 hours after each ifosfamide infusion, days 1-3
Ifosfamide, I.V., 1.33 g/m^2/day, days 1-3
Mitoxantrone (Novantrone®), I.V., 8 mg/m^2, day 1
Etoposide, I.V., 65 mg/m^2/day, days 1-3

Repeat cycle every 28 days

Pro-MACE

Prednisone, P.O., 60 mg/m^2, days 1-14
Methotrexate, I.V., 1.5 g/m^2, day 14
Leucovorin calcium, I.V., 50 mg/m^2 q6h x 5 doses beginning 24 h after methotrexate dose, day 14
Doxorubicin (Adriamycin®), I.V., 25 mg/m^2, days 1 & 8
Cyclophosphamide, I.V., 650 mg/m^2, days 1 & 8
Etoposide, I.V., 120 mg/m^2, days 1 & 8

Repeat cycle every 28 days

Pro-MACE-CytaBOM

Prednisone, P.O., 60 mg/m^2, days 1-14
Doxorubicin (Adriamycin®), I.V., 25 mg/m^2, day 1
Cyclophosphamide, I.V., 650 mg/m^2, day 1
Etoposide, I.V., 120 mg/m^2, day 1
Cytarabine, I.V., 300 mg/m^2, day 8
Bleomycin, I.V., 5 units/m^2, day 8
Vincristine (Oncovin®), I.V., 1.4 mg/m^2 (max: 2 mg), day 8
Methotrexate, I.V., 120 mg/m^2, day 8
Leucovorin calcium, P.O., 25 mg/m^2 q6h x 4 doses, day 9

Repeat cycle every 21 days

Malignant Melanoma

BCDT

Carmustine (BCNU), I.V., 150 mg/m^2, day 1
Cisplatin, I.V., 25 mg/m^2, days 1-3, 21-23
Dacarbazine, I.V., 220 mg/m^2, days 1-3, 21-23

Tamoxifen, P.O., 10 mg bid, days 1-42

BHD

Carmustine (BCNU), I.V., 100-150 mg/m², day 1

Repeat cycle every 42 days

Hydroxyurea, P.O., 1480 mg/m², days 1-5
Dacarbazine, I.V., 100-150 mg/m², days 1-5

Repeat cycle every 21 days

DTIC-ACTD

Dacarbazine, I.V., 750 mg/m², day 1
Dactinomycin, I.V., 1 mg/m², day 1

Repeat cycle every 28 days

VBC

Vinblastine, I.V., 6 mg/m², days 1 & 2
Bleomycin, I.V., 15 units/m²/day continuous infusion, days 1-5
Cisplatin, I.V., 50 mg/m², day 5

Repeat cycle every 28 days

VDP

Vinblastine, I.V., 5 mg/m², days 1 & 2
Dacarbazine, I.V., 150 mg/m², days 1-5
Cisplatin (Platinol®), I.V., 75 mg/m², day 5

Repeat cycle every 21-28 days

Multiple Myeloma

AC (DC)

Doxorubicin (Adriamycin®), I.V., 30 mg/m², day 1
Carmustine, I.V., 30 mg/m², day 1

Repeat cycle every 21-28 days

BCP

Carmustine (BCNU), I.V., 75 mg/m², day 1
Cyclophosphamide, I.V., 400 mg/m², day 1
Prednisone, P.O., 75 mg, days 1-7

Repeat cycle every 28 days

EDAP

Etoposide, I.V., 100-200 mg/m², days 1-4
Dexamethasone, P.O./I.V., 40 mg/m², days 1-5
Cytarabine (Ara-C), 1000 mg, day 5
Cisplatin (Platinol®), I.V., 20 mg continuous infusion, days 1-4

MeCP

Methyl-CCNU, P.O., 100 mg/m², day 1

Repeat cycle every 56 days

Cyclophosphamide, I.V., 600 mg/m², day 1
Prednisone, P.O., 40 mg/m²/day, days 1-7

Repeat cycle every 28 days

MP

Melphalan, P.O., 8 mg/m², days 1-4
Prednisone, P.O., 40 mg/m²/day, days 1-7

Repeat cycle every 28 days

M-2

Vincristine, I.V., 0.03 mg/kg (max: 2 mg), day 1
Carmustine, I.V., 0.5 mg/kg, day 1
Cyclophosphamide, I.V., 10 mg/kg, day 1
Melphalan, P.O., 0.25 mg/kg, days 1-4
Prednisone, P.O., 1 mg/kg/day, then taper next 14 days, days 1-7

Repeat cycle every 35 days

VAD

Vincristine, I.V., 0.4 mg/day continuous infusion, days 1-4
Doxorubicin (Adriamycin®), I.V., 9-10 mg/m²/day continuous infusion, days 1-4
Dexamethasone, P.O., 40 mg, days 1-4, 9-12, 17-20

Repeat cycle every 25-35 days

VBAP

Vincristine, I.V., 1 mg, day 1
Carmustine (BCNU), I.V., 30 mg/m², day 1
Doxorubicin (Adriamycin®), I.V., 30 mg/m², day 1
Prednisone, P.O., 100 mg, days 1-4

Repeat cycle every 21 days

VCAP

Vincristine, I.V., 1 mg, day 1
Cyclophosphamide, P.O., 100 mg/m^2, days 1-4
Doxorubicin (Adriamycin®), I.V., 25 mg/m^2, day 2
Prednisone, P.O., 60 mg/m^2, days 1-4

Repeat cycle every 28 days

Single-Agent Regimens

DEX

Dexamethasone, 20 mg/m^2 every morning for 4 days beginning on days 1, 9, and 17, every 14 days for 3 cycles
Interferon alfa-2b, S.C., 3 million units 3 times/week for maintenance therapy in patients with significant response to initial chemotherapy treatment

Ovarian Cancer

Epithelial

CC

Carboplatin, I.V., 300 mg/m^2, day 1
Cyclophosphamide, I.V., 600 mg/m^2, day 1

Repeat cycle every 28 days

CDC

Carboplatin, I.V., 300 mg/m^2, day 1
Doxorubicin, I.V., 40 mg/m^2, day 1
Cyclophosphamide, I.V., 500 mg/m^2, day 1

Repeat cycle every 28 days

CHAP

Cyclophosphamide, I.V., 300-500 mg/m^2, day 1
Hexamethylmelamine, P.O., 150 mg/m^2, days 1-7
Doxorubicin (Adriamycin®), I.V., 30-50 mg/m^2, day 1
Cisplatin (Platinol®), I.V., 50 mg/m^2, day 1

Repeat cycle every 28 days

CP

Cyclophosphamide, I.V., 600 mg/m^2, day 1
Cisplatin (Platinol®), I.V., 75-100 mg/m^2, day 1

Repeat cycle every 21 days

PAC (CAP)

Cisplatin (Platinol®), I.V., 50 mg/m^2, day 1
Doxorubicin (Adriamycin®), I.V., 50 mg/m^2, day 1
Cyclophosphamide, I.V., 750 mg/m^2, day 1

Repeat cycle every 21 days x 8 cycles

PT

Cisplatin (Platinol®), I.V., 75 mg/m^2 (after Taxol®), day 1
Taxol®, I.V., 135 mg/m^2, day 1

Repeat cycle every 21 days

Single-Agent Regimen

Paclitaxel, I.V., 135 mg/m^2 continuous infusion, over 24 hours
Patient must be premedicated with:
Dexamethasone 20 mg P.O., 12 and 6 h prior
Diphenhydramine 50 mg I.V., 30 min prior
Cimetidine 300 mg I.V., or ranitidine 50 mg I.V., 30 min prior

Germ Cell

BEP

Bleomycin, I.V., 30 units, days 2, 9, 16
Etoposide, I.V., 100 mg/m^2, days 1-5
Cisplatin (Platinol®), I.V., 20 mg/m^2, days 1-5

VAC

Vincristine, I.V., 1.2-1.5 mg/m^2 (max: 2 mg) weekly for 10-12 weeks, or every 2 weeks for 12 doses
Dactinomycin (Actinomycin D), I.V., 0.3-0.4 mg/m^2, days 1-5
Cyclophosphamide, I.V., 150 mg/m^2, days 1-5

Repeat every 28 days

Pancreatic Cancer

FAM

Fluorouracil, I.V., 600 mg/m^2/wk, weeks 1, 2, 5, 6, 9
Doxorubicin (Adriamycin®), I.V., 30 mg/m^2/wk, weeks 1, 5, 9
Mitomycin C, I.V., 10 mg/m^2/wk, weeks 1, 9

FMS (SMF)

Fluorouracil, I.V., 600 mg/m^2, days 1, 8, 29 & 36
Mitomycin C, I.V., 10 mg/m^2, day 1
Streptozocin, I.V., 1 g/m^2, days 1, 8, 29 & 36

Repeat cycle every 56 days

SD

Streptozocin, I.V., 500 mg/m^2, days 1-5
Doxorubicin, I.V., 50 mg/m^2, days 1 & 22

Repeat cycle every 42 days

Renal Cancer

Single-Agent Regimens

Aldesleukin (rIL-2), various dosing regimens — please refer to the literature
Interferon alfa-2b, various dosing regimens — please refer to the literature
Floxuridine, S.C., 0.1 mg/kg, days 1-14

Repeat cycle every 21 days

Vinblastine, I.V., 1.2 mg/m^2 continuous infusion, days 1-4

Sarcoma

Bony Sarcoma

AC

Doxorubicin (Adriamycin®), I.V., 75-90 mg/m^2 96-h continuous infusion
Cisplatin, I.A./I.V., 90-120 mg/m^2, 6 days

Repeat cycle every 28 days

CYVADIC

Cyclophosphamide, I.V., 600 mg/m^2, day 1
Vincristine, I.V., 1.4 mg/m^2 (max: 2 mg) weekly x 6 weeks, then on day 1 of future cycles
Doxorubicin (Adriamycin®), I.V., 15 mg/m^2/day continuous infusion, days 1-4
Dacarbazine (DTIC), I.V., 250 mg/m^2/day continuous infusion, days 1-4

Repeat cycle every 21-28 days

HDMTX

Methotrexate, I.V., 8-12 g/m^2
Leucovorin calcium, I.V./P.O., 15-25 mg q6h for at least 10 doses beginning 24 h after methotrexate dose; courses repeated weekly for 2-4 weeks, alternating with various cancer chemotherapy combination regimens

IMAC

Ifosfamide, I.V., 1.2 g/m^2/day continuous infusion, days 1-5
Mesna, I.V., 400 mg/m^2 bolus prior to ifosfamide infusion day 1, then 1.2 g/m^2/day continuous infusion days 1-5 concurrent with ifosfamide, then 600 mg/m^2 continuous infusion over 12 hours after ifosfamide infusion, days 1-5
Doxorubicin (Adriamycin®), I.V., 15 mg/m^2/day continuous infusion, days 2-5
Cisplatin, I.V./I.A., 120 mg/m^2 continuous infusion over 24 hours, day 7

Repeat cycle every 28 days

VAIE

Vincristine, I.V., 1.5 mg/m^2/day, days 1 & 5
Doxorubicin (Adriamycin®), I.V., 20 mg/m^2/day continuous infusion, days 1-4
Ifosfamide, I.V., 1800 mg/m^2/day, days 1-5
Etoposide, I.V., 50 mg/m^2/day, days 1-5

Repeat cycle every 21 days

VADRIAC — High Dose

Vincristine, I.V., 1.5 mg/m^2/day, days 1 & 5
Cyclophosphamide, I.V., 2.1 g/m^2/day, days 1 & 2

Doxorubicin (Adriamycin®), I.V., 25 mg/m^2/day continuous infusion, days 1-3

Repeat cycle every 21 days

Soft-Tissue Sarcoma

CYADIC

Cyclophosphamide, I.V., 600 mg/m^2, day 1
Doxorubicin (Adriamycin®), I.V., 15 mg/m^2/day continuous infusion, days 1-4
Dacarbazine (DTIC), I.V., 250 mg/m^2/day continuous infusion, days 1-4

Repeat cycle every 21-28 days

CYVADIC

Cyclophosphamide, I.V., 500 mg/m^2, day 1
Vincristine, I.V., 1.4 mg/m^2 (max: 2 mg), days 1 & 5
Doxorubicin (Adriamycin®), I.V., 50 mg/m^2, day 1
Dacarbazine (DTIC), I.V., 250 mg/m^2, days 1-5

Repeat cycle every 21 days

ICE

Ifosfamide, I.V., 2000 mg/m^2, days 1-3
Carboplatin, I.V., 300-600 mg/m^2, day 3
Etoposide, I.V., 100 mg/m^2, days 1-3

ID

Ifosfamide, I.V., 5 g/m^2 continuous infusion over 24 hours, day 1
Mesna, I.V., 1 g/m^2 bolus prior to ifosfamide infusion, then 4 g/m^2 continuous infusion over 32 hours, day 1
Doxorubicin, I.V., 40 mg/m^2, day 1

Repeat cycle every 21 days

MAID

Mesna, I.V., 500 mg/m^2 bolus 15 min prior to ifosfamide infusion, then q3h x 3, days 1-3
Doxorubicin (Adriamycin®), I.V., 20 mg/m^2 continuous infusion over 24 h, days 1-3
Ifosfamide, I.V., 2500 mg/m^2 over 1 h, days 1-3
Dacarbazine*, I.V., 300 mg/m^2 continuous infusion over 24 h, days 1-3

Repeat cycle every 28 days

*Adriamycin and dacarbazine may be mixed in the same bag.

VAC

Vincristine, I.V., 2 mg/m^2 (max: 2 mg) per week on weeks 1-12
Dactinomycin, I.V., 0.015 mg/kg (max: 0.5 mg) every 3 months for 5-6 courses, days 1-5
Cyclophosphamide, P.O., 2.5 mg/kg/day for 2 years

PEDIATRIC REGIMENS

ALL, Induction

DVP

Daunorubicin, I.V., 25 mg/m^2, days 1, 8
Vincristine, I.V., 1.5 mg/m^2 days 1, 8, 15, 22
Prednisone, P.O., 40 mg/m^2, days 1-29

PVDA

Prednisone, P.O., 40 mg/m^2, days 1-29
Vincristine, I.V., 1.5 mg/m^2, days 1, 8, 15, 22
Daunorubicin, I.V., 25 mg/m^2, days 1, 8
Asparaginase, I.M., 10,000 units/m^2, days 2, 4, 6, 8, 10, 12, 15, 17, 19

VPA

Vincristine, I.V., 1.5 mg/m^2, days 1, 8, 15, 22
Daunorubicin, I.V., 25 mg/m^2, days 1, 8
Asparaginase, I.M., 10,000 units/m^2, days 2, 4, 6, 8, 10, 12, 15, 17, 19

AML, Induction

DA

Daunorubicin, I.V., 45-60 mg/m^2 continuous infusion, days 1-3
Cytarabine (Ara-C), I.V., 100 mg/m^2, q12h for 5-7 days

DAT

Daunorubicin, I.V., 45 mg/m^2 continuous infusion, days 1-3
Cytarabine (Ara-C), I.V., 100 mg/m^2 continuous infusion, days 1-7

Thioguanine, P.O., 100 mg/m², days 1-7

DAV

Daunorubicin, I.V., 30 mg/m² continuous infusion, days 1-3
Cytarabine (Ara-C), I.V., 250 mg/m² continuous infusion, days 1-5
Etoposide (VePesid®), I.V., 200 mg/m² continuous infusion, days 5-7

VAPA

Vincristine, I.V., 1.5 mg/m², days 1, 5
Doxorubicin (Adriamycin®), I.V., 30 mg/m² continuous infusion, days 1, 2, 3
Prednisone, P.O., 40 mg/m², days 1-5
Cytarabine (Ara-C), I.V., 100 mg/m² continuous infusion, days 1-7

Brain Tumors

CDDP/VP

Cisplatin, I.V., 90 mg/m², day 1
Etoposide, I.V., 150 mg/m², days 2, 3

MOP

Mechlorethamine (nitrogen mustard), I.V., 6 mg/m², days 1, 8
Vincristine (Oncovin®), I.V., 1.4 mg/m², days 1, 8
Procarbazine, P.O., 100 mg/m², days 1-14

PCV

Procarbazine, P.O., 60 mg/m², days 18-21
Methyl-CCNU, P.O., 110 mg/m², day 1
Vincristine, I.V., 1.4 mg/m², days 8-29

POC

Prednisone, P.O., 40 mg/m², days 1-14
Methyl-CCNU, P.O., 100 mg/m², day 2
Vincristine, I.V., 1.5 mg/m², days 1, 8, 15

Repeat cycle every 6 weeks

"8 in 1"

Methylprednisolone, I.V., 300 mg/m², day 1
Vincristine, I.V., 1.5 mg/m², day 1
Methyl-CCNU, P.O., 75 mg/m², day 1
Procarbazine, P.O., 75 mg/m²/day, day 1
Hydroxyurea, P.O., 1500 or 3000 mg/m², day 1
Cisplatin, I.V., 60 or 90 mg/m², day 1
Cytarabine, I.V., 300 mg/m², day 1
Cyclophosphamide, I.V., 300 mg/m² **or**
dacarbazine (DTIC), I.V., 150 mg/m², day 1

Hodgkin's Lymphoma

ABVD

Doxorubicin (Adriamycin®), I.V., 25 mg/m², days 1, 15
Bleomycin, I.V., 10 units/m², days 1-15
Vinblastine, I.V., 6 mg/m², days 1, 15
Dacarbazine (DTIC), I.V., 375 mg/m², days 1, 15

Repeat cycle every 28 days

COMP

Cyclophosphamide, I.V., 500 mg/m², days 1-8
Vincristine (Oncovin®), I.V., 1.4 mg/m², days 1, 8
Methotrexate, I.V., 40 mg/m², days 1, 2
Prednisone, P.O., 40 mg/m², days 1-15

COPP

Cyclophosphamide, I.V., 500 mg/m², days 1-8
Vincristine (Oncovin®), I.V., 1.4 mg/m², days 1, 8
Procarbazine, P.O., 100 mg/m², days 1-15
Prednisone, P.O., 40 mg/m², days 1-15

MOPP

Mechlorethamine (nitrogen mustard), I.V., 6 mg/m², days 1, 8
Vincristine (Oncovin®), I.V., 1.4 mg/m², days 1, 8
Procarbazine, P.O., 100 mg/m², days 1-15
Prednisone, P.O., 40 mg/m², days 1-15

Repeat cycle every 28 days

OPA

Vincristine (Oncovin®), I.V., 1.5 mg/m², days 1, 8, 15
Prednisone, P.O., 60 mg/m², days 1-15
Doxorubicin (Adriamycin®), I.V., 40 mg/m², days 1, 15

OPPA

Vincristine (Oncovin®), I.V., 1.5 mg/m^2, days 1, 8, 15
Procarbazine, P.O., 100 mg/m^2, days 1-15
Prednisone, P.O., 60 mg/m^2, days 1-15
Doxorubicin (Adriamycin®), I.V., 40 mg/m^2, days 1, 15

Repeat cycle every 28 days

Osteosarcoma

HDMTX

Methotrexate, I.V., 12 g/m^2, weekly for 2-12 weeks
Leucovorin calcium rescue, P.O./I.V., 15 mg/m^2 q6h for 10 doses beginning 30 hours after the beginning of the 4-hour methotrexate infusion
(serum methotrexate levels must be monitored)

MTXCP-PDAdr

Methotrexate, I.V., 12 g/m^2, weekly for 2-12 weeks
Leucovorin calcium rescue, P.O./I.V., 15 mg/m^2 q6h for 10 doses beginning 30 hours after the beginning of the 4-hour methotrexate infusion
(serum methotrexate levels must be monitored)
Cisplatin (Platinol®), I.V., 100 mg/m^2, day 1
Doxorubicin (Adriamycin®), I.V., 37.5 mg/m^2, days 2, 3

MTXCP-PDAdrI

Methotrexate, I.V., 12 g/m^2, weekly for 2-12 weeks
Leucovorin calcium rescue, P.O./I.V., 15 mg/m^2 q6h for 10 doses beginning 30 hours after the beginning of the 4-hour methotrexate infusion
(serum methotrexate levels must be monitored)
Cisplatin (Platinol®), I.V., 100 mg/m^2, day 1
Doxorubicin (Adriamycin®), I.V., 37.5 mg/m^2, days 2, 3
Ifosfamide, I.V., 1.6 mg/m^2, days 1-5

Sarcomas (Bony and Soft-Tissue)

ICE

Ifosfamide, I.V., 2 g/m^2, days 2, 3, 4
Carboplatin, I.V., 300-600 mg/m^2, day 1
Etoposide, I.V., 100 mg/m^2, days 2, 3, 4

VAC + Adr

Vincristine, I.V., 1.5 mg/m^2 (max: 2 mg)
Dactinomycin, I.V., 0.5-1.5 mg/m^2, days 1-5, every other week
Cyclophosphamide, I.V., 500-1500 mg/m^2
Doxorubicin (Adriamycin®), I.V., 35-60 mg/m^2

VACAdr-IfoVP

Vincristine, I.V., 1.5 mg/m^2 (max: 2 mg), weekly
Dactinomycin, I.V., 1.5 mg/m^2 (max: 2 mg), every other week
Doxorubicin (Adriamycin®), I.V., 60 mg/m^2 continuous infusion over 24 hours
Cyclophosphamide, I.V., 1-1.5 g/m^2
Ifosfamide, I.V., 1.6-2 g/m^2, days 1-5
Etoposide, I.V., 150 mg/m^2, days 1-5

VAdrC

Vincristine, I.V., 1.5 mg/m^2 (max: 2 mg)
Doxorubicin (Adriamycin®), I.V., 35-60 mg/m^2
Cyclophosphamide, I.V., 500-1500 mg/m^2

Wilms' Tumor

VAD

Vincristine, I.V., 1.5 mg/m^2, every other week
Dactinomycin, I.V., 0.4 mg/m^2, every other week alternating with doxorubicin, I.V., 25 mg/m^2, every other week

Repeat for a total of 6 months

VAD2

Vincristine, I.V., 1.5 mg/m^2
Dactinomycin, I.V., 0.15 mg/kg, days 1-5
Doxorubicin, I.V., 20 mg/m^2, days 1-3

For calculating pediatric doses of chemotherapy agents, as a general rule 1 m^2 corresponds to about 30 kg of ideal body weight. **For children weighing <15 kg or with surface area <0.6 m^2**, the dose per m^2 of an agent listed herein should be divided by 30 and multiplied by the weight of the child (in kg) to obtain the correct dose.

CANCER PAIN MANAGEMENT

(Adapted from the Agency for Healthcare Policy and Research, Publication No. 94-0593, March, 1994)

Recommended Clinical Approach

A. **Ask** about pain regularly. **Assess** pain systematically.

B. **Believe** the patient and family in their reports of pain and what relieves it.

C. **Choose** pain control options appropriate for the patient, family, and setting.

D. **Deliver** interventions in a timely, logical, coordinated fashion.

E. **Empower** patients and their families. **Enable** patients to control their course to the greatest extent possible.

WHO three-step analgesic ladder

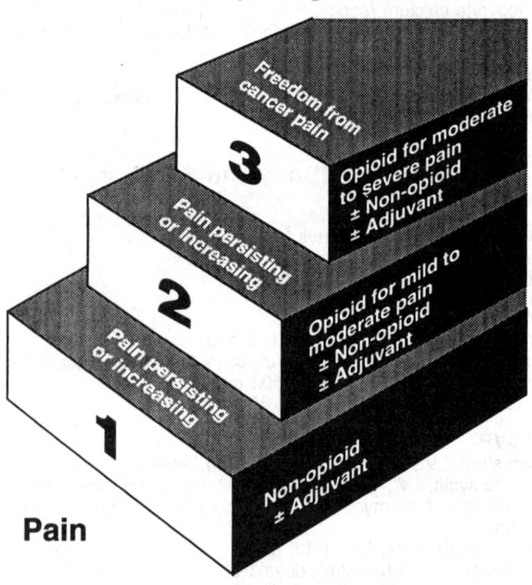

Continuing Pain Management

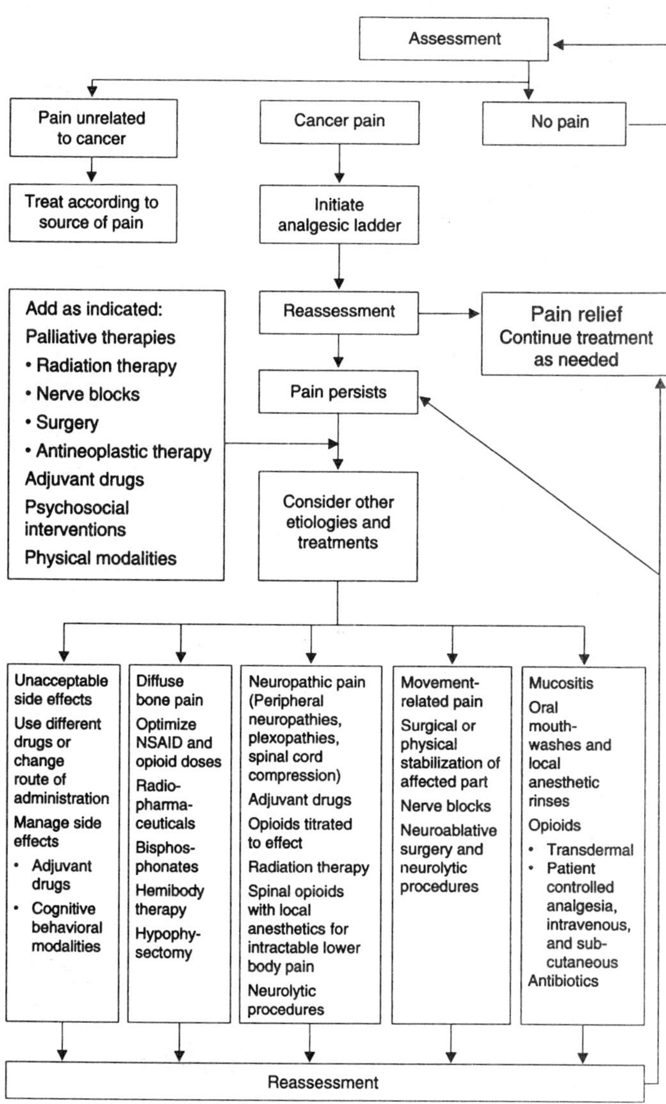

CHEMOTHERAPY COMPATIBILITY CHART

LEGEND

C = Physically & chemically compatible
P = Physically compatible for at least two hours at room temperature
S = Physically compatible for at least 5 min. in syringe
I = Incompatible
BLANK Information not available

	Blemomycin	Carboplatin	Carmustine	Chlorpromazine	Cimetidine	Cisplatin	Cyclophosphamide	Cytarabine	Dacarbazine	Dactinomycin	Daunorubicin	Dexamethasone	Diphenhydramine	Doxorubicin	Droperidol	Etoposide	Filgrastim	Floxuridine
Blemomycin						S	S					C	C	S	S		P	
Carboplatin																C	P	C
Carmustine									P								P	
Chlorpromazine					I	P	P	P					S	P	S		P	
Cimetidine				I		P	P	P				C	P	P	P		P	
Cisplatin	S			P	P		C					P	P	S	S	C	P	C
Cyclophosphamide	S			P	P	C						P	P	S	S	C	P	
Cytarabine				P	P						C	P	P		P	C	P	
Dacarbazine			P							P							P	
Dactinomycin									P								I	
Daunorubicin								C				I				C	P	
Dexamethasone	C				C	P	P	P			I		I	I			P	
Diphenhydramine	C			S	P	P	P	P				I		P	S		P	
Doxorubicin	S			P	P	S	S					I	P		S		P	
Droperidol	S			S	P	S	S	P					S	S			P	
Etoposide		C				C	C	C			C						I	C
Filgrastim	P	P	P	P	P	P	P	P	P	I	P	P	P	P	P	I		P
Floxuridine		C				C										C	P	
Fludarabine	P	P	P	I	P	P	P	P	P	P	I	P	P	P	P	P	P	P
Fluorouracil	C	I				S	C	I						S	I	C	I	C
Furosemide	S			I	C	S	P	P				P		I	I		I	
Gentamicin	C				C		P	I									P	
Haloperidol					P												P	
Heparin	C			I	P	S	S	I	I		I	P	P	I	I		I	C
Hydrocortisone	I			P				I			P	P	I	I	P		P	
Dydromorphone				S	S	P	P	P				I	S	P			P	
Hydroxyzine				S	S	P	P	P					S		S	P	P	
Idarubicin					P		P	P				I	P		P	I	P	
Ifosfamide		C				C										C	P	
Insulin, Regular					C			I										
Leucovorin	S					C	S							S	I		P	C
Lorazepam					P	P	P	P						P			P	
Melphalan	P	P	P	I	P	P	P	P	P	P	P	P	P	P	P	P	P	P
Meperidine				S	S							P	S		S		P	
Mesna		I				I											P	
Methotrexate	P			I	P	P	P	P	P			P	P	P	I		P	
Methylprednisolone					P	P	P	I						P			I	
Metoclopramide	S			S	P	S	P	P				P	P	S	S		P	
Mitomycin	S					S	S							S	S		I	
Mitoxantrone							C	C									P	
Morphine				S	P	P	P	P				P	S	P	S		P	
Ondansetron	P	P	P	P	P	P	P	P	P	P	P	P	P	P	P	P	P	P
Paclitaxel	P	P		I	P	P	P	P	P			P	P	P	P	P		P
Potassium Chloride				P	P			P				P	P		P	P	P	
Prochlorperazine				S	P	P	P	P				P	S	P	S		I	
Promethazine				S	P	P	P	P					S	P	S		P	
Ranitidine				S		P	P	P				C	P	P			P	
Sargramostim	P	P	P	I	P	P	P	P	P	P		P	P	P	P	P		P
Thiotepa						I											I	
Total Parenteral Nutrition					P			P										
Vinblastine						S	S							P	S		P	
Vincristine	C					S	S	P						S	S		P	
Vinorelbine	P	P	P	P	P	P	P	P	P	P	P	P	P		P	P	P	P

(continued)

LEGEND: C = Physically & chemically compatible; P = Physically compatible for at least two hours at room temperature; S = Physically compatible for at least 5 min. in syringe; I = Incompatible; BLANK Information not available	Fludarabine	Fluorouracil	Furosemide	Gentamicin	Haloperidol	Heparin	Hydrocortisone	Hydromorphone	Hydroxyzine	Idarubicin	Ifosfamide	Insulin, Regular	Leucovorin	Lorazepam	Melphalan	Meperidine	Mesna	Methotrexate
Blemomycin	P	C	S	C		C	I						S		P			P
Carboplatin	P	I									C				P		I	
Carmustine	P														P			
Chlorpromazine	I		I			I	P	S	S						I	S		I
Cimetidine	P		C	C	P	P		S	S	P		C		P	P	S		P
Cisplatin	P	S	S			S		P	P		C		C	P	P		I	P
Cyclophosphamide	P	C	P	P		S		P	P	P			S	P	P			P
Cytarabine	P	I	P	I		I	I	P	P	P		I		P	P			P
Dacarbazine	P					I									P			P
Dactinomycin	P														P			
Daunorubicin	I					I	P								P			
Dexamethasone	P		P			P	P	I		I					P	P		P
Diphenhydramine	P					P	I	S	S	P					P	S		P
Doxorubicin	P	S	I			I	I	P					S	P	P			P
Droperidol	P	I	I			I	P		S	P			I		P	S		I
Etoposide	P	C							P	I	C				P			
Filgrastim	P	I	I	P	P	I	P	P	P	P	P		P	P	P	P	P	P
Floxuridine	P	C				C							C		P			
Fludarabine		P	P	P	P	P	P	P	I		P			P	P	P	P	P
Fluorouracil	P		S			S	P				C		C		P			C
Furosemide	P	S		I		P	P			I			S		S	I		S
Gentamicin	P		I			I		P		I		P			P	P		
Haloperidol	P					I									P			
Heparin	P	S	P	I	I		I			I		P	S		P	I		S
Hydrocortisone	P	P	P			P				I		P			P	P		
Dydromorphone	P			P					S						P			P
Hydroxyzine	I							S							P	S	P	P
Idarubicin			I	I		I	I							I	P	I		I
Ifosfamide	P	C													P		C	
Insulin, Regular				P		P	P									P		
Leucovorin		C	S			S												S
Lorazepam	P									I					P			P
Melphalan	P	P	S	P	P	P	P	P	P	P	P			P		P	P	P
Meperidine	P		I	P		I	P		S	I		P			P			
Mesna	P								P		C				P			
Methotrexate	P	C	S			S		P	P	I			S	P	P			
Methylprednisolone	P					S	P						S		P	P		P
Metoclopramide	P	S	I			S	P		S	P		P	S		P	S		P
Mitomycin		S	S			S							S		P			P
Mitoxantrone	P	C					P								P			
Morphine	P		S	P		P	P		S			P			P	I		P
Ondansetron	P	I	I	P	P	P	P	C	P		P			I	P	P	P	P
Paclitaxel		P	P	P	P	P	P	P	I		P			P		P	P	P
Potassium Chloride	P	P	P			P	P			P		P			P	P		
Prochlorperazine	I		I			P	I	I	S						P	S		P
Promethazine	P		I			I	I	S	S							P		I
Ranitidine	P		C	P		C		S	I	P		C		P	P	S		P
Sargramostim		P	P	P	I	P	I	I	I	P	P			I		P	P	P
Thiotepa															P			
Total Parenteral Nutrition		C	P	P		P				P		P				P		
Vinblastine	P	S	I			I							S		P			P
Vincristine	P	P	I			S				I			S		P			P
Vinorelbine	P	I	I	P	P	P	P	P	P	P	P		P	P	P	P	P	P

(continued)

LEGEND

C = Physically & chemically compatible
P = Physically compatible for at least two hours at room temperature
S = Physically compatible for at least 5 min. in syringe
I = Incompatible
BLANK Information not available

	Methylprednisolone	Metoclopramide	Mitomycin	Mitoxantrone	Morphine	Ondansetron	Paclitaxel	Potassium Chloride	Prochlorperazine	Promethazine	Ranitidine	Sargramostim	Thiotepa	Total Parenteral Nutrition	Vinblastine	Vincristine	Vinorelbine
Blemomycin		S	S			P	P					P			C	C	P
Carboplatin						P	P					P					P
Carmustine						P						P					P
Chlorpromazine		S			S	P	I	P	S	S	S	I					P
Cimetidine	P	P			P	P	P	P	P	P		P		P			P
Cisplatin	P	S	S		P	P	P		P	P	P	P	I		S	S	P
Cyclophosphamide	P	P	S	C	P	P	P		P	P	P	P			S	S	P
Cytarabine	I	P		C	P	P	P	P	P	P	P	P		P		P	P
Dacarbazine						P	P					P					P
Dactinomycin						P						P					P
Daunorubicin						P											P
Dexamethasone		P			P	P	P	P	P		C	P					P
Diphenhydramine		P			S	P	P	P	S	S	P	P					P
Doxorubicin	P	S	S		P	P	P		P	P	P	P			P	S	
Droperidol		S	S		S	P	P	P	S	S		P			S	S	P
Etoposide						P	P	P				P					P
Filgrastim	I	P	I	P	P	P		P	I	P	P		I		P	P	P
Floxuridine						P	P					P					P
Fludarabine	P	P		P	P	P		P	I	P	P				P	P	P
Fluorouracil		S	S	C		I	P	P				P		C	S	P	I
Furosemide		I	S		S	I	P	P	I	I	C	P		P	I	I	I
Gentamicin					P	P	P				P	P		P			P
Haloperidol						P	P					I					P
Heparin	S	S	S		P	P	P	P	P	I	C	P		P	I	S	P
Hydrocortisone	P	P		P	P	P	P	P	I	I		I					P
Dydromorphone						C	P		I	S	S	I					P
Hydroxyzine		S			S	P	I		S	S	I	I					P
Idarubicin		P						P			P	P		P		I	P
Ifosfamide						P	P					P					P
Insulin, Regular		P			P			P			C			P			
Leucovorin	S	S	S												S	S	
Lorazepam						I	P				P	I					P
Melphalan	P	P	P	P	P	P		P	P	P	P		P		P	P	P
Meperidine	P	S			I	P	P	P	S	S	S	P		P			P
Mesna						P	P					P					P
Methotrexate	P	P	P		P	P	P		P	I	P	P			P	P	P
Methylprednisolone		P			P	I	I	I				I					I
Metoclopramide	P		S		S	P	P	P	S	S	S	P		P	S	S	P
Mitomycin		S				P						I			P	P	I
Mitoxantrone						P	I	C				P					P
Morphine	P	S				C	P	P	S	S	S	I		P			P
Ondansetron	I	P	P	P	C		P	P	P	P	P	I			P	P	P
Paclitaxel	I	P		I	P	P		P	P		P				P	P	
Potassium Chloride	I	P		C	P	P	P		P	S	P	P					P
Prochlorperazine		S			S	P	P	P		S	S	P					P
Promethazine		S			S	P		S	S		S	P					P
Ranitidine		S			S	P	P	P	S	S		P		P			P
Sargramostim	I	P	I	P	I	I		P	P	P	P			P	P	P	
Thiotepa																	I
Total Parenteral Nutrition		P			P						P	P					
Vinblastine		S	P			P	P					P				S	P
Vincristine		S	P			P	P					P			S		P
Vinorelbine	I	P	I	P	P	P		P	P	P	P		I		P	P	

DOSE EQUIVALENTS FOR OPIOID ANALGESICS IN OPIOID-NAIVE ADULTS ≥50 kg*

Drug	Approximate Equianalgesic Dose		Usual Starting Dose for Moderate to Severe Pain	
	Oral	Parenteral	Oral	Parenteral
Opioid Agonist†				
Hydromorphone‡ (Dilaudid®)	7.5 mg q3-4h	1.5 mg q3-4h	6 mg q3-4h	1.5 mg q3-4h
Levorphanol (Levo-Dromoran®)	4 mg q6-8h	2 mg q6-8h	4 mg q6-8h	2 mg q6-8h
Meperidine (Demerol®)	300 mg q2-3h	100 mg q3h	NA	100 mg q3h
Methadone (Dolophine®, others)	20 mg q6-8h	10 mg q6-8h	20 mg q6-8h	10 mg q6-8h
Morphine‡	30 mg q3-4h (repeat around-the-clock dosing) 60 mg q3-4h (single dose or intermittent dosing)	10 mg q3-4h	30 mg q3-4h	10 mg q3-4h
Morphine, controlled-release‡ (MS Contin®, Oramorph®)	90-120 mg q12h	NA	90-120 mg q12h	NA
Oxycodone (OxyContin®, others)	40-60 mg q12h	N/A	10-20 mg q12h	N/A
Oxymorphone‡ (Numorphan®)	NA	1 mg q3-4h	NA	1 mg q3-4h
Combination Opioid/NSAID Preparations				
Codeine (with aspirin or acetaminophen)	180-200 mg q3-4h	130 mg q3-4h	60 mg q3-4h	60 mg q2h (I.M., S.C.)
Hydrocodone (in Lorcet®, Lortab®, Vicodin®, others)	30 mg q3-4h	NA	10 mg q3-4h	NA
Oxycodone (Roxicodone®, also in Percocet®, Percodan®, Tylox®, others)	30 mg q3-4h	NA	10 mg q3-4h	TNA

*__Caution:__ Recommended doses do not apply for adult patients with body weight <50 kg. For recommended starting doses for adults <50 kg body weight, see following table of Dose Equivalents for Opioid Analgesics in Opioid-Naive Adults <50 kg.

†**Caution:** Recommended doses do not apply to patients with renal or hepatic insufficiency or other conditions affecting drug metabolism and kinetics.

‡**Caution:** For morphine, hydromorphone, and oxymorphone, rectal administration is an alternate route for patients unable to take oral medications. Equianalgesic doses may differ from oral and parenteral.

DOSE EQUIVALENTS FOR OPIOID ANALGESICS IN OPIOID-NAIVE ADULTS <50 kg

Drug	Approximate Equianalgesic Dose		Usual Starting Dose for Moderate to Severe Pain	
	Oral	Parenteral	Oral	Parenteral
Opioid Agonist*				
Hydromorphone† (Dilaudid®)	7.5 mg q3-4h	1.5 mg q3-4h	0.06 mg/kg q3-4h	0.015 mg/kg q3-4h
Levorphanol (Levo-Dromoran®)	4 mg q6-8h	2 mg q6-8h	0.04 mg/kg q6-8h	0.02 mg/kg q6-8h
Meperidine (Demerol®)	300 mg q2-3h	100 mg q3h	NA	0.75 mg/kg q2-3h
Methadone (Dolophine®, others)	20 mg q6-8h	10 mg q6-8h	0.2 mg/kg q6-8h	0.1 mg/kg q6-8h
Morphine‡	30 mg q3-4h (repeat around-the-clock dosing) 60 mg q3-4h (single dose or intermittent dosing)	10 mg q3-4h	0.3 mg/kg q3-4h	0.1 mg/kg q3-4h
Morphine, controlled-release†,§ (MS Contin®, Oramorph®)	90-120 mg q12h	NA	NA	NA
Combination Opioid/NSAID Preparations				
Codeine (with aspirin or acetaminophen)	180-200 mg q3-4h	130 mg q3-4h	0.5-1 mg/kg q3-4h	NA
Hydrocodone (in Lorcet®, Lortab®, Vicodin®, others)	30 mg q3-4h	NA	0.2 mg/kg q3-4h	NA
Oxycodone (Roxicodone®, also in Percocet®, Percodan®, Tylox®, others)	30 mg q3-4h	NA	0.2 mg/kg q3-4h	NA

***Caution:** Recommended doses do not apply to patients with renal or hepatic insufficiency or other conditions affecting drug metabolism and kinetics.

†**Caution:** For morphine, hydromorphone, and oxymorphone, rectal administration is an alternate route for patients unable to take oral medications. Equianalgesic doses may differ from oral and parenteral doses because of pharmacokinetic differences. **Note:** A short-acting opioid should normally be used for initial therapy of moderate to severe pain.

§Transdermal fentanyl (Duragesic®) is an alternative option. Transdermal fentanyl dosage is not calculated as equianalgesic to a single morphine dosage. See the package insert for dosing calculations. Doses >25 mcg/hour should not be used in opioid-naive patients.

DOSING DATA FOR ACETAMINOPHEN AND NSAIDs

Drug	Usual Dose for Adults >50 kg Body Weight	Usual Dose for Adults* <50 kg Body Weight
Acetaminophen and Over-the-Counter NSAIDs		
Acetaminophen†	650 mg q4h	10-15 mg/kg q4h
	975 mg q6h	15-20 mg/kg q4h (rectal)
Aspirin‡	650 mg q4h	10-15 mg/kg q4h
	975 mg q6h	15-20 mg/kg q4h (rectal)
Ibuprofen (Motrin®, others)	400-600 mg q6h	10 mg/kg q6-8h
Prescription NSAIDs		
Carprofen (Rimadyl®)	100 mg tid	
Choline magnesium trisalicylate (Trilisate®)§	1000-1500 mg tid	25 mg/kg tid
Choline salicylate (Arthropan®)§	870 mg q3-4h	
Diflunisal (Dolobid®)¶	500 mg q12h	
Etodolac (Lodine®)	200-400 mg q6-8h	
Fenoprofen calcium (Nalfon®)	300-600 mg q6h	
Ketoprofen (Orudis®)	25-60 mg q6-8h	
Ketorolac tromethamine (Toradol)#	10 mg q4-6h to a maximum of 40 mg/d	
Magnesium salicylate (Doan's®, Magan®, Mobidin®, others)	650 mg q4h	
Meclofenamate sodium (Meclomen®)•	50-100 mg q6h	
Mefenamic acid (Ponstel®)	250 mg q6h	
Naproxen (Naprosyn®)	250-275 mg q6-8h	5 mg/kg q8h
Naproxen sodium (Anaprox®)	275 mg q6-8h	
Sodium salicylate	325-650 mg q3-4h	
Parenteral NSAIDs		
Ketorolac tromethamine#,♦ (Toradol®)	60 mg initially, then 30 mg q6h; intramuscular dose not to exceed 5 days	

*Acetaminophen and NSAID dosages for adults weighing <50 kg should be adjusted for weight.

†Acetaminophen lacks the peripheral anti-inflammatory and antiplatelet activities of the other NSAIDs

‡The standard against which other NSAIDs are compared. May inhibit platelet aggregation for ≥1 week and may cause bleeding.

§May have minimal antiplatelet activity.

¶Administration with antacids may decrease absorption

#For short-term use only.

•Coombs'-positive autoimmune hemolytic anemia has been associated with prolonged use.

♦Has the same GI toxicities as oral NSAIDs.

Note: Only the above NSAIDs have FDA approval for use as simple analgesics, but clinical experience has been gained with other drugs as well.

DRUGS AND ROUTES OF ADMINISTRATION NOT RECOMMENDED FOR TREATMENT OF CANCER PAIN

Class	Drug	Rationale for Not Recommending
Antagonist	Naloxone Naltrexone	May precipitate withdrawal. Limit use to treatment of life-threatening respiratory depression.
Anxiolytics alone	Benzodiazepine (eg, alprazolam)	Analgesic properties not demonstrated except for some instances of neuropathic pain. Added sedation from anxiolytics may limit opioid dosing.
Combination preparations	Brompton's cocktail	No evidence of analgesic benefit to using Brompton's cocktail over single opioid analgesics.
	DPT (meperidine, promethazine, and chlorpromazine)	Efficacy is poor compared with that of other analgesics; high incidence of adverse effects.
Opioid agonist-antagonists	Pentazocine Butorphanol Nalbuphine	Risk of precipitating withdrawal in opioid-dependent patients. Analgesic ceiling. Possible production of unpleasant psychomimetic effects (eg, dysphoria, hallucinations).
Opioids	Meperidine	Short (2-3 hour) duration; repeated administration may lead to CNS toxicity (tremor, confusion, or seizures). High oral doses required to relieve severe pain, and these increase the risk of CNS toxicity.
Partial agonist	Buprenorphine	Analgesic ceiling; can precipitate withdrawal
Sedative/ hypnotic drugs alone	Barbiturates Benzodiazepines	Analgesic properties not demonstrated. Added sedation from sedative/hypnotic drugs limits opioid dosing.
Miscellaneous	Cannabinoids	Side effects of dysphoria, drowsiness, hypotension, and bradycardia preclude its routine use as an analgesic.
	Cocaine	Has demonstrated no efficacy as an analgesic or coanalgesic in combination with opioids.

Routes of Administration	Rationale for Not Recommending
Intramuscular (I.M.)	Painful. Absorption unreliable. Should not be used for children or patients prone to develop dependent edema or in patients with thrombocytopenia.
Transnasal	The only drug approved by the FDA for transnasal administration at this time is butorphanol, an agonist-antagonist drug which generally is not recommended. (See opioid agonist-antagonists above).

EXTRAVASATION MANAGEMENT OF CHEMOTHERAPEUTIC AGENTS

Risk Factors for Extravasation

- Vascular disease
- Elderly patients
- Vascular obstruction
- Vascular ischemia
- Prior radiation
- Small vessel diameter
- Venous spasms
- Traumatic catheter or needle insertion
- Decreased lymphatic drainage in mastectomy patients

Purpose

To minimize harm caused to the patient by the extravasation of vesicant chemotherapeutic agents through prompt detection and treatment.

Procedure

1. Stop administration of the chemotherapeutic agent.

2. Leave the needle in place.

3. Aspirate any residual drug and blood in the I.V. tubing, needle, and suspected extravasation site.

4. For all drugs except mechlorethamine (nitrogen mustard), remove the needle.

5. Apply cold pack if the extravasated drug is amsacrine, doxorubicin, daunorubicin, or mechlorethamine. Apply a hot pack if the extravasated drug is etoposide, teniposide, navelbine, vinblastine, vincristine, or vindesine. Refer to individual drug in Alphabetical Listing of Drugs for appropriate management.

6. Notify the physician who ordered the chemotherapy of the suspected extravasation. Institute the attached recommended interventions unless countermanded by the physician.

7. Document the date, time, needle size and type, insertion site, drug sequence, drug administration technique, approximate amount of drug extravasated, management, patient complaints, appearance of site, physician notification, and follow-up measures.

8. The extravasation site should be evaluated by the physician as soon as possible after the extravasation and periodically thereafter as indicated by symptoms.

9. For inpatients, assess the site every day for pain, erythema, induration, or skin breakdown. For outpatients, contact the patient daily for 3 days for assessment of the site, and weekly thereafter until the problem is resolved.

10. The plastic surgery service should be consulted by the physician if pain and/or tissue breakdown occur.

Amsacrine/Daunorubicin/Doxorubicin/Epirubacin/Idarubicin

1. Apply cold pack immediately for 1 hour; repeat qid for 3-5 days.[1,2]

2. Dimethyl sulfoxide (DMSO) 50% to 99% (w/v) solution: Apply 1.5 mL to site every 6 hours for 14 days; allow to air dry, do not cover.[3]

3. Injection of sodium bicarbonate is contraindicated.[4]

4. Injection of hydrocortisone is of doubtful benefit.[4,5]

Mechlorethamine (nitrogen mustard)

1. Mix 4 mL of 10% sodium thiosulfate with 6 mL of sterile water for injection.
2. Inject 4 mL of this solution into the existing I.V. line.
3. Remove the needle.
4. Inject 2-3 mL of the solution subcutaneously clockwise into the infiltrated area using a 25-gauge needle. Change the needle with each new injection.
5. Apply ice immediately for 6-12 hours.

Mitomycin

1. Data is not currently available regarding potential antidotes and the application of heat or cold.
2. The site should be observed closely. These injuries frequently cause necrosis. A plastic surgery consult may be required.
3. Dimethyl sulfoxide (DMSO) 50% to 99% (w/v) solution: Apply 1.5 mL to site every 6 hours for 14 days; allow to air dry, do not cover.[3]

Etoposide/Teniposide/Navelbine/Vinblastine/Vincristine/Vindesine[6]

1. Inject 3-5 mL of hyaluronidase (150 units/mL) subcutaneously clockwise into the infiltrated area using a 25-gauge needle. Change the needle with each injection.
2. Apply heat immediately for 1 hour; repeat qid for 3-5 days.
3. Application of cold is contraindicated.
4. Injection of hydrocortisone is contraindicated.

Footnotes

1. Dorr RT, Alberts DS, and Stone A, "Cold Protection and Heat Enhancement of Doxorubicin Skin Toxicity in the Mouse," *Cancer Treat Rep*, 1985, 69:431-7.
2. Larson D, "What Is the Appropriate Management of Tissue Extravasation by Antitumor Agents?" *Plastic & Reconstr Surg*, 1985, 75:397-402.
3. Oliver IW, Aisner J, Hament A, et al, "A Prospective Study of Topical Dimethyl Sulfoxide for Treating Anthracycline Extravasation," *J Clin Onc*, 1988, 6:1732-5.
4. Dorr RT, Alberts DS, and Chen HS, "Limited Role of Corticosteroids in Ameliorating Experimental Doxorubicin Skin Toxicity in the Mouse," *Canc Chemother and Pharmacol*, 1980, 5:17-20.
5. Coleman JJ, Walker AP, and Didolkar MS, "Treatment of Adriamycin Induced Skin Ulcers: A Prospective Controlled Study," *J Surg Oncol*, 1983, 22:129-35.
6. Dorr RT and Alberts DS, "Vinca Alkaloid Skin Toxicity Antidote and Drug Disposition Studies in the Mouse," *JNCI*, 1985, 74:113-20.

EXTRAVASATION TREATMENT OF OTHER DRUGS

Medication Extravasated	Cold/ WarmPack	Antidote
Vasopressors		
Dobutamine Dopamine Epinephrine Norepinephrine Phenylephrine	None	Phentolamine (Regitine®) Mix 5 mg with 9 mL of NS Inject a small amount of this dilution into extravasated area. Blanching should reverse immediately. Monitor site. If blanching should recur, additional injections of phentolamine may be needed.
I.V. Fluids and Other Medications		
Aminophylline Calcium Dextrose, 10% Electrolyte solutions Esmolol Magnesium sulfate Metoprolol Nafcillin Parenteral nutrition preparations Phenytoin Potassium Radiocontrast media Sodium solutions	Cold	Hyaluronidase (Wydase®) 1. Add 1 mL NS to 150-unit vial to make 150 units/mL 2. Mix 0.1 mL of above with 0.9 mL NS in 1 mL syringe to make final concentration = 15 units/mL 3. Inject 5 injections of 0.2 mL each with a 25-gauge needle into area of extravasation

TOXICITIES OF CHEMOTHERAPEUTIC AGENTS

Drug	Radiation-Recall Reactions	Ocular Toxicity	Pulmonary Toxicity	Cardiotoxicity	Hepatotoxicity	Cumulative Myelosuppression	Peripheral Neuropathy	CNS Depression	Alopecia
Allopurinol		x							
Altretamine							x		
Ara-C					x			x	
Azathioprine					x				
BCNU (carmustine)			x		x	x			x
Bleomycin	x		x						x
Busulfan		x	x		x				
Carboplatin						x	x		
CCNU (lomustine)			x		x				
Chlorambucil		x	x		x				
Cisplatin		x			x		x		
Cladribine						x			
Corticosteroids		x							
Cyclophosphamide		x	x	x*	x				x
Cytarabine		x	x						
Dactinomycin	x		x		x				x
Daunomycin				x†					
2'-Deoxycoformycin		x							
Docetaxel (Taxotere®)		x					x		x
Doxorubicin	x	x	x	x†	x				x
Etoposide	x		x		x				x
Floxuridine				x	x				x

(continued)

Drug	Radiation-Recall Reactions	Ocular Toxicity	Pulmonary Toxicity	Cardiotoxicity	Hepatotoxicity	Cumulative Myelosuppression	Peripheral Neuropathy	CNS Depression	Alopecia
Fludarabine			x			x			
Fluorouracil		x		x‡	x			x	x
G-CSF			x						
Gemcitabine									
Hydroxyurea	x								x
Idarubicin				x†					
Ifosfamide			x					x	x
Interferon		x	x						
Irinotecan			x						x
L-asparaginase			x		x			x	
Melphalan			x			x			
Mercaptopurine					x				
Methotrexate	x	x	x						x
Methyl-CCNU (semustine)			x			x			
Mithramycin		x							
Mitomycin-C		x	x			x			
Mitotane		x							
Mitoxantrone				x†					
Nitrogen mustard		x							x
Nitrosoureas		x							

(continued)

Drug	Radiation-Recall Reactions	Ocular Toxicity	Pulmonary Toxicity	Cardiotoxicity	Hepatotoxicity	Cumulative Myelosuppression	Peripheral Neuropathy	CNS Depression	Alopecia
Paclitaxel (Taxol®)				x			x		
Procarbazine			x			x		x	
Streptozocin					x				
Tamoxifen		x	x						
Teniposide			x						
Topotecan			x			x	x		x
Trimetrexate	x								
Vinblastine	x	x	x		x		x		x
Vincristine		x	x				x		x
Vinorelbine			x				x		

Adapted from Patterson W and Perry MC, "Chemotherapeutic Toxicities: A Comprehensive Overview," *Contemporary Oncology*, 1993, 3(7):58-61.

G-CSF = granulocyte-colony stimulating factor.

*At high dose

†Dose-related

‡Idiosyncratic

ADRENERGIC AGONISTS, CARDIOVASCULAR

Drug	Hemodynamic Effects			
	CO	TPR	Mean BP	Renal Perfusion
Amrinone	↑	↓	<–>	↑
Dobutamine	↑	↓	↑	<–>
Dopamine	↑	+/–*	<–>/↑*	↑*
Epinephrine	↑	↓	↑	↓
Isoproterenol	↑	↓	↓	+/–†
Metaraminol	↓	↑	↑	↓
Milrinone	↑	↓	<–>	↑
Norepinephrine	<–>/↓	↑	↑	↓
Phenylephrine	↓	↑	↑	↓

↑ = increase ↓ = decrease, <–> = no change, * = dose dependent

†In patients with cardiogenic or septic shock, renal perfusion commonly increases; however, in the normal patient, renal perfusion may be reduced with isoproterenol.

Drug	Hemodynamic Effects			
	α1	β1	β2	Dopamine
Dobutamine (Dobutrex®)	+	++++	++	0
Dopamine (Inotropin®)	++++	++++	++	++
Epinephrine (Adrenalin®)	++++	++++	++	++
Isoproterenol (Isuprel®)	0	++++	++++	0
Norepinephrine (Levophed®)	++++	++++	0	0

ANGIOTENSIN-CONVERTING ENZYME INHIBITORS

Comparisons of Indications and Adult Dosages

Drug	Hypertension	CHF	Renal Dysfunction	Dialyzable	Tablet Strengths (mg)
Benazepril	20-80 mg qd qd-bid Maximum: 80 mg qd	Not FDA approved	Cl_{cr} <30 mL/min: 5 mg/day initially Maximum: 40 mg qd	Yes	5, 10, 20, 40
Captopril	25-150 mg qd bid-tid Maximum: 450 mg qd	6.25-100 mg tid Maximum: 450 mg qd	Cl_{cr} 10-50 mL/min: 75% of usual dose Cl_{cr} <10 mL/min: 50% of usual dose	Yes	12.5, 25, 50, 100
Enalapril	5-40 mg qd qd-bid Maximum: 40 mg qd	2.5-20 mg bid Maximum: 20 mg bid	Cl_{cr} 30-80 mL/min: 5 mg/day initially Cl_{cr} <30 mL/min: 2.5 mg/day initially	Yes	2.5, 5, 10, 20
(Enalaprilat*)	(0.625 mg, 1.25 mg, 2.5 mg q6h Maximum: 5 mg q6h)	(Not FDA approved)	Cl_{cr} <30 mL/min: 0.625 mg)	(Yes)	(2.5 mg/2 mL vial)
Fosinopril	10-40 mg qd Maximum: 80 mg qd	10-40 mg qd	No dosage reduction necessary	Not well dialyzed	10, 20
Lisinopril	10-40 mg qd Maximum: 80 mg qd	5-20 mg qd	Cl_{cr} 10-30 mL/min: 5 mg/day initially Cl_{cr} <10 mL/min: 2.5 mg/day initially	Yes	5, 10, 20, 40
Losartan**	25-100 mg qd or bid		No adjustment needed	No	25, 50
Moexipril	7.5-30 mg qd qd-bid Maximum: 30 mg qd	Not FDA approved	Cl_{cr} <30 mL/min: 3.75 mg/day initially Maximum: 15 mg/day	Unknown	7.5, 15
Quinapril	10-80 mg qd qd-bid	5-20 mg bid	Cl_{cr} 30-60 mL/min: 5 mg/day initially Cl_{cr} <10 mL/min: 2.5 mg qd initially	Not well dialyzed	5, 10, 20, 40
Ramipril	2.5-20 mg qd qd-bid	2.5-20 mg qd	Cl_{cr} <40 mL/min: 1.25 mg/day Maximum: 5 mg qd	Unknown	1.25, 2.5, 5
Trandolapril	2-4 mg qd maximum: 8 mg/d qd-bid	Not FDA approved	Cl_{cr} <30 mL/min: 0.5 mg/day initially	No	1 mg, 2 mg, 4 mg
Valsartan**	80-160 mg qd		Decrease dose only if Cl_{cr} <10 mL/minute	No	

*Enalaprilat is the only available ACEI in a parenteral formulation.

**Angiotensin II antagonist

Dosage is based on 70 kg adult with normal hepatic and renal function.

Comparative Pharmacokinetics

Drug	Prodrug	Lipid Solubility	Absorption (%)	Serum $t_{1/2}$ (h)	Serum Protein Binding (%)	Elimination	Onset of Hypotensive Action (h)	Peak Hypotensive Effects (h)	Duration of Hypotensive Effects (h)
Benazepril	Yes	No data	37	10-12	>95	Primarily renal, some biliary	0.5-1	0.5-1	24
Benazeprilat									
Captopril	No	Not very lipophilic	75	<2	25-30	Metabolism to disulfide, then renally	0.25-0.5	0.5-1.5	6-12
Enalapril	Yes	Lipophilic	60 (53-73)	1.3	50-60	Renal	1	4-6	24
Enalaprilat				11			0.25	3-4	~6
Fosinopril	Yes	Very lipophilic	36	12	>95	Renal 50% Hepatic 50%	1	~3	24
Fosinoprilat									
Lisinopril	No	Very hydrophilic	25 (6-60)	12	0	Renal	1	~7	24
Moexipril	Yes	No data		2-9	≥50	Urine 13% Feces 53%	1		24
Quinapril	Yes	No data	60	0.8	97	Renal 61% Hepatic 37%	1	1	24
Quinaprilat				2					
Ramipril	Yes	Somewhat lipophilic	50-100	1-2	73	Renal	1-2	1	24
Ramiprilat				13-17	56				
Trandolapril	Yes	Very lipophilic	10-70	0.6-1.1	80	Hepatic Renal	0.5	2-4	≥24
Trandolaprilat			40-60	16-24	94				

ANTACID DRUG INTERACTIONS

Drug	Antacid				
	Al Salts	Ca Salts	Mg Salts	$NaHCO_3$	Mg/Al
Allopurinol	↓				
Anorexiants				↑	
Benzodiazepines	↑		↓	↓	↓
Calcitriol			x*		x*
Captopril					↓
Cimetidine	↓		↓		↓
Corticosteroids	↓		↓		↓
Digoxin	↓		↓		
Flecainide				↑	
Indomethacin	↓		↓		↓
Iron	↓	↓	↓	↓	↓
Isoniazid	↓				
Ketoconazole				↓	↓
Levodopa					↑
Lithium				↓	
Naproxen	↑		↑	↓	↑
Nitrofurantoin			↓		
Penicillamine	↓		↓		↓
Phenothiazines	↓		↓		↓
Phenytoin		↓			↓
Quinidine		↑	↑		↑
Quinolones	↓	↓	↓		↓
Ranitidine	↓				↓
Salicylates				↓	↓
Sodium polystyrene sulfonate	x†		x†		x†
Sulfonylureas				↑	
Sympathomimetics				↑	
Tetracyclines	↓	↓	↓	↓	↓
Tolmetin				x‡	

Pharmacologic effect increased (↑) or decreased (↓) by antacids.

*Concomitant use in patients on chronic renal dialysis may lead to hypermagnesemia.

†Concomitant use may cause metabolic alkalosis in patients with renal failure.

‡Concomitant use not recommended by manufacturer.

ANTIARRHYTHMIC DRUGS

Vaughan Williams Classification of Antiarrhythmic Drugs Based on Cardiac Effects

Type	Drug(s)	Conduction Velocity*	Refractory Period	Automaticity
Ia	Disopyramide Procainamide Quinidine	↓	↑	↓
Ib	Lidocaine Mexiletine Moricizine† Tocainide	0/↓	↓	↓
Ic	Flecainide Indecainide Propafenone‡	↓↓	0	↓
II	Beta-blockers	0	0	↓
III	Amiodarone Bretylium Sotalol‡	0	↑↑	0
IV	Diltiazem Verapamil§	↓	↑	↓

*Variables for normal tissue models in ventricular tissue.

†Also has type Ia action to decrease conduction velocity more than most type Ib.

‡Also has type II, beta-blocking action.

§Variables for SA and AV nodal tissue only.

Vaughan Williams Classification of Antiarrhythmic Agents and Their Indications/Adverse Effects

Type	Drug(s)	Indication	Route of Administration	Adverse Effects
Ia	Disopyramide	AF, VT	P.O.	Anticholinergic effects CHF
	Procainamide	AF, VT, WPW	P.O./I.V.	GI, CNS, lupus, fever, hematological, anticholinergic effects
	Quinidine	AF, PSVT, VT, WPW	P.O./I.V.	Hypotension, GI, thrombocytopenia, cinchonism
Ib	Lidocaine	VT, VF, PVC	I.V.	CNS, GI
	Mexiletine	VT	P.O.	GI, CNS
	Tocainide	VT	P.O.	GI, CNS, pulmonary, agranulocytosis
Ic	Flecainide	VT	P.O.	CHF, GI, CNS, blurred vision
	Propafenone	VT	P.O.	GI, blurred vision, dizziness
	Moricizine	VT	P.O.	Dizziness, nausea, rash, seizures
II	Esmolol	VT, SVT	I.V.	CHF, CNS, lupus-like syndrome, hypotension, bradycardia, bronchospasm
	Propranolol	SVT, VT, PVC, digoxin toxicity	P.O./I.V.	CHF, bradycardia, hypotension, CNS, fatigue
III	Amiodarone	VT	P.O.	CNS, GI, thyroid, pulmonary fibrosis, liver, corneal deposits
	Bretylium	VT, VF	I.V.	GI, orthostatic hypotension, CNS
	Ibutilide	VT, VF	I.V.	Torsade de pointes, hypotension, branch bundle block, AV block, nausea, headache
	Sotalol	VT	P.O.	Bradycardia, hypotension, CHF, CNS, fatigue
IV	Diltiazem	AF, PSVT	P.O./I.V.	Hypotension, GI, liver
	Verapamil	AF, PSVT	P.O./I.V.	Hypotension, CHF, bradycardia, vertigo, constipation
Miscellaneous	Adenosine	SVT, PSVT	I.V.	Flushing, dizziness, bradycardia, syncope
	Digoxin	AF, PSVT	P.O./I.V.	GI, CNS, arrhythmias
	Magnesium	VT, VF	I.V.	Hypotension, CNS, hypothermia, myocardial depression

AF = atrial fibrillation; PSVT = paroxysmal supraventricular tachycardia; VT = ventricular tachycardia; WPW = Wolf-Parkinson-White arrhythmias; VF = ventricular fibrillation; SVT = supraventricular tachycardia.

Comparative Pharmacokinetic Properties of Antiarrhythmic Agents

Type	Drug(s)	Bioavailability (%)	Primary Route of Elimination	Volume of Distribution (L/kg)	Protein Binding (%)	Half-Life	Therapeutic Range (mcg/mL)
Ia	Disopyramide	70-95	Hepatic/Renal	0.8-2	50-80	4-8 h	2-6
	Procainamide	75-95	Hepatic/Renal	1.5-3	10-20	2.5-5 h	4-15
	Quinidine	70-80	Hepatic	2-3.5	80-90	5-9 h	2-6
Ib	Lidocaine	20-40	Hepatic	1-2	65-75	60-180 min	1.5-5
	Mexiletine	80-95	Hepatic	5-12	60-75	6-12 h	0.75-2
	Tocainide	90-95	Hepatic	1.5-3	10-30	12-15 h	4-10
Ic	Encainide*	85-95 20-30	Hepatic/Renal	2.5-4	70-80	8-11 h 1-3 h	—
	Flecainide	90-95	Hepatic/Renal	8-10	35-45	12-30 h	0.3-2.5
	Propafenone*	11-39	Hepatic	2.5-4	85-95	12-32 h 2-10 h	—
	Moricizine	34-38	Hepatic	6-11	92-95	1-6 h	—
II	Esmolol	Refer to Beta-Blocker Comparison Chart					
	Propranolol	Refer to Beta-Blocker Comparison Chart					
III	Amiodarone	22-28	Hepatic	70-150	95-97	15-100 d	1-2.5
	Bretylium	15-20	Renal	4-8	Negligible	5-10 h	0.5-2
	Sotalol	90-95	Renal	1.6-2.4	Negligible	12-15 h	—
IV	Diltiazem	80-90	Hepatic/Renal	1.7	77-85	4-6 h	0.05-0.2
	Verapamil	20-40	Hepatic	1.5-5	95-99	4-12 h	>50 ng/mL

*__Top__ numbers reflect **poor** metabolizers and **bottom** numbers reflect **extensive** metabolizers

ANTICONVULSANTS BY SEIZURE TYPE

Seizure Type	Age	Commonly Used	Alternatives
Primarily generalized tonic-clonic seizures	1-12 mo	Carbamazepine* Phenytoin Phenobarbital	Valproate
	1-6 y	Carbamazepine* Phenytoin Phenobarbital	Valproate
	6-11 y	Carbamazepine	Valproate Phenytoin Phenobarbital Lamotrigine†
Primarily generalized tonic-clonic seizures with absence or with myoclonic seizures	1 mo - 18 y	Valproate	Phenytoin‡ Phenobarbital‡ Carbamazepine‡
Absence seizures	Any age	Ethosuximide	Valproate Clonazepam Diamox Lamotrigine†
Myoclonic seizures	Any age	Valproate Clonazepam	Phenytoin† Phenobarbital†
Tonic and atonic seizures	Any age	Valproate	Phenytoin† Clonazepam Phenobarbital†
Partial seizures	1-12 mo	Phenobarbital	Carbamazepine Phenytoin
	1-6 y	Carbamazepine	Phenytoin Phenobarbital Valproate† Lamotrigine† Gabapentin
	6-18 y	Carbamazepine	Lamotrigine Phenytoin Phenobarbital Tiagabine Topiramate Valproate†
Infantile spasms		Corticotropin (ACTH)	Prednisone† Valproate† Clonazepam† Diazepam†

†Not FDA approved for this indication.

‡Phenytoin, phenobarbital, carbamazepine will not treat absence seizures. Addition of another anticonvulsant (ie, ethosuximide) would be needed.

ANTIDEPRESSANT AGENTS

Comparison of Usual Dosage, Mechanism of Action, and Adverse Effects of Antidepressants

Drug	Usual Dosage (mg/d)	Reuptake Inhibition		Adverse Effects					
		N	S	ACH	Drowsiness	Orthostatic Hypotension	Cardiac Arrhythmias	GI Distress	Weight Gain
First-Generation Antidepressants *Tricyclic Antidepressants*									
Amitriptyline (Elavil®, Endep®)	100-300	Moderate	High	4+	4+	4+	3+	0	4+
Clomipramine† (Anafranil®)	100-250	Moderate	High	4+	4+	2+	3+	1+	4+
Desipramine (Norpramin®, Pertofrane®)	100-300	High	Low	1+	2+	2+	2+	0	1+
Doxepin (Adapin®, Sinequan®)	100-300	Low	Moderate	3+	4+	2+	2+	0	4+
Imipramine (Janimine®, Tofranil®)	100-300	Moderate	Moderate	3+	3+	4+	3+	1+	4+
Nortriptyline (Aventyl®, Pamelor®)	50-200	Moderate	Low	2+	2+	1+	2+	0	1+
Protriptyline (Vivactil®)	15-60	Moderate	Low	2+	1+	2+	3+	0	0
Trimipramine (Surmontil®)	100-300	Low	Low	4+	4+	3+	3+	0	4+
Monoamine Oxidase Inhibitors									
Phenelzine (Nardil®)	15-90	—	—	2+	2+	2+	1+	1+	3+
Tranylcypromine (Parnate®)	10-40	—	—	2+	1+	2+	1+	1+	2+
Second-Generation Antidepressants *Older Second-Generation Antidepressants*									
Amoxapine (Asendin®)	100-400	Moderate	Low	2+	2+	2+	2+	0	2+
Maprotiline (Ludiomil®)	100-225	Moderate	Low	2+	3+	2+	2+	0	2+
Trazodone (Desyrel®)	150-500	Very low	Moderate	0	4+	3+	1+	1+	2+
Newer Second-Generation Antidepressants									
Bupropion (Wellbutrin®)	300-450‡	Very low§	Very low§	0	0	0	1+	1+	0
Third-Generation Antidepressants *Selective Serotonin Reuptake Inhibitors*									
Fluoxetine (Prozac®)	10-40	Very low	High	0	0	0	0	3+¶	0
Fluvoxamine (Luvox®)	100-300	Very low	Very high	0	0	0	0	3+¶	0
Paroxetine (Paxil®)	20-50	Very low	Very high	1+	1+	0	0	3+¶	1+
Sertraline (Zoloft®)	50-150	Very low	Very high	0	0	0	0	3+¶	0

Comparison of Usual Dosage, Mechanism of Action, and Adverse Effects of Antidepressants *(continued)*

Drug	Usual Dosage (mg/d)	Reuptake Inhibition		Adverse Effects					
		N	S	ACH	Drowsiness	Orthostatic Hypotension	Cardiac Arrhythmias	GI Distress	Weight Gain
Serotonin/Norepinephrine Reuptake Inhibitors									
Venlafaxine# (Effexor®)	75-375	Very high	Very high	1+	1+	0	1+	3+¶	0
Atypical Antidepressants with 5HT2 Receptor Antagonist Properties									
Mirtazapine (Remeron®)**	15-45	Very low	Very low	1+	2+	0	0	3+	0
Nefazodone (Serzone®)**	300-600	Very low	High	1+	1+	0	0	1+	0

Key: N = norepinephrine; S = serotonin; ACH = anticholinergic effects (dry mouth, blurred vision, urinary retention, constipation); 0 - 4+ = absent or rare - relatively common.

†Not approved by FDA for depression

‡Not to exceed 150 mg/dose to minimize seizure risk

§Norepinephrine and serotonin reuptake inhibition is minimal, but inhibits dopamine reuptake

¶Nausea is usually mild and transient

Comparative studies evaluating the adverse effects of venlafaxine in relation to other antidepressants have not been performed

** These agents work primarily through antagonizing the postsynaptic 5HT2 receptor.

ANTIFUNGAL AGENTS

Activities of Various Agents Against Specific Fungi

Fungus	Itraconazole	Flucytosine*	Amphotericin B	Miconazole	Ketoconazole	Nystatin	Fluconazole	Griseofulvin
Aspergillus	x	—	x	—	—	—	?	—
Blastomyces	x	—	x	—	x	—	?	—
Candida	x	x	x	x	x	x	x	—
Chromomycosis	x	—	—	—	—	—	?	—
Coccidioides	x	—	x	x	x	—	x	—
Cryptococcus	x	x	x	x	x	—	x	—
Epidermophyton	—	—	—	—	x	—	—	x
Histoplasma	x	—	x	—	x	—	x	—
Microsporum	—	—	—	—	x	—	—	x
Mucor	—	—	x	—	—	—	—	—
Paracoccidioides	—	—	—	x	x	—	—	—
Phialophora	—	—	—	—	x	—	—	—
Pseudoallescheria	—	—	—	x	—	—	—	—
Rhodotorula	—	—	x	—	—	—	—	—
Sporothrix	x	—	x	—	—	—	?	—
Trichophyton	x	—	—	—	x	—	—	x

ANTIPSYCHOTIC AGENTS

Antipsychotic Agent	Equivalent Dosages (approx) (mg)	Usual Adult Daily Maintenance Dose (mg)	Sedation (Incidence)	Extrapyramidal Side Effects	Anticholinergic Side Effects	Cardiovascular Side Effects
Acetohexamine	20	60-120	Moderate	High	Low	Low
Chlorpromazine	100	200-1000	High	Moderate	Moderate	Moderate/high
Chlorprothixene	100	75-600	High	Moderate	Moderate	Moderate
Clozapine	50	300-900	High	Low	High	High
Fluphenazine	2	0.5-40	Low	High	Low	Low
Haloperidol	2	1-15	Low	High	Low	Low
Loxapine	10	25-250	Moderate	High	Low	Low
Mesoridazine	50	30-400	High	Low	High	Moderate
Molindone	15	15-225	Low	High	Low	Low
Olanzapine	N/A	10-15	High	Low	High	High
Perphenazine	10	16-48	Low	High	Low	Low
Pimozide	0.3-0.5	1-10	Moderate	High	Moderate	Low
Promazine	200	40-1200	Moderate	Moderate	High	Moderate
Risperidone	N/A	4-16	Low	Low	Low	Low
Thioridazine	100	200-800	High	Low	High	Moderate/high
Thiothixene	5	5-40	Low	High	Low	Low/moderate
Trifluoperazine	5	2-40	Low	High	Low	Low

NA = not available

BENZODIAZEPINES

Agent	Peak Blood Levels (oral) (h)	Protein Binding (%)	Volume of Distribution (L/kg)	Major Active Metabolite	Half-Life (parent) (h)	Half-Life* (metabolite) (h)	Adult Oral Dosage Range
Anxiolytic							
Alprazolam (Xanax®)	1-2	80	1.1	No	12-15	—	0.75-4 mg/d
Chlordiazepoxide (Librium®)	2-4	90-98	0.3	Yes	5-30	24-96	15-100 mg/d
Diazepam (Valium®)	0.5-2	96	1.1	Yes	20-80	50-100	4-40 mg/d
Lorazepam (Ativan®)	1-6	88-92	1.3	No	10-20	—	2-4 mg/d
Oxazepam (Serax®)	2-4	86-96	0.6-2	No	5-20	—	30-120 mg/d
Sedative/Hypnotic							
Estazolam (ProSom™)	2	93	—	No	10-24	—	1-2 mg
Flurazepam (Dalmane®)	0.5-2	97	—	Yes	Not significant	40-114	15-60 mg
Quazepam (Doral®)	2	>95	5	Yes	25-41	28-114	7.5-15 mg
Temazepam (Restoril®)	2-3	96	1.4	No	10-40	—	15-30 mg
Triazolam (Halcion®)	1	89-94	0.8-1.3	No	2.3	—	0.125-0.25 mg
Miscellaneous							
Clonazepam (Klonopin®)	1-2	86	1.8-4	No	18-50 h	—	1.5-20 mg/d
Clorazepate (Tranxene®)	1-2	80-95	—	Yes	Not significant	50-100 h	15-60 mg
Midazolam (Versed®)	0.4-0.7†	>95	0.8-6.6	No	2-5 h	—	NA

* = significant metabolite.
† = I.V. only.
NA = not available.

BETA-BLOCKERS

Agent	Adrenergic Receptor Blocking Activity	Lipid Solubility	Protein Bound (%)	Half-Life (h)	Bioavailability (%)	Primary (Secondary) Route of Elimination	Indications	Usual Dosage
Acebutolol (Sectral®)	$beta_1$	Low	15-25	3-4	40 7-fold*	Hepatic (renal)	Hypertension, arrhythmias	P.O.: 400-1200 mg/d
Atenolol (Tenormin®)	$beta_1$	Low	<5-10	6-9†	50-60 4-fold*	Renal (hepatic)	Hypertension, angina pectoris, acute MI	P.O.: 50-200 mg/d; I.V.: 5 mg x 2 doses
Betaxolol (Kerlone®)	$beta_1$	Low	50-55	14-22	84-94	Hepatic (renal)	Hypertension	P.O.: 10-20 mg/d
Bisoprolol (Zebeta®)	$beta_1$	Low	26-33	9-12	80	Renal (hepatic)	Hypertension	P.O.: 2.5-5 mg
Carteolol (Cartrol™)	$beta_1$ $beta_2$	Low	20-30	6	80-85	Renal	Hypertension	P.O.: 2.5-10 mg/d
Esmolol (Brevibloc®)	$beta_1$	Low	55	0.15	NA 5-fold*	Red blood cell	Supraventricular tachycardia, sinus tachycardia	I.V. infusion: 25-300 mcg/kg/min
Labetalol (Trandate®, Normodyne®)	$alpha_1$ $beta_1$ $beta_2$	Moderate	50	5.5-8	18-30 10-fold*	Renal (hepatic)	Hypertension	P.O.: 200-2400 mg/d; I.V.: 20-80 mg at 10-min intervals up to a maximum of 300 mg **or** continuous infusion of 2 mg/min
Metoprolol (Lopressor®)	$beta_1$	Moderate	10-12	3-7	50 10-fold*	Hepatic/ renal	Hypertension, angina pectoris, acute MI	P.O.: 100-450 mg/d; I.V.: Post-MI 15 mg Angina: 15 mg then 2-5 mg/hour Arrhythmias: 0.2 mg/kg
Nadolol (Corgard®)	$beta_1$ $beta_2$	Low	25-30	20-24	30 5-8 fold*	Renal	Hypertension, angina pectoris	P.O.: 40-320 mg/d
Penbutolol (Levatol™)	$beta_1$ $beta_2$	High	80-98	5	≅100	Hepatic (renal)	Hypertension	P.O.: 20-80 mg/d
Pindolol (Visken®)	$beta_1$ $beta_2$	Moderate	57	3-4†	90 4-fold*	Hepatic (renal)	Hypertension	P.O.: 20-60 mg/d

(continued)

Agent	Adrenergic Receptor Blocking Activity	Lipid Solubility	Protein Bound (%)	Half-Life (h)	Bioavailability (%)	Primary (Secondary) Route of Elimination	Indications	Usual Dosage
Propranolol (Inderal®, various)	$beta_1$ $beta_2$	High	90	3-5†	30 20-fold*	Hepatic	Hypertension, angina pectoris, arrhythmias	P.O.: 40-480 mg/d; I.V.: Reflex tachycardia 1-10 mg
Propranolol long-acting (Inderal-LA®)	$beta_1$ $beta_2$	High	90	9-18	20-30 fold*	Hepatic	Hypertropic subaortic stenosis, prophylaxis (post-MI)	P.O.: 180-240 mg/d
Sotalol (Betapace® Oral)	$beta_1$ $beta_2$	Low	0	12	90-100	Renal	Ventricular arrhythmias/ tachyarrhythmias	P.O. 160-320 mg/d
Timolol (Blocadren®)	$beta_1$ $beta_2$	Low to moderate	<10	4	75 7-fold*	Hepatic (renal)	Hypertension, prophylaxis (post-MI)	P.O.: 20-60 mg/d P.O.: 20 mg/d

Dosage is based on 70 kg adult with normal hepatic and renal function

Note: All $beta_1$ selective agents will inhibit $beta_2$ receptors at higher doses.

*Interpatient variations in plasma levels.

†Half-life increased to 16-27 h in creatinine clearance of 15-35 mL/min and >27 h in creatinine clearances <15 mL/min.

Selected Properties of Beta-Adrenergic Blocking Drugs

Drug	Relative $Beta_1$ Selectivity	Beta-Blockade Potency Ratio*	ISA	MSA
Acebutolol	+	0.3	+	+
Atenolol	+	1	–	–
Betaxolol	+		0	+
Bisoprolol	+		0	0
Carteolol	–		++	0
Esmolol	+	0.02	–	–
Labetalol	–		0	0
Metoprolol	+	1	–	–
Nadolol	–	2-9	–	–
Penbutolol	–		+++	+
Pindolol	–	6	++	+
Propranolol	–	1	–	++
Sotalol	–	0.3	–	–
Timolol	–	6	–	–

*Propranolol = 1

ISA = intrinsic sympathomimetic activity, MSA = membrane stabilizing activity.

CALCIUM CHANNEL BLOCKERS

Calcium Channel Blockers Comparative Actions

Agent	Actions					
	A-V Conduction Node	SA Node Automaticity	Contractility	Heart Rate	Cardiac Output	Peripheral Vascular Resistance
Dihydropyridines						
Nifedipine (Procardia®)	NE	0	0-SD*	0-SI	MI	PD
Amlodipine (Norvasc®)	0	0	0-SI	NE	SI	PD
Felodipine (Plendil®)	0	0	0-SI	0-SI	SI	PD
Isradipine (DynaCirc®)	0	0	0-SI	NE	SI	PD
Nicardipine (Cardene®)	0-SI	0	0-SI	0-SI	MI	PD
Nimodipine (Nimotop®)	NA	NA	NA	NA	NA	NA
Phenylalkylamines						
Verapamil (Calan®, Isoptin®)	NE	MD	MD	SE	SE	MD
Benzothiazepines						
Diltiazem (Cardizem®)	NE	SD	SD	SD	SE	SD
Miscellaneous						
Bepridil (Vascor®)	NE	SD	SD	SD	0	SD

*Drug may worsen symptoms of congestive heart failure due to systolic dysfunction (ejection fraction <40%)

MD = moderate decrease, MI = moderate increase, NA = not available, NE = negligible effect, PD = pronounced decrease, SD = slight decrease, SE = slight effect (increase or decrease), SI = slight increase

Calcium Channel Blockers Comparative Pharmacokinetics

Agent	Bioavailability (%)	Protein Binding (%)	Onset (min)	Peak (h)	Half-Life (h)	Volume of Distribution	Route of Metabolism	Route of Excretion
Dihydropyridines								
Nifedipine (prototype) (Adalat®, Procardia®/Procardia XL®)	Immediate/ sustained release 45-70/86	92-98	20	Immediate/ sustained release 0.5/6	2-5	ND	Liver, inactive metabolites	60%-80% urine, feces, bile
Amlodipine (Norvasc®)	52-88	97	6 h	6-9	33.8	21 L/kg	Liver, inactive metabolites, not a significant first-pass metabolism/presystemic metabolism	Bile, gut wall
Felodipine (Plendil®)	10-25	>99	3-5 h	2.5-5	10-36	10.3 L/kg	Liver, inactive metabolites, extensive metabolism by several pathways including cytochrome P-450, extensive first-pass metabolism/presystemic metabolism	70% urine, 10% feces
Isradipine (DynaCirc®)	15-24	97	120	0.5-2.5	8	2.9 L/kg	Liver, inactive metabolites, extensive first-pass metabolism	90% urine, 10% feces
Nicardipine (Cardene®)	35	>95	20	0.5-2	2-4	ND	Liver, saturable first-pass metabolism	60% urine, 35% feces
Nimodipine (Nimotop®)	13	>95	ND	≤1	1-2	0.43 L/kg	Liver, inactive metabolites, high first-pass metabolism	Urine
Phenylalkylamines								
Verapamil (prototype) (Calan®/ Calan® SR, Isoptin®/Isoptin® SR, Verelan®)	20-35	83-92	30	1-2.2	3-7	4.5-7 L/kg	Liver	70% urine, 16% feces

(continued)

Agent	Bioavailability (%)	Protein Binding (%)	Onset (min)	Peak (h)	Half-Life (h)	Volume of Distribution	Route of Metabolism	Route of Excretion
Benzothiazepines								
Diltiazem (prototype) (Cardizem®/ Cardizem® CD, Dilacor® XR)	40-67	70-80	30-60	Immediate/ sustained release 2-3/6-11	Immediate/ sustained release 3.5-6/5-7	ND	Liver; drugs which inhibit/ induce hepatic microsomal enzymes may alter disposition	Urine
Miscellaneous								
Bepridil (Vascor®)	59	>99	60	2-3	24	ND	Liver	70% urine, 22% feces

ND = no data.

Calcium Channel Blockers FDA-Approved Indications

Agent	Hypertension	Subarachnoid Hemorrhage	Arrhythmias	Angina
Dihydropyridines				
Nifedipine (prototype) (Adalat®, Procardia®/ Procardia XL®)	Sustained release only			Vasospastic and chronic stable
Amlodipine (Norvasc®)	X			Vasospastic and chronic stable
Felodipine (Plendil®)	X			
Isradipine (DynaCirc®)				
Nicardipine (Cardene®)	X			Chronic stable
Nimodipine (Nimotop®)		X		
Phenylalkylamines				
Verapamil (prototype) (Calan®/Calan® SR, Isoptin®/ Isoptin® SR, Verelan®)	X		X, I.V. — supraventricular arrhythmias	Unstable, vasospastic, and chronic stable
Benzothiazepines				
Diltiazem (prototype) (Cardizem®/Cardizem® CD, Dilacor® XR, Tiazac™)	X, Sustained release only		X, I.V. — supraventricular arrhythmias	Vasospastic and chronic stable
Miscellaneous				
Bepridil (Vascor®)				Chronic stable

CARDIOVASCULAR AGENTS

Adrenergic Agonists Hemodynamic Effects

Drug	Hemodynamic Effects							
	CO	TPR	Mean BP	Renal Perfusion	α_1	β_1	β_2	Dopamine Receptors
Dobutamine (Dobutrex®)	↑	↓	↑	<–>	+	++++	++	0
Dopamine (Intropin®)	↑	=/–†	<–>/↑†	↑†	++++	++++	++	++
Epinephrine (Adrenalin®)	↑	↓	↑	↓	++++	++++	++	0
Isoproterenol (Isuprel®)	↑	↓	↓	+/–‡	0	++++	++++	0
Norepinephrine (Levophed®)	<–>/↓	↑	↑	↓	++++	++++	0	0

↑ = increase, ↓ = decrease, <–> = no change, † = dose dependent

‡ In patients with cardiogenic or septic shock, renal perfusion commonly increases, however, in the normal patient, renal perfusion may be reduced with isoproterenol.

Usual Hemodynamic Effects of Intravenous Agents Commonly Used for the Treatment of Acute/Severe Heart Failure

Drug	Dose	HR	MAP	PCWP	CO	SVR
Amrinone	5-10 mcg/kg/min	0/↑	0/↓	↓	↑	↓
Dobutamine	2.5-20 mcg/kg/min	0/↑	0/↑	↓	↑	↓
Dopamine	1-3 mcg/kg/min	0	0	0	0/↑	↓
	3-10 mcg/kg/min	↑	↑	0	↑	0
	>10 mcg/kg/min	↑	↑	↑	↑	↑
Furosemide	20-80 mg, repeated as needed up to 4-6 times/day	0	0	↓	0	0
Milrinone	0.375-0.75 mcg/kg/min	0/↑	0/↓	↓	↑	↓
Nitroglycerin	0.1-2 mcg/kg/min	0/↑	0/↓	↓	0/↑	0/↓
Nitroprusside	0.25-3 mcg/kg/min	0/↑	0/↓	↓	↑	↓

HR = heart rate, MAP = mean arterial pressure, PCWP = pulmonary capillary wedge pressure, CO = cardiac output, SVR = systemic vascular resistance

↑ = increase, ↓ = decrease, 0 = no change

CORTICOSTEROIDS

Corticosteroids, Systemic Equivalencies Comparison

Glucocorticoid	Approximate Equivalent Dose (mg)	Routes of Administration	Relative Anti-inflammatory Potency	Relative Mineralocorticoid Potency	Half-life	
					Plasma (min)	Biologic (h)
Short-Acting						
Cortisone	25	P.O., I.M.	0.8	2	30	8-12
Hydrocortisone	20	I.M., I.V.	1	2	80-118	
Intermediate-Acting						
Prednisone	5	P.O.	4	1	60	18-36
Prednisolone	5	P.O., I.M., I.V., intra-articular, intradermal, soft tissue injection	4	1	115-212	
Triamcinolone	4	P.O., I.M., intra- articular, intrasynovial, intradermal, soft tissue injection	5	0	200+	
Methylprednisolone	4	P.O., I.M., I.V.	5	0	78-188	
Long-Acting						
Dexamethasone	0.75	P.O., I.M., I.V., intra-articular, intradermal, soft tissue injection	25-30	0	110-210	36-54
Betamethasone	0.6-0.75	P.O., I.M., intra- articular, intrasynovial, intradermal, soft tissue injection	25	0	300+	

Corticosteroids, Topical

Steroid		Vehicle
Lowest Potency (may be ineffective for some indications)		
0.1%	Betamethasone	cream
0.2%	Betamethasone	cream
0.05%	Desonide	cream, ointment, lotion
0.04%	Dexamethasone (Decaspray®)†	aerosol
0.1%	Dexamethasone (Decadron® Phosphate, Decaderm®)†	cream
1%	Hydrocortisone	cream, ointment, lotion
2.5%	Hydrocortisone	cream, ointment
0.25%	Methylprednisolone acetate (Medrol®)	ointment
1%	Methylprednisolone acetate (Medrol®)	ointment
Low Potency		
0.01%	Betamethasone valerate (Valisone®, reduced strength)	cream
0.1%	Clocortolone (Cloderm®)	cream
0.01%	Fluocinolone acetonide (Synalar®)†	cream, solution, shampoo, oil
0.025%	Flurandrenolide (Cordran®, Cordran® SP)†	cream, ointment
0.2%	Hydrocortisone valerate (Westcort®)	cream
0.025%	Triamcinolone acetonide (Kenalog®)†	cream, ointment
Intermediate Potency		
0.025%	Betamethasone benzoate	cream, gel, lotion
0.1%	Betamethasone valerate (Valisone®)†	cream, ointment, lotion
0.05%	Desoximetasone (Topicort® LP)	cream
0.025%	Fluocinolone acetonide†	cream, ointment
0.05%	Flurandrenolide (Cordran®, Cordran® SP)†	cream, ointment, lotion
0.05%	Fluticasone propionate	cream
0.025%	Halcinonide (Halog®)	cream, ointment
0.1%	Mometasone furoate	cream, ointment, lotion
0.1%	Triamcinolone acetonide (Kenalog®)†	cream, ointment
High Potency		
0.1%	Amcinonide (Cyclocort®)	cream, ointment
0.05%	Betamethasone dipropionate (Diprosone®)	cream, ointment, lotion
0.25%	Desoximetasone (Topicort®)	cream, ointment
0.2%	Fluocinolone (Synalar-HP®)	cream
0.05%	Fluocinonide (Lidex®)†	cream, ointment
0.1%	Halcinonide (Halog®)	cream, ointment, solution
0.5%	Triamcinolone acetonide†	cream, ointment
Very High Potency		
0.05%	Augmented betamethasone dipropionate (Diprolene®)	Ointment
0.05%	Clobetasol propionate (Temovate®)	Cream, ointment
0.05%	Diflorasone diacetate (Florone®, Maxiflor®)	Gel, ointment
0.05%	Halobetasol propionate	Cream, ointment

†Fluorinated.

CYCLOPLEGIC MYDRIATICS

Agent	Peak Mydriasis	Peak Cycloplegia	Time to Recovery
Atropine	30-40 min	1-3 h	>14 d
Cyclopentolate	25-75 min	25-75 min	24 h
Homatropine	30-90 min	30-90 min	6 h-4 d
Scopolamine	20-30 min	30 min-1 h	5-7 d
Tropicamide	20-40 min	20-35 min	1-6 h

GLAUCOMA DRUG THERAPY

Ophthalmic Agent	Reduces Aqueous Humor Production	Increases Aqueous Humor Outflow	Average Duration of Action	Strengths Available
Miotics*				
Cholinesterase inhibitors				
Demecarium	No data	Significant	7 d	0.125%-0.25%
Echothiophate	No data	Significant	2 wk	0.03%-0.25%
Isoflurophate	No data	Significant	2 wk	0.025%
Physostigmine	No data	Significant	24 h	0.25%
Direct-acting				
Acetylcholine	Some activity	Significant	14 min	Injection 1%
Carbachol	Some activity	Significant	8 h	0.75%-3%
Pilocarpine	Some activity	Significant	5 h	0.5%, 1%, 2%, 3%, 4%
Mydriatics				
Sympathomimetics				
Dipivefrin	Some activity	Moderate	12 h	0.1%
Epinephrine	Some activity	Moderate	18 h	0.25%-2%
Miscellaneous				
Beta Blockers				
Betaxolol	Significant	Some activity	12 h	0.5%
Levobunolol	Significant	Some activity	18 h	0.5%
Metipranolol	Significant	Some activity	18 h	0.3%
Timolol	Significant	Some activity	18 h	0.25%, 0.5%
Carbonic Anhydrase Inhibitors				
Acetazolamide	Significant	No data	10 h	250 mg tab, 500 mg cap
Carteolol	Yes	No	12 h	1%
Dorzolamide	Yes	No	8 h	2%
Latanoprost		Yes	8-12 h	0.005%
Methazolamide	Significant	No data	14 h	50 mg

*All miotic drugs significantly affect accommodation.

HYPOGLYCEMIC DRUGS, COMPARISON OF ORAL AGENTS

Contraindications to Therapy and Potential Adverse Effects of Oral Antidiabetic Agents

	Sulfonylureas	Metformin	Acarbose
Contraindications			
Insulin dependency	A	A	A*
Pregnancy/lactation	A	A	A
Hypersensitivity to the agent	A	A	A
Hepatic impairment	R	A	R
Renal impairment	R	A	R
Congestive heart failure		A	
Chronic lung disease		A	
Peripheral vascular disease		A	
Steroid-induced diabetes	R	R	
Inflammatory bowel disease		A	A
Major recurrent illness	R	A	
Surgery	R	A	
Alcoholism	R	A	
Adverse Effects			
Hypoglycemia	Yes	No	No
Body weight gain	Yes	No	No
Hypersensitivity	Yes	No	No
Drug interactions	Yes	No	No
Lactic acidosis	No	Yes	No
Gastrointestinal disturbances	No	Yes	No

*Can be used in conjunction with insulin. A = absolute; R = relative

Comparative Pharmacokinetics of Sulfonylureas

Drug	Duration of Action (h)	Dose and Frequency (mg)	Metabolism
First Generation Agents			
Acetohexamide	8-24	250-1500 bid	Hepatic (60%) with active metabolite
Chlorpropamide	24-72	100-500 qd	Renal excretion (30%) and hepatic metabolism with active metabolites
Tolazamide	12-24	100-1000 qd or bid	Hepatic with active metabolites
Tolbutamide	6-24	500-3000 bid or tid	Hepatic
Second Generation Agents			
Glimepiride	24	1-4 mg qd	Hepatic
Glipizide	12-24	2.5-40 qd or bid	Hepatic
Glipizide GITS	24	5-10 qd	Hepatic
Glyburide	16-24	1.25-20 qd or bid	Hepatic with active metabolites

LAXATIVES, CLASSIFICATION AND PROPERTIES

Laxative	Onset of Action	Site of Action	Mechanism of Action
Saline			
Magnesium Citrate (Citroma®)	0.5-3 h	Small and large intestine	Attract/retain water in intestinal lumen increasing intraluminal pressure; cholecystokinin release
Magnesium Hydroxide (Milk of Magnesia)			
Sodium Phosphate/ Biphosphate Enema (Fleet® Enema)	2-15 min	Colon	
Irritant/Stimulant			
Senna (Senokot®)	6-10 h	Colon	Direct action on intestinal mucosa; stimulate myenteric plexus; alter water and electrolyte secretion
Bisacodyl Tab (Dulcolax®)	0.25-1 h		
Bisacodyl Supp (Dulcolax®)			
Castor Oil	2-6 h	Small intestine	
Cascara Aromatic Fluid Extract	6-10 h	Colon	
Bulk-Producing			
Methylcellulose	12-24 h (up to 72 h)	Small and large intestine	Holds water in stool; mechanical distention; malt soup extract reduces fecal pH
Psyllium (Metamucil®)			
Malt Soup Extract (Maltsupex®)			
Lubricant			
Mineral Oil	6-8 h	Colon	Lubricates intestine; retards colonic absorption of fecal water
Surfactants/Stool Softener			
Docusate (Colace®)	24-72 h	Small and large intestine	Detergent activity; facilitates admixture of fat and water to soften stool
Miscellaneous and Combination Laxatives			
Glycerin Supp	0.25-0.5 h	Colon	Local irritation; hyperosmotic action
Lactulose (Cephulac®)	24-48 h	Colon	Delivers osmotically active molecules to colon
Docusate/ Casanthranol (Peri-Colace®)	8-12 h	Small and large intestine	Casanthranol – mild stimulant; docusate – stool softener
Polyethylene Glycol – Electrolyte Solution (GoLYTELY®)	30-60 min	Small and large intestine	Nonabsorbable solution which acts as an osmotic agent
Sorbitol 70%	24-48 h	Colon	Delivers osmotically active molecules to colon

LIPID-LOWERING AGENTS

Effects on Lipoproteins

Drug	Total Cholesterol (%)	LDLC (%)	HDLC (%)	TG (%)
Atorvastatin	↓25-45	↓40-60	↑5-8	↓19-37
Bile-acid resins	↓20-25	↓20-35	→	↑5-20
Fibric acid derivatives	↓10	↓10 (↑)	↑10-25	↓40-55
HMG-CoA RI (statins)	↓15-35	↓20-40	↑2-15	↓7-25
Nicotinic acid	↓25	↓20	↑20	↓40

Comparative Dosages of Agents Used to Treat Hyperlipidemia

Antilipemic Agent*	Usual Daily Dose	Average Dosing Interval
HMG-CoA Reductase Inhibitors		
Atorvastatin	10-80 mg	qd
Fluvastatin	20-40 mg	hs
Lovastatin	20-40 mg	hs
Pravastatin	20-40 mg	hs
Simvastatin	10-20 mg	hs
Fibric Acid Derivatives		
Clofibrate	2000 mg	qid
Gemfibrozil	1200 mg	bid
Miscellaneous Agents		
Niacin	6 g	tid
Bile Acid Sequestrants		
Colestipol	30 g	bid
Cholestyramine	24 g	tid-qid

Dosage is based on 70 kg adult with normal hepatic and renal function.

NARCOTIC AGONISTS

Comparative Pharmacokinetics

Drug	Onset (min)	Peak (h)	Duration (h)	Half-Life (h)	Average Dosing Interval (h)		Equianalgesic Doses* (mg)	
							I.M.	Oral
Alfentanil	Immediate	ND	ND	1-2	—	—	ND	NA
Buprenorphine	15	1	4-8	2-3			0.4	—
Butorphanol	I.M.: 30-60 I.V.: 4-5	0.5-1	3-5	2.5-3.5	3	(3-6)	2	—
Codeine	P.O.: 30-60 I.M.: 10-30	0.5-1	4-6	3-4	3	(3-6)	120	200
Fentanyl	I.M.: 7-15 I.V.: Immediate	ND	1-2	1.5-6	1	(0.5-2)	0.1	NA
Hydrocodone	ND	ND	4-8	3.3-4.4	6	(4-8)	ND	ND
Hydromorphone	P.O.: 15-30	0.5-1	4-6	2-4	4	(3-6)	1.5	7.5
Levorphanol	P.O.: 10-60	0.5-1	4-8	12-16	6	(6-24)	2	4
Meperidine	P.O./I.M./S.C.: 10-15 I.V.: ≤5	0.5-1	2-4	3-4	3	(2-4)	75	300
Methadone	P.O.: 30-60 I.V.: 10-20	0.5-1	4-6 (acute) >8 (chronic)	15-30	8	(6-12)	10	20
Morphine	P.O.: 15-60 I.V.: ≤5	P.O./I.M./S.C.: 0.5-1 I.V.: 0.3	3-6	2-4	4	(3-6)	10	60# (acute) 30 (chronic)
Nalbuphine	I.M.: 30 I.V.: 1-3	1	3-6	5		—	10	—
Naloxone†	2-5	0.5-2	0.5-1	0.5-1.5		—	—	—
Oxycodone	P.O.: 10-15	0.5-1	4-6	3-4	4	(3-6)	NA	30
Oxymorphone	5-15	0.5-1	3-6				1	10‡
Pentazocine	15-20	0.25-1	3-4	2-3	3	(3-6)		

NEUROMUSCULAR BLOCKING AGENTS

Comparative Neuromuscular Blocking Dosages*

Agent	Comparative Dosages (mcg/kg)	Recommended Bolus Dose	Recommended I.V. Infusion Rates
Short-Acting Agents			
Mivacurium (Mivacron®)	80-90	150 mcg/kg	1-15 mcg/kg/min
Rocuronium (Zemuron®)	300	0.6-1.2 mg/kg	10-40 mcg/kg/min
Succinylcholine	300	25-75 mg (1-2 mg/kg)	2.5 mg/min
Intermediate-Acting Agents			
Atracurium (Tracrium®)	225	400-500 mcg/kg	2-15 mcg/kg/min
Cisatracurium (Nimbex®)	100	150-200 mcg/kg	1-5 mcg/kg/minute
Pancuronium (Pavulon®)	60	40-100 mcg/kg	50-100 mcg/kg/h
Vecuronium (Norcuron®)	50-60	80-100 mcg/kg	0.8-1.2 mcg/kg/min
Long-Acting Agents			
Doxacurium (Nuromax®)	25-30	50 mcg/kg	Not applicable
Pipecuronium (Arduan®)	45	50-100 mcg/kg	Not applicable
Tubocurarine	500	100-600 mcg/kg	Not applicable

*Dosages in a 70 kg adult patient with normal renal and hepatic function.

Comparative Pharmacokinetic Parameters for Neuromuscular Blocking Agents in Adult Patients With Normal Renal and Hepatic Function

Agent	Volume of Distribution (central compartment)	Onset of Action	Duration of Action	Half-Life	Body Clearance
Short-Acting Agents		**1-2 min**	**10-20 min**		
Mivacurium (Mivacron®)	0.15-0.25 L/kg	2 min	17 min	16.9 min	3.3 L/kg/h 55 mL/kg/min
Rocuronium (Zemuron®)	0.22-0.25 L/kg	0.7-1 min	31-67 min	84-90 min	2.7 L/kg/min
Succinylcholine	Unknown	1-1.5 min	5-10 min	Unknown	Unknown
Intermediate-Acting Agents		**2-3 min**	**40-60 min**		
Atracurium (Tracrium®)	0.16-0.18 L/kg (0.04-0.06 L/kg)	2 min	30 min	20-21 min	5.3-6.1 mL/kg/min
Cisatracurium (Nimbex®)	0.133 L/kg	2 min	30 min	22-31 min	4.5-5.7 mL/kg/min
Pancuronium (Pavulon®)	0.26-0.28 L/kg (0.05-0.12 L/kg)	1-5.2 min	60 min	114-140 min	1.8-1.9 mL/kg/min
Vecuronium (Norcuron®)	0.19-0.25 L/kg (0.05-0.11 L/kg)	1.5 min	30 min	58-80 min	3.0-5.2 mL/kg/min
Long-Acting Agents		**4-6 min**	**90-180 min**		
Doxacurium (Nuromax®)	0.22±0.11 L/kg	6 min	83 min	99±54 min	2.67±0.09 mL/kg/min
Pipecuronium (Arduan®)	0.31±0.1 L/kg	3-5 min	70 min	137±68 min	2.3±0.04 mL/kg/min
Tubocurarine	0.22-0.39 L/kg	6 min	80 min	3.9 h	Unknown

NITRATES

Nitrates	Dosage Form	Onset (min)	Duration
Nitroglycerin	I.V.	1-2	3-5 min
	Sublingual	1-3	30-60 min
	Translingual spray	2	30-60 min
	Oral, sustained release	40	4-8 h
	Topical ointment	20-60	2-12 h
	Transdermal	40-60	18-24 h
Isosorbide dinitrate	Sublingual and chewable	2-5	1-2 h
	Oral	20-40	4-6 h
	Oral, sustained release	Slow	8-12 h
Isosorbide mononitrate	Oral	60-120	5-12h

Adapted from Corwin S and Reiffel JA, "Nitrate Therapy for Angina Pectoris," *Arch Intern Med*, 1985, 145:538-43 and Franciosa JA, "Nitroglycerin and Nitrates in Congestive Heart Failure," *Heart and Lung*, 1980, 9(5):873-82.

*Hemodynamic and antianginal tolerance often develops within 24-48 hours of continuous nitrate administration.

NONSTEROIDAL ANTI-INFLAMMATORY AGENTS

Comparative Dosages, and Pharmacokinetics

Drug	Maximum Recommended Daily Dose (mg)	Time to Peak Levels (h)*	Half-life (h)
Propionic Acids			
Fenoprofen (Nalfon®)	3200	1-2	2-3
Flurbiprofen (Ansaid®)	300	1.5	5.7
Ibuprofen	3200	1-2	1.8-2.5
Ketoprofen (Orudis®)	300	0.5-2	2-4
Naproxen (Naprosyn®)	1500	2-4	12-15
Naproxen sodium (Anaprox®)	1375	1-2	12-13
Acetic Acids			
Diclofenac sodium delayed release (Voltaren®)	225	2-3	1-2
Diclofenac potassium immediate release (Cataflam®)	200	1	1-2
Etodolac (Lodine®)	1200	1-2	7.3
Indomethacin (Indocin®)	200	1-2	4.5
Indomethacin SR	150	2-4	4.5-6
Ketorolac (Toradol®)	I.M.: 120† P.O.: 40	0.5-1	3.8-8.6
Sulindac (Clinoril®)	400	2-4	7.8 (16.4)‡
Tolmetin (Tolectin®)	2000	0.5-1	1-1.5
Fenamates (Anthranilic Acids)			
Meclofenamate (Meclomen®)	400	0.5-1	2 (3.3)§
Mefenamic acid (Ponstel®)	1000	2-4	2-4
Nonacidic Agent			
Nabumetone (Relafen®)	2000	3-6	24
Oxicam			
Piroxicam (Feldene®)	20	3-5	30-86

Dosage is based on 70 kg adult with normal hepatic and renal function.

*Food decreases the rate of absorption and may delay the time to peak levels.

†150 mg on the first day.

‡Half-life of active sulfide metabolite.

§Half-life with multiple doses.

SULFONAMIDE DERIVATIVES

The following table lists commonly prescribed drugs which are either sulfonamide derivatives or are structurally similar to sulfonamides. Please note that the list may not be all inclusive.

Commonly Prescribed Drugs

Classification	Specific Drugs
Antimicrobial Agents	Mafenide acetate (Sulfamylon®) Silver sulfadiazine (Silvadene®) Sodium sulfacetamide (Sodium Sulamyd®) Sulfadiazine Sulfamethizole Sulfamethoxazole (ie, Bactrim™ and co-trimoxazole) Sulfisoxazole (Gantrisin®)
Diuretics, Carbonic Anhydrase Inhibitors	Acetazolamide (Diamox®) Dichlorphenamide (Daranide®) Methazolamide (Neptazane®)
Diuretics, Loop	Bumetanide (Bumex®) Furosemide (Lasix®) Torsemide (Demadex®)
Diuretics, Thiazide	Bendroflumethiazide Benzthiazide Chlorothiazide (Diuril®) Chlorthalidone (Hygroton®) Cyclothiazide (Anhydron®) Hydrochlorothiazide (Dyazide®, HydroDIURIL®, Maxzide®) Hydroflumethiazide Indapamide (Lozol®) Methyclothiazide (Enduron®) Metolazone (Diulo®, Zaroxolyn®) Polythiazide Quinethazone Trichlormethiazide
Hypoglycemic Agents, Oral	Acetohexamide (Dymelor®) Chlorpropamide (Diabinese®) Glipizide (Glucotrol®) Glyburide (DiaBeta®, Micronase®) Tolazamide (Tolinase®) Tolbutamide (Orinase®)
Other Agents	Sulfasalazine (Azulfidine®)

GENERAL RECOMMENDATIONS ON IMMUNIZATION

Summary

The need for a single childhood immunization schedule prompted the unification of previous vaccine recommendations made by the American Academy of Pediatrics (AAP) and the Advisory Committee on Immunization Practices (ACIP). In addition to presenting the newly recommended schedule for the administration of vaccines during childhood, this report addresses the previous differences between the AAP and ACIP childhood vaccination schedules and the rationale for changing previous recommendations.

Recommendation

Because immune response is not affected by administering the third dose of OPV at as early as 6 months of age, and because earlier scheduling can ensure a higher rate of completion of the OPV primary series at a younger age, the third dose of OPV should be administered routinely at 6 months of age. Vaccination at as late as 18 months of age remains an acceptable alternative.

IMMUNIZATION GUIDELINES

Although there are small numbers of patients for whom specific vaccines are definitely contraindicated, it is likely that far greater numbers of patients fail to receive needed vaccines because of misconceptions concerning contraindications to adult immunizations. Some of the most common of these misconceptions are listed in the following table.

Conditions Which Are Not Considered to Be Contraindications to Vaccinations

- Reaction to a previous DTP dose that involved only soreness, redness, or swelling in the area of the vaccination site or temperature of less than 105°F (40.5°C)
- Mild acute illness with low-grade fever or mild diarrheal illness in an otherwise well child
- Current antimicrobial therapy or the convalescent phase of illness
- Prematurity
- Pregnancy of mother or other household contact
- Recent exposure to an infectious disease
- Breast-feeding
- A history of nonspecific allergies or relatives with allergies
- Allergies to penicillin or any other antibiotic, except anaphylactic reactions to neomycin or streptomycin
- Allergies to duck meat or duck feathers
- Family history of convulsions in persons considered for pertussis or measles vaccination
- Family history of sudden infant death syndrome in children considered for DTP vaccination
- Family history of an adverse event, unrelated to immunosuppression, following vaccination

Contraindications to Immunization

Minor illness is not a contraindication to vaccination, especially if the patient has a minor upper respiratory infection or allergic rhinitis. Delay of immunization should be considered if expected or potential vaccine side effects may accentuate or be accentuated by an underlying illness. Note that fever is not itself a contraindication to vaccination, however, if fever is associated with other signs of serious underlying illness, vaccination should be deferred until the patient has recovered. Moderate or severe illness, with or without fever, is considered a contraindication to DTP administration, as signs and symptoms associated with the underlying illness may be incorrectly attributed to the DTP vaccine.

Contraindications and Precautions to Subsequent Vaccination With Diphtheria and Tetanus Toxoids and Pertussis Vaccine (DTP)

Classification/Response to DTP Vaccination
Contraindications
• An immediate anaphylactic reaction
• Encephalopathy occurring within 7 days after vaccination
Precautions
• Fever ≥105°F (≥40.5°C) that is not attributed to another identifiable cause occurring within 48 hours after vaccination
• Collapse or shock-like state (ie, a hypotonic-hyporesponsive episode) occurring within 48 hours after vaccination
• Persistent, inconsolable crying lasting ≥3 hours and occurring within 48 hours after vaccination
• Convulsions with or without fever occurring within 3 days after vaccination

Recommended Childhood Immunization Schedule
United States, January - December 1997

Vaccines[1] are listed under the routinely recommended ages. Bars indicate range of acceptable ages for vaccination. Shaded bars indicate catch-up vaccination; at 11-12 years of age, hepatitis B vaccine should be administered to children not previously vaccinated, and Varicella vaccine should be administered to children not previously vaccinated who lack a reliable history of chicken pox.

Age ► / Vaccine ▼	Birth	1 mo	2 mos	4 mos	6 mos	12 mos	15 mos	18 mos	4-6 yrs	11-12 yrs	14-16 yrs
Hepatitis B[2,3]	Hep-1										
		Hep B-2			Hep B-3					Hep B[3]	
Diphtheria, Tetanus, Pertussis[4]			DTaP or DTP	DTaP or DTP	DTaP or DTP		DTaP or DTP[4]		DTaP or DTP	Td	
H. influenzae type b[5]			Hib	Hib	Hib[5]	Hib[5]					
Polio[6]			Polio[6]	Polio	Polio[6]				Polio		
Measles, Mumps, Rubella[7]						MMR			MMR[7] or	MMR[7]	
Varicella[8]						Var				Var	

[1] This schedule indicates the recommended age for routine administration of currently licensed childhood vaccines. Some combination vaccines are available and may be used whenever administration of all components of the vaccine is indicated. Providers should consult the manufacturers' package inserts for detailed recommendations.

[2] **Infants born to HBsAg-negative mothers** should receive 2.5 mcg of Merck vaccine (Recombivax HB®) or 10 mcg of SmithKline Beecham (SB) vaccine (Engerix-B®). The 2nd dose should be administered ≥1 month after the 1st dose. **Infants born to HBsAg-positive mothers** should receive 0.5 mL Hepatitis B Immune Globulin (HBIG) within 12 hours of birth, and either 5 mcg of Merck vaccine (Recombivax HB®) or 10 mcg of SB vaccine (Engerix-B®) at a separate site. The 2nd dose is recommended at 1-2 months of age and the 3rd dose at 6 months of age. **Infants born to mothers whose HBsAg status is unknown** should receive either 5 mcg of Merck vaccine (Recombivax HB®) or 10 mcg of SB vaccine (Engerix-B®) within 12 hour of birth. The 2nd dose of vaccine is recommended at 1 month of age and the 3rd dose at 6 months of age. Blood should be drawn at the time of delivery to determine the mother's HBsAg status; if it is positive, the infant should receive HBIG as soon as possible (no later than 1 week of age). The dosage and timing of subsequent vaccine doses should be based upon the mother's HBsAg status.

[3] Children and adolescents who have not been vaccinated against hepatitis B in infancy may begin the series during any childhood visit. Those who have not previously received 3 doses of hepatitis B vaccine should initiate or complete the series at the 11-12 year-old visit. The 2nd dose should be administered at least 1 month after the 1st dose, and the 3rd dose should be administered at least 4 months after the 1st dose and at least 2 months after the 2nd dose.

[4] DTaP (diphtheria and tetanus toxoids and acellular pertussis vaccine) is the preferred vaccine for all doses in the vaccination series, including completion of the series in children who have received ≥1 dose of whole-cell DTP vaccine. Whole-cell DTP is an acceptable alternative to DTaP. The 4th dose of DTaP may be administered as early as 12 months of age, provided 6 months have elapsed since the 3rd dose, and if the child is considered unlikely to return at 15-18 months of age. Td (tetanus and diphtheria toxoids, absorbed, for adult use) is recommended at 11-12 years of age if at least 5 years have elapsed since the last dose of DTP, DTaP, or DT Subsequent routine Td boosters are recommended every 10 years.

[5] Three *H. influenzae* type b (Hib) conjugate vaccines are licensed for infant use. If PRP-OMP (PedvaxHIB™ [Merck]) is administered at 2 and 4 months of age, a dose at 6 months is not required. After completing the primary series, any Hib conjugate vaccine may be used as a booster.

[6] Two poliovirus vaccines are currently licensed in the U.S.; inactivated poliovirus vaccine (IPV) and oral poliovirus vaccine (OPV). The following schedules are all acceptable by the ACIP, the AAP, and the AAFP, and parents and providers may choose among them:

1. IPV at 2 and 4 months; OPV at 12-18 months and 4-6 years
2. IPV at 2, 4, 12-18 months, and 4-6 years
3. OPV at 2, 4, 6-18 months, and 4-6 years

The ACIP routinely recommends schedule 1. IPV is the only poliovirus vaccine recommended for immunocompromised persons and their household contacts.

[7] The 2nd dose of MMR is routinely recommended at 4-6 years of age or at 11-12 years of age, but may be administered at any visit, provided at least 1 month has elapsed since receipt of the 1st dose and that both doses are administered at or after 12 months of age.

[8] Susceptible children may receive Varicella vaccine (Var) at any visit after the first birthday, and those who lack a reliable history of chickenpox should be immunized during the 11-12 year-old visit. Children ≥13 years of age should receive 2 doses, at least 1 month apart.

Adapted from the American Academy of Pediatrics and American Academy of Family Practice Physicians, Advisory Committee on Immunization Practices and the Centers for Disease Control.

RECOMMENDATIONS OF THE ADVISORY COMMITTEE ON IMMUNIZATION PRACTICES (ACIP)

Recommended Accelerated Immunization Schedule for Infants and Children <7 Years of Age Who Start the Series Late* or Who Are >1 Month Behind in the Immunization Schedule† (ie, children for whom compliance with scheduled return visits cannot be assured)

Timing	Vaccine(s)	Comments
First visit (≥4 mo)	DTP‡, DTaP, IPV, Hib‡§, hepatitis B, MMR (should be given as soon as child is age 12-15 mo)	All vaccines should be administered simultaneously at the appropriate visit.
Second visit (1 mo after first visit)	DTP‡, Hib‡§, hepatitis B	
Third visit (1 mo after second visit)	DTP‡, DTaP, IPV, Hib‡§	
Fourth visit (6 wk after third visit)	OPV	
Fifth visit (≥6 mo after third visit)	DTaP‡ or DTP, Hib‡§, hepatitis B	
Additional visits		
4-6 y	DTaP‡ or DTP, OPV, MMR	Preferably at or before school entry
14-16 y	Td	Repeat every 10 years throughout life

DTP = diphtheria-tetanus-pertussis.

DTaP = diphtheria-tetanus-acellular pertussis.

Hib = *Haemophilus influenzae* type b conjugate.

MMR = measles-mumps-rubella.

IPV = Inactivated poliovirus vaccine

OPV = poliovirus vaccine, live oral, trivalent.

Td = tetanus and diphtheria toxoids (for use among persons ≥7 years of age).

Modified from *MMWR Morb Mortal Wkly Rep*, 1994, 43(RR-1).

*If initiated in the first year of life, administer DTP doses 1, 2, and 3 and OPV doses 1, 2, and 3 according to this schedule; administer MMR when the child reaches 12-15 months of age.

†See individual ACIP recommendations for detailed information on specific vaccines.

‡Two DTP and Hib combination vaccines are available (DTP/HbOC [Tetramune®]; and PRP-T [ActHIB®, OmniHIB®] which can be reconstituted with DTP vaccine produced by Connaught). DTaP preparations are currently recommended only for use as the fourth and/or fifth doses of the DTP series among children 15 months through 6 years of age (before the seventh birthday). DTP and DTaP should not be used on or after the seventh birthday.

§The recommended schedule varies by vaccine manufacturer. For information specific to the vaccine being used, consult the package insert and ACIP recommendations. Children beginning the Hib vaccine series at age 2-6 months should receive a primary series of three doses of HbOC[HibTITER®] (Lederle-Praxis), PRP-T [ActHIB®, OmniHIB®] (Pasteur Merieux; SmithKline Beecham; Connaught), or a licensed DTP-Hib combination vaccine; **or** two doses of PRP-OMP [PedvaxHIB®] (Merck, Sharp, and Dohme). An additional booster dose of any licensed Hib conjugate vaccine should be administered at 12-15 months of age **and** at least 2 months after the previous dose. Children beginning the Hib vaccine series at 7-11 months of age should receive a primary series of two doses of an HbOC, PRP-T, PRP-OMP-containing vaccine. An additional booster dose of any licensed Hib conjugate vaccine should be administered at 12-18 months of age **and** at least 2 months after the previous dose. Children beginning the Hib vaccine series at ages 12-14 months should receive a primary series of one dose of an HbOC, PRP-T, or PRP-OMP-containing vaccine. An additional booster dose of any licensed Hib conjugate vaccine should be administered 2 months after the previous dose. Children beginning the Hib vaccine series at ages 15-59 months should receive one dose of any licensed Hib vaccine. Hib vaccine should not be administered after the fifth birthday except for special circumstances as noted in the specific ACIP recommendations for the use of Hib vaccine.

Recommended Immunization Schedule for Persons ≥7 Years of Age Not Vaccinated at the Recommended Time in Early Infancy*

Timing	Vaccine(s)	Comments
First visit	Td†, IPV‡, MMR§, and hepatitis B¶	Primary poliovirus vaccination is not routinely recommended for persons ≥18 years of age
Second visit (6-8 wk after first visit)	Td, IPV, MMR§·#, hepatitis B¶	
Third visit (6 mo after second visit)	Td, OPV, hepatitis B¶	
Additional visits	Td	Repeat every 10 years throughout life

MMR = measles-mumps-rubella.

IPV = inactivated poliovirus vaccine

OPV = poliovirus vaccine, live oral, trivalent.

Td = tetanus and diphtheria toxoids (for use among persons ≥7 years of age).

Modified from *MMWR Morb Mortal Wkly Rep*, 1994, 43(RR-1).

*See individual ACIP recommendations for details.

†The DTP and DTaP doses administered to children <7 years of age who remain incompletely vaccinated at age ≥7 years should be counted as prior exposure to tetanus and diphtheria toxoids (eg, a child who previously received two doses of DTP needs only one dose of Td to complete a primary series for tetanus and diphtheria).

‡When polio vaccine is administered to previously unvaccinated persons ≥18 years of age, inactivated poliovirus vaccine (IPV) is preferred. For the immunization schedule for IPV, see specific ACIP statement on the use of polio vaccine.

§Persons born before 1957 can generally be considered immune to measles and mumps and need not be vaccinated. Rubella (or MMR) vaccine can be administered to persons of any age, particularly to nonpregnant women of childbearing age.

¶Hepatitis B vaccine, recombinant. Selected high-risk groups for whom vaccination is recommended include persons with occupational risk, such as healthcare and public safety workers who have occupational exposure to blood, clients and staff of institutions for the developmentally disabled, hemodialysis patients, recipients of certain blood products (eg, clotting factor concentrates), household contacts and sex partners of hepatitis B virus carriers, injecting drug users, sexually active homosexual and bisexual men, certain sexually active heterosexual men and women, inmates of long-term correctional facilities, certain international travelers, and families of HB_sAg-positive adoptees from countries where HBV infection is endemic. Because risk factors are often not identified directly among adolescents, universal hepatitis B vaccination of teenagers should be implemented in communities where injecting drug use, pregnancy among teenagers, and/or sexually transmitted diseases are common.

#The ACIP recommends a second dose of measles-containing vaccine (preferably MMR to assure immunity to mumps and rubella) for certain groups. Children with no documentation of live measles vaccination after the first birthday should receive two doses of live measles-containing vaccine not less than 1 month apart. In addition, the following persons born in 1957 or later should have documentation of measles immunity (ie, two doses of measles-containing vaccine [at least one of which being MMR], physician-diagnosed measles, or laboratory evidence of measles immunity): a) those entering post-high school educational settings; b) those beginning employment in healthcare settings who will have direct patient contact; and c) travelers to areas with endemic measles.

Recommended Schedule of Vaccinations for Adolescents Ages 11-12 Years

Immunologic	Indications	Vaccine	Dose	Frequency	Route
Hepatitis A vaccine	Adolescents who are at increased risk of hepatitis A infection or its complications	Havrix®*; VAQTA®*	720 EL.U.†/0.5 mL‡ 25 units/0.5 mL	A total of two doses at 0§, 6-12 mo A total of two doses at 0, 6-18 mo	I.M. I.M.
Hepatitis B vaccine	Adolescents not vaccinated previously for hepatitis B	Recombivax HB®*; Engerix-B®*	5 mcg/0.5 mL 10 mcg/0.5 mL	A total of three doses at 0, 1-2, 4-6 mo A total of three doses at 0, 1-2, 4-6 mo	I.M. I.M.
Influenza vaccine	Adolescents who are at increased risk for complications caused by influenza or who have contact with persons at increased risk for these complications	Influenza virus vaccine#	0.5 mL	Annually (September-December)	I.M.
Measles, mumps, and rubella vaccine (MMR®)	Adolescents not vaccinated previously with two doses of measles vaccine at ≥12 months of age	MMR® II*	0.5 mL	One dose	S.C.
Pneumococcal polysaccharide vaccine	Adolescents who are at increased risk for pneumococcal disease or its complications	Pneumococcal vaccine polyvalent#	0.5 mL	One dose	I.M. or S.C.
Tetanus and diphtheria toxoids (Td)	Adolescents not vaccinated within the previous 5 years	Tetanus and diphtheria toxoids, adsorbed (for adult use)#	0.5 mL	Every 10 y	I.M.
Varicella virus vaccine	Adolescents not vaccinated previously and who have no reliable history of chickenpox	Varivax®*	0.5 mL	One dose•	S.C.

Modified from *MMWR Morb Mortal Wkly Rep*, 1996, 45(RR-13).

*Manufacturer's product name.

†Enzyme-linked immunosorbent assay (ELISA) unit.

‡Alternative dosage and schedule of 360 EL.U./0.5 mL and a total of three doses administered at 0, 1, and 6-12 months.

§0 months represents timing of the initial dose, and subsequent numbers represent months after the initial dose.

#Generic name.

•Adolescent ≥13 years of age should be administered a total of two doses (0.5 mL/dose) subcutaneously at 0 and 4-8 weeks.

Minimum Age for Initial Vaccination and Minimum Interval Between Vaccine Doses, by Type of Vaccine

Vaccine	Minimum *Age* for First Dose*	Minimum *Interval* From Dose 1 to 2*	Minimum *Interval* From Dose 2 to 3*	Minimum *Interval* From Dose 3 to 4*
DTP (DT)†	6 wk‡	4 wk	4 wk	6 mo
Combined DTP-Hib	6 wk	1 mo	1 mo	6 mo
DTaP*	6 wk			6 mo
Hib (primary series)				
HbOC	6 wk	1 mo	1 mo	§
PRP-T	6 wk	1 mo	1 mo	§
PRP-OMP	6 wk	1 mo	§	
OPV			6 wk	
IPV¶	6 wk	4 wk	6 mo#	
MMR	12 mo•	1 mo		
Hepatitis B	Birth	1 mo	2 mo♦	
Varicella-zoster	12 mo	4 wk		

DTP = diphtheria-tetanus-pertussis.

DTaP = diphtheria-tetanus-acellular pertussis.

Hib = *Haemophilus influenzae* type b conjugate.

IPV = inactivated poliovirus vaccine.

MMR = measles-mumps-rubella.

OPV = poliovirus vaccine, live oral, trivalent.

Modified from *MMWR Morb Mortal Wkly Rep*, 1994, 43(RR-1).

*These minimum acceptable ages and intervals may not correspond with the optimal recommended ages and intervals for vaccination. See tables for the current recommended routine and accelerated vaccination schedules.

†DTaP can be used in place of the fourth (and fifth) dose of DTP for children who are at least 15 months of age. Children who have received all four primary vaccination doses before their fourth birthday should receive a fifth dose of DTP (DT) or DTaP at 4-6 years of age before entering kindergarten or elementary school **and** at least 6 months after the fourth dose. The total number of doses of diphtheria and tetanus toxoids should not exceed six each before the seventh birthday.

‡The American Academy of Pediatrics permits DTP to be administered as early as 4 weeks of age in areas with high endemicity and during outbreaks.

§The booster dose of Hib vaccine which is recommended following the primary vaccination series should be administered no earlier than 12 months of age **and** at least 2 months after the previous dose of Hib vaccine.

¶See text to differentiate conventional inactivated poliovirus vaccine from enhanced-potency IPV.

#For unvaccinated adults at increased risk of exposure to poliovirus with <3 months but >2 months available before protection is needed, three doses of IPV should be administered at least 1 month apart.

•Although the age for measles vaccination may be as young as 6 months in outbreak areas where cases are occurring in children<1 year of age, children initially vaccinated before the first birthday should be revaccinated at 12-15 months of age and an additional dose of vaccine should be administered at the time of school entry or according to local policy. Doses of MMR or other measles-containing vaccines should be separated by at least 1 month.

♦This final dose is recommended no earlier than 4 months of age.

Summary of ACIP Recommendations on Immunization of Immunocompromised Adults*

Vaccine†	Routine (Not Immunocompromised)	HIV Infection/AIDS	Severely Immunocompromised (Non-HIV Related)‡	Asplenia	Renal Failure	Diabetes
Routine Infant Immunizations						
DTP (ST or T)§	Recommended	Recommended	Recommended	Recommended	Recommended	Recommended
OPV	Recommended	Contraindicated	Contraindicated	Recommended	Recommended	Recommended
eIPV	Use if indicated	Recommended	Recommended	Use if indicated	Use if indicated	Use if indicated
MMR (MR, M, or R)	Recommended	Recommended/ Considered¶	Contraindicated	Recommended	Recommended	Recommended
Hib	Recommended	Recommended	Recommended	Recommended	Recommended	Recommended
Hepatitis B#	Recommended	Recommended	Recommended	Recommended	Recommended	Recommended
Other Childhood Immunizations						
Pneumococcal•	Use if indicated	Recommended**	Recommended**	Recommended**	Recommended††	Recommended
Influenza♦	Use if indicated	Recommended	Recommended	Recommended	Recommended	Recommended

Clin Pharm, 1993, 12:675-84.

*A "recommended" entry indicates that the vaccine is recommended as part of the routine schedule or the medical condition represents an indication for use of the vaccine. A "use if indicated" entry indicates that the immunosuppression category is not a contraindication to use of the vaccine if it is otherwise indicated. A "contraindicated" entry indicates that the medical condition is an absolute or relative contraindication to use of the vaccine. A "considered" entry indicates that a decision to use the vaccine should include consideration of the individual patient's risk of disease and the likely effectiveness of the vaccine. See section on Principles for Vaccinating Immunocompromised Persons for a discussion of categories of immunosuppression.

†DTP = diphtheria and tetanus toxoids and pertussis vaccine adsorbed; DT = diphtheria and tetanus toxoids adsorbed; T = tetanus toxoid; OPV = oral poliovirus vaccine live; eIPV = enhanced inactivated poliovirus vaccine; MMR = measles, mumps, and rubella virus vaccine live; and Hib = *Haemophilus* b conjugate vaccine.

‡Severe immunosuppression can be the result of congenital immunosuppression, human immunodeficiency virus (HIV) infection, leukemia, lymphoma, aplastic anemia, generalized malignancy, or therapy with alkylating agents, antimetabolites, radiation, or large amounts of corticosteroids.

§Includes boosters of acellular pertussis-containing vaccine.

¶See discussion of MMR in text.

#Hepatitis B virus vaccine is now recommended for all infants.

•Recommended for persons 2 years of age or older.

♦Not recommended for infants younger than 6 months of age.

**Reimmunize every 6 years.

††Reimmunize every 3-5 years.

Summary of ACIP Recommendations on Immunization of Immunocompromised Adults*

Vaccine	Routine (Not Immunocompromised)	HIV Infection/ AIDS	Severely Immunocompromised (Non-HIV related)*	After Solid-Organ Transplant Recipient or Chronic Immunosuppressive Therapy	Asplenia	Renal Failure	Diabetes	Alcoholism and Alcoholic Cirrhosis
Td	Recommended	Recommended	Recommended	Recommended	Recommended	Recommended	Recommended	Recommended
MMR (MR/M/R)†	Use if indicated	Recommended/ considered‡	**Contraindicated**	**Contraindicated**	Use if indicated	Use if indicated	Use if indicated	Use if indicated
Hepatitis B	Use if indicated	Use if indicated	Use if indicated	Use if indicated	Use if indicated	Recommended§	Use if indicated	Use if indicated
Hib	Not recommended	Considered¶	Recommended	Recommended	Recommended	Use if indicated	Use if indicated	Use if indicated
Pneumococcal	Recommended if ≥65 years of age	Recommended	Recommended	Recommended	Recommended	Recommended	Recommended	Recommended
Meningococcal	Use if indicated	Use if indicated	Use if indicated	Use if indicated	Recommended	Use if indicated	Use if indicated	Use if indicated
Influenza	Recommended if ≥65 years of age	Recommended	Recommended	Recommended	Recommended	Recommended	Recommended	Recommended

Modified from Centers for Disease Control and Prevention, Recommendations of the Advisory Committee on Immunization Practices: Use of Vaccines and Immunoglobulins in Persons With Altered Immunocompetence, *MMWR Morb Mortal Wkly Rep*, 1993, 42(RR-5):1-18.

*Severe immunosuppression can be the result of congenital immunodeficiency, leukemia, lymphoma, generalized malignancy, or therapy with alkylating agents, antimetabolites, radiation, or large amounts of corticosteroids.

†MMR = measles, mumps, and rubella virus vaccine; M = measles only; M/R = measles and rubella only.

‡See discussion of MMR in section on human immunodeficiency virus (HIV) and the acquired immunodeficiency syndrome (AIDS).

§Patients with renal failure on dialysis should have their anti-HB_s response tested after vaccination, and those who do not respond should be revaccinated.

#See discussion of HIV.

Summary of ACIP Recommendations on Nonroutine Immunization of Immunocompromised Persons*

Vaccine†	(Not Immunocompromised)	HIV Infection or AIDS	Severely Immunocompromised (Non-HIV related)‡	Solid-Organ Transplant Recipient Receiving Chronic Immunosuppressive Therapy	Asplenia, Renal Failure, Diabetes, Alcoholism, and Alcoholic Cirrhosis
Live Vaccines					
BCG	Use if indicated	**Contraindicated**	**Contraindicated**	**Contraindicated**	Use if indicated
OPV	Use if indicated	**Contraindicated**	**Contraindicated**	**Contraindicated**	Use if indicated
Vaccinia	Use if indicated	**Contraindicated**	**Contraindicated**	**Contraindicated**	Use if indicated
Typhoid, TY21a	Use if indicated	**Contraindicated**	**Contraindicated**	**Contraindicated**	Use if indicated
Yellow fever§	Use if indicated	**Contraindicated**	**Contraindicated**	**Contraindicated**	Use if indicated
Killed or Inactivated Vaccines					
IPV	Use if indicated	Use if indicated	Use if indicated	Use if indicated	Use if indicated
Cholera	Use if indicated	Use if indicated	Use if indicated	Use if indicated	Use if indicated
Plague	Use if indicated	Use if indicated	Use if indicated	Use if indicated	Use if indicated
Typhoid, inactivated	Use if indicated	Use if indicated	Use if indicated	Use if indicated	Use if indicated
Rabies	Use if indicated	Use if indicated	Use if indicated	Use if indicated	Use if indicated
Anthrax	Use if indicated	Use if indicated	Use if indicated	Use if indicated	Use if indicated

Modified from Centers for Disease Control and Prevention, Recommendations of the Advisory Committee on Immunization Practices: Use of Vaccines and Immunoglobulins in Persons With Altered Immunocompetence, *MMWR Morb Mortal Wkly Rep*, 1993, 42(RR-5):1-18.

†BCG = Bacille Calmette-Guérin; OPV = oral poliovirus vaccine; IPV = inactivated poliovirus vaccine; HIV = human immunodeficiency virus; AIDS = acquired immunodeficiency syndrome.

‡Severe immunosuppression also can be the result of congenital immunodeficiency, leukemia, lymphoma, aplastic anemia, generalized malignancy, or therapy with alkylating agents, antimetabolites, radiation, or large amounts of corticosteroids.

§Yellow fever vaccine should be considered for patients when exposure to yellow fever cannot be avoided (see text).

Summary of ACIP Recommendations on Use of Immune Globulins in Immunocompromised Persons*

Immune Globulin	Not Immunocompromised	HIV Infected	Severely Immunocompromised†
IG	Recommended for infants and susceptible adults exposed to measles	Recommended for symptomatic patients exposed to measles regardless of immunization status Recommended for persons with exposure to hepatitis A or who will travel to HAV-endemic areas	Recommended for patients exposed to measles regardless of immunization status
VZIG‡	May be used for exposed susceptible adults and exposed susceptible pregnant women, and infants <28 days	Recommended for susceptible infants and adults after significant exposure to V-Z	Recommended for adults after significant exposure to V-Z
TIG	Recommended for those with serious wounds and <3 doses of tetanus toxoid	Same as for nonimmunocompromised	Same as for nonimmunocompromised
HBIG	Recommended for prophylaxis in susceptible persons with percutaneous, sexual, or mucosal exposure to HBV	Same as for nonimmunocompromised	Same as for nonimmunocompromised
HRIG	Recommended for postexposure prophylaxis of persons not previously vaccinated against rabies	Same as for nonimmunocompromised	Same as for nonimmunocompromised

Modified from Centers for Disease Control and Prevention, Recommendations of the Advisory Committee on Immunization Practices: Use of Vaccines and Immunoglobulins in Persons With Altered Immunocompetence, *MMWR Morb Mortal Wkly Rep*, 1993, 42(RR-5):1-18.

*IG = immune globulin; HIV = human immunodeficiency virus; VZIG = varicella-zoster IG; TIG = tetanus IG; HBIG = hepatitis B IG; HRIG = human rabies IG; V-Z = varicella-zoster; HBV = hepatitis B virus.

†Severe immunosuppression also can be the result of congenital immunodeficiency, leukemia, lymphoma, aplastic anemia, generalized malignancy, or therapy with alkylating agents, antimetabolites, radiation, or large amounts of corticosteroids.

‡See section on Use of Immune Globulins for a discussion of issues to be considered before use of VZIG.

Licensed Vaccines and Toxoids Available in the United States, by Type and Recommended Routes of Administration

	Type	Route
Adenovirus*	Live virus	Oral
Anthrax†	Inactivated bacteria	Subcutaneous
Bacillus of Calmette and Gu (BCG)	Live bacteria	Intradermal/ percutaneous
Cholera	Inactivated bacteria	Subcutaneous or intradermal‡
Diphtheria-tetanus-pertussis (DTP)	Toxoids and inactivated whole bacteria	Intramuscular
DTP-*Haemophilus influenzae* type b conjugate (DTP-Hib)	Toxoids, inactivated whole bacteria, and bacterial polysaccharide conjugated to protein	Intramuscular
Diphtheria-tetanus-acellular pertussis (DTaP)	Toxoids and inactivated bacterial components	Intramuscular
Hepatitis A	Inactivated virus	Intramuscular
Hepatitis B	Purified viral antigen	Intramuscular
Haemophilus influenzae type be conjugate (Hib)§	Bacterial polysaccharide conjugated to protein	Intramuscular
Influenza	Inactivated virus or viral components	Intramuscular
Japanese encephalitis	Inactivated virus	Subcutaneous
Measles	Live virus	Subcutaneous
Measles-mumps-rubella (MMR)	Live virus	Subcutaneous
Meningococcal	Bacterial polysaccharides of serotypes A/C/Y/W-135	Subcutaneous
Mumps	Live virus	Subcutaneous
Pertussis†	Inactivated whole bacteria	Intramuscular
Plague	Inactivated bacteria	Intramuscular
Pneumococcal	Bacterial polysaccharides of 23 pneumococcal types	Intramuscular or subcutaneous
Poliovirus vaccine		
Inactivated (IPV)	Inactivated viruses of all 3 serotypes	Subcutaneous
Oral (OPV)	Live viruses of all 3 serotypes	Oral
Rabies	Inactivated virus	Intramuscular or intradermal¶
Rubella	Live virus	Subcutaneous
Tetanus	Inactivated toxin (toxoid)	Intramuscular#
Tetanus-diphtheria (Td or DT)•	Inactivated toxins (toxoids)	Intramuscular#
Typhoid		
Parenteral	Inactivated bacteria	Subcutaneous♦
Ty21a oral	Live bacteria	Oral
Varicella	Live virus	Subcutaneous
Yellow fever	Live virus	Subcutaneous

Modified from *MMWR Morb Mortal Wkly Rep*, 1994, 43(RR-1).

*Available only to the U.S. Armed Forces.

†Distributed by the Division of Biologic Products, Michigan Department of Public Health.

‡The intradermal dose is lower than the subcutaneous dose.

§The recommended schedule for infants depends on the vaccine manufacturer; consult the package insert and ACIP recommendations for specific products.

¶The intradermal dose of rabies vaccine, human diploid cell (HDCV), is lower than the intramuscular dose and is used only for pre-exposure vaccination. **Rabies vaccine, adsorbed (RVA) should not be used intradermally.**

#Preparations with adjuvants should be administered intramuscularly.

•Td-tetanus and diphtheria toxoids for use among persons ≥7 years of age. Td contains the same amount of tetanus toxoid as DTP or DT, but contains a smaller dose of diphtheria toxoid. DT = tetanus and diphtheria toxoids for use among children <7 years of age.

♦Booster doses may be administered intradermally unless vaccine that is acetone-killed and dried is used.

Immune Globulins and Antitoxins* Available in the United States, by Type of Antibodies and Indications for Use

Immunobiologic	Type	Indication(s)
Botulinum antitoxin	Specific equine antibodies	Treatment of botulism
Cytomegalovirus immune globulin, intravenous (CMV-IGIV)	Specific human antibodies	Prophylaxis for bone marrow and kidney transplant recipients
Diphtheria antitoxin	Specific equine antibodies	Treatment of respiratory diphtheria
Immune globulin (IG)	Pooled human antibodies	Hepatitis A pre- and postexposure prophylaxis; measles postexposure prophylaxis
Immune globulin, intravenous (IGIV)	Pooled human antibodies	Replacement therapy for antibody deficiency disorders; immune thrombocytopenic purpura (ITP); hypogammaglobulinemia in chronic lymphocytic leukemia; Kawasaki disease
Hepatitis B immune globulin (HBIG)	Specific human antibodies	Hepatitis B postexposure prophylaxis
Rabies immune globulin (HRIG)†	Specific human antibodies	Rabies postexposure management of persons not previously immunized with rabies vaccine
Tetanus immune globulin (TIG)	Specific human antibodies	Tetanus treatment; postexposure prophylaxis of persons not adequately immunized with tetanus toxoid
Vaccinia immune globulin (VIG)	Specific human antibodies	Treatment of eczema vaccinatum, vaccinia necrosum, and ocular vaccinia
Varicella-zoster immune globulin (VZIG)	Specific human antibodies	Postexposure prophylaxis of susceptible immunocompromised persons, certain susceptible pregnant women, and perinatally exposed newborn infants

Modified from *MMWR Morb Mortal Wkly Rep*, 1994, 43(RR-1).

*Immune globulin preparations and antitoxins are administered intramuscularly unless otherwise indicated.

†HRIG is administered around the wounds in addition to the intramuscular injection.

Guidelines for Spacing the Administration of Immune Globulin Preparations* and Vaccines Containing Live Measles, Mumps, or Rubella Virus

SIMULTANEOUS ADMINISTRATION

Immunobiologic Combination	Recommended Minimum Interval Between Doses
Immune globulin and vaccine	Should generally not be administered simultaneously.† If simultaneous administration of measles-mumps-rubella (MMR), measles-rubella, and monovalent measles vaccine is unavoidable, administer at different sites and revaccinate or test for seroconversion after the recommended interval.

NONSIMULTANEOUS ADMINISTRATION

Immunobiologic Administered		Recommended Minimum Interval Between Doses
First	**Second**	
Immune globulin	Vaccine	Dose related†
Vaccine	Immune globulin	2 weeks

*Blood products containing large amounts of immune globulin (such as serum immune globulin, specific immune globulins [eg, TIG and HBIG], intravenous immune globulin [IGIV], whole blood, packed red cells, plasma, and platelet products).

†The duration of interference of immune globulin preparations with the immune response to the measles component of the MMR, measles-rubella, and monovalent measles vaccine is dose-related.

Suggested Intervals Between Administration of Immune Globulin Preparations for Various Indications and Vaccines Containing Live Measles Virus*

Indication	Dose (including mg IgG/kg)	Time Interval (mo) Before Measles Vaccination
Tetanus (TIG) prophylaxis	I.M.: 250 units (10 mg IgG/kg)	3
Hepatitis A (IG) prophylaxis		
Contact prophylaxis	I.M.: 0.02 mL/kg (3.3 mg IgG/kg)	3
International travel	I.M.: 0.06 mL/kg (10 mg IgG/kg)	3
Hepatitis B prophylaxis (HBIG)	I.M.: 0.06 mL/kg (10 mg IgG/kg)	3
Rabies immune globulin (HRIG)	I.M.: 20 IU/kg (22 mg IgG/kg)	4
Varicella prophylaxis (VZIG)	I.M.: 125 units/10 kg (20-40 mg IgG/kg) (maximum: 625 units)	5
Measles prophylaxis (IG) Standard (ie, nonimmunocompromised contact)	I.M.: 0.25 mL/kg (40 mg IgG/kg)	5
Immunocompromised contact	I.M.: 0.50 mL/kg (80 mg IgG/kg)	6
Blood transfusion		
RBCs, washed	I.V.: 10 mL/kg (negligible IgG/kg)	0
RBCs, adenine-saline added	I.V.: 10 mL/kg (10 mg IgG/kg)	3
Packed RBCs (Hct 65%)†	I.V.: 10 mL/kg (60 mg IgG/kg)	6
Whole blood cells (Hct 35%-50%)†	I.V.: 10 mL/kg (80-100 mg IgG/kg)	6
Plasma/platelet products	I.V.: 10 mL/kg (160 mg IgG/kg)	7
Replacement therapy for immune deficiencies	I.V.: 300-400 mg/kg (as IGIV)‡	8
Treatment of		
Immune thrombocytopenic purpura§	I.V.: 400 mg/kg (as IGIV)	8
Immune thrombocytopenic purpura§	I.V.: 1000 mg/kg (as IGIV)	10
Kawasaki disease	I.V.: 2 g/kg (as IGIV)	11

*This table is not intended for determining the correct indications and dosage for the use of immune globulin preparations. Unvaccinated persons may not be fully protected against measles during the entire suggested time interval, and additional doses of immune globulin and/or measles vaccine may be indicated after measles exposure. The concentration of measles antibody in a particular immune globulin preparation can vary by lot. The rate of antibody clearance after receipt of an immune globulin preparation also can vary. The recommended time intervals are extrapolated from an estimated half-life of 30 days of passively acquired antibody and an observed interference with the immune response to measles vaccine for 5 months after a dose of 80 mg IgG/kg.

†Assumes a serum IgG concentration of 16 mg/mL.

‡Measles vaccination is recommended for most HIV-infected children who do not have evidence of severe immunosuppression, but it is contraindicated for patients who have congenital disorders of the immune system.

§Formerly referred to as idiopathic thrombocytopenic purpura.

Modified from *MMWR Morb Mortal Wkly Rep*, 1996, 45(RR-12).

MISCELLANEOUS VACCINATION INFORMATION

Guidelines for Spacing Live and Killed Antigen Administration

Antigen Combinations	Recommended Minimum Interval Between Doses
≥2 killed antigens	None. May be given simultaneously or at any interval between doses.
Killed and live antigens	None. May be given simultaneously or at any interval between doses. (Exception: Concurrent administration of cholera and yellow fever vaccines should be avoided. Separate these vaccines by at least 3 weeks.)
≥2 live antigens	4 weeks minimum interval if not administered simultaneously. (Recent receipt of OPV is not a contraindication to MMR.) Vaccines associated with systemic reactions (cholera and parenteral typhoid or influenza and DTP in young children) should be given on separate occasions.

Passive Immunization Agents — Immune Globulins

Immune Globulin	Dosage		Route
Hepatitis B (H-BIG®)			I.M.
percutaneous inoculation	0.06 mL/kg/dose (within 24 hours) (5 mL max)		
perinatal	0.5 mL/dose (within 12 hours of birth)		
sexual exposure	0.06 mL/kg/dose (within 14 days of contact) (5 mL max)		
Immune globulin (IG)			I.M.*
hepatitis A prophylaxis	0.02 mL/kg/dose (as soon as possible or within 2 weeks after exposure) (single exposure)		
hepatitis B	0.06 mL/kg/dose (H-BIG® should be used)		
measles†	0.25 mL/kg/dose (max 15 mL/dose) (within 6 days of exposure)		
	0.5 mL/kg/dose (max 15 mL/dose) (immunocompromised children)		
Rabies‡	20 IU/kg/dose (within 3 days)		
Tetanus (serious, contaminated wounds; <3 previous tetanus vaccine doses)	250-500 units/dose		I.M.
Varicella-zoster§ (VZIG)	Within 48 hours but not later than 96 hours after exposure		I.M.¶
	0-10 kg	125 units = 1 vial	
	10.1-20 kg	250 units = 2 vials	
	20.1-30 kg	375 units = 3 vials	
	30.1-40 kg	500 units = 4 vials	
	>40 kg	625 units = 5 vials	

*Deep I.M. in the gluteal region for large doses only. Deltoid muscle or the anterolateral aspect of the thigh are preferred sites for injection. No greater than 5 mL/site in adults or large children; 1-3 mL/site in small children and infants. Maximum dose: 20 mL at one time.

†IG prophylaxis may not be indicated in a patient who has received IGIV within 3 weeks of exposure.

‡½ of dose used to infiltrate the wound with the remaining ½ of dose given I.M. Rabies immune globulin is not recommended in previously HDCV immunized patients.

§Infants born to women who develop varicella within 5 days before or 48 hours after delivery should receive 125 units I.M. as a single dose.

¶No greater than 2.5 mL of VZIG/one injection site. Doses >2.5 mL should be divided and administered at different sites.

Guidelines for Spacing the Administration of Immune Globulin (IG) Preparations and Vaccines

Immunobiologic Combinations		Recommended Minimum Interval Between Doses
Simultaneous Administration		
IG and killed antigen		None. May be given simultaneously at different sites or at any time between doses.
IG and live antigen		Should generally not be given simultaneously. If unavoidable to do so, give at different sites and revaccinate or test for seroconversion in 3 months. Example: MMR should not be given to patients who have received immune globulin within the previous 3 months.
Nonsimultaneous Administration		
First	**Second**	
IG	Killed antigen	None
Killed antigen	IG	None
IG	Live antigen	6 weeks, and preferably 3 months
Live antigen	IG	2 weeks

*The live virus vaccines, OPV, and yellow fever are exceptions to these recommendations. Either vaccine may be administered simultaneously or any time before or after IG without significantly decreasing antibody response.

Recommended for Routine Immunization of HIV-Infected Children — United States

	Known HIV Infection	
Vaccine	Asymptomatic	Symptomatic
DTP	Yes	Yes
OPV	No*	No*
IPV	Yes	Yes
MMR	Yes	Yes
HbCV	Yes	Yes
Pneumococcal	Yes	Yes
Influenza	No†	Yes

*Should be replaced with inactivated polio vaccine.

†Not contraindicated.

ADVERSE EVENTS AND VACCINATION

Reportable Events Following Vaccination

Vaccine/Toxoid		Event	Interval From Vaccination
DTP, DTaP, DTP-HiB, P, DT, Td, TT	A.	Anaphylaxis or anaphylactic shock	7 days
	B.	Encephalopathy (or encephalitis)	7 days
	C.	Any sequela (including death) of above events	No limit
	D.	Events described in manufacturer's package insert as contraindications to additional doses of vaccine	See package insert
Measles and mumps in any combination; MMR, MR, M	A.	Anaphylaxis or anaphylactic shock	7 days
	B.	Encephalopathy (or encephalitis)	15 days
	C.	Residual seizure disorder	15 days
	D.	Any sequela (including death) of above events	No limit
	E.	Events described in manufacturer's package insert as contraindications to additional doses of vaccine	See package insert
Rubella in any combination: MMR, MR, R	A.	Chronic arthritis	42 days
	B.	Anaphylaxis or anaphylactic shock	7 days
	C.	Encephalopathy (or encephalitis)	15 days
	D.	Residual seizure disorder	15 days
	E.	Any sequela (including death) of above events	No limit
	F.	Events described in manufacturer's package insert as contraindications to additional doses of vaccine	See package insert
Oral polio	A.	Paralytic polio	
(OPV)		• in a nonimmunodeficient recipient	30 days
		• in an immunodeficient recipient	6 months
		• in a vaccine-associated community case	No limit
	B.	Any sequela (including death) of above events	No limit
	C.	Events described in manufacturer's package insert as contraindications to additional doses of vaccine	See package insert
Inactivated polio (IPV)	A.	Anaphylaxis or anaphylactic shock	7 days
	B.	Any sequela (including death) of above events	No limit
	C.	Events described in manufacturer's package insert as contraindications to additional doses of vaccine	See package insert

The Reportable Events Table (RET) reflects what is reportable by law (42 USC 300aa-25) to the Vaccine Adverse Event Reporting System (VAERS) including conditions found in the manufacturers package insert. In addition, individuals are encouraged to report **any** clinically significant or unexpected events (even if you are not certain the vaccine caused the event) for **any** vaccine, whether or not it is listed on the RET. Manufacturers are also required by regulation (21CFR 600.80) to report to the VAERS program all adverse events made known to them for any vaccine.

Effective March 1995. Revised 21 May 1996.

PREVENTION OF HEPATITIS A THROUGH ACTIVE OR PASSIVE IMMUNIZATION

Recommendations of the Advisory Committee on Immunization Practices (ACIP)

December 27, 1996, Vol. 45, No. RR-15

PROPHYLAXIS AGAINST HEPATITIS A VIRUS INFECTION

Recommended Doses of Immune Globulin (IG) for Hepatitis A Pre-exposure and Postexposure Prophylaxis

Setting	Duration of Coverage	IG Dose*
Pre-exposure	Short-term (1-2 months)	0.02 mL/kg
	Long-term (3-5 months)	0.06 mL/kg†
Postexposure	—	0.02 mL/kg

*IG should be administered by intramuscular injection into either the deltoid or gluteal muscle. For children <24 months of age, IG can be administered in the anterolateral thigh muscle.

†Repeat every 5 months if continued exposure to HAV occurs.

Recommended Dosages of Havrix®*

Vaccinee's age (yrs)	Dose (EL.U.)†	Volume (mL)	No. doses	Schedule (mos)‡
2-18	720	0.5	2	0, 6-12
>18	1440	1.0	2	0, 6-12

*Hepatitis A vaccine, inactivated, SmithKline Beecham Biologicals

†ELISA units

‡0 months represents timing of the initial dose; subsequent numbers represent months after the initial dose.

Recommended Dosages of VAQTA®*

Vaccinee's age (yrs)	Dose (U)†	Volume (mL)	No. doses	Schedule (mos)‡
2-17	25	0.5	2	0, 6-18
>17	50	1.0	2	0, 6

*Hepatitis A vaccine, inactivated, Merck & Company, Inc.

†Units

‡0 months represents timing of the initial dose; subsequent numbers represent months after the initial dose.

PREVENTION OF MALARIA[1]

		Drug	Adult Dosage	Pediatric Dosage
Chloroquine-sensitive areas				
Drug of choice:		Chloroquine phosphate[2]	300 mg base (500 mg salt) P.O., once/week beginning 1 week before and continuing for 4 weeks after last exposure	5 mg/kg base (8.3 mg/kg salt) once/ week, up to adult dose of 300 mg base
Chloroquine-resistant areas[3]				
Drug of choice:[4]		Mefloquine[2,5,6]	P.O.: 250 mg once/week[7]	15-19 kg: 1/4 tablet 20-30 kg: 1/2 tablet 31-45 kg: 3/4 tablet >45 kg: 1 tablet
	or	Doxycycline[2,8,9]	100 mg daily	>8 y: 2 mg/kg/d P.O., up to 100 mg/d
	or	Chloroquine phosphate[2]	as above	as above
		plus pyrimethamine-sulfadoxine[10] for presumptive treatment[11]	Carry a single dose (3 tablets) for self-treatment of febrile illness when medical care is not immediately available	<1 y: 1/4 tablet 1-3 y: 1/2 tablet 4-8 y: 1 tablet 9-14 y: 2 tablets
		or **plus** proguanil[12] (in Africa south of the Sahara)	200 mg daily during exposure and for 4 weeks afterwards	<2 y: 50 mg daily 2-6 y: 100 mg daily 7-10 y: 150 mg daily 10 y: 200 mg daily

[1]At present, no drug regimen guarantees protection against malaria. If fever develops within a year (particularly within the first 2 months) after travel to malarious areas, travelers should be advised to seek medical attention. Insect repellents, insecticide-impregnated bed nets, and proper clothing are important adjuncts for malaria prophylaxis.

[2]For prevention of attack after departure from areas where *P vivax* and *P ovale* are endemic, which includes almost all areas where malaria is found (except Haiti), some experts, in addition, prescribe primaquine phosphate 15 mg base (26.3 mg/d or, for children, 0.3 mg base/kg/d during the last 2 weeks of prophylaxis. Others prefer to avoid the toxicity of primaquine and rely on surveillance to detect cases when they occur, particularly when exposure was limited or doubtful. Primaquine phosphate can cause hemolytic anemia, especially in patients whose red cells are deficient in glucose-6-phosphate dehydrogenase. This deficiency is most common in Blacks, Orientals, and Mediterranean peoples. Patients should be screened for G-6-PD deficiency before treatment. Primaquine should not be used during pregnancy.

[3]Chloroquine-resistant *P falciparum* infections have been reported in all areas that have malaria except Central America west of Panama Canal Zone, Mexico. Haiti, the Dominican Republic, and the Middle East (including Egypt). In pregnancy, chloroquine prophylaxis has been used extensively and safely, but the safety of other prophylactic antimalarial agents in pregnancy is unclear. Therefore, travel during pregnancy to chloroquine-resistant areas should be discouraged. For chloroquine-resistant parasitemia ≥10%, exchange transfusion has been used (Miller KD, et al, *N Engl J Med*, 321:65, 1989; Saddler M, et al; Vachon F, et al; Miller KD, et al, *N Engl J Med*, 322:58, 1990). Mefloquine is not recommended for use during pregnancy according to the current FDA labeling agreement; however, a review of mefloquine use in pregnancy from clinical trials and reports of inadvertent use of mefloquine during pregnancy suggested its use is not associated with adverse fetal or pregnancy outcomes, such as birth defects, still birth, and spontaneous abortions. Consequently, mefloquine may be considered for use by healthcare providers for prophylaxis in women who are pregnant or likely to become so when exposure to chloroquine-resistant *P. falciparum* is unavoidable. Because information on use in first trimester is limited, providers are asked to report exposures to CDC Malaria Section (770-488-7760).

[4]For prophylaxis where both chloroquine and pyrimethamine/sulfadoxine resistance coexist, mefloquine is the usual drug of choice. In areas with mefloquine-resistant plasmodium, such as Thailand, doxycycline is recommended.

[5]In the USA, a 250 mg tablet of mefloquine contains 228 mg of mefloquine base. Outside the USA, each 274 mg tablet contains 250 mg base.

[6]The pediatric dosage has not been approved by the FDA, and the drug has not been approved for use during pregnancy. Women should take contraceptive precautions while taking mefloquine and for 2 months after the last dose. Mefloquine is not recommended for children weighing less than 15 kg, or for patients taking beta blockers, calcium channel blockers, or other drugs that may prolong or otherwise alter cardiac conduction. Patients with a history of seizures or psychiatric disorders and those whose occupations require fine coordination or spatial discrimination should probably avoid mefloquine (*The Medical Letter*, 32:13, 1990).

[7]Beginning 1 week before travel and continuing weekly for the duration of stay and for 4 weeks after leaving.

[8]An approved drug, but considered investigational for this condition by the U.S. Food and Drug Administration.

[9]Beginning 1 day before travel and continuing for the duration of stay and for 4 weeks after leaving. The FDA considers use of tetracyclines as antimalarials to be investigational. Use of tetracyclines is contraindicated in pregnancy and in children younger than 8 years of age. Physicians who prescribe doxycycline as malaria chemoprophylaxis should advise patients to use an appropriate sunscreen (*The Medical Letter*, 31:59, 1989) to minimize the possibility of a photosensitivity reaction and should warn women that *Candida* vaginitis is a frequent adverse effect.

[10]*Fansidar* tablets contain 25 mg of pyrimethamine and 500 mg of sulfadoxine.

[11]Resistance to *Fansidar* should be anticipated in Southeast Asia, Bangladesh, Oceania, the Amazon basin, and in east Africa. Use of *Fansidar* is contraindicated in patients with a history of sulfonamide or pyrimethamine intolerance. In pregnancy at term and in infants less than 2 months old, pyrimethamine-sulfadoxine may cause hyperbilirubinemia

[12]Proguanil (Paludrine® — Ayerst, Canada; ICI, England), which is not available in the USA but is widely available overseas, is recommended mainly for use in Africa south of the Sahara. Failures in prophylaxis with chloroquine and proguanil have, however, been reported in travelers to Kenya (Barnes AJ, *Lancet*, 338:1338, 1991).

RECOMMENDATIONS FOR TRAVELERS

Vaccine Advice for Travelers

Vaccine	Indication	Dose	Comments
Cholera	The risk to tourists is very low	Refer to product labeling	The currently licensed parenteral vaccine (prepared from killed bacteria) has limited effectiveness, often causes reactions, and is generally not recommended for travelers
Hepatitis B vaccine	Not ordinarily recommended for foreign travel, except for medical personnel whose work could require handling of body fluids, or for people who expect to have sexual contacts, receive medical or dental care, or stay for >6 months in areas such as Southeast Asia or sub-Saharan Africa, where hepatitis B is highly endemic	I.M.: 3 doses over 2-6 (preferable) months	Hepatitis B vaccine is less effective when injected into the gluteal area, and should be injected into the deltoid muscle
Japanese encephalitis vaccine	Travelers who anticipate spending a month or longer in rural rice-growing areas where they will be heavily exposed to mosquitoes. Countries where the disease may be a problem include Bangladesh, Cambodia, China, India, Indonesia, Korea, Laos, Malaysia, Meaner (Burma), Nepal, Pakistan, the Philippines, Singapore, Sri Lanka, Taiwan, Thailand, Vietnam, and eastern areas of Russia.	Primary series of 3 doses given over 2-4 (preferable) weeks.	Formalin-activated, purified mouse-brain-derived vaccine
Measles vaccine	People born after 1956 who have not received 2 doses of measles vaccine (after their first birthday) and do not have a physician-documented history of infection or laboratory evidence of immunity should receive before traveling anywhere	Single dose of measles (or measles-mumps-rubella) vaccine at least 2 weeks before or 3 months after immune globulin	

(continued)

Vaccine	Indication	Dose	Comments
Meningococcal vaccine	Only for tourists traveling to areas where epidemics are occurring. Epidemics occur frequently in sub-Saharan Africa from December to June, and also in northern India and Nepal. Saudi Arabia requires a certificate of immunization for pilgrims to Mecca.	Single dose	
Polio vaccine	Adult travelers to tropical or developing countries who have not previously been immunized against polio	Adults: If protection is needed within 4 weeks, a single dose of enhanced inactivated polio vaccine (eIPV) or trivalent (live) oral polio vaccine (OPV) is recommended. Travelers who have previously completed a primary series should receive a booster of OPT or eIPV.	OPV rarely can cause vaccine-induced polio, particularly in previously unimmunized adults
Rabies vaccine	Travelers with an occupational risk of exposure or those traveling for extended periods in endemic areas	3 injections of vaccine over 3-4 weeks	
Tetanus and diphtheria toxoids	Tetanus-diphtheria toxoid (Td) booster every 10 years. Especially for travelers going to developing countries and to Russia and the Ukraine, where a large outbreak of diphtheria has been occurring in recent years.		

(continued)

Vaccine	Indication	Dose	Comments
Typhoid vaccine	Travel to rural areas of tropical countries, where typhoid tends to endemic, or to any area where an outbreak was occurring	P.O.: One capsule every other day for a total of 4 capsules, beginning at least 2 weeks before departure Parenteral: AKD and HP: Adults and children ≥10 y: Two doses of 0.5 mL S.C. administered at ≥4-week intervals Children <10 y: Two doses of 0.25 mL S.C. administered at ≥4-week intervals Vi: Adults and children ≥2 y: I.M.: 0.5 mL single dose	Killed bacteria parenteral vaccine is not fully protective and causes 1-2 days of pain at the site of injection sometimes accompanied by fever, malaise, and headache. Live oral vaccine reported to provide equally effective, longer than parenteral vaccine and have less adverse effects. Antibiotics should be avoided, if possible, for 1 week before and 3 weeks after oral typhoid vaccine.
Yellow fever vaccine	Travelers to rural areas in the yellow fever endemic zones, which include most of tropical South America and most of Africa between 15°N and 15°S. Some countries in Africa require a certificate of yellow fever vaccination from all entering travelers. Other countries in Africa, South America, and Asia require evidence of vaccination from travelers coming from infected or endemic areas.	Boosters are given every 10 years.	Attenuated live virus vaccine. Need to administer 10 days prior to entry in countries requiring yellow fever vaccination certification.

More than one vaccine can be given at the same time.
Immunocompromised or pregnant patients generally should not receive live virus vaccines, but measles vaccine is recommended for HIV-infected patients.

ANTIMICROBIAL PROPHYLAXIS

Antimicrobial Prophylaxis in Surgical Patients

Nature of Operation	Likely Pathogens	Recommended Drugs	Adult Dosage Before Surgery*
CLEAN			
Cardiac			
Prosthetic valve and other open-heart surgery	*S. epidermidis, S. aureus, Corynebacterium,* enteric gram-negative bacilli	Cefazolin **or** vancomycin‡	1 g I.V.
Vascular			
Arterial surgery involving the abdominal aorta, a prosthesis, or a groin incision	*S. aureus, S. epidermidis,* enteric gram-negative bacilli	Cefazolin **or** vancomycin‡	1 g I.V.
Lower extremity amputation for ischemia	*S. aureus, S. epidermidis,* enteric gram-negative bacilli, clostridia	Cefazolin **or** vancomycin‡	1 g I.V.
Neurosurgery			
Craniotomy	*S. aureus, S. epidermidis*	Cefazolin **or** vancomycin‡	1 g I.V.
Orthopedic			
Total joint replacement, internal fixation of fractures	*S. aureus, S. epidermidis*	Cefazolin **or** vancomycin‡	1 g I.V.
Ocular§	*S. aureus, S. epidermidis,* streptococci, enteric gram-negative bacilli, *Pseudomonas*	Gentamicin **or** tobramycin **or** combination of neomycin, gramicidin, and polymyxin B	Multiple drops topically over 2-24 h
		cefazolin	100 mg subconjunctivally at end of procedure
CLEAN-CONTAMINATED			
Head and neck			
Entering oral cavity or pharynx	*S. aureus,* streptococci, oral anaerobes	Cefazolin **or**	1 g I.V.
		clindamycin	600 mg I.V.
Gastroduodenal*			
High risk, gastric bypass, or percutaneous endoscopic gastrostomy only	Enteric gram-negative bacilli, gram-positive cocci	Cefazolin	1 g I.V.
Biliary tract*			
High risk only	Enteric gram-negative bacilli, enterococci, clostridia	Cefazolin	1 g I.V.
Colorectal*	Enteric gram-negative bacilli, anaerobes	Oral: Neomycin plus erythromycin base	1 g of each at 1 PM, 2 PM, and 11 PM the day before the operation¶
		Parenteral: Ceftizoxime	1 g I.V.
Appendectomy*	Enteric gram-negative bacilli, anaerobes	Ceftizoxime	1 g I.V.

(continued)

Nature of Operation	Likely Pathogens	Recommended Drugs	Adult Dosage Before Surgery
Vaginal or abdominal hysterectomy*	Enteric gram-negative bacilli, anaerobes, group B streptococci, enterococci	Cefazolin **or** Ceftizoxime	1 g I.V. 1 g I.V.
Cesarean section	Same as for hysterectomy	High risk only: Cefazolin	1 g I.V. after cor clamping
Abortion	Same as for hysterectomy	First trimester in patients with previous pelvic inflammatory disease:	
		Aqueous penicillin G	1 million units I.V.
		or	
		doxycycline	100 mg P.O. 1 hour before abortion, then 200 mg P.O. 30 minutes after abortion
		Second trimester:	
		Cefazolin	1 g I.V.
DIRTY			
Ruptured viscus	Enteric gram-negative bacilli, anaerobes, enterococci	Ceftizoxime with or without	1 g q8h I.V.
		gentamicin	1.5 mg/kg q8h I.V.
		or	
		clindamycin	600 mg I.V. q6h
		plus gentamicin	1.5 mg/kg q8h I.V.
Traumatic wound#	*S. aureus*, group A streptococci, clostridia	Cefazolin	1 g q8h I.V.

*Parenteral prophylactic antimicrobials for clean and clean-contaminated surgery can be given as a single intravenous dose just before the operation. Cefazolin can also be given intramuscularly. For prolonged operations, additional intraoperative doses should be given every 4-8 hours for the duration of the procedure. For "dirty" surgery, therapy should usually be continued for 5-10 days.

‡For hospitals in which methicillin-resistant *S. aureus* and *S. epidermidis* frequently cause wound infection, or for patients allergic to penicillins or cephalosporin.

§In addition, at the end of the operation many ophthalmologists give a subconjunctival injection of an aminoglycoside such as gentamicin (10-20 mg), with or without a cephalosporin such as cefazolin (100 mg).

¶After appropriate diet and catharsis.

#For bite wounds, in which likely pathogens may also include oral anaerobes, *Eikenella corrodens* (humans), and *Pasteurella multocida* (dog and cat), some *Medical Letter* consultants recommend use of amoxicillin-clavulanic acid (Augmentin®) or ampicillin/sulbactam (Unasyn®).

CEPHALOSPORINS BY GENERATION

First Generation	2nd Generation	3rd Generation	4th Generation
Cefadroxil (Duricef®)*	Cefaclor (Ceclor®)*	Cefixime (Suprax®)*	Cefepime (Maxipime®)†
Cefazolin (Ancef®)	Cefamandole (Mandol®)	Cefperazone (Cefobid®)†	
Cephalexin (Keflex®)*	Cefmetazole (Zefazone®)	Cefotaxime (Claforan®)	
Cephalothin (Keflin®)	Cefonicid (Monocid®)	Cefpodoxime (Vantin®)*	
Cephapirin (Cefadryl®)	Ceforanide (Precef®)	Ceftizoxime (Cefizox®)	
Cephradine (Anspor®)*	Cefotetan (Cefotan®)	Ceftriaxone (Rocephin®)	
	Cefoxitin (Mefoxin®)	Ceftazidime (Fortaz)†	
	Cefprozil (Cefzil®)*		
	Cefuroxime (Zinacef®)*		
	Cefuroxime axetil (Ceftin®)		
	Loracarbef (Lorabid®)		

*Oral dosage form available

†Anti-pseudomonal activity notable

Note: Other brand names or generic products may be available

OCCUPATIONAL EXPOSURE TO HIV

Provisional Public Health Service Recommendations for Chemoprophylaxis After Occupational Exposure to HIV, by Type of Exposure and Source Material — 1996

Type of Exposure	Source Material*	Antiretroviral Prophylaxis†	Antiretroviral Regimen‡
Percutaneous	Blood§		
	Highest risk	Recommend	ZDV + 3TC + IDV
	Increased risk	Recommend	ZDV + 3TC, ± IDV¶
	No increased risk	Offer	ZDV + 3TC
	Fluid containing visible blood, other potentially infectious fluid#, or tissue	Offer	ZDV + 3TC
	Other body fluid (eg, urine)	Not offer	
Mucous membrane	Blood	Offer	ZDV + 3TC, ±IDV¶
	Fluid containing visible blood, other potentially infectious fluid,# or tissue	Offer	ZDV, ± 3TC
	Other body fluid fluid (eg, urine)	Not offer	
Skin, increased risk•	Blood	Offer	ZDV + 3TC, ± IDV¶
	Fluid containing visible blood, other potentially infectious fluid,# or tissue	Offer	ZDV, ± 3TC
	Other body fluid fluid (eg, urine)	Not offer	

Adapted from *MMWR Morb Mortal Wkly Rep*, 1996, 4S:469-72.

*Any exposure to concentrated HIV (eg, in a research laboratory or production facility) is treated as percutaneous exposure to blood with highest risk.

†*Recommend* — postexposure prophylaxis (PEP) should be offered to the exposed worker with counseling (see MMWR report). *Offer* — PEP should be offered to the exposed worker with counseling (see MMWR report). *Not offer* — PEP should not be offered because these are not occupational exposures to HIV.

‡Regimens: zidovudine (ZDV), 200 mg three times a day; lamivudine (3TC), 150 mg two times a day; indinavir (IDV), 800 mg three times a day (if IDV is not available, saquinavir may be used, 600 mg three times a day). Prophylaxis is given for 4 weeks. For full prescribing information, see package inserts.

§*Highest risk* — **both** larger volume of blood (eg, deep injury with large diameter hollow needle previously in source patient's vein or artery, especially involving an injection of source-patient's blood) **and** blood containing a high titer of HIV (eg, source with acute retroviral illness or end-stage AIDS; viral load measurement may be considered, but its use in relation to PEP has not been evaluated). *Increased risk* —**either** exposure to larger volume of blood **or** blood with a high titer of HIV. *No increased risk* — **neither** exposure to larger volume of blood **nor** blood with a high titer of HIV (eg, solid suture needle injury from source patient with asymptomatic HIV infection).

¶Possible toxicity of additional drug may not be warranted (see MMWR report).

#Includes semen; vaginal secretions; cerebrospinal, synovial, pleural, peritoneal, pericardial, and amniotic fluids.

•For skin, risk is increased for exposures involving a high titer of HIV, prolonged contact, an extensive area, or an area in which skin integrity is visibly compromised. For skin exposures without increased risk, the risk for drug toxicity outweighs the benefit of PEP.

PREVENTION OF BACTERIAL ENDOCARDITIS

Recommendations by the American Heart Association (*JAMA*, 1997, 277:1794-801)

Consensus Process - The recommendations were formulated by the writing group after specific therapeutic regimens were discussed. The consensus statement was subsequently reviewed by outside experts not affiliated with the writing group and by the Science Advisory and Coordinating Committee of the American Heart Association. These guidelines are meant to aid practitioners but are not intended as the standard of care or as a substitute for clinical judgment.

Table 1. Cardiac Conditions*

Endocarditis Prophylaxis Recommended
High-risk Category
Prosthetic cardiac valves, including bioprosthetic and homograft valves
Previous bacterial endocarditis
Complex cyanotic congenital heart disease (eg, single ventricle states, transposition of the great arteries, tetralogy of Fallot)
Surgically constructed systemic pulmonary shunts or conduits
Moderate-risk Category
Most other congenital cardiac malformations (other than above and below)
Acquired valvar dysfunction (eg, rheumatic heart disease)
Hypertrophic cardiomyopathy
Mitral valve prolapse with valvar regurgitation and/or thickened leaflets
Endocarditis Prophylaxis Not Recommended
Negligible-risk Category (no greater risk than the general population)
Isolated secundum atrial septal defect
Surgical repair of atrial septal defect, ventricular septal defect, or patent ductus arteriosus (without residua beyond 6 months)
Previous coronary artery bypass graft surgery
Mitral valve prolapse without valvar regurgitation†
Physiologic, functional, or innocent heart murmurs
Previous Kawasaki disease without valvar dysfunction
Previous rheumatic fever without valvar dysfunction
Cardiac pacemakers (intravascular and epicardial) and implanted defibrillators

*This table lists selected conditions but is not meant to be all-inclusive.

†Individuals who have a mitral valve prolapse associated with thickening and/or redundancy of the valve leaflets may be at increased risk for bacterial endocarditis, particularly men who are 45 years of age or older.

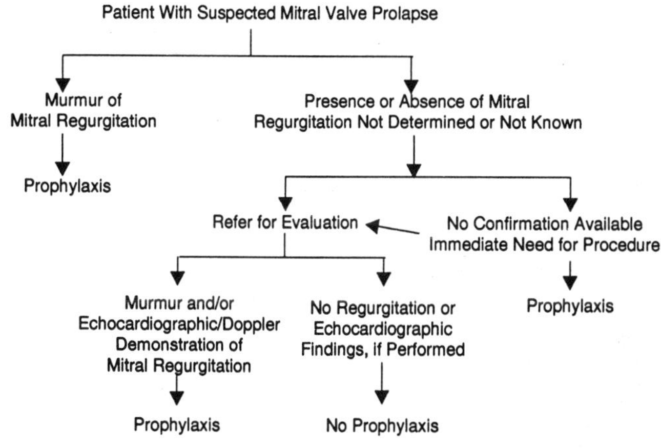

Table 2. Dental Procedures and Endocarditis Prophylaxis

Endocarditis Prophylaxis Recommended*
Dental extractions
Periodontal procedures including surgery, scaling and root planing, probing, and recall maintenance
Dental implant placement and reimplantation of avulsed teeth
Endodontic (root canal) instrumentation or surgery only beyond the apex
Subgingival placement of antibiotic fibers or strips
Initial placement of orthodontic bands but not brackets
Intraligamentary local anesthetic injections
Prophylactic cleaning of teeth or implants where bleeding is anticipated
Endocarditis Prophylaxis Not Recommended
Restorative dentistry† (operative and prosthodontic) with or without retraction cord‡
Local anesthetic injections (nonintraligamentary)
Intracanal endodontic treatment; post placement and buildup
Placement of rubber dams
Postoperative suture removal
Placement of removable prosthodontic or orthodontic appliances
Taking of oral impressions
Fluoride treatments
Taking of oral radiographs
Orthodontic appliance adjustment
Shedding of primary teeth

*Prophylaxis is recommended for patients with high- and moderate-risk cardiac conditions
†This includes restoration of decayed teeth (filling cavities) and replacement of missing teeth.
‡Clinical judgment may indicate antibiotic use in selected circumstances that may create significant bleeding.

Table 3. Recommended Standard Prophylactic Regimen for Dental, Oral, or Upper Respiratory Tract Procedures in Patients Who Are at Risk*

Endocarditis Prophylaxis Recommended
Respiratory tract
Tonsillectomy and/or adenoidectomy
Surgical operations that involve respiratory mucosa
Bronchoscopy with a rigid bronchoscope
Gastrointestinal tract*
Sclerotherapy for esophageal varices
Esophageal stricture dilation
Endoscopic retrograde cholangiography with biliary obstruction
Biliary tract surgery
Surgical operations that involve intestinal mucosa
Genitourinary tract
Prostatic surgery
Cystoscopy
Urethral dilation
Endocarditis Prophylaxis Not Recommended
Respiratory tract
Endotracheal intubation
Bronchoscopy with a flexible bronchoscope, with or without biopsy†
Tympanostomy tube insertion
Gastrointestinal tract
Transesophageal echocardiography†
Endoscopy with or without gastrointestinal biopsy†
Genitourinary tract
Vaginal hysterectomy†
Vaginal delivery†
Cesarean section
In uninfected tissues:
Urethral catheterization
Uterine dilatation and curettage
Therapeutic abortion
Sterilization procedures
Insertion or removal of intrauterine devices
Other
Cardiac catheterization, including balloon angioplasty
Implanted cardiac pacemakers, implanted defibrillators, and coronary stents
Incision or biopsy or surgically scrubbed skin
Circumcision

*Prophylaxis is recommended for high-risk patients, optional for medium-risk patients
†Prophylaxis is optional for high-risk patients

Table 4. Prophylactic Regimens for Dental, Oral, Respiratory Tract, or Esophageal Procedures

Situation	Agent	Regimen* Adults	Children
Standard general prophylaxis	Amoxicillin	2 g	50 mg/kg orally 1 h before procedure
Unable to take oral medications	Ampicillin	2 g I.M./I.V.	50 mg/kg I.M./I.V. within 30 min before procedure
Allergic to penicillin	Clindamycin or	600 mg	20 mg/kg orally 1 h before procedure
	Cephalexin† or cefadroxil† or	2 g	50 mg/kg orally 1 h before procedure
	Azithromycin or clarithromycin	500 mg	15 mg/kg orally 1 h before procedure
Allergic to penicillin and unable to take oral medications	Clindamycin or	600 mg	20 mg/kg I.V. within 30 min before procedure
	Cefazolin†	1 g	25 mg/kg I.M./I.V. within 30 min before procedure

*Total children's dose should not exceed adult dose

†Cephalosporins should not be used in individuals with immediate-type hypersensitivity reaction (urticaria, angioedema, or anaphylaxis) to penicillins

Table 5. Prophylactic Regimens for Genitourinary/Gastrointestinal (Excluding Esophageal) Procedures*

Situation	Agents*	Regimen† Adults	Children
High-risk‡ patients	Ampicillin plus gentamicin	Ampicillin 2 g I.M. or I.V. plus gentamicin 1.5 mg/kg (not to exceed 120 mg) within 30 min of starting the procedure; 6 h later, ampicillin 1 g I.M./I.V. or amoxicillin 1 g orally	Ampicillin 50 mg/kg I.M./I.V. (not to exceed 2 g) plus gentamicin 1.5 mg/kg within 30 min of starting the procedure; 6 h later, ampicillin 25 mg/kg I.M./I.V. or amoxicillin 25 mg/kg orally
High-risk‡ patients allergic to ampicillin/amoxicillin	Vancomycin plus gentamicin	Vancomycin 1 g I.V. over 1-2 h plus gentamicin 1.5 mg/kg I.M./I.V. (not to exceed 120 mg); complete injection/infusion within 30 min of starting the procedure	Vancomycin 20 mg/kg I.V. over 1-2 h plus gentamicin 1.5 mg/kg I.M./I.V.; complete injection/infusion within 30 min of starting the procedure
Moderate-risk§ patients	Amoxicillin or ampicillin	Amoxicillin 2 g orally 1 h before procedure, or ampicillin 2 g I.M./I.V within 30 min of starting the procedure	Amoxicillin 50 mg/kg orally 1 h before procedure, or ampicillin 50 mg/kg I.M./I.V. within 30 min of starting the procedure
Moderate-risk§ patients allergic to ampicillin/amoxicillin	Vancomycin	Vancomycin 1 g I.V. over 1-2 h; complete infusion within 30 min of starting the procedure	Vancomycin 20 mg/kg I.V. over 1-2 h; complete infusion within 30 min of starting the procedure

*Total children's dose should not exceed adult dose

†No second dose of vancomycin or gentamicin is recommended

‡High-risk: Patients are those who have prosthetic valves, a previous history of endocarditis (even in the absence of other heart disease, complex cyanotic congenital heart disease, or surgically constructed systemic pulmonary shunts or conduits.

§Moderate-risk: Individuals with certain other underlying cardiac defects. Congenital cardiac conditions include the following uncorrected conditions: Patent ductus arteriosus, ventricular septal defect, primum atrial septal defect, coarctation of the aorta, and bicuspid aortic valve. Acquired valvar dysfunction and hypertrophic cardiomyopathy are also moderate risk conditions.

PROPHYLAXIS FOR PATIENTS EXPOSED TO COMMON COMMUNICABLE DISEASES

Disease	Exposure	Prophylaxis/Management
Invasive *Haemophilus influenza* disease	Close contact with an infected child for more than 4 hours	Give rifampin 20 mg/kg orally once daily for 4 days (600 mg maximum daily dose) to entire family with at least one household contact less than 48 months old. Contraindication: Pregnant contacts.
Hepatitis A	Direct contact with an infected child, or sharing of food or utensils	Give 0.02 mL/kg immune globulin (IG) within 7 days of exposure.
Hepatitis B	Needlestick (used needle) Mucous membrane exposure with blood or body fluid Direct inoculation of blood or body fluid into open cut, lesion, or laceration	**Known source and employee status unknown: test patient for HB_sAg and employee for anti-HB_s**. If patient is HB_sAg negative and the patient does not have non-A, non-B hepatitis, do nothing. If patient is HB_sAg negative and has non-A, non-B hepatitis, **offer** ISG (optional). If patient is HB_sAg positive, give HBIG and hepatitis B vaccine within 48 hours of exposure. Employee antibody status may not be available for up to a week, so the above should be given as soon as patient's antigen status is known. Occasionally, the patient's antigen status will be unavailable for more than 24 hours. In these cases, HBIG should be given if the patient is high risk (ie, Asian immigrants, institutionalized patients, homosexuals, intravenous drug abusers, hemodialysis patients, patients with a history of hepatitis). If the employee is anti-HB_s negative, give the second and third doses of hepatitis B vaccine. **Known source if employee documented anti-HB_s positive:** If source has non-A, non-B hepatitis, offer ISG (optional). If employee is believed to be anti-HB_spositive due to vaccination, has received 3 doses of vaccine, and has not had an anti-HB_s test done, draw serum for anti-HB_s

(continued)

Disease	Exposure	Prophylaxis/Management
Measles	15 minutes or more in the same room with a child with measles from 2 days before the onset of symptoms to 4 days after the appearance of the rash	Children who have not been vaccinated and have not had natural infection should be isolated from the 7th through the 18th day after exposure and/or for 4 days after the rash appears. Those who have not been vaccinated should be vaccinated within 72 hours of exposure if no contraindication exists, or receive immune globulin (IG) 0.25 mL/kg I.M. for immunocompetent individuals and 0.5 mL/kg (maximum 15 mL) for immunosuppressed individuals. Children who are younger than 15 months of age should be revaccinated at 15 months of age but at least 3 months after receipt of vaccine or IG. Older individuals who have received IG should be vaccinated 3 months later.
Meningococcal disease	Household contact or direct contact with secretions	Household, day care center, and nursery school children should receive rifampin prophylaxis for 2 days. Dosages are given every 12 hours for a total of 4 doses. Dosage is 10 mg/kg/dose for children ages 1 month to 12 years (maximum 600 mg/dose), 5 mg/kg/dose for infants less than 1 month of age, and 600 mg/dose for adults. Contraindication: Pregnant contacts **Because prophylaxis is not always effective, exposed children should be monitored for symptoms.** **Employee exposure: Anyone who develops a febrile illness should receive prompt medical evaluation. If indicated, antimicrobial therapy should be administered.**

Disease	Exposure	Prophylaxis/Management
Pertussis	Housed in the same room with an infected child or spent 15 minutes in the playroom with the infected child	**Prophylaxis:** Contacts less than 7 years old who have had at least 4 doses of pertussis vaccine should receive a booster dose of DTP, unless a dose has been given within the past 3 years, and should receive erythromycin 40-50 mg/kg/day orally for 14 days. Contacts less than 7 years old who are not immunized or who have received less than 4 doses of DTP should have DTP immunization initiated or continued according to the recommended schedule. Children who have received their third dose 6 months or more before exposure should be given their fourth dose at this time. Erythromycin should also be given for 14 days. Contacts 7 years of age and above should receive prophylactic erythromycin (maximum of 1 g/day) for 10-14 days. All exposed patients should be watched closely for respiratory symptoms for 14 days after exposure has stopped because immunity conferred by the vaccine is not absolute and the efficacy of erythromycin in prophylaxis has not been established.
Tuberculosis	Housed in the same room with a child with contagious tuberculosis (tuberculosis is contagious if the child has a cough plus AFB seen on smear plus cavitation on CXR)	Place PPD immediately and 10 weeks after exposure. Start on INH. Consult Infectious Diseases if seroconversion occurs.
Varicella-zoster	1 hour or more in the same room with a contagious child from 24 hours before vesicles appear to when all vesicles are crusted, which is usually 5 to 7 days after vesicles appear. In household exposure, communicability is 48 hours before vesicles appear.	**Immunocompetent** children who have not been vaccinated or had natural infection, should have titers drawn only if they will still be hospitalized for more than 10 days after exposure. If titers are negative, they should be isolated from 10 to 21 days after exposure and/or until all lesions are crusted and dry. If VZIG was given the child should be isolated from 10 to 28 days after exposure. **Immunocompromised** children who have not been vaccinated or had natural infection should first have titers drawn, and then receive VZIG (varicella-zoster immune globulin) **1 vial/10 kg I.M.** up to a maximum of 5 vials as soon as possible but at most 96 hours after exposure. Fractional doses are not recommended. If titers are positive, nothing further need be done. If titers are negative, the child should be isolated from 10 to 28 days after exposure and should be monitored very carefully for tite appearance of vesicles so that treatment can be initiated. VZIG is available from the Blood Bank.

RECOMMENDATIONS FOR PROPHYLAXIS AGAINST TUBERCULOSIS

Multidrug-Resistant (MDR) Tuberculosis

By September 1992, clusters of MDR TB were reported in 14 U.S. hospitals and one prison system (*Ann Int Med*, 1993, 118-77): some organisms resistant to seven drugs (INH, RIF, KM, ETB, ethionamide, SM, rifabutin); nosocomial transmission in seven hospitals and one prison; MDR TB diagnosed in 241 patients, 17 healthcare workers (HCW); most transmission among AIDS patients (interval between exposure and diagnosis 1-3.5 months, diagnosis to death 4-16 weeks, mortality 72% to 89%); TBn skin test conversions in 18% to 50% of HCW. One HIV-negative HCW has died (*MMWR Morb Mortal Wkly Rep*, 1992, 41(RR11):52).

Any patient suspected of TB should be isolated (private room, negative pressure. HCW entering should wear high-efficiency masks (disposable particulate respirators) [for details (essential): *MMWR Morb Mortal Wkly Rep*, 1990, 39(RR17):14].

INH Preventive Therapy

No age limit applies for these six groups:

1. HIV-positive (risk of active disease 10%/year), AIDS 170 x ↑, HIV positive 113 x ↑) and previous risk factor for HIV infection and are suspected of having HIV infection.

2. Household members of persons with recently diagnosed tuberculous disease (risk 2% to 4% for first year); risk for infants and children may be twice that for adults

3. Newly infected persons; tuberculin test conversion within past 2 years (risk 3.3% first year)

4. Past tuberculosis, not treated with adequate chemotherapy (INH, rifampin, or alternatives)

5. Positive tuberculin reactors with chest x-ray consistent with nonprogressive tuberculous disease (risk 0.5% to 5%/year)

6. Positive tuberculin reactors with specific predisposing underlying conditions: illicit injection drug use (*MMWR Morb Mortal Wkly Rep*, 1989, 38:236), silicosis, diabetes mellitus, prolonged adrenocorticoid medication (>15 mg prednisone per day), immunosuppressive medication, hematologic diseases (Hodgkin's, leukemia), endstage renal disease, clinical condition with substantial rapid weight loss or chronic undernutrition, previous gastrectomy *(Am Rev Resp Dis*, 1986, 134:355)

Drug Resistance

Areas of high prevalence of INH resistance include Korea and Southeast Asian countries. U.S. isolates (1991) >8% resistant to ≥1 drug, 3% resistant (R) INH + RIF. Only 11 states had INH/RIF(R) isolates (NY 40% INH/RIF(R), NJ 6%).

Dosing Recommendations

INH and rifampin should be taken in a single early morning dose on an empty stomach. Directly observed therapy (DOT) recommended (↑ likelihood of cure). ~20% of patients are noncompliant (a major cause of resistance).

Specific Circumstances/ Organism	Comments	Regimen
Category I. Exposure (Household members and other close contacts of potentially infectious cases) (Exposee tuberculin test negative)*		
Neonate	Rx essential	INH (10 mg/kg/d) for 3 months, then repeat tuberculin test (TBnT). If mother's smear negative and infant's TBnT negative and chest x-ray (CXR) are normal, stop INH. In the United Kingdom, BCG is then given (*Lancet*, 1990, 2:1479), unless mother is HIV positive. If infants repeat TBnT is positive and/or CXR abnormal (hilar adenopathy and/or infiltrate), administer INH + RIF (10-20 mg/kg/d) (or streptomycin) for a total of 6 months. If mother is being treated, separation from mother is not indicated.
Children <5 y	Rx indicated	As for neonate first 3 months. If repeat TBnT is negative, stop. If repeat TBnT is positive, continue INH for a total of 9 months. If INH is not given initially, repeat TBnT at 3 months; if positive, treat with INH for 9 months (see Category II below).
Older children and adults	No rx	Repeat TBnT at 3 months, if positive, treat with INH for 6 months (see Category II below).
Category II. Infection Without Disease (Positive tuberculin test)*		
Regardless of age (see INH Preventive Therapy)	Rx indicated	INH (5 mg/kg/d, maximum: 300 mg/d for adults, 10 mg/kg/d not to exceed 300 mg/d for children). Results with 6 months of treatment are nearly as effective as 12 months (65% vs 75% reduction in disease). *Am Thoracic Society* (6 months), *Am Acad Pediatrics*, 1991 (9 months). If CXR is abnormal, treat for 12 months. In HIV-positive patient, treatment for a minimum of 12 months, some suggest longer. Monitor transaminases monthly (*MMWR Morb Mortal Wkly Rep* 1989, 38:247).
Age <35 y	Rx indicated	Reanalysis of earlier studies favors INH prophylaxis (if INH-related hepatitis case fatality rate is<1% and TB case fatality is ≥6.7%, which appears to be the case, monitor transaminases monthly (*Arch Int Med*, 1990, 150:2517).
INH-resistant organisms likely	Rx indicated	Data on efficacy of alternative regimens is currently lacking. Regimens include ETB + RIF daily for 6 months. PZA + RIF daily for 2 months, then INH + RIF daily until sensitivities from index case (if available) known, then if INH-CR, discontinue INH and continue RIF for 9 months, otherwise INH + RIF for 9 months (this latter is *Am Acad Pediatrics*, 1991 recommendation).
INH + RIF resistant organisms likely	Rx indicated	Efficacy of alternative regimens is unknown; PZA (25-30 mg/kg/d P.O.) + ETB (15-25 mg/kg/d P.O.) (at 25 mg/kg ETB, monitoring for retrobulbar neuritis required), for 6 months unless HIV positive, then 12 months; PZA + ciprofloxacin (750 mg P.O. bid) or ofloxacin (400 mg P.O. bid) x 6-12 months *(MMWR Morb Mortal Wkly Rep*, 1992, 41(RR11):68).

INH = isoniazid; RIF = rifampin; KM = kanamycin; ETB = ethambutol

SM = streptomycin; CXR = chest x-ray; Rx = treatment

See also guidelines for interpreting PPD in "Skin Testing for Delayed Hypersensitivity" in the Appendix.

*Tuberculin test (TBnT). The standard is the Mantoux test, 5 TU PPD in 0.1 mL diluent stabilized with Tween 80. Read at 48-72 hours measuring maximum diameter of induration. A reaction ≥5 mm is defined as positive in the following: positive HIV or risk factors, recent close case contacts, CXR consistent with healed TBc. ≥10 mm is positive in foreign-born in countries of high prevalence, injection drug users, low income populations, nursing home residents, patients with medical conditions which increase risk (see above, preventive treatment). ≥15 mm is positive in all others (*Am Rev Resp Dis*, 1990, 142:725). Two-stage TBnt: Use in individuals to be tested regularly (ie, healthcare workers). TBn reactivity may decrease over time but be boosted by skin testing. If unrecognized, individual may be incorrectly diagnosed as recent converter. If first TBnT is reactive but <10 mm, repeat 5 TU in 1 week, if then ≥10 mm = positive, not recent conversion (*Am Rev Resp Dis*, 1979, 119:587).

USPHS/IDSA GUIDELINES FOR THE PREVENTION OF OPPORTUNISTIC INFECTIONS IN PERSONS INFECTED WITH HUMAN IMMUNODEFICIENCY VIRUS: A SUMMARY

(*MMWR Morb Mortal Wkly Rep*, 1995 44(RR-8))

DRUG REGIMENS FOR ADULTS AND ADOLESCENTS

Prophylaxis for First Episode of Opportunistic Disease in HIV-Infected Adults and Adolescents

		Preventive Regimens	
Pathogen	**Indication**	**First Choice**	**Alternatives**
Strongly Recommended as Standard of Care			
*Pneumocystis carinii**	CD4+ count <200/μL or unexplained fever for ≥2 weeks or oropharyngeal candidiasis	TMP-SMX 1 DS P.O. qd (AI)	TMP-SMX, 1 SS P.O. qd (AI) or 1 DS P.O. tiw (AII); dapsone, 50 mg P.O. bid or 100 mg P.O. qd (AI); dapsone, 50 mg P.O. qd, **plus** pyrimethamine, 50 mg P.O. qw, **plus** leucovorin, 25 mg P.O. qw (AI); dapsone, 200 mg P.O. qw, **plus** pyrimethamine, 75 mg P.O. qw, **plus** leucovorin, 25 mg P.O. qw (AI); aerosolized pentamidine, 300 mg qm via Respirgard II nebulizer (AI)
Mycobacterium tuberculosis†			
Isoniazid-sensitive	TST reaction ≥5 mm **or** prior positive TST result without treatment **or** contact with case of active tuberculosis	Isoniazid, 300 mg P.O., **plus** pyridoxine, 50 mg P.O. qd x 12 mo (AI); **or** isoniazid, 900 mg P.O., **plus** pyridoxine, 50 mg P.O. biw x 12 mo (BIII)	Rifampin, 600 mg P.O. qd x 12 mo (BII)
Isoniazid-resistant	Same as above; high probability of exposure to isoniazid-resistant tuberculosis	Rifampin, 600 mg P.O. qd x 12 mo (BII)	Rifabutin, 300 mg P.O. qd x 12 mo (CIII)
Multidrug-resistant (isoniazid and rifampin)	Same as above; high probability of exposure to multidrug-resistant tuberculosis	Choice of drugs requires consultation with public health authorities	None
Toxoplasma gondii ‡	IgG antibody to *Toxoplasma* and CD4+ count <100/μL	TMP-SMX, 1 DS P.O. qd (AII)	TMP-SMX, 1 SS P.O. qd **or** 1 DS P.O. tiw (AII); dapsone, 50 mg P.O. qd, **plus** pyrimethamine, 50 mg P.O. qw, **plus** leucovorin, 25 mg P.O. qw (AI)
Recommended for Consideration in All Patients			
Streptococcus pneumoniae§	All patients	Pneumococcal vaccine, 0.5 mL I.M. x 1 (BIII)	None
Mycobacterium avium complex¶	CD4+ count <75/μL	Rifabutin, 300 mg P.O. qd (BII)	Clarithromycin, 500 mg P.O. bid (CIII); azithromycin, 500 mg P.O. tiw (CIII)
Not Recommended for Most Patients; Indicated for Consideration *Only* in Selected Populations or Patients			
Bacteria	Neutropenia	Granulocyte colony-stimulating factor 5-10 mcg/kg S.C. qd x 2-4 wk,**or** granulocyte-macrophage colony-stimulating factor, 250 mcg/m^2, I.V. over 2 h qd x 2-4 wk (CIII)	None
Candida species	CD4+ count <50 μL	Fluconazole, 100-200 mg P.O. qd (CI)	Ketoconazole, 200 mg P.O. qd (CIII)
Cryptococcus neoformans#	CD4+ count <50 μL	Fluconazole, 100-200 mg P.O. qd (BI)	Itraconazole, 200 mg P.O. qd (CIII)
Histoplasma capsulatum#	CD4+ count <50 μL, endemic geographic area	Itraconazole, 200 mg P.O. qd (CIII)	Fluconazole, 200 mg P.O. qd (CIII)
Coccidioides immitis#	CD4+ count <50 μL, endemic geographic region	Fluconazole, 200 mg P.O. qd (CIII)	Itraconazole, 200 mg P.O. qd (CIII)

(continued)

Pathogen	Indication	Preventive Regimens: First Choice	Preventive Regimens: Alternatives
CMV•	CD4+ count <50 µL and CMV antibody positivity	Oral ganciclovir, 1 g P.O. tid (CIII; only preliminary data available)	None
Unknown (herpes viruses?)♦	CD4+ count <200 µL	Acyclovir, 800 mg P.O. qid (CIII)	Acyclovir, 200 mg P.O. tid/qid (CIII)
Recommended for Consideration††			
Hepatitis B virus§	All susceptible (anti-HB_c-negative) patients	Engerix-B®, 20 mcg I.M. x 3 (BIII); **or** Recombivax HB®, 10 mcg I.M. x 3 (BIII)	None
Influenza virus§	All patients (annually, before influenza season)	Whole or split virus, 0.5 mL I.M./y (BIII)	Rimantadine, 100 mg P.O. bid (CIII); **or** amantadine, 100 mg P.O. bid (CIII)‡‡

Note: Not all of the recommended regimens reflect current Food and Drug Administration-approved labeling. Anti-HB_c = antibody to hepatitis B core antigen; biw = twice weekly; CMV = cytomegalovirus; DS = double-strength tablet; qm = monthly; qw = weekly; ss - single-strength tablet; tiw = three times weekly; TMP-SMX = trimethoprim-sulfamethoxazole; and TST = tuberculin skin test. The Respirgard II nebulizer is manufactured by Marquest, Englewood, CO; Engerix-B® by SmithKline Beecham, Rixensart, Belgium; and Recombivax HB® by Merck & Co, West Point, PA. Letters and Roman numerals in parentheses after regimens indicate the strength of the recommendation and the quality of the evidence supporting it (see text).

*Patients receiving dapsone should be tested for glucose-6-phosphate dehydrogenase deficiency. A dosage of 50 mg qd is probably less effective than a dosage of 100 mg qd. The efficacy of parenteral pentamidine (eg, 4 mg/kg/qm) is uncertain. Inadequate data are available on the efficacy and safety of atovaquone or clindamycin/primaquine. Sulfadoxine/pyrimethamine (Fansidar®, Laboratory Corporation of America, Nutley, NJ) is rarely used because it can elicit severe hypersensitivity reactions. TMP-SMX and dapsone/pyrimethamine (and possibly dapsone alone) appear to be protective against toxoplasmosis. TMP-SMX may reduce the frequency of some bacterial infections. Patients receiving therapy for toxoplasmosis with sulfadiazine/pyrimethamine are protected against *P. carinii* pneumonia and do not need TMP-SMX.

†Directly observed therapy is required for 900 mg of isoniazid biw; isoniazid regimens should include pyridoxine to prevent peripheral neuropathy. Exposure to multidrug-resistant tuberculosis may require prophylaxis with two drugs; consult public health authorities. Possible regimens include pyrazinamide plus either ethambutol or a fluoroquinolone.

‡Protection against *T. gondii* is provided by the preferred antipneumocystitis regimens. Pyrimethamine alone probably provides little, if any, protection. Dapsone alone cannot be recommended on the basis of currently available data.

§Data are inadequate concerning clinical benefit of vaccines against *S. pneumoniae*, influenza virus, and hepatitis B virus in HIV-infected persons, although it is logical to assume that those patients who develop antibody responses will derive some protection. Some authorities are concerned that immunizations may stimulate the replication of HIV. Prophylaxis with TMP-SMX may provide some clinical benefit by reducing the frequency of bacterial infections, but the prevalence of *S. pneumoniae* resistant to TMP-SMX is increasing. Hepatitis B vaccine has been recommended for all children and adolescents and for all adults with risk factors for hepatitis B infection. For additional information regarding vaccination against hepatitis B and vaccination and antiviral therapy against influenza.

¶Data on 500 mg of clarithromycin P.O. bid have been presented but have not yet been thoroughly analyzed. Data on the efficacy and safety of azithromycin prophylaxis are not yet available.

[#There may be a few unusual occupational or other circumstances under which prophylaxis should be considered; consult a specialist.

•Data on oral ganciclovir are still being evaluated; the durability of its effect is unclear. Acyclovir is not protective against CMV.

♦Data regarding the efficacy of acyclovir for prolonging survival are controversial; if acyclovir is beneficial, the biologic basis for the effect and the optimal dose and timing of therapy are uncertain.

††These immunizations or chemoprophylactic regimens are not targeted against pathogens traditionally classified as opportunistic but should be considered for use in HIV-infected patients. While the use of those products is logical, their clinical efficacy has not been validated in this population.

‡‡During outbreaks of influenza A.

Prophylaxis for Recurrence of Opportunistic Disease (After Chemotherapy for Acute Disease) in HIV-Infected Adults and Adolescents

Pathogen	Indication	Preventive Regimens First Choice	Preventive Regimens Alternatives
Recommended for Life as Standard of Care			
Pneumocystis carinii	Prior *P. carinii* pneumonia	TMP-SMX 1 DS P.O. qd (AI)	TMP-SMX, 1 SS P.O. qd (AI) or 1 DS P.O. tiw (AII); dapsone, 50 mg P.O. bid **or** 100 mg P.O. qd (AI); dapsone, 50 mg P.O. qd, **plus** pyrimethamine, 50 mg P.O. qw, **plus** leucovorin, 25 mg P.O. qw (AI); dapsone, 200 mg P.O. qw, **plus** pyrimethamine, 75 mg P.O. qw, **plus** leucovorin, 25 mg P.O. qw (AI); aerosolized pentamidine, 300 mg qm via Respirgard II nebulizer (AI)
Toxoplasma gondii *	Prior toxoplasmic encephalitis	TMP-SMX 1 DS P.O. qd and sulfadiazine, 1-1.5 g P.O. q6h, **plus** pyrimethamine, 25-75 mg P.O. qd, **plus** leucovorin, 10-25 mg P.O. qd-qid (AII)	Clindamycin, 300-450 mg P.O. q6-8h, **plus** pyrimethamine, 25-75 mg P.O. qd, **plus** leucovorin, 10-25 mg P.O. qd-qid (AII)
Mycobacterium avium complex†	Documented disseminated disease	Clarithromycin, 500 mg P.O. bid, **plus** one or more of the following: ethambutol, 15 mg/kg P.O. qd; rifabutin, 300 mg P.O. qd; ciprofloxacin, 500-750 mg P.O. bid (BIII)	Azithromycin, 500 mg P.O. qd, **plus** one or more of the following: ethambutol, 15 mg/kg P.O. qd; clofazimine 100 mg P.O. qd; rifabutin, 300 mg P.O. qd; ciprofloxacin, 500-750 mg P.O. bid (BIII)
Cytomegalovirus‡	Prior end-organ disease	Ganciclovir, 5-6 mg/kg I.V. 5-7 d/w or 1000 mg P.O. tid (AI); **or** foscarnet, 90-120 mg/kg I.V. qd (AI)	Sustained-release implants used investigationally
Cryptococcus neoformans	Documented disease	Fluconazole, 200 mg P.O. qd (AI)	Itraconazole, 200 mg P.O. qd (BIII); amphotericin B, 0.6-1 mg/kg I.V. qw-tiw (AI)
Histoplasma capsulatum	Documented disease	Itraconazole, 200 mg P.O. bid (AII)	Amphotericin B, 1 mg/kg I.V. qw (AI); fluconazole, 200-400 mg P.O. qd (BIII)
Coccidioides immitis	Documented disease	Fluconazole, 200 mg P.O. qd (AII)	Amphotericin B, 1 mg/kg I.V. qw (AI); itraconazole, 200 mg P.O. bid (AII); ketoconazole, 400-800 mg P.O. qd (BII)
Salmonella species (nontyphi)§	Bacteremia	Ciprofloxacin 500 mg P.O. bid for several months (BII)	None
Recommended Only if Subsequent Episodes Are Frequent or Severe			
Herpes simplex virus	Frequent/severe recurrences	Acyclovir, 200 mg P.O. tid **or** 400 mg P.O. bid (AI)	None
Candida species (oral, vaginal, or esophageal)	Frequent/severe recurrences	Fluconazole, 100-200 mg P.O. qd (AI)	Ketoconazole, 200 mg P.O. qd (BII); itraconazole, 100 mg P.O. qd (BII); clotrimazole troche, 10 mg P.O. 5 times/d (BII); nystatin, 5 x 10^5 units P.O. 5 times/d (CIII)

Note: Not all of the recommended regimens reflect current Food and Drug Administration-approved labeling. DS = double-strength tablet; qm = monthly; qw = weekly; SS = single-strength tablet; tiw = three times weekly; and TMP-SMX = trimethoprim-sulfamethoxazole. The Respirgard II nebulizer is manufactured by Marquest, Englewood, CO. Letters and Roman numerals in parentheses after regimens indicate the strength of the recommendation and the quality of the evidence supporting it (see text).

*Only pyrimethamine/sulfadiazine confers protection against *P. carinii* pneumonia.

†The long-term efficacy of any regimen is not well established. Many multiple-drug regimens are poorly tolerated. Drug interactions (eg, those seen with clarithromycin/rifabutin) can be problematic. Rifabutin has been associated with uveitis, especially when given at daily doses of >300 mg or along with fluconazole or clarithromycin.

‡Ganciclovir and foscarnet delay relapses by only modest intervals (often only 4-8 weeks). Ocular implants with sustained-release ganciclovir appear promising.

§Efficacious eradication of *Salmonella* has been demonstrated only for ciprofloxacin.

DRUG REGIMENS FOR CHILDREN

Prophylaxis for First Episode of Opportunistic Disease in HIV-Infected Infants and Children

Pathogen	Indication	Preventive Regimens: First Choice	Preventive Regimens: Alternatives
Strongly Recommended as Standard of Care			
*Pneumocystis carinii**	All infants 1-4 mo old born to HIV-infected women; HIV-infected or HIV-indeterminate infants <12 mo old; HIV-infected children 1-5 y old with CD4⁺ count <500/µL or CD4⁺ percentage of <15%; HIV-infected children 6-12 y old with CD4⁺ count <200/µL or CD4⁺ percentage <15%	TMP-SMX 150/750 mg/m^2/d in 2 divided doses P.O. tiw on consecutive days (AII); acceptable alternative schedules for same dosage (AII); single dose P.O. tiw on consecutive days, 2 divided doses P.O. qd, or 2 divided doses P.O. tiw on alternate days	Aerosolized pentamidine (children ≥5 y old), 300 mg qm via Respirgard II nebulizer (CIII); dapsone (children ≥1 mo old), 2 mg/kg (not to exceed 100 mg) P.O. qd (CIII); I.V. pentamidine, 4 mg/kg every 2-4 weeks (CIII)
Mycobacterium tuberculosis			
Isoniazid-sensitive	TST reaction ≥5 mm **or** prior positive TST result without treatment **or** contact with case of active tuberculosis	Isoniazid, 10-15 mg/kg (maximum, 300 mg) P.O. **or** I.M. qd x 12 mo **or** 20-30 mg/kg (maximum, 900 mg) P.O. biw x 12 mo (BIII)	Rifampin, 10-20 mg/kg (maximum, 600 mg) P.O. **or** I.V. qd x 12 mo (BII)
Isoniazid-resistant	Same as above; high probability of exposure to isoniazid-resistant tuberculosis	Rifampin, 10-20 mg/kg (maximum, 600 mg) P.O. **or** I.V. qd x 12 mo (BII)	Uncertain
Multidrug-resistant (isoniazid and rifampin)	Same as above; high probability of exposure to multidrug-resistant tuberculosis	Choice of drugs requires consultation with public health authorities	None
Varicella-zoster virus	Significant exposure to varicella with **no** history of varicella	VZIG, 1 vial (1.25 mL)/10 kg (maximum, 5 vials) I.M., given ≤96 h after exposure, ideally within 48 h (AI) (Children routinely receiving IVIG should receive VZIG if the last dose of IVIG was given >14 d before exposure)	None
Various pathogens	HIV exposure/infection	Immunizations¶	None
Recommended for Consideration in All Patients			
Toxoplasma gondii†	IgG antibody to *Toxoplasma* with severe immunosuppression (CD4⁺ count <100/µL) (Prophylaxis may be considered at higher CD4⁺ counts in the youngest infants, but no relevant data are available)	TMP-SMX, 150/750 mg/m^2/d in 2 divided doses P.O. tiw on consecutive days (CIII); acceptable alternative schedules for same dosage (CIII); single dose P.O. tiw on consecutive days, 2 divided doses P.O. qd, or 2 divided doses P.O. tiw on alternate days	Dapsone (children ≥1 mo old), 2 mg/kg **or** 15 mg/m^2(maximum, 25 mg) P.O. qd, **plus** pyrimethamine, 1 mg/kg P.O. qd, **plus** leucovorin, 5 mg P.O. every 3 days (CIII)
Not Recommended for Most Patients; Indicated for Consideration *Only* in Selected Populations or Patients			
Invasive bacterial infections	Hypogammaglobulinemia	IVIG, 400 mg/kg qm (AI)	None
Candida species‡	Severe immunosuppression	Nystatin (100,000 units/mL), 4-6 mL P.O. q6h; **or** topical clotrimazole, 10 mg P.O. 5 times/d (CII)	Ketoconazole, 5-10 mg/kg P.O. q12-24h (CI); fluconazole, 2-8 mg/kg P.O. qd (CI)
Cryptococcus neoformans	Severe immunosuppression	Fluconazole, 2-8 mg/kg P.O. qd (BI)	Itraconazole, 2-5 mg/kg P.O. q12-24h (CIII)
Histoplasma capsulatum	Severe immunosuppression, endemic geographic area	Itraconazole, 2-5 mg/kg P.O. q12-24h (CIII)	Fluconazole, 2-8 mg/kg P.O. qd (CIII)
Coccidioides immitis	Severe immunosuppression, endemic geographic area	Fluconazole, 2-8 mg/kg P.O. qd (CIII)	Itraconazole, 2-5 mg/kg P.O. q12-24h (CIII)
CMV§	CD4⁺ count <50 µL and CMV antibody positivity	Children 6-12 y; oral ganciclovir under investigation	None

(continued)

Pathogen	Indication	Preventive Regimens: First Choice	Preventive Regimens: Alternatives
Influenza A virus	High risk of exposure (eg, institutional outbreak)	Rimantadine or amantadine, 5 mg/kg qd (maximum, 150 mg) in 2 divided doses P.O. for children <10 y old; for children ≥10 y old, 5 mg/kg up to 40 kg, then 200 mg in 2 divided doses P.O. qd	None

Note: Not all of the recommended regimens reflect current Food and Drug Administration-approved labeling. biw = twice weekly; CMV = cytomegalovirus; IVIG = intravenous immune globulin; qm = monthly; tiw = three times weekly; TMP-SMX = trimethoprim-sulfamethoxazole; and VZIG = varicella-zoster immune globulin. The Respirgard II nebulizer is manufactured by Marquest, Englewood, CO. Letters and Roman numerals in parentheses after regimens indicate the strength of the recommendation and the quality of the evidence supporting it (see text).

*The efficacy of parenteral pentamidine (eg, 4 mg/kg qm) is controversial. TMP-SMX and dapsone/pyrimethamine (and possible dapsone alone) appear to be protective against toxoplasmosis, although relevant data have not been prospectively collected. Daily treatment with TMP-SMX reduces the frequency of some bacterial infections. Patients receiving sulfadiazine/pyrimethamine for toxoplasmosis are protected against*P. carinii* pneumonia and do not need TMP-SMX.

†Protection against *T. gondii* is provided by the preferred antipneumocystitis regimens. Dapsone alone cannot be recommended on the basis of currently available data. Pyrimethamine alone probably provides little, if any, protection.

‡Ketoconazole and fluconazole are preferred for prophylaxis of esophagitis and severe mucocutaneous infection.

§Data on oral ganciclovir are still being evaluated; durability of its effect is unclear. Acyclovir is not protective against CMV.

¶The following table shows the immunization schedule for HIV-exposed/infected infants is strongly recommended as the standard of care.

Age (mo)	Immunization (dose)
Newborn	Hep B (1)*
1	Hep B (2)
2	DTP (1), Hib (1)†
3	EIPV (1)†
4	DTP (2), Hib (2)†
5	EIPV (2)†
6	DTP (3), Hib (3), Hep B (3)†‡§
7	Influenza (1)¶
8	Influenza (2)¶
12	Hib (3 or 4)‡, MMR#
15	EIPV (3), DTaP (4)•
18	DTaP (4)•
24	Pneumococcal, 23-valent♦

Note: DTaP = diphtheria and tetanus toxoids with acellular pertussis; DTP = diphtheria-tetanus-pertussis; EIPV = enhanced inactivated polio vaccine; Hep B = hepatitis B; Hib = *Haemophilus influenzae* type b; and MMR = measles-mumps-rubella. This schedule differs from that recommended for immunization of immunocompetent children in the following ways: (1) EIPV replaces oral polio vaccine, and the first two doses of EIPV may be given at 3-5 months instead of 2-4 months; (2) the second dose of Hep B vaccine is given at 1 month; and (3) pneumococcal vaccine is recommended. This schedule is designed to deliver vaccine to HIV-infected children as early as possible and to limit the number of injections to two per visit.

*Infants born to mothers positive for hepatitis B surface antigen should receive hepatitis B immune globulin within 12 hours of birth in addition to Hep B vaccine.

†DTP and Hib vaccines are available together or separately. With the combined DTP-Hib vaccine, a single injection on each occasion is sufficient and can be given at 2, 4, and 6 months. Administration of EIPV as a second injection at 2 and 4 months can replace separate immunizations at 3 and 5 months.

‡The need for a third dose of Hib vaccine depends on which formulation was used previously. Regardless of whether the primary series requires two or three doses, a booster dose is required at 12-15 months.

§If DTP and Hib are given as separate injections at 6 months, the third dose of Hep B vaccine may be postponed until the next visit.

¶Primary immunization against influenza for children <9 years of age requires two doses of vaccine, the first of which can be given as early as 6 months of age. Subsequent vaccination should be undertaken annually, before the influenza season.

#HIV-infected children should receive prophylactic immunoglobulin after exposure to measles, whether or not they have been vaccinated against measles.

•DTaP can be administered at either 15 or 18 months. Alternatively, a fourth dose of DTP can be given as early as 12 months.

♦Some authorities recommend revaccination for HIV-infected children vaccinated ≥6 years previously.

Prophylaxis for Recurrence of Opportunistic Disease (After Chemotherapy for Acute Disease) in HIV-Infected Infants and Children

Pathogen	Indication	Preventive Regimens: First Choice	Preventive Regimens: Alternatives
Recommended for Life as Standard of Care			
Pneumocystis carinii	Prior *P. carinii* pneumonia	TMP-SMX 150/750 mg/m^2/d in 2 divided doses P.O. tiw on consecutive days (AI); acceptable alternative schedules for same dosage (AI); single dose P.O. tiw on consecutive days, 2 divided doses P.O. qd, or 2 divided doses P.O. tiw on alternate days	Aerosolized pentamidine (children ≥5 y old), 300 mg qm via Respirgard II nebulizer (AI); dapsone (children ≥1 mo old), 2 mg/kg (not to exceed 100 mg) P.O. qd (CIII); I.V. pentamidine, 4 mg/kg every 2-4 weeks (CIII)
*Toxoplasma gondii**	Prior toxoplasmic encephalitis	Sulfadiazine, 85-120 mg/kg in 2-4 divided doses P.O. qd **plus** pyrimethamine, 1 mg/kg or 15 mg/m^2 (maximum 25 mg) P.O. qd, **plus** leucovorin, 5 mg P.O. every 3 days (AII)	Clindamycin, 20-30 mg/kg in 4 divided doses P.O. qd, **plus** pyrimethamine, 1 mg/kg P.O. qd, **plus** leucovorin, 5 mg P.O. every 3 days (AII)
Mycobacterium avium complex†	Prior disease	Clarithromycin, 30 mg/kg in 2 divided doses P.O. qd, **plus** at least one of the following: ethambutol, 15-25 mg/kg P.O. qd; clofazimine, 50-100 mg P.O. qd; rifabutin, 300 mg P.O. qd; ciprofloxacin, 20-30 mg/kg in 2 divided doses P.O. qd (CIII)	None
Cryptococcus neoformans	Documented disease	Fluconazole, 2-8 mg/kg P.O. qd (CIII)	Itraconazole, 2-5 mg/kg P.O. q12-24h (CIII); amphotericin B, 0.5-1.5 mg/kg I.V. qw-tiw (AI)
Histoplasma capsulatum	Documented disease	Itraconazole, 2-5 mg/kg P.O. q12-48h (CIII)	Fluconazole, 2-8 mg/kg P.O. qd (CIII); amphotericin B, 1 mg/kg I.V. qw (AI)
Coccidioides immitis	Documented disease	Fluconazole, 2-8 mg/kg P.O. qd (CIII)	Amphotericin B, 1 mg/kg I.V. qw (AI)
Cytomegalovirus‡	Prior end-organ disease	Ganciclovir, 10 mg/kg in 2 divided doses I.V. qd for 1 wk, then 5 mg/kg I.V. qd; **or** foscarnet, 60-120 mg/kg I.V. qd (AI)	None
Salmonella species (nontyphi)§	Bacteremia	TMP/SMX, 150/750 mg/m^2 in 2 divided doses P.O. qd for several months (CIII)	Ampicillin, 50-100 mg in 4 divided doses P.O. qd (CIII); chloramphenicol, 50-75 mg/kg in 4 divided doses P.O. qd (CIII) (For children >6 y old, consider ciprofloxacin, 30 mg in 2 divided doses P.O. qd (CIII))
Recommended Only if Subsequent Episodes Are Frequent or Severe			
Invasive bacterial infections	More than 2 infections in 1 y period	IVIG, 400 mg/kg qm (AI)	TMP/SMX, 150/750 mg/m^2 P.O. qd (AI) (CIII)
Herpes simplex virus	Frequent/severe recurrences	Acyclovir, 600-1000 mg in 3-5 divided doses P.O. qd (CIII)	
Candida species	Frequent/severe recurrences	Ketoconazole, 5-10 mg/kg P.O. q12-24h; **or** fluconazole, 2-8 mg/kg P.O. qd (BI)	

Note: Not all of the recommended regimens reflect current Food and Drug Administration-approved labeling. IVIG = intravenous immune globulin; qm = monthly; qw = weekly; tiw = three times weekly; and TMP-SMX = trimethoprim-sulfamethoxazole. The Respirgard II nebulizer is manufactured by Marquest, Englewood, CO. Letters and Roman numerals in parentheses after regimens indicate the strength of the recommendation and the quality of the evidence supporting it (see text).

*Only pyrimethamine/sulfadiazine confers protection against *P. carinii* pneumonia. Although the clindamycin/pyrimethamine regimen is an alternative for adults, it has not been tested in children. However, these drugs are safe and are used for other infections.

†Ciprofloxacin should not be given to children <6 years of age. Rifabutin (5 mg/kg P.O. qd) may be given to children <6 years of age when a suspension becomes available.

‡Oral ganciclovir has not been studied in children.

§Choice of drug should be determined by susceptibilities of the organism isolated.

ANIMAL AND HUMAN BITES GUIDELINES

Wound Management

Irrigation: Critically important; irrigate all penetration wounds using 20 mL syringe, 19 gauge needle and >250 mL 1% povidone iodine solution. This method will reduce wound infection by a factor of 20. When there is high risk of rabies, use viricidal 1% benzalkonium chloride in addition to the 1% povidone iodine. Irrigate wound with normal saline after antiseptic irrigation.

Debridement: Remove all crushed or devitalized tissue remaining after irrigation; minimize removal on face and over thin skin areas or anywhere you would create a worse situation than the bite itself already has; do not extend puncture wounds surgically — rather, manage them with irrigation and antibiotics.

Suturing: Close most dog bites if <8 hours (<12 hours on face); do not routinely close puncture wounds, or deep or severe bites on the hands or feet, as these are at highest risk for infection. Cat and human bites should not be sutured unless cosmetically important. Wound edge freshening, where feasible, reduces infection; minimize sutures in the wound and use monofilament on the surface.

Immobilization: Critical in all hand wounds; important for infected extremities.

Hospitalization/I.V. Antibiotics: Admit for I.V. antibiotics all significant human bites to the hand, especially closed fist injuries, and bites involving penetration of the bone or joint (a high index of suspicion is needed). Consider I.V. antibiotics for significant established wound infections with cellulitis or lymphangitis, any infected bite on the hand, any infected cat bite, and any infection in an immunocompromised or asplenic patient. Outpatient treatment with I.V. antibiotics may be possible in selected cases by consulting with infectious disease.

Laboratory Assessment

Gram's Stain: Not useful prior to onset of clinically apparent infection; examination of purulent material may show a predominant organism in established infection, aiding antibiotic selection; not warranted unless results will change your treatment.

Culture: Not useful or cost effective prior to onset of clinically apparent infection.

X-Ray: Whenever you suspect bony involvement, especially in craniofacial dog bites in very small children or severe bite/crush in an extremity; cat bites with their long needle like teeth may cause osteomyelitis or a septic joint, especially in the hand or wrist.

Immunizations

Tetanus: All bite wounds are contaminated. If not immunized in last 5 years, or if not current in a child, give DPT, DT, Td, or TT as indicated. For absent or incomplete primary immunization, give 250 units tetanus immune globulin (TIG) in addition.

Rabies: In the U.S. 30,000 persons are treated each year in an attempt to prevent 1-5 cases. Domestic animals should be quarantined for 10 days to prove need for prophylaxis. High risk animal bites (85% of cases = bat, skunk, raccoon) usually receive treatment consisting of:

- human rabies immune globulin (HRIG): 20 units/kg I.M. (unless previously immunized with HDCV)
- human diploid cell vaccine (HDCV): 1 mL I.M. on days 0, 3, 7, 14, and 28 (unless previously immunized with HDCV - then give only first 2 doses)

Consult with Infectious Disease before ordering rabies prophylaxis.

Bite Wounds and Prophylactic Antibiotics

Parenteral vs Oral: If warranted, consider an initial I.V. dose to rapidly establish effective serum levels, especially if high risk, delayed treatment, or if patient reliability is poor.

Dog Bite:

1. Rarely get infected (~5%)
2. Infecting organisms: Staph coag negative, staph coag positive, alpha strep, diphtheroids, beta strep, *Pseudomonas aeruginosa*, gamma strep, *Pasteurella multocida*

3. Prophylactic antibiotics are seldom indicated. Consider for high risk wounds such as distal extremity puncture wounds, severe crush injury, bites occurring in cosmetically sensitive areas (eg, face), or in immunocompromised or asplenic patients.

Cat Bite:

1. Often get infected (~25% to 50%)
2. Infecting organisms: *Pasteurella multocida* (first 24 hours), coag positive staph, anaerobic cocci (after first 24 hours)
3. Prophylactic antibiotics are indicated in all cases.

Human Bite:

1. Intermediate infection rate (~15% to 20%)
2. Infecting organisms: Coag positive staph α, β, γ strep, *Haemophilus*, *Eikenella corrodens*, anaerobic streptococci, *Fusobacterium*, *Veillonella*, bacteroides.
3. Prophylactic antibiotics are indicated in almost all cases except superficial injuries.

See attached table for prophylactic antibiotic summary.

Bite Wound Antibiotic Regimens

	Dog Bite	Cat Bite	Human Bite
Prophylactic Antibiotics			
Prophylaxis	No routine prophylaxis, consider if involves face or hand, or immunosuppressed or asplenic patients	Routine prophylaxis	Routine prophylaxis
Prophylactic antibiotic	Amoxicillin	Amoxicillin	Amoxicillin
Penicillin allergy	Doxycycline if >10 y or co-trimoxazole	Doxycycline if >10 y or co-trimoxazole	Doxycycline if >10 y or erythromycin and cephalexin*
Outpatient Oral Antibiotic Treatment (mild to moderate infection)			
Established infection	Amoxicillin and clavulanic acid	Amoxicillin and clavulanic acid	Amoxicillin and clavulanic acid
Penicillin allergy (mild infection only)	Doxycycline if >10 y	Doxycycline if >10 y	Cephalexin* or clindamycin
Outpatient Parenteral Antibiotic Treatment (moderate infections – single drug regimens)			
	Ceftriaxone	Ceftriaxone	Cefotetan
Inpatient Parenteral Antibiotic Treatment			
Established infection	Ampicillin + cefazolin	Ampicillin + cefazolin	Ampicillin + clindamycin
Penicillin allergy	Cefazolin*	Ceftriaxone*	Cefotetan* or imipenem
Duration of Prophylactic and Treatment Regimens			
Prophylaxis: 5 days			
Treatment: 10-14 days			

*Contraindicated if history of immediate hypersensitivity reaction (anaphylaxis) to penicillin.

ANTIBIOTIC TREATMENT OF ADULTS WITH INFECTIVE ENDOCARDITIS

Table 1. Suggested Regimens for Therapy of Native Valve Endocarditis Due to Penicillin-Susceptible Viridans Streptococci and *Streptococcus bovis* (Minimum Inhibitory Concentration ≤0.1 μg/mL)*

Antibiotic	Dosage and Route	Duration (weeks)	Comments
Aqueous crystalline penicillin G sodium	12-18 million units/24 h I.V. either continuously or in 6 equally divided doses	4	Preferred in most patients older than 65 y and in those with impairment of the eighth nerve or renal function
or			
Ceftriaxone sodium	2 g once daily I.V. or I.M.†	4	
Aqueous crystalline penicillin G sodium	12-18 million units/24 h I.V. either continuously or in 6 equally divided doses	2	When obtained 1 hour after a 20- to 30-minute I.V. infusion or I.M. injection, serum concentration of gentamicin of approximately 3 μg/mL is desirable; trough concentration should be <1 μg/mL
With gentamicin sulfate‡	1 mg/kg I.M. or I.V. every 8 hours	2	
Vancomycin hydrochloride§	30 mg/kg/24 h I.V. in 2 equally divided doses, not to exceed 2 g/24 h unless serum levels are monitored	4	Vancomycin therapy is recommended for patients allergic to β-lactams; peak serum concentrations of vancomycin should be obtained 1 h after completion of the infusion and should be in the range of 30-45 μg/mL for twice-daily dosing

*Dosages recommended are for patients with normal renal function. For nutritionally variant streptococci, see Table 3. I.V. indicates intravenous; I.M., intramuscular.

†Patients should be informed that I.M. injection of ceftriaxone is painful.

‡Dosing of gentamicin on a mg/kg basis will produce higher serum concentrations in obese patients that in lean patients. Therefore, in obese patients, dosing should be based on ideal body weight. (Ideal body weight for men is 50 kg + 2.3 kg per inch over 5 feet, and ideal body weight for women is 45.5 kg + 2.3 kg per inch over 5 feet.) Relative contraindications to the use of gentamicin are age >65 years, renal impairment, or impairment of the eighth nerve. Other potentially nephrotoxic agents (eg, nonsteroidal anti-inflammatory drugs) should be used cautiously in patients receiving gentamicin.

§Vancomycin dosage should be reduced in patients with impaired renal function. Vancomycin given on a mg/kg basis will produce higher serum concentrations in obese patients than in lean patients. Therefore, in obese patients, dosing should be based on ideal body weight. Each dose of vancomycin should be infused over at least 1 h to reduce the risk of the histamine-release "red man" syndrome.

Table 2. Therapy for Native Valve Endocarditis Due to Strains of Viridans Streptococci and *Streptococcus bovis* Relatively Resistant to Penicillin G (Minimum Inhibitory Concentration >0.1 μg/mL and <0.5 μg/mL)*

Antibiotic	Dosage and Route	Duration (week)	Comments
Aqueous crystalline penicillin G sodium	18 million units/24 h I.V. either continuously or in 6 equally divided doses	4	Cefazolin or other first-generation cephalosporins may be substituted for penicillin in patients whose penicillin hypersensitivity is not of the immediate type.
With gentamicin sulfate†	1 mg/kg I.M. or I.V. every 8 h	2	
Vancomycin hydrochloride§	30 mg/kg/24 h I.V. in 2 equally divided doses, not to exceed 2 g/24 h unless serum levels are monitored	4	Vancomycin therapy is recommended for patients allergic to β-lactams

*Dosages recommended are for patients with normal renal function. I.V. indicates intravenous; I.M., intramuscular.

†For specific dosing adjustment and issues concerning gentamicin (obese patients, relative contraindications), see Table 1 footnotes.

‡For specific dosing adjustment and issues concerning vancomycin (obese patients, length of infusion), see Table 1 footnotes.

Table 3. Standard Therapy for Endocarditis Due to Enterococci*

Antibiotic	Dosage and Route	Duration (week)	Comments
Aqueous crystalline penicillin G sodium	18-30 million units/24 h I.V. either continuously or in 6 equally divided doses	4-6	4-week therapy recommended for patients with symptoms <3 months in duration; 6-week therapy recommended for patients with symptoms >3 months in duration.
With gentamicin sulfate†	1 mg/kg I.M. or I.V. every 8 h	4-6	
Ampicillin sodium	12 g/24 h I.V. either continuously or in 6 equally divided doses	4-6	
With gentamicin sulfate†	1 mg/kg I.M. or I.V. every 8 hours	4-6	
Vancomycin hydrochloride†‡	30 mg/kg/24 h I.V. in 2 equally divided doses, not to exceed 2 g/24 h unless serum levels are monitored	4-6	Vancomycin therapy is recommended for patients allergic to β-lactams; cephalosporins are not acceptable alternatives for patients allergic to penicillin
With gentamicin sulfate†	1 mg/kg I.M. or I.V. every 8 h	4-6	

*All enterococci causing endocarditis must be tested for antimicrobial susceptibility in order to select optimal therapy. This table is for endocarditis due to gentamicin- or vancomycin-susceptible enterococci, viridans streptococci with a minimum inhibitory concentration of >0.5 μg/mL, nutrionally variant viridans streptococci, or prosthetic valve endocarditis caused by viridans streptococci or *Streptococcus bovis*. Antibiotic dosages are for patients with normal renal function. I.V. indicates intravenous; I.M., intramuscular.

†For specific dosing adjustment and issues concerning gentamicin (obese patients, relative contraindications), see Table 1 footnotes.

‡For specific dosing adjustment and issues concerning vancomycin (obese patients, length of infusion), see Table 1 footnotes.

Table 4. Therapy for Endocarditis Due to Staphylococcus in the Absence of Prosthetic Material*

Antibiotic	Dosage and Route	Duration	Comments
	Methicillin-Susceptible Staphylococci		
Regimens for non-β-lactam-allergic patients			
Nafcillin sodium or oxacillin sodium	2 g I.V. every 4 h	4-6 wk	Benefit of additional aminoglycosides has not been established
With optional addition of gentamicin sulfate†	1 mg/kg I.M. or I.V. every 8 h	3-5 d	
Regimens for β-lactam-allergic patients			
Cefazolin (or other first-generation cephalosporins in equivalent dosages)	2 g I.V. every 8 h	4-6 wk	Cephalosporins should be avoided in patients with immediate-type hypersensitivity to penicillin
With optional addition of gentamicin†	1 mg/kg I.M. or I.V. every 8 hours	3-5 d	
Vancomycin hydrochloride‡	30 mg/kg/24 h I.V. in 2 equally divided doses, not to exceed 2 g/24 h unless serum levels are monitored	4-6 wk	Recommended for patients allergic to penicillin
	Methicillin-Resistant Staphylococci		
Vancomycin hydrochloride‡	30 mg/kg/24 h I.V. in 2 equally divided doses; not to exceed 2 g/24 h unless serum levels are monitored	4-6 wk	

*For treatment of endocarditis due to penicillin-susceptible staphylococci (minimum inhibitory concentration ≤0.1 μg/mL), aqueous crystalline penicillin G sodium (Table 1, first regimen) can be used for 4-6 weeks instead of nafcillin or oxacillin. Shorter antibiotic courses have been effective in some drug addicts with right-sided endocarditis due to *Staphylococcus aureus*. I.V. indicates intravenous; I.M., intramuscular.

†For specific dosing adjustment and issues concerning gentamicin (obese patients, relative contraindications), see Table 1 footnotes.

‡For specific dosing adjustment and issues concerning vancomycin (obese patients, length of infusion), see Table 1 footnotes.

Table 5. Treatment of Staphylococcal Endocarditis in the Presence of a Prosthetic Valve or Other Prosthetic Material*

Antibiotic	Dosage and Route	Duration (week)	Comments
Regimen for Methicillin-Resistant Staphylococci			
Vancomycin hydrochloride†	30 mg/kg/24 h I.V. in 2 or 4 equally divided doses, not to exceed 2 g/24 h unless serum levels are monitored	≥6	
With rifampin‡	300 mg orally every 8 h	≥6	Rifampin increases the amount of warfarin sodium required for antithrombotic therapy.
And with gentamicin sulfate§¶	1 mg/kg I.M. or I.V. every 8 h	2	
Regimen for Methicillin-Susceptible Staphylococci			
Nafcillin sodium or oxacillin sodium†	2 g I.V. every 4 h	≥6	First-generation cephalosporins or vancomycin should be used in patients allergic to β-lactam. Cephalosporins should be avoided in patients with immediate-type hypersensitivity to penicillin or with methicillin-resistant staphylococci.
With rifampin‡	300 mg orally every 8 h	≥6	
And with gentamicin sulfate§¶	1 mg/kg I.M. or I.V. every 8 h	2	

*Dosages recommended are for patients with normal renal function. I.V. indicates intravenous; I.M., intramuscular.

†For specific dosing adjustment and issues concerning gentamicin (obese patients, relative contraindications), see Table 1 footnotes.

‡Rifampin plays a unique role in the eradication of staphylococcal infection involving prosthetic material; combination therapy is essential to prevent emergence of rifampin resistance.

§For a specific dosing adjustment and issues concerning gentamicin (obese patients, relative contraindications), see Table 1 footnotes.

¶Use during initial 2 weeks.

Table 6. Therapy for Endocarditis Due to HACEK Microorganisms (*Haemophilus parainfluenzae, Haemophilus aphrophilus, Actinobacillus actinomycetemcomitans, Cardiobacterium hominus, Eikenella corrodens,* and *Kingella kingae*)*

Antibiotic	Dosage and Route	Duration (week)	Comments
Ceftriaxone sodium†	2 g once daily I.V. or I.M.†	4	Cefotaxime sodium or other third-generation cephalosporins may be substituted
Ampicillin sodium‡	12 g/24 h I.V. either continuously or in 6 equally divided doses	4	
With gentamicin sulfate§	1 mg/kg I.M. or I.V. every 6 h	4	

*Antibiotic dosages are for patients with normal renal function. I.V. indicates intravenous; I.M. intramuscular.

†Patients should be informed that I.M. injection of ceftriaxone is painful.

‡Ampicillin should not be used if laboratory tests show β-lactamase production.

§For specific dosing adjustment and issues concerning gentamicin (obese patients, relative contraindications), see Table 1 footnotes.

Note: Tables 1-6 are from Wilson WR, Karchmer AW, Dajani AS, et al, "Antibiotic Treatment of Adults With Infective Endocarditis Due to Streptococci, Enterococci, Staphylococci, and HACEK Microorganisms," *JAMA*, 1995, 274(21):1706-13, with permission.

ANTIMICROBIAL DRUGS OF CHOICE

The following table lists the antimicrobial drugs of choice for various infecting organisms. This was published in *The Medical Letter*. Users should not assume that all antibiotics which are appropriate for a given organism are listed or that those not listed are inappropriate. The infection caused by the organism may encompass varying degrees of severity, and since the antibiotics listed may not be appropriate for the differing degrees of severity, or because of other patient-related factors, it cannot be assumed that the antibiotics listed for any specific organism are interchangeable. This table should not be used by itself without first referring to *The Medical Letter*, an infectious disease manual, or the infectious disease department. Therefore, only use this table as a tool for obtaining more information about the therapies available.

Infecting Organism	Drug of First Choice	Alternative Drugs
Gram-Positive Cocci		
**Enterococcus*[1]		
endocarditis or other severe infection	Penicillin G or ampicillin + gentamicin or streptomycin	Vancomycin + gentamicin or streptomycin; teicoplanin;[2] quinupristin/dalfopristin[3]
uncomplicated urinary tract infection	Ampicillin or amoxicillin	Nitrofurantoin; a fluoroquinolone[4]
**Staphylococcus aureus* or *epidermidis*		
nonpenicillinase producing	Penicillin G or V[5]	A cephalosporin;[6,7] vancomycin; imipenem; clindamycin; a fluoroquinolone[4]
penicillinase-producing	A penicillinase-resistant penicillin[8]	A cephalosporin;[6,7] vancomycin; amoxicillin-clavulanic acid; ticarcillin-clavulanic acid; piperacillin/tazobactam; ampicillin-sulbactam; imipenem; clindamycin; a fluoroquinolone[4]
methicillin-resistant[9]	Vancomycin ± gentamicin ± rifampin	Trimethoprim-sulfamethoxazole; a fluoroquinolone;[4] minocycline[10]
Streptococcus pyogenes (group A) and groups C and G[11]	Penicillin G or V[5]	Clindamycin; erythromycin; a cephalosporin;[6,7] vancomycin; clarithromycin;[12] azithromycin
Streptococcus, group B	Penicillin G or ampicillin	A cephalosporin;[6,7] vancomycin; erythromycin
**Streptococcus*, viridans group[1]	Penicillin G ± gentamicin	A cephalosporin;[6,7] vancomycin
Streptococcus bovis[1]	Penicillin G	A cephalosporin;[6,7] vancomycin
Streptococcus, anaerobic or *Peptostreptococcus*	Penicillin G	Clindamycin; a cephalosporin;[6,7] vancomycin
Streptococcus pneumoniae[13] (pneumococcus)	Penicillin G or V[5,13]	A cephalosporin;[6,7] erythromycin; vancomycin ± rifampin; trimethoprim-sulfamethoxazole; azithromycin; clarithromycin;[12] clindamycin; chloramphenicol;[14] a tetracycline;[10] quinupristin/dalfopristin[3]
Gram-Negative Cocci		
Moraxella (Branhamella) catarrhalis	Trimethoprim-sulfamethoxazole	Amoxicillin/clavulanic acid; erythromycin; clarithromycin;[12] azithromycin; a tetracycline;[10]cefuroxime; [6]cefotaxime;[6] ceftizoxime;[6] ceftriaxone;[6] cefuroxime axetil;[6] cefixime;[6] a fluoroquinolone[4]
**Neisseria gonorrhoeae* (gonococcus)	Ceftriaxone[6]or cefixime[6]	Cefotaxime;[6]a fluoroquinolone;[4]spectinomycin; penicillin G
Neisseria meningitidis[15] (meningococcus)	Penicillin G	Cefotaxime;[6] ceftizoxime;[6] ceftriaxone;[6]chloramphenicol;[14] a sulfonamide[16]
Gram-Positive Bacilli		
Bacillus anthracis (anthrax)	Penicillin G	An erythromycin, a tetracycline[10]
Bacillus cereus, subtilis	Vancomycin	Imipenem; clindamycin

(continued)

Infecting Organism	Drug of First Choice	Alternative Drugs
Clostridium perfringens[17]	Penicillin G	Clindamycin; metronidazole; imipenem; a tetracycline;[10] chloramphenicol[14]
Clostridium tetani[18]	Penicillin G	A tetracycline[10]
Clostridium difficile[19]	Metronidazole	Vancomycin; bacitracin
Corynebacterium diphtheriae[20]	An erythromycin	Penicillin G
Corynebacterium, JK group	Vancomycin	Penicillin G + gentamicin; erythromycin
Listeria monocytogenes	Ampicillin ± gentamicin	Trimethoprim-sulfamethoxazole
Enteric Gram-Negative Bacilli		
**Bacteroides*		
oropharyngeal strains[21,22]	Penicillin G or clindamycin	Cefoxitin;[6] metronidazole; chloramphenicol;[14] cefotetan;[6] ampicillin/sulbactam
gastrointestinal strains	Metronidazole	Clindamycin; imipenem; ticarcillin/clavulanic acid; piperacillin/tazobactam; cefoxitin;[6] cefotetan;[6] ampicillin/sulbactam; piperacillin; chloramphenicol;[14] ceftizoxime;[6] cefmetazole[6]
**Campylobacter fetus*	Imipenem	Gentamicin
**Campylobacter jejuni*	A fluoroquinolone[4] or erythromycin	A tetracycline;[10] gentamicin
**Enterobacter*	Imipenem[23]	Cefotaxime;[6,23] ceftizoxime;[6,23] ceftriaxone[6,23] or ceftazidime;[6,23] gentamicin, tobramycin, or amikacin; trimethoprim-sulfamethoxazole; ticarcillin,[24] mezlocillin,[24] or piperacillin;[24] aztreonam;[23] a fluoroquinolone[4]
**Escherichia coli*[25]	Cefotaxime, ceftizoxime, ceftriaxone, or ceftazidime[6,23]	Ampicillin ± gentamicin, tobramycin, or amikacin; carbenicillin,[24] ticarcillin,[24] mezlocillin,[24] or piperacillin; [24] gentamicin, tobramycin, or amikacin; amoxicillin/clavulanic acid;[23] ticarcillin/clavulanic acid;[24] piperacillin/tazobactam;[24] ampicillin/sulbactam;[23] trimethoprim/sulfamethoxazole; imipenem;[23] aztreonam;[23] a fluoroquinolone;[4] another cephalosporin[6,7]
**Helicobacter pylori*[26]	Tetracycline hydrochloride[10] + metronidazole + bismuth subsalicylate	Tetracycline hydrochloride + clarithromycin[12] + bismuth subsalicylate; amoxicillin + metronidazole + bismuth subsalicylate
**Klebsiella pneumoniae*[25]	Cefotaxime, ceftizoxime, ceftriaxone, or ceftazidime[6,23]	Imipenem;[23] gentamicin, tobramycin, or amikacin; amoxicillin/-clavulanic acid;[23] ticarcillin/clavulanic acid;[24] piperacillin/tazobactam;[24] ampicillin/sulbactam;[23] trimethoprim-sulfamethoxazole; aztreonam;[23] a fluoroquinolone;[4] mezlocillin[24] or piperacillin;[24] another cephalosporin[6,7]
**Proteus mirabilis*[25]	Ampicillin[27]	A cephalosporin;[6,7,23] ticarcillin,[24] mezlocillin,[24] or piperacillin;[24] gentamicin, tobramycin, or amikacin; trimethoprim-sulfamethoxazole; imipenem;[23] aztreonam;[23] a fluoroquinolone;[4] chloramphenicol[14]

(continued)

Infecting Organism	Drug of First Choice	Alternative Drugs
Proteus, indole-positive (including *Providencia rettgeri*, *Morganella morganii*, and *Proteus vulgaris*)	Cefotaxime, ceftizoxime, ceftriaxone, or ceftazidime[6,23]	Imipenem;[23] gentamicin, tobramycin, or amikacin; carbenicillin,[24] ticarcillin,[24] mezlocillin,[24] piperacillin;[24] amoxicillin/clavulanic acid;[23] ticarcillin/clavulanic acid;[24] piperacillin/tazobactam;[24] ampicillin/sulbactam;[23] aztreonam;[23] trimethoprim-sulfamethoxazole; a fluoroquinolone[4]
**Providencia stuartii*	Cefotaxime, ceftizoxime, ceftriaxone, or ceftazidime[6,23]	Imipenem;[23] ticarcillin/clavulanic acid;[24] piperacillin/tazobactam;[24] gentamicin, tobramycin, or amikacin; carbenicillin;[24] ticarcillin,[24] mezlocillin,[24] or piperacillin;[24] aztreonam;[23] trimethoprim-sulfamethoxazole; fluoroquinolone[4]
**Salmonella typhi*[28]	A fluoroquinolone[4] or ceftriaxone[6]	Chloramphenicol;[14] trimethoprim-sulfamethoxazole; ampicillin; amoxicillin
*other *Salmonella*[29]	Cefotaxime[6] or ceftriaxone[6] or a fluoroquinolone[4]	Ampicillin or amoxicillin; trimethoprim-sulfamethoxazole; chloramphenicol[14]
**Serratia*	Cefotaxime, ceftizoxime, ceftriaxone, or ceftazidime[6,30]	Gentamicin or amikacin; imipenem;[30] aztreonam;[30] trimethoprim-sulfamethoxazole; carbenicillin,[31] ticarcillin,[31] mezlocillin,[31] or piperacillin;[31] a fluoroquinolone[4]
**Shigella*	A fluoroquinolone[4]	Trimethoprim-sulfamethoxazole; ampicillin; ceftriaxone[6]
**Yersinia enterocolitica*	Trimethoprim-sulfamethoxazole	A fluoroquinolone;[4] gentamicin, tobramycin, or amikacin; cefotaxime or ceftizoxime[6]
Other Gram-Negative Bacilli		
**Acinetobacter*	Imipenem[23]	Amikacin, tobramycin, or gentamicin; ticarcillin,[24] mezlocillin,[24] or piperacillin;[24] ceftazidime;[23] trimethoprim-sulfamethoxazole; a fluoroquinolone;[4] minocycline;[10] doxycycline[10]
**Aeromonas*	Trimethoprim-sulfamethoxazole	Gentamicin or tobramycin; imipenem; a fluoroquinolone[4]
Bartonella		
Agent of bacillary angiomatosis (*Bartonella henselae* or *quintana*)[32]	An erythromycin	Doxycycline[10]
Cat scratch bacillus (*Bartonella henselae*)[32,33]	Ciprofloxacin[34]	Trimethoprim-sulfamethoxazole; gentamicin; rifampin
Bordetella pertussis (whooping cough)	An erythromycin	Trimethoprim-sulfamethoxazole; ampicillin
**Brucella*	A tetracycline[10] + streptomycin or gentamicin	A tetracycline[10] + rifampin; chloramphenicol[14] ± streptomycin; trimethoprim-sulfamethoxazole ± gentamicin; rifampin + a tetracycline[10]
**Burkholderia cepacia*	Trimethoprim-sulfamethoxazole	Ceftazidime;[6] chloramphenicol[14]
Calymmatobacterium granulomatis (granuloma inguinale)	A tetracycline[10]	Streptomycin or gentamicin; trimethoprim-sulfamethoxazole; erythromycin
**Eikenella corrodens*	Ampicillin	An erythromycin; a tetracycline; amoxicillin/clavulanic acid; ampicillin/sulbactam; ceftriaxone
**Francisella tularensis* (tularemia)	Streptomycin	Gentamicin; a tetracycline;[10] chloramphenicol[14]
**Fusobacterium*	Penicillin G	Metronidazole; clindamycin; cefoxitin;[6] chloramphenicol[14]

(continued)

Infecting Organism	Drug of First Choice	Alternative Drugs
Gardnerella vaginalis (bacterial vaginosis)	Oral metronidazole[35]	Topical clindamycin or metronidazole; oral clindamycin
**Haemophilus ducreyi* (chancroid)	Erythromycin or ceftriaxone or azithromycin	A fluoroquinolone[4]
**Haemophilus influenzae*		
meningitis, epiglottitis, arthritis, and other serious infections	Cefotaxime or ceftriaxone[6]	Cefuroxime[6] (but not for meningitis); chloramphenicol [14]
upper respiratory infections and bronchitis	Trimethoprim-sulfamethoxazole	Cefuroxime;[6] amoxicillin/clavulanic acid; cefuroxime axetil;[6] cefaclor;[6] cefotaxime;[6] ceftizoxime;[6] ceftriaxone;[6] cefixime;[6] ampicillin or amoxicillin; a tetracycline;[10] clarithromycin;[12] azithromycin; a fluoroquinolone[4]
Legionella species	Erythromycin ± rifampin	Clarithromycin;[12] azithromycin; ciprofloxacin;[34] trimethoprim-sulfamethoxazole
Leptotrichia buccalis	Penicillin G	A tetracycline;[10] clindamycin; erythromycin
Pasteurella multocida	Penicillin G	A tetracycline;[10] a cephalosporin;[6,7] amoxicillin/clavulanic acid; ampicillin/sulbactam
**Pseudomonas aeruginosa*		
urinary tract infection	A fluoroquinolone[4]	Carbenicillin, ticarcillin, piperacillin, or mezlocillin; ceftazidime;[6] imipenem; aztreonam; tobramycin; gentamicin; amikacin
other infections	Ticarcillin, mezlocillin, or piperacillin + tobramycin, gentamicin, or amikacin[36]	Ceftazidime,[6] imipenem, or aztreonam + tobramycin, gentamicin, or amikacin; ciprofloxacin[34]
Pseudomonas mallei (glanders)	Streptomycin + a tetracycline[10]	Streptomycin + chloramphenicol[14]
**Pseudomonas pseudomallei* (melioidosis)	Ceftazidime[6]	Chloramphenicol[14] + doxycycline[10] + trimethoprim-sulfamethoxazole; amoxicillin/clavulanic acid; imipenem
Spirillum minus (rat bite fever)	Penicillin G	A tetracycline;[10] streptomycin
**Stenotrophomonas maltophilia (Pseudomonas maltophilia)*	Trimethoprim-sulfamethoxazole	Minocycline;[10] ceftazidime; [6] a fluoroquinolone[4]
Streptobacillus moniliformis (rat bite fever, Haverhill fever)	Penicillin G	A tetracycline;[10] streptomycin
Vibrio cholerae (cholera)[37]	A tetracycline[10]	Trimethoprim-sulfamethoxazole; a fluoroquinolone[4]
Vibrio vulnificus	A tetracycline[10]	Cefotaxime[6]
Yersinia pestis (plague)	Streptomycin	A tetracycline;[10] chloramphenicol;[14] gentamicin
Acid Fast Bacilli		
**Mycobacterium tuberculosis*[38]	Isoniazid + rifampin + pyrazinamide ± ethambutol or streptomycin[14]	Ciprofloxacin or ofloxacin;[34] cycloserine;[14] capreomycin[14] or kanamycin[14] or amikacin;[14] ethionamide;[14] clofazimine;[14] aminosalicylic acid[14]
**Mycobacterium kansasii*	Isoniazid + rifampin ± ethambutol or streptomycin[14]	Clarithromycin;[12] ethionamide;[14] cycloserine[14]
**Mycobacterium avium* complex	Clarithromycin[12] or azithromycin + one or more of the following: ethambutol; rifabutin; ciprofloxacin[34]	Rifampin; clofazimine;[14] amikacin[14]
prophylaxis	Rifabutin or clarithromycin[12]	Azithromycin

(continued)

Infecting Organism	Drug of First Choice	Alternative Drugs
Mycobacterium fortuitum complex	Amikacin + doxycycline[10]	Cefoxitin;[6] rifampin; a sulfonamide
Mycobacterium marinum (balnei)[39]	Minocycline[10]	Trimethoprim-sulfamethoxazole; rifampin; clarithromycin;[12] doxycycline[10]
Mycobacterium leprae (leprosy)	Dapsone + rifampin ± clofazimine	Minocycline;[10] ofloxacin;[34,40] sparfloxacin;[41] clarithromycin[12,42]
Actinomycetes		
Actinomyces israelii (actinomycosis)	Penicillin G	A tetracycline;[10] erythromycin; clindamycin
Nocardia	Trimethoprim-sulfamethoxazole	Sulfisoxazole; amikacin;[14] a tetracycline;[10] imipenem; cycloserine[14]
Chlamydiae		
Chlamydia psittaci (psittacosis, ornithosis)	A tetracycline[10]	Chloramphenicol[14]
Chlamydia trachomatis		
(trachoma)	Azithromycin	A tetracycline[10] (topical plus oral); a sulfonamide (topical plus oral)
(inclusion conjunctivitis)	Erythromycin (oral or I.V.)	A sulfonamide
(pneumonia)	Erythromycin	A sulfonamide
(urethritis, cervicitis)	Doxycycline[10] or azithromycin	Erythromycin; ofloxacin;[34] sulfisoxazole; amoxicillin
(lymphogranuloma venereum)	A tetracycline[10]	Erythromycin
Chlamydia pneumoniae (TWAR strain)	A tetracycline[10]	Erythromycin; clarithromycin;[12] azithromycin
Ehrlichia		
Ehrlichia chaffeensis	A tetracycline[10]	
Agent of human granulocytic ehrlichiosis[43]	A tetracycline[10]	
Mycoplasma		
Mycoplasma pneumoniae	Erythromycin or a tetracycline[10]	Clarithromycin;[12] azithromycin
Ureaplasma urealyticum	Erythromycin	A tetracycline;[10] clarithromycin;[12]
Rickettsia — Rocky Mountain spotted fever, endemic typhus (louse-borne), scrub typhus, trench fever, scrub typhus, Q fever	A tetracycline[10]	Chloramphenicol;[14] a fluoroquinolone[4]
Spirochetes		
Borrelia burgdorferi (Lyme disease)[44]	Doxycycline[10] or amoxicillin	Cefuroxime axetil;[6] ceftriaxone;[6] cefotaxime;[6] penicillin G; azithromycin; clarithromycin[12]
Borrelia recurrentis (relapsing fever)	A tetracycline[10]	Penicillin G
Leptospira	Penicillin G[5]	A tetracycline[10]
Treponema pallidum (syphilis)	Penicillin G	A tetracycline;[10]ceftriaxone[6]

(continued)

Infecting Organism	Drug of First Choice	Alternative Drugs
Treponema pertenue (yaws)	Penicillin G	A tetracycline[10]

*Resistance may be a problem; susceptibility tests should be performed.

1. Disk sensitivity testing may not provide adequate information; beta-lactamase assays and dilution tests for susceptibility should be used in serious infection.

2. An investigational drug in the U.S.A. (*Targocid* by Hoechst Marion Roussel).

3. An investigational drug in the U.S.A. available through Rhôone-Poulenc Rorer (610-454-3071).

4. For most infections, ofloxacin or ciprofloxacin. For urinary tract infections, norfloxacin, lomefloxacin, or enoxacin can be used. Ciprofloxacin and ofloxacin are available for intravenous use. None of these agents is recommended for children or pregnant women.

5. Penicillin V is preferred for oral treatment of infections caused by non-penicillinase-producing staphylococci and other gram-positive cocci. For initial therapy of severe infections, penicillin G, administered parenterally, is first choice. For somewhat longer action in less severe infections due to group A streptococci, pneumococci or *Treponema pallidum,* procaine penicillin G, an intramuscular formulation, is given once or twice daily. Benzathine penicillin G, a slowly absorbed preparation, is usually given in a single monthly injection for prophylaxis of rheumatic fever, once for treatment of group A streptococcal pharyngitis and once or more for treatment of syphilis.

6. The cephalosporins have been used as alternatives to penicillin in patients allergic to penicillins, but such patients may also have allergic reactions to cephalosporins.

7. For parenteral treatment of staphylococcal or nonenterococcal streptococcal infections, a "first-generation" cephalosporin such as cephalothin or cefazolin can be used; for staphylococcal endocarditis, some *Medical Letter* consultants prefer cephalothin. For oral therapy, cephalexin or cephradine can be used. The "second-generation" cephalosporins, cefamandole, cefprozil, cefuroxime, cefuroxime axetil, cefonicid, cefotetan, cefmetazole, cefoxitin, and loracarbef are more active than the first-generation drugs against gram-negative bacteria. Cefuroxime and cefamandole are active against ampicillin-resistant strains of *H. influenzae,* but cefamandole has been associated with prothrombin deficiency and occasional bleeding. Cefoxitin, cefotetan, and cefmetazole are active against *B. fragilis,* but cefotetan and cefmetazole have also been associated with prothrombin deficiency. The "third-generation" cephalosporins cefotaxime, cefoperazone, ceftizoxime, ceftriaxone, and ceftazidime have greater activity than the second-generation drugs against enteric gram-negative bacilli. Ceftazidime has poor activity against many gram-positive cocci and anaerobes, and ceftizoxime has poor activity against penicillin-resistant *S. pneumoniae* (Haas DW, et al, *Clin Infect Dis,* 1995, 20:671). Cefixime and cefpodoxime are oral cephalosporins with more activity than second-generation cephalosporins again facultative gram-negative bacilli; they have no useful activity against anaerobes or *Pseudomonas aeruginosa,* and cefixime has no useful activity against staphylococci. With the exception of cefoperazone (which, like cefamandole, can cause bleeding) and ceftazidime, the activity of all currently available cephalosporins against *Pseudomonas aeruginosa* is poor or inconsistent.

8. For oral use against penicillinase-producing staphylococci, cloxacillin or dicloxacillin is preferred; for severe infections, a parenteral formulation of nafcillin or oxacillin should be used. Ampicillin, amoxicillin, bacampicillin, carbenicillin, ticarcillin, mezlocillin, and piperacillin are not effective against penicillinase-producing staphylococci. The combination of clavulanic acid with amoxicillin or ticarcillin, sulbactam with ampicillin, and tazobactam with piperacillin are active against these organisms.

9. Many strains of coagulase-positive staphylococci and coagulase-negative staphylococci are resistant to penicillinase-resistant penicillins; these strains are also resistant to cephalosporins and imipenem.

10. Tetracyclines are generally not recommended for pregnant women or children younger than 8 years old.

11. For serious soft-tissue infection due to group A streptococci, clindamycin may be more effective than penicillin. Group A streptococci may, however, be resistant to clindamycin; therefore, some *Medical Letter* consultants suggest using both clindamycin and penicillin to treat serious soft-tissue infections. Group A streptococci may also be resistant to erythromycin, azithromycin, and clarithromycin.

12. Not recommended for use in pregnancy.

13. Strains frequently show intermediate or high-level resistance to penicillin. Infections caused by strains with intermediate resistance to penicillin may respond to cefotaxime or ceftriaxone. Cefuroxime or high doses of penicillin may be effective for pneumonia. Highly resistant strains and, before susceptibility is known, all patients with meningitis should be treated with vancomycin with or without rifampin in addition to a cephalosporin. In patients allergic to penicillin, erythromycin, azithromycin, or clarithromycin are often useful for respiratory infections; but vancomycin with or without rifampin is recommended for meningitis. Some strains of *S. pneumoniae* are resistant to erythromycin, clindamycin, trimethoprim-sulfamethoxazole, clarithromycin, azithromycin, and chloramphenicol. All strains tested so far are susceptible to quinupristin/dalfopristin.

14. Because of the possibility of serious adverse effects, this drug should be used only for severe infections when less hazardous drugs are ineffective.

15. Rare strains of *N. meningitidis* are resistant or relatively resistant to penicillin. Rifampin is recommended for prophylaxis in close contacts of patients infected by sulfonamide-resistant organisma.

16. Sulfonamide-resistant strains are frequent in the U.S.A.; sulfonamides should be used only when susceptibility is established by susceptibility tests.

17. Debridement is primary. Large doses of penicillin G are required. Hyperbaric oxygen therapy may be a useful adjunct to surgical debridement in management of the spreading, necrotic type.

18. For prophylaxis, a tetanus toxoid booster and, for some patients, tetanus immune globulin (human) are required.

19. In order to decrease the emergence of vancomycin-resistant enterococci in hospital, many *Medical Letter* consultants now recommend use of metronidazole first in treatment of most patients with *C. difficile* colitis, with oral vancomycin used only for seriously ill patients or those who do not respond to metronidazole. Also see *Medical Letter,* 1989, 31:94.

20. Antitoxin is primary; antimicrobials are used only to halt further toxin production and to prevent the carrier state.

21. *Bacteroides* species from the oropharynx may be resistant to penicillin; for patients seriously ill with infections that may be due to these organisms, or when response to penicillin is delayed, clindamycin should be used.

22. When infection is in the central nervous system, metronidazole is generally recommended.

23. In severely ill patients, most *Medical Letter* consultants would add gentamicin, tobramycin, or

amikacin.

24. In severely ill patients, most *Medical Letter* consultants would add gentamicin, tobramycin, or amikacin (but see footnote 36).

25. For an acute, uncomplicated urinary tract infections, before the infecting organism is known, the drug of first choice is trimethoprim-sulfamethoxazole.

26. Eradication of *H. pylori* with various antibacterial combinations, usually given concurrently with an H_2-receptor blocker or proton pump inhibitor has led to rapid healing of active peptic ulcers and low recurrence rates (Walsh JH and Peterson WL, *N Engl J Med,* 1995, 333:984).

27. Large doses (6 g or more/day) are usually necessary for systemic infections. In severely ill patients, some *Medical Letter* consultants would add gentamicin, tobramycin, or amikacin.

28. Ampicillin or amoxicillin may be effective in milder cases. Ciprofloxacin or amoxicillin is the drug of choice for *S. typhi* carriers.

29. Most cases of *Salmonella* gastroenteritis subside spontaneously without antimicrobial therapy.

30. In severely ill patients, most consultants would add gentamicin or amikacin.

31. In severely ill patients, most *Medical Letter* consultants would add gentamicin or amikacin (but see footnote 36).

32. Adal KA, et al, *N Engl J Med,* 1994, 330:1509.

33. Role of antibiotics is not clear (Margileth AM, *Pediatr Infect Dis J,* 1992, 11:474).

34. Usually not recommended for use in children or pregnant women.

35. Metronidazole is effective for bacterial vaginosis even though it is not usually active against *Gardnerella in vitro.*

36. Neither gentamicin, tobramycin, netilmicin, or amikacin should be mixed in the same bottle with carbenicillin, ticarcillin, mezlocillin, or piperacillin for intravenous administration. When used in high doses or in patients with renal impairment, these penicillins may inactivate the aminoglycosides.

37. Antibiotic therapy is an adjunct to and not a substitute for prompt fluid and electrolyte replacement.

38. For more details, see *Medical Letter,* 1995, 37:67.

39. Most infections are self-limited without drug treatment.

40. Ji B, et al, *Antimicrob Agents Chemother,* 1994, 38:662.

41. An investigational drug in the U.S.A.

42. Chan GP, et al, *Antimicrob Agents Chemother,* 1994, 38:515.

43. Bakken JS, et al, *JAMA,* 1994, 272:212.

44. For treatment of early infection in nonpregnant adults, doxycycline is preferred; for fully developed infection with arthritis or meningitis, ceftriaxone is preferred.

BACTERIAL MENINGITIS PRACTICAL GUIDELINES FOR MANAGEMENT

Empirical Therapy of Purulent Meningitis
(In cases in which a highly penicillin-resistant pneumococcus (MIC ≥2 mg/L) is suspected, vancomycin should be added)

Predisposing Factor	Common Organisms	Therapy
Age		
0-4 wk	*Escherichia coli*, group B streptococci, *Listeria monocytogenes*, *Klebsiella* sp	Ampicillin plus cefotaxime; or ampicillin plus an aminoglycoside
4-12 wk	*E. coli*, group B streptococci, *L. monocytogenes*, *Haemophilus influenzae*, *Streptococcus pneumoniae*, *Neisseria meningitidis*	Ampicillin plus a third generation cephalosporin*
3 mo - 18 y	*H. influenzae*, *N. meningitidis*, *S. pneumoniae*	Third generation cephalosporin*, or ampicillin plus chloramphenicol
18-50 y	*S. pneumoniae*, *N. meningitidis*	Third generation cephalosporin* ± ampicillin†
>50 y	*S. pneumoniae*, *N. meningitidis*, *L. monocytogenes*, gram-negative bacilli	Ampicillin plus a third generation cephalosporin*
Immunocompromised state	*S. pneumoniae*, *N. meningitidis*, *L. monocytogenes*, gram-negative bacilli (including *Pseudomonas aeruginosa*)	Vancomycin plus ampicillin plus ceftazidime‡
Basilar skull fracture	*S. pneumoniae*, *H. influenzae*, group A β-hemolytic streptococci	Third generation cephalosporin*
Postneurosurgery; head trauma	*Staphylococcus aureus*, *S. epidermidis*, gram-negative bacilli (including *P. aeruginosa*)	Vancomycin plus ceftazidime‡
Cerebrospinal fluid shunt	*S. epidermidis*, *S. aureus*, gram-negative bacilli (including *P. aeruginosa*), *Propionibacterium acnes*	Vancomycin plus ceftazidime‡

From *Drugs*, 1995, 50 (5):838-53.

MIC = minimum inhibitory concentration.

*Cefotaxime or ceftriaxone.

†If *Listeria* is thought to be a likely etiological agent.

‡Add gentamicin in proven *P. aeruginosa* meningitis.

Antimicrobial Therapy of Bacterial Meningitis of Known Etiology

Organism	Standard	Alternative
Haemophilus influenzae		
β-lactamase negative	Ampicillin	Third generation cephalosporin* or chloramphenicol or aztreonam
β-lactamase positive	Third generation cephalosporin*	Chloramphenicol or aztreonam or fluoroquinolone†
Neisseria meningitidis	Benzylpenicillin (penicillin G) or ampicillin	Third generation cephalosporin* or chloramphenicol
Streptococcus pneumoniae penicillin MIC		
<0.1 mg/L	Benzylpenicillin or ampicillin	Third generation cephalosporin* or chloramphenicol or vancomycin
0.1-1 mg/L	Third generation cephalosporin§	Vancomycin or imipenem*
≥2 mg/L	Vancomycin‡	Imipenem§ or meropenem¶
Enterobacteriaceae	Third generation cephalosporin*	Aztreonam or fluoroquinolone† or co-trimoxazole (trimethoprim plus sulfamethoxazole)

(continued)

Organism	Standard	Alternative
Pseudomonas aeruginosa	Ceftazidime#	Aztreonam# or fluoroquinolone†·#
Listeria monocytogenes	Ampicillin# or benzylpenicillin#	Co-trimoxazole
S. agalactiae	Ampicillin# or benzylpenicillin#	Third generation cephalosporin* or vancomycin
Staphylococcus aureus		
methicillin-sensitive	Nafcillin or oxacillin	Vancomycin
methicillin-resistant	Vancomycin‡	
S. epidermidis	Vancomycin‡	

From *Drugs*, 1995, 50 (5):838-53.
MIC = minimum inhibitory concentration.
*Cefotaxime or ceftriaxone.
†Contraindicated in patients <18 years of age.
‡Consider addition of rifampicin (rifampin).
§Associated with an increased incidence of seizures.
¶Not yet licensed in the U.S. for clinical use.
#Consider addition of an aminoglycoside.

Recommended Dosages of Antimicrobial Agents for Meningitis in Adults, Infants, and Children With Normal Renal and Hepatic Function (Therapy is given intravenously unless otherwise indicated)

Antimicrobial Agent	Total Daily Dose (Dosage Interval in Hours) Adults (g)	Infants and Children (mg/kg)
Amikacin*	15 mg/kg (8)	15-20 (8)
Ampicillin	12 (4)	200-300 (6)
Aztreonam	6-8 (6-8)	
Benzylpenicillin (penicillin G)	24 MU (4)	0.25 MU/kg (4-6)
Cefotaxime	8-12 (4-6)	200 (6-8)
Ceftazidime	6 (8)	125-150 (8)
Ceftriaxone	4 (12-24)	80-100 (12-24)
Chloramphenicol†	4-6 (6)	75-100 (6)
Ciprofloxacin	800 mg (12)	
Co-trimoxazole¶	10 mg/kg (12)	10 (12)
Gentamicin*	3-5 mg/kg (8)	7.5 (8)
Imipenem	2 (6)	
Nafcillin	9-12 (4)	200 (6)
Oxacillin	9-12 (4)	
Rifampicin (rifampin)‡	600 mg (24)	10-20 (12-24)§
Tobramycin*	3-5 mg/kg (8)	7.5 (8)
Vancomycin*·#	2-3 (8-12)	50-60 (6)

From *Drugs*, 1995, 50 (5):838-53.
*Need to monitor peak and trough serum concentrations.
†Higher doses recommended for pneumococcal meningitis.
‡Oral administration.
§Maximum daily dose of 600 mg.
¶Dosage based on trimethoprim component.
#May need to monitor cerebrospinal fluid concentrations in severely ill patients.

INTERPRETATION OF GRAM'S STAIN RESULTS GUIDELINES

These guidelines are not definitive but presumptive for the identification of organisms on Gram's stain. Treatment will depend on the quality of the specimen and appropriate clinical evaluation.

Gram-Negative Bacilli (GNB)	**Example**
Enterobacteriaceae	*E coli* *Serratia* sp *Klebsiella* sp *Enterobacter* sp *Citrobacter* sp
Pseudomonas aeruginosa	
Xanthomonas maltophilia	
Nonfermentative GNB	
Haemophilus influenzae	
Bacteroides fragilis group	
If fusiform (long and pointed)	*Fusobacterium* sp *Capnocytophaga* sp
Gram-Negative Cocci (GNC)	
Diplococci, pairs	*Neisseria meningitidis* *Neisseria gonorrhoeae* *Moraxella (Branhamella) catarrhalis*
Coccobacilli	*Acinetobacter* sp
Gram-Positive Bacilli (GPB)	
Diphtheroids (small pleomorphic)	*Corynebacterium* sp *Propionibacterium*
Large, with spores	*Clostridium* sp *Bacillus* sp
Branching, beaded, rods	*Nocardia* sp *Actinomyces* sp
Other	*Listeria* sp *Lactobacillus* sp
Gram-Positive Cocci (GPC)	
Pairs, chains, clusters	*Staphylococcus* sp *Streptococcus* sp *Enterococcus* sp
Pairs, lancet-shaped	*S. pneumoniae*

KEY CHARACTERISTICS OF SELECTED BACTERIA

Gram-Negative Bacilli (GNB)	Example
Lactose-positive	*Citrobacter* sp* (Enterobacteriaceae) *Enterobacter* sp* (Enterobacteriaceae) *Escherichia coli* (Enterobacteriaceae) *Klebsiella pneumoniae* (Enterobacteriaceae)
Lactose-negative/oxidase-negative	*Acinetobacter* sp *Morganella morganii* *Proteus mirabilis*: indole negative *Proteus vulgaris*: indole positive *Providencia* sp *Salmonella* sp *Serratia* sp† (Enterobacteriaceae) *Shigella* sp *Xanthomonas maltophilia*
Lactose-negative/oxidase-positive	*Aeromonas hydrophila* (may be lactose positive) *Alcaligenes* sp *Flavobacterium* sp *Moraxella* sp‡ *Pseudomonas aeruginosa* Other *Pseudomonas* sp
Anaerobes	*Bacteroides* sp (*B. fragilis*) *Fusobacterium* sp
Other	*Haemophilus influenzae* (coccobacillus)
Gram-Positive Baccili (GPB)	
Anaerobes	*Lactobacillus* sp *Eubacterium* sp *Clostridium* sp (spores) *Bifidobacterium* sp *Actinomyces* sp (branching, filamentous) *Propionibacterium acnes*
Bacillus sp	*B. cereus, B. subtilis* (large with spores)
Branching, beaded; partial acid-fast positive	*Nocardia* sp
CSF, blood	*Listeria monocytogenes*
Rapidly growing mycobacteria	*M. fortuitum* *M. chelonei*
Vaginal flora, rarely blood	*Lactobacillus* sp
Often blood culture contaminants	Diphtheroids (may be *Corynebacterium* sp)
Resistant to many agents except vancomycin	*C. jeikeium*
Other	*Actinomyces* sp (branching, beaded)
Gram-Negative Cocci (GNC)	
Diplococci, pairs	*Capnocytophaga* sp *Fusobacterium* sp (fusiform) *Moraxella catarrhalis* *Neisseria meningitidis* *Neisseria gonorrhoeae*
Coccobacili	*Acinetobacter* sp
Anaerobes	*Veillonella* sp
Gram-Positive Cocci (GPC)	
Catalase-negative	*Streptococcus* sp (chains) *Micrococcus* sp (usually insignificant)
Catalase-positive	*Staphylococcus* sp (pairs, chains, clusters)
Coagulase-negative	Coagulase-negative staphyloccoci (CNS)
Bloods	*S. epidermidis* or CNS
Urine	*S. saprophyticus* (CNS)
Coagulase-positive	*S. aureus*
Anaerobes	*Peptostreptococcus* sp
Fungi	
Molds	
Sparsely septate hyphae	Zygomycetes (eg, *Rhizopus* sp and *Mucor*)
Septate hyphae brown pigment	Phaeohyphomycetes, for example, *Alternaria* sp *Bipolaris* sp *Curvularia* sp *Exserohilum* sp
Nonpigmented (hyaline)	Hyalophomycetes, for example *Aspergillus* sp (*A. fumigatus, A. flavus*) Dermatophytes *Fusarium* sp *Paecilomyces* sp *Penicillium* sp

(continued)

Gram-Negative Bacilli (GNB)	Example
Thermally dimorphic (yeast in tissue; mold *in vitro*)	*Blastomyces dermatitidis* *Coccidioides immitis* *Histoplasma capsulatum* (slow growing) *Paracoccidioides brasilliensis* *Sporothrix schenckii*
Yeast	*Candida* sp (germ tube positive = *C. albicans* *Cryptococcus* sp (no pseudohyphae) *C. neoformans* *Rhodotorula, Saccharomyces* sp *Torulopsis glabrata* *Trichosporon* sp
Virus	Influenza Hepatitis A, B, C, D Human immunodeficiency virus Rubella Herpes Cytomegalovirus Respiratory syncytial virus Epstein-Barr
Chlamydiae	*Chlamydia trachomatis* *Chlamydia pneumoniae* (TWAR) *Chlamydia psitiaci*
Rickettsiae	
Ureaplasma	
Mycoplasma	*Mycoplasma pneumoniae* *Mycoplasma hominis*
Spirochetes	*Treponema pallidum* *Borrelia burgorferi*
Mycobacteria	*Mycobacterium tuberculosis* *Mycobacterium intracellulare*

Most Common Blood Culture Contaminants
Alpha-hemolytic streptococci
Bacillus sp
Coagulase-negative staphylococci
Diphtheroids
Lactobacilli
Micrococcus sp
Propionibacterium sp

*May be lactose-negative.

†May produce red pigment and appear lactose-positive initially.

‡May be either bacillary or coccoid.

RECOMMENDATIONS FOR PREVENTING THE SPREAD OF VANCOMYCIN RESISTANCE

Recommendations of the Hospital Infection Control Practices Advisory Committee (HICPAC)
(*MMWR Morb Mortal Wkly Rep*, 1995, 44(RR-12))

Prudent Vancomycin Use

Vancomycin use has been reported consistently as a risk factor for infection and colonization with VRE and may increase the possibility of the emergence of vancomycin-resistant *S. aureus* (VRSA) and/or vancomycin-resistant *S. epidermidis* (VRSE). Therefore, all hospitals and other healthcare delivery services, even those at which VRE have never been detected, should a) develop a comprehensive, antimicrobial-utilization plan to provide education for their medical staff (including medical students who rotate their training in different departments of the healthcare facility), b) oversee surgical prophylaxis, and c) develop guidelines for the proper use of vancomycin (as applicable to the institution).

Guideline development should be part of the hospital's quality-improvement program and should involve participation from the hospital's pharmacy and therapeutics committee; hospital epidemiologist; and infection-control, infectious-disease, medical, and surgical staffs. The guidelines should include the following considerations:

1. Situations in which the use of vancomycin is appropriate or acceptable

   - For treatment of serious infections caused by beta-lactam-resistant gram-positive microorganisms; vancomycin may be less rapidly bactericidal than are beta-lactam agents for beta-lactam-susceptible staphylococci

   - For treatment of infections caused by gram-positive microorganisms in patients who have serious allergies to beta-lactam antimicrobials

   - When antibiotic-associated colitis fails to respond to metronidazole therapy or is severe and potentially life-threatening

   - Prophylaxis, as recommended by the American Heart Association, for endocarditis following certain procedures in patients at high risk for endocarditis

   - Prophylaxis for major surgical procedures involving implantation of prosthetic materials or devices (eg, cardiac and vascular procedures and total hip replacement) at institutions that have a high rate of infections caused by MRSA or methicillin-resistant *S. epidermidis*. A single dose of vancomycin administered immediately before surgery is sufficient unless the procedure lasts >6 hours, in which case the dose should be repeated. Prophylaxis should be discontinued after a maximum of two doses.

2. Situations in which the use of vancomycin should be discouraged

   - Routine surgical prophylaxis other than in a patient who has a life-threatening allergy to beta-lactam antibiotics

   - Empiric antimicrobial therapy for a febrile neutropenic patient, unless initial evidence indicates that the patient has an infection caused by gram-positive microorganisms (eg, at an inflamed exit site of Hickman catheter) and the prevalence of infections caused by MRSA in the hospital is substantial

   - Treatment in response to a single blood culture positive for coagulase-negative *Staphylococcus*, if other blood cultures taken during the same time frame are negative (ie, if contamination of the blood culture is likely).

Because contamination of blood cultures with skin flora (eg, *S. epidermidis*) could result in inappropriate administration of vancomycin, phlebotomists and other personnel who obtain blood cultures should be trained to minimize microbial contamination of specimens.

- Continued empiric use for presumed infections in patients whose cultures are negative for beta-lactam-resistant gram-positive microorganisms
- Systemic or local (eg, antibiotic lock) prophylaxis for infection or colonization of indwelling central or peripheral intravascular catheters
- Selective decontamination of the digestive tract
- Eradication of MRSA colonization
- Primary treatment of antibiotic-associated colitis
- Routine prophylaxis for very low-birthweight infants (ie, infants who weigh <1500 g)
- Routine prophylaxis for patients on continuous ambulatory peritoneal dialysis or hemodialysis
- Treatment (chosen for dosing convenience) of infections caused by beta-lactam-sensitive gram-positive microorganisms in patients who have renal failure
- Use of vancomycin solution for topical application or irrigation

3. Enhancing compliance with recommendations

   - Although several techniques may be useful, further study is required to determine the most effective methods for influencing the prescribing practices of physicians
   - Key parameters of vancomycin use can be monitored through the hospital's quality assurance/improvement process or as part of the drug-utilization review of the Pharmacy and Therapeutics Committee and the medical staff

Selected Options for Changing Therapy Owing to Treatment Failure or Drug Intolerance*

Initial Regimen	Subsequent Regimen Options
Treatment Failure	
Zidovudine†	Zidovudine/didanosine ± protease inhibitor
	Zidovudine/lamivudine ± protease inhibitor
	Didanosine ± protease inhibitor
	Didanosine/stavudine ± protease inhibitor
Didanosine	Zidovudine/lamivudine ± protease inhibitor
	Zidovudine/didanosineprotease inhibitor
	Stavudine/protease inhibitor
Zidovudine/didanosine	Zidovudine/lamivudine ± protease inhibitor
	Stavudine/protease inhibitor
Zidovudine/zalcitabine	Zidovudine/lamivudine ± protease inhibitor
	Stavudine/protease inhibitor
	Didanosine/proteas inhibitor
Zidovudine/lamivudine	Didanosine/protease inhibitor
	Stavudine/protease inhibitor
	Didanosine/stavudine
	Lamivudine/stavudine
Drug Intolerance‡	
Zidovudine†	Didanosine
	Didanosine/stavudine
	Lamivudine/stavudine
	Stavudine
Didanosine	Zidovudine/lamivudine
	Lamivudine/stavudine
	Stavudine/protease inhibitor
Zidovudine/zalcitabine	
Intolerance to zidovudine	Didanosine
	Didanosine/protease inhibitor
	Didanosine/stavudine
	Stavudine/protease inhibitor

(continued)

Initial Regimen	Subsequent Regimen Options
Intolerance to zalcitabine	Zidovudine/lamivudine ± protease inhibitor
Zidovudine/lamivudine	Didanosine/protease inhibitor Stavudine/protease inhibitor Didanosine/stavudine

*For patients whose initial regimen includes a protease inhibitor, subsequent regimens should include at least 2 new drugs chosen from among nucleoside analogues, non-nucleoside reverse transcriptase inhibitors (if available), and protease inhibitors (one should be selected for which there is likely to be little or no cross-resistance to the initial protease inhibitor).

†Considered a suboptimal regimen; all patients on zidovudine monotherapy should be re-evaluated.

‡A protease inhibitor could be added to the nucleoside analogue regimens listed.

Adapted from *JAMA*, July 10, 1996, Vol 276, No. 2.

RECOMMENDATIONS OF THE ADVISORY COUNCIL ON THE ELIMINATION OF TUBERCULOSIS

(*MMWR*, 1993, 42(RR-7):1-8)

REGIMEN OPTIONS FOR THE INITIAL TREATMENT OF TB AMONG CHILDREN AND ADULTS

TB Without HIV Infection

Option 1

Administer daily INH, RIF, and PZA for 8 weeks followed by 16 weeks of INH and RIF daily or 2-3 times/week* in areas where the INH resistance rate is not documented to be <4%. EMB or SM should be added to the initial regimen until susceptibility to INH and RIF is demonstrated. Continue treatment for at least 6 months and 3 months beyond culture conversion. Consult a TB medical expert if the patient is symptomatic or smear or culture positive after 3 months.

Option 2

Administer daily INH, RIF, PZA and SM or EMB for 2 weeks followed by 2 times/ week* administration of the same drugs for 6 weeks (by DOT‡), and subsequently, with 2 times/week administration of INH and RIF for 16 weeks (by DOT). Consult a TB medical expert if the patient is symptomatic or smear or culture positive after 3 months.

Option 3

Treat by DOT, 3 times/week* with INH, RIF, PZA, and EMB or SM for 6 months†. Consult a TB medical expert if the patient is symptomatic or smear or culture positive after 3 months.

TB With HIV Infection

Options 1, 2, or 3 can be used, but treatment regimens should continue for a total of 9 months and at least 6 months beyond culture conversion.

*All regimens administered 2 times/week or 3 times/week should be monitored by DOT for the duration of therapy.

†The strongest evidence from clinical trials is the effectiveness of all four drugs administered for the full 6 months. There is weaker evidence that SM can be discontinued after 4 months if the isolate is susceptible to all drugs. The evidence for stopping PZA before the end of 6 months is equivocal for the 3 times/week regimen, and there is no evidence on the effectiveness of this regimen with EMB for less than the full 6 months.

‡DOT - directly observed therapy.

Dosage Recommendations for the Initial Treatment of TB Among Children*

Drugs	Children (daily)	Children (2 times/week)	Children (3 times/week)
Isoniazid	10-20 mg/kg Max: 300 mg	20-40 mg/kg Max: 900 mg	20-40 mg/kg Max: 900 mg
Rifampin	10-20 mg/kg Max: 600 mg	10-20 mg/kg Max: 600 mg	10-20 mg/kg Max: 600 mg
Pyrazinamide	15-30 mg/kg Max: 2 g	50-70 mg/kg Max: 4 g	50-70 mg/kg Max: 3 g
Ethambutol†	15-25 mg/kg Max: 2.5 g	50 mg/kg Max: 2.5 g	25-30 mg/kg Max: 2.5 g
Streptomycin	20-30 mg/kg Max: 1 g	25-30 mg/kg Max: 1.5 g	25-30 mg/kg Max: 1 g

*Children ≤12 years of age.

†Ethambutol is generally not recommended for children whose visual acuity cannot be monitored (<6 years of age). However, ethambutol should be considered for all children with organisms resistant to other drugs, when susceptibility to ethambutol has been demonstrated, or susceptibility is likely.

Dosage Recommendation for the Initial Treatment of TB Among Adults

Drugs	Adults (daily)	Adults (2 times/week)	Adults (3 times/week)
Isoniazid	5 mg/kg Max: 300 mg	15 mg/kg Max: 900 mg	15 mg/kg Max: 900 mg
Rifampin	10 mg/kg Max: 600 mg	10 mg/kg Max: 600 mg	10 mg/kg Max: 600 mg
Pyrazinamide	15-30 mg/kg Max: 2 g	50-70 mg/kg Max: 4 g	50-70 mg/kg Max: 3 g
Ethambutol†	5-25 mg/kg Max: 2.5 g	50 mg/kg Max: 2.5 g	25-30 mg/kg Max: 2.5 g
Streptomycin	15 mg/kg Max: 1 g	25-30 mg/kg Max: 1.5 g	25-30 mg/kg Max: 1 g

SUSPECTED ORGANISMS BY SITE OF INFECTION FOR EMPIRIC THERAPY

Urinary Tract	
Community acquired	*E. coli*, other gram-negative rods, *S. aureus*, *S. epidermidis*, *S. faecalis*
Nosocomial	Resistant gram-negative rods, enterococci
Respiratory Tract	
Pneumonia	
Community acquired	
normal adult	*S. pneumoniae*, virus, *Mycoplasma* (atypical)
normal child	*S. pneumoniae*, *H. influenzae*
aspiration	Aerobic and anaerobic mouth flora
alcoholic	*S. pneumoniae*, *Klebsiella*, anaerobes (below the belt)
COPD	*S. pneumoniae*, *H. influenzae*
Nosocomial	
aspiration	Mouth anaerobes, gram-negative aerobic rods, *S. aureus*
neutropenic	Fungi, gram-negative aerobic rods, *S. aureus*
HIV-infected	Fungi, *P. carinii*, *Legionella*, *Nocardia*, *S. pneumoniae*
Epiglottis	*H. influenzae*
Acute sinusitis	*S. pneumoniae*, *H. influenzae*, *M. catarrhalis (B. catarrhalis)*
Chronic sinusitis	Anaerobes, *S. aureus*
Bronchitis, otitis	*S. pneumoniae*, *H. influenzae*, *M. catarrhalis (B. catarrhalis)*
Pharyngitis	Group A streptococci
Skin and Soft Tissue	
Cellulitis	Group A streptococci, *S. aureus*
I.V. site	*S. aureus*, *S. epidermidis*
Surgical wound	*S. aureus*, gram-negative rods
Diabetic ulcer	*S. aureus*, gram-negative aerobic rods, anaerobes
Furuncle	*S. aureus*
Intra-abdominal	Anaerobes (*B. fragilis)*, *E. coli*, enterococci
Cardiac	
Endocarditis	
subacute	*S. viridans*
acute	
I.V. drug user	*S. aureus*, gram-negative aerobic rods, *S. faecalis*, fungi
prosthetic valve	*S. epidermidis*
Gastric	
Gastroenteritis	*Salmonella*, *Shigella*, *H. pylori*, *C. difficile*, ameba, *G. lamblia*, viral, *E. coli*
Bone/Joint	
Osteomyelitis/septic arthritis	*S. aureus*, gram-negative aerobic rods
Central Nervous System	
Meningitis	
<2 mo	*E. coli*, group B streptococci, *Listeria*
2 mo to 12 y	*H. influenzae*, *S. pneumoniae*, *N. meningitidis*
adult and nosocomial	*S. pneumoniae*, *N. meningitidis*, gram-negative aerobic rods
postneurosurgery	*S. aureus*, gram-negative rods

TREATMENT OF SEXUALLY TRANSMITTED DISEASES

Type or Stage	Drug of Choice	Dosage	Alternatives
CHLAMYDIA TRACHOMATIS			
Urethritis, cervicitis, conjunctivitis, or proctitis (except lymphogranuloma venereum)			
	Azithromycin **or**	1 g oral once	Ofloxacin[2] 300 mg oral bid x 7 d; erythromycin 500 mg oral qid x 7 d
	Doxycycline[1,2]	100 mg oral bid x 7 d	
Infection in pregnancy			
	Erythromycin[3]	500 mg oral qid x 7 d[4]	Amoxicillin 500 mg oral tid x 10 d; azithromycin[5] 1 g oral once
Neonatal			
Ophthalmia	Erythromycin	12.5 mg/kg oral or I.V. qid x 14 d	
Pneumonia	Erythromycin	12.5 mg/kg oral or I.V. qid x 14 d	Sulfisoxazole[6] 100 mg/kg/d oral or I.V. in divided doses x 14 d
Lymphogranuloma venereum			
	Doxycycline[1,2]	100 mg oral bid x 21 d	Erythromycin[3] 500 mg oral qid x 21 d
GONORRHEA[7]			
Urethral, cervical, rectal, or pharyngeal			
	Cefpodoxime 200 mg as a single dose; ceftriaxone	125 mg I.M. once	Cefixime 400 mg oral once; ciprofloxacin[2] 500 mg oral once; ofloxacin[2] 400 mg oral once; spectinomycin 2 g I.M. once[8]
Ophthalmia (adults)[9]			
	Ceftriaxone	1 g I.M. once **plus** saline irrigation	
Bacteremia, arthritis, and disseminated[10,11]			
	Ceftriaxone	1 g I.V. daily x 7-10 days, or for 2-3 d, followed by cefixime 400 mg oral bid or ciprofloxacin 500 mg oral bid to complete 7-10 d total therapy	Ceftizoxime or cefotaxime, 1 g I.V. q8h for 2-3 days or until improved, followed by cefixime 400 mg oral bid or ciprofloxacin 500 mg oral bid to complete 7-10 d total therapy
Neonatal			
Ophthalmia	Cefotaxime **or**	25 mg/kg I.V. or I.M. q8-12h x 7 d, **plus** saline irrigation	Penicillin G[12] 100,000 units/kg/d I.V. in 4 doses x 7 d, **plus** saline irrigation
	Ceftriaxone	125 mg I.M. once, **plus** saline irrigation	
Bacteremia, arthritis, and disseminated	Cefotaxime	25-50 mg/kg I.V. q8-12h x 7-14 d	Penicillin G[12] 75,000-100,000 units/kg/d I.V. in 4 doses x 7-14 d
Children (<45 kg)			
Urogenital, rectal, and pharyngeal	Ceftriaxone	125 mg I.M. once	Spectinomycin[13] 40 mg/kg I.M. once; amoxicillin[12] 50 mg/kg oral once **plus** probenecid 25 mg/kg (max: 1 g) oral once
Bacteremia, arthritis, and disseminated	Ceftriaxone **or**	50-100 mg/kg/d (max: 2 g) I.V. x 7-14 d	Penicillin G[12] 150,000-250,000 units/kg/d I.V. x 7-14 d
	Cefotaxime	50-200 mg/kg/d I.V. in 2-4 doses x 7-14 d	

(continued)

Type or Stage	Drug of Choice	Dosage	Alternatives
SEXUALLY ACQUIRED EPIDIDYMITIS			
	Ofloxacin	300 mg bid x 10 d	Ceftriaxone 250 mg I.M. once **followed by** doxycycline[1] 100 mg oral bid x 10 d
PELVIC INFLAMMATORY DISEASE			
hospitalized patients	Cefoxitin **or**	2 g I.V. q6h**plus** gentamicin 2 mg/kg I.V. once **followed by** gentamicin 1.5 mg/kg I.V. q8h until improved **followed by** doxycycline[2] 100 mg oral bid to complete 14 days[14]	Clindamycin 900 mg I.V. q8h
	Cefotetan **either one plus**	2 g I.V. q12h	
	Doxycycline[2] **followed by**	100 mg I.V. q12h, until improved	
	Doxycycline[2]	100 mg oral bid to complete 14 days	
outpatients	Cefoxitin **plus**	2 g I.M. once[2] 400 mg oral bid x 14 d **plus** metronidazole 500 mg oral bid x 14 d **or** clindamycin 450 oral qid x 14 d	Ofloxacin
	Probenecid **or**	1 g oral once	
	Ceftriaxone **either one followed by**	250 mg I.M. once	
	Doxycycline[2]	100 mg oral bid x 14 d	
VAGINAL INFECTION			
Trichomoniasis			
	Metronidazole[15]	2 g oral once	Metronidazole 375 mg or 500 mg oral bid x 7 d
Bacterial vaginosis			
	Metronidazole gel 0.75%	5 g intravaginally bid x 5 d	Metronidazole 500 mg oral bid x 7 d
Vulvovaginal candidiasis			
	Topical butoconazole, clotrimazole, miconazole, terconazole, or tioconazole[17]		Metronidazole 2 g oral once[16]; fluconazole 150 mg oral once
SYPHILIS			
Early (primary, secondary, or latent <1 y)			
	Penicillin G benzathine	2.4 million units I.M. once[18]	Doxycycline[2] 100 mg oral bid x 14 d
Late (more than 1 year's duration, cardiovascular, gumma, late-latent)			
	Penicillin G benzathine	2.4 million units I.M. weekly x 3 wk	Doxycycline[2] 100 mg oral bid x 4 wk
Neurosyphilis[19]			
	Penicillin G	2-4 million units I.V. q4h x 10-14 d	Penicillin G procaine 2.4 million units I.M. daily **plus** probenecid 500 mg qid oral, both x 10-14 d
Congenital			
	Penicillin G **or**	50,000 units/kg I.M. or I.V. q8-12h for 10-14 d	
	Penicillin G procaine	50,000 units/kg I.M. daily for 10-14 d	
CHANCROID[20]			
	Erythromycin[3] **or**	500 mg oral qid x 7 d	Ciprofloxacin[2] 500 mg oral bid x 3 d
	Ceftriaxone **or**	250 mg I.M. once	

(continued)

Type or Stage	Drug of Choice	Dosage	Alternatives
	Azithromycin	1 g oral once	
HERPES SIMPLEX			
First episode genital			
	Acyclovir	400 mg oral tid x 7-10 d	Acyclovir 200 mg oral 5 times/d x 7-10 d
First episode proctitis			
	Acyclovir	800 mg oral tid x 7-10 d	Acyclovir 400 mg oral 5 times/d x 7-10 d
Recurrent			
	Acyclovir[21]	400 mg oral tid x 5 d	
Severe (hospitalized patients)			
	Acyclovir	5 mg/kg I.V. q8h x 5-7 d	
Prevention of recurrence[22]			
	Acyclovir	400 mg oral bid	Acyclovir 200 mg oral 2-5 times/d

[1]Or tetracycline 500 mg oral qid or minocycline 100 mg oral bid.

[2]Contraindicated in pregnancy.

[3]Erythromycin estolate is contraindicated in pregnancy.

[4]In the presence of severe gastrointestinal intolerance, decrease to 250 mg qid and extend duration to 14 days.

[5]Safety in pregnancy not established.

[6]Only for infants older than 4 weeks.

[7]All patients should also receive a course of treatment effective for *Chlamydia*.

[8]Recommended only for use during pregnancy in patients allergic to beta-lactams. Not effective for pharyngeal infection.

[9]An oral fluoroquinolone, such as ciprofloxacin for 3-5 days, probably would also be effective, but experience is limited.

[10]If the infecting strain of *N. gonorrhoeae* has been tested and is known to be susceptible to penicillin or the tetracyclines, treatment may be changed to penicillin G 10 million units I.V. daily, amoxicillin 500 mg orally qid, doxycycline 100 mg orally bid, or tetracycline 500 mg orally qid.

[11]Endocarditis requires at least 3-4 weeks of parenteral therapy.

[12]If infecting strain of *N. gonorrhoeae* has been tested and is known to be susceptible.

[13]Not effective for pharyngeal infection.

[14]Or clindamycin 450 mg oral qid to complete 14 days.

[15]Metronidazole should be avoided during the first trimester of pregnancy; 2 g oral (single dose) may be given after the first trimester.

[16]Higher relapse rate, but useful for patients who may not comply with multiple-dose therapy.

[17]For preparations and dosage, see *The Medical Letter*, 36:81, 1994; avoid single-dose therapy.

[18]Some experts recommend repeating this regimen after 7 days, especially in patients with HIV infection.

[19]Patients allergic to penicillin should be desensitized.

[20]All regimens, especially single-dose ceftriaxone, are less effective in HIV-infected patients.

[21]Not highly effective for treatment of recurrences, but may help some patients if started early.

[22]Preventive treatment should be discontinued for 1-2 months once a year to reassess the frequency of recurrence.

REFERENCE VALUES FOR ADULTS

Automated Chemistry (CHEMISTRY A)

Test	Values	Remarks
SERUM PLASMA		
Acetone	Negative	
Albumin	3.2-5 g/dL	
Alcohol, ethyl	Negative	
Aldolase	1.2-7.6 IU/L	
Ammonia	20-70 mcg/dL	Specimen to be placed on ice as soon as collected
Amylase	30-110 units/L	
Bilirubin, direct	0-0.3 mg/dL	
Bilirubin, total	0.1-1.2 mg/dL	
Calcium	8.6-10.3 mg/dL	
Calcium, ionized	2.24-2.46 mEq/L	
Chloride	95-108 mEq/L	
Cholesterol, total	≤220 mg/dL	Fasted blood required – normal value affected by dietary habits This reference range is for a general adult population
HDL cholesterol	40-60 mg/dL	Fasted blood required – normal value affected by dietary habits
LDL cholesterol	65-170 mg/dL	LDLC calculated by Friewald formula... which has certain inaccuracies and is invalid at trig levels >300 mg/dL
CO_2	23-30 mEq/L	
Creatine kinase (CK) isoenzymes		
CK-BB	0%	
CK-MB (cardiac)	0%-3.9%	
CK-MM (muscle)	96%-100%	
CK-MB levels must be both ≥4% and 10 IU/L to meet diagnostic criteria for CK-MB positive result consistent with myocardial injury.		
Creatine phosphokinase (CPK)	8-150 IU/L	
Creatinine	0.5-1.4 mg/dL	
Ferritin	13-300 ng/mL	
Folate	3.6-20 ng/dL	
GGT (gamma-glutamyltranspeptidase)		
male	11-63 IU/L	
female	8-35 IU/L	
GLDH	To be determined	
Glucose (2-h postprandial)	Up to 140 mg/dL	
Glucose, fasting	60-110 mg/dL	
Glucose, nonfasting (2-h postprandial)	60-140 mg/dL	
Hemoglobin A_{1c}	8	
Hemoglobin, plasma free	<2.5 mg/100 mL	
Hemoglobin, total glycosolated (Hb A_1)	4%-8%	
Iron	65-150 mcg/dL	
Iron binding capacity, total (TIBC)	250-420 mcg/dL	
Lactic acid	0.7-2.1 mEq/L	Specimen to be kept on ice and sent to lab as soon as possible
Lactate dehydrogenase (LDH)	56-194 IU/L	
Lactate dehydrogenase (LDH) isoenzymes		
LD_1	20%-34%	
LD_2	29%-41%	
LD_3	15%-25%	
LD_4	1%-12%	
LD_5	1%-15%	
Flipped LD_1/LD_2 ratios (>1 may be consistent with myocardial injury) particularly when considered in combination with a recent CK-MB positive result		
Lipase	23-208 units/L	

(continued)

Test	Values	Remarks
Magnesium	1.6-2.5 mg/dL	Increased by slight hemolysis
Osmolality	289-308 mOsm/kg	
Phosphatase, alkaline		
adults 25-60 y	33-131 IU/L	
adults 61 y or older	51-153 IU/L	
infancy-adolescence	Values range up to 3-5 times higher than adults	
Phosphate, inorganic	2.8-4.2 mg/dL	
Potassium	3.5-5.2 mEq/L	Increased by slight hemolysis
Prealbumin	>15 mg/dL	
Protein, total	6.5-7.9 g/dL	
SGOT (AST)	<35 IU/L (20-48)	
SGPT (ALT) (10-35)	<35 IU/L	
Sodium	134-149 mEq/L	
Transferrin	>200 mg/dL	
Triglycerides	45-155 mg/dL	Fasted blood required
Urea nitrogen (BUN)	7-20 mg/dL	
Uric acid		
male	2.0-8.0 mg/dL	
female	2.0-7.5 mg/dL	
CEREBROSPINAL FLUID		
Glucose	50-70 mg/dL	
Protein		
adults and children	15-45 mg/dL	CSF obtained by lumbar puncture
newborn infants	60-90 mg/dL	

On CSF obtained by cisternal puncture: About 25 mg/dL

On CSF obtained by ventricular puncture: About 10 mg/dL

Note: Bloody specimen gives erroneously high value due to contamination with blood proteins

URINE

(24-hour specimen is required for all these tests unless specified)

Test	Values	Remarks
Amylase	32-641 units/L	The value is in units/L and **not** calculated for total volume
Amylase, fluid (random samples)		Interpretation of value left for physician, depends on the nature of fluid
Calcium	Depends upon dietary intake	
Creatine		
male	150 mg/24 h	Higher value on children and during pregnancy
female	250 mg/24 h	
Creatinine	1000-2000 mg/24 h	
Creatinine clearance (endogenous)		
male	85-125 mL/min	A blood sample must accompany urine specimen
female	75-115 mL/min	
Glucose	1 g/24 h	
5-hydroxyindoleacetic acid	2-8 mg/24 h	
Iron	0.15 mg/24 h	Acid washed container required
Magnesium	146-209 mg/24 h	
Osmolality	500-800 mOsm/kg	With normal fluid intake
Oxalate	10-40 mg/24 h	
Phosphate	400-1300 mg/24 h	
Potassium	25-120 mEq/24 h	Varies with diet; the interpretation of urine electrolytes and osmolality should be left for the physician
Sodium	40-220 mEq/24 h	
Porphobilinogen, qualitative	Negative	

(continued)

Test	Values	Remarks
Porphyrins, qualitative	Negative	
Proteins	0.05-0.1 g/24 h	
Salicylate	Negative	
Urea clearance	60-95 mL/min	A blood sample must accompany specimen
Urea N	10-40 g/24 h	Dependent on protein intake
Uric acid	250-750 mg/24 h	Dependent on diet and therapy
Urobilinogen	0.5-3.5 mg/24 h	For qualitative determination on random urine, send sample to urinalysis section in Hematology Lab
Xylose absorption test		
children	16%-33% of ingested xylose	
adults	>4 g in 5 h	
FECES		
Fat, 3-day collection	<5 g/d	Value depends on fat intake of 100 g/d for 3 days preceding and during collection
GASTRIC ACIDITY		
Acidity, total, 12 h	10-60 mEq/L	Titrated at pH 7

BLOOD GASES

	Arterial	Capillary	Venous
pH	7.35-7.45	7.35-7.45	7.32-7.42
pCO_2 (mm Hg)	35-45	35-45	38-52
pO_2 (mm Hg)	70-100	60-80	24-48
HCO_3 (mEq/L)	19-25	19-25	19-25
TCO_2 (mEq/L)	19-29	19-29	23-33
O_2 saturation (%)	90-95	90-95	40-70
Base excess (mEq/L)	-5 to +5	-5 to +5	-5 to +5

Complete Blood Count

	Hgb (g/dL)	Hct (%)	MCV (fL)	MCH (pg)	MCHC (%)	RBC (x 10^6/mm^3)	RDW	Plts (x 10^3/mm^3)
0-3 d	15-20	45-61	95-115	31-37	29-37	4-5.9	<18	250-450
1-2 wk	12.5-18.5	39-57	86-110	28-36	28-38	3.6-5.5	<17	250-450
1-6 mo	10-13	29-42	74-96	25-35	30-36	3.1-4.3	<16.5	300-700
7 mo - 2 y	10.5-13	33-38	70-84	23-30	31-37	3.7-4.9	<16	250-600
2-5 y	11.5-13	34-39	75-87	24-30	31-37	3.9-5	<15	250-550
5-8 y	11.5-14.5	35-42	77-95	25-33	31-37	4-4.9	<15	250-550
13-18 y	12-15.2	36-47	78-96	25-35	31-37	4.5-5.1	<14.5	150-450
Adult male	13.5-16.5	41-50	80-100	26-34	31-37	4.5-5.5	<14.5	150-450
Adult female	12-15	36-44	80-100	26-34	31-37	4-4.9	<14.5	150-450

WBC and Diff

	WBC (x 10^3/mm^3)	Segmented Neutrophils	Band Neutrophils	Eosinophils	Basophils	Lymphocytes	Atypical Lymphs	Monocytes	# of NRBCs
0-3 d	9-35	32-62	10-18	0-2	0-1	19-29	0-8	5-7	0-2
1-2 wk	5-20	14-34	6-14	0-2	0-1	36-45	0-8	6-10	0
1-6 mo	6-17.5	13-33	4-12	0-3	0-1	41-71	0-8	4-7	0
7 mo - 2 y	6-17	15-35	5-11	0-3	0-1	45-76	0-8	3-6	0
2-5 y	5.5-15.5	23-45	5-11	0-3	0-1	45-76	0-8	3-6	0
5-8 y	5-14.5	32-54	5-11	0-3	0-1	28-48	0-8	3-6	0
13-18 y	4.5-13	34-64	5-11	0-3	0-1	25-45	0-8	3-6	0
Adults	4.5-11	35-66	5-11	0-3	0-1	24-44	0-8	3-6	0

Sedimentation Rate, Westergren
- Children: 0-20 mm/hour
- Adult male: 0-15 mm/hour
- Adult female: 0-20 mm/hour

Sedimentation Rate, Wintrobe
- Children: 0-13 mm/hour
- Adult male: 0-10 mm/hour
- Adult female: 0-15 mm/hour

Reticulocyte Count
- Newborns: 2%-6%
- 1-6 mo: 0%-2.8%
- Adults: 0.5%-1.5%

REFERENCE VALUES FOR CHILDREN

Chemistry

Test	Age	Value
Albumin	0-1 y	2-4 g/dL
	1 y to adult	3.5-5.5 g/dL
Ammonia	Newborns	90-150 µg/dL
	Children	40-120 µg/dL
	Adults	18-54 µg/dL
Amylase	Newborns	0-60 units/L
	Adults	30-110 units/L
Bilirubin, conjugated, direct	Newborns	<1.5 mg/dL
	1 mo to adult	0-0.5 mg/dL
Bilirubin, total	0-3 d	2-10 mg/dL
	1 mo to adult	0-1.5 mg/dL
Bilirubin, unconjugated, indirect		0.6-10.5 mg/dL
Calcium	Newborns	7-12 mg/dL
	0-2 y	8.8-11.2 mg/dL
	2 y to adult	9-11 mg/dL
Calcium, ionized, whole blood		4.4-5.4 mg/dL
Carbon dioxide, total		23-33 mEq/L
Chloride		95-105 mEq/L
Cholesterol	Newborns	45-170 mg/dL
	0-1 y	65-175 mg/dL
	1-20 y	120-230 mg/dL
Creatinine	0-1 y	≤0.6 mg/dL
	1 y to adult	0.5-1.5 mg/dL
Glucose	Newborns	30-90 mg/dL
	0-2 y	60-105 mg/dL
	Children to adults	70-110 mg/dL
Iron	Newborns	110-270 µg/dL
	Infants	30-70 µg/dL
	Children	55-120 µg/dL
	Adults	70-180 µg/dL
Iron binding	Newborns	59-175 µg/dL
	Infants	100-400 µg/dL
	Adults	250-400 µg/dL
Lactic acid, lactate		2-20 mg/dL
Lead, whole blood		<30 µg/dL
Lipase	Children	20-140 units/L
	Adults	0-190 units/L
Magnesium		1.5-2.5 mEq/L
Osmolality, serum		275-296 mOsm/kg
Osmolality, urine		50-1400 mOsm/kg
Phosphorus	Newborns	4.2-9 mg/dL
	6 wk to ≤18 mo	3.8-6.7 mg/dL
	18 mo to 3 y	2.9-5.9 mg/dL
	3-15 y	3.6-5.6 mg/dL
	>15 y	2.5-5 mg/dL
Potassium, plasma	Newborns	4.5-7.2 mEq/L
	2 d to 3 mo	4-6.2 mEq/L
	3 mo to 1 y	3.7-5.6 mEq/L
	1-16 y	3.5-5 mEq/L
Protein, total	0-2 y	4.2-7.4 g/dL
	>2 y	6-8 g/dL
Sodium		136-145 mEq/L
Triglycerides	Infants	0-171 mg/dL
	Children	20-130 mg/dL
	Adults	30-200 mg/dL
Urea nitrogen, blood	0-2 y	4-15 mg/dL
	2 y to adult	5-20 mg/dL

(continued)

Uric acid	Male	3-7 mg/dL
	Female	2-6 mg/dL

ENZYMES

Alanine aminotransferase (ALT)	0-2 mo	8-78 units/L
(SGPT)	>2 mo	8-36 units/L
Alkaline phosphatase (ALKP)	Newborns	60-130 units/L
	0-16 y	85-400 units/L
	>16 y	30-115 units/L
Aspartate aminotransferase (AST)	Infants	18-74 units/L
(SGOT)	Children	15-46 units/L
	Adults	5-35 units/L
Creatine kinase (CK)	Infants	20-200 units/L
	Children	10-90 units/L
	Adult male	0-206 units/L
	Adult female	0-175 units/L
Lactate dehydrogenase (LDH)	Newborns	290-501 units/L
	1 mo to 2 y	110-144 units/L
	>16 y	60-170 units/L

BLOOD GASES

	Arterial	Capillary	Venous
pH	7.35-7.45	7.35-7.45	7.32-7.42
pCO_2 (mm Hg)	35-45	35-45	38-52
pO_2 (mm Hg)	70-100	60-80	24-48
HCO_3 (mEq/L)	19-25	19-25	19-25
TCO_2 (mEq/L)	19-29	19-29	23-33
O_2 saturation (%)	90-95	90-95	40-70
Base excess (mEq/L)	-5 to +5	-5 to +5	-5 to +5

THYROID FUNCTION TESTS

T_4 (thyroxine)	1-7 d	10.1-20.9 μg/dL
	8-14 d	9.8-16.6 μg/dL
	1 mo to 1 y	5.5-16 μg/dL
	>1 y	4-12 μg/dL
FTI	1-3 d	9.3-26.6
	1-4 wks	7.6-20.8
	1-4 mo	7.4-17.9
	4-12 mo	5.1-14.5
	1-6 y	5.7-13.3
	>6 y	4.8-14
T_3 by RIA	Newborns	100-470 ng/dL
	1-5 y	100-260 ng/dL
	5-10 y	90-240 ng/dL
	10 y to adult	70-210 ng/dL
T_3 uptake		35%-45%
TSH	Cord	3-22 μU/mL
	1-3 d	<40 μU/mL
	3-7 d	<25 μU/mL
	>7 d	0-10 μU/mL

CALCULATIONS FOR TOTAL PARENTERAL NUTRITION THERAPY — ADULT PATIENTS

Condition	Calorie Requirement (kcal/kg/d)	Protein Requirement (g/kg/d)
Resting state (adult medical patient)	20-30	0.8-1
Uncomplicated postop patients	·25-35	1-1.3
Depleted patients	30-40	1.3-1.7
Hypermetabolic patients (trauma, sepsis, burns)	35-45	1-5.2

1 g protein yields 4 kcal/g
1 g fat yields 9 kcal/g
1 g dextrose yields 3.4 kcal/g
1 g nitrogen = 6.25 g protein

Electrolytes Required/Day

	mEq/d
Sodium	60-120
Potassium	60-120
Chloride	100-150
Magnesium	10-24
Calcium	10-20
Phosphate	20-50 mmol/d
Sulfate	10-24
Acetate	60-150
Bicarbonate	Should not be added

Estimated Energy Requirements

Basal Energy Expenditure (BEE)	
Harris Benedict equation	
males	$BEE_{mal} = 66.67 + (13.75 \times kg) + (5 \times cm) - (6.76 \times y)$
females	$BEE_{fem} = 665.1 + (9.56 \times kg) + (1.85 \times cm) - (4.68 \times y)$
Total daily energy expenditure (TDE)	**TDE = (BEE) [(activity factor) + (injured factor)]**
Activity factor	Confined to bed = 1.2 Out of bed = 1.3
Injury factor	Surgery: Minor operations = 1-1.1 Major operations = 1.1-1.2
	Infection: Mild = 1-1.2 Moderate = 1.2-1.4 Severe = 1.4-1.6
	Skeletal trauma = 1.2-1.35
	Head injury (treated with corticosteroids) = 1.6
	Blunt trauma = 1.15-1.35
	Burns ≤20% body surface area (BSA) = 2 20%-30% BSA = 2-2.2 >30% BSA = 2.2

Estimated Fluid Requirements

30-35 mL/kg/d
or
mL/d = 1500 mL for first 20 kg of body weight + 20 mL/kg for body weight >20 kg

MEDIAN HEIGHTS AND WEIGHTS AND RECOMMENDED ENERGY INTAKE*

Age (y) or Condition	Weight (kg)	Weight (lb)	Height (cm)	Height (in)	REE† (kcal/d)	Average Energy Allowance (kcal)‡ Multiples of REE	/kg	/d§
Infants								
0-0.5	6	13	60	24	320		108	650
0.5-1	9	20	71	28	500		98	850
Children								
1-3	13	29	90	35	740		102	1300
4-6	20	44	112	44	950		90	1800
7-10	28	62	132	52	1130		70	2000
Male								
11-14	45	99	157	62	1440	1.70	55	2500
15-18	66	145	176	69	1760	1.67	45	3000
19-24	72	160	177	70	1780	1.67	40	2900
25-50	79	174	176	70	1800	1.60	37	2900
51+	77	170	173	68	1530	1.50	30	2300
Female								
11-14	46	101	157	62	1310	1.67	47	2200
15-18	55	120	163	64	1370	1.60	40	2200
19-24	58	128	164	65	1350	1.60	38	2200
25-50	63	138	163	64	1380	1.55	36	2200
51+	65	143	160	63	1280	1.50	30	1900
Pregnant								+0
1st trimester								+300
2nd trimester								+300
3rd trimester								+300
Lactating								
1st 6 months								+500
2nd 6 months								+500

*From *Recommended Dietary Allowances*, 10th ed, Washington, DC: National Academy Press, 1989.
†Calculation based on FAO equations, then rounded.
‡In the range of light to moderate activity, the coefficient of variation is ±20%.
§Figure is rounded.

DESENSITIZATION PROTOCOLS

PENICILLIN DESENSITIZATION PROTOCOL: MUST BE DONE BY PHYSICIAN!

Acute penicillin desensitization should only be performed in an intensive care setting. Any remedial risk factor should be corrected. All β-adrenergic antagonists such as propranolol or even timolol ophthalmic drops should be discontinued. Asthmatic patients should be under optimal control. An intravenous line should be established, baseline electrocardiogram (EKG) and spirometry should be performed, and continuous EKG monitoring should be instituted. Premedication with antihistamines or steroids is not recommended, as these drugs have not proven effective in suppressing severe reactions but may mask early signs of reactivity that would otherwise result in a modification of the protocol.

Protocols have been developed for penicillin desensitization using both the oral and parenteral route. As of 1987 there were 93 reported cases of oral desensitization, 74 of which were done by Sullivan and his collaborators. Of these 74 patients, 32% experienced a transient allergic reaction either during desensitization (one-third) or during penicillin treatment after desensitization (two-thirds). These reactions were usually mild and self-limited in nature. Only one IgE-mediated reaction (wheezing and bronchospasm) required discontinuation of the procedure before desensitization could be completed. It has been argued that oral desensitization may be safer than parenteral desensitization, but most patients can also be safely desensitized by parenteral route.

During desensitization any dose that causes mild systemic reactions such as pruritus, fleeting urticaria, rhinitis, or mild wheezing should be repeated until the patient tolerates the dose without systemic symptoms or signs. More serious reactions such as hypotension, laryngeal edema, or asthma require appropriate treatment, and if desensitization is continued, the dose should be decreased by at least 10-fold and withheld until the patient is stable.

Once desensitized, the patient's treatment with penicillin must not lapse or the risk of an allergic reaction increases. If the patient requires a β-lactam antibiotic in the future and still remains skin test-positive to penicillin reagents, desensitization would be required again.

Several patients have been maintained on long-term, low-dose penicillin therapy (usually bid-tid) to sustain a chronic state of desensitization. Such individuals usually require chronic desensitization because of continuous occupationally related exposure to β-lactam drugs.

Order for placement/availability at the bedside in the event of a hypersensitivity reaction during scratch/skin testing and desensitization:

Hydrocortisone: 100 mg IVP
Diphenhydramine: 50 mg IVP
Epinephrine: 1:1000 S.C.

Several investigators have demonstrated that penicillin can be administered to history positive, skin test positive patients if initially small but gradually increasing doses are given. However, patients with a history of exfoliative dermatitis secondary to penicillin should not be re-exposed to the drug, even by desensitization.

Desensitization is a potentially dangerous procedure and should be only performed in an area where immediate access to emergency drugs and equipment can be assured.

Begin between 8-10 AM in the morning.

Follow desensitization as indicated for penicillin G or ampicillin.

AMPICILLIN
Oral Desensitization Protocol

1. Begin 0.03 mg of ampicillin
2. Double the dose administered every 30 minutes until complete
3. Example of oral dosing regimen:

Dose #	Ampicillin (mg)
1	0.03
2	0.06
3	0.12
4	0.23

(continued)

Dose #	Ampicillin (mg)
5	0.47
6	0.94
7	1.87
8	3.75
9	7.5
10	15
11	30
12	60
13	125
14	250
15	500

PENICILLIN G PARENTERAL
Desensitization Protocol: Typical Schedule

Injection No.	Benzylpenicillin Concentration (units/mL)	Volume and Route (mL)*
1†	100	0.1 I.D.
2	↓	0.2 S.C.
3		0.4 S.C.
4		0.8 S.C.
5†	1,000	0.1 I.D.
6	↓	0.3 S.C.
7		0.6 S.C.
8†	10,000	0.1 I.D.
9	↓	0.2 S.C.
10		0.4 S.C.
11		0.8 S.C.
12†	100,000	0.1 I.D.
13	↓	0.3 S.C.
14		0.6 S.C.
15†	1,000,000	0.1 I.D.
16	↓	0.2 S.C.
17		0.2 I.M.
18		0.4 I.M.
19	Continuous I.V. infusion (1,000,000 units/h)	

*Administer progressive doses at intervals of not less than 20 minutes.

†Observe and record skin wheal and flare response to intradermal dose.

Abbreviations: I.D. = intradermal, S.C. = subcutaneous, I.M. = intramuscular, I.V. = intravenous.

PENICILLIN
Oral Desensitization Protocol

Step*	Phenoxymethyl Penicillin (units/mL)	Amount (mL)	Dose (units)	Cumulative Dosage (units)
1	1000	0.1	100	100
2	1000	0.2	200	300
3	1000	0.4	400	700
4	1000	0.8	800	1500
5	1000	1.6	1600	3100
6	1000	3.2	3200	6300
7	1000	6.4	6400	12,700
8	10,000	1.2	12,000	24,700
9	10,000	2.4	24,000	48,700
10	10,000	4.8	48,000	96,700
11	80,000	1	80,000	176,700
12	80,000	2	160,000	336,700
13	80,000	4	320,000	656,700
14	80,000	8	640,000	1,296,700

Observe patient for 30 minutes

(continued)

Step*	Phenoxymethyl Penicillin (units/mL)	Amount (mL)	Dose (units)	Cumulative Dosage (units)
Change to benzylpenicillin G I.V.				
15	500,000	0.25	125,000	
16	500,000	0.50	250,000	
17	500,000	1	500,000	
18	500,000	2.25	1,125,000	

*Interval between steps, 15 min

ALLOPURINOL
Successful Desensitization for Treatment of a Fixed Drug Eruption

	Oral Dose of Allopurinol
Days 1-3	50 mcg/day
Days 4-6	100 mcg/day
Days 7-9	200 mcg/day
Days 10-12	500 mcg/day
Days 13-15	1 mg/day
Days 16-18	5 mg/day
Days 19-21	10 mg/day
Days 22-24	25 mg/day
Days 25-27	50 mg/day
Day 28	100 mg/day

Prednisone 10 mg/day through desensitization and 1 month after reaching dose of 100 mg allopurinol

Modified from *J Allergy Clin Immunol*, 1996, 97:1171-2.

AMPHOTERICIN B

Challenge and Desensitization Protocol

1. Procedure supervised by physician
2. Epinephrine, 1:1000 wt/vol, multidose vial at bedside
3. Premixed albuterol solution at bedside for nebulization
4. Endotracheal intubation supplies at bedside with anesthesiologist on standby
5. Continuous cardiac telemetry with electronic monitoring of blood pressure
6. Continuous pulse oximetry
7. Premedication with methylprednisolone, 60 mg, I.V. and diphenhydramine, 25 mg I.V.
8. Amphotericin B (Fungizone®)* administration schedule
   a. 10^{-6} dilution, infused over 10 minutes
   b. 10^{-5} dilution, infused over 10 minutes
   c. 10^{-4} dilution, infused over 10 minutes
   d. 10^{-3} dilution, infused over 10 minutes
   e. 10^{-2} dilution, infused over 10 minutes
   f. 10^{-1} dilution (1 mg), infused over 30 minutes
   g. 30 mg in 250 mL 5% dextrose, infused over 4 hours

From Kemp SF and Lockey RF, "Amphotericin B: Emergency Challenge in a Neutropenic, Asthmatic Patient With Fungal Sepsis," *J Allergy Clin Immunol*, 1995, 96(3):425-7.

*Mixtures were prepared in 10 mL 5% dextrose by hospital intensive care unit pharmacy, unless otherwise noted.

CIPROFLOXACIN DESENSITIZATION

Modified from *J Allergy Clin Immunol*, 1996, 97:1426-7.

Premedicated with diphenhydramine hydrochloride, ranitidine, and prednisone 1 hour before the desensitization.

The individual doses were administered at 15-minute intervals. Because the patient was intubated in the intensive care unit, vital signs were continually monitored. The patient's skin was inspected for development of urticaria, and his chest was auscultated for wheezing every 10 minutes. No rash, hypotension, or wheezing developed during desensitization. The procedure took 4 hours, and once finished, the patient had received an equivalent to his first scheduled dose (400 mg twice daily). The second dose was given 4 hours later, followed by routine administration of 400 mg every 12 hours, with a small dose (25 mg intravenously) between therapeutic doses to maintain a drug level in the blood. The patient subsequently received 4 weeks of ciprofloxacin treatment without difficulty.

Desensitization Regimen for Ciprofloxacin

Ciprofloxacin Concentration (mg/mL)	Volume Given (mL)	Absolute Amount (mg)	Cumulative Total Dose (mg)
0.1	0.1	0.01	0.01
0.1	0.2	0.02	0.03
0.1	0.4	0.04	0.07
0.1	0.8	0.08	0.15
1	0.16	0.16	0.31
1	0.32	0.32	0.63
1	0.64	0.64	1.27
2	0.6	1.2	2.47
2	1.2	2.4	4.87
2	2.4	4.8	9.67
2	5	10	19.67
2	10	20	39.67
2	20	40	79.67
2	40	80	159.67
2	120	240	399.67

Drug volumes <1 mL were mixed with normal saline solution to a final volume of 3 mL and then slowly infused; the other doses were administered over 10 minutes, except the last dose (240 mg in 120 mL), which was given with an infusion pump over 20 minutes.

INSULIN DESENSITIZATION

Lilly's appropriate diluting fluid, sterile saline, or distilled water, to which 1 mL of the patient's blood or the addition of 1 mL of 1% serum albumin (making a 0.1% solution) for each 10 mL of stock diluent, is a satisfactory diluent. The albumin in the blood or serum albumin solution is necessary to retain the integrity of the higher dilutions by preventing adsorption to glass or plastic. Dilution is stable 30 days under refrigeration or room temperature, but should be used within 24 hours due to a lack of preservative.

1. Make a 1:1 dilution of single species (beef, pork, or human) insulin (50 units/mL).
2. Add 0.5 mL of the above dilution to 4.5 mL of diluent (5 units/mL).
3. Add 0.5 mL of the 5 units/mL dilution to 4.5 mL of diluent (0.5 unit/mL).
4. Add 0.5 mL of the 0.5 unit/mL dilution to 4.5 mL of diluent (0.05 unit/mL).
5. Add 0.5 mL of the 0.05 unit/mL dilution to 4.5 mL of diluent (0.005 unit/mL).

The 5 vials containing 50, 5, 0.5, 0.05, and 0.005 units/mL are ready for skin testing or desensitization procedures.

One may start desensitization by giving 0.02 mL of 0.05 unit/mL concentration (1/1000 unit) intradermally. If no reaction occurs, administer 0.04 and 0.08 mL of the same concentration at 30-minute intervals.

The procedure continues proceeding to the next greater concentration (0.5 unit/mL) and giving 0.02, 0.04, and 0.08 mL at 30-minute intervals.

In the same manner proceed through the 5 units/mL and 50 units/mL concentrations with the exception that these injections should be given subcutaneously.

Note: If a reaction is noted, back up 2 steps and try to proceed forward again.

If the patient reacts to the initial injection, it will be necessary to utilize the lower concentration (0.005 units/mL) to initiate the procedure.

It is essential that manifestations of allergic reactions not be obscured. Therefore, antihistamines or steroids should not be used during desensitization except to treat severe allergic reactions. The use of these agents may obscure mild to moderate reactions to the lower doses and result in more severe reactions as doses increase, leading to failure of the desensitization program.

RIFAMPIN and ETHAMBUTOL
Oral Desensitization in Mycobacterial Disease

Time from Start (h:min)	Rifampin (mg)	Ethambutol (mg)
0	0.1	0.1
00:45	0.5	0.5
01:30	1	1
02:15	2	2
03:00	4	4
03:45	8	8
04:30	16	16
05:15	32	32
06:00	50	50
06:45	100	100
07:30	150	200
11:00	300	400
Next day		
6:30 AM	300 twice daily	400 three times/day

From *Am J Respir Crit Care Med*, 1994, 149:815-7.

SKIN TESTS

Delayed Hypersensitivity (Anergy)

Delayed cutaneous hypersensitivity (DCH) is a cell-mediated immunological response which has been used diagnostically to assess previous infection (eg, purified protein derivative (PPD), histoplasmin, and coccidioidin) or as an indicator of the status of the immune system by using mumps, *Candida*, tetanus toxoid, or trichophyton to test for anergy. Anergy is a defect in cell-mediated immunity that is characterized by an impaired response, or lack of a response to DCH testing with injected antigens. Anergy has been associated with several disease states, malnutrition, and immunosuppressive therapy, and has been correlated with increased risk of infection, morbidity, and mortality.

Many of the skin test antigens have not been approved by the FDA as tests for anergy, and so the directions for use and interpretation of reactions to these products may differ from that of the product labeling. There is also disagreement in the published literature as to the selection and interpretation of these tests for anergy assessment, leading to different recommendations for use of these products.

General Guidelines

Read these guidelines before using any skin test.

Administration

1. Use a separate sterile TB syringe for each antigen. Immediately after the antigen is drawn up, make the injection intradermally in the flexor surface of the forearm.
2. A small bleb 6-10 mm in diameter will form if the injection is made at the correct depth. If a bleb does not form or if the antigen solution leaks from the site, the injection must be repeated.
3. When applying more than one skin test, make the injections at least 5 cm apart.
4. Do any serologic blood tests before testing or wait 48-96 hours.

Reading

1. Read all tests at 24, 48, and 72 hours. Reactions occurring before 24 hours are indicative of an immediate rather than a delayed hypersensitivity.
2. Measure the diameter of the induration in two directions (at right angles) with a ruler and record each diameter in millimeters. Ballpoint pen method of measurement is the most accurate.
3. Test results should be recorded by the nurse in the Physician's Progress Notes section of the chart, and should include the millimeters of induration present, and a picture of the arm showing the location of the test(s).

Factors Causing False-Negative Reactions

1. Improper administration, interpretation, or use of outdated antigen
2. Test is applied too soon after exposure to the antigen (DCH takes 2-20 weeks to develop.)
3. Concurrent viral illnesses (eg, rubeola, influenza, mumps, and probably others) or recent administration of live attenuated virus vaccines (eg, measles)
4. Anergy may be associated with:
   a. Immune suppressing chronic illnesses such as diabetes, uremia, sarcoidosis, metastatic carcinomas, Hodgkin's, acute lymphocytic leukemia, hypothyroidism, chronic hepatitis, and cirrhosis.
   b. Some antineoplastic agents, radiation therapy, and corticosteroids. If possible, discontinue steroids at least 48 hours prior to DCH skin testing.
   c. Congenital immune deficiencies.
   d. Malnutrition, shock, severe burns, and trauma.
   e. Severe disseminated infections (miliary or cavitary TB, cocci granuloma, and other disseminated mycotic infections, gram-negative bacillary septicemia).
   f. Leukocytosis (>15,000 cells/mm^3).

Factors Causing False-Positive Reactions

1. Improper interpretation
2. Patient sensitivity to minor ingredients in the antigen solutions such as the phenol or thimerosal preservatives
3. Cross-reactions between similar antigens

Candida **1:1000**
Dose = 0.1 mL intradermally (30% of children <18 months of age and 50% >18 months of age respond)
Can be used as a control antigen

Coccidioidin 1:1000
Dose = 0.1 mL intradermally (apply with PPD **and** a control antigen)

Mercury derivative used as a preservative for spherulin.

Histoplasmin 1:1000

Dose = 0.1 mL intradermally (yeast derived)

Multitest CMI (*candida*, diphtheria toxoid, tetanus toxoid, *Streptococcus*, old tuberculin, *Trichophyton*, *Proteus* antigen, and negative control)

Press loaded unit into the skin with sufficient pressure to puncture the skin and allow adequate penetration of all points.

Mumps 40 cfu per mL

Dose = 0.1 mL intradermally (contraindicated in patients allergic to eggs, egg products, or thimerosal)

Dosage as Part of Disease Diagnosis

Tuberculin Testing

Purified Protein Derivative (PPD)

Preparation	Dilution	Units/0.1 mL
First strength	1:10,000	1
Intermediate strength	1:2000	5
Second strength	1:100	250

The usual initial dose is 0.1 mL of the intermediate strength. The first strength should be used in the individuals suspected of being highly sensitive. The second strength is used only for individuals who fail to respond to a previous injection of the first or intermediate strengths.

A positive reaction is 10 mm induration or greater except in HIV-infected individuals where a positive reaction is 5 mm or greater of induration.

Adverse Reactions

In patients who are highly sensitive, or when higher than recommended doses are used, exaggerated local reactions may occur, including erythema, pain, blisters, necrosis, and scarring. Although systemic reactions are rare, a few cases of lymph node enlargement, fever, malaise, and fatigue have been reported.

To prevent severe local reactions, never use second test strengths as the initial agent. Use diluted first strengths in patients with known or suspected hypersensitivity to the antigen.

Have epinephrine and antihistamines on hand to treat severe allergic reactions that may occur.

Treatment of Adverse Reactions

Severe reactions to intradermal skin tests are rare and treatment consists of symptomatic care.

Skin Testing

All skin tests are given intradermally into the flexor surface of one arm.

Purified protein derivative (PPD) is used most often in the diagnosis of tuberculosis. *Candida, Trichophyton,* and mumps skin tests are used most often as controls for anergy.

Dose: The usual skin test dose is as follows:

Antigen		Standard Dose	Concentration
PPD	1 TU	0.1 mL	1 TU — highly sensitive patients
	5 TU	0.1 mL	5 TU — standard dose
	250 TU	0.1 mL	250 TU — anergic patients in whom TB is suspected
Candida		0.02 mL	
Histoplasmin		0.1 mL	Seldom used. Serology is preferred method to diagnose histoplasmosis.
Mumps		0.1 mL	
Trichophyton		0.02 mL	

Interpretation:

Skin Test	Reading Time	Positive Reaction
PPD	48-72 h	**≥5 mm considered positive for:** • close contacts to an infectious case • persons with abnormal chest x-ray indicating old healed TB • persons with known or suspected HIV infection **≥10 mm considered positive for:** • other medical risk factors • foreign born from high prevalence areas • medically underserved, low income populations • alcoholics and intravenous drug users • residents of long-term care facilities (including correctional facilities and nursing homes) • staff in settings where disease would pose a hazard to large number of susceptible persons **≥15 mm considered positive for:** • persons without risk factors for TB
Candida	24-72 h	5 mm induration or greater
Histoplasmin	24-72 h	5 mm or greater
Mumps	24-36 h	5 mm or greater
Trichophyton	24-72 h	5 mm induration or greater

Recommended Interpretation of Skin Test Reactions

Reaction	Local Reaction	
	After Intradermal Injections of Antigens	After Dinitrochlorobenzene
1+	Erythema >10 mm and/or induration >1-5 mm	Erythema and/or induration covering <½ area of dose site
2+	Induration 6-10 mm	Induration covering >½ area of dose site
3+	Induration 11-20 mm	Vesiculation and induration at dose site or spontaneous flare at days 7-14 at the site
4+	Induration >20 mm	Bulla or ulceration at dose site or spontaneous flare at days 7-14 at the site

Penicillin Allergy

The recommended battery of major and minor determinants used in penicillin skin testing will disclose those individuals with circulating IgE antibodies. This procedure is therefore useful to identify patients at risk for immediate or accelerated reactions. Skin tests are of no value in predicting the occurrence of non-IgE-mediated hypersensitivity reactions to penicillin such as delayed exanthem, drug fever, hemolytic anemia, interstitial nephritis, or exfoliative dermatitis. Based on large scale trials, skin testing solutions have been standardized.

Antihistamines, tricyclic antidepressants, and adrenergic drugs, all of which may inhibit skin test results, should be discontinued at least 24 hours prior to skin testing. Antihistamines with long half-lives (hydroxyzine, terfenadine, astemizole, etc) may attenuate skin test results up to a week, or longer after discontinuation.

When properly performed with due consideration for preliminary scratch tests and appropriate dilutions, skin testing with penicillin reagents can almost always be safely accomplished. Systemic reactions accompany about 1% of positive skin tests; these are usually mild but can be serious. **Therefore skin tests should be done in the presence of a physician and with immediate access to medications and equipment needed to treat anaphylaxis.**

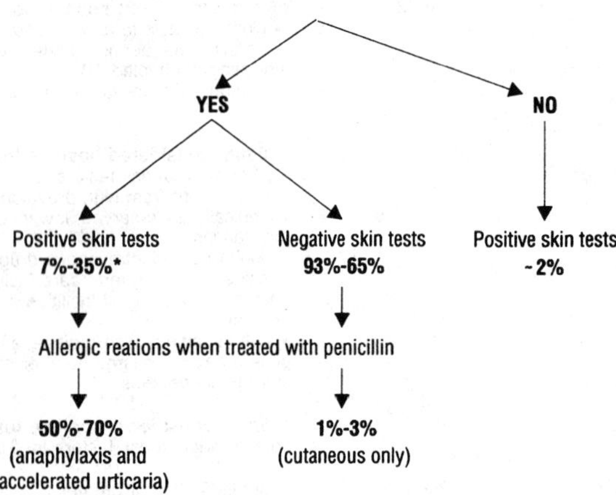

*One study found 65% positive

Prevalence of positive and negative skin tests and subsequent allergic reactions in patients treated with penicillin (based on studies using both penicilloyl-polylysine and minor determinant mixture as skin test reagents).

Penicillin Skin Testing Protocol

Skin tests evaluate the patient for the presence of penicillin IgE — sensitive mast cells which are responsible for anaphylaxis and other immediate hypersensitivity reactions. Local or systemic allergic reactions rarely occur due to skin testing, therefore, a tourniquet, I.V., and epinephrine should be at the bedside. The breakdown products of penicillin provide the antigen which is responsible for the allergy. Testing is performed with benzylpenicilloyl-polylysine (Pre-Pen®), the major determinant, penicillin G which provides the minor determinants and the actual penicillin which will be administered.

Controls are important if the patient is extremely ill or is taking antihistamines, codeine, or morphine. Normal saline is the negative control. Morphine sulfate, a mast cell degranulator, can be used as a positive control, if the patient is not on morphine or codeine. Histamine is the preferred positive control, however, is not manufactured in a pharmaceutical formulation anymore. A false-positive or false-negative will make further skin testing invalid.

Control Solutions

Normal saline = negative control
Morphine sulfate (10 mg/100 mL 0.9% NaCl, 0.1 mg/mL) = positive control

Test Solutions

Order the necessary solutions as 0.5 mL in a tuberculin syringe. **Note:** May need to order 2 syringes of each — one for scratch testing and one for intradermal skin testing.

I. **Pre-Pen®: Benzylpenicilloyl-polylysine (0.25 mL ampul) = MAJOR DETERMINANT**
   A. Undiluted Pre-Pen®
   B. 1:100 concentration
      To make: Dilute 0.1 mL of Pre-Pen® in 10 mL of 0.9% NaCl
   C. 1:10,000 concentration
      (Only necessary in patients with a history of anaphylaxis)
      To make: Dilute 1 mL of the 1:100 solution in 100 mL of 0.9% NaCl

II. **Penicillin G sodium/potassium = MINOR DETERMINANT**
   A. 5000 units/mL concentration
   B. 5 units/mL concentration
      (Only necessary in patients with a history of anaphylaxis)

To make: Dilute 0.1 mL of a 5000 units/mL solution in 100 mL of 0.9% NaCl

III. **Penicillin product to be administered — if not penicillin G**

A. **Ampicillin** 2.5 mg/mL concentration
To make: Dilute 250 mg in 100 mL of 0.9% NaCl

B. **Nafcillin** 2.5 mg/mL concentration
To make: Dilute 250 mg in 100 mL of 0.9% NaCl

Order for placement/availability at the bedside in the event of a hypersensitivity reaction during scratch/skin testing and desensitization:

Hydrocortisone: 100 mg IVP
Diphenhydramine: 50 mg IVP
Epinephrine: 1:1000 S.C.

Scratch/Skin Testing Protocol: Must Be Done by Physician!

1. Begin with the control solutions (ie, normal saline and morphine).

2. Administer **scratch tests** in the following order (beginning with the most dilute solution):

Pre-Pen®	Syringes: C,B,A
Penicillin G	Syringes: E,D
Ampicillin/Nafcillin	Syringe: F

The inner volar surface of the forearm is usually used.

A nonbleeding scratch of 3-5 mm in length is made in the epidermis with a 20-gauge needle.

If bleeding occurs, another site should be selected and another scratch made using less pressure.

A small drop of the test solution is then applied and rubbed gently into the scratch using an applicator, toothpick, or the side of the needle.

The scratch test site should be observed for the appearance of a wheal, erythema, and pruritis.

A positive reaction is signified by the appearance within 15 minutes of a pale wheal (usually with pseudopods) ranging from 5-15 mm or more in diameter.

As soon as a positive response is elicited, or 15 minutes has elapsed, the solution should be wiped off the scratch.

If the scratch test is negative or equivocal (ie, a wheal of <5 mm in diameter with little or no erythema or itching appears), an intradermal test may be performed.

If significant reaction, treat and proceed to desensitization.

3. Administer **intradermal tests** in the following order (beginning with the most dilute solution):

Pre-Pen®	Syringes: C,B,A
Penicillin G	Syringes: E,D
Ampicillin/Nafcillin	Syringe: F

Intradermal tests are usually performed on a sterilized area of the upper outer arm at a sufficient distance below the deltoid muscle to permit proximal application of a tourniquet if a severe reaction occurs.

Using a tuberculin syringe with a 3/8-5/8 inch 26- to 30-gauge needle, an amount of each tet solution sufficient to raise the smallest perceptible blob (usually 0.01 0.02 mL) is injected immediately under the surface of the skin.

A separate needle and syringe must be used for each solution.

Each test and control site should be at least 15 cm apart.

Positive reactions are manifested as a wheal at the test site with a diameter at least 5 mm larger than the saline control, often accompanied by itching and a marked increase in the size of the bleb.

Skin responses to penicillin testing will develop within 15 minutes.

If no significant reaction, may challenge patient with reduced dosage of the penicillin to be administered.

Physician should be at the bedside during this challenge dose!

If significant reaction, treat and begin desensitization.

PEDIATRIC ALS ALGORITHM BRADYCARDIA

Fig. 1: Pediatric bradycardia decision tree. ABCs indicates airway, breathing, and circulation; ALS, advanced life support; E.T., endotracheal; I.O., intraosseous; and I.V., intravenous.

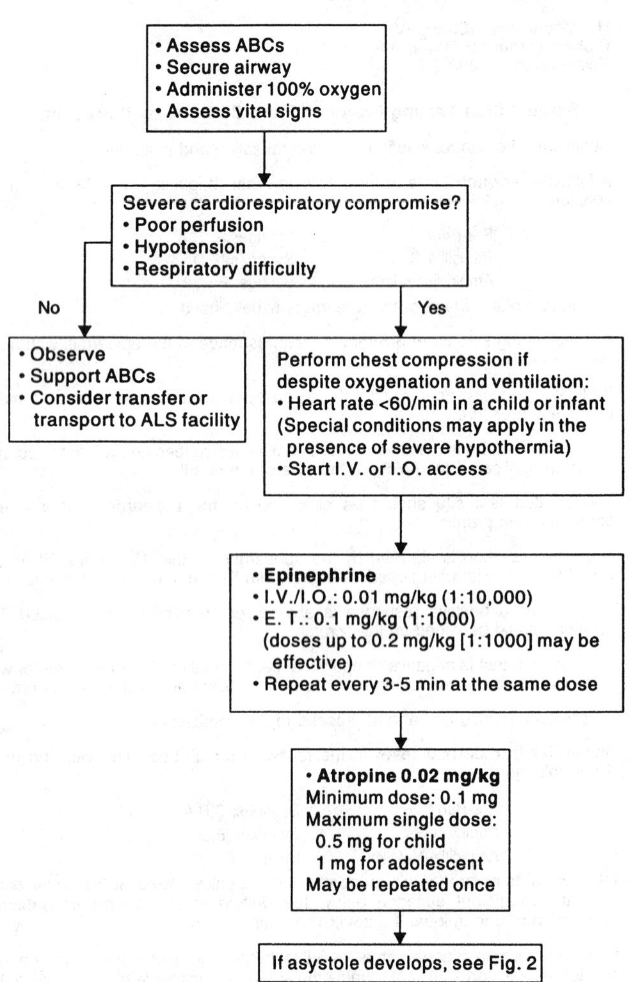

Used with permission: Emergency Cardiac Care Committee and Subcommittees, American Heart Association, "Guidelines for Cardiopulmonary Resuscitation and Emergency Care, IV: Pediatric Advanced Life Support," *JAMA*, 1992.

PEDIATRIC ALS ALGORITHM
Asystole and Pulseless Arrest

Fig. 2: Pediatric asystole and pulseless arrest decision tree. CPR indicates cardiopulmonary resuscitation; E.T., endotracheal; I.O., intraosseous; and I.V., intravenous.

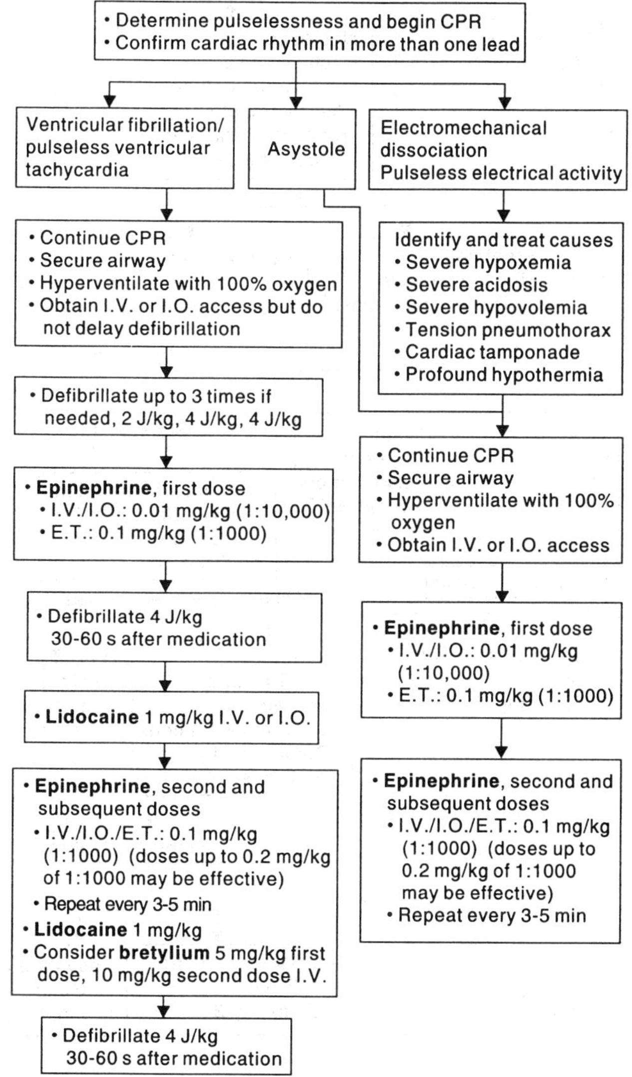

Used with permission: Emergency Cardiac Care Committee and Subcommittees, American Heart Association, "Guidelines for Cardiopulmonary Resuscitation and Emergency Care, IV: Pediatric Advanced Life Support," *JAMA*, 1992.

ADULT ACLS ALGORITHM
Emergency Cardiac Care

Fig. 1: Universal algorithm for adult emergency cardiac care (ECC)

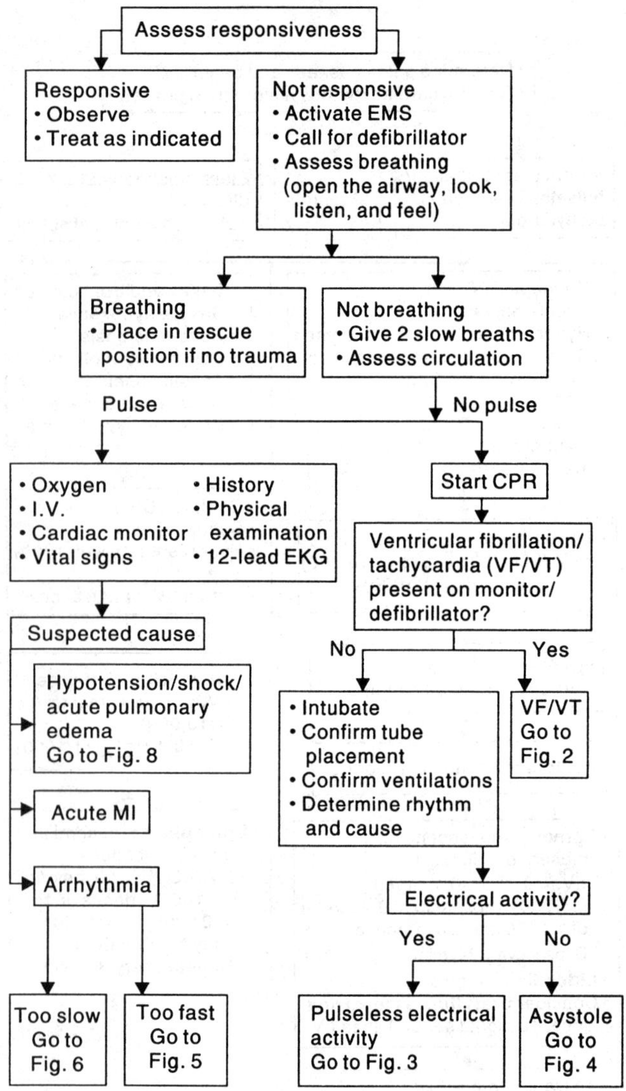

Used with permission: Emergency Cardiac Care Committee and Subcommittees, American Heart Association, "Guidelines for Cardiopulmonary Resuscitation and Emergency Care, III: Adult Advanced Cardiac Life Support," *JAMA*, 1992, 268:2199-2241.

ADULT ACLS ALGORITHM
V. Fib and Pulseless V. Tach

Fig. 2: Adult algorithm for ventricular fibrillation and pulseless ventricular tachycardia (VF/VT)

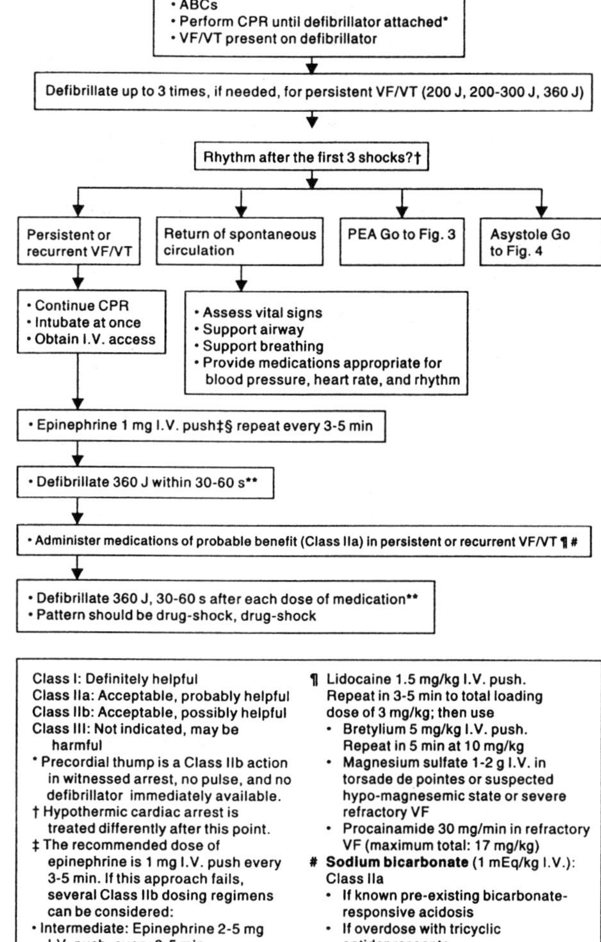

Class I: Definitely helpful
Class IIa: Acceptable, probably helpful
Class IIb: Acceptable, possibly helpful
Class III: Not indicated, may be harmful

* Precordial thump is a Class IIb action in witnessed arrest, no pulse, and no defibrillator immediately available.

† Hypothermic cardiac arrest is treated differently after this point.

‡ The recommended dose of epinephrine is 1 mg I.V. push every 3-5 min. If this approach fails, several Class IIb dosing regimens can be considered:
- Intermediate: Epinephrine 2-5 mg I.V. push, every 3-5 min
- Escalating: Epinephrine 1 mg-3 mg-5 mg I.V. push (3 min apart)
- High: Epinephrine: 0.1 mg/kg I.V. push, every 3-5 min

§ **Sodium bicarbonate (1 mEq/kg)** is Class I if patient has known pre-existing hyperkalemia

** Multiple sequenced shock (200 J, 200-300 J, 360 J) are acceptable here (Class I), especially when medications are delayed

¶ Lidocaine 1.5 mg/kg I.V. push. Repeat in 3-5 min to total loading dose of 3 mg/kg; then use
- Bretylium 5 mg/kg I.V. push. Repeat in 5 min at 10 mg/kg
- Magnesium sulfate 1-2 g I.V. in torsade de pointes or suspected hypo-magnesemic state or severe refractory VF
- Procainamide 30 mg/min in refractory VF (maximum total: 17 mg/kg)

Sodium bicarbonate (1 mEq/kg I.V.):
Class IIa
- If known pre-existing bicarbonate-responsive acidosis
- If overdose with tricyclic antidepressants
- To alkalinize the urine in drug overdoses

Class IIb
- If intubated and continued long arrest interval
- Upon return of spontaneous circulation after long arrest interval

Class III
- Hypoxic lactic acidosis

Used with permission: Emergency Cardiac Care Committee and Subcommittees, American Heart Association, "Guidelines for Cardiopulmonary Resuscitation and Emergency Care, III: Adult Advanced Cardiac Life Support," *JAMA*, 1992, 268:2199-2241.

ADULT ACLS ALGORITHM
Pulseless Electrical Activity

Fig. 3: Adult algorithm for pulseless electrical activity (PEA) (electromechani dissociation [EMD]).

PEA includes:
- Electromechanical dissociation (EMD)
- Pseudo-EMD
- Idioventricular rhythms
- Ventricular escape rhythms
- Bradyasystolic rhythms
- Postdefibrillation idioventricular rhythms

- Continue CPR
- Intubate at once
- Obtain I.V. access
- Assess blood flow using Doppler ultrasound

↓

Consider possible causes (Parentheses = possible therapies and treatments)
- Hypovolemia (volume infusion)
- Hypoxia (ventilation)
- Cardiac tamponade (pericardiocentesis)
- Tension pneumothorax (needle decompression)
- Hypothermia
- Massive pulmonary embolism (surgery, **thrombolytics**)
- Drug overdoses such as tricyclics, digitalis, beta blockers, calcium channel blockers
- Hyperkalemia*
- Acidosis†
- Massive acute myocardial infarction

↓

Epinephrine 1 mg I.V. push*‡, repeat every 3-5 min

↓

- If absolute bradycardia (<60 beats/min) or relative bradycardia, give **atropine** 1 mg I.V.
- Repeat every 3-5 min up to a total of 0.04 mg/kg§

Class I: Definitely helpful
Class IIa: Acceptable, probably helpful
Class IIb: Acceptable, possibly helpful
Class III: Not indicated, may be harmful

* **Sodium bicarbonate** 1 mEq/kg is Class I if patient has known pre-existing hyperkalemia

† **Sodium bicarbonate** 1 mEq/kg:
Class IIa
- If known pre-existing bicarbonate-responsive acidosis
- If overdose with tricyclic antidepressants
- To alkalinize the urine in drug overdoses

Class IIb
- If intubated and long arrest interval
- Upon return of spontaneous circulation after long arrest interval

Class III
- Hypoxic lactic acidosis

‡ The recommended dose of **epinephrine** is 1 mg I.V. push every 3-5 min. If this approach fails, several Class IIb dosing regimens can be considered.
- Intermediate: **Epinephrine** 2-5 mg I.V. push every 3-5 min
- Escalating: **Epinephrine** 1 mg-3 mg-5 mg I.V. push (3 min apart)
- High: **Epinephrine** 0.1 mg/kg I.V. push every 3-5 min

§ Shorter **atropine** dosing intervals are possibly helpful in cardiac arrest (Class IIb)

ADULT ACLS ALGORITHM
Asystole

Fig. 4: Adult asystole treatment algorithm.

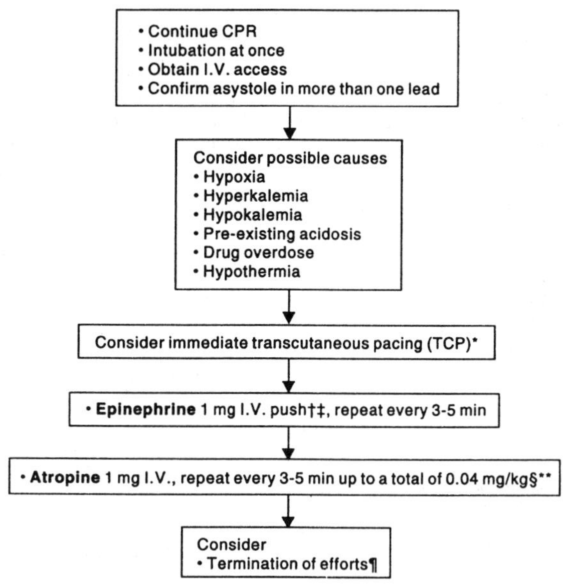

Class I: Definitely helpful
Class IIa: Acceptable, probably helpful
Class IIb: Acceptable, possibly helpful
Class III: Not indicated, may be harmful

* TCP is a Class IIb intervention. Lack of success may be due to delays in pacing. To be effective, TCP must be performed early, simultaneously with drugs. Evidence does not support routine use of TCP for asystole.

† The recommended dose of **epinephrine** is 1 mg I.V. push every 3-5 min. If this approach fails, several Class IIb dosing regimens can be considered:
- Intermediate: **Epinephrine** 2-5 mg I.V. push every 3-5 min
- Escalating: **Epinephrine** 1 mg-3 mg-5 mg I.V. push (3 min apart)
- High: **Epinephrine** 0.1 mg/kg I.V. push every 3-5 min

‡ Sodium bicarbonate 1 mEq/kg is Class I if patient has known pre-existing hyperkalemia

§ Shorter atropine dosing intervals are Class IIb in asystolic arrest

** Sodium bicarbonate 1 mEq/kg:
Class IIa
- If known pre-existing bicarbonate responsive acidosis
- If overdose with tricyclic antidepressants
- To alkalinize the urine in drug overdoses

Class IIb
- If intubated and continued long arrest interval
- Upon return of spontaneous circulation after long arrest interval

Class III
- Hypoxic lactic acidosis

¶ If patient remains in asystole or other agonal rhythm after successful intubation and initial medications and no reversible causes are identified, consider termination of resuscitative efforts by a physician. Consider interval since arrest.

Used with permission: Emergency Cardiac Care Committee and Subcommittees, American Heart Association, "Guidelines for Cardiopulmonary Resuscitation and Emergency Care, III: Adult Advanced Cardiac Life Support," *JAMA*, 1992, 268:2199-2241.

ADULT ACLS ALGORITHM
Tachycardia

Fig. 5: Adult tachycardia algorithm.

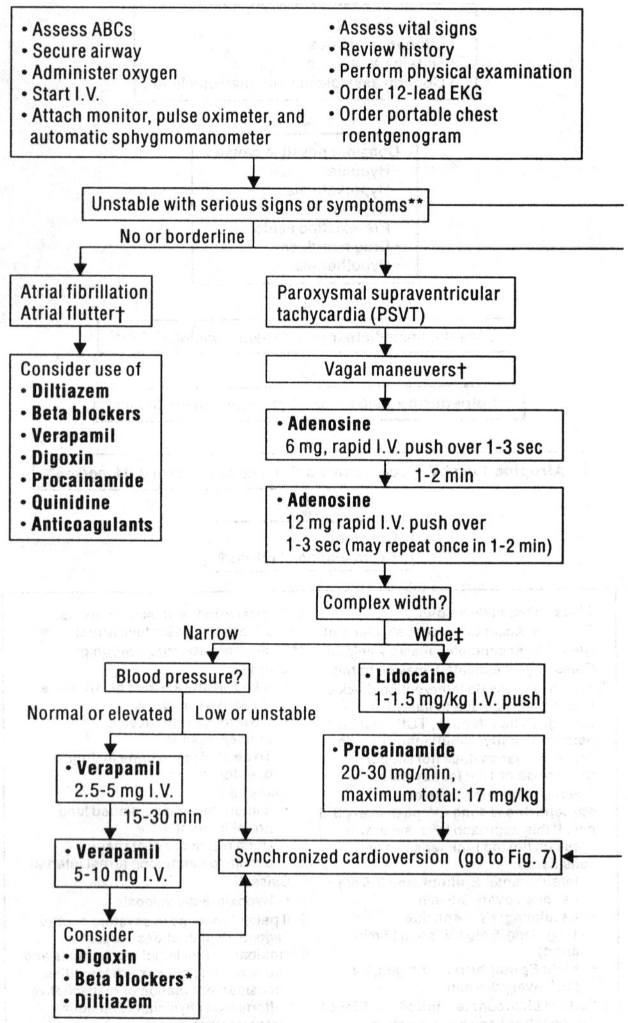

* Use extreme caution with beta blockers after verapamil

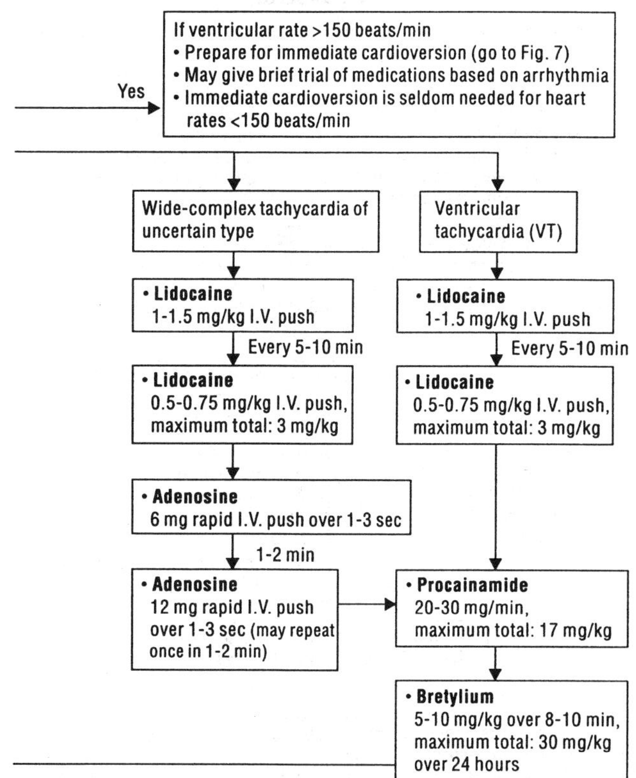
If ventricular rate >150 beats/min
• Prepare for immediate cardioversion (go to Fig. 7)
• May give brief trial of medications based on arrhythmia
• Immediate cardioversion is seldom needed for heart rates <150 beats/min
Yes
Wide-complex tachycardia of uncertain type
Ventricular tachycardia (VT)
• Lidocaine 1-1.5 mg/kg I.V. push
Every 5-10 min
• Lidocaine 0.5-0.75 mg/kg I.V. push, maximum total: 3 mg/kg
• Lidocaine 1-1.5 mg/kg I.V. push
Every 5-10 min
• Lidocaine 0.5-0.75 mg/kg I.V. push, maximum total: 3 mg/kg
• Adenosine 6 mg rapid I.V. push over 1-3 sec
1-2 min
• Adenosine 12 mg rapid I.V. push over 1-3 sec (may repeat once in 1-2 min)
• Procainamide 20-30 mg/min, maximum total: 17 mg/kg
• Bretylium 5-10 mg/kg over 8-10 min, maximum total: 30 mg/kg over 24 hours

** Unstable condition must be related to the tachycardia. Signs and symptoms may include chest pain, shortness of breath, decreased level of consciousness, low blood pressure (BP), shock, pulmonary congestion, congestive heart failure, acute myocardial infarction.

† Carotid sinus pressure is contraindicated in patients with carotid bruits; avoid ice water immersion in patients with ischemic heart disease.

‡ If the wide-complex tachycardia is known with certainty to be PSVT and BP is normal/elevated, sequence can include **verapamil.**

Used with permission: Emergency Cardiac Care Committee and Subcommittees, American Heart Association, "Guidelines for Cardiopulmonary Resuscitation and Emergency Care, III: Adult Advanced Cardiac Life Support," *JAMA*, 1992, 268:2199-2241.

ADULT ACLS ALGORITHM
Bradycardia

Fig. 6: Adult bradycardia algorithm (with the patient not in cardiac arrest).

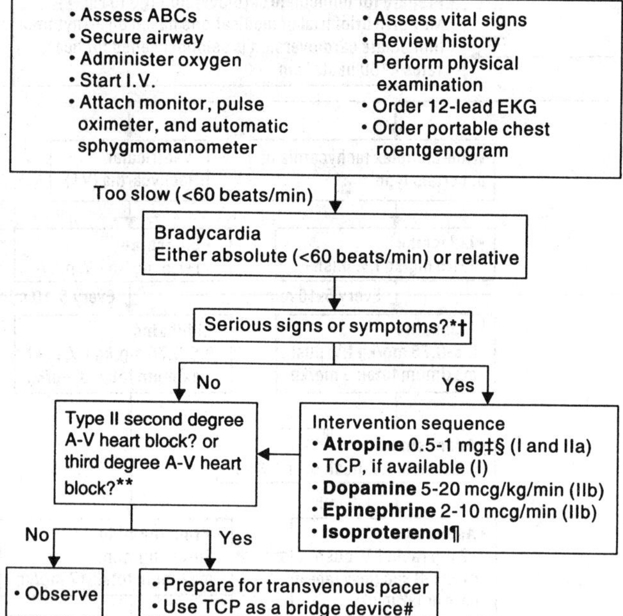

* Serious signs or symptoms must be related to the slow rate. Clinical manifestations include:
Symptoms (chest pain, shortness of breath, decreased level of consciousness), and
Signs (low BP, shock, pulmonary congestion, CHF, acute MI)

† Do not delay TCP while awaiting I.V. access or for **atropine** to take effect if patient is symptomatic.

‡ Denervated transplanted hearts will not respond to **atropine**. Go at once to pacing, **catecholamine** infusion, or both.

§ **Atropine** should be given in repeat doses in 3-5 min up to a total of 0.04 mg/kg. Consider shorter dosing intervals in severe clinical conditions. It has been suggested that atropine should be used with caution in atrioventricular (A-V) block at the His-Purkinje level (type II A-V block and new third degree block with wide QRS complexes) (Class IIb).

Never treat third degree heart block plus ventricular escape beats with **lidocaine.

¶ **Isoproterenol** should be used, if at all, with extreme caution. At low doses it is Class IIb (possibly helpful); at higher doses it is Class III (harmful).

Verify patient tolerance and mechanical capture. Use analgesia and sedation as needed.

Used with permission: Emergency Cardiac Care Committee and Subcommittees, American Heart Association, "Guidelines for Cardiopulmonary Resuscitation and Emergency Care, III: Adult Advanced Cardiac Life Support," *JAMA*, 1992, 268:2199-2241.

ADULT ACLS ALGORITHM
Electrical Conversion

Fig. 7: Adult electrical cardioversion algorithm (with the patient not in cardiac arrest).

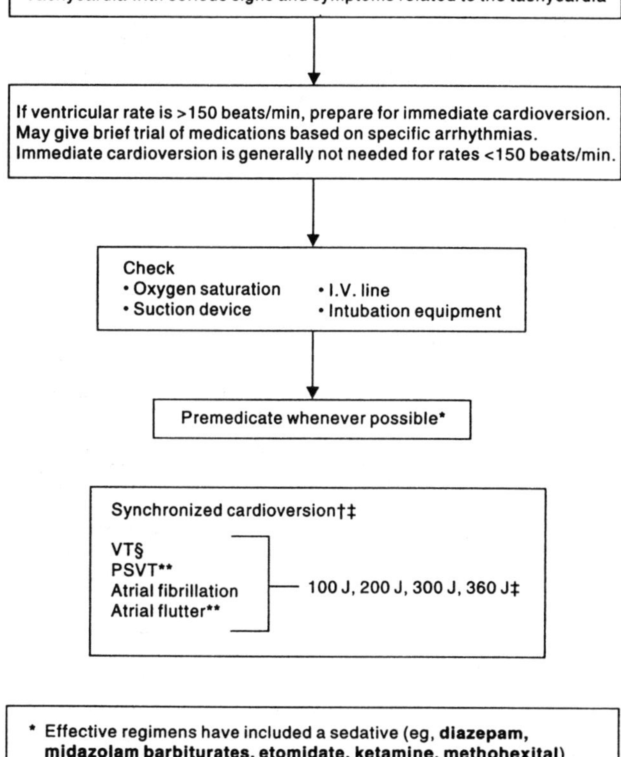

Tachycardia with serious signs and symptoms related to the tachycardia
If ventricular rate is >150 beats/min, prepare for immediate cardioversion.
May give brief trial of medications based on specific arrhythmias.
Immediate cardioversion is generally not needed for rates <150 beats/min.
Check
• Oxygen saturation
• Suction device
• I.V. line
• Intubation equipment
Premedicate whenever possible*
Synchronized cardioversion†‡
VT§
PSVT**
Atrial fibrillation
Atrial flutter**
100 J, 200 J, 300 J, 360 J‡

* Effective regimens have included a sedative (eg, **diazepam, midazolam barbiturates, etomidate, ketamine, methohexital**) with or without an analgesic agent (eg, **fentanyl, morphine, meperidine**). Many experts recommend anesthesia if service is readily available.

† Note possible need to resynchronize after each cardioversion.

‡ If delays in synchronization occur and clinical conditions are critical, go to immediate unsynchronized shocks.

§ Treat polymorphic VT (irregular form and rate) like VF: 200 J, 200-300 J, 360 J.

** PSVT and atrial flutter often respond to lower energy levels (start with 50 J).

Used with permission: Emergency Cardiac Care Committee and Subcommittees, American Heart Association, "Guidelines for Cardiopulmonary Resuscitation and Emergency Care, III: Adult Advanced Cardiac Life Support," *JAMA*, 1992, 268:2199-2241.

ADULT ACLS ALGORITHM
Hypotension, Shock

Fig. 8: Adult algorithm for hypotension, shock, and acute pulmonary edema.

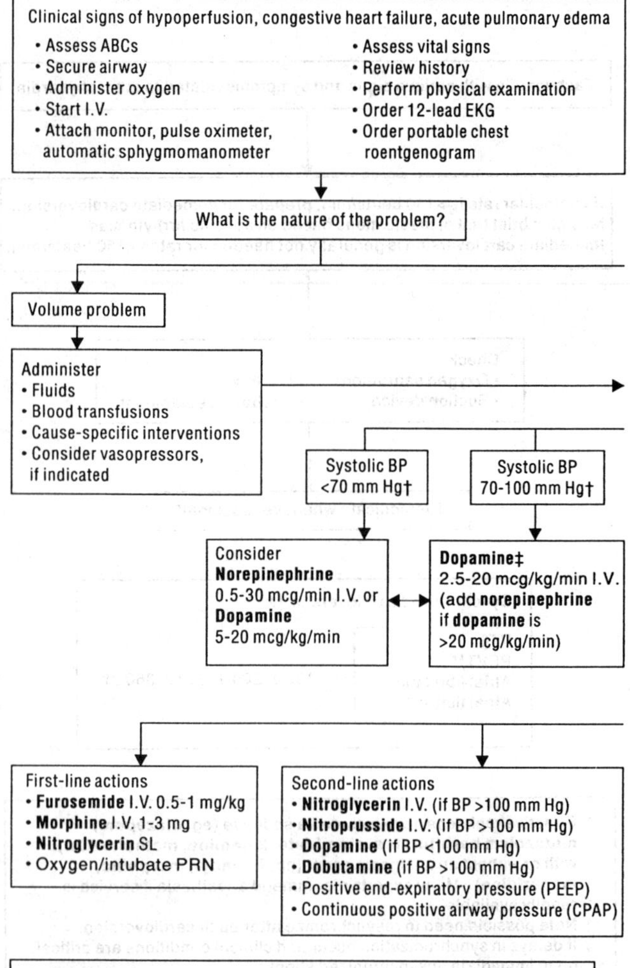

Clinical signs of hypoperfusion, congestive heart failure, acute pulmonary edema
• Assess ABCs
• Secure airway
• Administer oxygen
• Start I.V.
• Attach monitor, pulse oximeter, automatic sphygmomanometer
• Assess vital signs
• Review history
• Perform physical examination
• Order 12-lead EKG
• Order portable chest roentgenogram
What is the nature of the problem?
Volume problem
Administer
• Fluids
• Blood transfusions
• Cause-specific interventions
• Consider vasopressors, if indicated
Systolic BP <70 mm Hg†
Systolic BP 70-100 mm Hg†
Consider Norepinephrine 0.5-30 mcg/min I.V. or Dopamine 5-20 mcg/kg/min
Dopamine‡ 2.5-20 mcg/kg/min I.V. (add norepinephrine if dopamine is >20 mcg/kg/min)
First-line actions
• Furosemide I.V. 0.5-1 mg/kg
• Morphine I.V. 1-3 mg
• Nitroglycerin SL
• Oxygen/intubate PRN
Second-line actions
• Nitroglycerin I.V. (if BP >100 mm Hg)
• Nitroprusside I.V. (if BP >100 mm Hg)
• Dopamine (if BP <100 mm Hg)
• Dobutamine (if BP >100 mm Hg)
• Positive end-expiratory pressure (PEEP)
• Continuous positive airway pressure (CPAP)

* Base management after this point on invasive hemodynamic monitoring if possible.

† Fluid bolus of 250-500 mL normal saline should be tried. If no response, consider sympathomimetics.

‡ Move to **dopamine** and stop **norepinephrine** when BP improves. Avoid **dopamine** (consider **dobutamine**) if no signs of hypoperfusion.

§ Add **dopamine** and avoid **dobutamine** when systolic BP <90 mm Hg.

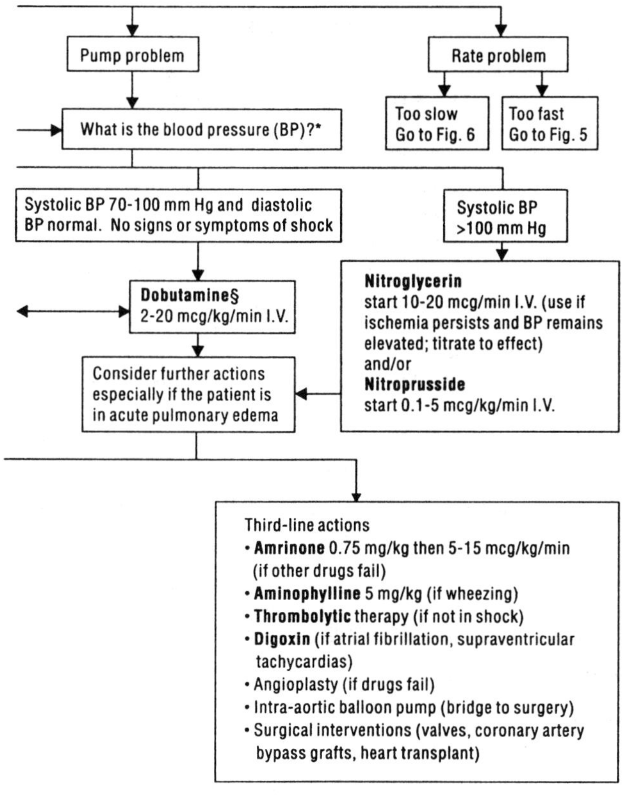

Used with permission: Emergency Cardiac Care Committee and Subcommittees, American Heart Association, "Guidelines for Cardiopulmonary Resuscitation and Emergency Care, III: Adult Advanced Cardiac Life Support," *JAMA*, 1992, 268:2199-2241.

NATIONAL ASTHMA EDUCATION AND PREVENTION PROGRAM

EXPERT PANEL REPORT II: GUIDELINES FOR THE DIAGNOSIS AND MANAGEMENT OF ASTHMA

February 1997

STEPWISE APPROACH FOR MANAGING ASTHMA IN ADULTS AND CHILDREN >5 YEARS OF AGE: CLASSIFY SEVERITY

Goals of Asthma Treatment

- Prevent chronic and troublesome symptoms (eg, coughing or breathlessness in the night, in the early morning, or after exertion)
- Maintain (near) "normal" pulmonary function
- Maintain normal activity levels (including exercise and other physical activity)
- Prevent recurrent exacerbations of asthma and minimize the need for emergency department visits or hospitalizations
- Provide optimal pharmacotherapy with minimal or no adverse effects
- Meet patients' and families' expectations of and satisfaction with asthma care

Clinical Features Before Treatment*

Symptoms**	Nighttime Symptoms	Lung Function
STEP 4: Severe Persistent		
•Continual symptoms •Limited physical activity •Frequent exacerbations	Frequent	•FEV_1/PEF ≤60% predicted •PEF variability >30%
STEP 3: Moderate Persistent		
•Daily symptoms •Daily use of inhaled short-acting $beta_2$-agonist •Exacerbations affect activity •Exacerbations ≥2 times/week; may last days	>1 time/week	•FEV_1/PEF >60% - 80% predicted •PEF variability >30%
STEP 2: Mild Persistent		
•Symptoms >2 times/week but <1 time/day •Exacerbations may affect activity	>2 times/month	•FEV_1/PEF ≥80% predicted •PEF variability 20% - 30%
STEP 1: Mild Intermittent		
•Symptoms ≤2 times/week •Asymptomatic and normal PEF between exacerbations •Exacerbations brief (from a few hours to a few days); intensity may vary	≤2 times/month	•FEV_1/PEF ≥80% predicted •PEF variability ≤20%

*The presence of one of the features of severity is sufficient to place a patient in that category. An individual should be assigned to the most severe grade in which any feature occurs. The characteristics noted in this figure are general and may overlap because asthma is highly variable. Furthermore, an individual's classification may change over time.

**Patients at any level of severity can have mild, moderate, or severe exacerbations. Some patients with intermittent asthma experience severe and life-threatening exacerbations separated by long periods of normal lung function and no symptoms.

STEPWISE APPROACH FOR MANAGING ASTHMA IN ADULTS AND CHILDREN OLDER THAN 5 YEARS OF AGE: TREATMENT

Preferred treatments are in bold print.

Long-Term Control	Quick Relief	Education
	STEP 4: Severe Persistent	
Daily medications: • **Anti-inflammatory: Inhaled corticosteroid (high dose)** AND • Long-acting bronchodilator: Either **long-acting inhaled beta$_2$-agonist**, sustained-release theophylline, or long-acting beta$_2$-agonist tablets AND • Corticosteroid tablets or syrup long term (2 mg/kg/ day, generally do not exceed 60 mg per day).	• Short-acting bronchodilator: **Inhaled beta$_2$-agonists** as needed for symptoms. • Intensity of treatment will depend on severity of exacerbation; see "Managing Exacerbations" • Use of short-acting inhaled beta$_2$-agonists on a daily basis, or increasing use, indicates the need for additional long-term control therapy.	Steps 2 and 3 actions plus: • Refer to individual education/counseling
	STEP 3: Moderate Persistent	
Daily medication: • Either — **Anti-inflammatory: Inhaled corticosteroid (medium dose)** OR — **Inhaled corticosteroid (low-medium dose)** and add a long-acting bronchodilator, especially for nighttime symptoms: Either **long-acting inhaled beta$_2$-agonist**, sustained-release theophylline, or long-acting beta$_2$-agonist tablets. • If needed — Anti-inflammatory: **Inhaled corticosteroids (medium-high dose) AND** — **Long-acting bronchodilator,** especially for nighttime symptoms; either **long-acting inhaled beta$_2$-agonist,** sustained release theophylline, or long-acting beta$_2$-agonist tablets.	• Short-acting bronchildilator: **Inhaled beta$_2$-agonists** as needed for symptoms. • Intensity of treatment will depend on severity of exacerbation; see "Managing Exacerbations." • Use of short-acting inhaled beta$_2$-agonists on a daily basis, or increasing use, indicates the need for additional long-term control therapy.	Step 1 actions plus: • Teach self-monitoring • Refer to group education if available • Review and update self-management plan
	STEP 2: Mild Persistent	
One daily medication: • **Anti-inflammatory:** Either **inhaled corticosteroid** (low doses) or **cromolyn or nedocromil** (children usually begin with a trial of cromolyn or nedocromil). • Sustained-release theophylline to serum concentration of 5-15 mcg/ mL is an alternative, but not preferred, therapy. Zafirlukast or zileuton may also be considered for patients ≥12 years of age, although their position in therapy is not fully established.	• Short-acting bronchodilator: **Inhaled beta$_2$-agonists** as needed for symptoms. • Intensity of treatment will depend on severity of exacerbation; see "Managing Exacerbations." •Use of short-acting inhaled beta$_2$-agonists on a daily basis, or increasing use, indicates the need for additional long-term control therapy.	Step 1 actions plus: • Teach self-monitoring • Refer to group education if available • Review and update self-management plan

(continued)

Long-Term Control	Quick Relief	Education
	STEP 1: Mild Intermittent	
• No daily medication needed.	• Short-acting bronchodilator: **Inhaled beta$_2$-agonists** as needed for symptoms. • Intensity of treatment will depend on severity of exacerbation; see "Managing Exacerbations" • Use of short-acting inhaled beta$_2$-agonists more than 2 times/week may indicate the need to initiate long-term control therapy	• Teach basic facts about asthma •Teach inhaler/spacer/holding chamber technique • Discuss roles of medications •Develop self-management plan •Develop action plan for when and how to take rescue actions, especially for patients with a history of severe exacerbations • Discuss appropriate environmental control measures to avoid exposure to known allergens and irritants

↓ Step down
Review treatment every 1-6 months; a gradual stepwise reduction in treatment may be possible.

↑Step up
If control is not maintained, consider step up. First, review patient medication technique, adherence, and environmental control (avoidance of allergens or other factors that contribute to asthma severity.)

Note:

- **The stepwise approach presents general guidelines to assist clinical decisionmaking; it is not intended to be a specific prescription. Asthma is highly variable; clinicians should tailor specific medication plans to the needs and circumstances of individual patients.**
- Gain control as quickly as possible; then decrease treatment to the least medication necessary to maintain control. Gaining control may be accomplished by either starting treatment at the step most appropriate to the initial severity of the condition or starting at a higher level of therapy (eg, a course of systemic corticosteroids or higher dose of inhaled corticosteroids).
- A rescue course of systemic corticosteroids may be needed at any time and at any step.
- Some patients with intermittent asthma experience severe and life-threatening exacerbations separated by long periods of normal lung function and no symptoms. This may be especially common with exacerbations provoked by respiratory infections. A short course of systemic corticosteroids is recommended.
- At each step, patients should control their environment to avoid or control factors that make their asthma worse (eg, allergens, irritants); this requires specific diagnosis and education.

ESTIMATED COMPARATIVE DAILY DOSAGES FOR INHALED CORTICOSTEROIDS

ADULTS

Drug	Low Dose	Medium Dose	High Dose
Beclomethasone dipropionate	168-504 mcg	504-840 mcg	>840 mcg
42 mcg/puff	(4-12 puffs — 42 mcg)	(12-20 puffs — 42 mcg)	(>20 puffs — 42 mcg)
84 mcg/puff	(2-6 puffs — 84 mcg)	(6-10 puffs — 84 mcg)	(>10 puffs — 84 mcg)
Budesonide Turbuhaler	200-400 mcg	400-600 mcg	>600 mcg
200 mcg/dose	(1-2 inhalations)	(2-3 inhalations)	(>3 inhalations)
Flunisolide	500-1000 mcg	1000-2000 mcg	>2000 mcg
250 mcg/puff	(2-4 puffs)	(4-8 puffs)	(>8 puffs)
Fluticasone	88-264 mcg	264-660 mcg	>660 mcg
MDI: 44, 110, 220 mcg/puff	(2-6 puffs — 44 mcg)	(2-6 puffs — 110 mcg)	(>6 puffs — 110 mcg)
	or		or
	(2 puffs — 110 mcg)		(>3 puffs — 220 mcg)
DPI: 50, 100, 250 mcg/dose	(2-6 inhalations — 50 mcg)	(3-6 inhalations — 100 mcg)	(>6 inhalations — 100 mcg)
Triamcinolone acetonide	400-1000 mcg	1000-2000 mcg	>2000 mcg
100 mcg/puff	(4-10 puffs)	(10-20 puffs)	(>20 puffs)

CHILDREN

Drug	Low Dose	Medium Dose	High Dose
Beclomethasone dipropionate	84-336 mcg	336-672 mcg	>672 mcg
42 mcg/puff	(2-8 puffs)	(8-16 puffs)	(>16 puffs)
84 mcg/puff			
Budesonide Turbuhaler	100-200 mcg	200-400 mcg	>400 mcg
200 mcg/dose		(1-2 inhalations — 200 mcg)	(>2 inhalations — 200 mcg)
Flunisolide	500-750 mcg	1000-1250 mcg	>1250 mcg
250 mcg/puff	(2-3 puffs)	(4-5 puffs)	(>5 puffs)
Fluticasone	88-176 mcg	176-440 mcg	>440 mcg
MDI: 44, 110, 220 mcg/puff	(2-4 puffs — 44 mcg)	(4-10 puffs — 44 mcg)	(>4 puffs — 110 mcg)
		or	
		(2-4 puffs — 110 mcg)	
DPI: 50, 100, 250 mcg/dose	(2-4 inhalations — 50 mcg)	(2-4 inhalations — 100 mcg)	(>4 inhalations — 100 mcg)
Triamcinolone acetonide	400-800 mcg	800-1200 mcg	>1200 mcg
100 mcg/puff	(4-8 puffs)	(8-12 puffs)	(>12 puffs)

NOTES:

- **The most important determinant of appropriate dosing is the clinician's judgment of the patient's response to therapy.** The clinician must monitor the patient's response on several clinical parameters and adjust the dose accordingly. The stepwise approach to therapy emphasizes that once control of asthma is achieved, the dose of mediation should be carefully titrated to the minimum dose required to maintain control, thus reducing the potential for adverse effect.
- The reference point for the range in the dosages for children is data on the safety on inhaled corticosteroids in children, which, in general, suggest that the dose ranges are equivalent to beclomethasone dipropionate 200-400 mcg/day (low dose), 400-800 mcg/day (medium dose), and >800 mcg/day (high dose).
- Some dosage may be outside package labeling.
- Metered-dose inhaler (MDI) dosages are expressed as the actuator dose (the amount of drug leaving the actuator and delivered to the patient), which is the labeling required in the United States. This is different from the dosage expressed as the valve dose (the amount of drug leaving the valve, all of which is not available to the patient), which is used in many European countries and in some of the scientific literature. Dry powder inhaler (DPI) doses (eg, Turbuhaler) are expressed as the amount of drug in the inhaler following activation.

ESTIMATED CLINICAL COMPARABILITY OF DOSES FOR INHALED CORTICOSTEROIDS

Data from *in vitro* and in clinical trials suggest that the different inhaled corticosteroid preparations are not equivalent on a per puff or microgram basis. However, it is entirely clear what implications these differences have for dosing recommendations in clinical practice because there are few data directly comparing the preparations. Relative dosing for clinical comparability is affected by differences in topical potency, clinical effects at different doses, delivery device, and bioavailability. The Expert Panel developed recommended dose ranges for different preparations based on available data and the following assumptions and cautions about estimating relative doses needed to achieve comparable clinical effect.

- **Relative topical potency using human skin blanching**
  - The standard test for determining relative topical anti-inflammatory potency is the topical vasoconstriction (MacKenzie skin blanching) test.
  - The MacKenzie topical skin blanching test correlates with binding affinities and binding half-lives for human lung corticosteroid receptors (see table below) (Dahlberg, et al, 1984; Hogger and Rohdewald 1994).
  - The relationship between relative topical anti-inflammatory effect and clinical comparability in asthma management is not certain. However, recent clinical trials suggest that different in vitro measures of anti-inflammatory effect is not certain. However, recent clinical trials suggest that different in vitro measures of anti-inflammatory effect correlate with clinical efficacy (Barnes and Pedersen 1993; Johnson 1996; Kamada, et al, 1996; Ebden, et al, 1986; Leblanc, et al, 1994; Gustaffson, et al, 1993; Lundback, et al, 1993; Barnes, et al, 1993; Fabbri, et al, 1993; Langdon and Capsey, 1994; Ayres, et al, 1995; Rafferty, et al, 1985; Bjorkander, et al, 1982, Stiksa, et al, 1982; Willey, et al, 1982.)

Medication	Topical Potency (Skin Blanching)*	Corticosteroid Receptor Binding Half-Life	Receptor Binding Affinity
Beclomethasone dipropionate (BDP)	600	7.5 hours	13.5
Budesonide (BUD)	980	5.1 hours	9.4
Flunisolide (FLU)	330	3.5 hours	1.8
Fluticasone propionate (FP)	1200	10.5 hours	18.0
Triamcinolone acetonide (TAA)	330	3.9 hours	3.6

*Numbers are assigned in reference to dexamethasone, which has a value of "1" in the MacKenzie test.

- **Relative doses to achieve similar clinical effects**
  - Clinical effects are evaluated by a number of outcome parameters (eg, changes in spirometry, peak flow rates, symptom scores, quick-relief $beta_2$-agonist use, frequency of exacerbations, airway responsiveness).
  - The daily dose and duration of treatment may affect these outcome parameters differently (eg, symptoms and peak flow may improve at lower doses and over a shorter treatment time than bronchial reactivity) (van Essen-Zandvliet, et al, 1992; Haahtela, et al, 1991)
  - Delivery systems influence comparability. For example, the delivery device for budesonide (Turbuhaler) delivers approximately twice the amount of drug to the airway as the MDI, thus enhancing the clinical effect (Thorsson, et al, 1994); Agertoft and Pedersen, 1993).
  - Individual patients may respond differently to different preparations, as noted by clinical experience.
  - Clinical trials comparing effects in reducing symptoms and improving peak expiratory flow demonstrate:
  - BDP amd BUD achieved comparable effects at similar microgram doses by MDI (Bjorkander, et al, 1982; Ebden, et al, 1986; Rafferty, et al, 1985).
  - BDP achieved effects similar to twice the dose of TAA on a microgram basis.

STEPWISE APPROACH FOR MANAGING INFANTS AND YOUNG CHILDREN (5 YEARS OF AGE AND YOUNGER) WITH ACUTE OR CHRONIC ASTHMA SYMPTOMS

Long-Term Control	Quick Relief
STEP 4: Severe Persistent	
• Daily anti-inflammatory medicine — High-dose inhaled corticosteroid with spacer/holding chamber and face mask — If needed, add systemic corticosteroids 2 mg/kg/day and reduce to lowest daily or alternate-day dose that stabilizes symptoms	•Bronchodilator as needed for symptoms (see step 1) up to 3 times/day
STEP 3: Moderate Persistent	
• Daily anti-inflammatory medication. Either: — Medium-dose inhaled corticosteroid with spacer/holding chamber and face mask OR Once control is established: — Medium-dose inhaled corticosteroid and nedocromil OR — Medium-dose inhaled corticosteroid and long-acting bronchodilator (theophylline)	• Bronchodilator as needed for symptoms (see step 1) up to 3 times/day
STEP 2: Mild Persistent	
• Daily anti-inflammatory medication. Either: — Cromolyn (nebulizer is preferred; or MDI) or nedocromil (MDI only) tid-qid — Infants and young children usually begin with a trial of cromolyn or nedocromil OR — Low-dose inhaled corticosteroid with spacer/holding chamber and face mask	• Bronchodilator as needed for symptoms (see step 1)
STEP 1: Mild Intermittent	
• No daily medication needed	• Bronchodilator as needed for symptoms $\leq$2 times/week. Intensity of treatment will depend upon severity of exacerbation (see "Managing Exacerbations"). Either: — Inhaled short-acting beta$_2$-agonist by nebulizer or face mask and spacer/ holding chamber or — Oral beta$_2$-agonist for symptoms • With viral respiratory infection: — Bronchodilator ever 4-6 hours up to 24 hours (longer with physician consult) but, in general, repeat no more than once every 6 weeks — Consider systemic corticosteroid if current exacerbation is sever OR patient has history of previous severe exacerbations

↓ Step Down
Review treatment every 1-6 months. If control is sustained for at least 3 months, a gradual stepwise reduction in treatment may be possible.

↑ Step Up
If control is not achieved, consider step up. But first: review patient medication technique, adherence, and environmental control (avoidance of allergens or other precipitant factors)

NOTES:

- **The stepwise approach presents guidelines to assist clinical decision making. Asthma is highly variable; clinicians should tailor specific medication plans to the needs and circumstances of individual patients.**

THERAPY RECOMMENDATIONS

- Gain control as quickly as possible; then decrease treatment to the least medication necessary to maintain control. Gaining control may be accomplished by either starting treatment at the step most appropriate to the initial severity of their condition or by starting at a higher level of therapy (eg, a course of systemic corticosteroids or higher dose of inhaled corticosteroids).
- A rescue course of systemic corticosteroid (prednisolone) may be needed at any time and step.
- In general, use of short-acting beta$_2$-agonist on a daily basis indicates the need for additional long-term control therapy.
- It is important to remember that there are very few studies on asthma therapy for infants.
- Consultation with an asthma specialist is recommended for patients with moderate or severe persistent asthma in this age group. Consultation should be considered for all patients with mild persistent asthma.

Management of Asthma Exacerbations: Home Treatment*

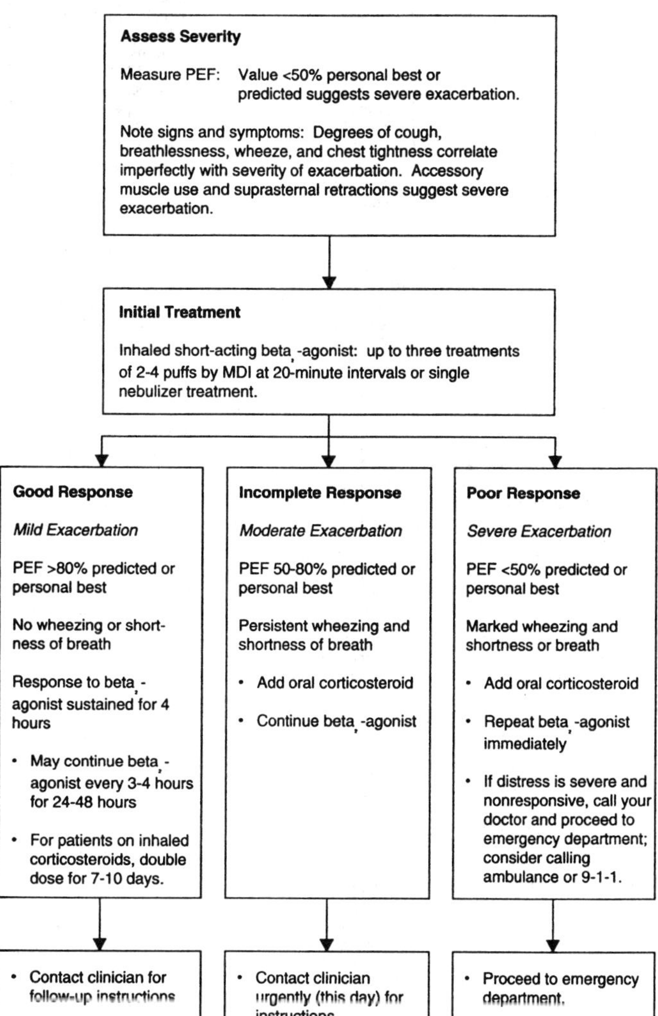

Assess Severity
Measure PEF: Value <50% personal best or predicted suggests severe exacerbation.
Note signs and symptoms: Degrees of cough, breathlessness, wheeze, and chest tightness correlate imperfectly with severity of exacerbation. Accessory muscle use and suprasternal retractions suggest severe exacerbation.
Initial Treatment
Inhaled short-acting beta$_2$-agonist: up to three treatments of 2-4 puffs by MDI at 20-minute intervals or single nebulizer treatment.
Good Response
Mild Exacerbation
PEF >80% predicted or personal best
No wheezing or shortness of breath
Response to beta$_2$-agonist sustained for 4 hours
• May continue beta$_2$-agonist every 3-4 hours for 24-48 hours
• For patients on inhaled corticosteroids, double dose for 7-10 days.
Incomplete Response
Moderate Exacerbation
PEF 50-80% predicted or personal best
Persistent wheezing and shortness of breath
• Add oral corticosteroid
• Continue beta$_2$-agonist
Poor Response
Severe Exacerbation
PEF <50% predicted or personal best
Marked wheezing and shortness or breath
• Add oral corticosteroid
• Repeat beta$_2$-agonist immediately
• If distress is severe and nonresponsive, call your doctor and proceed to emergency department; consider calling ambulance or 9-1-1.
• Contact clinician for follow-up instructions
• Contact clinician urgently (this day) for instructions.
• Proceed to emergency department.

* Patients at high risk of asthma-related death should receive immediate clinical attention after initial treatment. Additional therapy may be required.

Management of Asthma Exacerbations: Emergency Department and Hospital-Based Care

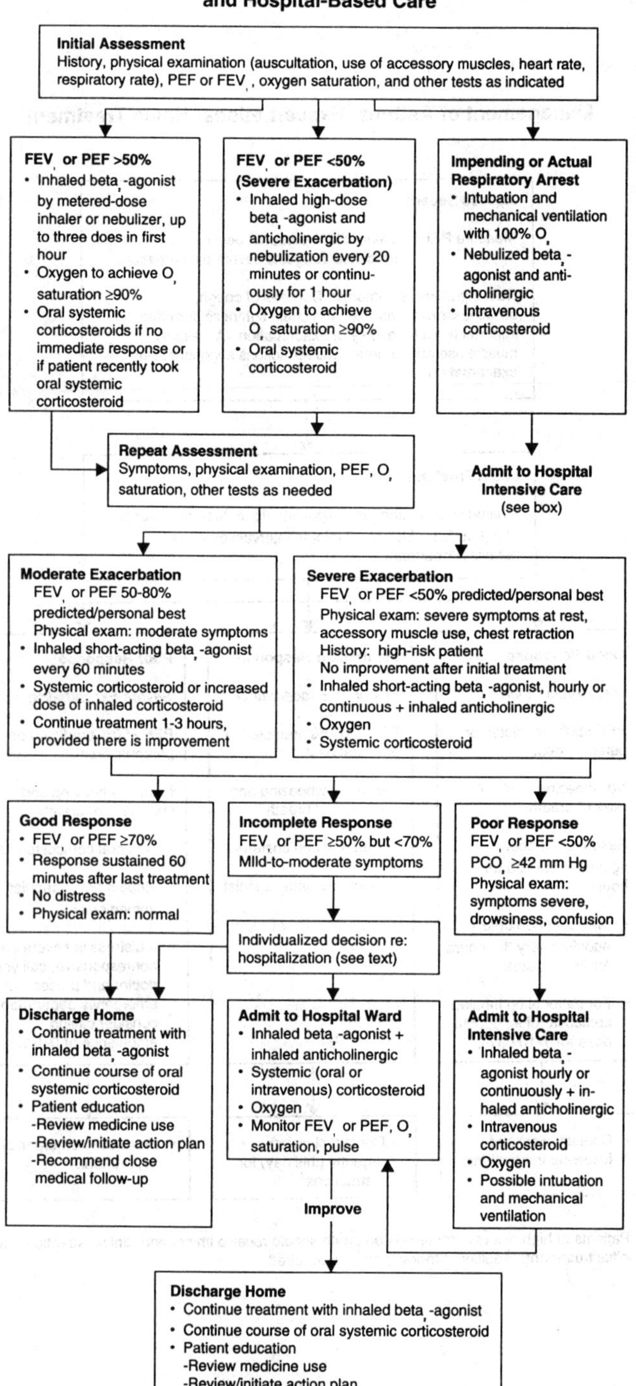

Initial Assessment
History, physical examination (auscultation, use of accessory muscles, heart rate, respiratory rate), PEF or FEV_1, oxygen saturation, and other tests as indicated
FEV_1 or PEF >50%
• Inhaled $beta_2$-agonist by metered-dose inhaler or nebulizer, up to three does in first hour
• Oxygen to achieve O_2 saturation ≥90%
• Oral systemic corticosteroids if no immediate response or if patient recently took oral systemic corticosteroid
FEV_1 or PEF <50% (Severe Exacerbation)
• Inhaled high-dose $beta_2$-agonist and anticholinergic by nebulization every 20 minutes or continuously for 1 hour
• Oxygen to achieve O_2 saturation ≥90%
• Oral systemic corticosteroid
Impending or Actual Respiratory Arrest
• Intubation and mechanical ventilation with 100% O_2
• Nebulized $beta_2$-agonist and anticholinergic
• Intravenous corticosteroid
Repeat Assessment
Symptoms, physical examination, PEF, O_2 saturation, other tests as needed
Admit to Hospital Intensive Care (see box)
Moderate Exacerbation
FEV_1 or PEF 50-80% predicted/personal best
Physical exam: moderate symptoms
• Inhaled short-acting $beta_2$-agonist every 60 minutes
• Systemic corticosteroid or increased dose of inhaled corticosteroid
• Continue treatment 1-3 hours, provided there is improvement
Severe Exacerbation
FEV_1 or PEF <50% predicted/personal best
Physical exam: severe symptoms at rest, accessory muscle use, chest retraction
History: high-risk patient
No improvement after initial treatment
• Inhaled short-acting $beta_2$-agonist, hourly or continuous + inhaled anticholinergic
• Oxygen
• Systemic corticosteroid
Good Response
• FEV_1 or PEF ≥70%
• Response sustained 60 minutes after last treatment
• No distress
• Physical exam: normal
Incomplete Response
FEV_1 or PEF ≥50% but <70%
Mild-to-moderate symptoms
Poor Response
FEV_1 or PEF <50%
PCO_2 ≥42 mm Hg
Physical exam: symptoms severe, drowsiness, confusion
Individualized decision re: hospitalization (see text)
Discharge Home
• Continue treatment with inhaled $beta_2$-agonist
• Continue course of oral systemic corticosteroid
• Patient education
-Review medicine use
-Review/initiate action plan
-Recommend close medical follow-up
Admit to Hospital Ward
• Inhaled $beta_2$-agonist + inhaled anticholinergic
• Systemic (oral or intravenous) corticosteroid
• Oxygen
• Monitor FEV_1 or PEF, O_2 saturation, pulse
Admit to Hospital Intensive Care
• Inhaled $beta_2$-agonist hourly or continuously + inhaled anticholinergic
• Intravenous corticosteroid
• Oxygen
• Possible intubation and mechanical ventilation
Improve
Discharge Home
• Continue treatment with inhaled $beta_2$-agonist
• Continue course of oral systemic corticosteroid
• Patient education
-Review medicine use
-Review/initiate action plan
-Recommend close medical follow-up

CONTRAST MEDIA REACTIONS, PREMEDICATION FOR PROPHYLAXIS AGAINST

(American College of Radiology Guidelines for Use of Nonionic Contrast Media)

It is estimated that approximately 5% to 10% of patients will experience adverse reactions to administration of contrast dye (less for nonionic contrast). In approximately 1000-2000 administrations, a life-threatening reaction will occur.

A variety of premedication regimens have been proposed, both for pretreatment of "at risk" patients who require contrast media and before the routine administration of the intravenous high osmolar contrast media. Such regimens have been shown in clinical trials to decrease the frequency of all forms of contrast medium reactions. Pretreatment with a 2-dose regimen of methylprednisolone 32 mg, 12 and 2 hours prior to intravenous administration of HOCM (ionic), has been shown to decrease mild, moderate, and severe reactions in patients at increased risk and perhaps in patients without risk factors. Logistical and feasibility problems may preclude adequate premedication with this or any regimen for all patients It is unclear at this time that steroid pretreatment prior to administration of ionic contrast media reduces the incidence of reactions to the same extent or less than that achieved with the use of nonionic contrast media alone. Information about the efficacy of nonionic contrast media combined with a premedication strategy, including steroids, is preliminary or not yet currently available. For high-risk patients (ie, previous contrast reactors), the combination of a pretreatment regimen with nonionic contrast media has empirical merit and may warrant consideration. Oral administration of steroids appears preferable to intravascular routes, and the drug may be prednisone or methylprednisolone. Supplemental administration of H_1 and H_2 antihistamine therapies, orally or intravenously, may reduce the frequency of urticaria, angioedema, and respiratory symptoms. Additionally, ephedrine administration has been suggested to decrease the frequency of contrast reactions, but caution is advised in patients with cardiac disease, hypertension, or hyperthyroidism. No premedication strategy should be a substitute for the ABC approach to preadministration preparedness listed above. Contrast reactions do occur despite any and all premedication prophylaxis. The incidence can be decreased, however, in some categories of "at risk" patients receiving high osmolar contrast media plus a medication regimen. For patients with previous contrast medium reactions, there is a slight chance that recurrence may be more severe or the same as the prior reaction, however, it is more likely that there will be no recurrence.

A general premedication regimen is

Methylprednisolone	32 mg orally at 12 and 2 hours prior to procedure
Diphenhydramine	50 mg orally 1 hour prior to the procedure

An alternative premedication regimen is

Prednisone	50 mg orally 13, 7, and 1 hour before the procedure
Diphenhydramine	50 mg orally 1 hour before the procedure
Ephedrine	25 mg orally 1 hour before the procedure (except when contraindicated)

Indication for nonionic contrast are

Previous reaction to contrast — premedicate*
Known allergy to iodine or shellfish
Asthma, especially if on medication
Myocardial instability or CHF
Risk for aspiration or severe nausea and vomiting
Difficulty communicating or inability to give history
Patients taking beta-blockers
Small children at risk for electrolyte imbalance or extravasation
Renal failure with diabetes, sickle cell disease, or myeloma
At physician or patient request

*Life-threatening reactions (throat swelling, laryngeal edema, etc), consider omitting the intravenous contrast.

CONVULSIVE STATUS EPILEPTICUS

Recommendations of the Epilepsy Foundation of America's Working Group on Status Epilepticus

(*JAMA*, 1993, 270:854-9)

Convulsive status epilepticus is an emergency that is associated with high morbidity and mortality. The outcome largely depends on etiology, but prompt and appropriate pharmacological therapy can reduce morbidity and mortality. Etiology varies in children and adults and reflects the distribution of disease in these age groups. Antiepileptic drug administration should be initiated whenever a seizure has lasted 10 minutes. Immediate concerns include supporting respiration, maintaining blood pressure, gaining intravenous access, and identifying and treating the underlying cause. Initial therapeutic and diagnostic measures are conducted simultaneously. The goal of therapy is rapid termination of clinical and electrical seizure activity; the longer a seizure continues, the greater the likelihood of an adverse outcome. Several drug protocols now in use will terminate status epilepticus. Common to all patients is the need for a clear plan, prompt administration of appropriate drugs in adequate doses, and attention to the possibility of apnea, hypoventilation, or other metabolic abnormalities.

Precipitants of Status Epilepticus

Precipitants	Children ≤16 y, %	Adults >16 y, %
Cerebrovascular	3.3	25.2
Medication change	19.8	18.9
Anoxia	5.3	10.7
Ethanol/drug-related	2.4	12.2
Metabolic	8.2	8.8
Unknown	9.3	8.1
Fever/infection	35.7	4.6
Trauma	3.5	4.6
Tumor	0.7	4.3
Central nervous system infection	4.8	1.8
Congenital	7.0	0.8

Diagnostic Studies in Status Epilepticus*

Initial (emergent) studies

- Glucose, electrolytes, BUN
- Oximetry or arterial blood gases
- Antiepileptic drug levels
- Lumbar puncture
- Complete blood count
- Urinalysis

Second-phase studies (follow stabilization)

- Liver function studies
- Toxicology screen
- EEG
- Brain imaging with CT or MRI scan

*BUN = blood urea nitrogen; EEG = electroencephalogram; CT = computed tomographic; MR = magnetic resonance imaging.

Major Drugs Used to Treat Status Epilepticus: I.V. Doses, Pharmacokinetics, and Major Toxicities

	Diazepam	Lorazepam	Phenytoin	Phenobarbital
Adult I.V. dose, mg/kg [total dose]	0.15-0.25	0.1 [4.8]	15-20	20
Pediatric I.V. dose, mg/kg [total dose]	0.1-1	0.05-0.5 [1.4 mg]	20	20
Pediatric per rectum dose, mg/kg	0.5 mg/kg (maximum: 20 mg)	–	–	–
Maximal administration rate, mg/min	5	2	50	100
Time to stop status, min	1-3	6-10	10-30	20-30
Effective duration of action, h	0.25-0.5	>12-24	24	>48
Elimination half-life, h	30	14	24	100
Volume of distribution, L/kg	1-2	0.7-1	0.5-0.8	0.7
Potential side effects				
Depression of consciousness	10-30 min	Several hours	None	Several days
Respiratory depression	Occasional	Occasional	Infrequent	Occasional
Hypotension	Infrequent	Infrequent	Occasional	Infrequent
Cardiac arrhythmias	-	-	In patients with heart disease	-

Suggested Timetable for the Treatment of Status Epilepticus*

Time (min)	Action†
0-5	Diagnose status epilepticus by observing continued seizure activity or one additional seizure
	Give oxygen by nasal cannula or mark; position patient's head for optimal airway patency; consider intubation if respiratory assistance is needed
	Obtain and record vital signs at onset and periodically thereafter; control any abnormalities as necessary; initiate EKG monitoring
	Establish an I.V.; draw venous blood samples for glucose level, serum chemistries, hematology studies, toxicology screens, and determinations of antiepileptic drug levels
	Assess oxygenation with oximetry or periodic arterial blood gas determinators
6-9	If hypoglycemia is established or a blood glucose determination is unavailable, administer glucose; in adults, give 100 mg of thiamine first, followed by 50 mL of 50% glucose by direct push into the I.V.; in children, the dose of glucose is 2 mL/kg of 25% glucose
10-20	Administer either 0.1 mg/kg of lorazepam at 2 mg/min or 0.2 mg/kg of diazepam at 5 mg/min by I.V.; if diazepam is given, it can be repeated if seizures do not stop after 5 min; if diazepam is used to stop the status, phenytoin should be administered next to prevent recurrent status
21-60	If status persists, administer 15-20 mg/kg of phenytoin no faster than 50 mg/min in adults and 1 mg/kg/min in children by I.V.; monitor EKG and blood pressure during the infusion; phenytoin is incompatible with glucose-containing solutions — the I.V. should be purged with normal saline before the phenytoin infusion
>60	If status does not stop after 20 mg/kg of phenytoin, give additional doses of 5 mg/kg to a maximal dose of 30 mg/kg
	If status persists, give 20 mg/kg of phenobarbital by I.V. at 100 mg/min; when phenobarbital is given after a benzodiazepine, the risk of apnea or hypopnea is great and assisted ventilation is usually required
	If status persists, give anesthetic doses of drugs such as phenobarbital or pentobarbital; ventilatory assistance and vasopressors are virtually always necessary.

*Time starts at seizure onset. Note that a neurological consultation is indicated if the patient does not wake up, convulsions continue after the administration of benzodiazepine and phenytoin, or confusion exists at any time during evaluation and treatment. Data modified from Treiman.

†EKG : electrocardiogram; I.V.: intravenous line

DIABETES MELLITUS TREATMENT

Insulin-Dependent Diabetes Mellitus

Treatment goals that emphasize glycemic control have been recommended by the American Diabetes Association (see table).

Glycemic Control for People With Diabetes

Biochemical Index	Nondiabetic	Goal	Action Suggested
Preprandial glucose	<115	80-120	<80 >140
Bedtime glucose (mg/dL)	<120	100-140	<100 >160
Hb A_{1C} (%)	<8	<7	>8

These values are for nonpregnant individuals.
Action suggested depends on individual patient circumstances, Hb A_{1C} referenced to a nondiabetic range of 4% to 6% (mean 5%, SD 0.5%).

Noninsulin-Dependent Diabetes Mellitus

Pharmacological Therapy of NIDDM - Consensus Statement

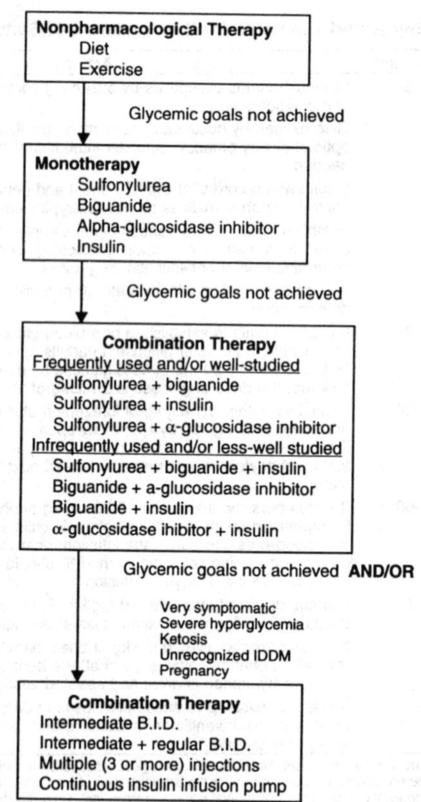

HEART FAILURE: MANAGEMENT OF PATIENTS WITH LEFT-VENTRICULAR SYSTOLIC DYSFUNCTION

Adapted from U.S. Department of Health & Human Services, the Agency for Healthcare Policy and Research (ACHPR) Publication No. 94-0613, June, 1994

Medications Commonly Used for Heart Failure

Drug	Initial Dose (mg)	Target Dose (mg)	Recommended Maximal Dose (mg)	Major Adverse Reactions
Thiazide Diuretics Chlorthalidone Hydrochlorothiazide	25 qd	As needed	50 qd	Postural hypotension, hypokalemia, hyperglycemia, hyperuricemia, rash; rare severe reaction includes pancreatitis, bone marrow suppression, and anaphylaxis
Loop Diuretics Bumetanide Ethacrynic acid Furosemide	0.5-1 qd 50 qd 10-40 qd	As needed	10 qd 200 bid 240 bid	Same as thiazide diuretics
Thiazide-Related Diuretic Metolazone	2.5*	As needed	10 qd	Same as thiazide diuretics
Potassium-Sparing Diuretics Amiloride Spironolactone Triamterene	5 qd 25 qd 50 qd	As needed	40 qd 100 bid 100 bid	Hyperkalemia (especially if administered with ACE inhibitor), rash, gynecomastia (spironolactone only)
ACE Inhibitors† Captopril	6.25-12.5 tid	50 tid	100 tid	Hypotension, hyperkalemia, renal insufficiency, cough, skin rash, angioedema, neutropenia
Enalapril	2.5 bid	10 bid	20 bid	
Fosinopril	10 qd	As needed	40 qd	
Lisinopril	5 qd	20 qd	40 qd	
Quinapril	5 bid	20 bid	20 bid	
Ramipril	2.5 qd	As needed	20 qd	
Digoxin	0.125 qd	As needed	As needed	Cardiotoxicity, confusion, nausea, anorexia, visual disturbances
Hydralazine	10-25 tid	75 tid	100 tid	Headache, nausea, dizziness, tachycardia. lupus-like syndrome
Isosorbide dinitrate	10 tid	40 tid	80 tid	Headache, hypotension, flushing

*Given as a single test dose initially.

†ACE inhibitors which have FDA approval to treat CHF

Note: ACE = angiotensin-converting enzyme

HELICOBACTER PYLORI TREATMENT

Multiple Drug Regimens for the Treatment of *H. pylori* Infection

Drug	Dosages*	Duration of Therapy
Regimen 1†		
Bismuth subsalicylate (Pepto-Bismol®)	Two 262 mg tablets 4 times/day	2 weeks
plus		
Metronidazole (Flagyl®)	250 mg 3 or 4 times/day	2 weeks
plus		
Tetracycline (various) or amoxicillin (Amoxil®, others)	250-500 mg 4 times/day	2 weeks
plus		
Histamine H_2-receptor antagonist	Full dose‡ at bedtime	4-6 weeks
Regimen 2		
Metronidazole (Flagyl®)	500 mg 3 times/day	12-14 days
plus		
Amoxicillin (Amoxil®, others)	750 mg 3 times/day	12-14 days
plus		
Histamine H_2-receptor antagonist	Full dose†at bedtime	6-10 weeks
Regimen 3		
Bismuth subsalicylate (Pepto-Bismol®)	Two 262 mg tablets 4 times/day	2 weeks
plus		
Tetracycline (various)	500 mg 4 times/day	2 weeks
plus		
Clarithromycin (Biaxin™)	500 mg 3 times/day	2 weeks
plus		
Histamine H_2-receptor antagonist	Full dose† after evening meal	6 weeks
Regimen 4		
Omeprazole (Prilosec™)	20 mg twice daily	2 weeks
plus		
Amoxicillin (Amoxil®, others)	1 g twice daily or 500 mg 4 times/day	2 weeks
Regimen 5		
Omeprazole (Prilosec™)	20 mg twice daily	2 weeks
plus		
Clarithromycin (Biaxin™)	250 mg twice a day or 500 mg 2 or 3 times/day	2 weeks
Regimen 6		
Ranitidine bismuth citrate (Tritec™)	400 mg twice daily	4 weeks
plus		
Clarithromycin (Biaxin™)	500 mg 3 times/day	2 weeks

*All therapies are oral and begin concurrently.

†Marketed as Helidac®, a packet containing 262.4 mg bismuth subsalicylate, 25 mg metronidazole and 500 mg tetracycline; an H_2-antagonist must be purchased separately.

‡Full dose refers to the dosage used to treat acute ulcers, not to the maintenance dose.

THERAPY OF HYPERLIPIDEMIA

(*JAMA*, 1993, 269(23), 3015-23)

Risk Status Based on Presence of CHD Risk Factors Other Than Low-Density Lipoprotein Cholesterol*

Positive Risk Factors

Male ≥45 y

Female ≥55 y or premature menopause without estrogen replacement therapy

Family history of premature CHD (definite myocardial infarction or sudden death before 55 y of age in father or other male first-degree relative, or before 65 y of age in mother or other female first-degree relative)

Current cigarette smoking

Hypertension (blood pressure ≥140/90 mm Hg†, or taking antihypertensive medication)

Low HDL cholesterol (<35 mg/dL† [0.9 mmol/L])

Diabetes mellitus

Negative Risk Factor‡

High HDL cholesterol (≥60 mg/dL [1.6 mmol/L])

*High risk, defined as a net of two or more coronary heart disease (CHD) risk factors, leads to more vigorous intervention, shown in Figures 1 and 2. Age (defined differently for men and women) is treated as a risk factor because rates of CHD are higher in the elderly than in the young, and in men than in women of the same age. Obesity is not listed as a risk factor because it operates through other risk factors that are included (hypertension, hyperlipidemia, decreased high-density lipoprotein [HDL] cholesterol, and diabetes mellitus), but it should be considered a target for intervention. Physical inactivity is similarly not listed as a risk factor, but it too should be considered a target for intervention, and physical activity is recommended as desirable for everyone. High risk due to coronary or peripheral atherosclerosis is addressed directly in Figure 3.

†Confirmed by measurements on several occasions.

‡If the HDL cholesterol level is ≥60 mg/dL (1.6 mmol/L), subtract one risk factor (because high HDL cholesterol levels decrease CHD risk)

Initial Classification Based on Total Cholesterol and HDL Cholesterol Levels*

Cholesterol Level		Initial Classification
Total Cholesterol		
<200 mg/dL	(5.2 mmol/L)	Desirable blood cholesterol
200-239 mg/dL	(5.2-6.2 mmol/L)	Borderline-high blood cholesterol
≥240 mg/dL	(6.2 mmol/L)	High blood cholesterol
HDL Cholesterol		
<35 mg/dL	(0.9 mmol/L)	Low HDL cholesterol

HDL indicated high-density lipoprotein.

Summary of the Second Report of the National Cholesterol Education Program (NCEP) Expert Panel on Detection, Evaluation, and Treatment of High Blood Cholesterol in Adults (Adult Treatment Panel II)

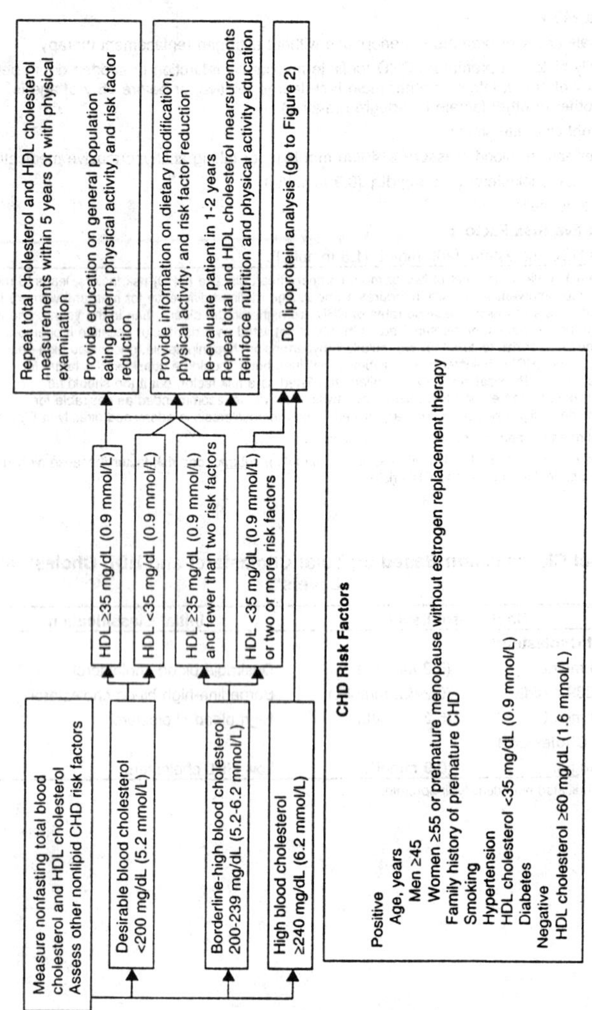

Fig. 1 - Primary prevention in adults without evidence of coronary heart disease (CHD). Initial classification is based on total cholesterol and high-density lipoprotein (HDL) cholesterol levels.

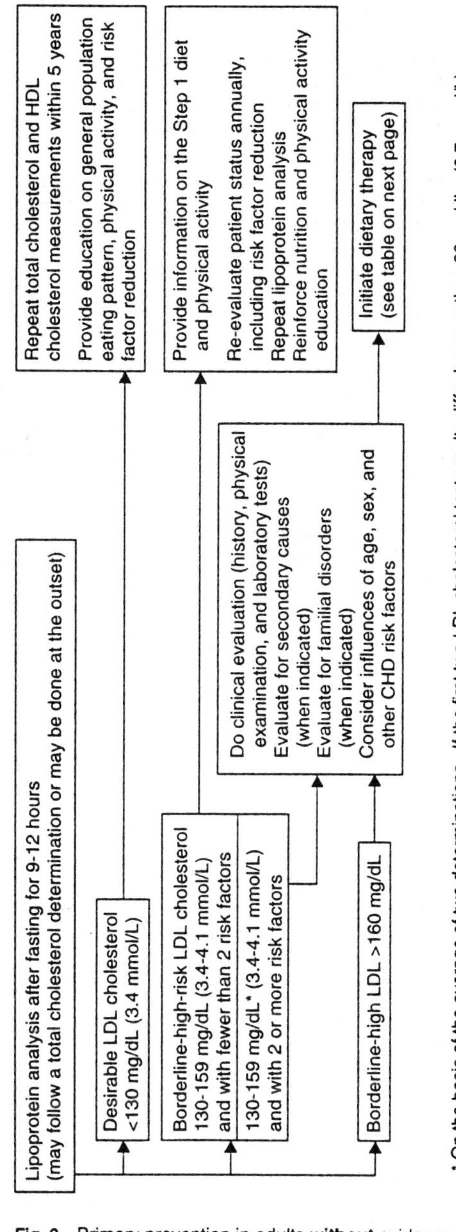

Fig. 2 - Primary prevention in adults **without** evidence of coronary heart disease (CHD). Subsequent classification is based on low-density lipoprotein (LDL) cholesterol level.

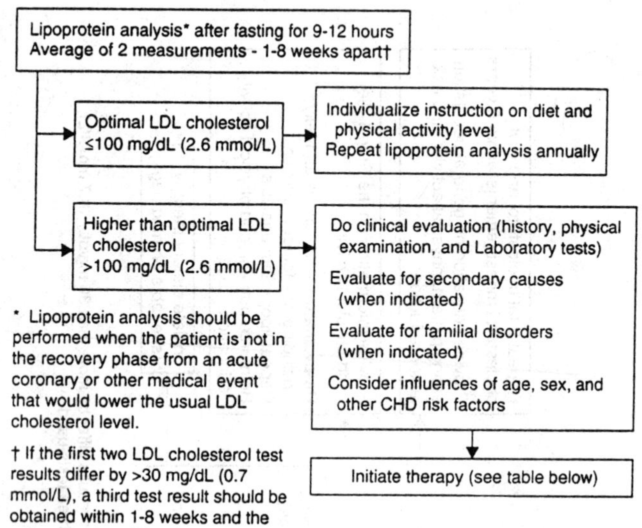
Lipoprotein analysis* after fasting for 9-12 hours
Average of 2 measurements - 1-8 weeks apart†
Optimal LDL cholesterol
≤100 mg/dL (2.6 mmol/L)
Individualize instruction on diet and physical activity level
Repeat lipoprotein analysis annually
Higher than optimal LDL cholesterol
>100 mg/dL (2.6 mmol/L)
Do clinical evaluation (history, physical examination, and Laboratory tests)
Evaluate for secondary causes (when indicated)
Evaluate for familial disorders (when indicated)
Consider influences of age, sex, and other CHD risk factors
Initiate therapy (see table below)

* Lipoprotein analysis should be performed when the patient is not in the recovery phase from an acute coronary or other medical event that would lower the usual LDL cholesterol level.

† If the first two LDL cholesterol test results differ by >30 mg/dL (0.7 mmol/L), a third test result should be obtained within 1-8 weeks and the average value of the 3 tests used.

Fig. 3 - Secondary prevention in adults **with** evidence of coronary heart disease (CHD). Classification is based on low-density lipoprotein (LDL) cholesterol level.

Treatment Decisions Based on LDL Cholesterol Level*

Patient Category	Initiation Level	LDL Goal
Dietary Therapy		
Without CHD and with fewer than two risk factors	≥160 mg/dL (4.1 mmol/L)	<160 mg/dL (4.1 mmol/L)
Without CHD and with two or more risk factors	≥130 mg/dL (3.4 mmol/L)	<130 mg/dL (3.4 mmol/L)
With CHD	>100 mg/dL (2.6 mmol/L)	≤100 mg/dL (2.6 mmol/L)
Drug Treatment		
Without CHD and with fewer than two risk factors	≥190 mg/dL (4.9 mmol/L)	<160 mg/dL (4.1 mmol/L)
Without CHD and with two or more risk factors	≥160 mg/dL (4.1 mmol/L)	<130 mg/dL (3.4 mmol/L)
With CHD	≥130 mg/dL (3.4 mmol/L)	≤100 mg/dL (2.6 mmol/L)

*LDL: low-density lipoprotein; CHD: coronary heart disease

Classification of Serum Triglyceride Levels

Classification	Serum Triglyceride Concentration
Normal	≤200 mg/dL
Borderline-high	200-400 mg/dL
High	400-1000 mg/dL
Very high	>1000 mg/dL

NCEP Stepped Approach for Dietary Modification

Nutrient	Step 1 Diet (% total kcal)	Step 2 Diet (% total kcal)
Total fat	<30	<30
saturated	<10	<7
polyunsaturated	Up to 10	Up to 10
monounsaturated	10-15	10-15
Carbohydrates	50-60	50-60
Protein	10-20	10-20
Cholesterol	<300 mg/d	<200 mg/d
Total calories	qs to maintain desirable wt	qs to maintain desirable wt

THERAPY OF HYPERTENSION

Classification of Hypertension in the Young by Age Group*

Age Group	High Normal (90-94th Percentile) mm Hg	Significant Hypertension (95-99th Percentile) mm Hg	Severe Hypertension (>99th Percentile) mm Hg
Newborns (systolic)			
7 d		96-105	≥106
8-30 d		104-109	≥110
Infants (≤2 y)			
systolic	104-111	112-117	≥118
diastolic	70-73	74-81	≥82
Children			
3-5 y			
systolic	108-115	116-123	≥124
diastolic	70-75	76-83	≥84
6-9 y			
systolic	114-121	122-129	≥130
diastolic	74-77	78-85	≥86
10-12 y			
systolic	122-125	126-133	≥134
diastolic	78-81	82-89	≥90
13-15 y			
systolic	130-135	136-143	≥144
diastolic	80-85	86-91	≥92
Adolescents (16-18 y)			
systolic	136-141	142-149	≥150
diastolic	84-91	92-97	≥96

*Adapted from the "Report of the Second Task Force on Blood Pressure Control in Children, 1987. Note that adult classifications differ.

The Fifth Report of the Joint National Committee on Detection, Evaluation, and Treatment of High Blood Pressure (JNC V) (*Arch Intern Med*, 1993:153)

Classification of Blood Pressure for Adults Aged 18 Years and Older*

Category	Systolic (mm Hg)	Diastolic (mm Hg)
Normal†	<130	<85
High normal	130-139	85-89
Hypertension‡		
Stage 1 (mild)	140-159	90-99
Stage 2 (moderate)	160-179	100-109
Stage 3 (severe)	180-209	110-119
Stage 4 (very severe)	≥210	≥120

*Not taking antihypertensive drugs and not acutely ill. When systolic and diastolic pressures fall into different categories, the higher category should be selected to classify the individual's blood pressure status. For instance, 160/92 mm Hg should be classified as stage 2, and 180/120 mm Hg should be classified as stage 4. Isolated systolic hypertension is defined as a systolic blood pressure ≥140 mm Hg and a diastolic blood pressure <90 mm Hg and staged appropriately (eg, 170/85 mm Hg is defined as stage 2 isolated systolic hypertension).

In addition to classifying stages of hypertension on the basis of average blood pressure levels, the clinician should specify presence or absence of target-organ disease and additional risk factors. For example, a patient with diabetes and a blood pressure of 142/94 mm Hg, plus left ventricular hypertrophy should be classified as having "stage 1 hypertension with target-organ disease (left ventricular hypertrophy) and with another major risk factor (diabetes)." This specificity is important for risk classification and management.

†Optimal blood pressure with respect to cardiovascular risk is <120 mm Hg systolic and <80 mm Hg diastolic. However, unusually low readings should be evaluated for clinical significance.

‡Based on the average of two or more readings taken at each of two or more visits after an initial screening.

Recommendations for Follow-up Based on Initial Set of Blood Pressure Measurements for Adults

Initial Screening Blood Pressure (mm Hg)*		
Systolic	**Diastolic**	**Follow-up Recommended†**
<130	<85	Recheck in 2 y
130-139	85-89	Recheck in 1 y‡
140-159	90-99	Confirm within 2 mo
160-179	100-109	Evaluate or refer to source of care within 1 mo
180-209	110-119	Evaluate or refer to source of care within 1 wk
≥210	≥120	Evaluate or refer to source of care immediately

*If the systolic and diastolic categories are different, follow recommendation for the shorter time follow-up (eg, 160/85 mm Hg should be evaluated or referred to source of care within 1 month).

†The scheduling of follow-up should be modified by reliable information about past blood pressure measurements, other cardiovascular risk factors, or target-organ disease.

‡Consider providing advice about life-style modifications.

Pharmacologic Treatment

The decision to initiate pharmacologic treatment in individual patients requires consideration of several factors: severity of blood pressure elevation, TOD, and presence of other conditions and risk factors.

Lifestyle modifications:
Weight reduction
Moderation of alcohol intake
Regular physical activity
Reduction of sodium intake
Smoking cessation

Inadequate response*

Continue lifestyle modifications
Initial pharmacologic selection:
Diuretics or beta blockers are preferred because reduction in morbidity and mortality has been demonstrated.

ACE inhibitors, calcium antagonists, alpha-receptor blockers, and alpha/beta blocker have not been tested nor shown to reduce morbidity and mortality.

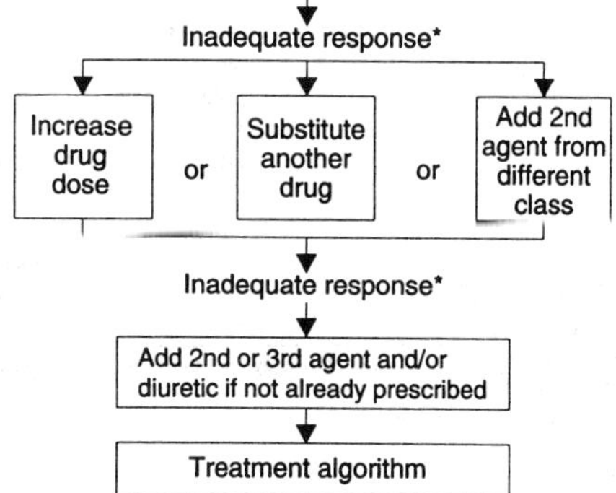

Antihypertensive Drug Therapy: Individualization Based on Special Considerations (Guidelines for Selecting Initial Therapy)*

Clinical Situation	Preferred	Requires Special Monitoring	Relatively or Absolutely Contraindicated
Cardiovascular			
Angina pectoris	B-blockers, calcium antagonists		Direct vasodilators
Bradycardia/heart block, sick-sinus syndrome			B-blockers, labetalol, verapamil, diltiazem
Cardiac failure (systolic)	Diuretics, ACE inhibitors		B-blockers, calcium antagonists, labetalol
Cardiac failure (diastolic)	B-blockers, calcium antagonists		
Hypertrophic cardiomyopathy with severe diastolic dysfunction	B-blockers, diltiazem, verapamil		Diuretics, ACE inhibitors, α_1-blockers, hydralazine, minoxidil
Hyperdynamic circulation	B-blockers		Direct vasodilators
Peripheral vascular occlusive disease		B-blockers	
After myocardial infarction	Non-ISA B-blockers**		Direct vasodilators
Renal			
Bilateral renal arterial disease or severe stenosis in artery to solitary kidney			ACE inhibitors
Renal insufficiency			
Early (serum creatinine, 130-221 μmol/L [1.5-2.5 mg/dL]			Potassium-sparing agents, potassium supplements
Advanced (serum creatinine, ≥221 μmol/L [≥2.5 mg/dL]	Loop diuretics	ACE inhibitors	Potassium-sparing agents, potassium supplements
Other			
Asthma/COPD			B-blockers, labetalol
Cyclosporine-associated hypertension	Nifedipine, labetalol	Verapamil†, nicardipine†, diltiazem†	
Depression		α_2-agonists	Reserpine
Diabetes mellitus	α-blockers		
Type I (insulin dependent)		B-blockers	
Type II		B-blockers, diuretics	
Dyslipidemia		B-blockers, diuretics	
Liver disease		Labetalol	Methyldopa
Pregnancy			
Preeclampsia	Methyldopa, hydralazine		Diuretics, ACE inhibitors
Chronic hypertension	Methyldopa		ACE inhibitors
Vascular headache	B-blockers		

*ACE = angiotensin-converting enzyme; ISA = intrinsic sympathomimetic activity; COPD = chronic obstructive pulmonary disease

†Can increase serum levels of cyclosporine

**IDS blockers = acebutolol, cardilol, and penbutolol

General Treatment Principles in the Treatment of Hypertensive Emergencies

Principle	Considerations
Admit the patient to the hospital, preferably in the intensive care unit. Monitor vital signs appropriately.	• Establish intravenous access and place patient on a cardiac monitor. • Place a femoral intra-arterial line and pulmonary arterial catheter, if indicated, to assess cardiopulmonary function and intravascular volume status.
Perform rapid but thorough history and physical examination.	• Determine cause of, or precipitating factors to, hypertensive crisis if possible (remember to obtain a medication history including Rx, OTC, and illicit drugs). • Obtain details regarding any prior history of hypertension (severity, duration, treatment), as well as other coexisting illnesses. • Assess the extent of hypertensive end organ damage. • Determine if a hypertensive urgency or emergency exists.
Determine goal blood pressure based on premorbid level, duration, severity and rapidity of increase of blood pressure, concomitant medical conditions, race, and age.	• Acute decreases in blood pressure to normal or subnormal levels during the initial treatment period may reduce perfusion to the brain, heart, and kidneys, and must be avoided except in specific instances (ie, dissecting aortic aneurysm) • Gradually establish a normal (or reasonable) blood pressure over the next 1 to 2 weeks.
Select an appropriate antihypertensive regimen depending on the individual patient and clinical setting.	• Initiate a controlled decrease in blood pressure. Avoid concomitant administration of multiple agents that may cause precipitous falls in blood pressure. • Select the agent with the best hemodynamic profile based on the primary treatment goal. • Avoid diuretics and sodium restriction during the initial treatment period unless there is a clear clinical indication (ie, CHF, pulmonary edema). • Avoid sedating antihypertensives in patients with hypertensive encephalopathy, CVA, or other CNS disorders in whom mental status must be monitored. • Use caution with direct vasodilating agents that induce reflex tachycardia or increase cardiac output in patients with coronary heart disease, history of angina or myocardial infarction, or dissecting aortic aneurysm. • Preferably choose an agent that does not adversely affect glomerular filtration rate or renal blood flow. • Preferably choose agents that have favorable effects on cerebral blood flow and its autoregulation, especially patients with hypertensive encephalopathy or CVAs. • Select the most efficacious agent with the fewest adverse effects based on the underlying cause of the hypertensive crisis and other individual patient factors.
Initiate a chronic antihypertensive regimen after the patient's blood pressure is stabilized	• Begin oral antihypertensive therapy once goal blood pressure is achieved before gradually tapering parenteral medications. • Select the best oral regimen based on cost, ease of administration, adverse effect profile, and concomitant medical conditions.

Oral Agents Used in the Treatment of Hypertensive Urgencies and Emergencies

Drug	Dose	Onset	Cautions
Captopril*	P.O.: 25 mg, repeat as required	15-30 min	Hypotension, renal failure in bilateral renal artery stenosis
Clonidine	P.O.: 0.1-0.2 mg, repeated every hour as needed to a total dose of 0.6 mg	30-60 min	Hypotension, drowsiness, dry mouth
Labetalol	P.O.: 200-400 mg, repeat every 2-3 h	30 min to 2 h	Bronchoconstriction, heart block, orthostatic hypotension

*There is no clearly defined clinical advantage in the use of sublingual over oral routes of administration with these agents.

Recommendations for the Use of Intravenous Antihypertensive Drugs in Selected Hypertensive Emergencies

Condition	Agent(s) of Choice	Agent(s) to Avoid or Use With Caution	General Treatment Principle
Hypertensive encephalopathy	Nitroprusside, labetalol, diazoxide	Methyldopa, reserpine	Avoid drugs with CNS sedating effects
Acute intracranial or subarachnoid hemorrhage	Nicardipine*, nitroprusside, trimethaphan	Beta blockers	Careful titration with a short-acting agent
Cerebral infarction	Nicardipine*, nitroprusside, labetalol, trimethaphan	Beta blockers, minoxidil, diazoxide	Careful titration with a short-acting agent. Avoid agents that may decrease cerebral blood flow.
Head trauma	Esmolol, labetalol	Methyldopa, reserpine, nitroprusside, nitroglycerin, hydralazine	Avoid drugs with CNS sedating effects, or those that may increase intracranial pressure
Acute myocardial infarction, myocardial ischemia	Nitroglycerin, nicardipine* (calcium channel blockers), labetalol	Hydralazine, diazoxide, minoxidil	Avoid drugs which cause reflex tachycardia and increased myocardial oxygen consumption
Acute pulmonary edema	Nitroprusside, nitroglycerin, loop diuretics	Beta blockers (labetalol), minoxidil, methyldopa	Avoid drugs which may cause sodium and water retention and edema exacerbation
Renal dysfunction	Hydralazine, calcium channel blockers	Nitroprusside, ACE inhibitors, beta blockers (labetalol)	Avoid drugs with increased toxicity in renal failure and those that may cause decreased renal blood flow.
Eclampsia	Hydralazine, labetalol, nitroprusside†	Trimethaphan, diuretics, diazoxide (diazoxide may cause cessation of labor)	Avoid drugs that may cause adverse fetal effects, compromise placental circulation, or decrease cardiac output.
Pheochromocytoma	Phentolamine, nitroprusside, beta blockers (eg, esmolol) only after alpha blockade (phentolamine)	Beta blockers in the absence of alpha blockade, methyldopa, minoxidil	Use drugs of proven efficacy and specificity. Unopposed beta blockade may exacerbate hypertension.
Dissecting aortic aneurysm	Nitroprusside and beta blockade, trimethaphan	Hydralazine, diazoxide, minoxidil	Avoid drugs which may increase cardiac output.
Postoperative hypertension	Nitroprusside, nicardipine*, labetalol	Trimethaphan	Avoid drugs which may exacerbate postoperative ileus.

*The use of nicardipine in these situations is by the recommendation of the author based on a review of the literature.

†Reserve nitroprusside for eclamptic patients with life-threatening hypertension unresponsive to other agents due to the potential risk to the fetus (cyanide and thiocyanate metabolites may cross the placenta).

Parenteral Agents Used in the Treatment of Hypertensive Emergencies

Drug	Mechanism of Action	Onset	Duration	Dosage	Adverse Effect and Cautionary Statements
Direct Acting Vasodilators					
Diazoxide Hyperstat®	Produces direct smooth muscle relaxation resulting in decreased blood pressure	1-5 min	6-12 h	50-150 mg as I.V. bolus, repeated, or 15-30 mg/min by I.V. infusion	Hypotension, tachycardia, aggravation of angina pectoris, nausea and vomiting, fluid retention, hyperglycemia with repeated injections
Hydralazine (Apresoline®)	Direct vasodilatation of arterioles (little effect on veins) causing decreased systemic resistance	I.V.: 10-30 min I.M.: 20-30 min	2-6 h	10-20 mg as I.V. bolus 10-40 mg I.M.	Tachycardia, headache, vomiting, aggravation of angina pectoris, local thrombophlebitis
Nitroglycerin (Tridil®)	Peripheral vasodilatation by direct action on venous and arteriolar smooth muscle, thus decreasing peripheral resistance	1-5 min	3-5 min	5-200 mcg/min as I.V. infusion	Headache, tachycardia, nausea and vomiting; requires special delivery system due to PVC binding; tolerance may develop with use ≥24 hours
Sodium nitroprusside (Nipride®)	Relaxation of vascular smooth muscle with dilation of peripheral arteries and veins	Instantaneous	2-3 min	0.25-10 mcg/kg/min as I.V. infusion; maximal dose for 10 minutes only	Hypotension, tachycardia, nausea, vomiting, muscle twitching; increased risk of thiocyanate/cyanide toxicity with renal and hepatic insufficiency; must shield from light
Adrenergic Agonists					
Esmolol (Brevibloc®)	Competitively blocks $beta_2$ and $beta_2$ adrenergic stimulation ($beta_2$ at high doses only)	2-10 min	10-30 min	I.V. infusion: LD: 500 mcg/kg x 1, then 50 mcg/kg/min x 4 min MD: 50-200 mcg/kg/min	Asymptomatic hypotension, bradycardia, phlebitis, dizziness, peripheral ischemia; extreme caution in patients with hyperreactive airway disease; usually useful only as adjunctive agent

(continued)

Drug	Mechanism of Action	Onset	Duration	Dosage	Adverse Effect and Cautionary Statements
Labetalol (Normodyne®, Trandate®)	Competitively blocks $alpha_1$, $beta_1$, and $beta_2$, adrenergic sites	5-10 min	3-6 h	20-80 mg as I.V. bolus every 10 min; 2 mg/min as I.V. infusion	Bronchoconstriction, heart block, orthostatic hypotension, vomiting; may not be effective in patients receiving α- or B-antagonist
Methyldopa (Aldomet®)	False transmitter stimulates central inhibitory α-adrenergic receptors resulting in decreased sympathetic outflow to peripheral vasculature and heart	30-60 min	12-24 h	250-1000 mg as I.V. infusion q6h	Drowsiness, peripheral edema, dry mouth, orthostatic hypotension, bradycardia, hemolytic anemia
Phentolamine (Regitine®)	Competitively blocks (α-adrenergic receptors to produce brief antagonism of epinephrine and norepinephrine)	1-2 min	15-30 min	5-15 mg as I.V. bolus	Tachycardia, orthostatic hypotension, arrhythmias, nausea, vomiting, paradoxical pressor response; may cause ischemic cardiac events, including MI
Calcium Channel Blocking Agent					
Nicardipine (Cardene®)	Inhibits the transmembrane influx of calcium ions into smooth muscle and cardiac muscle, thus producing vascular smooth muscle relaxation and coronary vasodilatation	1-5 min	3-6 h	Initial I.V. infusion of 5 mg/h up to 15 mg/h; after BP goal achieved, decrease to 3 mg/h	Hypotension, headache, tachycardia, nausea, vomiting; limited experience with use in hypertensive emergency
Angiotensin Converting Enzyme (ACE) Inhibitor					
Enalaprilat (Vasotec®)	Competitive ACE inhibition; prevents conversion of angiotensin I to angiotensin II (a potent vasoconstrictor)	15-60 min	12-24 h	0.625-1.25 mg IVPB q6h	Hypotension, chest pain, tachycardia, headache, hyperkalemia, neutropenia; caution in patients with impaired renal function or hypovolemia; limited experience with use in hypertensive emergencies

MANAGEMENT OF OVERDOSAGES

Poison Control Center Antidote Chart

Antidote	Poison/Drug	Indications	Dosage	Comments
Acetylcysteine (Mucomyst®)	Acetaminophen	Unknown quantity ingested and <24 hours have elapsed since the time of ingestion or unable to obtain serum acetaminophen levels within 12 hours of ingestion. >7.5 g acetaminophen acutely ingested Serum acetaminophen level >140 μg/mL at 4 hours postingestion Ingested dose >140 mg/kg	Dilute to 5% solutions with carbonated beverage, fruit juice, or water and administer orally. **Loading:** 140 mg/kg for 1 dose **Maintenance:** 70 mg/kg for 17 doses, starting 4 hours after the loading dose and given every 4 hours	SGOT, SGPT, bilirubin, prothrombin time, creatinine, BUN, blood sugar, and electrolytes should be obtained daily if a toxic serum acetaminophen level has been determined. **Note:** Activated charcoal has been shown to absorb acetylcysteine *in vitro* and may do so in patients. Serum acetaminophen levels may not peak until 4 hours postingestion, and therefore, serum levels should not be drawn earlier.
Amyl nitrate, sodium nitrate, sodium thiosulfate (cyanide antidote package)	Cyanide	Begin treatment at the first sign of toxicity if exposure is known or strongly expected.	Break ampul of amyl nitrate and allow patient to inhale for 15 seconds, then take away for 15 seconds. Use a fresh ampul every 3 minutes. Continue until injection of sodium nitrate (3% solution) 300 mg (0.15-0.33 mL/kg over 5 minutes in pediatric patients) can be injected at 2.5-5 mL/minute. Then immediately inject 12.5 g 25% sodium thiosulfate, slow I.V. (1.65 mL/kg in children).	If symptoms return, treatment may be repeated at half the normal dosages. For pediatric dosing see package insert. Do **not** use methylene blue to reduce elevated methemoglobin levels. Oxygen therapy may be useful when combined with sodium thiosulfate therapy.
Antivenin (*Crotalidae*) polyvalent (equine origin)	Pit viper bites (rattlesnakes, cotton-mouths, copperheads)	Mild, moderate, or severe symptoms and history of envenomation by a pit viper **Mild:** Local swelling, (progressive) pain, no systemic systems **Moderate:** Ecchymosis and swelling beyond the bite site, some systemic symptoms and/or lab changes **Severe:** Profound edema involving entire extremity, cyanosis, serious systemic involvement, significant lab changes	**Mild:** 3-5 vials of antivenin in 250-500 mL NS **Moderate:** 6-10 vials of antivenin in 500 mL NS **Severe:** Minimum of 10 vials in 500-1000 mL NS Administer over 4-6 hours. Additional antivenin should be given on the basis of clinical response and continuing assessment of severity of the poisoning.	Draw blood for type and crossmatch, hematocrit, BUN, electrolytes, CBC, platelets, coagulation profile. Do **not** administer heparin for possible allergic reaction. A tetanus shot should also be given.

(continued)

Antidote	Poison/Drug	Indications	Dosage	Comments
Atropine	Organophosphate and carbamate insecticides, mushrooms containing muscarine (inocybe or clitocybe)	Myoclonic seizures, severe hallucinations, weakness, arrhythmias, excessive salivation, involuntary urination, and defecation	**Children:** I.V.: 0.05 mg/kg **Adults:** I.V.: 1-2 mg Repeat dosage every 10 minutes until patient is atropinized (normal pulse, dilated pupils, absence of rales, dry mouth)	Caution should be used in patients with narrow-angle glaucoma, cardiovascular disease, or pregnancy. Plasma and/or erythrocyte cholinesterase levels will be depressed from normal. Atropine should only be used when indicated; otherwise, use may result in anticholinergic poisoning. For organophosphate poisoning, large doses of atropine may be required.
Calcium EDTA (calcium disodium versenate)	Lead	Symptomatic patients or asymptomatic children with blood levels >50µg/dL	50-75 mg/kg/day deep I.M. or slow I.V. infusion in 3-6 divided doses for up to 5 days	If urine flow is not established, hemodialysis must accompany calcium EDTA dosing. In most cases, the I.M. route is preferred.
Calcium gluconate	Hydrofluoric acid (HF), magnesium	Calcium gluconate gel 2.5% for dermal exposures of HF <20% concentration S.C. injections of calcium gluconate for dermal exposures of HF in >20% concentration or failure to respond to calcium gluconate gel	Massage 2.5% gel into exposed area for 15 minutes. Infiltrate each square centimeter of exposed area with 0.5 mL of 10% calcium gluconate S.C. using a 30-gauge needle. 1 mL/kg I.V. of a 10% solution for magnesium toxicity (intra-arterial injection)	Injections of calcium gluconate should not be used in digital area. With exposures to dilute concentrations of HF, symptoms may take several hours to develop. Calcium gluconate gel is not currently available. Contact your regional poison control center for compounding instructions.
Deferoxamine (Desferal®)	Iron	Serum iron >350 µg/dL. Inability to obtain serum iron in a reasonable time and patient is symptomatic.	**Mild symptoms:** I.M.: 10 mg/kg up to 1 g every 8 hours **Severe symptoms:** I.V.: 10-15 mg/kg/hour not to exceed 6 g in 24 hours; rates up to 35 mg/kg have been given.	Passing of vin rose-colored urine indicates free iron was present. Therapy should be discontinued when urine returns to normal color. Monitor for hypotension, especially when giving deferoxamine I.V.

(continued)

Antidote	Poison/Drug	Indications	Dosage	Comments
Digoxin immune Fab (ovine), (Digibind®)	Digoxin, digitoxin, oleander, foxglove, lily-of-the-valley (?), red squill (?)	Life-threatening cardiac arrhythmias, progressive bradyarrhythmias, second or third degree heart block unresponsive to atropine, serum digoxin level >5 ng/mL, potassium levels >5 mEq/L, or ingestion of >10 mg in adults (or 4 mg in children).	Multiply serum digoxin concentration at steady-state level by 5.6 and multiply the result by the patient's weight in kilograms, divide this by 1000 and divide the result by 0.6. This gives the dose in number of vials to use. For other dosing methods, see package insert.	Monitor potassium levels, continuous EKG. **Note:** Digibind® interferes with serum digoxin/digitoxin levels.
Dimercaprol (BAL in oil)	Arsenic, lead, mercury, gold, trivalent antimony, methyl bromide, methyl iodide	Any symptoms due to arsenic exposure All patients with symptoms or asymptomatic children with blood levels >70 mcg/d Any symptoms due to mercury and patient unable to take D-penicillamine	3-5 mg/kg/dose deep I.M. every 4 hours until GI symptoms subside and patient switched to D-penicillamine 3-5 mg/kg/dose deep I.M. every 4 hours for 2 days then every 4-12 hours for up to 7 additional days 3-5 mg/kg/dose deep I.M. every 4 hours for 48 hours, then 3 mg/kg/dose every 6 hours, then 3 mg/kg/dose every 12 hours for 7 more days	Patients receiving dimercaprol should be monitored for hypertension, tachycardia, hyperpyrexia, and urticaria. Used in conjunction with calcium EDTA in lead poisoning.
Ethanol	Ethylene glycol or methanol	Ethylene glycol or methanol blood levels >20 mg/dL Blood levels not readily available and suspected ingestion of toxic amounts Any symptomatic patient with a history of ethylene glycol or methanol ingestion	**Loading dose:** I.V.: 7.5-10 mL/kg 10% ethanol in D_5W over 1 hour **Maintenance dose:** I.V.: 1.4 mL/kg/hour of 10% ethanol in D_5W. Maintain blood ethanol level of 100-200 mg/dL.	Monitor blood glucose, especially in children, as ethanol may cause hypoglycemia. Do not use 5% ethanol in D_5W as excessive amounts of fluid would be required to maintain adequate ethanol blood levels. If dialysis is performed, adjustment of ethanol dosing is required.
Flumazenil (Romazicon®)	Benzodiazepine	As adjunct to conventional management/ diagnosis of benzodiazepine overdose	I.V.: 0.2 mg over 30 seconds; wait another 30 seconds, and then give an additional 0.3 mg over 30 seconds. Additional doses of 0.5 mg over 30 seconds at 1-minute intervals up to a cumulative dose of 3 mg.	Onset of reversal usually within 1-2 minutes. Contraindicated in patients with epilepsy, increased intracranial pressure, or coingestion of seizuregenic agents (ie, cyclic antidepressant).

(continued)

Antidote	Poison/Drug	Indications	Dosage	Comments
Glucagon	Propranolol: Hypoglycemic agents	Propranolol-induced cardiac dysfunction Treatment of hypoglycemia	S.C., I.M., or I.V.: 0.5-1 mg May repeat after 15 minutes	Requires liver glycogen stores for hyperglycemic response. Intravenous glucose must also be given in treatment of hypoglycemia.
Leucovorin (citrovorum factor, folinic acid)	Methotrexate, trimethoprim, pyrimethamine, methanol, trimetrexate	Methotrexate-induced bone marrow depression (methotrexate serum level >1 x 10^{-5} mmol/L); may also be useful in pyrimethamine-trimethoprim bone marrow depression	Dose should be equal to or greater than the dose of methotrexate ingested. Usually 10-100 mg/m^2 is given I.V. or orally every 6 hours for 72 hours.	Most effective if given within 1 hour after exposure. May not be effective to prevent liver toxicity. Monitor methotrexate levels. May enhance the toxicity of fluorouracil.
Methylene blue	Methemoglobin inducers (ie, nitrites, phenazopyridine)	Cyanosis Methemoglobin level >30% in an asymptomatic patient	I.V.: 1-2 mg/kg (0.1-0.2 mL/kg) per dose over 2-3 minutes. May repeat doses as needed clinically. Injection can be given as 1% solution or diluted in normal saline.	Treatment can result in falsely elevated methemoglobin levels when measured by a co-oximeter. Large doses (>15 mg/kg) may cause hemolysis.
Naloxone (Narcan®)	Opiates (eg, heroin, morphine, codeine)	Coma or respiratory depression from unknown cause or from opiate overdose	Give 0.4-2.0 mg I.V. bolus. Doses may be repeated if there is no response, up to 10 mg.	For prolonged intoxication, a continuous infusion may be used. See package insert for details or table previously presented in this text titled "Drugs to be Utilized in the Toxic Patient With Altered Mental Status.".
D-penicillamine (Cuprimine®)	Arsenic, lead, mercury	Following BAL therapy in symptomatic acutely poisoned patients Asymptomatic patients with excess lead burden Patient symptomatic from mercury exposure or excessive levels	100 mg/kg/day up to 2 g in 4 divided doses for 5 days 1-2 g/day in 4 divided doses for 5 days **Children:** 100 mg/kg/day up to 1 g/day in 4 divided doses. Given for 3-10 days. **Adults:** P.O.: 250 mg 4 times/day	Possible contraindication for patients with penicillin allergy. Monitor heavy metal levels daily in severely poisoned patients. Monitor CBC and renal function in patients receiving chronic D-penicillamine therapy. Dosages given are for short-term acute therapy only.

(continued)

Antidote	Poison/Drug	Indications	Dosage	Comments
Physostigmine salicylate (Antilirium®)	Atropine and anticholinergic agents, cyclic antidepressants Intrathecal baclofen	Myoclonic seizures, severe arrhythmias Refractory seizures or arrhythmias unresponsive to conventional therapies	**Children:** Slow I.V. push: 0.5 mg. Repeat as required for life-threatening symptoms **Adults:** Slow I.V. push: 0.5-2 mg Same as above	Dramatic reversal of anticholinergic symptoms after I.V. use. Should not be used just to keep patient awake. **Contraindications:** Asthma, gangrene; physostigmine use in cyclic antidepressant-induced cardiac toxicity it controversial. **Extreme caution** is advised — should be considered only in the presence of life-threatening anticholinergic symptoms.
Pralidoxime (2-PAM, Protopam®)	Organophosphate, insecticides, tacrine	An adjunct to atropine therapy for treatment of profound muscle weakness, respiratory depression, muscle twitching	**Children:** 25-50 mg/kg in 250 mL saline over 30 minutes **Adults:** I.V.: 2 g at 0.5 g/minute or infused in 250 mL NS over 30 minutes	Most effective when used in initial 24-36 hours after the exposure. Dosage may be repeated in 1 hour followed by every 8 hours if indicated.
Phytonadione (vitamin K_1)	Coumarin derivatives, indandione derivatives	Large acute ingestion of warfarin rodenticides; chronic exposure or greater than normal prothrombin time	**Children:** I.M.: 1-5 mg. With severe toxicity, vitamin K_1 may be given I.V. **Adults:** I.M.: 10 mg	Vitamin K therapy is relatively contraindicated for patients with prosthetic heart valves unless toxicity is life-threatening.
Protamine sulfate	Heparin	Severe hemorrhage	Maximum rate of 5 mg/minute up to a total dose of 200 mg in 2 hours. 1 mg of protamine neutralizes 90 units of beef lung heparin or 115 units of pork intestinal heparin.	Monitor partial thromboplastin time or activated coagulation time. Effect may be immediate and can last for 2 hours. Monitor for hypotension.
Pyridoxine (vitamin B_6)	Isoniazid monomethyl-hydrazine-containing mushrooms (Gyromitra); acrylamide, hydrazine	Unknown overdose or ingested isoniazid (INH) amount >80 mg/kg	I.V. pyridoxine in the amount of INH ingested or 5 g if amount is unknown given over 30-60 minutes.	Cumulative dose of pyridoxine is arbitrarily limited to 40 g in adults and 20 g in children.
Succimer (Chemet®)	Lead, arsenic, mercury	Asymptomatic children with venous blood lead 45-69 µg/dL. Not FDA approved for adult lead exposure or other metals.	P.O.: 10 mg/kg or 350 mg/m^2 every 8 hours for 5 days. Reduce to 10 mg/kg or 350 mg/m^2 every 12 hours for an additional 2 weeks.	Monitor liver function; emits "rotten egg" sulfur odor.

From Rush Poison Control Center, Rush-Presbyterian-St Luke's Medical Center, Chicago, IL 60612.

MANAGEMENT OF OVERDOSES

Toxin	Vital Signs	Mental Status	Symptoms	Physical Exam	Laboratories
Acetaminophen	Normal	Normal	Anorexia, nausea, vomiting	RUQ tenderness, jaundice	Elevated LFTs
Cocaine	Hypertension, tachycardia, hyperthermia	Anxiety, agitation, delirium	Hallucinations	Mydriasis, tremor, diaphoresis. seizures, perforated nasal septum	EKG abnormalities, increased CPK
Cyclic antidepressants	Tachycardia, hypotension, hyperthermia	Decreased, including coma	Confusion, dizziness	Mydriasis, dry mucous membranes, distended bladder, decreased bowel sounds, flushed, seizures	Long QRS complex, cardiac dysrhythmias
Iron	Early: Normal; Late: Hypotension, tachycardia	Normal; lethargic if hypotensive	Nausea, vomiting, diarrhea, abdominal pain, hematemesis	Abdominal tenderness	Heme + stool and vomit, metabolic acidosis, EKG and x-ray findings, elevated serum iron (early); child: hyperglycemia, leukocytosis
Opioids	Hypotension, bradycardia, hypoventilation, hypothermia	Decreased, including coma	Intoxication	Miosis, absent bowel sounds	Abnormal ABGs
Salicylates	Hyperventilation, hyperthermia	Agitation; lethargy, including coma	Tinnitus, nausea, vomiting, confusion	Diaphoresis, tender abdomen	Anion gap metabolic acidosis, respiratory alkalosis, abnormal LFTs, and coagulation studies
Theophylline	Tachycardia, hypotension, hyperventilation, hyperthermia	Agitation, lethargy, including coma	Nausea, vomiting. diaphoresis, tremor, confusion	Seizures, arrhythmias	Hypokalemia, hyperglycemia, metabolic acidosis, abnormal EKG

TOXICOLOGY INFORMATION

Initial Stabilization of the Patients

The recommended treatment plan for the poisoned patient is not unlike general treatment plans taught in advanced cardiac life support (ACLS) or advanced trauma life support (ATLS) courses. In this manner, the initial approach to the poisoned patient should be essentially similar in every case, irrespective of the toxin ingested, just as the initial approach to the trauma patient is the same irrespective of the mechanism of injury. This approach, which can be termed as routine poison management, essentially includes the following aspects.

- Stabilization: ABCs (airway, breathing, circulation; administration of glucose, thiamine, oxygen, and naloxone
- History, physical examination leading toward the identification of class of toxin (toxidrome recognition)
- Prevention of absorption (decontamination)
- Specific antidote, if available
- Removal of absorbed toxin (enhancing excretion)
- Support and monitoring for adverse effects

Drug	Effect	Comment
25-50 g **dextrose** ($D_{50}W$) intravenously to reverse the effects of drug-induced hypoglycemia (adult) 1 mL/kg $D_{50}W$ diluted 1:1 (child)	This can be especially effective in patients with limited glycogen stores (ie, neonates and patients with cirrhosis)	Extravasation into the extremity of this hyperosmolar solution can cause Volkmann's contractures
50-100 mg intravenous **thiamine**	Prevent Wernicke's encephalopathy	A water-soluble vitamin with low toxicity; rare anaphylactoid reactions have been reported
Initial dosage of **naloxone** should be 2 mg in adult patients preferably by the intravenous route, although intramuscular, subcutaneous, intralingual, and endotracheal routes may also be utilized. Pediatric dose is 0.1 mg/kg from birth until 5 years of age	Specific opioid antagonist without any agent properties	It should be noted that some semisynthetic opiates (such as meperidine or propoxyphene) may require higher initial doses for reversal, so that a total dose of 6-10 mg is not unusual for the adults. If the patient responds to a bolus dose and then relapses to a lethargic or comatose state, a naloxone drip can be considered. This can be accomplished by administering two-thirds of the bolus dose that revives the patient per hour or injecting 4 mg naloxone in 1 L crystalloid solution and administering at a rate of 100 mL/hour 0.4 mg/hour)
Oxygen, utilized in 100% concentration	Useful for carbon monoxide, hydrogen, sulfide, and asphyxiants	While oxygen is antidotal for carbon monoxide intoxication, the only relative toxic contraindication is in paraquat intoxication (in that it can promote pulmonary fibrosis)
Flumazenil	Benzodiazepine antagonist	Not routinely recommended due to increased risk of seizures

Laboratory Evaluation of Overdose

Unknown ingestion: Electrolytes, anion gap, serum osmolality, arterial blood gases, serum drug concentration

Known ingestion: Labs tailored to agent

Toxins Affecting the Anion Gap

Drugs Causing Increased Anion Gap (>12 mEq/L)

Nonacidotic
- Carbenicillin
- Sodium salts

Metabolic Acidosis
- Acetaminophen (ingestion >75-100 g)
- Acetazolamide
- Amiloride
- Ascorbic acid
- Benzalkonium chloride
- Benzyl alcohol
- Beta-adrenergic drugs
- Bialaphos
- 2-butanone
- Carbon monoxide
- Centrimonium bromide
- Chloramphenicol
- Colchicine
- Cyanide
- Dapsone
- Dimethyl sulfate
- Dinitrophenol
- Endosulfan
- Epinephrine (I.V. overdose)
- Ethanol
- Ethylene dibromide
- Ethylene glycol
- Fenoprofen
- Fluoroacetate
- Formaldehyde
- Fructose (I.V.)
- Glycol ethers
- Hydrogen sulfide
- Ibuprofen (ingestion >300 mg/kg)
- Inorganic acid
- Iodine
- Iron
- Isoniazid
- Ketamine
- Ketoprofen
- Metaldehyde
- Metformin
- Methanol
- Methenamine mandelate
- Monochloracetic acid
- Nalidixic acid
- Naproxen
- Niacin
- Papaverine
- Paraldehyde
- Pennyroyal oil
- Pentachlorophenol
- Phenelzine
- Phenformin (off the market)
- Phenol
- Phenylbutazone
- Phosphoric acid
- Potassium chloroplatinite
- Propylene glycol
- Salicylates
- Sorbitol (I.V.)
- Strychnine
- Surfactant herbicide
- Tetracycline (outdated)
- Theophyllinei
- Tienilic acid
- Toluene
- Tranylcypromine
- Vacor
- Verapamil

Drugs Causing Decreased Anion Gap (<6 mEq/L)

Acidosis
- Ammonium chloride
- Bromide
- Iodide
- Lithium
- Polymyxin B
- Tromethamine

Drugs Causing Increased Osmolar Gap

(by freezing-point depression, gap is >10 mOsm)

- Ethanol*
- Ethylene glycol*
- Glycerol
- Hypermagnesemia (>9.5 mEq/L)
- Isopropanol* (acetone)
- Iodine (questionable)
- Mannitol
- Methanol*
- Propylene glycol
- Severe alcoholic ketoacidosis or lactic acidosis
- Sorbitol*

*Toxins increasing both anion and osmolar gap.

Toxins Associated With Oxygen Saturation Gap

(>5% difference between measured and calculated value)

- Carbon monoxide
- Cyanide (questionable)
- Hydrogen sulfide (possible)
- Methemoglobin

Acetaminophen Toxicity

The Toxicology Laboratory is also very useful for determining levels of toxin in body fluids. Often these drug levels will guide therapy. For example, use of the Rumack-Matthew nomogram for acute acetaminophen poisoning can direct N-acetylcysteine therapy if the serum acetaminophen level falls above the treatment line.

Acetaminophen Toxicity Nomogram

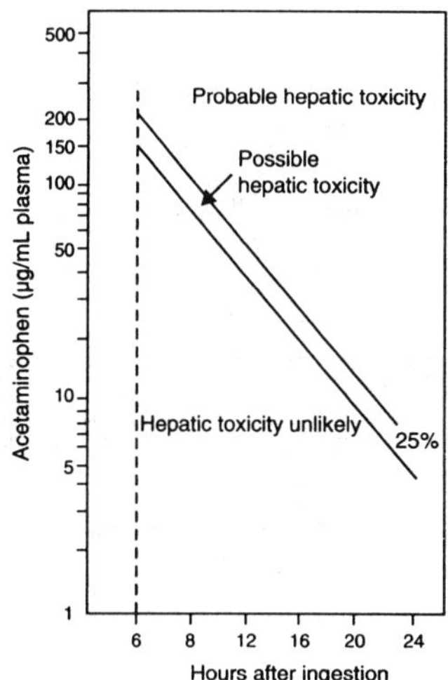

Ibuprofen Toxicity Nomogram

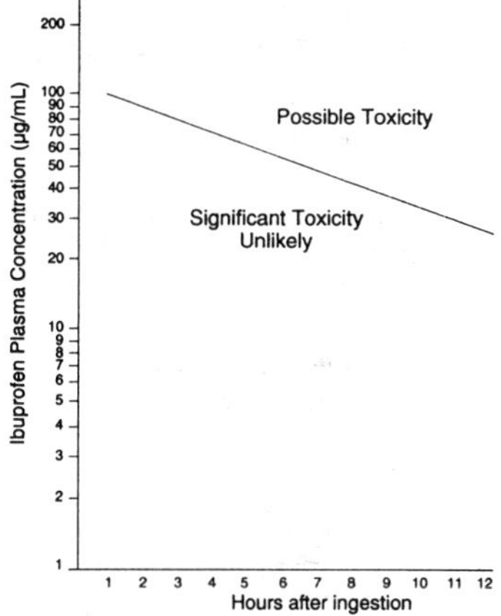

Ibuprofen nomogram, (From Hall AH, Smolinske SC, Stover B, et al, "Ibuprofen Overdose in Adults," *J Toxicol Clin Toxicol*, 1992, 30:34.)

Serum Salicylate Intoxication

Similarly, the Done nomogram is somewhat useful in predicting salicylate toxicity in pediatric patients. Neither nomogram should be utilized with chronic ingestions. Recently, a nomogram has been devised for theophylline ingestion; see the following nomogram.

History and Physical Examination

While the history and physical examination is the cornerstone of clinical patient management, it takes on special meaning with regard to the toxic patient. While

Serum Salicylate Level and Severity of Intoxication
Single Dose Acute Ingestion Nomogram

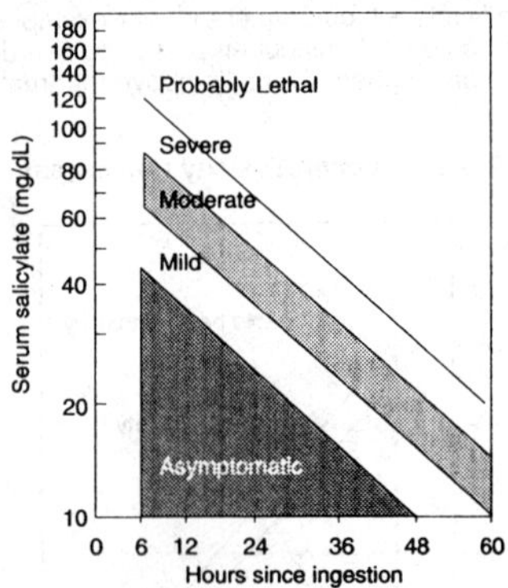

Done nomogram for salicylate poisoning. Note that this nomogram is not accurate for chronic ingestions nor for acute ingestions with enteric coated tabs. Clinical laboratory signs and symptoms are best indicators for assessments. (From Done AK, "Salicylate Intoxication: Significance of Measurements of Salicylate in Blood in Cases of Acute Ingestions," *Pediatrics*, 1960, 26:800; copyright American Academy of Pediatrics, 1960.)

Serum Theophylline Overdose

Nonsmokers

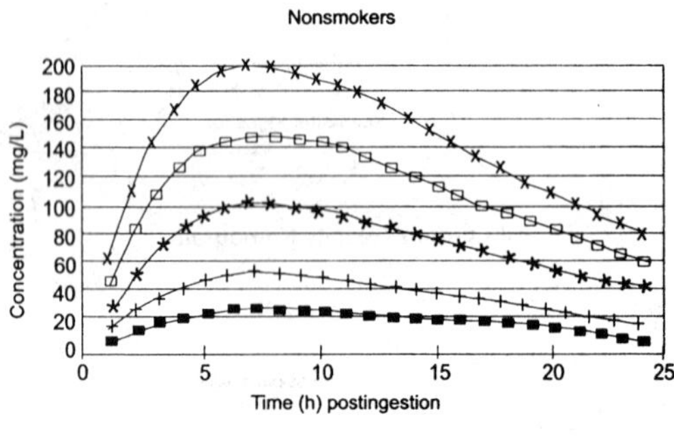

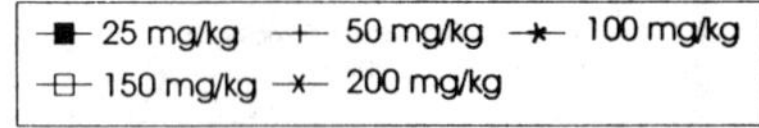

Serum Theophylline Overdose

Smokers and Children

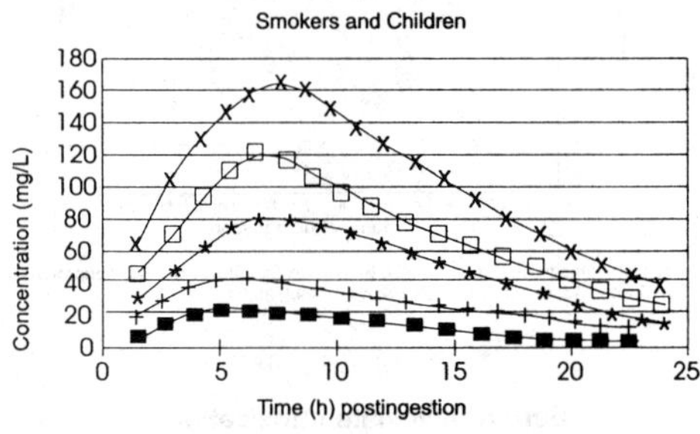

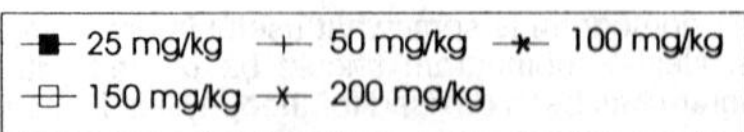

Nomogram for overdose of sustained-release theophylline in 1) nonsmoking adults, and 2) smokers and children. (Courtesy of Frank Paloucek, PharmD, College of Pharmacy, University of Illinois, Chicago.)

taking a history may be a more direct method of the determination of the toxin, quite often is is not reliable. Information obtained may prove minimal in some cases and could be considered partial or inaccurate in suicide gestures and addicts. A quick physical examination often leads to important clues about the nature of the toxin. These clues can be specific symptom complexes associated with certain toxins and can be referred to as "toxidromes". See the following table.

Prevention of Absorption

Toxic substances can enter the body through the dermal, ocular, pulmonary, parenteral, and gastrointestinal routes. The basic principle of decontamination involves appropriate copious irrigation of the toxic substances relatable to the route of exposure. For example, with ocular exposure, this can be done with normal saline for 30-40 minutes through a Morgan therapeutic lens. With alkali exposures, the pH should be checked until the runoff of the solution is either neutral or slightly acidic. Skin decontamination involves removal of the toxin with nonabrasive soap. This should especially be considered for organophosphates, methylene chloride, dioxin, radiation, hydrocarbons, and herbicide exposure. Separate drainage areas should be obtained for the contaminated runoff.

Since >80% of incidents of accidental poisoning in children occur through the gastrointestinal tract, a thorough knowledge of gastric decontamination is essential. There are essentially four modes of gastric decontamination, of which three are physical removal (emesis, gastric lavage, and whole bowel irrigation). Activated charcoal associated with a cathartic is the fourth mode for preventing absorption.

Methods of Enhanced Elimination of Toxic Substances/Drugs

Emesis with Syrup of Ipecac

Indications

- Use within 1 hour of ingestion
- Hydrocarbons with "dangerous additives"
- Heavy metals
- Toxic insecticides

Contraindications

- Children <6 months of age
- Nontoxic ingestion
- Lack of gag reflex
- Caustic/corrosive ingestions
- Hemorrhagic diathesis
- Sharp object ingestion
- Prior vomiting
- Ingestion of pure petroleum distillate

Dose: + 15 mL H_2O

Children:	6-12 months: 10 mL
	1-5 years: 15 mL
	>5 years: 30 mL
Adults:	30 mL

Note: Ipecac use is becoming less frequently recommended since <30% of the stomach is usually emptied and its use may delay the use of activated charcoal.

Gastric Lavage

Indications

- Use within 1 hour of ingestion
- Comatose patient with significant ingestion without contraindications
- Failure to respond to ipecac
- Large quantities of toxins

Contraindications

- Seizures
- Nontoxic ingestion
- Significant hemorrhagic diathesis
- Caustic ingestions, hydrocarbons
- Usually unable to use large enough tube in children <12 years of age

Note: Lavage is not routinely recommended except for recent and very large ingestions of noncontraindicated toxins since it is believed to actually push a significant portion of drug into the intestine and may delay administration of activated charcoal.

Enhancement of Elimination

Only recently has this aspect of poison management received more than cursory attention in practice and in the literature. The standard practice for enhancement of elimination consisted primarily of forced diuresis in order to excrete the toxin. However, the past 10 years experience has produced a radical change in the approach to this and therefore, a more focused methodology to eliminating absorbed toxins. Essentially, there are three methods by which absorbed toxins may be eliminated: recurrent adsorption with multiple dosings of activated charcoal, use of forced diuresis in combination with possible alkalinization of the urine, and use of dialysis or charcoal hemoperfusion.

Activated Charcoal Indications

Indications

- Single dose for agents known to be bound
- Multiple dose for drugs with favorable characteristics: Small volume of distribution (<1 L/kg), low plasma protein binding, biliary or gastric secretion, active metabolites that recirculate, drugs that exhibit a large free fraction (eg, dapsone, carbamazepine, digitalis, methotrexate, phenobarbital, salicylates, theophylline, tricyclic antidepressants), unchanged, lipophilic, long half-life

Recently, multiple dosing of activated charcoal ("pulse dosing") has been advocated as a method for removal of absorbed drug. This procedure has been demonstrated to be efficacious in drugs that re-enter the gastrointestinal tract through enterohepatic circulation (ie, digitoxin, carbamazepine, glutethimide) and with drugs that diffuse from the systemic circulation into the gastrointestinal tract due to formation of a concentration gradient ("the infinite sink" hypothesis).

Toxins Eliminated by Multiple Dosing of Activated Charcoal (MDAC)

Amitriptyline
Amoxapine
Baclofen (?)
Benzodiazepines (?)
Bupropion (?)
Carbamazepine*
Chlordecone
Cyclosporine
Dapsone
Diazepam
Digoxin
Glutethimide
Maprotiline
Meprobamate
Methotrexate
Methyprylon
Nadolol
Nortriptyline
Phencyclidine
Phenobarbital*
Phenylbutazone
Phenytoin (?)
Piroxicam
Propoxyphene
Salicylates (?)*
Theophylline*
Valproic acid*

*Only agents routinely recommended for removal with MDAC.

Contraindications

- Absence of hypoactive bowel sounds
- Caustic ingestions
- Drugs without effect: Acids, alkalis, alcohols, boric acid, cyanide, iron, heavy metals, lithium, insecticides

Dose

Children and Adults: 50-100 g initially or 1 g/kg weight; repeat doses of 25 g or 0.5 g/kg every 2-4 hours

Most effective at 1-hour postingestion but can remove at >1-hour postingestion

Doses subsequent to first may be admixed with water rather than a cathartic such as sorbitol to avoid diarrhea and consequent electrolyte disturbances.

Whole Bowel Irrigation–propylene glycol based solutions

Initial dose of charcoal is necessary prior to use. Avoid pretreatment with ipecac.

Indications

- Iron, lead, lithium
- Agents not bound by charcoal
- Modified or sustained-release dosage forms
- Body packers

Contraindications

- Bowel perforation
- Obstruction
- Ileus
- Gastrointestinal bleed

Dose

Maximum: 5-10 L
Toddlers/preschool: 250-500 mL/hour or 35 mL/kg
Adults: 1-2 L/hour
Terminate when rectal effluent = infusate = clear

Urinary Ion Trapping–to alkalinize the urine

Indications

- Salicylates
- Phenobarbital

Toxins Eliminated by Forced Saline Diuretics	Toxins Eliminated by Alkaline Diuresis
Bromidex	2,4-D chlorphenoxyacetic acid
Chromium	Fluoride
Cimetidine (?)	Isoniazid (?)
Cis-platinum	Mephobarbital
Cyclophosphamide	Methotrexate
Hydrazine	Phenobarbital
Iodide	Primidone
Iodine	Quinolones antibiotic
Isoniazid (?)	Salicylates
Lithium	Uranium
Methyl iodide	
Potassium chloroplatinite	
Thallium	

Dose

Sodium bicarbonate 1-2 mEq/kg every 3-4 hours or 100 mEq $NaHCO_3$ in 1 L $D_5{}^1/{}_4$NS at 200 mL/hour (desired urine pH: 7.6-7.8)

A urine flow of 3-5 mL/kg/hour should be achieved with a combination of isotonic fluids or diuretics. Although several drugs can exhibit enhanced elimination through an acidic urine (quinine, amphetamines, PCP, nicotine, bismuth, ephedrine, flecainide), the practice of acidifying the urine should be discouraged in that it can produce metabolic acidosis and promote renal failure in the presence of rhabdomyolysis. **Note:** Use caution in alkalinizing urine of children to avoid fluid overdose.

Hemodialysis

Indications

Drugs with favorable characteristics

- Low molecular weight (<500 daltons)
- Ionically charged
- H_2O soluble
- Low plasma protein binding (<70%-80%)
- Small volume of distribution (<1 L/kg)
- Low tissue binding
- Methanol, ethylene glycol, boric acid

Drugs and Toxins Removed by Hemodialysis

Acetaminophen
Acyclovir
Amanita phalloides (?)
Amantadine (?)
Ammonium chloride
Amphetamine
Anilines
Atenolol
Boric acid
Bromides

Bromisoval
Calcium
Captopril (?)
Carbromal
Carisoprodol
Chloral hydrate
Chlorpropamide
Chromium
Cimetidine (?)
Cyclophosphamide
Dapsone
Disopyramide
Enalapril (?)
Ethanol
Ethylene glycol
Famotidine (?)
Fluoride
Folic acid
Formaldehyde
Foscarnet sodium
Gabapentin
Glycol ethers
Hydrazine (?)
Hydrochlorothiazide
Iodides
Isoniazid
Isopropanol
Ketoprofen
Lithium
Magnesium
Meprobamate
Metal-chelate compounds
Metformin (?)
Methanol
Methaqualone
Methotrexate
Methyldopa
Methylprylone
Monochloroacetic acid
Nadolol
Oxalic acid
Paraldehyde
Phenelzine (?)
Phenobarbital
Phosphoric acid
Potassium
Procainamide
Quinidine
Ranitidine (?)
Rifabutin
Salicylates
Sotalol
Strychnine
Thallium
Theophylline
Thiocyanates
Tranylcypromine sulfate (?)
Verapamil (?)

Hemoperfusion

Indications

Drugs with favorable characteristics:

- Affinity for activated charcoal
- Tissue binding
- High rate of equilibration from peripheral tissues to blood

Examples: Barbiturates. carbamazepine, ethchlorvynol, methotrexate, phenytoin, theophylline

Drugs and Toxins Removed by Hemoperfusion (Charcoal)

Amanita phalloides (?)
Atenolol (?)
Bromisoval
Bromoethylbutyramide
Caffeine
Carbamazepine
Carbon tetrachloride (?)
Carbromal
Chloral hydrate (trichloroethanol)
Chloramphenicol
Chlorpropamide
Colchicine (?)
Creosote (?)
Dapsone
Diltiazem (?)
Disopyramide
Ethchlorvynol
Ethylene oxide
Glutethimide
Lindane
Meprobamate
Methaqualone
Methotrexate
Methsuximide
Methyprylon (?)
Metoprolol (?)
Nadolol (?)
Oxalic acid (?)
Paraquat
Phenelzine (?)
Phenobarbital
Phenytoin
Podophyllin (?)
Procainamide (?)
Quinidine (?)
Rifabutin (?)
Sotalol (?)
Thallium
Theophylline
Verapamil (?)

Exchange transfusion is another mode of extracorporeal removal of toxins that can be utilized in neonatal infant drug toxicity. It may be especially useful for barbiturate, iron, caffeine, sodium nitrite, or theophylline overdose.

TOXIDROMES

Toxin	Vital Signs	Mental Status	Symptoms	Physical Exam	Laboratories
Acetaminophen	Normal	Normal	Anorexia, nausea, vomiting	RUQ tenderness, jaundice	Elevated LFTs
Cocaine	Hypertension, tachycardia, hyperthermia	Anxiety, agitation, delirium	Hallucinations	Mydriasis, tremor, diaphoresis. seizures, perforated nasal septum	EKG abnormalities, increased CPK
Cyclic antidepressants	Tachycardia, hypotension, hyperthermia	Decreased, including coma	Confusion, dizziness	Mydriasis, dry mucous membranes, distended bladder, decreased bowel sounds, flushed, seizures	Long QRS complex, cardiac dysrhythmias
Iron	Early: Normal; Late: Hypotension, tachycardia	Normal; lethargic if hypotensive	Nausea, vomiting, diarrhea, abdominal pain, hematemesis	Abdominal tenderness	Heme + stool and vomit, metabolic acidosis, EKG and x-ray findings, elevated serum iron (early); child: hyperglycemia, leukocytosis
Opioids	Hypotension, bradycardia, hypoventilation, hypothermia	Decreased, including coma	Intoxication	Miosis, absent bowel sounds	Abnormal ABGs
Salicylates	Hyperventilation, hyperthermia	Agitation; lethargy, including coma	Tinnitus, nausea, vomiting, confusion	Diaphoresis, tender abdomen	Anion gap metabolic acidosis, respiratory alkalosis, abnormal LFTs, and coagulation studies
Theophylline	Tachycardia, hypotension, hyperventilation, hyperthermia	Agitation, lethargy, including coma	Nausea, vomiting. diaphoresis, tremor, confusion	Seizures, arrhythmias	Hypokalemia, hyperglycemia, metabolic acidosis, abnormal EKG

Examples of Toxidromes

Toxidromes	Pattern	Example of Drugs	Treatment Approach
Anticholinergic	Fever, ileus, flushing, tachycardia, urinary retention, inability to sweat, visual blurring, and mydriasis. Central manifestations include myoclonus, choreoathetosis, toxic psychosis with lilliputian hallucinations, seizures, and coma.	Antihistamines Baclofen Benztropine Jimson weed Methylpyroline Phenothiazines Propantheline Tricyclic antidepressants	Physostigmine for life-threatening symptoms only; may predispose to arrhythmias*
Cholinergic	Characterized by salivation, lacrimation, urination, defecation, gastrointestinal cramps, and emesis ("sludge"). Bradycardia and bronchoconstriction may also be seen.	Carbamate Organophosphates Pilocarpine	• Atropine* • Pralidoxime for organophosphate insecticides*
Extrapyramidal	Choreoathetosis, hyperreflexia, trismus, opisthotonos, rigidity, and tremor	Haloperidol Phenothiazines	• Diphenhydramine • Benztropine
Hallucinogenic	Perceptual distortions, synthesis, depersonalization, and derealization	Amphetamines Cannabinoids Cocaine Indole alkaloids Phencyclidine	Benzodiazepine
Narcotic	Altered mental status, unresponsiveness, shallow respirations, slow respiratory rate or periodic breathing, miosis, bradycardia, hypothermia	Opiates Dextromethorphan Pentazocine Propoxyphene	Naloxone*

(continued)

Toxidromes	Pattern	Example of Drugs	Treatment Approach
Sedative/Hypnotic	Manifested by sedation with progressive deterioration of central nervous system function. Coma, stupor, confusion, apnea, delirium, or hallucinations may accompany this pattern.	Anticonvulsants Antipsychotics Barbiturates Benzodiazepines Ethanol Ethchlorvynol Fentanyl Glutethimide Meprobamate Methadone Methocarbamol Opiates Quinazolines Propoxyphene Tricyclic antidepressants	• Naloxone* • Flumazenil; usually not recommended due to increased risk of seizures* • Urinary alkalinization (barbiturates)
Seizuregenic	May mimic stimulant pattern with hyperthermia, hyperreflexia, and tremors being prominent signs	Anticholinergics Camphor Chlorinated hydrocarbons Cocaine Isoniazid Lidocaine Lindane Nicotine Phencyclidine Strychnine Xanthines	• Antiseizure medications • Pyridoxine for isoniazid* • Extracorporeal removal of drug (ie, lindane, camphor, xanthines) • Physostigmine for anticholinergic agents*

(continued)

Toxidromes	Pattern	Example of Drugs	Treatment Approach
Serotonin	Confusion, myoclonus, hyperreflexia, diaphoresis, tremor, facial flushing, diarrhea, fever, trismus	Clomipramine Fluoxetine Isoniazid L-tryptophan Paroxetine Phenelzine Sertraline Tranylcypromine Drug combinations include: • MAO inhibitors with L-tryptophan • Fluoxetine or meperidine • Fluoxetine with carbamazepine or sertraline • Clomipramine and meclobemide • Trazadol and buspirone • Paroxetine and dextromethorphan	Withdrawal of drug/benzodiazepine
Solvent	Lethargy, confusion, dizziness, headache, restlessness, incoordination, derealization, depersonalization	Acetone Chlorinated hydrocarbons Hydrocarbons Naphthalene Trichloroethane Toluene	Avoid catecholamines

(continued)

Toxidromes	Pattern	Example of Drugs	Treatment Approach
Stimulant	Restlessness, excessive speech and motor activity, tachycardia, tremor, and insomnia — may progress to seizure. Other effects noted include euphoria, mydriasis, anorexia, and paranoia.	Amphetamines Caffeine (xanthines) Cocaine Ephedrine/pseudoephedrine Methylphenidate Nicotine Phencyclidine	Benzodiazepines
Uncoupling of oxidative phosphylation	Hyperthermia, tachypnea, diaphoresis, metabolic acidosis (usually)	Aluminum phosphide Aspirin/Salicylates 2,4-Dichlorophenol Di-n-Butyl Phthalate Dinitrophenols Dinitro cresols Hexachlorobutadiene Phosphorus Pentachlorophenol Tin (?) Zinc phosphide	Sodium bicarbonate to treat metabolic acidosis Patient cooling techniques Avoidance of atropine or salicylate agents Hemodialysis may be required for acidosis treatment

From Nice A, Leikin JB, Maturen A, et al, "Toxidrome Recognition to Improve Efficiency of Emergency Urine Drug Screens," *Ann Emerg Med*, 1988, 17:676-80.
*See the Poison Control Center Antidote Chart.

ACUTE INTERMITTENT PORPHYRIA, HEREDITARY COPROPORPHYRIA, AND VARIEGATE PORPHYRIA, CATEGORIES OF SAFE AND UNSAFE DRUGS

Unsafe	Safe
Alcohol	Acetaminophen
Barbiturates	Aspirin
Carbamazepine	Atropine
Danazol	Bromides
Ergots	Glucocorticoids
Ethchlorvynol	Insulin
Glutethimide	Narcotic analgesics
Griseofulvin	Penicillin and derivatives
Mephenytoin	Phenothiazines
Meprobamate	Streptomycin
Methyprylon	
Phenytoin	
Pyrazolones	
Succinimides	
Sulfonamide antibiotics	
Synthetic estrogens and progestins	
Valproic acid	

ADVERSE HEMATOLOGIC EFFECTS, DRUGS ASSOCIATED WITH

Drug	Red Cell Aplasia	Thrombo-cytopenia	Neutro-penia	Pancyto-penia	Hemolysis
Acetazolamide		+	+	+	
Allopurinol			+		
Amiodarone	+				
Amphotericin B				+	
Amrinone		++			
Asparaginase		+++	+++	+++	++
Barbiturates		+		+	
Benzocaine					++
Captopril			++		+
Carbamazepine		++	+		
Cephalosporins			+		++
Chloramphenicol		+	++	+++	
Chlordiazepoxide			+	+	
Chloroquine		+			
Chlorothiazides		++			
Chlorpropamide	+	++	+	++	+
Chlortetracycline				+	
Chlorthalidone			+		
Cimetidine		+	++	+	
Codeine		+			
Colchicine				+	
Cyclophosphamide		+++	+++	+++	+
Dapsone					+++
Desipramine		++			
Digitalis		+			
Digitoxin		++			
Erythromycin		+			
Estrogen		+		+	
Ethacrynic acid			+		
Fluorouracil		+++	+++	+++	+
Furosemide		+	+		
Gold salts	+	+++	+++	+++	
Heparin		++		+	
Ibuprofen			+		+
Imipramine			++		
Indomethacin		+	++	+	
Isoniazid		+		+	
Isosorbide dinitrate					+
Levodopa					++
Meperidine		+			
Meprobamate		+	+	+	
Methimazole			++		
Methyldopa		++			+++
Methotrexate		+++	+++	+++	++
Methylene blue					+
Metronidazole			+		
Nalidixic acid					+
Naproxen				+	
Nitrofurantoin			++		+
Nitroglycerine		+			
Penicillamine		++	+		
Penicillins		+	++	+	+++
Phenazopyridine					+++
Phenothiazines		+	++	+++	+
Phenylbutazone		+	++	+++	+
Phenytoin		++	++	++	+
Potassium iodide		+			
Prednisone		+			
Primaquine					+++
Procainamide			+		

(continued)

Drug	Red Cell Aplasia	Thrombo-cytopenia	Neutro-penia	Pancyto-penia	Hemolysis
Procarbazine		+	++	++	+
Propylthiouracil		+	++	+	+
Quinidine		+++	+		
Quinine		+++	+		
Reserpine		+			
Rifampicin		++	+		+++
Spironolactone			+		
Streptomycin		+		+	
Sulfamethoxazole with trimethoprim			+		
Sulfonamides	+	++	++	++	++
Sulindac	+	+	+	+	
Tetracyclines		+			+
Thioridazine			++		
Tolbutamide		++	+	++	
Triamterene					+
Valproate	+				
Vancomycin			+		

+ = rare or single reports.

++ = occasional reports.

+++ = substantial number of reports.

Adapted from D'Arcy PF and Griffin JP, eds, *Iatrogenic Diseases*, New York, NY: Oxford University Press, 1986, 128-30.

BREAST-FEEDING AND DRUGS

Adapted from American Academy of Pediatrics Committee on Drugs: "Transfer of Drugs and Other Chemicals Into Human Milk," *Pediatrics*, 1994, 93:137-50.

The following questions and options should be considered when prescribing drug therapy to lactating women (1) Is the drug therapy really necessary? Consultation between the pediatrician and the mother's physician can be most useful. (2) Use the safest drug, for example, acetaminophen rather than aspirin for analgesia. (3) If there is a possibility that a drug may present a risk to the infant, consideration should be given to measurement of blood concentrations in the nursing infant. (4) Drug exposure to the nursing infant may be minimized by having the mother take the medication just after she has breast-fed the infant and/or just before the infant is due to have a lengthy sleep period.

In tables 1-6, the fact that a pharmacologic or chemical agent does not appear on the lists is not meant to imply that it is not transferred into human milk or that it does not have an effect on the infant; it only indicates that there were no reports found in the literature.

Table 1. Drugs That Are Contraindicated During Breast-Feeding

Drug	Reason for Concern, Reported Sign or Symptom in Infant, or Effect on Lactation
Bromocriptine	Suppresses lactation; may be hazardous to the mother
Cocaine	Cocaine intoxication
Cyclophosphamide	Possible immune suppression; unknown effect on growth or association with carcinogenesis; neutropenia
Cyclosporine	Possible immune suppression; unknown effect on growth or association with carcinogenesis
Doxorubicin*	Possible immune suppression; unknown effect on growth or association with carcinogenesis
Ergotamine	Vomiting, diarrhea. convulsions (doses used in migraine medications)
Lithium	One-third to one-half therapeutic blood concentration in infants
Methotrexate	Possible immune suppression; unknown effect on growth or association with carcinogenesis; neutropenia
Phencyclidine (PCP)	Potent hallucinogen
Phenindone	Anticoagulant; increased prothrombin and partial thromboplastin time in one infant; not used in the United States

*Drug is concentrated in human milk

Table 2. Drugs of Abuse: Contraindicated During Breast-Feeding*

Amphetamine†	Marijuana
Cocaine	Nicotine (smoking)
Heroin	Phencyclidine

The Committee on Drugs strongly believes that nursing mothers should not ingest any compounds listed in Table 2. Not only are they hazardous to the nursing infant, but they are also detrimental to the physical and emotional health of the mother. This list is obviously not complete; no drug of abuse should be ingested by nursing mothers even though adverse reports are not in the literature.

†Drug is concentrated in human milk

Table 3. Radioactive Compounds That Require Temporary Cessation of Breast-Feeding*

Drug	Recommended Time for Cessation of Breast-Feeding
Copper 64 (^{64}Cu)	Radioactivity in milk present at 50 h
Gallium 67 (^{67}Ga)	Radioactivity in milk present for 2 wk
Indium 111 (^{111}In)	Very small amount present at 20 h
Iodine 123 (^{123}I)	Radioactivity in milk present up to 36 h
Iodine 125 (^{125}I)	Radioactivity in milk present for 12 d
Iodine 131 (^{131}I)	Radioactivity in milk present 2-14 d, depending on study
Radioactive sodium	Radioactivity in milk present 96 h
Technetium-99m (^{99m}Tc), ^{99m}Rc macroaggregates, ^{99m}Tc O4	Radioactivity in milk present 15 h to 3 d

*Consult nuclear medicine physician before performing diagnostic study so that radionuclide that has shortest excretion time in breast milk can be used. Before study, the mother should pump her breast and store enough milk in freezer for feeding the infant; after study, the mother should pump her breast to maintain milk production but discard all milk pumped for the required time that radioactivity is present in milk. Milk samples can be screened by radiology departments for radioactivity before resumption of nursing.

Table 4. Drugs Whose Effect on Nursing Infants is Unknown But May be of Concern

Psychotropic drugs, the compounds listed under antianxiety, antidepressant, and antipsychotic categories, are of special concern when given to nursing mothers for long periods. Although there are no case reports of adverse effects in breast-feeding infants, these drugs do appear in human milk and thus conceivably after short-term and long-term central nervous system function.

Antianxiety	Antidepressant	Antipsychotic
Diazepam	Amitriptyline	Chlorpromazine
Lorazepam	Amoxapine	Chlorprothixene
Midazolam	Desipramine	Haloperidol
Perphenazine	Dothiepin	Mesoridazine
Prazepam*	Doxepin	
Quazepam	Fluoxetine	**Miscellaneous**
Temazepam	Fluvoxamine	Chloramphenicol
	Imipramine	Metoclopramide*
	Trazodone	Metronidazole
		Tinidazole

*Drug is concentrated in human milk

Table 5. Drugs That Have Been Associated With Significant Effects on Some Nursing Infants and Should be Given to Nursing Mothers With Caution*

Drug	Reported Effect
Aspirin (salicylates)	Metabolic acidosis (one case)
Clemastine	Drowsiness, irritability, refusal to feed, high-pitched cry, neck stiffness (one case)
Mesalamine	Diarrhea (one case)
Phenobarbital	Sedation; infantile spasms after weaning from milk-containing phenobarbital, methemoglobinemia (one case)
Primidone	Sedation, feeding problems
Sulfasalazine (salicylazosulfapyridine)	Bloody diarrhea (one case)

*Measure blood concentration in the infant when possible.

Table 6. Maternal Medication Usually Compatible With Breast-Feeding

Acebutol
Acetaminophen
Acetazolamide
Acitretin
Acyclovir*
Alcohol (ethanol)
Allopurinol
Amoxicillin
Antimony
Atenolol
Atropine
Azapropazone (apazone)
Aztreonam
B_1 (thiamine)
B_6 (pyridoxine)
B_{12}
Baclofen
Barbiturate
Bendroflumethiazide
Bishydroxycoumarin (Dicumarol®)
Bromide
Butorphanol
Caffeine
Captopril
Carbamazepine
Carbimazole
Cascara
Cefadroxil
Cefazolin
Cefotaxime
Cefoxitin
Cefprozil
Ceftazidime
Ceftriaxone
Chloral hydrate
Chloroform
Chloroquine
Chlorothiazide
Chlorthalidone
Cimetidine*
Cisapride
Cisplatin
Clindamycin
Clogestone
Clomipramine
Codeine
Colchicine
Contraceptive pill with estrogen and progesterone
Cycloserine
D (vitamin)
Danthron
Dapsone
Dexbrompheniramine maleate with d-isoephedrine
Digoxin
Diltiazem
Dipyrone
Disopyramide
Domperidone
Dyphylline*
Enalapril
Erythromycin*
Estradiol
Ethambutol
Ethanol
Ethosuximide
Fentanyl
Flecainide
Flufenamic acid
Fluorescein
Folic acid
Gold salts
Halothane
Hydralazine
Hydrochlorothiazide
Hydroxychloroquine*
Ibuprofen
Indomethacin
Iodides
Iodine
Iodine (povidone-iodine/vaginal douche)
Iopanoic acid
Isoniazid
K_1 (vitamin)
Kanamycin
Ketorolac
Labetalol
Levonorgestrel
Lidocaine
Loperamide
Magnesium sulfate
Medroxyprogesterone
Mefenamic acid
Methadone
Methimazole (active metabolite of carbimazole)
Methocarbamol
Methyldopa
Methprylon
Metoprolol*
Metrizamide
Mexiletine
Minoxidil
Morphine
Moxalactam
Nadolol*
Nalidixic acid
Naproxen
Nefopam
Nifedipine
Nitrofurantoin
Norethynodrel
Norsteroids
Noscapine
Oxprenolol
Phenylbutazone
Phenytoin
Piroxicam
Prednisone
Procainamide
Progesterone
Propoxyphene
Propranolol
Propylthiouracil
Pseudoephedrine*
Pyridostigmine
Pyrimethamine
Quinidine
Quinine
Riboflavin
Rifampin
Scopolamine
Secobarbital
Senna
Sotalol
Spironolactone
Streptomycin
Sulbactam
Sulfapyridine
Sulfisoxazole
Suprofen
Terbutaline
Tetracycline
Theophylline
Thiopental
Thiouracil
Ticarcillin
Timolol
Tolbutamide
Tolmetin
Trimethoprim and sulfamethoxazole
Triprolidine
Valproic acid
Verapamil
Warfarin
Zolpidem

*Drug is concentrated in human milk

CYTOCHROME P-450 AND DRUG INTERACTIONS

Drugs Causing Inhibitory and Inductive Interactions

Inhibitory (Enhancement of Interacting Drug Effect)	Inductive (Impairment of Interacting Drug Effect)
Amiodarone (Cordarone®)	Anticonvulsants
Cimetidine (Tagamet®)	Chronic ethanol use
Erythromycin	Cigarette smoking
Ethanol intoxication	Rifampin (Rifadin®, Rimactane®)
Fluconazole	
Isoniazid (Laniazid®, Nydrazid®)	
Itraconazole	
Ketoconazole	
Neuroleptics	
Oral contraceptives	
Psoralen dermatologics	
Quinidine	
Quinolone antibiotics	
SSKIs	
Tricyclic antidepressants	

Low-Therapeutic-Index Drugs

Hepatic Oxidation (cytochrome P-450 mediated clearance)

Antiarrhythmic drugs
Anticonvulsants
Antineoplastic/immunosuppressive drugs
Oral anticoagulants
Theophylline

Drugs Metabolized by CYPIID6 That May Interact and Result in Toxicity

Tricyclic Antidepressants	Phenothiazines
Imipramine (Janimine®, Tofranil®)	Perphenazine (Trilafon®)
Clomipramine (Anafranil®)	Thioridazine (Mellaril®)
Amitriptyline (Elavil®, Endep®)	
Desipramine (Norpramin®, Pertofrane®)	
Nortriptyline (Aventyl®, Pamelor®)	

Drugs Metabolized by CYPIID6 That May Interact and Have Decreased or Altered Effect

Antiarrhythmics	B-Adrenergic Receptor Blockers
Flecainide (Tambocor®)	Metoprolol (Lopressor®, Toprol XL®)
Encainide (Enkaid®)	Timolol (Blocadren®)
Propafenone *Rythmol®)	
Mexiletine (Mextil®)	**Analgesics**
	Codeine

Drugs That Inhibit CYPIID6

Any substrate listed in above tables
Quinidine
Haloperidol (Haldol®)

LOW POTASSIUM DIET

Potassium is a mineral found in most all foods except sugar and lard. It plays a role in maintaining normal muscle activity and helps to keep body fluids in balance. Too much potassium in the blood can lead to changes in heartbeat and can lead to muscle weakness. The kidneys normally help to keep blood potassium controlled, but in kidney disease or when certain drugs are taken, dietary potassium must be limited to maintain a normal level of potassium in the blood.

The following guideline includes 2-3 g of potassium per day.

1. **Milk Group:** Limit to one cup serving of milk or milk product (yogurt, cottage cheese, ice cream, pudding).

2. **Fruit Group:** Limit to two servings daily from the low potassium choices. Watch serving sizes. Avoid the high potassium choices.

   Low Potassium
   Apple, 1 small
   Apple juice, applesauce 1/2 cup
   Apricot, 1 medium or 1/2 cup canned in syrup
   Blueberries, 1/2 cup
   Cherries, canned in syrup 1/3 cup
   Cranberries, cranberry juice 1/2 cup
   Fruit cocktail, canned in syrup 1/2 cup
   Grapes, 10 fresh
   Lemon, lime 1 fresh
   Mandarin orange, canned in syrup 1/2 cup
   Nectar: apricot, pear, peach 1/2 cup
   Peach, 1 small or 1/2 cup canned with syrup
   Pear, 1 small or 1/2 cup canned with syrup
   Pineapple, 1/2 cup raw or canned with syrup
   Plums, 1 small or 1/2 cup canned with syrup
   Tangerine, 1 small
   Watermelon, 1/2 cup

   High Potassium
   Avocado
   Banana
   Cantaloupe
   Cherries, fresh
   Dried fruits
   Grapefruit, fresh and juice
   Honeydew melon
   Kiwi
   Mango
   Nectarine
   Orange, fresh and juice
   Papaya
   Prunes, prune juice
   Raisins

3. Avoid use of the following salt substitutes due to their high potassium contents: Adolph's, Lawry's Season Salt Substitute, No Salt, Morton Season Salt Free, Nu Salt, Papa Dash, and Morton Lite Salt.

ORAL DOSAGES THAT SHOULD NOT BE CRUSHED

There are a variety of reasons for crushing tablets or capsule contents prior to administering to the patient. Patients may have nasogastric tubes which do not permit the administration of tablets or capsules; an oral solution for a particular medication may not be available from the manufacturer or readily prepared by pharmacy; patients may have difficulty swallowing capsules or tablets; or mixing of powdered medication with food or drink may make the drug more palatable.

Generally, medications which should not be crushed fall into one of the following categories:

- **Extended-Release Products.** The formulation of some tablets is specialized as to allow the medication within it to be slowly released into the body. This is sometimes accomplished by centering the drug within the core of the tablet, with a subsequent shedding of multiple layers around the core. Wax melts in the GI tract. Slow-K® is an example of this. Capsules may contain beads which have multiple layers which are slowly dissolved with time.

- **Medications Which Are Irritating to the Stomach.** Tablets which are irritating to the stomach may be enteric coated which delays release of the drug until the time when it reaches the small intestine. Enteric-coated aspirin is an example of this.

- **Foul Tasting Medication.** Some drugs are quite unpleasant in their taste and the manufacturer, to increase their palatability will coat the tablet in a sugar coating. By crushing the tablet, this sugar coating is lost and the patient tastes the unpleasant tasting medication.

- **Sublingual Medication.** Medication intended for use under the tongue should not be crushed. While it appears to be obvious, it is not always easy to determine if a medication is to be used sublingually. Sublingual medications should indicate on the package that they are intended for sublingual use.

- **Effervescent Tablets.** These are tablets which, when dropped into a liquid, quickly dissolve to yield a solution. Many effervescent tablets, when crushed, lose their ability to quickly dissolve.

Recommendations

1. It is not advisable to crush certain medications.
2. Consult individual monographs prior to crushing capsule or tablet.
3. If crushing a tablet or capsule is contraindicated, consult with your pharmacist to determine whether an oral solution exists or can be compounded.
4. Refer to individual drug monograph for crushing information.

Summary of Drug Formulations That Preclude Crushing

Type	Reason(s) for the Formulation
Enteric-coated	Designed to pass through the stomach intact with drug released in the intestines to: • prevent destruction of drug by stomach acids • prevent stomach irritation • delay onset of action
Extended release	Designed to release drug over an extended period of time. Such products include: • multiple layered tablets releasing drug as each layer is dissolved • mixed release pellets that dissolve at different time intervals • special matrixes that are themselves inert but slowly release drug from the matrix
Sublingual buccal	Designed to dissolve quickly in oral fluids for rapid absorption by the abundant blood supply of the mouth
Miscellaneous	Drugs that: • produce oral mucosa irritation • are extremely bitter • contain dyes or inherently could stain teeth and mucosal tissue

TYRAMINE CONTENT OF FOODS

Food	Allowed	Minimize Intake	Not Allowed
Beverages	Milk, decaffeinated coffee, tea, soda	Chocolate beverage, caffeine-containing drinks, clear spirits	Acidophilus milk, beer, ale, wine, malted beverages
Breads/cereals	All except those containing cheese	None	Cheese bread and crackers
Dairy products	Cottage cheese, farmers or pot cheese, cream cheese, ricotta cheese, all milk, eggs, ice cream, pudding (except chocolate)	Yogurt (limit to 4 oz per day)	All other cheeses (aged cheese, American, Camembert, cheddar, Gouda, gruyere, mozzarella, parmesan, provolone, romano, Roquefort, stilton
Meat, fish, and poultry	All fresh or frozen	Aged meats, hot dogs, canned fish and meat	Chicken and beef liver, dried and pickled fish, summer or dry sausage, pepperoni, dried meats, meat extracts, bologna, liverwurst
Starches — potatoes/rice	All	None	Soybean (including paste)
Vegetables	All fresh, frozen, canned, or dried vegetable juices except those not allowed	Chili peppers, Chinese pea pods	Fava beans, sauerkraut, pickles, olives, Italian broad beans
Fruit	Fresh, frozen, or canned fruits and fruit juices	Avocado, banana, raspberries, figs	Banana peel extract
Soups	All soups not listed to limit or avoid	Commercially canned soups	Soups which contain broad beans, fava beans, cheese, beer, wine, any made with flavor cubes or meat extract, miso soup
Fats	All except fermented	Sour cream	Packaged gravy
Sweets	Sugar, hard candy, honey, molasses, syrups	Chocolate candies	None
Desserts	Cakes, cookies, gelatin, pastries, sherbets, sorbets	Chocolate desserts	Cheese-filled desserts
Miscellaneous	Salt, nuts, spices, herbs, flavorings, Worcestershire sauce	Soy sauce, peanuts	Brewer's yeast, yeast concentrates, all aged and fermented products, monosodium glutamate, vitamins with Brewer's yeast

VITAMIN K CONTENT IN SELECTED FOODS

The following lists describe the relative amounts of vitamin K in selected foods. The abbreviations for vitamin K is "H" for high amounts, "M" for medium amounts, and "L" for low amounts.

Foods*	Portion Size†	Vitamin K Content
Coffee brewed	10 cups	L
Cola, regular and diet	3½ fl oz	L
Fruit juices, assorted types	3½ fl oz	L
Milk	3½ fl oz	L
Tea, black, brewed	3½ fl oz	L
Bread, assorted types	4 slices	L
Cereal, assorted types	3½ oz	L
Flour, assorted types	1 cup	L
Oatmeal, instant, dry	1 cup	L
Rice, white	½ cup	L
Spaghetti, dry	3½ oz	L
Butter	6 Tbsp	L
Cheddar cheese	3½ oz	L
Eggs	2 large	L
Margarine	7 Tbsp	M
Mayonnaise	7 Tbsp	H
Oils		
Canola, salad, soybean	7 Tbsp	H
Olive	7 Tbsp	M
Corn, peanut, safflower, sesame, sunflower	7 Tbsp	L
Sour cream	8 Tbsp	L
Yogurt	3½ oz	L
Apple	1 medium	L
Banana	1 medium	L
Blueberries	⅔ cup	L
Cantaloupe pieces	⅔ cup	L
Grapes	1 cup	L
Grapefruit	½ medium	L
Lemon	2 medium	L
Orange	1 medium	L
Peach	1 medium	L
Abalone	3½ oz	L
Beef, ground	3½ oz	L
Chicken	3½ oz	L
Mackerel	3½ oz	L
Meatloaf	3½ oz	L
Pork, meat	3½ oz	L
Tuna	3½ oz	L
Turkey, meat	3½ oz	L
Asparagus, raw	7 spears	M
Avocado, peeled	1 small	M
Beans, pod, raw	1 cup	M
Broccoli, raw and cooked	½ cup	H
Brussel sprout, sprout and top leaf	5 sprouts	H
Cabbage, raw	1½ cups shredded	H
Cabbage, red, raw	1½ cups shredded	M
Carrot	⅔ cup	L
Cauliflower	1 cup	L
Celery	2½ stalks	L
Coleslaw	¾ cup	M
Collard greens	½ cup chopped	H
Cucumber peel, raw	1 cup	H

(continued)

Foods*	Portion Size†	Vitamin K Content
Cucumber, peel removed	1 cup	L
Eggplant	1 1/4 cups pieces	L
Endive, raw	2 cups chopped	H
Green scallion, raw	2/3 cup chopped	H
Kale, raw leaf	3/4 cup	H
Lettuce, raw, heading, bib, red leaf	1 3/4 cups shredded	H
Mushroom	1 1/2 cups	L
Mustard greens, raw	1 1/2 cups	H
Onion, white	2/3 cup chopped	L
Parsley, raw and cooked	1 1/2 cups chopped	H
Peas, green, cooked	2/3 cup	M
Pepper, green, raw	1 cup chopped	L
Potato	1 medium	L
Pumpkin	1/2 cup	L
Spinach, raw leaf	1 1/2 cups	H
Tomato	1 medium	L
Turnip greens, raw	1 1/2 cups chopped	H
Watercress, raw	3 cups chopped	H
Honey	5 Tbsp	L
Jell-O® Gelatin	1/3 cup	L
Peanut butter	6 Tbsp	L
Pickle, dill	1 medium	M
Sauerkraut	1 cup	M
Soybean, dry	1/2 cup	M

*List is a partial listing of foods. For more complete information, refer to references 1-2.

†Portions in chart calculated from estimated portions provided in reference 4.

References:
[1]Booth SL, Sadowski JA, Weihrauch JL, et al, "Vitamin K_1 (Phylloquinone) Content of Foods a Provisional Table," *J Food Comp Anal*, 1993, 6:109-20.
[2]Ferland G, MacDonald DL, and Sadowski JA, "Development of a Diet Low in Vitamin K_1 (Phylloquinone)," *J Am Diet Assoc*, 1992, 92, 593-7.
[3]Hogan RP, "Hemorrhagic Diathesis Caused by Drinking an Herbal Tea," *JAMA*, 1983, 249:2679-80.
[4]Pennington JA, *Bowes and Church's Food Values of Portions Commonly Used*, 15th ed, JP Lippincott Co, 1985.

THERAPEUTIC CATEGORY & KEY WORD INDEX

(Continued)

ANTIHYPOGLYCEMIC AGENT

ANTIHYPERGLYCEMIC AGENT

ANTI-INFLAMMATORY AGENT

ANTI-INFLAMMATORY AGENT, INHALANT

VITAMIN A DERIVATIVE

VITAMIN, FAT SOLUBLE

VITAMIN, TOPICAL

VITAMIN, WATER SOLUBLE

CANADIAN/MEXICAN BRAND NAME INDEX